SYNDROMES

Rapid Recognition and
Perioperative Implications

SYNDROMES

Rapid Recognition and Perioperative Implications

Editors

Bruno Bissonnette, MD
Professor of Anesthesiology
University of Toronto
Director of Neurosurgical Anesthesiology
Staff Anesthesiologist
The Hospital for Sick Children
Toronto, Ontario, Canada

Igor Luginbuehl, MD
Assistant Professor
University of Toronto
Staff Anesthesiologist
The Hospital for Sick Children
Toronto, Ontario, Canada

Bruno Marciniak, MD
Praticien Hospitalier
Anesthésiste Réanimateur
Department d'Anesthésie Réanimation Chirurgicale
Clinique de Chirurgie Infantile et Orthopédie
Hôpital Jeanne de Flandre
Centre Hospitalier et Universitaire de Lille
Lille, France

Bernard J. Dalens, MD
Professeur Associé d'Anesthésiologie et
Réanimation
Université Laval
Praticien Hospitalier
Centre Hospitalier Université Laval
Québec, Québec, Canada

McGRAW-HILL
Medical Publishing Division

New York   Chicago   San Francisco   Lisbon   London   Madrid
Mexico City   Milan   New Delhi   San Juan   Seoul
Singapore   Sydney   Toronto

The McGraw·Hill Companies

Syndromes: Rapid Recognition and Perioperative Implications

Copyright © 2006 by the McGraw-Hill Companies, Inc. All rights reserved. Printed in the United States of America. Except as permitted under the United States Copyright Act of 1976, no part of this publication may be reproduced or distributed in any form or by any means, or stored in a database or retrieval system, without the prior written permission of the publisher.

1 2 3 4 5 6 7 8 9 0 CCW / CCW 9 8 7 6

ISBN: 0-07-135455-7

This book was set in Times Roman by TechBooks, Inc.
The editors were James F. Shanahan and Peter J. Boyle.
The production supervisor was Catherine H. Saggese.
The text designer was Marsha Cohen/Parallelogram Graphics.
The cover design was by Cathleen Elliott, from a concept by Bruno Bissonnette;
     photo © Jim Dowdalls/Photo Researchers, Inc.
The illustrations were edited by Drs. Ruth Luginbuehl-Oelhafen and Igor Luginbuehl.
The index was prepared by Drs. Anne Hébrard and Bruno Marciniak and family.
Courier Westford was printer and binder.

This book is printed on acid-free paper.

Library of Congress Cataloging-in-Publication Data
Syndromes : rapid recognition and perioperative management / editor, Bruno Bissonnette.—1st ed.
     p. ; cm.
   Includes bibliographical references and index.
   ISBN 0-07-135455-7
   1. Syndromes.   I. Bissonnette, Bruno.
   [DNLM: 1. Signs and Symptoms.   2. Diagnostic Techniques and Procedures.
3. Perioperative Care.   4. Syndrome. WB 143 S992 2005]
RC69.S96 2005
616.07′5—dc22   2005047945

To all the children of the world with special perioperative needs

CONTENTS

Color plates appear between pages 464 and 465.

CONTRIBUTORS

SPECIAL CONTRIBUTORS

David Bracco, MD
Assistant professeur d'Anesthésiologie et de Réanimation
Département d'Anesthésiologie et de Réanimation
Hôpital Notre-Dame
Centre Hospitalier de l'Université de Montréal
Montréal, Québec, Canada

Cheong Keng Fatt, MB, BS, M Med(Anaes.), MBA
Associate Professor
National University of Singapore
Senior Consultant and Clinical Director
Department of Anesthesia
National University Hospital
Singapore

Anne Hébrard, MD
Praticien Hospitalier
Anesthésiste-Réanimateur
Department d'Anesthésie Réanimation Chirurgicale 2
Clinique de Chirurgie Infantile et Orthopédie
Hôpital Jeanne de Flandre
Centre Hospitalier et Universitaire de Lille
Lille, France

Francis Veyckemans
Professeur d'Anesthésiologie et de Reanimation
Chef du Service d'Anesthésiologie
Cliniques Universitaire St. Luc
Brussels, Belgium

CONTRIBUTORS

Lola Adewale, MBBS
Consultant Pediatric Anesthetist
Department of Anesthesia
Birmingham Children's Hospital
Birmingham, United Kingdom

Ross Barlow, MD
Assistant Professor
University of Toronto
Staff Anesthesiologist
The Hospital for Sick Children
Toronto, Ontario, Canada

Edmund D. Carver, MBBS, MRCP, FRCA
Consultant Anesthetist
Birmingham Children's Hospital
Birmingham, United Kingdom

Steven H. Cray, MBBS, FRCA
Consultant Pediatric Anesthetist
Birmingham Children's Hospital
Birmingham, United Kingdom

Annette Davis, MBChB, FRCA
Consultant Pediatric Anesthetist
Royal Liverpool Children's NHS Trust
Liverpool, United Kingdom

John G. B. Emery, MBBS, FRCA
Consultant in Pediatric Anesthesia
Department of Anesthesia
University Hospital
Queen's Medical Centre
Nottingham, United Kingdom

Ross Fairgrieve, MBChB, FRCA
Consultant Anesthetist
Royal Hospital for Sick Children
Glasgow, United Kingdom

Jean Claude Granry, MD
Professor d'Anesthésiologie et Réanimation
Département d'Anesthésie-Réanimation
Centre Hospitalier Universitaire d'Angers
Angers, France

Corinne Gurtner, MD, FMH, DEAA
Spécialiste en Anesthésie-Réanimation FMH et Médecine
    Intensive FMH
Médecin-chef
Département d'Anesthésie-Réanimation
Hôpital de Sion
Sion, Switzerland

Jason Hayes, MD, FRCPC
Assistant Professor of Anesthesia
University of Toronto
Staff Anesthesiologist
The Hospital for Sick Children
Toronto, Ontario, Canada

David Ho, MD, MBBS, FANZCA
Consultant Anesthetist
Royal Children's Hospital, Brisbane
Herston, Queensland, Australia

Lucie Lebel, MD, FRCPC
Staff Anesthesiologist
Hôpital St-François d'Assise,
Centre Hospitalier Universitaire de Québec
Québec, Québec, Canada

Mark Levine, MBBCh, FRCPC
Assistant Professor of Anesthesia
University of Toronto
Staff Anesthetist
The Hospital for Sick Children
Toronto, Ontario, Canada

John Magner, MBBChBAO, FCARCSI
Clinical Research Fellow
St. Vincent's University Hospital
Dublin, Ireland

Conan L. McCaul, MBBChBAO, FFARCSI
Consultant in Anesthesia and Intensive Care Medicine
Waterford Regional Hospital
Waterford, Ireland

Joe Mellor, BSc, MBBS, FRCA
Consultant in Pediatric Cardiothoracic
    Anesthesia
Leeds Teaching Hospitals
Leeds, United Kingdom

Basem Naser, MBBS, FRCPC
Assistant Professor
University of Toronto
Director of Acute Pain Service
Staff Anesthesiologist
The Hospital for Sick Children
Toronto, Ontario, Canada

Anne Nicholson, MBBS, FANZCA
Consultant Pediatric Anesthetist
Royal Children's Hospital
Melbourne, Victoria, Australia

Martin Parry, BSc, MBBS, FRCA
Consultant Pediatric Anesthetist
Royal College of Anesthetists Tutor
Department of Anesthesia
Brighton and Sussex University
    Hospitals NHS Trust
Royal Alexandra Hospital for Sick Children
Brighton, East Sussex, United Kingdom

Hweeleng Pua, MBBS, MMed(Anaes)
Consultant Anesthesiologist
University of Singapore
Staff Anesthesiologist
Department of Anesthesia
National University Hospital
Singapore

Parvine Sadeghi, MD
Clinical Assistant Professor
Miami Children's Hospital
University of Miami
Miami, Florida, United States

Eric Philip Segar, MBChB, DCH, FRCA
Consultant Anesthetist
Bristol Royal Hospital for Children
Bristol, United Kingdom

Dale F. Szpisjak, MD
Assistant Professor
Department of Anesthesiology and
    Critical Care Medicine
Uniformed Services University of
    the Health Sciences
Bethesda, Maryland, United States

Daniel Trachsel, MD
Clinical Consultant
Specialist in Pediatrics and Pneumology
University Children's Hospital
Basel, Switzerland

Victor C. Un, MBChB, DA(UK), FRCA, FRCPC
Staff Anesthesiologist
Department of Anesthesia
North York General Hospital
Toronto, Ontario, Canada

ILLUSTRATION CONTRIBUTORS

Bruno Bissonnette, MD
Professor of Anesthesiology
University of Toronto
Director of Neurosurgical Anesthesiology
Staff Anesthesiologist
The Hospital for Sick Children
Toronto, Ontario, Canada

Igor Luginbuehl, MD
Assistant Professor
University of Toronto
Staff Anesthesiologist
The Hospital for Sick Children
Toronto, Ontario, Canada

Stephanie A. Holowka, MRT(R), MRT(MR)
Medical Radiation Technologist
Diagnostic Imaging
The Hospital for Sick Children
Toronto, Ontario, Canada

Adrian Bösenberg, MBChB(Cape Town), DA(SA), FCA(SA)
Professor and Second Chair
Department of Anesthesia
Faculty Health Sciences
University of Cape Town
Cape Town, South Africa

Christopher R. Forrest, MD, MSc, FRCS(C), FACS
Associate Professor
Division of Plastic Surgery
Department of Surgery
University of Toronto
Head, Division of Plastic Surgery
Medical Director
Centre for Craniofacial Care and Research
The Hospital for Sick Children
Toronto, Ontario, Canada

Bernice Krafchick, MD, FRCPC
Professor of Medicine
University of Toronto
Division of Dermatology
The Hospital for Sick Children
Toronto, Ontario, Canada

Elise Héon, MD, FRCSC
Professor of Ophthalmology
Ophthalmologist-in-Chief
Mira Godard Chair in Vision and Research
Department of Ophthalmology
The Hospital for Sick Children
Toronto, Ontario, Canada

FOREWORD 1:
An Anesthesiologist's
Perspective

In the past most infants and children with syndromes had anesthesia and surgery in children's hospitals. These children entered the hospital a day or two before surgery. This gave the anesthesiologist time to see the patient a day or more before surgery, become familiar with the syndrome, understand the patient's problems, and make a plan to ensure safe and efficient completion of surgery and anesthesia. Modern medical care has increased the number of patients with syndromes who survive, often with serious problems that require repeated surgery. Because of the way medicine is practiced today, these patients usually arrive in the hospital (often a community general hospital) on the day of surgery and have not been seen or evaluated by an anesthesiologist up to that time. Many of these children have problems that are potentially life-threatening or associated with severe difficulties during the induction, maintenance, and awakening from anesthesia.

There are thousands of syndromes, and new ones are described every year. It is difficult to remember even a fraction of these syndromes and their features, especially if we anesthetize these patients only occasionally. Insufficient information about the patients and their syndromes often leads to cancellation of surgery, loss of income by the parents who had to take a day away from work, and significant inconvenience for the family and the hospital. Consequently, anesthesiologists (and other health professionals) need a concise, informative, and easy-to-read source of information about syndromes and the risks they pose to patients who require anesthesia and surgery or intensive care management.

Syndromes: Rapid Recognition and Perioperative Implications meets this need. Having this information not only will improve patient safety, it will also reassure physicians caring for patients affected with complex medical conditions. Because there will be fewer delays or cancellations of surgery and fewer complications, parents will be more satisfied with the care of their children.

Many syndromes are associated with serious or potentially serious problems in anesthesiology, including cardiovascular disease, inability to extend the neck, inability to open the mouth, or the potential for increased intracranial pressure. By having the facts readily available about these pre-existing, complex medical conditions, anesthesiologists and other healthcare professionals will be able to ask the right questions of the family and of other physicians involved in the care of the patient. Parents often have significant knowledge about their child's problems but, under the stress of the situation, will often forget to mention them if not asked specifically. If physicians do not demonstrate proper knowledge about a condition, the parents of a child undergoing surgery may not have confidence that the "team" can provide safe care for their loved one. By understanding potential problems, the anesthesiologist will be able to plan accordingly and have available the right equipment (fiberoptic laryngoscope, light wand, etc.) or specialized assistance (someone to perform a tracheostomy) that may be required. For example, knowing that some syndromes are associated with severe acidosis and cardiac arrest during surgery would allow an anesthesiologist to modify the anesthesia technique and hopefully prevent these complications.

The organization of syndromes in this book allows anesthesiologists and others health professional to find information about a given medical condition rapidly. Each entry gives, at a glance, an overview of the syndrome and its major characteristics, genetic inheritance, pathophysiology, diagnosis, and clinical features. For the anesthesiologist, it provides the precautions before anesthesia, anesthetic considerations, and pharmacological implications. Relevant references are available. This rapid overview allows the anesthesiologist and others to have immediate access to the information needed to provide effective and safe care for these infants, children, and adults affected with pre-existing medical conditions and who are often very ill.

George Gregory, MD
Professor Emeritus
Department of Anesthesiology and Pediatrics
School of Medicine
University of California, San Francisco
San Francisco, California, United States

FOREWORD 2:
A Surgeon's Perspective

When we, as professionals, peruse a new medical book, most of us pay particular attention to the foreword, on which we depend for an independent overview and assessment of that book.

I am honored to have been requested by Professor Bruno Bissonnette, the editor and primary author, to write a foreword for this remarkable book, entitled *Syndromes: Rapid Recognition and Perioperative Implications*. It is my privilege to have known Professor Bissonnette personally since 1987, that is, ever since he was appointed to the staff of the Department of Anesthesia of the Hospital for Sick Children, Toronto.

Syndromes is timely as well as unique. In the present era of "same-day admission" there is no longer adequate time for preoperative assessment by the anesthesiologist who may be seeing the infant or child for the first time only shortly before the operative procedure is scheduled to begin.

Imagine yourself as the anesthesiologist being faced with the patient under such circumstances and noticing that "there is more to this patient's condition than meets the eye." Yet, at that time you do not know the nature of the pre-existing disorder, let alone know how that disorder may impact your administration of the anesthesia or the specific postoperative management required.

In a perfect world the nature of the pre-existing disorder would—whenever feasible—be conveyed to the anesthesiologist by the surgeon days, or even longer, before the proposed date of the operative procedure. Furthermore, this information could be shared with the family in order that they may understand the situation and sign a truly informed consent.

Consequently, there is an enormous need for a "user-friendly" reference wherein both the surgeon and anesthesiologist can rapidly and accurately recognize a pre-existent disorder and learn about its significance to perioperative management. The immediate availability of such an encyclopedic book can also prevent the undesirable phenomenon of the last-minute cancellation of the surgical procedure, with its resultant distress and frustration for the patient, family, and hospital staff. More importantly, the data in this unique book could help to prevent potential complications associated with the presence of the pre-existing disorder. This book thereby does the anesthetic and surgical professions a remarkable service in providing such precise and exhaustive information.

This wonderful book should be an essential addition to the personal libraries of anesthesiologists and surgeons who care for infants, children, and adults affected with special medical conditions. It should also be available in hospital libraries as well as at the desks of all operating room suites. It represents a monumental contribution to the increasingly complex fields of anesthesia and surgery.

Robert B. Salter, CC, OOnt, FRSC, MD, MS, FRCSC, FACS
Professor Emeritus of Surgery
University of Toronto
Department of Surgery, Division of Orthopedic Surgery
Senior Scientist Emeritus
The Research Institute
The Hospital for Sick Children
Toronto, Ontario, Canada

FOREWORD 3:
A Pediatrician's Perspective

Because of advances in medical technology and improvement of care, pediatricians are more and more often faced with complex chronic conditions or diseases. This concerns all the pediatric subspecialists, including pediatric intensivists. In fact, children with chronic conditions, particularly infants, have a more than threefold increased rate of hospitalization compared with the general pediatric population. Furthermore, around 30 to 45% of children admitted to the pediatric intensive care units (PICU) suffer from such diseases. The syndromes that are described in this new textbook represent a large part of these diseases. Finally, chronic conditions of congenital origin account for 4% of total deaths and for 15% of unscheduled PICU admissions.

Syndromes: Rapid Recognition and Perioperative Implications is a well-illustrated, quick-consultation reference. Each syndrome, listed in alphabetic order, is described in nine sections, plus essential references: main features ("at a glance") with their implication for anesthesia and intensive care, synonyms, historical facts when important, incidence, genetic inheritance, pathophysiology, diagnosis, precautions before anesthesia, anesthetic considerations, and pharmacological implications. Perhaps the most important sections of each entry are the last two, which summarize useful data often difficult to find rapidly: airway management, precautions to be taken for mobilization, fluid intake, and drug utilization (which drugs can be safely used and which must be avoided).

Why is this textbook useful? First, almost all these syndromes are orphan (or rare) diseases and thus are not well known by many pediatricians, who cannot be expected to memorize the 4500 listed syndromes. Moreover, surveys have indicated a lack of physician confidence in caring for children with special health care needs. The very concise description presented by Professor Bissonnette and the authors will help pediatricians recognize the key features of each syndrome. Second, many children with these syndromes may need invasive investigations and surgical procedures performed under sedation or anesthesia. This book indicates all the precautions required to avoid a possible last-minute cancellation and delay and guarantee safe perioperative management. Last but not least, the reader will have access to a very detailed thesaurus of all the syndromes discussed, their synonyms, and other conditions to be considered, in addition to numerous overview tables.

All pediatricians and residents, and more generally all health care providers, will find in this excellent book a quick and useful reference to improve the care for children who present with these syndromes and who frequently have special anesthetic care needs. No doubt this book merits translation into many languages, in order to provide help for physicians and children worldwide.

The authors and publisher are to be congratulated for producing such a thorough work.

Francis Leclerc, MD
Professor of Pediatrics
Director of the Pediatric Intensive Care Unit
University Hospital of Lille
Lille, France

FOREWORD 4:
A Patient's Perspective

I'm not sure who was more nervous: me or the resident of the large downtown Toronto teaching hospital who was given the unenviable task of learning about my medical condition—my syndrome—before a scheduled appointment with the regular specialist. I've never been keen on these sessions. They tend to make me feel more like a curiosity than an actual person. At the time, I was in my early 30s (I'm almost 50 now) and for years had been used as a teaching tool.

I remember one day a few years earlier when I had been lying in a bed at the same hospital after having had some tests done. In walked a gaggle of white-coated medicos, stethoscopes in pockets and a busy air about them. They were led by an imperious-looking gentleman who looked at me, said hello, introduced himself and asked if I would mind being the subject of a quiz he was about to give to the five interns accompanying him.

"Okay," I said.

He immediately lifted my gown and pointed to an 18-year-old surgical scar at my waist. "So," he queried, "whose work is this?"

Surprised, but not enough to be at a loss for words, I quickly chipped in, "Here's a hint. It's not Picasso."

After some uneasy laughter, one forthright soul piped up, "It's Dr. ——'s work."

"Correct. Good for you," said his leader.

And with that the white-coated gaggle moved on, speaking in low tones amongst themselves as they filed out of the room.

Now here I was again, though this time fully clothed and sitting in my wheelchair, wishing this resident would be as quick as his counterpart had been years earlier.

No such luck.

"So tell me about your condition."

I replied that it was a form of something called Arnold-Chiari.

"Oh," he said. "I've heard of that . . . I think."

Swell.

And so I went into my layman's description of Arnold-Chiari malformation, which was a very poor substitute for the precise description you'll find in this book. (A sample: "Defect in the formation of the lower portion of the medulla [posterior fossa]. . . . Can be associated, according to the type, with hydrocephalus, raised intracranial pressure, respiratory and cardiac center dysfunction. Infants may exhibit vomiting, mental impairment, and weakness. There is a possibility of limb paralysis. . . . Dizziness, weakness of the legs, headaches, double vision, or deafness may be present.")

"Oh," said the resident.

This was the incident that quickly came to mind when Professor Bruno Bissonnette and Dr. Igor Luginbuehl asked me to write a foreword for *Syndromes: Rapid Recognition and Perioperative Implications*. As Professor Bissonnette stated to me in his letter: "You should describe how patients affected with complex medical conditions and their families feel when confronted by the impression that medical professionals may not understand their medical condition. The value of this textbook will reside in its ability to help all physicians confronted with these conditions to come to a diagnosis rapidly and decide intelligently on the course of action."

So here goes: a quiz for the readers of this textbook.

What would you do if, instead of my being able to offer up an explanation of Arnold-Chiari myself, I was suddenly wheeled into the emergency department, unconscious, as happened in the mid-1990s when my condition unexpectedly deteriorated?

And what would you do if I were a child, being wheeled into emergency unit in the same physical state, and my parents were so panicked that all they were capable of doing was to utter the words: "Arnold-Chiari"?

In both cases, the future course of my life depends on the actions of professionals like you.

In the first case, quick-thinking people in my network got the information to the doctors on call. I was stabilized, then sent to another hospital for surgery a few days later. After months of rehabilitation I was able to reassemble the components of my life, albeit in a new shape. Most importantly, my daughter still had a father, my wife still had a husband, my students at a Toronto university still had a journalism instructor, my colleagues in the Canadian magazine industry still had a good editor they could hire. . . .

In the second case—my scenario only—what if information about Arnold-Chiari wasn't readily available to you?

I shudder just thinking about the possible consequences.

Stephen Trumper, BA, BAA
Executive Editor
National Post Business Magazine
Instructor, School of Journalism
Ryerson University
Toronto, Ontario, Canada

How to Use This Book

Syndromes: Rapid Recognition and Perioperative Implications offers an A-to-Z encyclopedic presentation of more than 2000 syndromes. Extensive cross-referencing of synonyms, variations, and international names further expands coverage to nearly 4500 entries. The presence of this icon ☞ preceding the name of a syndrome in the text indicates that it is also fully described under an alphabetical main entry in the book. Most syndromes are presented with 14 subdivisions, consisting of:

At a glance: Clinical information, with emphasis on the most important features.

Synonyms: A list of synonyms for each syndrome, facilitating identification in different parts of the world.

History: First recognition or description of the disease, with names, dates, and other pertinent information when available.

Incidence: An indication of the population most affected, international distribution, and number of cases reported in the literature to date is given. The prevalence of the disease is also mentioned when known.

Classification: Medical conditions with multiple subtypes. In most cases, a complete description of all subtypes is presented within the text.

Genetic inheritance: Current knowledge about the genetic basis of the syndrome, the locus of the gene, and inheritance pattern.

Pathophysiology: The underlying mechanisms potentially involved in the specific medical condition are described.

Diagnosis: Radiological and laboratory findings to help the user in the rapid recognition of each medical condition. Differential diagnoses may also be included.

Clinical aspects: A description of the clinical characteristics with an emphasis on the most frequent features and the main organ systems affected.

Precautions before anesthesia: Recommendations on medical consultations, preoperative radiographs, and functional and laboratory tests potentially needed.

Anesthetic considerations: Specific perioperative considerations, such as indications for premedication, airway management, vascular access, postoperative ventilation, etc. Emphasis is on the prevention of complications.

Pharmacological implications: Information about pharmacological interactions and potential contraindications associated with the use of specific medications.

Other conditions to be considered: A list (with synonyms) of potentially related medical conditions that could, from their clinical similarity with the main syndrome described, be considered as alternate diagnoses.

References: Pertinent references for further consultation.

Some syndromes described in this book are either extremely rare or not congenital in nature. However, we found it worthwhile to have them included in the text since we considered the information either important or interesting, or sometimes both.

The index (see How to Use the Index, p. 853) was developed by the authors to meet the needs of clinicians like themselves.

Aarskog Syndrome

At a glance: Short stature, round face, and hypertelorism. Cervical hypermotility and odontoid subluxation.

Synonyms: Aarskog-Scott Syndrome; Faciogenital Dysplasia; Faciodigitogenital Syndrome.

History: First described in 1970 by Dagfinn Aarskog, a Norwegian pediatric endocrinologist.

Incidence: Approximately 200 cases have been reported to date.

Genetic inheritance: Most likely X-linked recessive. Genetic heterogeneity or autosomal dominant inheritance with strong sex influence is possible.

Pathophysiology: Gene FGD1 (responsible for faciogenital dysplasia) encodes a guanine nucleotide exchange factor that specifically activates Cdc42, a member of the Rho family of guanosine triphosphatases (GTPases) involved in cellular signaling, migration, growth, and differentiation. Mutations to the FGD1 gene result in a human developmental disorder affecting specific skeletal structures, including elements of the face, cervical vertebrae, and distal extremities.

Diagnosis: Clinical features are recognizable at birth. Radiologic findings include cervical spine abnormalities with subluxation, facial abnormalities, phalangeal defects, and delayed bone age.

Clinical aspects: Patients present with anomalies of the face, genitalia, and limbs. Growth retardation usually becomes evident at age 2 to 4 years. Facial features may include a round face with hypertelorism, ophthalmoplegia, large cornea, hyperopic astigmatism, antimongoloid obliquity of the palpebral fissures, strabismus, and ptosis. The nose is short and stubby with anteverted nostrils. The philtrum is long with broad upper lip. Cleft lip/palate, a linear dimple below the lower lip, and enamel dysplasia are common. The midface is flattened secondary to maxillary hypoplasia and deformity of the anterior mandible. The ears are low-set, cup shaped, and floppy. Limb anomalies consist of short thumbs, digital contractures, syndactyly, clinodactyly, brachydactyly, camptodactyly, and simian creases. Abnormal genital findings include cryptorchidism, scrotal folds encircling the penis ventrally (shawl scrotum), and inguinal hernia. Associated heart defects have been described (e.g., pulmonary stenosis, ventricular septal defect). Mild developmental delay seems to be frequent. Other features are ligamentous laxity of the hands, knees, and feet, pectus excavatum, liver cirrhosis with portal hypertension, imperforated anus, macrocytic anemia, hemochromatosis, and broad flat feet with lymphedema.

Precautions before anesthesia: Evaluate for neck hypermobility and subluxation secondary to ligamentous laxity and malformations of cervical vertebrae (odontoid). Look for associated neurologic symptoms. Cervical spine radiographs may be helpful. Assess the airway for difficult tracheal intubation. Exclude associated heart defects (ECG, echocardiography). Ask for a chest radiograph and pulmonary function tests in presence of pectus excavatum. Blood workup should include a complete blood count to rule out anemia or thrombocytopenia (secondary to hypersplenism in the presence of liver cirrhosis), a coagulation status, and liver function tests in liver cirrhosis patients.

Anesthetic considerations: Potentially difficult airway management in case of mandibular deformity. Excessive hyperextension must be avoided because of risk for cervical luxation during tracheal intubation. In-line stabilization or fiberoptic intubation should be considered. Manipulate and position patients with great care (joint luxations) under general anesthesia. Carefully insert nasogastric tubes in the presence of portal hypertension to prevent hemorrhage from esophageal varices. Cooperation may be limited in the presence of mental retardation. Sedative and anxiolytic premedication and the presence of the primary caregiver for induction of anesthesia may be helpful.

Pharmacological implications: None, except in patients with associated congenital cardiac defects, in whom hemodynamically active drugs must be used with caution and antibiotic prophylaxis administered.

Other conditions to be considered:

☞**JUBERG-HAYWARD SYNDROME:** Familial bipolar syndrome characterized by short stature resulting from growth hormone deficiency. Affected individuals have microcephaly, cleft lip/palate, and deformities of the thumbs and limbs.

☞**ACROFACIAL DYSOSTOSIS NAGER TYPE:** Syndrome characterized primarily by malar hypoplasia, micrognathia, radial limb and thumb anomalies, and ear abnormalities.

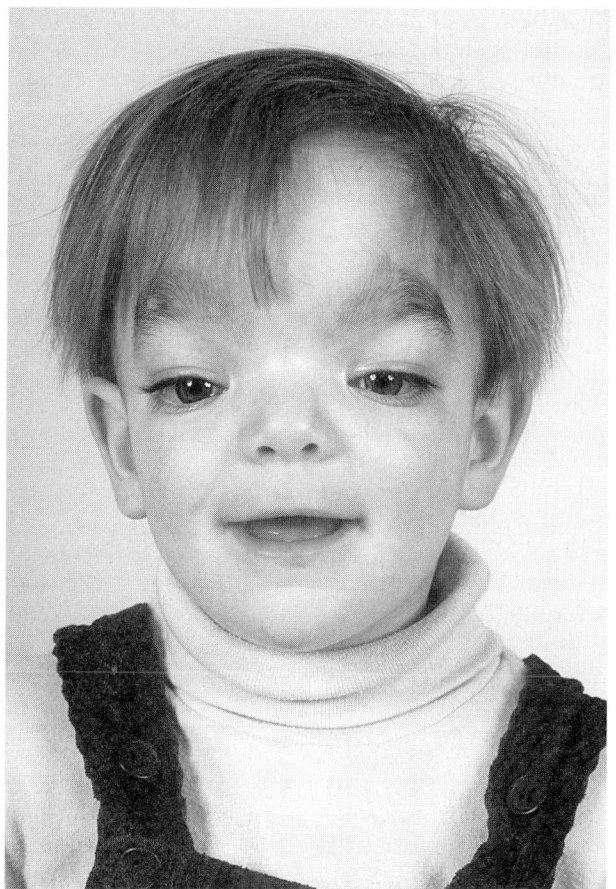

Aarskog syndrome Two-year-old boy with Aarskog syndrome shows round face with hypertelorism, strabismus, antimongoloid obliquity of the palpebral fissures, ptosis, a short stubby nose with anteverted nostrils, and a long philtrum.

REFERENCES:

Aarskog D: A familial syndrome of short stature associated with facial dysplasia and genital anomalies. *J Pediatr* 77:856, 1970.

Pasteris NG, Buckler J, Cadle AB, et al: Genomic organization of faciogenital dysplasia. *Genomics* 43:390, 1997.

Aase Syndrome

At a glance: Bilateral triphalangeal thumbs, congenital hypoplastic anemia, joint and skeletal deformities, delayed fontanelle closure, poor peripheral vascular access, possible ventricular septal defect.

Synonyms: Aase-Smith Variant; Aase Congenital Anemia; Blackfan-Diamond Anemia Variant.

History: First described in 1969 in two male siblings by Jon Morton Aase, an American pediatrician.

Genetic inheritance: Autosomal recessive transmission with normal chromosomes but also believed to possibly be autosomal dominant. Genetic basis of the disease is not known.

Pathophysiology: Decreased erythropoiesis. The anemia is caused by underdevelopment of the bone marrow.

Diagnosis: Based on bilateral triphalangeal thumbs at birth and anemia that usually presents at age 6 months.

Clinical aspects: Mild growth deficiency, third percentile. Congenital hypoplastic anemia tends to improve with age. Frequent transfusions are needed, often requiring chelation therapy. Bilateral triphalangeal thumbs. Narrow shoulder, radial hypoplasia, cleft lip/palate, and Dandy-Walker cyst may be present. Late closure of the fontanelles. Patients occasionally receive steroid therapy. Inability to fully extend the joints from birth (congenital contractures). Rarely spontaneous remission.

Precautions before anesthesia: Check hemoglobin and transfuse as needed. Check for systemic signs of iron overload, specifically hepatic cirrhosis and cardiac failure.

Anesthetic considerations: The hematocrit should be assessed preoperatively. Maintain oxygen-carrying capacity. Avoid myocardial depressants, especially with preexisting failure. Peripheral vascular access and placement of radial arterial catheter are difficult.

Pharmacological implications: No specific implications for this condition.

REFERENCES:

Muis M: Aase syndrome: Case report and review of the literature. *Eur J Pediatr* 145:153, 1986.

Yetgin S, Balci S, Irken G, et al: Aase-Smith syndrome. *Turk J Pediatr* 36:239, 1994.

Aase-Smith Syndrome

At a glance: Hydrocephalus (Dandy-Walker anomaly), cleft palate, severe joint contractures, congenital neuroblastoma, ventricular septal defects.

Synonyms: Distal Arthrogryposis Type IIB Syndrome; Triphalangeal Thumb-Hypoplastic Anemia Hydrocephalus Syndrome.

History: First described in 1968, in a father and two children, by Jon Morton Aase and David Weyhe Smith, American pediatricians.

Genetic inheritance: Autosomal dominant.

Diagnosis: Based on the clinical findings of severe joint contrac-tures and joint anomalies, and hydrocephalus with Dandy-Walker anomaly.

Clinical aspects: Cranial features may include hydrocephalus associated with a Dandy-Walker malformation, ptosis, external ear deformities, and limited mouth opening. Multiple ventricular septal defects have been reported. Severe joint contractures affect predominantly the fingers. Very thin and filiform fingers with absent knuckles. Limited extension of the elbows and knees. Clubfoot deformity. Congenital neuroblastoma has been reported.

Precautions before anesthesia: Obtain an echocardiogram to rule out cardiac lesions. Check for the presence of raised intracranial pressure (check fontanelle in infants). Ultrasound may be required to rule out neuroblastoma.

Anesthetic considerations: Very severe limitation of mouth opening. Expect airway management to be difficult. Maintain spontaneous ventilation until the airway has been secured. Careful positioning and padding are essential.

Pharmacological implications: Avoid neuromuscular blockers until the airway has been secured.

REFERENCE:

Patton MA, Sharma A, Winter RM: The Aase-Smith syndrome. *Clin Genet* 28:521, 1985.

Abetalipoproteinemia

At a glance: Rare congenital disorder that causes the body to not produce chylomicrons, low-density lipoprotein (LDL), and very-low-density lipoprotein (VLDL). Coagulation disorder, demyelination and ataxia, peripheral sensory neuropathy, retinitis pigmentosa, acanthocytosis, diminished response to local anesthetics.

Synonyms: Bassen-Kornzweig Syndrome; Acanthocytosis; Microsomal Triglyceride Transfer Protein Deficiency.

Incidence: Unknown. Males are approximately 1.5 times more often affected than females.

Genetic inheritance: Autosomal recessive. Abetalipoproteinemia is caused by mutations in the gene responsible for microsomal triglyceride transfer protein (MTP). MTP is thought to transfer lipids to the apo-β protein as it is translated, allowing it to attain the proper conformation for lipoprotein assembly. Gene locus is on chromosome 4q22-24.

Pathophysiology: Beta lipoproteins are lipoproteins of various molecular weights, with apo-100 (essential component of VLDL and LDL) and apo-48 (mainly in chylomicrons) as their principal subtypes. These lipoproteins bind to specific receptors on human cells, allowing exchange of lipids. Virtual absence of VLDLs and LDLs results in low levels of plasma cholesterol and triglycerides. However, cholesterol delivery to individual cells remains normal by an increased cholesterol-carrying capacity of the high-density lipoproteins (HDLs). Although the basal cortisol secretion in the adrenal cortex is normal, its maximal rate cannot be reached with corticotropin stimulation.

Diagnosis: Based on the clinical course, reduced plasma lipids (electrophoresis), and absent apo-β. A peripheral smear shows 50% acanthocytosis and hyperbilirubinemia (reduced red cell lifespan). Sural nerve biopsy reveals loss of large myelinated fibers.

Clinical aspects: Age of onset is the first year of life (gastrointestinal manifestations). Within the first 10 years, neurologic and ocular manifestations appear. Fat malabsorption (chronic diarrhea) is severe. Spinocerebellar ataxia, peripheral neuropathy, pigmented retinopathy, and ceroid myopathy are secondary to tocopherol transport defect in the blood. Muscle dysfunction resulting in pes cavus and kyphoscoliosis is common. Fatal cardiomyopathy has been described. Treatment is supportive only with fat-soluble vitamin supplements (A, D, E, K) and tocopherols. Use of triglyceride containing long-chain fatty acids has been attempted.

Precautions before anesthesia: Evaluate the extent of neurologic deficit. Check pulmonary function with SpO_2, FEV_1, and forced vital capacity; chest radiograph; arterial blood gas analysis. Laboratory investigations show anemia (resulting from iron and/or folate deficiency, autohemolysis) and prolonged prothrombin time (resulting from vitamin K deficiency, liver cirrhosis) but normal platelet function. Electrolyte changes may be present (because of potential adrenal dysfunction and vomiting and diarrhea as part of the fat malabsorption). Assess cardiac function (ECG, chest radiograph, echocardiogram for ventricular function). Hypoalbuminemia (caloric and protein malnutrition) and reduced α_1-acid glycoprotein levels may be present.

Anesthetic considerations: A rapid sequence induction technique is indicated in the presence of vomiting. High risk for cardiorespiratory failure in patients with severe lung and cardiac disease. Muscle weakness from myopathy and malnutrition may confound the problem. Regional anesthesia is contraindicated if coagulation is not within the normal range.

Pharmacological implications: Use of succinylcholine can be dangerous if neuropathy or myopathy is present (a fast nondepolarizing neuromuscular agent should be used; rocuronium can be a useful alternative for rapid sequence induction). Threshold for local anesthetic toxicity might be reduced because of general reduction in plasma proteins; hence the maximum safe dose should be strictly observed (or even reduced), especially with prolonged infusions.

REFERENCES:

Kane J, Havel R: Disorders of the biogenesis and secretion of lipoproteins containing the B apolipoproteins, in Scriver CR, Sly WS, Childs B, et al. (eds): *The Metabolic and Molecular Bases of Inherited Disease,* 7th ed. New York, McGraw Hill, 1995, p 1853.

Narcisi TM, Shoulders CC, Chester SA, et al: Mutations of the microsomal triglyceride-transfer-protein gene in abetalipoproteinemia. *Am J Hum Genet* 6:1298, 1995.

Triantafillidis JK, Kottaras G, Sgourous S, et al: Abetalipoproteinemia: Clinical and laboratory features, therapeutic manipulations, and follow-up study of three members of a Greek family. *J Clin Gastroenterol* 26:207, 1998.

Ablepharon-Macrostomia Syndrome (AMS)

At a glance: Quantitative and qualitative defects in development of the prosencephalic neural crest. Fish-like facial (mouth) appearance. Other craniofacial anomalies include triangularly shaped face, small nose, partial absence of tissue (coloboma) from the midportion of nostril walls. Heart, kidney, and liver anomalies are present, especially in neonates. Other features include skin and genitalia anomalies, absent eyelids, alopecia totalis, camptodactyly. Infants and children with AMS show delayed language development and mental retardation.

Incidence: AMS is an extremely rare congenital abnormality. Approximately six cases have been reported since McCarthy and West in 1977.

Genetic inheritance: Cause of AMS is unknown. Some of the cases suggest AMS is inherited as an autosomal recessive genetic trait. Autosomal dominant inheritance is possible because of a postulated relationship to the disorder in monozygotic twins from consanguineous parents. It seems most likely that AMS is, in fact, a new mutation autosomal disorder. The gene implicated may be located on chromosome 18, where a deletion has been found.

Pathophysiology: Unknown.

Diagnosis and clinical aspects: Diagnosis is made based on the clinical aspect of the newborn. The disorder is characterized by absence or hypoplasia of the lower eyelids (ablepharon/microblepharon), eyebrows, and eyelashes. Other eye features include corneal opacifications, nystagmus, and cryptophthalmos. An association with absent zygomatic arches has been described. Fusion defects of the mouth result in macrostomia with a fish-like mouth. The nose often is hypoplastic. The nipples may be absent or rudimentary and the genitalia ambiguous. The skin shows ichthyotic changes and redundant skin folds. Mental retardation with delayed development of expressive language is common. The primary goal of surgical treatment is preserving the cornea by early postnatal treatment, early lid reconstruction, and use of lubricants.

Precautions before anesthesia: Neonates should be carefully evaluated by echocardiography for associated heart, brain, or kidney abnormalities. In case of absent zygomatic arches, difficult airway management must be anticipated, especially with regard to tracheal intubation. Also evaluate for possible airway obstruction.

Anesthetic considerations and pharmacological implications: No anesthetic data about AMS and its anesthetic and pharmacological drug implications have been reported. The anesthesiologist must be aware of any associated abnormalities that will guide the choice of anesthetic technique and drugs. If a difficult tracheal intubation is anticipated, preservation of spontaneous ventilation is recommended until the airway is secured.

Other conditions to be considered:

☞**BARBER-SAY SYNDROME:** Hypertrichosis, atrophic skin, ectropion, macrostomia syndrome. Hypertelorism has been described. X-linked or autosomal dominant inheritance. Occasionally, cleft palate, primary hypospadias, shawl scrotum, and mild hearing loss are seen.

ABLEPHARON-ICHTHYOSIS: Similar to AMS, with excessive skin wrinkling, hyperkeratosis, periorbital tumors/cysts, and scalp defects.

REFERENCES:

Barber N, Say B, Bell RF, et al: Macrostomia, ectropion, atrophic skin, hypertrichosis and growth retardation. *Syndrome Ident* 8:6, 1982.

McCarthy GT, West CM: Ablepharon-macrostomia syndrome. *Dev Med Child Neurol* 19:659, 1977.

Pellegrino JE, Schnur RE, Boghosian-Sell L, et al: Ablepharon-macrostomia syndrome with associated cutis laxa: Possible localization to 18q. *Hum Genet* 97:532, 1996.

Acatalasia/Acatalasemia

At a glance: Inherited disorder with marked catalase deficiency resulting in enoral inflammation and teeth destruction.

Synonyms: Catalase Deficiency (CAT); Takahara Disease; Hypocatalasia.

History: Heterogeneous group of genetic disorders first discovered in 1948 by Takahara in Japan, an otolaryngologist who found that in cases of progressive oral gangrene, hydrogen peroxide applied to the ulcerated areas did not froth in the usual manner.

Incidence: The frequency of the gene is relatively high in Japan and is variable in the rest of the world. The frequency of heterozygotes is 0.09% in Hiroshima and Nagasaki but is on the order of 1.4% in other parts of Japan. Acatalasia also has been detected in Switzerland and Israel. Swiss and Israeli homozygotes show some residual catalase activity, suggesting the mutation is different from that responsible for the Japanese disease in which catalase activity is zero and no cross-reacting material has been identified.

Genetic inheritance: Believed to be an autosomal recessive disorder resulting from the virtual absence of catalase activity observed mainly in Japan and Switzerland. However, an autosomal dominant with polymorphism has been suggested. Gene map locus is 11p13 deletion.

Pathophysiology: Marked deficiency of catalase, which usually is present in red blood cells and other tissues. Catalase decomposes hydrogen peroxide and generates oxygen, protects tissues from oxidizing agents such as peroxide generated by bacteria (e.g., streptococci, pneumococci). Affected persons are unable to degrade exogenous or endogenous hydrogen peroxide, which accumulates in the periodontal tissues and leads to gingival hypoxemia with resultant ulceration and necrosis of soft and hard tissues. The Japanese variant (Takahara disease) is the symptomatic form, with the pathology confined to the oral cavity.

Diagnosis: Should be considered in the differential diagnosis of children with oral ulcerations. The patient's blood turns brown upon contact with hydrogen peroxide and lacks the generation of oxygen (bubbling). Catalase activity assays show low levels.

Clinical aspects: Children tend to be normal until eruption of the deciduous teeth, when deep necrotic periodontal or tonsillar ulcers with surrounding inflammation, dental caries, halitosis, loose teeth, and alveolar bone resorption begin to occur. Patients are rarely affected after puberty. Managed with surgical debridement, extraction of affected teeth, tonsillectomy, antibiotics, and meticulous oral hygiene. Except for potential loss of all teeth and parts of the alveolar bone, the overall prognosis in properly managed cases is good.

Precautions before anesthesia: Note the presence and location of any loose teeth and intraoral ulcerations.

Anesthetic considerations: Perform direct laryngoscopy carefully to prevent accidental dislodgment of loose teeth and trauma to periodontal or tonsillar ulcers. The latter may bleed easily and obstruct the view for endotracheal intubation. A cuffed endotracheal tube and/or throat pack are recommended to prevent irrigation fluid used during debridement from entering the airway. An awake extubation should minimize the risk of postextubation laryngospasm that may result from residual blood or secretions in a partially anesthetized patient.

Pharmacological implications: Avoid topical hydrogen peroxide, which is highly toxic to these patients.

REFERENCE:
Ogata M: Acatalasemia. *Hum Genet* 86:331, 1991.

Achalasia-Alacrima Syndrome

At a glance: The adrenocorticotropic hormone (ACTH) insensitivity syndrome is an inherited disorder, but in a small minority it is an acquired abnormality induced by the formation of antibodies that block ACTH receptors. In contrast to Addison syndrome, the renin–angiotensin–aldosterone axis functions normally.

Synonyms: Double A Syndrome; Adrenocorticotropic Insensitivity Syndrome.

Genetic inheritance: Autosomal recessive. Consists of several rare disorders with absent or markedly impaired adrenal response to ACTH. Most likely a variant of the Allgrove syndrome as shown by haplotype analysis.

Pathophysiology: Dysfunction or absence of ACTH receptors caused by a genetic defect or an acquired anomaly that induces formation of antibodies that block ACTH receptors.

Diagnosis: Based on the clinical findings of absent tears, dysphagia, and failure to thrive in infancy.

Clinical aspects: Absent tears in combination with achalasia. The disorder must be differentiated from ☞Allgrove or Triple A Syndrome (achalasia, alacrima, ACTH deficiency). Autonomic dysfunction has been reported as evidenced by electrophysiologic studies. Megaesophagus may occur.

Precautions before anesthesia: Check serum concentrations of electrolytes (mineralocorticoid deficiency), blood glucose, and ACTH. Obtain a history of vomiting, reflux, and dysphagia. Check for signs of autonomic dysfunction.

Anesthetic considerations: A rapid sequence induction technique is recommended because of the increased risk for gastroesophageal reflux. The likelihood of corneal abrasions is increased because of lack of tears. Possibility exists for autonomic dysfunction and cardiovascular instability in the absence of ACTH receptors.

Pharmacological implications: No known specific implication with this condition.

Other condition to be considered:

☞**ALLGROVE SYNDROME:** Inherited disease characterized by the triad of ACTH-resistant insufficiency, achalasia, and alacrima. It presents in the first decade of life with severe hypoglycemic episodes that may result in death. A mixed pattern of upper and lower motor neuropathy, sensory impairment, autonomic neuropathy, and mental retardation has been described.

REFERENCE:
Nussinson E, Hager H, Samara M, et al: Familial achalasia with absent tear production. *J Pediatr Gastrenterol Nutr* 7:284, 1988.

Achalasia-Microcephaly Syndrome

At a glance: Characterized by microcephaly, mental deficiency and early onset of symptoms of achalasia. Patients present with recurrent pulmonary aspirations and frequent respiratory infections.

Synonyms: Asherson Syndrome; Cricopharyngeal Achalasia.

Incidence/genetic inheritance: First described in 1978 in a Mexican family located in a small area in Northwest Mexico. There is no epidemiological study available to establish the incidence. Autosomal recessive inheritance is suggested.

Clinical aspects: Recurrent vomiting and pulmonary infections in a child with microcephaly, mental deficiency, achalasia.

Precautions before anesthesia: It is recommended to consider prophylaxis administration of sodium citrate to reduce the risk of pulmonary aspiration at time of induction of anesthesia. Evaluate serum electrolytes and arterial blood gases, if recurrent vomiting evident. A complete medical history and physical examination must be obtained to rule out the presence of reactive airways disease as a result of chronic aspiration. A chest x-ray and pulmonary function tests are indicated (when applicable).

Anesthetic considerations: Patients must be considered at significant risk for pulmonary aspiration of gastric contents. It is recommended to use an anesthesia technique to prevent this complication during induction of anesthesia and instrumentation of the airway. Reactive airway disease may be present as a result of chronic pulmonary aspiration. Intravascular volume depletion, serum electrolytes imbalances and arterial blood gases anomalies as a result of chronic vomiting must be corrected preoperatively in all patients.

Pharmacologic considerations: There are no known pharmacological implications in this medical condition. However, the use of anesthetic agents releasing histamine should be considered contraindicated in the presence of severe reactive airway disease.

REFERENCES:

Williams JJ, Sandlin CS, Dumars KW: New syndrome: Microcephaly associated with achalasia. *Am J Hum Genet* 30:106A, 1978.

Dumars KW, Williams JJ, Steele-Sandin C: Achalasia and microcephaly. *Am J Med Genet* 6:309–314, 1980.

Achard Syndrome

At a glance: Inherited disorder of the connective tissue, characterized mainly by brachycephaly, arachnodactyly, widespread dysostoses, increased ligament laxity, receding lower jaw (micrognathia), and joint laxity of the hands and feet.

History: First described in 1902 by Emile Charles Achard, a French internist.

Genetic inheritance: Autosomal dominant trait.

Diagnosis: Based on the clinical findings of brachnodactyly, micrognathia, and broad and brachycephalic skull.

Clinical aspects: Despite similarities, Achard syndrome and Marfan syndrome are different entities. Achard syndrome is a well-defined clinical entity characterized by widespread dysostoses most consistently affecting the tubular bones of the hands and feet, mandible, and calvaria, but it can occur anywhere in the skeleton. Ligament laxity manifests as hypermobility and/or subluxations of the joints (most commonly hands and feet) and increased lateral excursion of the patella. The skull is broad and brachycephalic, the lower jaw is small and receding, and the hands and feet show arachnodactyly. Body proportions are normal; however (in contrast to ☞Marfan Syndrome), most of these patients are known for not being tall. Patients with Achard syndrome lack the eye and heart abnormalities and the subnormal subcutaneous fat.

Precautions before anesthesia: Assess the airway for signs of difficult management.

Anesthetic considerations: Micrognathia may make airway management difficult. Spontaneous ventilation should be maintained until the airway has been secured. Careful patient positioning is required to avoid (sub)luxations of the joints.

Pharmacological implications: No known specific implications with this condition.

Other condition to be considered:

☞**MARFAN SYNDROME:** Familial disorder of generalized connective tissue abnormalities leading to connective tissue weakness associated with hyperextensible joints, dislocation of the lens, increased risk of valvular heart disease, risk of dissecting aortic aneurysm, and spontaneous pneumothorax.

REFERENCES:

Parish JG: Heritable disorders of connective tissues with arachnodactyly. *Proc R Soc Med* 53:515, 1960.

Duncan PA: The Achard syndrome. *Birth Defects Orig Artic Ser* 11:69, 1975.

Achard Thiers Syndrome

At a glance: Characterized by an insulin-resistant type 2 diabetes mellitus occurring primarily in postmenopausal women. It is associated with measurable increase in plasmatic androgen level.

Synonyms: Diabetic Bearded Women Syndrome; Adenoma Associated Virilism of Older Women.

History: First described in 1921 by Emile C. Achard, a French internist, and Joseph Thiers, a French Neurologist. The initial report of this medical condition was published in Paris in the Bulletin of the National Academy of Medicine.

Incidence: Occurs in postmenopausal females. The incidence remains unknown.

Genetic inheritance: Autosomal dominant or acquired.

Pathophysiology: Overproduction of male hormones androgens and other adrenocorticosteroid hormones (e.g., 11-oxysteroid) by the adrenal glands.

Diagnosis: Clinical presentation based on findings of hirsutism, virilization, hypertension, and abnormally high serum androgen levels in postmenopausal females.

Clinical aspects: Development of secondary male sexual traits, obesity, hypertension with subsequent end-organ cardiovascular disease.

Precautions before anesthesia: A complete medical history and physical examination must be obtained, especially the cardiovascular system. An ECG and echocardiography is recommended to eliminate the presence of a hypertrophic cardiomyopathy and cardiac disease as a result of long standing hypertension. A consultation with the endocrinology department is recommended. In the presence of severe obesity, the cardiorespiratory system must be evaluated to eliminate the potential effect of this complication and the possibility of chronic gastrointestinal reflux disease (GERD). The use of sodium citrate as prophylaxis for residual stomach content may be required prior to induction of general anesthesia.

Anesthetic considerations: Obesity may predispose patient to pulmonary aspiration of gastric contents during induction of general anesthesia, suggesting that a rapid sequence induction technique, when appropriate, may be indicated. The functional residual capacity may be compromised and postoperative ventilatory support required. Chronic hypertension may result in labile blood pressure control during anesthesia. Vascular access may be difficult as a result of obesity and subcutaneous tissue alterations.

Pharmacologic implications: Caution with sympathomimetics recommended.

REFERENCE:

Lubowe I: Achard-Thiers syndrome. *Arch Dermatol* 103:544, 1971.

Acheiropodia

At a glance: Characterized by bilateral congenital amputations of the upper and lower extremities and aplasia of the hands and feet. The specific pattern of malformations consist of a complete amputation of the distal epiphysis of the humerus, amputation of the distal part of the tibial diaphysis, and aplasia of the radius, ulna, fibula, and of the carpal, metacarpal, tarsal, metatarsal, and phalangeal bones.

Synonyms: Handless-Footless Families of Brazil; ACHP; Acheiropody.

Incidence/genetic inheritance: 1 in 250,000 births in Brazil. The highest incidence is observed among children born from consanguineous parents. Consanguinity has been found in 82% of parents. Autosomal recessive.

Clinical aspects: Bilateral congenital amputations of the upper and lower extremities and aplasia of the hands and feet, with the presence of Bohomoletz bone, i.e. an elongated small bone in the tip of the upper limb remnant, parallel to the axis of the humerus. However, the expressivity is rather variable and patients may or may not show this specific bone deformation characteristic of the disease.

Anesthetic considerations: There are no specific anesthetic considerations with this condition.

Pharmacological implications: There are no pharmacological implications.

REFERENCES:

Duboule D: The vertebrate limb: a model system to study the Hox/HOM gene network during development and evolution. *Bio Essays* 14:375, 1992.

Escamilla MA, DeMille MC, Benavides E, et al: A minimalist approach to gene mapping: locating the gene for acheiropodia, by homozygosity analysis. *Am J Hum Genet* 66:1995, 2000.

Achondrogenesis

At a glance: Very rare disorder characterized by extreme short-limbed dwarfism, lack of development of ribs, and other major bone formation. There are several subtypes of achondrogenesis. In general these forms are characterized by premature birth, fetal hydrops, normocephaly but an unusually soft cranial vault, and a short neck and trunk. Affected individuals have extremely short limbs, ribs, and vertebra. The disorder often is life-threatening either in utero or shortly after birth.

Synonyms: Chondrogenesis Imperfecta; Hypochondrogenesis; Lethal Neonatal Dwarfism; Lethal Osteochondrodysplasia; Neonatal Dwarfism.

Classification: Five subtypes of achondrogenesis have been described:

> Houston-Harris Type, achondrogenesis (type IA)
> Parenti-Fraccaro Type, achondrogenesis (type IB)
> Langer-Saldino Type, achondrogenesis (type II)
> Achondrogenesis, Type III
> Achondrogenesis, Type IV

Incidence and genetic inheritance: Achondrogenesis can be inherited as an autosomal or dominant recessive genetic trait. Achondrogenesis types IA, III, and IV are believed to be inherited as an autosomal recessive genetic trait. Achondrogenesis type IB is inherited as an autosomal recessive genetic trait with significant mutations in a gene called the *diastrophic dysplasia/sulfate transporter gene*. This gene encodes a sulfate transporter (DTDST). In addition, a deficiency in an enzyme responsible for the biologic activation of sulfate in children with type IB has been suggested. Achondrogenesis type II may be inherited by an autosomal recessive or dominant

genetic trait. The possibility of mutations of the gene (COL2A1) encoding type II collagen has been suggested.

Clinical aspects: There are several types of achondrogenesis. In general they are characterized by premature birth, fetal hydrops, normocephaly with cranial vault softness, and a short neck and trunk. Affected individuals have extremely short limbs, ribs, and vertebra, and other bones of the skeleton are not properly developed. Infants usually are born with a very prominent abdomen. Other features include a cleft palate, corneal clouding, ear deformities, and underdeveloped testicles and rectum.

Achondrogenesis type I affects individuals with abnormally small or short bones in the arms and/or legs (micromelia). The patient's head is normal, but the calvarial plates may be unusually soft. The two subtypes of achondrogenesis type I are *Houston-Harris type IA* and *Parenti-Fraccaro type IB*. The *Houston-Harris type* is characterized by premature birth, fetal hydrops, and polyhydramnios. After birth, the affected infant usually manifests micrognathia, low-bridged nose, extreme short stature that is identifiable at birth, very short limbs (micromelia), lack of development of the bones of the spine, and an extremely short neck. The infant usually is stillborn or dies shortly after birth. The *Parenti-Fraccaro type* is characterized by the presence of thin ribs subjected to spontaneous fractures during manipulation at birth. The patient presents as a short-limbed dwarf in whom the important short stature and short limb disorder is easily identifiable at birth. The respiratory system often is affected by respiratory insufficiency resulting from pulmonary hypoplasia. The child is born prematurely and most often presents a fetal hydrops. The skeleton system is significantly affected with inappropriate development, especially of the spine, arms and legs. The infants either are stillborn or usually die immediately after birth.

In *Langer-Saldino type (achondrogenesis type II),* the shape of the head usually is normal. The patient presents with marked micromelia dwarfism. However, the skull may be enlarged even in the presence of normal ossification. The absence of vertebral mineralization makes the patient susceptible to fractures. The sacrum and the ischial and pubic bones often are nonossified. Small iliac wings with concave borders give a characteristic shape to the pelvis. Very short but broad tubular bones associated with cupped metaphyses and short tubular bones give the extreme dwarfism appearance. Fetal hydrops, polyhydramnios, and hypochondrogenesis represent clinical variability. Rib fractures are very frequent in this syndrome. Cleft palate and cystic hygroma are reported. Barrel-shaped chest, short trunk, horizontal ribs, and distended abdomen are frequent features. This form of achondrogenesis may result in stillborn infants. In less severe cases, the baby may survive for 1 week or months.

Achondrogenesis type III is characterized by normal ribs and absence of fractures. The long bones (arms and legs) may seem normal but they appear mushroom-stemmed. Scientists believe achondrogenesis type III is a form of achondrogenesis type II and is not a distinct form of the disorder.

Achondrogenesis type IV is inherited as an autosomal recessive genetic trait. The long bones are normally developed at birth, the ribs do not appear to be susceptible to fractures, and their development is normal.

Anesthetic considerations: There are few occasions when anesthesia is implicated in the care of these infants because of the early lethality of the first two types. For patients requiring anesthesia, the main consideration is a difficult airway because of the micrognathia. The presence of pulmonary hypoplasia in type II may complicate mechanical ventilation. Positioning of these patients requires the most careful attention to prevent fractures of the ribs, vertebrae, and long tubular bones.

Other conditions to be considered:

☞**KNIEST SYNDROME** is characterized by extreme dwarfism with a shortened, barrel-shaped chest. The face is flat with bulging eyes. A flat nasal bridge, cleft palate, and repetitive ear infections have been described. Retinal detachment because of severe myopia has been reported. The arms and legs are very short and bowing. Usually enlargement of the joints causes pain and stiffness. Hernias, loss of hearing, and a collapsing trachea may occur.

CAMPTOMELIC SYNDROME is a rare congenital skeletal disorder inherited as an autosomal recessive genetic trait. It is characterized by dwarfism with bowing and an angular shape of the long bones of the legs. The shoulder and pelvic area often are abnormal. Patients usually have only 11 pairs of ribs instead of 12. Two forms of this disorder have been described: the *long-limbed form* and the *short-limbed form.*

☞**THANATOPHORIC DWARFISM** is another form of dwarfism characterized by an enlarged head, shortened bones in the arms and legs, small, short ribs and flattened vertebrae. An abnormally large amount of amniotic fluid is present, and very little fetal movement occurs before birth.

SHORT RIB SYNDROME is a form of short-limb dwarfism. The infant has cleft lip/palate, deformed ears, and a narrow chest with short ribs. The kidneys and genital organs often are affected. Brain malformations and absence of a gallbladder are common. This disorder is often life-threatening because of insufficient lung development.

☞**CHONDRODYSPLASIA: Grebe Syndrome** is a type of short-limbed dwarfism considered a type of achondrogenesis. However, it now is classified as a different chondrodysplasia disease. It is characterized by short-limbed dwarfism that affects both sexes. The disorder is evident from birth. The most characteristic features are extremely short limbs, with the legs more severely affected than the upper limbs. The hands are extremely short with toe-like fingers. The feet are in the valgus position. Polydactyly is seen in 50% of cases. Obesity occurs. Delayed mental development but mentally normal individual. Facies normal. Inherited as an autosomal recessive genetic trait.

REFERENCES:

Rittler M, Orioli IM: Achondrogenesis type II with polydactyly. *Am J Med Genet* 59:157, 1995.

Maroteaux P, Lamy M: Le diagnostic des nanismes chondro-dystrophiques chez les nouveau-nes. *Arch Franc Pediatr* 25:241, 1968.

Achondroplasia

At a glance: Achondroplasia is the most common form of short-limbed dwarfism. It is characterized by short-limbed dwarfism, macrocephaly, frontal bossing, a low nasal bridge, and midface hypoplasia. Skeletal malformations may include brachydactyly, lordosis, genu varum, and/or stenosis of the spine. Additional abnormalities may include limited extension of the elbows and hips, hypotonia, and frequent otitis media. In most cases achondroplasia appears sporadically.

Incidence and genetic inheritance: Achondroplasia appears to occur sporadically with no apparent family history. However, the possibility of familial transmission has been suggested, and inheritance as an autosomal dominant pattern with new dominant gene mutations has been reported. Advanced paternal age may be a contributing factor in cases of sporadic achondroplasia. In the absence of mutations, familial cases of achondroplasia have been reported as autosomal dominant inheritance but are much less common. Specific mutations of a gene known as *fibroblast growth factor receptor (FGFR)-3* are possible. The FGFR-3 gene is located on chromosome 4 (4p16.3).

Clinical aspects: Achondroplasia is a rare genetic disorder characterized by macrocephaly, frontal bossing, and depressed nasal bridge. The arms and legs usually are very short, and the trunk appears long in comparison. Rhizomelic dwarfism, unusually prominent abdomen and buttocks, and short hands with fingers usually assuming a "trident" or three-pronged position during extension are characteristic. The trident position is described by an index and middle finger typically close together and the ring finger and the pinkie close together, giving the hand a three-pronged (trident) appearance. The hands are generally short and broad. Infants typically have an arched or vaulted skull in response to the megaloencephaly, which is pathognomonic of the syndrome. The forehead is broad. Midface hypoplasia can be seen. The presence of dorsal kyphosis adds to the dwarfism appearance. Hydrocephalus may be present, so the risk of elevated intracranial pressure should be remembered. Compression of the brainstem because of foramen magnum stenosis may occur in some children and result in a life-threatening condition. The respiratory system may be associated with upper airway obstruction because of midface hypoplasia and short neck. Other features include hearing loss secondary to chronic recurrent otitis media. The incidence of obstructive sleep apnea has been reported because of the macroglossia, high arched palate, prominent mandible, and choanal stenosis. Tonsilloadenoidectomy may improve the symptoms. The cardiovascular system is not involved in this disease. However, as a result of airway obstruction, secondary pulmonary artery hypertension and right ventricular hypertrophy may develop. Obesity may develop in both genders. The mean male adult height is 131 cm and the mean female height is 124 cm. Children may have deformities of the rib cage, including excessive curvature or "cupping" of the ribs. Intellectually, achondroplasia does not cause any impairment or deficiencies in mental abilities. The life expectancy of infants older than 12 months is normal.

Anesthetic considerations: The presence of normal intelligence and proper social skills for their age should be considered in the management of the children, adolescents, and adults with the disorder. The most important anesthetic consideration should be the airway. The presence of choanal atresia or stenosis and macroglossia could make face-mask ventilation difficult. Direct laryngoscopy usually is not limited because of the prominent mandible, but the limitation of cervical mobility may make visibility of the larynx difficult. Associated with the potential presence of raised intracranial pressure, compression of the brainstem, foramen magnum stenosis, and limited mobility at the C1-C2 junction, the preparation for airway management requires proper planning. Fifty percent of patients present with spinal involvement, so proper monitoring of the spinal cord is indicated for induction, positioning, and maintenance of anesthesia. Use of somatosensory evoked potential should be considered, especially with surgical procedure requiring special positioning or mobilization of the cervical spine. The importance of monitoring resides in the changes that occur over time in comparison to baseline. Patients affected with pulmonary hypertension or right ventricular hypertrophy should be assessed preoperatively with care and proper anesthesia management applied for these conditions. If obesity is severe, the potential risk of gastrointestinal reflux must be kept in mind. Positioning of the patient may be influenced by the joint contracture and limited mobility. Proper padding of pressure points must be ensured.

Other conditions to be considered:

HYPOCHONDROPLASIA is a genetic disorder characterized by short-limbed dwarfism. Short stature often is not recognized until early to middle childhood or even until adulthood in some cases. Affected individuals may develop bowing of the legs during early childhood that often improves spontaneously with age. Additional features include macrocephaly, forehead bossing, and limited extension and rotation of the elbows. Mild mental retardation may be present in approximately 10 percent of cases. Sporadic cases with no apparent family history have been described. However, the disorder is familial and seems to be inherited as an autosomal dominant pattern.

REFERENCES:

Monedero P, Garcia-Pedrajas F, Coca I, et al: Is management of anesthesia for achondroplastic dwarfism really a challenge? *J Clin Anesth* 9:208, 1997.

McGlothen S: Anesthesia for cesarean section for achondroplastic dwarf: a case report. *AANA J* 68:305, 2000.

Cunningham MJ, Ferrari L, Kearse LA Jr, et al: Intraoperative somatosensory evoked potential monitoring in achondroplasia. *Paediatr Anaesth* 4:129, 1994.

Achoo Syndrome

At a glance: Twenty percent of the population sneezes when exposed to bright light. Look for nephropathic cystinosis.

Synonyms: Autosomal Dominant Compelling Helioophthalmic Outburst Syndrome; Photic Sneeze Reflex; Peroutka Sneeze Reflex.

Incidence and genetic inheritance: Incidence unknown. The syndrome probably is unrecognized in many individuals. May affect up to 20% of the Swedish population. Achoo syndrome is transmitted as an autosomal dominant trait.

Clinical aspects: May be a complication of slitlamp examination. Abnormal reflex sneezing secondary to bright light. May be associated with nephropathic cystinosis thought to be caused by crystal deposition in the cornea.

Anesthetic considerations: No known specific implications with this condition.

REFERENCE:

Beckman L, Nordenson I: Individual differences with respect to the sneezing reflex: An inherited physiological trait in man? *Hum Hered* 33:390, 1983.

Ackerman Syndrome

At a glance: Familial syndrome of fused pyramidal molar roots, hypotrichosis upper lip morphology without Cupid's bow but with a thickened and widened philtrum, and occasional juvenile glaucoma.

Synonyms: Pyramidal Molar Roots with Juvenile Glaucoma and Unusual Upper Lip; Juvenile Glaucoma with Unusual Upper Lip and Dental Roots Syndrome.

Genetic inheritance: Autosomal recessive.

Clinical aspects: Has been described in one family in which all siblings had pyramidal molar roots. Two siblings had glaucoma, and all had an unusual morphology of the upper lip without a Cupid's bow and a widened and thickened philtrum.

Anesthetic considerations: Avoid succinylcholine and other drugs that may increase intraocular pressure in the presence of glaucoma.

REFERENCE:

Ackerman JL, Ackerman AL, Ackerman A: Taurodont, pyramidal and fused molar roots associated with other anomalies in a kindred. *Am J Phys Anthropol* 38:681, 1973.

Acrocephalopolysyndactylous Dysplasia

At a glance: Polymalformative syndrome presenting with acrocephaly, cervical cavernous lymphangioma, multiple visceral malformations, short neck, and macroglossia. May be associated with Beckwith-Wiedemann syndrome in neonates.

Synonym: Elejalde Syndrome. (A different syndrome also called ☞Elejalde Syndrome has been described.) To avoid confusion, we recommend reserving this name for the syndrome described in section "E."

Incidence: Extremely rare abnormality of fetal development of unknown cause. Four cases have been reported.

Genetic inheritance: Autosomal recessive trait most possible. No genetic background or molecular data are available.

Diagnosis and clinical aspects: At birth, the diagnosis is made based on the clinical aspect: high birth weight, swollen and globular body, short neck with redundant skin folds, postaxial polydactyly, omphalocele, and enlarged liver and kidneys with renal dysplasia. Craniosynostosis has been described in one case.

Precautions before anesthesia: No published data on the anesthetic management or pharmacological implications in this syndrome are available. Precautions before anesthesia and anesthetic considerations must refer to data concerning omphalocele, renal failure, and craniosynostosis. In neonates, carefully look for any associated heart anomalies by echocardiography and rule out Beckwith-Wiedemann syndrome, which combines gigantism, macroglossia, hypoglycemia, and omphalocele. Evaluate for possible airway obstruction and difficult tracheal intubation related to short neck and macroglossia. Assess renal function with blood and urine analysis (electrolytes, urea, creatinine).

Anesthetic considerations: Fluid and electrolyte intake must be adapted to renal function. In case of suspected difficult tracheal intubation, maintenance of spontaneous ventilation is recommended until the airway has been secured. Alternative airway management options should be available (e.g., laryngeal mask airway, fiberoptic bronchoscope). In the presence of an omphalocele, intrathoracic, central venous, and intraabdominal pressures should be carefully monitored upon closure of the parietal defect.

Pharmacological implications: Drugs with predominantly renal elimination should be used cautiously. In case of suspected difficult tracheal intubation, neuromuscular blockers should be avoided until the airway has been secured. Avoid use of nitrous oxide during surgical repair of omphalocele because of risk for bowel distension.

REFERENCES:

Thornton CM, Stewart F: Elejalde syndrome: A case report. *Am J Med Genet* 69:406, 1997.

Nevin NC, Herron B, Armstrong MJ: An 18 week fetus with Elejalde syndrome (acrocephalopolydactylous dysplasia). *Clin Dysmorphol* 3:180, 1994.

Acrocephalopolysyndactyly Syndromes

At a glance: Complex association of faciocranial dysmorphism.
Classification and synonyms:

Acrocephalopolysyndactyly type I = Noack syndrome.
Acrocephalopolysyndactyly type II = Carpenter syndrome (most common)
Acrocephalopolysyndactyly type III = Sakati-Nyhan syndrome
Acrocephalopolysyndactyly type IV = Goodman syndrome

Genetic inheritance: Autosomal recessive. Gene locus unknown.
Pathophysiology: Unknown. May be related to accelerated maturation and premature differentiation of fibroblasts.
Diagnosis: Based on the clinical findings at birth and skull radiography of premature craniosynostosis of cranial sutures.
Precautions before anesthesia: The need to carefully assess the airway is obvious when treating a child. Midface hypoplasia with hypoplasia of the mandible may make mask fit difficult. During direct laryngoscopy, the larynx often cannot be visualized. Choanal atresia has been linked to these syndromes, so choanal patency should be checked before nasotracheal intubation. Radiographic studies of the cervical spine prior to anesthesia may be helpful. Airway strategies may include fiberoptic intubation, blind nasal intubation, or a laryngeal mask, but spontaneous ventilation and oxygenation must be maintained during these attempts. Neurosurgical complications of the acrocephalopolysyndactyly syndromes are progressive hydrocephalus, chronic tonsillar herniation, syringomyelia, and, although uncommon, respiratory standstill. Congenital heart disease must be ruled out, and pulmonary arterial pressure should be determined by echocardiography before the patient undergoes anesthesia. Check for visceral abnormalities before anesthesia.
Anesthetic considerations: Maintain spontaneous ventilation until the airway has been secured. The technical management of the airway must be prepared before induction of anesthesia. Surgical airway equipment and a surgeon experienced in airway management must be present in the operating room at all times.
Pharmacological implications: Succinylcholine and other neuromuscular relaxants can be used safely. Normal sensitivity to hypnotic and sedative drugs.

REFERENCES:
Nargozian C: Apert syndrome. Anesthetic management. *Clin Plast Surg* 18:227, 1991.
Sculerati N, Gottlieb MD, Chibbaro PD: Airway management in children with major craniofacial anomalies. *Laryngoscope* 108:1806, 1998.

ACROCEPHALOPOLYSYNDACTYLY TYPE I: NOACK SYNDROME

At a glance: Noack syndrome is very similar to Pfeiffer syndrome. Patients present with enlarged thumbs, duplication of the great toes, and moderate acrocephaly.
Synonym: Dominant type of acrocephalopolysyndactyly.
History: Named after Margot Noack, a 20th-century German physician.

Genetic inheritance: Inherited as an autosomal dominant condition.
Clinical aspects: The disease involves the hands and feet. Patients have enlarged thumbs and duplication of the great toes. Moderate acrocephaly. Considered identical to Pfeiffer syndrome.
Precautions before anesthesia: Evaluate the head and neck anatomy in consideration of airway management (reduced size of nasopharynx, maxilla, mandible, limited mouth opening, anomalies of the palate and tracheal cartilage, combined with cervical spine abnormalities may lead to difficult airway management). Radiographs of the cervical spine may be helpful in the evaluation process. Request echocardiography for patients with congenital cardiac lesions. Preoperative chest radiograph may be helpful. Preoperative blood workup should include a complete blood count, electrolytes, creatinine, and blood urea nitrogen (BUN). Keep in mind that the incidence of increased intracranial pressure is 15% with one fused suture and increases to 35% with two or more sutures affected.
Anesthetic considerations: Mental retardation may lead to poor cooperation upon separation from the parents or during induction of anesthesia. Difficult airway management should be expected. Maintenance of spontaneous ventilation and oxygenation during attempts to control the airway is strongly recommended. Be prepared to use alternative techniques to manage the airway (laryngeal mask, fiberoptic intubation). A surgeon familiar with surgical airway management and the necessary equipment should always be present in the operating room. Specific anesthetic measures are required in case of congenital heart disease or increased intracranial pressure. The eyes must be carefully protected because of the high risk for corneal damage as a result of proptosis.
Pharmacological implications: Sedative premedication in patients with increased intracranial pressure should be used with caution and under supervision of trained personnel only. Hypotensive anesthesia most often is achieved using volatile anesthetics, opioids, and/or sympathoadrenergic receptor-blocking drugs. Avoid nitrous oxide secondary to risk of venous air embolism. Antibiotic prophylaxis for subacute bacterial endocarditis may be necessary.

ACROCEPHALOPOLYSYNDACTYLY TYPE II: CARPENTER SYNDROME

At a glance: Craniosynostosis, acrocephaly, peculiar facies, syndactyly, short stature, midface or mandible hypoplasia, short neck, and high arched palate. Cardiac malformations.
History: First described by George Carpenter (1859–1910), a British physician.
Genetic inheritance: Autosomal recessive inheritance.
Clinical aspects: Typically evident at or shortly after birth. The head is acrocephalic and often called the "tower-shaped skull" (turricephaly), resulting from craniosynostosis including coronal, sagittal, and lambdoid sutures. Increased intracranial pressure may occur. The skull can appear brachycephalic (short and broad). Other features include facial anomalies of hypertelorism, mild downward slanting of the palpebral fissures, microcornea, corneal opacity, and optic atrophy. The nose appears dysplastic with depressed nasal bridge, the ears are low-set, and upper and lower jaws are hypoplastic with a narrow and high arched palate. The syndrome often is associated with brachydactyly, with absence of the middle phalanges, cutaneous syndactyly, and presence of supernumerary toes. Polydactyly is not as frequent. Congenital heart defects present in up to 50% of cases (atrial septal defect, ventricular septal defect, patent ductus arteriosus, tetralogy of Fallot, pulmonary stenosis, and transposition of great vessels have been reported). Mild-to-moderate obesity and cryptorchidism occur in affected males. Mental retardation

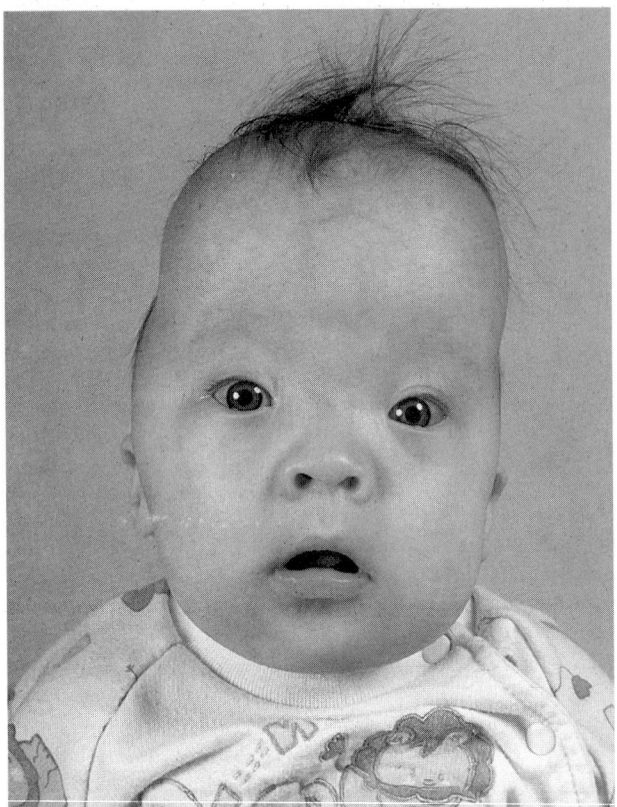

Acrocephalopolysyndactyly type II Acrocephaly in a 20-month-old girl with Carpenter syndrome.

most often is present, but some patients with normal intelligence have been reported.

Precautions before anesthesia: Evaluate the head and neck anatomy in consideration of airway management (reduced size of nasopharynx, maxilla, mandible, anomalies of the palate and tracheal cartilage, combined with cervical spine abnormalities, may lead to difficult airway management). Radiographs of the cervical spine may be helpful in the evaluation process. Request echocardiography for patients with congenital cardiac lesions. Because up to one third of the children have intraoperative respiratory problems (mainly significant wheezing in patients with recent airway infection), the threshold to cancel the procedure in these patients in the presence of an active or recent upper airway infection should be low. Preoperative chest radiograph may be helpful. Preoperative blood workup should include a complete blood count, electrolytes, creatinine, and BUN. Keep in mind that the incidence of increased intracranial pressure is 15% with one fused suture and increases to 35% with two or more sutures affected.

Anesthetic considerations: Mental retardation may lead to poor cooperation upon separation from the parents or during induction of anesthesia. Difficult airway management should be expected. Maintenance of spontaneous ventilation and oxygenation during attempts to control the airway is strongly recommended. Be prepared to use alternative techniques to manage the airway (laryngeal mask, fiberoptic intubation). A surgeon familiar with surgical airway management and the necessary equipment should always be present in the operating room. Specific anesthetic measures are required in case of congenital heart disease or increased intracranial pressure. The eyes must be carefully protected because of the high risk for corneal damage because of proptosis.

Pharmacological implications: Sedative premedication in patients with increased intracranial pressure should be used with caution and under supervision of trained personnel only. Hypotensive anesthesia most often is achieved using volatile anesthetics, opioids, and/or sympathoadrenergic receptor-blocking drugs. Avoid nitrous oxide because of the risk of venous air embolism. Antibiotic prophylaxis for subacute bacterial endocarditis may be necessary.

Other condition to be considered:

SUMMITT SYNDROME is a variant of Carpenter syndrome. Patients present with obesity and normal intelligence.

REFERENCES:

Robinson LK, James HE, Mubarak SJ, et al: Carpenter syndrome: Natural history and clinical spectrum. *Am J Med Genet* 20:461, 1985.

Carpenter G: Two sisters showing malformations of the skull and other congenital abnormalities. *Rep Soc Study Dis Child Lond* 1:110, 1901.

ACROCEPHALOPOLYSYNDACTYLY TYPE III: SAKATI-NYHAN SYNDROME

At a glance: Patients present with severe acrocephaly and distinctive leg defects (hypoplastic tibia, bowed femora, coxa valga). Other features include brachydactyly, duplication of the first toe, preaxial polydactyly, and congenital heart disease.

Synonyms: Acrocephalopolysyndactyly with Leg Hypoplasia; Sakati Syndrome.

History: First described by Nadia Sakati, William Leo Nyhan, and W.K. Tisdale, 20th-century American physicians.

Genetic inheritance: Autosomal dominant inheritance is most likely. Advanced parental age may be a risk factor.

Diagnosis: Radiographs confirm osseous anomalies.

Clinical aspects: Craniosynostosis and acrocephaly. Small face with prognathism, maxillary hypoplasia, dysplastic low-set ears, and short neck with low hairline are common findings. Congenital heart defects, preaxial polydactyly, and distinctive leg anomalies (coxa valga, bowed femora, hypoplastic tibia) are additional findings. No treatment of the underlying disorder is available.

Precautions before anesthesia: Evaluate the head and neck anatomy in consideration of airway management (reduced size of nasopharynx, maxilla, mandible, anomalies of the palate and tracheal cartilage, combined with cervical spine abnormalities may lead to difficult airway management). Radiographs of the cervical spine may be helpful in the evaluation process. Request echocardiography for patients with congenital cardiac lesions. Because up to one third of the children have intraoperative respiratory problems (mainly significant wheezing in patients with recent airway infection), the threshold to cancel the procedure in these patients in the presence of an active or recent upper airway infection should be low. Preoperative chest radiograph may be helpful. Preoperative blood workup should include a complete blood count, electrolytes, creatinine, and BUN. Keep in mind that the incidence of increased intracranial pressure is 15% with one fused suture and increases to 35% with two or more sutures affected.

Anesthetic considerations: Mental retardation may lead to poor cooperation upon separation from the parents or during induction of anesthesia. Difficult airway management should be expected. Maintenance of spontaneous ventilation and oxygenation during attempts to control the airway is strongly recommended. Be prepared to use alternative techniques to manage the airway (laryngeal mask, fiberoptic intubation). A surgeon familiar with surgical airway management and the necessary equipment should always be present in the operating room. Specific anesthetic measures might be required in the presence of congenital heart disease (antibiotic prophylaxis for subacute bacterial endocarditis may be required) or increased intracranial pressure. The eyes must be carefully protected because of the high risk for corneal damage because of proptosis.

Pharmacological implications: Sedative premedication in patients with increased intracranial pressure should be used with caution and under supervision of trained personnel only. Hypotensive anesthesia is most often achieved using volatile anesthetics, opioids and/or sympathoadrenergic receptor-blocking drugs. Avoid nitrous oxide secondary to the risk of venous air embolism. Antibiotic prophylaxis for subacute bacterial endocarditis may be necessary.

REFERENCE:

Sakati N, Nyhan W, Tisdale W: A new syndrome with acrocephalopolysyndactyly, cardiac disease, and distinctive defects of the ear, skin and lower limbs. *J Pediatr* 79:104, 1971.

ACROCEPHALOPOLYSYNDACTYLY TYPE IV: GOODMAN SYNDROME

At a glance: Extremely rare genetic disorder characterized by marked malformations of the head and face, polysyndactyly, and congenital heart defects, which may result in early death. Includes ulnar deviation with clinodactyly and camptodactyly. Believed to be a variant of Carpenter syndrome.

Synonyms: Acrodynia; Pink Disease; Feer Disease.

Nature: Since the cause was identified in 1955 (mercury-containing paint, especially latex paint), the incidence in the general population is decreasing.

Incidence: Incidence decreasing since 1955 in the general population because the causes are well identified (paint containing mercury, especially latex paint).

Genetic inheritance: Autosomal recessive inheritance.

Diagnosis: High mercury level in urine.

Clinical aspects: Acrocephaly secondary to craniosynostosis and syndactyly, clinodactyly, and camptodactyly. Ulnar deviation seems characteristic the association with congenital. Congenital heart defects has been reported: one child died of Eisenmenger syndrome. Hydrocephalus and raised intracranial pressure occur, especially in patients with several fused sutures.

Precautions before anesthesia: Evaluate the head and neck anatomy in consideration of airway management (reduced size of nasopharynx, maxilla, mandible, anomalies of the palate and tracheal cartilage, combined with cervical spine abnormalities, may lead to difficult airway management). Radiographs of the cervical spine may be helpful in the evaluation process. Request echocardiography for patients with clinical suspicion of congenital cardiac lesions. Preoperative chest radiograph may be helpful. Preoperative blood workup should include a complete blood count, electrolytes, creatinine, and BUN. Keep in mind that the incidence of increased intracranial pressure is 15% with one fused suture and more than 35% with two or more sutures affected.

Anesthetic considerations: Mental retardation may lead to poor cooperation upon separation from the parents or during induction of anesthesia. Difficult airway management should be expected. Maintenance of spontaneous ventilation and oxygenation during attempts to control the airway is strongly recommended. Be prepared to use alternative techniques to manage the airway (laryngeal mask, fiberoptic intubation). A surgeon familiar with surgical airway management and the necessary equipment should always be present in the operating room. Specific anesthetic measures might be required in the presence of congenital heart disease or increased intracranial

pressure. The eyes must be carefully protected because of the high risk for corneal damage as a result of proptosis.

Pharmacological implications: Sedative premedication in patients with increased intracranial pressure should be used with caution and under supervision of trained personnel only. Hypotensive anesthesia is most often achieved using volatile anesthetics, opioids, and/or sympathoadrenergic receptor-blocking drugs. Avoid nitrous oxide secondary to the risk of venous air embolism. Antibiotic prophylaxis for subacute bacterial endocarditis may be necessary.

REFERENCES:

Dinehart SM, Dillard R, Raimer SS, et al: Cutaneous manifestations of acrodynia (pink disease). *Arch Dermatol* 124:107, 1988.

Fuortes LJ, Weismann DN, Graeff ML, et al: Immune thrombocytopenia and elemental mercury poisoning. *J Toxicol Clin Toxicol* 33:449, 1995.

Acrocephalosyndactyly Syndromes

At a glance: Group of diseases characterized by craniofacial anomalies resulting from premature sutural craniosynostosis and hand and foot anomalies consisting primarily of brachydactyly, syndactyly, and polysyndactyly. A number of different subtypes exist but considerable phenotypic overlap occurs, so investigators now consider many of these syndromes to represent variants of the same disease. The classification into subtypes in the literature is conflicting. Furthermore, the classification of acrocephalosyndactyly versus acrocephalopolysyndactyly is regarded by many as a pseudo-distinction.

Definition: Acrocephalosyndactyly syndromes are characterized by craniosynostosis, dysmorphic facial features, and severe syndactyly of the hands and feet.

Classification: Acrocephalosyndactyly syndromes classically have been divided into five subtypes:

> Acrocephalosyndactyly Type I = Apert syndrome
> Acrocephalosyndactyly Type II = Apert-Crouzon syndrome (most common)
> Acrocephalosyndactyly Type III = Saethre-Chotzen syndrome
> Acrocephalosyndactyly Type V = Pfeiffer syndrome

Genetic inheritance: Autosomal dominant. Increased paternal age is considered a risk factor.

Pathophysiology: These syndromes result from mutations in the gene encoding FGFR-2. The responsible gene has been mapped to 10q26. The defect causes abnormal osseous development resulting in irregular bridging of the mesenchymal tissue that eventually forms bone. The cranium and distal extremities are predominantly affected.

Diagnosis: Based on clinical findings. Radiographic examinations confirm osseous abnormalities.

Precautions before anesthesia: Evaluate the head and neck anatomy in consideration of airway management (reduced size of nasopharynx, maxilla, mandible, anomalies of the palate and tracheal cartilage, combined with cervical spine abnormalities, may lead to difficult airway management). Radiographs of the cervical spine may be helpful in the evaluation process. Request echocardiography for patients with congenital cardiac lesions. Because up to one third of the children affected with these conditions present with intraoperative respiratory problems, recent upper respiratory infections might require cancellation of the procedure in these patients in the presence of an active or recent upper airway infection should be low. Preoperative chest radiograph may be helpful. Preoperative blood workup should include a complete blood count, electrolytes, creatinine, and BUN. Keep in mind that the incidence of increased intracranial pressure is 15% with one fused suture and increases to 35% with two or more sutures affected.

Anesthetic considerations: Mental retardation may lead to poor cooperation upon separation from the parents or during induction of anesthesia. Difficult airway management should be expected. Maintenance of spontaneous ventilation and oxygenation during attempts to control the airway is strongly recommended. Be prepared to use alternative techniques to manage the airway (laryngeal mask, fiberoptic intubation). A surgeon familiar with surgical airway management and the necessary equipment should always be present in the operating room. Specific anesthetic measures might be required in the presence of congenital heart disease or increased intracranial pressure. The eyes must be carefully protected because of the high risk for corneal damage as a result of proptosis.

Pharmacological implications: Sedative premedication in patients with increased intracranial pressure should be used with caution and under supervision of trained personnel only. Hypotensive anesthesia is most often achieved using volatile anesthetics, opioids, and/or sympathoadrenergic receptor-blocking drugs. Avoid nitrous oxide secondary to the risk of venous air embolism. Antibiotic prophylaxis for subacute bacterial endocarditis may be necessary.

ACROCEPHALOSYNDACTYLY TYPE I: APERT SYNDROME

At a glance: Characterized by agenesis or premature closure of the cranial sutures, midface hypoplasia, and symmetrical syndactyly of the hands and feet involving at least the second, third, and fourth digits. An extensive midline calvarial defect extends from the gabella to the posterior fontanelle. Partial cervical spine fusion is common and almost always involves C5-6. Numerous facial anomalies are seen. Heart defects may be associated.

Synonym: Vogt Cephalosyndactyly.

History: First reported in 1894 by S.W. Wheaton and extensively described in 1906 by Eugène Charles Apert, a French pediatrician.

Incidence: 1:65,000 to 1:160,000. Both sexes are equally affected. Apert syndrome accounts for approximately 5% of all craniosynostoses.

Genetic inheritance: Autosomal dominant. However, the majority is sporadic and results from new mutations. The syndrome results from mutations in the gene encoding FGFR-2. The gene has been mapped to 10q26. Higher paternal age seems to be a risk factor.

Pathophysiology: This genetic defect leads to abnormal osseous development resulting in irregular bridging of mesenchymal tissue that eventually transforms into bone. The cranium and distal extremities are predominantly affected.

Diagnosis: Based on clinical findings. Radiographs confirm osseous abnormalities.

Clinical aspects: The coronal sutures are most commonly involved, resulting in high forehead and flat facies. A horizontal groove above the supraorbital ridge and a break in the continuity of eyebrows are common. Facial dysmorphism is further characterized by spheno-ethmoido-maxillary hypoplasia, a short nose with bulbous tip, and depressed nasal bridge, prominent mandible, and a narrow and high arched palate (with cleft in approximately

30%). Choanal stenosis or atresia is frequent. Agenesis of the corpus callosum, malformations of the limbic system, encephaloceles, hydrocephalus, and abnormalities of the pyramidal tract have been described. The degree of mental retardation is variable. Fused cervical vertebrae occur in up to 70% of patients and most commonly involve C5 and C6, although they are often multiple. The limbs show the typical features of syndactyly (most often digits II, III, IV) with broad great toes and thumbs. The shoulder, elbow, and hip joints may be either ankylotic or even aplastic. Congenital cardiac lesions (e.g., patent ductus arteriosus, atrial septal defect, ventricular septal defect, pulmonary stenosis, tetralogy of Fallot, coarctation of the aorta) can be detected in up to 10% of these patients. Other features of the syndrome are genitourinary anomalies (e.g., vaginal atresia, clitoris hypertrophy, uterus bicornis, cryptorchidism, polycystic kidney disease, hydronephrosis, bladder neck stenosis), which occur in approximately 10% of patients. Esophageal atresia has been described in 2% of patients. Airway anomalies occur in up to 2% of patients and include tracheoesophageal fistula, abnormal tracheal cartilage (stiff or vertically fused tracheal rings, which may impair the ability to clear the trachea effectively from secretions), and absence of the right middle lobe or interlobar fissures of the lungs. A higher incidence of pyloric stenosis, imperforate anus, and biliary atresia has been reported in these patients compared with the normal population. There is no curative treatment for the disorder, and the prognosis depends on the severity of the condition. Early neurosurgical treatment does not prevent mental retardation.

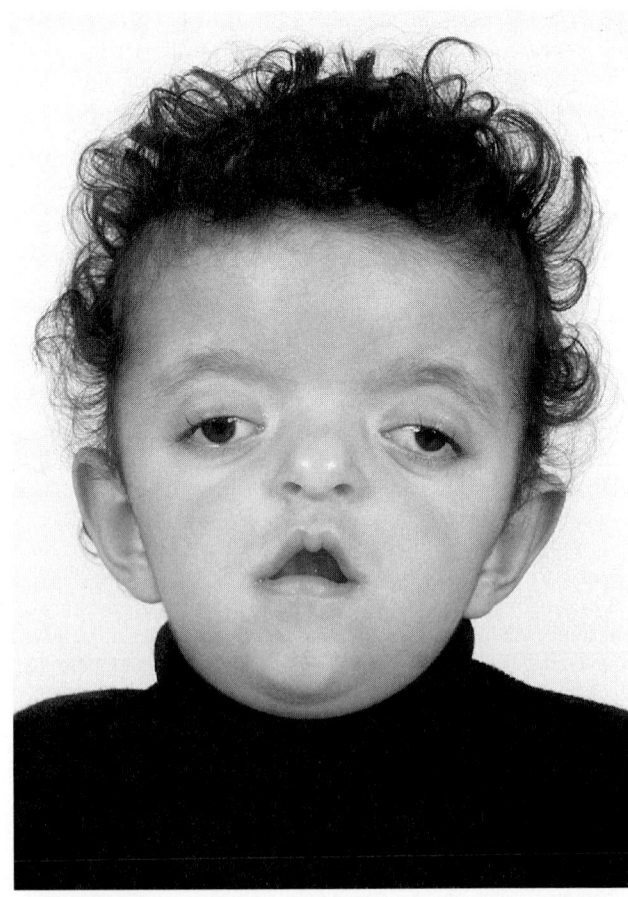

Apert syndrome   Typical facial appearance of an 18-month-old girl with Apert syndrome.

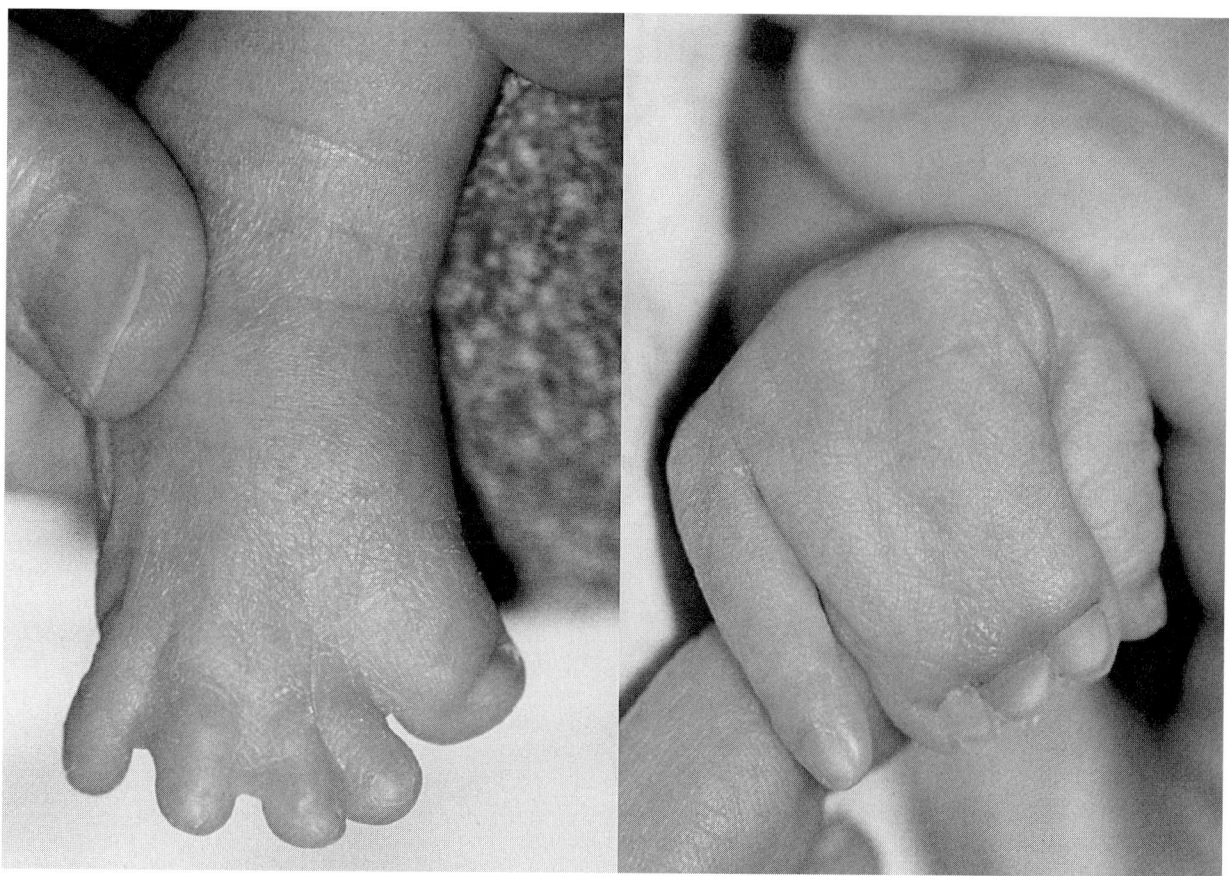

Apert syndrome   Syndactyly of the fingers and toes of a newborn boy with Apert syndrome.

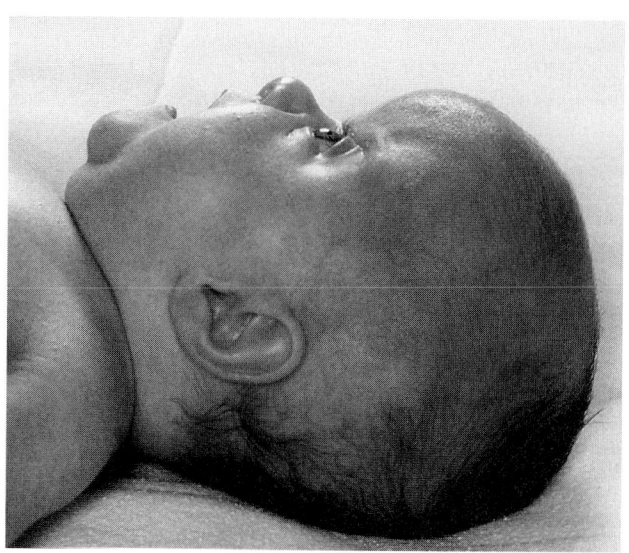

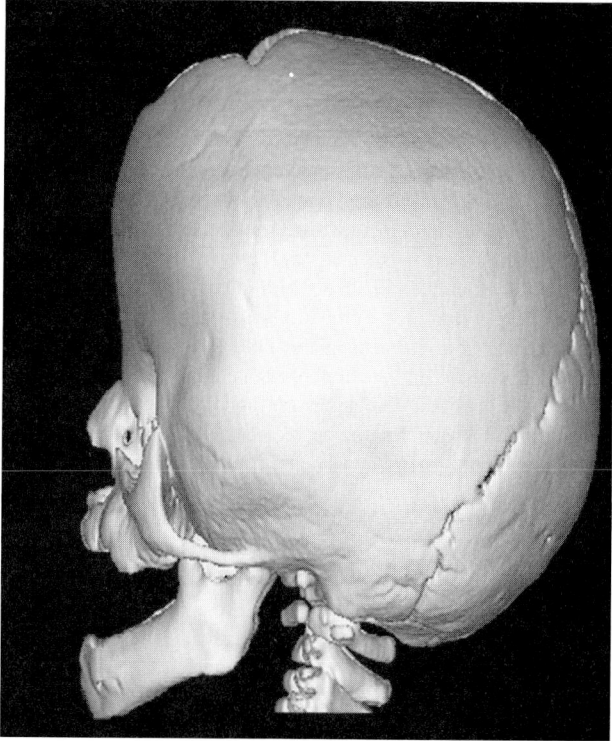

Apert syndrome   High forehead and flat face caused by midface hypoplasia result in the characteristic profile in a 6-month-old boy with Apert syndrome. CT scan (of a different patient) shows coronal craniosynostosis.

Precautions before anesthesia: Evaluate the head and neck anatomy in consideration of airway management (reduced size of nasopharynx, maxilla, mandible, anomalies of the palate and tracheal cartilage, combined with cervical spine abnormalities, may lead to difficult airway management). Radiographs of the cervical spine may be helpful in the evaluation process. Request echocardiography for patients with congenital cardiac lesions. Because up to one third of these children have intraoperative respiratory problems the presence of an active or recent upper airway infection will be highly significant. Preoperative chest radiograph may be helpful. Preoperative blood workup should include a complete blood count, electrolytes, creatinine, and BUN. Keep in mind that the incidence of increased intracranial pressure is 15% with one fused suture and more than 35% with two or more sutures affected.

Anesthetic considerations: Mental retardation may lead to poor cooperation upon separation from the parents or during induction of anesthesia. Difficult airway management should be expected. Maintenance of spontaneous ventilation and oxygenation during attempts to control the airway is strongly recommended. Be prepared to use alternative techniques to manage the airway (laryngeal mask, fiberoptic intubation). A surgeon familiar with surgical airway management and the necessary equipment should always be present in the operating room. Specific anesthetic measures may be required in the presence of congenital heart disease (antibiotic prophylaxis for subacute bacterial endocarditis may be required) or increased intracranial pressure. The eyes must be carefully protected because of the high risk for corneal damage as a result of proptosis. Current surgical technique for craniosynostosis consists of total cranial vault reconstruction, which carries a high risk of major blood loss (often significantly more than one circulating blood volume). Large-bore intravenous access with the possibility to transfuse rapidly is mandatory. However, vascular access in these patients often is challenging. Accurate evaluation of blood loss usually is difficult. Invasive hemodynamic monitoring with the possibility of regular intraoperative blood work sampling (complete blood count, blood gas analysis, electrolytes, coagulation parameters) is requested. Depending on the positioning of the patient, the risk of venous air embolism should be kept in mind and the need for central venous access considered. For this reason, nitrous oxide should not be used in these patients. To reduce the amount of homologous blood transfusions, preoperative hemodilution, intraoperative cell saver techniques, and induced arterial hypotension have been used. However, arterial hypotension might not be tolerated in patients with increased intracranial pressure in order to maintain cerebral perfusion pressure. Ventilation should be aimed at normocapnia or mild hypocapnia. Because of massive transfusion and the prolonged operative time, hypothermia in these usually small patients is not uncommon. Although mild hypothermia may offer some degree of cerebral protection, moderate hypothermia must be avoided. Postoperative ventilation may be necessary in the presence of significant facial edema associated with the surgical procedure. Securing the endotracheal tube with a suture rather than tape is preferable because accidental extubation can be fatal.

Pharmacological implications: Sedative premedication in patients with increased intracranial pressure should be used with caution and under supervision of trained personnel only. Hypotensive anesthesia is most often achieved using volatile anesthetics, opioids, and/or sympathoadrenergic receptor-blocking drugs. Avoid nitrous oxide secondary to the risk of venous air embolism. Antibiotic prophylaxis for subacute bacterial endocarditis may be necessary.

REFERENCES:

Nargozian C: Apert syndrome. Anesthetic management. *Clin Plast Surg* 18:227, 1991.

Elwood T, Sarathy PV, Geiduschek JM, et al: Respiratory complications during anaesthesia in Apert syndrome. *Paediatr Anaesth* 11:701, 2001.

ACROCEPHALOSYNDACTYLY TYPE II: CROUZON SYNDROME

At a glance: Craniofacial dysostosis syndrome with skull deformities similar to Apert syndrome but absent syndactyly. Characteristic features include exophthalmos, hypertelorism, beaked nose, maxillary hypoplasia, and micrognathia.

Synonyms: Craniofacial Dysostosis; Fibroblast Growth Factor Receptor II Deficiency (FGFR-2 Deficiency).

History: First described in 1912 by Octave Crouzon (1874–1938), a French neurologist.

Classification: Apert-Crouzon syndrome is characterized by the facial features of Crouzon and Apert-like syndactyly. The original classification was acrocephalosyndactyly type II, but it is now regarded as a variant of type I.

Incidence: 1:25,000 live births. Both genders are equally affected. It accounts for approximately 4.5% of all cases of craniosynostosis at birth.

Genetic inheritance: Autosomal dominant but de novo mutations in up to 50%. High penetrance with variable degree of expressivity. Several sporadic cases linked to paternal age. Gene map locus is 10q26.

Pathophysiology: Crouzon syndrome results from mutations in the gene encoding for FGFR-2. (However, Crouzon syndrome with acanthosis nigricans results from a mutation in the FGFR-3 gene.) The mutation increases the maturation rate of cells in the osteoblastic lineage. During fetal development, premature ossification with increased subperiosteal bone formation and premature ossification of the calvaria are responsible for the craniosynostosis. In mutant fetal calvaria cells, alkaline phosphatase is up to fourfold higher than normal. The mutation involves only one of the multiple tissue-specific isoforms involved in the osteogenesis of the frontal bones of the skull. This results in premature synostosis of the coronal, sagittal, and occasionally lambdoidal sutures beginning in the first year of life. The rate and order of fusion determine the extent of deformity.

Diagnosis: Clinical diagnosis is made at birth. Skull radiography shows bony abnormalities with premature coronal craniosynostosis. Many patients diagnosed in the past have been reclassified as acrocephalosyndactyly syndrome type III.

Clinical aspects: Coronal and sagittal sutures are most commonly involved. Maxillary hypoplasia, relative mandibular prognathism, parrot beaked nose (often with nasal obstruction) are typical. Ophthalmologic features include shallow orbits with proptosis, hypertelorism, and divergent strabismus. Short upper lip (occasionally with cleft) and high arched palate (occasionally with cleft), bifid uvula, and dental crowding are common, whereas macroglossia is less frequent. Mild-to-moderate mental retardation. Skull radiology shows pronounced digital impressions of the skull and a triangular shape of the optic foramen secondary to increased intracranial pressure resulting from progressive hydrocephalus. Almost three fourths of Crouzon patients have chronic herniation of the cerebellar tonsils, and one fourth has fused cervical vertebrae, which most commonly involves C2-3. Syndactyly is less severe than in Apert syndrome, with the thumbs and fifth fingers usually free. Broad tarsal bones or

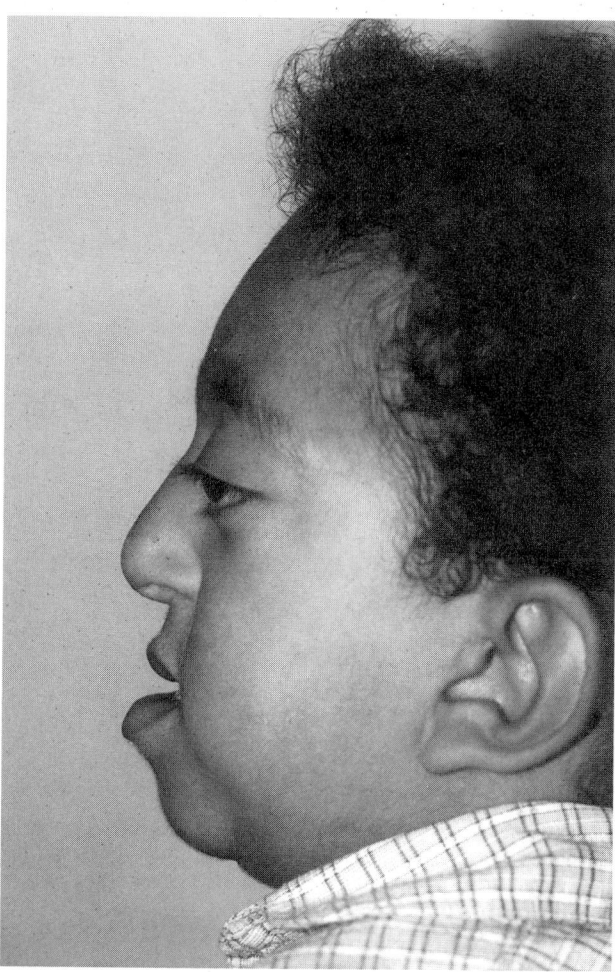

Acrocephalosyndactyly type II Adolescent boy shows characteristic facial features of acrocephalosyndactyly type II (Crouzon syndrome) with proptosis, midface hypoplasia, short upper lip and mandible, and low set ears.

fused tarsal bones may be present in addition to the aforementioned findings (so-called Jackson-Weiss syndrome, see *Other Conditions to Be Considered*). There is no treatment of the underlying disorder, and morbidity depends on the severity of the condition.

Precautions before anesthesia: The need to carefully assess the airway is obvious when treating a child. Midface hypoplasia with hypoplasia of the mandible can make mask fit difficult, and visualization of the vocal cords often is impossible with regular laryngoscopy. Choanal atresia has been linked to Crouzon syndrome, so choanal patency should be checked before induction. Nasal obstruction often results in obligatory mouth breathing. Radiographic studies of the cervical spine before anesthesia to demonstrate cervical vertebral fusion may be indicated. Cervical fusion limits neck extension. One case report describes a completely cartilaginous trachea with replacement of the cartilaginous rings by a continuous plate in a child with Crouzon syndrome. The patient continued to have respiratory problems despite choanal atresia repair and died of respiratory problems at age 23 months. Be aware of progressive hydrocephalus (14% incidence with only one fused suture), chronic tonsillar herniation (10% symptomatic), syringomyelia, and uncommonly respiratory standstill in these patients. Check for visceral abnormalities before anesthesia.

Anesthetic considerations: Mental retardation may lead to poor cooperation upon separation from the parents or during induction of anesthesia. Difficult airway management should be expected. Maintenance of spontaneous ventilation and oxygenation during attempts to control the airway is strongly recommended. Be prepared to use alternative techniques to manage the airway (laryngeal mask, fiberoptic intubation). A surgeon familiar with surgical airway management and the necessary equipment should always be present in the operating room. Specific anesthetic measures may be required in the presence of congenital heart disease (antibiotic prophylaxis for subacute bacterial endocarditis may be required) or increased intracranial pressure. The eyes must be carefully protected because of the high risk for corneal damage as a result of proptosis. Current surgical technique for craniosynostosis consists of total cranial vault reconstruction, which carries a high risk of major blood loss (often significantly more than one circulating blood volume). Large-bore intravenous access with the possibility to transfuse rapidly is mandatory. However, vascular access in these patients often is challenging. Accurate evaluation of blood loss usually is difficult. Invasive hemodynamic monitoring with the possibility of regular intraoperative blood work sampling (complete blood count, blood gas analysis, electrolytes, coagulation parameters) is requested. Depending on the positioning of the patient, the risk of venous air embolism should be kept in mind and the need for central venous access considered. For this reason, nitrous oxide should not be used in these patients. To reduce the amount of homologous blood transfusions, preoperative hemodilution, intraoperative cell saver techniques, and induced arterial hypotension have been used. However, arterial hypotension should not be tolerated in patients with increased intracranial pressure in order to maintain cerebral perfusion pressure. Ventilation should be aimed at normocapnia or mild hypocapnia. Because of massive transfusion and the prolonged operative time, hypothermia in these usually small patients is not uncommon. Although mild hypothermia may offer some degree of cerebral protection, moderate hypothermia must be avoided. Postoperative ventilation may be necessary in the presence of significant facial edema associated with the surgical procedure. Securing the endotracheal tube with a suture rather than tape is preferable because accidental extubation can be fatal.

Pharmacological implications: Sedative premedication in patients with increased intracranial pressure should be used with caution and under supervision of trained personnel only. Hypotensive anesthesia is most often achieved using volatile anesthetics, opioids, and/or sympathoadrenergic receptor-blocking drugs. Avoid nitrous oxide secondary to the risk of venous air embolism. Antibiotic prophylaxis for subacute bacterial endocarditis may be necessary.

Other condition to be considered:

☞**JACKSON-WEISS SYNDROME:** Either autosomal dominant inherited or sporadically occurring disorder characterized by craniosynostosis, midface hypoplasia, hypertelorism, strabismus, ptosis, and anomalies of the feet; hands usually are normal. The facial appearance has been linked to that in patients with Crouzon syndrome, although the absence of marked proptosis is an obvious difference. Similar to the other forms of acrocephalosyndactyly, the genetic defect has been linked to the FGFR-2 gene, which has been mapped to 10q26.

REFERENCES:

Cinalli G, Renier D, Sebag G, et al: Chronic tonsillar herniation in Crouzon's and Apert's syndromes: The role of premature synostosis of the lambdoid suture. *J Neurosurg* 83:575, 1995.

Devine P, Bhan M, Feingold M, et al: Completely cartilaginous trachea in a child with Crouzon syndrome. *Am J Dis Child* 138:40, 1984.

Sculerati N, Gottlieb MD, Zimbler MS, et al: Airway management in children with major craniofacial anomalies. *Laryngoscope* 108:1806, 1998.

ACROCEPHALOSYNDACTYLY SYNDROME TYPE III: SAETHRE-CHOTZEN SYNDROME

At a glance: Form of acrocephalosyndactyly characterized by variable craniosynostosis, dysmorphic facies, and minimal syndactyly of hands and feet.

Synonyms: Fibroblast Growth Factor Receptor II Deficiency; FGFR-2 Deficiency.

History: First described by H. Saethre, a Norwegian psychiatrist, in 1931 and by F. Chotzen, a German psychiatrist, in 1932.

Incidence: Not described but probably the most common heritable disorder involving coronal craniostenosis.

Genetic inheritance: Autosomal dominant with a high penetrance and highly variable expressivity. The responsible gene has been mapped to 7p21-p22.

Pathophysiology: The syndrome results from a mutation of the TWIST transcription gene, which encodes a basic helix–loop–helix transcription factor. This results in abnormal osseous development and irregular bridging in early bone formation, particularly affecting the cranium and the distal extremities. The gene mutation results in an increased maturation rate of cells in the osteoblastic lineage. During fetal development, premature ossification with increased subperiosteal bone formation and premature ossification of the calvaria are responsible for the craniosynostosis. In mutant fetal calvarial cells, alkaline phosphatase levels are up to fourfold higher than normal.

Diagnosis: Based on the clinical findings at birth. Skull radiographs confirm osseous abnormalities and premature coronal craniosynostosis.

Clinical aspects: The degree of craniosynostosis may be very mild. The coronal sutures are most commonly involved. Fusion of the plates often is asymmetrical. A flat and asymmetrical facies with a very low frontal hairline, palpebral ptosis, hypoplastic maxilla, high arched palate or cleft palate, and dental anomalies are common findings. Most children have normal intelligence, but hydrocephalus may occur. Syndactyly is of variable extent (most often involves fingers 2 and 3, usually with cutaneous syndactyly, but separate bone structures), as is brachydactyly. The thumbs are normal. Contractures of elbow and knee joints are not uncommon. Congenital heart defects and renal abnormalities with renal failure may be associated. There is no treatment of the underlying disorder, but prognosis usually is excellent.

Precautions before anesthesia: Evaluate the head and neck anatomy in consideration of airway management (reduced size of nasopharynx, maxilla, mandible, anomalies of the palate and tracheal cartilage, combined with cervical spine abnormalities, may lead to difficult airway management). Radiographs of the cervical spine may be helpful in the evaluation process. Request echocardiography for patients with congenital cardiac lesions. The incidence of intraoperative respiratory problems is high, and a patient presenting with recent upper respiratory tract infections may have the procedure cancelled. Preoperative chest radiograph may be helpful. Preoperative blood workup should include a complete blood count, electrolytes, creatinine, and BUN (renal problems not unusual). Keep in mind that the incidence of increased intracranial pressure is 15% with one fused suture and more than 35% with two or more sutures affected.

Anesthetic considerations: Mental retardation may lead to poor cooperation upon separation from the parents or during induction of anesthesia. Difficult airway management should be expected. Maintenance of spontaneous ventilation and oxygenation during attempts to control the airway is strongly recommended. Be prepared to use alternative techniques to manage the airway (laryngeal mask, fiberoptic intubation). A surgeon familiar with surgical airway management and the necessary equipment should always be present in the operating room. Specific anesthetic measures may be required in the presence of congenital heart disease (antibiotic prophylaxis for subacute bacterial endocarditis may be required) or increased intracranial pressure. The eyes must be carefully protected because of the high risk for corneal damage as a result of proptosis. Current surgical technique for craniosynostosis consists of total cranial vault reconstruction, which carries a high risk of major blood loss (often significantly more than one circulating blood volume). Large-bore intravenous access with the possibility to transfuse rapidly is mandatory. However, vascular access in these patients often is challenging. Accurate evaluation of blood loss usually is difficult. Invasive hemodynamic monitoring with the possibility of regular intraoperative blood work sampling (complete blood count, blood gas analysis, electrolytes, coagulation parameters) is requested. Depending on the positioning of the patient, the risk of venous air embolism should be kept in mind and the need for central venous access or rapid fluid administration may be considered. For this reason, nitrous oxide should not be used in these patients. To reduce the amount of homologous blood transfusions, preoperative hemodilution, intraoperative cell saver techniques, and induced arterial hypotension have been used. However, arterial hypotension should not be tolerated in patients with increased intracranial pressure in order to maintain cerebral perfusion pressure. Ventilation should be aimed at normocapnia or mild hypocapnia. Because of massive transfusion and the prolonged operative time, hypothermia in these usually small patients is not uncommon. Although mild hypothermia may offer some degree of cerebral protection, moderate hypothermia must be avoided. Postoperative ventilation may be necessary in the presence of significant facial edema associated with the surgical procedure. Securing the endotracheal tube with a suture rather than tape is preferable because accidental extubation can be fatal.

Pharmacological implications: In the presence of significant renal disease, drugs with predominately renal excretion must be administered in reduced doses. Sedative premedication in patients with increased intracranial pressure should be used with caution and under supervision of trained personnel only. Hypotensive anesthesia is most often achieved using volatile anesthetics, opioids, and/or sympathoadrenergic receptor-blocking drugs. Avoid nitrous oxide secondary to the risk of venous air embolism. Antibiotic prophylaxis for subacute bacterial endocarditis may be necessary.

REFERENCES:

Cinalli G, Renier D, Sebag G, et al: Chronic tonsillar herniation in Crouzon's and Apert's syndromes: The role of premature synostosis of the lambdoid suture. *J Neurosurg* 83:575, 1995.

Sculerati N, Gottlieb MD, Zimbler MS: Airway management in children with major craniofacial anomalies. *Laryngoscope* 108:1806, 1998.

ACROCEPHALOSYNDACTYLY TYPE V: PFEIFFER SYNDROME

At a glance: Sagittal craniostenosis associated with broad thumbs and toes (mostly second toe), variable maxillary retrusion, and

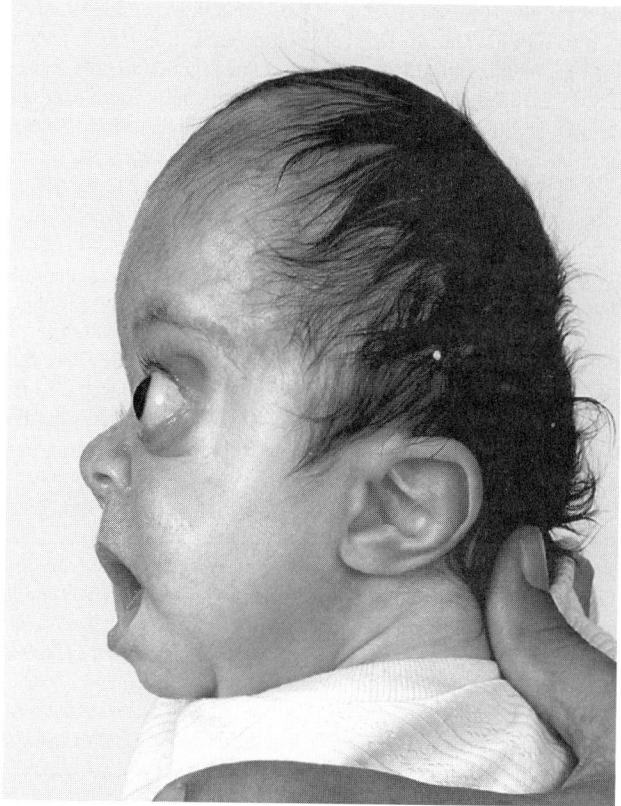

Acrocephalosyndactyly Type IV Newborn shows acrocephaly, shallow orbits with proptosis, and midface hypoplasia, all characteristic features of Pfeiffer syndrome.

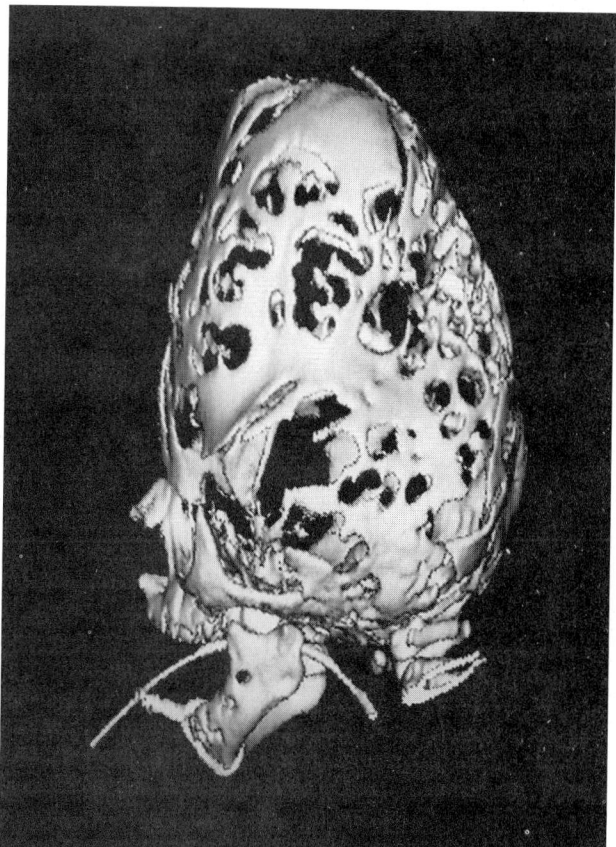

Acrocephalosyndactyly Type IV Lateral view of the head in a three-dimensional MRI-reconstruction of a (different) patient with acrocephalosyndactyly type V (Pfeiffer syndrome) shows significant osseous abnormalities with extremely thinned cranial vault (in many locations even with total absence of the bone), which is considered secondary to increased intracranial pressure that resulted in pressure atrophy of the bone. Midface hypoplasia and shallow orbits can be found in this patient. (Patient with endotracheal tube in situ.)

partial soft tissue syndactyly. There are three variants. Congenital heart disease most often presents. Mental deficiency and mandibular ankylosis occur. When associated with a congenital heart disease, the syndrome is called *Pfeiffer cardiocranial syndrome.*

Synonyms: Fibroblast Growth Factor Receptor I Deficiency.

Nature: Accelerated maturation of fibroblast-derived cells with premature bony suture closing. Heritable distinct craniosynostosis with growth and developmental retardation and congenital heart defects.

Incidence: Very rare.

Genetic inheritance: Autosomal recessive inheritance with intrafamilial variability. Complete penetrance and variable expressivity. Some sporadic cases. Gene map locus is 8p11.2-p11.1.

Pathophysiology: This genetic defect results in irregular bridging in the mesenchymal tissue that forms the bone. The cranium and distal extremities are predominantly affected. Mutation in the FGFR-1 gene and sometimes the FGFR-2 gene result in premature cell maturation and bony suture closure, as in Crouzon syndrome. During fetal development, premature ossification with increased extent of subperiosteal bone formation and premature ossification of the calvaria are responsible for the craniosynostosis. In mutant fetal calvaria cells, alkaline phosphatase is fourfold higher than normal.

Diagnosis: Based on clinical features, with congenital heart defect and sagittal craniosynostosis being the cardinal manifestations of the syndrome. Clinical diagnosis at birth (craniosynostosis with broad thumbs and great toes). Skull radiography showing premature coronal craniosynostosis.

Clinical aspects: Midface hypoplasia, with flat facies and proptosis, shallow orbits, down-slanting palpebral fissures, hypertelorism,

and strabismus. Associated with mild craniosynostosis (usually coronal and sagittal sutures) and acrocephaly. Limbs with broad thumb, broad great toe, and polysyndactyly. Cutaneous syndactyly (or polysyndactyly) involving the hands and feet. Radiology of the thumb shows a triangular or trapezoidal proximal phalanx, occasionally fused with distal phalanx. Varying degree of hearing loss, classified as moderate to severe in most patients. Generally, normal inner ear anatomy. Choanal atresia, submucosal cleft palate, cartilaginous trachea. Laryngomalacia, tracheomalacia, and bronchomalacia. Occasionally fused spinal vertebrae, usually at the cervical level. Associated anomalies include Arnold-Chiari malformation, odontoid hypoplasia, imperforate anus, and congenital heart disease (4%; atrial septal defect, ventricular septal defect, patent ductus arteriosus, tetralogy of Fallot, pulmonic stenosis, partial anomalous venous return).

Three clinical subtypes have been delineated with respect to prognosis:

Type I (classic) patients present with normal intelligence and good prognosis.

Type II patients present with cloverleaf skull, severe ocular proptosis, and ankylosis of the elbows. Associated problems include complete tracheal rings, resulting in tracheal stenosis, intestinal malrotation, and ☞Prune Belly syndrome.

Type III is manifested by the absence of cloverleaf skull but the presence of elbow ankylosis and a high morbidity in infancy (as described for type II). Additional features of Pfeiffer syndrome include hallux valgus deformity with a triangular proximal phalanx of the great toe and an enlarged first metatarsal bone. Cutaneous syndactyly of the second and third digits and shortening of the middle phalanges are often present in the hands and feet. Growth and developmental retardation (except for type I), sagittal craniosynostosis, micrognathia with mandibular ankylosis, congenital heart defects (septal defects, patent ductus arteriosus, tetralogy of Fallot, anomalous pulmonary venous return), tracheobronchial anomalies, large joint contractures, syndactyly, and genital anomalies are often present. As with other forms of craniosynostosis, it is thought that if the cranial anomaly remains untreated, many of these children will suffer from cortex-associated decrease of intelligence. Therefore, surgical management is initiated at a very early stage.

Types II and III have severe central nervous system involvement (hydrocephalus, mental retardation, seizures) associated with a very poor prognosis and a risk of dying early.

Precautions before anesthesia: Check choanal patency before induction of anesthesia. The potential for tracheal stenosis causing biphasic stridor is often associated. Chest radiograph should be obtained. Perform radiographic study of the cervical spine before anesthesia.

- Fusion of cervical vertebrae is present in 30% of patients with Pfeiffer syndrome. Careful diagnosis of odontoid hypoplasia is essential to facilitate positioning and to prevent damage during direct laryngoscopy. Children are at high risk for obstructive sleep apnea

- Goldee children the presence of or pulmonale should be excluded by polysomnography and cardiac echography. Preoperative and postoperative use of a nasopharyngeal airway should be considered. Hydrocephalus is often present. Increased intracranial pressure is caused by craniosynostosis in most cases. Assess potential for a difficult airway (limited mouth opening, micrognathia). Evaluate lower airway patency (tracheobronchial anomalies) via clinical history and chest radiography, including tomography or computed tomography (CT) scan. Evaluate presence, type, and severity of cardiac involvement. Determine presence of elevated intracranial pressure or hypsocephalous from the craniosynostosis. Laboratory investigations include complete blood count, electrolytes, chest radiography, ECG, and arterial blood gas analysis. Premedication is based on physical status and developmental age but should be avoided in patients with elevated intracranial pressure.

Anesthetic considerations: Mental retardation may lead to poor cooperation upon separation from the parents or during induction of anesthesia. Difficult airway management must be expected. Maintenance of spontaneous ventilation and oxygenation during attempts to control the airway is strongly recommended. Be prepared to use alternative techniques to manage the airway (laryngeal mask, fiberoptic intubation). A surgeon familiar with surgical airway management and the necessary equipment should always be present in the operating room. Specific anesthetic measures will be required in the presence of increased intracranial pressure. The eyes must

be carefully protected because of the high risk for corneal damage as a result of proptosis. Current surgical technique for craniosynostosis consists of total cranial vault reconstruction, which carries a high risk of major blood loss (often significantly more than one circulating blood volume). Large-bore intravenous access with the possibility to transfuse rapidly is mandatory. However, vascular access in these patients often is challenging. Accurate evaluation of blood loss usually is difficult. Invasive hemodynamic monitoring with the possibility of regular intraoperative blood work sampling (complete blood count, blood gas analysis, electrolytes and coagulation parameters) is requested. Depending on the positioning of the patient, the risk of venous air embolism should be kept in mind and the need for central venous access considered. For this reason, nitrous oxide should not be used in these patients. To reduce the amount of homologous blood transfusions, preoperative hemodilution, intraoperative cell saver techniques, and induced arterial hypotension have been used. However, arterial hypotension should not be tolerated in patients with increased intracranial pressure in order to maintain cerebral perfusion pressure. Ventilation should be aimed at normocapnia or mild hypocapnia. Because of massive transfusion and prolonged operative time, hypothermia in these usually small patients is not uncommon. Although mild hypothermia may offer some degree of cerebral protection, moderate hypothermia must be avoided. Postoperative ventilation may be necessary in the presence of significant facial edema associated with the surgical procedure. Securing the endotracheal tube with a suture rather than tape is preferable because accidental extubation can be fatal.

Pharmacological implications: Sedative premedication in patients with increased intracranial pressure should be used with caution and under supervision of trained personnel only. Hypotensive anesthesia is most often achieved using volatile anesthetics, opioids, and/or sympathoadrenergic receptor-blocking drugs. Avoid nitrous oxide secondary to the risk of venous air embolism.

Other condition to be considered:

☞**NOACK SYNDROME,** also called *acrocephalopolysyndactyly type I* or *dominant type of acrocephalopolysyndactyly,* involves the hands and feet. Patients have enlarged thumbs and duplication of the great toes. Moderate acrocephaly is present.

REFERENCES:

Digilio MC, Marino B, Borzaga U, Giannotti A, Dallapiccola B: Intrafamilial variability of Pfeiffer-type cardiocranial syndrome. *Am J Med Genet* 73:480, 1997.

Meyer P, Renier D, Blanot S, Orliaguet G, Arnaud E, Lajeunie E: Anesthesia and intensive care of craniostenosis and craniofacial dysmorphism in children. *Ann Fr Anesth Reanim* 16:152, 1997.

Scholtes JL, Thauvoy C, Moulin D, Gribomont BF. Craniofaciosynostosis: Anesthetic and perioperative management. Report of 71 operations. *Acta Anaesthesiol Belg* 36:176, 1985.

Acrofacial Dysostosis: An Overview

At a glance: Acrofacial dysostosis is an umbrella term for several apparently distinctive genetic modifications. The disorder is characterized by distinctive craniofacial malformations, especially involving severe mandibular hypoplasia and preaxial and postaxial limb defects.

Classification and synonyms: There are six types of acrofacial dysostosis.

Acrofacial dysostosis, ☞Nager type (mandibulofacial dysostosis, split-hand deformity-mandibulofacial dysostosis)

Acrofacial dysostosis lethal type of Rodriguez

Acrofacial dysostosis, Weyers type (☞Weyers syndrome II)

Acrofacial dysostosis postaxial, Miller type (☞Miller syndrome)

Acrofacial dysostosis, Catania type

Acrofacial dysostosis, Palagonia type

Incidence and genetic inheritance: All acrofacial dysostosis types are inherited as either autosomal dominant or recessive pattern.

Clinical aspects: *Nager acrofacial dysostosis* is a rare hereditary disorder marked by unusual facial development. Cleft lip/palate, defective development of bones in the jaw and arms, smaller than normal thumbs, hearing loss, and ear deformities are characteristics of this disorder.

Acrofacial dysostosis lethal type of Rodriguez is inherited as an autosomal recessive trait and is characterized by small stature, severe mandibular hypoplasia (micrognathia), phocomelia and oligodactyly of the upper limbs, absence of fistula, microtia, and cleft palate. Limb deficiencies are predominantly preaxial. The skin is thin and atrophic, vessels can be seen over the trunk, and elastosis perforans is present. There is a severe hypoplasia of the shoulder and pelvic girdles. Other features are severe internal organ anomalies, including arrhinencephaly and abnormal lung lobulation. The cardiovascular system presents congenital anomalies. The disorder is associated with early lethality. Most patients die of respiratory complications during the neonatal period, partly because of the presence of severe mandibular hypoplasia.

Weyers acrofacial dysostosis is present from birth, affects both sexes, and is characterized by postaxial polydactyly of the hands and feet, hexadactyly and fusion of fifth and sixth metatarsals and metacarpals and bony clefts of the mandibular symphysis. Other features include orodental anomalies, hypoplastic and dysplastic nails, short stature, micrognathia, small mouth, hypoplasia of the larynx. Congenital heart defect may be present.

Miller acrofacial dysostosis is thought to be inherited as an autosomal recessive trait and is apparent at birth. It is characterized by postaxial acrofacial dysostosis, which is defined by its postaxial limb deficiency. Craniofacial malformations, malar hypoplasia, severe micrognathia, cleft palate, small, protruding, "cup-shaped" ears, colobomas, drooping of the lower eyelids, and ectropion are seen. The limb abnormalities in infants and children may include severe hypoplasia, syndactyly, and/or absence of certain fingers and toes (e.g., fifth digits and, in some cases, fourth and third digits). Hypoplasia of the ulna and radius causes the forearms to appear unusually short.

Catania acrofacial dysostosis was reported in 1993 as a "new" form of acrofacial dysostosis. It is characterized by mild intrauterine growth retardation and postnatal shortness of stature, severe microcephaly, widow's peak, mandibulofacial dysostosis without cleft palate, mild preaxial, and especially more conspicuous postaxial upper limb involvement with short hands, simian creases, and mild interdigital webbing. Other features include genitourinary and gastrointestinal dysfunctions, such as hypospadias, cryptorchidism, and diversified hernias. Although the disorder is believed to be transmitted via an X-linked dominant inheritance, an autosomal dominant genetic transmission is highly possible considering that, in this report, the mother was severely affected. Most patients presented with extensive caries.

Palagonia acrofacial dysostosis affects patients who present with normal intelligence compared with the Sicilian type, Catania. This form of acrofacial dysostosis does not feature severe caries but rather oligodontia, short stature, frizzy hair with aplatis cutis verticis, mild cutaneous syndactyly of digits 2 to 5, and cleft lip/palate. Other features include abnormalities of the skeletal system, such as a small odontoid process and spina bifida occulta at S1. The inheritance pattern has been suggested to be X-linked dominant genetic transmission, but an autosomal dominant inheritance is favored by some.

Anesthetic considerations: The main consideration with any type of acrofacial dysostosis remains airway management. Preparation for difficult tracheal intubation is essential. A nasopharyngeal approach (fiberoptic) and/or laryngeal mask airway should be ready for use. Special intubation devices, such as fiberoptic laryngoscope, Bullard laryngoscope, and light wand, must be readily available. Spontaneous ventilation should be maintained until the airway is secure. The presence of an otorhinolaryngologist who can perform emergency tracheostomy must be planned in case all other attempts to secure the airway fail. Venous access can be difficult because of limb defects. The potential presence of cardiovascular and pulmonary problems must be assessed prior to induction of anesthesia.

Other conditions to be considered:

☞**TREACHER COLLINS SYNDROME** is characterized by underdevelopment of the malar, mandibular, and maxillary bones, slanted eyes, notching of lower eyelids, and a receding chin. Underdevelopment of the jaw may cause problems in swallowing or breathing in the newborn. Malformed ear pinna usually is present. The presence of a normal face with a beak-like nose, receding chin, and acute deafness are characteristic of people with Treacher Collins syndrome.

☞**GOLDENHAR SYNDROME** is a rare congenital disorder that includes partial absence of the upper eyelid or an unusual slant of the eyelid, asymmetry of the skull, sharply prominent forehead, absent or closed nostrils, and cleft palate.

☞**ORAL-FACIAL-DIGITAL SYNDROME** is a rare genetic disorder characterized by episodes of neuromuscular disturbances, split tongue, splits in the jaw, midline cleft lip, overgrowth frenulum, broad-based nose, epicanthic folds, polydactyly, and clinodactyly.

☞**JUBERG-HAYWARD SYNDROME** is a rare hereditary disorder characterized by cleft lip/palate, a smaller-than-normal-size head, deformities of the thumbs and toes, and growth hormone deficiency resulting in short stature.

HEMIFACIAL MICROSOMIA (HFM) SYNDROME affects 1:5000 births. It can be confused with a Treacher Collins-like syndrome. However, it is not genetic. The syndrome can cause abnormalities that are always uneven on both sides of the face, whereas both sides of the face appear equally affected in Treacher Collins syndrome. The facial nerve is frequently paralyzed in hemifacial microsomia. Features include mandibular underdevelopment, microtia, facial nerve paresis in 40% of patients, macrostomia, and underdevelopment of the cheek and eye on the affected side of the face. Less common are abnormalities of the vertebrae and ribs, cleft lip/palate, and heart and kidney abnormalities, which are very rare.

REFERENCES:

Opitz C, Stoll C, Ring P: Nager syndrome. Problems and possibilities of therapy. *J Orofac Orthop* 61:226, 2000.

Petit P, Moerman P, Fryns JP: Acrofacial dysostosis syndrome type Rodriguez: A new lethal MCA syndrome. *Am J Med Genet* 42:343, 1992.

Wessels MW, den Hollander NS, Cohen-Overbeek TE, et al: Prenatal diagnosis and confirmation of the acrofacial dysostosis syndrome type Rodriguez. *Am J Med Genet* 113:97, 2002.

Donnai D, Hugues HE, Winter RM: Postaxial acrofacial dysostosis (Miller) syndrome, in Donnai D, Winter RM (eds): *Congenital Malformation Syndromes.* London, Chapman & Hall, London, 1995, p 333.

Opitz JM, Mollica F, Sorge G, et al: Acrofacial dysostosis: Review and report of a previously undescribed condition: The autosomal or X-linked dominant Catania form of acrofacial dysostosis. *Am J Med Genet* 47:660, 1993.

Sorge C, Pavone L, Polizi A, et al: Another "new" form, the Palagonia type of acrofacial dysostosis in a Sicilian family. *Am J Med Genet* 69:388, 1997.

Acro-Fronto-Facio-Nasal Dysostosis Syndrome (Types I and II)

At a glance: Frontonasal dysostosis, retarded growth, and mental development. Brachycephaly, broad notched nasal tip, cleft lip/palate, and macrostomia. Polysyndactyly, camptodactyly, and hypoplasia of the distal phalanges of the hands. Iliac hypoplasia, short legs, and hypospadias.

Synonyms:

Type I: Postaxial Polysyndactyly, Frontonasal Dysostosis, and Cleft Lip/Palate; Cleft Lip/Palate with Frontonasal Dysostosis and Postaxial Polysyndactyly.

Type II: Naguib-Richieri-Costa Syndrome; Richieri-Costa-Montagnoli Syndrome; Hypertelorism, Hypospadias, and Polysyndactyly Syndrome.

Nature: The term *dysostosis* refers to a defect in the ossification process, which results in malformations of individual bones arising either isolated or multiple. Some patients also exhibit axial involution. The dysostosis predominantly involves the extremities. The most common forms are syndactyly or polydactyly, which may occur in combination with craniofacial or other abnormalities. Two types of this syndrome, each including only a small number of patients, have been described.

Incidence: Extremely rare congenital abnormality described in fewer than 10 patients of both sexes.

Genetic inheritance: An autosomal recessive trait has been suggested, although insufficient genetic background information or molecular data are available. However, normal chromosomes, parental consanguinity, and familial occurrence suggest an autosomal recessive inheritance is possible.

Pathophysiology: Unknown.

Diagnosis and clinical aspects: At birth, the diagnosis is suspected based on the clinical aspect characterized by facial and other anomalies: hypertelorism, eye anomalies, broad notched nasal tip, cleft lip/palate, camptodactyly, brachydactyly, and polysyndactyly of fingers and toes, anomalies of the feet, and hypospadias. Severe mental retardation is common.

Acrofrontofacionasal dysostosis I: Mental retardation, short stature, hypertelorism with eye anomalies, broad notched nasal tip, cleft lip/palate, postaxial camptobrachypolysyndactyly af-

fecting fingers and toes, fibular hypoplasia, and anomalies of the foot structure are the most common findings.

Acrofrontofacionasal dysostosis II: Hypertelorism, proptosis, ptosis, wide forehead, microbrachycephaly, broad nose with midline groove, hypospadias, syndactyly of the fingers, and broad thumbs and halluces.

Precautions before anesthesia: Obtain a thorough and careful examination for associated abnormalities of the heart (echocardiography) and kidneys (blood work, ultrasound). The patient's mental and neurologic status must be assessed to determine a thoughtful approach to premedication and induction. Evaluate for difficult airway and venous access.

Anesthetic considerations and pharmacological implications: There are no published data concerning anesthetic or pharmacological implications in this syndrome. Use of regional anesthesia and analgesia provides a reasonable alternative whenever applicable in these children. Proptosis makes the eyes vulnerable to injuries, so good protection and lubrication intraoperatively are recommended.

REFERENCES:

Richieri-Costa A, Colletto G, Gollop TR, et al: A previously undescribed autosomal recessive multiple congenital anomalies/mental retardation (MCA/MR) syndrome with frontonasal dysostosis, cleft lip/palate, limb hypoplasia and postaxial polysyndactyly; acro-fronto-facio-nasal dysostosis syndrome. *Am J Genet* 20:631, 1985.

Naguib KK: Hypertelorism, proptosis, ptosis, polysyndactyly, hypospadias and normal height in 3 sibs: A new syndrome? *Am J Med Genet* 29:35, 1988.

Teebi AS: Naguib-Richieri-Costa syndrome: Hypertelorism, hypospadias, and polysyndactyly syndrome [letter]. *Am J Med Genet* 44:115, 1992.

Acromesomelic Dysplasia

At a glance: Extremely short stature as a result of acromesomelic dysplasia of the limbs (forearms, forelegs, hands, feet). In general, patients present with normal intelligence. Joint dislocations may occur. Normal craniofacial and axial skeleton. Care with positioning.

Synonyms: Acromesomelic Dwarfism; AMD.

Classification:

Type I = Maroteaux (AMDM) type
Type II = Hunter-Thompson (AMDH) type
Type III = ☞Grebe (AMDG) type/Brazilian Achondrogenesis
Type IV = Brahimi Bacha type or Algerian type
Type V = Campailla Martinelli type or Italian type

Genetic inheritance: Autosomal recessive. The AMDM gene has not yet been identified, but a mutation at the location 9p13-q12 appears to be the most likely cause. In 1996 the AMDH gene was identified as a mutation in cartilage-derived morphogenetic protein 1 (CDMP-1), which has been mapped to 20q11.2.

Pathophysiology: The genetic mutation leads to abnormal linear growth of the skeleton.

Diagnosis: Characteristic clinical and radiographic features in infancy.

Clinical aspects:

TYPE I: MAROTEAUX TYPE (AMDM): Skeletal disorder that affects the limbs and the spine. Newborns affected with AMDM generally are of normal weight, length, and head circumference but can have short-appearing limbs. Older children and adults are significantly shorter than their peers, generally of normal intelligence, and are not expected to have any additional medical complications other than their skeletal changes.

TYPE II: HUNTER-THOMPSON TYPE (AMDH): The prevalence is unknown but it seems to be less frequent than the other types of acromesomelic dysplasia. Dwarfism is present at birth. The adult height is approximately 120 cm. The trunk is normally proportioned. Severe dwarfism is mostly limited to the limbs (extremely short stature), with the legs more severely affected than the arms. The middle segment (forearm with bowing of the radius and posterior dislocation of its head; lower leg with marked shortening of tibia and fibula) and distal segment (short hands and feet) show the most severe changes. Dislocation of the large joints (elbow, hip, knee, ankle) is frequently observed. The fingers usually are very short secondary to cuboidal shape of the metacarpals and shortening of the middle and proximal phalanges. Intelligence, facial appearance, and head circumference are normal. Corneal opacities may occur.

TYPE III: GREBE TYPE (AMDG): Short-limbed dwarfism affecting both sexes and evident from birth. The most characteristic features are extremely short limbs, with the legs more severely affected than the upper limbs. The hands are extremely short with toe-like fingers, and the feet are in valgus position. Polydactyly is present in 50% of patients. Facies is normal and obesity is common. Mental development is delayed, but patients ultimately are mentally normal.

TYPE IV: BRAHIMI BACHA TYPE: Spondylometaphyseal dysplasia, most often associated with severe metaphyseal changes and severe genua valgum.

TYPE V: CAMPAILLA MARTINELLI TYPE: Dwarfism with severe limb shortening, most pronounced in the forearms and lower legs, associated with dysplasia of the tubular bones of the hands and feet. Intelligence is normal.

Anesthetic considerations: Normal craniofacial and axial skeleton. Care with positioning of the limbs because of high risk for dislocations. No specific anesthetic considerations.

REFERENCE:

Langer LO, Beals RK, Solomon IL, et al: Acromesomelic dwarfism: Manifestations in childhood. *Am J Med Genet* 1:87, 1977.

Acromicric Dysplasia

At a glance: Disease characterized by severe growth retardation, mild facial anomalies, and markedly shortened hands and feet secondary to short and stubby metacarpals and phalanges.

Incidence and genetic inheritance: Approximately 30 cases have been reported. Most cases seem to be sporadic; however, vertical transmission also has been described. Because both sexes are affected, an autosomal dominant mode of inheritance is most likely. Acromicric dysplasia, geleophysic dysplasia, and Moore-Federmann syndrome may be allelic forms of the same disorder of different disturbances of the same metabolic pathway.

Pathophysiology: Histologic, histochemical, and electron microscopic examinations of the growth cartilage reveal lesions having disorganization of the growth zone with islands of cells, some showing signs of degeneration. Abnormal organization of collagen results in thick rims surrounding the cells and wide fibers in the interter-

ritorial matrix. Most chondrocytes contain large accumulations of glycogen.

Diagnosis: Based on the clinical features. Radiologic examination reveals short stubby metacarpals and phalanges with notching of the second metacarpal on the radial side and the fifth metacarpal on the ulnar side. The shapes of the epiphysis and metaphysis of the long bones are almost normal, except for a slight deformation of the femoral heads in some patients.

Clinical aspects: Mild facial anomalies, marked shortening of hands and feet, and growth retardation, which is severe in the majority of patients. Body length at birth is usually normal, but short stature becomes progressively evident with increasing age and reaches a final body height of approximate 130 cm. Mild dysmorphic features that are present at birth most often disappear later in life. Intelligence usually is normal. Joint mobility may be limited secondary to severe contractures. Other possible features include spine abnormalities, hoarse voice, and frequent infections of the ears and upper airway. Apart from short metacarpals and phalanges, a notch on the radial side of the second metacarpal, a notch on the ulnar side of the fifth metacarpal, and a notch along the internal border of the femoral heads, no other major radiographic abnormalities have been described. Storage phenomena (mucopolysaccharides), such as progressive thickening of the skin and mitral and aortic valves, and hepatomegaly have been described in a few patients. However, these storage phenomena seem to be more characteristic for ☞Geleophysic Dysplasia and ☞Moore-Federmann Syndrome.

Anesthetic considerations: Positioning may be difficult. Because of recurrent infections of the upper airway, careful preoperative examination should ensure that the patient's airway is optimized for the procedure. Chest radiograph may be required; if in doubt, echocardiography may help assess valvular and cardiac function.

REFERENCES:

Maroteaux P, Stanescu R, Stanescu V, et al: Acromicric dysplasia. *Am J Med Genet* 24:447, 1986.

Hennekam RCM, van Bever Y, Oorthuys JWE: Acromicric dysplasia and geleophysic dysplasia: similarities and differences. *Eur J Pediatr* 155:311, 1996.

Faivre L, Le Merrer M, Baumann, et al: Acromicric dysplasia: Long term outcome and evidence of autosomal dominant inheritance. *J Med Genet* 38:745, 2001.

Acrorenal-Mandibular Syndrome

At a glance: Limb malformation involving syndactyly, median clefts of the hands and feet, and aplasia and/or hypoplasia of the phalanges, metacarpals, and metatarsals.

Synonyms: Split-Hand and Split-Foot with Mandibular Hypoplasia; Acrorenal-Uterine-Mandibular Syndrome.

Incidence and genetic inheritance: Extremely rare congenital abnormality of unknown cause. Autosomal recessive.

Clinical aspects: At birth, the diagnosis is suspected on the clinical aspect, oligohydramnios, and intrauterine growth retardation. Features include severe ectrodactyly (split-hand, split-foot malformation) associated with genital and visceral abnormalities (uterus didelphys or unicornis, vaginal anomalies, polycystic kidney disease or hypoplastic kidneys, diaphragmatic hernia, absent lung lobes, lung segmentation defects). Scoliosis, pectus carinatum, and abnormal number of ribs and vertebral size have been reported. Severe mandibular hypoplasia and low-set ears may be additional features.

Anesthetic considerations: The presence of severe mandibular hypoplasia may indicate difficult airway management; difficult tracheal intubation must be anticipated. Electrolytes and fluid intake must be appropriately balanced in patients with renal insufficiency. Spontaneous ventilation should be maintained until the airway is secured. The dosage of drugs with predominantly renal excretion must be reduced according to the degree of renal insufficiency.

REFERENCE:
Evans JA, Phillips S, Reed M, et al: Severe acro-renal-uterine-mandibular syndrome. *Am J Med Genet* 93:67, 2000.

Acyl-CoA Dehydrogenase Deficiency Syndrome

At a glance: Acylated coenzyme A (acyl-CoA) dehydrogenases are a family of mitochondrial enzymes that catalyze the first dehydrogenation step in the beta oxidation of fatty acyl-CoA derivatives. Fatty acids provide important respiratory fuel for many tissues, including heart, brain, skeletal muscle, pancreas, placenta, brown adipose tissue, kidney, and liver. The disorder is inherited as an autosomal recessive trait. Metabolic acidosis, severe hypoglycemia without ketosis, and coma are frequent features of all types of acyl-CoA dehydrogenase deficiency syndrome. It also occurs during adulthood. Large amounts of glutaric acid in the blood and urine are caused by deficiency of the enzyme "multiple acyl-CoA dehydrogenase".

Classification: The family of acyl-CoA dehydrogenase deficiency syndromes contains eight members. The most frequent are the following five:

  Short-chain acyl-CoA dehydrogenase deficiency (SCAD)
  Medium-chain acyl-CoA dehydrogenase deficiency (MCAD)
  Long-chain acyl-CoA dehydrogenase deficiency (LCAD)
  Very-long-chain acyl-CoA dehydrogenase deficiency (VLCAD)
  Multiple acyl-CoA dehydrogenase deficiency (MADD)
  (Synonym: ☞Glutaric Acidemia Type II)

Incidence and genetic inheritance: All types are inherited as either autosomal dominant or recessive pattern.

Pathophysiology: All acyl-CoA dehydrogenase deficiencies catalyze the same initial dehydrogenation of the substrate at the beta-carbon atom and require electron transfer flavoprotein as an electron acceptor. They differ distinctly from each other with regard to the length and configuration of the hydrocarbon chain of their respective substrates and have accordingly received appropriate names. They are nuclear encoded and are synthesized as precursor proteins in the cytosol with an N-terminal leader peptide, which is cleaved off upon import to the mitochondria, producing a mature monomer. It has been genetically mapped on the 11q25. Analysis using a Northern blot system detected an approximately 2.1-kb ACAD8 transcript in all tissues examined, namely, heart, lung, brain, skeletal muscle, pancreas, placenta, liver, and kidney.

Clinical aspects: *Short-chain acyl-CoA dehydrogenase deficiency* (SCAD) is an extremely rare inherited disorder of fat metabolism often recognized as an organic acidemia disorder. All reported cases have occurred in females. A pattern of occurrence has not been defined. Severe metabolic acidosis and hyperammonemia are principal features of the disorder. There are two distinct types of SCAD. A *congenital form* is characterized by progressive hypotonia and or-

ganic acidemia. The clinical symptoms in infants associated with organic acidemia include poor feeding, frequent vomiting, failure to thrive, progressive muscle weakness, hypotonia, growth retardation, impaired mental development, and lethargy. Other features may include hypoglycemia, accumulation of excessive amounts of fatty acids in muscle and/or liver tissue, and severe hyperammonemia. Unusually low levels of carnitine in muscle tissue (secondary carnitine deficiency) may occur. In some infants the presence of cerebral edema and raised intracranial pressure, hepatosplenomegaly, liver steatosis, biliary cholestasis, and focal hepatocellular necrosis have been reported. It often is considered life-threatening. The *milder adult onset form* of this disorder affects the skeletal muscles and is characterized by severe muscle weakness. Muscle weakness probably is the result of accumulation of fatty acids leading to lipid storage myopathy. An abnormally low levels of the amino acid carnitine in muscle tissue (secondary carnitine deficiency) has been suggested. The association of high levels of acid in the urine and muscle weakness is considered pathognomonic.

Medium-chain acyl-CoA dehydrogenase deficiency (MCAD) is a very rare inherited metabolic disorder but is the most common disease in a group of disorders that involve abnormalities of fatty acid metabolism. It is inherited as an autosomal recessive genetic trait. The gene responsible is thought to be chromosome 1p. It is believed to affect males and females equally. In the general population, it occurs in approximately 1:50,000 live births. In Americans of Northwestern European origin, it may occur in 1:6400 to 1:46,000 individuals. In most cases, onset occurs during infancy, usually between the ages of 3 to 15 months. However, in some rare cases, symptoms may not become apparent until later in childhood. The clinical manifestations of the disease usually are present during infancy, most frequently between 3 to 15 months of age. However, in extremely rare situations, the onset of age may not be until later in childhood. It is characterized by a deficiency of the enzyme medium chain acyl-CoA dehydrogenase. This enzyme is most active in the liver, leukocytes, and fibroblasts and is necessary for oxidation medium-chain fatty acids. Metabolism failure can lead to abnormal accumulation of fatty acids in the liver and the brain. In infants, symptoms may include recurrent episodes of hypoglycemia, lethargy, muscle stiffness, pain and cramps, vomiting, and liver dysfunction (including coagulation disorders). These symptoms are most frequently triggered during extended periods of fasting. Infants usually appear normal until they are subjected to a period of 12 to 16 hours of fasting. Extended periods of fasting leads to hypoglycemia, coma, and life-threatening complications (e.g., severe metabolic acidosis). Infants may be affected with liver steatosis and hepatomegaly, hepatic dysfunction, and hyperammonemia. In addition, affected infants may show hypocarnitinemia that affects the mitochondria and leads to severe metabolic acidosis. Other clinical features include cerebral edema, raised intracranial pressure, and encephalopathy. Neuromotor development, such as learning to crawl, walk, and speak, can be delayed. In very rare cases, patients may present with aphasia, hypotonia, and failure to thrive. The cardiovascular system usually is not affected. Conduction block has been suggested but most probably is coincidental.

Long-chain acyl-CoA dehydrogenase deficiency (LCAD) is a rare genetic disorder of fatty acid metabolism (i.e., fatty acid oxidation disorder) that is transmitted as an autosomal recessive trait. The gene involved seems to be located on the long arm of chromosome 2 (2q34-q35). The onset of initial symptoms is apparent during the first year of life, with some affected patients showing symptoms during the neonatal period. However, a few cases with later symptom onset have been reported, including two children with initial episodes occurring at age 18 months and 8 years. It is characterized by severe hypoglycemia following a period of fasting or during an infection. Infants may present with an acute episode of respiratory depression, including respiratory arrest, and cardiac arrest. Lethargy and eventually coma have been reported. The hypoglycemic period usually is not associated with accumulation of ketone bodies (hypoketotic hypoglycemia). Additional characteristics include cardiomyopathy or hypertrophic heart, dysrhythmias, hepatomegaly, severe hypotonia, and dicarboxylic aciduria. Patients may experience episodes of extreme fatigue, muscle soreness or pain, and myoglobinuria. However, such "attacks," which may begin in the second decade of life or later, tend to occur after decreased dietary intake, emotional stress, or viral illness.

Very-long-chain acyl-CoA dehydrogenase deficiency (VLCAD) is a very rare disorder inherited by an autosomal recessive genetic trait. It is unique among the acyl-CoA dehydrogenases because of its size, structure, and intramitochondrial distribution. The very-long-chain acyl-CoA dehydrogenase differs from the other acyl-CoA dehydrogenases in that it is loosely bound to the mitochondrial inner membrane. It is characterized by hypoketotic hypoglycemia and hepatocellular disease. The cardiovascular system is affected mainly by cardiomyopathy, including hypertrophic cardiomyopathy. Pericardial effusion has been reported. The presence of cardiomyopathy is the most common cause of death in these patients. Exercise induces myoglobinemia and myoglobinuria. Laboratory evaluation demonstrates the presence of very-long-chain acyl-CoA dehydrogenase deficiency, marked lipid accumulation in many tissues, and hyperaminemia. Increased urinary adipate and sebacate may be observed.

Multiple-chain acyl-CoA dehydrogenase deficiency (MADD): Two forms of glutaric aciduria type II occur during different stages of life. Both forms are considered organic acidemias, characterized by excess acid in the blood and urine. (1) *Glutaricaciduria IIA* or *neonatal form of glutaricaciduria II* is a very rare, X-linked hereditary disorder characterized by large amounts of glutaric acids in blood and urine. It affects males only, with onset of symptoms at birth. The neonatal form of glutaricaciduria IIA is caused by deficiency of an element common to all three acyl-CoA dehydrogenase enzymes, so the disorder can also be called multiple acyl-CoA dehydrogenase deficiency. (2) *Glutaricaciduria IIB* (ethylmalonic adipicaciduria) is known as the adult form of glutaricaciduria II. *Glutaricaciduria IIB* affects males and females equally. This milder form of the disorder is inherited as an autosomal recessive trait. Metabolic acidosis and hypoketotic hypoglycemia occur during adulthood.

Anesthetic considerations: Preoperative fasting must be avoided in all acyl-CoA types. Patients should receive glucose supplementation perioperatively. The amount of glucose administered can be considerable during periods of stress, high metabolic demand, or metabolic decompensation. From 10 to 15 mg/kg/min may be required, and use of 10% dextrose solution is recommended. Repeated plasma glucose levels must be obtained regularly. Proper evaluation of cardiac function must be performed preoperatively. Cardiac echocardiography should be performed to rule out cardiomyopathy. The respiratory system should be assessed, especially in the presence of MCAD. The association of lethargy and severe hypotonia must be considered during administration of anesthesia.

Other conditions to be considered:

☞**GLUTARIC ACIDEMIA TYPE I** is a rare hereditary metabolic disorder caused by a deficiency of the enzyme glutaryl-CoA dehydrogenase. It is characterized by hypotonia, severe vomiting, and metabolic acidosis. The patient may present with neurologic signs of dystonia or athetosis. Mental retardation may occur. It is also known as a member of a group of disorders called *organic acidemias.*

☞**ORNITHINE CARBAMOYLTRANSFERASE DEFICIENCY** is a rare inherited metabolic disease and is one of six inherited urea cycle disorders. It is caused by a deficiency in the metabolism of ammonia into urea. These deficiencies cause hyperammonemia. It is characterized by a lack of appetite, vomiting, drowsiness, seizures, and/or coma. Hepatomegaly is possible.

UREA CYCLE ENZYME DEFICIENCIES (UCE) are a group of rare inherited metabolic disorders. The classifications for UCE are citrullinemia, arginosuccinic aciduria, arginase deficiency, N-acetyl glutamate synthetase deficiency, carbamyl phosphate synthetase deficiency, and ornithine transcarbamylase deficiency. The symptoms of all urea cycle disorders vary in severity and result in hyperammonemia. Symptoms include lack of appetite, vomiting, drowsiness, seizures, and/or coma. Hepatomegaly is often present.

☞**CARNITINE DEFICIENCY** is a rare metabolic disorder that may be inherited or it may occur as a result of organic acidemias such as short-chain acyl-CoA dehydrogenase deficiency. It is used as a carrier of muscular energy in the body. A deficiency of carnitine can cause extreme hypotonia, vomiting, confusion, and/or coma. It may be associated with hypoglycemia, chronic heart disease, and/or cardiac failure.

☞**REYE SYNDROME** is a rare disorder that predominantly affects children from approximately age 4 to 12 years. In some cases, it was initially suspected in infants or children with fatty acid oxidation disorders, including LCAD deficiency. It is primarily characterized by rapid accumulation of fat in the liver and acute encephalopathy. Associated symptoms include sudden onset of severe and persistent vomiting, elevated blood levels of hepatic transaminases, severe disorientation; seizures; and coma. Although the pathophysiology remains unknown, an association with salicylate use in children or adolescents during viral illnesses, particularly upper respiratory tract infections (e.g., influenza B) or varicella, has been suggested.

Adactylia

At a glance: Unilateral defects of the hand with absent portions of digits.

Synonym: Unilateral Terminal Transverse Defects of Hand.

Genetic inheritance: Autosomal dominant.

Clinical aspects: Unilateral defects of the hand with absent terminal portions of digits 2 to 5. Mildly hypoplastic thumb. Tiny nail remnants on digital stumps.

Anesthetic considerations: No known specific considerations with this condition.

REFERENCE:
Graham JM, Brown FE, Struckmeyer CL, et al: Dominantly inherited unilateral terminal transverse defects of the hand (adactylia) in twin sisters and one daughter. *Pediatrics* 78:103, 1986.

Adams Nance Syndrome

At a glance: Characterized by paroxysmal tachycardia, hypertension, syncope and seizures. It is associated with dominantly inherited microphthalmos, cataracts, and renal stones. Hyperglycinuria has been suggested as the responsible cause.

Incidence/genetic inheritance: This medical condition has been described in a brother and sister in 1967. There are very few cases reported in the literature. It is suggested to be inherited as an autosomal recessive trait.

Clinical aspects: Characterized by the clinical presentation of tachycardia, severe vascular hypertension, microphthalmos, visual loss, seizures, cataracts, and kidney stones. Other clinical features include cardiac conduction defects, paroxysmal tachycardia, nystagmus, glaucoma/buphthalmos, and xanthomas/lipomas. It is believed to be caused by a disturbance in glycine metabolism.

Precautions before anesthesia: It is recommended to obtain a cardiology consultation. A 12-lead ECG, chest x-ray, and possible echocardiography should be obtained. Evaluate for end-organ damage as a result of chronic hypertension. A complete cell blood count, electrolytes, BUN, creatine, and blood glucose levels should be measured before anesthesia. Patients are at risk for paroxysmal supraventricular tachycardia (usually sinus tachycardia) in the perioperative period. Severe hypertensive episodes may be encountered; maintenance of antihypertensive therapy must be maintained until the morning of anesthesia. Consider preoperative beta-blocker, calcium channel blocker, and/or angiotensin converting enzyme (ACE) inhibitor before general anesthesia. Hypertension must be controlled before elective surgery. Because of the presence of vascular hypertension, it is important to ensure that the intravascular volume is adequate before induction of anesthesia. A review of the medication used to control the seizure activities must be obtained. The antiseizure medication must be continued until the morning of surgery.

Anesthetic considerations: Cardiac conduction defects, i.e., paroxysmal supraventricular tachycardia and/or sinus tachycardia, and severe possible vascular hypertension are considered major potential complications during induction of anesthesia. Direct current or pharmacological cardioversion may become necessary and should be readily available. It may be necessary to treat hypertension perioperatively as well. Patients may have relative intravascular volume deficit as a result of hypertension and should be corrected before induction of anesthesia.

Pharmacologic implications: Avoid anesthetic agents leading to cardiovascular stimulation such as sympathomimetic agents that may initiate a hypertensive response and/or paroxysmal tachycardia perioperatively. Patients are usually premedicated with antihypertensive medications. The use of intravenous antiseizure medications should be considered during long surgical procedures.

REFERENCES:

Adams CW, Nance WE: Persistent tachycardia, paroxysmal hypertension, and seizures: Association with hyperglycinuria, dominantly inherited microphthalmia, and cataracts. *JAMA* 202:525, 1967.

Adams-Oliver Syndrome (AOS)

At a glance: Very rare inherited disorder characterized by defects of the scalp associated with multiple scarred and hairless areas that usually have dilated blood vessel directly under the skin. Scalp defects are present at birth. The extremities are either short (hypoplastic fingers and toes) or characterized by absent hands and lower legs. Congenital heart defect must be ruled out.

Synonyms: Congenital Scalp Defects with Distal Limb Reduction Anomalies; Absence Defect of Limbs, Scalp, and Skull.

History: Described in 1945 by Forrest H. Adams and C.P. Oliver, both American physicians.

Incidence: Rare congenital abnormality. Approximately 100 cases have been described. Both sexes are equally affected.

Genetic inheritance: In most families, the disorder clearly follows an autosomal dominant pattern of inheritance, but in some families the penetrance is reduced. No genetic background information or molecular data concerning the Adams-Oliver syndrome are available.

Pathophysiology: The pathophysiologic mechanism remains unknown, but a vascular pathogenesis with interruption of early embryonic blood supply to the subclavian arteries has been discussed.

Diagnosis: The diagnosis is made clinically with findings of a scalp defect combined with distal limb anomalies.

Clinical aspects: For some researchers, this syndrome represents one of many forms of ☞Aplasia Cutis Congenita. The congenital midline scalp defect often is solitary and associated with an underlying skull defect and dilated scalp veins converging to the skin defect. Typically, these lesions appear as small ulcerations that may heal spontaneously. Larger lesion may require surgery with skin grafting and often are associated with an underlying bone defect. In a small number of patients, these defects have resulted in death secondary to infection (fatal meningitis) or hemorrhage from the sagittal sinus. However, the clinical expression of this syndrome is highly variable. The defect of the cranium usually is not associated with nervous system abnormalities. Intellectual development seems normal. However, hydrocephalus, microcephaly, seizure disorder, and mental retardation have been reported in a few patients. Limb reduction anomalies (found in 80% of patients) are most commonly characterized by hypoplastic or absent distal phalanges and in some cases absence of the lower leg below the midcalf level. On the upper limb, the metacarpals or the fingers may be completely absent or the terminal phalanges of the fingers are hypoplastic. Other anomalies may include congenital heart defects (present in up to 13% of patients, e.g., tetralogy of Fallot, pulmonary atresia, double-outlet right ventricle, pulmonary vein stenosis, atrial septal defect), cerebral arteriovenous malformations, encephalocele, microphthalmia, cleft lip/palate, cutis marmorata telangiectatica congenita, ☞Epidermolysis Bullosa, thin and hyperpigmented skin, woolly hair, and supernumerary nipples. Bronchial and renal anomalies and portal hypertension have been described in a small number of patients.

Precautions before anesthesia: In neonates, look carefully for associated abnormalities. Cardiac malformations should be excluded by echocardiography. The anesthesiologist must be aware of the possible association with ☞Epidermolysis Bullosa. Look for possible complications of large or multiple scalp defects, such as infection (meningitis) or hemorrhage. Obtain complete blood count, electrolytes, creatinine, and BUN. Appropriate blood products must be available during surgical closure of large defects.

Anesthetic considerations: The main anesthetic consideration in these children is the association with congenital heart defects. Pulmonary hypertension without anatomical cardiac defects has been described. Placement of venous access and degree of invasive monitoring are determined by the extent of the planned surgery, expected blood loss, and associated anomalies (cardiac defects, pulmonary and portal hypertension).

Pharmacological implications: No pharmacological data on Adams-Oliver syndrome are available. In the presence of cardiac defects, subacute bacterial endocarditis prophylaxis may be required. In patients with renal anomalies or portal hypertension, the dosage and dosage interval for drugs with predominantly renal and hepatic elimination, respectively, may require adjustment.

Other conditions to be considered:

☞POLAND SYNDROME: Autosomal dominant, dextrocardia, hypoplasia or absence of the pectoralis muscle, hypoplastic ribs, hemivertebrae, unilateral syndactyly, hypoplastic muscles (e.g. serratus anterior, infraspinatus, deltoid). All features are unilateral and occur mostly (75%) on the right side. Males are affected three times more often than females.

☞**APLASIA CUTIS CONGENITA:** Macrocephaly, large, high forehead, unilateral facial palsy, mental retardation, congenital heart defect (e.g., ventricular septal defect, tetralogy of Fallot, valvular pulmonary stenosis), Autosomal dominant inheritance.

☞**SETLEIS SYNDROME:** Puckered periorbital skin, absent or multiple rows of eyelashes.

☞**JOHANSON-BLIZZARD SYNDROME:** Polymalformative syndrome characterized by nasal alar hypoplasia (beak-shaped), scalp defects, hypothyroidism, pancreatic achylia, and congenital deafness.

☞**GOLTZ SYNDROME:** Complex mesoectodermal hereditary disorder characterized by focal dermal atrophy with herniation of fat producing multiple papillomas, in association with skeletal, dental, ocular, and other anomalies.

☞**STREETER ANOMALY:** Constricting amniotic bands leading to amputation with scarring, distal syndactyly, cleft lip/palate, anencephaly, encephalocele, hydrocephaly, omphalocele, and gastroschisis. Other internal anomalies involve the heart, lungs, diaphragm, kidneys, and gonads.

☞**DELLEMAN OORTHUYS SYNDROME:** Multiple congenital anomaly syndrome mainly affecting the central nervous system, eyes, and skin.

REFERENCES:

Farrell SA, Warda LJ, LaFlair P, et al: Adams-Oliver syndrome: A case with juvenile chronic myelogenous leukemia and chylothorax. *Am J Med Genet* 47:1175, 1993.

Pereira-da-Silva L, Leal F, Santos GC, et al: Clinical evidence of vascular abnormalities at birth in Adams-Oliver syndrome: Report of two further cases [letter]. *Am J Med Genet* 94:75, 2000.

Zapata HH, Sletten LJ, Pierpont ME: Congenital cardiac malformations in Adams-Oliver syndrome. *Clin Genet* 47:80, 1995.

Addisonian Syndrome

At a glance: Progressive weakness, anemia, hypoglycemia, and hyperpigmentation of the skin. Vomiting, apneic spells, cyanosis, vascular collapse, and cardiovascular shock may be consequential.

Synonyms: Addison Disease; Adrenal Insufficiency; Adrenal Hypoplasia/Aplasia.

History: First described in 1849 by Thomas Addison, the English physician, in patients suffering from tuberculosis with suprarenal involvement.

Genetic inheritance: Most cases are sporadic, but depending on the etiology solid evidence exists for autosomal recessive and X-linked recessive forms.

Pathophysiology: Complete or partial deficit of mineralocorticoids and glucocorticoid hormones, excreted by the zonae fasciculata (aldosterone) and glomerulosa (glucocorticoids) of the adrenal cortex, caused by different mechanisms. Autoimmune mechanisms (which may be associated with other autoimmune diseases, e.g. chronic lymphocytic thyroiditis, hyperthyroidism, diabetes mellitus, celiac disease), adrenal aplasia, X-linked congenital adrenal hypoplasia, cytomegalic adrenocortical hypoplasia, familial hypoadrenocorticism, pituitary gland hypoplasia, isolated ACTH deficiency, X-linked adrenoleukodystrophy, and Waterhouse Friderichsen Syndrome (fulminant form caused by meningococcemia). Dysfunction of the adrenal cortex leads to interrupted hypothalamic and anterior pituitary gland feedback inhibition, resulting in continuous and uninhibited secretion of ACTH. Cleavage of the prohormone pro-opiomelanocortin in the adenohypophysis results in simultaneous secretion of ACTH and melanocyte-stimulating hormone (MSH). The elevated MSH level is responsible for the typical bronze hyperpigmentation in patients with primary adrenal insufficiency.

Diagnosis: Vomiting, cyanosis, apneic spells, hypoglycemia, seizures, and vascular collapse are the usual presenting symptoms of an adrenal crisis. Cardiovascular collapse may occur. Plasma and urinary concentrations of all adrenal steroids are low. Serum glucose level usually is low. Sodium plasma concentrations are decreased (but rarely <120 mmol/l) but potassium plasma concentrations are increased (but rarely >7.0 mmol/l). Moderate metabolic acidosis with plasma bicarbonate levels between 15 and 20 mmol/l is common. BUN typically is elevated. Urinary excretion of sodium and chloride is increased, whereas potassium excretion is decreased. Plasma cortisol levels—if measured before treatment—are low. However, the final diagnosis of adrenocortical insufficiency is based on the finding of an absent or decreased response in adrenal steroid synthesis to stimulation with external (intravenous or intramuscular) ACTH. Increased serum concentrations of cortisol and aldosterone are signs of a functional adrenal cortex. Under normal conditions, cortisol synthesis increases by a factor of two to five times above normal levels after administration of ACTH. Failure of aldosterone serum level to double within 30 minutes of ACTH administration indicates a problem with mineralocorticoid synthesis. A normal ACTH stimulation test result excludes the diagnosis of primary adrenocortical insufficiency. The adrenal glands may appear enlarged on abdominal CT scan or sonography in patients with Addison disease secondary to infection, hemorrhage, or malignancies involving the adrenals. Primary adrenal insufficiency results in atrophic adrenal glands secondary to inactivity. Idiopathic autoimmune adrenocortical insufficiency usually resulting from autoimmune lymphocytic infiltration of the adrenal cortex is the most common cause of Addisonian syndrome, accounting for approximately 80% of cases. Another significant percentage results from adrenal cortex destruction by tuberculosis.

Idiopathic autoimmune Addison disease may occur in isolation or in combination with other autoimmune diseases, such as diabetes mellitus type I, systemic lupus erythematosus, Hashimoto thyroiditis, Graves disease, vitiligo, alopecia (areata, totalis, universalis), pernicious anemia, myasthenia gravis, idiopathic hypophysitis, idiopathic hypoparathyroidism, primary biliary cirrhosis, and chronic active hepatitis. Other diseases may have the potential to cause Addisonian syndrome (e.g. tuberculosis, sarcoidosis, blastomycosis, histoplasmosis, cryptococcosis, meningococcemia, AIDS, cytomegalovirus infection). Hodgkin and non-Hodgkin lymphomas and metastases from different carcinomas (lung, breast, kidney) may affect the adrenal glands. Addisonian syndrome in patients with ☞Allgrove Syndrome is caused by a congenital adrenocortical unresponsiveness to ACTH. Several drugs may interfere with adrenal steroidogenesis (ketoconazole, busulfan, etomidate, aminoglutethimide) or ACTH storage in the pituitary (methadone). Addisonian syndrome has been described as a complication of pregnancy and anticoagulant therapy with heparin or warfarin resulting in adrenocortical hemorrhage. Heparin-induced (thrombocytopenia and) thrombosis may result in thrombosis of adrenal vessels followed by necrosis of the gland. An acute adrenal crisis can be precipitated by trauma, surgery, and significant physical and/or emotional stress. Another common cause of an adrenal crisis is the failure to appropriately replace steroids in patients receiving long-term steroid medication.

Clinical aspects: Progressive weakness, anemia, and hyperpigmentation are salient features. Pigmentation is caused by increased levels of ACTH. Laboratory findings depend on the type of hypoadrenalism: hyponatremia, hyperkalemia, metabolic acidosis, and anemia are present in primary adrenal insufficiency. Elevated BUN and creatinine concentrations are common and result from hypovolemia, decreased renal plasma flow, and decreased glomerular filtration rate. Fasting and increased sensitivity to insulin with increased peripheral glucose utilization may result in hypoglycemia. Hypoglycemia without electrolyte imbalance may occur in patients with secondary adrenal insufficiency.

Precautions before anesthesia: Treatment of known adrenal insufficiency is daily administration of cortisol and fludrocortisone. During stress, the dosages must be increased by 50 to 100%. Acute adrenal insufficiency is treated with 5 to 10% dextrose in isotonic saline. Hydrocortisone initially is given as a bolus, followed by an infusion until symptoms subside. Intramuscular injections of cortisone acetate are given daily and then progressively reduced when the patient's clinical status improves. The salt-retaining hormone desoxycorticosterone (DOCA) is administered daily to maintain electrolyte balance. Anesthetic management of patients with documented adrenal insufficiency must include provision of exogenous corticosteroids and focus on the adequacy of the dose supplemented. Serum electrolytes and blood glucose levels (fasting hypoglycemia is common) should be checked on a regular basis.

Anesthetic considerations: There is no direct influence of anesthetic agents (except etomidate) on the rise of cortisol in response to surgical stress (which is reduced or suppressed only by high central neuraxial blockade). Untreated or partially treated patients may develop an acute adrenal crisis, which is potentially lethal and requires the same treatment as the other forms of acute adrenal insufficiency.

Pharmacological implications: Careful titration of the anesthetic agents may be necessary because patients with Addisonian syndrome are prone to myocardial depression following administration of potent anesthetics.

Other conditions to be considered:

☞**ALLGROVE SYNDROME:** This is a genetic autosomal recessive disease characterized by the triad of ACTH-resistant insufficiency, achalasia, and alacrima. It presents in the first decade of life with severe hypoglycemic episodes that can result in death. Mixed pattern of upper and lower motor neuropathy, autonomic neuropathy, sensory impairment, and mental retardation.

☞**X-LINKED ADRENOLEUKODYSTROPHY:** Disorder characterized by progressive demyelinization of the central nervous system and peripheral adrenal insufficiency.

REFERENCES:

Weatherill D, Spence AA: Anaesthesia and disorders of the adrenal cortex. *Br J Anaesth* 56:741, 1984.

Stewart PM: Adrenal cortex and endocrine hypertension, in Larsen PR (ed): *Williams Textbook of Endocrinology,* 10th ed. Philadelphia, WB Saunders Company, 2003, p 491.

Adducted Thumbs Syndrome

At a glance: Stiff facies, open mouth, high arched palate with cleft. Craniostenosis and microcephaly. Swallowing difficulties and generalized myopathic hypotonia. Respiratory insufficiency that generally leads to death in early infancy.

Incidence and genetic inheritance: Approximately 10 cases have been reported. Inheritance seems to be autosomal recessive.

Pathophysiology: Dysmyelination characterized by excessive myelin-dependent gliosis, myelin solubilization, and transient formation of phospholipid-containing plaques on the brain's surface.

Diagnosis: Clinical features and absence of extension of the thumb during the Moro reflex.

Clinical aspects: Typical features are craniostenosis, microcephaly, large occiput, mental retardation, seizures, external ophthalmoplegia, myopathic stiff facies, low-set and large, malrotated ears, open mouth, microgenia, abnormal temporomandibular joints (anomaly of the processus condylaris and mandibulares), high arched palate with cleft, and velopharyngeal insufficiency are common findings. Swallowing difficulties (absent gag reflex) and generalized myopathic hypotonia are typical. Laryngomalacia, recurrent pneumonias, and pectus excavatum have been described in the majority of patients. The most characteristic sign is flexion and adduction of the thumbs with arthrogryposis of elbows, wrists, and knees. Respiratory insufficiency is mainly caused by the generalized myopathic hypotonia and the main reason for the poor prognosis with death in early infancy (only one patient has survived the first year of life). Muscle biopsy reveals unspecific signs of congenital myopathy (i.e., wide variation in the diameter of muscle fibers, normal distribution of type I and II fibers, increased number of centrally located nuclei, increased interstitial tissue, lack of signs of denervation).

Precautions before anesthesia: Obtain a history of developmental milestones, muscular hypotonia, recent chest infections, and swallowing difficulties. Assess respiratory function and obtain chest radiograph. Arterial blood gas analysis may be helpful under certain circumstances. Postoperative mechanical ventilation is likely given the poor muscle function and the associated respiratory problems (pneumonia, laryngomalacia).

Anesthetic considerations: Although difficult airway management would be expected given the facial anomalies described, no tracheal intubation problems have been reported in these children. Arthrogryposis may make vascular access and positioning difficult. Respiratory insufficiency likely will require intermittent positive pressure ventilation (IPPV) postoperatively.

Pharmacological implications: No data are available; however, avoiding depolarizing agents in patients with congenital myopathies is advisable.

Other conditions to be considered:

☞**MASA SYNDROME:** Syndrome characterized by acrocephaly, brachycephaly, flat occiput, and maxillary hypoplasia. The mouth is small and the upper lip is thin. Muscular hypertrophy of the legs and subluxation of the hip.

☞**ARTHROGRYPOSIS:** Spectrum of different syndromes characterized by persistent multiple limb contractures. Often associated with pharyngeal, cardiac, urinary, and gastric abnormalities. Often midline dysraphism abnormalities.

CHRISTIAN SYNDROME I (Christian-Andrews-Conneally-Muller Syndrome): Adducted thumbs syndrome with craniosynostosis, arthrogryposis, and cleft palate. Microcephaly, prominent occiput, hypertelorism, antimongoloid palpebral fissures, ophthalmoplegia, abnormal ear placement, and bifid uvula. Autosomal recessive.

☞**FREEMAN-SHELDON SYNDROME:** Genetic malformative disorder characterized by microstomia, flat midface with a small pinched mouth mimicking whistling, clubfoot, contracted muscles of the joints of the fingers, and hands malformations.

CONGENITAL CLASPED THUMBS: Extremely rare disorder that is inherited in either an autosomal dominant or an X-gonosomal manner. The congenitally clasped thumbs most likely are secondary to atrophy or absence of the abductor and extensor pollicis muscles and/or tendons. Ulnar deviation of the hands with flexed digits, kyphoscoliosis, clubfoot, generalized muscular hypotonia, and muscular hypotrophy are common findings.

REFERENCES:

Kunze J, Park W, Hansen KH, et al: Adducted thumb syndrome. Report of a new case and a diagnostic approach. *Eur J Pediatr* 141:122, 1983.

Christian JC, Andrews PA, Conneally PM, et al: The adducted thumbs syndrome: an autosomal recessive disease with arthrogryposis, dysmyelination, craniostenosis, and cleft palate. *Clin Genet* 2:95, 1971.

Fitch N, Levy EP: Adducted thumb syndromes. *Clin Genet* 8:190, 1975.

Adenosine Deaminase Deficiency

At a glance: Heterogeneous systemic disorder caused by the deficiency of adenosine deaminase (ADA) resulting primarily in severe combined (cellular and humoral) immunodeficiency but also systemic abnormalities.

Synonyms: Severe Combined Immunodeficiency Syndrome due to Adenosine Deaminase Deficiency; ADA Deficiency.

Incidence: Estimated to be approximately 1:1,000,000. Adenosine deaminase deficiency (ADAD) accounts for approximately 20% of all patients with severe combined immunodeficiency syndrome (SCID).

Genetic inheritance: Autosomal recessive. More than 50 mutations of ADA have been found. The genetic defect has been mapped to gene locus 20q13.11.

Pathophysiology: ADA catalyzes the irreversible conversion of adenosine and 2'-deoxyadenosine to inosine and 2'-deoxyinosine. Because of alternate bypass routes in the purine catabolic pathway, ADAD patients have normal concentrations of inosine and 2'-deoxyinosine. However, the concentrations of adenosine and 2'-deoxyadenosine are elevated, and accumulation of 2'-deoxyadenosine seems to be the main culprit in the development of ADA deficiency because its phosphorylation leads to deoxyadenosine triphosphate (dATP). The excessive amount of dATP (up to 200-fold increased concentrations have been reported) results in toxicity and leads to allosteric inhibition of ribonucleotide reductase, an enzyme involved in DNA synthesis. Immature T (and to a lesser degree B) lymphocytes show highest sensitivity to this toxicity (most likely as a consequence of their high turnover), which results in impaired cellular immunity and decreased synthesis of immunoglobulins. Some researchers are convinced that the neurologic abnormalities are caused by the same mechanism. Elevated levels of dATP also induce apoptosis in thymic lymphocytes and affect normal methylation processes.

Diagnosis: Early diagnosis is crucial so that severe and potentially fatal infections can be prevented. The absolute lymphocyte count is a useful diagnostic test for screening because lymphopenia is present at birth in nearly all patients with SCID. Because the enzyme defect is found in all body cells, dATP concentration in erythrocytes is considered a sensitive marker for the metabolic severity of ADAD; however, measurements are needed before any transfusions, enzyme replacement therapy, or bone marrow transplant is started.

Clinical aspects: The majority of ADAD patients present with SCID in the first 4 to 8 months of life, usually in combination with skeletal and neurologic anomalies. These patients often have a fatal outcome. However, up to 20% are diagnosed later in life, either in childhood or as adults with an immunodeficiency that evolves insidiously and mainly involves cellular immunity. It seems that little residual ADA activity (approximately 10% of normal) is sufficient to prevent profound immunodeficiency. The suggested classification has four groups:

1. *SCID,* which is diagnosed in the first year of life, presents with failure to thrive and recurrent (most often opportunistic) infections. Lymphopenia is profound (most severe of all forms of SCID), with absent cellular and humeral immune function.
2. *Delayed onset,* for which the diagnosis usually is made between 1 and several years of age. Patients present with clinical deterioration secondary to the combined immunodeficiency.
3. *Late onset,* for which diagnosis is made after the first decade of life, secondary to major immunologic and clinical deterioration (initially chronic chest infections, oral and vaginal candidiasis, viral warts, recurrent dermatomal zoster).
4. *Partial ADAD,* in which the patient is ADA deficient but otherwise healthy, with normal immune function.

In all patients with SCID, the thymus is severely hypoplastic, with a lack of corticomedullary distinction and thymocytes. Hassall corpuscles are either abortive or absent. Symptoms pointing to the diagnosis include recurrent and/or opportunistic infections with candida (oral candidiasis), respiratory syncytial virus, adenovirus, parainfluenza virus, cytomegalovirus, or pneumonia secondary to *Pneumocystis carinii.* Bacterial pneumonia, Gram-negative sepsis, and persistent diarrhea with failure to thrive are common and often the cause of death. Behavioral and neurologic problems (with severity proportional to dATP levels) are common in ADAD patients and may include hyperactivity/attention deficit disorders, aggressivity, sensorineural hearing loss, seizures, spasticity, athetosis, head lag, tremor, nystagmus, and decreased cognitive function and IQ. Renal problems have been reported in a number of patients and include proteinuria and transient proximal renal tubular acidosis. The kidneys often are enlarged, and histologic examination reveals mesangial sclerosis with thickening of the subendothelial layer of capillary walls, particularly in the juxtamesangial region. Some degree of (most likely progressive) glomerulosclerosis may be seen. Adenosine, which is elevated in ADAD, has significant effects on arteriolar resistance and renin secretion. Fibrosis of the adrenal cortex (especially in the subcapsular region) and the pituitary gland is a common finding. Adrenal insufficiency with a high risk of hypoglycemia, hyponatremia, and hypokalemia has been reported. Hypocalcemia is common. Osseous anomalies are characterized by prominent costochondral junctions, and microscopic examination shows chondroosseous dysplasia with disordered chondrocyte columns, hypertrophic chondrocytes in resting cartilage, ballooned lacunae, and abrupt transition of cartilage to bone. The skin often is edematous and appears hyperpigmented. Pulmonary alveolar proteinosis has been found in a few patients. Transfusion of normal erythrocytes leads to a temporary decrease in the serum adenosine concentration and an increase in lymphocyte count; however, retransfusions are required every few weeks to maintain ADA activity above a certain level. Covalent binding of modified bovine intestinal ADA to polyethylene glycol (polyethylene glycol-modified adenosine deaminase [PEG-ADA]) has been used successfully to partially correct the enzyme defect and thereby allow immune function to recover to a degree at least sufficient to prevent opportunistic infections. The risks and side effects are lower than with bone marrow transplantation; however, the costs reportedly are excessive. Gene therapy with viral vectors has been used with some success in a number of patients. Hemosiderosis with marked iron depositions in hepatocytes, Kupffer cells, and spleen is seen after chronic transfusions. The most prominent ADAD patient probably was the "Bubble Boy," a boy who lived in a germ-proof plastic enclosure to prevent infections until he died at age 12 years.

Precautions before anesthesia: Obtain a complete blood count (especially after recent bone marrow transplant) and check blood glucose and electrolyte levels (hypocalcemia, hypokalemia). Assess liver and kidney function and obtain a chest radiograph. Cooperation may be difficult because of hyperactivity, aggressivity, and/or cognitive impairment; sedative premedication may be advantageous. A recent transfusion leads to increased ADA-levels and provides at least some protection from infections. Alternatively, injection of PEG-ADA provides the same degree of protection. However, to ensure an optimal effect, the timing of the transfusion or injection should be correlated to the date of surgery.

Anesthetic considerations: Strict aseptic technique is mandatory to prevent infections. Vascular access may be difficult because of edematous skin. Graft-versus-host reaction after transfusion of non-irradiated blood has been described in these patients, so ensure the blood has been irradiated prior to administration. This step also applies to patients after bone marrow transplantation until full engrafting has been established. Check blood glucose concentration on a regular basis during the perioperative period.

Pharmacological implications: Vaccination with attenuated, living viruses must be avoided because patients may otherwise suffer from a severe infection.

Other conditions to be considered:

☞**OMENN SYNDROME:** Inherited form of SCID secondary to defective T lymphocytes and lack of B lymphocytes.

☞**PURINE NUCLEOSIDE PHOSPHORYLASE DEFICIENCY:** Inherited disease of purine catabolism resulting in deficient T cell immunity and, frequently, neurologic symptoms.

☞**NEZELOF SYNDROME:** Genetic form of thymus hypoplasia resulting in lack of competent T cells.

☞**DIGEORGE SYNDROME:** Genetic defect leading to a wide range of phenotypic presentations, mainly developmental defects in the outflow tract of the heart, hypoparathyroidism with hypocalcemia, and thymic hypoplasia/aplasia with immune defects.

REFERENCES:

Arredondo-Vega FX, Santisteban I, Daniels S, et al: Adenosine deaminase deficiency: Genotype-phenotype correlations based on expressed activity of 29 mutant alleles. *Am J Hum Genet* 63:1049, 1998.

Buckley RH, Schiff RI, Schiff SE, et al: Human severe combined immunodeficiency: Genetic, phenotypic, and functional diversity in one hundred eight infants. *J Pediatr* 130:378, 1997.

Ratech H, Greco A, Gallo G, et al: Pathologic findings in adenosine deaminase-deficient severe combined immunodeficiency. *Am J Pathol* 120:157, 1985.

Adie Syndrome

At a glance: Neurologic phenomenon in which one or less commonly both pupils are dilated and respond either slowly or not at all to light. It can be associated with autonomic nervous system instability (syncope, vagal hyporeflexia, postural hypotension), slow gastric emptying, and tendon hyporeflexia.

Synonyms: Holmes Adie Syndrome; Constitutional Areflexy-Tridoplegia Interna; Myotonic Pupil; Myotonic Pupillary Reaction; Pseudo Argyll-Robertson Syndrome; Weill-Reys Syndrome; Saenger Syndrome.

History: Described in 1931 by William John Adie, a British physician and neurologist. However, the disease was mentioned earlier by many others. John Hughlings Jackson described the disease at the end of the 19th century. Max Nonne, J. Strassberger, and Alfred Saenger described it just at the beginning of the 20th century. Georges Weill and L. Reys probably were the first to describe this disease as its own (nonsyphilitic) entity.

Genetic inheritance: Autosomal dominant.

Pathophysiology: The features of Adie syndrome are idiopathic but also may appear secondary to other disorders (e.g., diabetes, syphilis). The pupils are sensitive to methacholine (quaternary ammonium parasympathomimetic agent).

Diagnosis: The following signs are crucial for diagnosis: either unilateral or bilateral pupillotonia (tonic, sluggish reaction of pupil[s] to light) with light-near dissociation of accommodation (condition in which the pupillary reflex response to light is either absent or abnormal, while the near response is still intact) and hypoactive or absent tendon reflexes.

Clinical aspects: Evidence indicates Adie syndrome is actually the first sign of a gradually progressive, usually benign, autonomic dysfunction. Therefore, other signs of autonomic dysfunction must be sought.

Precautions before anesthesia: History should elicit symptoms of syncope, vagal hyporeflexia, postural hypotension, sweating abnormalities with patchy anhidrosis, bladder and bowel dysfunction, erectile and ejaculatory dysfunction, and delayed gastric emptying. Signs to elicit in addition to those pertaining to the eye may include blood pressure measurements in the lying and standing position (Schellong test). Investigations should include ECG, possibly 24-hour ECG, and results of carotid sinus massage or tilt-table provocation test for arrhythmia.

Anesthetic considerations: In patients with considerable autonomic dysfunction, profound bradycardia may occur in response to painful stimuli. Precautions (rapid sequence induction) must be taken if the patient is suspected of having a full stomach. Direct laryngoscopy may produce an unexpectedly large swing in arterial blood pressure, and this response may usefully be obtunded by adequate depth of anesthesia.

Pharmacological implications: Atropine or other anticholinergic drugs may be useful agents in patients prone to bradyarrhythmia.

REFERENCE:

Bacon PJ, Smith SE: Cardiovascular and sweating dysfunction in patients with Holmes-Adie syndrome. *J Neurol Neurosurg Psychiatry* 56:1096, 1993.

Adrenogenital Syndrome

At a glance: Congenital adrenal hyperplasia encompasses several autosomal recessive disorders with complete or partial deficiency of an enzyme involved in the cortisol or aldosterone synthesis.

Synonyms: Adrenal Virilism; Congenital Adrenal Hyperplasia.

Cholesterol

$\downarrow$ 17-Alpha-Hydroxylase

Pregnenolone $\rightarrow$ 17-Hydroxy-Pregnenolone $\rightarrow$ Dehydroepiandrosterone

$\downarrow$ 3-Beta-Hydroxy-Steroid-Dehydrogenase $\downarrow$ $\downarrow$

Progesterone $\rightarrow$ 17-Hydroxy-Progesterone $\rightarrow$ Androstenedione $\rightarrow$ Estrone

$\downarrow$ 21-Hydroxylase $\downarrow$ $\downarrow\uparrow$ $\downarrow\uparrow$

Deoxycorticosterone $\rightarrow$ 11-Deoxycortisol $\rightarrow$ Testosterone $\rightarrow$ **Estradiol**

$\downarrow$ $\downarrow$ 11-Beta-Hydroxylase $\downarrow\uparrow$

Corticosterone Cortisol **Dihydrotestosterone**

$\downarrow$ $\downarrow\uparrow$

18-Hydroxy-Corticosterone **Cortisone**

$\downarrow$

Aldosterone

Adrenal Steroid Biosynthesis

Incidence: Worldwide, the frequency of the classic form is estimated to be 1:5000 to 1:15,000. However, in Yupik Eskimos of Alaska, the disease occurs in up to 1:300 neonates.

Genetic inheritance: Most often autosomal recessive inheritance. Spontaneous mutations are possible.

Pathophysiology: The common finding in all of these cases is an elevated ACTH level resulting from significantly decreased negative feedback of cortisol on ACTH secretion in the pituitary gland. Congenital adrenal hyperplasia (CAH), which to the histopathologic finding of adrenal cortical hyperplasia, is the result of these elevated ACTH levels. Any of the steps involved in adrenal steroidogenesis can be affected. The classic form, which is responsible for more than 90% of all cases of CAH, is characterized by absent or decreased activity of the enzyme 21-hydroxylase. Whereas the classic form denotes the early diagnosed form of 21-hydroxylase deficiency, the nonclassic form denotes the same enzyme defect with late diagnosis (because of absent salt wasting and developmental abnormalities) and signs of hyperandrogenism. From 5 to 8% of CAH cases are caused by dysfunction of the enzyme 11-β-hydroxylase. In the remainder of patients with CAH, the affected enzyme is either 17α-hydroxylase or 3β-hydroxysteroid dehydrogenase.

Depending on the affected enzyme, the symptoms can vary widely. *Deficiency of 21-hydroxylase,* which converts 17α-hydroxyprogesterone to 11-deoxycortisol, results in accumulation of cortisol precursors that are metabolized to adrenal androgens (dehydroepiandrostenedione [DHEA] and androstenedione) instead. Absence of negative feedback on pituitary ACTH secretion, which is caused by a lack of cortisol, potentiates the symptoms. Clinically, the children may present in two forms: "simple virilization" or "salt wasting." At birth, female infants appear virilized with clitoral enlargement, labial fusion, and/or urogenital sinus. Left untreated, these signs can become even more prominent over time. Sexual development in male infants usually is normal, but excessive androgen production can result in sexual precocity. In up to 70% of all infants, "simple virilization" is accompanied by salt wasting because of a mineralocorticoid deficiency with hyponatremia, hyperkalemia, and hypotension (hypovolemia). Plasma renin activity is elevated, and signs of hypoaldosteronism may occur in the first weeks of life.

Deficiency in 11-β-hydroxylase, which is needed to convert 11-deoxycortisol and deoxycorticosterone (DOC) to cortisol and corticosterone, also results in decreased cortisol levels and increased ACTH levels. As a consequence, steroid precursors and androgens are markedly increased. Clinically, female patients may show the same genital ambiguity as in 21-hydroxylase deficiency, but most often the changes are subtler. Some patients are diagnosed in puberty, only because of menstrual irregularities and hirsutism in girls or severe acne in boys. Half of the patients, in contrast to patients with 21-hydroxylase deficiency, suffer from arterial hypertension, which most likely is caused by hypervolemia in response to excessive levels of DOC, although DOC levels and hypertension do not correlate well and some patients show signs of hypoaldosteronism.

The key enzyme in the steroidogenesis, *17α-hydroxylase* (which is responsible for hydroxylation of progesterone, the substrate for synthesis of cortisol, androgens, and estrogens), has 17,20-lyase activity, although the two activities can be separated from each other in vivo. Lyase is used to produce androgens (DHEA, androstenedione, testosterone) and estrogens. Plasma levels of progesterone and ACTH are increased, whereas the levels of cortisol, 11-deoxycortisol, 17α-hydroxyprogesterone, DHEA, testosterone, and estrogens are decreased. Mineralocorticoid synthesis is unaffected, and an increased substrate influx to this pathway results in increased levels of DOC and corticosterone with decreased plasma renin and aldosterone levels. Clinically, patients present around the time of expected puberty with hypogonadism, hypokalemia, and arterial hypertension. Female patients suffer from primary amenorrhea and absent secondary sexual characteristics. Male patients most often present with complete pseudohermaphroditism with female external genitalia, blind ending vagina, absent uterus and Fallopian tubes, and intraabdominal testes.

Deficiency of 3β-hydroxysteroid dehydrogenase is a very rare form of CAH. Synthesis of all adrenal steroids is affected, with decreased levels of progesterone, glucocorticoids, mineralocorticoids, androgens, and estrogens. However, evidence of mineralocorticoid deficiency may be absent in some patients. Most often, adrenal insufficiency in early infancy leads to the diagnosis, although cases with late diagnosis around puberty (girls with hirsutism and

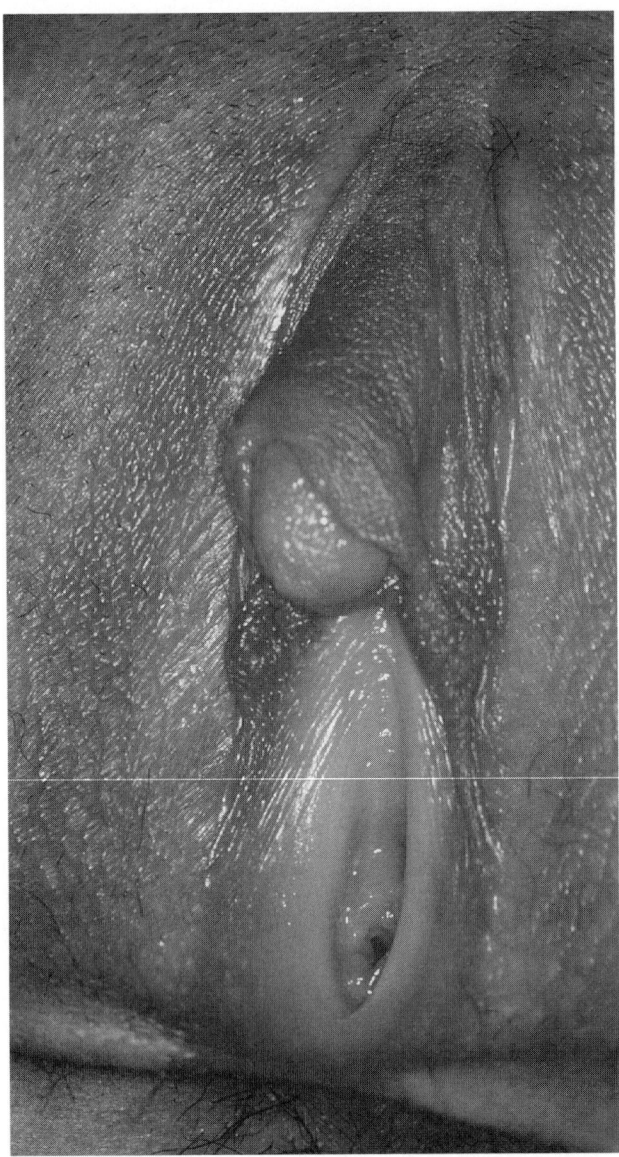

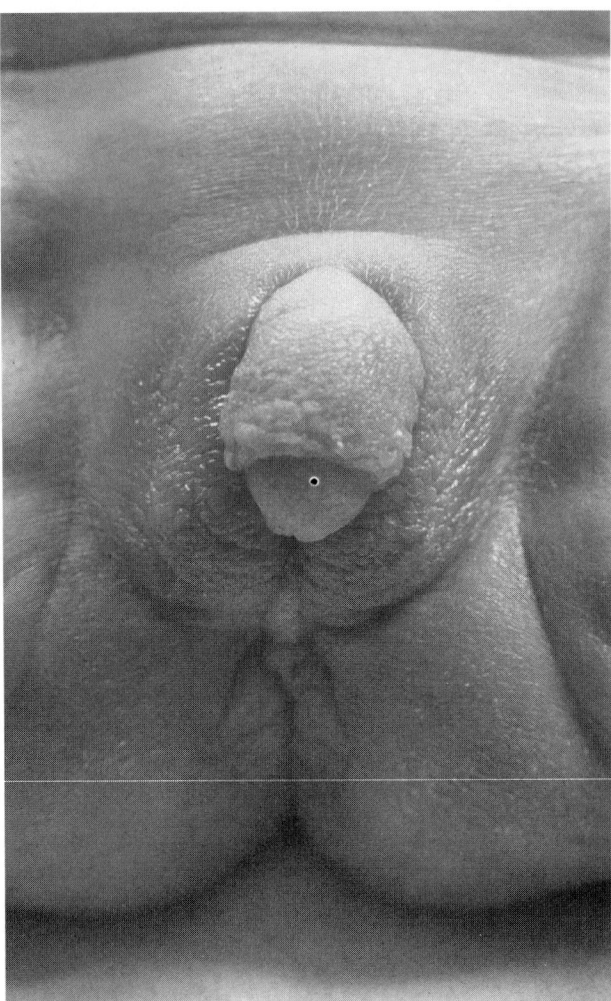

Adrenogenital syndrome   Clitoris hypertrophy in a female with adrenogenital syndrome.

Adrenogenital syndrome   Ambiguous genitalia in an infant with adrenogenital syndrome.

oligomenorrhea) have been described. Affected infant girls show virilization of the external genitalia (probably because of increased testosterone levels from peripheral conversion of DHEA). Boys can show the entire spectrum, from only slight derangement of the male genitalia (hypospadia) to almost normal external female genitalia (male pseudohermaphroditism).

Diagnosis: Clinical findings combined with measurements of the different enzyme plasma and urine levels confirm the diagnosis. ACTH testing with measurement of 17α-hydroxyprogesterone plasma levels at baseline and after 60 minutes has become the gold standard for diagnosis of 21-hydroxylase deficiency. The early-morning 17α-hydroxyprogesterone level can be used as a screening test.

Clinical aspects: Clinical manifestations of the disease relate to the degree of cortisol and/or aldosterone deficiency and, in some cases, to the accumulation of precursor adrenocortical hormone. Genital ambiguity, electrolyte disorders, and arterial hypertension or hypotension in infancy; absent or incomplete puberty in girls, with primary amenorrhea or oligomenorrhea and hirsutism;

precocial puberty; and marked acne in boys all may be signs of CAH.

Precautions before anesthesia: Check for glucose and electrolyte abnormalities. Patients usually undergo replacement therapy with hydrocortisone (10–25 mg/m²/day) or dexamethasone. Patients with salt wasting also receive mineralocorticoid substitution with fludrocortisone. The therapeutic goals are optimal replacement of the missing hormones and suppression of ACTH secretion with hyperandrogenemia to allow for normal skeletal maturation and growth. The lack of optimal dosage or patient compliance may easily result in obesity and reduced body height and fertility.

Anesthetic considerations: Correct any glucose and electrolyte abnormalities before taking the patient to the operating room. Invasive blood pressure monitoring with the additional option for blood sampling should be considered in patients scheduled for more extensive procedures or in patients with significant changes in preoperative electrolyte and/or blood glucose concentrations. Tight perioperative control of blood glucose is recommended.

Pharmacological implications: Continue hormone replacement therapy and consider additional perioperative stress dose of glucocorticoids. Avoid succinylcholine in patients with preexisting hyperkalemia. Consider prolonged duration of action of nondepolarizing muscle relaxants in patients with uncorrected hypokalemia.

Other conditions to be considered:

20,22-DESMOLASE DEFICIENCY (Congenital Lipoid Adrenal Hyperplasia; Cholesterol Desmolase Complex Defect): Autosomal recessive inheritance, with the mutation mapped to genes located on 15q23-q24, and 8p11.2. Conversion of cholesterol to pregnenolone is the first step in adrenal and gonadal steroidogenesis. Hydroxylation of cholesterol at positions 20 and 22, side-chain cleavage (SCC), and further conversion to pregnenolone require the presence of a complex mitochondrial mixed-function oxidase system, which initially was known as *20,22-desmolase* and now is designated *cytochrome P-450$_{SCC}$*. This first part in steroidogenesis is not only the rate-limiting step but also is the principal site of action of ACTH. This defect affects not only the adrenal but also the gonadal steroidogenesis. Because of the complete lack of steroids, this most severe form of congenital adrenal hyperplasia already is present in the neonatal period. It manifests as failure to thrive, diarrhea, vomiting, and salt wasting syndrome (hyponatremia and hypokalemia), which may be fatal if not treated early and results in important implications in the perioperative fluid regimen. Affected males usually have female external genitalia with male genital ducts (blind ending vagina and absence of the müllerian duct derivatives). Females with the disease have normal external and internal genital tracts.

The term *congenital lipoid adrenal hyperplasia* is explained by enlarged and lipid laden adrenals found at autopsy. Although successful replacement therapy has been described, most of these children do not survive infancy.

REFERENCES:

Donohoue P, Parker KL, Migeon CJ: Congenital adrenal hyperplasia, in Scriver CR, Beaudet AL, Sly WS, Valle D (eds): *The Metabolic and Molecular Basis of Inherited Disease*, 8th ed. New York, McGraw-Hill, 2001, p 4077.

Tajima T, Fujieda K, Kouda N, et al: Heterozygous mutation in the cholesterol side chain cleavage enzyme (P450scc) gene in a patient with 46,XY sex reversal and adrenal insufficiency. *J Clin Endocrinol Metab* 86:3820, 2001.

Adrenomyodystrophy

At a glance: Characterized by primary adrenal insufficiency, dystrophic myopathy, severe psychomotor retardation, fatty degeneration of the liver, megalocornea, chronic constipation, and terminal massive bladder ectasia. There are ACTH-producing microadenomas in the pituitary gland. It is suggested that this medical condition is different from adrenoleukodystrophy or glycerol kinase deficiency.

Incidence/genetic inheritance: The incidence remains unknown. It has been described in 1982 in two brothers, both of whom died in childhood. It is believed to be inherited as an X-linked recessive transmission.

Clinical aspects: Characterized by the presence of primary adrenal insufficiency, dystrophic myodystrophy, severe psychomotor retardation, megalocornea, terminal massive bladder ectasia, fatty liver degeneration, and chronic constipation. Other clinical features include osteoporosis, short stature, and/or dwarfism. The condition is lethal in infancy and childhood. Laboratory findings demonstrate an increase in plasmatic ACTH. Intravascular volume depletion and electrolyte imbalances may also be present. It is believed to be caused by ACTH-producing pituitary microadenomas.

Precautions prior to anesthesia: It is recommended to obtain an endocrinology consultation before anesthesia. It is likely that glucocorticoid replacement therapy will have been initiated and stress doses of glucocorticoids will be required perioperatively. Evaluate intravascular fluid status. Preoperative laboratory investigations should include serum electrolytes and glucose levels, cell blood count and differential, and liver enzyme function. A complete evaluation of the neuromuscular function and the severity of the dystrophic myopathy must be obtained. Because of the potential severity of the muscular involvement, it might be important to evaluate the pulmonary function (forced vital capacity [FVC], peak expiratory flow rate [PEFR], forced expiratory volume in one second [FEV1], FEV1/FRC ratio, arterial blood gas analysis, chest x-rays) when applicable.

Anesthetic considerations: Patients may be at risk for intraoperative hypotension and cardiovascular collapse due to inadequate cortisol stress response during induction of anesthesia or as a response to surgical stimulus. The potential association of hypovolemia and electrolyte disturbances must also be considered. The administration of supplement intravenous glucocorticoid doses is required preoperatively. Patients are also at increased risk for hyperkalemia resulting in arrhythmias and cardiac arrest following the administration of succinylcholine. Variable response to nondepolarizing muscle relaxants has been reported and proper neuromuscular monitoring must be used. Behavioral problems as a result of mental retardation may render the induction of anesthesia difficult. The use of preoperative anxiolytic and sedative medications might be appropriate when clinically indicated. Patients may be at risk for corneal abrasions secondary to megalocornea. Mechanical ventilation may be required postoperatively depending on the duration and type of surgery and degree of neuromuscular dysfunction.

Pharmacologic implications: The use of succinylcholine is considered a relative contraindication. Nondepolarizing muscle relaxants should be used, however, the possibility of prolonged effect must be prevented by the use of a peripheral nerve stimulator.

REFERENCE:

von Petrykowski W, Beckmann R, Bohm N, et al: Adrenal insufficiency, myopathic hypotonia, severe psychomotor retardation, failure to thrive, constipation, and bladder ectasia in 2 brothers: Adrenomyodystrophy. *Helv Paediat Acta* 37:387, 1982.

ADULT Syndrome

At a glance: ADULT is an acronym for *A*cro-*D*ermato-*U*ngual-*L*acrimal-*T*ooth. The main findings are hypodontia, very brittle and/or premature loss of permanent teeth, and ectrodactyly (split hands and feet). There is no evident impairment of general health in patients with ADULT syndrome.

Incidence and genetic inheritence: Extremely rare. Autosomal dominant with variable expression. No genetic background or molecular data are available.

Clinical aspects: The main findings are hypodontia and/or premature loss of permanent teeth, ectrodactyly (split hands and feet), occasionally with oligodactyly, dermal and/or osseous syndactyly. The breasts (glands and nipples) may be absent or hypoplastic. Absence or obstruction of the nasolacrimal ducts, sparse hair (alopecia areata, frontal baldness), skin atrophy, excessive freckling, and onychodysplasia may be seen. Radiologic findings: Ectrodactyly on x-ray films.

Anesthetic considerations: There is no evident impairment of general health in patients with ADULT syndrome. The main anesthetic consideration is the teeth. They are very brittle and may be easily broken or avulsed during direct laryngoscopy. Use of regional anesthesia and analgesia provides a reasonable alternative in patients with this syndrome.

Other conditions to be considered:

☞**ECTRODACTYLY-ECTODERMAL DYSPLASIA CLEFTING SYNDROME:** Autosomal dominant inherited syndrome with maxillary hypoplasia, mild malar hypoplasia, cleft lip/palate, choanal atresia, hearing loss, photophobia and blepharophimosis, dacryocystitis, cryptorchidism, hypogonadotropic hypogonadism renal agenesis or dysplasia, hydronephrosis, occasionally mental retardation, central diabetes insipidus.

LIMB MAMMARY SYNDROME: Very rare syndrome characterized by severe anomalies of the hands and feet in combination with hypoplasia or aplasia of the mammary gland and nipple. As in ADULT syndrome, the lacrimal duct can be atretic or obstructed, and the nails may be thickened and dystrophic. Hypodontia and cleft palate have been described. A later study placed the ADULT syndrome gene locus in the same chromosome region as the LMS locus, thereby suggesting the two conditions are allelic.

☞**AEC SYNDROME:** Disorder characterized by cleft lip/palate, unilateral or bilateral fusion of the eyelids, hair anomalies, onychodystrophy, hypohidrosis, and dental anomalies. The mutation has been mapped to 3q27, like all the aforementioned disorders.

☞**SCHINZEL SYNDROME:** Very rare autosomal dominant syndrome characterized by bone malformations and apocrine deficiency. Anesthetic management must consider difficult intubation, renal dysfunction, and the possibility of hyperthermia.

ABSENCE OF ULNA AND FIBULA WITH SEVERE LIMB DEFICIT (Al Awadi Teebi Farag Syndrome, Limb/Pelvis-Hypoplasia/Aplasia Syndrome; Al-Awadi Raas-Rothschild Syndrome; Schinzel Phocomelia Syndrome): Autosomal recessive with severe deficiency of all four limbs, including absent feet, hypoplastic femora, absent ulnae, absent fibulae, thoracic dystrophy, and pelvic deformity.

REFERENCES:

Propping P, Friedl W, Wienker TF, et al: ADULT syndrome allelic to limb mammary syndrome (LMS)? *Am J Med Genet* 90:179, 2000.

Propping P, Zerres K: ADULT syndrome: An autosomal dominant disorder with pigment anomalies, ectrodactyly, nail dysplasia and hypodontia. *Am J Med Genet* 45:642, 1993.

AEC Syndrome

At a glance: AEC is an acronym for *A*nkyloblepharon-*E*ctodermal Defects *C*left Lip/Palate. The disorder is characterized by cleft lip/palate, unilateral or bilateral fusion of the eyelids, hair anomalies, onychodystrophy, hypohidrosis, and dental anomalies.

Synonym: Hay Wells Syndrome.

Incidence: This form of ☞Ectodermal Dysplasia is very rare, with probably fewer than 20 cases described in the medical literature. Females and males are equally affected.

Genetic inheritance: AEC syndrome is inherited as an autosomal dominant trait. The gene defect has been mapped to 3q27, which encodes for tumor protein p63.

Diagnosis: Usually made with the typical clinical features and family history.

Clinical aspects: The face of these mentally normal patients usually is oval shaped with a broad nasal bridge. Partial or complete

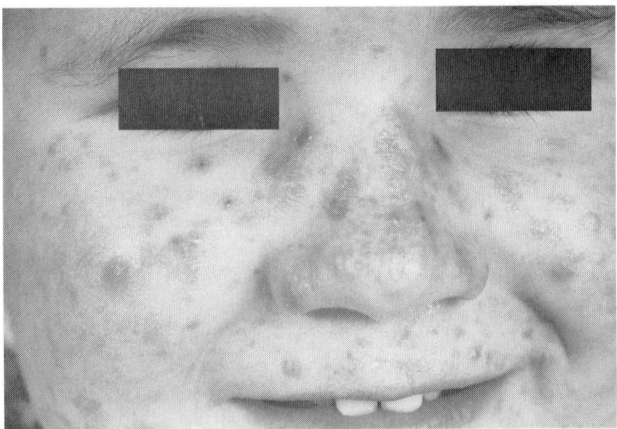

AEC syndrome Skin features in the face of a young boy suffering from AEC syndrome. see color plates.

fusion of the eyelids because of tissue bands (ankyloblepharon filiforme adnatum) and absent lacrimal puncta may be present at birth. Eyelashes may be sparse or absent. Photophobia and recurrent blepharoconjunctivitis are common. Auditory canals may be atretic or stenotic, resulting in conductive hearing loss. ☞Ectodermal Dysplasia usually presents with sparse, coarse, wiry scalp hair, which may progress to partial or even total alopecia, often secondary to recurrent scalp infections. The skin appears dry and cracking and often is hyperpigmented. Palmoplantar keratoderma is common in adults. Dystrophic or missing nails, mild hypohidrosis, and dental anomalies such as hypodontia, enamel defects, and abnormally shaped teeth are common findings. Cleft lip/palate with or without maxillary hypoplasia, cupped ears, syndactyly, hypospadias and/or micropenis, and short stature have been reported in some patients. Cardiac defects include ventricular septal defects and patent ductus arteriosus.

Precautions before anesthesia: Although no specific reports for this disease exist, because of mild depression of the immune system and hypoplasia/absence of the respiratory mucus glands, other forms of ectodermal dysplasia often are associated with a predisposition to respiratory tract infections, which can be life-threatening. To our knowledge, no such reports exist for AEC syndrome; nevertheless this potential should be kept in mind when assessing the patient.

Anesthetic considerations: Hypohidrosis usually is mild and likely will not result in increased body temperature during

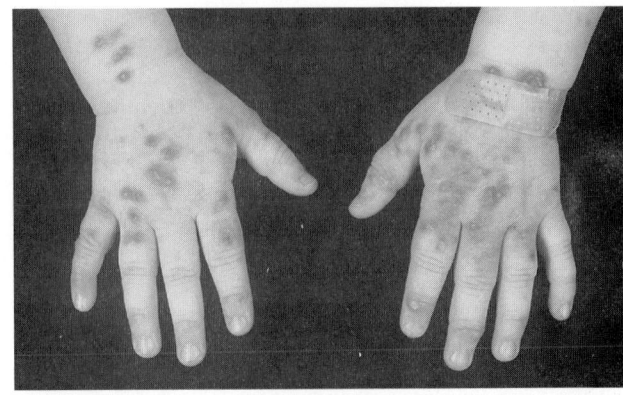

AEC syndrome Skin lesions on the hands and forearms of a toddler diagnosed with AEC syndrome.

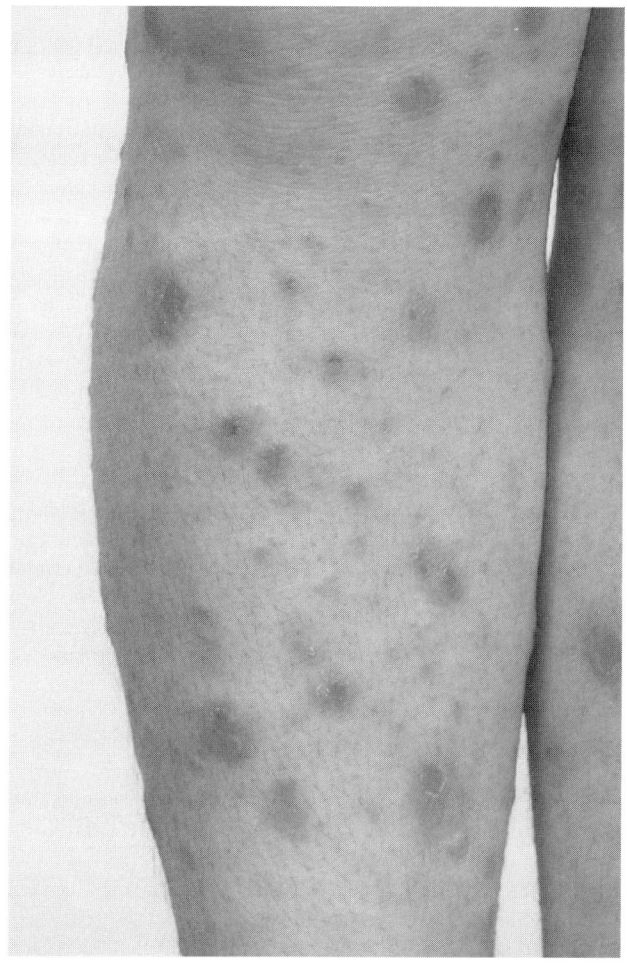

AEC syndrome Excoriated skin lesions on the lower leg of an adult patient with AEC syndrome.

plasia inherited as an autosomal dominant trait associating missing/irregular fingers and/or toes, abnormalities of the hair and glands, cleft lip/palate, unusual facial features, and abnormalities of the eyes and urinary tract, which can vary from mild to severe.

☞**HALLERMAN-STREIFF SYNDROME:** Genetic syndrome characterized by distinctive craniofacial malformations, including brachycephaly, bird-like facies with "parrot-beaked" nose, hypoplastic mandible, hypotrichosis, ocular abnormalities (congenital cataracts, microphthalmia), dental defects, skin atrophy (scalp, nasal area), and dwarfism.

☞**JOHANSON-BLIZZARD SYNDROME:** Polymalformative syndrome characterized by nasal alar hypoplasia (beak shaped), scalp defects, hypothyroidism, pancreatic achylia, and congenital deafness.

JORGENSON LENZ SYNDROME: Mild short stature, microcephaly, ptosis-blepharophimosis, facial asymmetry, prognathism, restricted joint mobility, radioulnar synostosis. The name of this syndrome is based on a single paper.

RAPP-HODGKIN HYPOHIDROTIC ECTODERMAL DYSPLASIA: Autosomal dominant inherited anhidrotic ectodermal dysplasia with cleft lip/palate, hypodontia, nail and hair anomalies, and alopecia in adulthood. The mouth of some of these patients has been described as small. Assessment prior to anesthesia is recommended. Some researchers consider this disorder a variant of AEC syndrome.

REFERENCES:
Hay RJ, Wells RS: The syndrome of ankyloblepharon, ectodermal defects and cleft lip and palate: an autosomal dominant condition. *Br J Dermatol* 94:287, 1976.

Speigel J, Colton A: AEC syndrome: Ankyloblepharon, ectodermal defects, and cleft lip and palate. *J Am Acad Dermatol* 12:810, 1985.

Weiss AH, Riscile G, Kousseff BG: Ankyloblepharon filiforme adnatum. *Am J Med Genet* 42:369, 1992.

anesthesia, but body temperature should be measured. Tracheal intubation may be difficult secondary to cleft lip/palate and maxillary hypoplasia. Hypoplasia or even absence of mucous glands in the respiratory tract has been reported in some cases of ectodermal dysplasia; therefore, humidified air should be used during general anesthesia.

Pharmacological considerations: No adverse drug reactions specific for this disease have been reported.

Other conditions to be considered:

☞**ADULT SYNDROME:** The main manifestations are hypodontia, very brittle and/or early loss of permanent teeth, and ectrodactyly (split hands and feet). General health of patients with ADULT syndrome does not seem to be impaired.

☞**CHRIST-SIEMENS-TOURAINE SYNDROME:** Genetic disorder characterized by the association of hypohidrosis, hypotrichosis, and defective dentition with peculiar facies. Consequences are related to thermoregulation and exocrine gland insufficiency.

CLOUSTON SYNDROME (☞Ectodermal Dysplasia): Autosomal dominant ectodermal dysplasia characterized by the triad of palmoplantar hyperkeratosis, nail dystrophy, and alopecia. Facial appearance, teeth, and sweating are normal.

☞**ECTRODACTYLY, ECTODERMAL DYSPLASIA, AND CLEFT LIP/PALATE (EEC) SYNDROME:** Rare form of ectodermal dys-

Agnathia-Holoprosencephaly

At a glance: The infant presents with agnathia associated with cleft lip/palate, hypertelorism, and dysregulation of the sympathetic nervous system. Holoprosencephaly is associated with agenesis of the corpus callosum.

Synonym: Dysgnathia Complex.

Nature: Agnathia-holoprosencephaly is a complex anomaly of the development of face and brain frequently associated with situs inversus and visceral anomalies.

Incidence: Extremely rare (probably <20 cases have been described).

Genetic inheritance: Agnathia-holoprosencephaly may be genetically determined as an autosomal recessive trait by a single recessive gene. Three reported cases had duplication of 6q and monosomy 18p.

Pathophysiology: Probably results from an inductive defect of the prechordal mesoderm or failure of migration of neural crest mesenchyme into the maxillary prominence during weeks 4 and 5 of gestation.

Diagnosis and clinical aspects: Agnathia-holoprosencephaly is a developmental field complex anomaly that affects the development of the face and brain and is frequently associated with situs inversus and visceral anomalies. At birth, the infant presents with agnathia and other craniofacial anomalies, such as cleft lip/palate, synotia (fusion of the ears in the midline below the chin), synophthalmia (cyclopia), or hypertelorism. Situs inversus must be ruled out. Magnetic resonance imaging (MRI) scans may demonstrate (alobar) holoprosencephaly with agenesis of the corpus callosum and other brain defects. Other anomalies may include visceral anomalies such as aglossia or microglossia, and microstomia, tracheoesophageal fistula, and congenital cardiac lesions. Prenatal ultrasound examination may reveal intrauterine growth retardation, agnathia (mandibular agenesis), or significant mandibular hypoplasia. Most patients do not survive the first year of life, but survival longer than 1 year has been described in isolated cases.

Precautions before anesthesia: Neonates should be carefully evaluated for associated visceral abnormalities. In particular, congenital cardiac lesions should be ruled out by echocardiography. Mental and neurologic status must be assessed for a thoughtful approach to induction. Evaluate for signs of airway obstruction and difficult airway management because of agnathia and other facial defects. Difficult tracheal intubation must be anticipated when treating a child.

Anesthetic considerations: Because of difficult airway management, spontaneous breathing should be maintained until the airway is secured. Fiberoptic intubation may be required or, depending on the procedure, a laryngeal mask airway can be used. However, be aware that mouth opening of less than 1 cm has been described in several cases.

Pharmacological implications: Anticholinergic drugs may assist in reducing secretions in cases of difficult airway management.

REFERENCES:

Ozden S, Bilgic R, Delikara N, et al: The sixth clinical report of a rare association: Agnathia-holoprosencephaly-situs inversus. *Prenat Diagn* 22:840, 2002.

Pauli RM, Pettersen JC, Arya S, et al: Familial agnathia-holoprosencephaly. *Am J Med Genet* 14:677, 1983.

Bixler D, Ward R, Gale DD: Agnathia-holoprosencephaly: A developmental field complex involving face and brain. Report of 3 cases. *J Craniofac Genet Dev Biol Suppl* 1:241, 1985.

Aicardi Syndrome

At a glance: Rare disorder characterized by partial or complete agenesis of the corpus callosum, infantile spasms (spasm-like epilepsy), mental retardation, and an ocular abnormality called *lacunae of the retina*. Often associated with other features such as microcephaly and porencephalic cysts. Onset generally is between age 3 to 5 months. The disorder affects only females.

Synonyms: Corpus Callosum Agenesis-Ocular Anomalies-Salaam Seizures Syndrome; Chorio-Retinal Anomalies-Corpus Callosum Agenesis-Infantile Spasms Syndrome; Corpus Callosum Agenesis-Chorio-Retinopathy-Infantile Spasms Syndrome; Corpus Callosum Agenesis-Chorio-Retinal Abnormality Syndrome.

History: Aicardi syndrome was first described in 1965 by Jean François Marie Aicardi, the French neurologist.

Incidence: Worldwide approximately 300 to 500 patients have been described.

Genetic inheritance: Transmitted as an X-linked dominant trait with embryonic lethality in hemizygous males; however, one male patient (47-XXY) with Aicardi syndrome has been reported. Gene locus at Xp22.

Pathophysiology: Unknown.

Diagnosis: Aicardi syndrome is most often diagnosed between age 3 and 5 months. Initially, affected girls seem to develop normally before they begin to have infantile spasms. Onset of infantile spasms at this age results from closure of the final neural synapses in the brain, a normal stage of brain development. The combination of myoclonic seizures with the characteristic EEG pattern (periodic, asynchronous discharges from both hemispheres but no hypsarrhythmia), lacunar chorioretinopathy, and complete (72%) or partial agenesis (28%) of the corpus callosum (with a high rising third ventricle) usually leads to the diagnosis. However, advances in MRI and CT scanning have shown that the absence (agenesis) of the corpus callosum may be less frequent than initially thought. Brain heterotopia has been demonstrated by pneumoencephalogram. Vertebral anomalies (especially cervical) are frequent. Costovertebral defects can be detected on conventional radiographs.

Clinical aspects: In addition to the clinical signs leading to the diagnosis, microcephaly, Dandy-Walker malformation, lissencephaly, polymicrogyria, porencephalic cysts, cortical ectopia and heterotopias, absent pineal gland, papillomata of the choroid plexus, and ventriculomegaly have been associated with Aicardi syndrome. Costovertebral defects, including hemivertebrae, kyphoscoliosis, and rib anomalies (extra, absent, or fused ribs, and/or other malformations), were present in 39% of patients. Cleft lip/palate and cavernous hemangioma have been reported.

Precautions before anesthesia: Obtain neck and chest radiographs to determine the presence of vertebral and costovertebral anomalies. Myoclonic seizures are frequent, and proper evaluation of the antiepileptic medication is necessary to decide if intravenous administration of antiseizure drugs is required in the perioperative period. Hydrocephalus and raised intracranial pressure must be ruled out prior to induction of anesthesia.

Anesthetic considerations: In the presence of cleft lip/palate, cervical vertebral anomalies, and/or a cavernous hemangioma, airway management may be difficult. Careful positioning is necessary because of vertebral and costovertebral anomalies (e.g., kyphoscoliosis). Perioperative care may include antiepileptic medication (e.g., barbiturates, benzodiazepines). High concentrations of volatile anesthetic should be avoided. In the presence of raised intracranial pressure, a rapid sequence induction (preferentially with rocuronium) to prevent regurgitation and aspiration should be considered. Recurrent regurgitation and aspiration may affect ventilation, especially in the presence of kyphoscoliosis. Maintenance of mild-to-moderate hypocapnia reduces intracranial pressure, but triggering of seizure activity must be avoided.

Pharmacological implications: Patients usually are given chronic antiseizure medication, which may result in induction of microsomal liver enzymes. Consequently, metabolism of similarly metabolized drugs may be accelerated.

Other conditions to be considered:

☞**SCHINZEL-GIEDION SYNDROME:** Distinct dysmorphic syndrome of congenital hydronephrosis, skeletal dysplasia (open cranial sutures, steep short skull, wide occipital synchondrosis), and severe developmental retardation. Coarse facies characterized by midface retraction, bulbing forehead, facial hemangiomas, short nose with anteverted nostrils, protruding large tongue, and hypertelorism. Patients usually die during infancy.

☞**WEST SYNDROME:** Disorder characterized by the triad of infantile spasms, interictal EEG pattern termed *hypsarrhythmia,* and mental retardation. This severe epilepsy syndrome is an age-dependent expression of a significantly damaged brain. The type of epilepsy observed in patients affected with Aicardi syndrome is sometimes referred to as *West syndrome*. Aicardi syndrome can be considered a "symptomatic" cause of West syndrome. Difficult airway management should not be expected because the anatomical anomalies of Aicardi syndrome (head, neck, chest) are not part of West syndrome.

☞**LENNOX-GASTAUT SYNDROME:** Severe form of epilepsy resulting in significant learning disabilities and impaired organization of movements.

REFERENCES:

Aicardi J, Chevrie JJ, Rousselie F. Le syndrome spasmes en flexion, agénésie calleuse, anomalies chorio-rétiniennes. *Arch Fr Pediatr* 26:1103, 1969.

Rosser T: Aicardi syndrome. *Arch Neurol* 60:1471, 2003.

Neidich JA, Nussbaum RL, Packer RJ, et al: Heterogeneity of clinical severity and molecular lesions in Aicardi syndrome. *J Pediatr* 116:911, 1990.

Aicardi-Goutieres Syndrome

At a glance: Characterized by progressive familial encephalopathy in infancy, calcification of the basal ganglia and chronic cerebrospinal fluid (CSF) lymphocytosis. This medical condition leads rapidly to a vegetative state and early death. It is considered to be a distinct type of leukodystrophy transmitted as an autosomal recessive trait.

Synonyms: Familial Infantile Encephalopathy with Calcification of Basal Ganglion.

Incidence/genetic inheritance: Forty cases have been reported in the literature, highest among consanguineous couples. It is considered a heterogenous autosomal recessive disorder. The gene map locus leads to 3p21.

Pathophysiology: calcification of basal ganglia and chronic cerebrospinal fluid lymphocytosis.

Diagnosis: Based on clinical presentation of progressive encephalopathy associated with chronic CSF elevation of lymphocytosis (pleocytosis), interferon-alpha, neopterin and biopterin, and 5-methyl THF. A CT or MRI scan shows frontal atrophy, white matter hypodensity, and calcification of lenticular nuclei. This medical condition resembles the neurological sequelae of congenital infection but with negative TORCH serology results.

Clinical aspects: Progressive infantile encephalopathy, extrapyramidal dyskinesia, porencephaly, holoprosencephaly, microcephaly, plagiocephaly, spastic quadriplegia, profound mental retardation, coloboma, hypertonia, rigidity, seizures, ptosis, leading to a vegetative state death usually by age 4 years. Other clinical features include visual disturbance with abnormal eye movement.

Precaution before anesthesia: A complete evaluation of the central nervous system (CNS), respiratory and cardiac dysfunctions must be obtained. Obtain a 12-lead ECG and echocardiography when necessary. The possibility for difficult airway management during face-mask ventilation and tracheal intubation must be considered. Obtain chest x-rays, arterial blood gas analysis, and pulmonary function tests, where applicable, to rule out potential restrictive and reactive pulmonary disease. Patients receiving antiseizure medications should be maintained until the morning of surgery.

Anesthetic considerations: High complication rate depending on severity of disease and degree of cardiac, respiratory, and neurologic dysfunction. Consider avoidance of elective surgery under general anesthesia. Expect a high degree of variability with respect to du-

ration of action of nondepolarizing muscle relaxants. Potential of hyperkalemia with succinylcholine administration. Difficult intubation must be anticipated in patients with microcephaly and retrognathia. Potentially difficult vascular access. Following prolonged surgical procedures, the use of mechanical ventilation and intensive care observation might be indicated.

Pharmacologic implications: Possible hyperkalemia with succinylcholine administration, expect possible prolongation of action with nondepolarizing muscle relaxants. Patients on chronic antiseizure medications may show signs of hepatic enzyme activations which might interfere with the pharmacokinetic of the anesthetic agents.

Other condition to be considered:

☞**TORCH:** An acronymic syndrome referring to a group of fetal infectious malformations. It stands for: *T*oxoplasmis, *O*ther agents, *R*ubella, *C*ytomegalovirus, and *H*erpex simplex. Common signs involve essentially intracranial anomalies such as intracerebral calcifications and seizure.

REFERENCES:

Crow YJ, Jackson AP, Roberts E, et al: Aicardi-Goutieres syndrome displays genetic heterogeneity with one locus (AGS1) on chromosome 3p21. *Am J Hum Genet* 67:213, 2000.

Mehta L, Trounce JQ, Moore JR, Young ID: Familial calcification of the basal ganglia with cerebrospinal fluid pleocytosis. *J Med Genet* 23:157, 1986.

Tolmie JL, Shillito P, Hughes-Benzie R, Stephenson JBP: The Aicardi-Goutieres syndrome (familial, early onset encephalopathy with calcifications of the basal ganglia and chronic cerebrospinal fluid lymphocytosis). *J Med Genet* 32:881, 1995.

Ainhum

At a glance: A narrow strip of hardened skin with constricting ring formation on the little toe at the level of digitoplantar fold, progressively leading to spontaneous amputation.

Synonym: Dactylosis Spontanea.

Genetic inheritance: Familial occurrence with autosomal dominant inheritance has been described, but many sporadic cases have been reported.

Clinical aspects: Ainhum is characterized by the occurrence of a circular constriction band most often located at the root of the fifth toe, rarely of a finger. As constriction progresses, the toe becomes disabled, and spontaneous amputation finally results. The disorder seems to be more frequent in Africa. Classic features of the affected area include hyperkeratosis, chronic dermatitis, ligamental destruction, and finally osteoporosis with cortical bone resorption. Although the origin of the disease remains to be elucidated, mechanical and/or inflammatory causes have been favored by many authors.

Anesthetic considerations: There are no specific considerations for this condition.

Other conditions to be considered:

PSEUDOAINHUM: Ainhum-like constriction bands that also may finally result in amputation of a digit (finger or toe) have been described in conjunction with neurogenic acroosteolysis, genodermatoses, and mutilating keratoderma.

☞STREETER ANOMALY: Constricting amniotic bands leading to amputation with scarring, distal syndactyly, cleft lip/palate, anencephaly, encephalocele, hydrocephaly, omphalocele, and gastroschisis. Other internal anomalies involve the heart, lungs, diaphragm, kidneys, and gonads.

☞**ADAMS-OLIVER SYNDROME:** Very rare inherited disorder characterized by defects of the scalp associated with multiple scarred and hairless areas that usually have dilated blood vessels directly under the skin. Scalp defects are present at birth. The extremities are either short (hypoplastic fingers and toes) or characterized by absent hands and lower legs. Congenital heart defect must be ruled out.

REFERENCES:

Genakos JJ, Cocores JA, Terris A: Ainhum (dactylolysis spontanea). Report of a bilateral case and literature review. *J Am Podiatr Med Assoc* 76:676, 1986.

Simon KMB: Ainhum, a family disease. *JAMA* 76:560, 1921.

Warter A, Audouin J, Sekou H: [Spontaneous dactylolysis or ainhum. Histopathologic study]. *Ann Pathol* 8:305, 1988.

Alacrima (Congenital)

At a glance: Complete absence of tears.

Genetic inheritance: Autosomal dominant.

Clinical aspects: Deficient lacrimation and punctate corneal abrasions from infancy. Hypoplasia of lacrimal glands.

Anesthetic considerations: Examine the eyes for preexisting corneal lesions and obtain a history of corneal abrasions. The eyes should be well lubricated during anesthesia to prevent corneal abrasions.

Other conditions to be considered: Alacrima can refer to a disorder in association with achalasia, addisonism, hyperuricemia, and ectodermal dysplasia.

☞**ACHALASIA-ALACRIMA SYNDROME:** Inherited disorder but in a small minority can be an acquired abnormality induced by the formation of antibodies that block ACTH receptors. Fluid and electrolyte disorders. In contrast to Addison disease, the renin–angiotensin–aldosterone axis functions normally. Regurgitation and aspiration occur upon induction.

☞**ALLGROVE SYNDROME:** Triple A syndrome is a genetic autosomal recessive disease characterized by the triad of ACTH-resistant insufficiency, achalasia, and alacrima. It appears in the first decade of life with severe hypoglycemic episodes, which can cause death. Mixed pattern of upper and lower motor neuropathy, sensory impairment, autonomic neuropathy, and mental retardation. Regurgitation and aspiration occur upon induction.

☞**CHRIST-SIEMENS-TOURAINE SYNDROME:** Genetic disorder characterized by the association of hypohidrosis, hypotrichosis, and defective dentition with peculiar facies. Consequences are related to thermoregulation and exocrine gland insufficiency.

☞**SCHINZEL-GIEDION SYNDROME:** Distinct dysmorphic syndrome of congenital hydronephrosis, skeletal dysplasia (open cranial sutures, steep short skull, wide occipital synchondrosis), and severe developmental retardation. Coarse facies characterized by midface retraction, bulbing forehead, facial hemangiomas, short nose with anteverted nostrils, protruding large tongue, and hypertelorism. Death usually occurs during infancy.

REFERENCE:

Mondino BJ, Brown SI: Hereditary congenital alacrima. *Arch Ophthalmol* 94:1478, 1976.

Alagille Syndrome

At a glance: This autosomal dominant association involves primarily the heart (ventricular septal defect, atrial septal defect), pulmonary artery stenoses, and hepatic dysfunction. Coagulation disorders can be important. The presence of a broad forehead and long, thin face are characteristic.

Synonyms: Cardiovertebral Syndrome; Alagille-Watson Syndrome; Watson-Miller Syndrome; Arteriohepatic Dysplasia (AHD); Cholestasis-Peripheral Pulmonary Stenosis; Hepatic Ductular Hypoplasia-Multiple Malformations Syndrome; Hepatofacioneuro-Cardiovertebral Syndrome.

Incidence: 1:100,000 live births.

Genetic inheritance: Autosomal dominant with highly variable expression. However, 15 to 50% of cases are new mutations. The defect has been assigned to chromosome 20 band p12.

Pathophysiology: Unknown.

Diagnosis: Based on the clinical findings, although there is wide variability in the manifestations of the disease. Diagnostic criteria require the presence of cholestasis and two of the following findings: characteristic facies, pulmonary artery stenosis, "butterfly" hemivertebrae, and posterior embryotoxon (thickening of Descemet membrane and corneal endothelium).

Clinical aspects: Presentation of Alagille syndrome is highly variable with respect to all the organ systems involved but consists mainly of prolonged neonatal jaundice or cardiac symptoms/signs. However, patients may be asymptomatic, or the jaundice may resolve by age 2 years. The spectrum of hepatic disease is highly variable. Pruritus may be the main symptom and often is invalidating. Liver biopsy reveals a paucity of intrahepatic bile ducts. Other features are hepatomegaly, obstructive liver disease, cirrhosis, splenomegaly, and truncal and facial telangiectasia. Deficiencies of fat-soluble vitamins are frequent and may result in coagulopathy (vitamin K), rickets (vitamin D), retinopathy (vitamin A, E), peripheral neuropathy, and myopathy (vitamin E). Liver function tests show elevated serum bile acid concentrations, conjugated hyperbilirubinemia, and elevated serum levels of alkaline phosphatase and γ-glutamyl transferase. The characteristic features of "cholestasis facies" are a round face with prominent ears, bulbous nose, and pointed chin. A prominent forehead, deeply set eyes, hypertelorism, straight nose, short philtrum, down-slanted palpebral fissures, micrognathia/retrognathia, and brachycephaly may occur. Cardiovascular anomalies are present in 95% of patients and may include peripheral pulmonic stenosis, systemic hypertension, atrial septal defect, ventricular septal defect, coarctation of the aorta, and tetralogy of Fallot. Musculoskeletal features involve the vertebrae ("butterfly" hemivertebrae denotes vertebrae, which are split sagittally into pairs because of failure of fusion of their anterior arches). Abnormal ribs, spina bifida occulta, delayed bone age, absent or abnormal ulnae, terminal hypoplasia of the fingers, and clinodactyly of the fifth finger may be seen. In association with posterior embryotoxon other ophthalmologic features can occur, such as strabismus secondary to paresis of ocular muscles, keratoconus (and other structural abnormalities of the cornea), eccentric or ectopic pupils, enophthalmos, and pigmentary retinopathy). Cerebrovascular complications may include ☞Moya-Moya Disease (progressive obliteration of the intracranial carotid arteries and formation of an extensive vascular network of dilated small branches). Other signs are regrouped as minor signs and include undescended/ectopic testes, ureteral anomalies, renal agenesis/hypoplasia/dysplasia, renal artery stenosis, intrauterine growth retardation, late puberty, hypogonadism, and mental retardation. Hepatocellular carcinoma and papillary thyroid carcinoma may occur as a late complication.

Precautions before anesthesia: Assess cardiac, hepatic, and renal function. In the presence of portal hypertension, development of esophageal varices should be considered. Evaluate cardiac anatomy and, given the high incidence of cardiac anomalies, an echocardiogram should be obtained. Nutritional status should be optimized because failure to thrive is a common finding.

Anesthetic considerations: Anesthesia and surgery may precipitate hepatic and renal failure in patients with advanced liver disease. Consequently, anesthetic management in the presence of liver disease should be directed to maintaining hepatic and renal blood flow. The facial features of the disease suggest airway management may be difficult, although this finding has not been reported to date. Central neuraxial blockade is contraindicated in the presence of coagulopathy.

Pharmacological implications: Endocarditis prophylaxis is required in patients with structural cardiac lesions. Rifampicin taken as an antipruritic agent can induce hepatic microsomal enzymes and consequently accelerate the metabolism of similarly eliminated drugs. Drugs with minimal hepatic and renal metabolism are preferred. Postoperative jaundice has been reported after a combined propofol/isoflurane anesthetic.

Other condition to be considered:

☞**CAROLI SYNDROME:** Rare congenital disorder of the intrahepatic bile ducts characterized by intrahepatic dilatation of the biliary tree, resulting from ductal plate malformation.

REFERENCES:

Choudry DK, Rehman MA, Schwartz RE, et al: The Alagille's syndrome and its anaesthetic considerations. *Paediatr Anaesth* 8:79, 1998.

Lykavieris P, Hadchouel M, Chardot C, et al: Outcome of liver disease in children with Alagille syndrome: A study of 163 patients. *Gut* 49:431, 2001.

Png K, Veyckemans F, De Kock M, et al: Hemodynamic changes in patients with Alagille's syndrome during orthotopic liver transplantation. *Anesth Analg* 89:1137, 1999.

Albinism

At a glance: Heterogeneous group of hereditable diseases of the melanin pigmentary system.

Classification:

OCULOCUTANEOUS ALBINISM

Type IA = Tyrosinase negative albinism
Type IB = Yellow mutant albinism
Type IC = Platinum albinism
Type II = Tyrosinase-positive albinism
Type III = Minimal pigment albinism
Type IV = Brown albinism
Type V = Rufus albinism
Type VIA = Hermansky-Pudlak syndrome
Type VIB = Chediak-Higashi syndrome
Type VII = Autosomal dominant albinism

OCULAR ALBINISM

Type I = Albinism autosomal recessive
Type II = Albinism Forsius-Ericksson syndrome

Type III = Albinism with sensorineural deafness
Type IV = Tietz syndrome

Genetic inheritance: Type I is an autosomal recessive disorder that is associated with a defect in the gene encoding for tyrosinase. Most of the other types are either autosomal dominant or sex-linked variants and are believed to be tyrosinase positive. Albinism does exist in all racial groups.

Pathophysiology: Oculocutaneous albinism is caused by congenital melanin metabolism defects. The common defect linking all forms of albinism affects the formation of melanosomes. Melanin biosynthesis is initiated by the catalytic oxidation of tyrosine to dopa (3-4-dihydroxyphenylalanine, a melanin precursor) by tyrosinase. This reaction requires dopa as a cofactor. Albinos are either tyrosinase positive or negative, and all subtypes can be identified by clinical and biochemical means. The degree of melanin depletion is used to classify the disease into different subtypes.

Diagnosis: Both ocular and cutaneous tissues are affected in this form of albinism, with diffuse leukodermia and variable pilosity disorders. The disease is potentially severe because patients may develop cutaneous carcinoma or melanoma with more or less early onset. Two types of oculocutaneous albinism have been identified, depending on the presence or absence of tyrosinase. The tyrosinase-negative form, also called *complete albinism type I,* is the most severe. Hypoplasia of the fovea, translucent iris, photophobia, nystagmus, decreased visual acuity, and inability of binocular vision are crucial to the diagnosis.

Clinical aspects: In addition to the features described, patients with oculocutaneous albinism have decreased pigmentation of skin and hair, whereas patients with ocular albinism have disease limited to the eyes. Albinism is not associated with impaired intelligence. In fact, an association with higher intellect may exist. Patients should be instructed to shield their eyes and skin from the sun.

Precautions before anesthesia: There are no specific problems for most types of oculocutaneous albino patients undergoing surgery or anesthesia. However, patients with ☞Chediak-Higashi Syndrome (Type VIB) or ☞Hermansky-Pudlak Syndrome (Type VIA) have considerable anesthetic considerations. In general terms, all other types require routine preoperative evaluation. However, evaluation of coagulation parameters is recommended.

Anesthetic considerations: Provided that Hermansky-Pudlak syndrome and Chediak-Higashi syndrome could be excluded, there should be no specific anesthetic contraindications. Occasionally, patients complain of photophobia because of the brightness of the light in the operating room.

Pharmacological implications: There are no specific indications or contraindications to anesthetic agents.

REFERENCES:

King R, Hearing VJ, Creel DJ, et al: Albinism, in Scriver CR, Beaudet AL, Sly WS, Valle D (eds): *The Metabolic And Molecular Basis of Inherited Disease,* 8th ed. New York, McGraw-Hill, 2001, p 5587.

Scheinfeld NS: Syndromic albinism: A review of genetics and phenotypes. *Dermatol Online J* 9:5, 2003.

OCULOCUTANEOUS ALBINISM TYPE VIA: HERMANSKY-PUDLAK SYNDROME

At a glance: Autosomal recessive inherited disorder associated with cardiomyopathy, restrictive lung disease, frequent abdominal pain, and severe coagulation disorder. Nystagmus and reduced visual acuity.

Synonym: Oculocutaneous Albinism–Hemorrhagic Diathesis Syndrome.

History: Described in 1959 by F. Hermansky and P. Pudlak, Czech internists.

Incidence: Highest incidence found in the Puerto Rican population (1:1800). A high incidence of a milder variant of Hermansky-Pudlak syndrome has been described in an isolated high mountain village in the southern Swiss Alps.

Genetic inheritance: The most common form of this autosomal recessive disorder (Hermansky-Pudlak syndrome type I) is caused by a mutation within the Hermansky-Pudlak syndrome gene 1 (HPS1) localized on chromosome 10q23. The HPS1 gene consists of 2100 bp and encodes a transmembrane protein locus that likely is a component of multiple cytoplasmic organelles, the granular fraction of melanocytes, and the cytoplasm of nonmelanotic cells. At least seven different types of Hermansky-Pudlak syndrome can be distinguished genetically.

Pathophysiology: It is associated with hypopigmentation and prolonged bleeding times because of a platelet storage pool defect. Accumulation of ceroid pigment in lysosomal organelles in leukocytes and cells of the reticuloendothelial system.

Diagnosis: Standard blood tests (including platelet count, bleeding time, prothrombin time, and activated partial thromboplastin time) fail to identify the platelet defect in HPS. However, electron microscopic examination of the platelets reveals the absence of dense bodies in the platelets, which is characteristic for the syndrome. Clinically, the combination of albinism and bleeding diathesis is indicative.

Clinical aspects: Hair color ranges from white to light brown. The irides may be translucent. Light skin color is associated with numerous freckles. Hypertrichosis of the eyelashes and trichomegaly on the arms and legs are found in approximately one third of affected individuals. Actinic keratosis and elastosis of the skin, lentigines, melanocytic nevi with dysplastic features, melanoma, squamous cell cancer, and basalioma are common findings secondary to increased susceptibility to ultraviolet light. Acanthosis nigricans-like lesions on the neck and in the axillae are found in almost one third of HPS1-positive patients. Bleeding diathesis is secondary to lack of platelet dense bodies (storage site of serotonin, calcium, and phosphate) and occurs despite normal platelet counts, normal prothrombin, and partial chromoplastin times. Bruising without adequate trauma and recurrent epistaxis are normally observed in more than 90% of patients. Other features include reduced visual acuity (in fact, the majority of these patients are legally blind), horizontal (and less commonly vertical) nystagmus, strabismus, and photophobia resulting from hypopigmentation of the iris and fundus. Severe pulmonary fibrosis, cardiomyopathy, inflammatory bowel disease (granulomatous colitis with severe bloody diarrhea, usually beginning in the second decade of life), and kidney disease occur secondary to ceroid accumulation. Cor pulmonale may occur secondary to pulmonary fibrosis. Approximately half of the patients die of complications related to pulmonary fibrosis (usually in the fourth decade of life); approximately 10% die of bleeding complications.

Precautions before anesthesia: Complete evaluation of the coagulation system, bleeding time (which can be normal in up to 25% of patients), and platelet count including a complete blood count (anemia secondary to bleeding) are essential. Most often the platelet count is in the normal range, but the ability of the platelets to adhere is nonexistent. Pulmonary function tests should be obtained, and a chest radiograph (or preferably a high-resolution CT scan) is manda-

tory to eliminate or assess the importance of the fibrosis. Consideration to postoperative ventilatory support should always be kept in mind and proper arrangement with the intensive care unit organized beforehand. If cardiomyopathy is suspected, an echocardiographic examination is strongly recommended. Assess for renal insufficiency (creatinine, BUN).

Anesthetic considerations: Excessive blood loss during surgery should be expected. Consequently, large-bore intravenous access is recommended. Regional anesthesia in general is relatively contraindicated, and central neuraxial anesthesia techniques should be considered a major contraindication. The risk of potential bleeding (even in the presence of minor surgery and normally not associated with bleeding) should not be underestimated, and appropriate blood products must be easily available. Some patients may be undergoing steroid therapy for gastrointestinal problems. Some reports indicate DDAVP (1-desamino-8-D-arginine vasopressin) has been used successfully to alleviate the bleeding issues to a certain degree.

Pharmacological implications: Because bleeding tendency is considerably increased after ingestion of aspirin, surgery should be delayed if possible. There are no specific pharmacological considerations.

Other conditions to be considered:

☞**GRISCELLI SYNDROME:** Albinism with immunodeficiency characterized by partial pigmentary dilution of the skin and hair (silvery gray hair), frequent infections, neurologic abnormalities, and fatal outcome caused by uncontrolled T lymphocyte and macrophage activation syndrome. Clinical features include the presence of large clumps of pigment in hair shafts and accumulation of melanosomes in melanocytes. Two types are described: type 1 with severe neurologic impairment and type 2 with immunologic deficiency.

☞**ELEJALDE SYNDROME:** Silver hair and severe dysfunction of the central nervous system (neuroectodermal melanolysosomal disease). Clinical features include silver-leaden hair, bronze skin after sun exposure, and neurologic involvement (seizures, severe hypotonia, mental retardation).

☞**CHEDIAK-HIGASHI SYNDROME:** Autosomal recessive disorder characterized by immunodeficiency, platelet dysfunction, and partial oculocutaneous albinism. It may present with axonal and demyelinating types of peripheral neuropathy that can be associated with central nervous system disorders.

CROSS SYNDROME (Cross-McKusick-Breen-Syndrome; Kramer Syndrome): Extremely rare autosomal recessive inherited syndrome (<20 cases have been described). Most symptoms are present at birth or develop shortly thereafter and may include very light skin color and silvery hair in combination with ophthalmologic (microphthalmia, corneal clouding, cataract, ectropion) and central nervous system anomalies (dolichocephaly, mental retardation, athetosis, ataxia, spastic paraplegia, tetraplegia). Gingival fibromatosis may develop at the age of emergence of the first teeth and may result in complete coverage of the teeth and become so significant that ventilation is impaired. Ventilation can be decreased further by a dysfunctional diaphragm.

REFERENCES:

Depinho RA, Kaplan KL: The Hermansky-Pudlak syndrome: Report of three cases and review of pathophysiology and management considerations. *Medicine* 64:192, 1985.

Hermansky F, Pudlak P: Albinism associated with hemorrhagic diathesis and unusual pigmented reticular cells in the bone marrow: Report of two cases with histochemical studies. *Blood* 14:162, 1959.

OCULOCUTANEOUS ALBINISM TYPE VIB: CHEDIAK-HIGASHI SYNDROME

At a glance: Autosomal recessive disorder characterized by immunodeficiency, platelet dysfunction, and partial oculocutaneous albinism. It may present with axonal and demyelinating types of peripheral neuropathy that can be associated with central nervous system disorders.

Synonyms: Chediak-Steinbrinck-Higashi Syndrome; Beguez Cesar Syndrome.

History: First described in 1943 by A. Beguez Cesar, the Cuban pediatrician. W. Steinbrinck, the German physician, A.M. Chediak, the Cuban physician, and O. Higashi, the Japanese pediatrician, reported their findings in 1948, 1952, and 1953, respectively.

Incidence: Very rare. Approximately 200 cases have been described worldwide. Most patients are of Spanish or South American descent.

Genetic inheritance: Autosomal recessive (caused by mutations in the lysosomal trafficking regulator gene Chediak-Higashi syndrome 1). Consanguinity is a risk factor. Defective melanosome transfer is a secondary phenomenon of a primary defect in a protein called *LYST* (lysosome trafficking regulator), which is crucial for vesicle trafficking, membrane dynamics, and receptor signaling. The majority of patients with Chediak-Higashi syndrome present with severe disease in childhood. These patients have a functionally null-mutant CHS1 allele, whereas patients with onset in adolescence or adulthood have missense-mutant alleles that most likely encode CHS1 polypeptides with partial function.

Diagnosis: Partial, tyrosinase-positive oculocutaneous albinism with formation of giant melanosomes suggests an even distribution of melanin is inhibited. Giant peroxidase-filled lysosomal granules can be detected in leukocytes, lymphocytes, natural killer cells, Schwann cells, and in certain cells of liver, spleen, pancreas, and kidneys. In fact, the diagnosis is made by the presence of these giant lysosomal granules found in neutrophils and bone marrow cells. The bleeding disorder is caused by a storage pool disease of the platelets with decreased content of ADP and serotonin, resulting in abnormal platelet aggregation and prolonged bleeding time. In addition to the features of albinism, photophobia, hypopigmentation, and loss of binocular vision, patients with Chediak-Higashi syndrome show marked susceptibility to infections. The neutrophils are predominately affected, and the coalescence of their lysosomes in forming giant lysosomes seems to inhibit neutropoiesis and lead to intramedullary granulocyte destruction with the clinical finding of neutropenia. Furthermore, the neutrophils have a severely decreased content of proteases, particularly elastase and cathepsin G. This neutrophil defect with decreased chemotaxis and incomplete degranulation in combination with abnormalities of the lymphocytes, natural killer cells, and the monocytes results in an ineffective immune system. Death often occurs in the first decade of life as a result of infection or bleeding, although survival into the second and third decade has been reported in milder cases. Patients surviving that long, however, are at risk for progression to an accelerated lymphoma-like phase characterized by diffuse lymphohistiocytic infiltration (often leading to hemophagocytosis) of bone marrow, lymph nodes, liver, and spleen. This infiltration of the bone marrow results in exacerbation of the existing neutropenia and new onset of anemia and thrombocytopenia, which is potentiated by the developing (hepato)splenomegaly. Although the process is not neoplastic in origin, the patient's prognosis is uniformly dismal.

Clinical aspects: Hypopigmentation affects the skin, hair, and eyes. Other findings include hepatosplenomegaly, jaundice, muscle weakness, cranial nerve palsies, neurodegeneration with intellectual decline, markedly delayed nerve conduction velocities, tremor, seizures, ataxia, and diffuse brain and spinal cord atrophy (as seen by CT and MRI). Approximately 10 to 15% of patients have a milder clinical phenotype and survive into adulthood but then often develop the same progressive neurologic dysfunction and intellectual decline described above. Thrombocytopenia and leukopenia are common, and immunodeficiency with impaired chemotaxis and bactericidal activity and abnormal natural killer cell function result in recurrent and sometimes life-threatening systemic pyogenic infections. Staphylococcal and streptococcal infections are the most common reasons for medical presentation. The accelerated phase may lead to mediastinal and hilar lymphadenopathy, jaundice, splenomegaly, hepatomegaly, gingivitis, and a pseudomembranous sloughing of the buccal mucosa. In a few patients, bone marrow transplantation provided the only available curative treatment, with best results obtained when the surgery was performed before patients were in the accelerated phase of the disease.

Precautions before anesthesia: Patients often present for surgical treatment of abscesses. They may be severely septic. A thorough history and examination should be performed to demonstrate hepatosplenomegaly, which is suggestive of serious end-stage disease. A complete blood count with leukocyte differentiation reveals cellular abnormalities. Platelet function tests and a bleeding time should routinely be obtained. Patients may be taking steroids. Treatment with high doses of ascorbic acid has been used with some beneficial effects. However, such high doses of vitamin C have been associated with renal impairment and calculi, so renal function should be checked in patients treated with this regimen. Neurologic and pulmonary function should be assessed preoperatively. If patients are in the accelerated phase of the disease, CT scan of the chest may reveal mediastinal lymphadenopathy with potential airway and vessel compression.

Anesthetic considerations: Excessive blood loss during surgery should be expected. Consequently, large-bore intravenous access is recommended. Regional anesthesia in general is relatively contraindicated, and central neuraxial anesthesia techniques should be considered a major contraindication. Even in the presence of a normal platelet count, function most likely is impaired. Because patients are highly susceptible to infections, every effort should be made to prevent iatrogenic infections. If mediastinal lymphadenopathy with airway compression is present, muscle relaxants must be avoided and spontaneous breathing maintained at all times.

Pharmacological implications: No specific pharmacological considerations exist, but they may be indicated to avoid use of neuromuscular relaxants, especially succinylcholine, if neuropathy is significant. Nonsteroidal antiinflammatory drugs should be avoided in the presence of already decreased platelet function. Avoid muscle relaxants in patients with symptomatic mediastinal lymphadenopathy.

Other conditions to be considered:

☞**GRISCELLI SYNDROME:** Albinism with immunodeficiency characterized by partial pigmentary dilution of the skin and hair (silvery gray hair), frequent infections, neurologic abnormalities, and fatal outcome caused by uncontrolled T lymphocyte and macrophage activation syndrome. Clinical features include the presence of large clumps of pigment in hair shafts and accumulation of melanosomes in melanocytes. Two types are described: type I with severe neurologic impairment and type II with immunologic deficiency.

☞**ELEJALDE SYNDROME:** Silver hair and severe dysfunction of the central nervous system (neuroectodermal melanolysosomal disease). Clinical features include silver-leaden hair, bronze skin after sun exposure, and neurologic involvement (seizures, severe hypotonia, mental retardation).

☞**HERMANSKY-PUDLAK SYNDROME:** Autosomal recessive inherited disorder associated with cardiomyopathy, restrictive lung disease, frequent abdominal pain, and severe coagulation disorder. Nystagmus and reduced visual acuity.

CROSS SYNDROME (Cross-McKusick-Breen-Syndrome; Kramer Syndrome): Extremely rare autosomal recessive inherited syndrome (<20 cases have been described). Most symptoms are present at birth or develop shortly thereafter and may include very light skin color and silvery hair in combination with ophthalmologic (microphthalmia, corneal clouding, cataract, ectropion) and central nervous system anomalies (dolichocephaly, mental retardation, athetosis, ataxia, spastic paraplegia, tetraplegia). Gingival fibromatosis may develop at the age of emergence of the first teeth and result in complete coverage of the teeth and become so significant that ventilation is impaired. Ventilation may be further decreased by a dysfunctional diaphragm.

REFERENCES:

Ulsoy H, Erciyes N, Ovali E, et al: Anesthesia in Chediak-Higashi syndrome—Case report. *Middle East J Anesthesiol* 13:101, 1995.

Scheinfeld NS: Syndromic albinism: A review of genetics and phenotypes. *Dermatol Online J* 9:5, 2003.

Albright-Butler Syndrome

At a glance: Patients present with renal tubular acidosis, nephrocalcinosis, and renal failure. Hypokalemia with muscle weakness and periodic paralysis is frequent. Polyuria, vomiting, and dehydration lead to fluid and electrolyte imbalances.

Synonyms: Primary Distal Renal Tubular Acidosis; Butler-Albright Syndrome.

Incidence: Undetermined. Females are slightly more often affected.

Genetic inheritance: Autosomal dominant; however, autosomal recessive and multiple dominant forms have been described. The disorder most often occurs sporadically.

Pathophysiology: The primary defect is a diminished ability to excrete hydrogen ions as ammonium and titratable acid in the distal renal tubule, despite a low plasma bicarbonate concentration. Acidosis is the result of the inability to excrete the full endogenous load of nonvolatile acids, while the generation of bicarbonate is minimal.

Diagnosis: Anorexia, vomiting, constipation, polyuria, dehydration, and growth retardation are the main symptoms. Nephrocalcinosis is an almost constant finding and may lead to interstitial nephritis and renal failure. Patients are unable to achieve a urine pH below 6.0.

Clinical aspects: Onset usually occurs after age 2 years. Failure to thrive is common. Acidosis is responsible for osteomalacia and pathologic fractures (secondary to decreased intestinal calcium resorption), growth retardation, and nephrocalcinosis with possible renal insufficiency. Hyperchloremia, hypokalemia, and low serum bicarbonate are responsible for polyuria. Hypokalemia may be severe enough to cause weakness and periodic paralysis-like symptoms. Twenty-five percent of patients may present as a metabolic emergency. Life-threatening dehydration can be associated with respiratory difficulties, flaccid paralysis, cardiac arrhythmias, coma, and circulatory collapse. Nerve deafness has been described.

Despite the potential severity of symptoms, the prognosis is good if treatment is established early enough to prevent renal damage.

Precautions before anesthesia: Extensive laboratory tests are required to evaluate electrolyte levels (in blood and urine), acid-base balance, and renal function. Administration of potassium to fully correct hypokalemia is recommended before any correction of acidosis is initiated in order to prevent a further fall in the potassium serum concentration triggered by an increase in plasma pH. Acidosis is corrected with slow administration of sodium bicarbonate. Hypocalcemia often is present, and correction of hypokalemia and acidosis may decrease serum calcium concentration further. Consequently, repeated boluses of intravenous calcium may be required to prevent tetany. Because the disease is congenital, bicarbonate supplements are a lifelong requirement. For patients undergoing anesthesia, replace oral intake with intravenous suppletmentation.

Anesthetic considerations: A central venous line can be useful for evaluating volume status but also for perioperative administration of concentrated electrolyte solutions. Volume expansion with normal saline solutions may paradoxically worsen the acidosis by further promoting renal bicarbonate losses.

Pharmacological implications: Acidosis and hypovolemia increase the sensitivity to muscle relaxants, so close monitoring of muscle relaxation is mandatory. Administration of thiazide diuretics may exacerbate a preexisting hypokalemia and so must be avoided. Use of succinylcholine is best avoided in the presence of muscle weakness secondary to the risk of a sudden and exaggerated hyperkalemic response.

Other conditions to be considered:

☞**DE TONI DEBRÉ FANCONI SYNDROME:** Rare acquired or inherited condition involving a generalized transport defect in the proximal tubules with renal losses of glucose, phosphate, calcium, uric acid, amino acids, and bicarbonates leading to short stature, osteomalacia, and renal failure.

☞**PERIODIC PARALYSIS:** Congenital abnormality in membrane electrolyte conductance leading to episodic muscle weakness.

☞**LIGHTWOOD SYNDROME:** Nonhereditary form of primary tubular acidosis presenting with hypercalcemia, hypercalciuria, and nephrocalcinosis.

☞**ADENOSINE DEAMINASE DEFICIENCY:** Heterogeneous systemic disorder caused by deficiency of ADA resulting primarily in severe combined (cellular and humoral) immunodeficiency but also systemic abnormalities.

☞**GITELMAN SYNDROME:** Inherited renal tubular defect resulting in urinary loss of magnesium, sodium, potassium, and chloride with otherwise normal kidneys.

☞**LOWE SYNDROME:** Genetically transmitted polymalformative syndrome characterized by the association of ocular problems with renal dysfunction and mental retardation.

☞**PHOSPHOENOLPYRUVATE CARBOXYKINASE DEFICIENCY:** Congenital metabolic disease leading to a defect in gluconeogenesis.

☞**PROPIONIC ACIDEMIA:** Inborn error of metabolism affecting mitochondrial catabolism of valine and isoleucine that left untreated results in ketoacidosis, lethargy, coma, and finally death.

☞**PYRUVATE CARBOXYLASE DEFICIENCY:** Mitochondrial disease impairing synthetic pathways and leading to hypoglycemia and severe lactic acidosis.

☞**TYROSINEMIA:** Elevated blood tyrosine levels are present in several clinical entities. The term *tyrosinemia* is used to describe several syndromes. In general, the association of liver and renal failure, marked edema, epistaxis, and distinctive cabbage-like odor are characteristic of the disease.

REFERENCES:

Caldas A, Broyer M, Dechaux M, et al: Primary distal tubular acidosis in childhood: Clinical study and long-term follow-up of 28 patients. *J Pediatr* 121:233, 1992.

Zakzouk SM, Sobki SH, Mansour F, et al: Hearing impairment in association with distal renal tubular acidosis among Saudi children. *J Laryngol Otol* 109:930, 1995.

Albright Hereditary Osteodystrophy

At a glance: Syndrome presenting with round face, short stature, short neck, and obesity. Subcutaneous and intracranial calcifications, seizures, and neuromuscular problems such as fatigue and muscle cramps. Pseudohypoparathyroidism and hypocalcemia.

Synonym: Pseudohypoparathyroidism Type IA. Strictly, Albright Hereditary Osteodystrophy relates to type IA only. However, for completeness, Pseudohypoparathyroidism Type IB is included here. Do not confuse Albright Hereditary Osteodystrophy with ☞McCune-Albright Syndrome.

Incidence: Exact incidence is unknown; however, in Japan the incidence is estimated to range from 3 to 4 per 1,000,000 live births.

Genetic inheritance: Autosomal dominant inheritance. In *type IA,* the genetic defect involves the α subunit of the stimulatory G protein (which is either defect or only produced in minimal amounts) that couples pathways for transmembrane signaling and enhances the production of cyclic adenosine monophosphate (cAMP). The gene encoding for this α subunit of the G protein (GNAS1) has been mapped to the long arm of chromosome 20 (20q13.2). Occasionally, a small terminal deletion on chromosome 2 may exist. Full expression occurs in patients with maternal transmission, whereas only partial expression occurs in paternally transmitted cases. All patients are heterozygous, leaving them with one normal allele for the α subunit, which is not only required for parathormone, but also for many other peptide hormones (e.g., adrenocorticotropin [ACTH], thyrotropin, glucagon, gonadotropins, antidiuretic hormone). Consequently, these patients may clinically exhibit some resistance to the effects of all these hormones. Although *type IB* also is autosomal dominant inherited, the underlying defect is different. The mutation has been mapped to 20q13.3 (i.e., close to the *GNAS1* gene region). Hormonal resistance appears to be caused by limited or absent responsiveness of the kidneys to parathormone. The skeletal lesions in these patients are evidence of an intact bone response to parathormone.

Pathophysiology: Increase in parathyroid hormone release and deficient end-organ responsiveness, either because of germline mutation in the gene encoding G α subunit, thus decreasing expression or function of G protein (type IA), or presumably a receptor defect (type IB).

Diagnosis: Hypocalcemia associated with hyperphosphatemia occurs in type IA but not in type IB. The activity of protein G is reduced in type IA but is normal in type IB. Hyperparathyroidism in combination with hypocalcemia is caused by either secondary hyperparathyroidism or pseudohyperparathyroidism. Administration of exogenous parathormone is used to assess the renal and osseous response. The concentration changes of calcium, phosphate, calcitriol, and cAMP in the plasma and of phosphate and cAMP in the urine are measured. Serum concentration for estrogen is low but

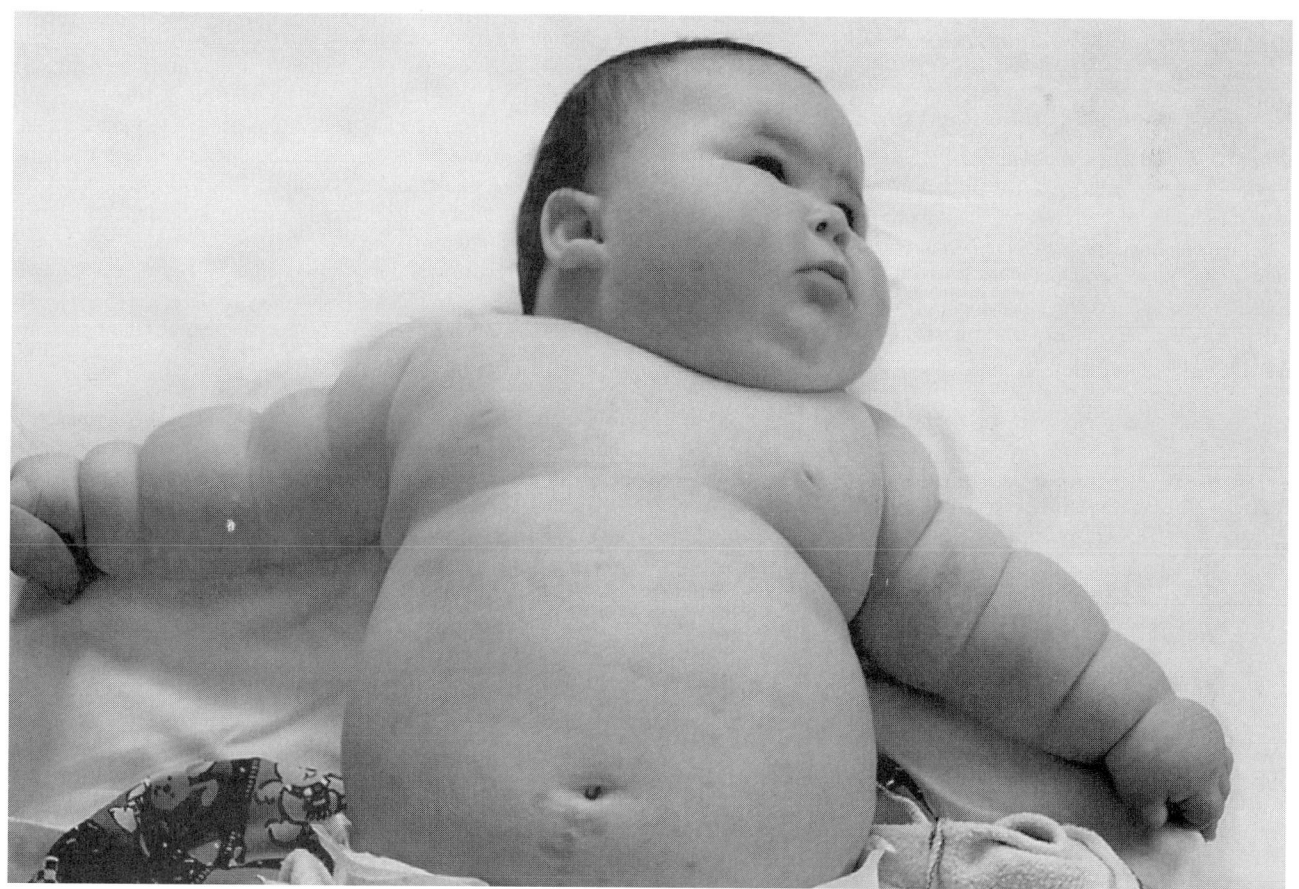

Albright hereditary osteodystrophy   This infant with obesity, round face, and short neck shows some of the typical features of this disorder.

concentrations of Luteinizing Hormone (LH) and Follicular Stimulating Hormone (FSH) are high (reflecting involvement of G protein in the actions of all these hormones). CT scan of the head may reveal calcifications of the choroid plexus and basal ganglia.

Clinical aspects: Morphologically, patients with pseudohyperparathyroidism type IA often present with a round face, short stature and neck, obesity, brachydactyly with short metacarpals, mental retardation, cataract, and delayed tooth eruption with enamel hypoplasia. Intracranial and subcutaneous calcifications, neuromuscular problems such as fatigue and muscle cramps, and seizures are common. Other endocrinologic signs may include pseudohypoparathyroidism with parathyroid hyperplasia, hypocalcemic tetany, hypothyroidism, (secondary to thyrotropin resistance), deficient prolactin release, partial resistance to antidiuretic hormone, and arterial hypertension. Oligomenorrhea (secondary to gonadotropin resistance), seizures, and impaired olfaction have been described in pseudohyperparathyroidism type IA.

Precautions before anesthesia: Chronic hypocalcemia is treated by oral calcium and vitamin D supplements. Assess the airway for difficult intubation secondary to facial anomaly. Surgery should be postponed until serum calcium concentration reaches normal levels. If surgery is urgent, intravenous calcium therapy must be given under continuous ECG monitoring.

Anesthetic considerations: Respiratory and/or metabolic alkalosis must be avoided because it further decreases the ionized serum calcium concentration. Arterial blood gases and pH should be monitored regularly in the perioperative period. No data are available concerning the anesthetic technique. Regional anesthesia is an option; however, mental retardation and osseous anomalies may result in difficulties.

Pharmacological implications: Citrate in blood transfusions but also administration of fresh-frozen plasma and albumin-containing solutions may result in hypocalcemia. Close monitoring and intravenous bolus doses of calcium chloride or calcium gluconate are required.

Other condition to be considered:

☞**McCune-Albright Syndrome:** This disorder presents with the triad of polyostotic fibrous dysplasia, café au lait skin pigmentation, and autonomous endocrine hyperfunction. The most common form of autonomous endocrine hyperfunction is gonadotropin-independent precocious puberty, but affected individuals also may suffer from hyperthyroidism, hypercorticism, pituitary gigantism, and/or acromegaly. Nonendocrine abnormalities include hypophosphatemia, chronic liver disease, tachycardia, and rarely sudden death, possibly from cardiac arrhythmias.

References:

Spiegel A: The molecular basis of disorders caused by defects in G proteins. *Horm Res* 47:89, 1997.

Ringel MD, Schwindinger WF, Levine MA: Clinical implications of genetic defects in G proteins. The molecular basis of McCune-Albright syndrome and Albright hereditary osteodystrophy. *Medicine* 75:171, 1996.

Alexander Syndrome

At a glance: A degenerative disorder of the nervous system caused by leukodystrophy. Affects mostly males and usually begins at approximately 6 months of age. Symptoms include mental and physical retardation, enlargement of the brain and head, spasticity (arms and legs), and seizures.

Synonyms: Demyelinogenic Leukodystrophy; Dysmyelinogenic Leukodystrophy; Fibrinoid Leukodystrophy; Fibrinoid Degeneration of Astrocytes; Megalencephaly with Hyaline Panneuropathy; Macrocephaly with Feeble Mindedness and Encephalopathy with Peculiar Deposits.

History: First described in 1949 by William Stuart Alexander, a British pathologist.

Incidence: Unknown. Fewer than 100 cases have been reported. No racial preferences have been reported. Males are affected approximately 2.5 times more often than females.

Genetic inheritance: Alexander syndrome is a transmissible astrocytic abnormality with varying expression. It is thought to be inherited in an autosomal dominant way, but de novo mutations have been described. The genetic defect has been mapped to 17q21 and 11q13, and more than 20 different mutations have been identified. These genes encode for glial fibrillary acidic protein (GFAP), which is the main intermediate filament protein synthesized in mature astrocytes. Most likely, GFAP in Alexander syndrome is defective and hinders the normal interaction between astrocytes and oligodendrocytes, finally resulting in dysmyelination and demyelination.

Pathophysiology: Cause unknown. Nonneoplastic white matter expansion with neuronal dysfunction and astrocyte proliferation associated with demyelination occur. An association of an astrocyte response to an exogenous stimulus (e.g., diphtheria-tetanus-pertussis vaccination) has been hypothesized. Histopathology shows widespread reactive gliosis and hyaline inclusions in astrocytes, so-called *Rosenthal fibers* (RFs). RFs consist mainly of big aggregations of α B-crystallin (a stress protein), heat shock protein, and glial fibrillary acidic protein. They are often found in subpial, periventricular, and perivascular brain areas. Their occurrence in brainstem and spinal cord is less frequent. The distribution of RFs is closely correlated with areas of demyelination and loss of oligodendroglia. Although extensive and progressive frontal white matter demyelination occurs, no inflammatory cells can be found. These areas may degenerate into brain lacunae. Signs of storage disease are absent.

Diagnosis: Brain biopsy and histology demonstrate perivascular hyaline, eosinophilic, and argyrophilic RFs. Abnormal astrocytes with functional demyelination is the prominent feature. Brain imaging is useful only for the infantile form of Alexander syndrome. It shows progressive white matter reduction and cystic changes predominantly in the frontal lobes. No enzyme defect has been identified. Progressive megalencephaly (very large head) during the first year of life is a very common finding. The disease is associated with progressive spasticity and dementia. Molecular genetic testing is available to confirm the diagnosis of Alexander syndrome, so a brain biopsy is no longer mandatory. Prenatal diagnosis is possible.

Clinical aspects: *Infantile type:* This is the most common type of Alexander syndrome. Onset usually is between 6 and 24 months of age. Failure to thrive, vomiting, hyperreflexia, hydrocephalus secondary to aqueductal stenosis, megalencephaly with frontal bossing, psychomotor retardation and regression, and loss of intellect, followed by spasticity and intractable seizures, are seen. A few cases of hydrocephalus result from nonobstructive ventriculomegaly. Death usually occurs by age 6 years.

Juvenile type: Onset is in childhood (age 4–10 years but sometimes later), with a slower progression than in the infantile form. Macrocephaly bulbar and pseudobulbar signs may predominate. Intellectual function often is preserved despite the presence of RFs. Vomiting, ataxia, speech problems, spasticity, and painful muscle spasms are common findings. Death usually occurs within 10 years after disease onset.

Adult type: This form of Alexander disease not only is the least common but also is the most variable form. It may resemble the juvenile form, but onset is later in life (usually in the third or fourth decade) and progression is slower. Survival is highly variable and ranges from a few to several years. Clinical signs may fluctuate and include sleep disturbances with sleep apnea, bulbar and/or pseudobulbar signs (dysphagia, dysarthria, palatal myoclonus), ataxia, dysmetria, nystagmus, seizures, dysfunction of the autonomic nervous system (e.g., hypothermia, abnormal sweating, orthostatic hypotension, urinary retention), and gait disturbances (hemiparesis or tetraparesis, spasticity). The clinical course of this form is comparable to that of multiple sclerosis.

Beside the infantile form, the distinction of a *neonatal type* with very early onset and rapid progression has been suggested. This form shows very stereotyped symptoms that are partly different from the infantile form: early, often intractable and generalized seizures, hydrocephalus with raised intracranial pressure resulting from aqueductal stenosis secondary to pathologic astroglia proliferation. There is an obvious lack in developmental progression, but spasticity and ataxia are not prominent features. Cerebrospinal fluid protein content is elevated. The typical neuroradiologic findings (e.g., severe white matter affection with frontotemporal predominance, involvement of basal ganglia, periventricular enhancement) are present.

Precautions before anesthesia: Evaluate the extent of neurologic involvement: degree of paraparesis, intracranial pressure, and bulbar palsy. Check for the presence of intracranial hypertension; determine history of antiepileptic medication. Determine adequacy of pulmonary function for possibility of recurrent pulmonary aspiration and pneumonia. Obtain a chest radiograph (recurrent aspiration). Laboratory workup should include a complete blood count, electrolytes, glucose, and often arterial blood gas analysis. Check for signs of failure to thrive/malnutrition. Premedication probably is not required in the infantile population, but if premedication is necessary, hypercapnia and consequently a further increase in intracranial pressure must be avoided. Furthermore, keep in mind that patients with the adult form may suffer from sleep apnea. These patients are prone to airway complications postoperatively (aspiration, atelectasis, pneumonia). Depending on the extent of the planned procedure, postoperative mechanical ventilation may be required.

Anesthetic considerations: The airway must be secured (endotracheal intubation) in the presence of diminished airway reflexes and/or history of recurrent regurgitation and aspiration. A rapid sequence intubation is recommended. In the presence of increased intracranial pressure, a total intravenous anesthesia technique seems to be advantageous. Careful positioning with supportive padding is important in the presence of extensive spasticity/contractures. Anesthetic requirements and recovery may be altered if mental retardation is evident. Opioid use should be judicious. Antisialogue medications may be indicated if secretions are copious. Continue preoperative antiepileptic medication on the day of surgery and restart them—if necessary parenterally—immediately in the postoperative period. Be aware of possible perioperative seizures. The patient should not be extubated before he/she is fully awake. Airway complications result from poor pharyngeal muscle control.

Pharmacological implications: To prevent an exaggerated hyperkalemic response, do not administer succinylcholine if there is evidence of demyelination. Meperidine, ketamine, and enflurane are relatively contraindicated in patients with known seizures. Phenothiazines, butyrophenones, metoclopramide, and other dopaminergic blockers should be avoided because they may increase extrapyramidal movement disorders. Serotonin antagonists (5-HT$_3$ receptor

antagonists) are believed to be appropriate because they do not have antidopaminergic effects.

Other conditions to be considered: See ☞Leukodystrophies for an overview table.

☞**CANAVAN SYNDROME:** Progressive leukodystrophy caused by spongy degeneration of the central nervous system. It is uniformly fatal within 18 months after onset of symptoms.

☞**METACHROMATIC LEUKODYSTROPHY:** Inherited disorder of myelin metabolism with progressive loss of white matter in the central and peripheral nervous systems.

☞**PELIZAEUS-MERZBACHER SYNDROME:** Very rare slowly progressive dysmyelinating disease affecting, in a diffuse pattern, the cerebrum, cerebellum, brainstem, and spinal cord. Two types are described: X-linked (infantile form) and autosomal dominant (preadulthood form). Clinical features include stridor, muscle spasticity, and nystagmus. Often fatal in the first year of life from respiratory complications.

☞**X-LINKED ADRENOLEUKODYSTROPHY:** Disorder characterized by progressive demyelinization of the central nervous system and peripheral adrenal insufficiency.

☞**SCHILDER SYNDROME:** Rare, progressive, lethal disease of the central nervous system that affects mostly children. Characterized by adrenal atrophy and diffuse central demyelination. Presents with progressive dementia, spasticity, cortical blindness, deafness, hemiplegia, quadriplegia, ataxia, pyramidal signs, retrobulbar neuritis, and pseudobulbar palsy. Seizures. Onset in late childhood. Most patients die within few months after onset.

☞**ZELLWEGER SYNDROME:** Disorder characterized by the congenital absence of functioning peroxisomes (cellular structures responsible for elimination of toxic substances) resulting in a cerebrohepatorenal syndrome. The disease affects brain development, particularly myelination. Most important features include hepatomegaly, polycystic kidney disease, visual disturbances, and high plasma levels of iron and copper. Other features include muscular hypotonia already noticeable at birth, mental retardation, seizures, coagulopathy, and dysphagia with recurrent aspiration. Congenital heart defects have been described. Life expectancy is approximately 6 months.

REFERENCES:

Besley GT, Elpeleg ON, Shaag A, et al: Prenatal diagnosis of caravan disease. Problems and dilemmas. *J Inherit Metab Dis* 22:263, 1999.

Springer S, Erlewein R, Naegele T, et al: Alexander disease— Classification revisited and isolation of a neonatal form. *Neuropediatrics* 31:86, 2000.

Pridmore CL, Baraitser M, Harding B, et al: Alexander's disease: Clues to diagnosis. *J Child Neurol* 8:134, 1993.

Alkaptonuria (AKU)

At a glance: Deficiency of homogentisic acid oxidase leads to discoloration and staining of tissues. Sudden dark urine should alert the clinician of the possible presence of homogentisic acid. Valvular heart disease and myocardial ischemia may occur in adults.

Synonyms: Homogentisic Acid Oxidase Deficiency; Homogentisate 1,2-Dioxygenase; Alkaptonuria; Hereditary Ochronosis.

Incidence: 1:250,000 live births, with a higher incidence reported from Slovakia and the Dominican Republic.

Genetic inheritance: Autosomal recessive. The mutation has been mapped to the homogentisate 1,2-dioxygenase locus on 3q21-q23. Both sexes are equally affected, but the course of the disease is more severe in men.

Pathophysiology: The enzyme homogentisic acid oxidase is required to crack open the benzol ring of phenylalanine and tyrosine to allow for further degradation. Lack of this enzyme leads to increased amounts of homogentisic acid (ortho-meta-dihydroxyphenylacetic acid), which is mainly excreted in high concentrations in the urine; the rest is oxidized and polymerized by polyphenol oxidase to toxic benzoquinone acetic acid that irreversibly binds to collagen. Exposition of the urine to air results in oxidation of homogentisate to a pigment-like substance, which is responsible for the color change to brown-black. This reaction can be significantly accelerated by alkalinization of the urine. If the urine is sufficiently acidotic, the discoloration can be so subtle and slow that the disease is not recognized until the affected patient presents with ochronosis and/or arthrotic symptoms. Yet a brown-black discoloration of the diapers most often is the first sign of this disorder. Rapid renal clearance of homogentisate does not prevent it (and related metabolites) from slow deposition in cartilage and connective tissues throughout the body. However, the sclerae and the cartilage of ears and nose usually do not show a detectable blue-black discoloration until adulthood. Polymerization of homogentisate to benzoquinone acetic acid and its deposition into these tissues is responsible for the dark staining, called *ochronosis,* and affects the intervertebral discs, tendons, and cartilage of the (large) joints. After age 30 years, these depositions may lead to degeneration of the cartilage and a clinical picture similar to that of rheumatoid arthritis.

Diagnosis: Urine turns black upon exposition to air secondary to the high concentration of homogentisic acid. A pathognomonic sign of this disorder is the dark blue (or brown-black) staining of the sclerae and cartilage, which is most obvious on nose and ears, but also occurs in joints, which later in life may lead to periarticular calcifications. Radiologic changes of the spine (including ruptured intervertebral discs) have been reported and may resemble osteoarthritis. The presence of pigments can be detected in sweat and on clothes.

Clinical aspects: The only manifestation in childhood is darkening of urine upon standing. In adulthood, there is progressive darkening of collagenous tissues and cartilage (ochronosis), including the sclerae. Osteoarthritic signs, a sign of premature cartilage degeneration in these patients, usually begin in the fourth decade of life. Arthritis involves the spine, hips, and knees and is progressively disabling. There may be a higher incidence of valvular heart disease caused by ochronosis (e.g., aortic and mitral valves). Myocardial infarction because of calcification of the coronaries seems to be more common in these patients compared to the normal population. Urolithiasis is more common in these patients. No effective treatment is known, although a high dose of ascorbic acid (1 g/day) have shown some beneficial effects. A study showed that nitisinone, a drug that has been used to treat hereditary tyrosinemia type I, can reduce the production of homogentisic acid, but the long-term safety and efficacy of this drug have not been established. Drastically reduced protein intake has been favorable to a certain degree in reducing the unwanted metabolites, but the efforts were not in relation to the benefits.

Precautions before anesthesia: Cardiac function should be assessed clinically and by ECG. Echocardiography may be required in selected cases (adults) to rule out valvular and/or coronary heart disease. Alkaptonuria per se but also high doses of ascorbic acid may lead to nephrolithiasis, so renal function should be checked, particularly in patients receiving ascorbic acid.

Anesthetic considerations: Children with this condition rarely have clinical symptoms, and no particular problems with anesthesia are expected. Adults may have valvular heart disease warranting antibiotic prophylaxis for subacute bacterial endocarditis and appropriate modification of the anesthetic plan. Epidural and spinal anesthesia may be difficult to perform because of significant lumbosacral arthritis and ankylosis.

Pharmacological implications: No agents are specifically contraindicated. However, drugs with predominantly renal elimination should be avoided or used at a reduced dose in the presence of renal insufficiency.

REFERENCES:

Touart DM, Sau P: Cutaneous deposition diseases. Part II. *J Am Acad Dermatol* 39:527, 1998.

Wolff JA, Barshop B, Nyhan WL, et al: Effects of ascorbic acid in alkaptonuria: alterations in benzoquinone acetic acid and an ontogenic effect in infancy. *Pediatr Res* 26:140, 1989.

Phornphutkul C, Introne WJ, Perry MB, et al: Natural history of alkaptonuria. *N Engl J Med* 347:2111, 2002.

Allan-Herndon Syndrome

At a glance: Although most neonates and infants with this disorder appear to develop normally in the first few months of life, the presence of poor muscle tone most often already is present at birth. By age 6 months, hypotonia, inability to hold up the head, and severe muscle atrophy are detectable. Severe mental retardation is associated with multiple congenital anomalies.

Synonyms: Allan-Herndon-Dudley Syndrome; AHDS; X-Linked Mental Retardation with Hypotonia.

Genetic inheritance: X-linked recessive. Gene located in Xq21.

Diagnosis: Based on clinical features and family history.

Clinical aspects: Only males are affected. Except for hypotonia, these boys appear normal at birth. When the child is approximately 6 months old, the parents often notice that the child is unable to hold up the head. Motor development is severely impaired so that the ability to walk is achieved either very late or not at all. Generalized muscular atrophy, which is associated with myopathic findings on histologic examination, becomes obvious in early infancy. Later in infancy, spastic paraplegia with joint contractures, hyperreflexia with clonus, ataxia, athetosis, and dysarthria become increasingly more obvious. Scoliosis may occur. Mental retardation usually is severe. Craniofacial anomalies may include elongation and bitemporal narrowing of the head with enlarged and dysplastic ears. Pectus excavatum has been described in many of these boys.

Precautions before anesthesia: Assess the degree of scoliosis, pectus excavatum, and joint contractures. If scoliosis or pectus excavatum is severe, assess pulmonary function and obtain a chest radiograph, arterial blood gas analysis, and pulmonary function tests if possible. Echocardiography may be indicated if there are any concerns about heart function (cor pulmonale).

Anesthetic considerations: The presence of severe mental retardation suggests a lack of cooperation, and sedation in the older child prior to induction of anesthesia may be required. Careful positioning and padding are required because of contractures. Depending on the degree of scoliosis and pectus excavatum, postoperative mechanical ventilation may be required. As in any patient with signs of muscular hypotonia and/or myopathy, depolarizing muscle relaxants should be used only with caution. Whether these patients have a predisposition to malignant hyperthermia is unknown, but it may be wise to provide a trigger-free anesthesia.

Pharmacological implications: None reported; however, an exaggerated hyperkalemic response to succinylcholine should be expected. No data on the predisposition to malignant hyperthermia are available, so use of succinylcholine probably is best reserved for special situations.

Other conditions to be considered:

☞**FRAGILE X SYNDROME:** The most common form of X-linked mental retardation (XLMR). Affects males more often and more severely than females. Only subtle dysmorphic features. Behavioral issues may be more pronounced.

☞**JUBERG-MARSIDI SYNDROME:** X-linked recessive inherited syndrome characterized by severe mental retardation, deafness, failure to thrive, microgenitalism, and early death.

☞**HAPPY PUPPET SYNDROME:** Rare disorder characterized by developmental delay, ataxia, dysmorphic facial features, and seizures associated with a happy, sociable disposition.

☞**MASA SYNDROME:** Extremely rare inherited disorder that is one of several disorders known as the XLMR syndromes.

RENPENNING SYNDROME: Extremely rare form of X-linked (moderate-to-severe) mental retardation. It has been linked to Xp11.2-p11.4. Other findings may include short stature, moderate microcephaly, prognathism, and small testes. Affected patients may use repetitive speech and show an aggressive behavior. Longevity seems not to be impaired, and female carriers do not show any heterozygous signs.

ESCALANTE SYNDROME: Same features as Renpenning syndrome associated with macroorchidism.

SUTHERLAND-HAAN SYNDROME (Sutherland-Haan X-Linked Mental Retardation Syndrome; X-Linked Mental Retardation with Spastic Diplegia): Extremely rare form of X-linked severe mental retardation. Features of the disorder include short stature, spastic diplegia, significant congenital heart defects, and craniofacial abnormalities (microcephaly, cleft palate or high arched palate, abnormal ears, bulbous nose, broad nasal bridge, malar hypoplasia, micrognathia, small mouth). No reports exist about anesthesia in these patients, but difficult airway management seems likely.

REFERENCES:

Bialer MG, Lawrence L, Stevenson RE, et al: Allan-Herndon-Dudley syndrome: Clinical and linkage studies on a second family. *Am J Med Genet* 43:491, 1992.

Schwartz CE, Ulmer J, Brown A, et al: Allan-Herndon syndrome. II. Linkage to DNA markers in Xq21. *Am J Hum Genet* 47:454, 1990.

Kalscheuer VM, Freude K, Musante L, et al: Mutations in the polyglutamine binding protein 1 gene cause X-linked mental retardation. *Nat Genet* 35:313, 2003.

Allgrove Syndrome

At a glance: Autosomal recessive inherited disease characterized by the triad of ACTH-resistant adrenal insufficiency, achalasia, and alacrima. It presents in the first decade of life with severe hypoglycemic episodes, which can result in death. A mixed pattern of upper and lower motor neuropathy, sensory impairment, autonomic neuropathy, and mental retardation is common.

Synonyms: Achalasia-Addisonianism-Alacrima Syndrome (AAA); Triple A Syndrome; Hypoadrenalism with Achalasia.

Incidence: No exact numbers are available, but the disorder is extremely rare. No gender or racial predilection has been reported.

Genetic inheritance: Autosomal recessive. Consanguinity is a well-known risk factor. The genetic defect has been mapped to 12q13, a region close to the type II keratin gene cluster, which may explain why patients with Allgrove syndrome often have hyperkeratosis palmoplantaris.

Diagnosis: Any patient who presents with a combination of alacrima and achalasia (may present as failure to thrive) should undergo complete testing of the pituitary–adrenal axis to rule out adrenal insufficiency. Baseline ACTH and cortisol levels should be measured and an ACTH stimulation test performed. Most often, mineralocorticoid production is not affected, but several cases with mineralocorticoid deficiency have been reported. Thus, serum levels of sodium, potassium, aldosterone, and renin may be helpful in establishing the diagnosis. Esophageal motility tests can be used to show dysphagia because this sign is present in almost all patients. Plasma antiadrenal antibodies are not a feature of this disorder, and their presence should instead point the investigations to ☞Addisonian Syndrome.

Clinical aspects: Alacrima is the earliest and most consistent clinical sign of Allgrove syndrome (tearless crying) and may lead to severe keratopathy and corneal ulcerations. However, a hypoglycemic seizure is the most common initial presentation, and unrecognized adrenal crisis is still the leading cause of death in this population. Hyperpigmentation of the skin, developmental delay, seizures (not hypoglycemic), dysphagia (achalasia), hypernasal speech (secondary to velopharyngeal incompetence), and microcephaly are frequent findings. The face often has been described as long and thin, with a long philtrum, narrow upper lip, and down-turned mouth. Even in the absence of dysphagia, almost all patients show some degree of esophageal dysmotility. Megaesophagus is a potential complication. A history of vomiting, reflux, and dysphagia is frequent and may be responsible for failure to thrive. Autonomic dysfunction presents with abnormal sweating, abnormal pupillary reflexes with anisocoria, and poor heart rate variability with postural hypotension. Other neurologic manifestations may include polyneuropathy with sensory and motor components, hyperreflexia, ataxia, muscle weakness parkinsonism (in adults), impaired visual evoked potentials, and mild mental retardation. Bulbospinal amyotrophy has been described in several patients. Because autonomic dysfunction and amyotrophy both are common, some researchers have suggested that autonomic dysfunction and amyotrophy both be added to the eponym, making it a AAAAA (5A) instead of AAA (3A) syndrome. Hyperkeratosis palmoplantaris has been found in many affected individuals. Abdominal CT may reveal atrophy of the adrenal glands. Autopsy in one patient showed gross atrophy of the zona fasciculata and reticularis of the adrenals, whereas the zona glomerulosa was normal.

Precautions before anesthesia: Recurrent aspiration is a well-known complication in these patients with achalasia and mental retardation and may result in acute bronchopneumonia with fatal consequences. Preoperative chest radiograph should be obtained, and pulmonary function test may be indicated for selected patients (especially when recurrent aspiration occurs). Review the glucocorticoid replacement therapy and obtain a blood glucose profile. In addition, preoperative blood workup should include a complete blood count and electrolytes because mineralocorticoid deficiency has been reported in some patients. To prevent hypoglycemia, patients should be started on a dextrose-containing solution at the beginning of the preoperative fasting period. The oral glucocorticoid replacement dose should be given on the day of surgery, and additional intravenous doses may be required in the perioperative period to cover for the stress, depending on the extent of the procedure.

Anesthetic considerations: Patients are candidates for a rapid sequence induction because of gastroesophageal reflux, dysphagia, and recurrent vomiting. There is an increased risk of corneal abrasions because of the lack of tears, so the eyes should be well lubricated and the eyelids taped shut after induction of anesthesia. Autonomic dysfunction may result in hemodynamic instability. Cardiovascular shock secondary to adrenal crisis is possible, as is severe hypoglycemia resulting in sudden death. Consequently, frequent perioperative measurements of blood glucose are mandatory. Invasive blood pressure monitoring is helpful for early diagnosis of hemodynamic instability and simultaneously allows for frequent blood sampling.

Pharmacological implications: No known specific implications with this condition.

Other conditions to be considered:

☞**ACHALASIA-ALACRIMA SYNDROME:** ACTH insensitivity syndrome is an inherited disorder but in a small minority can be an acquired abnormality induced by the formation of antibodies that block ACTH receptors. Fluid and electrolytes disorders occur. In contrast to Addison disease, the renin–angiotensin–aldosterone axis functions normally.

☞**ADDISONIAN SYNDROME:** Progressive weakness, anemia, hypoglycemia, and hyperpigmentation of the skin. Vomiting, apneic spells, cyanosis, vascular collapse, and cardiovascular shock may be consequential.

☞**X-LINKED ADRENOLEUKODYSTROPHY:** Disorder characterized by progressive demyelinization of the central nervous system and peripheral adrenal insufficiency.

REFERENCES:

Chu ML, Berlin D, Axelrod FB: Allgrove syndrome: Documenting cholinergic dysfunction by autonomic tests. *J Pediatr* 129:156, 1996.

Gazarian M, Cowell CT, Boenney M, et al: The "4A" syndrome: Adrenocortical insufficiency associated with achalasia, alacrima, autonomic and other neurological abnormalities. *Eur J Pediatr* 154:18, 1995.

Moore PS, Couch RM, Perry YS: Allgrove syndrome: An autosomal recessive syndrome of ACTH insensitivity, achalasia and alacrima. *Clin Endocrinol (Oxf)* 34:107, 1991.

Alopecia-Contractures-Dwarfism Mental Retardation Syndrome

At a glance: Alopecia and severe growth retardation associated with thoracic kyphoscoliosis, bilateral dislocated hips, and joint contractures (elbows, fingers, knees). The presence of turridolichocephaly and prominent nose are clues that assist in the diagnosis.

Synonym: ACD Mental Retardation Syndrome.

Incidence: Fewer than 10 cases have been reported.

Genetic inheritance: Autosomal recessive. Consanguinity has been reported in the parents of at least two patients.

Diagnosis: Turridolichocephaly and a prominent nose associated with severe growth retardation and alopecia are the most frequent features.

Clinical aspects: The most common clinical findings are turridolichocephaly, prominent nose, large and soft ears, alopecia (partialis or totalis), severe growth retardation with thoracic kyphoscoliosis, bilateral dislocation of the hips, joint contractures, and mild syndactyly with a short fifth digit. Telecanthus and marked myopia are present in some patients. Mental retardation is severe, with an IQ of approximately 40. Enamel dysplasia results in severe and multiple cavities. Less frequent features include ichthyosis, hidrotic ectodermal dysplasia, hypolacrimation, hypohidrosis, optic nerve atrophy with photophobia, autoimmune thyroiditis, multiple skeletal anomalies (fusions of elbows, carpals, metacarpals, spine), and recurrent respiratory infections.

Precautions before anesthesia: Assess clinically the degree of kyphoscoliosis and obtain pulmonary function tests if the degree of kyphoscoliosis is significant. Obtain a chest radiograph. Arterial blood gas analysis may be helpful in assessing ventilation in the presence of recurrent aspirations/infections and/or kyphoscoliosis. Check the mobility of the neck because vertebral fusion may result in difficult tracheal intubation if the fusion affects the cervical spine. If kyphoscoliosis is severe, postoperative mechanical ventilation may be necessary.

Anesthetic considerations: Mental retardation often results in limited cooperation, and sedation prior to induction of anesthesia may be helpful. Careful direct laryngoscopy is needed to prevent damage to already compromised teeth. Careful positioning of the patient is required in view of kyphoscoliosis and joint contractures. Avoid aggressive warming of the patient if hypohidrosis is present. Keep the eyes well lubricated during anesthesia (hypolacrimation). Vascular access may be challenging, depending on the severity of the skin changes.

Pharmacological implications: There are no specific implications with this condition.

REFERENCES:

Schinzel A: A case of multiple skeletal anomalies, ectodermal dysplasia, and severe growth and mental retardation. *Helv Paediatr Acta* 35:243, 1980.

Dumic M, Cvitanovic M, Ille J, et al: Syndrome of short stature, mental deficiency, microcephaly, ectodermal dysplasia, and multiple skeletal anomalies. *Am J Med Genet* 93:47, 2000.

Alpers Disease

At a glance: Very rare progressive neurologic disorder, predominantly involving the gray matter, and characterized by spasticity and myoclonia. Dementia ensues combined with hepatic cirrhosis. Poor prognosis, generally within a few months. Possible exacerbation by stress or infection.

Synonyms: Progressive Sclerosing Poliodystrophy; Alpers Huttenlocher Syndrome; Alpers Diffuse Degeneration of Cerebral Gray Matter with Hepatic Cirrhosis; Alpers Progressive Infantile Poliodystrophy; Christensen Disease; Christensen-Krabbe Disease; Diffuse Cerebral Degeneration in Infancy; Progressive Cerebral Poliodystrophy; Progressive Neuronal Degeneration of Childhood with Hepatic Cirrhosis.

History: First recognized by Alfons Maria Jakob and first described by Bernard Alpers in 1931.

Incidence: Fewer than 50 cases have been described. Both genders are equally affected.

Genetic inheritance: Autosomal recessive. Certain affected individuals may inherit the genetic predisposition for the disorder. However, some researchers do not believe in a genetic cause, and increasing evidence indicates that Alpers syndrome may be a manifestation of childhood prion disease.

Pathophysiology: Acute impairment of mitochondrial function leading to a potentially reversible cytotoxic cerebral edema could play an important pathogenetic mechanism in Alpers syndrome. Mitochondrial mutations or deletions may cause a defect in the electron transport chain and consequently impaired oxidative phosphorylation, oxidative stress, and metabolic disturbances.

Diagnosis: Onset is early in life, with convulsions (most often in the second year of life). The diagnosis of Alpers syndrome usually follows a thorough clinical examination followed by special investigations. Abnormal electroencephalography (high-amplitude slow waves in combination with lower-amplitude polyspikes), progressive brain atrophy on CT or MRI, microcephaly, loss of visual evoked potentials, and abnormal liver function tests point to the diagnosis of Alpers syndrome. Histopathologic examination of the brain reveals spongiform degeneration and microcystic lesions with loss of neurons and demyelination, reactive cortical gliosis, and accumulation of lipids. Severe loss of almost all granular cells and persistent Purkinje cells can be found in the cerebellar cortex. The cerebral lesions can be unilateral or bilateral and predominately affect the occipital and parietal cortex, but cerebellum, brainstem, and basal ganglia also are involved. Widespread necrosis may involve the hippocampus, thalamus, substantia nigra, and amygdala.

Clinical aspects: Alpers disease usually begins in early childhood, predominantly affects the cerebral gray matter, and is characterized by progressive dementia and/or regression (loss of milestones), growth retardation, audiovisual impairment (blindness is possible), intractable seizures, myoclonus, ataxia, spasticity, areflexia, nystagmus, hypotonia, partial paralysis, dysphagia, and often liver damage. Liver involvement usually is a late sign and may result in jaundice, liver failure, and hepatic cirrhosis. Liver transplant does not result in clinical improvement and is not recommended at this point. Clinical exacerbation of seizures during stress (surgery) or infections has been described. Several biochemical abnormalities have been described in patients with Alpers disease, including dysfunction of the citric acid cycle, decreased levels of cytochromes a and aa3, decreased utilization of pyruvate, and deficiency of pyruvate dehydrogenase. As the disease progresses, many children become hypotonic, anemic, and thrombocytopenic. Progressive psychomotor deterioration (commonly with status epilepticus) in combination with acute hepatic failure finally terminates the course of this disease, often before age 3 years. Hypotension and sudden cardiorespiratory arrest have been reported.

Precautions before anesthesia: Evaluate neurologic function (clinical, history, EEG, CT/MRI). Evaluate liver involvement (clinically, ultrasound, CT and/or MRI, laboratory tests including coagulation). Obtain a complete blood count because anemia and thrombocytopenia are common in advanced stages of the disease. Retrognathia and chest deformities have been reported. Check for difficult tracheal intubation. Dysphagia may result in recurrent aspiration pneumonia, so a chest radiograph is recommended.

Anesthetic considerations: Patients have a high risk of aspiration most likely because of swallowing difficulties related to the neurologic findings. Rapid sequence induction is recommended. Central neuraxial anesthesia should be avoided in the presence of clotting abnormalities. Careful intraoperative positioning is required (contractures, thin subcutaneous tissue secondary to malnutrition/growth retardation).

Pharmacological implications: Consider interactions among antiepileptic medications, liver function, and anesthetic drugs. Given the fact that these children may have some degree of paralysis, succinylcholine should be used cautiously because an exaggerated hyperkalemic response is possible.

Other conditions to be considered:

☞**GANGLIOSIDOSIS TYPE II:** Heritable lysosomal storage disorder with ganglioside accumulation leading to severe neurologic impairment and premature death.

☞**NEURONAL CEROID LIPOFUSCINOSES:** Hereditary progressive neurodegenerative disorders with mental retardation, visual loss, and seizures. Neuronal ceroid lipofuscinoses probably are the most common class of neurodegenerative disease in children.

☞**LEIGH SYNDROME:** Severe progressive necrotizing encephalopathy caused by a mitochondrial disorder impeding oxidative phosphorylation.

REFERENCES:

Gauthier-Villars M, Landrieu P, Cormier-Daire V, et al: Respiratory chain deficiency in Alpers syndrome. *Neuropediatrics* 32:150, 2001.

Kayihan N, Nennesmo I, Ericzon B-G, et al: Fatal deterioration of neurological disease after orthotopic liver transplantation for valproic acid-induced liver damage. *Pediatr Transplant* 4:211, 2000.

Ulmer S, Flemming K, Hahn A, et al: Detection of acute cytotoxic changes in progressive neuronal degeneration of childhood with liver disease (Alpers-Huttenlocher syndrome) using diffusion-weighted MRI and MR spectroscopy. *J Comput Assist Tomogr* 26:641, 2002.

α_1-Antitrypsin Deficiency (AATD)

At a glance: α_1-Antitrypsin deficiency (AATD) is a relatively common inherited disorder. It primarily presents with early-onset panacinar lung emphysema and with liver cirrhosis in a minority of the patients. Cardiac arrest in association with general anesthesia has been described.

Synonyms: α_1-Antiprotease Deficiency; Hereditary Pulmonary Emphysema; AATD.

Incidence: Worldwide, approximately 1:2000 to 1:4000 newborns have AATD. This disorder is found in all ethnic groups but most frequently in Caucasians.

Genetic inheritance: AATD is inherited in an autosomal recessive pattern. In the majority of patients, the parents are carriers (heterozygous for the defect) but show no symptoms of the disease. A gene called *SERPINA1* (*Ser*ine [or cysteine] *p*roteinase *in*hibitor, clade A [AAT], member *1*) is responsible for production of AAT and has been mapped to 14q32.1.

The *SERPINA1* gene comes in many alleles (>100 different phenotypic variants of AATD have been identified). Most people (approximately 90%) are homozygous for the M version (PiMM, where Pi = *p*roteinase *in*hibitor), which is characterized by normal levels of AAT (serum levels 20–60 mmol/l). Two altered alleles of the *SERPINA1* gene result in moderately low to very low AAT levels and are called the S and Z allele, respectively. Individuals with a PiZZ (AAT serum level 3.3–7 mmol/l) or PiSZ phenotype are at high risk to develop AATD. In fact, the PiZZ phenotype is responsible for almost all the cases of AAT-related emphysema and liver disease. In general, individuals with a PiMS or PiSS genotype can produce enough AAT to prevent lung damage. In general, a serum level of approximately 11 mmol/l and higher is considered sufficient to prevent lung damage. However, patients with the PiMZ genotype (carrier) who smoke are at increased risk for lung disease. In a rare variant, termed the *00 (null-null) phenotype,* no AAT is produced.

Pathophysiology: AAT is a glycoprotein with a molecular weight of 54 kDa. It is produced in hepatocytes and mononuclear phagocytes. The genetic defect in AATD alters the molecule (misfolding secondary to substitution of alanine for valine at amino acid residue 213 and substitution of lysine for glutamate at amino acid residue 342 of AAT) such that, although synthesized, it cannot be released from the endoplasmic reticulum, where a significant part is degraded but the rest accumulates in the form of insoluble intracellular globular inclusions. The inclusion can easily be identified on routine (H and E) and periodic acid-Schiff (PAS)–stained liver biopsies (except in the Pi00 genotype, where AAT production is completely absent). AAT serum levels in PiZZ patients are approximately 10 to 15% of normal values, meaning that 85 to 90% of AAT produced remains intracellularly, of which a significant part is degraded; the rest accumulates. The major function of AAT is inhibition of several mainly neutrophil-derived proteases, particularly at sites of inflammation where high amounts of active serine proteases (elastase, trypsin, cathepsin G, proteinase 3) are released from infiltrating polymorphonuclear cells. (Obviously, the synonymous but more general term α_1-antiproteinase deficiency is more appropriate; nevertheless AATD is the commonly used name for the disease.) AAT normally is released from hepatocytes into the blood circulation, where it circulates unbound and diffuses into pulmonary interstitial and alveolar lining fluids. Neutrophil elastase, which normally is released during phagocytosis of organisms or particles in the alveoli, is inactivated by AAT. The resulting imbalance between proteases and antiproteases in the lungs is responsible for unimpeded destruction of elastin and collagen in the alveolar walls. This process results in progressive panacinar lung emphysema initially with distension of the alveolus and the alveolar duct, but it also affects the respiratory bronchioles. This process is more pronounced at the base of the lungs. Because smokers have an increased number of neutrophils and macrophages (and therefore increased elastase levels) in the alveoli but they also have decreased antielastase activity (oxidants in cigarette smoke inhibit AAT), destruction is amplified by smoking. Why only 10 to 15% of patients with the PiZZ phenotype develop liver disease, which seems to be associated with accumulation of AAT in hepatocytes in the form of insoluble globules, is unknown. This theory is supported by the observation that patients with the 00 (null-null) phenotype (completely absent AAT synthesis) may suffer from emphysema like patients with the ZZ and SZ phenotype, but they do not show signs of cirrhosis or liver cancer. However, other genetic factors and a specific sensitivity in some patients seem to be involved in the pathogenesis of liver disease. Antitrypsin acts as an acute phase protein, and its serum level may increase significantly in response to inflammation and fever. Prevention and early treatment of these symptoms in PiZZ homozygote infants seems important. Serum levels also may increase in association with neoplasias, pregnancy, and oral contraceptives.

Diagnosis: On routine serum electrophoresis, more than 90% of the α_1-globulin fraction is made up of AAT. Hence, a missing α_1-peak is suggestive of AATD. However, direct measurement of serum AAT levels is possible, and patients with low or borderline serum AAT levels should undergo phenotyping to confirm the diagnosis

of AATD. A direct test for the presence or absence of the PiZ allele is available and more sensitive. The severity of emphysema is best documented with standard pulmonary function tests. The majority of patients are diagnosed with AATD secondary to their symptoms and often present with moderate-to-severe airflow obstruction with a reduction in forced expired volume in the first second (FEV$_1$) to 30 to 40%. Increased lung volumes (a consequence of increased residual volume because of air trapping) and reduced vital capacity usually are present. Prenatal diagnosis of AATD is available.

Clinical aspects: In the first 2 decades of life, liver disease is the main manifestation of AATD; lung problems evolve later in life (see below). Among adolescents with the PiZZ phenotype, lung function appears to be normal. Lung disease usually does not present until the late fourth or early fifth decade of life. It starts with intermittent symptoms such as dyspnea initially on strenuous exertion only (cardinal symptom), wheezing, chronic cough, and spirometric evidence of obstructive airway disease. Many patients initially are falsely labeled as having asthma. Bronchiectases and pulmonary cysts may occur later in life. Occasionally, the pulmonary disease is rapidly progressive, most often seen in patients with preexisting liver disease secondary to AATD. Panacinar emphysema is characterized by hyperinflated, hyperlucent lung bases and bullae formation on chest x-ray film, all secondary to destruction of normal lung tissue. Oligemia resulting from the rarefaction or lack of regular branching vessels also has been used as a criterion. Clinical features that indicate the possibility of AATD and should trigger further evaluation include emphysema and recurrent bronchitis in younger adults (age 30–45 years), particularly in nonsmokers and patients with a positive family history for emphysema of the basal lung areas and occasionally adult-onset asthma. The decline in FEV$_1$ in healthy adults is estimated to be approximately 30 ml/year, but may be as high as 300 ml/year in adults with the PiZZ phenotype. Mortality rate is inversely proportional to the decline in FEV$_1$. Emphysema is the cause of death in almost three fourths of AATD patients; the majority of patients die before age 60 years. This is especially true for patients who were diagnosed with AATD because of symptoms and not as a result of a screening process. Most patients initially respond to bronchodilator therapy (β-adrenergic drugs, inhaled steroids). Oral corticosteroids usually are reserved for acute exacerbations with increased cough and sputum production. Theophylline has been used in the past but is no longer the first-line treatment. However, some patients may experience a relief in their degree of dyspnea, so some pneumologists advocate a therapeutic trial in a subgroup of patients. Weekly intravenous replacement therapy of AAT (made from pooled, purified, human plasma protein concentrate) is available. Restoration of serum and alveolar AAT concentrations to protective levels seems to have beneficial effects, but the treatment is expensive. In any patient presenting with chronic liver disease, not only AAT serum levels but also the Pi phenotype should be determined, as AAT serum concentration alone may be misleading because AAT is also an acute phase protein (see *Pathophysiology*) and may be falsely elevated. The clinical range of liver disease is wide and includes neonatal cholestasis, neonatal or juvenile micronodular cirrhosis, chronic hepatitis, and hepatocellular carcinoma (more common in males). However, only approximately 10 to 15% of neonates with the PiZZ phenotype show signs of liver disease, most commonly starting as cholestatic jaundice, which in most cases resolves in the first months of life. It also may result in fatal liver failure, esophageal varices, and bleeding complications. Chronic liver disease accounts for approximately 10% of deaths related to AATD. Hepatosplenomegaly may persist even after jaundice resolves and may result in hypersplenism with thrombocytopenia. Liver transplant has been used successfully to treat not only liver failure but also the enzyme defect. Patients with end-stage lung disease can be treated with lung or combined heart-lung transplant.

Precautions before anesthesia: Lung function should be assessed by spirometry to determine forced vital capacity and FEV_1. Measuring lung volumes (ideally by plethysmography) and diffusing capacity may be required for special circumstances. Chest radiograph is strongly recommended. Hepatic function (serum concentrations of transaminases, bilirubin, albumin; activated partial thromboplastin time; international normalized ratio) should be assessed in all patients with low or borderline levels of AAT. A complete blood cell count including platelets (hypersplenism) should be obtained because of potential bleeding issues (e.g., esophageal varices, bleeding ulcers). Given the reduced pulmonary function and the increased risk for airway complications in most of these patients, lung function and respiratory tract infections should be optimized and treated before the patient undergoes anesthesia. Review and evaluate bronchodilator therapy (β-adrenergic agents, inhaled steroids) to maximize lung function. Cor pulmonale can be present in patients with long-standing pulmonary disease. If in doubt, ECG and transthoracic echocardiography should be performed. Because fever and infections result in elevated serum AAT levels in healthy individuals but mainly increased intracellular levels in AATD patients, avoid anesthesia under these circumstances, although it probably does not affect the short-term course of the disease.

Anesthetic considerations: AATD patients are subject to all the complications typical for patients with chronic obstructive pulmonary disease (pneumonia, pneumothorax, acute airway obstruction, respiratory failure) well known from chronic cigarette smoking. (Hyper)reactive airway disease poses a significant risk in these patients. Significant air trapping requiring emergency sternotomy and cardiopulmonary bypass secondary to cardiac arrest has been described in AATD patients undergoing heart-lung transplant. If permitted by the surgical procedure, maintenance of spontaneous ventilation (mask or laryngeal mask airway) probably is advantageous in these patients. Three pediatric AATD cases have been reported. General anesthesia (two with halothane; one case not specified) administered for minor surgical procedures resulted in accelerated hepatic failure and death of the patients. The exact cause of fatal deterioration could not be determined, but general anesthesia (halothane?) was considered the main culprit.

Pharmacological implications: Use of halothane in patients with AATD-related liver disease probably is not advisable. Nonsteroidal antiinflammatory drugs should be used carefully in the presence of liver disease (bleeding complications). Stress ulcer prophylaxis may be indicated, depending on the kind of surgery.

Other conditions to be considered:

☞**KARTAGENER SYNDROME:** Inherited polymalformative syndrome characterized by bronchiectasis, situs inversus, and chronic sinusitis.

☞**MUCOVISCIDOSIS:** Congenital multiorgan disease affecting mainly the lungs, liver, and pancreas. Frequent lung infections, hemoptysis, intolerance to exercise, presence of clubbing fingers suggesting pulmonary hypertension, rectal prolapse, and nasal polyps.

REFERENCES:

Crystal RG: Alpha-1-antitrypsin deficiency, emphysema, and liver disease: Genetic basis and strategies for therapy. *J Clin Invest* 85:1343, 1990.

Myles PS, Weeks AM: Alpha 1-antitrypsin deficiency: Circulatory arrest following induction of general anesthesia. *Anaesth Intens Care* 20:358, 1992.

Burke JA, Kiesel JL, Blair JD: α1-Antitrypsin deficiency and liver disease in children. *Am J Dis Child* 130:621, 1976.

Alpha-Ketoglutarate Dehydrogenase Deficiency

At a glance: Characterized by hypotonia, metabolic acidosis, and hyperlactatemia immediately after birth. The life expectancy is limited to about 30 months of age. Death is caused by neurologic deterioration. Other clinical features include axial hypotonia with no head control until late in childhood. Metabolic acidosis with acute episodes of acidotic decompensation and sometimes hypoglycemia may occur during infections. Low plasmatic molar ratios of ketone bodies in neonate with congenital lactic acidosis have been suggested as an indicator of dysfunction of the tricarboxylic acid cycle.

Synonyms: Alpha-KGD deficiency; 2-Alpha-ketoglutarate dehydrogenase deficiency; Oxoglutaric aciduria; Oxoglutarate dehydrogenase.

Incidence/genetic inheritance: There are no epidemiological studies to establish the incidence. A total of 9 infants with isolated alpha-ketoglutarate dehydrogenase deficiency have been reported in the literature. All reported cases are from Northern Africa, mostly Algeria and Tunisia. It is believe that this medical condition is inherited as an autosomal recessive trait.

Pathophysiology: Alpha-ketoglutarate dehydrogenase is an enzyme of the Krebs cycle that catalyzes the oxidation of alpha-ketoglutarate to succinyl CoA. It is one of 3 alpha-ketoacid dehydrogenase enzymes, the others being pyruvate dehydrogenase and branched-chain ketoacid dehydrogenase. Each of these enzymes is a complex of multiple units. Each unit has 3 distinct subunits. The E1 (alpha-ketoacid decarboxylase), E2 (dihydrolipoyl transacetylase) and E3 (dihydrolipoyl dehydrogenase or lipoamide dehydrogenase) are identical in all 3 alpha-ketoacid dehydrogenases. Alpha-ketoglutarate dehydrogenase, fumarase, and succinate dehydrogenase are the only enzymes of the human Krebs cycle in which a single enzyme deficiency state has been defined.

Clinical aspects: The clinical presentation includes severe hypotonia, metabolic acidosis, congenital lactic acidosis, early childhood death. Laboratory investigations reveal hyperlactatemia and alpha-ketoglutarate dehydrogenase deficiency.

Anesthetic considerations: An arterial blood gas analysis, serum electrolytes, cell blood count and differential must be obtained preoperatively. Patients presenting severe neurological dysfunction may present with seizure activities, airway problems and postoperative complications. Intraoperative cardiovascular instability is possible as a result of electrolyte disturbances. It is essential to correct any intravascular volume deficit and electrolyte imbalances before all elective surgical procedures. Intravenous fluid solutions that contain lactate must be avoided. Postoperative admission to an ICU or a constant care facility may be indicated depending on the severity of the case and the type of surgical procedure performed.

Pharmacological implications: Variable and prolonged response to neuromuscular relaxants should be expected and the use of a peripheral nerve stimulator is recommended to assess degree of neuromuscular blockade during general anesthesia. In the presence of severe hypotonia, it is recommended to avoid the use of succinyl-choline.

REFERENCES:
Guffon N, Lopez-Mediavilla C, Dumoulin R, et al: 2-Ketoglutarate de-hydrogenase deficiency, a rare cause of primary hyperlactataemia: Report of a new case. *J Inherit Metab Dis* 16:821–830, 1993.
Kohlschutter A, Behbehani A, Langenbeck Uet, al: A familial progressive neurodegenerative disease with 2-oxoglutaric aciduria. *Europ J Pediat* 138:32–37, 1982.

Alpha-Mannosidosis

At a glance: Characterized by Hurler-like facial features, moderate-to-severe mental retardation, recurrent pulmonary infections, reduced hearing, immunodeficiency, skeletal abnormalities, and primary central nervous system disease, mainly ataxia. It is also frequently associated with corneal opacities, aseptic destructive arthritis, and metabolic myopathy. Communicating hydrocephalus can occur in individuals of any age. Cardiac and renal complications are rarely encountered. Alpha-mannosidosis is insidiously progressive. Individuals may live into the sixth decade.

Synonyms: Lysosomal Alpha-D-mannosidase Deficiency; Alpha-Mannosidase B Deficiency; Mannosidosis.

Incidence: Very little is known about the prevalence of alpha-mannosidosis. A study from Australia reported prevalence of one in 500,000. A study from Norway reported six individuals in a population of four million. The disease is not specific to any ethnic group, as individuals from all parts of the world have been described .

Genetic inheritance: It is inherited as an autosomal recessive trait.

Classification: There are three types of alpha-mannosidosis that be suggested:

TYPE I (MILD JUVENILE): Mild form delineated by clinical recognition of the disease after age ten years, with absence of skeletal abnormalities, myopathy, and slow progression.

TYPE II (MILD INFANTILE): Moderate form with clinical recognition before age ten years, with presence of skeletal abnormalities, myopathy, and slow progression.

TYPE III (SEVERE INFANTILE): Severe form with obvious progression, leading to early death from primary central nervous system involvement or infection.

Pathophysiology: Alpha-mannosidosis is one of a group of very rare inherited disorders known as glycoprotein and related storage diseases. These disorders are caused by a defect in the breakdown of complex molecules in the cells, as a result of an enzyme deficiency. The enzyme that is lacking is known as alpha-D-mannosidase. The molecules that are not broken down are stored in the small components within cells known as lysosomes.

Diagnosis: The diagnosis relies on demonstration of deficient acid alpha-mannosidase enzyme activity in peripheral blood leukocytes or other nucleated cells such as fibroblasts, amniocytes, or the trophoblast. The diagnosis can be confirmed by measuring the presence of urinary oligosaccharides. Alpha-mannosidase is needed for the catabolism of many oligosaccharides and glycoproteins.

Clinical aspects: Infiltration of tissues with oligosaccharides and glycoproteins results in vomiting, hepatosplenomegaly, large head, thick calvaria, low anterior hairline, coarse facial features (Hurler-like), thick eyebrows, flat nose, large ears, macroglossia, widely spaced teeth, gingival hypertrophy deafness, lens opacities, prognathism, tall stature, ataxia, and muscular hypotonia. Other clini-cal features include lumbar gibbus, big hands and feet, dysostosis multiplex, bowed femurs, storage cells in bone marrow, vacuolated lymphocytes, pancytopenia, recurrent respiratory tract infections, immunoglobulin deficiency, hypogammaglobulinemia, antiplatelet antibodies, antineutrophil antibodies, low haptoglobin level, and severe mental retardation (adult form). Pectus carinatum, skeletal abnormalities, dilated cerebral ventricles and raised intracranial pressure, spondylolysis and spondylolisthesis of L5 on S1.

Anesthetic considerations: Upper airway obstruction is a major consideration in these patients. The airway management will be comparable to patient affected with Hurler syndrome. A potentially difficult airway management, including direct laryngoscopy and tracheal intubation must be anticipated and proper equipment prepared. Spontaneous respiration must be maintained until confirmation that ventilation can be ensured with face-mask ventilation or when confirmation of lung ventilation after tracheal intubation. The use of awake fiberoptic intubation with or without a laryngeal mask airway is highly recommended. Obtain cell blood count and differential, a 12-lead ECG, chest x-ray, and 2D echocardiography in all patients when possible. The pulmonary system must be assessed carefully for the presence of restrictive and/or reactive airway disease. Obtain an arterial blood gas determination and pulmonary function tests when the patient is cooperative. The use of preoperative bronchodilator therapy must be considered. Patients may be uncooperative depending on level of mental retardation, making induction of anesthesia difficult. The use of preoperative sedation and/or anxiolytic is not advisable in severely affected patients. Each patient must be evaluated individually before sedation is given. Centroneuraxial regional anesthesia is relatively contraindicated in patients with moderate to severe spinal deformities. Attainment of intravenous access may be difficult. Patients may experience bleeding disorders with the presence of antiplatelet antibodies. Obtain coagulation studies preoperatively.

Other conditions to be considered: There are approximately 50 diseases known as lysosomal storage diseases. In addition to alpha mannosidosis and a related disorder, beta mannosidosis, the lysosomal storage disorders include Fabry disease, Gaucher disease, cystinosis, aspartyl glycosaminuria, mucopolysaccharidoses, mucolipidoses, and many others.

REFERENCES:
Michelakakis H, Dimitriou E, Mylona-Karayanni C, Bartsocas CS: Phenotypic variability of mannosidosis type II: Report of two Greek siblings. *Genetic Counseling* 3:195–199, 1992.
Tollersrud OK, Berg T, Healy P, et al: Purification of bovine lysosomal alpha-mannosidase, characterization of its gene and determination of two mutations that cause alpha-mannosidosis. *Europ J Biochem* 246:410–419, 1997.

Alport Syndrome

At a glance: Generalized inherited disorder of basement membranes that involves type IV collagen, characterized by hematuria and progressive neurosensory deafness. Predominant in males. Ocular signs can be present. Renal failure occurs frequently.

Synonym: Familial Hematuric Nephritis with Neurosensory Deafness.

History: First described in 1902 by L.B. Guthrie, the English Physician. It was not until 1927 that Arthur Cecil Alport, a South African physician, recognized the association of renal failure and progressive deafness.

Incidence: Geographic variability. It is the most common form of hereditary glomerular disease and is estimated to account for approximately 2.5 to 3% of all cases of pediatric end-stage renal disease. Males are affected more often and more severely than females as the majority of cases are X-linked inherited, which usually affects females only mildly.

Genetic inheritance: In 85% of patients, inheritance is X-linked caused by mutation on Xq22.3 affecting the gene encoding the α-5 chain of basement membrane collagen COL4A5 (see *Pathophysiology*). In the remaining 15%, inheritance is autosomal recessive (caused by mutation in either the COL4A3 or COL4A4 gene, which have been mapped to 2q36-q37 and 2q36-q37, respectively. Autosomal dominant inheritance has been described in isolated cases.

Pathophysiology: In the early stages of Alport syndrome, the glomeruli show segmental proliferation and/r sclerosis. An increase in mesangial matrix often is combined with a foamy appearance of glomerular and tubular epithelial cells secondary to intracellular depositions of fat and mucopolysaccharides. Progression of the disease results in extensive glomerulosclerosis, tubular atrophy, and tubulointerstitial fibrosis. Electron microscopy allows detection of irregular thickening of the glomerular and tubular basement membrane. One of the main components of the basement membranes is type IV collagen, which consists of six subunits, a1 to a6. In Alport syndrome, depending on the mode of inheritance, subunit a3, a4, or a5 is altered, which all occur almost exclusively in basement membranes of the kidney, the cochlea, and the eye. This situation explains the unique distribution of the disease.

Diagnosis: Based on the presence of three of the four major signs: familial history of microhematuria, typical lesions of the glomerular basement membrane, sensorineural deafness, and characteristic ocular abnormalities (anterior lenticonus, spherophakia, cataract, perimacular degeneration).

Clinical aspects: Generally, the disorder is more severe in males. Initially, patients most often present only with persistent hematuria (microhematuria with intermittent gross hematuria) starting in early childhood and a positive family history for hematuria. Other renal features include proteinuria, hypertension, and renal failure (occurs in >90% of male patients but only 3% of female patients after age 25 years). However, the typical histologic findings may not yet be present in young children. End-stage renal failure, sensorineural, high-frequency hearing loss (in >80% of males and >50% of females), and ophthalmic lesions appear later in life (usually between age 20 and 40 years). Other features may include hypoparathyroidism, thrombocytopenia, ichthyosis, and diffuse leiomyomatosis. This diffuse leiomyomatosis is typical in a subgroup of patients with the X-linked form of Alport syndrome, occurs in older children, and affects the tracheobronchial system and the esophagus. The condition in the former results in recurrent upper airway infections, cough, stridor, and even dyspnea, but in the latter may lead to dysphagia and vomiting. Bowel involvement with constipation has been reported. Genital leiomyomatosis (vulva and clitoris) in girls has been described. Fatal complications and extensive surgery (including esophagectomy) have been described in patients with diffuse leiomyomatosis.

Precautions before anesthesia: Preoperative blood workup should include a complete blood count (renal anemia, thrombocytopenia) and serum concentrations of electrolytes, urea, creatinine, calcium, phosphate, and protein. Check the degree of proteinuria. Assess the severity of hearing loss. Severe thrombocythemia is a rare finding but should be treated preoperatively if severe and

may be a contraindication to central neuraxial blockades. Assess the airway for signs of stridor, cough, and dyspnea and rule out tracheobronchial leiomyomatosis. Patients may have received treatment for asthma. If in doubt, obtain a radiograph or CT scan of the chest.

Anesthetic considerations: Depending on the extent of the procedure, invasive blood pressure monitoring may be required. If diffuse leiomyomatosis is present or suspected, a rapid sequence induction technique is recommended. If the airway is involved, spontaneous ventilation must be maintained, and continuous positive airway pressure may be beneficial. Hypoparathyroidism requires regular control of calcium and phosphate serum concentrations in the perioperative period.

Pharmacological implications: Perioperative fluid management and drug doses should be adapted to renal function. Anesthetic drugs without renal metabolism are preferable. Aminosides should be used with care because of potential negative effects on renal function and hearing loss.

Other conditions to be considered:

    Fechtner Syndrome (Macrothrombocytopathy, Nephritis, Deafness, and Leukocyte Inclusion Syndrome; Alport Syndrome with Leukocyte Inclusions and Macrothrombocytopenia): Characterized by a combination of nephritis (with symptoms ranging from microhematuria to end-stage renal failure), high-frequency sensorineural deafness, congenital cataracts, macrothrombocytopenia, and inclusion bodies in neutrophils and eosinophils.

    ☞Epstein Syndrome: High-frequency sensorineural deafness and renal disease similar to that found in Alport syndrome. Macrothrombocytopenia results in prolonged bleeding time and impaired platelet aggregation in response to collagen.

REFERENCES:

Alport AC: Hereditary familial congenital haemorrhagic nephritis. *Br Med J* 1:504, 1927.

Gross O, Netzer KO, Lambrecht R, et al: Meta-analysis of genotype-phenotype correlation in X-linked Alport syndrome: Impact on clinical counselling. *Nephrol Dial Transplant* 17:1218, 2002.

Liapis H, Gokden N, Hmiel P, et al: Histopathology, ultrastructure, and clinical phenotypes in thin glomerular basement membrane disease variants. *Hum Pathol* 33:836, 2002.

Alström Syndrome

At a glance: Inherited syndrome with diabetes mellitus; cardiac, hepatic, and renal involvement; and progressive visual and hearing loss.

History: First described in 1959 by Carl Henry Alström, Bertil Hallgren, L.B. Nilsson, and H. Asander, all Swedish physicians.

Incidence and genetic inheritance: Approximately 200 patients with Alström syndrome have been reported since the first description in 1959. The genetic defect of this autosomal recessive inherited disorder has been mapped to 2p13-p12.

Clinical aspects: The syndrome results in progressive pigmentary retinopathy (cone–rod dystrophy) and often cataract. Early loss of central vision (in contrast to loss of peripheral vision first in retinitis pigmentosa) results in nystagmus. Light perception usually is lost by age 20 years. Generally mild-to-moderate obesity, advanced bone age, growth retardation with short stature secondary to growth hormone deficiency, and sensorineural hearing loss (mild-to-moderate) are additional features. Alström syndrome can be difficult to diagnose, and noninsulin-dependent diabetes mellitus developing in late childhood/early adulthood may finally lead to the diagnosis. Insulin resistance seems to be responsible for the decreased glucose tolerance and diabetes mellitus. Unresponsiveness of target organs to the action of other hormones (vasopressin, gonadotropins, ACTH) has been suspected. Later in life, patients suffer from progressive chronic nephropathy with renal insufficiency, hepatic failure, atherosclerosis, and congestive heart failure secondary to dilated cardiomyopathy (myocardial fibrosis has been demonstrated at autopsy and on myocardial biopsies, which is not necessarily related to coronary artery disease). However, an increasing percentage (up to 35%) of patients with infantile cardiomyopathy has been described in the last years. Adolescent and adult forms also exist and affect approximately 25% of patients, usually manifesting between adolescence and age 40 years. Severe pulmonary interstitial fibrosis with pulmonary hypertension has been reported. Hypersecretory lungs is a less common finding. Abnormal liver function test results in early childhood are common. The disease often progresses to hepatic cirrhosis and hepatic failure in the second or third decade of life. Other liver findings reported include chronic, nonspecific, lymphocytic hepatitis; patchy hepatic necrosis; and hepatosplenomegaly with ascites and portal hypertension. The first signs of renal disease may be polyuria and polydipsia as a result of a tubular defect secondary to interstitial fibrosis. Renal biopsy often reveals diffuse glomerulosclerosis, tubular atrophy, and interstitial fibrosis. End-stage renal disease is a late finding but often occurs before age 20 years. Urologic problems affect more than 50% of patients and are characterized by detrusor-urethral dyssynergia, which may result in lower abdominal and perineal pain. Symptoms include incontinence, retention, and recurrent urinary tract infections. Male hypogonadotropic hypogonadism has been described and results in low plasma testosterone levels secondary to low plasma gonadotropin concentrations. These males often have small external genitalia and inadequate secondary sexual development at puberty, often associated with gynecomastia. Subclinical hypothyroidism has been described. Approximately one third of Alström syndrome patients have a varying degree of kyphoscoliosis. Although some patients with mental retardation have been described, these patients most often are mentally normal.

Precautions before anesthesia: Patients require extensive workup before they undergo anesthesia. Echocardiography should be performed to determine the degree of cardiomyopathy and pulmonary hypertension. Pulmonary function tests and chest radiograph are required secondary to pulmonary interstitial fibrosis. Hepatic and renal assessment may consist of abdominal ultrasound and blood workup, which should include a complete blood count (renal anemia, thrombocytopenia secondary to splenomegaly), arterial blood gas analysis, serum levels of electrolytes, transaminases, γ-glutamyltranspeptidase, creatinine, BUN, urate, and blood glucose. Obtain a blood glucose profile and review the recent history for blood glucose levels. These patients often have gastroesophageal reflux disease.

Anesthetic considerations: Communication may be difficult because of visual and hearing impairment, so patients may be stressed. Sedative premedication may be helpful. A rapid sequence induction technique is recommended. Pulmonary hypersecretion requires access to the endotracheal tube at all times in case suctioning is necessary. Check blood glucose concentration preoperatively, with a standard approach to diabetes mellitus recommended. Expect patients

(although not described) to be hemodynamically labile because of suspected resistance to antidiuretic hormone, ACTH, and other hormones on the one hand and because of cardiovascular disease and renal failure on the other hand. Postoperative mechanical ventilation may be required because of cardiomyopathy and pulmonary disease and should be arranged beforehand.

Pharmacological implications: Drug choice and dosage should take into account the severity of hepatic and renal insufficiency. Avoid drugs with negative inotropic effects.

Other conditions to be considered:

☞**BARDET-BIEDL SYNDROME:** Mental retardation, pigmentary retinopathy, polydactyly, obesity, renal anomalies, hypogenitalism.

☞**COHEN SYNDROME:** Inherited disorder characterized by hypotonia, obesity, prominent incisors, and nonprogressive psychomotor retardation.

☞**KEARNS-SAYRE SYNDROME:** Mitochondrial encephalomyopathy characterized by progressive external ophthalmoplegia, atypical retinitis pigmentosa, and cardiomyopathy.

☞**MELAS SYNDROME:** *M*itochondrial myopathy, *e*ncephalopathy, *l*actic *a*cidosis, *s*troke-like episodes (MELAS) is a progressive neurodegenerative disorder. The typical presentation includes features such as mitochondrial encephalomyopathy, lactic acidosis, and stroke-like episodes. Other features include diabetes mellitus and deafness.

REFERENCES:

Benso C, Hadjadj E, Conrath J, et al: Three new cases of Alström syndrome. *Graefes Arch Clin Exp Ophthalmol* 240:622, 2002.

Macari F, Lautier C, Girardet A, et al: Refinement of genetic localization of the Alström syndrome on chromosome 2p12-13 by linkage analysis in a North African family. *Hum Genet* 103:658, 1998.

Russell-Eggitt IM, Clayton PT, Coffey R, et al: Alström syndrome. Report of 22 cases and literature review. *Ophthalmology* 105:1274, 1998.

Amelogenesis Imperfecta

At a glance: Inherited condition that affects the enamel of the teeth, making them soft and thin. The teeth are easily damaged and appear yellow because the dentin is visible through the thin enamel.

Incidence and genetic inheritance: 1:20,000 live births for the most common form (enamel hypocalcification, see *Clinical Aspects*). Most often autosomal dominant inheritance, with the defect mapped to 4q21 and 4q11-q21. However, some forms are X-linked dominant with the defect located on Xp22 and Xq22-28, and other forms are autosomal recessive.

Clinical aspects: Both the primary and the secondary dentitions are affected. Two types of amelogenesis imperfecta have been described:

1. Hereditary enamel hypocalcification, where the amount of enamel is normal but the degree of calcification is insufficient. This is the most frequent type of enamel dysplasia.
2. Hereditary enamel hypoplasia, where the quality of the enamel is normal but the quantity is deficient.

The enamel defect becomes obvious soon after the teeth erupt and is lost soon thereafter. In the case of enamel hypocalcification, the enamel can easily be scraped off the teeth. Anterior open bite is

present in approximately two thirds of patients. The clinical course in the autosomal recessive form is more severe than in the other forms. This can be confirmed by radiologic and histologic findings.
Anesthetic considerations: Obtain history and document loose teeth. Teeth are soft and may be easily damaged, especially during laryngoscopy.
Other conditions to be considered:
☞**Trichodentoosseous Syndrome:** Features of this autosomal dominant inherited disorder are enamel hypoplasia and hypocalcification, combined with curly, dry hair.
Amelogenesis Imperfecta, Hypomaturation-Hypoplasia-Type with Taurodontism Syndrome: Clinically very similar but genetically slightly different. The dental changes seen in this syndrome are identical to those occurring in trichodentoosseous syndrome, but hair changes and osteosclerosis are absent.
☞**Laryngo-Onycho-Cutaneous Syndrome:** Severe progressive multisystem disorder involving the skin (dermal granula and ulcerations) and larynx (vocal cord granuloma), often lethal during childhood.

REFERENCES:
Backman B, Holmgren G: Amelogenesis imperfecta: A genetic study. *Hum Hered* 38:189, 1988.

Rajpar MH, Harley K, Laing C, et al: Mutation of the gene encoding the enamel-specific protein, enamelin, causes autosomal-dominant amelogenesis imperfecta. *Hum Mol Genet* 10:1673, 2001.

Amelo-Onychohypohidrotic Syndrome

At a glance: Disorder that results in the combination of teeth and nail anomalies with hypohidrosis.
Incidence and genetic inheritance: Extremely rare, autosomal dominant inherited disorder described in two families.
Clinical aspects: Hypoplastic, hypocalcified enamel of teeth; onycholysis and subungual hyperkeratosis; hypohidrosis.
Anesthetic considerations: Obtain history and document loose teeth. Careful direct laryngoscopy is required to prevent damage to fragile teeth. Hypohidrosis may result in temperature disturbances, and atropine should be used carefully.

REFERENCE:
Witkop CJ Jr, Brearley LJ, Gentry WC Jr: Hypoplastic enamel, onycholysis, and hypohidrosis inherited as an autosomal dominant trait. A review of ectodermal dysplasia syndromes. *Oral Surg Oral Med Oral Pathol* 39:71, 1975.

Amenorrhea-Galactorrhea Syndrome (AGS)

At a glance: Disorder characterized by galactorrhea and amenorrhea.
Synonyms and Classification: Amenorrhea-Galactorrhea-Hyperprolactinemia Syndrome.

Type I = Chiari-Frommel Syndrome: persistent AGS after giving birth.

Type II = Ahumada-Del Castillo Syndrome (Argonz del Castillo-Ahumada Syndrome; Amenorrhea-Galactorrhea FSH Decrease Syndrome; Nonpuerperal Galactorrhea-Amenorrhea Syndrome): AGS not associated with pregnancy. Estrogen deficiency and decreased urinary gonadotropin levels.

Type III = Forbes-Albright Syndrome: AGS caused by chromophobe prolactin-producing adenoma of the pituitary.

Genetic inheritance: Autosomal dominant.
Pathophysiology: Tumors resembling chromophobe adenomas of the pituitary gland with eosinophilic granulation on tetrachrome staining.
Clinical aspects: Secondary amenorrhea with galactorrhea. Enlargement of the sella turcica.
Anesthetic considerations: No known specific anesthetic considerations for this syndrome.

REFERENCE:
Rimoin DL, Schimke RN: *Genetic Disorders of the Endocrine Glands.* St. Louis, CV Mosby, 1971.

Amish Hair–Brain Syndrome

At a glance: Inherited syndrome with mild psychomotor retardation, hypogonadism, short stature, brittle hair.
Synonyms: Amish Brittle Hair Syndrome; BIDS; Brittle Hair, Intellectual Deficit, Decreased Fertility, and Short Stature Syndrome.
Incidence and genetic inheritance: Initially described in 25 children of an Amish kindred with autosomal recessive transmission.
Clinical aspects: The most striking signs are brittle hair and short stature. The hair defect is secondary to a markedly reduced cystine content resulting in lack of sulfur-rich matrix proteins. The microscopic appearance of the hair shows an irregular and grooved surface. The same underlying defect seems to be responsible for nail dystrophy (brittle, short nails).
The intellectual deficit usually is mild. Reduced fertility is secondary to hypogonadism.
Anesthetic considerations: Obtain a full history of the patient's neurologic status. Depending on the severity of mental retardation, the patient may benefit from anxiolytic premedication. No specific anesthetic considerations.
Other conditions to be considered:
☞**Brittle Hair and Mental Deficit Syndrome:** Genetic disorder characterized by abnormal hair fibers and mental deficiency.
☞**Pollitt Syndrome:** Inherited syndrome with developmental delay and trichorrhexis nodosa.
☞**Netherton Syndrome:** Most likely autosomal recessive transmitted inborn error of metabolism that manifests with bamboo hair, atopic diathesis, congenital ichthyosiform erythroderma, and hypogammaglobulinemia.

REFERENCES:
Allen RJ: Neurocutaneous syndromes in children. *Postgrad Med* 50:83, 1971.

Jackson CE, Weiss L, Watson JH: "Brittle" hair with short stature, intellectual impairment and decreased fertility: An autosomal recessive syndrome in an Amish kindred. *Pediatrics* 54:201, 1974.

Amyoplasia Congenita

At a glance: Rare congenital disorder constituting about one third of cases of ☞Arthrogryposis Multiplex Congenita characterized by multiple contractures of joints.

Synonyms: Guérin-Stern Syndrome; Otto Syndrome; Rocher-Sheldon Syndrome; Rossi Syndrome; Congenital Arthromyodysplastic Syndrome; Myodysplasia Foetalis Deformans; Myodystrophia Foetalis Deformans.

Nature: Congenital disorder that may result from an intrauterine vascular accident affecting the fetal spinal cord.

Genetic inheritance: Sporadic cases. Incidence is approximately 1:10,000 live births. Higher incidence is found in twins.

Pathophysiology: Unknown. Two forms have been described:

1. *Neuropathic form* in which anterior horn cells are reduced in number, pyramidal tract and motor roots are demyelinated, and axons in peripheral nerves are reduced.
2. *Myopathic form* in which joint deformities result from lack of movements in utero.

Diagnosis: Based on clinical findings at birth in a child with contracture of numerous joints in a flexed position (arthrogryposis), hypoplasia of the attached musculature, and development of multiple pterygia in affected joints. In approximately two thirds of patients, all four limbs are affected; in approximately one fourth of patients, the lower extremities are more severely affected than the arms; and in the remaining cases, the arms are more severely affected than the lower extremities. The term *amyoplasia* refers to replacement of muscles by fibrous tissue in different areas.

Clinical aspects: Intelligence in these patients is normal. Common features involve the head and neck (low-set ears, ptosis, limited eye movements laterally and upward, abnormal retinal pigmentation, flattened nose, round facies, frontal midline capillary hemangioma, micrognathia, cleft palate), skeleton (scoliosis, dislocated hips, internally rotated and adducted shoulders, fixed extended elbows, wrist deformities consisting of flexion and ulnar deviation, talipes varus, syndactyly, camptodactyly, amputation of digits), gastrointestinal tract (gastroschisis, intestinal atresia, hypertrophic pyloric stenosis, gastric ulcers), and chest (hypoplastic lungs, diaphragmatic hernia, hydrothorax). Lymphedema has been observed.

Precautions before anesthesia: Evaluate respiratory function (clinical, chest radiographs, pulmonary function tests if possible, arterial blood gases analysis, CT scans). Assess for difficult airway management (micrognathia, cleft palate).

Anesthetic considerations: Tracheal intubation may be difficult and may require adapted anesthetic management. Spontaneous ventilation should be maintained until the airway is secured. If significant, pleural effusions should be drained preoperatively. Postoperative mechanical ventilatory support may be necessary and should be arranged beforehand. Careful intraoperative positioning is mandatory and can be challenging secondary to limited joint mobility. Complications resulting from positioning, such as pressure sores and fractures, have been described. Venous access can be difficult with all the contractures. Avoid bag-mask ventilation in the presence of diaphragmatic hernia.

Pharmacological implications: Muscle deficiency and respiratory function may require lower doses of muscle relaxants. Opioids should be used judiciously. No relation between malignant hyperthermia and arthrogryposis syndromes has been demonstrated. However, hyperpyrexia and hypermetabolism have been described in association with volatile anesthetics, although these reactions were thought to be distinct from malignant hyperthermia.

Other conditions to be considered: See ☞Arthrogryposis Multiplex Congenita for a summary.

REFERENCES:

Sells JM, Jaffe KM, Hall JG: Amyoplasia, the most common type of arthrogryposis: The potential for good outcome. *Pediatrics* 97:225, 1996.

Shenoy MU, Marlow N, Stewart RJ: Amyoplasia congenita and intestinal atresia: A common etiology. *Acta Paediatr* 88:1405, 1999.

Hopkins PM, Ellis FR, Halsall PJ: Hypermetabolism in arthrogryposis multiplex congenita. *Anaesthesia* 46:374, 1991.

Amyotrophic Lateral Sclerosis

At a glance: Degenerative motor neuron disease evolving to progressive muscle weakness resulting in paralysis.

Synonyms: ALS; Lou Gehrig Disease (named after a famous American baseball player with New York Yankees who succumbed to amyotrophic lateral sclerosis in 1941).

History: Described in 1869 by Jean-Martin Charcot, a French neurologist.

Incidence: Annually, approximately five new cases per 100,000 in the general population, mainly male patients (male-to-female ratio 1.5:1) age 40 to 60 years.

Genetic inheritance: Etiology is not known. Approximately 10% of cases are inherited in an autosomal dominant fashion. The remaining cases are believed to be caused by an unknown slow virus infection. Despite extensive searches for infectious causative agents, no viral or bacterial etiology has been identified. Oxidative stress may be relevant.

Pathophysiology: Degenerative motor neuron disease may include cortical neuron degeneration (primary lateral sclerosis), central nuclei (pseudobulbar palsy), and/or motor neurons (progressive spinal amyotrophia). The hypothesis that excitotoxicity, oxidative stress, and mitochondrial dysfunction are involved in the process of neuronal cell death is supported at least in part by research reporting discovery of mutations of superoxide dismutase-1 in approximately 10% of patients with familial ALS. Anterior horn cells in the spinal cord and cranial motor nerves are predominantly involved in ALS. Patients may present with bulbar palsy or (commonly symmetrical and distal) weakness of single or multiple muscle groups of the limbs. The primarily bulbar form of ALS is associated with a worse prognosis with regard to severity and survival time. Fasciculations of the intrinsic hand muscles, which are an early and characteristic sign, later progress to weakness and atrophy and eventually spread proximally to the forearms and shoulder girdle muscles. Typically, both upper and lower motor neurons are affected. Clinically limb or tongue fasciculations, hyperreflexia, clonus, and spasticity are found. An inflammatory response with activated microglia, reactive astrocytes, and IgG antibodies can be found in affected areas of the spinal cord. However, how these changes are related to neuronal cell death is not known. Autoimmune phenomena may be involved in the pathogenesis of ALS. Corticospinal and corticobulbar tracts may show signs of wallerian degeneration.

Diagnosis: Progressive adult-onset muscular weakness with muscular spasms and fasciculations (although a few cases have been reported in children). Initially, the disease is localized but rapidly spreads to all muscles. In addition to the clinical examination, electromyography studies are used to identify lower motor neuron dysfunction. Long-lasting, polyphasic fasciculation potentials and signs of chronic partial denervation are characteristic of ALS.

Clinical aspects: Initially the disease may present with fasciculations of the intrinsic hand muscles, which later change to weakness and atrophy and then spread proximally to the shoulder girdle. However, involvement of the various muscle groups is inhomogeneous. As the disease progresses, atrophy and weakness involve most of the skeletal muscles, including those of the tongue, pharynx, larynx, and chest. Swallowing problems, with frequent choking and bronchopulmonary aspirations, are common. The sensibility is not affected. Serum creatine phosphokinase levels are normal, no cardiac involvement is seen, and intellectual function remains unchanged. Loss of autonomic control with orthostatic hypotension and tachycardia has been described. Extraocular muscles, bladder, and anal sphincter muscles typically are spared. Some patients with cancer exhibit a symptom complex similar to ALS as part of a paraneoplastic syndrome. Some researchers have reported decreased levels of insulin-like growth factor-1 (IGF-1) in patients with ALS. Patients with ALS may benefit from treatment with recombinant human IGF-1, although survival remains the same. Riluzole is a benzothiazole glutamate antagonist medication that may prolong tracheostomy-free survival but not overall survival. Because no effective therapy exists to date, the prognosis remains grim. Death usually results from pulmonary complications within 5 to 10 years after the first symptoms.

Precautions before anesthesia: Impairment of respiration, altered response to muscle relaxants, and predisposition of aspiration affect anesthetic management. Obtain a complete history, particularly with regard to muscle wasting and previous complications, especially respiratory failure and anesthesia-related complications. Obtain lung function tests (vital capacity, maximum minute ventilation, forced expiratory flow). Assess cardiac function and request a cardiology consultation if pulmonary hypertension cannot be ruled out. Blood workup should include serum electrolytes (potassium). Consider regional anesthesia (when indicated) if lung function is significantly jeopardized; however, keep in mind that an epidural anesthesia with a sensory level at T5 will decrease the vital capacity by almost 15% and may impede respiratory function and gas exchange. Postoperative mechanical ventilatory support almost always is required after major surgery and should be arranged beforehand.

Anesthetic considerations: There is a very high incidence of respiratory complications because of neuromuscular dysfunction. Although respiratory drive is considered normal in ALS, respiratory function and reserve are significantly compromised. Because the disease involves several cranial nerves, airway protection may not be adequate. Patients should always be considered high-risk candidates for aspiration. Consequently, a rapid sequence induction is recommended. The trachea should not be extubated before the patient is fully awake because of poor airway control and ventilatory muscles.

Pharmacological implications: Avoid succinylcholine because an exaggerated hyperkalemic response is possible. The sensitivity and duration of action of nondepolarizing muscle relaxants is markedly increased, so reduced doses are required and relaxation should be controlled with a peripheral nerve stimulator. To avoid using neuromuscular blocking agents, small doses of volatile anesthetic agents often are sufficient to achieve adequate surgical relaxation in ALS patients. Hemodynamic instability has been reported with halogenated agents. Because of autonomic nervous system involvement, the dose of atropine may be higher than normal to successfully treat bradycardia. Riluzole is primarily metabolized by

liver isoenzyme cytochrome P-450. Metabolism and elimination of other drugs using the same pathway may be altered.

Other conditions to be considered:

☞**DERMATOMYOSITIS AND POLYMYOSITIS:** Both diseases belong to a group of connective tissue disorders known as *idiopathic inflammatory myopathies.* They are a multisystem disease characterized by necrotizing inflammatory myopathy of striated muscles and a skin rash, both of unknown etiology.

☞**MYASTHENIA GRAVIS:** Neuromuscular disorder characterized by muscle weakness and rapid muscle fatigue. Usually apparent during adulthood, but onset can occur at any age. Most individuals present with eyelid ptosis, diplopia, and excessive muscle fatigue following exercise. Other features commonly include dysarthria, dysphagia, and proximal limb weakness. Approximately 10 percent develop potentially life-threatening complications resulting from severe respiratory depression (myasthenic crisis).

☞**PROGRESSIVE BULBAR PALSY OF CHILDHOOD:** Motor neuropathy affecting lower six cranial nerves but sparing the limbs. Deafness. X-linked or autosomal recessive. Age of onset is late childhood. Other features include excessive drooling, dysarthria, recurrent pulmonary aspiration, and pneumonia evolving to pulmonary failure. Limb involvement and pyramidal tract signs may develop later. Mortality within the first 2 decades of life.

REFERENCES:

Beach TP, Stone WA, Hamelberg W: Circulatory collapse following succinylcholine: Report of a patient with diffuse lower motor neuron disease. *Anesth Analg* 50:431, 1971.

Festoff BW, Suo Z, Citron BA: Prospects for the pharmacotherapy of amyotrophic lateral sclerosis: Old strategies and new paradigms for the third millennium. *CNS Drugs* 17:699, 2003.

Hara K, Sakura S, Saito Y, et al: Epidural anesthesia and pulmonary function in a patient with amyotrophic lateral sclerosis. *Anesth Analg* 83:878, 1996.

Andermann Syndrome

At a glance: Familial syndrome characterized by agenesis of the corpus callosum, mental retardation, and progressive sensorimotor neuropathy.

Synonym: Charlevoix Disease.

Incidence: Originally described in French Canadians from Charlevoix County, Quebec, Canada. Traced back to a couple married in Quebec City in the 17th century. The incidence in the Saguenay and Lac St.-Jean region in the province of Quebec has been estimated as 1:2100 live births. The carrier rate is 1:23 inhabitants.

Genetic inheritance: Autosomal recessive. The gene defect has been mapped to 15q13-q15.

Pathophysiology: Electromyography shows absence of sensory action potentials, slight reduction in motor nerve conduction velocity, and signs of denervation and reinnervation in the distal muscles of the lower extremities. Muscle biopsy shows angular fibers and atrophy. Overall pathologic picture is suggestive of a chronic demyelinating neuropathy.

Diagnosis: Characteristic features include brachycephaly with a long, triangular, asymmetrical facies with hypoplastic maxilla, large mandibular angle, high arched palate, protruding tongue, and prominent chin with a long lip to chin distance. Bilateral blepharoptosis, hypertelorism, nystagmus, mild ophthalmoplegia, and abnormal visual evoked potentials have been described. The clinical course provides valuable clues to the diagnosis. CT scans show total or partial agenesis of the corpus callosum.

Clinical aspects: Unremarkable neonatal period followed by hypotonia and slowing of motor development, starting at age 4 to 6 months. Although some patients can walk, by age 10 to 13 years they are wheelchair-bound or bed-bound. Areflexia, paraparesis, psychosis, and seizures are observed. Other features include diffuse hypotonia, absence of deep tendon reflexes, flexion contractures in the metacarpophalangeal joints, low-set thumbs, pes equinovarus, hammertoe deformity, syndactyly of the toes, and sensory neuropathy in a glove and stocking distribution. Progressive scoliosis becomes apparent with older age and may lead to severely restrictive lung function. Moderate mental retardation with an IQ ranging from 45 to 60 in the majority of cases.

Precautions before anesthesia: Evaluate pulmonary function (clinical, chest radiographs, CT, pulmonary function test, arterial blood gas analysis). Echocardiography should be performed if cor pulmonale and pulmonary hypertension are suspected. Assess the airway for difficult airway management. Evaluate neurologic function (clinical, full history, electroencephalogram, CT, MRI). Postoperative ventilatory support may be necessary and should be arranged beforehand.

Anesthetic considerations: No literature is available. Potentially difficult airway management in view of facial abnormalities. Spontaneous ventilation should be maintained until the airway is secured. Patients may not tolerate general anesthesia if respiratory function is severely reduced.

Pharmacological implications: Because of increased sensitivity to muscle relaxants, avoid depolarizing muscle relaxants and use nondepolarizing agents cautiously under the control of a peripheral nerve stimulator. Consider interaction between anesthetic drugs and antiepileptic treatment.

Other conditions to be considered: Numerous syndromes are associated with agenesis of the corpus callosum. The following list is not all-conclusive.

☞**AICARDI SYNDROME:** Combination of myoclonic seizures with characteristic EEG pattern, lacunar chorioretinopathy, and (complete or partial) agenesis of the corpus callosum is characteristic of this X-linked dominant inherited syndrome.

☞**SCHINZEL ACROCALLOSAL SYNDROME:** Very rare autosomal recessive, complex polymalformative disease with predominant neurologic and skeletal anomalies.

☞**FG SYNDROME:** X-linked form of mental retardation associated with complete or partial agenesis of the corpus callosum and minor facial, skeletal, and gastrointestinal anomalies.

☞**CEREBRORENODIGITAL SYNDROME:** Autosomal recessive inherited syndrome with corpus callosum agenesis, Dandy-Walker malformation, mental retardation, paraparesis or quadriparesis.

☞**DANDY-WALKER MALFORMATION:** Congenital anomaly of the cerebellum and fourth ventricle characterized by hypoplasia of the cerebellum and hydrocephalus resulting from cystic expansion of the fourth ventricle in the posterior fossa.

☞**HARD SYNDROME:** Very rare, severe autosomal recessive, quickly lethal acronymic syndrome with major neurologic impairment. Common features include *h*ydrocephalus, *a*gyria, and *r*etinal *d*ysplasia. It is characterized by type II lissencephaly in association with retinal dysplasia, obstructive hydrocephalus, and agenesis of the corpus callosum. Affected infants typically have severe growth failure, severe microcephaly, seizures, microphthalmia, and cataracts. Some affected infants have an occipital encephalocele.

☞**OPITZ-FRIAS SYNDROME:** Genetic disorder characterized by craniofacial anomalies, ocular hypertelorism, cleft lip/palate, epicanthal folds, and a wide, flat nasal bridge. Affected males present cryptorchidism, bifid scrotum, and/or hypospadias. The most significant anomalies are the presence of cleft in the larynx and trachea, pulmonary hypoplasia, dysphagia, and respiratory obstruction. Hypoplasia or agenesis of the corpus callosum, kidney abnormalities, cardiac defects, and mental retardation have been reported.

☞**PSAUME SYNDROME (Papillon Psaume Syndrome; OFD Type I):** Congenital X-linked syndrome lethal for males, characterized by orofacial and digital defects associated with cardiac and renal anomalies.

☞**RUBINSTEIN-TAYBI SYNDROME:** Rare syndrome characterized by craniofacial anomalies and complex multiple malformations, including cardiac, digestive, and respiratory.

REFERENCES:

De Braekeleer M, Dallaire A, Mathieu J: Genetic epidemiology of sensorimotor polyneuropathy with or without agenesis of the corpus callosum in northeastern Quebec. *Hum Genet* 91:223, 1993.

Hauser E, Bittner R, Liegl, C, et al: Occurrence of Andermann syndrome out of French Canada: Agenesis of the corpus callosum with neuronopathy. *Neuropediatrics* 24:107, 1993.

Larbrisseau A, Vanesse M, Brochu P, et al: The Andermann syndrome: Agenesis of the corpus callosum associated with mental retardation and progressive sensorimotor neuronopathy. *Can J Neurol Sci* 11:257, 1984.

Andersen Cardiodysrhythmic Periodic Paralysis Syndrome

At a glance: Characterized by the clinical triad of potassium-sensitive periodic paralysis (low, normal, or high potassium levels), ventricular arrhythmias (bigeminy, long QT interval, ectopy, bidirectional ventricular tachycardia), and dysmorphic facial features. Sudden death has been reported. Andersen syndrome must not be confused with Andersen disease (glycogen storage disease type IV).

Synonyms: Andersen Syndrome; Long QT Syndrome Type 7 (LQT7); Cardiodysrhythmic type of Potassium-Sensitive Periodic Paralysis.

Incidence: Exact incidence is unknown but probably fewer than 150 cases have been described.

Genetic inheritance: Autosomal dominant condition with clinical features of periodic paralysis and prolonged QT syndrome but genetically distinct from these conditions. However, sporadic cases have been reported, and the penetrance is highly variable. More than one gene may be involved. Research determined that Andersen cardiodysrhythmic periodic paralysis syndrome (ACPPS) is caused by mutations in the KCNJ2 gene. This gene has been mapped to 17q23 and encodes the inward rectifier K^+ channel Kir2.1, which is expressed in cardiac and skeletal muscle, explaining the combination of cardiac and skeletal muscle involvement.

Pathophysiology: Other forms of periodic paralysis result from mutations in skeletal muscle-specific Na^+, K^+, and Ca^{2+} channels. ACPPS is unique among the channelopathies because of the combination of a skeletal and a cardiac muscle phenotype. The potassium-sensitive periodic paralysis can be associated with hypokalemia, hyperkalemia, or normokalemia. Periodic paralysis occurs with different types of cardiac arrhythmias, most commonly prolonged QT syndrome and ventricular arrhythmias (ventricular bigeminy, bidirectional ventricular tachydysrhythmia, nonsustained ventricular tachycardia, frequent ventricular ectopy).

Diagnosis: Clinical triad of potassium-sensitive periodic paralysis, ventricular ectopy, and dysmorphic features are characteristic and allow for an early diagnosis. To prevent sudden cardiac death, cardiac evaluation with serial EKGs and measurements of QTc interval are essential and should be performed early for all patients undergoing workup for periodic paralysis. A prolonged QTc (QTc = QT/$\sqrt{RR}$) is present in most patients with ACPPS and is considered by some researchers to be a diagnostic sign. In general, the degree of facial dysmorphism does not correlate with the severity of heart and/or muscle involvement; often the dysmorphic features are mild. The age at onset of periodic paralysis varies from 4 to 18 years. Patients usually have proximal weakness that may exacerbate upon a hypokalemic challenge with intravenous glucose and insulin. However, because fluctuations in serum K^+ levels may trigger/exacerbate cardiac arrhythmias in these patients, provocative testing for hypokalemic or hyperkalemic periodic paralysis is contraindicated in ACPPS patients.

Clinical aspects: Dysmorphic features may include short stature, low-set ears (40%), hypertelorism (36%), broad nasal root, micrognathia (50%), prognathism, cleft palate or high arched palate (10%), clinodactyly (70%), syndactyly (11%), and scoliosis (11%). The main neurologic sign is periodic paralysis, which is not necessarily related to hyperkalemia or hypokalemia and usually presents with proximal muscle weakness (and not myotonia). Cardiac manifestations most often are prolonged QT syndrome and symptomatic or asymptomatic ventricular tachycardias. Patients have a higher risk for sudden cardiac death, although the incidences of syncope and cardiac arrest are significantly lower than in patients with type 1 and 2 long QT syndrome. ☞Long QT Syndrome is present in more than 70% of Andersen syndrome patients with the KCNJ2 mutation, and ventricular arrhythmias occur in 64%. Triggers for periodic paralysis are inconsistent but may include rest after activities, periods of inactivity, and sleep. Fasting, but also eating a large meal, and becoming chilled are other common triggers. Chemical fumes and vapors containing hydrocarbons (paint, gasoline, car exhaustion) have been described as triggers in some patients. Even for an individual patient, potassium shifts during attacks of weakness are inconsistent. This finding indicates that at one point paralysis may be caused by hypokalemia (most common form 55%), but the next time it may be triggered by hyperkalemia (22%). Potassium-sensitive ACPPS patients may become weak and develop QTc prolongation when they are hypokalemic. Carbonic anhydrase inhibitors are used in this form of periodic paralysis to reduce the frequency and severity of the attacks.

Precautions before anesthesia: Careful history and examination to determine the presence and potential triggers of proximal weakness. Determine association of K^+ level and weakness (which may be variable) if possible. Complete cardiovascular evaluation and consultation with a cardiologist should be obtained, including ECG to calculate the QTc interval. Consider continuation of all cardiac medications, particularly beta blockers. Preoperative blood workup should include electrolyte (K^+, Ca^{2+}) and blood glucose levels. Carefully evaluate the airway in view of micrognathia, prognathia, and high arched palate because they may result in difficult airway management. If scoliosis is severe (but most often is mild), lung function tests and echocardiography may be indicated, and arrangements for postoperative mechanical ventilation may be required. Pulmonary, hepatic, and thyroid function tests are recommended if the patient has been receiving amiodarone treatment for more than 1 year or shows specific symptoms.

Anesthetic considerations: Judicious sedative premedication may be useful to reduce sympathetic output and prevent QT interval prolongation. Avoid histamine-releasing drugs and halothane. Ensure the patient is deeply anesthetized prior to intubation and consider extubation while the patient still is under deep anesthesia (assuming no anatomical considerations or difficulties with airway management). Beta blockers to treat tachyarrhythmias should be available. Check serum electrolytes (K^+) frequently in the perioperative period. Although no reports about anesthetic management have been published, based upon knowledge from other forms of periodic paralysis, not administering succinylcholine in order to prevent rapid changes in the K^+ serum level and malignant hyperthermia seems prudent.

Pharmacological implications: Consider possible interactions between anesthetic drugs and cardiac medications. Patients may be receiving amiodarone and acetazolamide treatment. Appropriate drugs must be available for management of arrhythmias, particularly beta blockers (e.g., esmolol). See ☞Long QT Interval for an extensive list of drugs that affect the QT interval.

Other conditions to be considered:

☞**LONG QT SYNDROME:** Congenital or acquired adrenergic-induced ventricular arrhythmias.

☞**PERIODIC PARALYSIS:** Congenital abnormality in membrane electrolyte conductance leading to episodic muscle weakness.

☞**THYROTOXIC PERIODIC PARALYSIS:** Acquired disorder characterized by intermittent episodes of muscle weakness alternating with periods of normal muscular function. Occurs during hyperthyroidism and thyrotoxicosis. Hypokalemia is present during attacks. May be precipitated by low plasma concentration of insulin. Occurs predominantly in Asian males but also has been found in Latin American males.

REFERENCES:

Sansone V, Griggs RC, Meola G, et al: Andersen's syndrome: A distinct periodic paralysis. *Ann Neurol* 42:305, 1997.

Tristani-Firouzi M, Jensen JL, Donaldson MR, et al: Functional and clinical characterization of KCNJ2 mutations associated with LQT7 (Andersen syndrome). *J Clin Invest* 110:381, 2002.

Tawil R, Ptacek LJ, Pavlakis SG, et al: Andersen's syndrome: Potassium-sensitive periodic paralysis, ventricular ectopy, and dysmorphic features. *Ann Neurol* 35:326, 1994.

Angel-Shaped Phalangoepiphyseal Dysplasia (ASPED)

At a glance: Often referred to as *peripheral dysostosis.* Marked hyperextensibility of the fingers and precocious osteoarthritis of the hips. Characteristically, the middle phalanges represent an "angel-shaped phalanx," which results from modification of the epiphysis, diaphysis, and metaphysis, resembling the little angels used to decorate a Christmas tree.

Incidence and genetic inheritance: Extremely rare; exact incidence unknown. Autosomal dominant.

Clinical aspects: Clinical features and distinctive findings on radiologic examination of the phalanges. Angel-shaped phalanx results from a disturbance in the development of the epiphysis, diaphysis, and metaphysis resembling the little angels used to decorate a

Christmas tree. The wings are formed by a diaphyseal cuff, the skirt by a cone-shaped epiphysis, and the head by the distal pseudoepiphysis. Hyperextensibility of the fingers and precocious arthritis of the hips (coxarthrosis). Hypodontia (congenital absence of up to five teeth) is often present.

Anesthetic considerations: Positioning may be difficult, depending on the procedure and degree of coxarthrosis. Careful direct laryngoscopy is required in the presence of dental anomalies.

Other conditions to be considered:

☞**ARKLESS-GRAHAM SYNDROME:** Short hands and feet, short stature, and brachycephaly. Distinct facies characterized by prominent mandible (protruding jaw); small, broad, upturned nose with flat nasal bridge; and small mouth. Other features include skin, genital, dental, and musculoskeletal abnormalities. Mental retardation is present in 90% of children and can be severe.

☞**PSEUDOHYPOPARATHYROIDISM:** Very rare disorder characterized by renal and/or bony anomalies caused by insensitivity to parathyroid hormone.

REFERENCES:

Warashina H, Sakano S, Kitamura S, et al: Total hip arthroplasty for a patient with angel-shaped phalango-epiphyseal dysplasia (ASPED). A case report. *Nagoya J Med Sci* 65:103, 2002.

Graham JM Jr, Krakow D, Tolo VT, et al: Radiographic findings and Gs-alpha bioactivity studies and mutation screening in acrodysostosis indicate a different etiology from pseudohypoparathyroidism. *Pediatr Radiol* 31:2, 2001.

Giedion A, Prader A, Fliegel C, et al: Angel-shaped phalango-epiphyseal dysplasia (ASPED): Identification of a new genetic bone marker. *Am J Med Genet* 47:765, 1993.

Aniridia

At a glance: It is estimated that approximately one third of patients with sporadic aniridia will develop a Wilms tumor, and approximately half of patients with aniridia, genitourinary anomalies (e.g., hypospadias), and mental retardation will develop a Wilms tumor. The association with genitourinary anomalies and mental retardation is known as ☞WAGR Syndrome. Most patients have prominent lips and macrognathia. Other features may include congenital cataracts, nystagmus, ptosis, and blindness. The presence of ptosis and generalized hypotonia in a subgroup of patients suggests a susceptibility to malignant hyperthermia.

Incidence: Estimated between 1:60,000 and 1:100,000 live births. All races are affected.

Genetic inheritance: Both hereditary and sporadic forms exist. Approximately 30% of cases arise spontaneously. The usual form of inheritance is an autosomal dominant trait, but autosomal recessive transmission has been suggested for the rare Gillespie syndrome. There are two genetic loci for aniridia: aniridia type 1 (AN1) results from a defect on the short arm of chromosome 2; aniridia type 2 (AN2) has been related to a defect on 11p13. Aniridia as an isolated ocular malformation is an autosomal dominant disorder caused by a mutation in the *PAX6* (paired box gene family) gene located on 11p13. Although patients with a positive family history for aniridia do not have an increased risk for Wilms tumor, patients without a positive family history for aniridia (sporadic cases) have a 30% risk of developing Wilms tumor.

Pathophysiology: Aniridia is related to a primary arrest in the neuroectodermal development and a secondary disturbance of the three neural crest waves from the mesenchyme. Functional develop-

ment of the anterior segment is a complex interrelationship between neural ectoderm and the neural crest waves mesenchyme. Cellular and/or biochemical aberrations may result in malformation or regression of different layers of the anterior segment of the eye. The iris stroma is hypoplastic, and the extent of the defect ranges from slit-like lesions of the iris stroma only visible under slitlamp examination to coloboma-like defects and almost complete absence of the iris stroma. The root of the iris, however, is most often visible on gonioscopy. Aniridia has been produced experimentally in mice with maternal vitamin A deficiency.

Diagnosis: At birth, the iris is reduced to a small tube. In general, vision is decreased, with numerous other contributing anomalies including light scatter, corneal and lenticular opacities, severe glaucoma, nystagmus, optic nerve agenesis, and foveal hypoplasia.

Clinical aspects:

ANIRIDIA AND ABSENT PATELLA: This combination has been reported in three generations of one family. Bilateral cataracts and glaucoma complicated by aniridia and hypoplastic or aplastic patellae.

☞**GILLESPIE SYNDROME:** Typical presentation is discovery of fixed dilated pupils in a hypotonic infant. Neurologic signs include marked motor delay, hypotonia, disabling ataxia, and usually mental retardation. The combination with tetralogy of Fallot and/or cardiomyopathy has been reported.

ANIRIDIA, MICROCORNEA, AND SPONTANEOUSLY REABSORBED CATARACT: This combination has been described in three generations of one family. Patients have a poor prognosis of ocular function because of a high incidence of cataracts, glaucoma, corneal pannus, nystagmus, and foveal hypoplasia.

ANIRIDIA, PARTIAL, WITH UNILATERAL RENAL AGENESIS AND PSYCHOMOTOR RETARDATION: Congenital glaucoma, telecanthus, and frontal bossing; unilateral renal agenesis and mental retardation.

Precautions before anesthesia: If the clinical findings are limited to the eye, no specific considerations arise from this syndrome, except use of an anesthetic technique that does not cause further increase in intraocular pressure in patients with glaucoma. In contrast, some patients have cardiomyopathy, tetralogy of Fallot, generalized hypotonia, and scoliosis. Preoperative echocardiography is recommended to determine the lesions and their hemodynamic significance. The presence of Wilms tumor requires further diagnostic measures, such as abdominal ultrasound, CT scanning, and/or MRI. Preoperative blood workup should include a complete blood count (anemia), electrolytes, and assessment of renal function (creatinine, BUN). Mental and neurologic status (decreased vision/blindness) must be assessed for a thoughtful approach to premedication and induction.

Anesthetic considerations: Considerations are in reference to pediatric eye surgery and are the same for normal children as those with syndromes associated with congenital aniridia. Avoid measures that increase intraocular pressure and be aware of oculocardiac reflex. In patients with congenital cardiac lesions, the anesthetic approach must consider their hemodynamic consequences and the drug effects. Large-bore intravenous access and invasive blood pressure monitoring are recommended in patients undergoing surgery for Wilms tumor removal.

Pharmacological implications: Presence of ptosis and generalized hypotonia in Gillespie syndrome may suggest a susceptibility to malignant hyperthermia. Consequently, it would be prudent to avoid triggering drugs. Due to glaucoma, patients may be taking beta blockers (e.g., timolol, to reduce production of aqueous humor), parasympathomimetics (e.g., pilocarpine, to lower outflow resistance of aqueous humor), and carbonic anhydrase inhibitors (e.g., acetazolamide, to reduce secretion of aqueous humor), or a combination of these drugs. Even though these drugs are applied locally (except acetazolamide), they may have systemic side effects, which should be kept in mind while providing anesthesia.

Other conditions to be considered: The following syndromes are associated with Wilms tumor:

☞**WAGR SYNDROME:** Unusual association of Wilms tumor, ocular signs, and mental retardation.

☞**DENYS-DRASH SYNDROME:** Manifests in small children and consists of the triad of congenital nephropathy, Wilms tumor, and ambiguous genitalia.

☞**BECKWITH-WIEDEMANN SYNDROME:** Most often sporadically occurring syndrome with exomphalos, macroglossia, gigantism, and hypoglycemia resulting from hyperinsulinism.

☞**PERLMAN SYNDROME:** Neonatal gigantism accompanied by visceromegaly (especially renal dysplasia or tumour) and at risk for hypoglycemia. This condition consists of nephromegaly, renal dysplasia, Wilms tumor, macrosomia, hypotonia, cryptorchidism, and multiple facial dysmorphism (round full face, micrognathia, macrosomia).

REFERENCES:
Davis LM, Stallard R, Thomas GH: Two anonymous DNA segments distinguish the Wilms tumor and aniridia loci. *Science* 241:840, 1988.

Jotterand V, Boisjoly HM, Harnois C: 11p13 deletion, Wilms' tumour, and aniridia: unusual genetic, non-ocular and ocular features of three cases. *Br J Ophthalmol* 74:568, 1990.

Yanagidate F, Dohi S, Iizawa A: Anaesthetic management for a patient with WAGR syndrome. *Anaesthesia* 56:1215, 2001.

Ankyloblepharon Filiforme Adnatum and Cleft Palate

At a glance: This entity is an ectodermal dysplasia defect associated with a cleft lip/palate. It is most often associated with congenital filiform fusion of the eyelids.

Synonym: Congenital Filiform Fusion of the Eyelids with Cleft Palate and/or Cleft Lip.

Incidence and genetic inheritance: Ankyloblepharon filiform fusion of eyelids has been reported in approximately 30 cases. The association with cleft lip/palate has been described in fewer than 10 cases. The inheritance pattern is autosomal dominant with incomplete penetrance and variable expressivity. It is not certain whether this represents a separate mutation. No genetic background or molecular data are available.

Clinical aspects: In ankyloblepharon filiforme adnatum, the eyelid margins are partially or completely fused together with a normal horizontal fissure. The child presents with ectodermal defects: seborrhea of the scalp or elsewhere.

Anesthetic considerations: There is no evident impairment of general health in patients with this disorder. Three cases have been associated with trisomy 18 (Edwards syndrome), and the combination with hydrocephalus and a myelomeningocele has been described in one case.

Other conditions to be considered:

☞**AEC SYNDROME:** Autosomal dominant inherited disorder caused by a mutation in the tumor protein p63 gene located on 3q27. It is associated with normal intelligence, ankyloblepharon filiforme adnatum, atresia of the tear duct, sparse or absent eyelashes,

maxillary hypoplasia, cleft lip/palate, hypodontia or oligodontia, broad nasal bridge, atretic external auditory canal, and conductive hearing loss. Cardiac findings include ventricular septal defect and patent ductus arteriosus. Hypospadias and micropenis have been described in males. Dermatologic signs include palmoplantar hyperkeratosis, hyperpigmentation, scalp erosions, dystrophic nails, and sparse scalp and body hair with patchy alopecia. Depending on the procedure, subacute bacterial endocarditis prophylaxis may be required.

☞**CHANDS:** Autosomal recessive inherited disorder presenting with curly hairs, hypoplastic nails, and eyelid fusion.

☞**ECTRODACTYLY, ECTODERMAL DYSPLASIA, AND CLEFT LIP-PALATE (EEC) SYNDROME:** Autosomal dominant inherited syndrome with maxillary hypoplasia, mild malar hypoplasia, cleft lip/palate, choanal atresia, hearing loss, photophobia and blepharophimosis, dacryocystitis, cryptorchidism, hypogonadotropic hypogonadism renal agenesis or dysplasia, hydronephrosis, occasionally mental retardation, central diabetes insipidus.

☞**ADULT SYNDROME:** Main findings are hypodontia, very brittle and/or premature loss of permanent teeth, and ectrodactyly (split hands and feet). There is no evident impairment of general health in patients with ADULT syndrome.

REFERENCES:
Akkermans CH, Stern LM: Ankyloblepharon filiforme adnatum. *Br J Ophthalmol* 63:129, 1979.

Hay RJ, Wells RS: The syndrome of ankyloblepharon, ectodermal defects and cleft lip and palate: An autosomal dominant condition. *Br J Dermatol* 94:287, 1976.

Evans DGR, Evans ID, Donnai, D, et al: Ankyloblepharon filiforme adnatum in trisomy 18 Edwards syndrome. *J Med Genet* 27:720, 1990.

Antley-Bixler Syndrome

At a glance: Inherited syndrome with craniofacial dysmorphism and skeletal and other anomalies. Frequently associated with respiratory failure in the neonatal period.

Synonyms: Multisynostotic Osteodysgenesis with Long Bone Fractures; Trapezoidocephaly-Synostosis Syndrome.

History: First description in 1975 by Ray M. Antley and David Bixler, two American physicians.

Genetic inheritance: Inherited as an autosomal recessive genetic trait. A few cases may be sporadic or transmitted as an autosomal dominant trait. Parental consanguinity is a known risk factor.

Pathophysiology: The flavoprotein POR (cytochrome *P*-450 [*oxido*]*r*eductase) is the electron donor for all microsomal P-450 enzymes. Mutations in this POR gene could be demonstrated in patients with Antley-Bixler syndrome. The lack or malfunction of POR may result in accumulation of drugs and environmental toxins usually metabolized by hepatic cytochrome P-450, which may result in levels high enough to cause teratogenicity. Fluconazole is one drug that has been implicated in the pathogenesis of Antley-Bixler syndrome. This genetic defect has been mapped to 7q.11.2. The role of a mutation in the FGF-2 gene, which initially was suspected to be the cause of this disorder, now seems less certain. Abnormalities of the steroid biogenesis have been reported and seem to be at least partly responsible for the genital anomalies found in female patients.

Diagnosis: Based on clinical findings of trapezoidocephaly and multiple skeletal fusion. Craniofacial anomalies result in severe upper airway obstruction that can lead to death secondary to respiratory failure at birth or in the first weeks of life in approximately 50% of cases.

Clinical aspects: Multiple malformations predominately involve the head: severe midface hypoplasia, frontal bossing, craniosynostosis, brachycephaly, low-set dysplastic ears, small nose with low nasal bridge, anteverted nares, and choanal atresia are common. Acrocephaly, flat supraorbital ridges, proptosis, down-slanted palpebral fissures, hypertelorism, paresis of ocular muscles, cleft soft palate with bifid uvula, microstoma, and long philtrum are less common findings. Skeletal findings include narrowing of the rib cage, abnormal vertebrae, pelvic anomalies (narrow iliac wings), absent or abnormal (bowing) femora, radioulnar and radiohumeral synostosis, restricted joint mobility secondary to contractures, camptodactyly, arachnodactyly, talipes varus or valgus, and multiple fractures. Congenital fractures (in some cases multiple) have been described. Congenital cardiac defects (e.g., atrial septal defect), anomalies of the urinary tract (renal agenesis) and external female genitalia (vaginal atresia, hypoplastic labia majora, agglutinated labia minora), and imperforate anus may occur. Intellectual status can be normal, but variable degrees of mental retardation and hydrocephalus have been reported.

Precautions before anesthesia: Evaluate the airway carefully (clinically, radiographically, eventually use fiberoptic examination). Check overall joint mobility (particularly neck mobility and mouth opening). Determine neurologic status and rule out cardiac anomalies (clinically, echocardiographically, electrocardiographically). Check renal function (creatinine, BUN).

Anesthetic considerations: Airway management (mask ventilation, direct laryngoscopy, tracheal intubation) can be difficult because of facial malformations, as reflected by high mortality in the first weeks of life secondary to respiratory complications. Choanal atresia may require emergency tracheostomy at birth. Maintenance of spontaneous ventilation and oxygenation during attempts to control the airway is highly recommended. Be prepared to use alternative techniques to manage the airway (laryngeal mask, fiberoptic intubation). A surgeon familiar with surgical airway management and the necessary equipment should always be present in the operating room. Specific anesthetic measures are required in case of congenital heart disease or increased intracranial pressure. The eyes must be carefully protected because of the high risk for corneal damage as a result of proptosis. Intraoperative fluid regimen and anesthetic drugs choice must be adapted to renal function.

Pharmacological implications: Prophylactic antibiotics as indicated in case of cardiac lesions.

Other conditions to be considered:

☞**ACROCEPHALOSYNDACTYLY SYNDROMES:** Group of diseases characterized by craniofacial anomalies resulting from premature sutural craniosynostosis and hand and foot anomalies, primarily consisting of brachydactyly, syndactyly, and polysyndactyly. Although a number of different subtypes exists, considerable phenotypic overlap exists, and investigators now consider many of these syndromes to be variants of the same disease. Classification into subtypes reported in the literature is conflicting. Furthermore, classification of acrocephalosyndactyly versus acrocephalopolysyndactyly is regarded by many as a pseudodistinction.

REFERENCES:

Fluck CE, Tajima T, Pandey AV, et al: Mutant P450 oxidoreductase causes disordered steroidogenesis with and without Antley-Bixler syndrome. *Nat Genet* 36:228, 2004.

Bradley JP, Kawamoto HK, Taub P, et al: Antley-Bixler syndrome: Correction of facial deformities and long-term survival. *Plast Reconstr Surg* 111:1454, 2003.

LeBard SE, Thiemann LJ: Antley-Bixler syndrome: A case report and discussion. *Paediatr Anaesth* 8:89, 1998.

APECED Syndrome

At a glance: APECED is an acronym for *a*utoimmune *p*ol*y*endocrinopathy, *c*andidiasis, *e*ctodermal *d*ystrophy. This autoimmune syndrome is composed of multiple endocrinopathies associated with various other signs, including hepatitis and eye abnormalities. Can lead to premature death.

Synonyms: Whitaker Syndrome; Autoimmune Polyendocrinopathy Syndrome, type I; Polyglandular Autoimmune Syndrome Type I; Hypoadrenocorticism Hypoparathyroidism Moniliasis.

Incidence: Very rare syndrome. Occurs more frequently in Finland, where the prevalence in the general population is estimated to be 1:25,000 in the general population. Depending on the source, females are affected up to twice as often as males.

Genetic inheritance: Autosomal recessive and autosomal dominant inheritance are observed. This disorder may not be inherited as a simple mendelian recessive but may be autoimmune in nature.

Pathophysiology: Maps to 21q22.3. A mutation in the AIRE (autoimmune regulator) gene is responsible for pathogenesis of APECED syndrome.

Diagnosis: Determined by the presence of two of the three major clinical symptoms: (1) hypoparathyroidism (present in almost 80% of patients), (2) corticoadrenal hyperplasia or hypoplasia (>70%), and/or (3) chronic mucocutaneous candidiasis. It affects children and adults younger than 35 years and can be lethal in infancy or childhood.

Clinical aspects: Mucocutaneous candidiasis is most often the first symptom and usually appears between 3 and 5 years of age. Over the next 5 years, hypoparathyroidism very likely occurs, whereas adrenal insufficiency often takes another 5 years to become clinically manifest. This is the most common order and time frame; however, wide variations are possible, and the different organ manifestations of this disease can occur independent of each other. More than three fourths of APECED patients develop chronic hypoparathyroidism, which can lead to tetany with carpopedal spasms (Trousseau sign), Chvostek sign, acral paresthesias, laryngospasm, mild encephalopathy, seizures, cataracts, and papilledema. The ECG may show QT interval prolongation and ventricular arrhythmias. Signs of mineralocorticoid and glucocorticoid deficiency often occur simultaneously, although their onsets can be up to 3 years apart. Initial symptoms are chronic fatigue, weakness, anorexia, and orthostatic hypotension. Hyperpigmentation as a sign of primary adrenal insufficiency can be helpful for the differential diagnosis. Weight loss and arterial hypotension (not only associated with orthostasis) usually are late signs of Addisonian syndrome. Beside the endocrine features, patients may have hypogonadism (more frequent in women), insulin-dependent diabetes mellitus, hypoaldosteronism, and pituitary defects. Other organs affected may include the eye (keratopathy, keratoconjunctivitis, cataract, photophobia), teeth (enamel hypoplasia), skin (vitiligo, ectodermal dystrophy, alopecia, chronic mucocutaneous candidiasis), and gastrointestinal tract (malabsorption, diarrhea, chronic atrophic gastritis, pernicious anemia, chronic active hepatitis, cholelithiasis, asplenia).

Cerebral vascular anomalies and intracranial calcifications have been reported. Laboratory investigations may detect pernicious anemia, multiple autoantibodies, and abnormal phosphate and calcium metabolism.

Precautions before anesthesia: Evaluate endocrine status clinically and with laboratory investigations, including blood and urine electrolytes (phosphate and calcium), blood glucose, thyroid function tests, and echocardiography. Obtain a complete blood count (anemia). Evaluate cardiac status (clinical, ECG). Evaluate hepatic function in case of chronic hepatitis (clinical, laboratory investigations including coagulation tests, abdominal ultrasound).

Anesthetic considerations: Intraoperative fluid replacement must be adapted to adrenal function and preexisting electrolyte shifts. Strict asepsis is needed considering the immunologic status of these patients.

Pharmacological implications: Avoid hepatotoxic drugs. In case of hepatic failure, adapt the dosage of drugs with predominately hepatic elimination. Serum protein levels may be decreased and result in an increased fraction of free (active) drug concentration. Reduction in the dosage of drugs with high protein binding may be necessary. Perioperative steroid stress coverage may be required.

Other conditions to be considered:

AUTOIMMUNE POLYENDOCRINE DISEASE TYPE II (Schmidt Syndrome): Affects mainly middle-aged females and is characterized by the combination of Addisonian syndrome, autoimmune thyroid disease, and/or insulin-dependent diabetes mellitus. In contrast to APECED syndrome, which is more frequent, hypoparathyroidism is not a feature of this disorder. Inheritance most likely is autosomal dominant.

☞ADDISONIAN SYNDROME: Progressive weakness, anemia, hypoglycemia, and hyperpigmentation of the skin. Vomiting, apneic spells, cyanosis, vascular collapse, and cardiovascular shock may be consequential.

REFERENCES:

Halonen M, Eskelin P, Myhre AG, et al: AIRE mutations and human leukocyte antigen genotypes as determinants of the autoimmune polyendocrinopathy-candidiasis-ectodermal dystrophy phenotype. *J Clin Endocrinol Metab* 87:2568, 2002.

Whitaker JA, Landing BH, Esselborn VM, et al: Syndrome of familial juvenile hypoadrenocorticism, hypoparathyroidism and superficial moniliasis. *J Clin Endocrinol Metab* 16:1374, 1956.

Aplasia Cutis Congenita

At a glance: Most-often inherited disorder with circumscribed or more extensive skin lesions that also may involve underlying tissues. Neurologic and cardiac anomalies have been described.

Synonyms: Congenital Scalp Defect; Congenital Defects of Skull and Scalp.

Incidence: More than 500 cases have been described in the literature. No racial or sexual predilection has been reported.

Genetic inheritance: Autosomal dominant with great expression variability. However, autosomal recessive and sporadic cases also have been reported.

Pathophysiology: Beside genetic factors, several other mechanisms probably are involved. Amniotic bands resulting from early rupture of the amniotic membranes are considered responsible for a couple of cases of aplasia cutis congenita (ACC). Other mechanisms discussed in the pathogenesis of this disorder are environmental fac-

tors (e.g., toxins and teratogens [maternal cocaine abuse, misoprostol, methimazole during pregnancy], intrauterine infections) and early embryonic vascular abnormalities with compromised blood flow to a circumscribed area of the skin.

Diagnosis: Based on clinical findings. Skin lesions can occur anywhere on the body but are found most often on the scalp. More than 80% of solitary lesions are found on the scalp.

Clinical aspects: Noninflammatory and well-demarcated lesions have different shapes, with diameters ranging from 0.5 to 10 cm and dilated scalp veins radiating from the periphery of scalp defect. The defect often is located in the area of the vertex of the skull. In a few cases, almost complete absence of skin and skull bone (partial acrania) has been reported and associated with high mortality (infection, hemorrhage). The aspect of the lesions is quite variable because it depends upon the stage of uterine development when the insult occurs. Defects caused early in gestation may be healed before birth and appear as an atrophic transparent membrane or a fibrotic scar. However, defects that develop later in gestation may present as ulcerations of variable depth. Although most defects are limited to the epidermis, occasionally the ulcerations are deep and involve the underlying subcutaneous, periosteal, and osseous tissues or even the meninges. On the scalp, the alopecic and scarred area usually is surrounded by a rim of abnormal hair growth, known as the *hair collar sign*. Small defects usually heal under formation of an atrophic scar, and underlying osseous lesions close spontaneously within the first year of life. However, extensive or multiple lesions may require surgical excision and plastic surgery (skin grafting, tissue expanders, flaps) to close the defects. Aside from the formation of atrophic scars, truncal and limb defects heal surprisingly well. Other findings may include chest with pectus excavatum, supernumerary nipples, and ☞Poland Syndrome. Congenital cardiac lesions, such as tetralogy of Fallot, pulmonary valvular atresia, and ventricular septal defects, have been described in some patients. Various neurologic anomalies include mental retardation, seizures, spasticity, hemiparesis, encephalocele or exencephaly, porencephaly, and schizencephaly. Other features may affect the eyes (strabismus, microphthalmia) and genitourinary tract (cryptorchidism, renal duplication). Cutis marmorata telangiectatica congenita and dermatoglyphic abnormalities may be associated with ACC.

Precautions before anesthesia: Assess cardiac function in case of congenital lesions (clinically, ECG, echocardiography). Obtain information about eventual bone defects associated with skin lesions. Evaluate neurologic status (clinical, history, EEG). Preoperative blood workup should include renal parameters (electrolytes, creatinine, BUN).

Anesthetic considerations: Avoid manipulations to affected skin areas to prevent trauma (risk of hemorrhage, particularly for scalp lesions) or infection. If skin lesions are extensive, peripheral venous access may be difficult. Congenital cardiac lesions may require specific anesthetic technique.

Pharmacological implications: Prophylactic antibiotics in case of cardiac anomalies may be required. Antiepileptic medications may interfere with elimination of similarly metabolized drugs. Cautious intraoperative fluid regimen is required in case of significant renal dysfunction.

Other conditions to be considered:

BRONSPIEGEL ZELNICK SYNDROME: Extremely rare (<5 cases have been described), autosomal recessive inherited form of aplasia cutis. Initially characterized by the findings of ACC, symptoms of intestinal lymphangiectasia arise in infancy

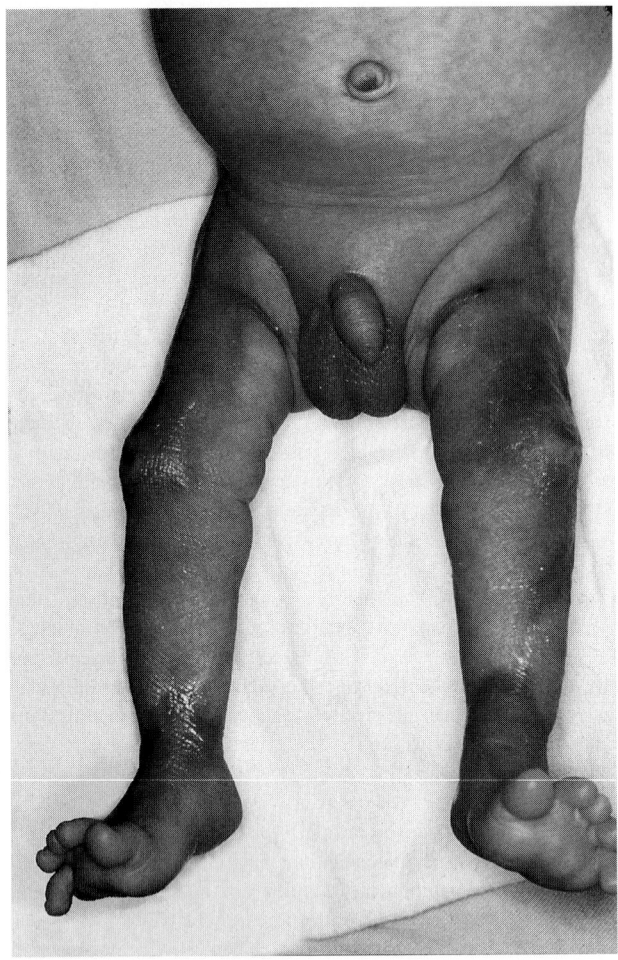

Aplasia cutis congenita Skin defects in a boy with aplasia cutis congenita. See color plates.

or early childhood with hypoproteinemia, generalized edema, humoral immune deficiency, lymphopenia, and malabsorption.

☞**ADAMS-OLIVER SYNDROME:** Very rare inherited disorder characterized by defects of the scalp associated with multiple scarred and hairless areas that usually have dilated blood vessels directly under the skin. Scalp defects are present at birth. The extremities are either short (hypoplastic fingers and toes) or characterized by absent hands and lower legs. Congenital heart defect must be ruled out.

☞**CUTIS MARMORATA TELANGIECTATICA CONGENITA:** Congenital cutaneous disorder with persistent cutis marmorata, telangiectasia, and phlebectasia. Often reported in association with a variety of other congenital anomalies.

☞**EPIDERMAL NEVUS SYNDROME:** Genetically transmitted neurodermatosis characterized by epidermal nevi, odontodysplasia, mental retardation, and various malformations.

☞**EPIDERMOLYSIS BULLOSA:** Group of inherited bullous disorders characterized by blister formation in response to mechanical trauma.

☞**JOHANSON-BLIZZARD SYNDROME:** Polymalformative syndrome characterized by nasal alar hypoplasia (beak-shaped), scalp defects, hypothyroidism, pancreatic achylia, and congenital deafness.

☞**GOLTZ SYNDROME:** Complex mesoectodermal hereditary disorder characterized by focal dermal atrophy with herniation of fat-producing multiple papillomas, in association with skeletal, dental, ocular, and other anomalies.

☞**SETLEIS SYNDROME:** Puckered periorbital skin; absent or multiple rows of eyelashes.

☞**STREETER ANOMALY:** Constricting amniotic bands leading to amputation with scarring, distal syndactyly, cleft lip/palate, anencephaly, encephalocele, hydrocephaly, omphalocele, and gastroschisis. Other internal anomalies involve the heart, lungs, diaphragm, kidneys, and gonads.

REFERENCES:

Ribuffo D, Costantini M, Gullo P, et al: Aplasia cutis congenita of the scalp, the skull, and the dura. *Scand J Plast Reconstr Surg Hand Surg* 37:176, 2003.

Martinez-Lage JF, Almagro MJ, Lopez Hernandez F, et al: Aplasia cutis congenita of the scalp. *Childs Nerv Syst* 18:634, 2002.

Kelly BJ, Samolitis NJ, Xie DL, et al: Aplasia cutis congenita of the trunk with fetus papyraceus. *Pediatr Dermatol* 19:326, 2002.

Apolipoprotein C-II Deficiency

At a glance: Inborn error of metabolism characterized by deficiency of a cofactor necessary for activation of lipoprotein lipase. Diabetes mellitus, pancreatitis, and epigastric pain are often associated. It does not exclude the possibility of angina in early age and congestive heart failure.

Synonym: Hyperlipoproteinemia Type IB.

Genetic inheritance: Autosomal recessive. Mutations in the apolipoprotein C-II (APOC2) gene, which has been mapped to 19q13.2, are considered responsible for the disorder.

Pathophysiology: Apolipoprotein C-II is a cofactor for activation of lipoprotein lipase, the enzyme that hydrolyzes triglycerides in plasma and transfers fatty acids to tissues. Deficiency of apolipoprotein C-II leads to marked elevation of plasma triglycerides and chylomicronemia.

Diagnosis: Based on clinical findings and the presence of chylomicrons in fasting plasma. Fasting triglyceride levels are characteristically greater than 10 mmol/l.

Clinical aspects: Despite hypertriglyceridemia, patients usually do not seem to be at risk for premature development of atherosclerosis. Recurrent bouts of pancreatitis are common and may result in life-threatening necrotizing pancreatitis. Eruptive xanthomas are seen in the skin, and mild hepatosplenomegaly may occur. Frequent episodes of epigastric pain are common. Patients may develop diabetes mellitus. A diet low in long-chain fatty acids can be helpful in reducing symptoms. However, a severe infantile form of apolipoprotein C-II deficiency with massive hyperchylomicronemia and severe encephalopathy has been described in a 5-week-old girl from consanguineous parents. Symptoms included lethargy, macrocephaly, marked hepatosplenomegaly, and severely hyperlipemic blood with significant hypercholesterolemia and hypertriglyceridemia. Cranial MRI revealed marked cerebral atrophy with extradural and intraocular fatty deposits. Developmental delay and other neurologic abnormalities were severe and did not improve despite appropriate diet, which resulted in normalization of the plasma lipid profile. This child was homozygous for apolipoprotein deficiency II, which explains the severity of the disease.

Precautions before anesthesia: Patients may have diabetes mellitus. The possibility of angina pectoris occurring at an early age cannot be excluded. Congestive heart failure must be excluded and treated appropriately if present.

Anesthetic considerations: Anesthesia management for this condition has not been described, but no particular difficulties should be anticipated. A patient with evidence of diabetes mellitus or coronary heart disease should receive anesthetic management according to standard protocols used for each underlying medical condition.

Pharmacological implications: Propofol has been associated with postoperative pancreatitis and probably should not be used in these patients.

Other conditions to be considered:

☞**BERARDINELLI-SEIP SYNDROME:** Inherited disorder with hyperinsulinemia resulting from insulin resistance combined with lipodystrophy and acromegaloid features.

☞**HYPERLIPOPROTEINEMIA TYPE I:** Inherited inborn error of metabolism characterized by a massive accumulation of chylomicrons and triglycerides in plasma resulting in recurrent abdominal pain and hepatosplenomegaly.

HYPERLIPIDEMIA TYPE IIA: Genetic disorder of lipid metabolism causing accumulation of cholesterol, thus increasing the risk of cardiovascular diseases. Hypercholesterolemia, Low-Density Lipoprotein—LDL—Receptor Disorder.

☞**KOBBERLING DUNNIGAN SYNDROME:** Genetically transmitted metabolic disorder characterized by partial lipodystrophy, insulin resistance leading to glucose intolerance, and hypertriglyceridemia. Affects children and young adults. Onset is slow, manifested by progressive loss of subcutaneous fat. Other features include hypocomplementemia, glomerulonephritis, and autoimmune disorders. Affects mostly women.

☞**PHYTOSTEROLEMIA:** Rare inherited disorder characterized by congenital hypercholesterolemia, presenting clinically with tendon xanthomas, premature coronary artery disease, and atherosclerosis.

REFERENCES:

Wilson CJ, Oliva CP, Maggi F, et al: Apolipoprotein C-II deficiency presenting as a lipid encephalopathy in infancy. *Ann Neurol* 53:807, 2003.

Bijvoet SM, Bruin T, Kastelein JJ: The familial hyperchylomicronaemia syndrome. *Neth J Med* 42:36, 1993.

Ohno M, Ishibashi S, Nakao K, et al: A neonatal case of apolipoprotein C-II deficiency. *Eur J Pediatr* 148:550, 1989.

Argininemia

At a glance: Urea cycle disorder that leads to hyperammonemia and neurologic symptoms, which are less severe than in other forms of urea cycle abnormalities.

Synonyms: Arginase Deficiency; Hyperargininemia; ARG1 Deficiency.

Incidence: Unknown. No sexual predilection.

Genetic inheritance: Autosomal recessive. Numerous mutations have been mapped to 6q23.

Pathophysiology: The hepatic urea cycle is the major pathway for metabolism and elimination of proteins and amino acids. Arginase is the mediator of the terminal step in the urea cycle, explaining the relatively mild clinical expression of the disease. Multiple allelic variants exist. The two isoenzymes of arginase—arginase-I (found

in the liver) and arginase-II (located in the kidneys)—are specified by separate gene loci, called ARG1 (located on 6q23) and ARG2 (on 14q24.1-q24.3). The arginase-I isoenzyme contributes 98% of the arginase activity in the liver, and its absence is the cause of argininemia. Isoenzyme type II is inducible, and its activity may increase up to fourfold in patients suffering from argininemia. Arginase-II is used to metabolize arginine (released from hepatocytes) to produce urea and ornithine. While this urea is excreted, the newly synthesized ornithine returns to the liver and is incorporated in the urea cycle. Hyperammonemia in arginase deficiency can be severe but most often is mild to moderate because arginase-II can take over a certain degree of arginase-I function and because arginine (containing two nitrogen molecules) still can be released by the liver and then cleared by the kidneys. The first reason is that formed arginine, which contains two waste nitrogen molecules, can be released from the hepatocyte and excreted in urine.

Diagnosis: Generally based on clinical findings of delayed development, protein intolerance, and spasticity. However, these symptoms are unspecific, and the diagnosis may be difficult and missed for a significant period of time. Diagnosis is confirmed by a red cell arginase assay. Prenatal diagnosis is possible using DNA analysis.

Clinical aspects: Onset typically is during the neonatal period. Main features include failure to thrive, signs of hyperammonemia (anorexia, irritability, tachypnea, lethargy, vomiting), and additional neurologic signs (progressive spastic quadriplegia, seizures, mental retardation, hyperactivity). Coma and cerebral edema may occur. Usually mild hepatomegaly can occur. Laboratory findings include hyperammonemia, hyperarginemia, di-amino-aciduria (arginuria, lysinuria, cystinuria, ornithinuria), oroticaciduria, pyrimidinuria, and elevated amino acid levels in the cerebrospinal fluid (arginine, ornithine, aspartate, threonine, glycine, methionine). Stress and infection can trigger an attack.

Precautions before anesthesia: Assess neurologic function and review the electroencephalogram. Check liver function (clinically and with laboratory investigations such as transaminases, γ-glutamyltransferase, bilirubin levels, coagulation tests, proteins). Check for signs of hypovolemia in case of recurrent vomiting; check electrolytes.

Anesthetic considerations: Perioperative nutrition should aim for high carbohydrate intake and low protein intake to prevent arginine load. To prevent a catabolic state, avoid longer fasting periods and/or cover them with dextrose-containing intravenous solutions. Prevent oral, pharyngeal, and gastrointestinal bleeding (because of risk of hyperammonemia from absorption of blood) and consider a nasogastric tube for aspiration and irrigation.

Pharmacological implications: Consider interactions among antiepileptic medications, liver function, and anesthetic drugs. Patients often are taking benzoate or phenylacetate (phenylbutyrate), which provide alternative routes for elimination of waste nitrogen. Transamination of benzoate leads to hippurate, which is easily excreted by the kidneys. Conversion of phenylacetate to phenylacetyl-CoA allows for conjugation with glutamine to form phenylacetyl glutamine. Both pathways result in elimination of ammonia. Phenylbutyrate offers the advantage of better taste for oral administration than phenylacetate.

Other conditions to be considered:

☞**CITRULLINEMIA:** Syndrome arising from argininosuccinate synthetase deficiency leading to hyperammonemia and neurologic consequences.

☞**HHH SYNDROME:** Genetically transmitted inborn error of metabolism resulting from a defect in the transport of ornithine into the mitochondrial matrix, clinically characterized by early growth retardation, learning disabilities, periodic confusion, and ataxia.

☞**METHYLMALONIC ACIDEMIA:** Heterogeneous inborn error of metabolism leading to metabolic acidosis and accumulation of methylmalonic acid and its by-products.

☞**N-ACETYLGLUTAMATE SYNTHETASE DEFICIENCY:** Congenital mitochondrial disorder that affects the metabolism of ammonium and results in hyperammonemia.

☞**ORNITHINE CARBAMOYLTRANSFERASE DEFICIENCY:** Rare genetic disorder characterized by complete or partial lack of the enzyme ornithine transcarbamylase. Lack of this enzyme results in excessive hyperammonemia, which is a known neurotoxin. Clinically, patients present with vomiting, refusal to eat, progressive lethargy, and coma.

☞**PROPIONIC ACIDEMIA:** Inborn error of metabolism affecting the mitochondrial catabolism of valine and isoleucine. Untreated, the disorder results in ketoacidosis, lethargy, coma, and finally death.

REFERENCES:

Iyer R, Jenkinson CP, Vockley JG, et al: The human arginases and arginase deficiency. *J Inherit Metab Dis* 21(suppl 1):86, 1998.

Prasad AN, Breen JC, Ampola MG, et al: Argininemia: A treatable genetic cause of progressive spastic diplegia simulating cerebral palsy: Case reports and literature review. *J Child Neurol* 12:301, 1997.

Santos Silva E, Martins E, Cardoso ML, et al: Liver transplantation in a case of argininaemia. *J Inherit Metab Dis* 24:885, 2001.

Arginosuccinic Acid Lyase Deficiency

At a glance: Rare inherited enzymatic disorder characterized by severe hyperammonemia. Affected infants clinically present with vomiting, lack of appetite and failure to thrive, progressive lethargy, severe hypotonia, and coma. This entity is part of a group of disorders called *urea cycle disorders* (described later).

Synonyms: Arginosuccinic Aciduria; ASL Deficiency; Arginino Succinase Deficiency; ASA Deficiency.

Incidence and genetic inheritance: Inherited as an autosomal recessive genetic transmission.

Pathophysiology: Argininosuccinate lyase is one of six enzymes that play a role in the metabolism of nitrogen from the body, preventing accumulation of amino acids from metabolic protein waste and development of hyperammonemia.

Clinical aspects: Severity varies among patients. A severe form of the disorder, characterized by *complete absence* of the enzyme, usually is present in the neonatal period and is called the *severe form*. A milder form of the disorder, characterized by *partial absence* of the enzyme, affects infants later during infancy or early childhood. A *late-onset form*, which occurs in adults, has been identified. Hyperammonemia is the main characteristic of this disease. The *severe form* of argininosuccinic aciduria occurs 24 to 72 hours after birth, usually after feeding. This form of the disease is clinically characterized by refusal to eat, severe failure to thrive, lethargy, vomiting, and neurologic irritability, often suggesting seizures. Affected infants may experience respiratory abnormalities, cerebral edema, and hepatomegaly. Hyperammonemic coma has been reported. If it is left untreated for more than 72 hours, neurologic abnormalities such as severe developmental delays and mental retardation are trademarks of surviving infants. Death is always inevitable for those not treated immediately. In infants with *partial enzyme deficiency,* onset of the disorder usually occurs later during infancy or childhood. Clinically, the symptomatology includes failure to grow and thrive, protein-free diet, ataxia, lethargy, and vomiting. Other features include dry brittle hair that may result in alopecia. These infants may alternate between periods of wellness and hyperammonemia. Hyperammonemic coma and life-threatening complications are potential complications.

Anesthetic considerations: Considerations are several. The children may require anesthesia while they are in systemic failure. Careful preoperative assessment of cardiovascular and neurologic status is important. Acute metabolic encephalopathy, associated with severe cerebral edema and significant raised intracranial pressure, may be present at induction. The possibility of subclinical seizure activities during anesthesia must be considered. Administration of intravenous antiepilepsy medication should be kept in mind. Severe hepatomegaly and respiratory abnormalities are among the anesthetic considerations. Administration of high-calorie fluid, without protein, must be given preoperatively. The potential risks of pulmonary aspiration after gastrointestinal surgery may lead to acute respiratory decompensation because of high protein load. Severe metabolic acidosis must be treated immediately. The decision to administer general anesthesia can be made based only on the patient's general health condition. The most important precautions must be taken to prevent sudden cardiovascular depression and loss of systemic vascular resistance in patients already presenting without any systemic reserve.

Other conditions to be considered:

UREA CYCLE DISORDERS are a group of rare disorders that affect the urea cycle. The consequence of this enzymatic disorder leads to a failure in the biochemical processes of nitrogen conversion to urea. The symptoms of all urea cycle disorders vary in severity and result from severe hyperammonemia. It is clinically characterized by a lack of appetite, vomiting, drowsiness, seizures, and eventually coma. Hepatomegaly may be present. Life-threatening complications may result if the disorder is not treated immediately. In addition to *argininosuccinic aciduria,* the other urea cycle disorders are carbamyl phosphate synthetase deficiency; argininosuccinate synthetase deficiency (☞citrullinemia); ornithine transcarbamylase deficiency; arginase deficiency and ☞N-acetylglutamate synthetase deficiency.

☞**REYE SYNDROME** is a rare childhood disorder characterized by liver failure, encephalopathy, hypoglycemia, and hyperammonemia. The disorder usually follows a viral infection. Administration of aspirin to children recovering from chicken pox or influenza has been implicated. Deficiencies of urea cycle enzymes may have a role in the development of Reye syndrome. Symptoms include vomiting, diarrhea, tachypnea, irritability, fatigue, and behavioral changes. Neurologic symptoms may be life-threatening and include seizures, stupor, and coma.

ORGANIC ACIDEMIAS are a rare group of inherited metabolic disorders characterized by accumulation of amino acids in response to failure of enzymatic reactions. It is clinically characterized by hypotonia, poor feeding, vomiting, lethargy, and seizures. The symptoms may progress to coma and life-threatening complications if the disorders are not treated. A genetic transmission has been suggested for these disorders.

REFERENCES:

Lee B, Goss J: Long-term outcome of urea cycle disorders. *J Pediatr* 138:S-62, 2001.

Kamoun P, Fensom AH, Shin YS, et al: Prenatal diagnosis of urea cycle diseases: A survey of European cases. *Am J Med Genet* 55:247, 1995.

Arkless-Graham Syndrome

At a glance: Short stature, hands and feet, and brachycephaly. Distinct facies characterized by prominent mandible, small, broad nose with flat nasal bridge, and small mouth. Other abnormalities affect skin, genitals, teeth, and musculoskeletal system. Mental retardation is present in 90% of children and can be severe.

Synonyms: Acrodysostosis Syndrome; Maroteaux-Malamut Syndrome.

Genetic inheritance: Chromosome studies have been normal. An autosomal dominant inheritance pattern has been described in two families. Sporadic cases have been described. The average parental age was slightly increased compared to the general parent population, which suggests advanced parental age is a risk factor for the condition.

Pathophysiology: Unknown. Some researchers consider the disorder to be a normocalcemic variant of pseudohypoparathyroidism.

Diagnosis: Based on clinical features, with absence of endocrine abnormalities distinguishing it from pseudohypoparathyroidism. Epiphyseal stippling on radiologic examination is a constant finding in infancy.

Clinical aspects: The most common manifestations (present in >75% of patients) include mental retardation and/or learning difficulties, hypoplasia of the nose (short, broad nose with depressed nasal bridge) and the maxilla (often with prognathism), peripheral dysostosis, hyperplasia of the first ray of the foot, acromesomelic brachymelia, and decreased interpedicular distance of the vertebrae. A small mouth and marked hearing loss are other common findings. On radiologic examination advanced skeletal maturation is seen in combination with cone-shaped epiphyses, peripheral dysostosis, and abnormal metacarpophalangeal pattern profile. The hands and feet appear small secondary to shortening of the tubular bones. Poor growth results in brachymelic dwarfism.

Precautions before anesthesia: Mental retardation and hearing loss may make the management of these patients difficult. Sedative or anxiolytic premedication and the presence of the primary caregiver during induction may be helpful. Careful assessment of the airway in consideration of difficult airway management (hypoplastic maxilla, vertebral anomalies) is needed. Blood workup should include electrolytes, particularly calcium and phosphate levels to rule out pseudohypoparathyroidism.

Anesthetic considerations: Hypoplasia of the maxilla may lead to airway obstruction under anesthesia. Maintenance of spontaneous ventilation until the airway has been secured is recommended. Significant restrictions of hands, feet, and spine mobility may make positioning difficult and requires careful padding.

Pharmacological implications: Avoid neuromuscular blockers until the airway has been secured.

Other conditions to be considered:

☞**ALBRIGHT HEREDITARY OSTEODYSTROPHY:** Syndrome presenting with round face, short stature, short neck, and obesity. Subcutaneous and intracranial calcifications, seizures, and neuromuscular problems such as fatigue and muscle cramps. Pseudohypoparathyroidism and hypocalcemia.

REFERENCES:

Hernandez RM, Miranda A, Kofman-Alfaro S: Acrodysostosis in two generations: An autosomal dominant syndrome. *Clin Genet* 39:376, 1991.

Butler MG, Rames LJ, Wadlington WB: Acrodysostosis: Report of a 13-year-old boy with review of literature and metacarpophalangeal pattern profile analysis. *Am J Med Genet* 30:971, 1988.

Arnold-Chiari Syndrome

At a glance: Depending on the type, the disorder can be associated with hydrocephalus, raised intracranial pressure, and respiratory and cardiac center dysfunction. Infants may exhibit vomiting, weakness, and mental impairment.

Synonyms: Cerebromedullary Malformation Syndrome.

Definition: In 1883, John Cleland, a British poet and anatomist, first described the abnormality of the brainstem and cerebellum. The two German pathologists Hans Chiari in 1891 and Julius Arnold in 1894 further detailed this anomaly in children with hydrocephalus. The term *Arnold-Chiari syndrome* (ACS) was coined in 1907 by the students of Arnold (not honoring Cleland's work). It comprises a variety of anatomical abnormalities resulting from a bony defect in the posterior fossa and upper cervical spine. This process results in herniation of the cerebellar vermis and choroid plexus through the foramen magnum, with elongation of the medulla and fourth ventricle, and noncommunicating hydrocephalus.

Classification:

Type I: Displacement of the often elongated cerebellar tonsils through the foramen magnum into the cervical spinal canal. The medulla oblongata may be slightly displaced, kinked, or compressed. The vermis cerebelli and the fourth ventricle most often are not or are only mildly involved. The degree of hydrocephalus, hydromelia (distension of the central canal), and syringomyelia (distension of the paracentral cavities) is variable. Myelomeningocele is not a feature of this type of ACS; however, other cranial and vertebral abnormalities occur in approximately one fourth of patients and may include atlantooccipital fusion, abnormal positioning of the odontoid process, ☞Klippel-Feil Syndrome, cervical ribs, fused thoracic ribs, and kyphoscoliosis. This type of ACS is also called the *adult type* because many of the patients were not (and often still are not) diagnosed before the second or third decade of life in the era before CT and MRI.

Type II: Usually manifested by severe hydrocephalus and myelomeningocele in infancy. Radiologically, type II is characterized by a relatively small posterior fossa, which results in elongation of the pons and the fourth ventricle into the spinal canal, displacement of the medulla oblongata, and crowding of the cervical cord roots into an upward course (upward herniation). Kinking of the medulla at the cervicomedullary junction occurs in more than 50% of cases. This form of ACS is frequently associated with other anomalies of the central nervous system, such as aqueductal stenosis with occlusive hydrocephalus (often presenting after repair of myelomeningocele, dysgenesis of the corpus callosum, syringomyelia, hydromyelia, ☞Diastematomyelia, and tethered cord). Other anomalies affect the first two cervical vertebrae (incomplete segmentation and/or malrotation).

Type III and Type IV: These two types are extremely rare.

Type III refers to the combination of cervical spina bifida with cerebellar herniation through the foramen magnum. The Type IV designation has been used by some researchers to describe severe cerebellar hypoplasia without cerebellar displacement through the foramen magnum.

Incidence: Approximately 1:1000 live births. ACS type II is present in almost all children with myelomeningocele and becomes symptomatic in approximately 20% of the children during infancy. A slight predilection for females has been reported.

Genetic inheritance: A few cases of Arnold-Chiari syndrome with an autosomal recessive inheritance associated with myelomeningocele and prenatal onset have been reported in the literature.

Pathophysiology: Generally, this malformation appears to be multifactorial and fundamentally the same as anencephaly and spina bifida. Caudal fixation of the cord and traction on the brainstem during growth may play a role. The importance of abnormal fluid pressures during development of the neural tube cannot be excluded. Another possible etiology is overexpansion of the nervous system within the bony vertebrae.

Diagnosis: Early hydrocephalus associated with Arnold-Chiari syndrome usually occurs when myelomeningocele causes paralysis below the level of the lesion. These babies usually present for primary closure in the first few days of life. Many surgeons electively insert a ventriculoperitoneal shunt at the time of repair because most patients will become symptomatic within the first month of life. Late presentation usually is symptomatic of posterior fossa hydrocephalus, which is confirmed by CT or MRI.

Clinical aspects: There is a wide variety of symptoms. Patients suffering from *Type I ACS* often have a long-standing history of (suboccipital) headache. In hindsight, these patients often were labeled as clumsy. The degree of tonsillar ectopia and the severity of neurologic symptoms usually are directly correlated. Tonsillar herniation of more than 12 mm into the spinal canal almost always is symptomatic. A trauma, although minor in most cases, often precedes the onset of symptoms. Ophthalmologic symptoms include photophobia, diplopia, and retrobulbar pain. Vertigo and dizziness, nystagmus, and hearing problems have been reported. Spinal cord dysfunction affects almost all patients with syringomyelia and approximately two thirds of patients without syringomyelia. Compression of the spinal cord may result in paresthesias, ataxia, weakness or paralysis, and bowel and bladder control problems. Compression of the medulla may cause dysphagia, dysphasia, cranial nerve palsies, apnea, palpitations, and sudden cardiac death. Vocal cord paralysis with stridor, aspiration, and respiratory distress have been described. At any age, patients may have abnormal response to hypoxia and/or hypercarbia secondary to brainstem dysfunction.

In *Type II ACS*, neonates or infants most often present with rapid progressive neurologic deterioration. The symptoms usually occur after the first 2 weeks of life. Life-threatening symptoms may occur and be associated with dysfunction of the medulla oblongata (respiratory center) and cranial nerves IX and X. In fact, small hemorrhagic infarctions in the medulla of these patients are not an uncommon finding. In infancy, respiratory distress with inspiratory stridor and episodic apnea is a common sign and may indicate impending brainstem compression. Obstructive apnea may be the result of bilateral vocal cord palsy. Dysphagia with absent gag reflex may lead to recurrent aspirations and further compromise ventilation. Weakness and painful spasticity may involve all four extremities. Scoliosis may already be present. If symptoms start later in childhood, onset is more gradual and may include syncope, nystagmus, ataxia, hyperreflexia, weakness of the arms, or spastic quadriparesis. Gas-

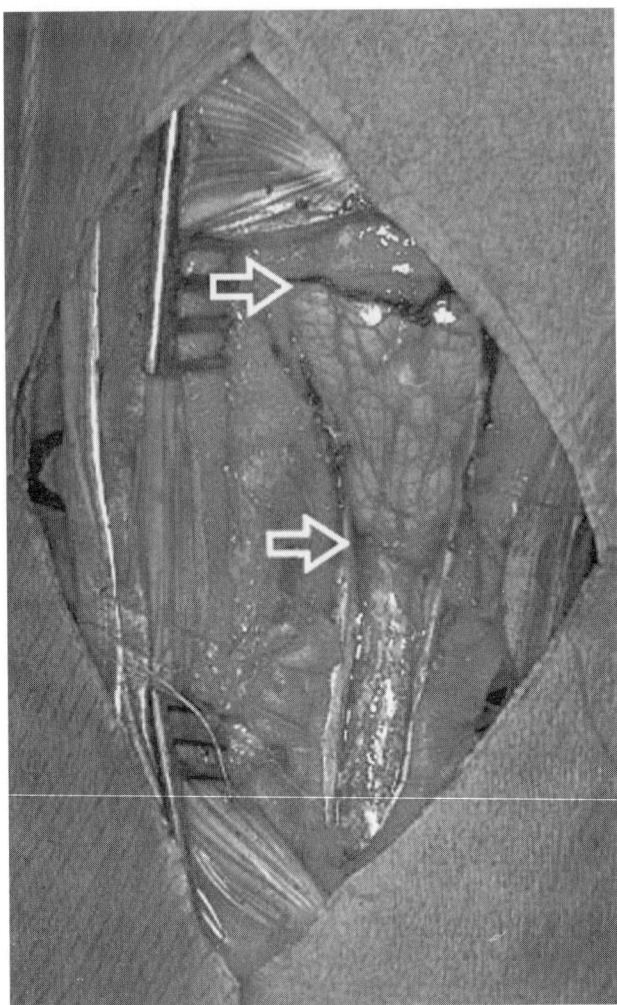

Arnold-Chiari syndrome Caudal displacement of the cerebellar tonsils (between *arrows*) into the opened spinal canal (dorsal laminae removed) in a patient undergoing surgery for Arnold-Chiari syndrome.

troesophageal reflux disease and depressed cough reflex may result in recurrent aspirations. Morbidity and mortality from ACS type II (as a result of hindbrain dysfunction) is significant. The mortality rate of ACS type II is approximately 15% during infancy, and long-term survival rarely exceeds 50%.

Precautions before anesthesia: The time of presentation may involve evaluation of a premature infant and assessment of other abnormalities. The association with myelomeningocele affects preoperative assessment and the anesthetic plan, particularly difficulties with regard to positioning for intubation. Infection and paralysis are other issues associated with myelomeningocele. Preoperative assessment should include an evaluation for signs of increased intracranial pressure and brainstem and/or cervical cord compression. If recurrent aspiration is a problem, preoperative chest radiograph and arterial blood gas analysis are recommended. Occasionally, patients require preoperative tracheal intubation because of recurrent aspiration. Obtain ECG to check for arrhythmias.

Anesthetic considerations: Anesthetic considerations include prematurity and heat conservation, ventilation pressures, and glucose requirements. The presence of myelomeningocele requires

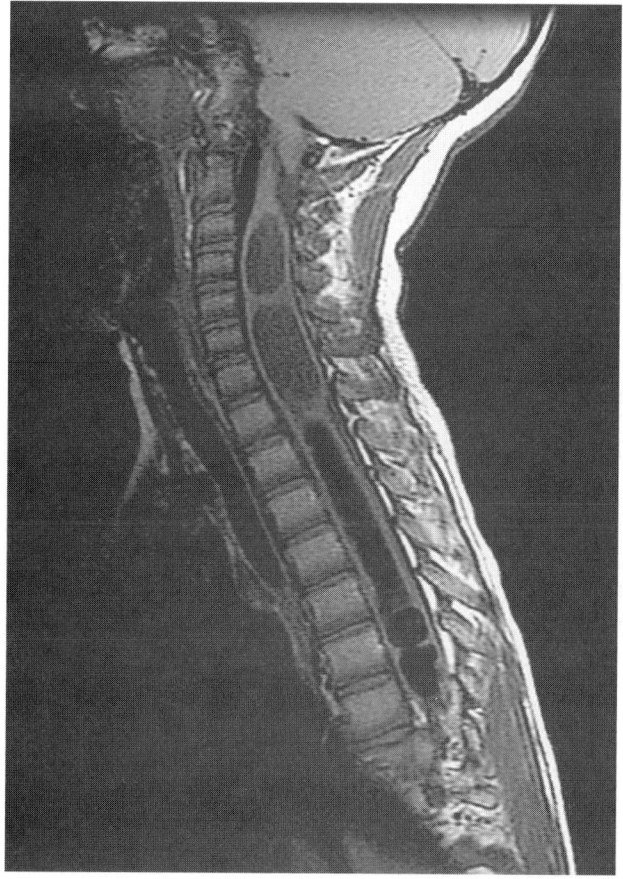

Arnold-Chiari syndrome The CT scan of a patient with Arnold-Chiari syndrome shows herniation of the cerebellar tonsils in the upper cervical spinal canal and the presence of a significant syringomyelia (different patient).

a custom-made pillow with a hole to prevent pressure on the myelomeningocele during intubation. Alternatively, the patient can be intubated in the left lateral decubitus position. Intracranial hypertension requires special anesthetic consideration: invasive arterial monitoring and mild hyperventilation combined with other means to reduce intracranial pressure (e.g., mannitol) may be necessary, and an intravenous anesthetic technique seems beneficial. Careful positioning is mandatory because these patients are in the prone position for the operation. Extreme flexion and extension of the head may result not only in brainstem compression but also in endobronchial intubation and extubation, respectively. Intraoperative cardiovascular collapse with resistant arterial hypotension and bigeminy associated with brainstem compression for bleeding control of a lacerated sinus has been reported. If the level of the surgical field is above the level of the heart, bear in mind the possibility of venous air embolism. A rapid sequence induction technique is recommended in the presence of dysphagia, recurrent aspirations, and/or gastroesophageal reflux, Ventilatory abnormalities with abnormal responses to hypoxia and hypercapnia may persist postoperatively. Postoperative mechanical ventilation may be necessary. On rare occasions, vocal cord paralysis and/or reduced gag reflex may require tracheostomy and gastrostomy to secure the airway.

Pharmacological implications: Succinylcholine seems not to cause exaggerated hyperkalemia in the presence of paralysis from myelomeningocele. Mannitol and other agents to reduce intracranial

pressure may be required. Nitrous oxide probably is best avoided in these patients secondary to increased cerebral blood flow and the risk of venous air embolism.

REFERENCES:
Tanaka M, Harukuni I, Naito H: Intraoperative cardiovascular collapse in an infant with Arnold-Chiari malformation, *Paediatr Anaesth* 7:163, 1997.

Wu YW, Chin CT, Chan KM, et al: Pediatric Chiari I malformations: Do clinical and radiologic features correlate? *Neurology* 53:1271, 1999.

Milhorat TH, Chou MW, Trinidad EM, et al: Chiari I malformation redefined: Clinical and radiographic findings for 364 symptomatic patients. *Neurosurgery* 44:1005, 1999.

Arrhythmogenic Right Ventricular Dysplasia

At a glance: Most-often inherited disease of the myocardium resulting in cardiomyopathy and risk of sudden death in otherwise healthy young adults.

Synonyms: Arrhythmogenic Right Ventricular Cardiomyopathy; ARVC.

Incidence: Rare. Predominance in males. Arrhythmogenic right ventricular dysplasia (ARVD) is estimated to account for up to 5% of unexpected sudden deaths in individuals younger than 65 years and 3 to 4% of sudden deaths occurring during sports. The prevalence is unknown, and estimates range from 1.5:1000 to 4.5:1000 in the general population.

Genetic inheritance: Autosomal dominant, with mutations mapped to chromosome 14. However, depending on the gene/chromosome involved, eight different types of ARVD have been described. Type 1 is the most common form. Autosomal recessive and sporadic forms have been described.

Pathophysiology: Abnormal development of the right ventricle results in fibrous and fatty deposits in the free wall of the right ventricular myocardium. The subepicardial and mediomural layers are predominately affected; the subendocardial area may be preserved. Uhl anomaly is a severe form of ARVD in which the myocardium is severely dysplastic and the epicardium and endocardium are closely applied, resulting in the so-called "parchment ventricle." The left ventricle may be involved in severe forms. The interventricular septum usually is preserved. Two pathologic types of ARVD have been described.

1. The *fibrofatty form* is characterized by a mixture of fat and fibrous tissue, myocardial thinning, and atrophy of the myocytes. The degeneration typically affects a triangular area (so-called "triangle of dysplasia"), which comprises the right ventricular infundibulum, the lateral apical region, and the right ventricular outflow tract. In the majority of cases, the myocardium shows lymphocytic infiltrates, which may extend to left ventricular areas. Approximately half of patients show a right ventricular aneurysm at autopsy.

2. The second form is the *fatty form,* in which the right ventricular myocardium is replaced partly or almost entirely by adipose tissue. Lymphocytic infiltrates most often are missing, and left ventricular involvement is uncommon.

The main clinical consequences arising from these degenerative changes are various forms of arrhythmias caused by abnormalities in depolarization, repolarization, and conduction.

Diagnosis: Based on ECG findings (e.g., T-wave inversion on right-sided chest leads, right bundle branch block at rest, and isolated QRS prolongation in leads V_1–V_3). One of the main findings on echocardiography is dilatation of the right ventricle. Fatty infiltration of the myocardium can often be seen. At a later stage, sacculations or aneurysms of the right ventricular free wall in combination with right ventricular thinning and wall-motion abnormalities can be found. Endomyocardial biopsy and MRI may be useful to confirm the diagnosis. Valvular heart disease, active myocarditis, metabolic cardiomyopathy, and coronary artery disease must be excluded. Based on the classification and the criteria of the European Society of Cardiology and the ISFC Working Group on Cardiomyopathies and Dysplasia, the diagnosis of ARVD is confirmed if two major criteria, or one major plus two minor criteria, or four minor criteria from different groups are present (see Table A-1, p. 69).

Clinical aspects: The disease may be asymptomatic in the early stages, with well-preserved exercise tolerance. Arrhythmias are often associated with left bundle branch block and usually are well tolerated. Arrhythmias may be triggered by stress, but they also can occur at rest or even during sleep. Most often these arrhythmias present as palpitations, syncope, or less frequently as sudden death. Basically all forms of ventricular arrhythmias are possible, ranging from asymptomatic isolated extrasystoles to sustained and hemodynamically significant right ventricular tachycardia with left bundle branch block, which is the most common presenting form. However, the origins of arrhythmias are not limited to the right ventricle: supraventricular tachycardias, including atrial extrasystoles, flutter, and fibrillation, have been described as the initial symptom. Ventricular failure usually is not part of the presentation. Echocardiography and angiography demonstrate regional or global abnormalities of right ventricular structure and function. Treatment may include class I antidysrhythmics, amiodarone, beta blockers, and use of an automatic implantable cardioverter-defibrillator (AICD).

Precautions before anesthesia: Full assessment of the cardiovascular system, including clinical examination, chest radiograph, ECG, and echocardiography. Obtain a history of palpitations, syncopes, and the triggering events. Correct any electrolyte disturbances before the patient is brought to the operating room. Ensure optimal treatment of dysrhythmias and congestive cardiac failure. Note the presence or absence of an AICD and consult the cardiologist about potential problems arising from electrocauterization. Continue antidysrhythmic drugs in the perioperative period.

Anesthetic considerations: Choose the anesthetic technique that does not provoke dysrhythmias. Avoid anxiety, hypercapnia, hypoxia, acidosis, and hypokalemia. Treat any dysrhythmias promptly. Administer fluids carefully to prevent deterioration of cardiac function. Risk of ventricular dysrhythmias requires the ability for cardioversion. Maintain a low threshold for invasive monitoring. Ensure a deep level of anesthesia before intubation. Cautious use of electrocauterization in the presence of an AICD is advised (check with the cardiologist if uncertain).

Pharmacological implications: Halothane is relatively contraindicated because of sensitization of the myocardium to circulating catecholamines and its negative inotropic effect. Avoid drugs with any potential to cause tachycardia and dysrhythmias (e.g., pancuronium is relatively contraindicated).

Other condition to be considered:

☞**BRUGADA SYNDROME:** Familial syndrome of spontaneous idiopathic ventricular fibrillation, which probably is one of the most frequent causes of sudden death in patients with normal hearts.

REFERENCES:

Fontaine G, Fontaliran F: Arrhythmogenic right ventricular dysplasia. *Annu Rev Med* 50:17, 1999.

Fontaine G, Aouate P, Fontaliran F: Arrhythmogenic right ventricular dysplasia, torsades de pointes and sudden death. New concepts. *Ann Cardiol Angeiol (Paris)* 46:531, 1997.

Arthrogryposis (Arthrogryposis Multiplex Congenita)

At a glance: Spectrum of different syndromes characterized by persistent multiple limb contractures. Often associated with midline dysraphism abnormalities. Distal arthrogryposis type I and ☞Freeman-Sheldon Syndrome are the most common forms. Often associated with pharyngeal, cardiac, urologic, and gastric abnormalities.

Classification:

Distal Arthrogryposis, Type I: Characterized by distal involvement of hands and feet, medially overlapping fingers, clenched fists, camptodactyly, and clubfoot. Neurologic development is normal and Response to physical therapy usually is good.

Distal Arthrogryposis Type II: Heterogenous group. Congenital distal joint contractures are associated with numerous other anomalies.

Incidence: Varies from 0.3 to 3 cases per 1000 live births. No racial or sexual predilection has been reported (except for cases with X-linked transmission).

Genetic inheritance: Most cases are sporadic. Type 1 may be autosomal dominant inherited (chromosome 9), but autosomal recessive transmission has been reported. Some syndromes in which arthrogryposis is part of the clinical picture have X-linked transmission. Identical twins often are discordant for the condition, and the intrafamilial phenotype is highly variable.

Pathophysiology: The pathogenetic mechanism is a matter of debate. Most likely it is a combination of a central and a peripheral neuromuscular disease. Generalized fetal akinesia seems to be a significant risk factor, which also is favored by oligohydramnios, anomalies of the uterus, and twin pregnancies. Several etiologic theories have been postulated: hormonal, fetal blood supply, neurogenic or myogenic disturbances, toxins (e.g., alcohol or drugs such as phenytoin), and maternal infections (e.g., rubeola, rubella, coxsackievirus, enterovirus). Arthrogryposis is classified into four categories: myopathies, neuropathies, connective tissue disorders, and exogenous effects.

Diagnosis: There are few prenatal ultrasonic findings. The clinical diagnosis usually is made at birth, with the characteristic positioning, internal rotation at the shoulders, extension at the elbows, and flexion at the wrists. Severe equinovarus deformity of the feet usually is present. The face is round (although asymmetry is common) and often associated with a frontal midline capillary hemangioma, flat nasal bridge, and mild micrognathia. Depending on the cause of arthrogryposis, intelligence may be normal. Fetal akinesia

Table A-1   *Arrhythmogenic Right Verticular Dysplasia: Criteria*

Criteria	Major	Minor
Global and/or regional myocardial dysfunction and structural anomalies detected by echocardiography, ventriculography, MRI, or radionuclide scintigraphy	Severe dilatation and reduction of right ventricular ejection fraction with absent or only mild left ventricular involvement	Minor global right ventricular dilatation and/or mild reduction in right ventricular ejection fraction with normal left ventricular function
	Localized right ventricular aneurysms (akinetic or dyskinetic areas with diastolic bulging); severe right ventricular segmental dilatation	Mild right ventricular segmental dilatation; regional right ventricular hypokinesia
Repolarization abnormalities on the ECG		T-wave inversion on the right precordial leads beyond V_1 (in patients >12 yrs and no signs of right bundle branch block)
Depolarization and/or conduction abnormalities on the ECG	Epsilon waves or localized prolongation (>110 ms) of the QRS complex on the precordial leads (V_1–V_3)	Presence of late potentials on the signal-averaged ECG
Arrhythmias		Sustained or nonsustained left bundle branch block-type ventricular tachycardia (ECG, Holter ECG, exercise testing) More than 1000 ventricular extrasystoles with left bundle branch block morphology within 24 hrs proven by Holter ECG
Family history	Familial disease confirmed at necropsy or surgery	Positive family history for premature (age <35 yrs); sudden death from suspected arrhythmogenic right ventricular dysplasia; positive family history confirmed by clinical diagnosis based on the criteria presented in this table

may be associated with intrauterine growth retardation, craniofacial anomalies, and hypoplastic lungs. Two thirds of arthrogryposis patients have involvement of all four limbs (usually symmetrically), one fourth of patients have predominant involvement of the lower limbs, and the rest have involvement of mainly the upper limbs.

Clinical aspect: Numerous syndromes include at least some aspects of arthrogryposis. In general, the deformities are symmetrical, with increasing severity distally. Hands and feet are affected the most. Radioulnar synostosis and syndactyly may add to the deformities. Contractures and rigidity of the joints are common and may result in joint pterygia and dislocation of the large joints (e.g., hip, knee, shoulders, elbow). Mobility in the temporomandibular joint often is significantly decreased. Spinal canal stenosis, atlantoaxial instability, and/or fusion of cervical vertebrae have been described. Scoliosis is not uncommon and may result in abnormal lung function. Muscle atrophy, absence of muscles, and structural abnormalities of the muscles may be present. Peripheral sensation is most often normal. Other clinical findings may affect the head (mental retardation, seizures, craniosynostosis, mi-

crocephaly, eye anomalies), heart (congenital lesions, cardiomyopathy), lungs (laryngeal and/or tracheal clefts, tracheal stenosis, hypoplastic lungs, diaphragmatic dysfunction, hernia), urogenital system (renal anomalies, cryptorchidism, micropenis, absent labia, inguinal hernia), and skin (scalp defects, sparse or abundant subcutaneous tissue, absent skin creases on the flexor side of the joints, skin dimples over contractures, amniotic constriction bands, peripheral cyanosis).

Precautions before anesthesia: These patients are challenging cases for the anesthesiologist. They combine difficult airway (because of micrognathia, limited mobility of temporomandibular joints, atlantooccipital instability), difficult central and peripheral venous access (because of contractures), and risk of hyperpyrexia during and after anesthesia. Careful assessment of the airway is mandatory. Request echocardiography for any patient with suspected cardiac disease or with severe scoliosis. Lung function test may be required for patients with respiratory anomalies. Preoperative blood workup should include a complete blood count, electrolytes, and renal parameters (creatinine, BUN). Depending on the planned operation, postoperative mechanical ventilation may be required and should be organized in advance.

Anesthetic considerations: Patients may be mentally delayed, which may make communication and cooperation difficult. Anxiolytic and/or sedative premedication and the presence of the primary caregiver during induction may be helpful. Difficult airway management is likely, and spontaneous ventilation should be maintained until the airway has been secured. Primary fiberoptic intubation (awake or asleep) or placement of a laryngeal mask airway (LMA) under topical anesthesia followed by fiberoptic intubation through the LMA have been proposed and used successfully. Careful intraoperative positioning is required to prevent injuries and fractures, which may occur with minimal trauma.

Pharmacological implications: No relation between malignant hyperthermia and arthrogryposis syndromes has been demonstrated. Although hypermetabolism and hyperthermia have been described, they are not believed to be related to malignant hyperthermia. However, structural changes in the muscles may result in an exaggerated hyperkalemic response to succinylcholine. Chronic antiseizure treatment may interfere with the metabolism and elimination of other drugs that share the same metabolic pathways.

Other conditions to be considered:

DISTAL, X-LINKED ARTHROGRYPOSIS MULTIPLEX CONGENITAL (X-Linked Arthrogryposis, X-Linked Arthrogryposis Type I; Infantile X-Linked Spinal Muscular Atrophy): X-linked form of arthrogryposis (gene defect mapped to Xp11.3-q11.2) includes a lethal form with severe contractures, scoliosis, chest deformities, hypotonia, micrognathia, and death resulting from respiratory failure during the first 3 months of life. A moderate form with normal intelligence includes ptosis, microphallus, cryptorchidism, and inguinal hernia. A third form also with normal intelligence is mild and "resolutive" and includes moderate contractures, which improve dramatically with age.

ARTHROGRYPOSIS MULTIPLEX CONGENITA, DISTAL, TYPE IIB (Distal Arthrogryposis Type IIb; Freeman-Sheldon Syndrome Variant): Dominant form of arthrogryposis (genetic defect mapped to 11p15.5) with clinical features between arthrogryposis type 1 and Freeman-Sheldon syndrome. Clinically triangular-shaped face, attached earlobes, small mouth and mandible, and limb deformities. Some children have feeding problems at birth and require surgical revision of the oropharynx. Difficult intubation should be expected.

☞**PENA-SHOKEIR SYNDROME, TYPE I:** Autosomal recessive syndrome characterized by multiple ankyloses, camptodactyly, facial abnormalities (rigid face, small mouth, arched palate, micrognathia, short neck), pulmonary hypoplasia, and short-bowel syndrome. Neurologic involvement includes hydrocephalus, microgyria, and cerebellar hypoplasia. Often spontaneous abortion or stillbirth occurs. The presence of antibodies to fetal acetylcholine (ACh) receptors has been demonstrated in mothers of patients. The antibodies do not affect adult ACh receptors, and fetal ACh receptors are replaced by the adult type by week 33 of gestation. The presence of anti-ACh receptor antibodies leads to fetal akinesia/hypokinesia sequence in the offspring of an asymptomatic mother with myasthenia gravis.

X-LINKED FETAL AKINESIA SYNDROME: Rare, X-linked syndrome characterized by polyhydramnios, cerebral malformations (absence of corpus callosum, arrhinencephaly), and fetal hypotonia. Stillborn or death occurs during the first week of life.

ARTHROGRYPOSIS MULTIPLEX CONGENITA WITH WHISTLING FACE (Illum Syndrome): Rare autosomal recessive disorder that is lethal within the first months of life. Autopsy shows extensive calcium deposits in the central nervous system and in skeletal muscle. In addition to multiple congenital contractures, these children usually show severe neurologic dysfunction and autonomic nervous disease with excessive salivation, temperature instability, apnea, and bradycardia. Intubation reportedly is very difficult.

ARTHROGRYPOSIS OPHTHALMOPLEGIA RETINOPATHY (Arthrogryposis with Oculomotor Limitation and Electroretinal Abnormalities; Oculomelic Dysplasia): Rare autosomal dominant disease including arthrogryposis, limitation of eye movements, abnormal retinal pigmentation, and abnormal retinogram. Associated with hypertrophic pyloric stenosis.

ARTHROGRYPOSIS, ECTODERMAL DYSPLASIA, CLEFT LIP/PALATE, AND DEVELOPMENTAL DELAY: Very rare, X-linked syndrome associated with severe contractures, ectodermal dysplasia, cleft palate, and psychomotor and growth retardation.

ARTHROGRYPOSIS, RENAL DYSFUNCTION, AND CHOLESTASIS SYNDROME (ARC Syndrome): Very rare autosomal recessive or X-linked disease. Clinical association with severe cholestasis, arthrogryposis with anterior motor neuron degeneration, and renal tubular cell degeneration with nephrocalcinosis. Usually lethal within the first month.

ARTHROGRYPOSIS-LIKE SYNDROME (Kuskokwim Disease): Extremely rare, autosomal recessive disorder described in Alaskan Inuits. Results in multiple joint contractures with compensatory muscle hypertrophy.

GORDON SYNDROME (Distal Arthrogryposis Multiplex Congenita Type IIA; Camptodactyly, Cleft Palate, and Clubfoot Syndrome): Autosomal dominant distal arthrogryposis that includes clubfoot, camptodactyly of hands and feet, short stature, cleft lip/palate with pharyngeal malformation and pterygium colli, eyelid ptosis, exophthalmos, and vertebral anomalies. Feeding problems may be an issue. Difficult airway management should be expected.

JEQUIER KOZLOWSKI SKELETAL DYSPLASIA: Very rare syndrome including unusual craniofacial appearance, arthrogryposis, advanced bone age of the hips, and unique radiologic skeletal abnormalities.

KALYANRAMAN SYNDROME: Very rare disease resulting in arthrogryposis, epileptic seizures, and migrational brain disorders. MRI findings include polymicrogyria, pachygyria, and fused schizencephaly. Abnormal neuropsychological features, mental retardation, neurogenic electromyography changes, and partial or generalized seizures have been described.

MASSA CASAER CEULEMANS SYNDROME: Very rare disease characterized by arthrogryposis multiplex congenita secondary to lissencephaly type I. The prognosis is very poor. A similar association between arthrogryposis and type II lissencephaly (cobblestone lissencephaly) has been described, also with lethal prognosis within the first months of life.

ARTHROGRYPOSIS WITH OCULOMOTOR LIMITATION AND ELECTRORETINAL ABNORMALITIES (Oculomelic Amyoplasia): Autosomal dominant disease with arthrogryposis and aplasia of limb muscles replaced by bands of fibrous tissue. Additional findings include progressive ophthalmoplegia, abnormal macular pigmentation, and sometimes abnormal electroretinogram. Body height usually is normal.

☞**TRICHOOCULODERMOVERTEBRAL SYNDROME:** Rare autosomal recessive disorder characterized by ectodermal dysplasia (skin scaling and hyperchromic spots on all four limbs, hypohidrosis, excessive bruising after injuries or scratching, onychodysplasia nuclear cataract). Neurologic evaluation reveals brachycephaly and microcephaly. Cleft lip/palate, oligodontia, and enamel abnormalities have been reported.

STOLL ALEMBIK FINCK SYNDROME: Variant of trichooculodermovertebral syndrome with a tendency to excessive bruising and scarring after injuries and scratching.

☞**MULTIPLE SYNOSTOSES SYNDROME I (WL SYNDROME):** Autosomal dominant disorder characterized by bilateral limb dysplasia and multiple synostoses (elbows, wrist, metacarpal, finger, ankle), proximal symphalangism, and proximal and intermedial interphalangeal flexion creases. The metacarpals are short and broad. Symphalangism is progressive and tends to grow in ulnar-to-radial and proximal-to-distal directions. The nails are either hypoplastic or absent. As in other symphalangism syndromes, conductive deafness probably results from anomalies of the auditory ossicles (otosclerotic deafness). Strabismus and a broad, tubular-shaped nose are other hallmarks of this disorder. Vertebral abnormalities can lead to spinal canal stenosis and significant limitation in flexion and extension of the neck. Pectus excavatum has been described. Careful preoperative neurologic and cervical examination before anesthesia is recommended. Airway management may be difficult because of the neck anomalies. If chest deformity is significant, preoperative lung function tests and echocardiography may be indicated. Perform intubation either under cervical in-line stabilization or with a fiberoptic airway equipment. (The name *WL Syndrome* originates from the initials of the surnames of two fathers with children suffering from the disorder).

BRACHYDACTYLY-DISTAL SYMPHALANGISM SYNDROME (Sillence Syndrome): Autosomal dominant disorder with normal-to-tall body height, similar to multiple synostosis syndrome with distal (rather than proximal) synostosis, "Chess-pawn"-shaped distal phalanges, thoracolumbar scoliosis, and clubfoot.

VAN BIERVLIET HENDRICKX VAN ERTBRUGGEN SYNDROME (Craniofacial Dysostosis Arthrogryposis Progeroid Appearance): Extremely rare disease with intrauterine growth retardation and later dwarfism, craniofacial (partial absence of the mandibula, microstoma, low-set ears) and cerebral anomalies (mental retardation, agenesis of the corpus callosum and septum pellucidum, aqueduct stenosis), and arthrogryposis. The chest may be narrow and warrants further preoperative evaluation. Antenatal exposure to cytomegalovirus may be a risk factor.

REFERENCES:

Nguyen NH, Morvant EM, Mayhew JF: Anesthetic management for patients with arthrogryposis multiplex congenita and severe micrognathia: Case reports. *J Clin Anesth* 12:227, 2000.

Rozkowski A, Smyczek D, Birnbach DJ: Continuous spinal anesthesia for cesarean delivery in a patient with arthrogryposis multiplex congenita. A clinical report. *Reg Anesth* 21:477, 1996.

Szmuk P, Ezri T, Warters DR, et al: Anesthetic management of a patient with arthrogryposis multiplex congenita and limited mouth opening. *J Clin Anesth* 13:59, 2001.

Asymmetrical Short Stature Syndrome

At a glance: Associated with craniofacial, ocular, and skeletal anomalies. Intelligence is normal.

Incidence and genetic inheritance: Extremely rare; reported in only one family. Most likely autosomal dominant inheritance.

Clinical aspects: Short stature. Frontal bossing with a hypoplastic mandible. One leg is shorter than the other, with a pelvic tilt. Intelligence is normal.

Anesthetic considerations: Assess neck mobility because of the possibility of fused abnormal cervical vertebrae (radiograph, CT scan). Assess degree of difficulty of intubation in the presence of a hypoplastic mandible. Difficult airway management must be expected in the presence of fused cervical vertebrae and hypoplastic mandible. Avoid neuromuscular blockers to maintain spontaneous breathing until the airway has been secured.

REFERENCE:

Jung HH, Smith DW: Dominantly inherited asymmetric short stature with associated anomalies: A new syndrome. *Am J Hum Genet* 32:114A, 1980.

ATR-X Syndrome

At a glance: ATR-X is an acronym for *a*lpha-*t*halassemia, mental *r*etardation, *X*-linked syndrome. It is characterized by genital abnormalities, microcephaly, midface hypoplasia, severe mental retardation, neuromotor dysfunction, seizures, and hypotonia. Occasionally, the patient presents with a ventricular septal defect and gastrointestinal reflux.

Synonyms: X-Linked Mental Retardation Hypotonic Face Syndrome; XLMR Hypotonic Face Syndrome.

Genetic inheritance: Caused by mutations of the ATR-X gene. It is inherited as an X-linked dominant transmission, and only males are affected. α-Thalassemia/mental retardation syndrome also has been suggested to be a contiguous gene syndrome resulting from deletion in 16p.

Classification: There are four subtypes of α-thalassemia. In the presence of a defect on the one α-globin gene, the patient presents with no symptoms of anemia and requires no treatment. The patient is known as a *silent carrier*. If two α-globin genes are missing or damaged, the condition is known as α-thalassemia minor or α-thalassemia trait. In the case of three missing α-globin genes, the person has mild-to-moderately severe anemia, and this condition is termed *hemoglobin H disease* because it causes production of a heavy hemoglobin that is less stable than normal hemoglobin. The mild forms may not require any treatment. The more severe forms usually do not require treatment with blood transfusions except during periods of stress on the body (such as infection). If all four α-globin genes are missing, the child will die before birth. This hemoglobin sometimes is called *hemoglobin Bart*.

Incidence and genetic inheritance: X-linked inherited recessive disorder resulting from a defect in the gene encoding X-linked helicase-2. The helicases are involved in numerous intracellular functions, including DNA recombination and regulation of transcription. It also has been suggested to result from a deletion in the 16p gene.

Clinical aspects: Patients affected with this disorder present with significant postnatal growth deficiency and mental retardation with absent speech capability. The clinical characteristics describing this entity are numerous and include microcephaly, midface hypoplasia, low-set ears that are rotated posteriorly, low nasal bridge, carp-shaped mouth, full lips, and large protruding tongue. The cardiovascular system is most often affected with a perimembranous ventricular septal defect. The shape of the chest is abnormal because ribs are frequently missing. Most patients have hernias and gastroesophageal reflux. The genitourinary system shows hypospadias, small penis, shawl scrotum, cryptorchidism. Renal function demonstrates hydronephrosis and renal agenesis. Neurologically, besides severe mental retardation, spasticity and seizures activity resulting from cerebral atrophy are the most frequent features. Defects of the musculoskeletal system show kyphoscoliosis resulting from hemivertebrae, coxa valga of the pelvis, tapering fingers, fifth finger clinodactyly, and a talipes equinovarus prominent in the feet. The hematology system shows mild hypochromic microcytic anemia and a mild form of hemoglobin H disease. The disease presents with all hematologic characteristics of an α-thalassemia disease.

Precautions before anesthesia: Complete hematologic evaluation must be obtained before surgery. The hematocrit should be checked because of the high incidence of anemia. The cardiovascular system should be assessed and an echocardiogram obtained. Renal functions must be evaluated for kidney failure/dysfunction.

Anesthetic considerations: The presence of gastrointestinal reflux is common and the potential risk of pulmonary aspiration in older children must be kept in mind. Patients affected with renal agenesis or dysfunction present with difficult fluid and electrolyte management. The choice of anesthetic medication might be influenced by the problem. The presence of severe mental retardation and absence of speech make induction of anesthesia and postoperative management more difficult.

Pharmacological implications: Renal dysfunction affects the pharmacodynamics of anesthetic medication.

Other condition to be considered:

☞**THALASSEMIA:** Most frequent genetic disorder with a large geographic influence. Clinical signs result from hemolysis by chronic anemia. Clinical features include hepatosplenomegaly, bone deformations, and cardiac failure. Strict asepsis is needed. Most people who inherit thalassemia are Asian, Filipino, Mediterranean, Middle Eastern, or, less frequently, of African descent.

REFERENCES:

Gibbons RJ, Brueton L, Buckle VJ, et al: Clinical and hematological aspects of the X-linked alpha-thalassemia/mental retardation syndrome (ATR-X syndrome). *Am J Med Genet* 55:288, 1995.

McPherson EW, Clemens MM, Gibbons RJ, et al: X-linked alpha-thalassemia/mental retardation (ATR-X) syndrome: A new kindred with severe genital anomalies and mild hematological expression. *Am J Med Genet* 55:302, 1995.

Atypical Mole Syndrome (AMS)

At a glance: Genetic disorder characterized by the presence of abnormal nevi that predispose to melanoma development.

Synonyms: BK Mole Syndrome; Familial Atypical Mole Melanoma (FAMM) Syndrome; Familial Atypical Multiple Mole Melanoma (FAMMM) Syndrome; Hereditary Dysplastic Nevus Syndrome; Nevoid Melanoma Syndrome.

History: First reported in 1820 by W. Norris.

Incidence: Prevalence in white population of America and Europe is approximately 2 to 5%. In Sweden, 18% of white adults have atypical moles clinically but only 8% have the typical histologic features. No sex predilection. Atypical moles are rare in black, Asian, and Middle Eastern populations.

Genetic inheritance: Clinical history and family examinations suggest an autosomal dominant mode of inheritance. A first proposed assignment of a melanoma gene (CMM1) chromosome 1p36 was not confirmed. A second proposed gene (cell cycle regulator CDKN2A [P16], a cyclin-dependent kinase) has been mapped to chromosome 9p21, and this gene assignment has been confirmed. Germline mutations in this gene occur in approximately 20% of kindreds with familial atypical mole syndrome. Penetrance is variable. Exposure to ultraviolet light plays a role in the phenotypic expression of the syndrome.

Pathophysiology: Dysplastic nevi appear to be histogenetic precursors of melanomas.

Diagnosis: Clinically based on the presence and specific appearance of nevi. The National Institutes of Health Consensus Conference requires the following criteria to establish the diagnosis:

1. First-degree (e.g., parent, sibling or child) or second-degree relative (e.g., grandparent, grandchild, aunt, uncle) with malignant melanoma
2. Large number of nevi, often more than 50, some of which are atypical nevi
3. Nevi that demonstrate certain microscopic features

Histologic examination of dysplastic nevi shows compound nevi with evidence of abnormal growth. Nevus cell nests within the epidermis may be enlarged and show abnormal coalescence with adjacent nests. As part of this process, single nevus cells begin to replace the normal basal cell layer along the dermoepidermal junction. Cytologically, the atypical features consist of irregular, often angulated, nuclear contours frequently combined with hyperchromasia. Associated alterations occur in the superficial dermis, with sparse lymphocytic infiltrate, loss of melanin pigment from presumably destroyed nevus cells, phagocytosis of melanin pigment by dermal macrophages, and linear fibrosis surrounding the involved epidermal rete ridges. This atypical nevus syndrome phenotype is the most potent risk factor for melanoma in families and in the general population. Although most dysplastic nevi are stable lesions, transition to melanoma is well known and can occur within a few months. Atypical mole syndrome (AMS) represents the highest risk factor known for malignant melanoma. A 7-year followup of 14 families indicated affected individuals having at least two relatives with malignant melanoma have a 100% lifetime risk of developing a melanoma, whereas all other affected persons have a lifetime risk of approximately 18%. An increased risk for development of pancreatic cancer has been reported for some mutations. The synonymous name *BK moles* is derived from the initials of the surnames of the two families studied initially.

Clinical aspects: Multiple dysplastic nevi are the hallmark of AMS. In familial AMS, the lesions usually appear during the first decade of life. Typical features are present by the end of puberty. During adolescence, the nevi become dysplastic and more numerous. The nevi usually are larger than ordinary moles (6–15 mm) and have a different distribution over the body (in sun-exposed but also in non–sun-exposed areas) such as the scalp, buttocks, and female breasts. For the diagnosis, at least two atypical nevi must be present, although most often they are numerous. Clinically, atypical nevi are characterized by variable pigmentation and irregular, ill-defined borders. Pathologic changes of the nevi include irregular borders, a mixture of colors, indistinct margins, and a persistent macular component. If a black area develops within a nevus, the lesion should be excised to rule out a melanoma. Small and nondysplastic nevi appear by age 5 to 6 years.

Precautions before anesthesia: Melanoma can become metastatic mainly in the lymph nodes, brain, liver, lungs, and bone;

thus, a complete workup should be obtained if metastatic disease is suspected.

Anesthetic considerations: There are no specific considerations per se, except in the case of metastatic disease, where affected organs should be taken into account and the anesthesia plan tailored consequently.

Pharmacological implications: None reported (patients with AMS usually require a sunscreen with a sun protection factor of at least 15).

REFERENCES:

Greene MH, Clark WH, Tucker MA, et al: Acquired precursors of cutaneous malignant melanoma: The familial dysplastic nevus syndrome. *N Engl J Med* 312:91, 1986.

Gruis NA, Van der Velden PA, Bergman W, et al: Genetics of familial atypical multiple mole-melanoma (FAMMM) syndrome in The Netherlands: How far have we come? *Bull Cancer* 85:627, 1998.

Lynch HT, Brand RE, Hogg D, et al: Phenotypic variation in eight extended CDKN2A germline mutation familial atypical multiple mole melanoma-pancreatic carcinoma-prone families: The familial atypical mole melanoma-pancreatic carcinoma syndrome. *Cancer* 94:84, 2000.

Aughton Syndrome

At a glance: Extremely rare syndrome with dextrocardia and facial, ophthalmologic, and neurologic abnormalities.

Synonyms: Dextrocardia with Unusual Facies and Microphthalmia Syndrome.

Incidence and genetic inheritance: Two presumably unrelated Arab children, both born to consanguineous parents, have been described, suggesting that autosomal recessive transmission is most likely.

Clinical aspects: The two children had dextrocardia associated with sloping forehead, microphthalmia, prominent nose, micrognathia, and plantar folding. One child had a cleft palate, mental retardation, and choreoathetosis; the other child had vertebral fusion defects and supernumerary ribs.

Anesthetic considerations: Prior to anesthesia, associated malformations must be assessed. Difficult tracheal intubation should be expected secondary to the described malformations. Adequate anxiolysis often is helpful in the management of mentally retarded patients.

Other condition to be considered:

☞**GOLDENHAR SYNDROME:** Common birth defect of vascular origin involving first and second branchial arch derivatives, resulting mainly in facial and vertebral anomalies.

REFERENCES:

Aughton DJ: New syndrome? Clinical anophthalmia, dextrocardia, and skeletal anomalies in an infant born to consanguineous parents. *Am J Med Genet* 37:178, 1990.

Nachlieli T, Gershoni-Baruch R: Dextrocardia, microphthalmia, cleft palate, choreoathetosis, and mental retardation in an infant born to consanguineous parents. *Am J Med Genet* 42:458, 1992.

B

Babinski-Fröhlich Syndrome

At a glance: Partial destruction of hypothalamic nuclei resulting in hormonal dysfunction with obesity, growth retardation, and hypogonadism.

Synonyms: Adiposogenital Syndrome; Dystrophia Adiposo-Genitalis; Neuropituitary Dystrophy; Cerebral Adiposity; Pituitary Infantilism of Adults; Fröhlich Syndrome; Fröhlich Obesity; Morbus Fröhlich Syndrome; Launois-Cléret Syndrome.

Incidence: Unknown, but male prevalence.

Pathophysiology: Several organic lesions of the hypothalamus may cause this disorder, including tumors (craniopharyngioma), encephalitis, Friedreich ataxia, demyelinating diseases, and microcephaly. Originally described as delayed puberty, hypogonadism, and obesity associated with a tumor impinging on the hypothalamus. Presence of obesity indicates damage to the appetite-regulating regions of the hypothalamus. Hypothalamic dysfunction and hypopituitarism mainly affect the somatotropic hormones and the gonadotropins.

Clinical aspects: Obesity with prepubertal onset affecting breasts, abdomen, femoral regions, and hips. Delayed development of secondary sexual characteristics. Headache, visual impairment, mental retardation. Polyuria and polydipsia as a result of diabetes insipidus.

Diagnosis: Based on the clinical and biochemical features (low serum gonadotropin levels; positive vasopressin test for polyuria, if diabetes insipidus is present). Radiologic examinations may show delayed ossification of skeletal structures, suprasellar calcification or destruction, depending on the etiology.

Precautions before anesthesia: Dehydration as a consequence of diabetes insipidus requires preoperative fluid replacement and check of serum electrolytes. The patient may be anxious and uncooperative because of mental retardation and visual disturbances. Sedative premedication and/or the presence of the primary care giver for induction of anesthesia may be helpful.

Anesthetic considerations: Venous access can be difficult. Depending on the grade of obesity, a rapid sequence induction should be considered. Obesity and upper airway obstruction may render face-mask ventilation difficult.

Other condition to be considered:

☞PRADER-LABHART-WILLI SYNDROME: Infantile hypotonia, early childhood-onset obesity, hypogonadism, mental retardation.

REFERENCES:
Bruch H: The Froehlich's syndrome: Report of the original case. *Am J Dis Child* 58:1282, 1939.

Reichlin S: Neuroendocrinology, in Williams RH, Larsen RP (eds): *Williams' Textbook of Endocrinology*. 9th ed. Philadelphia, WB Saunders, 1998, p 165.

Bader Syndrome

At a glance: Presence of congenital tumors in the esophagus or mediastinum.

Synonym: Odontoma Dysphagia Syndrome.

Incidence and genetic inheritance: Less than 10 cases have been described. Autosormal dominant inheritance was suspected in 5 cases, while at least one case seemed to be sporadic.

Clinical aspects: Odontoma is an undifferentiated mass (hamartoma) arising from tooth germ or surrounding tissue. The three reported cases had multiple odontomas (odontomatosis) associated with severe dysphagia. The child reported by Bader died at the age of 6 years after esophageal surgery. Histology revealed leiomyomatosis of the muscularis propria of the stenotic esophagus. The child also had stenosis of the intrathoracic descendent aorta with calcifications, chronic interstitial myocarditis, pyelonephritis, and hepatic sclerosis. Another report describes a father and three children with multiple odontomas that were present at birth or became apparent in infancy. One child died of pneumonia at the age of 3 months. The father and one son also had severe dysphagia from stenosis and dysmotility of the inferior part of the esophagus. No other changes were reported.

Anesthetic considerations: Chronic aspirations may compromise pulmonary function. Possible cardiac, renal, and hepatic involvement should be assessed prior to intervention. Depending on the size and location of the odontomas, mask ventilation and intubation may be difficult.

REFERENCES:
Bader G: Odontomatosis (multiple odontomas). *Oral Surg Oral Med Oral Pathol* 23:770, 1967.

Schonberger W: Multiple odontomas (odontomatosis) and dysphagia in father and son—A syndromic connection? *Z Kinderheilkd* 117:101, 1974.

Schmidseder R, Hausamen JE. Multiple odontogenic tumors and other anomalies. An autosomal dominant inherited syndrome. *Oral Surg Oral Med Oral Pathol* 39:249, 1975.

BADS

At a glance: BADS is an acronym for *B*lack Locks with *A*lbinism and *D*eafness *S*yndrome. Newborns with white hair, eyebrows, and eyelashes (ermine-like camouflage), some black locks, and depigmented skin with some brown spots. Other features include nystagmus, photophobia, retinal depigmentation, and deafness. Mild mental retardation is possible.

Synonym: Ermine Phenotype (Pigmentary Disorder with Hearing Loss).

History: In 1979, Witkop described the association of albinism with black locks and congenital hearing loss.

Incidence: Extremely rare; less than 10 cases have been reported.

Genetic inheritance: Autosomal recessive.

Pathophysiology: Results from either a failure of migration of melanocytes or an autoimmune mechanism.

Diagnosis: Characteristic features include white hair, white eyebrows and eyelashes with scattered black tufts (black locks), reminiscent of the winter color change of the ermine (weasel) fur from brown-black to white, which affects the entire body, except for the distal half of the tail that remains brown-black. Sensorineural hearing loss is present.

Clinical aspects: Affected patients have vitiligo and patchy depigmentation, mild mental retardation, nystagmus, photophobia, retinal depigmentation. Early recognition of hearing impairment and protection from ultraviolet sunlight are the mainstay of management.

Precautions before anesthesia: The appropriate anesthetic plan should be communicated to the patient by relatives or a person fluent in sign language. The patient should bring his/her hearing aid to the operating room.

Anesthetic considerations: Cooperation may be limited, depending on the degree of mental retardation. Presence of the primary caregiver during induction and/or anxiolytic and sedative premedication may be helpful. In regards to the photosensitivity, the brightness of the operating room lights should be dimmed as much as possible. No specific anesthetic concerns related to this disorder are expected.

Pharmacological implications: No known specific implications.

Other condition to be considered:

ABCD SYNDROME: An acronym that stands for *Albinism, Black lock, Cell migration disorder of the neurocytes of the gut, and Deafness. It is considered an autosomal recessive inheritance condition, characterized pathologically by aganglionosis of large intestine, total absence of neurocytes and nerve fibers of small intestine, and total lack of sympathetic and parasympathetic innervation in small and large intestine. Usually lethal within the first months of life due to gastrointestinal dysfunction. The clinical features include albinism, macrosomnia, black lock at temporal occipital region, and retinal depigmentation. It is essential to evaluate the intravascular volume status, serum electrolytes, serum albumin, cell blood count, and coagulation profile. A chest x-ray and an ECG must be obtained to assess the respiratory and cardiac status.

REFERENCES:

O'Doherty NJ, Gorlin RJ: The ermine phenotype: Pigmentary-hearing loss heterogeneity. *Am J Med Genet* 30:945, 1988.

Witkop CJ Jr: Depigmentations of the general and oral tissues and their genetic foundations. *Ala J Med Sci* 16:330, 1979.

Ballard Syndrome

At a glance: Inherited brachydactyly syndrome not affecting other organ systems.

Synonyms: Brachydactyly, Combined types B and E; Pitt Williams Brachydactyly.

Incidence and genetic inheritance: Twelve members in five generations of a family with autosomal dominant inheritance of this subtype of brachydactyly have been described. The syndrome is named after the affected family.

Clinical aspects: Members of this family have shortened metacarpals and metatarsals IV and V. Broadened thumbs were described in some members, as well as dysplastic fingernails (grooved and koilonychia-like) on the affected fingers and toes. In 1951, Julia Bell classified the brachydactylies in five main groups (A–E). This present form of brachydactyly combines the features of type B and E. Type B involves index to little fingers and is characterized by a symmetrical deformity with hypoplasia or absence of the distal phalanges with absence or dysplasia of the affected nails. Changes on the ulnar side are more pronounced than changes on the radial side. In type E, one or more metacarpals are shortened, either with or without shortening of the metatarsals.

Anesthetic considerations: No anesthetic implications arise from the described features.

Other conditions to be considered: Brachydactyly is a common feature of many syndromes. Its significance results from the association with other abnormalities. If brachydactyly is found, a thorough clinical examination is warranted, looking for other malformations that might have specific implications for anesthesia.

REFERENCES:

Bell J: On brachydactyly and symphalangism: Introduction and classification of cases. *Treasury Hum Inherit* 5:1, 1951.

Pitt P, Williams I: A new brachydactyly syndrome with similarities to Julia Bell types B and E. *J Med Genet* 22:202, 1985.

Ballinger-Wallace Syndrome

At a glance: Maternally transmitted syndrome with diabetes mellitus (DM), neurosensory deafness, and ophthalmic abnormalities.

Synonyms: Maternally Inherited Diabetes Mellitus-Deafness Syndrome; Noninsulin-Dependent Diabetes Mellitus with Deafness.

Incidence: Unknown. DM affects 5% of the population in the Western world. It consists of a genetically heterogeneous group of disorders with glucose intolerance being the common clinical feature. More than 60 different hereditary DM syndromes have been described. Maternally inherited DM and deafness represents a unique syndrome within this grouping.

Genetic inheritance: The mitochondrial form of DM and deafness is inherited in a heterogeneous pattern. The syndrome has been associated with a 10.4-kb mitochondrial DNA (mtDNA) deletion and a mutation in nucleotide 3243, altering the mitochondrial tRNA for leucine. The deletion is unique because it is maternally transmitted, removes the light strand origin of mtDNA replication, inhibits mitochondrial protein synthesis, and is not associated with the hallmarks of other mtDNA deletion syndromes (ptosis, ophthalmoplegia, or muscle weakness).

Pathophysiology: The mtDNA deletion causes a defect in the mitochondrial oxidative phosphorylation, which impairs pancreatic islet cell function. Once the mitochondrial adenosine triphosphate (ATP) production of the islet cells falls below the level required for appropriate glucose "sensing," DM ensues. The exact mechanism of protein synthesis inhibition is unclear.

Diagnosis: Based on clinical features consistent with the disorder (see below). Pathologic glucose tolerance test, audiometry testing, and ophthalmic examination. The pedigree demonstrates maternal inheritance.

Clinical aspects: The syndrome is characterized by DM (non-insulin and insulin dependent with age of onset between 20 and 30 years), progressive bilateral neurosensory hearing loss, and impaired vestibular function (unsteady gait, dizziness). Ophthalmologic examination reveals pigmentary retinal degeneration (normal visual acuity with concentric narrowing of the visual fields) and eventually external ophthalmoplegia. Seizures and dysarthria have also been reported.

Precautions before anesthesia: Obtain a detailed clinical history and a thorough clinical examination to determine the systemic involvement of DM (coronary artery disease, arterial hypertension, nephropathy, neuropathy, retinopathy) and the degree of hearing loss and vestibular impairment. Review the treatment for DM (actual blood glucose level, glycemia control, diabetic medication regimen). Evaluate cardiac function (electrocardiography, exercise electrocardiography, echocardiogram), neurologic function (peripheral and autonomic neuropathy), and renal function (urea, creatinine, electrolytes, glomerular filtration rate). Blood work should include a complete blood count.

Anesthetic considerations: Diabetic patients have a higher perioperative morbidity and mortality compared to nondiabetic patients. Diabetic patients should receive priority on all scheduled operating lists. Perioperative monitoring of blood glucose and cardiac, pulmonary, and renal function is essential. Meticulous attention must be paid to patient positioning because of peripheral neuropathy, and increased propensity to tissue damage. Patients with autonomic neuropathy are unable to compensate for positional changes, and sympathectomy because of central neuraxial blockade may result in severe arterial hypotension. Remember that these patients are at increased risk for ileus and aspiration (especially patients suffering from diabetic ketoacidosis or autonomic neuropathy with delayed gastric emptying because of gastric atony) and require a rapid sequence induction. Use lactate-containing solutions (lactated Ringer solution) carefully (or avoid them altogether) because they may exacerbate a preexisting lactic acidosis in hyperglycemic states.

Pharmacological implications: Patients on preoperative long-acting sulfonylureas (glibenclamide) and metformin should be switched to short-acting sulfonylureas (glipizide, gliclazide, tolbutamide) 3 days before operation. Patients on long-acting insulin should be changed to a combination of short- and intermediate-acting insulins in the preoperative period. The choice of regimen for perioperative diabetic management depends on the type of diabetes (insulin or noninsulin dependent), preoperative diabetic control, and type of surgery. Patients controlled with diet or oral antidiabetic drugs usually will require insulin for moderate and major surgery. Insulin-dependent patients will require intravenous insulin for all but the most minor procedures. Two common approaches are used: separate infusions of insulin and glucose with potassium, or a single combined glucose-potassium insulin infusion (GPI). Both require regular blood sugar monitoring (1–2 hourly) and adjustment of infusion rates.

Other conditions to be considered:

☞**WOLFRAM SYNDROME:** Autosomal recessive inherited syndrome with the defect on the short arm of chromosome 4 often referred to as *DIDMOAD* (*d*iabetes *i*nsipidus, *d*iabetes *m*ellitus, *o*ptic *a*trophy, and *d*eafness) syndrome. However, only insulin-dependent DM and bilateral progressive optic atrophy are required for the diagnosis. DM commonly precedes the other signs of DIDMOAD and often develops earlier in these patients (age 3–10 years) when compared to Ballinger-Wallace syndrome. An inherited abnormality of thiamine metabolism may be responsible for the multisystemic manifestations of DIDMOAD syndrome. Some patients present with sideroblastic or megaloblastic anemia, neutropenia, or thrombocytopenia, which responded well to treatment with thiamin. Cardiomyopathy, hypothyroidism, mental retardation, nystagmus, and seizures may be present. Diabetes insipidus is caused by a loss of vasopressin neurons in the supraoptic nucleus and a defect in processing vasopressin precursors. In addition to the aforementioned precautions before anesthesia, the presence of diabetes insipidus may require preoperative correction and careful intraoperative and postoperative monitoring of the patient's fluid balance.

☞**ROGERS SYNDROME:** Autosomal recessive inherited disorder. Triad of thiamine-responsive anemia (macrocytic anemia, sometimes with moderate thrombocytopenia), DM, and sensorineural deafness. Some cases may have a situs inversus viscerum totalis or a cardiac septal defect. Preoperative evaluation may include echocardiography and subacute bacterial endocarditis prophylaxis. Situs inversus should be kept in mind for all invasive procedures.

REFERENCES:

Ballinger SW, Shoffner JM, Gebhart S, et al: Mitochondrial diabetes revisited [letter]. *Nat Genet* 7:458, 1994.

Ballinger SW, Shoffner JM, Hedaya EV, et al: Maternally transmitted diabetes and deafness associated with a 10.4 kb mitochondrial DNA deletion. *Nat Genet* 1:11, 1992.

Velho G, Byrne MM, Clement K, et al: Clinical phenotypes, insulin secretion, and insulin sensitivity in kindreds with maternally inherited diabetes and deafness due to mitochondrial tRNA Leu (UUR) gene mutation. *Diabetes* 45:487, 1996.

Bamforth-Lazarus Syndrome

At a glance: Extremely rare congenital genetic disorder combining cleft palate and hypothyroidism.

Synonyms: Bamforth Syndrome; Congenital Hypothyroidism, Spiky Hair, and Cleft Palate Syndrome.

Incidence and genetic inheritance: Only five children have been described. Autosomal recessive inheritance. The genetic defect affects the gene encoding thyroid transcription factor-2, which is, among other factors such as thyroid transcription factor-1, thyroid-stimulating hormone receptor genes, and Pax-8, implicated in the early thyroid organogenesis. The hair defect seems to be caused by a mutation in the *FOXE 1* gene. Gene map locus is 9q22.

Clinical aspects: Three children, two siblings and one single child, showed neonatal respiratory distress, presumably from upper airway obstruction. Facial features included choanal atresia, cleft palate, bifid epiglottis, and micrognathia. Congenital hypothyroidism and spiky hair were present at birth. Mild developmental delay was described in two and might have been related to hypothyroidism. Thyroid agenesis is possible. Other features included polyhydramnios in three cases and low-set ears.

Anesthetic considerations: Direct laryngoscopy and tracheal intubation may be difficult because of micrognathia and malformations of the palate and epiglottis. However, at least one child was mechanically ventilated, and no difficulties with intubation were reported. Choanal atresia precludes nasal intubation and respiratory distress can be marked in the neonatal period and require surgical treatment. Two children had recurrent aspirations and poor feeding, possibly because of pharyngeal dysmotility. Chronic lung disease may be present secondary to chronic aspirations and mechanical ventilation. These patients are on thyroid hormone replacement therapy. Despite adequate therapy, these patients are usually of short stature.

REFERENCES:

Bamforth JS, Hughes IA, Lazarus JH, et al: Congenital hypothyroidism, spiky hair, and cleft palate. *J Med Genet* 26:49, 1989.

Brancaccio A, Minichiello A, Grachtchouk M, et al. Requirement of the forkhead gene *FOXE 1*, a target of sonic hedgehog signaling, in hair follicle morphogenesis. *Hum Mol Genet* 13;2595, 2004.

Buntinex IM, Van Overmeire B, Desager K, et al: Syndromic association of cleft palate, bilateral choanal atresia, curly hair, and congenital hypothyroidism. *J Med Genet* 30:427, 1993.

Bangstad Syndrome

At a glance: Primordial bird-head nanism associated with progressive ataxia and multiple endocrinopathies.

Incidence and genetic inheritance: Only two siblings from non-consanguineous Norwegian parents have been described.

Clinical Aspects: At the time of description, the older individual was a 26-year-old man; his sister was 16 years old. Both had dwarfism and a characteristic bird-like facies. The two siblings were mentally retarded and suffered from progressive ataxia and epilepsy. Multiple endocrinopathies included goiter, primary gonadal insufficiency, and insulin-resistant diabetes mellitus. Thyroid-stimulating hormone was elevated in one, but both were clinically euthyroid. Age at onset of diabetes mellitus in the male was 16 years; the girl was not diabetic at the time of description. Parathyroid hormone, luteinizing hormone, follicle-stimulating hormone, and adrenocorticotropic hormone levels were elevated.

Anesthetic considerations: Assessment of the endocrinologic status is most important prior to anesthesia. Hypothyroidism should be treated prior to surgery. Diabetes mellitus should be optimized if necessary. Adrenal insufficiency should be suspected and, depending on the extent of the procedure, a stress dose of steroids should be considered. Relative resistance not only to insulin, but also to other external hormones might be expected. Depending on the extent of the facial abnormalities, airway management may be difficult.

REFERENCE:

Bangstad H-J, Beck-Nielsen H, Hother-Nielsen O, et al: Primordial bird-head nanism associated with progressive ataxia, early onset insulin-resistant diabetes, goiter, and primary gonadal insufficiency. *Acta Paediatr Scand* 78:488, 1989.

Banki Syndrome

At a glance: Inherited anomalies of bones and joints of the hands.

Incidence and genetic inheritance: In 1965, Z. Banki, a Hungarian physician, described the syndrome in three generations of the same Hungarian family. Assumed to be a unique, autosomal dominant inherited mutation.

Clinical aspects: Family members affected with the syndrome demonstrate fusion of the cuneiform and lunate bones of the wrist, clinometacarpia, brachymetacarpia, leptometacarpia, and clinodactyly. No other systemic manifestations of this condition occurred.

Anesthetic considerations: Care with positioning of the wrists during anesthesia because of decreased mobility and increased susceptibility of the wrist joints to trauma. Venous access may be difficult in hands.

REFERENCE:

Banki Z: Kombination erblicher Gelenk-und Knochenanomalien an der Hand. Zwei neue Röntgenzeichen. *Fortschr Röntgenstr* 103:598, 1965.

Bannayan-Zonana Syndrome

At a glance: Inherited disorder characterized by excessive growth prenatally and postnatally manifesting with macrocephaly and scaphocephaly with normal intelligence or mild mental retardation and multiple hamartomas (lipomas, intestinal polyps). As affected infants age, the growth rate slows down and commonly results in normal adult height.

Synonyms: Bannayan-Riley-Ruvalcaba Syndrome; Ruvalcaba-Myhre-Smith Syndrome.

Incidence: Unknown, but several case reports exist.

Genetic inheritance: Presumed autosomal dominant inheritance with male predominance (up to 80% of cases). Variability in the severity of the condition in affected individuals suggests allelic mutations or possible genetic heterogeneity. The gene for Bannayan-Zonana syndrome has been localized to the q22-23 region within the PTEN (phosphate and tensin) homologue locus of chromosome 10. The Bannayan-Zonana syndrome should be unified into a single entity with other similar, previously considered separate syndromes, namely, Riley-Smith, Ruvalcaba, Cowden, and Lhermitte-Duclos. Clinical and molecular data support the unification with the proposed new nomenclature PTEN-MATCHS syndrome.

Pathophysiology: Multiple hamartomas with various angiomatous, lymphangiomatous, and lipomatous constituents. Muscle biopsy demonstrates a lipid storage myopathy with increased depositions of lipid droplets in type I fibers. Type II fibers are smaller than normal. Lipid myopathy may result from a defect in long-chain fatty acid oxidation, which is caused by a deficiency of long-chain L-3-hydroxyacyl-CoA dehydrogenase.

Diagnosis: Clinical features and muscle biopsy. Electromyography is consistent with a myopathic condition.

Clinical aspects: Increased birth weight (>4 kg [8.8 lb]) and length (>97th percentile), with normal adult height are typical. Macrocephaly, macroencephaly, scaphocephaly, and delayed closure of fontanelles. Intracranial manifestations include increased incidence of intracranial tumors, hemangiomas, arteriovenous malformations, hemorrhage, and seizure activity. Extracranial arteriovenous malformations occur. Delayed psychomotor development with dyscoordination, myopathy, and hypotonia. Intelligence may be normal or mildly retarded. Increased salivation and drooling. Ophthalmologic features consist of strabismus (exotropia), hypertelorism, and pseudopapilledema. High-arched palate. Hashimoto thyroiditis has been reported in affected individuals. Pectus excavatum. Juvenile intestinal polyposis with increased risk of intussusception. Protein-losing enteropathy and hepatomegaly may occur. Intestinal and skin lipomas tend to regress with age. Thumbs and great toes are broad (clubbing). Skin manifestations include hemangiomas, multiple lipomas, telangiectases, café-au-lait spots, facial acanthosis nigricans-like discoloration, and cutis marmorata. Penis may be enlarged with spotted pigmentation of the glans. Thyroid and breast tumors may be malignant.

Precautions before anesthesia: Detailed clinical history and examination to evaluate the extent of systemic involvement: neurologic status, intracranial pathology (tumor, hemangiomata), signs of increased intracranial pressure, seizures (anticonvulsant therapy), and mental retardation (sedative premedication may be valuable in the absence of increased intracranial pressure); cardiovascular status (heart failure secondary to arteriovenous malformation, heart failure medication); and respiratory status (myopathy, hypotonia, degree of pectus excavatum, potential respiratory compromise). Evaluate the airway for potential difficulties (high-arched palate, macrocephaly). Anticholinergic premedication may be beneficial if salivation is excessive. Obtain blood work with complete blood count, electrolytes, urea, liver function tests, and thyroid function tests.

Anesthetic considerations: If difficult airway management is anticipated, an awake fiberoptic tracheal intubation (mental retardation may reduce cooperation) or inhalational induction should be considered. Standard neuroanesthetic techniques should be used if an intracranial pathology is present. Spikes in intracranial pressure should be avoided and every effort made to maintain cerebral perfusion pressure. A combination of intravenous induction (thiopental or propofol), opioids, muscle paralysis with controlled ventilation to normo- or mild hypocapnia, and maintenance with either isoflurane (<1 MAC) or target-controlled infusion of propofol. Position the head carefully (neutral position) and consider a slight head-up tilt position to assist cerebral venous drainage. Postoperative ventilation may be required for some patients (myopathy, hypotonia, pectus excavatum, neurologic symptoms, intracranial surgery).

Pharmacological implications: Patients receiving anticonvulsant medication should be continued on their regimen until surgery. Postoperatively the medications should be given parentally until oral intake resumes. Succinylcholine should be avoided if possible (myopathy with risk of hyperkalemia), and nondepolarizing neuromuscular blocking agents should be titrated to effect with a peripheral nerve stimulator. Thiopentone is the agent of choice for induction, but propofol, etomidate, and benzodiazepines are acceptable alternatives. Sedative premedication may be helpful, but should be avoided in patients with intracranial pathology (raised intracranial pressure, altered level of consciousness).

Other conditions to be considered:

Lhermitte-Duclos Syndrome: (Dysplastic Gangliocytoma of the Cerebellum; Benign Hypertrophy of the Cerebellum; Diffuse Ganglioneuroma of the Cerebellar Cortex; Neurocystic Blastoma; Hamartoblastoma, Cerebellar Gangliomatosis; Neurocytoma Myelinicum; Gangliocytoma Myelinicum Diffusum; Purkinjeoma.) Approximately 100 cases have been described. The patients present in young adult age with symptoms of cerebellar dysfunction (absent or only minimal signs in 50%), occlusive hydrocephalus, and signs of increased intracranial pressure. However, symptoms may be present shortly after birth. In approximately 60% of patients, Lhermitte-Duclos syndrome occurs isolated, whereas in the remaining 40% an association with Cowden syndrome can be diagnosed. Magnetic resonance imaging usually confirms the clinical diagnosis. Macroscopically, the cerebellar folia and cortex are enlarged. Histologic examination reveals replacement of the cerebellar internal granular cell layer by large dysplastic neuronal cell bodies resembling Purkinje cells. Prominent myelinated tracts with axonal enlargement in the outer molecular layer of the cerebellar cortex are considered typical.

☞Cowden Syndrome: A disorder characterized by multiple hamartomas and a risk of breast, thyroid and uterine neoplasias.

☞Riley-Smith Syndrome: Rare syndrome similar to the Bannayan-Zonana Syndrome characterized by macrocephaly, pseudopapilledema hemangiomata, and multiple lipomas. Subcutaneous hemangioma may be present at birth or appear later in childhood.

References:

Bannayan GA: Lipomatosis, angiomatosis, and macrencephalia. A previously undescribed congenital syndrome. *Arch Pathol* 92:1, 1971.

DiLiberti JH: Inherited macrocephaly-hamartoma syndromes. *Am J Med Genet* 79:284, 1998.

Sansal I, Sellers WR. The biology and clinical relevance of the PTEN tumor suppressor pathway. *J Clin Oncol* 22:2954, 2004.

Banti Syndrome

At a glance: Acquired syndrome with idiopathic portal hypertension and splenic anemia.

Synonyms: Banti-Senator Disease; Senator Syndrome; Spleen-Liver Syndrome; Chronic Congestive Splenomegaly; Hepatolienal Fibrosis; Noncirrhotic idiopathic portal hypertension.

Pathophysiology: Syndrome characterized by increased splenic and portal pressures resulting in portal hypertension of unknown etiology. Possible causes of portal hypertension include toxins, infections (bacterial/malaria), and immunologic or genetic factors. The portal hypertension is accompanied by splenomegaly and esophageal varices. Liver failure is an uncommon finding. Anemia and thrombocytopenia accompany the hypersplenism.

Diagnosis: Portal hypertension in the absence of any obvious etiology. Liver biopsy excludes hepatic causes. Extrahepatic portal vein obstruction must be excluded.

Clinical aspects: Idiopathic portal hypertension is most commonly found in Japan (female > male) and India (male > female). Patients usually present with bleeding from gastroesophageal varices in the absence of ascites, jaundice, or other signs of hepatic failure. Patients usually present for treatment of varices by sclerotherapy or portocaval anastomoses. Prognosis is usually good. Symptoms may include ascites, weakness, anemia, leukopenia, thrombocytopenia, and/or episodes of bleeding from the gastrointestinal tract.

Precautions before anesthesia: Intravascular volume, hemoglobin and platelet count must be evaluated and, depending on the procedure, corrected if necessary. Although liver function is usually normal, hepatic function should be evaluated.

Anesthetic considerations: Caution with passage of nasogastric tubes. Significant blood loss should be expected for abdominal operations (portal hypertension, thrombocytopenia). Rapid sequence induction may be considered if recent bleeding has occurred.

Pharmacological implications: Avoidance of halothane prevents its implication in the etiology of postoperative jaundice. Avoid drugs requiring hepatic metabolism in the presence of deranged liver function. Nonsteroidal antiinflammatory drugs affect platelet function and gastric mucosa and should be avoided or used with caution only.

References:

Bosch J, D'Amico G, Garcia-Pagon JC: Portal hypertension, in Schiff ER, Sorrell MF, Maddrey WC (eds): *Schiff's Disease of the Liver*, 9th ed. Philadelphia, Lippincott Williams and Wilkins, 2003; p 429.

Ohnishi K, Saito M, Terabayashi H, et al: Portal hemodynamics in idiopathic portal hypertension (Banti's syndrome). *Gastroenterology* 92:751, 1987.

Stankovics J, Nagy A, Mehes K, et al: Umbilical venous catheterization and development of Banti syndrome: The possible role of the factor V Leiden mutation. *Eur J Pediatr* 157:696, 1998.

Baraitser-Winter Syndrome

At a glance: Inherited syndrome with iris coloboma, ptosis, hypertelorism, mental retardation, broad nasal bridge, and short stature.

Synonym: Iris Coloboma, Ptosis, Hypertelorism, and Mental Retardation Syndrome.

Incidence: Unknown, but very rare.

Genetic inheritance: Autosomal recessive inheritance. The disease has been assigned to a pericentric inversion involving chromosome locus 2p12-q14.

Diagnosis: The typical clinical picture aids in making the diagnosis. Chromosomal studies may show the pericentric inversion on chromosome 2.

Clinical aspects: Global developmental delay with lissencephaly, pachygyria or polymicrogyria, and hypotonia are typical. Seizures have been reported. Colobomata affect the iris but also may involve the retina and the optic nerve. These may be the only features distinguishing this syndrome from Noonan syndrome. Hypertelorism, ptosis, prominent epicanthic folds, thickened, edematous eyelids, and heterochromia of the iris are further ophthalmologic features. Broad nasal bridge, long philtrum, thin upper lip, macrostomia, webbed neck, and short stature are other morphologic features. Some patients present with ventricular septal defect.

Precautions before anesthesia: The need for specific investigations must be guided by the clinical scenario. If Noonan syndrome is considered, echocardiography would be useful to exclude cardiac defects.

Anesthetic considerations: Developmental delay may affect the ability of patients to cooperate. Although no reports describing anesthetic management have been published, these patients should be considered to be at risk for malignant hyperthermia because of the close relationship with Noonan syndrome.

Pharmacological implications: Inhalational anesthetics and succinylcholine should be avoided because of possible malignant hyperthermia. Neuromuscular blockers should be used with caution in the presence of hypotonia.

Other conditions to be considered:

☞**NOONAN SYNDROME:** Rare genetic disorder with phenotypical similarity to Turner syndrome; however, the karyotype in Noonan syndrome is normal.

☞**KING-DENBOROUGH SYNDROME:** Autosomal dominant transmitted dysmorphic syndrome with susceptibility to malignant hyperthermia.

REFERENCES:

Baraitser M, Winter RM: Iris coloboma, ptosis, hypertelorism, and mental retardation: A new syndrome. *J Med Genet* 25:41, 1988.

Verloes A: Iris coloboma, ptosis, hypertelorism, and mental retardation: Baraitser-Winter syndrome or Noonan syndrome? *J Med Genet* 30:425, 1993.

Barber-Say Syndrome

At a glance: Hypertrichosis, atrophic skin, ectropion, and macrostomia.

Incidence: Less than 10 cases have been reported since 1982.

Genetic inheritance: Defective regulation or mutation of an unspecified gene may be responsible for this condition and for the ablepharon-macrostomia syndrome (AMS). Whether Barber-Say Syndrome is a totally separate entity or part of a clinical spectrum that includes the AMS, is unclear.

Pathophysiology: The exact mechanism resulting in abnormal development of the skin and its related structures remains to be determined.

Diagnosis: Clinical features. Characteristic signs of Barber-Say syndrome that distinguish it from AMS include bilateral ectropion and generalized hypertrichosis already present at birth. Skin biopsy shows a decreased number of elastic fibers with hypocollagenosis, atrophic epidermis, hyperkeratosis, and a thin reticular layer of dermis.

Clinical aspects: The syndrome is characterized by hypertrichosis and an unusual face with absent or sparse eyebrows, ocular hypertelorism, ocular telecanthus, and bilateral ectropion, or even absent eyelids. The nasal bridge is broad and the nostrils are anteverted. Macrostomia, thin lips, high-arched, narrow palate, and micrognathia and retrognathia. Dentition is normal, but tooth eruption may be delayed. Abnormal ear conchae with small or atretic external auditory meatus. Audiometry and auditory brainstem reflexes are normal. The chest is large with widely spaced, hypoplastic, inverted, or even absent nipples. Hypoplasia of mammary glands and labia

minora may occur. Abnormal laxity of the skin. Mild retardation of psychomotor development with reduced or normal IQ has been reported. Abdominal, renal, and cardiac ultrasound examination are normal. Results of hematologic, endocrinologic, and radiologic examinations usually are unremarkable.

Precautions before anesthesia: Venous access may be difficult because of the laxity and redundancy of the skin. Airway assessment (retrognathia/micrognathia and high-arched, narrow palate). Anticholinergic premedication may be advisable in the case of expected difficult airway management.

Anesthetic considerations: If difficult airway management is anticipated, an inhalational induction or awake fiberoptic tracheal intubation should be considered. Simple eye ointment for eye protection should be administered to both eyes to prevent corneal damage during anesthesia.

Pharmacological implications: No specific pharmacological considerations apply.

Other condition to be considered:

☞**ABLEPHARON-MACROSTOMIA SYNDROME:** Extremely rare congenital dysmorphic syndrome with predominantly facial anomalies. Heart, kidney and liver anomalies are also common.

REFERENCES:

Barber N, Say B, Bell RF, et al: Macrostomia, ectropion, atrophic skin, hypertrichosis, and growth retardation. *Syndr Ident* 8:6, 1982.

Mazzanti L, Bergamaschi R, Neri I, et al: Barber-Say syndrome: Report of a new case. *Am J Med Genet* 78:188, 1998.

Sod R, Izbizky G, Cohen-Salama M: Macrostomia, hypertelorism, atrophic skin, severe hypertrichosis without ectropion: Milder form of Barber-Say syndrome. *Am J Med Genet* 73:366, 1997.

Bardet-Biedl Syndrome

At a glance: Mental retardation, pigmentary retinopathy, polydactyly, obesity, renal anomalies, and hypogenitalism.

Synonym: Biedl Syndrome. Often incorrectly called (and confused with) Laurence-Moon-Bardet-Biedl Syndrome, which first should be called Laurence Moon Syndrome and second is a separate entity presenting with spastic paraplegia.

Incidence: Sex ratio 1:1. Increased in the Arab population of Kuwait (among the Bedouins) with an estimated (minimal) prevalence of 1:13,500.

Genetic inheritance: Autosomal recessive. Consanguinity of parents not uncommon. Several types of Bardet-Biedl syndrome (BBS) have been identified. BBS-1 is linked to 11q13 and BBS-2 maps to 16q21, whereas BBS-3, BBS-4, and BBS-5 map to 3p13–p12, 15q22.3–q23, and 2q31, respectively. BBS-6 is linked to a mutation on 20p12. Heterozygotes have an increased frequency of obesity, hypertension, diabetes mellitus, and renal disease. Hepatic fibrosis may occur in homozygotes.

Pathophysiology: Hypogonadism of central origin combined with a decreased level of growth hormone.

Diagnosis: Cardinal signs of the syndrome are obesity, hypogenitalism, polydactyly, mental retardation, and retinal dystrophy.

Clinical aspects: The different types of BBS vary mainly in their degree of mental retardation, obesity, and distribution of polydactyly (may occur on all four extremities, only on two, or even be absent). Polydactyly, brachydactyly, and syndactyly of hands and/or feet, but also short broad bones and flat joint surfaces of the metacarpophalangeal or metatarsophalangeal joints (short, broad feet) are common. Renal functional (renal insufficiency with increased fractional sodium excretion) and structural abnormalities (calyceal cysts, diverticula, clubbing and blunting, abnormal [fetal] lobulation). Intact urine acidification, no proteinuria, glycosuria, or hyperaminoaciduria. End-stage renal failure seems to be uncommon. Hypogenitalism in males with serum testosterone levels lower than the levels of compared obese but otherwise normal children. Testosterone level fails to respond to human chorionic gonadotropin therapy. Although infertility is common, some male patients reportedly are fertile. In females, vaginal atresia and hypoplasia of the uterus were reported. Diabetes mellitus, hypercholesterolemia, and arterial hypertension may be present. Cardiac anomalies (hypertrophy of the interventricular septum and left ventricle, dilated cardiomyopathy) are reported in up to 50% of patients. Hepatic fibrosis is common. Retinal dystrophy (only a few cases with typical retinitis pigmentosa) results in elevation of dark adaptation threshold with night blindness by approximately 4 years of age, progressing to visual problems during daytime at approximately 6 to 7 years of age. None of the patients older than 16 years had a best-corrected visual acuity higher than 0.1, and many were classified as legally blind. A higher frequency of hypodontia, small teeth with short roots, and higher buffering capacity of saliva was reported.

Precautions before anesthesia: Evaluation of renal and cardiac function. Check blood glucose level to exclude hyperglycemia.

Anesthetic considerations: Because of renal dysfunction, dehydration must be prevented. Cardiac function must be evaluated before and throughout anesthesia, with close followup of blood pressure, urinary output, and plasma glucose levels. As a consequence of obesity, the anesthesiologist must expect difficult vascular access, ventilation, and tracheal intubation. As a result of increased risk of aspiration (obesity, diabetes mellitus), decreased functional residual capacity, and increased closing capacity of the lungs (obesity), a rapid sequence induction with appropriate preoxygenation is recommended. Dental problems (small teeth with short roots) require special attention during direct laryngoscopy. If a regional anesthetic technique is planned, problems with identification of anatomical landmarks (obesity) can occur.

Pharmacological implications: Avoid drugs that increase blood glucose. Closely evaluate renal function before injection of drugs that undergo predominantly renal elimination.

Other conditions to be considered:

☞**LAURENCE-MOON SYNDROME:** Autosomal recessive inherited syndrome with mental retardation, congenital cardiac disease, pigmentary retinopathy, hypogenitalism, and spastic paraplegia.

☞**ALSTRÖM SYNDROME:** Inherited syndrome with progressive visual and hearing loss, diabetes mellitus, and cardiac, hepatic, and renal involvement.

☞**RUBINSTEIN-TAYBI SYNDROME:** Usually occurs sporadically; less often autosomal dominant inherited syndrome characterized by broad thumbs and halluces and dysmorphic facies. Mental and physical development delayed. Cardiac, vertebral, and other anomalies.

☞**BIEMOND SYNDROME TYPE II:** Inherited syndrome characterized by anomalies of the eyes and extremities and mental delay.

☞**COHEN SYNDROME:** Inherited disorder characterized by hypotonia, obesity, prominent incisors, and nonprogressive psychomotor retardation.

REFERENCES:

Beales PL, Elcioglu N, Woolf AS, et al: New criteria for improved diagnosis of Bardet-Biedl syndrome: Results of a population survey. *J Med Genet* 36;437, 1999.

Elbedour K, Zucker N, Zalzstein E, et al: Cardiac abnormalities in the Bardet-Biedl syndrome: Echocardiographic studies of 22 patients. *Am J Med Genet* 52;164, 1994.

Riise R, Andreasson S, Borgastrom M, et al: Intrafamilial variations of the phenotype in Bardet-Biedl syndrome. *Br J Ophthalmol* 81:378, 1997.

Barlow Syndrome

At a glance: Functional, constitutional or degenerative disorder of the mitral valve.

Synonyms: Mitral Valve Prolapse; Familial Mitral Regurgitation; Floppy Mitral Valve; Familial Myxomatous Valvular Disease; Myxomatous Mitral Valve Prolapse; Myxomatous Degeneration of the Mitral Valve.

Incidence: Mitral valve prolapse (MVP) is found in 3 to 5% of adults. The predominance in young female adults disappears in the older population.

Genetic inheritance: In the majority of idiopathic MVP cases, inheritance is autosomal dominant. In some cases, it is linked to chromosome 16p. Penetrance of MVP is variable.

Pathophysiology: In approximately 80% of cases (typically children or young females), MVP is considered a functional consequence of a valve–ventricle mismatch. In these patients, MVP and mitral regurgitation (MR) tend to resolve slowly over time, and the prognosis is generally good. In a minority of cases (20%), MVP is the result of progressive myxomatous degeneration of the mitral valve leaflets. These patients, mostly males, develop severe MR and eventually left ventricular dysfunction. With worsening MR, progressive pulmonary hypertension ensues. Valve replacement is needed after an average of approximately 25 years.

Diagnosis: Echocardiography, family history, and clinical examination. Secondary forms must be excluded.

Clinical aspects: Typical midsystolic click can be heard in approximately 80% of cases. Common features of functional MVP are recurrent chest pain, dyspnea episodes, palpitations, syncopes, and an increased anxiety level. Individuals with this form of MVP typically have a lean body stature. Complications from functional MVP are rare and include endocarditis, arrhythmias, and probably a slightly increased risk of thromboembolic events. Arrhythmias are of supraventricular origin, or they manifest as premature ventricular contractions. A higher incidence of preexcitation syndromes has been reported. Fortunately, malignant ventricular arrhythmias are rare. In an analysis of 50 patients with sudden cardiac death related to surgery and/or anesthesia, 47 (94%) had cardiac lesions on autopsy, but MVP was found in only one (2%). Atrial fibrillation is common in patients with progressive myxomatous degeneration. Symptoms and complications of pulmonary hypertension and left ventricular dysfunction become more pronounced in advanced disease stages. One child had a cerebrovascular event in a follow-up study of 119 children with MVP. Electrocardiographic recordings were abnormal in 63%, with premature ventricular contraction and T-wave inversion noted most commonly. There was no case of sudden death.

Precautions before anesthesia: Personal medical history should include palpitations, syncope, anesthesia, and current medication (e.g., beta-blocking agents, anxiolytics, anticoagulants). The electrocardiogram might identify patients with atrial fibrillation or preexcitation syndromes, but is unreliable in terms of predicting arrhythmias during anesthesia. Electrolytes should be in the normal range. Adequate anxiolysis reduces palpitations. The degree of MR and any additional cardiac anomalies should be known; when in doubt, echocardiography may be necessary.

Anesthetic considerations: Adequate intravascular filling reduces symptoms of functional MVP. However, fluid administration must be carefully titrated to prevent deterioration of MR. For the same reason, an increase of systemic afterload (vasoconstriction) must be prevented, and vasodilators might be considered as long as normotension is maintained. Maintaining a higher heart rate decreases left ventricular filling pressures during diastole, thus decreasing MR. The sensitivity of the myocardium to catecholamines usually is increased in advanced stages.

Pharmacological implications: Volatile anesthetics are safe in lower concentrations, but might cause myocardial depression with worsening left ventricular function at higher concentrations. Benzodiazepines are equally well tolerated, and no evidence contraindicates neuroblockers. In contrast, barbiturates should be avoided (at least in higher doses) because of their potential for myocardial depression. Ketamine is generally regarded as disadvantageous because of its sympathomimetic effects and consequent aggravation of MR. In addition, endocarditis prophylaxis in general is indicated in MVP, except for mild cases with no murmur and no MR.

Other conditions to be considered: MVP and MR are associated with various clinical conditions and syndromes. Coronary heart disease with or without rupture of the papillary muscle, congestive and hypertrophic cardiomyopathies, congenital heart disease (mostly atrial septal defect), and various connective tissue disorders, such as ☞Marfan syndrome, ☞Ehlers-Danlos syndrome, and ☞osteogenesis imperfecta, have been associated with MVP.

REFERENCES:

Bisset GS III, Schwartz DC, Meyer RA, et al: Clinical spectrum and long-term follow-up of isolated mitral valve prolapse in 119 children. *Circulation* 62:423, 1980.

Boudoulas H, Kolibash AJ, Baker P, et al: Mitral valve prolapse and the mitral valve prolapse syndrome: A diagnostic classification and pathogenesis of symptoms. *Am Heart J* 118:796, 1989.

Hanson EW, Neerhut RK, Lynch C 3rd. Mitral valve prolapse. *Anesthesiology* 85:178, 1996.

Barnes Syndrome

At a glance: Autosomal dominant disorder characterized by a small, bell-shaped thorax and laryngeal stenosis with iliac and pelvis dysplasia.

Synonym: Thoraco-Laryngo-Pelvic Dysplasia.

Incidence: Two families with two children each and one sporadic case have been described. The diagnosis was retrospectively suggested in a third family described with thoracopelvic dysostosis.

Genetic inheritance: Classic mendelian autosomal dominant inheritance with variable penetrance has been suggested.

Pathophysiology: Small lungs and a restrictive chest wall as a result of the thoracic dysplasia give rise to respiratory distress in the newborn. In addition, laryngeal stenosis might cause upper airway obstruction with increased work of breathing.

Diagnosis: Radiologic and clinical features, family history.

Clinical aspects: The typical triad consists of laryngeal stenosis, thoracic dysplasia with a small, bell-shaped chest wall, and a small pelvis. Affected individuals usually present with respiratory distress

at birth, and tracheal intubation was difficult in all. Tracheostomy was usually indicated for long-term ventilation. Tracheostomy was performed as an emergency procedure in one patient at 5 weeks of age because the child could not be reintubated after a failed extubation trial. This child later underwent successful laryngotracheoplasty. Because of the small thorax and pelvis, the abdomen appears big and protuberant in babies. Long-term outcome is not yet defined. Mortality is high; in fact, the oldest described individual who underwent thoracoplasty to increase the thoracic diameter in early childhood eventually died of cor pulmonale at 14 years of age. The children in the two families were delivered by cesarean section because of cephalopelvic disproportion (mother with small pelvis, who obviously suffered from a milder form of Barnes syndrome; however, tracheal intubation reportedly was difficult secondary to laryngeal stenosis).

Precautions before anesthesia: Ideally, tracheal intubation is done in the delivery room or the operating room with an ear-nose-throat or pediatric surgeon present in case urgent tracheostomy is needed. Considering the available literature, assessing older children for the presence of pulmonary hypertension prior to intervention seems prudent.

Anesthetic considerations: High positive pressures might be necessary for adequate ventilation because of the restrictive chest physiology, especially in the younger child. Pulmonary hypertension, if present, may not be well tolerated, and the increased right ventricular afterload because of positive pressure ventilation leads to a higher risk of right ventricular failure. Avoid acidosis and hypercapnia to keep pulmonary vascular resistance as low as possible, which is of particular risk during induction with difficult face-mask ventilation and/or failed attempts of tracheal intubation.

Pharmacological implications: In the presence of cor pulmonale, pulmonary vasoconstrictors should be avoided. If extubation is considered in patients with borderline respiratory function, a nerve stimulator should be used to prevent any residual paralysis.

Other conditions to be considered:

☞ELLIS VAN CREVELD SYNDROME: Genetic form of short-limbed dwarfism.

☞JEUNE SYNDROME: Jeune and Barnes syndromes share the predominant feature of thoracic hypoplasia but are genetically distinct. In Jeune syndrome, chest wall hypoplasia tends to be more severe. In contrast, laryngeal stenosis is not a feature of the Jeune phenotype.

☞SHORT RIB POLYDACTYLY SYNDROME TYPE II (Majewski Syndrome): Lethal entity characterized by median cleft lip, preaxial and postaxial polysyndactyly, short ribs and limbs, genital abnormalities, and anomalies of epiglottis and viscera. Other features include polycystic kidneys, transposition of the great vessels, and atretic lesions of the gastrointestinal and genitourinary systems.

☞SHORT RIB POLYDACTYLY SYNDROME TYPE I (Saldino-Noonan Syndrome): Lethal condition of newborns characterized by hydropic appearance, postaxial polydactyly, severely shortened and flipper-like limbs, and striking metaphyseal dysplasia of tubular bones. The pelvis resembles that of ☞Ellis van Creveld syndrome and ☞Jeune syndrome. As in type II (Majewski syndrome), polycystic kidneys, transposition of the great vessels, and atresic lesions of the gastrointestinal and genitourinary systems occur.

☞SHORT RIB POLYDACTYLY SYNDROME TYPE III (Verman-Naumoff Syndrome): Lethal entity characterized by a short cranial base, bulging forehead, depressed nasal bridge, flat occiput.

☞**BEEMER-LANGER SYNDROME:** Lethal entity presenting with hydrops, ascites, median cleft of the upper lip, narrow chest, and short, bowed limbs.

Other thoracic dysplasia syndromes, such as thanatophoric dwarfism, have been described rarely.

REFERENCES:

Burn J, Hall C, Marsden D, et al: Autosomal dominant thoraco-laryngopelvic dysplasia: Barnes syndrome. *J Med Genet* 23:345, 1986.

Gilchrist BF, Shroff V, DeLuca FG, et al: Management of thoracolaryngeal dysplasia. *Eur J Pediatr Surg* 6:231, 1996.

Wood E, Kearns D: Laryngotracheal stenosis in thoracolaryngopelvic dysplasia: Barnes syndrome. *Otolaryngol Head Neck Surg* 113:807, 1995.

Barrow-Fitzsimmons Syndrome

At a glance: Short limbs, abnormal face, and congenital heart disease.

Synonym: Cardiofacial Short Limbs Syndrome.

Incidence and genetic inheritance: Only one case has been described.

Clinical aspects: The child presented at birth with oxygenation failure caused by a severe congenital heart defect described as single ventricle with absent left ventricle, absent mitral valve, and truncus arteriosus. The boy also showed features of chondrodysplastic dwarfism with short limbs, cryptorchism, and facial anomalies, including prominent nasal bridge, epicanthal folds, and micrognathia. He died in the newborn period.

Anesthetic considerations: If tracheal intubation is warranted, anesthetic principles of hypoplastic left heart syndrome physiology apply, including careful titration of oxygenation to prevent pulmonary overcirculation and excessive hypoxemia with risk of myocardial failure. In addition, if an active management strategy is chosen, prostaglandin E_1 is needed until surgical systemic-to-pulmonary shunt is established. Facial anomalies may result in difficult airway management.

REFERENCE:

Barrow M, Fitzsimmons JS: A new syndrome. Short limbs, abnormal facial appearance, and congenital heart defect. *Am J Med Genet* 18:431, 1984.

Barth Syndrome

At a glance: Genetic disorder with dilated cardiomyopathy, neutropenia, and skeletal myopathy with muscle weakness.

Synonyms: Fatal Infantile X-Linked Cardiomyopathy; Cardioskeletal Myopathy with Neutropenia and Abnormal Mitochondria; Cardioskeletal Myopathy-Neutropenia; 3-Beta Methylglutaconic Aciduria, Type II.

Incidence: Rare, but families from various parts of the world have been described.

Genetic inheritance: Barth syndrome (BTHS) is ascribed to mutations in the G4.5 gene (tafazzin, TAZ), which is encoded on chromosome Xq28. The syndrome is transmitted in an X-linked recessive mode, and heterozygous females are healthy carriers because of skewed X-chromosome inactivation.

Pathophysiology: Electron microscopic examination reveals abnormal mitochondria in skeletal muscle, myocardium, liver, kidney, and myelocytes. Diminished cytochrome concentrations have been demonstrated in isolated mitochondria, presumably associated with defects in the respiratory chain reaction. Neutropenia results from arrested granulopoiesis at the myelocyte stage.

Diagnosis: Clinical picture, family history, muscle biopsy, and genetic analysis. In addition, mildly elevated levels of 3-methylglutaconate, 3-methylglutarate, and 2-ethylhydracrylate in the urine are common. Low L-carnitine levels have been described occasionally.

Clinical aspects: The hallmark of BTHS is a combination of dilated cardiomyopathy with endocardial fibroelastosis, neutropenia with severe infections, and skeletal myopathy with muscle weakness, sparing the extraocular and bulbar muscles. Onset of cardiomyopathy may be precipitous and the response to standard congestive heart failure treatment variable. The degree of myeloic dysfunction ranges from chronic severe neutropenia to sporadic episodes of neutropenia. Phenotypic expression of BTHS is variable. Forms with late onset and milder courses have been described, as have severe forms with lethal noncompaction of the left ventricular myocardium. Fasting ketone production is normal, but mild lactacidosis and hypoglycemia have been observed in some patients. One case report described rapid deterioration with L-carnitine; the patient subsequently showed dramatic improvement of cardiac function, growth, and neutrophil count with large doses of pantothenic acid. Before the advent of transplantation medicine, affected males died of cardiac failure or septic complications in infancy or early childhood. Now, survival for more than 7 years following heart transplantation has been reported.

Precautions before anesthesia: Cardiac dysfunction should be assessed and treatment optimized preoperatively. Personal history should include previous anesthesias, palpitations, syncopes, and current medication. Electrolytes must be within the normal range. For elective surgery, the patient should be free of current infections. If muscle weakness is clinically relevant, pulmonary function testing including measurement of maximum inspiratory pressures identifies those who might be at risk for prolonged mechanical ventilation after anesthesia.

Anesthetic considerations: Fluid administration and systemic vasoconstriction must be carefully titrated to optimize cardiac output and maintain blood pressure stability. Maintaining a high heart rate decreases left ventricular filling during diastole, thereby decreasing end-diastolic pressure and myocardial oxygen demand. Note that in advanced stages, myocardial sensitivity to catecholamines often is increased. Adequate glucose administration should be provided and glucose and lactate levels monitored. A strictly aseptic technique is mandatory to prevent infections in patients with neutropenia, which may already be present at birth.

Pharmacological implications: Volatile anesthetics are safe in lower concentrations, but may cause myocardial depression at higher concentrations. Benzodiazepines usually are well tolerated, but may cause hypotension if cardiac performance is marginal or if the patient is relatively volume depleted from chronic diuretic therapy. In contrast, barbiturates are better avoided for myocardial depression, and ketamine is generally regarded as disadvantageous because of its sympathomimetic effects and consequent increase in afterload. Succinylcholine is best avoided because of the potential risk of hyperkalemia in the presence of generalized myopathy. Although nondepolarizing muscle relaxants are not contraindicated, because of the generalized muscle weakness they should be used, if at all, in reduced doses and with a peripheral nerve stimulator only.

Other conditions to be considered: X-linked endocardial fibroelastosis and X-linked cardiomyopathy are regarded as different phenotypic expressions of the same disorder.

REFERENCES:

Cantlay AM, Shokrollahi K, Allen JT: Genetic analysis of the G4.5 gene in families with suspected Barth syndrome. *J Pediatr* 135:311, 1999.

Christodoulou J, McInnes RR, Jay V, et al: Barth syndrome: Clinical observations and genetic linkage studies. *Am J Med Genet* 50:264, 1994.

D'Adamo P, Fassone L, Gedeon A, et al: The X-linked gene G4.5 is responsible for different infantile dilated cardiomyopathies. *Am J Hum Genet* 61:862, 1997.

Bart-Pumphrey Syndrome

At a glance: Inherited syndrome with knuckle pads, leukonychia, and sensorineural deafness.

Incidence and genetic inheritance: Incidence unknown. In 1967, Bart and Pumphrey described the syndrome in a large kindred and three families. Autosomal dominant inheritance. The mutation seems to affect the *GJB2* gene encoding the gap junction protein connexin-26.

Clinical aspects: Hearing loss is caused by a cochlear defect. Features include knuckle pads and leukonychia (possible on fingers and toes). Keratosis palmoplantaris is common in older patients.

Anesthetic considerations: Considering hearing loss, adapted preoperative explanations should be given to the patients to prevent anxiety. Leukonychia can alter accuracy of pulse oximetry.

Other conditions to be considered:

☞**VOHWINKEL SYNDROME:** Congenital deafness with keratopachyderma and constrictions of fingers and toes.

☞**KERATOSIS ICHTYOSIS DEAFNESS (KID) SYNDROME:** A form of ectodermal dysplasia characterized by inflammation of the corneae (keratitis), skin scales, and deafness.

REFERENCES:

Bart RS, Pumphrey RE: Knuckle pads, leukonychia and deafness. A dominantly inherited syndrome. *N Engl J Med* 276:202, 1967.

Ramer JC, Vasily DB, Ladda RL: Familial leukonychia, knuckle pads, hearing loss and palmoplantar hyperkeratosis: an additional family with Bart-Pumphrey syndrome. *J Med Genet* 31:68, 1994.

Richard G, Brown N, Ishida-Yamamoto A, et al. Expanding the phenotypic spectrum of Cx26 disorders: Bart-Pumphrey syndrome is caused by a novel missense mutation in GJB2. *J Invest Dermatol* 123:856, 2004.

Bartter Syndrome

At a glance: Autosomal recessive transmitted secondary hyperaldosteronism with normal blood pressure and polyuria. Peculiar facies is common. Do not confuse with Schwarz-Bartter syndrome (also called syndrome of inappropriate antidiuretic hormone secretion [SIADH]).

Synonyms: Hypokalemic Alkalosis with Hypercalciuria Aldosteronism–Normal Blood Pressure Syndrome; Hypokalemic Alkalosis Juxtaglomerular Hyperplasia Syndrome.

History: Named after the American physician Frederic Crosby Bartter, who described this syndrome in 1962. However, 2 years earlier, P. Pronove had already described the disorder in a 5-year-old boy.

Incidence: Exact incidence is unknown, but is estimated to be approximately 1:1,000,000 to 10 in 1,000,000 live births. No racial or sexual predilection has been reported.

Genetic inheritance: Autosomal recessive.

Pathophysiology: Caused by mutation in the Na-K-2Cl cotransporter gene (located on 1p36); it also is caused by mutations in the K^+ channel (ROMK). The primary defect resides in active chloride reabsorption in the loop of Henle.

Diagnosis: Unusual form of secondary hyperaldosteronism in which hypertrophy and hyperplasia of the juxtaglomerular cells are associated with normal blood pressure and hypokalemic alkalosis in the absence of edema. The features are short stature, hyperactive renin-angiotensin system, lack of effect of angiotensin on blood pressure, renal potassium wasting, increased renal prostaglandin production, and occasionally hypomagnesemia. It can be simulated by habitual vomiting, as in anorexia nervosa.

Clinical aspects: The first consequence of the tubular defect in Bartter syndrome is polyuria, which is already present during fetal life. It is responsible for particular complications of pregnancy, such as polyhydramnios and premature delivery. Patients usually are symptomatic early in life (growth usually is below the age standards, and final height may be compromised). Clinical features include peculiar facies with large head, prominent forehead, triangular face, large pinnae, and large eyes. Renal failure is frequent and nephrocalcinosis, renal juxtaglomerular cell hypertrophy, and increased renal echogenicity with loss of corticomedullary differentiation have been described. Other signs include mental retardation generalized weakness, muscle cramps, tetany, amyotrophia, platelet aggregation defect, polydipsia polyuria, vomiting, and constipation.

Precautions before anesthesia: Evaluate muscular weakness (clinical, electromyogram) and renal function (laboratory, ultrasound, radionuclide imaging). Laboratory investigations should include electrolytes, arterial blood gas analysis (hypokalemic metabolic alkalosis), plasma aldosterone, and plasma renin (hyperactive renin-angiotensin system). An electrocardiogram may be obtained to evaluate for arrhythmias.

Anesthetic considerations: High aspiration risk because of gastric mobility perturbation. Preoperative medications should be continued for as long as possible and reintroduced as soon as possible. Intraoperative fluid regimen can increase hypokalemia and hyperventilation. Perioperative cardiac monitoring can be necessary in case of profound hypokalemia (even in chronic hypokalemia, where anesthesia provides less arrhythmias than in acute hypokalemia).

Pharmacological implications: Adapt muscle relaxants to muscular amyotrophy and hypotonia. Propofol should be avoided for prolonged anesthesia or sedation because of its effect on urinary acid excretion. Caution if insulin or bicarbonates are used (risk of hypokalemia).

Other conditions to be considered:

ANTENATAL HYPERCALCIURIC FORM OF BARTTER SYNDROME (Hyperprostaglandin E Syndrome): The abnormalities in this form of Bartter syndrome already present between the 24th and 30th week of gestation with fetal polyuria leading to polyhydramnios and often premature birth. The neonates suffer from hypokalemic metabolic alkalosis, severe salt wasting and hyperprosta-glandinuria. Marked hypercalciuria is essential for the diagnosis and may result in nephro-calcinosis and osteopenia. Serum-magnesium levels are mildly to moderately decreased. Growth is delayed. Treatment with inhibitors of prostaglandin synthesis may be life-saving. Caused by a defect in either NKCC2, the

Na-K-Cl cotransporter-2 (SLC12A1 or KCNJ1) located on 1p36, 15q15-q21.1, and 11q24.

☞**GITELMAN SYNDROME:** Inherited renal tubular defect resulting in urinary loss of magnesium, sodium, potassium and chloride in patients with otherwise healthy kidneys.

REFERENCES:

Bartter FC, Pronove P, Gill JR Jr, et al: Hyperplasia of the juxtaglomerular complex with hyperaldosteronism and hypokalemic alkalosis: A new syndrome. *Am J Med* 33:811, 1962.

Kannan S, Delph Y, Moseley HSL: Anaesthetic management of a child with Bartter's syndrome. *Can J Anaesth* 42:808, 1995.

Landau D, Shalev H, Ohaly M, et al: Infantile variant of Bartter syndrome and sensorineural deafness: A new autosomal recessive disorder. *Am J Med Genet* 59:454, 1995.

Basal Cell Carcinomas with Milia and Coarse, Sparse Hair Syndrome

At a glance: Basal cell carcinomas, multiple milia of face and limbs, increased sweating and facial pigmentation, and sparse scalp and body hair.

Incidence and genetic inheritance: Incidence is not known. Inheritance seems to be either autosomal dominant or X-linked dominant.

Clinical aspects: Main features are sparse and coarse scalp hair, sparse body hair, and multiple, often big milia on face and limbs, which tend to disappear around puberty. Basal cell carcinomas (most often multiple) develop in early adult life. Some patients complain about excessive sweating. Some researchers believe it is the same entity as ☞Bazex syndrome.

Anesthetic considerations: Atropine and other parasympatholytic drugs may reduce the excessive sweating, which could otherwise render taping for the endotracheal tube, the intravenous cannula, and ECG electrodes challenging. However, temperature must be controlled to prevent hyperthermia.

Other condition to be considered:

☞**BAZEX SYNDROME:** X-linked dominant inherited disorder characterized by follicular atrophoderma in combination with hypotrichosis, hypohidrosis, and nevoid basal cell carcinoma.

REFERENCES:

Oley CA, Sharpe H, Chenevix-Trench G: Basal cell carcinomas, coarse sparse hair, and milia. *Am J Med Genet* 43:799, 1992.

Vabres P, de Prost Y: Bazex-Dupre-Christol syndrome: A possible diagnosis for basal cell carcinomas, coarse sparse hair, and milia [letter]. *Am J Med Genet* 45:786, 1993.

Basan Syndrome

At a glance: Ectodermal dysplasia, absent dermatoglyphic pattern, changes in nails, simian crease, and abnormal sweating.

Incidence: Unknown. First described by M. Basan in 1965; since then a limited number of articles describing various patients with features of the syndrome have been published. However, clear distinction between epidermal ridge disorders remains difficult because of the heterogeneous nature of these conditions and the lack of an accepted classification system.

Genetic inheritance: Autosomal dominant inheritance. Genetic heterogeneity results in a spectrum of familial absence/dissociation of dermal ridge patterns.

Pathophysiology: The precise mechanisms leading to the wide phenotypic variations of the syndrome remain to be determined.

Diagnosis: Based on clinical examination, family history, and genetic analysis.

Clinical aspects: The syndrome is characterized by multiple congenital milia on the chin and neonatal vesicular/bullous lesions on the fingers and soles of the feet, which resolve during the first month of life. Ectodermal dysplasia with absence or abnormality of dermal ridge patterns, simian creases, and lack of sweat glands on the volar surfaces. The fingertips are tapered and there is an increased cold sensitivity on hands and feet. The nails are rough, with transverse groves and longitudinal ridges. The skin is smooth with a leather-like texture. No other congenital abnormalities are associated with the condition. Life expectancy appears to be normal.

Precautions before anesthesia: Premedication with anticholinergic agents (e.g., atropine) should be avoided in neonates and infants because the condition is associated with a reduced number of sweat glands, potentially resulting in pyrexia and abnormal body temperature regulation.

Anesthetic considerations: Temperature monitoring should be used in all cases. Vascular access in the extremities may be difficult as a consequence of the leather-like skin texture.

Pharmacological implications: Careful use of anticholinergic drugs in neonates.

Other condition to be considered:

☞**ECTODERMAL DYSPLASIA:** At least 150 other forms of Ectodermal Dysplasia are known.

REFERENCES:

Reed T, Schreiner RL: Absence of dermal ridge patterns: genetic heterogeneity. *Am J Med Genet* 16:81, 1983.

Richards W, Kaplan M: Anhidrotic ectodermal dysplasia. An unusual case of pyrexia in the newborn. *Am J Dis Child* 117:597, 1969.

Schaumann B, Alter M: *Dermatoglyphics in Medical Disorders*. New York, Springer-Verlag, 1976, p 89.

Basaran Yilmaz Syndrome

At a glance: A disease characterized by keratoderma, hypotrichosis, and leukonychia totalis.

Synonym: Keratoderma Hypotrichosis Leukonychia Syndrome.

Incidence and genetic inheritance: One Turkish female and her two daughters have been described.

Clinical aspects: The family presented with congenital hypotrichosis, dry skin, keratosis pilaris, and leukonychia totalis. Hair characteristics included trichorrhexis nodosa and trichoptilosis (longitudinal splitting of the distal end of the hair). The patients gradually developed palmoplantar keratoderma and hyperkeratotic lesions on their knees, elbows, and perianal area.

Anesthetic considerations: The described features of this syndrome were strictly confined to the skin, and no anesthetic implications are expected.

Other conditions to be considered: The syndrome must be distinguished from other forms of palmoplantar keratoderma (☞keratosis palmoplantaris with esophageal cancer; ☞Papillon-Lefevre syndrome, ☞Schopf-Schulz-Passarge syndrome), which may be associated with an increased risk of malignancies, especially of the esophagus or colon.

REFERENCE:
Basaran E, Yilmaz E, Alpsoy E, et al: Keratoderma, hypotrichosis and leukonychia totalis: A new syndrome? *Br J Dermatol* 133:636, 1995.

REFERENCE:
Battaglia A, Ferrari A, Orsitto E, et al: New autosomal recessive syndrome of mental retardation, coarse face, microcephaly and skeletal abnormalities. *Clin Dysmorphol* 5:41, 1996.

Bassoe Syndrome

At a glance: Form of autosomal recessive congenital muscular dystrophy.

Synonym: Congenital Muscular Dystrophy with Infantile Cataract and Hypogonadism.

History: In 1956 H.H. Bassoe described a syndrome of congenital muscular dystrophy, infantile cataract, and hypogonadism (in females, ovarian agenesis; in males, Klinefelter syndrome). Seven persons living in a small, isolated Norwegian village were identified.

Clinical aspects: Clinical signs include hypotonia, abnormal gait, expressionless face, cataract, amyotrophy/muscle agenesis, and small/atrophic testicles, which may result in late puberty or hypogonadism as a late sign. Less frequent signs include ptosis, kyphosis, hyperextensible joints, abnormally placed nipples, squinting/paresis of ocular muscles, and increased carrying angle of the elbows.

Anesthetic considerations: No literature about this condition associated with anesthesia is available, but certain considerations can be made. Because weakness of muscles can be extensive, the same precautions as for congenital muscular dystrophy are recommended. The disease requires a complete workup, including neurologic and motor milestones, family history, and previous medical problems. Respiratory function should be checked by chest radiography and arterial blood gas analysis. Preoperative physiotherapy likely will be beneficial. Postoperative mechanical ventilation may be necessary in severely affected patients. Delayed respiratory failure may occur. Plan to use regional anesthesia techniques where possible. Remember, the possibility of severe paucisymptomatic cardiac disease.

Pharmacological implications: Succinylcholine may cause rhabdomyolysis and cardiac arrest as a consequence of hyperkalemia.

REFERENCE:
Bassoe HH: Familial congenital muscular dystrophy with gonadal dysgenesis. *J Clin Endocrinol* 16:1614, 1956.

Battaglia Syndrome

At a glance: Coarse face, microcephaly, mental retardation, and epilepsy.

Incidence and genetic inheritance: Only two sibs have been described. Inheritance was suspected to be autosomal recessive.

Clinical aspects: Brother and sister presented with microcephaly, mental retardation, and epilepsy, which was refractory to medical treatment in the brother, but was sufficiently controlled in the sister. In addition, both individuals had hirsutism, a coarse face, scoliosis, and a retarded bone age.

Anesthetic considerations: Preanesthetic and postanesthetic management may be challenging because of an increased level of anxiety with mental retardation. Antiepileptic therapy may require preoperative adjustment, and drug interactions are common with certain antiseizure drugs. Severe scoliosis has its own anesthetic implications (difficult tracheal intubation, restrictive airway disease, cor pulmonale), which may require further considerations.

Bazex Syndrome

At a glance: X-linked dominant inherited syndrome characterized by follicular atrophoderma in combination with hypotrichosis, hypohidrosis, and nevoid basal cell carcinoma.

Synonyms: Bazex-Dupré-Christol Syndrome; Acrokeratosis Paraneoplastica; Follicular Atrophoderma-Basocellular Proliferations-Hypotrichosis Syndrome; Follicular Atrophoderma-Basal Cell Carcinoma Syndrome.

History: First described in 1966 by A. Bazex, A. Dupré, and B Christol in six members of the same family. In 1996 A. Kidd et al. reviewed all the cases reported at that time and estimated approximately 120 identified cases from 15 kindreds. Hitherto, only described in caucasians, although a very similar disorder was described in a Japanese family.

Genetic inheritance: X-linked dominant inheritance. Gene map locus Xq24-q27.

Diagnosis: Based on characteristic clinical features of affected patients and appearance of their hairs under scanning electron microscopy. In contrast to the frequently used term *follicular atrophoderma,* the histologic analysis of lesions does not demonstrate skin atrophy.

Clinical aspects: Individuals have pitting or so-called *multiple icepick marks* on the dorsum of their hands, the elbow, and occasionally the face, which are present from early infancy on. Histologic studies show that these areas of pitting, which are commonly termed *follicular atrophoderma,* do not demonstrate atrophy. Facial basal cell carcinomas develop between the ages of 15 and 25 years. Hypotrichosis is present in all cases, and scanning electron microscopy of the hair demonstrates a flattened and twisted appearance. Some patients may show a circumscribed absence of sweat glands. Pinched nose with hypoplastic alae and prominent columella was considered another characteristic manifestation. No other systemic abnormalities are associated.

Anesthetic considerations: No literature on this syndrome in association with anesthesia is available. No specific anesthetic considerations are expected.

Other conditions to be considered:

    CONGENITAL HYPOTRICHOSIS WITH MILIA SYNDROME (Hypotrichosis with Light-Colored Hair and Facial Milia): Autosomal dominant inherited syndrome with scalp hypotrichosis, facial milia, and reduction in hair shaft melanin.

    ☞**BASAL CELL CARCINOMAS WITH MILIA AND COARSE, SPARSE HAIR SYNDROME:** Basal cell carcinomas, multiple milia of face and limbs, increased sweating and facial pigmentation, sparse scalp and body hair.

    ☞**ROMBO SYNDROME:** Genetic disorder with facial follicular skin atrophy, milia and telangiectasis, absent eyelashes and eyebrows, and basal cell carcinomas later in life.

REFERENCES:
Bazex A, Dupré A, Christol B: Atrophodermic folliculaire, proliferations baso-cellulaires et hypotrichose. *Ann Derm Syph* 93:241, 1966.

Kidd A, Carson L, Gregory DW, et al: A Scottish family with Bazex-Dupré-Christol syndrome: Follicular atrophoderma, congenital hypotrichosis, and basal cell carcinomas. *J Med Genet* 33:493, 1996.

Vabres P, Lacombe D, Rabinowitz LG, et al: The gene for Bazex-Dupré-Christol syndrome maps to chromosome Xq. *J Invest Dermatol* 105:87, 1995.

Bazopoulou-Kyrkanidou Syndrome

At a glance: Craniofaciocervical osseous dysplasia associated with microstoma, short neck, and short midface. Congenital torticollis is frequently present.

Synonym: Cranio-Facio-Cervical Osteoglyphic Dysplasia.

Incidence and genetic inheritance: One sporadic case in Greece has been described.

Clinical aspects: The patient had progressive neck stiffness starting at the age of 6 years, followed by generalized destruction of the periodontium with intraosseous lucent lesions in cranium and vertebrae. Biopsy revealed osseous destruction and nonspecific chronic inflammation. As an adult, neck mobility was significantly reduced, and other described features included hypoplasia of the maxilla, microstomia, and cross-bite. Mental development was normal.

Anesthetic considerations: Main issue for anesthesia is severe neck rigidity and microstomia, which might make tracheal intubation very difficult. However, the propositus had several surgical interventions, and no anesthetic difficulties were reported.

REFERENCE:

Bazopoulou-Kyrkanidou E, Vrotsos I, Kyrkanides S, et al: Hyperbrachycephaly, short face, midface hypoplasia, fusion of cervical vertebrae, radiolucent bone defects and severe destruction of periodontium—A new syndrome: Craniofaciocervical osteoglyphic dysplasia. *Genet Couns* 5:257, 1994.

Beals Syndrome

At a glance: Genetic syndrome characterized by multiple osseous dysplasia, ear anomalies, and short stature.

Synonym: Auriculo-Osteodysplasia. Do not confuse with congenital contractural arachnodactyly, which sometimes is also referred to as *Beals syndrome.*

Incidence and genetic inheritance: Two families with autosomal dominant inheritance have been reported. Ratio of females to males is approximately 1:1. The genetic defect has not been identified.

Clinical aspects: Dysplasia of the radiocapitellar joint with or without dislocation of the radial head, characteristically shaped ears with elongated and attached earlobes, and an associated small lobule beneath are the hallmarks of this syndrome. Hip dislocation is more frequent in these families. Females tend to have masculine torsos. All affected individuals have a slightly reduced body height. Intelligence is normal.

Anesthetic considerations: Based on the described features, no specific implications for anesthesia are expected. However, positioning the patient requires care to prevent luxation of the affected joints, especially with use of neuromuscular blocking agents.

REFERENCE:

Beals RK: Auriculo-osteodysplasia: A syndrome of multiple osseous dysplasia, ear anomaly, and short stature. *J Bone Joint Surg Am* 49A:1541, 1967.

Beardwell Syndrome

At a glance: Genetic disorder with ankylosis of the spine and hyperkeratosis of palms and soles.

Synonym: Ankylosing Vertebral Hyperostosis with Tylosis.

Incidence and genetic inheritance: One Greek Cypriot family has been described. Because six members of the sibship had tylosis (hyperkeratosis punctata plantaris and palmaris) alone, two independent genetic traits may have been present.

Clinical aspects: All the affected individuals had ankylosing vertebral hyperostosis, including ossification of paraspinal ligaments and formation of large osteophytes. Most were asymptomatic; a few complained about low-grade back pain. Tylosis was present in all patients. One member had mild psoriasis. The osseous manifestations are basically identical to those found in diffuse idiopathic skeletal hyperostosis (DISH), and some researchers use Beardwell and Forestier syndrome synonymously. However, although onset of DISH (ankylosing hyperostosis, asymmetrical skeletal hyperostosis or senile ankylosing hyperostosis) before 50 years of age is exceedingly rare, affected individuals here were between 18 and 50 years old at the time of the report. DISH often is asymptomatic, but many of the different symptoms and complications reported are dependent on the location of the osteophytes. The symptoms may range from pain and stiffness to stridor and difficulties swallowing. Furthermore, a higher incidence of diabetes mellitus and other metabolic disorders has been reported.

Anesthetic considerations: Most of the individuals described by Beardwell were asymptomatic, and implications for anesthesia have not been described. However, anesthetic complications in DISH patients have been reported, for example, difficult tracheal intubation from deviation and stenosis of the trachea, decreased neck mobility, vocal cord paresis, and one case requiring emergency tracheostomy for severe airway obstruction caused by an osteophytic mass.

Other conditions to be considered:

FORESTIER DISEASE (Diffuse Idiopathic Skeletal Hyperostosis, DISH): The bony lesions are phenotypically similar. The incidence of DISH is higher, and it has been described in Caucasians and Africans.

☞**KERATOSIS PALMARIS ET PLANTARIS:** Other forms of palmoplantor hyperkeratosis are summarized under this title.

REFERENCES:

Beardwell A: Familial ankylosing vertebral hyperostosis with tylosis. *Ann Rheum Dis* 28:518, 1969.

Crosby ET, Grahovac S: Diffuse idiopathic skeletal hyperostosis: An unusual cause of difficult intubation. *Can J Anaesth* 40:54, 1993.

Kiss C, Szilagyi M, Paksy A, et al: Risk factors for diffuse idiopathic skeletal hyperostosis: A case-control study. *Rheumatology (Oxford)* 41:27, 2002.

Beare-Stevenson Syndrome

At a glance: Sporadic disorder with craniosynostosis, anogenital, and skin anomalies.

Synonym: Beare-Stevenson Cutis Gyrata Syndrome.

Incidence: About ten individuals have been described, including children of Caucasian and African descent.

Genetic inheritance: A new mutation on chromosome 10q26, transmitted in an autosomal dominant way, seems to be the most likely cause. This gene is also involved in other craniosynostosis syndromes (e.g., Crouzon syndrome, Apert syndrome, Pfeiffer syndrome). Only sporadic cases have been described. Mutations in fibroblast growth factor receptor-2 were found in some, but not all, patients.

Pathophysiology: Unknown.

Diagnosis: Made by clinical picture and family history.

Clinical aspects: Presents with a combination of craniofacial defects, ear malformations, skin anomalies, and anogenital defects. Craniosynostosis, choanal atresia, and a cleft or narrow palate are the prominent craniofacial features. Five patients had mild-to-severe cloverleaf skull, and one presented with acrocephaly. Neurologic malformations were limited to hydrocephalus in some of the patients with cloverleaf skull, and one patient also had agenesis of the corpus callosum. Upper airway obstruction caused respiratory distress postnatally in some cases. Skin anomalies presented with deep skin furrows (cutis gyrata) and acanthosis nigricans. Prominent umbilical stump or umbilical hernia have been reported, as have an anteriorly placed anus, cryptorchidism, and a bifid scrotum. Most children die early, usually of unknown causes or respiratory failure. The longest reported survival time is 13 years.

Precautions before anesthesia: Craniofacial anatomy must be assessed prior to anesthesia. Chest radiography is helpful to depict signs of recurrent aspirations. Some patients were described as having nonreactive pupils, which must be documented prior to the intervention.

Anesthetic considerations: Expect difficult tracheal intubation from narrow palate, clefts, choanal atresia, and mucosal tags of the alveolar gingiva. These children have died unexpectedly in the perioperative period, so they should be considered high-risk patients for anesthesia. If signs of increased intracranial pressures are present, adequate cerebral perfusion pressure must be maintained at all times. Whenever possible, regional anesthesia is preferable.

Pharmacological implications: If signs of decompensated hydrocephalus are present, for example, sunsetting of the eyes, drugs with a potential to increase intracranial pressure should be avoided.

Other conditions to be considered: The syndrome shares features with other ☞craniosynostosis syndromes, but the combination of the described features is considered unique.

REFERENCES:

Hall BD, Cadle RG, Golabi M, et al: Beare-Stevenson cutis gyrata syndrome. *Am J Med Genet* 44:82, 1992.

Przylepa KA, Paznekas W, Zhang M, et al: Fibroblast growth factor receptor 2 mutations in Beare-Stevenson cutis gyrata syndrome. *Nat Genet* 13:492, 1996.

Vargas RA, Maegama GH, Taucher SC, et al: Beare-Stevenson syndrome: Two South American patients with FGFR2 analysis. *Am J Med Genet* 121:41, 2003.

Beckwith-Wiedemann Syndrome

At a glance: Most often a sporadically occurring syndrome with exomphalos, macroglossia, gigantism, and hypoglycemia caused by hyperinsulinism.

Synonyms: Wiedemann-Beckwith Syndrome; Beckwith Syndrome; Wiedemann Syndrome; Wiedemann-Beckwith-Combs Syndrome; Infantile Gigantism; EMG Syndrome; Exomphalos-Macroglossia-Gigantism Syndrome; Familial Macroglossia-Omphalocele Syndrome; Macroglossia-Omphalocele-Visceromegaly Syndrome.

Incidence: 1:13,700 live births in West India. The incidence in other countries is approximately 1.5:100,000 live births.

Genetic inheritance: Most cases are sporadic; however, approximately 15% are inherited in an autosomal dominant mode with incomplete penetrance and variable expressivity. Failure of normal biparental inheritance of chromosome 11p15 (11p ter p15).

Pathophysiology: The 11p15 chromosome region contains a growth-promoting and a tumor-suppression gene. The genetic anomaly results in increased expression of the "insulin-like growth factor-2" gene IGF-2, which is responsible for the somatic overgrowth and predisposition to tumors. Altered placental endocrine physiology may play a role in producing many of the features already found during the neonatal period. Omphalocele, anomalies of intestinal rotation and fixation, and diaphragmatic eventration may be secondary to early visceromegaly.

Diagnosis: During pregnancy, polyhydramnios, and a very large placenta (up to twice the normal size) with increased length of the umbilical cord are characteristic. The birth weight for boys and girls is around the 95th and 75th percentile, respectively. Growth velocity is increased in the first 4 to 6 years of life (postnatal growth >90th percentile) and associated with advanced bone age, but

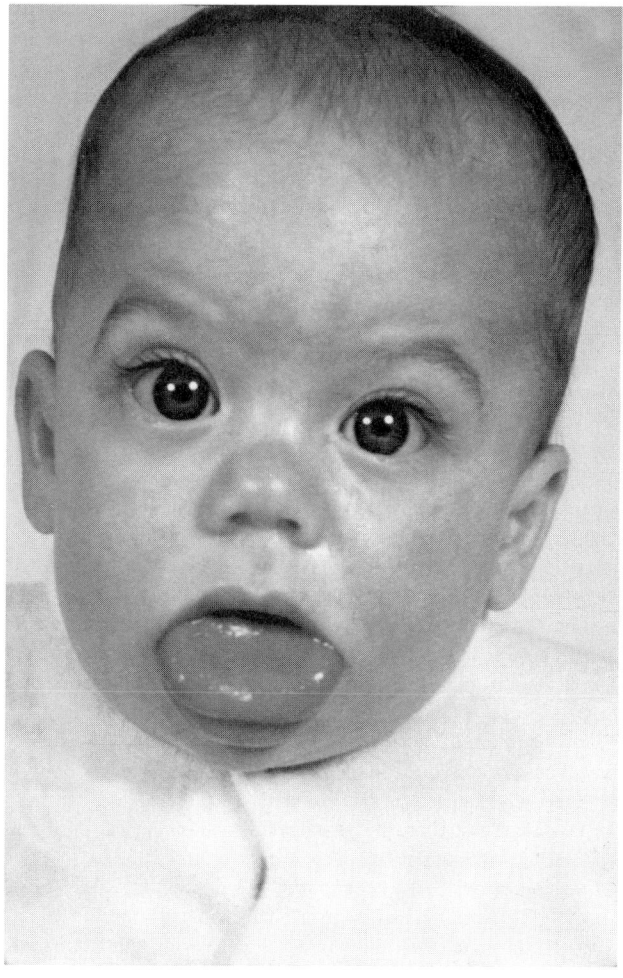

Beckwith-Wiedemann Syndrome   Pronounced macroglossia in a baby with Beckwith-Wiedemann syndrome.

normalization thereafter. Severe hypoglycemia is present in approximately 30 to 60% of newborns, with the highest incidence in the first 3 days of life. Macroglossia and omphalocele or umbilical defects, ear lobe grooves, and circular depression on the posterior rim of helix are other features.

Clinical aspects: Macroglossia is present in 98% of cases. Visceromegaly is characteristic: nephromegaly (with dysplasia of the renal medulla in 97%), splenomegaly (82%), and hepatomegaly (73%). Adrenocortical cytomegaly and pituitary amphophil hyperplasia have been reported. Intestinal malrotation with pyloric and/or ileal stenosis, imperforate anus, and atresia of the colon occasionally occur. Omphalocele and umbilical hernia may partially result from visceromegaly. Midface hypoplasia (hypoplastic maxilla) is associated with prominent occiput, ear anomalies, somatic gigantism, cryptorchidism, overgrowth of external genitalia, hypospadias, and bicornuate uterus. Conductive deafness may develop. Hemihypertrophy has been reported and is more often associated with malignant tumors (adrenal carcinoma, nephroblastoma [Wilms tumor], hepatoblastoma, thoracic neuroblastoma, rhabdomyosarcoma, congenital gastric teratoma) and require regular followups. The incidence of benign tumors (adrenal adenoma, myxoma, ganglioneuroma, carcinoid tumors) is increased. Hypoglycemia, if present in the neonatal period, may persist during the first years of life. Hypoglycemia is a result of relative hyperinsulinism associated with pancreatic islet hyperplasia. Mental retardation may result from neonatal hypoglycemia, but is otherwise rare (approximately 12% of patients). Hyperlipidemia, hypercholesterolemia, and hypocalcemia or hypercalcemia are commonly found. Sporadic cases with cardiomyopathy, congenital cardiac lesions (atrial septal defect, ventricular septal defect, hypoplastic left heart syndrome, tetralogy of Fallot, pulmonary artery stenosis), or cardiac hamartomas have been described. Infant mortality is high (up to 20%) and usually results from heart and respiratory failure.

Precautions before anesthesia: All patients must be checked for hypoglycemia and corrected if necessary (10% dextrose to provide 6–8 mg/kg/min of dextrose). Evaluate for difficult direct laryngoscopy and tracheal intubation as a result of macroglossia and maxillary hypoplasia. Echocardiography may be indicated. Surgery in children consists mainly of omphalocele repair, tumoral surgery and partial glossectomy.

Anesthetic considerations: The patient may be a giant premature baby, combining the risks of prematurity with those of macroglossia and its potential subsequent respiratory complications. Possible difficult tracheal intubation must be anticipated and a fiberoptic bronchoscope must be available immediately. Tracheomalacia resulted in failed extubation and subsequent tracheostomy in a case report of a 3-month-old boy. Use of laryngeal mask is relatively contraindicated because of the risks of regurgitation and aspiration. Close monitoring of glycemia and avoidance of hypoglycemia-inducing drugs are recommended throughout the perioperative period.

Pharmacological implications: Avoid nitrous oxide in cases of bowel obstruction. Depending on the presence and the pathophysiology of an associated cardiac lesion, drugs with negative inotropic or peripheral vasodilating action can be contraindicated. Subacute bacterial endocarditis prophylaxis may be required.

Other conditions to be considered:

☞**ANIRIDIA:** It is estimated that approximately one third of patients with sporadic aniridia will develop a Wilms tumor, whereas approximately half of patients with aniridia, genitourinary anomalies (e.g., hypospadias), and mental retardation will develop a Wilms tumor. Most patients have prominent lips and macrognathia. Other features may include congenital cataracts, nystagmus, ptosis, and

blindness. The presence of ptosis and generalized hypotonia in a subgroup of patients may suggest a susceptibility to malignant hyperthermia.

☞**WAGR SYNDROME:** Unusual association of Wilms tumor, ocular signs, and mental retardation.

☞**DENYS-DRASH SYNDROME:** Consists of the triad of congenital nephropathy, Wilms tumor, and ambiguous genitalia; manifests in small children.

REFERENCES:

Celiker V, Basgul E, Karagoz AH: Anesthesia in Beckwith-Widemann syndrome. *Paediatr Anaesth* 14:778, 2004.

Suan C, Ojeda R, Garcia-Perla JL, et al: Anesthesia and the Beckwith-Wiedemann syndrome. *Paediatr Anaesth* 6:231, 1996.

Weksberg R, Shuman C, Smith AC, Beckwith-Widemann syndrome. *Am J Med Genet C Semin Med Genet* 137:12, 2005.

Beemer-Langer Syndrome

At a glance: Genetic disorder characterized by multiple skeletal (and other) anomalies and death either in utero or in the early neonatal period as a result of respiratory failure.

Synonyms: Beemer-Langer Type Short Rib-Polydactyly Syndrome; Short Rib-Polydactyly Syndrome Type IV; SRPS Type IV; Polydactyly with Neonatal Chondrodystrophy, Type IV.

Incidence: Approximately 30 cases have been described.

Genetic inheritance: Autosomal recessive. The syndrome has been linked to a variety of genetic mutations, including an inversion on chromosome 17q21 or 17q23, an unbalanced translocation involving chromosome 6 and 22, and a balanced pericentric inversion on chromosome 4. Most karyotypes, however, are normal.

Pathophysiology: Unknown.

Diagnosis: Made by the clinical picture and family history.

Clinical aspects: Short ribs with pulmonary hypoplasia are associated with a variety of other malformations. Short tubular bones, perinatal hydrops, and macrocephaly are present in almost all children. Midline cleft with or without cleft palate, congenital heart disease, central nervous system malformations, and gastrointestinal and urogenital abnormalities are other frequently encountered features. The syndrome is generally lethal; most children die in utero or during early infancy as a result of respiratory insufficiency secondary to pulmonary hypoplasia.

Precautions before anesthesia: Because of the dismal prognosis, these patients are unlikely candidates for anesthesia. If interventions are indicated, the full extent of craniofacial and cardiac malformations must be assessed.

Anesthetic considerations: Anesthetic implications include potentially difficult airway management, oxygenation failure on the ventilator, and severe difficulties weaning from the ventilator. Considerations regarding the cardiovascular pathophysiology depend on the underlying cardiac defect. Assess renal function (creatinine, urea).

Pharmacological implications: Depending on the cardiac state, agents causing myocardial depression or resulting in changes of systemic and/or pulmonary vascular resistance should be used cautiously. Avoid drugs with predominantly renal elimination (or adjust the dose) in the presence of decreased renal function. Subacute bacterial endocarditis prophylaxis may be required.

Other Condition to Be Considered: Although polydactyly is unusual in Beemer-Langer syndrome, it is considered part of the four known ☞**Short Rib-Polydactyly Syndromes,** which all are transmitted in an autosomal recessive pattern, and all represent extreme and lethal forms of chondrodysplasia and dwarfism. Clearly separating the four different types from each other can be difficult or impossible. **Saldino-Noonan Syndrome** (Synonyms: Short Rib-Polydactyly Syndrome Type 1; Polydactyly With Neonatal Chondrodystrophy, Type I) **Majewski Syndrome** (Synonyms: Short Rib-Polydactyly Syndrome Type 2; Polydactyly With Neonatal Chondrodystrophy, Type II) **Verma-Naumoff Syndrome** (Synonyms: Short Rib-Polydactyly Syndrome Type 3; Polydactyly With Neonatal Chondrodystrophy, Type III)

REFERENCES:

Chen H, Mirkin D, Yang S: De novo 17q paracentric inversion mosaicism in a patient with Beemer-Langer type short rib-polydactyly syndrome with special consideration of short rib polydactyly syndromes. *Am J Med Genet* 53:165, 1994.

Myong N-H, Park J-W, Chi JG: Short-rib polydactyly syndrome, Beemer-Langer type, with bilateral huge polycystic renal dysplasia. *J Korean Med Sci* 13:201, 1998.

Vujanic GM, Hunt NCA: New case of Beemer-Langer syndrome. *Pediatr Dev Pathol* 3:281, 2000.

Beemer Lethal Malformation Syndrome

At a glance: Rapidly progressing, lethal-ending genetic syndrome with cardiac, neurologic, hematologic, and skeletal anomalies.

Synonym: Beemer-van Ertbruggen Syndrome.

Genetic inheritance: Unknown, but extremely rare; presumed autosomal recessive.

Diagnosis: Physical appearance, clinical course (lethal), radiologic imaging (dense bones), neuroradiologic imaging (hydrocephalus), echocardiography (double-outlet right ventricle), and complete blood count (thrombocytopenia).

Clinical aspects: Characterized by a variety of clinical abnormalities, which proved rapidly lethal in the reported cases. External examination reveals ambiguous external genitalia and a bulbous nose with broad nasal bridge. Skeletal bones are denser than normal. The condition is associated with severe cardiac malformations (double-outlet right ventricle). Neurologic examination and imaging demonstrate hydrocephalus. Blood screening reveals a thrombocytopenia.

Precautions before anesthesia: No reports about anesthesia in these patients exist. However, detailed preoperative assessment is required to determine the extent of cardiac and neurologic malformations. Cardiac consultation with electrocardiogram, echocardiogram, and blood gas analysis to delineate the cardiac lesion and determine the appropriate management is recommended. Neurologic consultation may include CT or MRI. Obtain a complete blood count. Thrombocytopenia may require platelet transfusions. The medical team and parents must have a clear treatment plan.

Anesthetic considerations: Anesthetic technique must be tailored to the underlying cardiac malformations. In addition, induction and maintenance of anesthesia must consider the increased intracranial pressure in the presence of hydrocephalus. Early endotracheal intubation and mild hyperventilation lower intracranial pressure. Thrombocytopenia precludes the use of regional techniques. Be prepared for prolonged postoperative ventilation and monitoring.

Pharmacological implications: Care must be taken when sedative and narcotic agents are administered in the presence of hydrocephalus and raised intracranial pressure. Because of their dose-dependent myocardial depressant effects, intravenous and inhalational agents must be carefully titrated to effect in the presence of cardiac malformations. Consider an opioid-based anesthetic technique. In the presence of increased intracranial pressure, isoflurane below 1 MAC is a suitable maintenance agent. The choice of intravenous induction agent is influenced by the cardiac lesion. Thiopentone, benzodiazepines, and propofol are acceptable options in the presence of raised intracranial pressure.

REFERENCE:

Beemer FA, von Ertbruggen I: Peculiar facial appearance, hydrocephalus, double-outlet right ventricle, genital anomalies and dense bones with lethal outcome. *Am J Med Genet* 19:391, 1984.

Begeer Syndrome

At a glance: Genetic disorder with mental retardation, cataract, deafness, and polyneuropathy.

Synonyms: Polyneuropathy Cataract Deafness Syndrome; Cataract Ataxia Deafness Retardation Syndrome.

Incidence and genetic inheritance: Only two sibs have been described. Autosomal recessive inheritance was suspected.

Clinical aspects: Two adult sisters with mild mental retardation and ataxia, presumably as a result of impaired proprioception, were described. Both siblings had congenital cataracts and were of short stature during childhood. Progressive sensorineural deafness developed in the third decade of life.

Anesthetic considerations: Appropriate anxiolysis may be helpful in the presence of developmental delay and hearing loss, but no other specific anesthetic implications are expected.

Other Condition to Be Considered:

☞**REARDON-WILSON-CAVANAGH SYNDROME:** Similar features are seen in this syndrome. However, in contrast to Beeger syndrome the onset of hearing loss is in infancy, and there is no association with congenital cataract.

REFERENCE:

Begeer JH, Scholte FA, van Essen AJ: Two sisters with mental retardation, cataract, ataxia, progressive hearing loss, and polyneuropathy. *J Med Genet* 28:884, 1991.

Behçet Syndrome

At a glance: Suspected autoimmune vasculitis with a genetic predisposition.

Synonym: Behçet Disease.

History: First described in 1937 by Dr. Helusi Behçet, a Turkish dermatologist.

Incidence: Prevalence is highest in Turkey (80–320:100,000 in the general population) and Asia (2–30:100,000 in the general population), but patients from many parts of the world have been described. Male gender is predominant, especially in severe Behçet disease.

Genetic inheritance: The majority of cases are sporadic, but familial forms are described. Behçet disease has been associated with HLA-B51 in 45 to 60% of cases, but the significance of this finding for the pathogenesis of Behçet disease is not established.

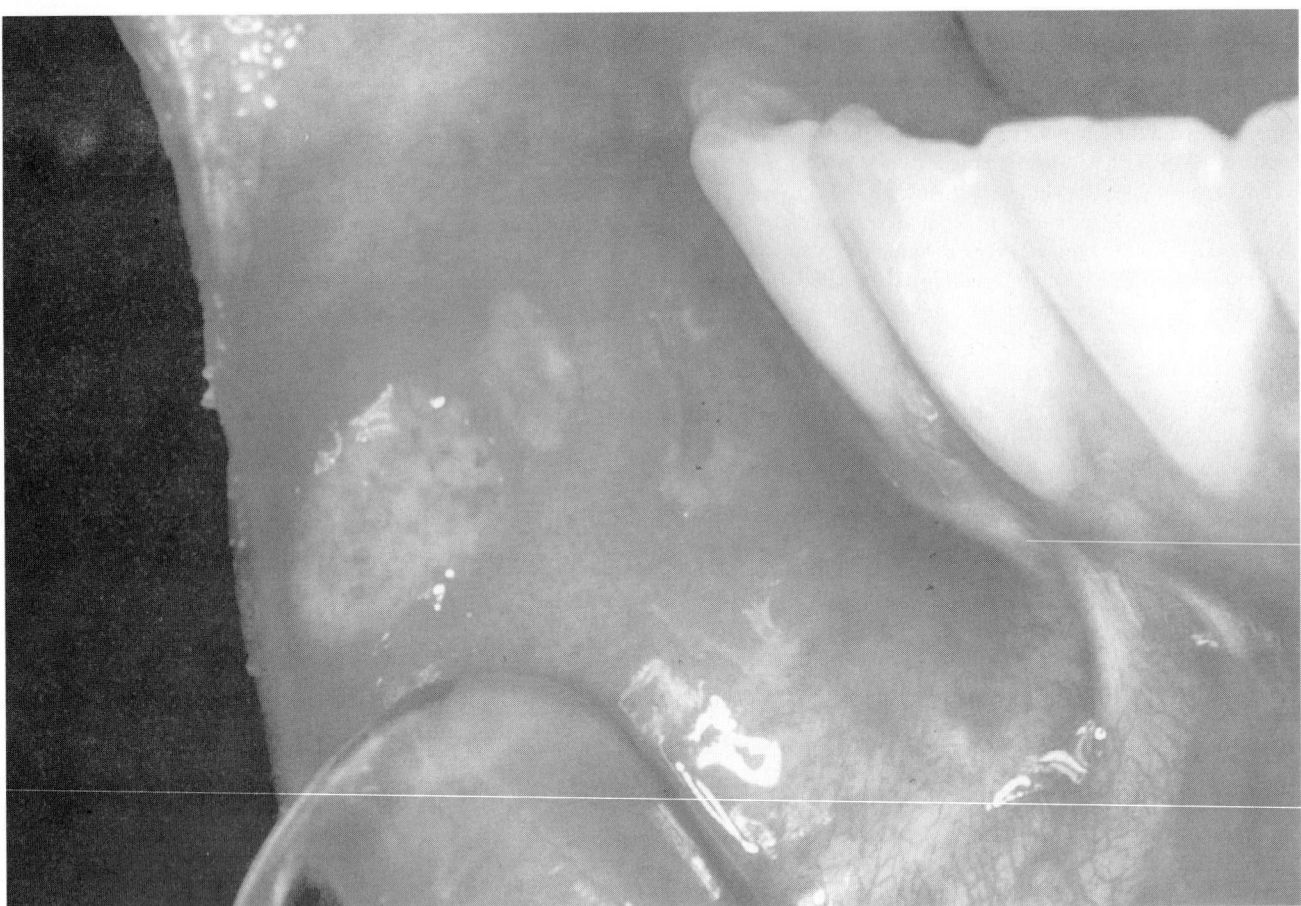

Behçet Disease   Ulcerations on the mucosa of the lower lip of a patient with Behçet disease. See color plates.

Pathophysiology: The cornerstone of the disease is a multisystemic vasculitis involving large and small vessels in various degrees. The underlying cause has not been defined, but an autoimmune pathogenesis, including an abnormal T-cell response to microbial antigens and cross-reaction toward body tissue, is suspected. Characteristically, skin pathergy is present or so-called positive, that is, an exaggerated reaction with formation of a papule or a pustula after minor trauma such as a needle puncture occurs. Although helpful (but not pathognomonic) for the diagnosis of Behçet disease, the majority of patients do not show this reaction.

Diagnosis: No specific tests are available. The diagnosis relies on the clinical picture, and criteria for establishing the diagnosis have been published by the International Study Group for Behçet's Disease.

Clinical aspects: Recurrent oral and genital ulcerations and uveitis or retinal vasculitis are the characteristic findings in Behçet disease. Systemic manifestation may affect joints, gut, kidney, lung, and the cardiovascular system. Lung involvement presents with pulmonary infarction, hemoptysis, recurrent pneumonia, bronchiolitis obliterans, organizing pneumonia, and pleurisy. Cardiovascular manifestations include pulmonary artery aneurysms, intracardiac thrombus formation with right-sided predominance, and deep venous thrombosis of large veins. Aneurysmatic changes and thrombosis have been described in many other sites, including gut and brain. The clinical course of Behçet disease is characterized by alternating periods of disease activity and remission. Therapy mainly consists of antiinflammatory and/or immunosuppressive therapy, usually including steroids with or without cyclophosphamide. Because of the risks and benefits, the therapeutic approach to clot formation must be evaluated individually. Mortality is low and usually is the consequence of a thrombotic or hemorrhagic complication.

Precautions before anesthesia: The possibility of systemic involvement has a significant impact on anesthesia. Chest radiography should be ordered to assess the extent of pulmonary manifestations. Cardiac and large-vessel involvement can be evaluated sonographically and should include the potential sites of central venous catheter insertion. Laboratory tests should include a complete blood count, coagulation profile, and routine chemistry. Drug history is important, especially to identify patients on anticoagulation or chronic steroid medication warranting perioperative stress prophylaxis.

Anesthetic considerations: Reported perioperative events include difficult tracheal intubation from oral scarring and two postoperative deaths from pulmonary hemorrhage in patients who underwent cardiac surgery for removal of an intracardiac thrombus. Intraoperative management should aim at reducing the risk of pulmonary hypertension and includes prevention of acidosis, hypercarbia, hypoxia, and pulmonary vasoconstrictors, and appropriate analgesia and depth of anesthesia. Pulmonary angiography is generally discouraged because of the increased risk of pulmonary vascular injury.

Pharmacological implications: If pulmonary vascular involvement is present, the risk of increasing pulmonary artery pressure should be minimized. Most inhaled anesthetics have the potential to reduce hypoxic pulmonary vasoconstriction and thus might be

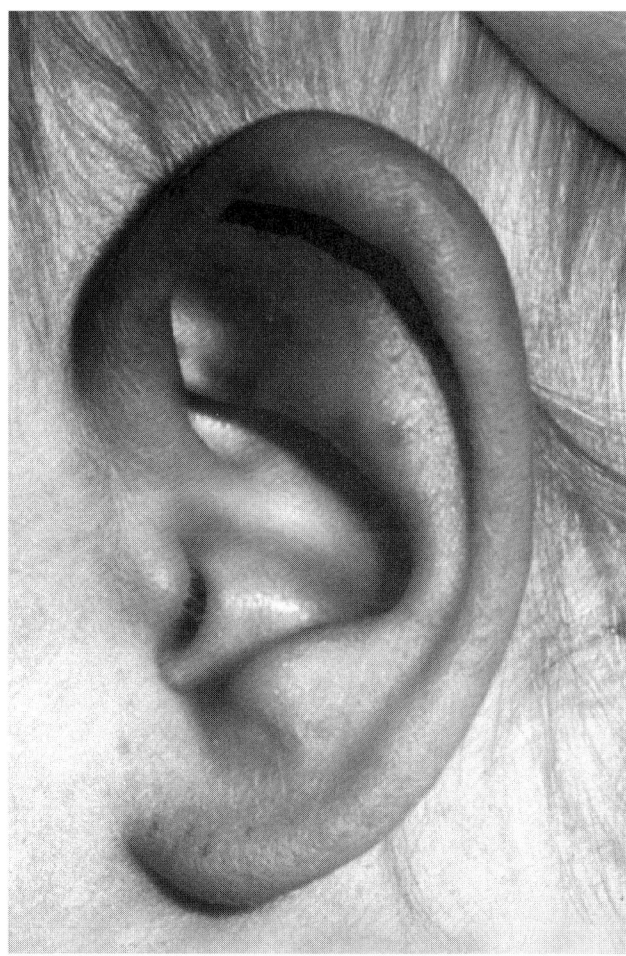

Behçet Disease Vasculitis with thrombosis leads to segmental hemorrhagic infarction of the ear in a patient with Behçet disease.

beneficial, whereas the majority of intravenous anesthetic agents have no effect on hypoxic pulmonary vasoconstriction. α-Adrenergic agents should be used cautiously. If the gut is involved, the risk of gastrointestinal bleeding and bowel perforation is increased, especially in patients on steroid medication. In this case, antacid drugs should be given perioperatively. Glaucoma in patients with Behçet disease has been described, but seems to be rare. If present, drugs that potentially increase intraocular pressure should be avoided (e.g., succinylcholine, ketamine).

Other conditions to be considered: Behçet disease is distinguished from a number of other autoimmune vasculitic diseases such as the following:

☞**SYSTEMIC LUPUS ERYTHEMATOSUS:** Chronic inflammatory, remitting, relapsing, multisystemic disorder of connective tissue, principally involving the skin, joints, kidneys, and serosal membranes.

☞**POLYARTERITIS NODOSA:** Autoimmune vasculitis affecting the small- and medium-size arteries. Any organ can be affected; however, polyarteritis nodosa most often involves the skin, joints, kidneys, gastrointestinal tract, and peripheral nerves. Consequently, the clinical picture is highly variable.

REFERENCES:

Al-Mutawa SA, Hegab SM: Behçet's disease. *Clin Exp Med* 4:103, 2004.

Erkan F, Gul A, Tasali E: Pulmonary manifestations of Behçet's disease. *Thorax* 56:572, 2000.

Kone-Paul I, Geisler I, Wechsler B, et al: Familial aggregation in Behçet's disease: High frequency in siblings and parents of pediatric probands. *J Pediatr* 135:89, 1999.

Behr Syndrome

At a glance: Genetic disorder with bilateral optic atrophy, mental retardation, and ataxia.

Synonyms: Infantile Optic Atrophy–Ataxia Syndrome; Optic Atrophia–Ataxia Syndrome.

Incidence: Unknown; both sexes seem to be equally affected.

Genetic inheritance: Families with several affected members have been described. An autosomal recessive mode of inheritance was suggested, but a significant genetic heterogeneity seems likely.

Pathophysiology: Unknown. Increased urine 3-methylglutaconate and 3-methylglutate levels have been reported in some individuals with a Behr-like syndrome. Histopathologically, central optic nerve atrophy and disarray of the normal structure of the lateral geniculate nuclei have been described.

Diagnosis: Based on the clinical features and family history. Autopsy of one patient showed central atrophy of the optic nerves and a total disarray of the normal laminar pattern of the lateral geniculate nucleus with dropout of neurons and gliosis. Numerous axonal spheroids were noted in the neuropil. Similar spheroids with cell loss and gliosis were also found in the thalamus and the pallida. A relationship of Behr syndrome with ☞Seitelberger syndrome (infantile neuroaxonal dystrophy) was suggested.

Clinical aspects: Characterized by early onset of bilateral optic nerve atrophy resulting in partial visual field defects, and neurologic symptoms including ataxia and spastic gait, mental retardation, nystagmus, epilepsy, positive Babinski sign, and urinary incontinence. The disease is most often progressive over an extended time, followed by a period of relative stability. Lower limb contractures develop in up to 70% of patients. These patients may present for lengthening of the Achilles tendon or release of the adductors.

Precautions before anesthesia: The severity of the clinical symptoms should be defined prior to anesthesia. In particular, a history of current medical treatment and efficacy for seizures should be obtained. Anxiolysis may be helpful in the management of patients with visual impairment and mental retardation. Pupillary reaction to light may be altered and should be documented prior to anesthesia.

Anesthetic considerations: No adverse experiences with anesthesia have been reported. Careful intraoperative positioning is needed, but can be difficult (contractures).

Pharmacological implications: Chronic antiseizure therapy may alter the pharmacokinetic of other drugs with hepatic metabolism.

Other conditions to be considered: Behr syndrome shares many features with the following conditions:

SPINOCEREBELLAR ATAXIA SYNDROMES: Such as: ☞Boucher-Neuhäuser Syndrome; ☞Friedreich Ataxia; ☞Infantile Onset Spinocere; Bettar Ataxia (IOSCA); ☞Machado-Joseph Disease; ☞Roussy-Levy Syndrome. Some authors regard Behr syndrome as a form of a spinocerebellar ataxia syndrome.

☞**SEITELBERGER SYNDROME:** Probably an autosomal recessive transmitted progressive degenerative encephalopathy with axonal swelling and spheroid axonal degeneration.

☞**Hallervorden-Spatz Disease:** Autosomal recessive inherited neurodegenerative syndrome that primarily affects the basal ganglia.

References:

Copeliovitch L, Katz K, Arbel N, et al: Musculoskeletal deformities in Behr syndrome. *J Pediatr Orthop* 21:512, 2001.

Horoupian DS, Zucker DK, Moshe S, et al: Behr syndrome: A clinicopathologic report. *Neurology* 29:323, 1979.

Thomas PK, Workman JM, Thage O: Behr's syndrome: A family exhibiting pseudodominant inheritance. *J Neurol Sci* 64:137, 1984.

Behrens-Baumann-Dust Syndrome

At a glance: Microphthalmos, Dandy-Walker anomaly, and ocular anomalies (optic disc atrophy, lid adhesion, and/or ankyloblepharon).

Synonym: Oculocerebral Dysplasia.

Incidence and genetic inheritance: Two sibs have been described. Autosomal recessive inheritance was suggested.

Clinical aspects: A 16-year-old girl with bilateral microphthalmos, aplasia of the right optic nerve, and a large cerebellar Dandy-Walker cyst was described. She was mentally normal, and no clinical consequences from the Dandy-Walker cyst were mentioned. Her 13-year-old brother had unilateral optic nerve aplasia with ipsilateral cryptophthalmus and contralateral microphthalmos. He suffered from significant mental retardation.

Anesthetic considerations: If a Dandy-Walker malformation is present with signs of compression and increased intracranial pressure, a lumbar puncture for spinal anesthesia is contraindicated and anesthetic management must address the problem of raised intracranial pressure. Adequate anxiolysis is often helpful in the management of mentally delayed patients, but in the presence of increased intracranial pressure may have more adverse than beneficial effects. No other specific anesthetic implications are expected from the described ophthalmologic features.

Reference:

Behrens-Baumann W, Dust G, Rittmeier K, et al: Oculo-cerebral dysplasia: Aplasia of the optic nerve with familial microphthalmos and cryptophthalmos. Clinical and computer tomography study. *Klin Monatsbl Augenheilkd* 179:90, 1981.

Bellini-Chiumello-Rimoldi Syndrome

At a glance: Genetic disorder with metaphyseal dysplasia that is more pronounced in the lower than in the upper extremities.

Synonyms: Metaphyseal Acrodysplasia; Wedge-Shaped Epiphysis of Knees; Metaphyseal Acroscyphodysplasia.

Incidence and genetic inheritance: Only two Italian and two Australian siblings and two unrelated cases, one from Italy and one from Morocco, have been described. Autosomal recessive inheritance was suggested.

Clinical aspects: Cup-shaped dysplasia of the metaphyses mainly of the knees with premature epiphyseal–metaphyseal fusion and gross deformation of the femoral condyles were described as char-

acteristic features. The radiologic aspect of the knees is specific, with the lower femoral and upper tibial epiphyses embedding themselves in their metaphyses, which results in the typical cup shape. Premature central epiphyseal–metaphyseal fusion and gross deformation of the femoral condyles (or even coalescence) may occur. Progressive coxa valga, bowed tibiae, and short stature are associated features. The upper extremities are less affected, but significant shortening of hand and finger bones can be found. Three of the four children described showed psychomotor retardation. In addition to the symptoms described, one child had mild scoliosis.

Anesthetic considerations: Positioning may be difficult and careful padding is required. No other defects were described, so no specific anesthetic implications are expected. Adequate anxiolysis may be helpful in the management of mentally impaired patients.

References:

Bellini F, Chiumello G, Rimoldi R, et al: Wedge-shaped epiphyses of the knees in two siblings: A new recessive rare dysplasia? *Helv Paediatr Acta* 39:365, 1984.

Kozlowski K, Meradji M, Beemer FA: Dutch variant of Bellini metaphyseal dysplasia: report of two siblings. *Australas Radiol* 39:282, 1995.

Verloes A, Le Merrer M, Farriaux JP, et al: Metaphyseal acroscyphodysplasia. *Clin Genet* 39:362, 1991.

Bencze Syndrome

At a glance: Autosomal dominant transmitted disorder with strabismus and hemifacial hyperplasia.

Synonym: Hemifacial Hyperplasia with Strabismus.

Incidence and genetic inheritance: Only a few cases have been described in the world literature, and the true incidence is unknown. Autosomal dominant inheritance is suspected.

Clinical aspects: Hemifacial hyperplasia involves the facial bones and facial soft tissue. Growth of the neurocranium is unaffected. The eyeball of the affected side is of normal size, but two of the three generations in the first described family had ipsilateral, uncorrectable amblyopia and/or convergent or alternating strabismus. Dentition was accelerated on the affected side. In the opinion of Bencze et al., hemifacial hyperplasia and eye features were genetically connected. In a second family that was described later, the phenotypic spectrum was expanded to include submucous cleft palate. Intelligence in this latter family reportedly was normal.

Anesthetic considerations: Although hemifacial hyperplasia is mild in many cases, involvement of the tongue, tonsils, and neck has been described in some cases. Severe respiratory distress can develop, similar to infants with extensive cystic hygroma. Therefore, a thorough clinical assessment of the upper airway is mandatory prior to anesthesia.

Other conditions to be considered: Other syndromes of hemifacial hyperplasia with or without bone involvement have been reported worldwide, first by Beck in 1836. However, these cases did not include eye features. In addition, syndromes of hemihypertrophy involving other body parts, such as ☞Klippel-Trénaunay syndrome, are well known.

References:

Bencze J, Schnitzler A, Walawska J: Dominant inheritance of hemifacial hyperplasia associated with strabismus. *Oral Surg Oral Med Oral Pathol* 35:489, 1973.

Sculerati N, Jacobs JB: Congenital facial hemihypertrophy: A report of a case with airway compromise. *Head Neck Surg* 8:124, 1985.

Berardinelli-Seip Syndrome

At a glance: Inherited disorder with hyperinsulinemia caused by insulin resistance combined with lipodystrophy and acromegaloid features.

Synonyms: Berardinelli-Seip-Lawrence Syndrome; Berardinelli Syndrome; Seip Syndrome; Seip-Lawrence Syndrome; Congenital Generalized Lipodystrophy; (Congenital) Lipoatrophic Diabetes; Lipodystrophy-Acromegaloid Gigantism Syndrome.

Incidence: Estimated prevalence is 0.2–0.3:100,000 in the general population.

Genetic inheritance: Autosomal recessive disorder. Two genetic loci (11q13 and 9q34) are associated with the syndrome.

Pathophysiology: No unifying pathogenetic mechanism has been identified. The insulin receptor seems to be normal.

Diagnosis: Based on the clinical picture, including hyperinsulinemia and in some cases a positive family history. Berardinelli-Seip syndrome commonly refers to the congenital form of generalized lipodystrophy, whereas Seip-Lawrence syndrome usually refers to the acquired form (in which the anabolic syndrome is more variable and immunologic disturbances more common; see also *Other Conditions to Be Considered*).

Clinical aspects: Hallmarks of Berardinelli-Seip syndrome are a near-absent adipose tissue present already at birth or in early infancy and a congenital (nonketoacidotic) insulin resistance with variable degrees of glucose intolerance and diabetes mellitus. The insulin resistance with hyperinsulinemia results in an anabolic syndrome resulting in increased growth velocity, advanced bone age, muscular hypertrophy and masculine body build, acromegaloid stigmata, enlarged genitalia in infancy (labial hypertrophy and sexual precocity, polycystic ovaries), abundant scalp hair and hypertrichosis, and organomegaly (often with visceral organs showing twice the normal weight). The anabolic syndrome is further exacerbated by a voracious appetite. Associated features are liver cirrhosis, esophageal varices, and hypertriglyceridemia with risk of pancreatitis. Acanthosis nigricans, which is variable but often marked and extensive, seems to be a constant sign of Berardinelli-Seip syndrome (as seen in other syndromes with pronounced insulin resistance). It is most often located in the extensional areas (elbows, knees) and in places exposed to wear and tear (axilla, neck, waist). Scoliosis and cystic bone lesions are found in some patients. Mental retardation is not a constant feature but is present in approximately 50% of patients. Cardiovascular involvement (arterial hypertension, hypertrophic cardiomegaly, coronary heart disease) is the leading cause of early death. Medical management consists of moderate restriction of caloric intake (preferably with short-chain fatty acids), insulin as indicated, and antihyperlipidemic drug therapy.

Precautions before anesthesia: No reports describing anesthesia in these patients have been published. However, two features require special attention: diabetes mellitus and cardiovascular involvement. The latter rarely causes problems in childhood, but the risk of coronary ischemia must be considered in young adult patients. If in doubt, at least a chest radiograph and electrocardiogram should be obtained, and chronic cardiac medication must be evaluated. Abrupt discontinuation of angina pectoris medication can precipitate an ischemic episode. Assess hepatic and pancreatic function preoperatively.

Anesthetic considerations: Management of the metabolic and cardiovascular derangements follows standard approach. If there are any signs of coronary heart disease, attention should be paid to provide adequate sedation and analgesia. Any increase in myocardial oxygen demand should be avoided (increase in afterload, contractility, or heart rate). Toddlers are at increased risk for developing potentially dangerous hyperplasia of the pharyngeal tonsils and adenoids. Macroglossia has been described in some patients. Maintaining airway patency may be challenging.

Pharmacological implications: In patients with coexisting heart disease, volatile anesthetics are safe in lower concentrations but may cause myocardial depression with worsening left ventricular function at higher concentrations. Benzodiazepines usually are well tolerated, and there is no evidence contraindicating muscle relaxants. In contrast, because of their potential negative inotropic effects, propofol and barbiturates should either be avoided or used in low doses only in patients with significant cardiomyopathy. Ketamine is generally regarded as disadvantageous because of its sympathomimetic effects resulting in increased oxygen requirements. Drugs with predominant hepatic clearance should be avoided in patients with liver failure.

Other conditions to be considered:

ACQUIRED GENERALIZED LIPODYSTROPHY: Refers to an identical syndrome with later onset, often preceded by a well-defined illness, usually an infection. Acquired generalized lipodystrophy tends to be associated with worse liver disease and a more rapid development of diabetes mellitus.

PARTIAL LIPOATROPHY SYNDROMES: A number of partial lipoatrophy syndromes have been described (☞Köbberling-Dunnigan Syndrome; Familial Lipodystrophy of Limbs and Lower Trunk; Lipodystrophic Diabetes; and Reverse Partial Lipodystrophy). In some patients, genetic analysis identified an associated locus on chromosome 1q21-22. Loss of subcutaneous adipose tissue usually begins in puberty, sparing chin, neck, axilla, and back, resulting in a cushingoid appearance. Adipose tissue may accumulate intraabdominally. Metabolic abnormalities are similar to those described in Berardinelli-Seip syndrome.

☞**APOLIPOPROTEIN C-II DEFICIENCY** (Synonym: Familial Hyperlipoproteinemia type IB): An inborn error of metabolism characterized by the deficiency in a necessary cofactor for the activation of lipoprotein lipase. Diabetes mellitus, pancreatitis, or epigastric pain does not exclude the possibility of congestive heart failure and angina in early age.

☞**HYPERLIPOPROTEINEMIA TYPE I** (Synonyms: Bürger-Grütz Syndrome; Essential Familial Hyperlipemia; Exogenous Hypertriglyceridemia; Fat-Induced Hyperlipemia; Fredrickson Type I Hyperlipoproteinemia; Hyperchylomicronemia; Hyperlipidemia I; Hyperlipoproteinemia Type I; Idiopathic Familial Hyperlipemia; Lipoprotein Lipase Deficiency, Familial Retention Hyperlipemia): Inherited inborn error of metabolism characterized by a massive accumulation of chylomicrons and triglycerides in plasma resulting in recurrent abdominal pain and hepatosplenomegaly.

☞**HYPERLIPIDEMIA TYPE IIA:** A genetic disorder of lipid metabolism causing accumulation of cholesterol and thus increasing the risk of cardiovascular diseases. Hypercholesterolemia, Low Density Lipoprotein–LDL–Receptor Disorder.

☞**PHYTOSTEROLEMIA:** (Synonym: Sitosterolemia): A rare inherited disorder characterized by congenital hypercholesterolemia, presenting clinically with tendon xanthomas, premature coronary artery disease and atherosclerosis.

REFERENCES:

Bjornstad PG, Foerster A, Ihlen H: Cardiac findings in generalized lipodystrophy. *Acta Paediatr Suppl* 413:39, 1996.

Capeau J, Magre J, Lascols O, et al: Diseases of adipose tissue: genetic and acquired lipodystrophies. *Biochem Soc Trans* 33:1073, 2005.

Seip M, Trygstad O: Generalized lipodystrophy, congenital and acquired (lipoatrophy). *Acta Paediatr Suppl* 413:2, 1996.

Berdon Syndrome

At a glance: Inherited syndrome characterized by microcolon, intestinal hypoperistalsis, dilated small bowel loops and constipation, urinary retention, giant bladder (megacystis), and hydronephrosis.

Synonyms: Megacystis-Microcolon-Intestinal Hypoperistalsis Syndrome (MMIHS); MMIH Syndrome.

Incidence: Rare, but a number of MMIHS cases in families of various ethnic backgrounds have been described.

Genetic inheritance: Mode of transmission is autosomal recessive, with a female predominance of 4:1. Two candidate genes for MMIHS have been located on chromosome 15q24.

Pathophysiology: Unknown. Some studies suggest a role of the β-4/α-3 neuronal nicotinic acetylcholine receptor unit. Histologically, the longitudinal smooth muscle fibers of the gut wall are thin with degenerative vacuoles and increased collagen deposits.

Diagnosis: Based on clinical picture and family history.

Clinical aspects: Characteristic features of MMIHS are a microcolon with dilated, hypoperistaltic small bowel loops and a large bladder that can be associated with a dilatation of the upper urinary tract. In most cases, the myenteric and submucosal plexus are normal. The abdominal wall might be hypotonic and thin walled, as in prune belly syndrome. One family with MMIHS occurrence in the daughter and isolated prune belly syndrome in the son has been described. One child who died shortly after birth showed cleft palate, severe micrognathia, and a truncus arteriosus communis overriding both ventricles. Another child had multiple cardiac rhabdomyomata at autopsy. Also, one case of MMIHS in trisomy 18 has been reported, but the colon in this child showed aganglionosis. Even with surgery, mortality is high, but some success with intestinal transplantation has been reported.

Precautions before anesthesia: Children need a thorough clinical assessment. Although rare, cardiac involvement should be excluded prior to anesthesia.

Anesthetic considerations: Multiple surgical interventions have been reported, but no anesthetic complications were mentioned. Tracheal intubation might be difficult in the presence of cleft palate and micrognathia. Expect a weak cough as a result of abdominal wall hypoplasia. Postoperative mechanical ventilation may be necessary.

Pharmacological implications: Neuromuscular blockade should be used cautiously and monitored with a peripheral nerve stimulator. Long-term opioid medication should be avoided because of the inhibiting effect on smooth muscles in gut and bladder wall.

Other condition to be considered:

CHRONIC IDIOPATHIC INTESTINAL PSEUDOOBSTRUCTION: MMIHS must be differentiated from this milder autosomal dominant form, which can be associated with megacystis but results in only minor symptoms prior to adolescence.

REFERENCES:

Kohler M, Pease PW, Upadhyay V. Megacystis-microcolon-intestinal hypoperistalsis syndrome (MMIHS) in siblings: case report and review of the literature. *Europ J Pediatr Surg* 14:362, 2004.

Puri P, Shinkai M: Megacystis microcolon intestinal hypoperistalsis syndrome. *Semin Pediatr Surg* 14:58,2005.

Rolle U, O'Briain S, Pearl RH, et al: Megacystis-microcolon-intestinal hypoperistalsis syndrome: Evidence of intestinal myopathy. *Pediatr Surg Int* 18:2, 2002.

Berk-Tabatznik Syndrome

At a glance: Sporadic syndrome with cervical vertebral anomalies and optic atrophy.

Synonym: Congenital Optic Atrophy and Brachytelephalangy.

Incidence and genetic inheritance: Extremely rare; only two sporadic cases have been described.

Clinical aspects: Initially described in a 16-year-old girl with congenital optic atrophy, posterior hemivertebrae with cervical kyphosis, and hypoplasia of distal phalanges. The second child with this syndrome had short stature, hypoplasia of the cervical vertebral bodies, and some degree of mental retardation, which possibly was attributable to visual and auditory impairment. Spastic quadriparesis was present in both cases.

Anesthetic considerations: The extent of cervical vertebral malformations should be assessed because they can result in difficult airway management. Spastic quadriparesis may result in difficult positioning, so careful padding is required. Because of mild mental retardation and visual and hearing impairment, preoperative anxiolysis is recommended. The presence of the primary care-giver for induction of anesthesia may be helpful. Neither individual had other malformations.

Other condition to be considered:

☞BEHR SYNDROME: Genetic disorder with bilateral optic atrophy, mental retardation, and ataxia.

REFERENCE:

Hartwell EA, Robinson LK, Robinson LH, et al: Congenital optic atrophy and brachytelephalangy: The Berk-Tabatznik syndrome. *Am J Med Genet* 29:383, 1988.

Bernard-Soulier Syndrome

At a glance: Genetic disorder characterized by giant platelets, mild-to-moderate thrombocytopenia, abnormal platelet function, and bleeding disproportionate to the reduced number of platelets.

Synonyms: Giant Platelet Syndrome; Familial Macrothrombocytopenia; Deficiency of Platelet Glycoprotein Ib; Hemorrhagiparous Thrombocytic Dystrophy.

History: First described in 1948 by Jean Bernard and Jean-Pierre Soulier, French hematologists.

Incidence: Probably less than 1:1,000,000 in the general population.

Genetic inheritance: Autosomal recessive. Genetic research located the GP-1BA gene on 17pter-p12 for the classic Bernard-Soulier syndrome (type A) and the GP-1BB gene on 22q11.2 for type B.

Pathophysiology: The mutation results in a deficiency of platelet membrane glycoprotein (GP) Ib (GP-1BA), GP-Is (glycocalicin), GP-V, and GP-IX. (Glycocalicin results from proteolytic cleavage of GP-1BA.) These factors are responsible for the interaction between von Willebrand factor and the platelet membrane and are essential for normal platelet adhesion in the early phase of primary hemostasis. Furthermore, the giant platelets show altered binding of factors V and XI and do not develop regular coagulation activity upon contact with collagen.

Diagnosis: Bleeding tendency noted during childhood. Clinical picture and morphologic features of the platelets on blood smear examination, which shows increased size (giant platelets may have a diameter up to 8 μm) with dense granulomeres, resulting in a pseudonucleated or lymphocytoid aspect.

Clinical aspects: Moderate-to-severe bleeding of purpuric type (bruising, epistaxis, menorrhagia). Bleeding time is prolonged, but clot retraction and platelet aggregation by adenosine diphosphate and collagen are normal. Heterozygous family members may show approximately half the normal levels of platelet GP Ib-IX-V expression; however, they suffer from only mild bleeding diatheses, if at all. Affected patients have a history of frequent episodes of epistaxis, gingival and cutaneous bleeding, and hemorrhage associated with trauma. Platelet counts may range from very low ($<30,000/\mu$L) to marginally low or normal ($\sim200,000/\mu$L). In individual patients it may fluctuate considerably over a period of years. Skin bleeding time may range from only marginally prolonged (5–10 minutes) to more than 20 minutes. The severity of symptoms may progressively worsen or become alleviated throughout puberty and adult life. Splenectomy apparently has been beneficial in moderating thrombocytopenia and the severity of clinical symptoms.

Precautions before anesthesia: Check platelet count and bleeding time. Bleeding tendency is variable (some patients remain asymptomatic until later adulthood), but can be severe during surgery, trauma, or pregnancy. Evaluate hematologic status (complete blood count, bleeding time, platelet function tests, prothrombin time, partial thromboplastin time). Activated recombinant factor VII (rFVIIa) and fresh plasma concentrate should be immediately available in the event they are required.

Anesthetic considerations: Avoid central neuraxial blocks. Direct laryngoscopy and tracheal intubation must be atraumatic. General supportive measures and specific treatment of bleeding episodes. Severe hemorrhagic shock occurs spontaneously or secondary to surgery. High-dose recombinant factor VIIa has been used to correct bleeding and was postulated to act on platelets in the absence of tissue factor to activate factors IX and X and thus enhance thrombin generation. Transfusion of platelet-rich plasma is another technique that has been used successfully to stop severe hemorrhage.

Pharmacological implications: Consider use of desmopressin acetate (DDAVP) and antifibrinolytics. Avoid drugs or products adversely affecting platelet function, such as nonsteroidal antiinflammatory drugs and hydroethyl starch. Halothane and sevoflurane (and dibucaine) may affect platelet function. Antifibrinolytics may or may not be beneficial.

Other conditions to be considered:

THROMBOPATHIC THROMBOCYTOPENIA: Although this disorder is similar to the Bernard-Soulier syndrome, the inheritance is autosomal dominant.

☞**GLANZMANN THROMBASTHENIA:** This autosomal recessive transmitted bleeding disorder is characterized by prolonged bleeding time, absence of platelet aggregation, and impaired clot retraction as a consequence of a dysfunction or deficiency of platelet membrane glycoprotein complex IIb-IIIa.

GRAY PLATELET SYNDROME: Rare platelet disorder characterized by a marked decrease or absence of platelet-specific α-granules. These are the most abundant cell organelles in platelets containing more than 20 different proteins, of which platelet factor-4, thromboglobulin, platelet-derived growth factor, thrombospondin, and homologues of von Willebrand factor are the most important. The term *gray platelet* is derived from the gray microscopic appearance of these platelets, which is a result of their increased size in combination with the reduced number of granules. Inheritance most likely is autosomal dominant. Initially, the defect seemed to be limited to the megakaryocytic cell line, but new research in an affected family showed also a secretory disorder in the neutrophil blood cell line (alkaline phosphatase and others), resulting in gray neutrophils.

MONTREAL PLATELET SYNDROME: Resembles Bernard-Soulier syndrome in many aspects. Platelet gigantism is caused by superabundant platelet membranes and an abnormal change in shape. However, in contrast to Bernard-Soulier syndrome, GP I levels seem to be normal.

The following syndromes (May-Hegglin anomaly, Sebastian syndrome, Fechtner syndrome, Epstein syndrome) called *platelet storage pool defects or platelet-type von Willebrand disease* all are caused by a mutation on gene map locus 22q11.2, which has been found to be the *nonmuscle myosin heavy-chain-9 (MYH9)* gene.

MAY-HEGGLIN ANOMALY (Macrothrombocytopenia with Leukocyte Inclusions; Dohle Leukocyte Inclusions with Giant Platelets): Autosomal dominant inherited bleeding disorder characterized by the triad of giant platelets, thrombocytopenia, and large leukocyte inclusion bodies. Gene map locus is 22q11.2-q13. The pathophysiology is poorly understood but seems to be related to a defect in the microtubular system, which results in abnormal maturation and fragmentation of megakaryocytes. The lifespan of platelets appears to be normal. The inclusion bodies are called *Dohle bodies,* are often spindle shaped, and consist of cytoplasmic RNA. They may represent paracrystalline arrays of depolymerized ribosomes. Although thrombocytopenia occurs in half of these patients, severe bleeding is rare and many patients are asymptomatic. Successful craniotomy with DDAVP (desmopressin) therapy has been reported.

SEBASTIAN SYNDROME: The presence of macrothrombocytopenia with neutrophil inclusion bodies is reminiscent of May-Hegglin anomaly, but ultrastructural analysis of the inclusion bodies reveals their similarity with the ones found in Fechtner syndrome (see below). In fact, Sebastian and Fechtner syndrome differ from each other only by the features of Alport syndrome (deafness and nephritis). Inheritance is autosomal dominant. The defect is also located on the long arm of chromosome 22 (22q11.2).

FECHTNER SYNDROME (Macrothrombocytopathy, Nephritis, Deafness, and Leukocyte Inclusion Syndrome; Alport Syndrome with Leukocyte Inclusions and Macrothrombocytopenia): The name of this autosomal dominant transmitted syndrome is derived from the surname of the family first described with this disorder. Like May-Hegglin anomaly and Sebastian syndrome, the defect of this syndrome is located on the long arm of chromosome 22 (22q11.2). Clinically, it is characterized by a combination of nephritis (with symptoms ranging from microhematuria to end-stage renal failure), high-frequency sensorineural deafness, congenital cataracts, macrothrombocytopenia, and inclusion bodies in neutrophils and eosinophils. Although the aspect of the inclusion bodies under the light microscope is similar to the inclusion bodies seen in May-Hegglin Anomaly, ultrastructurally they are different. The abnormal size of the platelets seems to be a result of an abnormality in the cytoskeleton of megakaryocytes interfering with the demarcation membrane system and the normal expulsion of platelets.

☞**EPSTEIN SYNDROME:** The gene map locus of this autosomal dominant transmitted syndrome is also on the long arm of chromosome 22 (22q11.2). High-tone sensorineural deafness and renal disease are similar to that found in ☞Alport syndrome. Macrothrombocytopenia results in prolonged bleeding time and impaired platelet aggregation in response to collagen. The giant platelet formation seems to be the result of a degenerative process in megakaryocytes, which leads to nuclear regression and cytoplasmic fragmentation.

REFERENCES:

Burns ER: Platelet studies in the pathogenesis of thrombocytopenia in May-Hegglin anomaly. *Am J Pediatr Hematol Oncol* 13:431, 1991.

Caen JP, Nurden AT, Jeanneau C, et al: Bernard-Soulier syndrome: A new platelet glycoprotein abnormality. Its relationship with platelet adhesion to subendothelium and with the factor VIII von Willebrand protein. *J Lab Clin Med* 87:587, 1976.

Coller BS, Zarrabi MH: Platelet membrane studies in the May-Hegglin anomaly. *Blood* 58:279, 1981.

Sehbai AS, Abraham J, Brown VK: Perioperative management of a patient with May-Hegglin anomoly requiring craniotomy. *Am J Hematol* 79:303, 2005.

Drouin A, Favier R, Masse JM, et al: Newly recognized cellular abnormalities in the gray platelet syndrome. *Blood* 98:1382, 2001.

Seri M, Savino M, Bardo D, et al. Epstein syndrome: another renal disorder with mutations in the nonmuscle myosin heavy chain 9 gene. *Hum Genet* 110:182, 2002.

Balduini CL, Lolascon A, Savoia A: Inherited thrombocytopenias: from genes to therapy. *Haematologica* 87:860, 2002.

Ozelo MC, Sivirin P, Larina L: Use of recombinant factor VIIa in the management of severe bleeding episodes in patients with Bernard-Soulier syndrome. *Ann Hematol* Jul 26, 2005 (E-pub ahead of print).

Rodriguez V, Nichols WL, Charleswarth JE, et al. Sebastian Vlatelet syndrome: a hereditary macrothrombocytopenia. *Mayo Clin Proc* 78:1416, 2003.

Heynen MJ, Blockmans D, Verwilghen RL, et al: Congenital macrothrombocytopenia, leukocyte inclusions, deafness and proteinuria: Functional and electron microscopic observations on platelets and megakaryocytes. *Br J Haematol* 70:441, 1988.

Peterson LC, Rao KV, Crosson JT, et al: Fechtner syndrome: A variant of Alport's syndrome with leukocyte inclusions and macrothrombocytopenia. *Blood* 65:397, 1985.

Bernhardt-Roth Syndrome

At a glance: Entrapment neuropathy of the lateral femoral cutaneous nerve resulting in discomfort and numbness.

Synonym: Familial Meralgia Paraesthetica.

Incidence and genetic inheritance: Uncommon; limited to case reports of familial occurrence in several families. Sigmund Freud and one of his sons were affected by this disorder. Autosomal dominant transmission. Most cases of meralgia paresthetica however are acquired.

Clinical aspects: Compression of the lateral femoral cutaneous nerve at the level of Poupart ligament or in the fascia lata soon after entering the thigh beneath the lateral end of the inguinal ligament. Numbness and discomfort over the lateral aspect of the thigh, accompanied by decreased objective sensation to touch, pain, and sometimes temperature.

Anesthetic considerations: Caution in transfer and positioning the patient. Avoid further compression over the areas through which the nerve travels, that is, over the lateral aspect of the inguinal ligament and the lateral aspect of the thigh.

REFERENCES:

Massey EW: Familial occurrence of meralgia paraesthetica [letter]. *Arch Neurol* 35:182, 1978.

Massey EW: Meralgia paraesthetica in a child. *J Pediatr* 93:325, 1978.

Siu TL, Chandran KN: Neurolysis for meralgia paresthetica: an operative series of 45 cases. *Surg Neurol* 63:19, 2005.

Best Disease

At a glance: Inherited, gradually starting, progressive, polymorphic macular degeneration.

Synonyms: Vitelliform Macular Dystrophy; Polymorphic Vitelline Macular Degeneration; Juvenile Vitelliform Macular Dystrophy.

Incidence: Unknown. Several large kindreds have been reported in the literature, with one gene source being traced back to the 17th century in Sweden.

Genetic inheritance: Autosomal dominant inheritance. Gene linkage studies demonstrated the gene responsible for Best disease is located on chromosome 11q13. However, later work illustrated the genetic heterogeneity of the condition and described several allelic variants. One case of nonpenetrance of Best disease has been reported.

Pathophysiology: Characterized by a gross yellow or orange discoid subretinal lesion in the macula. Histopathologic findings on postmortem specimens showed excessive lipofuscin accumulation in the retinal pigment epithelial cells and the subretinal pigment epithelial cell space. The final stage of retinal pigment epithelial atrophy, uncommon before the age of 40 years, may result in a choroidal neovascularization membrane with further loss in visual acuity.

Diagnosis: Usually diagnosed between 3 and 16 years of age, with a mean age at manifestation of 6 years. The diagnosis is based on the characteristic appearance of a discoid lesion in the macula, which usually is bilateral, but may be asymmetric. The mass described in the macular area initially has the appearance of the intact yolk of a fried egg and seems to be present at birth. Progression of the disease with abnormal pigmentation then results in a picture called *scrambling the egg*. Photoreceptor loss occurs in the affected area, and the origin of the accumulated material is thought to derive from degenerated pigment epithelial cells of the retina. Patients and carriers of the disorder have abnormal responses in the electrooculogram. Electroretinographic responses remain normal.

Clinical aspects: Fundoscopy reveals the changes usually before visual impairment exists. Therefore visual acuity usually is normal at first manifestation, but the condition tends to be progressive over many years and results in abnormal pigmentation, chorioretinal atrophy, and gradual visual impairment. No systemic manifestations of the condition have been noted. No effective treatment for this disease is known. Although rare, marked loss of central vision may render patients legally blind. Choroidal neovascularization can be controlled by laser treatment.

Precautions before anesthesia: No specific precautions are required.

Anesthetic considerations: Especially in younger patients undergoing ophthalmic examination under general anesthesia, oculocardiac reflex with profound bradycardia should be expected. Treatment is twofold and includes first stopping the stimulation and second, if still necessary, anticholinergic drugs. No other specific precautions are required.

Pharmacological implications: No known specific pharmacological implications.

Other conditions to be considered:

☞**STARGARDT SYNDROME:** Inherited and rapidly progressive macular degeneration with juvenile onset.

CENTRAL SEROUS RETINOPATHY (Central Serous Chorioretinopathy): Retinal pigment epithelial disorder generally occurring in patients younger than 50 years and presenting with unilateral, acute decrease of visual acuity.

REFERENCES:

Braley AE: Dystrophy of the macula. *Am J Ophthalmol* 61:1, 1966.

Gorman S, Flaherty WA, Fishman GA, et al: Histopathologic findings in Best's vitelliform macular dystrophy. *Arch Ophthalmol* 106:1261, 1988.

Bethlem Myopathy

At a glance: Genetic disorder consisting of a benign congenital myopathy and contractures.

Synonym: Benign Congenital Muscular Dystrophy.

Incidence: Unknown. Since the original report of the condition in 1977 by J. Bethlem and G.K. Van Wijngaarden, the myopathy has been described in at least nine pedigrees from various geographical locations, including the Netherlands, Poland, and Canada. The largest pedigree with the disorder was of French-Canadian ancestry in which the disease was traced back through seven generations.

Genetic inheritance: Autosomal dominant. Gene map locus is most often 21q22.3, but in some patients is 2q37, suggesting a locus heterogeneity within Bethlem myopathy.

Pathophysiology: Genetic linkage studies suggest Bethlem myopathy is caused by mutations in the genes encoding the three constituent α-chain subunits of type VI collagen. Microfibrillar type VI collagen is believed to play a role in bridging cells with the extracellular matrix.

Diagnosis: Made by clinical features consistent with the condition. Electromyography demonstrates a myopathic pattern. Muscle biopsy reveals nonspecific features of a myopathy. Nerve conduction is normal, and creatinine phosphokinase serum levels are normal or mildly elevated.

Clinical aspects: Characterized by a benign limb girdle myopathy with mild-to-moderate weakness and wasting of muscles. Onset is in early infancy or childhood (age 2–5 years) with a benign course and slow progression, leaving some of the affected patients only minimally impaired in old age. However, many patients require a wheelchair after 50 years of age, and some die of respiratory failure as a consequence of progressive respiratory muscle weakness, particularly of the diaphragm. Proximal and extensor muscles are more affected than distal and flexor muscles. Early flexion contractures involve the elbows, ankles, interphalangeal joints of the last four fingers, and planta pedis. Congenital torticollis may be present. Cardiac and respiratory involvement usually is not a feature of this condition.

Precautions before anesthesia: Detailed clinical history and examination are required to determine the exact nature of the myopathy and the progression of the condition. Evaluate the severity of any flexion deformities and congenital torticollis. Obtain family history of previous anesthetic complications (hyperthermic response). Blood work should include creatinine phosphokinase and electrolytes.

Anesthetic considerations: Airway management, including direct laryngoscopy and tracheal intubation, may be difficult in the presence of fixed flexion deformities of neck muscles or congenital torticollis (awake fiberoptic intubation or inhalational induction in children followed by fiberoptic intubation may be required). Positioning and venous access may be difficult because of flexion deformities. Although congenital myopathies have been associated with malignant hyperthermia, the evidence supporting this causal relationship is poor. No case reports of malignant hyperthermia reaction in Bethlem myopathy have been published. Nevertheless, caution should be exercised when using known trigger agents, and full monitoring (including core and peripheral temperature) should be used in the perioperative period. Depending on the degree of muscle weakness and the procedure, postoperative mechanical ventilation may be required.

Pharmacological implications: Avoidance of known trigger agents may be advisable until more information about the condition is available. Nondepolarizing muscle relaxants, if used, should be titrated to effect using a peripheral nerve stimulator. The benign myopathy associated with this condition, which makes it unique among the other congenital myopathies, suggests an exaggerated response to these agents is unlikely. Due to the risk of a hyperkalemic response, succinylcholine should not be used in patients with significant muscle weakness. Anticholinergic premedication is recommended if fiberoptic intubation is planned.

Other conditions to be considered:

☞**ULLRICH DISEASE:** An autosomal recessive disorder characterized by muscular weakness and orthopedic findings. Abnormal cellular immunity may be present.

☞**LIMB-GIRDLE TYPE OF MUSCULAR DYSTROPHY:** This is an inherited symmetric muscular weakness, initially of the lower limbs, with slow progression and associated cardiac anomalies.

☞**EMERY-DREIFUSS MUSCULAR DYSTROPHY:** X-linked form of muscular dystrophy with an onset at approximately 5 years of age and includes cardiac anomalies.

HAUPTMANN-TANNHAUSER MUSCULAR DYSTROPHY: Symptoms are similar to Emery-Dreifuss muscular dystrophy, but inheritance is autosomal dominant instead of X-linked.

REFERENCES:

Bethlem J, Van Wijngaarden GK: Benign myopathy, with autosomal dominant inheritance. A report on three pedigrees. *Brain* 99:91, 1976.

Lampe AK, Bushby KM: Collagen VI related muscle disorders. *J Med Genet* 42:673, 2005.

Speer MC, Tandan R, Rao PN, et al: Evidence for locus heterogeneity in the Bethlem myopathy and linkage to 2q37. *Hum Mol Genet* 5:1043, 1996.

Biemond Syndrome Type I

At a glance: Inherited syndrome with mental retardation, cerebellar ataxia, nystagmus, strabismus, and brachydactyly.

Synonym: Brachydactyly-Nystagmus-Cerebellar Ataxia Syndrome.

Incidence and genetic inheritance: Only a few cases have been reported (four generations in one family). Transmitted as an autosomal dominant trait.

Clinical aspects: Mental retardation, nystagmus, strabismus, and shortening of the metacarpal and metatarsal bones. The posterior column ataxia is characterized by reduced sensory action potentials in nerve conduction tests and ataxia secondary to cerebeliar atrophy.

Anesthetic considerations: No reports exist about this syndrome in the context of anesthesia. Mental retardation can affect the cooperation of the patient, and sedative premedication and/or the presence of the primary care-giver for induction of anesthesia may be helpful.

REFERENCES:

Biemond A: Brachydactylie, nystagmus en cerebellaire ataxis als familiar syndrome. *Ned Tijdschr Geneesk* 78:1423, 1934.

Nachmanoff DB, Segal RA, Dawson DM, et al: Hereditary ataxia with sensory neuronopathy: Biemond's ataxia. *Neurology* 48:273, 1997.

Biemond Syndrome Type II

At a glance: Inherited syndrome characterized by anomalies of the eyes and extremities and mental delay.

Incidence and genetic inheritance: Extremely rare syndrome in which both autosomal dominant and recessive inheritance have been suggested, although the recessive mode is favored.

Clinical aspects: Stigmata of this syndrome are mental retardation, iris colobomata or aniridia, obesity, short stature, postaxial polydactyly, and hypogenitalism. Occasionally, absent incisor teeth, hydrocephalus, arachnoid cysts, cryptorchidism, and hypospadias are found.

Anesthetic considerations: No reports exist about this syndrome in the context of anesthesia. Mental retardation can affect the cooperation of the patient, and sedative premedication and/or the presence of the primary care-giver for induction of anesthesia may be helpful.

Other conditions to be considered:

☞**BARDET-BIEDL SYNDROME:** Characterized by mental retardation, pigmentary retinopathy, polydactyly, obesity, renal anomalies, and hypogenitalism.

☞**LAURENCE-MOON SYNDROME:** Autosomal recessive inherited syndrome with mental retardation, congenital cardiac disease, pigmentary retinopathy, hypogenitalism, and spastic paraplegia.

☞**ALSTRÖM SYNDROME:** Inherited syndrome with progressive visual and hearing loss, diabetes mellitus, and cardiac, hepatic, and renal involvement.

☞**RUBINSTEIN-TAYBI SYNDROME:** Most often occurs sporadically and less often autosomal dominantly inherited. Characterized by broad thumbs and halluces and dysmorphic facies. Mental and physical development delayed. Cardiac, vertebral, and other anomalies.

REFERENCE:

Verloes A, Temple IK, Bonnet S, et al: Coloboma, mental retardation, hypogonadism, and obesity: Critical review of the so-called Biemond syndrome type 2, updated nosology, and delineation of three "new" syndromes. *Am J Med Genet* 69:370, 1997.

Bietti Crystalline Corneoretinal Dystrophy

At a glance: Genetic disorder characterized by deposits of small crystals in the peripheral cornea and the retina resulting in visual impairment.

Synonym: Bietti Tapetoretinal Degeneration with Marginal Corneal Dystrophy.

Incidence: Rare disease in the occident, but relatively common in China.

Genetic inheritance: Autosomal recessive disorder. The mutation most likely is located on 4q35. New research found mutations in the *CYP4V2* gene, which is encoding a protein belonging to a novel member of the cytochrome P450 family. Parental consanguinity is frequently observed.

Pathophysiology: Underlying systemic disorder of the lipid metabolism has been suggested but never proven.

Diagnosis: Refractile deposits found in both paracentral and peripapillary retina and marginal cornea are the most common features of this syndrome. Electrodiagnostic testing shows pathologic changes in the electrooculogram and decreased scotopic and photopic responses in the electroretinogram. Skin biopsies and histologic examination of tissue from corneal and conjunctival biopsies have shown crystal-like cholesterol or cholesterol-ester and complex lipid inclusions in fibroblasts. Similar inclusions are present in circulating lymphocytes.

Clinical aspects: Patients usually become symptomatic in the third decade of life, manifested by reduced visual acuity and other visual symptoms. Occurrence of this disorder in children has only recently been reported. Clinically, degeneration of the retinal pigment epithelium with glistening intraretinal fundal dots can be found in combination with choroidal vessel sclerosis, marginal corneal dystrophy, and visual field constriction. Patients also complain about progressive hemeralopia (night blindness).

Precautions before anesthesia: No specific anesthetic considerations concerning this syndrome, and there is no evident impairment of general health.

Anesthetic considerations: The same considerations apply as for healthy children undergoing eye surgery. Especially in younger patients undergoing ophthalmic examination under general anesthesia, oculocardiac reflex with profound bradycardia should be expected. The treatment is twofold and includes first stopping the stimulation and second, if still necessary, anticholinergic drugs.

Pharmacological implications: No known pharmacological implications.

REFERENCES:

Jiao X, Munier FL, Iwata F, et al: Genetic linkage of Bietti crystalline corneoretinal dystrophy to chromosome 4q35. *Am J Hum Genet* 67:1309, 2000.

Kaiser-Kupfer MI, Chan CC, Markello TC, et al: Clinical biochemical and pathologic correlations in Bietti's crystalline dystrophy. *Am J Ophthalmol* 118:569, 1994.

Shan M, Dong B, Zhao X, et al. Novel mutations in the CYP4V2 gene associated with Bietti crystalline corneoretinal dystrophy. *Mol Vis* 11:738, 2005.

Bjornstad Syndrome

At a glance: Genetic disorder with pili torti and sensorineural deafness.

Synonym: Pili Torti and Nerve Deafness Syndrome.

Incidence and genetic inheritance: Approximately 37 cases have been described. Autosomal recessive with gene map locus on 2q34-36.

Clinical aspects: Deafness is evident in the first years of life. The severity stabilizes by puberty. Abnormalities of hair (alopecia, or coarse, dry, lusterless, fragile hair) are present and mainly of cosmetic concern. Microscopic examination of the hair shaft shows flattening at irregular intervals and a 180-degree twisting around its axis. Diagnosis is confirmed by optical and scanning electron microscopy. Mental retardation or hypogonadism in some patients.

Anesthetic considerations: No specific anesthetic implications should arise from this disorder. Benzodiazepine premedication may decrease the anxiety of these patients with severe deafness given that communication may be difficult. Parental presence at induction may be helpful for a fearful child who is unable to communicate well. Constant reassurance by the parent or signing for older patients is necessary during induction and upon emergence from anesthesia.

REFERENCES:

Lubianca Neto JF, Lu L, Eavey RD, et al: The Bjornstad syndrome (sensorineural hearing loss and pili torti) disease gene maps to chromosome 2q34-36. *Am J Hum Genet* 62:1107, 1998.

Richards KA, Mancini AJ: Three members of a family with pili torti and sensorineural hearing loss: The Bjornstad syndrome. *J Am Acad Dermatol* 46:301, 2002.

Seelvag E: Pili torti and sensorineural hearing loss: A follow-up of Bjornstad's original patients and a review of the literature. *Eur J Dermatol* 10:91, 2000.

Blackfan-Diamond Syndrome

At a glance: Congenital hypoplastic anemia manifesting in the first year of life. Increased risk for leukemia.

Synonyms: Diamond-Blackfan Anemia; Congenital Hypoplastic Anemia; Congenital Pure Red Cell Anemia/ Aplasia; Chronic Congenital Aregenerative Anemia; Chronic Erythroblastopenia; Constitutional Erythroid Hypoplasia; Erythrogenesis Imperfecta; Estren-Dameshek Variant of Fanconi Anemia.

History: First described in 1938 by the two American pediatricians Kenneth Daniel Blackfan and Louis Klein Diamond.

Incidence: Several hundred cases have been reported in the literature. Annual incidence is approximately 5:1,000,000 live births.

Genetic inheritance: Most often autosomal dominant, but autosomal recessive transmission with normal chromosomes has been described (parental consanguinity is a risk factor). Approximately

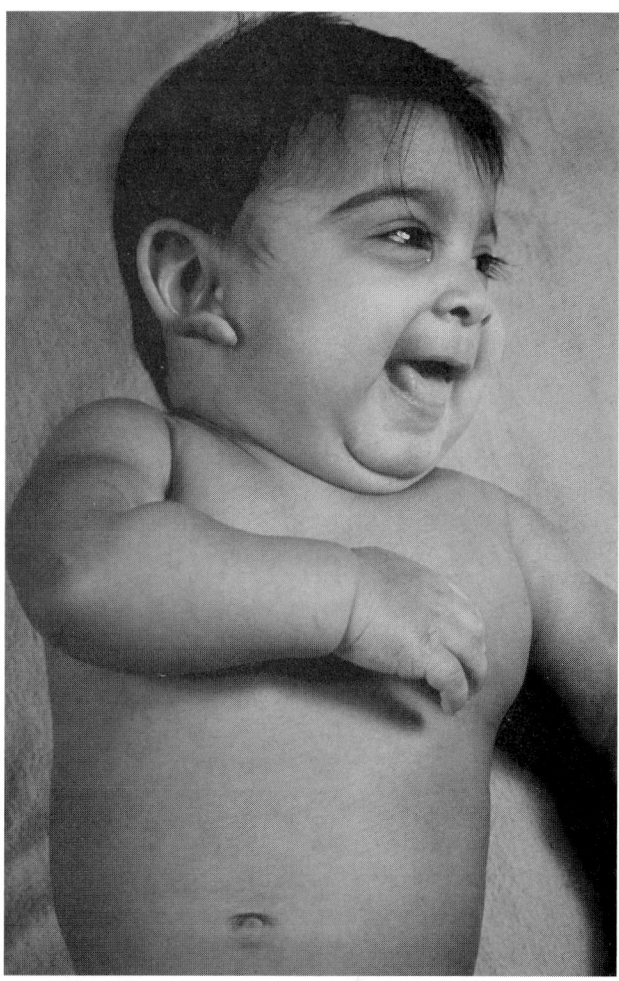

Blackfan-Diamond Syndrome Seven-month-old boy with Blackfan-Diamond syndrome has anomalies of the ear and a short neck because of fusion of the cervical vertebrae.

25% of cases can be linked to a mutation of the ribosomal protein S19 (RBS19) with gene map locus 19q13.3. The function of this protein has not been elucidated.

Pathophysiology: Uncertain, but may be secondary to a defect of pluripotent stem cell differentiation into erythroid progenitor cells (response to erythropoietin may be altered).

Diagnosis: Typically, the initial signs are pallor and dyspnea during breast-feeding or bottle feeding. Diagnosis usually is made by 6 months of age (70–90% of patients present by the first 3 months of life, but only 13% are anemic at birth): severe macrocytic anemia, high hemoglobin F levels for patient's age, reticulocytopenia (usually <1%), normal white cell count, and normal-to-elevated platelets. As a consequence of complete cessation of erythropoiesis, many patients do not have an elevated mean corpuscular volume initially. However, these patients become macrocytic once recovery of erythropoiesis occurs. Bone marrow aspiration shows decreased erythroid precursors with less than 5% of nucleated cells being erythroblasts. Hepatosplenomegaly may occur in up to 40% of affected children and, because it is reversible after transfusion, it most likely reflects heart failure. Although not pathognomonic, increased levels of erythrocyte adenosine deaminase can frequently be detected. Serum and urine erythropoietin levels are elevated. Approximately

67% of patients respond initially to steroids and approximately 40% require regular transfusions. Allogenic bone marrow transplant may be a therapeutic option for steroid-resistant patients but remains controversial because the disease is not malignant and secondary response of these patients to steroids is well known.

Clinical aspects: Congenital hypoplastic anemia. Relapse is often associated with infections. Patients may be transfusion dependent from time of diagnosis if they are resistant to steroids or become secondarily transfusion dependent once steroid resistance develops. Chelation therapy with deferoxamine is often required with chronic transfusions. Associated anomalies with this disease occur in approximately 40% of patients and may include growth retardation, facial abnormalities (microcephaly or macrocephaly, wide fontanelle, micrognathia, arched or cleft palate, macroglossia, thickening of the upper lip), ocular abnormalities (microphthalmos, strabismus, hypertelorism, epicanthal folds, blue sclerae, cataracts, glaucoma), thumb abnormalities (absent, bifid, subluxed, supernumerary), and renal abnormalities (absent, duplicated, or horseshoe kidneys). Other symptoms and findings include congenital heart defects, abnormal weakness and fatigue, pale skin, protruding scapulae, and webbing or abnormal shortening of the neck because of fused cervical vertebrae.

Precautions before anesthesia: Check hematocrit and transfuse as needed. Check for systemic signs of iron overload, specifically hepatic fibrosis/cirrhosis and myocardial failure. Check hepatic and renal function (laboratory, ultra-sound). Evaluate possibility of difficult tracheal intubation.

Anesthetic considerations: Maintain oxygen-carrying capacity. Direct laryngoscopy or tracheal intubation can be difficult in case of facial and cervical abnormalities and may require adapted anesthetic management. Postoperative cardiac and respiratory monitoring may be necessary.

Pharmacological implications: Hepatic metabolism of drugs may be reduced in patients with chronic transfusions. Halothane probably is best avoided. Avoid myocardial depressant drugs in the presence of preexisting cardiac failure. Prophylactic antibiotherapy as in immunodeficient patients. Muscle relaxant should be avoided until the airway is secured.

Other conditions to be considered:

☞**AASE SYNDROME:** Autosomal recessive inherited syndrome characterized by bilateral triphalangeal thumbs and anemia usually presenting at approximately 6 months of age.

☞**FANCONI ANEMIA:** Spontaneous chromosomal aberrations associated with hypocellular marrow, pancytopenia, and constitutional aplastic anemia presenting in the first years of life associated with growth retardation.

☞**CONGENITAL DYSERYTHROPOIETIC ANEMIAS:** Although these anemias are aregenerative, bone marrow biopsy does not show a quantitative loss of cell line precursors because the underlying defect affects the maturation of these cells.

TRANSIENT ERYTHROBLASTOPENIA OF CHILDHOOD (TEC): Acquired red cell aplasia that most likely is infectious (parvovirus B19) or toxic in origin and may appear in small epidemics. In 90% of cases, the age at presentation is older than 1 year. Some patients may experience neutropenia. TEC is accompanied by cessation of erythropoiesis, so the mean corpuscular volume is not increased initially. However, during the recovery phase, which is characterized by a marked reticulocytosis, the mean corpuscular volume becomes elevated. Recovery usually starts within 1 to 2 months from onset.

AUTOIMMUNE ERYTHROBLASTOPENIA: Acquired disease that is very rare in the pediatric population. Most often it is diagnosed in association with an autoimmune hemolytic anemia caused by cold-reactive antibodies most commonly following a mycoplasma pneumonia or infectious mononucleosis. Drugs that may induce an autoimmune hemolytic anemia include penicillins, cephalosporins, erythromycin, acetaminophen, methyldopa, and procainamide.

REFERENCES:

Ball SE, McGuckin CP, Jenkins G, et al: Diamond-Blackfan anaemia in the UK: analysis of 80 cases from a 20-year birth cohort. *Br J Haematol* 94:645, 1996.

Manglani M, Lokeshwar MR, Sharma R: Diamond-Blackfan anemia: report of 6 cases. *Indian Pediatr* 40:355, 2003.

Walters MC, Abelson HT: Pediatric hematology. Interpretation of the complete blood count. *Pediatr Clin North Am* 43:599, 1996.

Bladder Exstrophy

At a glance: Major congenital disorder resulting in abnormal development of the cloacal membrane with failure of fusion of the entire lower abdominal wall, including lower urinary tract, external genitalia, and symphysis pubis.

Incidence: Incidence varies from 1:20,000 to 1:30,000 live births, with a prevalence of 3.3:100,000 live births and a male-to-female ratio of 2:1 to 3:1. The recurrence risk for sibs is approximately 1%, with a one in 70 recurrence risk for offspring of affected subjects.

Genetic inheritance: Bladder exstrophy most likely is a multifactorially inherited anomaly. Only 20 cases of familial bladder exstrophy have been reported. One report of a pair of monozygotic twins—one with bladder exstrophy, the other with no congenital abnormalities—has been described. The authors of this report concluded that the condition was not purely genetically determined.

Pathophysiology: Abnormal development of cloacal membrane during the fifth and sixth weeks of embryonic life impedes normal mesodermal movement and prevents midline fusion of the musculoskeletal elements of the infraumbilical anterior abdominal wall.

Diagnosis: Prenatal diagnosis using ultrasonography is the method of choice. A reliable diagnosis can be obtained before 20 weeks of gestation based on the absence of a bladder, normal kidneys, a semisolid mass protruding from the lower abdominal wall, and a low insertion of the umbilical cord into the abdomen. Clinical appearance and familial history (rare).

Clinical aspects: Prenatal diagnosis usually is made between 12 and 20 weeks of gestation. Failure of fusion of the cloacal membrane results in a complete lower anterior abdominal wall defect. This malformation is characterized by exstrophy of the bladder with a small bladder plate, lower urinary tract defect (urethra and bladder neck), abnormal external genitalia, open symphysis pubis, and nonfused lower abdominal wall. The kidneys are usually normal in appearance. The defect may involve the lower gastrointestinal tract and the spinal canal. Other anomalies can be associated. Most affected males develop severe sexual dysfunction because of a short penis and erection abnormalities.

Precautions before anesthesia: Neonates require a full preoperative assessment to determine the extent of the bladder exstrophy and the presence of any other associated congenital abnormalities. Laboratory investigations should include a complete blood count, blood glucose, urea, and electrolytes, including calcium and phosphate. Renal and liver function tests, a clotting screen, and cross-matching of blood should be obtained. The cardiovascular status and state of fluid hydration should be assessed because the condition is associated with marked fluid losses prior to correction. Older children likely will have undergone several operations and will benefit from sedative premedication. Latex allergy may be a problem in children who have undergone several urologic or plastic reconstructive procedures. Use of a latex-free anesthesia and surgery equipment is recommended.

Anesthetic considerations: Standard preparation for all neonates undergoing major surgery, including arterial and central venous line. Repair of bladder exstrophy involves prolonged surgery with major blood loss and significant fluid requirements. Epidural analgesic techniques (caudal or lumbar approach) may be appropriate if the defect does not involve the spinal canal. Postoperatively, the neonate will require a period of ventilation and careful fluid management. Measures to maintain body temperature should be taken.

Pharmacological implications: Perioperative prophylaxis with steroids and/or antihistaminics (H_1 and H_2 blocker) may be considered for patients with known latex allergy.

Other conditions to be considered:

EXSTROPHY OF THE CLOACA SEQUENCE: Most severe form of the exstrophy complex. Results from a developmental defect of the mesenchyme that causes a midline defect of the lower abdominal structures, exposing the bladder and a large portion of the bowel through the anterior abdominal wall. The patient usually presents with failed fusion of the symphysis pubis, often associated with incomplete development of the lumbosacral vertebrae leading to hydromelia. Omphalocele may coexist. In males, diphallus with bifid scrotum is usually present. Females often have duplication and occasionally vaginal atresia or agenesis. Other features include renal anomalies such as polycystic kidneys and renal agenesis.

OEIS COMPLEX (Omphalocele-Exstrophy-Imperforate Anus-Spinal Defects): Inherited disorder resulting from an autosomal recessive trait. Patients present with an omphalocele, exstrophy-epispadias sequence, and pubic diastasis. An imperforated anus is often associated. Spinal defects because of failed fusion of vertebrae are always present. This rare complex is thought to be the most severe end of a spectrum of birth defects.

REFERENCES:

Messelink EJ, Aronson DC, Knuist M, et al: Four cases of bladder exstrophy in two families. *J Med Genet* 31:490, 1994.

Baird AD, Mathews RI, Gearheart JP: The use of combined bladder and epispadias repair in boys with classic bladder exstrophy: outcomes, complications and consequences. *J Urol* 174:1421, 2005.

Mourtzinos A, Borer JG: Current management of bladder exstrophy. *Curr Urol Rep* 5:137, 2004.

Bland-White-Garland Syndrome

At a glance: Congenital anomaly of the left coronary artery.
Synonyms: *A*nomalous *L*eft *C*oronary *A*rtery from the *P*ulmonary *A*rtery; ALCAPA.
Incidence: 1:300,000 live births (0.25–0.5% of all cardiac malformations).
Genetic inheritance: Not an inherited disorder.
Pathophysiology: Because the left coronary artery arises from the pulmonary trunk, perfusion of the left heart must be provided by the pulmonary artery or from collaterals of the right coronary artery. Myocardial perfusion remains normal in the early neonatal period when pulmonary pressure is high. As pulmonary pressure and resistance decrease by 1 to 2 months of age, myocardial perfusion becomes insufficient and ischemia or even myocardial infarction with global ventricular failure occurs. Depending upon the importance of collateral vessels between the right and left coronary arteries, left-to-right shunting of oxygenated blood from the right coronary artery to the left coronary artery and into the pulmonary artery may create a "myocardial steal," resulting in increased ischemic insult to the anterolateral myocardium with global left ventricular dilatation and dysfunction. Papillary muscle infarction and/or mitral annular dilatation may result in secondary mitral valve regurgitation. Left atrial dilation and finally pulmonary venous congestion ensue, adding congestive symptoms to those of angina pectoris.

Diagnosis: Infants present with respiratory distress, feeding intolerance, and failure to thrive. Congestive heart failure in an infant with either no murmur on auscultation or the murmur of mitral insufficiency is suspicious for ALCAPA. The electrocardiogram may reveal anterolateral myocardial ischemia or infarction. Thallium myocardial perfusion scintigraphy or echocardiography assists in the diagnosis of this specific malformation. Aortic angiography provides the final confirmation and is a good tool for assessing the collateral vessels. The diagnosis is generally made during the first year of life, but occasionally may become manifest later in childhood or even in adulthood. Sudden death has been reported in these patients following exertion.

Clinical aspects: Rapidly progressive deterioration of physical condition, including dyspnea, expectorations, perspiration, tachycardia, and refusal to drink with failure to thrive. The patient may have angina pectoris associated with feeding. It has been estimated that 90% of untreated patients die in the first year of life. The lesion is sometimes discovered during investigation for heart murmur (although a murmur is not a constant finding) or chest pain in late childhood or adulthood.

Precautions before anesthesia: Obtain full history of cardiopulmonary symptoms of the patient. Evaluate cardiac function with electrocardiogram, chest radiography, echocardiography, left cardiac catheterization, and coronary angiography (ejection fraction, left ventricular diameter, pulmonary artery pressure and saturation, arterial saturation).

Anesthetic considerations: Symptomatic infants undergoing surgery to correct their coronary anomaly will have pulmonary venous congestion, a diminished cardiac output, decreased contractility as a result of chronic ischemia of the myocardium, and, frequently, myocardial infarction and some degree of subendocardial fibrosis. Avoid factors that reduce pulmonary vascular resistance (alkalosis, hypocapia, hyperoxia), since this may result in increased coronary steal. There is a high risk of ventricular arrhythmias. The clinical condition of the patient may be variable. The experience with this pathology in children is limited because of the rarity of the condition; however, the same principles used for treatment of severe coronary heart disease in adults are applicable. Special attention must be paid to fluid administration to ensure adequate cardiac output without causing pulmonary edema.

Pharmacological implications: Avoid agents with negative inotropic effect, especially volatile anesthetics in high concentrations. Intravenous induction and high-dose opioid technique seem to be the technique of choice. Weaning from cardiopulmonary bypass should be expected to be eventful. High doses of catecholamines may be required to augment cardiac output.

REFERENCES:

Kleinschmidt S, Grueness V, Molter G: The Bland-White-Garland syndrome. Clinical picture and anaesthesiological management. *Paediatr Anaesth* 6:65, 1996.

Nicholson WJ, Schuler B, Lerakis S, Helmy T: Anomalous origin of the coronary arteries from the pulmonary trunk in two separate patients with a review of clinical implications and current treatment recommendations. *Am J Med Sci* 328:112, 2004.

Blepharophimosis, Ptosis, and Epicanthus Inversus Syndrome

At a glance: Hereditary syndrome affecting the eyelids, with the clinical symptom triad of blepharophimosis, ptosis, and epicanthus inversus (fold curving in the mediolateral direction inferior to the inner canthus).

Synonyms: Hereditary Blepharophimosis-Ptosis-Epicanthus Inversus Syndrome; Blepharophimosis Sequence; Blepharophimosis Syndrome; Blepharophimosis-Ptosis-Epicanthus Inversus-Primary Amenorrhea Syndrome; Blepharophimosis-Ptosis-Epicanthus Inversus-Telecanthus Complex; Blepharoptosis-Blepharophimosis-Epicanthus Inversus-Telecanthus Syndrome; Blepharophimosis-Ptosis-Epicanthus Syndrome with (BPES I)/without (BPES II) Ovarian Failure.

Incidence: Rare syndrome with unknown incidence.

Genetic inheritance: Autosomal dominant transmitted disorder, but 50% of cases occur without a family history. In sporadic cases, there seems to be an apparent maternal (but not paternal) age effect. Two types of the syndrome exist: Blepharophimosis, Ptosis, and Epicanthus Inversus Syndrome (BPES) type I with infertility in affected females is transmitted by affected males to their offspring, and BPES type II with normal fertility is transmitted by females and males. Female infertility in BPES type I is a predominant symptom and the distinction between the two types is important for genetic counseling. Infertility is inherited as an autosomal dominant sex-limited trait. Infertility seems to be associated with a nonsense mutation of the gene encoding a Forkhead transcription factor, Forkhead L2 (FOXL2), which seems to be involved in ovarian follicle stiumulation and steroid biosynthesis. The two entities are further differentiated by incomplete penetrance in BPES type II only and by difference in the sex ratios of affected children. The gene locus has been mapped to 3q22.3-23.

Pathophysiology: Unknown.

Diagnosis: Made by clinical picture and family history.

Clinical aspects: Literally, blepharophimosis means narrowing of the eyelid. In BPES, the horizontal palpebral aperture is reduced and associated with eyelid dysplasia, ptosis, telecanthus, and epicanthus inversus. Affected females with BPES type I have a small uterus with primary amenorrhea, infertility, and primary ovarian failure as a result of hypoplastic ovaries. Breast development is normal, pubic and axillary hair is scant but normal in distribution. Gonadotropin levels are elevated, estrogen and progesterone levels decreased. A low nasal bridge may be an additional finding and mental retardation may occur, especially in sporadic cases.

Precautions before anesthesia: No specific anesthetic precautions are required because there is no evident impairment of general health in BPES. However, older female patients with BPES type I may have premature osteoporosis and require caution with positioning.

Anesthetic considerations: Considerations are not different from healthy patients undergoing the same procedure. Especially in younger patients undergoing ophthalmic examination under general anesthesia, oculocardiac reflex with profound bradycardia should be expected. The treatment is twofold and includes first stopping the stimulation and second, if still necessary, anticholinergic drugs.

Pharmacological implications: No known pharmacological implications.

Other conditions to be considered: Other blepharophimosis-ptosis syndromes including the following:

☞**ACRO-FRONTO-FACIO-NASAL DYSOSTOSIS SYNDROME (Type I and II):** Frontonasal dysostosis, retarded growth, and mental development. Brachycephaly, broad notched nasal tip, and cleft lip/palate and macrostomia. Polysyndactyly, camptodactyly, and hypoplasia of the distal phalanges of the hands. Iliac hypoplasia, short legs and hypospadias.

☞**BLEPHAROPTOSIS WITH MYOPIA AND ECTOPIA LENTIS:** Genetic disease with features limited to the eye and its appendices.

☞**FRYDMAN COHEN KARMON SYNDROME:** Inherited syndrome with blepharophimosis, ptosis, short stature, and syndactyly.

DE DIE SMULDERS-DROOG-VAN DIJK SYNDROME: Blepharophimosis, nasal groove, and growth retardation.

JORGENSON-LENZ SYNDROME: Mildly shortened stature, microcephaly, ptosis-blepharophimosis, facial asymmetry, prognathism, restricted joint mobility, and radioulnar synostosis. The name of this syndrome is based on a single paper.

OHDO-MADOKORO-SONODA SYNDROME (Blepharophimosis Syndrome, Ohdo Type): Blepharophimosis, ptosis, mental retardation, congenital heart disease, and hypoplastic teeth.

SIMOSA-PENCHASZADEH-BUSTOS SYNDROME (Simosa Craniofacial Syndrome; Blepharophimosis Telecanthus Microstomia Syndrome): High forehead, elongated and flattened face, arched and sparse eyebrows, short palpebral fissures. Microstomia, high and narrow palate. Intelligence normal. Facies similar to the "whistling face syndrome" (☞Freeman-Sheldon syndrome). Potential difficult airway management.

ELSCHNIG SYNDROME (Rodini-Richieri-Costa Syndrome; Blepharocheilodontic): Blepharoptosis, cleft palate, ectropion and dental anomalies.

REFERENCES:

Pisarska MD, Bae J, Klein C, Hsueh AJ: Forkhead 12 is expressed in the ovary and represses the promotor activity of the steroidogenic acute regulatory gene. Endocrinology 145:3424, 2004.

Zlotogora J, Sagi M, Cohen T: The blepharophimosis, ptosis, and epicanthus inversus syndrome: Delineation of two types. *Am J Hum Genet* 35:1020, 1983.

Blepharoptosis with Myopia and Ectopia Lentis

At a glance: Genetic disease with features limited to the eye and its appendices.

Incidence: Extremely rare abnormality, but exact incidence is not known.

Genetic inheritance: Inheritance is autosomal dominant. No genetic background or molecular data are available.

Pathophysiology: It has been suggested that a connective tissue defect of sclera and zonule, combined with a disinsertion of the levator palpebrae aponeurosis, is the common factor underlying the clinical features.

Diagnosis: Presents with the triad of congenital blepharoptosis, high-grade myopia, and ectopia lentis.

Clinical aspects: Blepharoptosis, abnormally long globes, abnormally long upper eyelids, and a well-maintained function of the levator characterize this syndrome.

Precautions before anesthesia: No specific anesthetic precautions are required.

Anesthetic considerations: Considerations are not different from healthy children undergoing the same procedure. Especially in younger patients undergoing ophthalmic examination under general anesthesia, oculocardiac reflex with profound bradycardia should be expected. The treatment is twofold and includes first stopping the stimulation and second, if still necessary, anticholinergic drugs. No other specific precautions are required.

Pharmacological implications: No known pharmacological implications.

Other conditions to be considered: Other blepharophimosis-ptosis syndromes such as the following:

☞**ACRO-FRONTO-FACIO-NASAL DYSOSTOSIS SYNDROME (Type I and II):** Frontonasal dysostosis, retarded growth, and mental development. Brachycephaly, broad notched nasal tip, and cleft lip/palate and macrostomia. Polysyndactyly, camptodactyly, and hypoplasia of the distal phalanges of the hands. Iliac hypoplasia, short legs, and hypospadias.

☞**BLEPHAROPTOSIS PTOSIS AND EPICANTHUS INVERSUS SYNDROME:** Hereditary syndrome affecting the eyelids with the clinical symptom triad of blepharophimosis, ptosis, and epicanthus inversus (fold curving in the mediolateral direction inferior to the inner canthus).

☞**FRYDMAN COHEN KARMON SYNDROME:** Inherited syndrome with blepharophimosis, ptosis, short stature, and syndactyly.

DE DIE SMULDERS-DROOG-VAN DIJK SYNDROME: Blepharophimosis, nasal groove, and growth retardation.

JORGENSON-LENZ SYNDROME: Mildly shortened stature, microcephaly, ptosis-blepharophimosis, facial asymmetry, prognathism, restricted joint mobility, and radioulnar synostosis. The name of this syndrome is based on a single paper.

OHDO-MADOKORO-SONODA SYNDROME (Blepharophimosis Syndrome, Ohdo Type): Blepharophimosis, ptosis, mental retardation, congenital heart disease, and hypoplastic teeth.

SIMOSA-PENCHASZADEH-BUSTOS SYNDROME (Simosa Craniofacial Syndrome; Blepharophimosis Telecanthus Microstomia Syndrome): High forehead, elongated and flattened face, arched and sparse eyebrows, short palpebral fissures. Microstomia, high and narrow palate. Intelligence normal. Facies similar to the "whistling face syndrome" (Freeman-Sheldon syndrome). Potential difficult airway management.

REFERENCE:
Gillum WN, Anderson RL: Dominantly inherited blepharoptosis, high myopia, and ectopia lentis. *Arch Ophthalmol* 100:282, 1982.

Bloom Syndrome

At a glance: Autosomal recessive inherited disorder characterized by prenatal and postnatal growth retardation, photosensitivity, telangiectasias, skin pigment anomalies, and increased risk of malignancies most likely as a consequence of chromosomal instability.

Synonyms: Congenital Telangiectatic Erythema; Bloom-Torre-Machacek Syndrome.

Incidence: 1:160,000 live births. More common in Ashkenazi Jews from Eastern Europe.

Genetic inheritance: Autosomal recessive. Gene map locus 15q26.1.

Pathophysiology: The protein BLM encoded by the normal gene acts in the maintenance of genomic stability. A mutation in this gene results in Bloom Syndrome. Spontaneous chromosome breakage with exchanges between homologous chromosome segments lead to increased sister chromatid exchanges and are assumed to be responsible for the phenotype and the predisposition to neoplasias.

Diagnosis: Clinical signs plus chromosomal and DNA analysis. Amniocentesis for amniotic fluid cell culture with assessment of the number of sister chromatid exchanges allows prenatal diagnosis.

Clinical aspects: Prenatal and postnatal growth retardation are hallmarks of this syndrome and usually the first reason to seek medical attention. Clinical signs include dolichocephaly and malar hypoplasia resulting in a "bird-like" face, photosensitivity with telangiectasias in the face and other sun-exposed areas (butterfly-like midface distribution; plaques or macules in other locations), and café-au-lait spots. Pulmonary fibrosis, bronchiectasis, cardiomyopathy, primary hypogonadism and mental retardation are variable findings. Adult-onset diabetes mellitus may occur in the second or third decade of life. Immunocompromise is caused by decreased levels of IgM and IgA and can result in life-threatening gastrointestinal and respiratory infections. Predisposition to neoplasias is another important feature, with an up to 300-fold increased risk of malignancies compared to the normal population (especially lymphomas, leukemias, squamous cell carcinomas, and gastrointestinal adenocarcinomas). Approximately 20% of patients will experience one (or more) neoplasia(s), which may present as early as 4 years of age but is most common in the mid-twenties for leukemias and lymphomas and in the mid-thirties for solid tumors. Patients are at risk for developing diabetes mellitus in the second or third decade of life.

Precautions before anesthesia: Obtain a full history. Check blood glucose profile and levels in case of diabetes mellitus. Rule out mediastinal mass in the presence of lymphoma or leukemia. Check respiratory and cardiac function (clinical, chest radiography, echocardiography, arterial blood gas analysis, pulmonary function tests).

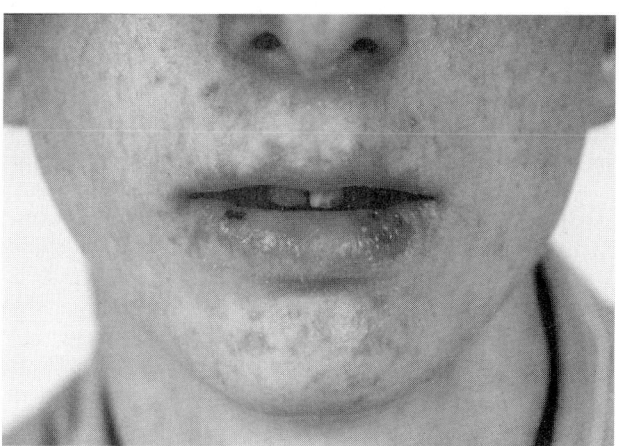

Bloom Syndrome Perioral and facial telangiectasias in a boy with Bloom syndrome. See color plates.

Anesthetic considerations: Strict asepsis for these patients is mandatory and reverse isolation must be considered. Enforce aggressive pulmonary toilet in the presence of bronchiectases. Perioperative cardiac and respiratory monitoring should be considered.

Pharmacological implications: Avoid myocardial depressant drugs in the presence of cardiomyopathy. Consider prophylactic antibiotics as in immunodeficient patients.

Other conditions to be considered:

☞**PORPHYRIAS:** a group of disorders characterized by enzymatic defects in the heme biosynthesis. Depending on the primary location of the defect, the porphyrias are classified as erythropoietic and hepatic forms.

☞**COCKAYNE SYNDROME:** Characteristics of this autosomal recessive inherited disease are dwarfism, precociously senile appearance, pigmentary retinal degeneration, optic atrophy, progressive sensorineural deafness, sensitivity to sunlight, and mental retardation. Disproportionately long limbs with large hands and feet and flexion contractures of joints are usual skeletal features.

☞**ROTHMUND-THOMSON SYNDROME:** Poikiloderma, alopecia or sparse hair, dystrophic teeth and nails, saddle nose, short stature, skeletal defects, juvenile cataract, premature aging, and high incidence of cutaneous and noncutaneous malignancies characterize this autosomal recessive inherited disorder.

☞**SYSTEMIC LUPUS ERYTHEMATOSUS:** A chronic, inflammatory multisystemic disorder of the connective tissue, principally involving the skin, joints, kidneys, and serosal membranes.

REFERENCES:

German J: Bloom's syndrome. XX. The first 100 cancers. *Cancer Genet Cytogenet* 93:100, 1997.

Kaneko H, Kondo N: Clinical features of Bloom syndrome and function of the causative gene, BLM helicase. *Expert Rev Mol Diagn* 4:393, 2004.

Keller C, Keller KR, Shew SB, et al: Growth deficiency and malnutrition in Bloom syndrome. *J Pediatr* 134:472, 1999.

Blue Diaper Syndrome

At a glance: Genetic disorder with defective transport for L-tryptophan resulting in blue urine.

Synonyms: Familial Hypercalcemia and Indicanuria; Drummond Syndrome; Familial Hypercalcemia with Nephrocalcinosis and Indicanuria; Tryptophan Malabsorption Syndrome.

Incidence: Very rare with a frequency of 1:1117 consecutive patients studied for detection of inborn error of metabolism.

Genetic inheritance: Either autosomal recessive or X-linked recessive inheritance.

Pathophysiology: Caused by a deficiency of a substrate-specific intestinal membrane transport system for L-tryptophan. The defect is located in the brush-border membrane of epithelial cells in the small intestine and kidney tubules, similar to Hartnup disease, cystinuria, iminoglycinuria, and lysine malabsorption syndrome.

Diagnosis: Blue discoloration of the diapers starting in early infancy is secondary to bacterial degradation of tryptophan, producing indigo blue by enzymatic conversion of indolic compounds in the urine. Severe and prolonged hypercalcemia is frequent. Excess tryptophan is measured in the feces of the child, and increased tryptophan derivatives (indole acetic acid, indole lactic acid) found in the urine are of intestinal origin. These derivatives result from an increased concentration of tryptophan in the intestinal lumen. The plasma concentration of tryptophan is normal, but the increase following oral L-tryptophan intake is less than normal. Renal clearance of tryptophan is normal. In one report, the blue-greenish stool discoloration was attributed to a pigment derived from *Pseudomonas aeruginosa.*

Clinical aspects: Hypercalcemia and nephrocalcinosis are associated with failure to thrive, recurrent unexplained fever, infection, irritability, and constipation. Prognosis is unfavorable if complicated by nephrocalcinosis. Ocular abnormalities, such as microcornea, hypoplasia of the optic disc, and abnormal eye movements, have been described. The indoluria may look like the one in Hartnup syndrome, but a specific hyperaminoaciduria exists.

Precautions before anesthesia: Evaluation of hydration, renal function, and hypercalcemia. Treatment of potentially associated infections. Rule out paralytic ileus.

Anesthetic considerations: A case of perioperative death has been reported after a mastoidectomy in an infant, but no data on the anesthetic technique used are available. Regional anesthesia can be performed. Because of a tendency toward dehydration, anesthetic drugs that may mask a low circulating volume and lead to vascular collapse should be avoided. Appropriate hydration and urinary output must be enforced. Paralytic ileus results in increased risk of regurgitation and aspiration during induction. Consequently, a rapid sequence induction is mandatory.

Pharmacological implications: Avoid drugs with predominantly renal elimination (or consider reduced dose) in the presence of decreased kidney function.

Other conditions to be considered:

☞**HARTNUP SYNDROME/DISEASE:** Autosomal recessive disorder caused by a defective transport of tryptophan and other neutral (i.e., monoamine-monocarboxylic) amino acids in the small intestine and kidneys. Patients may present with a pellagra-like skin condition, cerebellar ataxia, and gross aminoaciduria.

☞**DIAMINOPENTANURIA:** Increased renal clearance of cystine, lysine, arginine, and ornithine secondary to a dysfunction of the reabsorptive capacity of the renal tubules. In addition, defective intestinal absorption results in increased degradation of these amino acids by bacteria in the intestine.

☞**HYPERPROLINEMIA:** Autosomal recessive inherited disorder with decreased renal tubular reabsorption of glycine and the imino acids proline and hydroxyproline. Patients with type II disease may be taking antiseizure medication, so epileptogenic drugs should be avoided.

☞**LYSINURIC PROTEIN INTOLERANCE:** Autosomal recessive disease characterized by defective transport of the dibasic amino acids.

PURPLE URINE BAG SYNDROME (PUBS Syndrome): Tryptophan (L-tryptophan) is a rarely used antidepressant drug. It decomposes in the gut to form indoxyl sulfate, which is absorbed and secreted in the urine (indican). Urinary organisms, such as *Proteus* and *Klebsiella*, have indoxyl sulfatase activity to metabolize indican to indigo, particularly in alkaline urine. In the other suggested pathway, once indoxyl sulfate comes in contact with air, it is oxidized to insoluble indigo, which causes the deep purple discoloration of the urine, the catheter, and the urine bag. Enteritis, pancreatic insufficiency, ileus, peritonitis (increased production), renal insufficiency (diminished excretion), bile acids, and steroidal conjugates also can cause a purple discoloration of the urine. Other reports suggest the color results from an interaction between indigo crystals in the urine and indirubin dissolved in the plastic bag for the urine. Most often, except for the scary color, this finding has no clinical relevance.

REFERENCES:

Chen Y, Wu L, Xiong Q: The ocular abnormalities of blue diaper syndrome. *Metab Pediatr Syst Ophthalmol* 14:73, 1991.

Drummond KN, Michael AF, Ulstrom RA, et al: The blue diaper syndrome: familial hypercalcemia with nephrocalcinosis and indicanuria. A new familial disease, with definition of the metabolic abnormality. *Am J Med* 37:928, 1964.

Libit SA, Ulstrom RA, Doeden D: Fecal *Pseudomonas aeruginosa* as a cause of the blue diaper syndrome. *J Pediatr* 81:546, 1972.

Blue Rubber Bleb Nevus Syndrome

At a glance: Multiple cutaneous and noncutaneous (mainly gastrointestinal tract) venous malformations, which can result in discomfort and hemorrhage.

Synonym: Bean Syndrome.

Incidence: Unknown, but extremely rare. Men and women are equally affected. Occurs in all races, although caucasians seem to be more frequently affected.

Genetic inheritance: Most cases are sporadic, but autosomal dominant inheritance has been described.

Diagnosis: Hemangiomas typically occur on the trunk, upper extremities, perineum, and in the gastrointestinal tract (from mouth to anus), but they can principally occur everywhere in the body (oral cavity hemangiomas may occur in up to 60% of patients). They are associated with nocturnal pain and hyperhydrosis in the affected skin areas.

Clinical aspects: The rubber-like hemangiomas may be tender but usually are easily compressible and refill promptly after compression. They are highly variable in size (from a few millimeters to many centimeters), color (from red to black), morphology (from flat to elevated to pedunculated nodules), and number (from a few to hundreds). Bleeding from the skin lesions is rare in the absence of trauma; however, anemia (iron deficiency anemia) and death as a result of gastrointestinal bleeding may occur, although most commonly the bleeding is slow, chronic, and occult. Intussusception, volvulus, and bowel infarction have been described. Lesions involving the bones and joints are less common, but can cause profound discomfort and deformity, loss of function, and spontaneous fractures. Central nervous system involvement (seizures, ataxia, dementia), although rare, can be fatal (hemorrhage). Cerebellar medulloblastoma has been associated with this syndrome. Pregnancy seems to have the potential to exacerbate bleeding from gastrointestinal lesions.

Precautions before anesthesia: Check hemoglobin. Assess extremities for hemangiomas prior to obtaining intravascular access or performing peripheral regional anesthesia and evaluate the airway for presence of hemangiomas that may obstruct the view or bleed during airway management.

Anesthetic considerations: Anticipate the need for transfusion. Perform gentle direct laryngoscopy and tracheal intubation, especially in the presence of oral hemangiomas. Avoid esophageal instrumentation (nasogastric or orogastric tubes) in the presence of gastrointestinal hemangiomas.

Pharmacological implications: No known pharmacological implications.

Other conditions to be considered:

☞**KLIPPEL-TRENAUNAY SYNDROME:** Form of vascular malformation with congenital aplasia and/or dysplasia of specific parts of the vascular system in association with bony and soft tissue hypertrophy.

☞**MAFFUCCI SYNDROME:** Congenital disorder characterized by dyschondroplasia of one or more limbs, multiple enchondromas, and soft tissue hemangiomas.

VENOUS LAKES: Lesions present as dark blue to violaceous, easily compressible papules caused by ectasia of venules. They predominantly occur on chronically sun-exposed skin (most often located on the ears or lips of elderly patients). The lesions are harmless and have no clinical significance; however, they play an important role in the differential diagnosis of more severe lesions with a potentially similar aspect (melanoma, basalioma, or squamous cell carcinoma), as thrombosis is frequently present in these lesions.

REFERENCES:

Andersen JM: Blue rubber bleb nevus syndrome. *Curr Treat Options Gastroenterol* 4:433, 2001.

Kanai M, Noike M, Masaki C, et al: Severe gastrointestinal bleeding during pregnancy in a case of blue rubber bleb nevus syndrome. *Semin Thromb Hemast* 31:284, 2005.

Requena L, Sangueza OP: Cutaneous vascular anomalies. Part I. Hamartomas, malformations, and dilation of preexisting vessels. *J Am Acad Dermatol* 37:523, 1997.

Book Syndrome

At a glance: A rare form of ectodermal dysplasia with premolar aplasia, hyperhidrosis, premature cavities, and premature whitening of the hair.

Synonyms: *P*remolar Aplasia, *H*yperhidrosis, and Premature *C*avities Syndrome; PHC Syndrome.

Incidence: Extremely rare.

Genetic inheritance: Autosomal dominant with high penetrance.

Pathophysiology: Unknown, but PHC syndrome belongs to the heterogeneous group of ectodermal dysplasias that includes more than 150 diseases with various inheritance modes and genetic heterogenicity. In ectodermal dysplasia, the initial factor seems to be a perturbation of epithelial morphogenesis.

Diagnosis: Premature whitening of the hair with characteristic dental defects and a family with similar history.

Clinical aspects: Dental affection is the most frequent sign. Anodontia or oligodontia can affect all teeth, but missing premolars are the most characteristic. Abnormal dental position and tooth shape anomaly may be observed. Premature whitening of hair can appear even in childhood and may be associated with poorly formed dermatoglyphs and distal digital creases. Increased sweating of the hands and feet are very frequent (hyperhidrosis).

Precautions before anesthesia: No other disorders are associated with this particular syndrome. However, because of a mild depression of the immune system and a defect in the respiratory mucous glands, other forms of ectodermal dysplasia often show a predisposition to respiratory tract infections, which are potentially life-threatening. No such reports exist specifically for this syndrome, but nevertheless should be kept in mind when assessing the patient. Evaluate dental position, aspect, and mobility, and severity of hyperhidrosis.

Anesthetic considerations: No reports of anesthetic experience with these patients are available. Patients may present for surgical management of hyperhidrosis. Extremity lesions can interfere with pulse oximetry. Direct laryngoscopy must be done very carefully considering the dental anomalies.

Pharmacological implications: Hyperhidrosis must be evaluated before use of parasympatholytic drugs (flush, hyperthermia more frequent with atropine).

Other conditions to be considered: Far more than 100 different forms of ectodermal dysplasia are known; only a few are mentioned here to show the wide variety of this entity.

RAPP-HODGKIN HYPOHIDROTIC ECTODERMAL DYSPLASIAS: Autosomal dominant inherited anhidrotic ectodermal dysplasia with cleft lip/palate, hypodontia, hair anomalies and alopecia in adulthood, and nail anomalies.

☞**CHRIST-SIEMENS-TOURAINE SYNDROME:** Inherited disease characterized by absence of sweat glands (anhidrosis, distorted heat regulation), and sebaceous glands (xerosis), hypotrichosis, poor dental development, and facial abnormalities (prominent forehead, thick lips, saddle nose).

☞**PSAUME SYNDROME (Orofaciodigital Syndrome Type I):** A syndrome with X-linked dominant transmission or sporadic (75%) occurrence with oral (tongue and dental anomalies, cleft lip/palate), facial (hypertelorism, telecanthus, micrognathia), digital (brachydactyly, syndactyly, duplication of hallux), cerebral (cerebellar atrophy, agenesis of the corpus callosum, Dandy-Walker malformation, mild mental retardation), and renal anomalies (polycystic kidney disease). Almost all affected patients are females, although some affected males have been reported.

☞**ELLIS-VAN CREVELD SYNDROME:** Autosomal recessive inherited syndrome with congenital cardiac defects, pulmonary hypoplasia because of a small chest, dwarfism, polydactyly, nail dystrophy, and dystonias.

CLOUSTON SYNDROME (☞**Ectodermal Dysplasias):** Autosomal dominant ectodermal dysplasia characterized by the triad of palmoplantar hyperkeratosis, nail dystrophy, and alopecia. Facial appearance, teeth, and sweating are normal.

☞**INCONTINENTIA PIGMENTI:** X-linked dominant genodermatosis with skin pigmentation changes that are often associated with ocular, dental, central nervous abnormalities and malignancies (Wilms tumor, retinoblastoma, myeloid leukemia, rhabdomyosarcoma).

☞**ECTRODACTYLY ECTODERMAL DYSPLASIAS CLEFTING SYNDROME:** Autosomal dominant inherited anomaly complex characterized by ectrodactyly of hands and feet, ectodermal dysplasia, and cleft lip/palate.

☞**GORLIN-GOLTZ SYNDROME:** Autosomal dominant transmitted neurocutaneous syndrome characterized by facial, skin, and skeletal abnormalities and later (usually after puberty) occurrence of multiple basal cell carcinomas.

☞**SETLEIS SYNDROME:** Characterized by an aged leonine face with absent or multiple rows of eyelashes, redundant facial soft tissue, and rubbery feel to facial skin. Characteristic bitemporal skin marks and association with imperforate anus.

☞**CHANDS:** Autosomal recessive inherited disorder presenting with curly hairs, hypoplastic nails, and eyelid fusion.

☞**OCULODENTODIGITAL DYSPLASIA:** Ectodermal dysplasia with autosomal dominant inheritance characterized by mental retardation, microcephaly, microphthalmia, glaucoma, enamel hypoplasia, syndactyly, camptodactyly, and hypotrichosis.

PACHYONYCHIA CONGENITA (Jadassohn-Lewandowsky Syndrome) (focal [nummular] type of ☞**Keratosis palmaris et plantaris):** Genetic disorder with onychogryposis, hyperkeratosis of the palms, soles, knees, and elbows. Tiny cutaneous horns in many areas and leukoplakia of the oral mucosa.

☞**CRANIODIAPHYSEAL DYSPLASIA:** Bone disorder characterized by marked hyperostosis of the craniofacial bones and diaphyseal expansion of the tubular bones resulting in significant clinical complications.

☞**SCHOPF-SCHULTZ-PASSARGE SYNDROME:** Autosomal recessive inherited keratosis palmoplantaris with cystic eyelids, hypodontia, and hypotrichosis. Increased frequency of tumors of exocrine glands.

☞**CARNEVALE-HERNANDEZ-CASTILLO-TORRES SYNDROME:** Extremely rare syndrome characterized by triphalangeal thumbs, brachy (syn-) dactyly, and occasionally ectrodactyly of the feet and hands.

☞**MONILETHRIX:** Genetic effect limited to the hair and occasionally the skin but does not belong to the group of ectodermal dysplasias.

☞**TRICHODENTO-OSSEOUS SYNDROME:** Features of this autosomal dominant inherited disorder are enamel hypoplasia and hypocalcification, combined with curly, dry hair. Clinically very similar but genetically slightly different is the amelogenesis imperfecta, hypomaturation-hypoplasia-type with taurodontism syndrome. The dental changes seen in this syndrome are identical to those found in trichodento-osseous syndrome, but hair changes and osteosclerosis are absent.

☞**TRICHO-RHINO-PHALANGEAL DYSPLASIA TYPE II:** Most often autosomal dominant inherited syndrome with mental retardation, microencephaly, multiple exostoses, musculoskeletal dysplasia, and redundant skin.

☞**XERODERMA, TALIPES, AND ENAMEL DEFECT SYNDROME:** Ectodermal dysplasia combined with congenital heart disease.

☞**ODONTOTRICHOMELIC SYNDROME:** Genetic syndrome with anomalies of limbs, ears, eyes, and ectodermal structures.

☞**TOOTH AND NAIL SYNDROME:** Rare autosomal dominant ectodermal dysplasia characterized by defects of the nail plates of the fingers (onychorrhexis) and toes (koilonychia). Familial hypodontia with normal hair and sweat gland function.

NAEGELI ECTODERMAL DYSPLASIA (Naegeli-Franceschetti-Jadassohn Syndrome): Autosomal dominant inherited disease limited to the ectoderm (hypohidrosis, palmoplantar keratoderma, lack of dermatoglyphics [fingerprint lines], characteristic reticular hyperpigmentation on neck, chest and abdomen, onychodystrophy and yellowish spots on the enamel). Other organ systems reportedly are not affected; in particular, mental retardation has not been described as a feature of this disease.

ONYCHOTRICHODYSPLASIA WITH NEUTROPENIA: Extremely rare disorder caused by an autosomal recessive mutation. Clinical signs include onychotrichodysplasia, chronic neutropenia, and mild mental retardation. However, patients with normal intelligence have been reported. Trichorrhexis nodosa with bamboo-like appearance of the hair results in brittle hair. The chronic neutropenia may be part of the so-called *lazy leukocyte syndrome*. No case reports related to anesthesia have been found, but strict asepsis seems mandatory in the perioperative care to prevent infections.

REFERENCES:

Book JA: Clinical and genetic studies of hypodontia. I. Premolar aplasia, hyperhidrosis, and cavities prematura. A new hereditary syndrome in man. *Am J Hum Genet* 2:240, 1950.

Salinas CF, Sahn EE, Richards MA, Hutchins HS Jr: Congenitally missing teeth and severe hyperhidrosis: Book syndrome or a new ectodermal dysplasia syndrome? *Dysmorph Clin Genet* 6:59, 1992.

Verhage J, Habbema L, Vrensen GF, et al: A patient with ony-chotrichodysplasia, neutropenia and normal intelligence. *Clin Genet* 31:374, 1987.

Kozlowski K, Tsuruta T, Kameda Y, et al: New forms of neonatal death dwarfism. Report of 3 cases. *Pediatr Radiol* 10:155, 1981.

Winship I, Cremin B, Beighton P: Boomerang dysplasia. *Am J Med Genet* 36:440, 1990.

Boomerang Dysplasia

At a glance: Genetic disorder. A form of lethal neonatal dwarfism in which the long bones have a boomerang shape, resulting in skeletal dysplasia.

Incidence: Unknown. Approximately eight reported cases worldwide since Kozlowski's first description of the disorder in 1981.

Genetic inheritance: Precise genetics are unknown, but it has been suggested that X-linked recessive inheritance may occur. (There seems to be a male preponderance.) Consanguinity of the parents was not reported in any of the cases.

Pathophysiology: The mutation seems to affect the *FLNB* (*Filamin Bela*) gene located on 3p 14.3. *FLNB* acts primarily on stabilization of action within the cell and as such is involved in enchondral ossification, vertibral segmentation and the formation of joints.

Diagnosis: Characteristic clinical features and radiologic abnormalities consistent with the phenotypical description of the syndrome. Demonstration of histologic changes in the bone and cartilage may be an adjunct to clinical diagnosis; however, they may be similar to those seen in atelosteogenesis.

Clinical aspects: Congenital dwarfism with marked shortness and deformity of all four limbs is the most striking feature of this condition. Defects of the frontal bones in combination with an encephalocele have been reported. The nose has a flat and broad nasal root, a hypoplastic nasal septum and slanted nares. Cleft palate, malar hypoplasia, micrognathia, and short neck have been observed. Radiographically, the long bones may be absent, hypoplastic, or characteristically curved and flat, giving the condition its name boomerang dysplasia. Absent radii and fibulae, hypoplastic ilia, and absent pubic bones are other consistent findings. Retarded ossification of the spine and digits occurs. Boomerang dysplasia is a universally fatal condition; all reported patients died within the first hours of birth.

Precautions before anesthesia: All patients died within the first hours of birth so they are highly unlikely to present for anesthesia. Standard assessment as for all neonatal cases would apply. Airway management could be difficult (micrognathia, cleft palate, short neck), and premedication with an antisialagogue agent could be helpful.

Anesthetic considerations: If airway difficulty is anticipated, either awake fiberoptic tracheal intubation or inhalational induction of anesthesia followed by conventional or fiberoptic tracheal intubation should be considered.

Pharmacological implications: No specific pharmacological considerations.

Other Conditions to Be Considered:

☞**Chondrodysplasia Giant Cell Type (Atelosteogenesis I):** Autosomal dominant inherited, also a lethal form of chondrodysplasia is characterized by rhizomelic limb shortening.

☞**Larsen Syndrome:** A congenital dysmorphic syndrome associated with characteristic anomalies of face, hands and feet and multiple congenital dislocations. Spine, airway and cardiac anomalies result in significantly increased perioperative risk.

References:
Bicknell LS, Morgan T, Bonafe L, et al: Mutations in FLNB cause boomerang dysplasia. *J Med Genet* 42:e43, 2005.

Börjeson-Forssman-Lehmann Syndrome

At a glance: An inherited syndrome with mental deficiency and endocrine disorder.

Synonym: Börjeson Syndrome.

History: First described in 1962 by M. Börjeson, H. Forssman, and J. O. Lehmann.

Genetic inheritance: Transmitted as an X-linked recessive trait, thus, predominantly males are affected, although heterozygous female carriers may manifest certain, although much more variable, features of the disease (suggesting X-linked incomplete recessive inheritance). Gene map locus is Xq26-q27. The mutations seem to affect the *PHF6* gene (plant homeodomain zinc-finger transcription factor gene), which is involved in DNA-transcription.

Diagnosis: Based on the clinical appearance. Characteristic facial appearance (round, fatty face with large, protruding tongue, large but normally formed ears, relative microcephaly, prominent brow ridge, deep-set eyes, ptosis) associated with mental retardation and epileptic attacks. No known biochemical or cytogenetic markers.

Clinical aspects: Mild-to-severe intellectual handicap, epilepsy, hypogonadism (hypogonadotropic hypogonadism with delayed second-degree sexual characteristics), hypometabolism, marked obesity, swelling of subcutaneous facial tissue, short neck, short stature and narrow palpebral fissure. Hyperkyphosis that increases with age was reported.

Precautions before anesthesia: The patient's history should be evaluated in relation to seizures, current anticonvulsant therapy, and complications resulting from the therapy in particular. Plasma anticonvulsant levels may require determination and the dose optimized to ensure adequate levels. Marked obesity necessitates systematic review of associated cardiovascular and respiratory diseases. The airway should be assessed because difficulty in direct laryngoscopy is not uncommon in these patients. Cardiac function should be evaluated carefully, as one case of a 19-year-old patient who presented for heart transplantation secondary to dilated cardiomyopathy was reported. Cardiac function should be assessed in the presence of morbid obesity (to exclude pulmonary hypertension) and hypometabolism with electrocardiogram, chest radiography, echocardiography, and, if necessary, radionuclide imaging. Carefully evaluate respiratory function in the presence of hyperkyphosis (including lung function tests). H_2-antagonist therapy may be indicated to reduce the risk of pulmonary aspiration. Premedication with respiratory depressant drugs should be avoided in morbidly obese patients. Recommended laboratory investigations include complete blood count, electrolytes, arterial blood gas analysis, urea, and occasionally anticonvulsant plasma levels.

Anesthetic considerations: Difficult cooperation as a result of mental retardation is possible. Marked obesity makes vascular access difficult and desaturation on induction more likely than in nonobese patients. Adequate preoxygenation should be given prior to induction of anesthesia. In the morbidly obese in whom difficult tracheal intubation is anticipated, direct laryngoscopy under topical anesthesia may be helpful. If the larynx is visualized, a rapid sequence induction should be performed to prevent desaturation and minimize risk of pulmonary aspiration. If the larynx cannot be visualized, an awake fiberoptic tracheal intubation is the safest approach. Mechanical ventilation is preferred over spontaneous breathing as tidal volume breathing falls within the closing volume range and commonly results in hypoxemia. A regional anesthesia technique, such as spinal or epidural anesthesia, requires reduced doses of local anesthetics (75–80% of regular dose). Continuous oxygen therapy, physiotherapy, and deep venous thrombosis prophylaxis with early mobilization (if possible) are required in the postoperative period. Triggers that potentiate the occurrence of seizures must be avoided. Hypothermia is a risk factor in patients with hypometabolism and temperature monitoring is mandatory. Facilities to warm the patient (convective forced air warming devices, warming blankets) should be used. Intravenous fluids and inhaled gases should be warmed.

Pharmacological implications: Anticonvulsant therapy should be continued up to the morning of surgery. Factors that may trigger seizures must be avoided (enflurane with hypocapnia, methohexital, ketamine). Propofol is best avoided until the possible association of propofol with perioperative seizures is resolved. Larger doses of vecuronium may be required for patients on chronic phenobarbital therapy because of hepatic enzyme induction. Aspiration prophylaxis should be given. However, reduced doses of neuromuscular blockers may be required to achieve complete relaxation with pre-existing hypotonia. In any case, a peripheral nerve stimulator should be used to monitor muscle relaxation. Anticholinergics may be helpful when a difficult intubation is anticipated. Obese patients have increased plasma pseudocholinesterase levels and may require increased doses of suxamethonium. However, hypometabolic patients have an increased sensitivity to narcotics and anesthetic agents.

Other conditions to be considered:

☞**PRADER-LABHART-WILLI SYNDROME:** Autosomal dominant transmitted disease characterized by infantile hypotonia, hypogonadism, and obesity.

☞**BARDET-BIEDL SYNDROME:** Autosomal recessive inherited disorder characterized by mental retardation, pigmentary retinopathy, polydactyly, obesity, and hypogenitalism.

☞**COHEN SYNDROME:** Disorder characterized by nonprogressive psychomotor retardation, facial, musculoskeletal and ophthalmologic abnormalities, and autosomal recessive inheritance.

REFERENCES:

Visootsak J, Rosner B, Dykens E, et al: Clinical and behavioral features of patients with Borjeson-Forssman-Lehmann syndrome with mutations in PHF6. *J Pediatr* 145:819, 2004.

Turner G, Lower KM, White SM, et al: The clinical picture of the Borjeson-Forssman-Lehmann syndrome in males and heterozygous females with PHF6 mutations. *Clin Genet* 65:226, 2004.

Kaplinsky E, Perandones C, Galiana MG, et al: Börjeson-Forssman-Lehmann syndrome and dilated cardiomyopathy: A previously unreported association. *Can J Cardiol* 17:80, 2001.

Borrone Dermato-Cardio-Skeletal Syndrome

At a glance: Genetic disorder resulting in progressive skin, heart, bone, and joint abnormalities.

Incidence: Only one case report describing two brothers with the syndrome has been published.

Genetic inheritance: Unclear, but postulated to be either autosomal recessive or X-linked recessive. The two brothers were the offspring of healthy parents from a small Italian village, and consanguinity was denied.

Pathophysiology: Involvement of the skin, bone, joints, and heart suggests a disorder of proteins of the extracellular matrix. Laboratory studies demonstrated that fibroblast production of collagen type I was normal, but other disorders of the protein matrix of connective tissue may exist.

Diagnosis: Clinical and radiologic findings consistent with the syndrome (see *Clinical Aspects*). Biochemical and pathologic studies excluded known metabolic diseases. Skin biopsy shows chronic dermatitis with fibrosis, hyalinosis, metaplastic ossification, and infundibular follicular cysts. Gingival biopsy demonstrates fibromatosis. The diagnosis was made within the first year of life. In the clinical course, one brother is still alive at the age of 36 years with medically controlled heart failure. The second brother died at the age of 24 years as a consequence of progressive heart failure secondary to mitral valve prolapse.

Clinical aspects: Skin lesions include acne conglobata and thickening of the skin. Hypertelorism, low nasal bridge, subocular folds, prominent ears, teeth anomalies, and gingival hypertrophy result in a coarse facies. Musculoskeletal anomalies comprise osteolysis, kyphoscoliosis, brachydactyly, clinodactyly of the fifth finger, genu recurvatum, and flexion contractures of the large joints. Radiologic findings include vertebrae with reduced sagittal diameter, anterior beaking, and abnormalities consistent with Scheuermann osteochondritis. Feet and hands demonstrate osseous lacunae and cortical erosions. Mitral valve prolapse may lead to heart failure. Psychomotor and intellectual development are normal. Bilateral inguinal hernias were reported.

Precautions before anesthesia: Assess cardiac function, flexion deformities, oral dentition, and gingival margins. Cardiac assessment should include a cardiac consultation with clinical examination, electrocardiogram, chest radiography, and echocardiography. Complete blood count and electrolytes (because of diuretic therapy) should be checked preoperatively.

Anesthetic considerations: Venous access may be difficult because of thickening of the skin. The limbs must be positioned carefully in the presence of flexion deformities with adequate padding and support at all pressure areas. The choice of induction and maintenance agents for anesthesia depends on the severity of the cardiac involvement. The basic aims in mitral valve prolapse with regurgitation should be to maintain preload, prevent bradycardia, limit myocardial depression, and reduce afterload, if possible. A narcotic technique using fentanyl with muscle relaxation and supplemental inhalational agent is preferable. In addition to standard anesthetic monitoring, depending on the extent of the surgical procedure, an arterial line, a Swan-Ganz catheter, and/or transesophageal echocardiography may be indicated.

Pharmacological implications: Care should be taken when using agents that have significant effects on myocardial contractility and systemic vascular resistance. Routine cardiac medication should be continued perioperatively. Appropriate antibiotic endocarditis prophylaxis coverage should be administered.

REFERENCE:

Borrone C, Di Rocco M, Crovato F, et al: New multisystemic disorder involving heart valves, skin, bones, joints in two brothers. *Am J Med Genet* 46:228, 1993.

Boucher-Neuhäuser Syndrome

At a glance: A form of spinocerebellar ataxia associated with chorioretinal dystrophy and hypogonadotropic hypogonadism.

Incidence: Unknown. Only 19 cases from 10 families have been reported in the literature. The syndrome remains poorly recognized and probably underreported.

Genetic inheritance: Pleiotropic single-gene disorder with an autosomal recessive pattern of inheritance.

Pathophysiology: The tissues involved are all of neuroectodermal origin; however, the exact link between the three features is unclear. The nature of the gene involved and its specific role in the pathophysiology are unknown. The absence of a response to luteinizing hormone also suggests disturbed pituitary function. The abnormal pattern of the thyroid-stimulating hormone and prolactin response to thyrotropin-releasing hormone plus the growth hormone response to gonadotropin-releasing factor and insulin-induced hypoglycemia also point to a hypothalamic involvement.

Diagnosis: Clinical findings consistent with the syndrome. No specific diagnostic tests are available. CT and/or MRI scans show evidence of cerebellar atrophy. Serum levels of luteinizing hormone, follicle-stimulating hormone, estrogen, and testosterone are abnormally low. Electroretinography is abnormal, with a marked reduction in the amplitude of both rods and cones. Fluorescein angiography demonstrates filling of the major choroidal vessels in the atrophic regions combined with an extensive loss in the choriocapillaris.

Clinical aspects: Characterized by hypogonadotropic hypogonadism. Usually this disorder is diagnosed at the onset of puberty (primary amenorrhea, poor development of sexual organs, sparse growth of secondary hair, short stature, delayed puberty, delayed bone age, infertility), spinocerebellar ataxia (with a variable age of onset; impaired balance, ataxic gait, mild dysmetria on finger-to-nose testing, but marked dysmetria on heel-to-shin testing, nystagmus, bilateral extensor plantar responses), and choroidal dystrophy (variable age of onset, diffuse and slowly progressive, with involvement of the choriocapillaris, retinal pigment epithelium, and outer retina, resulting in loss of visual acuity with a dense ring scotoma and a spared central field). Muscle strength, sensibility, and proprioception are normal.

Precautions before anesthesia: Clinical history and examination to evaluate the progression of the condition.

Anesthetic considerations: No specific anesthetic considerations.

Pharmacological implications: Patients are often on sex hormone replacement therapy (testosterone, estrogen, oral contraceptives). Depending on the procedure, deep vein thrombosis prophylaxis is recommended because of estrogen replacement therapy. No other specific pharmacological considerations.

Other conditions to be considered:

☞**GORDON HOLMES SYNDROME:** Genetic disorder with hypogonadism and progressive cerebellar ataxia.

☞**KALLMANN SYNDROME:** Inherited syndrome characterized by hypogonadotropic hypogonadism and anosmia caused by agenesis of the olfactory bulbs, often combined with other birth defects (cardiac anomalies, cleft lip/palate, renal anomalies).

Other forms of spinocerebellar ataxia, such as the following:

☞**MACHADO-JOSEPH DISEASE:** Form of autosomal dominant inherited spinocerebellar ataxia with clinical onset usually in adulthood but occasionally in adolescence.

☞**INFANTILE-ONSET SPINOCEREBELLAR ATAXIA (IOSCA):** Some researchers also used the term *spinocerebellar ataxia* (SCA) type 8 for this disease, but the term has not been uniformly accepted. IOSCA is an inherited spinocerebellar ataxia with onset usually in the first 2 years of life.

☞**ROUSSY-LEVY SYNDROME:** Autosomal dominant spinocerebellar degeneration. Appears in early childhood and progresses slowly. Implications concerning regional anesthesia and spinal neurologic monitoring.

☞**FRIEDREICH ATAXIA:** Inherited disorder that leads to progressive dysfunction of the cerebellum (ataxia, nystagmus), spinal cord, and peripheral nerves.

REFERENCES:

Limber ER, Bresnick GH, Lebovitz RM, et al: Spinocerebellar ataxia, hypogonadotropic hypogonadism, and choroidal dystrophy (Boucher-Neuhauser syndrome). *Am J Med Genet* 33:409, 1989.

Rump P, Hamel BC, Pinckers AJ, et al: Two sibs with chorioretinal dystrophy, hypogonadotrophic hypogonadism, and cerebellar ataxia: Boucher-Neuhauser syndrome. *J Med Genet* 34:767, 1997.

Ogawa S, Aikawa S, Kato T, et al: Prominent expression of spinocerebellar ataxia type-I (SCA1) gene encoding ataxin-1 in LH-producing cells, Lbeta T2. *J Reprod Dev* 50:557, 2004.

Bouveret Syndrome

At a glance: Gastric outlet obstruction caused by a large gallstone blocking the pylorus or duodenum.

Incidence: Unknown; fewer than 200 cases reported.

Genetic inheritance: Acquired condition.

Pathophysiology: Acute cholecystitis results in adhesion formation between the gallbladder and intestine. The large gallstone causes ischemia of the cystic wall. Necrosis results, allowing passage of the stone through a cholecystenteric fistula to any adherent bowel but, in more than 66% of the cases, to the duodenum. However, duodenal obstruction constitutes only 3% of all cases of gall-stone ileus.

Diagnosis: Usually made during operation but more recently at endoscopy or on CT scan. The diagnosis is supported by air in the biliary tree in the presence of a gastric outlet obstruction.

Clinical aspects: History of cholecystitis is present in approximately half of patients. Signs and symptoms are those of small bowel obstruction, nausea, vomiting, epigastric pain, and abdominal distension. Only 50 to 70% of patients present with the characteristic features of intestinal obstruction, which may result from continuous impacting and disimpacting of the stone during its passage distally. Relief of symptoms after the stone becomes mobile again may suggest gastroenteritis, especially with the common finding of diarrhea. However, as the diameter of the small bowel becomes smaller distally and the gallstone bigger by accumulation of intestinal contents, the impaction finally is complete and irreversible. Approximately 66% of all impacted gallstones are found in the ileum; only approximately 4% successfully pass the ileocecal valve and cause colonic obstruction. Gastrointestinal hemorrhage may occur from duodenal ulceration or erosion of cystic artery (one case). Vomiting leads to dehydration and electrolyte disturbances (hypochloremic, hypokalemic metabolic alkalosis). Anemia may be present as a consequence of occult loss or gastrointestinal hemorrhage.

Precautions before anesthesia: Check volume status and correct hypovolemia, hemoglobin, electrolytes, and acid-base status preoperatively. Investigate coexisting diseases as indicated. Pass a nasogastric tube, which can be removed for induction, to decompress the stomach.

Anesthetic considerations: Ileus and full stomach. Aspirate nasogastric tube prior to rapid sequence induction. High abdominal incision in patients with preexisting lung disease predisposes to postoperative pulmonary complications; thoracic epidural analgesia may be advantageous. Consider other therapeutic options, such as endoscopic stone removal, endoluminal YAG-laser lithotripsy, or extracorporal shockwave lithotripsy.

Pharmacological implications: No known specific implications.

REFERENCES:

Lobo DN, Jobling JC, Balfour TW. Gallstone ileus: Diagnostic pitfalls and therapeutic successes. *J Clin Gastroenterol* 30:72, 2000.

Swift SE, Spencer JA. Gallstone ileus: CT findings. *Clin Radiol* 53:451, 1998.

Maiss J, Hochberger J, Hahn EG, et al: Successful laserlithotripsy in Bouveret's syndrome using a new frequency doubled doublepulse Nd: YAG laser (FREDDY). *Scand J Gastroenterol* 39:791, 2004.

Bowen Syndrome

At a glance: The displayed features suggest autosomal trisomy, particularly trisomy 18. However, there is no chromosome abnormality. Neurologic signs include severe hypotonia, psychomotor retardation, seizures, inability to suck, and absent neonatal reflexes. Distinctive "lightbulb"-shaped head. Cardiac defects may include patent ductus arteriosus, aortic abnormalities and septal defects.

Synonym: Bowen Syndrome of Multiple Malformations.

Incidence: Two families have been described, one with associated Zellweger syndrome.

Genetic inheritance: Autosomal recessive.

Pathophysiology: Unknown.

Diagnosis: Based on a constellation of clinical features and biochemical findings: abnormal liver function tests, including hypothrombinemia, elevated serum iron levels and iron saturation, elevated cerebraspinal fluid protein levels, and proteinuria. Diagnosis is confirmed by the absence of peroxisomes in fibroblasts and decreased dihydroxyacetone phosphate acyltransferase activity and plasmalogen content in blood cells and fibroblasts.

Clinical aspects: Patients rarely live beyond 1 year of age (mean age at death is approximately 12 weeks). Neurologic signs include severe hypotonia, psychomotor retardation, inability to suck, agenesis of the corpus callosum, and absent neonatal reflexes. Patients have low-set ears, small mandible, and glaucoma. Cardiac defects may include patent ductus arteriosus, aortic abnormalities, and septal defects. Other features can include enlarged clitoris, hypospadias, and finger flexion.

Precautions before anesthesia: Patients are unlikely to present for major surgery because of the dismal prognosis. The usually severe neurologic problems may require palliative feeding by insertion of a G-tube, which often can be achieved with infiltration of local anesthetics supplemented with ketamine or low dose inhalational anesthetics by mask if required. Preoperative evaluation of the neurologic sequelae of the syndrome and renal function. Preop-

erative fasting will not be tolerated, and measures for appropriate intravenous fluids and supplementation should be undertaken.

Anesthetic considerations: Direct laryngoscopy and tracheal intubation can be difficult because of the small mandible and may require adapted anesthetic management.

Pharmacological implications: Endocarditis prophylaxis is required if cardiac abnormalities are present. Agents that depend on hepatic or renal excretion should be used with care. Use of neuromuscular blockers may not be necessary because of the profound hypotonia; ketamine is a useful supplement if any further anesthesia is required.

Other conditions to be considered:

RHIZOMELIC TYPE OF ☞**Chondrodysplasia Punctata:** Inherited disease with a defect in the biosynthesis of peroxisomes and plasmalogen.

☞**X-LINKED ADRENOLEUKODYSTROPHY:** Inherited disease with accumulation of very-long-chain fatty acids resulting in demyelination and inflammation in the white matter of the brain combined with reduced adrenal steroid synthesis.

REFERENCES:

Bowen P, Lee CSN, Zellweger H, et al: A familial syndrome of multiple congenital defects. *Bull Johns Hopkins Hosp* 114:402, 1964.

Kelley RI: Review: The cerebrohepatorenal syndrome of Zellweger, morphologic and metabolic aspects. *Am J Med Genet* 16:503, 1983.

Bowen-Conradi Syndrome

At a glance: Autosomal recessive transmitted disease resulting in death in the first year of life secondary to neurologic disease and airway problems.

Synonym: Bowen-Hutterite Syndrome.

Incidence: Approximately 43 cases have been reported in the literature. 39 of them were Hutterite patients and 4 were from other populations. The estimated incidence in the Hutterite population is 1:355 live births.

Genetic inheritance: Autosomal recessive trait. Comprehensive pedigree records have enabled researchers to determine that all six of the Hutterite families are related to a kindred extending back to the 1770s. The Hutterites subdivided into three Leute groups after arriving in North America in the late 1800s. Cases recognized from colonies in northern and southern Alberta, South Dakota, and southern Manitoba suggest the gene for this condition may be widely distributed among this population. Consanguinity was present within this pedigree. The gene locus has been mapped to 12p13.3.

Pathophysiology: The gene responsible for this syndrome and the underlying pathophysiology has not been determined. The exact cause of death in these neonates remains unclear, but the combination of severe neurologic impairment and airway abnormalities has been implicated.

Diagnosis: Clinical course, physical appearance, and familial history. Bowen-Conradi syndrome is morphologically very similar to trisomy 18, however, chromosome analysis is normal in the former.

Clinical aspects: Major features are proportional intrauterine growth retardation and low birth weight, microcephaly, dolichocephaly, sloping forehead, severe micrognathia, retroglossia, narrow pharynx, prominent nose, rocker-bottom feet, mild joint movement limitations, and undescended testes. Neonates with this condition have a significant neurologic deficit with poor muscle tone, feeding, and crying, and developmental delay. The average age at death is 13 months (range 1 day to 9 years).

Precautions before anesthesia: Obtain a full clinical assessment of the airway (micrognathia, retroglossia, narrow pharynx), the degree of neurologic impairment (hypotonia, feeding difficulties, aspiration, impairment of pharyngeal and laryngeal reflexes), the respiratory system (pneumonia, hypoventilation secondary to hypotonia, sleep apnea or obstructive episodes), and nutritional status. Laboratory investigations should include a complete blood count, urea and electrolytes, and arterial blood gases (indicator of pulmonary function).

Anesthetic considerations: Difficult direct laryngoscopy and tracheal intubation should be anticipated in all cases. All the necessary adjuncts for management of the difficult airway should be prepared before induction of anesthesia. Inhalational induction with spontaneous respiration prior to tracheal intubation or an awake fiberoptic intubation technique are the safest approaches. In extreme instances, a tracheostomy may be required prior to surgery. Use of regional anesthesia techniques is not specifically contraindicated and will decrease the need for opioids with their respiratory depressant side effects. A postoperative period of elective mechanical ventilation may be necessary because of hypotonia, abnormal ventilatory control, and poor respiratory function. After tracheal extubation, patients will require continued cardiovascular, respiratory, and neurologic monitoring in a high-dependency area because of the risk of apnea and airway obstruction.

Pharmacological implications: Care should be taken when administering sedative, inhalational, opioid, or muscle-relaxing drugs because these children are highly sensitive to the action of each of these agents. Muscle relaxants can be used (always in conjunction with a nerve stimulator), but probably are unnecessary because of the preexisting general hypotonia associated with the condition.

Other condition to be considered:

☞PENA-SHOKEIR SYNDROME TYPE 2 (SYNONYMS: CEREBRO-OCULO-FACIO-SKELETAL SYNDROME; COFS SYNDROME): Rapidly progressive neurological disorder leading to brain atrophy with calcifications, cataracts, microcornea, optic atrophy, progressive joint contractures and growth failure.

REFERENCES:

Gupta A, Phadke SR: Bowen-Conradi syndrome in an Indian infant: first non-Hutterite case. *Clin Dysmorphol* 10:155, 2001.

Lamont RE, Loredo-Osti J, Roslin NM, et al: A locus for Bowen-Conradi syndrome maps to chromosome region 12p13.3. *Am J Med Genet A* 132:136, 2005.

Lowry RB, Innes AM, Bernier FP, et al: Bowen-Conradi syndrome: a clinical and genetic study. *Am J Med Genet A* 120:423, 2003.

Brachmann-De Lange Syndrome

At a glance: A severe and characteristic syndrome of craniofacial malformations associated with neurological impairment.

Synonyms: Cornelia De Lange Syndrome; De Lange Syndrome; Typus Degenerativus Amstelodamensis.

History: First described by the German physician Winfried Robert Clemens Brachmann in 1916. In 1933, the Dutch pediatrician Cornelia Catharina de Lange reported two more cases and called the disorder "Typus degenerativus Amstelodamensis".

Incidence: 1:10,000–40,000 live births.

Genetic inheritance: Autosomal dominant, transmission has been described, however most cases are sporadic. The defect has been mapped to the *Nipped-B-like (NIPBL)* gene on 5p13.1.

Pathophysiology: Unknown.

Diagnosis: Based on the clinical findings of characteristic facies in association with prenatal and postnatal growth retardation and mental retardation.

Clinical aspects: About one-third of these children are born prematurely and present with prenatal and postnatal growth retardation resulting in short adult stature (growth hormone deficiency was found in some patients). Feeding problems often result in failure to thrive. Mild to moderate mental retardation and hypertonicity are common. Deafness and seizures may occur. Ophtalmological problems may include myopia, ptosis, microcornea, aniridia, strabismus, and nystagmus. Behavior problems are a common problem in these children and present as hyperactivity, aggression, and self-inflicted injuries, sometimes comparable to an "autism-like" behavior. The malformations are complex and involve the head (microcephaly and brachycephaly) and a short neck with nuchal webbing. The facial features may include low anterior hairline, bushy eyebrows often with synophrys, low-set ears, depressed nasal bridge, anteverted nares, micrognathia, long philtrum with thin upper lip, cleft lip, high-arched or cleft palate, downturned corners of the mouth and widely spaced teeth (often with delayed eruption). The voice is initially often low-pitched, which resolves as the children grow. Hirsutism and cutis marmorata are frequent. Skeletal involvement may include scoliosis, limited elbow extension, and dislocation of the radial head, phoco- or micromelia, and anomalies of the usually small hands and feet (oligodactyly, clinodactyly, partial syndactyly). Thoracic features that have been described are small nipples, short sternum, and supernumerary ribs. Other findings can include congenital heart defects (in up to 15% of patients; most commonly atrial and ventricular septal defects, pulmonary stenosis, tetralogy of Fallot), hypopituitarism, and congenital diaphragmatic hernia. Gastrointestinal problems are common and comprise gastroesophageal reflux (in up to two-thirds of patients; Barrett esophagus and esophageal scarring have been reported) with recurrent aspirations and pneumonias frequently resulting in respiratory problems, pyloric stenosis, intestinal malrotation and volvulus. Urogenital anomalies that may affect renal function are also common and include hydronephrosis, renal dysplasia and cysts, and vesicoureteral reflux. Furthermore, hypoplastic external genitalia, cryptorchidism and hypospadias have been described on a regular base. Thrombocytopenia and increased pain tolerance due to decreased pain sensation have been reported in several patients.

Precautions before anesthesia: Evaluate neurological function (clinically, electroencephalogram) and check efficacy of seizure treatment. Evaluate airway anatomy (clinically, radiologically, or by fiberoptic examination, if deemed necessary). Rule out congenital cardiac defects (clinically, electrocardiogram, echocardiography). Laboratory investigations should include a complete blood count (thrombocytopenia), electrolytes, creatinine and urea. Patient cooperation may be limited, and sedative/anxiolytic premedication and/or the presence of the primary caregiver for induction of anesthesia may be helpful.

Anesthetic considerations: Direct laryngoscopy and tracheal intubation can be difficult due to micrognathia and short neck. Maintain spontaneous ventilation until the airway has been secured. Awake fiberoptic intubation should be considered. There is an increased risk of aspiration. Patients with a history of congenital

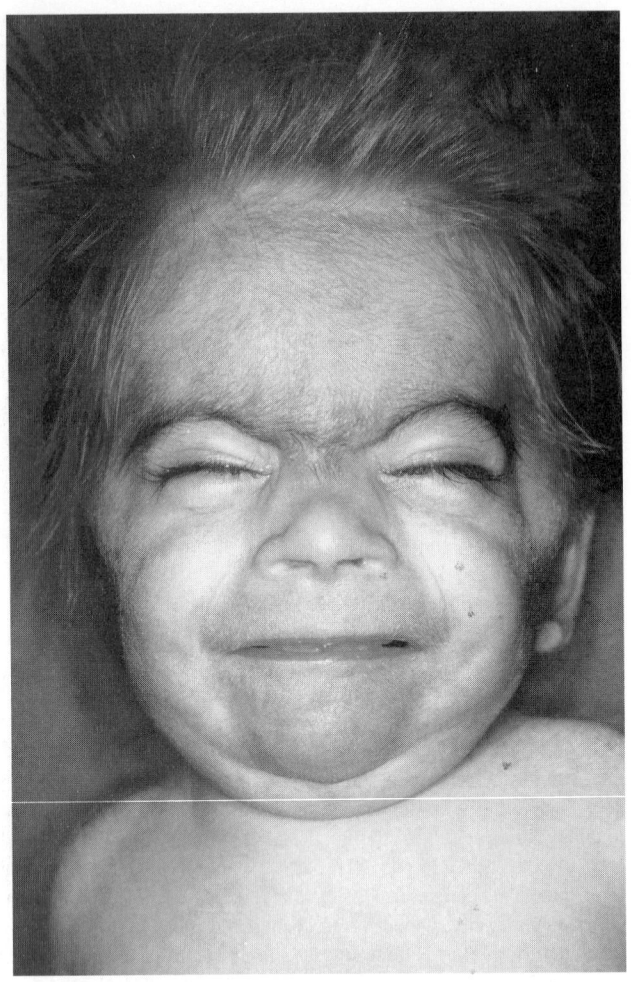

Bushy eyebrows, depressed nasal bridge, long philtrum, thin upper lip, and microcephaly in a boy with Brachmann-de Lange syndrome.

diaphragmatic hernia may have increased pulmonary artery pressures and care should be taken not to further increase pulmonary vascular resistance (maintain inotropy and avoid acidosis, hypercapnia and hypoxia). Careful intraoperative positioning and padding are required because of the skeletal anomalies.

Pharmacological implications: Subacute bacterial endocarditis prophylaxis may be required. Consider drug interactions and altered drug metabolism with antiepileptic treatment.

Other conditions to be considered:

☞**COFFIN-SIRIS SYNDROME:** A congenital syndrome with growth and mental retardation, feeding difficulties, digital anomalies and coarse facies.

☞**FETAL ALCOHOL SYNDROME:** a disorder characterized by a series of physical, mental and neurobehavioral birth defects resulting from chronic alcohol consumption during pregnancy.

☞**FRYNS SYNDROME:** A very rare polymalformative syndrome reported by Fryns in 1979 and characterized by diaphragmatic hernia and unusual facies. The proportion of patients who survive the neonatal period represents 14% of reported cases. Majority are stillborn or die in early neonatal period.

☞**HOLT-ORAM SYNDROME:** Genetically transmitted malformation syndrome characterized by congenital thenar hypoplasia and the association of a congenital heart disease (ventricular and atrial

septal defect) and upper limb malformation (underdevelopment of bones and/or extra bones).

REFERENCES:

Gillis LA, McCallum J, Kaur M, et al: NIPBL mutational analysis in 120 individuals with Cornelia de Lange syndrome and evaluation of genotype-phenotype correlations. *Am J Hum Genet* 75:610, 2004.

Russell KL, Ming JE, Patel K, et al: Dominant paternal transmission of Cornelia de Lange syndrome: a new case and review of 25 previously reported familial recurrences. *Am J Med Genet* 104:267, 2001.

Tsusaki B, Mayhew JF: Anaesthetic implications of Cornelia de Lange syndrome. *Paediatr Anaesth* 8:181, 1998.

Brachydactyly-Ectrodactyly Syndrome with Fibular Aplasia or Hypoplasia

At a glance: Genetic disorder resulting in complex dysostosis with distal limb deformities.

Incidence and genetic inheritance: Only two case reports with a total of nine possible affected individuals have been described. Postulated to be autosomal dominant inheritance with low penetrance and variable expressivity, although the exact pattern of inheritance is rather complex and not fully understood. The reported cases have been from two unrelated Italian families with no history of consanguinity.

Clinical aspects: The propositus, a 25-year-old woman, presented with brachydactyly and ectrodactyly of the feet, metacarpal and phalangeal hypoplasia, and aplasia or hypoplasia of the fibula. A second cousin demonstrated only milder acromelic defects. A similar pattern of variable skeletal deformities was described in seven members of an unrelated Italian family. No other major defects were noted. Radiologic examination showed hypoplasia of ulnae, styloid processes, metacarpal bones, and phalanges. The femora were normal, but the fibulae were replaced by retrotibial rudiments and the tibiae were hypoplastic. The tarsal bones were fused and the metatarsal bones and proximal phalanges grossly deformed.

Anesthetic considerations: Venous access may be difficult because of limb deformities. Careful padding is required.

Other conditions to be considered:

☞**DU PAN SYNDROME:** a genetic disorder characterized by complex brachydactyly and fibular hypoplasia.

☞**SCHINZEL SYNDROME:** an inherited disorder characterized by bone malformations and apocrine deficiency.

REFERENCES:

Genuardi M, Zollino M, Bellussi A, et al: Brachy-ectrodactyly and absence or hypoplasia of the fibula: An autosomal dominant condition with low penetrance and variable expressivity. *Clin Genet* 38:321, 1990.

Lewin SO, Opitz JM: Fibular a/hypoplasia: Review and documentation of the fibular developmental field. *Am J Med Genet Suppl* 2:215, 1986.

Evans JA, Reed MH, Greenberg CR: Fibular aplasia with ectrodactyly. *Am J Med Genet* 113:52, 2002.

Brachymorphism-Onychodysplasia-Dysphalangism Syndrome

At a glance: Presumed genetic disorder causing short stature, hand abnormalities, and mild intellectual impairment.

Synonym: BOD Syndrome.

Incidence and genetic inheritance: Only about 10 cases have been reported in the literature. The exact mode of inheritance is unclear but is postulated to be autosomal dominant. Although the syndrome has features in common with Coffin-Siris syndrome, it is distinguishable by a milder phenotype and less severe intellectual impairment.

Clinical aspects: Features include intrauterine, proportionate growth retardation, postnatal dwarfism, hypoplastic or aplastic fifth digits, hypoplastic or aplastic fingernails, and abnormal phalanges. All affected individuals have facial dysmorphism with a large mouth, pointed chin, broad nose, and flat malar area. Some patients have mild intellectual impairment and microcephaly. Radiologic findings include aplasia, hypoplasia, or fusion of the fifth digit or toe and brachymesophalangism. One of the affected individuals had cystic adenomatoid malformation of the lungs, however, this does not appear to be a consistent feature of the syndrome. Life expectancy is normal.

Anesthetic considerations: Careful intraoperative positioning is needed, but can be difficult. Venous access may be difficult. Pulse oximetry can be difficult. Patients with mild intellectual impairment may benefit from sedative premedication. The facial dysmorphism of the syndrome usually is not associated with difficult airway management.

Other condition to be considered:

☞COFFIN SIRIS SYNDROME: Probably autosomal dominant transmitted syndrome with developmental delay, hypoplasia of the fifth digit nails and phalanges, sparse scalp hair, bushy eyebrows, wide mouth, hirsutism, and prominent or hypertrophied lips.

REFERENCES:

Senior B: Impaired growth and onychodysplasia: Short children with tiny toenails. *Am J Dis Child* 122:7, 1971.

Verloes A, Bonneau D, Guidi O, et al: Brachymorphism-onychodysplasia-dysphalangism syndrome. *J Med Genet* 30:158, 1993.

Branchial Myoclonus with Spastic Paraparesis and Cerebellar Ataxia Syndrome

At a glance: Genetic disorder resulting in familial branchial myoclonus, spastic paraparesis, and cerebellar ataxia.

Incidence: Approximately 13 cases have been reported. The original description in 1988 reported a family with six affected individuals in two generations. No other definite case reports have been published.

Genetic inheritance: Autosomal dominant.

Pathophysiology: The precise mechanism leading to this progressive degenerative condition remains poorly understood. The levels of the serotonin metabolite 5-hydroxyindoleacetic acid in the cerebrospinal fluid (CSF) are low, and an abnormality in serotonin-mediated neurotransmission has been proposed as a possible cause.

Diagnosis: Made by clinical features consistent with the syndrome. CT and MRI scans demonstrate severe atrophy of medulla, brainstem, and cervical spinal cord, and mild atrophy of the cerebral and cerebellar cortex, with normal pons and olives. CSF studies reveal a markedly reduced concentration in the serotonin metabolite 5-hydroxyindoleacetic acid. Visual auditory and somatosensory evoked responses, electroencephalo- and electromyogram are normal.

Clinical aspects: Characterized by a rhythmic branchial myoclonus (affecting palate, pharynx, larynx, lower face, and neck) resulting in dysphagia, dysphonia, choking spells, spastic paraparesis (preserved, muscle strength brisk reflexes, normal sensation), cerebellar ataxia (truncal), nystagmus, and normal mental status. The age at onset usually is between 30 and 50 years. The condition is progressive, leading to death or severe disability within 5 to 10 years of onset.

Precautions before anesthesia: Detailed history and examination are necessary to determine the progression of neurologic impairment (bulbar palsy, degree of spastic paraparesis and cerebellar ataxia). Assess speech, swallowing, and glottic competency (gastrostomy feeding, tracheostomy). Pulmonary assessment (especially with a history of frequent aspiration episodes) by chest radiography, spirometry, and arterial blood gas analysis. Evaluate motor impairment (wheelchair bound).

Anesthetic considerations: There is an increased risk of aspiration as a result of laryngeal incompetence (consider awake fiberoptic or a rapid sequence induction for tracheal intubation). Spastic paraparesis may lead to fixed limb deformities with difficulty in positioning and venous access. These patients have normal sensation in affected limbs (and hence normal analgesic requirements). The potential risk for postoperative ventilation, tracheostomy, and feeding gastrostomy should be considered.

Pharmacological implications: Suxamethonium should be avoided (hyperkalemia, rhabdomyolysis, arrhythmia, myoglobinuria, cardiac arrest). Acid aspiration prophylaxis is recommended (H_2 blockers, antacids). Treatment with 5-hydroxytryptophan and carbidopa at highest tolerated doses may improve ataxia, but not myoclonus.

REFERENCES:

De Yebenes JG, Vazquez A, Rabano J, et al: Hereditary branchial myoclonus with spastic paraparesis and cerebellar ataxia: A new autosomal dominant disorder. *Neurology* 38:569, 1988.

Howard RS, Greenwood R, Gawler J, et al: A familial disorder associated with palatal myoclonus, other brainstem signs, tetraparesis, ataxia and Rosenthal fiber formation. *J Neurol Neurosurg Psychiatry* 56:977, 1993.

Branchio-Oculo-Facial Syndrome

At a glance: Inherited malformative syndrome characterized by low birth weight, distinctive craniofacial malformations, and atrophic skin lesion.

Synonyms: BOF Syndrome; BOFS; Hemangiomatous Branchial Cleft-Lip Pseudocleft Syndrome; Imperforate Nasolacrimal Duct and Premature Aging Syndrome; Lip Pseudocleft-Hemangiomatous Branchial Cyst Syndrome; Branchial Clefts with Characteristic

Facies, Growth Retardation, Imperforate Nasolacrimal Duct, and Premature Aging; Lee-Root-Fenske Syndrome.

Genetic inheritance: Autosomal dominant.

Pathophysiology: Unknown.

Diagnosis: Based on the clinical findings of typical face associated with growth retardation.

Clinical aspects: Features of this disorder involve the head (microcephaly, small forehead, micrognathia, malar hypoplasia, broad or divided nasal tip, depressed nasal bridge, short nasal septum, cleft lip and palate, lip pits, dental abnormalities), the ears (microtic, low-set and/or posteriorly rotated, overfolded with hypoplastic superior helix, posterior and preauricular pit, supraauricular sinuses, conductive hearing loss secondary to fusion of the middle ear ossicles), the eyes (hypertelorism, ptosis, upslanting palpebral fissures, strabismus, telecanthus, microphthalmia, anophthalmia, iris and retinal coloboma, cataract, lacrimal duct obstruction, myopia), the kidneys (renal agenesis, cystic kidney disease), the skeleton (kyphosis, hyperlordosis, hypoplastic thumbs, polydactyly, clinodactyly), the skin (aplasia cutis congenita, subcutaneous scalp cysts, hemangiomatous branchial clefts, supernumerary nipples, hypoplastic fingernails, premature graying of hair) and the central nervous system (mild mental retardation, agenesis of cerebellar vermis). Postnatal growth deficiency is present in approximately 50% of cases.

Precautions before anesthesia: Evaluate for signs of difficult airway management (clinic, radiography). Assess renal function (clinically, ultrasound, laboratory). Mental retardation and impaired hearing may limit patient cooperation. Sedative and/or anxiolytic premedication as well as the presence of the primary care-giver for induction of anesthesia may be helpful.

Anesthetic considerations: Mask ventilation and endotracheal intubation should expected to be difficult and an adapted anesthetic management may be required.

Pharmacological implications: Intraoperative fluid regimen and anesthetic drug choice should be adapted to renal function. Maintain spontaneous ventilation until the airway has been secured.

REFERENCES:

Lee WK, Root AW, Fenske N: Bilateral branchial cleft sinuses associated with intrauterine and postnatal growth retardation, premature aging, and unusual facial appearance: a new syndrome with dominant transmission. *Am J Med Genet* 11:345, 1982.

Lin AE, Semina EV, Daack-Hirsch S, et al: Exclusion of the branchio-oto-renal syndrome locus (EYA1) from patients with branchio-oculo-facial syndrome. *Am J Med Genet* 91:387, 2000.

Trummer T, Muller D, Schulze A et al: Branchio-oculo-facial syndrome and branchio-otic/branchio-oto-renal syndromes are distinct entities. *J Med Genet* 39:71, 2002.

Branchio-Skeleto-Genital Syndrome

At a glance: Genetic disorder resulting in anomalies of branchial arch, skeleton, and genitalia.

Synonyms: BSG Syndrome; El Sahy-Waters Syndrome.

Incidence: Unknown. Only one case report of three boys from a single family.

Genetic inheritance: Presumed autosomal recessive trait. All the affected brothers were offspring of a first-cousin couple in a family pedigree with a history of consanguinity. Variable expression of the syndrome is thought to occur, as two other siblings had mental retardation, but no other features of the condition.

Pathophysiology: Several laboratory investigations to determine the nature of the chromosomal or metabolic errors failed to delineate a cause. Histologic and radiologic analysis of the dental cysts showed they were dentigerous (an odontogenic cyst surrounding the crown of an impacted tooth). Teeth from these patients had an unusual form of dentine dysplasia, mainly affecting the bulbar areas, which had not been described previously.

Diagnosis: Clinical course, morphologic appearance, radiology of mandible and maxilla (with multiple dental cysts), and oral histopathology of teeth (abnormal dentine dysplasia).

Clinical aspects: Features include mental retardation, seizures, brachycephalic skull, cervical fusion between second and third vertebrae, Schmorl nodes (i.e., herniations of the intervertebral disc through the vertebral endplate) in the lumber area, pectus excavatum, and penoscrotal hypospadias. Children have class III malocclusions with hypoplasia of the maxilla resulting in relative mandibular prognathism, a bifid uvula or partial cleft palate. Multiple dental cysts are present in the maxilla and mandible with misalignment of all the teeth of the upper jaw. Nasal bones are broad and flat, with a wide nasal tip and flared alar cartilages. All patients had hypertelorism, nystagmus of the right eye on right and left gaze, and divergent strabismus and slight ptosis of the right eye. Incomplete expression of the syndrome may be associated with mental retardation, but normal morphology.

Precautions before anesthesia: Obtain a full history of problems associated with the syndrome: mental retardation (sedative premedication may be advantageous), seizures (anticonvulsant therapy and efficacy), and degree of pectus excavatum. Evaluate the airway for potential difficulties (poor dentition, limited neck mobility, class III malocclusion, cleft palate). Consider anticholinergic premedication to decrease airway secretions if fiberoptic intubation is planned. Obtain a complete blood count.

Anesthetic considerations: If difficult airway management is anticipated, an awake fiberoptic tracheal intubation (mental retardation may reduce cooperation) or inhalational induction with maintained spontaneous ventilation should be considered. Regional anesthesia techniques can be used, especially for urologic procedures, provided no other specific contraindications are present (e.g., thrombocytopenia in patients taking sodium valproate).

Pharmacological implications: Muscle relaxants should be avoided until the airway has been secured. Avoid potentially epileptogenic drugs such as methohexital, ketamine, and enflurane. Sodium valproate may cause hepatic dysfunction, thrombocytopenia, and pancreatitis. Several of the commonly used anticonvulsant agents can cause sedation and hepatic enzyme induction resulting in altered pharmacokinetic and pharmacodynamic responses to various anesthetic agents. Patients receiving anticonvulsant medication should be continued on their regimen until surgery, and medications should be given parentally postoperatively until oral intake is tolerated.

REFERENCES:

El Sahy NI, Reid Waters W. The branchio-skeletal-genital syndrome. A new hereditary syndrome. *Plast Reconst Surg* 48:542, 1971.

Wedgwood DL, Curran JB, Lavelle CL, Trott JR: Cranio-facial and dental anomalies in the Branchio-Skeleto-Genital (BSG) syndrome with suggestions for more appropriate nomenclature. *Br J Oral Surg* 21:94, 1983.

Brauer Syndrome

At a glance: Genetic disorder with characteristic facial skin changes.

Synonyms: Focal Facial Dermal Dysplasia (FFDD) type I; Bitemporal Aplasia Cutis Congenita; Hereditary Symmetrical Aplastic Nevi of Temples.

Incidence: Undetermined. Since the original description in 1929 by August Brauer, a German physician, only a few papers have been published reporting kindreds of variable size (one family has more than 155 affected members) with the condition. The disorder is pre-dominantely expressed in males. One sporadic case has been reported in a Mexican-American male infant.

Genetic inheritance: Autosomal dominant inheritance, with possible variable expressivity. All of the three large reported kindreds demonstrated father-to-son transmission. Some investigators have suggested that Brauer and Setleis (FFDD type II) syndrome may be a single disorder with autosomal dominant inheritance with variable expressivity and reduced penetrance.

Pathophysiology: Histologic analysis of the lesions demonstrates a mesodermal dysplasia characterized by loss of subcutaneous fat and almost complete continuity between the epidermis and underlying skeletal muscle. Areas of skin puckering are caused by hypoplasia of the corium and subcutaneous fat.

Diagnosis: Physical appearance, family history, characteristic histologic appearance of skin lesion biopsy.

Clinical aspects: Manifestations of the condition are generally limited to the skin. Wrinkling or puckering of the skin at the temple region (original description noted similarity to obstetric "forceps marks"). Occasionally, guttate areas cover middle forehead and chin. Usually, the affection is bilateral, and only two of the original 38 patients described by Brauer had a unilateral occurrence. One case report of a 2-month-old child suggested a possible association between the syndrome and tetralogy of Fallot, although no other related cardiac anomalies have been described. Brauer and Setleis (focal facial dermal dysplasia type II) syndromes have been suggested by some authors to be the same condition.

Precautions before anesthesia: Preoperative assessment is important to determine the presence of a cardiac condition. No other specific precautions prior to anesthesia have been reported.

Anesthetic considerations: No specific complications during anesthesia have been reported. However, some reports suggest the epidermis overlying the lesions may be more susceptible to injury following trauma. Extra care with padding of the affected region for protection from pressure and trauma during anesthesia may be necessary.

Pharmacological implications: No known pharmacological implications.

Other Condition to Be Considered:

☞**SETLEIS SYNDROME:** Most likely autosomal dominant transmitted disorder with variable expressivity and reduced penetrance. Characterized by skin changes limited to the head, resulting in an aged leonine appearance.

REFERENCES:

Kowalski DC, Fenske NA: The focal facial dermal dysplasia: Report of a kindred and a proposed new classification. *J Am Acad Dermatol* 27:575, 1992.

Masuno M, Imaizumi K, Makita Y, et al: Autosomal dominant inheritance in Setleis syndrome. *Am J Med Genet* 57:57, 1995.

Tay YK, Morelli JG, Weston WL: Focal facial dermal dysplasia: report of a case with associated cardiac defects. *Br J Dermatol* 135:607, 1996.

Brittle Hair and Mental Deficit Syndrome

At a glance: Genetic disorder characterized by abnormal hair fibers and mental deficiency.

Synonym: Sabinas Brittle Hair Syndrome.

Incidence: Unknown. Affected families have been found only in the remote village of Sabinas in northern Mexico.

Genetic inheritance: Most likely autosomal recessive inheritance. Affected families demonstrate parental consanguinity with the occurrence in siblings of both sexes, both of which support autosomal recessive inheritance.

Pathophysiology: Examination of hair fibers demonstrates a reduction in the cuticular layer and a collapsed cortex. The cystine content of the hair is reduced, and the copper-to-zinc ratio is increased. No specific histopathologic changes in the central nervous system have been described.

Diagnosis: Made by clinical appearance and by morphologic and biochemical abnormalities of hair fibers. Affected newborns may be identified by persistent scalp hypotrichosis.

Clinical aspects: Characterized by dry, brittle, fragile hair, developmental delay, and normal stature. Affected newborns may be identified by persistent scalp hypotrichosis. In the postpubertal period, individuals have reduced or virtually absent pubic and axillary hair. Onychodystrophy was noted in some patients. A variable degree of mental retardation has been described. The condition may be similar to ☞Pollitt syndrome and ☞Amish hair–brain syndrome. Both of these syndromes demonstrate autosomal recessive inheritance, abnormal hair, and associated mental retardation. However, the exact interrelationship of these three syndromes is unclear. New research found genetic heterogeneity between Amish-hair-brain syndrome on the one hand and Politt and Brittle hair deficit syndrome on the other hand.

Anesthetic considerations: Obtain a full history of the patient's neurologic status. Patients may benefit from sedative premedication or, depending on the severity of their mental retardation, from the presence of the primary care-giver for induction of anesthesia.

Other conditions to be considered:

☞**AMISH HAIR–BRAIN SYNDROME:** Inherited syndrome with mild psychomotor retardation, hypogonadism, short stature, and brittle hair.

☞**POLLITT SYNDROME:** Inherited syndrome with developmental delay and trichorrhexis nodosa.

☞**NETHERTON SYNDROME:** Most likely autosomal recessive transmitted inborn error of metabolism manifesting as bamboo hair, atopic diathesis, congenital ichthyosiform erythroderma, and hypogammaglobulinemia.

REFERENCES:

Arbisser AI, Scott CI, Howell RR, et al: A syndrome manifested by brittle hair with morphologic and biochemical abnormalities, developmental delay and normal stature. *Birth Defects Orig Artic Ser* 12:219, 1976.

Howell RR, Arbisser AI, Parsons DS, et al: The Sabinas syndrome. *Am J Hum Genet* 33:957, 1981.

Nakabayashi K, Amann D, Ren Y, et al: Identification of CTorf11 (TTDN1) gene mutations and genetic heterogeneity in nonphotosensitive trichothiodystrophy. *Am J Hum Genet* 76:510, 2005.

Bronze Baby Syndrome

At a glance: Rare disorder characterized by development of a gray-brown discoloration that may persist for months in neonates undergoing phototherapy for neonatal hyperbilirubinemia.

Synonym: Neonatal Jaundice.

Genetic inheritance: None.

Pathophysiology: Combination of hepatocellular dysfunction and increased bilirubin products from photodestruction during phototherapy. The exact source of the pigment is unknown; it may be a photoisomer of natural bilirubin. Phototherapy with bilirubin acts as a catalyst, forming photoproducts from copper-bound porphyrins, causing skin discoloration.

Diagnosis: Age and clinical course (appearance of the discoloration with the use of phototherapy), liver biopsy (hepatocellular dysfunction with decreased excretion of bile constituents and photooxidation products at the level of bile canaliculi). Causative factor for the hyperbilirubinemia should be determined by appropriate tests.

Clinical aspects: Discoloration usually improves over time. Outcome usually is benign in cases where the hyperbilirubinemia is caused by icterus neonatorum, although the prognosis depends on the causative liver disease. Risk of bilirubin encephalopathy may be increased.

Precautions before anesthesia: Exclude other causes of discoloration (e.g., cyanosis, gray baby syndrome from chloramphenicol overdose). Evaluate severity of hepatic dysfunction and determine the underlying cause of impairment. Kernicterus should be excluded and appropriate treatment instituted (exchange transfusion, phenobarbital). Preoperative investigations should include a complete blood count, liver function tests, coagulation studies, arterial blood gas analysis, urea, and creatinine.

Anesthetic considerations: Anesthetic issues related to neonatal period should be considered (immaturity of various systems, differences in pharmacokinetics and pharmacodynamics). Adequate hydration should be maintained in patients with significant hyperbilirubinemia to prevent development of renal failure. Administer vitamin K. If prothrombin time is abnormal, clotting factors should be available. Hypotension should be avoided to minimize the reduction in hepatic perfusion. Anesthetic management of the neonate must take into account the causative factor for the development of hyperbilirubinemia. The perioperative risk is significantly increased in the presence of kernicterus. Factors known to precipitate seizures in neonates should be avoided (e.g., hypoxia, hypercarbia, hyponatremia, hypoglycemia).

Pharmacological implications: Hepatocellular dysfunction prolongs the elimination half-life of drugs excreted via the biliary system (e.g., pancuronium, vecuronium). Atracurium or cisatracurium is the drug of choice for paralysis. Halothane should be avoided in view of a theoretical risk of hepatitis, especially since sevoflurane is available for inhalational induction. Anesthetic agents that are proconvulsants should be avoided.

REFERENCES:
Ashley JR, Littler CM, Burgdorf WH, et al: Bronze baby syndrome. *J Am Acad Dermatol* 12:325, 1985.

Bertini G, Dani C, Fonda C, et al. Bronze baby syndrome and the risk of kernicterus. *Acta Paediatr* 94:968, 2005.

Rubaltelli FF, Da Riol R, D'Amore ES, Jori G: The bronze baby syndrome: evidence of increased tissue concentration of copper porphyrins. *Acta Paediatr* 85:381, 1996.

Brown-Vialetto-Van Laere Syndrome

At a glance: Genetic disorder characterized by bilateral sensorineural deafness and variable but progressive cranial and spinal motor nerve involvement.

Synonyms: Pontobulbar Palsy with Deafness; Progressive Bulbar Palsy with Perceptive Deafness; Progressive Bulbar Palsy with Sensorineural Deafness.

Incidence: Unknown, but more than 30 cases have been reported in the literature with an unconfirmed number of affected siblings and relatives.

Genetic inheritance: Originally thought to be autosomal recessive transmitted, but later suggested to be genetically heterogeneous with autosomal recessive and dominant transmission or the result of a mutant gene carried on the X-chromosome. Both familial and sporadic cases have been reported.

Pathophysiology: Muscle biopsy sections demonstrate atrophic fibers scattered equally between type I and II fibers. Histologically, silver staining shows loss of axons in intravascular nerve bundles. Sural nerve biopsy shows a depletion of nerve fibers and fibrosis in the perineurium. Electron microscopy reveals nonspecific changes characteristic of denervated muscle fibers. Cranial nerves and nuclei show a marked loss of both myelin and axons with gliosis. Electrophysiologic testing of affected muscle groups shows widespread and symmetrical denervation at the level of the lower motor neuron suggesting a pathologic process affecting the motor neuron or proximal part of the motor nerve roots. An upper motor neuron component was also detected in certain muscle groups.

Diagnosis: Characteristic clinical findings, clinical course, electrophysiologic testing, muscle and nerve biopsy, and histopathologic analysis.

Clinical aspects: The onset is usually in childhood, and the course tends to be irregularly progressive. The presenting symptom is usually a perceptive hearing loss caused by bilateral sensorineural deafness of slow or rapid onset. This is followed by signs of lower cranial nerve motor palsies. Intercurrent illness or physiologic stress, including surgery or pregnancy, may precipitate or exacerbate the condition. The severity of the condition varies from mild to severe, resulting in death. Neurologic involvement includes bulbar palsy, loss of cranial and spinal motor nerve function, wasting and fasciculation of the tongue, widespread muscle wasting with weakness and hypotonia most obviously in neck and lower limb girdle. Coordination and sensation remain intact. Respiratory complications include nocturnal hypoventilation because of marked diaphragmatic weakness (forced vital capacity [FVC] is severely reduced) and obstructive sleep apnea. Bulbar nerve involvement causes laryngeal and pharyngeal dyscoordination, nasal speech, and dysphagia with failure to protect the laryngeal inlet resulting in aspiration episodes. Scoliosis and cervical subluxation have been reported.

Precautions before anesthesia: Full neurologic assessment (degree of bulbar involvement), chest radiography, respiratory function tests (in advanced cases, the FVC is often reduced to <1 liter), arterial blood gas analysis (hypercapnia). Consider postoperative need for mechanical ventilation. Cervical spine radiograph may be indicated if any signs or a suspicion for cervical subluxation exists.

Anesthetic considerations: Bulbar nerve palsy may predispose to aspiration in the perioperative period. There is a high risk of diminished respiratory reserve and respiratory complications such as aspiration, pneumonia, nocturnal hypoventilation, and hypercarbia. Bilateral deafness may make communication during the perioperative period difficult. Regional anesthesia may be appropriate (maintained consciousness, limited respiratory depression, reduced risk of aspiration). A rapid sequence induction technique is recommended, however keep in mind that cervical subluxation requires special attention during airway management and positioning. In-line stabilization and/or fiberoptic tracheal intubation limits cervical movements. Consider placement of a nasogastric tube, gastrostomy tube, or a longterm intravenous line for parenteral nutrition.

Pharmacological implications: Be careful with sedative premedication and opioid analgesic agents. There is a high risk of respiratory depression and loss of protective reflexes. Titration of nondepolarizing muscle relaxants to clinical effect using a peripheral nerve stimulator is recommended. Ensure the nerve stimulator is used in a nonaffected nerve-muscle unit. Although no specific reports of anesthetic management of these cases have been published, avoidance of suxamethonium probably is wise. Consider acid aspiration prophylaxis in the presence of significant bulbar palsy.

Other condition to be considered:

☞**Progressive Bulbar Palsy of Childhood (Fazio-Londe disease):** an inherited condition characterized by progressive paralysis of muscles innervated by cranial nerves. Significant atrophy of muscles innervated by cranial nerves and the corticobubar tracts occurs.

REFERENCES:

Dipti S, Childs AM, Livingston JH, et al: Brown-Vialetto-Van Laere syndrome; variability in age at onset and disease progression highlighting the phenotypic overlap with Fazio-Londe disease. *Brain Dev* 27:443, 2005.

Megarbane A, Desguerres I, Rizkallah E, et al: Brown-Vialetto-Van Laere syndrome in a large inbred Lebanese family: Confirmation of autosomal recessive inheritance? *Am J Med Genet* 92:117, 2000.

Sathasivam S, O'Sullivan S, Nicolson A, et al: Brown-Yialetto-Van Laere syndrome: Case report and literature review. *Amyotroph Lateral Scler Other Motor Neuron Disord* 1:277, 2000.

Brugada Syndrome

At a glance: A familial disorder characterized by spontaneous idiopathic ventricular fibrillation that probably is one of the most frequent causes of sudden death in patients with a structurally normal heart.

Synonyms: Idiopathic Ventricular Fibrillation; Right Bundle Branch Block, ST-Segment Elevation, and Sudden Death Syndrome.

Incidence: Prevalence is estimated to be 1:10,000 to 5:10,000 in the general population in western countries. Higher frequency (1:2500) may be found in eastern countries.

Genetic inheritance: Autosomal dominant. Approximately 3/4 of clinically affected individuals are males.

Pathophysiology: Caused by mutations in the gene encoding the α-subunit of the voltage-gated sodium channel type V (SCN5A). A reentrant mechanism has been evocated. Loss of the dome of the action potential occurs because of an ion imbalance during phase 1 of the action potential. Increasing the potassium current increases ST-segment elevation, whereas interventions increasing calcium current diminish ST-segment elevation and vice versa.

Diagnosis: Based on the typical electrocardiographic pattern of ST-segment elevation in leads V_1 to V_3 and incomplete or complete right bundle branch block. Genetic studies can confirm the diagnosis, but a negative result does not exclude the diagnosis.

Clinical aspects: Syncope and cardiac arrest, typically occurring in the third and fourth decade of life, usually at rest or during sleep. However, all ages can be symptomatic. Classification of patients is not clearly established, but history of syncope and spontaneous electrocardiographic modifications seems to bear a bad prognosis. Intracardiac defibrillators have been used successfully.

Precautions before anesthesia: Obtain full familial and personal history. Evaluate cardiac status (clinical, electrocardiogram). Evaluate perioperative electrolyte levels (Na, Ca, K).

Anesthetic considerations: Successful anesthetic management of patients with Brugada syndrome has been described for general and regional anesthesia. Resuscitation devices must be present at all times (internal or external defibrillator). Perioperative cardiac monitoring is imperative. In high-risk patients (syncope and spontaneous electrocardiographic modifications), benefit of preoperative intracardiac defibrillator implantation must be considered.

Pharmacological implications: Perioperative fluid regimen must carefully consider the absolute necessity of electrolyte equilibrium. Calcium blockers should be avoided. Amiodarone has been used successfully in some patients.

Other condition to be considered:

☞**Arrhythmogenic Right Ventricular Dysplasia:** Most often inherited disease of the myocardium resulting in cardiomyopathy and risk of sudden death in otherwise healthy young adults.

REFERENCES:

Edge CJ, Blackman DJ, Gupta K, et al: General anaesthesia in a patient with Brugada syndrome. *Br J Anaesth* 89:788, 2002.

Grant AO: Electrophysiological basis and genetics of Brugada syndrome. *J Cardiovasc Electrophysiol* 16(Suppl 1):521, 2005.

Priori SG, Napolitano C, Gasparini M, et al: Natural history of Brugada syndrome: Insights for risk stratification and management. *Circulation* 105:1342, 2002.

Bruyn-Scheltens Syndrome

At a glance: A variant of hereditary spastic paraparesis characterized by spasticity, amyotrophy of the extremities, and urinary malformations.

Synonyms: Silver Syndrome; Silver Spastic Paraplegia Syndrome; Spastic Paraparesis with Amyotrophy of Hands and Feet.

Incidence: Approximately 12 affected families have been described in the literature.

Genetic inheritance: Autosomal dominant, although autosomal recessive transmission has been suggested for some cases. The genetic defect has been mapped to 11q12-q14.

Pathophysiology: Unknown.

Diagnosis: Made based on the family history and the clinical findings of gait disturbances with spastic paraparesis of the legs, and severe amyotrophy of the small hand muscles.

Clinical aspects: The age at the onset of symptoms is very variable (first to seventh decade of life). Gait disturbances are the predominant and often first sign of the disorder. Foot deformities (pes cavus) with hyperreflexia of the leg and positive Babinski sign may develop during the course of the disease. Amyotrophy of the intrinsic hand muscles with marked muscle weakness and wasting can occur uni- or bilaterally and mainly affects the thenar and dorsalis interosseus 1 muscles. (Rarely, it may also involve the feet). Generally, sensation is preserved, except for an occasionally mild reduction in vibration sense in the lower limbs in older patients. Neurophysiological studies favor anterior horn cell or motor nerve root involvement rather than a generalized neuropathy. In particular, no evidence of concurrent median or ulnar neuropathy could be found. However, median motor nerve conduction velocities may be mildly reduced. Other features may include urinary urgency, urinary incontinence and sphincter disturbances. In patients with the autosomal recessive inherited type of this disorder, amyotrophy often begins in the first decade of life and spasticity dominates over paraparesis. Severe muscle wasting of the thenar and hypothenar muscles may often coexist with amyotrophy below the level of the knees and pes cavus deformity.

Precautions before anesthesia: Evaluate neurologic status (clinically, full history, electromyography) and degree of muscle wasting.

Anesthetic considerations: Careful intraoperative positioning and padding is needed. Regional anesthesia is not contraindicated, but requires clear explanations should be given to the patient and family.

Pharmacological implications: Muscle relaxants are not contraindicated but weakness can be misinterpreted at end of procedure. Succinylcholine is probably best avoided due to neuropathy and amyotrophy.

Other conditions to be considered:

ANTINOLO NIETO BORREGO SYNDROME: Autosomal dominant inherited disorder with skin hypoplasia and demyelinating peripheral neuropathy. Regional anesthesia should probably be avoided (primarily for medico-legal purposes).

ABDALLAT DAVIS FARRAGE SYNDROME (Synonyms: Neurocutaneous Syndrome Abdallat Type; Spastic Paraplegia with Pigmentary Abnormalities): Disorder characterized by albinism, patchy skin pigmentation and insensitivity to pain that must be considered in postoperative care.

BAHEMUKA BROWN SYNDROME (Synonym: Spastic Paraplegia with Facial Cutaneous Lesions): Autosomal recessive inherited disorder with spastic paraplegia and irregular (decreased or increased) skin pigmentation.

REFERENCES:

Bruyn RPM, Scheltens P, Lycklama a Nijeholt J, et al: Autosomal recessive paraparesis with amyotrophy of the hands and feet. *Acta Neurol Scand* 87:443, 1993.

Warner TT, Patel H, Proukakis C, et al: A clinical, genetic and candidate gene study of Silver syndrome, a complicated form of hereditary spastic paraplegia. *J Neurol* 251:1068, 2004.

Windpassinger C, Wagner K, Petek E, et al: Refinement of the Silver syndrome locus on chromosome 11q12–q14 in four families and exclusion of eight candidate genes. *Hum Genet* 114:99, 2003.

Budd-Chiari Syndrome

At a glance: Acquired multifactorial condition caused by postsinusoidal hepatic venous outflow obstruction and ascites. The cause of the obstruction may be related to hypercoagulability of the blood, infections, cancer, and other conditions, which may be acute, chronic, or asymptomatic. The leading cause (in up to 40% of cases), however, is "idiopathic."

Synonyms: Chiari Syndrome; Venoocclusive Disease of the Liver.

Incidence: More than 4000 cases have been described.

Genetic inheritance: No genetic basis has been described. The etiology is multifactorial; a causative factor is frequently not identified. Risk factors include myeloproliferative disease, polycythemia rubra vera, thrombophilia, including factor V Leiden, paroxysmal nocturnal hemoglobinuria, lupus anticoagulant, protein C deficiency, antithrombin III deficiency, α_1-antitrypsin deficiency, oral contraceptive medication, pregnancy, malignancy, systemic and local infection, autoimmune disease, trauma, sarcoidosis, and membranous webs.

Pathophysiology: The symptoms result from decreased hepatic venous outflow, which may be secondary to an obstruction of small hepatic venules (e.g., following hepatotoxin ingestion), major hepatic veins (caused by hypercoagulable states, malignancy, or other conditions), or the inferior vena cava between the hepatic veins and the right atrium (e.g., caused by a membranous web, thrombosis, progression of renal adenocarcinoma, or compression from outside). Obstruction to flow results in portal hypertension and hepatocellular damage. Cirrhosis and portal hypertension eventually develop. The two-year mortality rate in untreated disease is 20 to 40%.

Diagnosis: The most important diagnostic tool is ultrasonography with the pathognomonic finding of absent hepatic vein images, intrahepatic collaterals enlargement of the caudate lobe of the liver, and lack of portal venous, hepatic, and inferior vena cava blood flow. Alternatively, hepatic venography or MRI may be used.

Clinical aspects: Depending on the level of the obstruction, 3 types of Budd-Chiari syndrome can be distinguished:

Type I: occlusion of the inferior vena cava with or without secondary hepatic vein occlusion.

Type II: occlusion of major hepatic veins.

Type III: obstruction of small centrilobular venules (also called veno-occlusive disease). Very rare in infants and young children. It may present as either fulminant hepatic failure associated with pain, hepatomegaly, jaundice, ascites, and rapid deterioration of hepatic function with encephalopathy requiring acute intervention, or acute nonfulminant Budd-Chiari syndrome associated with pain, ascites, and hepatomegaly. Chronic Budd-Chiari syndrome with insidious onset of abdominal discomfort and ascites because of portal hypertension is also possible. Occlusion of the inferior vena cava may cause edema of the lower limbs and varicose veins of the legs and lower trunk. Patients may present with esophageal varices. Management of Budd-Chiari syndrome may include liver transplantation, particularly in fulminant forms, formation of cavoatrial or mesoatrial shunts, and use of thrombolytic agents. Transjugular intrahepatic parto-systemic shunts (TIRS) is becoming popular to decompress the portal venous system.

Precautions before anesthesia: Preoperative investigation should be aimed at determining the extent of liver and other concomitant organ disease in addition to the effects of therapy (e.g., diuretics, anticoagulants, chemotherapy). In severe disease, multisystem involvement is seen. The operative risk is low if hepatic synthetic function is maintained. Coagulopathy secondary to diminished clotting factor production and thrombocytopenia from hypersplenism may be present. Coagulation abnormalities should be corrected (vitamin K, fresh-frozen plasma, platelets, desmopressin acetate as indicated) if there is active bleeding. It is reasonable to correct severe coagulation abnormalities in the absence of ongoing bleeding if invasive vascular access is planned. Blood examination should include sodium, potassium, chloride, creatinine, blood urea nitrogen, arterial blood gas analysis, liver enzymes, albumin, coagulation profile (prothrombin time, partial prothrombin time, international normalized ratio) a complete blood count, chest radiography, and an electrocardiogram. Echocardiography may be indicated, depending on the clinical presentation and the planned surgical intervention. Preoperative drainage of significant pleural and/or pericardial effusions should be considered.

Anesthetic considerations: The chosen anesthetic technique should aim to maintain hepatic blood flow and perfusion. Intravascular depletion and electrolyte abnormalities caused by diuretic therapy may be present. Portal hypertension predisposes to esophageal varices and upper gastrointestinal bleeding. Consequently, nasogastric tubes should be placed with caution. Restrictive lung disease secondary to pleural effusions and ascites predispose to atelectasis and hypoxemia. Pulmonary hypertension and hepatopulmonary syndrome are occasionally seen. Gastric emptying may be delayed, so precautions against aspiration should be considered. Intracranial pressure may be increased in decompensated disease. Perioperative anticoagulation may be required in patients with hypercoagulable states.

Pharmacological implications: Drug pharmacokinetics may be affected by impaired hepatic extraction and metabolism, altered volumes of distribution, and altered plasma protein binding. Renal impairment may coexist.

REFERENCES:

Menon KV, Shah V, Kamath PS: The Budd-Chiari syndrome. *N Engl J Med* 350:578, 2004.

Strunin L: Anesthetic management of patients with liver disease, in Millward-Sadler GH, Wright R, Arthur MJP (eds): *Wright's Liver and Biliary Disease*. London, WB Saunders, 1992, p 1381.

Ziser A, Plevak DJ, Wiesner RH, et al: Morbidity and mortality in cirrhotic patients undergoing anesthesia and surgery. *Anesthesiology* 90:42, 1999.

Burton Syndrome

At a glance: Genetic disorder leading to skeletal dysplasia.

Synonym: Kniest-like Dysplasia with Pursed Lips and Ectopia Lentis.

Incidence: Only three cases reported in the literature.

Genetic inheritance: First described in two siblings, one male and one female. A second case in a 2-year-old girl subsequently was reported. Mode of inheritance is uncertain, but autosomal recessive or gonadal mosaicism is most likely.

Pathophysiology: Iliac bone biopsy reveals markedly abnormal cartilage matrix in certain areas with large clumps of aggregated collagen fibrils. The growth plates are shorter than normal; however, the resultant calcified cartilage and bone trabeculae appear normal. Electron microscopy confirms the presence of broad-banded, aggregated collagen fibers, 10 to 30 times broader than normal, scattered throughout the cartilage matrix.

Diagnosis: Based on the characteristic clinical and radiologic findings. The analysis of bone biopsy specimens reveals distinctive abnormalities in the cartilage matrix.

Clinical aspects: Characterized by short stature (< 3rd percentile), shortness and bowing of limbs, bell-shaped thorax with flaring of lower ribs, short neck, rhizomelia, talipes equinovarus, mild craniofacial disproportion, stiffness, and swelling of wrists and knees. Other features include microstomia high-arched palate, pursed lips, and ectopia lentis. Radiologic findings of platyspondyly with cervical kyphosis resulting in decreased neck mobility, pectus carinatum, increased lumbosacral angle, bowing and shortening of the lower limbs, dumbbell-shaped long bones, short diaphyses, flared metaphyses and metaphyseal sclerosis, delayed ossification of the femoral heads and dysplastic femoral necks, wide short ribs, short and broad pelvis with narrow sacrosciatic notches, and brachydactyly are present. Unlike Kniest dysplasia, coronal clefts are absent. Psychomotor development appears normal for age.

Precautions before anesthesia: Preoperative assessment should include a full history and examination. Careful assessment of the airway to determine the potential for difficult airway management (microstomia, cervical kyphosis and limitation of neck movements reported by age 1.5 years). Radiologic investigation to assess neck stability may be required in the presence of cervical vertebral dysplasia. Anticholinergic premedication to decrease secretions can be of value in the younger age group, particularly if difficult airway management and/or fiberoptic intubation is anticipated. Use lung function tests to assess respiratory function.

Anesthetic considerations: Induction of anesthesia must take into consideration the potential for difficult airway management (small mouth, reduced neck mobility). A gaseous induction with halothane or sevoflurane may be advisable with a selection of devices available for control of the airway and tracheal intubation. During anesthesia, the neck should be maintained in a neutral or slightly extended position with adequate neck support at all times. Although not reported as being a problem in infants with this syndrome, respiratory insufficiency following anesthesia may be a potential risk in these children as they become older and the degree of thoracic dystrophy increases. Preoperative assessment and the nature of the surgery should enable the anesthesiologist to determine if postoperative respiratory support will be required. The patient should be positioned carefully with adequate padding and support to all areas because of fixed deformities in the limbs and neck. Regional anesthesia is not contraindicated, but because of the vertebral abnormalities and joint stiffness associated with this syndrome central neuraxial anesthesia could be difficult to perform and should be reserved for patients in whom the benefits outweigh the risks of other alternative forms of pain relief.

Pharmacological implications: No known specific pharmacological implications.

Other conditions to be considered:

KNIEST DYSPLASIA: Autosomal dominant inherited collagen type II disorder resulting in defective cartilage with craniofacial and spinal abnormalities. ☞(**Kniest Syndrome**).

☞**FREEMAN-SHELDON SYNDROME:** An inherited disorder characterized by microstomia (small, pinched mouth mimicking whistling), club feet and contractures of fingers.

☞**DIASTROPHIC DYSPLASIA:** An autosomal recessive inherited form of short limb dwarfism associated with spinal anomalies.

☞**SCHWARTZ-JAMPEL SYNDROME:** An inherited disorder manifesting with muscle stiffness (hypertrophied muscle) and mild, nonprogressive muscle weakness (myotonia). Onset is usually in the first year of life.

☞**LARSEN SYNDROME:** A congenital dysmorphic syndrome associated with characteristic anomalies of hands and feet and multiple congenital dislocations. Anomalies of spine, airway and heart occur.

REFERENCES:

Burton BK, Sumner T, Langer LO Jr, et al: A new skeletal dysplasia: Clinical, radiologic, and pathologic findings. *J Pediatr* 109:642, 1986.

Lo IF, Roebuck DJ, Lam ST, et al: Burton skeletal dysplasia: The second case report. *Am J Med Genet* 79:168, 1998.

Buschke-Ollendorff Syndrome

At a glance: An inherited disorder characterized by disseminated connective tissue nevi and osteopoikilosis.

Synonyms: Curth Syndrome; Schreus Syndrome; Disseminated Dermatofibrosis with Osteopoikilosis; Dermato-Osteopoikilosis; Dermatofibrosis Lenticularis Disseminata with Osteopoikilosis; Osteopathia Condensans Disseminata.

History: Named after Abraham Buschke (1868–1943), a German dermatologist and Helen Ollendorff Curth (born 1899), a German-American dermatologist, who first described the disorder in 1928.

Incidence: Approximately 1:20,000 live births.

Genetic inheritance: Autosomal dominant with incomplete penetrance.

Pathophysiology: Unknown.

Diagnosis: Characterized by slightly yellowish papules and nodules distributed symmetrically or asymmetrically on the trunk and extremities with induration of the skin and subcutaneous tissues. These skin changes are also called dermatofibrosis lenticularis dis-

seminata. Radiographs show circumscribed sclerotic areas near the epiphyses and metaphyses of many bones, particularly of the pelvis and extremities.

Clinical aspects: Patients can have short stature and often present with hoarseness. Clinical signs concern essentially the skin (dermatofibrosis lenticularis disseminata, palmoplantar hyperkeratosis, connective tissue nevi) and locomotor organs (epiphyseal, diaphyseal or metaphyseal anomalies, osteopoikilosis, osteosclerosis, melorheostosis (cortical thickening of the long bones often associated with pain), stiff joints, muscle fibrosis and contractures). Other features can include otosclerosis, cleft lip palate and insulin-dependent diabetes.

Precautions before anesthesia: Evaluate osteomuscular repercussions (clinical, radiographs, laboratory investigations including phosphocalcic metabolism).

Anesthetic considerations: Only a few implications concerning venous/regional anesthesia puncture sites that can be covered by skin lesions. Cautious intraoperative positioning and padding is needed.

Pharmacological implications: No known pharmacological implications.

Other condition to be considered:

GUNAL-SEBER-BASARAN SYNDROME (Dacryocystitis-Osteopoikilosis): Autosomal dominant with pigmented nevi, osteosclerosis, or osteopetrosis and defect of lacrimal system that may be considered in case parasympatholytic drugs are used.

REFERENCES:

Buschke A, Ollendorff-Curth H: Ein Fall von Dermatofibrosis lenticularis disseminata und Osteopathia condensans disseminata. *Dermatol Wochenschrift (Hamburg)* 86:257, 1928.

Kawamura A, Ochiai T, Tan-Kinashita M, Suzuki H: Buschke-Ollendorff syndrome: three generations in a Japanese family. *Pediatr Dermatol* 22:133, 2005.

Nevin NC, Thomas PS, Davis RI, et al: Melorheostosis in a family with autosomal dominant osteopoikilosis. *Am J Med Genet* 82:409, 1999.

C

C Syndrome

At a glance: A rare polymalformative syndrome characterized by a triangular-shaped head that is already present at birth, combined with cardiac, digestive, and skeletal anomalies.

Synonyms: Opitz Trigonocephaly Syndrome; Trigonocephaly "C" Syndrome; Trigonocephaly Syndrome. ("C" in the name of this syndrome refers to the initial of one of the first patients originally described by Opitz).

History: First described in 1969 by J.M. Opitz, a contemporary German-American geneticist.

Incidence: Approximately 40 cases have been described in the literature.

Genetic inheritance: Most likely autosomal recessive inheritance.

Pathophysiology: Unknown; malformation of the head is a result of premature union of the skull bones.

Diagnosis: Based on clinical findings of skull malformation combined with peculiar facies (narrow, pointed forehead, flat and broad nasal bridge with a short nose, epicanthus) and multiple cardiac, digestive, and skeletal anomalies.

Clinical aspects: These patients present with short stature, skin laxity, and failure to thrive (generalized hypotonia and poor sucking reflex). The main features involve the head and neck (short neck, trigonocephaly, biparietal widening of the head, metopic craniosynostosis, microcephaly, agenesis of the corpus callosum, micrognathia, low-set and posteriorly rotated ears, epicanthal folds, upward slanted palpebral fissures, strabismus, anteverted nares, flat and broad nasal bridge, short nose, high arched and deeply furrowed palate, oral frenula, thick anterior alveolar ridges, macrostomia); the central nervous system (hypotonia, seizures, psychomotor retardation); the heart (tetralogy of Fallot, ventricular septal defect, patent ductus arteriosus, Eisenmenger syndrome); the lungs (abnormal segmentation of the lungs); the gastrointestinal system (visceral angiomatosis, omphalocele, hepatomegaly); the genitourinary tract (prominent clitoris and labia majora, cryptorchidism, renal cortical cysts, hydronephrosis); and the skeleton (hyperextensible joints, fused sternal ossification centers, scoliosis, anomalous ribs, radial head dislocation, postaxial polydactyly, clinodactyly, terminal transverse limb reduction, metacarpal hypoplasia, hip dislocation). Clotting disorders and abnormally placed nipples are frequent findings. Approximately half of the patients die within the first year of life.

Precautions before anesthesia: Evaluate neurologic function (clinically, electroencephalography, computed tomography scanning, and/or magnetic resonance imaging). Check cardiac function (clinically, echocardiography, chest radiography, electrocardiography, and/or cardiac catheterization if necessary). Assess for signs of difficult airway management and evaluate respiratory function secondary to anomalies of the chest, skeleton, and abdominal muscles (clinically, pulmonary function test, chest radiography, and arterial blood gases analysis). Check kidney and liver function (clinically, sonography, laboratory tests). Preoperative laboratory investigation should include a complete blood count, electrolytes, creatinine, blood urea nitrogen, and coagulation tests. Postoperative mechanical ventilation may be necessary and should be arranged in advance.

Anesthetic considerations: Airway management may be difficult due to micrognathia and short neck and may require adapted anesthetic techniques such as primary fiberoptic tracheal intubation or intubation through a laryngeal mask (blind or with fiberoptic guidance). Joint laxity and preexisting dislocations require careful intraoperative positioning. Regional anesthesia is not contraindicated, but can be difficult to realize due to skeletal abnormalities and should be done only if coagulation status and platelet count are within normal limits.

Pharmacological implications: Consider interaction between antiepileptic and anesthetic drugs. Prophylactic antibiotics in case of cardiac lesions may be required. In order to maintain spontaneous breathing, neuromuscular blockers should be avoided until the airway has been secured. Anesthetic drug choice should be adapted to cardiac, hepatic, and renal function.

Other condition to be considered:

C-LIKE SYNDROME (Bohring Syndrome; Bohring-Opitz Syndrome; Opitz Trigonocephaly-like Syndrome): Fewer than 10 cases have been described. In contrast to C-syndrome, these patients present with intrauterine growth retardation, flexion deformities of the arms with dislocation of the radial heads, cleft lip/palate, exophthalmos with retinal anomalies, and hirsutism predominately on the forehead. In all the cases reported to date, no clear inheritance pattern could be found for this disorder. They seem to be sporadic, although autosomal recessive inheritance has been suggested.

REFERENCES:

Azimi C, Kennedy SJ, Chitayat D, et al: Clinical and genetic aspects of trigonocephaly: A study of 25 cases. *Am J Med Genet* 117A:127, 2003.

Greenhalgh KL, Newbury-Ecob RA, Lunt PW, et al: Siblings with Bohring-Opitz syndrome. *Clin Dysmorph* 12:15, 2003.

Opitz JM, Johnson RC, McCreadie SR, et al: The C syndrome of multiple congenital anomalies. *Birth Defects Orig Artic Ser* 2:161, 1969.

Cacchi-Ricci Disease

At a glance: A most often asymptomatic, sporadically occurring disorder resulting in cystic dilatation of the collecting tubules of the kidneys. Complications include urinary tract infections, hematuria, nephrocalcinosis, and, rarely, renal dysfunction.

Synonyms: Medullary Sponge Kidney (MSK); Precaliceal Canalicular Ectasia; Ricci-Cacchi Syndrome.

History: Described in 1948 and named after R. Cacchi, an Italian urologist, and V. Ricci, an Italian radiologist.

Incidence: Up to one in 200 urograms may show signs of Cacchi-Ricci syndrome (CRS). The actual incidence in the general population is not exactly known (because it may be asymptomatic), but the estimated incidence ranges from 1:5000–10,000. CRS has been found in 13% of 800 patients with calcium urolithiasis, with a higher frequency in women (19%) than in men (12%). However, in most series, men are more frequently affected than women, but morbidity seems to be higher in females. No racial predilection has been reported.

Genetic inheritance: Most cases are sporadic, although a few familial cases have been described.

Pathophysiology: The exact pathophysiology is unknown. However, most researchers consider CRS to be a developmental defect affecting the formation of the collecting tubules, whereas others consider it a primary progressive degeneration of the collecting tubules manifesting later on in life. The kidney size is usually normal or slightly enlarged. Histopathologic examination reveals cystic dilatation of the distal collecting tubules. Proximally, these cysts often communicate with the collecting tubules, while distally they are connected to the papillary ducts or the renal calyx. The cysts often contain calculi.

Diagnosis: Made on radiologic findings (sonography, plain radiography, intravenous urography, computed tomography scanning) and/or confirmed by histopathology (renal biopsy). Nephrocalcinosis is a common finding and often is the symptom that results in discovery of the disease (abdominal radiographs taken during evaluation of urinary tract infections or abdominal pain). Most patients remain asymptomatic throughout their life, but a minority of patients develop symptoms (typically in the second or third decade of life) that often are related to complications such as infection, hematuria, and nephrocalcinosis rather than to the CRS itself. The disease process may affect only one medullary pyramid in one or both kidneys or involve several medullary pyramids diffusely in both kidneys.

Clinical aspects: Common features are pain (38%), ureteral colics (28%), polyuria (28%), urinary tract infections, or hematuria. Often it is an incidental finding during evaluation of the abdomen or the urinary tract for other reasons. In the absence of complications, the overall renal function is and remains normal. Other features can include hypercalciuria (common), hyperuricosuria, urolithiasis, acidification of the urine, or impairment of urinary concentration. If renal involvement is segmental, surgical resection may be beneficial. A higher incidence of Wilms tumor and other abdominal malignancies has been reported in patients diagnosed with CRS during childhood. Regular followup in this population is mandatory.

Precautions before anesthesia: Assess renal function and evaluate for recurrent urinary tract infections and hematuria. In the absence of complications, CRS does not require therapy. However, the progression of nephrocalcinosis needs regular followup. In case of renal dysfunction, check arterial blood pressure and obtain blood work, including a complete blood count (anemia) and serum concentrations of electrolytes, creatinine, and blood urea nitrogen.

Anesthetic considerations: No specific anesthetic considerations are expected to arise from this disorder, except for the few cases with renal insufficiency.

Pharmacological implications: Cautious intravenous fluid management and adjusted dosage of predominately renally excreted drugs in case of renal dysfunction. Avoid nephrotoxic drugs.

Other conditions to be considered: Medullary sponge kidney has been reported in association with congenital hypertrophic pyloric stenosis, distal renal tubular acidosis, hyperparathyroidism and the following disorders:

☞**BECKWITH-WIEDEMANN SYNDROME:** Most often sporadic occurring syndrome with exomphalos, macroglossia, gigantism, and hypoglycemia due to hyperinsulinism.

☞**CAROLI SYNDROME:** A congenital disorder of the intrahepatic bile ducts characterized by intrahepatic dilatation of the biliary tree, resulting from ductal plate malformation.

☞**EHLERS-DANLOS SYNDROME:** Heterogeneous group of inherited connective tissue disorders, characterized by joint hyperlaxity, skin extensibility, and tissue fragility.

☞**MARFAN SYNDROME:** A familial disorder of generalized connective tissue abnormalities leading to connective tissue weakness with hyperextensible joints, dislocation of the lens, increased risk of valvular/aortic disease, and spontaneous pneumothorax.

AUTOSOMAL DOMINANT POLYCYSTIC KIDNEY DISEASE (Polycystic Kidney Disease type III): Affects middle-aged to older adults. Progressive renal failure as the cysts become larger. Rarely seen prenatally or in children. Patients may have berry aneurysms of the cerebral arteries—a genetic disorder frequently producing renal failure in childhood. It is the most common genetically determined childhood cystic disease of the kidneys. Congenital malformation of the collecting tubules.

REFERENCES:

Cacchi R, Ricci V: Sopra una rara e forse ancora non descritta affezione cistica della piramidi renali ("rene a spugna"). *Atti della Societat Italiana di Urologia* 21:59, 1948.

Thomas E, Witte Y, Thomas J, et al: Cacchi and Ricci's disease. Radiology, epidemiology and biology. *Prog Urol* 10:29, 2000.

Thomsen HS, Levine E, Meilstrup JW, et al: Renal cystic diseases. *Eur Radiol* 7:1267, 1997.

CADASIL

At a glance: A polymorphic neurologic syndrome with recurrent infarctions in the white matter resulting in a wide range of neurologic symptoms (depression, dementia, seizures, pseudobulbar paralysis). CADASIL is an acronym for *c*erebral *a*utosomal *d*ominant *a*rteriopathy with *s*ubcortical *i*nfarcts and *l*eukoencephalopathy.

Synonyms: Hereditary Multi-Infarct Dementia; Familial Vascular Leukoencephalopathy.

Incidence: More than 50 affected families have been described. No sexual predilection has been reported.

Genetic inheritance: Autosomal dominant. The gene defect has been mapped to the NOTCH3 gene (which encodes a transmembrane receptor with a large number of epidermal growth factor-like repeats), located on 19p13.2-p13.1.

Pathophysiology: Not clearly understood. The disease is related to mutations in the NOTCH3 gene. Dense osmiophilic granular material in contact with arteriolar smooth muscle cells can be revealed by electron microscopy.

Diagnosis: Based on clinical findings characterized by the acronymic association and a positive family history. Prominent signal abnormalities on magnetic resonance imaging include hyperintense lesions on T2-weighted images of the subcortical white matter, especially in the anterior part of the temporal lobes, the periventricular portion of the occipital lobes, and the basal ganglia. Small linear and punctate lacunas can be detected in the periventricular white matter, brainstem, thalamus, external capsule, and corpus callosum. Based on the abnormal accumulation of NOTCH3-positive material within small vessels, immunostaining of skin biopsy samples using a monoclonal antibody specific for NOTCH3 is the basis of a reliable and easy diagnostic test. Skin biopsy revealing granular osmiophilic material can be used for the diagnosis.

Clinical aspects: The onset of symptoms occurs generally in young adults of both sexes, with complete penetrance of the disorder between 30 and 40 years of age. The most consistent findings are cerebrovascular ischemic episodes (most often classic transient ischemic attacks or lacunar strokes, but occasionally insidious deficits developing over several days). Recurrent subcortical ischemic events occur in more than 80% of patients, and a progressive or stepwise subcortical dementia with pseudobulbar palsy can be found in almost one third of the patients. Clinical symptoms result from (nonarteriosclerotic, nonamyloidotic) vasoocclusive cerebral infarcts in the white matter that can cause a wide range of neurologic signs: relapsing strokes, seizures, pseudobulbar palsy, gait anomalies, dementia, urinary incontinence, hemiparesis or hemiplegia, and even tetraplegia. Sensorineuronal dysfunctions may lead to speech defect, deafness, visual loss, and insensitivity to pain. The behavior is severely affected and may present as mood disorders, manic episodes, depression, and dementia. Approximately 60% of patients have cognitive deficits, almost 40% have migraine (usually with aura), and 10% have epilepsy. The mean age at death of males is approximately 53 years versus 59 years for females.

Precautions before anesthesia: Obtain a full neurologic status and history (review electroencephalography reports, computed tomography scans, and magnetic resonance images). Some patients may be on acetazolamide therapy, so preoperative acid-base status and serum electrolytes should be checked. If mental retardation is clinically significant, anxiolytic and sedative premedication and/or presence of the primary caregiver for induction of anesthesia may be helpful.

Anesthetic considerations: Maintaining cerebral perfusion pressure and unobstructed cerebral venous drainage (avoid Trendelenburg position), preventing hypocapnia, and avoiding cerebral vasoconstrictive drugs (e.g., propofol) are the main goals of anesthesia. Regional anesthesia is not contraindicated per se (although some patients are on acetylsalicylic acid), but central neuraxial blockade should probably be avoided given the neurologic symptoms. If used, however, care should be taken to maintain mean arterial pressure.

Pharmacological implications: Consider the interaction between anesthetic and antiepileptic drugs. Avoid epileptogenic drugs. In patients with hemiparesis/hemiplegia or tetraplegia, succinylcholine should be avoided because of a possible exaggerated hyperkalemic response due to muscular denervation.

Other conditions to be considered:

☞**MOYAMOYA SYNDROME:** A progressive disease that affects the cerebral vasculature. The disease is characterized by narrowing and/or complete obstruction of the carotids. Headaches, various vision problems, mental retardation, paralysis, seizures, and psychiatric problems may occur. Cerebral hemorrhage (subarachnoid), cerebral infarction, severe headaches, speech disorders, and sudden onsets of recurrent paralysis are part of the presentation and most often occur in juvenile Moyamoya patients.

REFERENCES:
Dieu JH, Veyckemans F: Perioperative management of a CADASIL type arteriopathy patient. *Br J Anaesth* 91:442, 2003.

Inzitari D, Sarti C: Screening for CADASIL mutations. *Stroke* 34:205, 2003.

Markus HS, Martin RJ, Simpson MA, et al: Diagnostic strategies in CADASIL. *Neurology* 59:1134, 2002.

CAHMR Syndrome

At a glance: Extremely rare syndrome with mental retardation, hypertrichosis, and cataract. CAHMR is an acronym that stands for *ca*taract, *h*ypertrichosis, and *m*ental *r*etardation.

Incidence and genetic inheritance: Two cases in one family (a boy and a girl) have been described. Inheritance is considered autosomal recessive, given that the parents of the two patients were healthy first cousins.

Clinical aspects: Both children had congenital lamellar cataracts, a narrow and high arched palate, and generalized hypertrichosis, predominately affecting the back, shoulders, and sides of the face. Other reported features include microdontia, pectus excavatum, and mental retardation.

Anesthetic considerations: Expect tracheal intubation to be difficult secondary to the narrow, high arched palate. Depending on the degree of pectus excavatum, pulmonary and cardiac function may be affected. In order to obtain a good signal on the electrocardiogram, the skin in the area where the electrodes are placed may require shaving. To prevent skin burns, the same applies for the electrocautery plate.

REFERENCE:
Temtamy SA, Sinbawy AH: Cataract, hypertrichosis, and mental retardation (CAHMR): A new autosomal recessive syndrome. *Am J Med Genet* 41:432, 1991.

Calderon Gonzalez-Cantu Syndrome

At a glance: Mental retardation associated with skin and hair anomalies.

Synonym: Hair Defect with Photosensitivity and Mental Retardation.

Incidence and genetic inheritance: Three cases have been described (three sisters). Autosomal recessive.

Clinical aspects: Include stubby, coarse, sparse, fragile scalp hair, eyelashes, and eyebrows; photosensitivity; mental retardation was described as nonprogressive. Decreased body hair and recurrent infections have been described.

Anesthetic considerations: The features of the syndrome do not suggest that any specific precautions are necessary.

REFERENCE:
Calderon R, Gonalez-Cantu N: Kinky hair, photosensitivity, broken eyebrows and eyelashes and non-progressive mental retardation. *J Pediatr* 95:1007, 1979.

CAMFAK Syndrome

At a glance: This congenital syndrome presents with craniofacial, skeletal, and neurologic anomalies and might be an early form of Cockayne syndrome. CAMFAK is an acronym for *ca*taract, *m*icrocephaly, *fa*ilure to thrive, and *k*yphoscoliosis.

Incidence and genetic inheritance: Extremely rare, with probably fewer than 15 cases described. Autosomal recessive.

Clinical aspects: Severe mental and growth retardation, microcephaly and micrognathia with bird-like facies (with similarities to ☞Seckel Syndrome), spasticity, cerebellar hypoplasia, cerebral and cerebellar microcalcifications, central and peripheral demyelination, cataracts, enophthalmos, kyphoscoliosis, ☞Arthrogryposis, bilateral hip dislocations, and camptodactyly.

Anesthetic considerations: The presence of micrognathia indicates potentially difficult airway management. Maintain spontaneous ventilation and avoid neuromuscular blockers until the airway has been secured. Patient positioning and vascular access may be difficult due to spasticity and arthrogryposis. If kyphoscoliosis is clinically significant, preoperative lung function tests, arterial blood gas analysis, and echocardiography may be indicated. Regional anesthesia is not contraindicated per se. However, given the clinical findings, it seems technically challenging (limited cooperation and difficult positioning). Furthermore, in a progressive demyelinating disease, the authors would not recommend a central neuraxial anesthesia technique. Anxiolytic and sedative premedication (careful in patients with cardiopulmonary compromise due to kyphoscoliosis) and the presence of the primary caregiver during induction of anesthesia may be helpful. Kyphoscoliosis with associated respiratory dysfunction increases the risk of postoperative mechanical ventilation, which should be arranged for in advance.

Other conditions to be considered:

☞**COCKAYNE SYNDROME:** A complex congenital genetic disorder characterized by the association of dwarfism, deafness, microcephaly, facies similar to progeria syndrome, ataxia, photosensitivity and eye malformations, retinal atrophy, and renal insufficiency with premature aging and atherosclerosis.

☞**SECKEL SYNDROME:** Syndrome involving a form of primordial dwarfism with a characteristic head shape ("bird-like") and pongidoid microcephaly (also called "chimpanzee brain"). Other features include large ears, sparse hair, joint defects, clubfoot, trident hands, and mental retardation.

☞**PENA-SHOKEIR SYNDROME TYPE II:** A rapidly progressive neurologic disorder leading to brain atrophy with calcifications, cataracts, microcornea, optic atrophy, progressive joint contractures, and growth failure.

REFERENCE:

Talwar D, Smith SA: CAMFAK syndrome: A demyelinating inherited disease similar to Cockayne syndrome. *Am J Med Genet* 34:194, 1989.

Czeizel A, Lowry RB: Syndrome of cataract, mild microcephaly, mental retardation and perthes-like changes in sibs. *Acta Paediat Hung* 30:343, 1990.

Camptodactyly Syndrome, Guadalajara Types I and II

At a glance: Camptodactyly syndrome associated with other skeletal anomalies and mild mental retardation.

Synonym: Type I: Faciothoracoskeletal Syndrome.

Incidence and genetic inheritance: Approximately 10 cases have been described to date. Autosomal recessive inheritance with parental consanguinity is a significant risk factor.

Clinical aspects: Common findings in Guadalajara type I and II are intrauterine growth retardation, short stature, abnormal vertebral size, pelvis anomaly, pectus excavatum or carinatum, camptodactyly, microphthalmos, and mental retardation.

Guadalajara type I: In addition to the aforementioned signs, these patients have seizures, microcephaly and brachycephaly, flat facies, microcornea, telecanthus, epicanthic folds, blepharophimosis, anteverted nares, prognathism, microstoma, dental malocclusion, anodontia, restricted joint mobility, and metacarpal anomalies.

Guadalajara type II: Additional findings in these patients are microcephaly, short neck, low-set ears, ptosis, hypertelorism, thin lips, retrognathia and micrognathia, scoliosis, ulnar deviation of the fingers, and hypoplastic patellae.

Anesthetic considerations: The described features suggest airway management may be difficult. Careful intraoperative positioning is needed. Consider interactions between anesthetic drugs and antiepileptic treatment.

REFERENCES:

Cantu JM, Garcia-Cruz, D, Gil-Viera J, et al: Guadalajara camptodactyly syndrome type II. *Clin Genet* 28:54, 1985.

Cantu JM, Rivera H, Nazara Z, et al: Guadalajara camptodactyly syndrome: A distinct probably autosomal recessive disorder. *Clin Genet* 18:153, 1980.

Figuera LE, Ramirez-Duenas ML, Garcia-Cruz D, et al: Guadalajara camptodactyly syndrome type I: A corroborative family. *Clin Genet* 43:11, 1993.

Camurati-Engelmann Syndrome

At a glance: Musculoskeletal syndrome leading to enhanced bone formation, hyperostosis, and sclerosis of the diaphyses of the long bones.

Synonyms: Progressive Diaphyseal Dysplasia; Engelmann Disease; Osteopathia Hyperostotica Scleroticans Multiplex Infantalis.

Incidence: The exact incidence is unknown. To date, approximately 200 cases have been described. No racial predilection.

Genetic inheritance: Autosomal dominant. Camurati-Engelmann syndrome (CES) is caused by mutations in the β_1 transforming growth factor gene (TGFB1) located on 19q13.1-q13.3. A variant exists in which TGFB1 is not altered.

Pathophysiology: Growth suppression of fibroblasts and proliferation of osteoblasts lead to characteristic thickening of bony cortices on periosteal surfaces and in the medullary canal. Initially, the disorder occurs in femur and tibia, but then progressively spreads to other bones.

Diagnosis: Based on clinical findings. Confirmed by radiology. Muscle biopsy reveals atrophy, but is unspecific.

Clinical aspects: The disease typically presents with severe bone pain (especially in the legs), gait anomalies (waddling and broad-based) and difficulties in running, easy fatigability, and reduced muscle mass with proximal muscle weakness in childhood or adolescence, but onset in the third decade has been described. The changes begin bilaterally in femur and/or tibia, resulting in massive endosteal and periosteal thickening of the diaphyseal corticalis (diaphyseal sclerosis). As the disease progresses, other skeletal findings occur, such as diaphyseal widening, Erlenmeyer flask deformity, coxa and genua valga, joint contractures, sclerosis of the skull base, the mandible, posterior parts of vertebrae, kyphosis, and scoliosis. Head and neck involvement may occur later in the course of the disease and include frontal bossing, proptosis, enlargement of the mandible, frequent headache, and cranial nerve impingements (in more than one third of patients) that may result in deafness (conductive and/or sensorineural), optic nerve compression (papilledema has been described), visual impairment, glaucoma, diplopia, and facial palsy. The patients usually appear slim to cachectic, sometimes referred to as marfanoid habitus. Delayed dentition with severe caries, delayed puberty, hepatosplenomegaly secondary to extramedullary hematopoiesis (thought to be a consequence of narrowing of the medullary cavities) are features that have occasionally been described. Steroids have been shown not only to alleviate the pain but also to halt or even reverse the underlying findings in many patients. Nonsteroidal antiinflammatory drugs are also used for pain control.

Precautions before anesthesia: Obtain a complete blood count (including platelets) to rule out bone marrow insufficiency. In patients with hepatosplenomegaly, liver function should be checked (transaminases, bilirubin, albumin, coagulation profile). In later stages of the disease, mouth opening and neck mobility should be checked carefully because airway management could be complicated by changes in the mandible and the neck. Assess the extent of cranial neuropathies and muscular weakness. Depending on the procedure, prolonged postoperative mechanical ventilation may be required if kyphosis/scoliosis and muscle weakness are significant. Preoperative pulmonary function tests and an echocardiography (cor pulmonale) may be indicated in selected patients. Expect communication difficulties in the presence of deafness and visual impairment. Sedative and/or hypnotic premedication and/or presence of the primary caregiver during induction of anesthesia may be helpful for these patients to alleviate their stress.

Anesthetic considerations: Be prepared for difficult airway management in patients with long-standing disease. Maintain spontaneous ventilation until the airway has been secured. Regional anesthesia is not contraindicated (given normal coagulation and platelet count), but positioning may be difficult due to contractures. In particular, central neuraxial blockade can be challenging (vertebral anomalies, kyphosis, scoliosis), although spinal anesthesia has been used successfully for caesarean section in a patient with CES. The anomalies may cause unpredictable spreading of local anesthetics, and a continuous technique (spinal or epidural) with the possibility of titration probably is preferable. Particular attention should be paid to corneal protection in the presence of exophthalmos (lubricate the eyes and tape them shut). Cardiomyopathy has been described in some related syndromes, but to our knowledge not in CES.

Pharmacological implications: Corticosteroid therapy is frequent and perioperative supplementation may be required. Avoid neuromuscular blockers until the airway has been secured.

Other conditions to be considered:

RIBBING DISEASE (Hereditary Multiple Diaphyseal Sclerosis): This autosomal recessive inherited disorder of the extremities shares some similarities with CES. In fact, some authors have suggested that CES and Ribbing disease are phenotypic variations of the same disorder. However, the onset is usually later in life (postpuberty). Diaphyseal osteosclerosis and hyperostosis are often unilateral (or bilateral, but then with asymmetrical and asynchronous course) with the tibia almost always affected and limited to one or maximally four long bones. Skull involvement is not a feature of Ribbing disease. Bone pain, swelling, and tenderness may be present. Radiographic features include osteosclerosis and hyperostosis of the tubular bones.

☞**CRANIODIAPHYSEAL DYSPLASIA:** A bone disorder characterized by marked hyperostosis of the craniofacial bones and diaphyseal expansion of the tubular bones resulting in significant clinical complications.

☞**KENNY-CAFFEY SYNDROME:** A hereditary skeletal dysplasia resulting in proportionate dwarfism characterized by thickening of the inner cortex with stenosis of the medullary cavities of the tubular bones.

☞**PYLE DISEASE:** An inherited bone dysplasia affecting the enchondral growth of long bones, which results in failure of

modeling and causes increased circumference of the ends of the shafts.

REFERENCES:

Makita Y, Nishimura G, Ikegawa S, et al: Intrafamilial phenotypic variability in Engelmann disease (ED): are ED and Ribbing disease the same entity? *Am J Med Genet* 91:153, 2000.

Nowicki RW, Norris A: Caesarean section in a patient with Engelmann's disease. *Anaesthesia* 54:1118, 1999.

Vaughn SP, Broussard S, Hall CR: Confirmation of the mapping of the Camurati-Engelmann locus to 19q13.2 and refinement to a 3.2-cM region. *Genomics* 66:119, 2000.

Canavan Syndrome

At a glance: A progressive leukodystrophy caused by spongy degeneration of the central nervous system. The clinical triad of hypotonia, macrocephaly, and lack of head control in an infant more than 3 to 5 months old is suspicious for this disorder.

Synonyms: Canavan-Van Bogaert-Bertrand Disease; Canavan Sclerosis; Van-Bogaert-Bertrand Syndrome; Van-Bogaert-Bertrand Spongy Degeneration Syndrome; Cerebral White Matter Spongy Degeneration; Spongy Degeneration of the Nervous System; Familial Spongy Degeneration; Encephalopathia Spongiotica; Acetylaspartic Aciduria; Progressive Degenerative Subcortical Encephalopathy; Aminoacylase-2 Deficiency; ACY2 Deficiency; Aspartoacylase Deficiency.

Incidence: Although the disorder has been described in all ethnic groups, the highest incidence has been reported in Ashkenazi Jews, in whom it occurs in approximately 1:13,000 live births.

Genetic inheritance: Autosomal recessive. The disease is caused by mutations of the aspartoacylase gene, which has been mapped to 17pter-p13.

Pathophysiology: Aspartoacylase deficiency leads to a buildup of N-acetylaspartate. This defect results in demyelination of the white matter of the internal and external capsule, corpus callosum, subcortical white matter, and posterior fossa.

Diagnosis: It is based on clinical features and the demonstration of significantly elevated N-acetylaspartate levels in urine, blood, cerebrospinal fluid, and the brain (detected by magnetic resonance spectroscopy). Neuroradiologic studies show white matter degeneration in affected areas. Brain histology shows spongy degeneration (unspecific), but is usually not required for the diagnosis. Electron microscopy reveals swelling of the astrocytes and abnormalities of the mitochondria. Cultured skin fibroblasts show reduced aspartoacylase activity.

Clinical aspects: Three different forms of Canavan disease (CD) have been described (neonatal, infantile, and late-onset form). The infantile form seems to be the most common form, and only the rate of disease progression is highly variable. Onset is usually in early infancy at 2 to 4 months of age with loss of the already acquired milestones, while death occurs most often within the first decade of life (although death by approximately 18 months of age is not uncommon). However, survival into the teens has also been reported, and one patient survived for more than 30 years. Patients initially present with poor head control due to hypotonia or atonia of the neck muscles. Hypotonia soon becomes generalized and changes to spastic diplegia or quadriplegia as the disease progresses, ending in late decerebrate or decorticate posturing. Generalized seizures are common. Ocular features include optic atrophy, nystagmus, and finally blindness. Closure of the anterior fontanelle is delayed, and macrocephaly is a common finding. Patients usually are deaf. Copious oral secretions and gastroesophageal reflux can occur. No effective treatment is available. Therapies are mainly symptomatic (e.g., seizure control, physiotherapy). Gene therapies are currently under investigation.

Precautions before anesthesia: The patient's seizure control should be assessed and medications altered, if necessary. A chest radiograph is recommended if recurrent or recent aspiration is an issue. Consider premedication with a nonparticulate antacid, H_2-antagonist, or proton pump inhibitor. Avoid antidopaminergic medications because they can exacerbate existing extrapyramidal movement disorders. Sedative and anxiolytic premedication and the presence of the primary caregiver during induction of anesthesia may be considered. Anticholinergic drugs (e.g., atropine, glycopyrrolate) can be helpful in reducing oral secretions. Depending on the type of procedure, postoperative mechanical ventilation may be required.

Anesthetic considerations: A rapid sequence induction technique is recommended. Given the copious secretions and the gastroesophageal reflux disease, patients should be intubated to protect the airway from aspirations. Principal anesthetic considerations are related to seizure control, prevention of aspiration, and airway complications. Carefully evaluate for generalized hypotonia postoperatively.

Pharmacological implications: Chronic antiseizure therapy may change the elimination of anesthetic and other drugs. Avoid medications that reduce the seizure threshold or interfere with the antiepileptic treatment. Avoid succinylcholine in patients with spastic diplegia or quadriplegia due to the risk of an exaggerated hyperkalemic response.

Other conditions to be considered: (An overview table can be found under ☞Leukodystrophies).

☞**ALEXANDER SYNDROME:** A degenerative and progressive disorder of the nervous system caused by leukodystrophy. Affects mainly males and usually begins at approximately 6 months of age. Symptoms include mental and physical retardation, enlargement of the brain and head, spasticity (arms and legs), and seizures.

☞**METACHROMATIC LEUKODYSTROPHY:** An inherited disorder of myelin metabolism with progressive loss of white matter in the central and peripheral nervous system.

☞**PELIZAEUS-MERZBACHER SYNDROME:** A very rare slowly progressive dysmyelinating disease affecting in a diffuse pattern the cerebrum, cerebellum, brainstem, and spinal cord. Two types are described: X-linked (infantile form) and autosomal dominant (preadulthood form). Clinical features include stridor, muscle spasticity, and nystagmus. Often fatal in the first year of life because of respiratory complications.

☞**X-LINKED ADRENOLEUKODYSTROPHY:** A disorder characterized by progressive demyelinization of the central nervous system and peripheral adrenal insufficiency.

☞**SCHILDER SYNDROME:** A rare, progressive, lethal disease of the central nervous system that affects mostly children and is characterized by adrenal atrophy and diffuse central demyelination. Presents with progressive dementia, spasticity, cortical blindness, deafness, hemiplegia, quadriplegia, ataxia, pyramidal signs, seizures, retrobulbar neuritis, and pseudobulbar palsy. Onset in late childhood. Most patients die within a few months after onset.

☞**ZELLWEGER SYNDROME:** A disorder characterized by the congenital absence of functioning peroxisomes (cellular structures responsible for elimination of toxic substances) resulting in a cerebrohepatorenal syndrome. The disease affects the brain development, particularly myelination. The most important features include hepatomegaly, polycystic kidney disease, visual disturbances, and high plasma levels of iron and copper. Other features include muscular hypotonia already noticeable at birth, mental retardation, seizures, coagulopathy, and dysphagia with recurrent aspiration. Congenital heart defects have been described. Life expectancy is approximately 6 months.

REFERENCES:

Feigenbaum A, Moore R, Clarke J, et al: Canavan disease: Carrier-frequency determination in the Ashkenazi Jewish population and development of a novel molecular diagnostic assay. *Am J Med Genet* 124A: 142, 2004.

Tobias JD: Anaesthetic considerations for the child with leukodystrophy. *Can J Anaesth* 39:394, 1992.

Traeger EC, Rapin I: The clinical course of Canavan disease. *Pediatr Neurol* 18:207, 1998.

Cantalamessa-Baldini-Ambrosi Syndrome

At a glance: A rare multiorgan syndrome with short stature, hypogonadism, severe mental retardation, and mitral valve prolapse.

Synonym: Hypogonadism Mitral Valve Prolapse Mental Retardation Syndrome.

Incidence: The exact incidence is not known, but this disorder is extremely rare.

Genetic inheritance: Not conclusive. Both X-linked recessive and autosomal recessive inheritance have been suggested.

Diagnosis: Based on clinical findings of primary hypogonadism, mitral valve prolapse, and mental retardation. Most patients with mitral valve prolapse have a midsystolic click followed by a late systolic murmur; however, echocardiography is needed to confirm the diagnosis.

Clinical aspects: Patients typically are obese, of short stature with a short neck, and suffer from a variable degree of mental retardation. The palate is often narrow and vaulted. Mitral regurgitation is frequent. Patients have primary hypogonadism with small and atrophic testes, delayed puberty, gynecomastia and decreased body hair. In otherwise healthy patients, symptoms of mitral valve prolapse may include fatigue, dyspnea, exercise intolerance, chest pain, headache, sleep disorders, anxiety and panic attacks, and irritable bowel signs. The etiology of these symptoms is not well understood but most likely is multifactorial, including autonomic dysfunction with adrenergic hyperresponsiveness and an abnormal renin-angiotensin-aldosterone response to volume depletion. Patients often present with a low resting blood pressure, which seems to be associated with low intravascular volume that may often lead to dizziness and syncope.

Precautions before anesthesia: Cardiac arrhythmias are common (88%) in asymptomatic pediatric patients with mitral valve prolapse. At least a 12-lead electrocardiogram and/or preferably a Holter monitoring (24 hours) are recommended preoperatively. Antiarrhythmic therapy may be required. Electrolytes, particularly magnesium, should be checked and normalized if necessary. Cardiac function and the severity of mitral regurgitation should be assessed by echocardiography.

Anesthetic considerations: Be aware of the possibility of cardiac arrhythmias. Obesity implies decreased functional residual capacity and less reserve for hypoxia, increased airway pressures, difficult vascular access, and a higher overall rate of postoperative complications. Potentially difficult direct laryngoscopy. In the presence of significant mitral incompetence, goal-directed hemodynamic management should be considered.

Pharmacological implications: Subacute bacterial endocarditis prophylaxis is usually recommended if mitral valve prolapse is associated with thickened leaflets and/or mitral regurgitation.

REFERENCES:

Bobkowski W, Siwinska A, Gorzna H, et al: Dysrhythmias documented by 48-hour electrocardiographic monitoring in children with mitral valve prolapse. *Pediatr Pol* 71:493, 1996.

Cantalamessa L, Baldini M, Ambrosi B, et al: A syndrome of primary gonadal failure, short stature, mitral valve prolapse, and mental retardation. *Am J Med Genet* 33:117, 1989.

Cantu Syndrome

At a glance: A congenital multisystem syndrome leading to macrocephaly, cardiac anomalies, osteodysplasia, and hypertrichosis.

Synonyms: Cantu Sanchez Corona Hernandes Syndrome; Craniofaciocardioskeletal Syndrome.

Incidence: Extremely rare. Fewer than 30 cases have been reported in the literature.

Genetic inheritance: Most cases are sporadic. De novo autosomal dominant as well as X-linked dominant transmission have been discussed. Microdeletions seem to be the most likely cause of this disorder. Phenotypic variability exists. No sexual predilection.

Pathophysiology: Unknown. Histologic analysis of multiple organs is nonspecific.

Diagnosis: Based on the clinical findings of mild mental deficiency and the distinct malformations. Storage disorders must be excluded.

Clinical aspects: The principle features are short stature, osteochondrodysplasia, macrocephaly with frontal bossing, exophthalmos and hypertelorism, macroglossia, cardiac anomalies (e.g., concentric hypertrophic cardiomyopathy, septal defects, pericardial effusions, and cardiomegaly), joint hyperextensibility, cutis laxa with wrinkled palms and soles, and hypertrichosis. Skeletal anomalies include abnormally small vertebral bodies, wide ribs, narrow chest, and slender long bones. Computed tomography scanning or magnetic resonance imaging of the head may reveal bilateral calcifications of the arteriae thalamostriatae and enlargement of the lateral ventricles and external cerebrospinal fluid spaces. Pyloric stenosis and elevated serum alkaline phosphatase levels have been described. A single case of pulmonary hypertension responsive to steroid therapy has been reported.

Precautions before anesthesia: Anesthesia care has not been described, although at least one child did undergo cardiac surgery. Cardiomegaly on chest radiographs is indicative of cardiac involvement and requires further evaluation including echocardiography. Airway examination should include oral cavity inspection, as a number of patients have a large, bulky tongue. Mental retardation may result in increased anxiety and limited cooperation. Sedative and anxiolytic premedication and the presence of the primary caregiver during induction of anesthesia may be helpful.

Anesthetic considerations: Direct laryngoscopy can be difficult (macroglossia), and spontaneous ventilation must be preserved un-

til the airway has been secured. Consider draining hemodynamically significant pericardial effusions preoperatively (or at least after induction of anesthesia). Vascular access can be difficult in the presence of cutis laxa. Central neuraxial blockade is not contraindicated per se, however, cooperation may be limited (mental retardation) and access difficult due to vertebral anomalies. Care should be taken with regard to intraoperative positioning of patients with hyperelastic joints. Careful protection of the eyes (lubrication and taped shut) must be provided because patients are at high risk for corneal damage due to exophthalmos.

Pharmacological implications: Avoid neuromuscular blockers until the airway has been secured. Subacute bacterial endocarditis prophylaxis may be required.

Other conditions to be considered:

☞**COSTELLO SYNDROME:** A syndrome characterized by postnatal growth deficiency, coarse facies, redundant skin on the neck, acanthosis nigricans, developmental delay, and papillomata.

DE BARSY MOENS DIERCKS SYNDROME: Extremely rare disorder inherited as an autosomal recessive trait. The main characteristics are frontal bossing, large prominent ears, athetosis, cloudy cornea, hypotonia and hyperlaxity of small joints, and/or short stature.

REFERENCES:

Engels H, Bosse K, Ehrbrecht A, et al: Further case of Cantu syndrome: Exclusion of cryptic subtelomeric chromosome aberrations. *Am J Med Genet* 111:205, 2002.

Lazalde B, Sanchez-Urbina R, Nuno-Arana I, et al: Autosomal dominant inheritance in Cantu syndrome (congenital hypertrichosis, osteochondrodysplasia, and cardiomegaly). *Am J Med Genet* 94:421, 2000.

Robertson SP, Kirk E, Bernier F, et al: Congenital hypertrichosis, osteochondrodysplasia, and cardiomegaly: Cantu syndrome. *Am J Med Genet* 85:395, 1999.

CAPOS Syndrome

At a glance: A very rare congenital neurologic syndrome that presents in infancy. CAPOS is an acronym for *c*erebellar ataxia with *a*reflexia, *p*es cavus, *o*ptic atrophy, and *s*ensorineural hearing loss.

Incidence and genetic inheritance: Three cases (mother and two children) have been described. Autosomal dominant or maternal mitochondrial inheritance has been suggested.

Clinical aspects: In the cases described to date, a nonspecific recurrent febrile illness triggers acute onset of neurologic symptoms with generalized hypotonia and cerebellar ataxia in previously healthy infants between the age of 12 and 24 months. Initially, full recovery between episodes is possible. Other features include progressive, nonreversible optic nerve atrophy, nystagmus, sensorineural hearing loss, and pes cavus.

Anesthetic considerations: Anesthesia has not been reported in this syndrome. Assess neuromuscular function. Avoid aminoglycosides and other ototoxic drugs in the presence of preexisting hearing loss.

REFERENCE:

Nicolaides P, Appleton RE, Fryer A: Cerebellar ataxia, areflexia, pes cavus, optic atrophy, and sensorineural hearing loss (CAPOS): A new syndrome. *J Med Genet* 33:419, 1996.

Congenital Disorders of Glycosylation

At a glance: Congenital disorders of glycosylation (CDG) refers to a group of multisystemic disorders characterized by dysmorphism, coagulation disorders and psychomotor retardation. Multiple subtypes exist, of which type Ia is by far the most common.

Synonyms: Carbohydrate-Deficient Glycoprotein Syndromes (former name).

CDG type Ia	Phosphomannomutase II deficiency
	Olivopontocerebellar atrophy of neonatal onset
	Sialotransferrin development deficiency syndrome
	Jaeken syndrome
CDG type Ib	Phosphomannose isomerase deficiency
CDG type IIc	Leukocyte adhesion deficiency syndrome types I and II (II: ☞Rambam-Hasharon syndrome)

Classification: There are basically two types of protein glycosylation: N-glycosylation and O-glycosylation. N-glycosylation comprises an assembly pathway (in the cytosol and the endoplasmic reticulum) and a processing pathway (in the endoplasmic reticulum and the Golgi complex). O-glycosylation is more complex but lacks a processing pathway. Of the 16 known defects, 12 affect N-glycosylation (eight are assembly defects [CDG Ia-Ih] and four are processing defects [CDG IIa-IId]) and four affect the O-glycosylation.

Incidence: Approximately 350 patients with CDG type Ia (by far the most common type) have been reported worldwide. Half of these cases are estimated to have occurred in Scandinavia. For the other types of CDG, the number of reported patients varies between one and 30 for each type of CDG type I and II.

Genetic inheritance: Autosomal recessive, except for the multiple exostoses syndrome, which is autosomal dominant inherited.

Pathophysiology: CDG are due to defects in the synthesis of the glycan moiety of glycoproteins and other glycoconjugates. It results in a defective attachment of carbohydrates to proteins due to mutations affecting the N-glycosylation or O-glycosylation. In CDG type I, lipid-linked oligosaccharide assembly and transfer is affected. In CDG type II, trimming of the protein-bound oligosaccharide or the sugar attachment to it is affected.

Diagnosis: Clinical findings and electrophoretic patterns of serum transferrin (serum transferring isoelectrofocusing) is the gold standard for N-glycosylation defects. The lack of negatively charged sialic acid (a component of transferring) results in a cathodal shift in the electrophoresis, which is considered diagnostic, although a normal pattern does not exclude CDG. Multiple subtypes exist (see Table C-1), of which CDG type Ia is the most common. Depending on the subtype, coagulation disorders may result in a prothrombotic or bleeding tendency.

Clinical aspects: *Conditions associated with a defect in N-glycosylation:*

The clinical features differ between the subtypes. The disorders may affect the head and neck (prominent forehead, large ears, strabismus, nystagmus, myopia, retinopathy pigmentosa, flat nasal bridge, thin upper lip, cleft palate), heart (hypertrophic obstructive cardiomyopathy, cardiac failure, exudative pericarditis, pericardial effusions), blood (prolonged prothrombin time, factor XI deficiency, antithrombin III deficiency, thrombocytosis, platelet hyperaggregability, neutrophil dysfunction, decreased levels of immunoglobulins A and G), central nervous system (psychomotor retardation, generalized hypotonia, cerebral and cerebellar abnormalities, ataxia, hyporeflexia, seizures, stroke-like episodes, olivopontine hypoplasia, ☞Dandy-Walker Syndrome, peripheral neuropathy), skin (orange-peel skin, fat pads, inverted nipples, erythematous changes), endocrine system (hypothyroidism, hypogonadism), liver and gastrointestinal tract (hepatic fibrosis/cirrhosis, hepatomegaly, hypalbuminemia, ascites, failure to thrive, intestinal lymphangiectases, small bowel villous atrophy, abnormal intestinal permeability and enterocyte lipid transport, associated with abnormal glycosylation of intestinal glycoproteins, diarrhea, vomiting), and kidneys (renal cysts, proximal tubulopathy, nephritic syndrome). Other features include pleural effusions, osteopenia, recurrent fractures, kyphosis, dystrophic limbs, weakness, and joint contractures. The clinical picture of CDG type Ib differs markedly from the other forms of CDG, presenting as a protein-losing enteropathy, hyperinsulinemic hypoglycemia, and thrombosis or bleeding disorder. Generalized hypotonia is the only neurologic abnormality in CDG type Ib. Mannose substitution in these patients is an effective treatment. Death in early infancy has been described in a few patients with CDG.

In CDG type IIc, patients present with moderate-to-severe psychomotor retardation, seizures, hypotonia, strabismus, and feeding difficulties. These patients are prone to recurrent infections due to deficient neutrophil motility and can have the so-called *Bombay blood phenotype,* in which the patient inherits two recessive alleles of the H gene and therefore does not express the "H" protein on the erythrocyte surface. Because the "H" protein is a precursor of the "A" and "B" antigens in the ABO system, patients lack these antigens (they have blood group O_h). These patients can basically receive blood only from another Bombay phenotype person. Because this anomaly is very rare, arrangements for blood transfusions must be made well in advance.

Conditions associated with a defect in O-glycosylation:

☞**Ehlers Danlos Syndrome:** A heterogeneous group (9 types have been described) of inherited connective tissue disorders, characterized by joint hyperlaxity, skin extensibility and tissue fragility. A variant with progeroid features is caused by glucuronyltransferase/N-acetyl-D-hexosaminyltransferase deficiency.

☞**HARD Syndrome** (Acronym for: *H*ydrocephalus, *A*gyria, *R*etinal *D*ysplasia): A very rare and severe autosomal recessive, rapidly lethal syndrome with major neurological impairment. It is characterized by type II lissencephaly in association with retinal dysplasia, obstructive hydrocephalus, and agenesis of the corpus callosum. Affected infants typically have severe growth failure, severe microcephaly, seizures, microphthalmia, and cataracts. In addition, some affected infants have an occipital encephalocele.

Muscle Eye Brain Syndrome: This autosomal recessive inherited syndrome has many features in common with HARD Syndrome. It was first described by the Finnish physician Pirkko Santavuori in 1977. The main findings are congenital brain anomalies (pachygyria, polymicrogyria, hydrocephalus, and lissencephaly) with mental

Table C-1

CDG Type	CDG Subtype	Defect	Enzyme Defect	Clinical Presentation
I	Ia	N-glycosylation (assembly)	Phosphomannomutase II deficiency	Multisystem disease, hyperglycemia (see text)
	Ib	N-glycosylation (assembly)	Phosphomannose isomerase deficiency	Hyperinsulinemic hypoglycemia
	Ic	N-glycosylation (assembly)	Glycosyltransferase I deficiency	Hypotonia, strabismus, seizures
	Id	N-glycosylation (assembly)	Mannosyltransferase VI deficiency	Severe psychomotor retardation, brain anomalies, microcephaly, hypsarrhythmia
	Ie	N-glycosylation (assembly)	Dolichylphosphate-mannose synthase I deficiency	Severe psychomotor retardation, seizures, microcephaly
	If	N-glycosylation (assembly)	Lec35 deficiency	Severe encephalopathy, dwarfism, erythematous skin disorder
	Ig	N-glycosylation (assembly)	Mannosyltransferase VIII deficiency	Facial dysmorphism, psychomotor retardation, hypotonia, seizures, microcephaly
	Ih	N-glycosylation (assembly)	Glycosyltransferase II deficiency	Hepatomegaly, protein-losing enteropathy, ascites, hypalbuminemia
II	IIa	N-glycosylation (processing)	N-acetylglucosaminyl-transferase II deficiency	Craniofacial dysmorphism, psychomotor retardation, epilepsy, skeletal anomalies, coagulation factor XI deficiency
	IIb	N-glycosylation (processing)	Glucosidase I deficiency	Facial dysmorphism, hypotonia, seizures
	IIc	N-glycosylation (processing)	GDP-fucose transporter deficiency	Craniofacial dysmorphism, severe psychomotor and growth retardation, recurrent bacterial infections
	IId	N-glycosylation (processing)	β-1,4-Galactosyltransferase I deficiency	Psychomotor retardation, Dandy-Walker syndrome, myopathy
Progeroid variant of Ehlers-Danlos syndrome		O-glycosylation	β-1,4-Galactosyltransferase VII deficiency	Psychomotor retardation, macrocephaly, progeria
Multiple exostoses syndrome		O-glycosylation	Glucuronyltransferase/-N-acetyl-D-hexosaminyl-transferase deficiency	Multiple osteochondromas in long bones
HARD syndrome		O-glycosylation	O-Mannosyltransferase I	Severe psychomotor retardation, brain and eye anomalies, muscle dystrophy
Muscle eye brain syndrome		O-glycosylation	O-Mannosyl-β-1,2-N-acetylglucosaminyl-transferase I	Severe psychomotor retardation and muscle weakness, seizures

CDG, Congenital disorder of glycosylation.

retardation and abnormal electroencephalogram, joint contractures, muscular dystrophy leading to generalized hypotonia and weakness (with increased levels of serum creatinine phosphokinase), and ocular lesions (retinal hypoplasia, glaucoma) resulting in impaired vision.

Multiple Exostoses Syndrome: Hereditary Multiple Exostoses (HME) is the only CDG that is inherited in an autosomal dominant fashion, although sporadic occurrence is responsible for approximately 10% of patients! Three different types of this disorder are known, each one resulting from a different genetic defect. The genetic defects of Type I, II, and III have been mapped to 8q24.11-q24.13, 11p12-p11, and 19p, respectively. The disorder is characterized by multiple epiphyseal exostoses of the long bones and the digits. Most of these exostoses do not grow any further once the patient has reached puberty, and treatment is often not required, however, in severe cases, the tumors may result in deformities of the forearms, spine, pelvis, knees, and ankles, or impose upon blood vessels, nerves, and tendons and, besides the locally destructive effects, also cause severe pain.

Precautions before anesthesia: Cardiac, renal, thyroid, and hepatic function should be assessed preoperatively. Pericardial and pleural effusions should be sought and drained preoperatively if significant. Obtain a complete coagulation status. Check history for seizures and treatment efficiency. Patients may be severely developmentally delayed, sedative premedication, and/or presence of the primary caregiver for induction of anesthesia may be helpful. Ensure that the patient either does not have the Bombay phenotype or that compatible blood products are available for a procedure with potential blood loss.

Anesthetic considerations: In CDG type Ia, there is a prothrombotic tendency, whereas in CDG type IIa there is a bleeding tendency. Impaired cardiac function may occur secondary to cardiomyopathy and pericardial effusions. Kyphosis, recurrent fractures, and contractures can make patient positioning difficult and require special attention.

Pharmacological implications: Chronic use of seizure medications and abnormalities of renal, hepatic, and thyroid function affect the metabolism and excretion of some anesthetic drugs. Drugs that reduce the seizure threshold or interfere with the antiepileptic treatment should be avoided. Avoid succinylcholine because of potentially exaggerated hyperkalemic response.

REFERENCES:
Aebi M, Helenius A, Schenk B, et al: Carbohydrate-deficient glycoprotein syndromes become congenital disorders of glycosylation: An updated nomenclature for CDG. *Glycoconj J* 16:669, 1999.

Jaeken J: Komrower Lecture. Congenital disorders of glycosylation (CDG): It's all in it! *J Inherit Metab Dis* 26:99, 2003.

Van Geet C, Jaeken J, Freson K, et al: Congenital disorders of glycosylation type Ia and IIa are associated with different primary haemostatic complications. *J Inherit Metab Dis* 24:477, 2001.

Carbon Baby Syndrome

At a glance: A form of progressive mucocutaneous pigmentation caused by singly dispersed melanosomes within keratinocytes.
Synonyms: Universal Acquired Melanosis; Progressive Black Carbon Hyperpigmentation of Infancy.
Incidence and genetic inheritance: Two case reports. Inheritance pattern is undetermined.

Clinical aspects: Diffuse and progressive hyperpigmentation that becomes generalized is present from early infancy on. Facial features include sparse scalp hair with decreased pigmentation, broad cheeks, long and bulbous nose, anomalies of the external female genitalia, and mental retardation. Histologic examination of the skin reveals a so-called "negroid pattern" in the epidermal melanosomes.
Anesthetic considerations: Mental retardation may result in increased anxiety and limited cooperation. Sedative and anxiolytic premedication and the presence of the primary caregiver during induction of anesthesia may be helpful. No other specific anesthetic considerations. Rule out other (more common) diseases that may cause abnormal pigmentation. In the neonate, diffuse discoloration may be caused by adrenal insufficiency and should be excluded prior to surgery or anesthesia. A transient gray-brown color can be seen following phototherapy for hyperbilirubinemia.

REFERENCE:
Ruiz-Maldonado R, Tamayo L, Fernandez-Diez J: Universal acquired melanosis. The carbon baby. *Arch Dermatol* 114:775, 1978.

Cardiogenital Syndrome

At a glance: An extremely rare and frequently lethal disease in infants characterized by cardiac and urogenital anomalies.
Synonyms: Genital Anomaly-Cardiomyopathy Syndrome; Najjar Syndrome.
Incidence and genetic inheritance: Fewer than 10 patients have been described. Autosomal recessive inheritance has been suggested (although to date this disorder has been described only in boys). Parental consanguinity seems to be a significant risk factor.
Clinical aspects: Urogenital features, which include hypospadias/epispadias, micropenis, testicular atrophy, and a bifid hypoplastic scrotum, are most likely caused by a primary testicular failure. Cardiomyopathy is frequent (myofiber disarray), and cardiac dysfunction may be rapidly progressive and severe in early infancy. Death usually results from cardiac failure. Additional features include anodontia, protruding lips, decreased sweating, decreased body hair, and mental retardation.
Anesthetic considerations: Anesthesia care has not been reported in this syndrome. Cardiac function should be assessed by echocardiography. A 12-lead electrocardiogram may show cardiac conduction defects. Serum electrolytes should be checked and disturbances corrected. Cardiac dysfunction should set a low threshold for invasive monitoring, and inotropic support may be required. Arrhythmias may occur. Decreased sweating may lead to abnormal thermoregulation. Mental retardation may result in increased anxiety and limited cooperation. Sedative and anxiolytic premedication and the presence of the primary caregiver during induction of anesthesia may be helpful.

REFERENCES:
Najjar SS, Der Kaloustian VM, Ardati KO: Genital anomaly and cardiomyopathy: A new syndrome. *Clin Genet* 26:371, 1984.

Najjar SS, Der Kaloustian VM, Nassif SI: Genital anomaly, mental retardation, and cardiomyopathy: A new syndrome? *J Pediatr* 83:286, 1973.

Thomas IT, Jewett T, Lantz P, et al: Najjar syndrome revisited. *Am J Med Genet* 47:1151, 1993.

Carey-Fineman-Ziter Syndrome

At a glance: Congenital syndrome characterized by a combination of Moebius syndrome and Pierre Robin sequence.

Synonym: Myopathy; Moebius Robin Syndrome.

Incidence: Fewer than 10 cases have been described. No sexual predilection.

Genetic inheritance: Autosomal recessive.

Pathophysiology: Not completely understood. Electromyography shows fasciculations and small motor units. Nerve conduction velocity and serum creatinine kinase are normal. Muscle biopsy shows a variation in fiber size, evidence of degeneration and regeneration, and a predominance of type II fibers.

Diagnosis: Based on clinical findings of the characteristic facies and muscular weakness. Neuromuscular investigations may confirm the diagnosis.

Clinical aspects: Microstomia and micrognathia occur secondary to partial absence of the mandible. Microcephaly, ptosis, ophthalmoplegia, downward slanting of the palpebral fissures, thin upper lip with long philtrum, arched palate or cleft palate, and absence or hypoplasia of the tongue may be observed. The pectoral muscles are absent or hypoplastic. Muscle weakness secondary to nonspecific primary myopathy predominantly affects the limbs, although facial weakness with an expressionless face has been described. Skeletal features include scoliosis, brachydactyly, varus deformity, and talipes equinovarus. Bulbar dysfunction can occur. Variants of this disease with central hypoventilation have been described. Laryngostenosis has been described in one patient. Intelligence is normal.

Precautions before anesthesia: Examination should be directed toward evaluation of the airway, degree of muscle weakness, and identification and treatment of active pulmonary infection (recurrent aspirations). Check for central hypoventilation syndrome. Depending on the procedure, postoperative mechanical ventilation may be required.

Anesthetic considerations: Anesthesia in these patients has not been described. However, the facial features suggest airway management most likely will be difficult. Maintain spontaneous ventilation until the airway has been secured. Although patients are at increased risk for aspiration because of bulbar palsy, a rapid sequence intubation technique cannot safely be accomplished in the presence of a potentially difficult airway. Alternatively, awake fiberoptic intubation can be used.

Pharmacological implications: Avoid neuromuscular blockers until the airway has been secured. Succinylcholine is best avoided in myopathic syndromes. Expect patients to be very sensitive to the respiratory depressant effects of anesthetic drugs.

Other conditions to be considered:

☞**MOEBIUS SYNDROME:** A rare developmental disorder characterized by facial paralysis already present at birth. Facial nerve development is absent, and the sixth (abducens) and seventh (facialis) cranial nerves are most often affected. Other features include numerous abnormalities of the orofacial region and malformations of the limbs. Mental retardation occurs in approximately 10% of patients.

☞**PIERRE ROBIN SYNDROME:** A syndrome with multiple etiologies resulting from mandibular aplasia. Characterized by the association of cleft palate, glossoptosis, and micrognathia.

BRADDOCK CAREY SYNDROME (Thrombocytopenia Robin Sequence): Features are similar and associated with thrombocytopenia, deafness, short stature, and absent scalp hair. Extremely rare disorder (described in two girls only) with a characteristic dysmorphism (microcephaly, facial anomalies with Pierre Robin sequence, agenesis of the corpus callosum, enamel hypoplasia, and chronic thrombocytopenia, although megakaryocytes can be adequate) already present in the neonatal period. Mental retardation with developmental and growth delay was noted in both patients.

REFERENCES:

Carey JC, Fineman RM, Ziter FA: The Robin sequence as a consequence of malformation, dysplasia and neuromuscular syndromes. *J Pediatr* 101:858, 1982.

Ryan A, Marshall T, FitzPatrick DR: Carey-Fineman-Ziter (CFZ) syndrome: Report on affected sibs. *Am J Med Genet* 82:110, 1999.

Verloes A, Bitoun P, Heuskin A, et al: Mobius sequence, Robin complex, and hypotonia: severe expression of brainstem disruption spectrum versus Carey-Fineman-Ziter syndrome. *Am J Med Genet A* 127: 277, 2004.

Carmi Syndrome

At a glance: A form of junctional epidermolysis bullosa that is associated with pyloric atresia and often results in death in the first year of life.

Synonyms: Epidermolysis Bullosa Lethalis with Pyloric Atresia; Aplasia Cutis Congenita with Gastrointestinal Atresia.

Incidence: Approximately 70 cases have been reported. Junctional epidermolysis bullosa accounts for approximately 1% of all epidermolysis bullosa cases.

Genetic inheritance: Autosomal recessive. The genetic defects have been mapped to 17q11-qter and chromosome 2.

Pathophysiology: In junctional epidermolysis bullosa, blister formation in the plane of the lamina lucida results in separation of the epidermis from the basal lamina. The hemidesmosome content in the lamina lucida of these patients often is significantly reduced in quantity and quality (structural anomalies). The bullae per se heal without superficial scarring; however, erosions provide an easy portal of entry for bacteria, which trigger inflammation and marked fibrosis. Intestinal obstruction can result from separation of the intestinal mucosal layer, which is followed by a secondary inflammatory reaction and fibrosis, causing obliteration of the intestinal lumen. The condition has been postulated to result from a mutation in two of the integrin genes (integrin alpha-6 and integrin beta-4), which appears to affect the integrity of the basement membrane, the hemidesmosomes, and the control of the normal scarring process during wound healing. The sequence of events is initiated by separation of the epidermis or intestinal mucosal layers from the basal lamina. The resulting inflammatory reaction triggers massive fibrosis involving the deep layers of the tissue and leading to damage of skin and obstruction of the intestinal lumen. If aplasia cutis congenita is present, mixed skin lesions with blisters and patchy lack of skin can be seen.

Diagnosis: Based on the clinical findings of epidermolysis bullosa or aplasia cutis congenita associated with gastrointestinal signs. Transmission electron microscopy and immunofluorescence mapping can be used to confirm the diagnosis. Elevated amniotic fluid α-fetoprotein levels have been described in some cases.

Clinical aspects: Polyhydramnios in the last trimester and premature delivery occur frequently. The skin may initially appear normal, but there may already be areas of blistering and skin loss. Bullae form easily in response to minor trauma. In the first year of life, a pathognomonic, chronic perinasal, and/or perioral crusted lesion may appear. One study reported mixed skin lesions, including blisters and a patchy lack of skin, in all affected infants. All skin layers are involved and show marked dystrophic changes. Nails may be either absent or severely dystrophic. Almost all patients have intestinal obstructions, especially membranous pyloric atresia or stenosis. Intestinal obstruction results from proliferative connective tissue changes. Pyloric atresia presents with nonbilious vomiting, which may be projectile. Esophageal atresia has been described. Epidermolysis bullosa-like lesions may affect the respiratory tract and cause acute respiratory failure. Commonly associated anomalies include aplasia cutis congenita (43%) and obstruction at the ureterovesical junction (14%), which may lead to bilateral hydronephrosis. The high mortality of up to 80% in the first year of life is most often due to systemic sepsis (from skin infections) and/or chronic diarrhea with protein-losing gastroenteropathy, which occurs despite successful surgical correction of gastrointestinal atresia.

Precautions before anesthesia: Assess for, and correct if necessary, dehydration, anemia, hypoproteinemia, and serum electrolyte abnormalities in the presence of diarrhea and protein-losing enteropathy. Hypokalemic metabolic alkalosis may be present. Assess airway patency and renal function. Adequate premedication may prevent struggling with an uncooperative patient and thus help reduce resultant skin damage.

Anesthetic considerations: The goal is to prevent trauma to skin and mucosal surfaces by appropriate positioning and padding. Because shearing forces potentially cause the most damage, monitoring should not include the use of adhesive gels or tapes. The sticky surround of the electrocardiogram electrodes must be removed. Alternatively, needle electrodes have been used successfully. Intravenous (and other) cannulas can be sutured in place. Wrapping the limbs in soft padding prior to use of automated blood pressure recording devices helps prevent skin lesions. The pressure from an anesthetic face mask may be damaging, so it should be held gently just above the face. Soft face masks with an air cuff seal and generous use of Vaseline cream (to reduce shearing forces to the skin) may be advantageous. Likewise, oropharyngeal airways should be used only if absolutely necessary. Whenever possible, endotracheal intubation is avoided because of the risk of inducing laryngotracheobronchial bullae formation, which may result in proximal airway obstruction. If required, intubation should be done as gently as possible with a well-lubricated, undersized tube. Once intubated, any movement of the endotracheal tube must be prevented (e.g., changing head position, coughing) and endotracheal suctioning must be avoided, if possible. Use of intravenous ketamine (e.g., in combination with propofol or midazolam) in a spontaneously breathing patient has been described, as have various techniques involving maintenance of anesthesia via volatile agents delivered through head boxes or gently applied face masks. Hypothermia may develop rapidly, so temperature should be carefully monitored, and warming devices such as convective forced-air warmers should be used.

Pharmacological implications: Patients may be on (systemic or topical) phenytoin therapy because its use reportedly decreases collagenase activity, increases fibroblast contractility and trauma tolerance, and accelerates wound healing. Anabolic and glucocorticoid steroids are sometimes used in this condition, so extra steroid coverage may be required in the perioperative period.

Other conditions to be considered:

☞**EPIDERMOLYSIS BULLOSA:** A genetic disorder characterized by cutaneous blistering and scarring following already minor trauma. The more than 20 different subtypes of the disease have been grouped into three main categories: epidermolysis bullosa simplex, dystrophic epidermolysis bullosa, and junctional epidermolysis bullosa.

☞**PEMPHIGUS:** Rare autoimmune blistering disease that affects the skin and mucous membranes. Patients have circulating antibodies to an intercellular cement substance of the basal membrane.

REFERENCES:

Holzman RS, Worthen HM, Johnson KL: Anesthesia for children with junctional epidermolysis bullosa (lethalis). *Can J Anaesth* 34:395, 1987.

Maman E, Maor E, Kachko L, et al: Epidermolysis bullosa, pyloric atresia, aplasia cutis congenita: Histopathological delineation of an autosomal recessive disease. *Am J Med Genet* 78:127, 1998.

Morrel DS, Fine JD: Junctional epidermolysis bullosa with pyloric stenosis. *Pediatr Dermatol* 18:539, 2001.

Carnevale-Canun-Mendoza Syndrome

At a glance: Autosomal dominant disease combining osteolysis, amyotrophy, and nephropathy.

Synonyms: Multicentric Osteolysis Nephropathy; Hereditary Osteolysis of Carpal Bones with Nephropathy.

Incidence and genetic inheritance: Approximately 100 cases have been reported worldwide. Autosomal dominant inheritance has been described, but many cases seem to be de novo mutations.

Clinical aspects: Diagnosis can be made within the first year of life. However, clinical appearance is variable and involves the head (triangular face, exophthalmia, corneal clouding, micrognathia, retrognathia), the skeleton (onset with arthritis-like episodes affecting primarily the ankles [tarsal bones] and wrists [carpal bones], radiologically resulting in osteolytic changes with progressive deformities and later complete osteolysis and a variable degree of disability secondary to restricted joint mobility, with additional skeletal features of multifocal osteolyses, pes cavus, narrow diaphyses, metacarpal anomalies, and camptodactyly), and the muscles (amyotrophy, cachectic build, electromyographic abnormalities). Arterial hypertension and renal disease resulting from arteriolar intima proliferation and media hypertrophy. Focal glomerulosclerosis and proteinuria have been described. Renal insufficiency may start in the second or third decade of life. Death resulting from azotemia in these patients has occurred. One patient suffered from valvular pulmonary stenosis. Some patients are described as having a marfanoid habitus.

Anesthetic considerations: To our knowledge, anesthesia has not been described in this condition. Renal function and blood pressure should be evaluated preoperatively. These patients most likely already are taking or should begin receiving antihypertensive medication. Facial features suggest airway management may be difficult. Avoid neuromuscular blockers and maintain spontaneous ventilation until the airway has been secured. Use of succinylcholine has not been evaluated, and the risk of malignant hyperthermia is unknown. Trigger agents should not be used or should be used with caution only in the presence of a myopathy. Abnormal response to neuromuscular blockers is possible. Renal failure may alter the metabolism and excretion of some anesthetic agents. Preoperative blood work should include a complete blood count, serum electrolytes, blood urea nitrogen, and creatinine. Avoid sudden and significant decreases in arterial blood pressure.

REFERENCES:

Carnevale A, Canun S, Mendoza L, et al: Idiopathic multicentric osteolysis with facial anomalies and nephropathy. *Am J Med Genet* 26:877, 1987.

Costa MM, Santos H, Santos MJ, et al: Idiopathic multicentric osteolysis: A rare disease mimicking juvenile chronic arthritis. *Clin Rheumatol* 15:97, 1996.

Shinohara O, Kubota C, Kimura M, et al: Essential osteolysis associated with nephropathy, corneal opacity, and pulmonary stenosis. *Am J Med Genet* 15:482, 1991.

Carnevale-Hernandez-Castillo-Torres Syndrome

At a glance: A disorder that results in anatomical anomalies of the hands and feet.

Synonym: Triphalangeal Thumbs and Brachyectrodactyly Syndrome.

Incidence and genetic inheritance: The few cases reported relate to four kindreds mainly from Mexico. It occurs either sporadically or as an autosomal dominant inherited syndrome with highly variable expression.

Clinical aspects: The syndrome is diagnosed based on the clinical findings of congenital anomalies of the hands and feet. These findings are principally restricted to the extremities and include triphalangeal thumbs, brachy(syn)dactyly of the index fingers and third toes and occasionally ectrodactyly of the hands and feet. Short stature, ectrodactyly (more often of the feet than of the hands), and onychodystrophy occasionally occur.

Anesthetic considerations: Anesthesia for patients with this condition has not been reported. The mainly peripheral nature of the features and the absence of associated organ dysfunction suggest no specific precautions should be necessary.

REFERENCES:

Carnevale A, Hernandez M, del Castillo V: A new syndrome of triphalangeal thumbs and brachyectrodactyly. *Clin Genet* 18:244, 1980.

Silengo MC, Biagioli M, Bell GL, et al: Triphalangeal thumb and brachy-ectrodactyly syndrome: Confirmation of autosomal dominant inheritance. *Clin Genet* 31:13, 1987.

Zenteno JC, Aguinaga M, Chavez V, et al: Triphalangeal thumb and brachyectrodactyly syndrome: An uncommon entity with evidence of geographic distribution. *Clin Genet* 50:152, 1996.

Carnevale-Krajewska-Fischetto Syndrome

At a glance: Genetic disorder with facial features, hip dislocation, and diminished abdominal musculature.

Synonym: Ptosis Strabismus Diastasis.

Incidence and genetic inheritance: Extremely rare. The two brothers described had consanguineous parents, hence autosomal recesssive inheritance has been suggested.

Clinical aspects: Diagnosis is based on the clinical findings. Facial features include depressed nasal bridge, hypertelorism, blepharophimosis, blepharoptosis, and paresis of ocular muscles with strabismus. The ears are low set with a folded helix, and the external auditory canal may be atretic or absent. Vision and hearing may be impaired. The palate may be arched and narrow. Hip dysplasia leads to dislocation. Aplasia or hypoplasia of the abdominal muscles results in diastasis. Pronation and supination are limited, but flexion and extension in the elbow are normal. Short stature, mild mental retardation, and cryptorchidism present in both patients.

Anesthetic considerations: Anesthesia in these patients has not been described. The presence of a narrow, arched palate may make tracheal intubation difficult. Abdominal muscle defects may lead to postoperative ventilation problems. Postoperative mechanical ventilation may therefore be required. Patient cooperation may be limited secondary to mental retardation and impaired hearing and vision. Sedative and anxiolytic premedication and the presence of the primary caregiver during induction of anesthesia may be helpful.

REFERENCE:

Carnevale F, Krajewska G, Fischetto R, et al: Ptosis of eyelids, strabismus, diastasis recti, hip defect, cryptorchidism, and developmental delay in two sibs. *Am J Med Genet* 33:186, 1989.

Carney Complex

At a glance: Carney complex consists of spotty skin pigmentation in association with multiple neoplasias (mainly cardiac and endocrine tumors). The two types of Carney complex are type I and type II. Both types show the same clinical features.

Synonyms: Myxoma-Spotty Pigmentation-Endocrine Overactivity; Carney Syndrome.

History: Initially, the term NAME syndrome (acronym for *n*evi, *a*trial myxomas, *m*yxoid neurofibroma, *e*phelides) was proposed for this condition. Later, the term LAMB syndrome (acronym for *l*entigines, *a*trial myxomas, *m*ucocutaneous myxomas, *b*lue nevi) was suggested. Both syndromes now are part of the Carney complex. The American physician J.A. Carney reviewed several of these cases in 1985 and suggested a common pathogenetic link between the clinical findings.

Incidence: In the United States, cardiac myxomas occur with a frequency of 5–10:10,000, of which approximately 7% are associated with Carney syndrome. The syndrome can present at any age and in either sex. No sexual predilection has been found.

Genetic inheritance: Autosomal dominant with variable penetrance. Because type I has been researched more thoroughly, we discuss this type here. It is caused by mutations of the PRKAR1A gene (*p*rotein *k*inase, c-*A*MP-dependent, *r*egulatory, type *I*, *a*lpha, also called tissue specific extinguisher 1), which is an important regulator of the serine-threonine kinase activity catalyzed by the protein kinase A holoenzyme, and has been mapped to 17q22-q24. The exact function of PRKAR1A in cell cycle regulation, growth, and/or proliferation in general and Carney complex syndrome in particular remains to be elucidated, but a function as a tumor suppressor gene has been discussed.

Pathophysiology: Cardiac myxomas, while histologically benign, may cause embolic phenomena, valvular obstruction, and heart failure. Myxomas are also found in the thyroid and adrenal glands, brain, breasts, and testes. Nonmyxomatous tumors, such as Sertoli cell tumors of the testis, pituitary adenomas, and psammomatous melanotic schwannomas, may occur. Primary pigmented nodular adrenocortical disease, a characteristic micronodular form of bilateral adrenal hyperplasia, causes a unique, inherited form of Cushing syndrome. Thyroid and pituitary dysfunction have been observed.

Systemic symptoms may be caused by overproduction of the proinflammatory cytokine interleukin-6 by myxoma cells.

Diagnosis: Based on the clinical findings of pigmented skin lesions associated with neoplasias (particularly myxomas). The mean age at the time of diagnosis is 10 to 20 years.

Clinical aspects: Skin manifestations include dark pigmented skin lesions (lentigines). Although they can be found anywhere on the body, they typically are located in the center of the face (i.e., periorally, perinasally, periorbitally, and in the sclerae). The finding of lentigines on the lips in association with a myxoma or an endocrine disorder/tumor should prompt further examinations to rule out Carney complex. Urogenital (vulvar) lentigines also are considered characteristic for this disorder. Cardiac myxomas may be solitary or multiple and can occur in any cardiac chamber, although almost 90% occur in one of the atria. The left atrium accounts for 80% of all atrial myxomas. After resection they may recur (approximately in 10–20% of cases) at the same or different intracardiac and/or extracardiac sites. Cardiac myxomas account for 25% of deaths in patients with Carney complex. A history of neurologic deficits or transient ischemic attacks may be present if tumor embolization has occurred. Systemic manifestations such as fever, arthralgia, elevated erythrocyte sedimentation rate, and lupus-like rashes may accompany some myxomas. Extracardiac myxomas (of breast, testis, thyroid, brain, adrenal gland) and nonmyxomatous tumors (e.g., Sertoli cell and Leydig cell tumor of the testis, pituitary adenomas, and psammomatous melanotic schwannomas [mainly esophagus and stomach, but also along the paraspinal sympathetic ganglia]) have been described. Pituitary adenomas may result in hyperprolactinemia and acromegaly.

Precautions before anesthesia: Anesthesia management will be influenced by the presence of cardiac involvement and the type of endocrinopathy. Initial biochemical endocrine assessment should consist of venous thyroxine/thyroid-stimulating hormone, cortisol, and growth hormone levels. Abnormalities should be further assessed by an endocrinologist. Renal function and glucose and electrolyte levels should be checked. Echocardiography should be performed to determine the presence, size, number, localization, and hemodynamic significance of cardiac myxomas. Results of electrocardiography usually are normal unless valvular dysfunction is present. The presence of back pain and/or radiculopathy may indicate a spinal tumor and warrants further (predominantly radiologic) investigation.

Anesthetic considerations: Cardiac myxomas may cause low cardiac output by valvular obstruction. Hypoxemia may occur secondary to tumor embolization and intracardiac right-to-left shunts via a patent foramen ovale. Intraoperative transesophageal echocardiography may be useful in guiding volume management and inotropic support. Pulmonary artery catheterization is relatively contraindicated (especially with right-sided intracardiac myxomas). The hemodynamic effects of the myxoma may be position dependent. Cardiovascular collapse on induction of anesthesia and sudden death have been reported. Preoperative pharmacological control of endocrinopathy is indicated. Close perioperative control of blood glucose levels in the presence of diabetes (Cushing syndrome, acromegaly) is mandatory. Airway management could be difficult if the features of acromegaly are pronounced (macroglossia, prominent jaw). Hypertension and hypokalemia may occur in association with Cushing syndrome and warrant correction.

Pharmacological implications: Antibiotic prophylaxis may be indicated in the presence of valvular involvement. Anticoagulation does not appear to reduce the incidence of embolic events from myxomas. Patients who are receiving or have undergone previous medical or surgical treatment for Cushing syndrome may require perioperative steroidal supplementation.

Other condition to be considered:

☞**MULTIPLE ENDOCRINE NEOPLASIA:** Consists of benign, and sometimes malignant tumors (often multiple in a tissue) of the parathyroids, enteropancreatic neuroendocrine system, anterior pituitary gland, and other tissues. Skin angiofibromas and skin collagenomas are common.

REFERENCES:

Mortiz HA, Azad SS: Right atrial myxoma: Case report and anaesthetic considerations. *Can J Anaesth* 36:212, 1989.

Wilkes D, McDermott DA, Basson CT: Clinical phenotypes and molecular genetic mechanisms of Carney complex. *Lancet Oncol* 6:501, 2005.

Szokol JW, Franklin M, Murphy GS, et al: Left ventricular mass in a patient with Carney's complex. *Anesth Analg* 95:874, 2002.

Carnitine Deficiency

At a glance: A disorder that results from decreased carnitine concentrations in plasma and tissues preventing mitochondria from adequate beta oxidation. Primary and secondary defects have been described. The manifestations are cardiomyopathy, encephalopathy, and myopathy.

Synonyms: Systemic Carnitine Deficiency; Primary Carnitine Deficiency.

Incidence: For primary defects, the incidence is as high as 1 in 40,000 live births (Japan). The incidence for secondary causes is unknown.

Genetic inheritance: Autosomal recessive. Evidence exists that primary carnitine deficiency is caused by mutations in the *SLC22A5* (*sol*ute *c*arrier family 22 [organic cation transporter] member 5) gene, which has been mapped to 5q33.1. *SLC22A5* is also called *OCTN2* (organic cation/carnitine transporter 2) gene. Heterozygotes for primary carnitine deficiency have a higher risk of late-onset cardiac hypertrophy than normal individuals.

Pathophysiology: Carnitine is derived from diet, but is also endogenously synthesized from lysine in the liver and kidneys. It is taken up from the plasma into peripheral tissues by a high-affinity, sodium-dependent carnitine cotransporter. Primary carnitine deficiency results from a decreased function of this cotransporter, leading to low intracellular and high urine carnitine levels. Biologic effects of carnitine deficiency do not occur unless the carnitine levels are at least below 20% of the norm. Carnitine is required for intracellular esterification of long-chain fatty acids, and its absence inhibits their entry into mitochondria. Beta oxidation of long-chain fatty acids and ketone bodies and energy production are consequently impaired. Carnitine further plays a role in increasing the ratio between free and acylated coenzyme A (acyl-CoA) by binding and assisting in the elimination of acyl residues. The resulting intramitochondrial accumulation of acyl-CoA esters in carnitine deficiency affects the pathways of the intermediary metabolism (e.g., Krebs cycle, pyruvate oxidation), which all require CoA. Low muscle carnitine levels in the presence of normal serum levels characterize myopathic carnitine deficiency, which is limited to the muscle only. It seems to result from a defect in the muscle carnitine transporter. Secondary carnitine deficiency may be seen in organic acidemia, disorders of fatty acid oxidation (e.g., medium-chain acyl-CoA dehydrogenase deficiency), in preterm infants, especially those receiving total parenteral nutrition without carnitine supplementation, Fanconi renal tubulopathy, and in patients taking valproic acid (decreased renal tubular reabsorption of carnitine) or zidovudine.

Diagnosis: Both primary and secondary carnitine deficiency may present as sudden death. Older children frequently present with symptoms of heart failure as a result of progressive cardiomyopathy that typically does not respond to diuretic therapy or inotropic agents. Symptoms may progress rapidly. Younger children may present with hypoglycemic and hypoketotic encephalopathy, which may be triggered by fasting or intercurrent illness. A skin biopsy can be used to confirm reduced carnitine transport in fibroblasts that express the transporter, which is diagnostic of primary deficiency. Muscle biopsy may be required for diagnosis of secondary disorders.

Clinical aspects: Most commonly the disorder affects the heart (progressive cardiomyopathy with cardiomegaly), but it also affects the central nervous system (encephalopathy with lethargy, somnolence, coma, sensorimotor neuropathy, muscle weakness and hypotonia) and the eyes (pigmented retinopathy). Other features may include hepatomegaly, abdominal pain, vomiting and diarrhea. Laboratory findings may include hypoglycemia, decreased levels of carnitine in plasma, liver, and muscle, high fasting plasma fatty acids, hyperammonemia, and absence of ketonuria. A complete blood count may reveal a hypochromic, microcytic anemia.

Precautions before anesthesia: Assess cardiac rhythm and function by electrocardiography, echocardiography, and/or radionucleotide techniques. Elective surgery should be deferred in the presence of impaired cardiac function or arrhythmias because carnitine supplementation can improve cardiac function, muscle strength, and ketone production. However, carnitine therapy in long-chain fatty acid oxidation defects is controversial because long-chain acylcarnitines may have toxic effects and have proarrhythmogenic effects, which may result in sudden cardiac death. Obtain blood work for a complete blood count, serum electrolyte levels, prothrombin and partial thromboplastin times, and kidney and liver function. Check acid-base status in the presence of prolonged vomiting/diarrhea.

Anesthetic considerations: Avoid prolonged preoperative fasting and start a dextrose-containing infusion at the beginning of the fasting period. Ensure normal glucose levels perioperatively by repeated measurements and further administration of intravenous dextrose as necessary. Ensure carnitine supplementation has been taken as usual.

Pharmacological implications: Avoid valproic acid and zidovudine. Succinylcholine probably is best avoided if myopathic features are present or suspected.

Other conditions to be considered:

☞**Carnitine Palmitoyltransferase Deficiency:** Carnitine palmitoyltransferase (CPT) deficiency is a group of disorders caused by defects in the enzymes CPT I or II. CPT I is the most common human lipid myopathy. The metabolic myopathy can be triggered by effort, anesthesia, or stress and results in episodes of rhabdomyolysis and myoglobinuria.

☞**Isovaleric Acidemia:** A genetic disorder affecting the branched chain organic acids, the most frequent form of leucine metabolism disorders. It results in accumulation of isovaleric acid (and its metabolites), leading to vomiting, dehydration, severe metabolic acidosis, and neurologic manifestations.

☞**Methylmalonic Acidemia:** A heterogeneous inborn error of metabolism affecting the amino acid metabolism, leading to

metabolic acidosis and accumulation of methylmalonic acid and its by-products.

☞**Propionic Acidemia:** An inborn error of metabolism affecting the mitochondrial catabolism of valine and isoleucine. Untreated it results in ketoacidosis, lethargy, coma, and finally death.

References:

Rinaldo P, Stanley CA, Hsu BY, et al: Sudden neonatal death in carnitine transporter deficiency. *J Pediatr* 131:304, 1997.

Rowe RW, Helander E: Anesthetic management of a patient with systemic carnitine deficiency. *Anesth Analg* 71:295, 1990.

Wang Y, Korman SH, Ye J, et al: Phenotype and genotype variation in primary carnitine deficiency. *Genet Med* 3:387, 2001.

Carnitine Palmitoyltransferase Deficiency

At a glance: Carnitine palmitoyltransferase (CPT) deficiency is a group of disorders caused by defects in the enzymes CPT I or II. Type I is the most common human lipid myopathy. The metabolic myopathy can be triggered by effort, anesthesia/surgery, or stress and results in episodes of rhabdomyolysis and myoglobinuria.

Synonyms: Metabolic Myopathy and Carnitine Palmitoyltransferase Deficiency.

Incidence: CPT deficiency is the most common metabolic cause of recurrent myoglobinuria.

Genetic inheritance: Autosomal recessive. Three polymorphisms and more than 20 mutations have been identified in the *CPT2* gene among patients with CPT II deficiency, with the responsible genetic defect mapped to 1p32. The mutations for the hepatic and muscle isoforms of CPT I are located on 11q13 and 22q13.3, respectively.

Pathophysiology: CPT I and II exist as two functionally distinct mitochondrial enzymes, embedded in the outer (CPT I) and inner (CPT II) mitochondrial membranes. Both are involved in facilitation of the transmembranous transport of fatty acids into the mitochondria.

Diagnosis: Skin/muscle biopsy may be required to confirm the diagnosis. Prompt diagnosis can help to avoid risk factors and to prevent rhabdomyolysis and renal failure secondary to myoglobinuria.

Clinical aspects: CPT I exists in hepatic and muscle isoforms. To date, only hepatic CPT deficiency has been reported to cause clinical symptoms. In infancy, hepatic CPT I normally presents as recurrent hypoketotic, hypoglycemic coma triggered by fasting, exercise, intercurrent illness, cold stress, or a high-fat/low-carbohydrate diet. Additional findings during these acute episodes include metabolic acidosis, hepatomegaly with raised transaminases, hyperammonemia, and seizures. CPT I is normally not associated with cardiomyopathy or myopathy, although arrhythmias have been reported in pediatric patients, particularly in the infantile form. The results of liver function tests may remain pathologic for a few weeks before normalization is reestablished. CPT II deficiency is most commonly manifested in adulthood as intermittent episodes of myoglobinuria and myalgia occurring after exercise, fasting, sleep deprivation, (febrile) intercurrent illnesses, and anesthesia/surgery. Acute renal failure and cardiac arrest secondary to anesthesia-related rhabdomyolysis have been described. Between attacks, the patients may be asymptomatic, and electromyography, serum creatine kinase activity, and the response of serum lactate to ischemic exercise usually are normal. A rare infantile form of CPT II deficiency may present as fatal hypoglycemia with coma and/or with multiorgan involvement (cardiomyopathy, hepatic failure, and muscle weakness).

Precautions before anesthesia: Liver and renal function and serum levels of electrolytes, carnitine, glucose, creatine kinase, and ammonia should be assessed preoperatively. Twelve-lead and/or Holter electrocardiography may be required if the history or examination suggests arrhythmias. In case of cardiomyopathy, echocardiography is recommended. The preoperative fasting period should be kept as short as possible. The recommendation is to start a dextrose-containing infusion at the beginning of the fasting period. Sedative and anxiolytic premedication may be helpful in reducing perioperative stress.

Anesthetic considerations: Acute deteriorations including coma and rhabdomyolysis may be precipitated by fasting, hypoglycemia, and perioperative stress. The minimum allowable duration of fasting should be considered, and patients should be given dextrose-containing intravenous fluids to prevent hypoglycemia. CPT-deficient patients may be susceptible to malignant hyperthermia: one group of researchers found that a subset of individuals in patients with known malignant hyperthermia phenotype had a primary deficiency of carnitine palmitoyltransferase and that others had a milder enzyme deficiency secondary to the primary defect in malignant hyperthermia. Regional anesthesia for intraoperative and postoperative analgesia significantly reduces the stress response and provides reasonable alternatives to general anesthesia and exposure to potential trigger agents. Dehydration should be avoided.

Pharmacological implications: Malignant hyperthermia trigger agents should be avoided.

Other conditions to be considered:

☞**CARNITINE DEFICIENCY:** A disorder caused by decreased carnitine concentrations in plasma and tissues preventing mitochondria from adequate beta oxidation. Primary and secondary defects have been described. The manifestations are cardiomyopathy, encephalopathy, and myopathy.

☞**MYOADENYLATE DEAMINASE DEFICIENCY:** Either primary genetic disease affecting the muscle purine nucleotide metabolism or secondary to another neuromuscular or metabolic disease. It is found in up to 2% of muscle biopsies submitted for pathologic examination.

☞**PHOSPHOGLYCERATE KINASE DEFICIENCY:** A rare congenital enzymatic defect in glycolysis, mainly affecting the muscles and erythrocytes.

☞**REYE SYNDROME:** May present similar to infantile CPT I. A potentially life-threatening, multifactorial syndrome resulting from a previous viral infection treated by aspirin and a genetic sensibility. Dehydration, intracranial hypertension, and liver failure must be considered. Presentation includes vomiting, lethargy, irrational behavior, and delirium. Tachypnea, jaundice, fever, and coma suggest end-stage disease. Reye syndrome usually appears 3 to 5 days after the onset of chickenpox rash.

REFERENCES:

Katsuya H, Misumi M, Ohtani Y, et al: Postanesthetic acute renal failure due to carnitine palmityl transferase deficiency. *Anesthesiology* 68:945, 1988.

Neuvonen PT, van den Berg AA: Postoperative coma in a child with carnitine palmitoyltransferase I deficiency. *Anesth Analg* 92:646, 2001.

Vladutiu GD, Hogan K, Saponara I, et al: Carnitine palmitoyl transferase deficiency in malignant hyperthermia. *Muscle Nerve* 16:485, 1993.

Carnosinemia

At a glance: An inherited metabolic disorder characterized by severe mental defect and myoclonic seizures.

Synonyms: (Serum-) Carnosinase Deficiency; Beta-Alanine-Pyruvate Aminotransferase; Hyper-Beta Carnosinemia

Incidence and genetic inheritance: Fewer than 10 cases have been described. Autosomal recessive transmission with the mutation located on 18q21.3. Parental consanguinity has been described in some of the cases.

Clinical aspects: Progressive neurologic disorder with variable phenotype associated with severe mental retardation, myoclonic seizures, tremor, and hypotonia caused by a defect in carnosinase activity. Central nervous system findings at autopsy may include severe axonal degeneration, loss of Purkinje fibers, and neuraxonal spheroids in the gray matter as a result of demyelinization and reactive fibrosis. Carnosine, a dipeptide of histidine and alanine, is found in significant concentrations in meat. A strictly meat-free diet can result in amelioration of the symptoms, but does not provide a cure. Deficiency of carnosinase results in high serum and urine levels of carnosine.

Anesthetic considerations: Anesthesia in these patients has not been described. Patient cooperation may be limited secondary to mental retardation. Sedative and anxiolytic premedication and the presence of the primary caregiver during induction of anesthesia may be helpful. Consider interaction between anesthetic drugs and antiepileptic treatment and avoid drugs that reduce the seizure threshold.

REFERENCES:

Willi SM, Zhang Y, Hill JB, et al: A deletion in the long arm of chromosome 18 in a child with serum carnosinase deficiency. *Pediatr Res* 41:210, 1997.

Wisniewski K, Fleisher L, Rassin D, et al: Neurological disease in a child with carnosinase deficiency. *Neuropediatrics* 12:143, 1981.

Caroli Disease and Caroli Syndrome

At a glance: A congenital disorder of the intrahepatic bile ducts characterized by intrahepatic dilatation of the biliary tree, which may result in cholangitis, cholelithiasis, sepsis, hepatic failure, and portal hypertension.

Synonyms: Congenital Dilatation of Intrahepatic Bile Ducts; Communicating Cavernous Ectasia of Intrahepatic Bile Ducts; Choledochal Cysts Type V (Todani classification).

Incidence: The exact incidence is not known but is considered to be very low (probably fewer than 200 cases described in the literature). Caroli syndrome occurs more frequently than Caroli disease (see *Clinical Aspects* for differentiation). Both forms are more common in females.

Genetic inheritance: Not precisely known. Autosomal recessive has been suggested for both Caroli disease and Caroli syndrome.

Pathophysiology: In Caroli disease, polycystic segmentation of the larger intrahepatic bile ducts (segmental, left and right) occurs, whereas in Caroli syndrome the ductal abnormalities are more widespread. Both forms are characterized by fibrosis of the portal tracts. Both Caroli disease and Caroli syndrome are thought to originate from a pathologic development in the formation of the ductal plate. The ductal plate originates from hepatocytes surrounding the intrahepatic portal vein branches. Further differentiation during fetal life results in the formation of small tubules, which coalesce to form the intrahepatic biliary tree. Failure of the ductal plate to differentiate are summarized as ductal plate malformations. The anomalous structure of the intrahepatic bile ducts leads to saccular or fusiform dilatation and ectasia with biliary stasis, cholelithiasis, cholangitis with intrahepatic abscesses, and recurrent sepsis.

Diagnosis: Diagnosis of exclusion. Fetal ultrasound examination of liver and kidneys during pregnancy has resulted in prenatal diagnosis of Caroli disease/syndrome. However, further radiologic investigations (computed tomography scanning, magnetic resonance imaging, cholangiography), endoscopic retrograde cholangiopancreatography, and liver biopsy may be required to confirm the diagnosis. Approximately half of the patients also have extrahepatic fusiform enlargement of the common hepatic and common bile duct.

Clinical aspects: The findings in Caroli disease are limited to ectasia or segmental dilatation of the larger intrahepatic ducts. In Caroli syndrome, which is more common than Caroli disease, the pathologic findings include smaller bile ducts and congenital hepatic fibrosis. Caroli disease frequently presents with complications as a result of cholangitis (fever, right upper quadrant pain). The first presentation of Caroli syndrome may result from complications of portal hypertension, most often upper gastrointestinal bleeding. Liver cirrhosis has been described. Overwhelming sepsis with death is not a rare complication for these patients. On examination, jaundice hepatomegaly, splenomegaly, and renal masses associated with renal disease may be found. Although presentation is most frequently in adulthood, childhood and neonatal cases have been described. Patients are at risk for progressive hepatic failure. Caroli disease/syndrome can coexist with medullary sponge kidney, medullary cystic kidney disease, and autosomal recessive polycystic kidney disease (renal cysts, interstitial fibrosis, potential for renal insufficiency). Occasionally, the disorder is limited to one liver lobe (commonly the left) or segment only, and hepatic lobectomy has been used to treat these cases. Liver transplantation has been used for severe cases with whole liver involvement. Compared to the normal population, an up to 100-fold increased risk of cholangiocarcinoma has been reported in these patients, with up to 24% of patients experiencing this type of malignancy at some point in their life.

Precautions before anesthesia: Preoperative blood work should include a complete blood count (anemia due to chronic infection, bleeding from esophageal varices, or renal failure), thrombocytopenia (secondary to hypersplenism), creatinine, blood urea nitrogen, and liver function tests (bilirubin and transaminases may be normal or only slightly increased).

Anesthetic considerations: Anesthetic management is determined by the degree of associated hepatic and renal dysfunction. Central neuraxial anesthesia is contraindicated in the presence of coagulopathy. The risk of surgery has not been specifically assessed in Caroli disease/syndrome. Whereas surgery likely will be tolerated well by patients with normal hepatic function, this usually does not apply to patients with compromised liver function. Anesthesia techniques should aim to maintain hepatic blood flow by preventing low arterial blood pressure and ensuring appropriate intravascular volume. Blood loss from abdominal surgery may be significant in the presence of portal hypertension, and large-bore intravenous access (preferentially in the upper body half), invasive monitoring, and blood products available for transfusion are required. A nasogastric tube must be inserted carefully to prevent trauma to

esophageal varices. Postoperative mechanical ventilation may be required.

Pharmacological implications: Broad-spectrum antibiotic coverage is indicated in the presence of active cholangitis. Coagulopathy should be corrected with vitamin K, fresh-frozen plasma, deamino-8-D-arginine vasopressin (DDAVP), and platelets as necessary. Renal dysfunction may require perioperative hemodialysis and/or pharmacologic intervention for potassium control. Hepatic and/or renal dysfunction may affect the volume of distribution, protein binding, and metabolism of drugs. Pseudocholinesterase activity can be altered. Drugs should be selected based on their known properties in the presence of hepatic and renal dysfunction. Nephrotoxic drugs should be avoided.

Other conditions to be considered:

☞**POLYCYSTIC LIVER DISEASE:** A form of hepatobiliary fibropolycystic disease characterized by an overgrowth of biliary epithelium and supportive connective tissue. Multiple cysts are present in the liver parenchyma. The condition usually is associated with polycystic kidney disease.

☞**POLYCYSTIC KIDNEY DISEASE:** Genetic disorder that frequently results in renal failure in childhood. It is the most common genetically determined childhood cystic disease of the kidneys. Congenital malformation of the collecting tubules.

INFANTILE POLYCYSTIC KIDNEY DISEASE: Autosomal recessive disorder with onset in the first year of life, characterized by generalized dilation of the collecting tubules resulting in fusiform cysts. Hepatic involvement with proliferation and dilation of the bile ducts leading to hepatic fibrosis occurs. Reported incidence is approximately 1.5–6: 1000 pediatric patients.

REFERENCES:

Levy AD, Rohrmann CA Jr, Murakata LA, et al: Caroli's disease: Radiologic spectrum with pathologic correlation. *AJR Am J Roentgenol* 179:1053, 2002.

Madjov R, Chervenkov P, Madjova V, Balev B: Caroli's Disease. Report of 5 cases and review of literature. *Hepatogastroenterology* 52:609, 2005.

Summerfield JA, Nagafuchi Y, Sherlock S, et al: Hepatobiliary fibropolycystic diseases. A clinical and histological review of 51 patients. *J Hepatol* 2:141, 1986.

Carpal Tunnel Syndrome

At a glance: A familial syndrome of constrictive median neuropathy caused by enlarged tendons and/or ligaments in the wrist, often resulting from inflammation.

Synonyms: Thenar Amyotrophy of Carpal Origin; Constrictive Median Neuropathy.

Genetic inheritance: Autosomal dominant. A high degree of penetrance within affected families has been described. Genetic linkage unknown.

Pathophysiology: Marked, noninflammatory thickening of the transverse carpal ligaments and/or flexor tendon sheaths, digital flexor tenosynovitis, constrictive median neuropathy, associated with thenar atrophy and weakness of the hand. Severe vitamin B_6 deficit is associated with this disorder, and supplemental vitamin B_6 improves the symptoms in some cases, even obviating surgery.

Diagnosis: Early age of onset (usually third decade of life, but much earlier onset has been described) of entrapment neuropathy. Progressive course with need for surgical relief. The clinical course of the entrapment neuropathy is characteristic and includes paresthesia in the distribution of the median nerve, nocturnal aggravation of symptoms, and thenar atrophy and hand weakness in long-standing cases. Electromyography can be used to confirm the diagnosis.

Clinical aspects: Symptoms may be reproduced by volar wrist percussion (Tinel sign), sustained wrist flexion (Phalen sign), or wrist extension (palmar prayer sign). Occurring in the context of familial aggregation and excluding secondary causes such as trauma, local edema (during pregnancy), tissue infiltration (myxedema, mucopolysaccharidosis, mucolipidosis, sarcoidosis, amyloidosis), or inflammatory tenosynovitis (rheumatoid arthritis, gout, systemic lupus erythematosus). Thickened transverse carpal ligament and digital flexor tenosynovitis are observed. Familial carpal tunnel syndrome is described in related persons suffering from amyloidosis, mucopolysaccharidosis, and mucolipidosis.

Anesthetic considerations: Local infiltration, regional anesthesia, and general anesthesia have all been used successfully.

REFERENCES:

David WS, Chaudhry V, Dubin AH, et al: Literature review: NervePace digital electroneurometer in the diagnosis of carpal tunnel syndrome. *Muscle Nerve* 27:378, 2003.

Gossett JG, Chance PF: Is there a familial carpal tunnel syndrome? An evaluation and literature review. *Muscle Nerve* 21:1533, 1998.

Cartilage-Hair Hypoplasia Syndrome

At a glance: A form of severe short-limbed dwarfism with hair anomalies, defective immunity, and erythrogenesis.

Synonym: Metaphyseal Chondrodysplasia McKusick type.

History: First recognized as a distinct entity in the Old Order Amish, a religious group in the United States, in 1965 by the American geneticist V.A. McKusick, who is also the founder and one of the editors of the "Online Mendelian Inheritance in Man" (OMIM) database.

Incidence: Clustering is found in Old Order Amish (1–2 in 1000 live births) and in certain areas of Finland (1 in 23,000 live births). It is very rare in other populations. No sexual predilection.

Genetic inheritance: Autosomal recessive with reduced penetrance. Caused by mutations of the mitochondrial RNA-processing endoribonuclease gene, which is located on 9p21-p12. This enzyme is responsible for cleavage of RNA in the mitochondrial DNA synthesis and for nucleolar cleaving of pre-rRNA.

Pathophysiology: Defective cellular proliferation has been described affecting predominantly T-cells (resulting in lymphopenia in almost two thirds of patients), but also involves B-cells (low serum concentrations of immunoglobulins A and/or G; in approximately one third of patients), neutrophils, and fibroblasts. This syndrome has been suggested to result from a generalized defect in cellular proliferation.

Diagnosis: Incomplete extension in the elbows, anterolateral chest deformity, genua varum, and excessive distal length of the fibula relative to the tibia are specific skeletal features. The major radiologic abnormalities are confined to the metaphyseal regions of tubular bones. Biopsy shows hypoplasia of cartilage to be the nature of the skeletal abnormalities.

Clinical aspects: Radiographs show metaphyseal dysostosis. The disorder may involve the cervical spine (odontoid hypoplasia), the skeleton (short stature secondary to dwarfism with an adult height usually <135 cm, flaring of the lower rib cage at the costochondral junction, scoliosis, lumbar hyper-lordosis, platyspondylia, narrowed interpeduncular distances, small pelvic inlet, limited elbow extension, metaphyseal dysplasia, fibular length exceeding tibial length distally, short hands, brachydactyly, joint hyperextensibility), the viscera (Hirschsprung disease, esophageal atresia, anal stenosis, malabsorption), the teeth (microdontia, anomalies of the incisors and premolars), and the hair and skin (sparse, fine, light colored hair, redundant skin folds around the neck and the extremities, hypopigmentation, onychodysplasia). Laboratory investigations may show macrocytic anemia, neutropenia, lymphopenia, and cellular immunodeficiency. Recurrent pulmonary and opportunistic infections in these patients are common (mainly *Candida albicans, Pneumocystis carinii*, and *Cytomegalovirus*). Patients are predisposed to a severe course of *Varicella* infection (multiple fatalities have been reported) and malignancies (in approximately 5% of patients, mainly non-Hodgkin lymphomas). Susceptibility to infections usually improves in adulthood. The higher mortality in these patients compared to the general population mainly refers to children and is a result of the compromised immune system.

Precautions before anesthesia: Obtain a complete blood count with differentiation of red and white cells. The degree of anemia may correspond to the degree of immune deficiency. Anemia usually is mild, however, severe forms of hypoplastic anemia of childhood have been reported. Assess the airway for difficult intubation. Recurrent pulmonary infections warrant careful evaluation of pulmonary function (chest radiograph, arterial blood gas analysis, pulmonary function test). Check cardiac function to delineate the extent of cardiac compromise secondary to chest deformities and scoliosis (electrocardiography, echocardiography). If any concerns exist regarding the stability of the cervical spine, radiologic examinations should be performed.

Anesthetic considerations: Strict aseptic technique during insertion of lines, performance of any regional blocks, and other invasive procedures is mandatory in the presence of immune deficiency. Lumbar spinal or epidural anesthesia may be difficult because of scoliosis, pronounced lumbar lordosis, and diminished interpeduncular distance. Venous access often is difficult because obesity is frequent in these patients. A very short neck (and potentially unstable cervical spine) may make access to the jugular vein difficult or impossible. In addition, exposure of the larynx may prove extremely difficult during conventional laryngoscopy in some patients with dwarfism secondary to a very short neck. In-line stabilization and extreme care are required for intubation of patients with unstable cervical spine. Alternatively, fiberoptic intubation (awake or asleep) may be used. Cases of significant ventilation problems secondary to tracheobronchial malacia with tracheal collapse on induction of anesthesia have been reported. Careful handling of the anomalous teeth is recommended to prevent dislocation. Patients with respiratory compromise often require postoperative mechanical ventilation, especially in the presence of thoracic deformities. Respiratory or metabolic acidosis may cause a profound rise in pulmonary artery pressures and should be avoided in patients with preexisting pulmonary hypertension. Hypercapnia (with respiratory acidosis) can easily result from inhalational anesthesia, and a manually assisted ventilation technique is recommended if difficult airway management is expected. Spontaneous ventilation must be preserved until the airway has been secured. Blood products must be irradiated in these patients to prevent a graft-versus-host reaction. Careful positioning secondary to skeletal anomalies with joint laxity is necessary.

Pharmacological implications: An inhalation induction or awake-fiberoptic intubation should be performed in patients with anticipated airway difficulties and muscle relaxants avoided until the airway has been secured. Caution with attenuated live vaccines because of potential risk of severe infection.

Other conditions to be considered:

☞METAPHYSEAL CHONDRODYSPLASIA, JANSEN TYPE: An extremely rare progressive disorder in which portions of the bones of the arms and legs develop abnormally with unusual cartilage formations and subsequent abnormal bulbous metaphyses (metaphyseal chondrodysplasia). Affected individuals exhibit unusually short arms and legs and short stature (short-limbed dwarfism), findings that typically become apparent during early childhood. Infants with Jansen-type metaphyseal chondrodysplasia may have characteristic facial abnormalities and additional skeletal malformations. Hypercalcemia is present.

☞METAPHYSEAL CHONDRODYSPLASIA, SCHMID TYPE: A very rare inherited disorder characterized by short stature with abnormally short arms and legs (short-limbed dwarfism). Other physical characteristics may include outward "flaring" of the lower rib cage, genua vara, pain in the legs, and/or hip deformities (coxa vara). Such abnormalities of the legs and hips typically result in an unusual "waddling" gait.

REFERENCES:

Makatie O, Sulisalo T, de la Chapelle A, et al: Cartilage-hair hypoplasia. *J Med Genet* 32:39, 1995.

Ridanpaa M, van Eenennaam H, Pelin K, et al: Mutations in the RNA component of RNase MRP cause a pleiotropic human disease, cartilage-hair hypoplasia. *Cell* 104:195, 2001.

Takkunen O, Cozanitis D, Halttunen P, et al: Tracheobronchomalacia in an adult with metaphyseal chondrodysplasia. *Ann Fr Anesth Reanim* 5:527, 1986.

Cartwright-Nelson-Fryns Syndrome

At a glance: An inherited disease with facial deformations, severe mental retardation, and acral limb deficiencies.

Synonym: Growth Retardation, Mental Retardation, Phalangeal Hypoplasia Syndrome.

Incidence and genetic inheritance: Extremely rare; autosomal recessive.

Clinical aspects: Features include malformations of the face (partial mandibular absence, narrow forehead, low hair line) and limbs (small feet and hands, terminal hypoplasia of the toes and fingers, small or absent toenails and fingernails) in combination with neurologic anomalies (severe mental retardation, seizures, generalized hypotonia). Intrauterine growth retardation and postnatal growth failure resulting in short stature have been reported.

Anesthetic considerations: Anesthesia in this disorder has not been described. The features of the syndrome suggest mask ventilation and direct laryngoscopy may be difficult. Chronic antiepileptic treatment can alter the metabolism of some anesthetic agents.

REFERENCE:

Cartwright J, Nelson M, Fryns JP: Pre- and postnatal growth retardation—severe mental retardation—acral limb deficiencies with

poorly keratinized nails. Another example of a distinct syndrome of inherited intrauterine dwarfism? *Genet Couns* 2:147, 1991.

Castleman Disease

At a glance: Lymphoproliferative disorder characterized by large, benign, hyperplastic lymph nodes (localized form, paucisymptomatic, and multicentric form).

Synonyms: Castleman Tumor; Angiofollicular Lymph Node Hyperplasia; Angiomatous Lymphoid Hamartoma; Lymphatic Hamartoma; Giant Lymph Node Hyperplasia; Giant Benign Lymphoma.

History: Named after B. Castleman, an American pathologist, who first described this condition in 1956.

Incidence: Rare. Localized form is more frequent than the multicentric form.

Classification: Three histologic variants (plasma cell, hyaline-vascular and mixed) and two clinical variants (localized and multicentric) exist. The hyaline-vascular variant accounts for approximately 90% of the cases. The localized form is more common than the multicentric form.

Pathophysiology: The etiology of this disease has not been fully determined. Current knowledge suggests the multicentric plasma cell variant is highly associated with an infection by human herpes virus 8 (HHV-8). In addition, these patients also seem to have an increased risk of developing other HHV-8-associated malignancies, such as (extranodal) B-cell non-Hodgkin lymphomas, multiple myeloma, and Kaposi sarcoma. The localized plasma cell and the mixed variant of Castleman disease are frequently found in patients who have a history of lymphoma. Interleukin-6 overproduction, either endogenously or virally encoded, has been made responsible for uncontrolled plasma cell proliferation in these two variants.

Diagnosis: Based on the characteristic lymph node histology and exclusion of other disorders resulting in lymph node swelling. The localized form is often asymptomatic or becomes symptomatic once the diameter of the lymph node is significant enough to cause local compression of important structures, such as airway, vessels, or nerves (resulting in pain). The multicentric form is always symptomatic because of high production of interleukin-6.

Clinical aspects: The localized variant of Castleman disease presents as a mass lesion. The mediastinum, abdomen, and neck are the sites most commonly affected. Lesions up to 16 cm in diameter have been reported. Constitutional symptoms are most commonly seen in the plasma cell and multicentric forms. Symptoms include asthenia, weight loss, fever, skin rash, hemolytic anemia, and/or hypergammaglobulinemia. Hepatomegaly and/or splenomegaly are present in approximately 75% of cases. In approximately 25% of patients, the disease may also present with features of ☞ PEP (*p*lasma cell dyscrasia, *e*ndocrinopathy, *p*olyneuropathy) syndrome. Amyloidosis has been described in a number of cases. Patients with multicentric disease are prone to infections and malignancies. Treatment is surgical excision where possible (localized variant). Surgery, steroids, and chemotherapy are mainly used for the multicentric variant, which has a poor prognosis. Paraneoplastic pemphigus vulgaris has been described in some patients suffering from Castleman disease. The disease in the pediatric population appears to have a more favorable course than in adults.

Precautions before anesthesia: Preoperative assessment should attempt to determine the direct and systemic effects of the lesion(s). Assess mediastinal or thoracic masses (chest radiographs, computed tomography scanning, diagnostic bronchoscopy), and ask about positional stridor and dyspnea to determine the degree of tracheobronchial compression and cardiovascular involvement. Pulmonary function tests can be useful for adults, but are less sensitive (and more difficult to obtain) in the pediatric population. Evaluate for adverse effects of chemotherapy.

Anesthetic considerations: Loss of airway patency and/or cardiovascular collapse may occur on induction in patients with mediastinal masses. Preserve spontaneous ventilation or at least avoid neuromuscular blocking agents if signs of airway or vascular compression are present. In some cases, changing the patient's position (e.g., from supine to lateral decubitus or prone position) and/or rigid bronchoscopy have been used successfully to (at least partially) resolve airway compression. Another concern is the loss of sympathetic tone on induction resulting in cardiopulmonary collapse secondary to a significant drop in pulmonary and systemic venous return. Positive pressure ventilation in the case of airway collapse may be helpful, but its hemodynamic effects will result in further exacerbation of cardiac filling. Regional or local anesthetic techniques are recommended whenever possible.

Pharmacological implications: Avoid neuromuscular blocking agents if signs of compression of the airway or major vessels are present. Adapted antibiotic therapy in case of immunosuppression may be required.

Other condition to be considered:

☞**PEP SYNDROME:** A plasma cell dyscrasia (bone marrow disorder) that causes multisystem disorders, including neuropathy, organ overgrowth, endocrine dysfunctions, and skin changes.

REFERENCES:

Palestro G, Turrini F, Pagano M, et al: Castleman's disease. *Adv Clin Pathol* 3:11, 1999.

Parez N, Bader-Meunier B, Roy CC, et al: Paediatric Castleman disease: Report of seven cases and review of the literature. *Eur J Pediatr* 158:631, 1999.

Wang J, Zhu X, Li R, et al: Paraneoplastic pemphigus associated with Castleman tumor: a commonly reported subtype of paraneoplastic pemphigus in china. *Arch Dermatol* 141:1285, 2005.

Castro-Gago-Pombo-Novo Syndrome

At a glance: Extremely rare syndrome with mainly face and hand anomalies.

Synonym: Microcephaly, Albinism, Digital Anomalies Syndrome.

Incidence and genetic inheritance: Fewer than 10 cases have been described. Autosomal recessive transmission.

Clinical aspects: Microcephaly, cerebral cortical atrophy with mental retardation, micrognathia, retrognathia, oculocutaneous albinism, and digital anomalies (hypoplasia of the distal phalanx of fingers I, III, and IV on the right side and I, III, and V on the left side, and agenesis of the distal part of the right first toe) have been described.

Anesthetic considerations: Anesthesia in this syndrome has not been described. The described features of micrognathia and retrognathia suggest that mask ventilation and direct laryngoscopy may be difficult. In that case, spontaneous ventilation should be maintained until the airway has been secured.

REFERENCE:

Castro-Gago M, Pombo M, Novo I, et al: Sindrome familiar de microcefalia con albinismo oculocutaneo y anomalias digitales. *Ann Esp Pediatr* 19:128, 1983.

Cat Cry Syndrome

At a glance: A syndrome associated with a high-pitched, cat-like cry in the newborn period, severe mental retardation, facial anomalies, scoliosis, muscular hypotonia and congenital cardiac defects.

Synonyms: Cri-du-Chat Syndrome; Lejeune Syndrome, Deletion of Short Arm of Chromosome 5; Monosomy 5p.

History: First described in 1963 by the French pediatrician Jérôme Jean L.M. Lejeune.

Incidence: Appears to be the most common human deletion syndrome, with an incidence of 1 in 15,000 to 1 in 50,000 live births. The frequency in patients with profound mental retardation (IQ<20) may be as high as 0.3%. A slight female predominance has been reported.

Genetic inheritance: The syndrome arises from a partial or total deletion of the short arm of chromosome 5. A loss of the critical 5p15.2 region gives rise to most of the clinical features. The vast majority of cases are sporadic resulting from new mutations. Some arise from unbalanced translocations or parental chromosomal rearrangements. The severity of the syndrome is related to the extent of the chromosome deletion.

Pathophysiology: Unknown.

Diagnosis: Based on the clinical picture plus molecular cytogenetic confirmation of 5p deletion with fluorescent in situ hybridization (FISH), which is considered the gold standard.

Clinical aspects: The name of the syndrome derives from the characteristic, high-pitched cry in infancy, which sounds similar to the mewing of a cat and is considered diagnostic for this disorder. The abnormal cry is mainly caused by anatomical anomalies of the larynx (long, curved and floppy epiglottis, laryngeal hypoplasia, laryngomalacia, asymmetric vocal cords, anterior approximation of the vocal cords with a large posterior commissure), however, in some patients the larynx was found to be structurally normal, which explains why some researchers believe that there may also be a neurological component involved in the abnormal cry. Mental retardation is most often severe. Central nervous findings include marked brainstem atrophy (mainly at the level of the pons) and cerebellar hypoplasia also involving the middle cerebellar peduncles. Generalized muscular hypotonia, poor sucking reflex, and respiratory distress may result in failure to thrive, which in combination with the commonly present intrauterine growth retardation results in postnatal growth retardation. The head usually is microcephalic with a round face due to full cheeks, downward slanting of the palpebral fissures, hypertelorism, low-set ears, depressed nasal bridge, micro- and/or retrognathia with a high-arched, narrow palate (cleft palate has also been described), and macrostomia. Up to 30% of these patients have congenital cardiac defects (most commonly atrial and/or ventricular septal defects, tetralogy of Fallot, pulmonary stenosis, and patent ductus arteriosus). Abdominal findings may include malrotation, megacolon, and inguinal hernias. The urogenital system may also be affected and findings include renal anomalies (e.g., renal agenesis, horsehoe kidney, hydronephrosis), hypospadias, cryptorchidism and testicular atrophy (although spermiogenesis is most often with intact). Skeletal features that have been reported are scoliosis, clubfoot, clinodactyly, and syndactyly of fingers and toes. Abnormal dermatoglyphics (e.g., simian crease) and premature graying of the hair may be present. Severely destructive behavioral problems (agression, self-mutilation) have been described repeatedly. Many patients die in early childhood mainly from respiratory distress (aspiration pneumonia) or the consequences of congenital cardiac defects.

Precautions before anesthesia: Preoperative assessment should focus on signs for difficult airway management. Echocardiography should be performed to rule out cardiac defects. A chest radiograph is recommended in the face of recurrent aspiration pneumonias. If pneumonias are common and scoliosis is severe, echocardiography should also look for signs of cor pulmonale. Proton-pump inhibitors or H_2-antagonists may be indicated to reduce gastric secretions. Assess kidney function (creatinine, blood urea nitrogen) and check serum electrolytes as well as a complete blood count. Patient cooperation is likely to be limited due to mental retardation and behavioral issues. Sedative premedication (careful if signs of cor pulmonale exist) and/or the presence of the primary caregiver for induction of anesthesia may be helpful.

Anesthetic considerations: Difficult direct laryngoscopy and tracheal intubation mainly resulting from micro-/retrognathia should be expected. Abnormal anatomy of the larynx may account for stridor and the cat-like cry in early infancy, but does probably not affect the ease of intubation. However, a smaller than expected endotracheal tube should be ready. Upper airway obstruction may result from the anatomical abnormalities in addition to muscular hypotonia indicating the potential need for prolonged postoperative mechanical ventilation. These patients have a high risk of gastroesophageal reflux and pulmonary aspiration, therefore a modified rapid sequence induction or awake fiberoptic intubation (which may be challenging in an uncooperative patient) have to be considered. Distinct cardiac defects require an adapted anesthesia technique. Other considerations concern difficulties in maintaining normothermia. The operating room should therefore be heated (especially during induction of anesthesia), and a forced-air convective warmer, heating blanket, and warmed infusions be used.

Pharmacological implications: There is no reported association with malignant hyperthermia or succinylcholine-induced hyperkalemia. Muscular hypotonia may cause an exaggerated or unpredictable response to neuromuscular blockers. The use of a peripheral nerve stimulator and titration of neuromuscular blockers to effect is therefore recommended. Subacute bacterial endocarditis prophylaxis may be required.

Other conditions to be considered:

☞**Happy Puppet Syndrome:** Characterized by severe developmental delay, speech impairment, movement dyskinesia, behavioral uniqueness of frequent laughter/smiling, apparent happy demeanor, and easily excitable personality, but short attention span. Seizures with onset before the age of 3 years. Prognathia, excessive chewing, and macroglossia. The craniofacial characteristics of cri-du-chat syndrome resemble this entity.

☞**Cat Eye Syndrome:** An inherited neurodevelopmental disorder with large phenotypic variability, ranging from nearly normal to severe malformations of many organs.

References:

Brislin RP, Stayer SA, Schwartz RE: Anaesthetic considerations for the patient with cri du chat syndrome. *Paediatr Anaesth* 5:139, 1995.

Cerruti Mainardi P, Perfumo C, Cali A, et al: Clinical and molecular characterisation of 80 patients with 5p deletion: genotype-phenotype correlation. *J Med Genet* 38:151, 2001.

Tamraz J, Rethore MO, Lejeune J, et al: [Brain morphometry using MRI in Cri-du-Chat Syndrome. Report of seven cases with review of the literature]. *Ann Genet* 36:75, 1993.

Cat Eye Syndrome

At a glance: An inherited neurodevelopmental disorder with large phenotypic variability, ranging from nearly normal to severe malformations of many organs.

Synonyms: Schmid-Fraccaro Syndrome; Partial Tetrasomy of Chromosome 22; Coloboma-Anal Atresia Syndrome; Ocular Coloboma-Imperforate Anus Syndrome.

History: In 1879 the Swiss ophthalmologist O. Haab was the first to describe a syndrome of anal atresia combined with coloboma. However, the extra chromosome 22 responsible for the syndrome was detected by W. Schmid from Zurich, Switzerland, and M. Fraccaro from Pavia, Italy, who named it cat eye syndrome (CES) because of the inferior coloboma (resulting in a vertical, cat-like pupil) and the downslanting palpebral fissures, although more than 50% of patients have no signs of coloboma.

Incidence: In Switzerland, the incidence has been estimated to be 1 in 50,000–150,000 live births. This most likely is representative of other countries, as no racial predilection has been reported.

Genetic inheritance: Autosomal dominant. Trisomy or tetrasomy 22 (22q11). The additional chromosome 22 generally arises de novo from one of the parents.

Pathophysiology: Not fully described.

Diagnosis: Clinical features (mainly coloboma, anal atresia, and preauricular pits/tags) may lead to the diagnosis. However, because of the wide clinical spectrum of this disorder, the final diagnosis is made by fluorescent in situ hybridization (FISH), which shows the presence of an extra marker chromosome derived from chromosome 22 (partial extra chromosome or duplication) containing two copies of the CES region.

Clinical aspect: Clinical variability is remarkable, with the spectrum of features ranging from only minimally affected individuals to those with the full picture of malformations and lethal outcome. Minimally affected patients may show only downslanting palpebral fissures and preauricular pits or tags. However, CES usually is characterized by the combination of coloboma of the iris (uni- or bilateral), total or partial coloboma of the choroidea and/or optic nerve, microphthalmia (most often unilateral), downslanting palpebral fissures, preauricular tags and/or pits, and anal atresia with rectovesical, rectovaginal, or rectovulvar fistulas in females and rectovesical, rectourethral, or rectoperineal fistulas in males. Other frequently encountered anomalies include renal anomalies (absence of one or both kidneys, supranumeric kidneys, renal hypoplasia, hydronephrosis) and congenital cardiovascular malformations (tetralogy of Fallot, total anomalous pulmonary venous drainage, persistent left superior vena cava, Eisenmenger complex) in more than one third of patients. Additional craniofacial stigmata may include aniridia, cataract, hypertelorism, strabismus, inner epicanthic folds, flat nasal bridge, choanal atresia, cleft lip and palate, mandibular hypoplasia, additional ear malformations (reduction of the auricles to several tags only and atresia of the external auditory canal), and hypothalamic growth hormone deficiency (without severe growth retardation). Skeletal anomalies may present as absence or synostosis of ribs, scoliosis, vertebral fusions, and limb malformations (radial aplasia, duplication of the hallux, absent toes and sirenomelia). Visceral anomalies include pulmonary segmentation defects, intestinal malrotation, biliary atresia, Hirschsprung disease, Meckel diverticulum, umbilical hernia, uterus hypoplasia and vaginal atresia in girls, and hypospadia in boys. Cases of CES in combination with spina bifida or myelomeningocele have been reported. Normal or only slightly delayed mental development is common, but in rare cases, patients with the full picture of the syndrome have severe mental retardation.

Precautions before anesthesia: Except for minimally affected patients, all patients will require surgery at some point (anal atresia, congenital heart malformations). Preoperative blood work should include a complete blood count, evaluation of renal function (blood urea nitrogen, creatinine), and hepatic function tests (transaminases, bilirubin, ammonia, albumin, coagulation profile). Cardiac lesions should be investigated by echocardiography and/or cardiac catheterization. Evaluate the airway clinically (possibly by radiography) for anesthetic management. Check for choanal atresia.

Anesthetic considerations: Micrognathia and limited mouth opening may make direct laryngoscopy and tracheal intubation difficult. Alternative airway management techniques may be necessary (e.g., awake fiberoptic intubation, [intubating] laryngeal mask airway). Choanal atresia precludes nasal intubation. Regional anesthetic techniques do not appear to be specifically contraindicated (given coagulation is normal), but central neuraxial blockade could be difficult secondary to vertebral anomalies. Limb malformations could make the blood pressure cuff difficult to apply. Radial aplasia may render radial artery cannulation difficult or impossible. Mental retardation may impair cooperation. Sedative and/or anxiolytic premedication and the presence of the primary caregiver during induction of anesthesia may be helpful.

Pharmacological implications: The selection of anesthetic agents is influenced by the degree of associated renal and hepatic dysfunction and the underlying cardiac lesion. Subacute bacterial endocarditis prophylaxis may be indicated.

Other condition to be considered:

☞**CAT CRY SYNDROME:** A syndrome associated with a high-pitched, cat-like cry in the newborn period, severe mental retardation, facial anomalies, scoliosis, muscular hypotonia and congenital cardiac defects.

REFERENCES:
Berends MJ, Tan-Sindhunata G, Leegte B, van Essen AJ: Phenotypic variability of Cat-Eye syndrome. *Genet Couns* 12:23, 2001.

Devavaram P, Seefelder C, Lillehei CW: Anaesthetic management of Cat Eye Syndrome. *Paediatr Anaesth* 11:746, 2001.

Rosias PPR, Sijstermans JMJ, Theunissen PMV, et al: Phenotypic variability of the cat eye syndrome, case report and review of the literature. *Genet Couns* 12:273, 2001.

Cataract-Alopecia-Sclerodactyly Syndrome

At a glance: Inherited condition affecting skin, eyes and digits.
Synonym: CASS.
Incidence and genetic inheritance: Described in only one family with 5 affected siblings on Rodrigues Island in the Indian ocean (approximately 1600 km east of Madagascar). Autosomal recessive.

Clinical aspects: Sclerodactyly, hyperkeratosis, digital contractures, and pseudo-Ainhum syndrome (digital constriction bands with autoamputation) associated with cataract and total alopecia.
Anesthetic considerations: Anesthesia in this condition has not been described. Theoretically, the digital features may limit the patient's ability to activate certain devices, such as a pump for patient controlled analgesia.
Other condition to be considered:

☞**AINHUM:** A narrow strip of hardened skin with constricting ring formation on the little toe at the level of digitoplantar fold progressively leading to spontaneous amputation.

REFERENCE:
Wallis C, Ip FSL, Beighton P: Cataracts, alopecia, and sclerodactyly: A previously apparently undescribed ectodermal dysplasia syndrome on the island of Rodrigues. *Am J Med Genet* 32:500, 1989.

Cataract-Microcornea-Syndrome

At a glance: Familial disorder with features limited to the eyes.
Incidence and genetic inheritance: Fewer than 25 patients have been described in the literature. Autosomal dominant.
Clinical aspects: Dysplastic malformation of the anterior segment of the eye characterized by the combination of congenital cataract and microcornea (diameter <11 mm). Occasionally, other ocular anomalies such as iris coloboma, sclerocornea, myopia, or Peters anomaly (central corneal opacity associated with abnormal corneal development that may result in cataract, adhesions of the iris to the cornea, and glaucoma) may be present.
Anesthetic considerations: No known specific anesthetic problems or other associated abnormalities.
Other condition to be considered:

☞**NANCE-HORAN SYNDROME:** A very rare congenital disorder combining cataract and dental anomalies.

REFERENCES:
Green JS, Johnson GJ: Congenital cataract with microcornea and Peters' anomaly as expressions of one autosomal dominant gene. *Ophthalmic Paediatr Genet* 7:187, 1986.

Salmon JF, Wallis CE, Murray AD: Variable expressivity of autosomal dominant microcornea with cataract. *Arch Ophthalmol* 106:505, 1988.

Catlin Marks

At a glance: Congenital syndrome consisting of symmetrical bony skull defects.
Synonyms: Parietal Foramina (Per-)Magna; Cranium Bifidum; 11p11.2 Deletion Syndrome.
History: It was W.M. Goldsmith in 1922 who chose the name Catlin Marks for this disorder because he observed this defect in several generations of a family named Catlin.
Incidence: While small parietal foramina are found in up to 70% of the population, large parietal foramina with a diameter of several centimeters are estimated to affect 1:15000–20000 live births.
Genetic inheritance: Autosomal dominant. The genetic defect has been mapped to 11p11.2, 5q34.q35.
Pathophysiology: Parietal foramina are caused by either mutations of the MSX2 gene (PFM-1, Parietal Foramina Magna gene

1; 5q34.q35) or by haploinsufficiency of the ALX4 gene (PFM-2; 11p11.2). These mutations will result in abnormal ossification of the membranous calvarium.

Diagnosis: Frequently asymptomatic. Patients have symmetrical oval defects of the parietal bone.

Clinical aspects: Considerable variation among and within families suffering from the condition. Circumscribed scalp aplasia, seizures, cleft lip and palate, and spina bifida occulta (cervical and lumbosacral) have been described. Cranium bifidum consists of wide fontanelles (anterior and posterior), which persist into childhood. The fontanelles tend to close in mid-childhood but may leave residual frontal or parietal foramina. Cranium bifidum may be associated with encephaloceles and structural vascular malformations of the brain.

Precautions before anesthesia: If central neuraxial anesthesia is planned, spinal radiographs and/or magnetic resonance imaging should be considered preoperatively given the possibility of spina bifida occulta.

Anesthetic considerations: Spina bifida occulta may increase the incidence of complications after central neuraxial anesthesia. Avoid anesthetic agents that lower the seizure threshold. Chronic antiseizure medication may alter the metabolism of some anesthetic agents.

Other condition to be considered:

☞**A**CROCEPHALOSYNDACTYLY **S**YNDROME **T**YPE **III** **(Saethre-Chotzen Syndrome):** Craniosynostosis with low frontal hairline, ptosis, and brachydactyly and cutaneous syndactyly of the fingers and of the second and third toes. Cranial abnormalities are variable. Other features may include cleft palate, hydrophthalmos, cardiac malformations, and contractures of the elbows and knees.

REFERENCES:

Chrzanowska K, Kozlowski K, Kowalska A: Syndromic foramina parietalia permagna. *Am J Med Genet* 6:401, 1998.

Spruijt L, Verdyck P, van Hul W, et al: A novel mutation in the MSX2 gene in a family with foramina parietalia permagna (FPP). *Am J Med Genet A* 139A:45, 2005.

Wuyts W, Cleiren E, Homfray T, et al: The ALX4 homeobox gene is mutated in patients with ossification defects of the skull (foramina parietalia permagna, OMIM 168500). *J Med Genet* 37:916, 2000.

Cavernous Sinus Syndrome

At a glance: Ophthalmoplegia, proptosis, and orbital congestion are the most frequent findings. It is caused by lesions of the cavernous sinus. Parasellar lesions including tumors, carotid artery aneurysms, and carotid-cavernous fistulas have been described.

Synonyms: Foix Syndrome; Jefferson Syndrome; Foix-Jefferson Syndrome.

Incidence: Approximately 5% of all ophthalmoplegias are the result of cavernous sinus syndrome.

Genetic inheritance: No genetic background.

Pathophysiology: The cavernous sinuses are paired. They contain the oculomotor nerves, carotid arteries, and their sympathetic plexus and are traversed by the ophthalmic branch of the trigeminal nerve. Tumors (primary or secondary), carotid artery aneurysms, carotid-cavernous fistulas, and inflammatory processes are the main causes of this disorder.

Diagnosis: The syndrome can be diagnosed clinically. Funduscopy shows optic disc edema and retinal hemorrhages, however, diagnostic imaging and laboratory studies are required to establish the nature of the lesion.

Clinical aspects: On examination, patients have ophthalmoplegia, orbital congestion, and proptosis. Cranial nerve palsies may be isolated or comprise a combination of third, fourth, and sixth cranial nerve palsies. Ophthalmoplegia may be painful. Ocular pulsation suggests a vascular fistula. There may be conjunctival congestion and arterialization of the conjunctival veins, diminished sensation in the ophthalmic branch of the trigeminal nerve, and decreased or absent corneal reflex. The pupil on the affected side is typically in mid-position and nonreactive to light.

Precautions before anesthesia: Patients should be assessed for raised intracranial pressure and potential endocrinopathy (both, hormonal over- and underproduction) associated with tumors in or around the sella turcica. Serum electrolyte and glucose levels should be measured. Where applicable, treatment of the endocrinopathy should be initiated prior to surgery.

Anesthetic considerations: Main anesthesia concerns are raised intracranial pressure (occasionally) and endocrine effects with associated organ dysfunction. Maintain a cerebral perfusion pressure of at least 60 mmHg, prevent seizures and fever, and adjust ventilation to aim for low normocapnia to mild hypocapnia. However, in the presence of vascular lesions, rapid increases in blood pressure must also be avoided.

Pharmacological implications: In the presence of increased intracranial pressure, drugs that increase cerebral blood flow should be avoided or used only at low concentrations/doses.

Other condition to be considered:

TOLOSA-**H**UNT **S**YNDROME: Refers to a cavernous-sinus syndrome caused by an idiopathic inflammatory lesion, an abnormal autoimmune response, or tumors/metastases in the area of the cavernous sinus. Symptoms most commonly occur at the beginning of the fifth decade of life and include chronic and severe (often unilateral) headache often preceding ophthalmoplegia. Mild fever, double vision, exophthalmos, ptosis, vertigo, chronic fatigue, and arthralgia may occur. Steroids have been used successfully; however, spontaneous remission is common (except when caused by tumors/metastases), as is recurrence. No sexual predilection has been reported.

REFERENCES:

Biousse V, Mendicino ME, Simon DJ, et al: The ophthalmology of intracranial vascular abnormalities. *Am J Ophthalmol* 125:527, 1998.

Keane JR: Cavernous sinus syndrome: Analysis of 151 cases. *Arch Neurol* 53:967, 1996.

Van Overbeeke JJ, Jansen JJ, Tulleken CA: The cavernous sinus syndrome. An anatomical and clinical study. *Clin Neurol Neurosurg* 90:311, 1988.

Cayler Syndrome

At a glance: Typical asymmetry during crying associated with visceral malformations.

Synonyms: Asymmetrical Crying Facies with Cardiac Defect; Cayler Type of Cardiofacial Syndrome; Hypoplasia of Depressor Anguli Oris Muscle with Cardiac Defect.

Incidence: Sporadic or familial disorder. Estimates vary between 0.63% and 0.82% of the general population. Male-to-female ratio 2:1.

Genetic inheritance: Either autosomal dominant or multifactorial. An association with pericentric inversion of chromosome 15 and with deletion of chromosome 22q11.2 has been reported.

Pathophysiology: Congenital hypoplasia or agenesis of the depressor anguli oris muscle on one side of the mouth results in facial asymmetry that is evident during crying.

Diagnosis: Based on clinical and/or electromyographic findings. Affected infants suck well without drooling from either corner of the mouth and have normal forehead wrinkling, eye closure, and nasolabial fold depth, all of which exclude facial nerve palsy.

Clinical aspects: Unilateral asymmetry of the face during crying, because of predominantly left-sided defects of the depressor anguli oris. Associated anomalies involve the head (mental retardation, microcephaly, cerebral cortical atrophy, prominent ears, micrognathia, retrognathia, cleft palate, anodontia), the heart (atrial septal defects, ventricular septal defects, conotruncal anomalies, and tetralogy of Fallot), and the viscera (respiratory distress, diaphragmatic hernia, polycystic kidneys, hydronephrosis, hypoplasia of kidneys, ectopic testes). Short stature has been described. Hypoparathyroidism and hypocalcemia have been reported in at least one patient.

Precautions before anesthesia: Thoroughly assess the patient for signs of cardiac lesions (clinically, echocardiography, electrocardiogram) and renal anomalies and insufficiency (ultrasound, blood work). Check for difficult airway management. Mental retardation may impair cooperation. Sedative and/or anxiolytic premedication and the presence of the primary caregiver during induction of anesthesia may be helpful.

Anesthetic considerations: Given the anatomical anomalies of the face, airway management must be expected to be difficult. The recommendation is to maintain spontaneous ventilation until the airway has been secured. Alternative airway management techniques should be considered (e.g., fiberoptic intubation, laryngeal mask airway). Congenital cardiac defects require specific anesthetic precautions and management.

Pharmacological implications: Avoid neuromuscular blockers until the airway has been secured. Subacute bacterial endocarditis prophylaxis may be necessary.

Other condition to be considered:

☞**DiGeorge Syndrome:** a genetic defect leading to a wide range of phenotypic presentations, mainly developmental defects in the outflow tracts of the heart, hypoparathyroidism with hypocalcemia, and thymic aplasia or hypoplasia with immune defects.

References:

Akcacus M, Ozkul Y, Gunes T, et al: Associated anomalies in asymmetric crying facies and 22q11 deletion. *Genet Couns* 14:325, 2003.

Cayler GG: An epidemic of congenital facial paresis and heart disease. *Pediatrics* 40:666, 1967.

Lin DS, Huang FY, Lin SP, et al: Frequency of associated anomalies in congenital hypoplasia of depressor anguli oris muscle: A study of 50 patients. *Am J Med Genet* 71:215, 1997.

CCGE Syndrome

At a glance: Extremely rare, inherited disorder combining malformations of head, heart, genitalia, and limbs. CCGE is an acronym for *c*left palate, *c*ardiac defect, *g*enital anomalies and *e*ctrodactyly.

Synonyms: Acrocardiofacial Syndrome; Richieri-Costa Orquizas Syndrome.

Incidence and genetic inheritance: Approximately five cases have been described. Autosomal recessive transmission has been suggested. Parental consanguinity was noted in at least one case.

Clinical aspects: Findings may involve the head and neck (scaphocephaly, high forehead, blepharophimosis, flattened nose and philtrum, small mouth and nostrils, micrognathia and/or retrognathia, narrow arched palate, cleft palate, thin lips, long and low-set ears, short neck), the heart (hypoplastic left heart syndrome, atrial septal defects, ventricular septal defects, coarctation of the aorta, patent ductus arteriosus, mitral valve prolapse), the central nervous system (mental retardation, cerebral atrophy, enlarged cisterna magna), the genitalia (hypospadias, micropenis, hypoplastic scrotum, cryptorchidism), and the limbs (oligodactyly, cleft hand, syndactyly of toes). Other features may include oligohydramnios and intrauterine growth retardation. Death in the first weeks of life occurred in more than half of patients and was caused by cardiac anomalies.

Anesthetic considerations: Anesthesia in this condition has not been described. Cardiac function and anatomy must be determined preoperatively (clinically, echocardiography, electrocardiography). Congenital cardiac lesions warrant specific anesthetic precautions and management. Facial features suggest airway management could be difficult.

Pharmacological implications: Subacute bacterial endocarditis prophylaxis may be necessary.

Other condition to be considered:

☞**Ectrodactyly, Ectodermal Dysplasia, and Clefting (EEC) Syndrome:** Autosomal dominant inherited syndrome with ectodermal dysplasia and craniofacial and urogenital anomalies. Occasionally, mental retardation and central diabetes insipidus are present.

References:

Giannotti A, Digilio MC, Mingarelli R, et al: An autosomal recessive syndrome of cleft palate, cardiac defect, genital anomalies, and ectrodactyly (CCGE). *J Med Genet* 32:72, 1995.

Guion-Almeida ML, Zechi-Ceide RM, Richieri-Costa A: Cleft lip/palate, abnormal ears, ectrodactyly, congenital heart defect, and growth retardation: Definition of the acro-cardio-facial syndrome. *Clin Dysmorph* 9:269, 2000.

Richieri-Costa A, Orquizas LC: Ectrodactyly, cleft lip/palate, ventricular septal defect, micropenis and mental retardation in a Brazilian child born to consanguineous parents. *Rev Bras Genet* 10:787, 1987.

Cecato-De Lima-Pinheiro Syndrome

At a glance: Extremely rare form of ectodermal dysplasia with eye, hair, skin, and teeth anomalies.

Synonym: Oculotrichodysplasia.

Incidence and genetic inheritance: Two cases from one family have been described. Autosomal recessive transmission has been suggested because the parents were first cousins and 11 other siblings were unaffected.

Clinical aspects: Diagnosis is made clinically and by scanning electron microscopy of the hair, which shows structural anomalies. Patients present with short stature. Other clinical features involve the eyes (retinopathy pigmentosa, sparse eyelashes and [lateral] eyebrows), the teeth (caries, widely spaced, small, pointy deciduous teeth), the nails (fragile and brittle, onychodysplasia), the hair (trichodysplasia, sparse scalp, axillary and pubic hair, generalized hypotrichosis), and the skin (dry, scaling).

Anesthetic considerations: Anesthesia in this condition has not been described. According to the symptoms, no specific anesthetic precautions are necessary. However, dental fragility predisposes to injury during airway manipulations and should be kept in mind.

Other conditions to be considered: Other forms of ☞Ectodermal Dysplasia: A rare group of inherited disorders which arises from disturbances in one or more ectodermal structures and their accessory appendages. The absence or deficient function of at least two derivatives of the ectoderm constitutes a form of ectodermal dysplasia. Each combination of defects represents another type of ectodermal dysplasia and has a specific name. At least 150 different forms of ectodermal dysplasia have been identified.

REFERENCE:

Cecatto-De-Lima L, Pinheiro M, Freire-Maia N: Oculotrichodysplasia (OTD): A new probably autosomal recessive condition. *J Med Genet* 25:430, 1988.

Celiac Disease

At a glance: A chronic malabsorptive disease of the small intestine resulting from ingestion of gluten.

Synonyms: Celiac Sprue; Gluten-Sensitive Enteropathy; Herter Disease; Herter-Heubner Disease.

Incidence: For symptomatic gluten-sensitive enteropathy, the incidence is 1:150–1000 in Europe, but a greater proportion of individuals (1:200–400) may have clinically silent disease. The incidence appears to be much lower in the black and Asian population, which is explained by a lower frequency of human leukocyte antigen (HLA)-DQ2 or HLA-DQ8.

Genetic inheritance: Multifactorial. The causative genetic component involves an assortment of major histocompatibility complex genes interacting with environmental factors. Celiac disease is the first HLA-associated disease for which the "at-risk genotypes" have been delineated. In the vast majority (>93%) of patients with celiac disease, genetic susceptibility has been associated with the HLA-DQ2 heterodimer, encoded by the DQA1*0501 and DQB1*02 genes. The remaining minority not expressing DQ2 is positive for DR4 and shows the DQ8 heterodimer, which is encoded by DQA1*0301/DQB1*0302 genes. The two heterodimers DQ2 and DQ8 are located on the surface of antigen-presenting cells and are involved in binding of peptides to be presented to CD4+ T lymphocytes. This association supports the importance of CD4+ T lymphocytes in the pathogenesis of celiac disease, as a T-cell–mediated inflammatory response in the proximal small bowel is made responsible for the intestinal problems.

Pathophysiology: The mucosal lesion represents an immunologically mediated injury triggered by gluten. The amino acid residue of gliadin triggers the abnormal immune response. Gluten is found in wheat, rye, barley, triticale, and oats. The alcohol-soluble prolamine fraction is the component of gluten that is responsible for the symptoms of celiac disease. Depending on the cereal, this prolamine fraction has different names: gliadin in wheat, secalin in rye, avenin in oats, and hordein in barley (newer research suggests avenin is tolerated). Tissue transglutaminase, the major target of autoantibodies in celiac disease, converts glutamine residues of gluten to glutamic acid. This deamination results in significantly increased DQ binding and T-cell recognition.

Diagnosis: Malabsorption usually begins at approximately 4 to 20 months of age (although later onset has been reported), but 10 to 20% of patients become "tolerant" to gluten during adolescence. The disease is permanent, even if no symptoms are present. The best combination of serologic tests for the diagnosis is anti-gliadin IgA, anti-gliadin IgG, and anti-endomysium IgA. The high serum count of intraepithelial lymphocytes suggests activated mucosal cell-mediated immunity. The final diagnosis of celiac disease must always rely on the results of an intestinal biopsy showing villous atrophy. Serologic tests usually are performed at the onset of clinical symptoms. If the results are positive, then an intestinal biopsy is indicated to confirm the diagnosis. Serologic tests can be used to control the response to treatment with a gluten-free diet.

Clinical aspects: Clinical signs start in early infancy a few weeks after a diet containing gluten is added to breast-feeding. Intestinal symptoms are variable, including diarrhea, nausea, vomiting, bloating, steatorrhea, and constipation. Other features include failure to thrive, anorexia, hypoprothrombinemia as a result of malabsorption of vitamin K, osteoporosis, defective enamel, skin rash (dermatitis herpetiformis Duhring; a papulovesicular skin condition), recurrent aphthous stomatitis, edema as a result of hypoproteinemia, decreased blood levels of vitamin A and E, anemia as a result of folate deficiency and/or iron deficiency, and rickets secondary to vitamin D malabsorption. Puberty may be delayed, and refractory epilepsy associated with brain calcifications has been reported in 5% of patients. Arthritis occurs frequently in adults (26%) and requires regular followup. Serum prolactin in patients with active celiac disease is significantly higher and can be correlated to the degree of mucosal atrophy. Celiac disease is more common in patients also suffering from other genetic or immune diseases (e.g., Down syndrome, selective IgA deficiency, IgA nephropathy, rheumatoid arthritis, thyroid diseases, insulin-dependent diabetes mellitus). Children with diabetes mellitus, even when asymptomatic, should be screened yearly for celiac disease. A significantly increased risk for intestinal adenocarcinomas, non-Hodgkin (T-cell) lymphomas, and squamous cell carcinomas of the oropharynx and esophagus has been reported in patients with long-standing celiac disease.

Precautions before anesthesia: Preoperative blood work should include a complete blood count (anemia), total serum protein and albumin (hypoproteinemia), serum electrolytes (including calcium), and coagulation parameters (vitamin K-dependent coagulation factors). Depending on the clinical manifestation (diarrhea, vomiting), the volume status must be assessed and corrected if necessary. For patients with diabetes mellitus, either a blood glucose profile should be obtained or their personal serum glucose diary should be reviewed (if available). For patients with abnormal thyroid function, a preoperative check is recommended.

Anesthetic considerations: Regional anesthesia techniques are not contraindicated per se, but a review of the coagulation status is highly recommended.

Pharmacological implications: The child must be managed as though he/she were hypovolemic and hypoproteinemic, so the dose of agents decreasing arterial blood pressure should be reduced. This also applies to drugs with high protein binding.

REFERENCES:

Devlin SM, Andrews CN, Beck PL: Celiac disease. CME update for family physicians. *Can Fam Physician* 50:719, 2004.

Fasano A, Berti I, Gerarduzzi T et al: Prevalence of celiac disease in at-risk and not-at-risk groups in the United States: A large multicenter study. *Arch Intern Med* 163:286, 2003.

Vidales MC, Zubillaga P, Zubillaga I, et al: Allele and haplotype frequencies for HLA class II (DQA1 and DQB1) loci in patients with celiac disease from Spain. *Hum Immunol* 65:352, 2004.

Cenani Syndactylism

At a glance: A disorder associated with osseous syndactyly and mesomelic brachymelia.

Synonyms: Cenani-Lenz Syndactyly; Cenani-Lenz Oligodactyly-Synostosis Syndrome.

History: Named after A. Cenani from Turkey and W. Lenz from Germany, two medical geneticists who described this disorder in 1967, although reports have described this syndrome as early as 1938.

Incidence and genetic inheritance: Extremely rare (fewer than 10 patients have been described). Most often transmission is autosomal recessive, however, quasidominant inheritance has also been described. In most cases, parental consanguinity is present.

Clinical aspects: The main findings are short stature, syndactyly/synostosis with abnormal phalanges, and fusion of the metacarpals resembling the "spoon hand" deformity of ☞Apert syndrome. The ulna and radius may be fused and shortened. The feet are usually less severely affected. Joint mobility may be restricted. Agenesis or hypoplasia of the kidneys, genital anomalies, cavernous hemangiomas, and supernumerary nipples have been observed occasionally. Facial features may include a high, wide, prominent forehead, hypertelorism, downslanting palpebral fissures, short nose with depressed nasal bridge, short but prominent philtrum, and malar hypoplasia.

Anesthetic considerations: Preoperative blood work should include a complete blood count (renal anemia) and levels of serum electrolytes, creatinine, and blood urea nitrogen. Airway anatomy should be assessed because airway management could potentially be difficult, depending on the degree of malar hypoplasia. Limb deformities and the site of surgery may limit (venous and arterial) vascular access sites. Careful intraoperative positioning and padding are required. Both fluid regimen and anesthetic drug doses should be adapted in the presence of renal dysfunction.

REFERENCES:

Cenani A, Lenz W: Totale Syndaktylie und totale radioulnare Synostose bei zwei Brüdern. Ein Beitrag zur Genetik der Syndaktylien. *Zeitschr Kinderheilk Berl* 101:181, 1967.

De Smet L, De Beere P, Fryns JP: Cenani-Lenz Syndrome in father and daughter. *Genet Couns* 7:153, 1996.

Temtamy SA, Ismail S, Nemat A: Mild facial dysmorphism and quasidominant inheritance in Cenani-Lenz syndrome. *Clin Dysmorph* 12:77, 2003.

Cennamo Gangemi Magli Syndrome

At a glance: A very rare syndrome combining ocular and neurologic signs.

Synonym: Hydrocephalus Cataract Microphthalmos Syndrome.

Incidence and genetic inheritance: Only a single case has been described. Autosomal recessive inheritance has been suggested because the parents were consanguineous.

Clinical aspects: Bilateral cataracts, microcornea, microphthalmos, hydrocephaly, high vaulted palate, generalized hypertonia and hyperreflexia have been described in a 9-month-old girl.

Anesthetic considerations: Anesthesia in this condition has not been described. Hydrocephalus is most likely associated with raised intracranial pressure. In this case, anesthesia should focus on normal ventilation or mild hyperventilation, preventing seizures and hyperthermia, and using a (preferably intravenous) anesthesia technique not resulting in increased cerebral blood flow.

REFERENCE:

Cennamo G, Gangemi M, Magli A: Hydrocephalus combined with congenital cataract and microphthalmia. *J Pediatr Ophthalmol Strabismus* 16:382, 1979.

Central Core Disease

At a glance: Congenital myopathy with a specific histologic pattern and high susceptibility to malignant hyperthermia.

Synonyms: Muscle Core Disease; Muscular Central Core Disease; Central Fibrillary Myopathy; Shy-Magee Syndrome.

Incidence: Accounts for approximately 15% of all congenital myopathies. No sexual predilection.

Genetic inheritance: Autosomal dominant trait with the gene locus mapped to 19q13.1, which is in close proximity to one of the genes for malignant hyperthermia (ryanodine receptor gene). Expression is variable.

Pathophysiology: Can be caused by at least 22 different mutations in the ryanodine receptor-1 gene (RyR1). According to one common hypothesis, these mutations could result in the formation of excessively leaky sarcoplasmic reticulum Ca^{2+} release channels. The ryanodine receptor is a protein involved in calcium release into the sarcoplasm from the sarcoplasmic reticulum. It has been postulated that after the exposition to trigger agents, the ryanodine receptor releases excessive amounts of calcium resulting in sustained muscle contraction and hypermetabolism.

Diagnosis: Requires muscle biopsy. The "central core" is a histopathologic description related to an area of low staining that extends the length of the muscle fibers and is devoid of mitochondria and other cell organelles. Type 1 muscle fibers are predominately affected. Nerve conduction studies are normal and electromyography is nonspecific. Normal plasma levels of creatinine phosphokinase do not rule out central core disease. Susceptibility to malignant hyperthermia is determined by in vitro contraction testing with halothane and caffeine.

Clinical aspects: There is a wide variation in the clinical spectrum of this disease. The myopathy is asymptomatic in some patients, but in others (although rarely) it can be severe. Most commonly, it already presents in infancy with hypotonia and delayed motor milestones. A history of decreased fetal movement and/or breech presentation is often given. However, the first signs of this disease can be a slowly progressive limb-girdle syndrome with onset in adolescence or an attack of malignant hyperthermia. Central core disease may not be symptomatic until late in life. Proximal muscle weakness is common and manifests as difficulties in walking or climbing the stairs. Deep tendon reflexes may be significantly reduced or even absent. Muscle wasting occurs. Skeletal abnormalities may be part of the clinical picture and include kyphoscoliosis, congenital hip dislocation, patella dislocation, feet deformities (pes planus, pes cavus), and joint contractures. Mandibular hypoplasia has been reported in a few cases. These patients are mentally normal.

Precautions before anesthesia: As in all myopathies, evaluate cardiac (increased incidence of mitral valve prolapse) and respiratory function (e.g., clinically, chest radiographs, echocardiography, radionuclide scintigraphy, pulmonary function tests, arterial blood gases analysis), particularly in the presence of kyphoscoliosis. Blood work should include serum levels of electrolytes (including calcium) and creatinine phosphokinase.

Anesthetic considerations: Patients are susceptible to malignant hyperthermia, and at least one death related to malignant hyperthermia has been reported. Until proven otherwise, these patients should be considered at high risk for malignant hyperthermia. Even asymptomatic family members should be considered at risk for malignant hyperthermia until susceptibility has been individually determined by in vitro muscle contraction studies. Regional anesthesia is preferred whenever possible. Depending on the degree of mandibular hypoplasia, airway management should be expected to be difficult. Careful intraoperative positioning is needed because of joint contractures and increased risk of dislocations at the same time.

Pharmacological implications: All malignant hyperthermia-triggering agents should be avoided, particularly succinylcholine and volatile anesthetic agents. Subacute bacterial endocarditis prophylaxis may be required in the presence of mitral valve prolapse with mitral regurgitation and/or thickened mitral leaflets.

Other conditions to be considered:

☞**CONGENITAL MYOPATHY WITH FIBER-TYPE DISPROPORTION:** A rare genetic myopathy already presenting at birth with hypotonia, muscle weakness, and high arched palate. Findings occurring later in life include short stature, progressive scoliosis, hip dislocation, and deformities of the feet.

☞**MYOTUBULAR MYOPATHY:** Congenital muscle disease characterized by generalized hypotonia, muscle weakness, and central nuclei on muscle biopsy (myotube-like aspect).

☞**NEMALINE ROD MYOPATHY:** A rare congenital and slowly progressive inherited neuromuscular disease usually apparent at birth and characterized by extreme hypotonia.

REFERENCES:

Curran JL, Hall WJ, Halsall PJ, et al: Segregation of malignant hyperthermia, central core disease and chromosome 19 markers. *Br J Anaesth* 83:217, 1999.

Islander G, Henriksson KG, Ranklev-Twetman E: Malignant hyperthermia susceptibility without central core disease (CCD) in a family where CCD is diagnosed. *Neuromuscul Disord* 5:125, 1995.

Sewry CA, Muller C, Davis M, et al: The spectrum of pathology in central core disease. *Neuromuscul Disord* 12:930, 2002.

Cephaloskeletal Dysplasia

At a glance: A brachymelic primordial disproportionate dwarfism associated with facial dysmorphism and neurologic impairment.

Synonyms: Microcephalic Osteodysplastic Primordial Dwarfism, Type I and III (MOPD I and III); Brachymelic Primordial Dwarfism; Taybi-Linder Syndrome (MOPD I); Low-Birth-Weight Dwarfism with Skeletal Dysplasia.

Incidence and genetic inheritance: Approximately 22 cases have been described. Autosomal recessive. Parental consanguinity has been reported for some cases.

Clinical aspects: Some features are shared with those of ☞Seckel Syndrome, however, dwarfism in MOPD I and III is disproportionate. Type I is characterized by short and bowed long bones. Typical findings in type III include elongated clavicles, cleft cervical vertebral arches, lumbar platyspondyly, enlarged metaphyses, and marked dysplasia of the pelvis. However, MOPD type I and III now are accepted as variants of the same disease.

Severe intrauterine (with oligohydramnios) and postnatal growth retardation are almost always present. The disease may affect head and neck (microcephaly, closed anterior fontanelle at birth, prominent occiput, sloping forehead, low-set and dysplastic ears, large protruding eyes, strabismus, big, prominent nose, mandibular hypoplasia, high vaulted narrow palate, unilateral choanal atresia, short neck), the urogenital tract (micropenis, cryptorchidism, obstructive hydronephrosis), the skeleton (hip dislocation, joint flexion deformities, flexion contractures in the big joints, short limbs, brachydactyly, clinodactyly of the fifth digit, delayed bone age, abnormal vertebral size and shape [cervical clefts, platyspondyly], flared iliac wings, shallow acetabula, delayed metaphyseal maturation, bowed femurs and humeri) and the central nervous system (delayed psychomotor development, seizures, micrencephaly, corpus callosum agenesis, gyral anomalies, enlarged lateral ventricles, hypoplastic cerebellum and frontal lobes, agenesis of the cerebellar vermis, heterotopias). Other features include alopecia, dry skin, bilateral simian creases, and decreased sweating. Tetralogy of Fallot and renal leakage have been described in one case. This disease is generally lethal within the first year of life. The oldest survivor died at 6.5 years of age. The recorded causes of death are most often infections, such as meningitis, meconium peritonitis, aphthous stomatitis, sepsis, and airway infections with pneumonia.

Anesthetic considerations: Anesthesia in this condition has not been described. Renal function should be assessed if hydronephrosis is present. The features of the disease suggest that mask ventilation and direct laryngoscopy may be difficult. Given the possible anomalies of the cervical spine, tracheal intubation should be performed in a way that forced reclination of the head is avoided. Decreased sweating may lead to abnormal thermoregulation in the perioperative period. Joint contractures may make patient positioning difficult. Central neuraxial anesthesia is not contraindicated, but may be difficult secondary to anatomical anomalies and difficulties with positioning. Patients are predisposed to seizures. Avoid drugs that lower the seizure threshold. Anticonvulsant medications and renal failure may alter the metabolism and excretion of some anesthetic agents.

Other conditions to be considered:

☞**CEREBRO-OCULO-SKELETO-RENAL SYNDROME:** A congenital syndrome combining dwarfism and ocular, cerebral, and renal symptoms. Lethal in infancy.

MICROCEPHALIC OSTEODYSPLASTIC PRIMORDIAL DWARFISM (MOPD) TYPE II: Approximately 20 cases have been described. Inheritance is autosomal recessive, with parental consanguinity being a causative factor in almost one third of the patients. Both sexes seem to be equally affected. Intrauterine and severe postnatal growth retardation with disproportionate dwarfism have been reported in almost all cases. Moderate mental retardation, microcephaly with a high forehead, dysplastic ears, prominent nose, mandibular hypoplasia, retarded ossification, narrow and high iliac wings, shallow acetabula, coxa vara, short and bowed humeri and femora, proximal femoral epiphyseolysis, enlarged metaphyses, metaphyseal flaring, triangular epiphyses, and clinodactyly are common findings. Occasionally, craniosynostosis, antimongoloid slanting of the palpebral fissures, and cryptorchidism can be diagnosed. Anomalies of inner organs appear not to be related to this syndrome, although one patient with hypoplasia of the anterior corpus callosum has been described. Anesthetic implications mainly arise from airway management, which may be difficult in the presence of mandibular hypoplasia. Positioning may be difficult secondary to the orthopedic features.

☞SECKEL SYNDROME: A form of primordial dwarfism with characteristic head shape ("bird-like") and pongidoid microcephaly (also called "chimpanzee brain"). Other features include large ears, sparse hair, joint defects, clubfoot, trident hands, mental retardation.

REFERENCES:

Majewski F, Goecke TO: Microcephalic osteodysplastic primordial dwarfism type II: Report of three cases and review. *Am J Med Genet* 80:25, 1998.

Sigaudy S, Toutain A, Moncla A, et al: Microcephalic osteodysplastic primordial dwarfism Taybi-Linder type: Report of four cases and review of the literature. *Am J Med Genet* 80:16, 1998.

Vichi GF, Currarino G, Wasserman RL, et al: Cephaloskeletal dysplasia (Taybi-Linder syndrome: Osteodysplastic primordial dwarfism type III): Report of two cases and review of the literature. *Pediatr Radiol* 30:644, 2000.

Cerebellar Hypoplasia

At a glance: Congenital defect of cerebellum with its neurologic symptomatology.

Incidence and genetic inheritance: Very rare, autosomal recessive.

Clinical aspects: In complete cerebellar aplasia, infants present at birth with hypotonia, tremor and nystagmus. Central respiratory depression has been described. Less severe forms are manifested by varying degrees of nonprogressive ataxia, tremor, nystagmus, speech disorder, areflexia/hyporeflexia, mental retardation, and paraparesis/quadriparesis. Patients may present at advanced age.

Anesthetic considerations: Anesthesia care for autosomal recessive cerebellar hypoplasia has not been described. Evaluate respiratory function (clinical, history, chest x-rays, computed tomography, pulmonary function test, arterial blood gas analysis). In Joubert syndrome, of which cerebellar hypoplasia has been a component, increased sensitivity to respiratory depressants has been reported. Extended postoperative respiratory monitoring is recommended. Possible increased sensitivity to opiates and other respiratory depressants should be expected.

REFERENCES:

Habre W, Sims C, D'Souza M: Anaesthetic management of children with Joubert syndrome. *Paediatr Anaesth* 7:251, 1997.

Mathews KD, Afifi AK, Hanson JW: Autosomal recessive cerebellar hypoplasia. *J Child Neurol* 4:189, 1989.

Megarbane A, Delague V, Salem N, et al: Autosomal recessive congenital cerebellar hypoplasia and short stature in a large inbred family. *Am J Med Genet* 87:88, 1999.

Cerebral Aneurysm-Cirrhosis Syndrome

At a glance: Familial syndrome with idiopathic nonarteriosclerotic cerebral calcifications (FINCC), cirrhosis, pulmonary emphysema and berry cerebral aneurysms.

Synonym: Berry Aneurysm; Cirrhosis; Pulmonary Emphysema; Cerebral Calcification.

Incidence: Unknown, but extremely rare. Only one case report of three affected male siblings has been published.

Genetic inheritance: In this family, FINCC with the additional features of cirrhosis, pulmonary emphysema, and berry cerebral aneurysms was thought to result from a complex pleiotropic mendelian mutation, either autosomal or X-linked recessive in nature. The parents were not consanguineous, and the family history was unremarkable.

Pathophysiology: Basic pathogenesis remains unknown, but an inborn error of metabolism may be responsible.

Diagnosis: Made based on the clinical features consistent with the syndrome. Computed tomography scanning or magnetic resonance imaging may reveal berry aneurysms of cerebral vessels (cerebral angiography), cerebral calcifications, and pulmonary bullae and cysts. A liver biopsy may show fatty degeneration and portal fibrosis preceding periportal and micronodular cirrhosis. Lung function tests and conventional chest radiographs may be helpful.

Clinical aspects: Include nonarteriosclerotic cerebral calcifications symmetrically involving the cortical and subcortical areas, the dentate nucleus, the basal ganglia and the thalamus, cerebral berry aneurysms (most commonly of the middle cerebral, anterior and posterior communicating arteries), liver abnormalities (cirrhosis with portal hypertension, hepatic failure, hepatic encephalopathy, hepatomegaly), clotting abnormalities, severe bilateral pulmonary emphysema, short stature, seizures starting in infancy, dysarthria, dysmetria, delayed motor development, and incoordination. Mental retardation was present in one of the three siblings. Of the three reported cases, one died of liver failure and portal hypertension at 3 years of age; the other two died secondary to ruptured cerebral aneurysms at ages 8 and 13 years, respectively.

Precautions before anesthesia: Obtain a thorough clinical history and examination to evaluate the extent of systemic involvement of the condition, with particular emphasis on the neurologic, hepatic, pulmonary, and hematologic systems. Preoperative blood work should include a complete blood count and serum concentrations of creatinine, urea, electrolytes, and blood glucose. Evaluate pulmonary function (chest radiographs, spirometry, gas diffusion studies, arterial blood gas analysis), hepatic function (liver function tests, coagulation profile, liver biopsy, portal hypertension), neurologic investigations (diagnostic imaging with cerebral angiography, electroencephalography), and cardiovascular status (diuretic therapy in liver failure may lead to intravascular volume depletion).

Anesthetic considerations: Liver failure, cirrhosis, and portal hypertension are all associated with a high risk for general anesthesia and surgery. Regional anesthesia may be an appropriate technique if significant respiratory and hepatic disease is present, provided the patient is cooperative and coagulation and platelet count are within acceptable ranges. Special considerations for anesthesia in liver failure include a rapid sequence induction secondary to decreased gastric emptying and encephalopathy, altered pharmacokinetics and pharmacodynamics of most anesthetic drugs, and avoidance of systemic hypotension (associated with a deterioration in liver function). Provide renal protection (hepatorenal syndrome and intravascular volume depletion are not uncommon), controlled ventilation (abnormal gas exchange, basilar atelectasis, and intrapulmonary arteriovenous shunting are frequent), treat coagulopathy (vitamin K, fresh-frozen plasma, platelets), and administer a dextrose-containing infusion (secondary to decreased glycogen reserves). Preventing excessive intraarterial pressure changes during induction and laryngoscopy is essential to avoid potential rupture or rebleeding of intracranial aneurysms. Intravenous induction (thiopentone or propofol) with neuromuscular blockers and a liberal dose of opioids and lidocaine is recommended to obtund the reflex response to intubation. Controlled ventilation to adjusted to yield normocapnia or mild hypocapnia is recommended, and maintenance of anesthesia is possible with either isoflurane (<1 minimum alveolar concentration) or a target controlled infusion with propofol. Neutral and slight head-up positioning should help cerebral venous drainage. Sudden rises and falls in intracranial pressure should be avoided, and every effort should be made to maintain cerebral perfusion pressure within the physiologic (or preoperative) range, particularly if cerebral autoregulation is compromised.

Pharmacological considerations: Avoid potentially hepatotoxic agents (e.g., halothane). Be careful with agents partially or completely metabolized and excreted by the liver. Elective patients with a prolonged prothrombin time should receive vitamin K. All preoperative medications should be continued (e.g., anticonvulsants, bronchodilators, steroids). Avoid nitrous oxide in the presence of marked pulmonary emphysema.

REFERENCE:

Kahn E, Markowitz J, Duffy L, et al: Berry aneurysms, cirrhosis, pulmonary emphysema, and bilateral symmetrical cerebral calcifications: A new syndrome. *Am J Med Genet Suppl* 3:343, 1987.

Cerebro-Oculo-Skeleto-Renal Syndrome

At a glance: A congenital syndrome combining dwarfism and ocular, cerebral, and renal symptoms. Lethal in infancy.
Synonym: Silengo-Lerone-Pelizza Syndrome.
Incidence and genetic inheritance: A single case of a boy has been reported. Pattern of genetic inheritance is undetermined.
Clinical aspects: Intrauterine and severe postnatal growth retardation are associated with multiple other symptoms involving the head and neck (microcephaly, congenital optic atrophy, nystagmus, flattened nose, thin lips), the central nervous system (dilated cerebral ventricles, electroencephalographic abnormalities with intractable seizures, porencephaly/schizencephaly, profound mental retardation, hyperreflexia), the skeleton (skeletal dysplasia with short rib cage, abnormalities of the pelvis and vertebrae), and the limbs (rhizomelic micromelia, short feet with brachydactyly). The patient also had renal failure that resulted in early death.

Anesthetic considerations: Anesthesia in this condition has not been described. Patients are prone to seizures and would therefore most likely receive antiepileptic therapy. Consider interaction and altered metabolism of anesthetic drugs secondary to chronic anti-seizure drug therapy. Renal failure has implications for fluid and electrolyte balance and the excretion of some anesthetic agents. Intraoperative positioning might be challenging. Mental retardation might impair cooperation. Sedative and/or anxiolytic premedication and the presence of the primary caregiver during induction of anesthesia might be helpful.
Other condition to be considered:
☞**CEPHALOSKELETAL DYSPLASIA:** A brachymelic primordial disproportionate dwarfism associated with facial dysmorphism and neurologic impairment.

REFERENCE:

Silengo MC, Lerone M, Pelizza A, et al: A new syndrome with cerebro-oculo-skeletal-renal involvement. *Pediatr Radiol* 20:612, 1990.

Cerebro-Reno-Digital Syndrome

At a glance: An inherited syndrome combining severe neurologic impairment, hepatic, and renal failure.
Synonym: Meckel-like Syndrome.
Incidence and genetic inheritance: Fewer than 10 cases have been described. Autosomal recessive inheritance.
Clinical aspects: The diagnosis is based on the clinical findings of cystic kidney dysplasia, fibrotic changes of the liver, and occipital encephalocele. Computed tomography scanning and/or magnetic resonance imaging reveals the other cerebral anomalies (see below in this section). This multipolar syndrome is lethal in childhood and involves the head and neck (low-set ears with abnormal helix, short palpebral fissures, small nose, anteverted nares, downturned mouth, high vaulted, narrow palate), the central nervous system (agenesis of the corpus callosum and cerebellar vermis, ☞Dandy-Walker Syndrome, occipital encephalocele, seizures, hypertonia, ataxia, paraparesis/quadriparesis, mental retardation, speech deficit), the eyes (ptosis, nystagmus, strabismus, visual loss, retinoschisis), and the limbs (polydactyly, brachydactyly of the toes). Other features may include renal hypoplasia, renal failure, hepatic fibrosis, and splenomegaly. The syndrome is basically a combination of the ☞Smith-Lemli Opitz syndrome and the ☞Meckel-Gruber syndrome.
Anesthetic considerations: Renal and hepatic function should be fully assessed (complete blood count, serum concentrations of electrolytes, creatinine, blood urea nitrogen, transaminases, alkaline phosphatase, gamma-glutamyl transferase, bilirubin, albumin, and coagulation status). Consider alterations in drug efficacy (altered protein binding of the drug may result in increased free fraction of the drug) and metabolism. The presence of hydrocephalus with raised intracranial pressure should be determined because it may require special anesthetic management. Consider interaction between antiepileptic medications and anesthetic drugs.
Other conditions to be considered:
☞**MECKEL-GRUBER SYNDROME:** Genetic disorder with the main features being encephalocele, polydactyly, and polycystic kidneys, but with a wide phenotypic variation.
☞**SMITH-LEMLI-OPITZ SYNDROME:** A syndrome characterized by the inability to synthesize cholesterol. It presents with

growth retardation, central nervous system anomalies (white matter), developmental delay, severe dysphagia, microcephaly, micrognathia, cleft palate, cataracts, ptosis, polysyndactyly and syndactyly of the second and third toes, and congenital heart defects (e.g., transposition of the great vessels). Congestive heart failure and liver failure are not uncommon.

REFERENCES:
Franceschini P, Licata D, Guala A, et al: Cerebro-reno-digital (Meckel-like) syndrome with limb malformations and acetabular spurs in two sibs: a new MCA syndrome? *Am J Med Genet A* 131:213, 2004.

Genuardi M, Dionisi-Vici C, Sabetta G, et al: Cerebro-reno-digital (Meckel-like) syndrome with Dandy-Walker malformation, cystic kidneys, hepatic fibrosis, and polydactyly. *Am J Med Genet* 47:50, 1993.

Lurie IW, Lazjuk GI, Korotkova IA, et al: The cerebro-reno-digital syndromes: A new community. *Clin Genet* 39:104, 1991.

Cerebrocortical Degeneration of Infancy

At a glance: A progressive form of cerebral degeneration of childhood.

History: Most likely a genetic disorder first described by Laurence and Cavanagh in 1968.

Incidence: Unknown. One case series of the disorder affecting two girls in one family, two boys in a second family, and one male in a third family has been reported.

Genetic inheritance: Likely autosomal recessive.

Pathophysiology: Progressive atrophy of the cerebral cortex already occurs in infancy and is basically confined to the gray matter. At the time of autopsy, all the brains of these patients showed severe ulegyria (i.e., scarring and atrophy of cerebral gyri secondary to a prenatal or perinatal injury) and a uniformly severe destruction of neurons in the cerebral cortex with astrocytic replacement and microglial invasion. The basal ganglia were relatively preserved, with loss of neurons limited to the thalamus. It has been hypothesized that a genetic predisposition to thiamine deficiency is responsible for the described features, as a similar form of degeneration could be found in calves with thiamin deficiency.

Diagnosis: Depends on the histologic findings at autopsy.

Clinical aspects: Affected patients appear normal at birth, with no history of traumatic or anoxic injury. However, developmental arrest presents in the first few months of life with progression to decerebrate rigidity. Seizures may occur. Death resulted from overwhelming infection.

Precautions before anesthesia: Patients may need anesthesia/sedation for diagnostic procedures (e.g., computed tomography scanning and/or magnetic resonance imaging). Assess neurologic status preoperatively and obtain history of seizures. Assess for pulmonary infections from recurrent aspirations.

Anesthetic considerations: Depending on the procedure, the respiratory status may be exacerbated in the presence of preexisting compromised respiratory function. Prolonged postoperative mechanical ventilation may be required.

Pharmacological implications: Antiepileptic treatment may result in interaction with anesthetic drugs and alter their metabolism. Avoid medications that lower the seizure threshold.

REFERENCES:
Laurence KM, Cavanagh JB: Progressive degeneration of the cerebral cortex in infancy. *Brain* 91:261, 1968.

Pill AH: Evidence of thiamine deficiency in calves affected with cerebrocortical necrosis. *Vet Rec* 81:178, 1967.

Cerebrocostomandibular Syndrome

At a glance: A syndrome of mental retardation, palatal defects, micrognathia, and severe costovertebral abnormalities. Often lethal in infancy.

Synonyms: Smith-Theiler-Schachenmann Syndrome; Rib Gap Syndrome; Rib Gap Defects with Micrognathia.

History: First described by D.W. Smith, K. Theiler, and G. Schachenmann in 1966.

Incidence: Approximately 60 cases have been described.

Genetic inheritance: Familial cases with both autosomal recessive and autosomal dominant patterns have been reported (clinically indistinguishable). However, sporadic cases have been described, and the disorder has been suggested to be genetically heterogeneous.

Pathophysiology: Unknown.

Diagnosis: Based on clinical or radiologic findings of facial malformations associated with severe costovertebral impairment (posterior rib gap defects are mandatory for the diagnosis).

Clinical aspects: The disease mainly involves the head and neck (brachycephaly, micrognathia, partial facial hypoplasia, multifocal growth retardation involving vomer, nasoseptal cartilage, and mandibular condyles, indicative of maxillomandibular growth arrest, short hard palate with central defect, absent soft palate and uvula, glossoptosis, webbed neck, posterior nuchal skin folds) and the skeleton (kyphoscoliosis, narrow rib cage, severe costovertebral abnormalities, multiple posterior rib gap defects filled with fibrovascular tissue resulting in flail chest, pectus carinatum). Mental retardation, neural tube defects, absence of the olfactory bulbs, impaired hearing, intrauterine and postnatal growth retardation, pulmonary hypoplasia with neonatal respiratory distress, and cardiac disease (ventricular septal defect) can be associated with this disorder. One case was reported with hypoplastic left heart syndrome, and another case involved omphalocele and cystic hygroma. In more than half of the patients, death occurs in the first year of life and usually results from respiratory complications.

Precautions before anesthesia: Assess respiratory function (clinically, chest radiographs, computed tomography scanning, arterial blood gas analysis). Stridor may indicate tracheal stenosis. Evaluate the anatomy with regard to airway management secondary to facial anomalies. Signs and symptoms of spinal cord compression secondary to kyphoscoliosis should be sought.

Anesthetic considerations: Anesthesia in this condition has not been described. However, because the facial anomalies in these patients have also been referred to as Pierre Robin anomaly, airway management should be expected to be difficult. Alternative airway management techniques should be available (e.g., fiberoptic bronchoscope, [intubating] laryngeal mask airway, retrograde intubation) and spontaneous ventilation maintained until the airway has been secured. Flail chest, restrictive lung disease, and tracheal lesions predispose to perioperative respiratory complications and may result in prolonged postoperative mechanical ventilation. Pulmonary hypoplasia and hyphoscoliasis could both result in increased right ventricular pressures and indicate the need for echocardiography. Tracheal stenosis may require a smaller than predicted endotracheal tube. Central neuraxial blockade should be expected to be difficult considering the vertebral anomalies.

Pharmacological implications: Muscle relaxants should be avoided until the airway has been secured. Subacute bacterial endocarditis prophylaxis may be necessary.

Other condition to be considered:

☞PIERRE ROBIN SYNDROME: A congenital syndrome with multiple etiologies characterized by mandibular hypoplasia/aplasia. It is characterized by the association of cleft palate, glossoptosis and micrognathia.

REFERENCES:

James PA, Aftimos S: Familial cerebro-costo-mandibular syndrome: A case with unusual prenatal findings and review. *Clin Dysmorphol* 12:63, 2003.

Kang YK, Lee SK, Chi JG: Maxillo-mandibular development in cerebrocostomandibular syndrome. *Pediatr Pathol* 12:717, 1992.

Kirk E, Ades L: Hypoplastic left heart in cerebrocostomandibular syndrome. *J Med Genet* 35:879, 1998.

Ceroid Storage Disease

At a glance: A metabolic disease resulting from accumulation of ceroid in the body leading to neurologic and hepatic impairment.

Synonym: Lipofuscin Storage Disease.

Incidence: Unknown. Only isolated case reports exist.

Genetic inheritance: Unknown.

Pathophysiology: Ceroid deposits are found in liver, spleen, intestinal mucosa, lymph nodes, bone marrow, and perithymic fat tissue. Ceroid is a granular, autofluorescent substance, also known as *lipofuscin*. It is thought to consist of cholesterol esters and glycolipids. It has been identified in human tissues, within neurons and large macrophage-like cells in association with several disease processes, for example, ☞Neuronal Ceroid Lipofuscinoses, including Batten Disease.

Diagnosis: Histologic features of affected tissues, in combination with clinical course.

Clinical aspects: Poor physical and mental development, progressive malabsorption, hepatosplenomegaly, liver cirrhosis, anemia, and thrombocytopenia can be observed. Laboratory changes described have included hyponatremia, hypocalcemia, hyperbilirubinemia, and prolonged clotting times. Death usually occurs in childhood.

Precautions before anesthesia: Assess renal and hepatic function and serum levels of electrolytes including calcium. Check complete blood count and obtain a clotting profile. Ideally, significant electrolyte changes are corrected preoperatively.

Anesthetic considerations: Anesthesia in this disorder has not been described. Portal hypertension is possible and may result in significant bleeding, particularly during abdominal surgery. Therefore, large-bore intravenous access is recommended. Insertion of a nasogastric tube should be performed carefully with a well-lubricated tube to avoid bleeding from possible esophageal varices. Regional anesthesia seems not to be contraindicated, however, ensure that coagulation and platelet count (thrombocytopenia secondary to hypersplenism) are within the acceptable range for regional anesthesia.

Pharmacological implications: Liver cirrhosis may not only result in altered metabolism of most anesthetic and other drugs but also affects the protein-binding, and consequently, the efficacy and toxicity of (highly protein-bound) drugs. The choice and dosage of drugs should consider hepatic and/or renal dysfunction.

Other conditions to be considered:

☞HERMANSKY-PUDLAK SYNDROME: Genetically transmitted metabolic disorder causing albinism, visual impairment, and platelet pool storage deficiency resulting in bleeding diathesis and lysosomal accumulation of ceroid lipofuscin with pulmonary fibrosis, inflammatory bowel disease, and renal insufficiency.

☞HALLERVORDEN-SPATZ DISEASE: Inherited disorder characterized by progressive degeneration of the central nervous system as a result of iron deposition in basal ganglia. Most commonly, it begins in childhood as a dystonic syndrome. Other features include distorting muscle contractions of the face, limbs, and trunk, choreoathetosis, muscle rigidity, spasticity, seizures, and dementia. Less common symptoms include painful muscle spasms, mental retardation, and visual impairment.

☞NEURONAL CEROID LIPOFUSCINOSES: A group of hereditary, progressive, neurodegenerative disorders with mental retardation, visual loss, and seizures. This group probably represents the most common class of neurodegenerative diseases in children.

REFERENCES:

Oppenheimer EH, Andrews EC: Ceroid storage disease in childhood. *Pediatrics* 27:931, 1959.

Ryan GB, Anderson RM, Menkes JH, et al: Lipofuscin (ceroid) storage disease of the brain: Neuropathological and neurochemical studies. *Brain* 93:617, 1970.

Ceruloplasmin Deficiency

At a glance: A group of genetic disorders affecting the expression of the ceruloplasmin gene leading to an iron storage disorder with hepatic failure and progressive dementia.

Classification: Hypoceruloplasminemia; Aceruloplasminemia.

Incidence: Unknown, but extremely rare.

Genetic inheritance: Autosomal recessive. A number of allelic variants exist. The responsible gene is located on chromosome 3q23-q24.

Pathophysiology: The multicopper oxidase ceruloplasmin plays an essential role in the normal iron homeostasis. Ceruloplasmin is mainly synthesized in hepatocytes (to a lesser degree also in astrocytes, Sertoli cells, and macrophages) and after incorporation of six copper atoms (holoceruloplasmin) secreted into the plasma. Ceruloplasmin is also an acute phase protein. The rate of ceruloplasmin synthesis or its secretion is not affected by copper, however, its lack results in an unstable, rapidly degraded apoprotein without oxidase activity. The critical physiologic defect in this disorder is the absence of enzymatically active holoceruloplasmin. Within cells, iron is stored as the ferric form Fe^{3+}, but is released as the ferrous form Fe^{2+}, which can react spontaneously with oxygen-containing compounds, resulting in oxidization to Fe^{3+} and release of highly reactive free radicals. Ceruloplasmin, a copper-containing, 132-kDa plasma metalloprotein, is also known as *ferroxidase,* which catalyzes the oxidation of Fe^{2+} to Fe^{3+} with the complete reduction of oxygen to water without releasing free radicals. Fe^{3+} is strongly bound to transferrin, which is basically the only way iron is transported through the body, and the combination of Fe^{2+}-oxidizing ceruloplasmin and Fe^{3+}-binding transferrin guards against the presence of free Fe^{2+} in the circulation, with consequent antioxidant protection. The normal oxidation rate of Fe^{2+} may be too slow to support a regular supply of Fe^{3+}, thus, ceruloplasmin may maintain a sufficient flow rate from storage Fe^{2+} to transferrin-Fe^{3+} by its ferroxidase action. Individuals with ceruloplasmin deficiency have hemosiderosis, shown by low serum iron, high serum ferritin (reflecting the degree of tissue iron overload), and iron accumulation in many tissues leading to neurologic abnormalities and diabetes, supporting ceruloplasmin's important role in the release of cellular iron. Although serum copper is low, urinary copper excretion is normal, and there is no abnormal accumulation of copper in hepatic or other tissues.

Diagnosis: The serum levels of ceruloplasmin, copper, and iron are decreased, whereas the serum level of ferritin is increased. Liver biopsy shows iron accumulation in hepatocytes and Kupffer cells. Computed tomography scanning and/or magnetic resonance imaging demonstrate the iron accumulation in the basal ganglia. Autopsy may confirm significant accumulation of iron and destruction in the basal ganglia, substantia nigra, and dentate nucleus. In addition, iron deposits can be found in neuronal and glial cells, whereas the cerebral cortex usually is not or only mildly affected.

Clinical aspects: The clinical presentation is variable. Symptoms usually start between the fourth and sixth decade of life. Diabetes mellitus is a result of pancreatic fibrosis and often the first sign of the disorder, so these patients already are insulin dependent when other features occur, such as peripheral retinal degeneration and blepharospasm, torticollis, chorea, dysarthria, dystonia, ataxia, and early onset of dementia. A mild anemia is common. Rarely, hepatic iron overload results in hepatic cirrhosis with portal hypertension.

Precautions before anesthesia: Obtain a complete blood count (anemia, thrombocytopenia). Check blood glucose levels and, in case of known diabetes mellitus, review the treatment (sulfonylureas versus insulin) and obtain a blood glucose profile of the last weeks. Assess for liver dysfunction and/or cirrhosis. In patients with long standing diabetes mellitus, renal function and an electrocardiogram should also be checked.

Anesthetic considerations: In patients with diabetes mellitus, a standard approach for this disease can be used, and regular perioperative checks of blood glucose are recommended. Portal hypertension is possible in these patients and may result in significant bleeding particularly during abdominal surgery. Hence, large-bore intravenous access is recommended. The insertion of a nasogastric tube should be performed carefully with a well-lubricated tube to avoid bleeding from possible esophageal varices. Regional anesthesia seems not to be contraindicated, however, ensure that coagulation and platelet count (thrombocytopenia secondary to hypersplenism) are within the acceptable range for regional anesthesia.

Pharmacological implications: Low-dose insulin infusion in combination with a glucose-containing intravenous solution usually is started preoperatively in insulin-dependent patients (alternatively, insulin can be administered subcutaneously). Hepatic insufficiency may not only result in altered metabolism of most anesthetic and other drugs, but also affect the protein-binding and consequently the efficacy and toxicity of (highly protein-bound) drugs. The choice and dosage of drugs should take potential hepatic dysfunction into consideration.

Other conditions to be considered:

☞**HEMOCHROMATOSIS:** Hereditary hemochromatosis is a disorder in which iron is excessively absorbed by the digestive tract and accumulates in body tissues, which progressively causes diabetes mellitus, joint disorders, cardiac arrhythmias and then heart failure, hepatic cirrhosis, skin color changes, and increased risk of cancer.

☞**WILSON DISEASE:** An inherited disease of copper metabolism characterized by liver cirrhosis and central nervous system findings. Prognosis is fatal if not recognized and treated. In contrast to ceruloplasmin deficiency, the absence or impaired function of a copper-transporting ATP-ase in Wilson disease disrupts the copper movement into the secretory pathway, which results in the decreased serum ceruloplasmin observed in these patients.

REFERENCES:

Harris ZL: Aceruloplasminemia. *J Neurol Sci* 207:108, 2003.

Okamoto N, Wada S, Oga T, et al: Hereditary ceruloplasmin deficiency with hemosiderosis. *Hum Genet* 97:755, 1996.

Xu X, Pin S, Gathinji M, Fuchs R, et al: Aceruloplasminemia: An inherited neurodegenerative disease with impairment of iron homeostasis. *Ann N Y Acad Sci* 1012:299, 2004.

Cervico-Oculo-Acoustic Syndrome

At a glance: A congenital condition affecting mostly females and consisting of deafness, vertebral fusion, and abducens palsy.

Synonyms: COA Syndrome; Wildervanck Syndrome.

History: First described by the Dutch geneticist L.S. Wildervanck in 1952.

Incidence: Approximately 85 cases have been described.

Genetic inheritance: Most cases appear to be sporadic, however, polygenic and X-linked dominant inheritance have been discussed.

Pathophysiology: Deafness is a result of a bony malformation of the inner ear. The ☞Klippel-Feil Syndrome (see Clinical Aspects) may involve fusion of cervical, thoracic, and/or lumbar vertebrae; however, fusion of C2-C3 is the most common form.

Diagnosis: Based on clinical findings of the (sometimes incomplete) triad of bilateral abducens paresis with ☞Duane retraction syndrome, deafness, and Klippel-Feil syndrome. Diagnostic imaging is used to confirm the vertebral anomalies.

Clinical aspects: Deafness may be sensorineural, conductive, or mixed. The neck has a webbed appearance, and there is a variable degree of cervical fusion (Klippel-Feil syndrome). Abducens nerve palsy with globe retraction on looking medially is present (Duane retraction syndrome). Additional abnormalities may include short stature, microcephaly, hydrocephalus, brainstem and cerebellar hypoplasia, occipital meningocele, structural facial asymmetry, facial palsy, strabismus, cleft palate, scoliosis, Sprengel deformity (elevated, hypoplastic scapula), spina bifida, preauricular, tags and pseudopapilledema. One case report describes ☞Diastematomyelia of the lower medulla and cervical cord that was accompanied by vermian hypoplasia and tonsillar herniation of the cerebellum resulting in triventricular hydrocephalus. Cardiac defects such as atrial and/or ventricular septal defects may be present. Intelligence usually is normal, but some patients with mental retardation have been reported.

Precautions before anesthesia: Patients with the Klippel-Feil syndrome are vulnerable to cervical cord injury during laryngoscopy and during head and neck movements. Evaluate the spine clinically, and obtain conventional radiographs and/or computed tomography scanning. Neurologic lesions occur most frequently at the cervicooccipital junction. Assess for increased intracranial pressure and congenital cardiac lesions (echocardiography may be required). In a minority of cases, lung and/or kidney problems have been described. In this case, lung function tests with blood gas analysis and/or a complete blood count with serum concentrations of electrolytes, creatinine, and blood urea nitrogen may be indicated.

Anesthetic considerations: Patients may have cervical instability and are at high risk for spinal cord injury during direct laryngoscopy, tracheal intubation, and positioning for surgery. The patient should be managed as an unstable cervical spine and should have inline stabilization for laryngoscopy and intubation. However, tracheal intubation may be difficult because of restricted neck movement. Given the risk of spinal lesions on intubation, awake fiberoptic intubation is the technique of choice. Alternatively, asleep fiberoptic intubation or (intubating) laryngeal mask can be used (particularly in children), however then the "real-time" neurologic monitoring of the awake patient is not available in this scenario. Use of continuous spinal cord monitoring (if available) is then recommended. Intraoperatively, the head and neck should be maintained in a position that has been determined preoperatively to be safe. Meticulous attention must be paid to positioning, particularly if the patient is to be turned prone. Recommendations are to use regional anesthesia whenever possible. Incremental central neuraxial techniques may be preferable to single-shot techniques to control block height. However, central neuraxial blocks may be difficult to perform in the presence of the anomalies described and are contraindicated in patients with increased intracranial pressure.

Pharmacological implications: Muscle relaxants should be avoided until the airway has been secured. In the presence of congenital cardiac lesions, subacute bacterial endocarditis prophylaxis may be necessary.

Other conditions to be considered:

☞**DUANE RETRACTION SYNDROME:** A neuroophthalmologic condition associated with abnormal ocular movement, usually not accompanied by other congenital anomalies.

☞**KLIPPEL-FEIL SYNDROME:** Syndrome characterized by the congenital fusion of any two of the seven cervical vertebrae resulting in shortness of the neck, restricted neck movements, and low posterior hair line.

☞**GOLDENHAR SYNDROME:** Common birth defect of vascular origin involving the first and second branchial arch derivatives resulting mainly in hemifacial microsomia with absent ear, eye, and vertebral anomalies. Usually associated with cardiovascular anomalies including ventricular septal defect, atrial septal defect, patent ductus arteriosus, tetralogy of Fallot, and coarctation of the aorta. Arnold-Chiari malformation and hydrocephalus have been reported.

REFERENCES:

Balci S, Oguz KK, Firat MM, et al: Cervical diastematomyelia in cervico-oculo-acoustic (Wildervanck) syndrome: MRI findings. *Clin Dysmorphol* 11:125, 2002.

Nagib MG, Maxwell RE, Chou SN: Identification and management of high-risk patients with Klippel-Feil syndrome. *J Neurosurg* 61:523, 1984.

O'Connor PJ, Moysa GL, Finucane BT: Thoracic epidural anesthesia for bilateral reduction mammoplasty in a patient with Klippel-Feil syndrome. *Anesth Analg* 92:514, 2001.

CHANDS

At a glance: Ectodermal dysplasia associated with ankyloblepharon. CHANDS is an acronym for *c*urly *h*air, *a*nkyloblepharon, and *n*ail *d*ysplasia, *s*yndrome.
Synonym: Baughman Syndrome.

Incidence and genetic inheritance: Fewer than 10 cases have been described. Autosomal recessive mode of inheritance with pseudodominance has been suggested. Consanguinity seems to be a risk factor.

Clinical aspects: The main clinical signs are listed in the acronym: curly hair, ankyloblepharon (fusion of the eyelids), and nail dysplasia (hypoplastic, hyperconvex, grooved). Other signs may include abnormal gait, ataxia, speech defect, hypermetropia, and strabismus. One case also had fibrous adhesions between maxilla and mandibula at the level of the premolars, but also from the buccal mucosa to the alveolar ridges, which basically resulted in the inability to open the mouth.

Anesthetic considerations: In the presence of interalveolar fusion and inability to open the mouth (in the case reported by Ohishi et al., interalveolar distance was 4 mm at birth), airway management is very difficult. In this report, surgery was postponed until 1 year of age because feeding (surprisingly) was not an issue. At the time of surgery, mouth opening was 6 mm preoperatively and 12 mm after cutting of the fibrous bands. Endotracheal intubation was performed, but the technique used had not been described. Either awake fiberoptic nasal intubation or, if this option is not available, tracheotomy under local anesthesia is the technique of choice. As illustrated by this case, separation of the mandibula and maxilla does not immediately improve the situation from an anesthetic point of view because ankylosis of the temporomandibular joints is present. Other anesthetic implications are limited to eye protection (in Ohishi's report, the eyelids were separated immediately after birth by an ophthalmologist, and apparently no anesthetic was given at that time).

Other condition to be considered:

☞**ECTODERMAL DYSPLASIAS (ED):** A group of inherited disorders characterized by disturbances in one or more ectodermal structures and their accessory appendages. The absent or deficient function of at least two derivatives of the ectoderm constitutes a form of ED.

More than 150 different forms of ED have been described.

REFERENCES:

Ohishi M, Kai S, Ozeki S, et al: Alveolar synechia, ankyloblepharon, and ectodermal disorders: An autosomal recessive disorder? *Am J Med Genet* 38:13, 1991.

Toriello HV: Alveolar synechia-ankyloblepharon-ectodermal defects likely CHANDS. *Am J Med Genet* 49:348, 1994.

Toriello HV, Lindstrom JA, Waterman DF, et al: Re-evaluation of CHANDS. *J Med Genet* 16:316, 1979.

Charcot-Marie-Tooth Disease

At a glance: A hereditary polyneuropathy condition presenting with distal weakness and muscular atrophy (myopathy).
Synonyms: Hereditary Motor and Sensory Neuropathy Type I; Peroneal Muscular Atrophy.
History: This disorder was first described in 1886 in Paris by the two French neurologists Jean Martin Charcot and Pierre Marie, who identified it as a primary muscle disease, and independently in Cambridge by the English physician Howard Henry Tooth, who correctly interpreted his findings as a primary neurologic disease.
Incidence: Estimates vary widely between 1:2500 and 1:10,000 live births. Charcot-Marie-Tooth syndrome type I (CMT I) accounts for approximately two thirds of all CMT cases, whereas CMT II

constitutes the residual one third. No racial or sexual predilection could be identified.

Genetic inheritance: CMT can be inherited in different patterns: autosomal dominant, autosomal recessive, and X-linked transmission have been described. The dominant form is the most common. Far more than 20 different mutations are known to cause CMT, and new ones are added on a regular basis. The two genes most commonly involved are the PMP22 (peripheral myelin protein 22) gene, located on 17p11.2, and the MPZ (myelin protein zero) gene, which has been mapped to 1q22.

Pathophysiology: The syndrome can be divided into two types based on electrophysiologic, clinical, and genetic features. *CMT I* is a demyelinating form of peripheral polyneuropathy characterized by decreased motor nerve conduction velocities, hypertrophy of peripheral nerves with typical onion bulb formation and segmental demyelination. As a result of a mutation in the PMP22 gene, the myelin that is formed is unstable and breaks down easily. Larger motor and sensory axons may be involved. *CMT II*, the so-called neuronal form, is characterized by normal or only slightly diminished motor nerve conduction velocities and normal myelination and nerve size. The pathoanatomical correlate is direct axonal death and Wallerian degeneration. Because most patients also have sensory nerve involvement, the disorders are now also summarized as *hereditary motor and sensory neuropathy type I* (see also "Hereditary Motor and Sensory Neuropathies (HMSN): Overview").

Diagnosis: Based on the clinical findings of distal muscle weakness and atrophy and supported and confirmed by nerve conduction studies and specialized genetic testing. Nerve biopsy is rarely indicated. Special rare types may require DNA analysis.

Clinical aspects: Although there is considerable variation in the age of onset, the severity and progression rate of symptoms and the clinical phenotype of all forms of CMT are generally similar. A minority of patients present at birth with hypotonia or later with motor delay. However, the majority of patients present later in life, usually within the first 2 decades. The most common complaint is distal leg weakness, which manifests as frequent tripping and muscle atrophy. Hand involvement follows in most cases. Pregnancy may exacerbate a preexisting weakness in 50% of patients with early-onset disease. The exacerbation is transient in one third of women, but unfortunately is progressive in the other two thirds. Cardiomyopathy and cardiac conduction abnormalities are seen occasionally. Clinical features may include foot dropping, pes cavus deformity, muscle cramping, steppage or equine gait, "champagne bottle" or stork legs, hammer toes, clawhand, and diminished or absent deep tendon reflexes. Pain and temperature sensation are normal. The diaphragm, phrenic nerve, and vocal cords are occasionally involved. Life expectancy usually is not affected, and confinement to the wheelchair is rare.

CHARCOT-MARIE-TOOTH DISEASE TYPE I:

Type IA: Approximately 90% of CMT I patients belong to this group. They all have in common a partial duplication of the PMP22 gene: clinical symptoms appear in the first or early in the second decade of life. In infants and children, the disease presents with patients walking on their toes and severe tightness of the heel cord. Occasionally, these patients are born with clubfoot. Gait anomalies, foot deformities, and loss of balance are the main complaints in these patients and the reason they seek medical help. Distal leg weakness predominantly affects the dorsiflexor muscles (innervated by the peroneal nerve), which may result in frequent tripping over objects lying on the floor. Accordingly, difficulties or inability to walk on the heels usually is one of the early signs of the disease. As the disease

progresses, weakness becomes more pronounced and results in foot drops with each step, forcing the patient to flex the hips more, which leads to the steppage or equine gait. The imbalance between intrinsic and extrinsic foot muscles may result in the formation of pes cavus. Peroneal muscle atrophy may lead to inverted "champagne bottle" or stork legs, but may be masked by a thicker layer of subcutaneous fat. At this stage, patients often complain about leg muscle cramps and lumbar back pain. Later, most often the hands also start to show signs of weakness and atrophy that may result in clawhand deformity (marked extension of the fingers in the metacarpophalangeal joints, while the distal and proximal interphalangeal joints are flexed) with serious handicapping in daily life. Involvement of the hand does not appear to be related to the degree of leg weakness. Decreased vibratory sense is common, and mild sensory loss in a stocking distribution is not uncommon. Enlargement of the nerves to the point that they can be seen or palpated occurs in about one fourth of patients and is more common in men, but it seems not to be related to the severity of the disease. Approximately 40% of patients have a tremor, which usually starts in the fourth decade of life. Symptoms of hip dysplasia usually begin in adolescence. Pulmonary symptoms have been reported in CMT patients. Spirometry values and static lung volumes are usually within normal limits, but testing of the inspiratory and expiratory muscles reveals a significantly decreased function.

VARIANTS OF CMT IA:

☞**Roussy Lévy Syndrome:** This phenotypic variant has some features in common with ☞Friedreich Ataxia and presents with pes cavus, distal limb weakness, areflexia, tremor in the hands, and distal sensory loss with ataxia. Genetic analysis in these patients has shown a duplication of the PMP22 gene.

Davidenkow Syndrome (Scapuloperoneal Atrophy): Scapuloperoneal muscle atrophy with pes cavus, areflexia, and distal sensory loss. Motor nerve conduction velocities are decreased, and hypertrophic changes of the nerves are present. These patients have the partial duplication of 17p11.2, supporting the fact that this is another variant of CMT IA.

Type IB: This group accounts for the residual 10% of CMT I patients, which share a point mutation in the MPZ gene. In comparison with CMT IA, symptoms start much earlier with delayed ability to walk, proximal leg weakness, and slower nerve conduction velocities than in CMT IA. Sural nerve biopsy reveals the demyelinating process with onion bulb formation.

VARIANTS OF CMT IB:

☞**Dejerine Sottas Syndrome/HMSN III:** Characterized by onset in infancy or early childhood with delayed motor development, rapid progression, and often profound nerve hypertrophy. This form is most often caused by either de novo point mutations in the PMP22 or MPZ gene.

Congenital Hypomyelination: Infantile hypotonia secondary to distal muscle weakness, areflexia, and very slow nerve conduction velocities. The combination with joint contractures and ☞**Arthrogryposis Multiplex** has been described. Sural nerve biopsy reveals hypomyelination without signs of active myelin breakdown. This form is caused by mutations in the MPZ gene.

CHARCOT-MARIE-TOOTH DISEASE TYPE II:

This genetically heterogenous form of CMT, also called the *neuronal type* of CMT, is clinically similar to CMT I (with the same wide variability). However, the age of onset is more variable and in general is later than in CMT I. Motor nerve conduction velocities are normal or only slightly diminished, the nerves show no signs of hypertrophy, and nerve biopsy lacks the typical onion bulb formation seen in CMT I. Distal leg weakness with muscular atrophy, pes cavus deformity, and steppage gait are similar to CMT I, while the hand muscles are less often affected and deep tendon reflexes are intact. Genetically, several different mutations have been identified and mapped to chromosomes 1, 3, and 7.

CMTX/X-Linked HMSN: In approximately 90%, CMTX is inherited in an X-linked dominant transmission; the remaining 10% show X-linked recessive transmission. The clinical signs are similar to those of CMT IA, but males are more severely affected than females. The significantly decreased nerve conduction velocity supports a demyelinating process.

Precautions before anesthesia: Assess the patient neurologically and ask about respiratory and cardiac problems. Pulmonary function tests including chest radiography and arterial blood gas analysis should be performed if respiratory involvement (secondary to respiratory muscle weakness) is suspected. An electrocardiogram is recommended for all patients, and an echocardiogram may be indicated depending on the clinical findings.

Anesthetic considerations: Anesthesia may exacerbate preexisting respiratory disease, and prolonged postoperative mechanical ventilation may be required. A peripheral nerve stimulator should be used to monitor neuromuscular blockade if muscle relaxants are to be used. However, care should be taken to place the electrodes on an unaffected nerve to prevent erroneous results. Regional anesthesia has been used successfully in multiple cases. Involvement of the autonomic nervous system may result in abnormal temperature regulation.

Pharmacological implications: The literature suggests the induction dose of thiopentone may need to be reduced in Charcot-Marie-Tooth disease. A small number of case reports indicate use of succinylcholine in CMT may result in hyperkalemia or malignant hyperthermia-like reactions. However, this finding has not been confirmed by a larger, retrospective series of a total of 161 procedures in 86 patients, of whom 48% received succinylcholine and 90% received malignant hyperthermia triggering agents without significant adverse effects. It has been suggested, however, that individuals with acute exacerbations of the disease represent a subset of patients who have altered responses to muscle relaxants and that, in such a scenario, succinylcholine should be avoided and other muscle relaxants used in small incremental doses with neuromuscular monitoring.

Other condition to be considered:

☞**Cowchock Syndrome:** An X-linked form of sensory and motor neuropathy characterized by atrophy of the peroneal muscles but also involving other distal muscles of the legs and arms.

REFERENCES:

Antognini JF: Anesthetic management in Charcot-Marie-Tooth disease. *Anesth Analg* 75:313, 1992.

Naguib M, Samarkandi AH: Response to atracurium and mivacurium in a patient with Charcot-Marie-Tooth disease. *Can J Anaesth* 45:56, 1998.

Tetzlaff JE, Schwendt I: Arrhythmia and Charcot-Marie-Tooth disease during anesthesia. *Can J Anaesth* 47:29, 2000.

CHARGE Syndrome

At a glance: A life-threatening, congenital syndrome of multiple abnormalities, consisting of coloboma, heart disease, choanal atresia, mental and growth retardation, genital and urinary anoma-

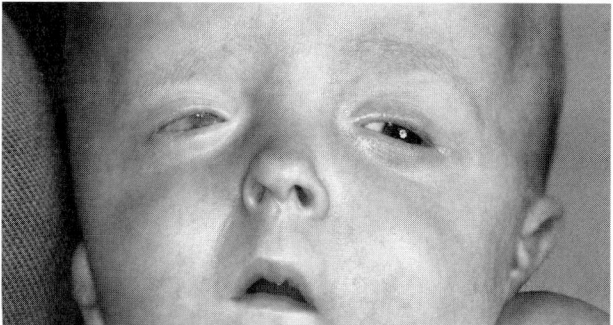

CHARGE Syndrome Eye anomalies in a 3-month-old boy with CHARGE syndrome. See color plates.

lies, and ear anomalies with deafness. The prognosis worsens if the disorder is associated with concomitant cyanotic congenital heart disease, central nervous system anomalies, and esophageal atresia. CHARGE is an acronym for *c*oloboma, *h*eart anomaly, choanal *a*tresia, mental and growth *r*etardation, *g*enital anomalies, and *e*ar anomalies.

Synonym: CHARGE Association.

Incidence: Approximately 1:13,000–15,000 live births. No sexual or racial predilection has been reported.

Genetic inheritance: More than 90% of the cases occur sporadically. Exposure to teratogenic substances (e.g., thalidomide, hydantoin), but also maternal diabetes mellitus have been suggested to

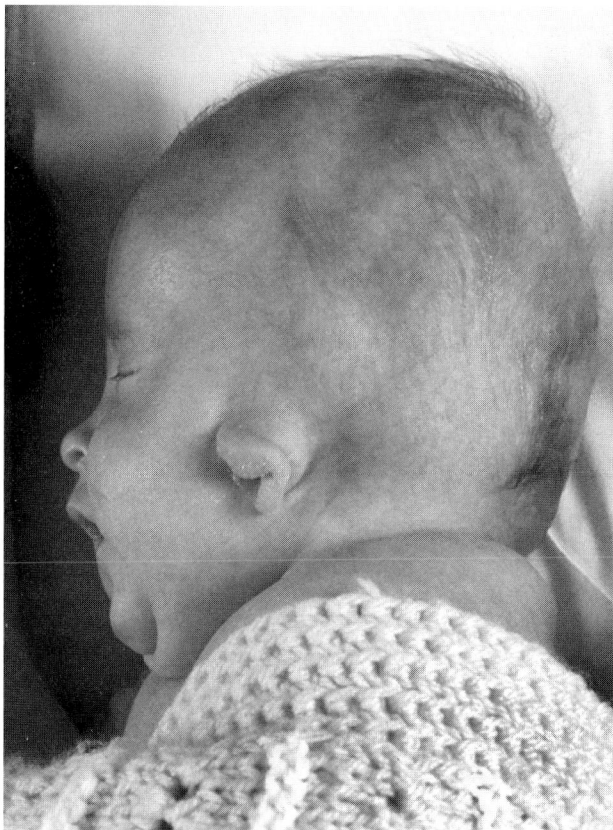

CHARGE Syndrome Anomaly of the ear in the same baby with CHARGE syndrome.

play a causative role. The residual cases are familial with autosomal recessive transmission.

Pathophysiology: CHARGE syndrome is a midline developmental defect attributed to an arrest in embryologic differentiation during early organogenesis. The mechanism has not been precisely identified, but may include failure of the cervical neural crest cells to migrate into the derivatives of the pharyngeal pouches and arches, deficient blastogenesis as a result of defective interaction between mesoderm and neural crest cells, and failure of mesoderm formation.

Diagnosis: None of the features in the CHARGE acronym are universally present. The clinical diagnosis is based on the presence of four of the seven features described in the acronym, including at least one major anomaly. Patients may present in the neonatal period with respiratory distress and feeding difficulties. Delayed presentation is usually associated with persistent nasal discharge, failure to thrive, audiovisual defects, and developmental delay.

Clinical aspects: Prenatal ultrasound may already reveal polyhydramnios, intrauterine growth retardation, and brain and heart anomalies. A wide range of features involve the heart (present in up to 80% of patients; cardiac defects such as atrial and ventricular septal defects, atrioventricular canal, conotruncal malformations, tetralogy of Fallot, hypoplastic left heart syndrome, patent ductus arteriosus, pulmonary stenosis, and coarctation of the aorta are common), the airway (choanal atresia is bilateral in 50% of cases and may present with respiratory distress in the neonatal period when bilateral; choanal stenosis is less common; laryngomalacia, laryngeal cleft, and subglottic stenosis are occasionally seen), the central nervous system (mild-to-moderate mental retardation is common; seizures are occasionally present; multiple cranial neuropathies such as facial nerve palsy, sensorineural hearing loss [the most common feature in CHARGE syndrome], glossopharyngeal and vagal nerve palsy with swallowing problems resulting in frequent aspirations, and hyposmia may be present; magnetic resonance imaging of the brain usually demonstrates cerebral atrophy, midline brain defects, forebrain anomalies, and occasionally hydrocephalus), the genitourinary system (vesicoureteral reflux, hydronephrosis, horseshoe kidney, absent kidney, genital hypoplasia [micropenis, hypospadias, cryptorchidism]), and the skeleton (hypotonia of the upper truncus, hemivertebrae, scoliosis, clinodactyly, and syndactyly). Tracheoesophageal fistula and esophageal atresia are present occasionally (in up to 20% of patients). Facial abnormalities may include a square face with asymmetry, dysplasia of the external and middle ear (Mondini defect), midface hypoplasia and micrognathia, nerve palsies, and cleft lip/palate, but usually are mild. Heart defects and postoperative pulmonary complications are the major cause of death.

Precautions before anesthesia: The presence of active lower respiratory tract infections should be determined and treated preoperatively. Renal function should be assessed (creatinine and blood urea nitrogen). Cardiac function and anatomy should be defined preoperatively by echocardiography. Check for seizure activity (electroencephalography). Prolonged postoperative mechanical ventilation may be required (laryngomalacia, frequent aspirations, truncal hypotonia). Preoperative and postoperative chest physiotherapy is often helpful. Because of mental retardation and hearing loss, cooperation may be limited. Sedative and/or anxiolytic premedication and the presence of the primary caregiver during induction of anesthesia may be helpful.

Anesthetic considerations: The presence of midface hypoplasia, micrognathia, anterior larynx, small mouth, and cleft lip and palate may make face-mask ventilation and tracheal intubation difficult. Airway management seems to become more difficult with age.

Laryngomalacia may require continuous positive airway pressure when a face mask is used. A smaller than expected tube size may be needed in the presence of subglottic stenosis. From an airway point of view, spontaneous ventilation should be maintained until the airway has been secured. However, because these patients have an increased risk of aspiration (even in the absence of a tracheoesophageal fistula), a rapid-sequence induction is preferable. The decision regarding priority (airway management vs. aspiration) depends on the clinical findings and patient history. Choanal atresia makes nasogastric tube and nasal airway management impossible. Special management is required in the presence of congenital cardiac lesions. Careful intraoperative positioning is needed.

Pharmacological implications: Muscle relaxants should be avoided until the airway has been secured. Subacute bacterial endocarditis prophylaxis may be needed, depending on the cardiac defect and the kind of procedure to be done. Chronic antiseizure medication may alter metabolism and elimination of some anesthetic drugs.

Other conditions to be considered:

☞**DiGeorge Syndrome:** A genetic defect leading to a wide range of phenotypic presentations, mainly developmental defects in the outflow tract of the heart, hypoparathyroidism with hypocalcemia, and thymic hypoplasia/aplasia with immune defects.

☞**Renal-Coloboma Syndrome:** A familial syndrome combining ocular, renal, and neurologic anomalies.

☞**Velocardiofacial Syndrome:** Includes typical facies and cardiac anomalies. Various other malformations can be associated (including endocrine and ophthalmic structures). It is a phenotypical variant of the DiGeorge syndrome.

☞**VA(C)TER(L)-Association:** The acronym describes *v*ertebral anomalies, *a*nal atresia, (*c*ardiac defects), *t*racheo*e*sophageal fistula, *r*enal anomalies and *l*imb anomalies. Other coexisting abnormalities must be excluded.

REFERENCES:

Stack CG, Wyse RK: Incidence and management of airway problems in the CHARGE Association. *Anaesthesia* 46:582, 1991.

Tellier AL, Cormier-Daire V, Abadie V, et al: CHARGE syndrome: Report of 47 cases and review. *Am J Med Genet* 76:402, 1998.

White DR, Giambra BK, Hopkin RJ, et al: Aspiration in children with CHARGE syndrome. *Int J Pediatr Otorhinolaryngol* 69:1205, 2005.

Charlie M Syndrome

At a glance: An exceptionally rare syndrome involving head and limbs.

Incidence and genetic inheritance: A single case has been described. Genetic inheritance has not been determined.

Clinical aspects: Bipolar disease involving head and neck (microcephaly, long large ears, microstomia, micrognathia and retrognathia, broad nose, short philtrum, cleft lip, thin lips, oligodontia) and limbs (metacarpal abnormalities, triphalangeal thumb, bifid great toe, brachydactyly, syndactyly [fingers], oligodactyly, foot anomalies, dysplastic toenails).

Anesthetic considerations: Anesthesia in this condition has not been described. However, the features of the disease suggest airway management most likely will be difficult. Spontaneous ventilation should be maintained until the airway has been secured. Alternative airway management techniques, such as fiberoptic intubation or (intubating) laryngeal mask, should be easily available.

REFERENCE:
Bonioli E, Sbolgi P, Bernaola E et al: The "Charlie M." syndrome: A new clinical entity? Description of a case. *Minerva Pediatr* 32:699, 1980.

Chauffard Syndrome

At a glance: A chronic inflammatory disease of variable severity that affects the joints and may involve the connective tissues and viscera.

Synonyms: Juvenile Rheumatoid Arthritis (JRA); Still Disease; Still Chauffard Disease. The International League of Associations of Rheumatologists Task Force on the Classification of Childhood Arthritis has proposed that the previously used terminology of *juvenile rheumatoid arthritis* be discarded and superseded by the umbrella term *juvenile idiopathic arthritis* (JIA).

Incidence: Approximately 10–20:100,000 children. A particularly high incidence has been described in Native Americans and in parts of Scandinavia. No sexual predilection exists, however, the oligoarticular and polyarticular forms tend to be more common in girls, whereas the systemic-onset form of the disease affects both genders equally.

Genetic inheritance: A complex genetic inheritance pattern is likely but is yet undefined.

Pathophysiology: The disease is caused by chronic synovial inflammation of unknown origin characterized by B-lymphocyte infiltration. Synovial proliferation seems to be the result of cytokines released by invading macrophages and T cells. Lymphocytic infiltration has been suggested to induce angiogenesis, thereby maintaining the disease process. Destruction of the joint cartilage and, later, of the bone is caused by the pannus. The etiology of the condition is unclear, but associations with particular HLA haplotypes (e.g., HLA-B27) have been observed.

Diagnosis: The previous American College of Rheumatology classification of JRA referred to oligoarticular arthritis, polyarticular arthritis, or systemic illness of at least 6 weeks' duration. In the current classification, JIA is defined as an arthritis occurring before 16 years of age, lasting for at least 6 weeks without an established cause and excludes psoriatic arthropathy and juvenile spondyloarthropathy. The diagnosis is made by exclusion of alternative conditions (e.g., malignancy or infection). The clinical course is variable and may resolve after a single episode, whereas systemic and articular flare-ups occur frequently in others.

Clinical aspects: The polyarticular form of Chauffard syndrome may occur in children at any age. The oligoarticular and the systemic-onset forms usually occur in early childhood, although later onset (including adolescence) has been described. Skeletal features include generalized osteopenia, joint involvement, either oligoarticular (1–4 joints, also called *pauciarticular)* or polyarticular (≥5 joints), with cartilage destruction preceding the bony involvement. Effusions in affected joints and radial deviation of the wrist may occur. Joint inflammation may be associated with muscle atrophy. Bony fusion of the cervical spine is common and most frequently occurs at the C2-C3 level secondary to apophyseal ankylosis. Atlantoodontoid instability may occur secondary to pannus formation in the joint, odontoid erosions, and ligamentous laxity. Dental malocclusion and mandibular hypoplasia associated with mandibular retrognathia are common and present in about one fourth of affected children. Limited mouth opening may occur in the absence of symptoms such as temporomandibular joint pain at rest or during function. Stridor may occur secondary to cricoarytenoiditis. Other findings may include uveitis, pericarditis, hepatosplenomegaly, lymphadenopathy, a pink, linear macular rash on trunk and extremities, anemia, and pulmonary interstitial fibrosis. Systemic features such as fever (often spiking several times a day and typically not responding to antipyretics), anorexia, encephalopathy, and hepatic dysfunction may occur during active systemic disease. Laboratory anomalies include leukocytosis, increased erythrocyte sedimentation rate, and seropositivity for rheumatoid factor (10%). Approximately 25% of patients are positive for antinuclear antibodies. Classic systemic Chauffard syndrome is an acute systemic illness generally without articular changes.

Precautions before anesthesia: History, examination, and investigations should aim to determine the complications arising from the disease and the treatment. Cervical spine stability should be assessed by clinical evaluation of cervical neuropathy and with flexion and extension radiographs. Obtain a complete blood count to detect (microcytic) anemia, and check hepatic (e.g., transaminases, bilirubin, coagulation factors, albumin) and renal function (creatinine, blood urea nitrogen). A chest radiograph, pulmonary function tests, and arterial blood gas analysis should be performed as indicated by clinical signs and symptoms. The need for postoperative mechanical ventilation should be anticipated in the presence of significant pulmonary disease. Toxic organ effects (e.g., renal, hepatic, hematologic changes) secondary to concomitant therapies should be determined. Electrocardiography and echocardiography should be performed if cardiac involvement (pericarditis, myocarditis) is suspected.

Anesthetic considerations: Limitation of mouth opening, cricoarytenoiditis, and cervical spine instability may all contribute to difficult airway management. Mouth opening may be inadequate to even facilitate laryngeal mask insertion. Multiple airway management techniques have been described, including awake or asleep fiberoptic intubation, intubating laryngeal mask, and laryngeal mask-guided fiberoptic intubation. Cardiac involvement may warrant invasive hemodynamic monitoring. Central neuraxial anesthesia is not contraindicated but may be technically difficult to perform mainly because of limitations in optimal positioning.

Pharmacological implications: Simultaneous medications may include nonsteroidal antiinflammatory agents, systemic steroids, cyclosporin, azathioprine, methotrexate, cyclophosphamide, chlorambucil, gold, sulfasalazine, erythropoietin, and immunoglobulins. Etanercept, an antagonist to tumor necrosis factor (TNF), seems to be a promising new drug for treatment of this disease. Many of these drugs may cause multiorgan toxicity and have established adverse drug–drug interactions. Specific anesthesia concerns include the dose-dependent inhibition of pseudocholinesterase activity by cyclophosphamide, which may prolong the effect of succinylcholine. Abrupt discontinuation of glucocorticoids may precipitate an adrenal crisis.

Other conditions to be considered:

☞**KAWASAKI DISEASE:** Self-limited vasculitic syndrome of unknown etiology characterized by fever, cervical adenopathies, and cardiac involvement (often lethal).

☞**SYSTEMIC LUPUS ERYTHEMATOSUS:** A disorder characterized by unpredictable exacerbation and remission of an inflammatory multisystemic disorder affecting the connective tissue. The circulation of immune complexes and activation of complement leads to involvement mainly of the skin, joints, kidneys, serosal membranes, lung, gastrointestinal tract, and heart.

REFERENCES:

Johnson K, Gardner-Medwin J: Childhood arthritis: Classification and radiology. *Clin Radiol* 57:47, 2002

Popat MT, Chippa JH, Russell R: Awake fibreoptic intubation following failed regional anaesthesia for caesarean section in a parturient with Still's disease. *Eur J Anaesthesiol* 17:211, 2000.

Smith BL: Anaesthesia for patients with juvenile chronic arthritis (Still's disease). *Anaesthesia* 53:314, 1998.

Chediak-Higashi Syndrome

At a glance: A frequently fatal disease of childhood characterized by the association of immune deficiency, partial oculocutaneous albinism, easy bruisability, bleeding, and recurrent infections.

Synonyms: Chediak-Steinbrinck-Higashi Syndrome; Beguez Cesar Syndrome; Oculocutaneous Albinism Type VIB.

History: First described by the Cuban pediatrician A. Beguez Cesar in 1943. The German physician W. Steinbrinck, the Cuban physician A.M. Chédiak, and the Japanese pediatrician O. Higashi reported their findings in 1948, 1952, and 1953, respectively.

Incidence: Approximately 200 cases have been described in the literature. Most affected patients are of Spanish or South American descent.

Genetic inheritance: Autosomal recessive. Caused by mutations in the lysosomal trafficking regular gene CHS1, which is located on 1q42.1-q42.2.

Pathophysiology: The defective melanosome transfer is a secondary phenomenon of a primary defect in the lysosome trafficking regulator (LYST) protein, a membrane-associated molecule that is important in protein docking and fusion and membrane stability. This is an imperfect oculocutaneous albinism with giant melanosomes. Giant peroxidase-filled lysosomal granules exist in leukocytes, and giant peroxidase-containing granules are present in Schwann cells.

Diagnosis: In addition to the features of albinism, photophobia, hypopigmentation, and loss of binocular vision, patients with Chediak-Higashi syndrome show marked susceptibility to infections. Death often occurs in the first decade of life as a result of infections, bleeding, and the accelerated lymphoma-like phase. However, survival into the second and third decade of life has been reported.

Clinical aspects: Staphylococcal and streptococcal infections are the most common reason for medical presentation. Immunosuppression can result in potentially life-threatening infections. Anemia, thrombocytopenia, and neutrophilia may develop. Other features can affect neurologic function with peripheral neuropathy and occasionally seizures. Most patients who survive their childhood frequently develop an accelerated phase of the disease characterized by lymphohistiocytic proliferation and hemophagocytic syndrome. In this accelerated phase, patients exhibit mediastinal and hilar lymphadenopathy, jaundice, hepatosplenomegaly, gingivitis, and a pseudomembranous sloughing of the buccal mucosa. Often this seems to be precipitated by viral infections, particularly the Epstein-Barr virus. Platelet function may be impaired before the accelerated phase of the disease because of functional platelet storage defects. Treatment with high doses of ascorbic acid has been beneficial in these patients. However, such high doses of vitamin C have been associated with renal impairment and calculi. Treatment with bone marrow transplantation has been performed.

Precautions before anesthesia: Patients may present for surgical treatment of abscesses. They may be severely septic. A thorough history and examination should be performed to confirm hepatosplenomegaly, which is suggestive of serious end-stage disease. A complete blood count reveals cellular abnormalities. Platelet function tests and bleeding time should be obtained, particularly when major surgery and/or central neuraxial blockade is contemplated. Kidney function (creatinine, blood urea nitrogen) should be assessed if the patient is taking high doses of vitamin C. Patients may be on long-term steroid therapy.

Anesthetic considerations: Strict precautions to prevent iatrogenic infections in these immunologically compromised patients should be taken. Regional anesthesia, particularly central neuraxial blockade, is relatively contraindicated in these patients in whom, even in the face of a normal count, platelet function most likely is impaired. If mediastinal lymphadenopathy is present, assess for signs of stridor, dyspnea and signs of cardiovascular compression and obtain a computed tomography scan of the chest to determine the degree of compression of the airway and/or major vessels, which may result in airway and cardiovascular collapse on induction of anesthesia. Maintenance of spontaneous ventilation is crucial in these patients.

Pharmacological implications: Consider interaction between antiepileptic treatment and anesthetic drugs. Succinylcholine should be avoided because of nerve lesions and the associated risk of exaggerated hyperkalemia. Avoid muscle relaxants in the presence of obstructing mediastinal lymphadenopathy. Consider giving perioperative stress doses of steroids in cases of long-term steroid treatment.

REFERENCES:

Ganschow R, Grabhorn E, Lemke J, et al: Cardiac failure in an infant with Chediak-Higashi syndrome: A hypothesis of the effect of diadenosine polyphosphates. *Pediatr Allergy Immunol* 13:307, 2002.

King R, Hearing VJ, Creel DJ, et al: Albinism, in: Scriver CR, Beaudet AL, Sly WS, Valle D (eds): *The Metabolic and Molecular Basis of Inherited Disease,* 8th ed. New York, McGraw-Hill, 2001, p 5587.

Ulsoy H, Erciyes N, Ovali E, et al: Anesthesia in Chédiak-Higashi syndrome—Case report. *Middle East J Anesthesiol* 13:101, 1995

Chemke-Oliver-Mallek Syndrome

At a glance: A bipolar syndrome involving eyes and extremities.

Synonym: Oculo-Digital Syndrome.

Incidence and genetic inheritance: A single case of a girl from consanguineous parents has been reported. Probably autosomal recessive transmission.

Clinical aspects: Disease involves the eyes with cataract, microphthalmos, retinal dysplasia, corneal clouding and visual loss and the limbs with irregular length of fingers, brachydactyly, terminal hypoplasia of fingers, clinodactyly of fifth finger, and absent, dysplastic, or small fingernails.

Anesthetic considerations: Anesthesia in this condition has not been described. The features of the disease do not suggest that specific anesthesia precautions are required.

REFERENCE:

Chemke J, Oliver M, Mallek D, et al: Multiple ophthalmic anomalies and digital hypoplasia. *J Genet Hum* 26:17, 1978.

Cherubism

At a glance: A nonneoplastic, fibroosseous disease characterized by bilateral, and painless enlargement of the jaws that give the patient a cherubic appearance.

Synonyms: CRBM; Familial Benign Giant Cell Tumor of the Jaw; Familial Multilocular Cystic Disease of the Jaw.

History: First described by Frangenheim in 1914 and completed by C. Jones in 1933.

Incidence: Approximately 280 cases have been reported in the literature.

Genetic inheritance: Autosomal dominant trait, with males affected twice as often as females. Penetrance in males is 100% versus only 50 to 70% in females. It may appear as solitary cases or in several members of the family, often in multiple generations. Sporadic cases have also been described. The responsible gene encodes SH3BP2 (*Src homology 3* [SH3] *binding protein 2*), which is located on 4p16.3. The SH3 region is a small protein domain and includes signaling proteins and cytoskeletal elements. These SH3 domains appear to function as mediators in protein–protein associations and regulation of cytoplasmic signaling.

Pathophysiology: Unknown. May be related to dental developmental processes in children, triggered by the eruption of secondary teeth.

Diagnosis: Made based on clinical findings of characteristic "cherub-like" facies caused most often by symmetrical fullness of the cheeks and jaws, resulting in a round face and retraction of the lower eyelids with exposure of the sclera below the rim of the iris. Radiologic examination shows multilocular cystic changes in mandible, maxilla, and ribs. Histologic examination of affected areas reveals replacement of the normal bony architecture by proliferating fibrous tissues, containing numerous multinucleated giant cells.

Clinical aspects: Patients may look normal in the first years of life. The initial changes are characterized by unilateral fullness of the cheeks, most often starting during the second or third year of life (but later onset is possible). Eventually, both mandibular rami and angles are involved, along with the maxilla. The growth rate is fastest during the first 2 years, then slows down and finally regresses during puberty. Hypertelorism is a constant sign. There is also an association with hyperplasia of cervical lymph nodes. The teeth are often loose and irregularly positioned. Extragnathic skeletal involvement is rare. Conservative management is recommended because it is a benign, self-limited condition. However, curettage of tissue hindering nasal breathing or function of the tongue may be indicated. Surgery may be requested for cosmetic reasons. Patients are mentally normal.

Precautions before anesthesia: Airway management is the main anesthetic problem in these patients. Thorough assessment is mandatory (e.g., check mouth opening, neck mobility, thyromental distance, Mallampati Score) to obtain an idea of what to expect. Skull radiographs may be helpful. Note the presence of any loose teeth.

Anesthetic considerations: Severe cases requiring surgical correction often present with marked enlargement of the mandible and maxilla. Mouth opening may be severely limited and the intraoral space significantly reduced because of enlargement of the bony structures. The teeth are often loose, and enoral ulcerations are not uncommon. Nasal intubation, either blind or better under fiberoptic bronchoscopic guidance, is preferred in such corrections to facilitate surgical correction. However, narrowing of the nasal airway is possible and should be ruled out before nasal intubation attempts. Preferably, awake fiberoptic intubation is done in patients with potential upper airway problems. Postoperative mechanical ventilation may be necessary to allow the surgical edema to subside before extubation.

Pharmacological implications: Muscle relaxants should not be administered until the airway has been secured.

Other conditions to be considered:

☞**RAMON SYNDROME:** An autosomal dominant inherited disorder with cherubism, dwarfism, spinal abnormalities (which may make intraoperative positioning difficult) and neurologic impairment, including mental retardation and seizures (whose therapy could interfere with the metabolism of anesthetic drugs).

CHERUBISM OPTIC ATROPHY SHORT STATURE SYNDROME (Al Gazali Khidr Prem Chandran Syndrome): Cherubism associated with dwarfism and visual impairment.

REFERENCES:

Battaglia A, Merati A, Magit A: Cherubism and upper airway obstruction. *Otolaryngol Head Neck Surg* 122:573, 2000.

Ozkan Y, Varol A, Turker N, et al: Clinical and radiological evaluation of cherubism: A sporadic case report and review of the literature. *Int J Pediatr Otorhinolaryngol* 67:1005, 2003.

Schultze-Mosgau S, Holbach LM, Wiltfang J: Cherubism: Clinical evidence and therapy. *J Craniofac Surg* 14:201, 2003.

CHILD Syndrome

At a glance: An inherited syndrome characterized by unilateral inflammatory nevus with strict midline demarcation sparing the face and ipsilateral defects involving all skeletal structures and internal organs. CHILD is an acronym for *congenital hemidysplasia* with *ichthyosiform erythroderma* and *limb defects*.

Synonyms: Unilateral Erythrokeratoderma; Unilateral Ectromelia; Unilateral Ichthyosiform Erythroderma; Unilateral Ichthyosiform Erythroderma with Ipsilateral Malformations.

History: Although Otto Sachs was the first to describe this disorder in an 8-year-old girl in 1903, R. Happle and colleagues were the first to use the acronymic designation "CHILD syndrome" in 1980.

Incidence: Approximately 30 cases have been reported.

Genetic inheritance: X-linked dominant trait with lethality in males. The responsible gene has been mapped to Xq28.

Pathophysiology: In view of the pattern of lateralization of the lesions, a postzygotic mutation appears to be more likely than a gametic half-chromatid mutation. It probably is caused by mutations in the NAD(P)H steroid dehydrogenase-like protein gene (NSDHL) and in the emopamil-binding protein gene (EBP), which is needed for cholesterol synthesis. Furthermore, skin fibroblasts from the affected area not only show a slower growth rate, but also a numerical and functional decrease in peroxisomes. This peroxisomal defect is limited to affected skin areas (peroxisomes in fibroblasts from unaffected skin are normal in number and function). This difference in growth rate seems to be associated with increased prostaglandin E_2 levels in affected skin areas because peroxisomes are involved in the metabolism of prostaglandins and fibroblast growth can be accelerated in vitro with prostaglandin synthesis inhibitors.

Diagnosis: The hallmark of this syndrome is a sharp midline demarcation of a unilateral, ichthyosiform erythroderma as a result of an inflammatory nevus. (Only one case with bilateral involvement

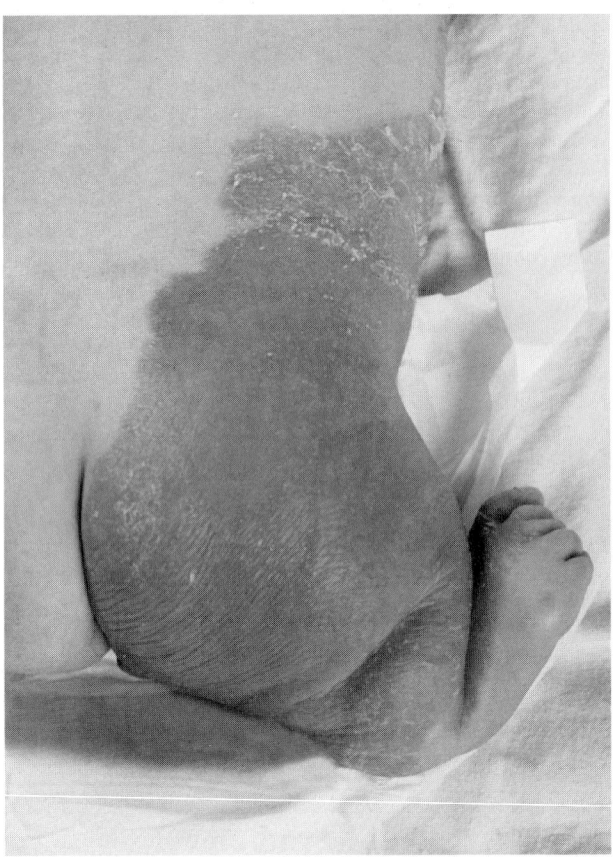

CHILD Syndrome Unilateral inflammatory nevus with hemidysplasia of the leg in a newborn with CHILD Syndrome. See color plates.

has been described.) This nevus spares the face. Many organs are asymmetrical, with hypoplasia on the side of ichthyosis. The right side of the body is more often affected than the left side. Histopathology of the involved epidermis is nonspecific and shows acanthosis, papillomatosis, and hyperkeratosis with parakeratosis. Biochemically, the involved fibroblasts show peroxisomal deficiency.

Clinical aspects: The disorder usually is either congenital or has its onset with persisting ichthyosis within the first month of life. Ipsilateral abnormalities on the side of ichthyosis are distinctive and affect the limbs (from hypoplasia of fingers to complete agenesis of the entire limb, onychodysplasia, webbing of elbows and knees), the bones (hypoplasia of skull, mandible, vertebrae, clavicles, ribs, scapulae), the central nervous system (mild mental retardation, ipsilateral brain hypoplasia, including brainstem, and cranial nerve anomalies), the heart (atrial and ventricular septal defects, single ventricle, single coronary ostium), the lungs (lung hypoplasia), and the kidneys (unilateral renal agenesis). Thyroid, adrenal, and genitourinary abnormalities and myelomeningocele have been described. Death most often results from cardiac lesions. No effective treatment for the dermatosis is known. Orthopedic (scoliosis), plastic, or prosthetic surgery may be required for specific anomalies. The prognosis depends on the presence and severity of internal and skeletal defects.

Precautions before anesthesia: A detailed review of all body systems is necessary because the disease is multisystemic. In particular, a systematic review of associated cardiovascular, respiratory, and neurologic disease is mandatory. Examination of the cardiovascular system for the presence, type, and severity of cardiac malfor-

mations may require electrocardiography, echocardiography, and cardiac catheterization. If scoliosis or unilateral lung hypoplasia is present, a detailed respiratory evaluation is necessary (i.e., chest radiograph, arterial blood gas analysis, pulmonary function tests). If mandibular hypoplasia is present, the airway should be assessed for potential difficulties with tracheal intubation. Laboratory investigations should include a complete blood count and serum concentrations of electrolytes, urea, creatinine, and thyroid hormones.

Anesthetic considerations: Anesthesia in these patients has not been reported. A regional anesthesia technique is recommended whenever possible. However, the performance of a central neuraxial block may be technically challenging in view of the abnormal vertebrae. Severe scoliosis can hinder proper positioning, and careful padding is necessary. Induction and maintenance of general anesthesia will be dictated by the presence, type, and severity of cardiac defects and the degree of pulmonary hypoplasia. Postoperative ventilation may be necessary if a high-dose narcotic technique was used for induction and maintenance of anesthesia (secondary to cardiac defects) or when significant respiratory impairment is present. Positive ventilation with the lowest peak airway pressure should be used in the presence of pulmonary hypoplasia to prevent barotrauma to the lungs. Both peripheral and central venous access can be difficult because of limb and/or clavicular anomalies.

Pharmacological implications: Subacute bacterial endocarditis prophylaxis may be required. If tracheal intubation is anticipated to be difficult in the presence of a hypoplastic mandible, muscle relaxants should not be used until the airway has been secured. Anesthetic drugs and perioperative fluid regimen should be adapted to renal function. Avoid heavy sedative premedication in the presence of significant respiratory impairment.

REFERENCES:

Bittar M, Happle R: CHILD syndrome avant la lettre. *J Am Acad Dermatol* 50:S34, 2004.

Happle R, Koch H, Lenz W: The CHILD syndrome: Congenital hemidysplasia with ichthyosiform erythroderma and limb defects. *Eur J Pediatr* 134:27, 1980.

Falek A, Heath CW Jr, Ebbin AJ, et al: Unilateral limb and skin deformities with congenital heart disease in two siblings: A lethal syndrome. *J Pediatr* 73:910, 1968.

Cholinesterase Deficiency

At a glance: A disorder caused by atypical or deficiency of pseudocholinesterase (PCE) leading to prolonged paralysis after administration of succinylcholine or mivacurium.

Synonyms: Pseudocholinesterase Deficiency; Plasma Cholinesterase Deficiency; Butyrylcholinesterase Deficiency; Cholinesterase II Deficiency; Succinylcholine Sensitivity; Suxamethonium Sensitivity.

Incidence: For homozygosity, the incidence is approximately 1:2,000–4,000, whereas the incidence for heterozygosity increases to up to 1:500. The gene for the dibucaine-resistant atypical cholinesterase appears to be widely distributed. Among Caucasians, males are affected almost twice as often as females. The frequency for heterozygosity is low among black people, Japanese and non-Japanese Orientals, South Americans, Australian aborigines, and Arctic Inuits (in general). However, there are a few Inuit populations (e.g., Alaskan Inuits) with an unusually high gene frequency for PCE deficiency. A relatively high frequency also was reported among Jews from Iran and Iraq, Caucasians from North America, Great Britain, Portugal, Yugoslavia, and Greece.

Genetic inheritance: Autosomal recessive. Genes encoding cholinesterase 1 (CHE1) and CHE2 have been mapped to 3q26.1-q26.2. One gene is silent, whereas the other is responsible for the defect in cholinesterase.

Pathophysiology: The inherited defect is caused by either the presence of an atypical PCE or complete absence of the enzyme. Cholinesterases are enzymes that facilitate hydrolysis of the esters of choline. Acetylcholine, the most commonly encountered of these esters, is the mediator of the whole cholinergic system. Acetylcholine is immediately inactivated "in situ" by a specific acetylcholinesterase in the ganglions of the autonomic nervous system (preganglionic and postganglionic in the parasympathetic nervous system and almost exclusively preganglionic in the sympathetic nervous system), in the synapses of the central nervous system, and in the neuromuscular junctions. The affinity of PCE is lower for acetylcholine, but higher for other esters of choline, such as butyrylcholine, benzoylcholine, and succinylcholine, and for aromatic esters (e.g., procaine, chloroprocaine, tetracaine). Normal PCE is produced in the liver, has a plasma half-life of 8 to 12 days, and can be found in plasma, erythrocytes, glial tissue, liver, pancreas, and bowel. When succinylcholine is used for anesthesia, its high plasma concentration immediately after intravenous injection decreases rapidly in normal individuals because of the rapid action of plasma PCE. In case of an atypical PCE or complete absence of PCE, the effect of the injected succinylcholine can last for up to 10 hours.

Diagnosis: The disorder is completely asymptomatic prior to the use of succinylcholine. The diagnosis is suspected in any patient with prolonged paralysis (>10 minutes) after succinylcholine administration. A nerve stimulator helps confirm the diagnosis by demonstrating the flaccidity of hand muscles. Laboratory tests use the property of the local anesthetic dibucaine, which can inhibit normal PCE activity in vitro, but has minimal effects on atypical enzymes. Normal PCE activity is reduced by nearly 80%, whereas the activity of atypical enzymes is reduced by only 20%. This defines the "dibucaine number" (DN), which represents the percentage inhibition of PCE by a fixed concentration of dibucaine under standardized conditions using benzoylcholine as the substrate. DN is calculated according to the following formula:

$$DN = 100 \times \left[1 - \frac{\text{PCE Activity with Dibucaine}}{\text{PCE Activity without Dibucaine}} \right]$$

DN ranges from 70 to 83 in normal individuals, 40 to 60 in heterozygous patients, and values below 30 in homozygous patients. Variants where the atypical enzyme was inhibited by sodium fluoride, but not by dibucaine have been reported. This can be confirmed by another test measuring the fluoride resistance (expressed as "fluoride number" [FN]; the formula used for calculation of DN also applies for FN), which decreases in patients presenting with the disorder. The normal range for FN is 56 to 65. The diagnosis can also be established by electrophoretic measurement of PCE plasma concentration.

Clinical aspects: Complications most commonly occur after injection of either succinylcholine or mivacurium and present with prolonged paralysis. Two forms of clinical presentation exist: (1) depolarizing block with tetanus that can be increased by anticholinesterases and (2) nondepolarizing block with fade in the train of four and a slight tetanus associated with posttetanic facilitation (dual block), in which case anticholinesterase agents are indicated

(prostigmine or neostigmine in combination with glycopyrrolate or atropine). Cardiac problems may include arrhythmia, ventricular fibrillation, and cardiac arrest as a result of succinylcholine. Neurologic manifestations include seizures, coma has been reported only following injection of procaine.

Laboratory investigations confirm reduced DN and/or decreased FN and decreased plasma PCE concentration.

Precautions before anesthesia: Check for previous anesthesia-related problems in the patient, the parents, and relatives. In case of prolonged motor block following administration of triggering agents (succinylcholine, mivacurium), blood samples must be obtained to measure DN and FN. Keep in mind that certain physiologic situations are associated with lower plasma PCE activity (newborn period and infancy, pregnancy, and increased age). Furthermore, decreased PCE activity has been reported in association with liver disease (e.g., cirrhosis, hepatitis), plasmapheresis, acute myocardial infarction, myxedema, and acute infections.

Anesthetic considerations: If the disease has not been diagnosed before anesthesia and prolonged motor block occurs, the treatment of choice is mechanical ventilation. Fresh blood or fresh-frozen plasma as a source of PCE is indicated only in case of cardiac complications.

Pharmacological implications: Succinylcholine, mivacurium, and amino-ester local anesthetics are contraindicated. Use of anticholinesterases must be discussed after evaluation and interpretation of the motor block (nerve stimulator). Certain drugs, such as pancuronium, metoclopramide, esmolol, chlorpromazine, bambuterol (a precursor of terbutaline), acetylcholinesterase inhibitors (neostigmine, pyridostigmine), echothiophate, steroids, and chemotherapeutic agents (cyclophosphamide), decrease PCE activity. In patients with partial deficiency of PCE, drugs that may cause an acquired decrease in PCE activity must be avoided.

REFERENCES:

Goudsouzian NG: Mivacurium in infants and children. *Paediatr Anaesth* 7:183, 1997.

Naik B, Hirshhorn S, Dharnidharka VR: Prolonged neuromuscular block due to cholinesterase depletion by plasmapheresis. *J Clin Anesth* 14:381, 2002.

Pasquariello CA, Schwartz RE: Plasma cholinesterase deficiency in a neonate. *Can J Anaesth* 40:529, 1993.

Chondrodysplasia Giant Cell Type

At a glance: A lethal form of chondrodysplasia characterized by rhizomelic limb shortening with giant cell chondrodysplasia.

Synonyms: Atelosteogenesis type I; Spondylohumerofemoral Hypoplasia.

Incidence and genetic inheritance: Extremely rare congenital disease (approximately 10 cases have been described), isolated cases only.

Clinical aspects: The diagnosis is made based on the clinical findings of micromelic dwarfism (distal hypoplasia of the humeri and femora), hypoplasia of the midthoracic spine, histology results (multiple degenerated chondrocytes that are encapsulated in fibrous tissue; resting cartilage appears intact, but hypocellular areas with multinucleated chondrocytes are interspersed with areas of normal cellularity), and radiologic signs. All reported cases have been stillborn or died soon after birth secondary to respiratory failure. Clinical features involve head and neck (facial hemangiomas, frontal bossing, prominent globes, edematous eyelids, depressed nasal bridge, nose and midface hypoplasia, micrognathia, cleft palate, short neck), the airway (laryngeal stenosis, small tunnel chest, missing ribs), the limbs (distal humeral and femoral hypoplasia, knee/elbow subluxation, talipes equinovarus, hypoplastic/absent fibulae, bowed radius/fibulae, phalangeal mineralization defects), and the axial skeleton (cervical fusion of vertebrae, midthoracic spine hypoplasia with platyspondyly, sagittal and coronal clefting). Encephaloceles have been reported.

Anesthetic considerations: Anesthesia in this condition has not been described. Cervical vertebral fusion and the facial features make airway management potentially difficult. The presence of laryngeal stenosis suggests that a smaller endotracheal tube may be required. Vascular access may be difficult.

Other conditions to be considered:

☞**THANATOPHORIC DWARFISM:** Severe form of micromelic dwarfism with narrow thorax. Death generally occurs in the first hours of life.

☞**DIASTROPHIC DYSPLASIA:** An autosomal recessive inherited form of short-limb dwarfism associated with spine anomalies.

REFERENCES:

Greally MT, Jewett T, Smith WL, et al: Lethal bone dysplasia in a fetus with manifestations of atelosteogenesis I and boomerang dysplasia. *Am J Med Genet* 47:1086, 1993.

Sillence DO, Lachman RS, Jenkins T, et al: Spondylohumerofemoral hypoplasia (giant cell chondrodysplasia): A neonatally lethal short-limb skeletal dysplasia. *Am J Med Genet* 13:7, 1982.

Yang SS, Roskamp J, Liu CT, et al: Two lethal chondrodysplasias with giant chondrocytes. *Am J Med Genet* 15:615, 1983.

Chondrodysplasia Grebe Type

At a glance: A rare form of autosomal recessive osteochondrodysplasia characterized by severe dwarfism with marked hypomelia and deformation.

Synonyms: Grebe Chondrodysplasia; Brazilian Achondrogenesis; Acromesomelic Dysplasia, Grebe Type; Acromesomelic Dwarfism; Achondrogenesis Type II.

Incidence: Fewer than 100 cases have been described. An increased frequency has been reported from Bahia, Brazil, where the gene frequency was evaluated to be 1:50, with a prevalence of 1:2000 live births.

Genetic inheritance: Autosomal recessive as a result of a mutation in the cartilage-derived morphogenetic protein-1 gene (CDMP1) located on 20q11.2.

Diagnosis: Based on the clinical findings of severe dwarfism with marked hypomelia and deformation of upper and lower limbs, with a proximo-distal gradient of severity. Radiographs show shortening and deformation of the forearm and foreleg bones, fusion of carpal and tarsal bones, and absence of proximal and middle phalanges and several metacarpal and metatarsal bones.

Clinical aspects: This disorder is limited to the skeleton and results in short limbs with the arms longer than the legs. The abnormalities are more severe distally: the humeri and femora are short but normally shaped, whereas radius/ulna and tibia/fibula are short and deformed, the carpal and tarsal bones and phalanges are rudimentary, and the metacarpals, metatarsals, and patellae are hypoplastic

or absent. The digits are consequently very short with a globular appearance connected with a soft-tissue bridge. Postaxial polydactyly and valgus deformity of hand and foot are common. The metatarsal, talus, cuneiform, and navicular bones may be fused. The axial skeleton is normal. An increased frequency of stillbirth and neonatal death has been reported. No mental retardation.

Precautions before anesthesia: Routine preoperative assessment. Check joint mobility for intraoperative positioning.

Anesthetic considerations: Anesthesia in this condition has not been described. The features of the disease suggest that vascular access may be difficult, and careful intraoperative positioning is required. Regional anesthesia is not contraindicated but should be expected to be difficult to perform due to positioning problems.

Pharmacological implications: There are no specific implications for this condition.

Other conditions to be considered:

☞**ACROMESOMELIC DYSPLASIA MAROTEAUX TYPE:** A very rare, autosomal recessive inherited disorder that seems to have its highest prevalence on the south Atlantic island of St. Helena (to which Napoleon was exiled in 1815). Dwarfism is severe and affects mainly the middle and distal parts of the limbs (progressive shortening of the tubular bones and bowing of radius and ulna) and the vertebrae (thoracic kyphosis).

☞**ACROMESOMELIC DYSPLASIA HUNTER-THOMPSON TYPE:** Extremely rare form of autosomal recessive inherited acromesomelic dysplasia characterized by severe dwarfism with the abnormalities limited to the limbs (more pronounced in the lower limbs). Multiple dislocations of the large joints with limited mobility are common. Patients are mentally normal. The same gene as in chondrodysplasia Grebe type is responsible for this disorder, although the mutation affects a different part of the gene. Intelligence seems to be normal in these patients, although the psychomotor milestones achieved may be delayed compared to the normal population.

REFERENCES:

Costa T, Ramsby G, Cassia F: Grebe Syndrome: Clinical and radiographic findings in affected individuals and heterozygous carriers. *Am J Med Genet* 75:523, 1998.

Thomas JT, Kilpatrick MW, Lin K, et al: Disruption of human limb morphogenesis by a dominant negative mutation in CDMP1. *Nat Genet* 17:58, 1997.

Chondrodysplasia-Pseudohermaphroditism Syndrome

At a glance: A severe form of congenital dwarfism, general chondrodysplasia, severe microcephaly with cerebellar vermis hypoplasia, hypoplastic iris, and coloboma of the optic disc.

Synonym: Nivelon-Mabille Syndrome.

Incidence and genetic inheritance: Two cases were reported worldwide by A. Nivelon and colleagues in 1992. Autosomal recessive inheritance has been suggested. The first sibling had normal female internal and external genitalia, whereas the karyotype was 46,XY. Pregnancy with the second child was terminated after antenatal diagnosis. The findings were similar except for a 46,XX karyotype.

Clinical aspects: Severe growth (already antenatal in origin) and mental retardation are present. Clinical features involve the head and central nervous system (thickened skull, microcephaly, hypoplasia/

agenesis of the cerebellar vermis, large ears, and everted upper lip), the skeleton (generalized chondrodysplasia, micromelia, short metacarpals and phalanges, which are widened in the midportion and distally, short iliac bones, broadened epiphyses, trapezoid vertebral bodies), and the eyes (deep set eyes, strabismus, miosis, short palpebral fissures, hypoplasia of the iris, coloboma of the optic disc, abnormal retinal vessels). Other features include pseudohermaphroditism and narrow chest with 11 pairs of ribs.

Anesthetic considerations: Anesthesia in this condition has not been described. The features of the disease suggest that restrictive lung disease may occur as a result of chest malformations. Intraoperative positioning may be difficult. The patient may have seizures, and pharmacologic treatment may interfere with the metabolism of some anesthetic drugs.

REFERENCE:

Nivelon A, Nivelon JL, Mabille JP, et al: New autosomal recessive chondrodysplasia-pseudohermaphroditism syndrome. *Clin Dysmorphol* 1:221, 1992.

Chondrodysplasia Punctata

At a glance: Refers to a heterogeneous group of disorders having in common ichthyosis and bony abnormalities probably as a result of abnormalities of steroidal biosynthesis. The international nomenclature and classification of osteochondrodysplasias categorized the subtypes of chondrodysplasia punctata as (1) rhizomelic type, (2) ☞Zellweger syndrome, (3) Conradi-Hünermann type, (4) X-linked recessive type, (5) brachytelencephalangic type, (6) tibialmetacarpal type, (7) vitamin K-dependent coagulation defect, and (8) other and acquired genetic disorders including warfarin embryopathy. Specific features of the most common individual types of chondrodysplasia punctata are given below.

Synonyms: Toriello-Higgins-Miller Syndrome; Chondrodystrophia Calcificans Congenita: Congenital Stippled Epiphyses.

Incidence: For rhizomelic chondrodysplasia punctata type I, the incidence in the general population has been estimated to be 1:100,000.

Genetic inheritance: Inherited as a sex-linked recessive trait and caused by a mutation in the arylsulfatase E (ARSE) gene. Known genes are located on Xp22.3 and Xp11.23-p11.22. Other syndromes can be inherited in an autosomal dominant or recessive fashion.

Diagnosis: Made clinically based on radiologic signs (calcified stippling of the hyaline cartilage and bones presenting in infancy and disappearing at 2–3 years of age) associated with multiple clinical signs such as limbs with short segments, dysmorphism with a hypoplastic nasal root, skin lesions, and cataracts. Laboratory assays can be used to demonstrate a deficiency in red blood cell plasmalogen, elevated plasma concentration of phytanic acid (although this depends on the food intake), and deficient plasmalogen biosynthesis and phytanic acid oxidation in skin fibroblasts.

Clinical aspects: This disorder is often associated with prematurity and can be lethal in early infancy. Hypotonia and asymmetry of the body are frequent. Other clinical features can involve the head and neck (brachycephaly, short neck, flat face, frontal bossing, coloboma of the iris, cataract, nystagmus, optic disc anomaly, flattened small nose with anteverted nares, partial absence of the mandible, short columella, long philtrum, tented upper lip, low-set ears with conductive deafness), the limbs (proximal shortening of humeri and femora [rhizomelia], micromelia, epiphyseal anoma-

lies, punctate calcifications of epiphyses, bowed diaphysis, brachydactyly, clinodactyly of the fifth finger, short great toe, small foot, metacarpal anomalies, dislocated hip and restricted joint mobility), the skeleton (flat cheek bones, punctate vertebrae, spina bifida occulta, abnormal vertebral size, pectus excavatum scoliosis), and the skin (absent scalp hair, ichthyosis, cutis marmorata, hypoplastic toenails). Other features that have been described are congenital cardiac lesions, respiratory distress, laryngeal abnormalities, dysplastic kidneys, hydronephrosis and megaureter, abnormal genitalia, splenomegaly, and liver enlargement.

RHIZOMELIC CHONDRODYSPLASIA (RCDP): Most often, this disorder is inherited in an autosomal recessive and rarely in an X-linked recessive fashion. It is caused by multiple peroxisomal abnormalities. Peroxisomes are ubiquitous cellular organelles involved in different cellular functions, such as β-oxidation of very-long-chain fatty acids (VLCFA), production of plasmalogen (involved in cell membrane integrity) and bile acids, gluconeogenesis, catabolism of purines and polyamines, and ethanol metabolism. The defect can be caused by either abnormally formed peroxisomes associated with several peroxisomal dysfunctions or by a defect involving only a single peroxisomal protein with normal peroxisomal structure. Based on biochemical findings, three forms of RCDP can be distinguished. In RCDP I, the defective gene has been identified as PEX7, which encodes for the peroxisomal type 2 targeting signal receptor (PTS2) and maps to 4p16-p14. The PTS2 defect affects multiple enzymes (peroxisomal 3-ketoacyl-CoA thiolase, alkyl-DHAP [dihydroxy acetone phosphate] synthase, DHAP-acyltransferase, and phytanoyl-CoA-hydroxylase). In RCDP II and III, the PEX-7 protein is normal, but a mutation affects the structural gene responsible for the specific enzyme, that is, dihydroxy acetone phosphate acyltransferase deficiency in RCPD II and alkyl-DHAP synthase deficiency in RCDP III. The plasmalogen level in erythrocytes is abnormal in all three types of RCDP. Enzyme activity measurements can be used to reliably diagnose RCDP prenatally. Clinical features are variable and may include congenital cataracts, micrognathia, cleft palate, low and broad nasal bridge, anteverted nares, respiratory insufficiency, short stature, rhizomelic limb shortening, metaphyseal splaying, joint contractures, vertebral anomalies (coronal clefting and kyphoscoliosis), failure to thrive, ichthyosis, cortical atrophy, delayed myelination (a result of deficiency of plasmalogens), seizures, sensorineural deafness, and severe mental retardation. The developmental quotient often is below 30. Although delayed, early developmental skills such as smiling and recognizing voices are achieved by most children. However, these children normally do not achieve the skill level of normal children 6 months of age. Because of the severe neurologic compromise, recurrent aspirations with recurrent respiratory tract infections are common. The chest may be small with restricted compliance. Cervical canal stenosis has been described in these patients and may result in tetraplegia. In more than half of the patients, death occurs before 2 years of age.

CONRADI-HÜNERMANN SYNDROME (Synonym: X-Linked Dominant Type of Chondrodysplasia Punctata): This form is caused by mutations in the delta-8-delta-7-sterol isomerase/emopamil binding protein and has been mapped to Xp11.23-p11.22. Clinical features are extremely variable and may include failure to thrive and anomalies of the head (☞Dandy-Walker malformation, ventriculomegaly, microphtalmus, glaucoma, cataracts, nystagmus, flat face, frontal bossing, and unilateral facial hypoplasia), the skeleton (short stature with asymmetric limb shortening, short neck, hemivertebrae, kyphoscoliosis, patellar dislocation, bilateral club feet), the skin (ichthyosis and "orange peel" skin, alopecia), the kidneys (hydronephrosis), and the lungs (tracheal calcifications and stenosis, restrictive lung disease with frequent respiratory complications). These patients may be mentally normal, however mild to moderate mental retardation has also been described. Atropine is contraindicated in patients with glaucoma. This syndrome has been related to ☞CHILD syndrome.

Precautions before anesthesia: Obtaining a full history and complete physical examination are imperative. Given the anatomical features of the disease, the patient needs to be carefully evaluated for possible difficulties in airway management. Evaluate cardiac (electrocardiogram, echocardiography) and renal function (creatinine, blood urea nitrogen) if necessary. Evaluate respiratory function (clinically, chest radiographs, pulmonary function tests, and arterial blood gas analysis).

Anesthetic considerations: Tracheal intubation can be difficult because of mandibular and laryngeal anomalies. Maintain spontaneous ventilation until the airway has been secured. Have smaller endotracheal tube sizes ready because of possible tracheal stenosis. Careful intraoperative positioning is required, but can be difficult because of multiple malformations. Because of the frequency of respiratory distress, particularly in neonates and infants, close perioperative (respiratory) monitoring is mandatory. Prolonged postoperative mechanical ventilation may be necessary. Regional anesthesia is not contraindicated but can be difficult to achieve. Venous and arterial access is often challenging. Consider the risk of dehydration in patients with severe ichthyosis.

Pharmacological implications: Muscle relaxants are not contraindicated, but should not be used before the airway has been secured. Subacute bacterial endocarditis prophylaxis may be required. Anesthetic drugs (particularly with predominantly renal elimination) and perioperative fluid management may require adaptation to renal function. However, it should be kept in mind that ichthyosis may result in increased fluid losses.

Other condition to be considered:

☞**NEURONAL CEROID LIPOFUSCINOSES:** A group of hereditary progressive neurodegenerative disorders with mental retardation, visual loss, and seizures. The neuronal ceroid lipofuscinoses probably are the most common class of neurodegenerative disease in children.

REFERENCES:

Braverman N, Lin P, Moebius FF, et al: Mutations in the gene coding 3-beta-hydroxysteroid-delta(8),delta(7)-isomerase cause X-linked dominant Conradi-Hunermann syndrome. *Nat Genet* 22:291, 1999.

International Working Group on Constitutional Diseases of Bone: International nomenclature and classification of the osteochondrodysplasias. *Am J Med Genet* 79:376, 1997.

Karoutsos S, Lansade A, Terrier G, et al: Chondrodysplasia punctata and subglottic stenosis. *Anesth Analg* 89:1322, 1999.

Moser A, Moser H, Kreiter N, et al: Life expectancy in rhizomelic chondrodysplasia punctata. *Am J Hum Genet* 59(S4):99, 1996.

Chorioretinal Dysplasia-Microcephaly-Mental Retardation Syndrome

At a glance: A syndrome associated with microcephaly, mental deficiency, and chorioretinal dysplasia.

Synonym: CDMMS; Microcephaly with Chorioretinopathy.

Incidence and genetic inheritance: Approximately 20 cases have been described in only about 10 families. Transmission is most likely autosomal dominant, although autosomal recessive inheritance has also been suggested.

Clinical aspects: The diagnosis is mainly based on the clinical findings of microcephaly, mild mental retardation, and chorioretinal dysplasia. Other features may include frontal bossing, lissencephaly, and lacunar retinal depigmentation. Microphthalmia, microcornea, and ocular pterygium have been described in one family. One reported family also had polycystic kidney disease, which was not thought to be associated with this syndrome.

Anesthetic considerations: Anesthesia in this condition has not been described. The features of the disease suggest patient cooperation may be limited. Anxiolytic and/or sedative premedication and the presence of the primary caregiver during induction of anesthesia may be helpful.

REFERENCES:

Hordijk R, Van de Logt F, Houtman WA, et al: Chorioretinal dysplasia-microcephaly-mental retardation syndrome: Another family with autosomal dominant inheritance. *Genet Couns* 7:113, 1996.

Sadler LS, Robinson LK: Chorioretinal dysplasia-microcephaly-mental retardation syndrome: Report of an American family. *Am J Med Genet* 47:65, 1993.

Choroideremia

At a glance: An inherited eye disorder characterized by progressive degeneration of the choroidea, retinal pigment epithelium, and neural retina.

Synonym: Progressive Tapetochoroidal Dystrophy.

Incidence: Less than 1:100,000 in the general population.

Genetic inheritance: X-chromosomal recessive transmission. Almost exclusively men are affected, but a few female cases have been described. The responsible gene has been mapped to Xq21.2.

Pathophysiology: A point mutation is responsible for impairment in geranyl transferase which affects vesicle transport in retinal cells in choroideremia. Affected males usually first note symptoms in adolescence, experiencing night blindness and peripheral visual field loss.

Diagnosis: Based on the clinical findings of progressive degeneration of the choroidea, with night blindness occurring in the teenage years. The differential diagnosis includes gyrate atrophy of the choroid, diffuse choriocapillaris atrophy and X-linked retinitis pigmentosa. The combination of inheritance mode, ophthalmic examination, visual field testing, and electroretinography (ERG) helps confirm the diagnosis.

Clinical aspects: The ERG in affected males may initially show a pattern of rod-cone degeneration. Fundoscopy reveals patchy areas of chorioretinal degeneration, usually beginning in the midperipheral areas of the fundus and manifesting as a ring scotoma. As these areas enlarge, the disease progresses to marked loss of the retinal pigment epithelium and the choriocapillaris, while deep choroidal vessels are preserved. Although the function and anatomy of the central macula is preserved until late in the disease process, affected men rarely retain any central vision beyond the seventh decade of life. Almost one third of these patients also have posterior subcapsular cataracts. Although choroideremia is essentially a retinal degenerative disease, associations with other clinical findings (severe mental retardation, agenesis of the corpus callosum, signs of encephalopathy, (sensorineural and conductive) hearing loss, distal motor neuropathy, and cleft lip and palate have been reported. No effective treatment exists.

Precautions before anesthesia: History should demonstrate the extent of retinal degeneration. Check for concomitant diseases as mentioned above.

Anesthetic considerations: In the presence of peripheral motor weakness, the effects of neuromuscular blockade may be enhanced and careful titration to effect will be necessary using a peripheral nerve stimulator. In the presence of severe weakness of the respiratory musculature, extubation at the end of a procedure may have to be delayed until full return of muscle function. The presence or absence of other neurologic findings may influence the anesthetic technique. Patients with this condition may be blind, and the psychological considerations pertaining to this situation should be kept in mind.

Pharmacological implications: Careful dosing of neuromuscular blockers is recommended in the presence of muscular weakness.

Other conditions to be considered:

X-Linked Retinitis Pigmentosa: Retinitis pigmentosa is the most common cause of inherited visual loss (approximately 1:4000 in the general population is affected). It usually begins between the second and fourth decade of life with night blindness and later is followed by tunnel vision. The rate and extent of progression are highly variable. More than 70 different genetic defects have been described, all resulting in retinitis pigmentosa. The X-linked form accounts for approximately 10% of cases. Differentiation from choroideremia may initially be difficult because the age at onset and the initial symptoms can be similar. However, ophthalmologic examination should easily determine the underlying disease.

☞**Stargardt Syndrome:** The most common form of inherited juvenile macular degeneration. Characterized by a reduction of central vision with preservation of peripheral vision. Onset is usually before 20 years of age. The macula presents with yellow-white spots of irregular shapes.

☞**Usher Syndrome:** A genetically heterogeneous condition associated with retinitis pigmentosa and deafness with variable age of onset. Multiple subtypes have been described.

Choroideremia Deafness Obesity (Ayazi Syndrome): This is the result of a contiguous gene deletion syndrome involving the choroideremia gene and the DFN3 gene (which encodes for X-linked deafness).

Choroideremia Hypopituitarism: Autosomal recessive transmitted disorder with short stature, ataxia, arterial hypertension, and dysfunction of the hypothalamo/hypophyseal axis, which must be considered for anesthetic management.

References:

MacDonald IM, Chen MH, Addison DJ, et al: Histopathology of the retinal pigment epithelium of a female carrier of choroideremia. *Can J Ophthalmol* 32:329, 1997.

Roberts MF, Fishman GA, Roberts DK, et al: Retrospective, longitudinal, and cross sectional study of visual acuity impairment in choroideraemia. *Br J Ophthalmol* 86:658, 2002.

Syed N, Smith JE, John SK, et al: Evaluation of retinal photoreceptors and pigment epithelium in a female carrier of choroideremia. *Ophthalmology* 108:711, 2001.

Christ-Siemens-Touraine Syndrome

At a glance: A heterogeneous genetic disorder caused by abnormal development of the ectodermal tissue and characterized by the association of hypohidrosis, hypotrichosis, defective dentition, peculiar facies, abnormal thermoregulation, and exocrine gland insufficiency.

Synonyms: Anhidrotic Ectodermal Dysplasia; Hypohidrotic Ectodermal Dysplasia.

History: This is the condition affecting the "Toothless Men of Sind," members of a Hindu kindred that resides in the vicinity of Hyderabad (the capital of Andhra Pradesh in India) and was described by Charles Darwin in 1875 and later by K.I. Thadani in 1934.

Incidence: Approximately 1:100,000 of the general population is affected.

Genetic inheritance: X-linked recessive. The disease is caused by a mutation in the ectodysplasin A gene (ED 1), which has been mapped to Xq12.2-q13.1. As a member of the tumor necrosis factor ligand superfamily, ectodysplasin is a membrane protein involved in signal transduction, promoting not only cell adhesion to the extracellular matrix, but also regulating the development of ectodermal appendages and epithelio–mesenchymal interactions. Although usually only men are affected and women act as carriers of the disease, the clinical picture in heterozygous females is highly variable, ranging from no symptoms to severe disease. Rarely, the disease is transmitted in an autosomal recessive or an autosomal dominant pattern.

Diagnosis: The clinical triad of anhidrosis (or hypohidrosis), hypotrichosis, and defective dentition is helpful for diagnostic purposes. Skin biopsy of the palm demonstrates the absence or hypoplasia of sweat glands.

Clinical aspects: Often the disorder presents in the first year of life with episodes of unexplained hyperpyrexia. Thermography can reveal abnormal skin temperature patterns consistent with altered peripheral vascular perfusion. The skin is abnormally dry (lack of sebum and sweat), and heat loss by evaporation is impaired secondary to hypoplastic/aplastic eccrine sweat glands. Associated features include characteristic facies (frontal bossing, saddle nose, flattened maxilla, small chin), fine, brittle, and scant hair (hypotrichosis), scant or absent eyelashes and eyebrows, onychodysplasia (spoon-shaped nails), aplastic/hypoplastic mammary glands with hypoplastic/absent nipples, and atopic-like dermatitis. Dental anomalies include hypodontia/anodontia, taurodontism (tooth with abnormally short roots and enlarged pulp chamber), and conical crowns. Lacrimation and meibomian glands may be absent or diminished. Respiratory tract mucous glands may be hypoplastic/aplastic, resulting in an increased propensity to bronchitis and pneumonia. Laryngeal incompetence with dry mucosal atrophy (often resulting in hoarse voice) is not uncommon and may contribute to recurrent chest infections. A variable degree of mental retardation may be present. Otherwise the prognosis is good, and survival to adulthood is common.

Precautions before anesthesia: Active infections, especially involving the chest, should be excluded as a cause of preoperative pyrexia. Evaluate anatomy for difficult tracheal intubation in view of the occurrence of hypoplastic maxilla and loose or missing teeth. Laryngeal incompetence may be suspected with a history of frequent coughing associated with meals. Evaluation by nasopharyngoscopy or contrast radiographs taken during swallowing has been suggested.

Anesthetic considerations: The facial anomalies with hypoplastic maxilla may make mask holding awkward and laryngoscopy and intubation difficult. In the presence of laryngeal incompetence, a rapid-sequence induction of anesthesia is recommended. If possible, a cuffed endotracheal tube should be used during general anesthesia to minimize the risk of regurgitation and pulmonary aspiration. Core temperature should be closely monitored during anesthesia. Avoidance of pyrexia is essential, therefore, warming devices should be used with care because thermoregulation in these patients is abnormal as a result of a significantly decreased ability to sweat. Although body temperature usually drops under anesthesia, cooling measures such as padded ice, cool intravenous solutions, or fans should be available. Use artificial tears or lubricating eyes ointment in patients with defective lacrimation and tape the eyes shut. The use of humidified gases during anesthesia to prevent excessive drying of the tracheobronchial tree is recommended.

Pharmacological implications: Atropine should be avoided because it may further decrease the ability to sweat, therefore resulting in increased body temperature. Maintain spontaneous ven-

tilation and avoid neuromuscular blockers until the airway has been secured.

Other condition to be considered:

☞**ECTODERMAL DYSPLASIA:** Rare group of inherited disorders that arise from disturbances in one or more ectodermal structures and their accessory appendages. The absence, or deficient function, of at least two derivatives of the ectoderm constitutes a form of ectodermal dysplasia. Each combination of defects represents another type of ectodermal dysplasia and has a specific name. At least 150 different forms of ectodermal dysplasia have been identified.

REFERENCES:

Gordon CP, Litz S: Multicore myopathy in a patient with anhidrotic ectodermal dysplasia. *Can J Anaesth* 39:966, 1992.

Halal F, Setton N, Wang NS: A distinct type of hidrotic ectodermal dysplasia. *Am J Med Genet* 38:552, 1991.

Kobielak K, Kobielak A, Roszkiewicz J, et al: Mutations in the EDA gene in three unrelated families reveal no apparent correlation between phenotype and genotype in the patients with an X-linked anhidrotic ectodermal dysplasia. *Am J Med Genet* 100:191, 2001.

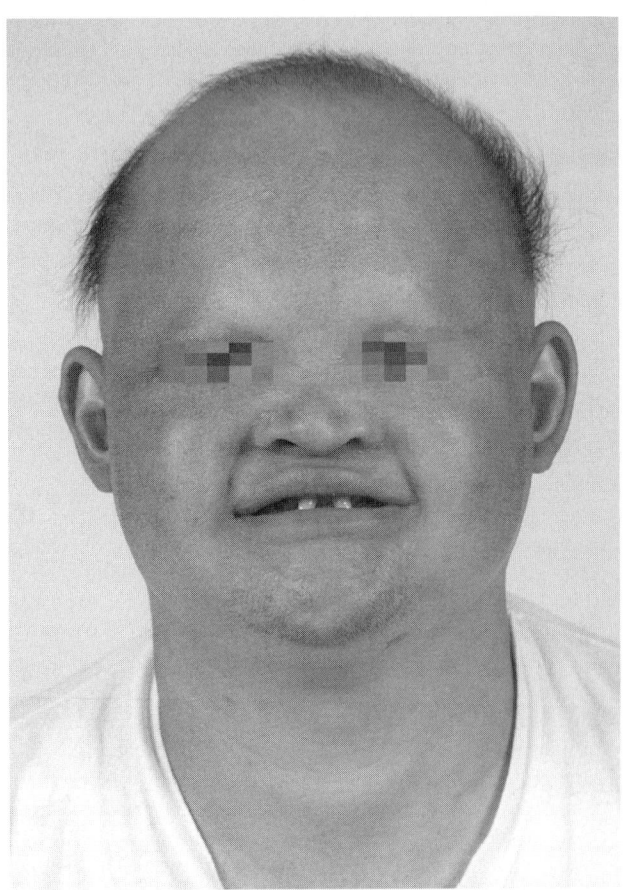 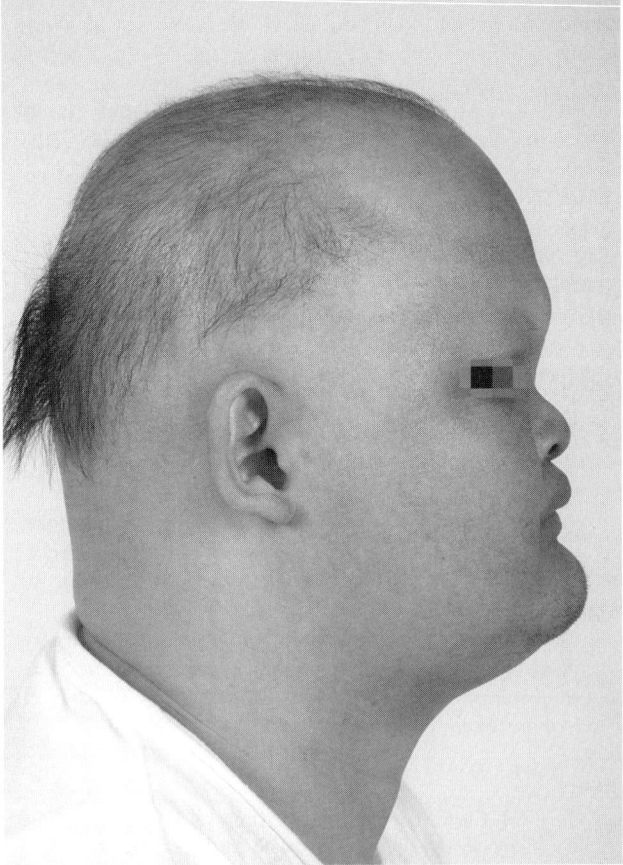

Christ-Siemens-Touraine Syndrome   This 19-year-old man with Christ-Touraine-Siemens syndrome has mild frontal bossing with dry and sparse scalp hair, prominent supraorbital ridges with scanty eyebrows, a depressed and wide nasal bridge (saddle nose), and high and wide cheekbones with a flattened maxilla. The lips are thickened, and the skin is dry with an atopic-like dermatitis. Partial anodontia is present.

Chronic Fatigue Syndrome

At a glance: An acquired clinical syndrome of severe disabling fatigue of at least 6 months' duration that affects both physical and mental functioning and is present at least 50% of the time.

Synonyms: Myalgic Encephalitis; Postviral Fatigue Syndrome; Chronic Fatigue Immune Dysfunction Syndrome; Postural Orthostatic Tachycardia Syndrome.

Incidence: Estimates range from 3–25:10,000 in the general population. Seems to be more common in females and in Caucasians.

Genetic inheritance: No evidence of a genetic basis.

Pathophysiology: Results of investigations are inconclusive. Suggested theories include impaired hypothalamic–pituitary–adrenal interactions and abnormalities of the central and peripheral nervous systems. Another hypothesis is based on impaired inflammatory cytokine production and cellular immunity, which may be linked to the symptoms of chronic fatigue syndrome (CFS) through changes in neurovascular regulation.

Diagnosis: Is based on clinical findings and requires the exclusion of other medical and psychiatric disorders, such as endocrinopathies (hypothyroidism, Addison disease), sleep apnea, narcolepsy, severe obesity, major depressive disorder, bipolar affective disorder, schizophrenia, chronic mononucleosis, malignancy, autoimmune disease, subacute infection, alcohol or substance abuse, or reactions to medications. To fulfill the Centers for Disease Control and Prevention (CDC) diagnostic criteria for CFS, a patient must satisfy two criteria. First, the patient must have chronic fatigue for a minimum of 6 months with other medical conditions excluded. Second, the patient must concurrently have four or more of the following: (1) substantial impairment of short-term memory or concentration, (2) sore throat, (3) tender lymph nodes, (4) muscle pain, (5) multijoint pain without swelling or tenderness, (6) headaches of a new type, pattern, or severity, (7) unrefreshing sleep, and (8) postexertional malaise lasting more than 6 hours. Symptoms must have persisted or recurred during 6 or more consecutive months of illness and must not have predated the fatigue.

Clinical aspects: As above. Remissions and relapses characterize the clinical course. Orthostatic hypotension consistent with postural orthostatic tachycardia syndrome is described in adolescents with this condition.

Precautions before anesthesia: No specific tests are required. The principal anesthetic concern is that the condition has not been misdiagnosed and an unrecognized condition is present (e.g., hypothyroidism).

Anesthetic considerations: Multiple anecdotal reports of exaggerated response to sedative hypnotics and anesthesia inducing agents exist. However, no systematic study of any anesthetic agents or techniques has been performed.

Pharmacological implications: Concomitant therapy may include corticosteroids which may require perioperative supplementation.

REFERENCES:

De Lorenzo F, Hargreaves J, Kakkar VV: Pathogenesis and management of delayed orthostatic hypotension in patients with chronic fatigue syndrome. *Clin Auton Res* 7:185, 1997.

Fukuda K, Straus SE, Hickie I, et al: The chronic fatigue syndrome: A comprehensive approach to its definition and study. International Chronic Fatigue Syndrome Study Group. *Ann Intern Med* 121:953, 1994.

Steele L, Dobbins JG, Fukuda K, et al: The epidemiology of chronic fatigue in San Francisco. *Am J Med* 105:83S, 1998.

Chronic Granulomatous Disease

At a glance: A genetically heterogenous, fatal immunodeficiency syndrome of childhood as a result of dysfunctional oxidative metabolism in the phagocytic cells, leading to recurrent and life-threatening bacterial and fungal infections.

Synonyms: Fatal Granulomatosis of Childhood; Chronic Granulomatous Disease of Childhood; Progressive Septic Granulomatosis; Cytochrome-b-Negative X-Linked Granulomatous Disease.

Incidence: Approximately 1:200,000–500,000 live births.

Genetic inheritance: In two thirds of cases, inheritance is X-linked recessive, with the responsible gene located on Xp21.1. In the remaining one third, transmission is autosomal recessive (Cytochrome-b-positive granulomatous disease), with the defect mapped to 7q11.23.

Pathophysiology: The production of antimicrobial reactive oxygen intermediates is impaired by a defective NADPH enzyme. The neutrophil phagocytic metabolic burst is impaired. Neutrophil chemotaxis and killing of organisms are defective. The disease is characterized by granulomas and recurrent infections by catalase-positive organisms. Typical organisms are *Aspergillus* (most common), *Candida, Staphylococcus, Pseudomonas, Salmonella, Nocardia, Serratia* species, and *Burkholderia cenocepacia*. Chronic granulomatous disease is caused by a defect of one of the subcomponents of the reduced nicotinamide adenine dinucleotide phosphate oxidase of neutrophils, monocytes, macrophages, and eosinophils. This situation results in a reduced ability to produce superoxide ions and hydrogen peroxide and is responsible for the significantly impaired ability to kill intracellular microorganisms.

Diagnosis: The most frequent presentation (75% of patients) are recurrent childhood infections. Granulocyte function can be assessed by the nitroblue tetrazolium test.

Clinical aspects: The disease manifests as skin infections, pneumonias, lung abscesses, lymphadenitis, diarrhea, perianal abscesses, hepatic, splenic, pancreatic, perinephritic, and subdiaphragmatic abscesses, osteomyelitis, and sepsis (15% of patients). An incidence of 3.7 severe infections requiring hospitalization per 100 patients and month has been reported. Granulomas in the skin, gastrointestinal tract, and genitourinary tract are characteristic and can result in esophageal, gastric outlet, intestinal, and ureteral obstruction. The most common indications for surgery include gastric outlet obstruction, hepatic abscesses, and enteric fistulas. Long-term antibiotic prophylaxis with trimethoprim-sulfamethoxazole has been successful in significantly reducing the incidence of severe bacterial infections, but fungal infections are increased. Itraconazole has been used successfully to reduce fungal infections. Therapy with γ-interferon reduces infections. Long-term complications include chronic lymphadenopathy (>80% of all patients), underweight and short stature (31% and 23%, respectively), chronic inflammatory processes (e.g., ulcerative stomatitis in almost 30%), chronic diarrhea (15%), and pulmonary fibrosis (10%). Approximately 20% of the patients die at a median age of 21 years from cardiopulmonary failure secondary to chronic or recurrent chest infections, but approximately 50% of patients survive the fourth decade of life, with a plateau after the third decade of life.

Precautions before anesthesia: Obtain a complete blood count. Check serum levels of electrolytes in patients with diarrhea. A chest radiograph is recommended in the presence of respiratory symptoms. For elective cases, patients with chronic pulmonary fibrosis should undergo pulmonary function tests (including arterial blood gas analysis).

Anesthetic considerations: Early aggressive antimicrobial and surgical treatment of infections has been recommended. Patients may present for surgery in septic states. Anesthesia care is determined by the nature of the presentation. A rapid-sequence induction is recommended in patients with gastrointestinal involvement. Based on the features of the disease, it does not appear that there are specific contraindications to any particular anesthesia technique. However, strict aseptic technique for all invasive procedures is mandatory. Among the numerous associated red cell antigens in the Kell blood group system, KX is the product of an X-linked gene and appears to be a precursor in the Kell biosynthetic pathway. The lack of KX on red cells results in significant changes in Kell antigenicity (called the *McLeod phenotype*). The leukocytes of boys with X-linked chronic granulomatous disease lack this KX antigen and consequently have defective bactericidal function. This situation may also result in delayed availability of blood products if transfusion is required. Checking with the blood bank in advance is recommended.

Pharmacological implications: Concurrent medications may include prophylactic antibiotics, antifungal drugs, and γ-interferon.

REFERENCES:

Johnston RB: Clinical aspects of chronic granulomatous disease. *Curr Opin Hematol* 8:17, 2001.

Liese J, Kloos S, Jendrossek V, et al: Long-term follow-up and outcome of 39 patients with chronic granulomatous disease. *J Pediatr* 137:687, 2000.

Wall RT, Buzzanell CA, Epstein TA, et al: Anesthetic considerations in patients with chronic granulomatous disease. *J Clin Anesth* 2:306, 1990.

Chudley Mental Retardation Syndrome

At a glance: An extremely rare disorder characterized by mental retardation, distinctive mouth, obesity, and hypogonadism.

Synonyms: Chudley-Lowry-Hoar Syndrome; Chudley Syndrome I.

Incidence and genetic inheritance: Extremely rare genetic disorder (fewer than 10 cases have been described) with expression only in male children. X-linked recessive inheritance with the gene locus between Xp21 and Xq26.

Clinical aspects: Moderate-to-severe mental retardation, short stature, mild obesity, hypogonadism (often also cryptorchidism), single palmar crease, and a low total finger ridge count. The distinctive face is characterized by microcephaly with bitemporal narrowness, almond-shaped palpebral fissures, depressed nasal bridge, anteverted nares, short and inverted V-shaped upper lip, high arched palate, and macrostomia.

Anesthetic considerations: Cooperation may be difficult because of mental retardation. Sedative and/or anxiolytic premedication and/or the presence of the primary caregiver during induction of anesthesia may be beneficial. Assess airway for difficult management. The large tongue may cause airway obstruction or make tra-

cheal intubation difficult. Venous access may be difficult because of obesity.

Other condition to be considered:

☞**PRADER-LABHART-WILLI SYNDROME:** An inherited disorder characterized by muscular hypotonia, early childhood-onset obesity, hypogonadism, and mental retardation.

REFERENCE:

Chudley AE, Lowry RB, Hoar DI; Mental retardation, distinct facial changes, short stature, obesity, and hypogonadism: A new x-linked mental retardation syndrome. *Am J Med Genet* 31:741, 1988.

Chudley-Rozdilsky-Houston Syndrome

At a glance: An extremely rare, inherited disorder characterized by multicore myopathy, musculoskeletal, endocrinological, and facial anomalies, hypogonadism, and mental retardation.

Synonyms: Multicore Myopathy with Mental Retardation, Short Stature, and Hypogonadotropic Hypogonadism; Chudley Syndrome II.

Incidence and genetic inheritance: This disorder has been described in only two siblings (a boy and a girl) of consanguineous parents. Autosomal recessive transmission has been suggested.

Clinical aspects: Characterized by a congenital, nonprogressive myopathy secondary to (proved histologically and electron microscopically) ☞Multicore myopathy, severe mental retardation, radiologic evidence of pituitary gland hypoplasia with short stature, hypogonadotropic hypogonadism, and generalized hypotrichosis. Musculoskeletal anomalies may include delayed bone maturation, osteopenia, lumbar hyperlordosis, limited joint mobility (particularly of the big joints, e.g., shoulders, elbows, hips, knees, ankles), clinodactyly, and evidence of mild but generalized muscle weakness. Facial anomalies may include microcephaly, thickening of the skull, hemifacial microsomia, enlarged frontal sinuses, microtia, atretic ear canal, hypertelorism, blepharoptosis, myopia, limited sagittal eye movements, high arched palate, and facial muscle weakness. Muscle biopsies reveal a high degree of variation in fiber size and occasionally fiber splitting. The multicores consist of numerous circumscribed, small areas of disorganization of the myofibrillar structure and decreased oxidative enzyme activity secondary to a lack of mitochondria. The long axis of the lesion is perpendicular or parallel to the long axis of the muscle fiber. These cores are usually smaller than central cores. For this reason they are also called *minicores*.

Anesthetic considerations: Thorough cardiac evaluation (including electrocardiogram and echocardiography) is recommended because multicore myopathy has been linked to cardiomyopathy in some cases. Similar to central core disease, malignant hyperthermia-triggering agents should be avoided in these patients. One case of unexplained fever and death has been described in an infant boy with multicore myopathy a few hours following cardiac catheterization with meperidine, hydroxyzine, and intravenous ketamine. Titrate neuromuscular blockers under peripheral nerve stimulator control or avoid them at all if possible. Succinylcholine is best avoided because it may trigger rhabdomyolysis, hyperkalemia, or even a malignant hyperthermia crisis. Sedative and/or anxiolytic premedication and/or the presence of the primary caregiver during induction of anesthesia may be beneficial in patients with mental retardation.

Other conditions to be considered:

☞**CENTRAL CORE DISEASE:** A congenital myopathy with a specific histologic pattern and high susceptibility to malignant hyperthermia.

☞**MULTICORE MYOPATHY:** A congenital muscular disease with nonprogressive muscle weakness. Cardiac involvement with congestive, restrictive or hypertropic cardiomyopathy has been described.

REFERENCE:

Chudley AE, Rozdilsky B, Houston CS, et al: Multicore disease in sibs with severe mental retardation, short stature, facial anomalies, hypoplasia of the pituitary fossa, and hypogonadotropic hypogonadism. *Am J Med Genet* 20:145, 1985.

Citrullinemia

At a glance: A clinically and biochemically heterogenous, inherited disorder caused by argininosuccinate synthetase deficiency that leads to hyperammonemia with neurologic consequences.

Synonym: Argininosuccinate Synthetase Deficiency.

Incidence: Unknown because no database exists and many cases may go undiagnosed. However, the overall incidence has been estimated to be approximately 1:250,000 people in the general population. The incidence of citrullinemia type II in Japan is approximately 1:100,000. No sexual predilection has been reported.

Genetic inheritance: Autosomal recessive, with frequent compound heterozygotes. Citrullinemia types I and III are caused by abnormalities of the gene for argininosuccinate synthetase, which is located on 9q34. The gene causing citrullinemia type II has been mapped to 7q21.3.

Pathophysiology: Under normal conditions, the enzyme argininosuccinate synthase (ASS) catalyzes the condensation of citrulline and aspartic acid to form argininosuccinic acid. Deficiency of ASS leads to marked elevation in the plasma citrulline concentration. There is a relative deficiency of ASS enzyme activity in citrullinemia type I and absent activity in type III. Patients with type II have an abnormality of hepatic argininosuccinate synthetase only, and liver biopsy uniformly shows liver steatosis. Citrulline also can be metabolized outside the liver, although to a lesser degree, because skin fibroblasts, brain, and kidney can express ASS. The reaction of citrulline with aspartic acid is associated with the elimination of one waste nitrogen molecule, while a second waste nitrogen molecule is incorporated into the urea cycle. Because this reaction is compromised, however, the overall capacity of the urea cycle in disposing nitrogen is cut roughly in half. Consequently, affected patients are at risk for developing hyperammonemia, which results in neurologic deterioration.

Diagnosis: Enzyme activity assays in cultured fibroblasts in types I and III or in liver cells in type II.

Clinical aspects: The most common form of the disease presents in the neonatal period with symptoms from hyperammonemia caused by protein intake at 24 to 72 hours of age. Poor feeding and lethargy progress to vomiting, irritability, impaired consciousness, tachypnea, seizures, and apnea. Intracranial pressure is usually increased because of cerebral edema. If unrecognized, the condition progresses to coma and finally death. Surviving infants usually show a lower intelligence quotient. However, some children present later with a subacute form of citrullinemia, which may manifest as mental retardation and other neurologic symptoms such as ataxia. They may show episodic vomiting and hyperammonemia triggered by minor illnesses or other catabolic episodes. The late-onset form of the disease, designated type II, occurs in late childhood or adulthood. Symptoms include enuresis, delayed menarche, insomnia, recurrent vomiting, tremors, episodes of confusion after meals, lethargy, hallucinations, behavioral changes, seizures, and brief episodes of coma. Independent of the type of citrullinemia, the majority of these patients die within a few years after symptom onset. Treatment in the neonatal period includes supportive therapy, intravenous glucose and insulin to suppress the protein catabolism, and use of sodium benzoate and phenylacetate to provide an alternative pathway for nitrogen excretion. Subsequent care depends upon restriction of protein intake to the minimal amount necessary for growth, use of α-keto analogues of essential amino acids, and arginine supplementation. Subsequent episodes of hyperammonemia, triggered by inappropriate diet, drugs (e.g., valproic acid, haloperidol), or illness causing decreased caloric intake and increased protein catabolism can be managed with intravenous glucose and arginine. Orthotopic liver transplantation has been used successfully to treat citrullinemia type II.

Precautions before anesthesia: Perform a neurologic examination and check for signs of increased intracranial pressure. Obtain a complete blood count and serum concentrations of electrolytes, glucose, and ammonia.

Anesthetic considerations: Be aware of the potential for precipitation of hyperammonemia associated with fasting, trauma, surgical stress, or gastrointestinal hemorrhage. In the presence of increased intracranial pressure, a rapid-sequence induction technique (preferably with rocuronium), mild hyperventilation, and intravenous agents or low-dose volatile anesthetics for maintenance are recommended. Prolonged mechanical ventilation may be necessary in patients with preoperative signs of respiratory distress or muscular hypotonia. Regional anesthesia may be advantageous not only from a pharmacologic point of view, but also because it allows assessment of neurologic function at any given time. However, spinal anesthesia must be avoided in the presence of increased intracranial pressure.

Pharmacological implications: Hyperammonemia may be triggered by interaction with various medications. A case report in the literature cites haloperidol specifically causing this reaction in citrullinemia. Sodium valproate has been shown to cause hyperammonemia in urea cycle disorders and should therefore be avoided. Presumably other drugs also can be responsible, so vigilance is essential. Perioperative nutrition should be poor in protein to prevent hyperammonemia.

Other conditions to be considered:

☞**ARGININEMIA:** An urea cycle disorder that leads to hyperammonemia and neurologic symptoms, which are less severe than in other forms of urea cycle abnormalities.

☞**HHH SYNDROME:** A genetically transmitted inborn error of metabolism caused by a defect in the transport of ornithine into the mitochondrial matrix, clinically characterized by early growth retardation, learning disabilities, periodic confusion, and ataxia.

☞**METHYLMALONIC ACIDEMIA:** A heterogeneous inborn error of metabolism leading to metabolic acidosis and accumulation of methylmalonic acid and its by-products.

☞**N-ACETYLGLUTAMATE SYNTHETASE DEFICIENCY:** Congenital mitochondrial disorder affecting the metabolism of ammonium resulting in hyperammonemia.

☞**Ornithine Carbamoyltransferase Deficiency:** A rare genetic disorder characterized by complete or partial lack of the enzyme ornithine transcarbamylase. The lack of this enzyme results in excessive hyperammonemia, which is a known neurotoxin. Clinically, these patients present with vomiting, refusal to eat, progressive lethargy, or coma.

☞**Propionic Acidemia:** An inborn error of metabolism affecting the mitochondrial catabolism of valine and isoleucine. Untreated, this situation results in ketoacidosis, lethargy, coma, and finally death.

References:

Beaudet AL, O'Brien WE, Bock HG et al: The human argininosuccinate synthetase locus and citrullinemia. *Adv Hum Genet* 15:161, 1986.

Haberle J, Pauli S, Linnebank M, et al: Structure of the human argininosuccinate synthetase gene and an improved system for molecular diagnostics in patients with classical and mild citrullinemia. *Hum Genet* 110:327, 2002.

Igarashi M, Kawana S, Iwasaki H, et al: Anesthetic management for a patient with citrullinemia and liver cirrhosis. *Masui* 44:96, 1995.

Cleft Hand and Absent Tibia Syndrome

At a glance: A syndrome that is characterized by cleft hand and tibial aplasia with ectrodactyly.

Synonyms: Aplasia of Tibia with Ectrodactyly; Tibial Aplasia with Split-Hand/Foot Deformity.

Incidence and genetic inheritance: In the general population, approximately 1:100,000 is affected. Despite the fact that consanguinity is common in the parents of affected children, inheritance is believed to be most often autosomal dominant with markedly reduced penetrance.

Clinical aspects: The syndrome consists of bilateral aplasia of the tibiae and split-hand/foot deformities (also called *lobster-claw deformity*). Other anomalies may include hypoplasia or aplasia of the ulnae, distal hypoplasia or bifurcation of the femora, aplasia of patellae, hypoplastic big toes, postaxial and intermediate polydactyly, and cup-shaped ears.

Anesthetic considerations: Evaluate the severity of the disease to prepare for intraoperative positioning. Venous access on hands and feet may be difficult.

Other conditions to be considered:

☞**Ectrodactyly:** Ectrodactyly describes a situation where at least one entire digit (both metacarpal/metatarsal and phalanges) is missing. It is a nonspecific term applied to a variety of malformations.

☞**Ectrodactyly, Ectodermal Dysplasia, and Cleft Lip-Palate (EEC) Syndrome:** Autosomal dominant inherited syndrome with facial (mild malar hypoplasia, maxillary hypoplasia, cleft lip and palate, choanal atresia), ocular and urogenital anomalies and occasionally mental retardation, and central diabetes insipidus.

References:

Majewski F, Kuster W, Ter Haar B, et al: Aplasia of tibia with split hand/foot deformity. Report of six families with 35 cases and considerations about variability and penetrance. *Hum Genet* 70:136, 1985.

Shenoy R, Kamath N: Bilateral congenital split hand with tibial aplasia. *Ind J Pediatr* 71:948, 2004.

Witters I, Devriendt K, Moerman P, et al: Bilateral tibial agenesis with ectrodactyly: Further evidence for autosomal recessive inheritance. *Am J Med Genet* 104:209, 2001.

Cleft-Limb-Heart Malformation Syndrome

At a glance: A syndrome possibly related to prematernal diabetes, with severe limb and craniofacial malformations and truncus arteriosus.

Synonyms: CLH Syndrome; Verloove-Vanhorick-Brubakk Syndrome.

Incidence and genetic inheritance: One case report of two siblings exists. Probably autosomal recessive transmission.

Clinical aspects: Clinical features involve the skeleton (deformities of both lower and upper limbs, short humeri and femora, tapering of the proximal femur with absence of the femoral head, deformed acetabula, lumbosacral spine deformation with four lumbar vertebral bodies, absence of the coccygeal bone and the calcaneus, absence of one metatarsal and metacarpal bone in both feet and hands with partial syndactyly of toes and fingers), facial deformities (micrognathia, small, low-set, malformed ears without external meatus, double cleft lip/palate), and the urogenital tract (malfunctioning horseshoe kidney, cryptorchidism). Other abnormalities include truncus arteriosus, bilateral bilobular lungs, and parathyroid aplasia. Both siblings had almost identical malformations, including the truncus arteriosus, and both died in the neonatal period.

Anesthetic considerations: Obtain a full cardiac assessment before anesthesia. Peripheral venous access may be difficult. Micrognathia and cleft palate may make airway management difficult. Maintain spontaneous ventilation until the airway has been secured. An increased ratio of pulmonary-to-systemic blood flow in truncus may result in severe congestive heart failure and requires specific anesthetic management. Subacute bacterial endocarditis prophylaxis may be indicated.

Reference:

Verloove-Vanhorick SP, Brubakk AM, Ruys JH: Extensive congenital malformations in two siblings: Maternal pre-diabetes or a new syndrome? *Acta Paediatr Scand* 70:767, 1981.

Cleft Palate Lateral Synechiae Syndrome

At a glance: A syndrome characterized by multiple intrabuccal synechiae associated with craniofacial malformations.

Synonym: CPLS Syndrome.

Incidence and genetic inheritance: Extremely rare genetic disorder (fewer than 10 cases have been described) with autosomal dominant inheritance.

Clinical aspects: Patients present with mental and growth retardation and hypotonia. Clinical features involve the head and neck with microcephaly, cleft palate, multiple, "cord-like" adhesions between the lateral aspects of the tongue, the floor of the mouth and the hard palate, protruding lips, hypoplastic or bifid uvula, micrognathia/retrognathia, beaked nose, short philtrum, malar hypoplasia, and lacrimal abnormalities.

Anesthetic considerations: Anesthesia in this condition has not been described. The described features suggest that face-mask ventilation may be difficult, and direct laryngoscopy and tracheal intubation may be impossible because of severely restricted mouth opening. Spontaneous ventilation should be preserved until the airway has been secured and alternative airway management techniques (e.g., awake fiberoptic nasal intubation) have to be considered.

REFERENCES:

Gassner I, Muller W, Rossler H et al: Familial occurrence of syngnathia congenita syndrome. *Clin Genet* 15:241, 1979.

Haramis HT, Apesos J: Cleft palate and congenital lateral alveolar synechia syndrome: Case presentation and literature review. *Ann Plast Surg* 34:424, 1995.

Nakata NM, Guion-Almeida ML, Richieri-Costa A: Cleft palate-lateral synechiae syndrome: Report on three new patients with additional findings and evidence for variability and heterogeneity. *Am J Med Genet* 47:330, 1993.

Cleidocranial Dysplasia

At a glance: Generalized skeletal dysplasia resulting in defects in the development of skull, clavicles, pelvis, and teeth.

Synonyms: Cleidocranial Dysostosis; Scheuthauer-Marie-Sainton Syndrome; Marie-Sainton Syndrome.

Incidence: More than 500 cases have been reported worldwide. No sexual predilection.

Genetic inheritance: Autosomal dominant. There is a wide variability in expression.

Pathophysiology: The disorder is caused by mutations in the transcription factor CBFA1 of the runt domain gene family. The responsible gene has been mapped to 6p21. This situation results in generalized dysplasia of bone and dental tissue. Initially it was postulated that the disease affects only the membranous bones (neurocranium, a portion of the clavicle, and some facial bones). However, we now know that cleidocranial dysplasia is a generalized skeletal dysplasia. There is growth retardation and a slight effect on skeletal maturation over time.

Diagnosis: Based on the clinical findings of skull, dental, pelvic, and clavicular malformations and confirmed with genetic mapping. Radiographs show persistently open skull sutures and fontanelle with bulging of the calvarium, short fifth finger middle phalanx, and characteristic bone changes.

Clinical aspects: The disease involves mainly the head and neck (brachycephaly, enlarged calvaria, frontal bossing with wide forehead and hypertelorism, wormian bones, large foramen magnum, hypoplasia or absence of frontal and paranasal sinuses, midfacial hypoplasia, micrognathia, nonunion of mandibular symphysis, high arched palate or cleft palate, delayed eruption of deciduous and permanent teeth, enamel and root hypoplasia, cavities, supernumerary teeth [up to 30 extra teeth have been described], and deafness) and the skeleton (short stature, spina bifida occulta, [unilateral or bilateral] hypoplastic [more often at the acromial than at the sternal end] or aplastic [rare] clavicles with the ability to appose the shoulders, narrow, bell-shaped thorax with short, oblique ribs, cervical ribs, small scapula with dysplastic acromial facets and supraspinatus fossae, hypoplastic pubic bones with widened symphysis pubis, hip dislocation, generalized joint laxity, brachydactyly, excessive length of metacarpal and metatarsal II (and V) bones secondary to extra

epiphyses, short middle phalanx of the fifth fingers, cup-shaped and hypoplastic distal phalanges with onychodysplasia). Respiratory distress occurs frequently.

Precautions before anesthesia: Because of the facial malformations and the abnormal and fragile teeth, the airway must be examined closely with regard to difficult management. Assessment of respiratory function (clinical examination, chest radiographs and/or computed tomography scanning, pulmonary function tests, arterial blood gas analysis) is required secondary to the usually narrow thorax, which results in decreased compliance and respiratory distress in early infancy. Cor pulmonale has not been described in this condition, but the potential for increased right ventricular pressure should be kept in mind.

Anesthetic considerations: Patients may have difficult airway management and be at risk for postoperative respiratory distress in the presence of reduced pulmonary reserves. Maintain spontaneous ventilation until the airway has been secured. Care with positioning is essential because of joint laxity and the tendency for dislocations. Keep spinal and vertebral anomalies in mind if considering central neuraxial blockade. Abnormal clavicles may make central venous access difficult (more so for subclavian than for internal jugular vein approach).

Pharmacological implications: Avoid neuromuscular blockers until the airway has been secured. Patients may have a reduced respiratory reserve if the thorax is significantly affected. Respiratory depressants should be used with care.

Other conditions to be considered:

☞**YUNIS-VARON SYNDROME:** Autosomal recessive inherited syndrome associated with generalized skeletal dysplasia and other features such as cardiac anomalies (tetralogy of Fallot, cardiomyopathy) and severe neurologic impairment (profound developmental delay, agenesis of the corpus callosum, arrhinencephaly). Death in the neonatal period is frequent.

☞**PYKNODYSOSTOSIS:** Inherited syndrome characterized by congenital osteosclerosis, short stature, frontal and occipital bossing, short wide hands, and multiple other anomalies.

REFERENCES:

Cooper SC, Flaitz CM, Johnston DA et al: A natural history of cleidocranial dysplasia. *Am J Med Genet* 104:1, 2001.

Golan I, Baumert U, Held P, et al: Radiological findings and molecular genetic confirmation of cleidocranial dysplasia. *Clin Radiol* 57:525, 2002.

Mundlos S: Cleidocranial dysplasia: Clinical and molecular genetics. *J Med Genet* 36:177, 1999.

Cleidorhizomelic Syndrome

At a glance: An exceptional genetic syndrome of characteristic rhizomelic short stature and lateral clavicular defect.

Synonym: Wallis-Zieff-Goldblatt Syndrome.

Incidence and genetic inheritance: One case report of an affected mother and son exists. Probably autosomal dominant inheritance.

Clinical aspects: Features include rhizomelic short stature, lateral clavicular defect (consisting of a bifid appearance of the lateral third caused by an abnormal processus arising from the fusion center), broad proximal and middle phalanges, and hypoplasia of the middle phalanges of the fifth fingers.

Anesthetic considerations: Careful intraoperative positioning is needed. Subclavian central venous access could be difficult secondary to clavicular anomalies.

REFERENCE:

Wallis C, Zieff S, Goldblatt J: Newly recognized autosomal dominant syndrome of rhizomelic shortness with clavicular defect. *Am J Med Genet* 31:881, 1988.

Cloverleaf Skull

At a glance: A congenital nonsyndromic abnormality with a characteristic trilobular aspect of the skull.

Synonym: Kleeblattschädel.

Incidence: Craniosynostosis occurs in approximately 1:2,100 live births in the general population. Cloverleaf skull (CLS) accounts for less than 1% of cases.

Genetic inheritance: All reported cases have been sporadic.

Pathophysiology: The abnormally shaped skull is caused by premature ossification of the coronal, sagittal, and lambdoid sutures. The metopic and squamous sutures do not fuse. It has been hypothesized that abnormal development of the periosteal vascular plexus alters the ossification and development of the skull. CLS may occur as an isolated finding, but is more commonly associated with ☞Thanatophoric Dwarfism, ☞Achondrogenesis, and Camptomelic Dysplasia. It is also seen in ☞Acrocephalopolysyndactyly (Carpenter Syndrome), and ☞Acrocephalosyndactyly Syndromes (Apert, Pfeiffer, and Crouzon Syndromes).

Diagnosis: Based on the clinical findings of trilobular skull aspect and craniosynostosis in radiologic examinations (conventional radiography, computed tomography scanning, and magnetic resonance imaging).

Clinical aspects: Neonatal death is frequent. Patients may have mental retardation. On examination, the skull has a trilobed appearance with high forehead, beaked nose, and depressed premaxillary region. Hydrocephalus is common. Raised intracranial pressure is seen in approximately 45% of patients with complex craniosynostoses. Other features involve the eyes (marked proptosis, exophthalmos, corneal ulcerations) and the limbs (elbow ankylosis, dysostosis multiplex, syndactyly of toes and fingers, restricted joint mobility). Abnormal vertebral size has occasionally been reported.

Precautions before anesthesia: The presence of raised intracranial pressure should be determined. If CLS is part of a syndrome or skeletal dysplasia, the patient should be investigated for features of that condition. Evaluate for difficult airway management.

Anesthetic considerations: Patients may have increased intracranial pressure. On the one hand, this situation makes a rapid-sequence induction (increased risk of vomiting) for tracheal intubation with controlled ventilation desirable. On the other hand, maintenance of spontaneous ventilation may be required until the airway has been secured if airway management is expected to be difficult. The final decision depends on the clinical situation. Careful eye protection is

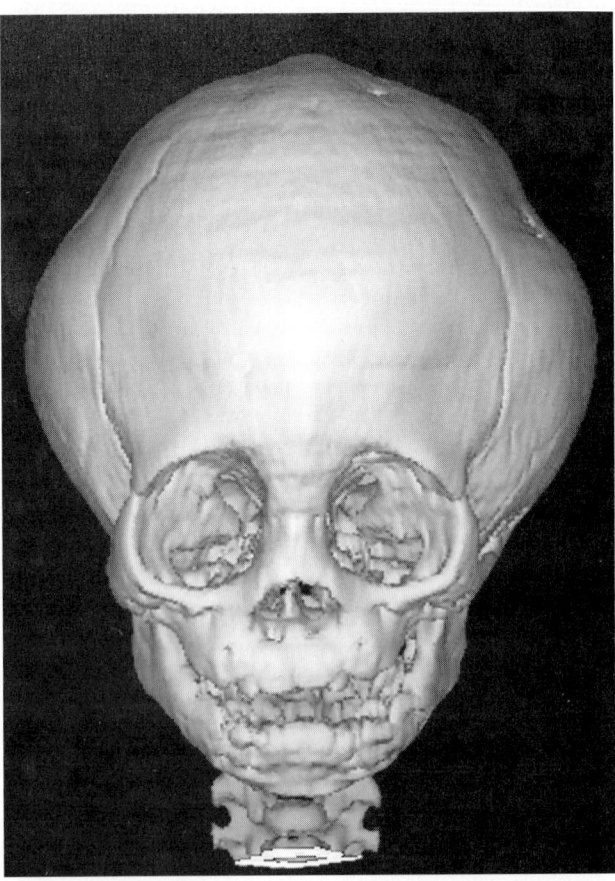

Cloverleaf Skull Airway management was very difficult in this 14-month-old boy with cloverleaf skull.

Cloverleaf Skull Three-dimensional reconstruction of the cranial computed tomography scan of the same boy gives a better impression of the underlying anomaly in cloverleaf skull.

required because of increased risk for corneal ulceration secondary to proptosis. Careful intraoperative positioning is needed because of orthopedic features.

Pharmacological implications: Succinylcholine and ketamine should be avoided if possible in the presence of already increased intracranial pressure.

Other conditions to be considered:

CLOVERLEAF SKULL AND BONE DYSPLASIA: CLS in combination with genital and chest anomalies that could increase respiratory risks.

☞**KOZLOWSKI WARREN FISHER SYNDROME:** Lethal form of CLS with genital anomalies and rhizomelic micromelia.

CLOVERLEAF SKULL WITH MICROMELIA AND THORACIC DYSPLASIA (Benallegue Lacete Syndrome): A frequently early lethal syndrome caused by respiratory distress as a result of thoracic cage hypoplasia.

☞**THANATOPHORIC DWARFISM:** Results from a sporadic defect in the fibroblast growth factor 3 gene, which is a transmembranous regulator. The disease is lethal usually shortly after birth secondary to respiratory failure (thoracic cage hypoplasia). The incidence is approximately 1:10,000 births, making it the most common lethal bone dysplasia.

OSTEOGLOPHONIC DYSPLASIA (Craniofacial Dysostosis with Fibrous Metaphyseal Defects): Short stature and stubby hands. There is acrocephaly and CLS deformities with frontal bossing.

☞**ACHONDROGENESIS:** A defect in the development of bone and cartilage. A rare type of dwarfism that usually is fatal at birth or soon thereafter. Very short trunk, arms, legs, and neck. The head appears large in relation to the trunk. Hypoplastic mandibula and narrow chest.

CAMPOMELIC DYSPLASIA (Camptomelic Dysplasia): Autosomal dominant inheritance. Incidence is about 1:2,000,000 live births. Short limb dwarfism with prenatal onset. Large anterior fontanelle, macrocephaly, micrognathia, hearing loss, cleft palate. Congenital heart defects (atrial and ventricular septal defects, tetralogy of Fallot), and respiratory failure because of hypoplastic thoracic cage result in early neonatal death.

CARPENTER SYNDROME (☞Acrocephalopolysyndactyly Type II): A condition characterized by craniosynostosis, acrocephaly, facial anomalies and syndactyly. Cardiac malformations have also been described.

APERT SYNDROME (☞Acrocephalosyndactyly Type I): Agenesis or premature closure of the cranial sutures, midface hypoplasia, and symmetrical syndactyly of the hands and feet involving at least the second, third, and fourth digits. Cervical spine fusion is common and almost always involves C5-C6. Numerous facial anomalies and heart defects may be associated.

PFEIFFER SYNDROME (☞Acrocephalosyndactyly type V): Sagittal craniostenosis associated with broad thumbs and toes (mostly second toe), variable maxillary retrusion, and partial soft tissue syndactyly characterize this syndrome. Congenital heart disease is most often present.

CROUZON SYNDROME (☞Acrocephalosyndactyly type II): A form of craniofacial dysostosis similar to Apert syndrome, but without syndactyly. Characteristic features include exophthalmos, maxillary hypoplasia, hypertelorism, and a beaked nose.

REFERENCES:

Crysdale WS, Kohli-Dang N, Mullins GC, et al: Airway management in craniofacial surgery: Experience in 542 patients. *J Otolaryngol* 16:207, 1987.

Ridgway EB, Weiner HL: Skull deformities. *Pediatr Clin North Am* 51:359, 2004.

Taylor WJ, Hayward RD, Lasjaunias P, et al: Enigma of raised intracranial pressure in patients with complex craniosynostosis: The role of abnormal intracranial venous drainage. *J Neurosurg* 94:377, 2001.

Clubfoot

At a glance: An intrauterine developmental malformation with a genetic component affecting the talus and resulting in medial and plantar deviation. Clubfoot is part of multiple syndromes.

Synonym: Talipes Equinovarus.

Incidence: Varies according to the racial group. One study reported an incidence of 1:1000 in Caucasians, 7:1000 in Polynesians, and 0.5:1000 in Japanese. Bilateral cases occur in 40%. The male-to-female ratio is approximately 2.5:1.

Genetic inheritance: It is thought to be due to the action of a major gene with additional contribution of multifactorial inheritance. Autosomal dominant inheritance has been suggested.

Pathophysiology: In some cases, electron microscopy has shown some evidence of neurogenic muscle disease, suggesting an innervation defect.

Diagnosis: Deformity of the talus with medial and plantar deviation of its neck. The ankle joint mortice is normal, and foot deviation follows the talar neck deformity.

Clinical aspects: Medial and plantar deviation of one or both feet (pes adductus, equinovarus, supinatus) can be diagnosed by ultrasound in utero. Postnatally, radiographic evaluation requires weight-bearing or simulated weight-bearing anteroposterior and lateral radiographs of the foot. The talus deformity consists of hypoplasia with plantar and medial deviation of the shortened talar neck with lateral rotation in the ankle mortice. Radiographs show medial subluxation of the navicular bone, which articulates with the medial aspect of the talus neck. Medial subluxation of the cuboid bone on the calcaneus head results in medial midfoot displacement. Additional findings include shortening and contractures of ligaments and joint capsules around the ankle mortice, and contracted and hypoplastic calf muscles.

Precautions before anesthesia: Search for evidence of coexistent diseases, such as Myelomeningocele, ☞Chondrodysplasia Punctata, ☞Arthrogryposis Multiplex Congenita, ☞Neurofibromatosis Generalizata, and many others.

Anesthetic considerations: Anesthesia may be performed with general, regional, or combined techniques. A regional approach may be preferred in the presence of a myopathy. Combined neurologic, electromyographic, and muscle biopsy studies show myopathic changes in up to 70% of clubfoot patients. This high rate of myopathic changes suggests regional anesthesia techniques may be preferred to prevent possible problems related to malignant hyperthermia.

Pharmacological implications: Careful use of succinylcholine and nondepolarizing neuromuscular blockers in the presence of myopathy and the use of a peripheral nerve stimulator is recommended.

REFERENCES:

Chapman C, Stott NS, Port R, et al: Genetics of club foot in Maori and Pacific people. *J Med Genet* 37:680, 2000.

Wang J, Palmer RM, Chung CS: The role of major gene in clubfoot. *Am J Hum Genet* 42:772, 1988.

Zanette G, Manani G, Pittoni G, et al: Prevalence of unsuspected myopathy in infants presenting for clubfoot surgery. *Paediatr Anaesth* 5:165, 1995.

COACH Syndrome

At a glance: An inherited syndrome characterized by the combination of hepatic fibrosis, early onset ataxia, cerebellar aplasia, oligophrenia, and coloboma. COACH is an acronym for *c*erebellar vermis aplasia, *o*ligophrenia, congenital *a*taxia, ocular *c*oloboma and *h*epatic fibrosis.

Incidence and genetic inheritance: Fewer than 20 cases have been described. Autosomal recessive inheritance. Parental consanguinity has been reported in some cases.

Clinical aspects: The diagnosis is based on moderate mental retardation associated with early-onset ataxia and hypotonia, inconstant coloboma, and hepatic cirrhosis in association with a positive family history. Imaging studies show cerebellar vermis hypoplasia or aplasia but normal supratentorial structures. Liver biopsy characteristically reveals periportal fibrosis, cholestasis, reduced number of intrahepatic bile ducts, and chronic inflammatory infiltrates. Other features may involve the head and neck (flat round face, hypertelorism, ptosis, optic nerve coloboma and optic disc atrophy, upturned nose, macrostomia, macroglossia, occipital encephalocele), the central nervous system (ataxia and hypotonia, later spasticity; the term "molar tooth" sign is used to describe the brainstem malformation with elongated superior cerebellar peduncles and pronounced interpeduncular fossa), the musculoskeletal system (postaxial polydactyly, slender skeleton), the kidneys (multiple medullary cysts, renal impairment), and the viscera (hepatomegaly splenomegaly, hepatic cirrhosis, and portal hypertension in 70% of patients). Episodic tachypnea and ventricular septal defect have been described. Death may result from complications of hepatic fibrosis, gastrointestinal bleeding, or kidney failure. Successful liver and combined liver and kidney transplantation have been reported.

Anesthetic considerations: Obtain a complete blood count (anemia secondary to gastrointestinal hemorrhage) and check serum levels of electrolytes. Thrombocytopenia secondary to portal hypertension with splenomegaly (hypersplenism) was described in one patient. Assess renal (creatinine, blood urea nitrogen) and hepatic function (transaminases, bilirubin, albumin, coagulation status). Reduced doses of muscle relaxant agents may be required. Consider alterations in the metabolism and elimination of drugs in the presence of hepatic and/or renal failure. The potential for airway obstruction, a result of macroglossia, requires preoperative evaluation. Careful insertion of nasogastric tubes is required because the majority of patients have esophageal varices. Bleeding from abdominal surgery may be increased in the presence of portal hypertension and coagulopathy. Large-bore intravenous access is therefore recommended. Consider subacute bacterial endocarditis prophylaxis in the presence of congenital cardiac lesions.

Other conditions to be considered:

☞**JOUBERT SYNDROME:** A genetic peroxisomal disorder characterized by cerebral malformations (vermis and brainstem) resulting in severe coordination (ataxia) and breathing (sleep apnea, hyperpnea) disorders.

ARIMA SYNDROME (Cerebro-Oculo-Hepato-Renal Syndrome): This syndrome is similar to Joubert syndrome, however, the Arima syndrome also presents with retinal dystrophy and visual tracking anomalies (oculomotor ataxia), renal failure, and liver dysfunction.

☞**LOKEN SENIOR SYNDROME:** An autosomal recessive inherited disorder characterized by rapidly progressive renal insufficiency (nephronophthisis), progressive retinitis pigmentosa, and ataxia. Manifestation during the first year of life. Blindness develops within the first 2 years of life.

☞**RENAL-COLOBOMA SYNDROME:** A familial syndrome combining ocular, renal, and neurologic anomalies.

REFERENCES:

Foell D, August C, Frosch M, et al: Early detection of severe cholestatic hepatopathy in COACH syndrome. *Am J Med Genet* 111:429, 2002.

Uemura T, Sanchez EQ, Ikegami T, et al: Successful combined liver and kidney transplant for COACH syndrome and 5-yr follow-up. *Clin Transplant* 19:717, 2005.

Verloes A, Lambotte C: Further delineation of a syndrome of cerebellar vermis hypo/aplasia, oligophrenia, congenital ataxia, coloboma and hepatic fibrosis. *Am J Med Genet* 32:227, 1989.

Coats Disease

At a glance: A disorder characterized by idiopathic progressive, retinal telangiectasia with intraretinal and/or subretinal exudation. Possible association with renal dysfunction and cranial malformations.

Synonyms: Congenital Retinal Telangiectasia; Leber Miliary Aneurysm Disease; Exudative Retinitis.

History: A progressive congenital retinopathy first described by the Scottish ophthalmologist George Coats in 1908.

Incidence: Unknown.

Genetic inheritance: Coats disease is a sporadic, nonhereditary condition. Males are affected three times more often than females. No racial or ethnic predilection has been reported.

Pathophysiology: The retinal capillary endothelium is abnormally permeable. Affected vessels show a marked thickening of the basement membrane and widespread loss of endothelial cells and pericytes with subsequent disintegration of the blood-retinal barrier. The retinal protein norrin may be deficient or abnormal. There are retinal telangiectasias and aneurysms of the capillaries, venules, and arterioles. Lipoproteinaceous exudations are found in intraretinal and subretinal areas.

Diagnosis: The age at onset has two peaks, one before 20 years of age and the second afterward. Most often, however, it is diagnosed at 7 to 10 years of age by the onset of retinal telangiectasias with intraretinal and/or subretinal exudation.

Clinical aspects: Coats disease is unilateral in more than 90% of cases and most frequently occurs in otherwise healthy patients. Bilateral occurrence is so rare that some researchers recommend questioning the diagnosis in these patients. The disease manifests as a deterioration in either central or peripheral vision. Rarely, Coats disease is associated with pathologic findings of the head and neck (microcephaly, intracranial calcifications, ataxia, depressed premaxillary region), the skin (absent scalp hair, syndactyly of fingers, dysplastic, grooved nails), and other ocular manifestations (paresis of ocular muscles, glaucoma). Renal impairment has been reported in some patients.

Precautions before anesthesia: In cases of isolated Coats disease, no specific anesthetic precautions are required. However, if there is an association with extraocular manifestations, anesthetic care is influenced by the nature and severity of these features. Renal function may need to be assessed (electrolytes, serum creatinine, blood urea nitrogen). Check for difficult airway management.

Anesthetic considerations: Tracheal intubation can be difficult.

Pharmacological implications: Renal dysfunction may affect elimination of drugs with predominantly renal excretion. Perioperative fluid regimen must be adapted to renal function. Avoid drugs that may increase intraocular pressure in the presence of glaucoma (e.g., atropine, succinylcholine).

Other conditions to be considered: Similar ocular features may be seen in retinitis pigmentosa, ☞Alport Syndrome, ☞Brachmann-de Lange Syndrome, ☞Epidermal Nevus Syndrome, ☞Hallermann-Streiff Syndrome, ☞Landouzy-Dejerine Dystrophy ☞Senior-Loken Syndrome, ☞Ullrich-Turner Syndrome, aplastic anemia, and in renal transplant patients. However, the most important differential diagnosis in pediatric patients is ☞Retinoblastoma, and failure to distinguish these two conditions will have serious consequences. Retinoblastoma usually is diagnosed at a younger age and does not have a sexual predilection. Retinoblastoma has a positive family history in approximately 10% and is bilateral in approximately 40% of patients, whereas Coats disease is unilateral in more than 90% of patients.

REFERENCES:

Shields JA, Shields CL: Review: Coats disease: The 2001 LuEsther T. Mertz lecture. *Retina* 22:80, 2002.

Shields JA, Shields CL, Honavar SG, et al: Clinical variations and complications of Coats' disease in 150 cases: The 2000 Sanford Gifford Memorial Lecture. *Am J Ophthalmol* 131:561, 2001.

Tolmie JL, Browne BH, McGettrick PM, et al: A familial syndrome with Coats' reaction retinal angiomas, hair and nail defects and intracranial calcification. *Eye* 2:297, 1988.

Cockayne Syndrome

At a glance: A complex inherited and congenital disorder characterized by the association of dwarfism, deafness, microcephaly, facial anomalies, ataxia, photosensitivity, retinal atrophy, and renal insufficiency with premature aging and atherosclerosis.

Synonyms: Deafness-Dwarfism-Retinal Atrophy; Dwarfism with Renal Atrophy and Deafness; Neill-Dingwall Syndrome; Progeroid Nanism.

History: First described by the English Physician Edward Alfred Cockayne in 1936.

Incidence: Occurs in approximately 1:200,000 live births. No ethnic or sexual predilection has been reported.

Genetic inheritance: Autosomal recessive. Cockayne syndrome (CS) type I (also called *type A*, see "Clinical Aspects") results from a defect in the CS type A or CSA or ERCC8 (*e*xcision *r*epair *c*ross-complementing rodent repair deficiency, *c*omplementation group 8) gene, which is located on chromosome 5. Cells carrying the mutated ERCC8 gene exhibit a hypersensitivity to ultraviolet light. After exposure to ultraviolet light, these cells fail to recover their ability to synthesize ribonucleic acid and to repair or excise and degrade lesions in deoxyribonucleic acid strands. In CS type II (type B), the mutation affects the transcription-coupled and global genome DNA excision repair gene ERCC6 (*e*xcision *r*epair *c*ross-complementing

rodent repair deficiency, *c*omplementation group 6), which has been mapped to 10q11.

Pathophysiology: A defective transcription-coupled repair of oxidative damages to the DNA contributes to developmental defects.

Diagnosis: In classic CS type I, the diagnosis is based on the clinical findings, whereas the "nonclassic" form is confirmed by DNA repair assays in lymphoblasts or skin fibroblasts. In older children, classic CS type I should be suspected in the presence of both major and three minor criteria. In infants or toddlers, the diagnosis is likely when one minor and both major criteria are fulfilled and abnormalities in DNA repair are present. The major criteria consist of (1) postnatal growth retardation (height and weight below the fifth percentile at 2 years of age resulting in "cachectic dwarfism" appearance) and (2) progressive neurologic dysfunction (early developmental delay and progressive deterioration). Intracranial pericapillary calcifications (in cortex and basal ganglia), leukodystrophy with scattered neuronal loss, and normal pressure hydrocephalus may be present. The seven minor criteria are (1) dermal photosensitivity (poikiloderma), (2) pigmentary retinopathy, blindness, and/or cataracts, (3) diffuse and segmental peripheral demyelination with decreased nerve conduction velocity, (4) sensorineural hearing loss, (5) sclerotic epiphyses, vertebral and pelvic abnormalities, thickening of the calvarium, (6) thin skin and brittle hair, sunken eyes, and stooped standing posture, and (7) dental cavities. In CS type II, the diagnosis is based on the findings of failure to thrive beginning right from birth with severely delayed gains in height and weight combined with absent or minimal progress in the neurologic development. Eye anomalies are frequent and include congenital cataracts and other structural ocular defects such as microphthalmos and microcornea.

Clinical aspects: Premature aging is the hallmark of all types of CS. CS I (type A or "classic" form) presents in infancy and is less severe than CS II (type B or "congenital" or "connatal" form), which presents earlier and is generally apparent already at birth. CS III (type C or "late-onset" form) presents later in life, and there is no universal agreement as to the existence of CS III. The *classic form (type I)* may involve the head and neck (microcephaly, thickened calvarium, intracranial calcifications, mandibular prognathism, loss of facial adipose tissue with wrinkled face, slender nose, malformed ears, sensorineural hearing loss, hypoplastic teeth with caries, delayed eruption of deciduous teeth), the nervous system (mental retardation, leukodystrophy, normal pressure hydrocephalus, seizures, nystagmus, ataxia, dysarthria, tremor, generalized weakness, peripheral neuropathy), the eyes ("salt and pepper" retinal pigmentation, optic nerve atrophy, strabismus, hypermetropia, corneal opacity, decreased lacrimation; development of cataracts before the age of 3 years is associated with a severe course of the disease and early mortality), the cardiovascular system (arterial hypertension, arrhythmias, premature atherosclerosis), the genitourinary tract (renal failure, proteinuria, cryptorchidism, micropenis), the musculoskeletal system (short stature, vertebral anomalies with kyphosis, small squared-off pelvis with hypoplastic iliac wings, mild-to-moderate limitation of joint movements, sclerotic phalangeal epiphyses), and the skin (precocious senile appearance [wrinkling], photosensitivity, scarring, poikiloderma, anhydrosis and dry skin, thin and dry hair, decreased subcutaneous adipose tissue, café-au-lait spots). Other features include hepatosplenomegaly with elevated liver enzyme serum concentrations. There is no increase in malignancies or susceptibility to infections. Death in CS I patients usually occurs early in the second decade of life. Growth failure in patients with congenital CS type II is obvious at birth (intrauterine and postnatal growth retardation) or shortly after birth. Neurologic development is either absent or severely delayed. Congenital cataracts or other structural ocular anomalies occur in up to one third of patients. Arthrogryposis and/or early joint contractures result in restricted movement and kyphoscoliosis. Death usually occurs before 10 years of age, often as a result of pneumonia. In several aspects, CS type II resembles the ☞Pena-Shokeir Syndrome Type II. A small subset of patients share some features of CS, but show normal growth and neurologic development. These patients have been assigned the diagnosis of "late-onset" CS or *CS type III*. However, the debate is ongoing whether CS type III is in fact a form of CS or an entirely different syndrome.

In fewer than 10 cases, CS was associated with ☞Xeroderma Pigmentosum (XP-CS). This rare variant shares signs of xeroderma pigmentosum with all the features of the classic form of CS.

Precaution before anesthesia: Obtaining a complete blood count and serum concentrations of electrolytes, creatinine, and urea is recommended. Advanced generalized and coronary atherosclerosis is part of the disease. An electrocardiogram (arrhythmias, ischemia) and a chest radiograph should be requested. Blood pressure control should be assessed. Evaluate the airway with regard to difficult management. Check for gastroesophageal reflux (frequent) and recurrent aspiration pneumonia. Developmental delay may limit patient cooperation. Sedative and/or anxiolytic premedication and the presence of the primary caregiver during induction of anesthesia may be helpful.

Anesthetic considerations: Difficult mask ventilation and direct laryngoscopy and tracheal intubation have been reported. The tracheal diameter may be less than expected, requiring a smaller than predicted endotracheal tube. Maintenance of spontaneous ventilation is desired until the airway has been secured. However, there may be an increased risk of aspiration because of gastroesophageal reflux, and a rapid-sequence induction technique would be preferred. The final decision depends mainly on the clinical findings (severity of facial dysmorphism on the one hand and of gastroesophageal reflux on the other hand). Decreased sweating may lead to thermoregulatory abnormalities. Restricted joint movement may lead to difficult vascular access and patient positioning. Eye protection with eye ointment and taping the eyes shut is imperative secondary to decreased lacrimation.

Pharmacological implications: In a single case report, a dose of nifedipine 2 mg given to a 10-kg female with Cockayne syndrome for control of systemic hypertension resulted in transient cerebral ischemia and loss of consciousness at a systolic blood pressure of 138 mmHg. Anesthesia-related drops in arterial blood pressure should therefore be treated aggressively. Atropine should be avoided because of deficient lacrimation. Consider interaction between anesthetic drugs and antiepileptic treatment and also decreased elimination of drugs with predominantly renal excretion.

Other conditions to be considered:

☞**Pena-Shokeir Syndrome Type II:** A rapidly progressive neurologic disorder leading to brain atrophy with calcifications, cataracts, microcornea, optic atrophy, progressive joint contractures, and growth failure.

☞**Xeroderma Pigmentosum:** A syndrome characterized by a defect in ultraviolet radiation induced DNA repair mechanisms. The DNA damage is cumulative and irreversible. This condition may be lethal in infancy or childhood.

References:

Nance MA, Berry SA: Cockayne syndrome: Review of 140 cases. *Am J Med Genet* 42:68, 1992.

Sasaki R, Hirota K, Masuda A: Nifedipine-induced transient cerebral ischemia in a child with Cockayne syndrome. *Anaesthesia* 52:1236, 1997.

Wooldridge WJ, Dearlove OR, Khan AA: Anaesthesia for Cockayne syndrome. Three case reports. *Anaesthesia* 51:478, 1996.

CODAS Syndrome

At a glance: A very rare syndrome combining multiple malformations involving head and skeleton. CODAS is an acronym for cerebral *o*cular *d*ental *a*uricular *s*keletal anomalies.

Incidence and genetic inheritance: Only three cases have been reported. Inheritance is undetermined; all three cases appear to be sporadic. Two girls and one boy have been affected, two of them are of Mennonite ancestry. Consanguinity was not reported in any of the cases.

Clinical aspects: All laboratory investigations including karyotype, metabolic screening, and studies of cholesterol biosynthesis and peroxisomes yielded normal results, and the underlying defect has not been identified. However, the features of the disease suggest that a collagen gene defect is involved. Clinical signs may involve the head and neck (microcephaly, overfolded ears with dysplastic helices, flat nose with vertically grooved nasal tip, short philtrum, abnormal enamel projections, gingiva hypertrophy), the central nervous system (developmental delay), the eyes (congenital cataracts, ptosis, nystagmus), the skeleton (delayed ossification of upper and lower extremities, odontoid hypoplasia, deformed vertebral bodies with coronal clefts, scoliosis, radiologic signs of spondyloepiphyseal dysplasia, generalized abnormalities of the ilium, joint dislocations, hypoplastic pectoral muscles, generalized hypotonia, restricted pronation and supination,) and the skin (alopecia).

Anesthetic considerations: Anesthesia in this condition has not been described. Odontoid abnormalities may be associated with instability of the cervical spine. Ascertain stability of the cervical spine both clinically and radiologically, but also assess the range of motion of the cervical spine (other vertebral anomalies). Perform direct laryngoscopy and tracheal intubation either with in-line stabilization or primarily with the fiberoptic bronchoscope. Careful intraoperative positioning is required to prevent joint dislocations. Developmental delay may limit patient cooperation. Sedative and/or anxiolytic premedication and the presence of the primary caregiver during induction of anesthesia may be helpful.

References:

De Almeida JC, Vargas FR, Barbosa-Neto JG, et al: CODAS syndrome: A new distinct MCA/MR syndrome with radiological changes of spondyloepiphyseal dysplasia. Another case report. *Am J Med Genet* 55:19, 1995.

Innes AM, Chudley AE, Reed MH, et al: Third case of cerebral, ocular, dental, auricular, skeletal anomalies (CODAS) syndrome, further delineating a new malformation syndrome: First report of an affected male and review of literature. *Am J Med Genet* 102:44, 2001.

Shebib SM, Reed MH, Shuckett EP, et al: Newly recognized syndrome of cerebral, ocular, dental, auricular, skeletal anomalies: CODAS syndrome—A case report. *Am J Med Genet* 40:88, 1991.

Coffin-Lowry Syndrome

At a glance: A syndrome of mental retardation and osteocartilaginous abnormalities with peculiar facies.

Synonyms: Coffin-Siris-Wegienka Syndrome (do not confuse with ☞Coffin Siris Syndrome, which is a different disease); Soft Hands Syndrome.

History: First described by Grange S. Coffin, an American pediatrician, Evelyn Siris, an American radiologist, and Laurence C. Wegienka, an American physician, in 1966. However, to avoid (further) confusions with ☞Coffin Siris Syndrome, it was decided to name the syndrome described here as Coffin Lowry Syndrome (after Robert Bryan Lowry, a British medical geneticist, who described a fourth family with the same findings in 1971).

Incidence: 1:50,000–100,000 live births. No sexual predilection, but the disease is more severe in males.

Genetic inheritance: X-linked semidominant inherited disorder caused by mutations in the gene coding for the RSK2 (ribosomal s6 kinase 2), a growth factor-regulated serine-threonine protein kinase (involved in promotion of mitosis and activation of genes) that has been mapped to Xp22.2-p22.1. However, research shows that only a minority of patients with this disorder actually have a mutation in the RSK2 gene.

Pathophysiology: Abnormal proteodermatan sulfate, glycolipid-like lysosomal granules, and vacuoles have been found in cultured skin fibroblasts. Accumulation of hyaluronate and hyperprolinemia have been reported in some patients.

Diagnosis: Based on the clinical association of growth and psychomotor retardation with hypotonia, progressive skeletal deformations, characteristic facial dysmorphism, and large soft hands.

Clinical aspects: There is a wide variability in the expression of the features of the syndrome. Involvement of the head and neck can present as thickened calvarium, small sinuses paranasales, flat occiput, delayed suture closure with large anterior fontanelle, prominent supraorbital ridges with bushy brows, downwardly slanted palpebral fissures, hypertelorism, blepharoptosis, large and prominent ears, large nose with broad base and elongated philtrum, mandibular prognathism, maxillary/midfacial hypoplasia, large mouth with big lips, and longitudinally furrowed tongue with a dorsal groove. The facial features are generally not present at birth, but become apparent by the second year of life, after which they become more pronounced. Dental anomalies are numerous and may include congenital absence of some teeth, delayed eruption, enamel hypoplasia, caries, early loss of teeth, abnormal size and shape, malposition, malalignments, and periodontal disease. Involvement of the musculoskeletal system presents as short thorax, bifid sternum, pectus excavatum or carinatum, vertebral dysplasia, kyphosis, scoliosis, delayed bone age, ligamental calcifications, hyperextensible joints, muscle atrophy, large and soft hands with simian crease, and tapering of the fingers. Cardiovascular involvement is frequent, with features including atrial septal defects, persistent ductus arteriosus, valvular anomalies (mitral valve prolapse, mitral regurgitation, tricuspid insufficiency), impaired cardiac function, right ventricular hypertrophy, restrictive cardiomyopathy, endomyocardial fibroelastosis, and ventricular arrhythmias. Central nervous system features consist of generalized hypotonia, which may be the earliest presenting sign and related to paroxysmal drop attacks (cataplexy or hyperexplexia). In addition, seizures, hydrocephalus, agenesis of the corpus callosum, abnormal gyration, faulty cortical lamination, calcification of the falx cerebri, sensorineural hearing loss, mental retardation, a tendency to obsessive-compulsive behavior, and cervical radiculopathy (secondary to calcification of the ligamentum flavum and consequent stenosis of the spinal canal) have been described. Inguinal and umbilical hernias and rectal and uterine prolapse appear to be common in these patients. Liver cirrhosis, recurrent respiratory infections, and emphysema have been described. Most of the clinical findings become more pronounced with increasing age.

Precautions before anesthesia: Structural and functional cardiac abnormalities should be identified preoperatively (echocardiogram, electrocardiogram, chest radiograph) because they are responsible for fatal outcome. Endomyocardial fibroelastosis may be asymptomatic, and a high index of clinical suspicion is needed with respect to cardiac involvement. Evaluate neurologic function (clinically, review electroencephalogram, computed tomography scans, and/or magnetic resonance images). Evaluate intubation anatomy and document dental anomalies. Assess liver, renal, and pulmonary function, although pulmonary function tests may be of limited value because of decreased patient compliance. Laboratory investigations should include a complete blood count, serum levels of electrolytes, creatinine, and blood urea nitrogen, and arterial blood gas analysis in selected patients. Frequent or chronic pulmonary infections combined with emphysema may require prolonged mechanical ventilation postoperatively. Developmental delay may limit patient cooperation. Sedative and/or anxiolytic premedication and the presence of the primary caregiver during induction of anesthesia may be helpful.

Anesthetic considerations: The facial features suggest airway management may be difficult. Cardiac involvement may warrant specific anesthesia techniques and invasive monitoring. Special attention is needed for the teeth. Patients are prone to seizures. Controlled ventilation with normocapnia or mild hypocapnia is recommended in the presence of untreated hydrocephalus. Careful intraoperative positioning is needed because of musculoskeletal involvement. Regional anesthesia is not contraindicated per se, but central neuraxial blockade may be difficult to perform and should be avoided in the presence of radiculopathy or hydrocephalus.

Pharmacological implications: Chronic use of many antiseizure medications may alter the metabolism of certain anesthetic agents. Subacute bacterial endocarditis prophylaxis may be required as indicated. In the presence of renal and/or hepatic insufficiency, drugs should be selected and dosed accordingly.

Other conditions to be considered:

☞**FRAGILE X SYNDROME:** A syndrome comprising X-linked mental retardation in children with prognathism, hypotonia, and autism and a characteristic, but variable facies (long face, high arched palate, malocclusion). Additional abnormalities may include hyperlordosis, heart defects, pectus excavatum, shortening of the tubular bones of the hands, and joint laxity.

☞**SOTOS SYNDROME:** Characterized by excessively rapid growth during the first year of life, acromegalic craniocerebral features (macrocephaly, prominent forehead) and a nonprogressive cerebral disorder with mental retardation. Other features include high arched palate and prognathism with premature eruption of teeth, hypotonia, hyperthyroidism or hypothyroidism, and delayed motor and cognitive development.

☞**WILLIAMS SYNDROME:** A syndrome characterized by peculiar elfin facies associated with infantile hypercalcemia, cardiac defects, and mild mental retardation. High frequency of sudden death.

ALPHA ☞**THALASSEMIA:** The clinical signs of this disorder are a result of hemolysis and chronic anemia. The clinical features include hepatosplenomegaly, bone deformations, and cardiac failure. Strict asepsis is needed.

REFERENCES:

Charles S, Passuti N, Rogez JM, et al: Fatal cardiac complications in a child operated on for severe scoliosis with a Coffin-Lowry syndrome. A propos of a case. *Chir Pediatr* 29:36, 1988.

Coffin GS: Postmortem findings in the Coffin-Lowry Syndrome. *Genet Med* 5:187, 2003.

Facher JJ, Regier EJ, Jacobs GH, et al: Cardiomyopathy in Coffin-Lowry syndrome. *Am J Med Genet* 128A:176, 2004.

Stephenson JB, Hoffman MC, Russell AJ, et al: The movement disorders of Coffin-Lowry syndrome. *Brain Dev* 27:108, 2005.

Coffin-Siris Syndrome

At a glance: A congenital syndrome with growth and mental retardation, feeding difficulties, digital anomalies, and coarse facies.

Synonyms: Fifth Digit Syndrome; Dwarfism-Onychodysplasia Syndrome; Short Stature-Onychodysplasia Syndrome.

History: First described by Grange S. Coffin, an American pediatrician, and Evelyn Siris, an American radiologist, in 1970. To avoid confusion with the Coffin Siris Wegienka Syndrome, it was decided to name the latter syndrome ☞Coffin Lowry Syndrome (after Robert Brian Lowry, a British medical geneticist, who described a fourth family with the findings of Coffin-Siris-Wegienka Syndrome in 1971).

Incidence: Since its first description, approximately 65 cases have been reported. The male-to-female ratio is approximately 1:4.

Genetic inheritance: The mode of inheritance is uncertain, but is most likely autosomal dominant. However, a case has been made suggesting autosomal recessive inheritance. It remains possible that inheritance may not be mendelian in nature. The genetic defect is thought to be in the 7q32-q34 region.

Diagnosis: Based on the clinical findings of developmental delay, mental retardation, hypoplasia of the fifth digit nail and terminal phalanges of hands and feet, sparse scalp hair, bushy eyebrows, wide mouth, hirsutism, and prominent or hypertrophied lips.

Clinical aspects: The constant finding is absence or hypoplasia of the distal and middle phalanges, especially those of the fifth digits of the hands and/or feet with aplasia/hypoplasia of the nail of the fifth digit (other digits may also be affected). The other main features that have been reported are low birth weight, failure to thrive (poor sucking and feeding difficulties), and recurrent respiratory tract infections. Central nervous system anomalies may include microcephaly, generalized hypotonia, developmental delay, and mild-to-moderate mental retardation, ☞Dandy-Walker Malformation, hypoplasia/aplasia of the corpus callosum, and abnormal and ectopic cerebellar nuclei. Sparse scalp hair, long eyelashes, and bushy eyebrows contrast with hirsutism. In addition, a wide mouth with prominent or thick lips, choanal atresia, flat nasal bridge, anteverted and wide nasal tip, and high arched palate (occasionally with cleft) are often present. Occasionally, ptosis, short philtrum, and macroglossia occur. Short stature with vertebral anomalies (kyphosis, scoliosis, spina bifida occulta, sacral dimple), joint laxity, small patellae, and delayed bone age are fairly frequent. A variety of associated cardiac defects have been described, including patent foramen ovale, tetralogy of Fallot, atrial and ventricular septal defects, patent ductus arteriosus, pulmonary stenosis, and persistent left superior vena cava. Diaphragmatic hernia has been reported in a few patients. Urogenital anomalies, such as hydronephrosis, congenital microureters with stenosis at the vesicoureteral junction, ectopic, small, or fused kidneys, cryptorchidism, hypospadias, and uterus aplasia have been described. Ocular anomalies are common and may include myopia, astigmatism, strabismus, nystagmus, and tear duct anomalies. Mild-to-severe hearing loss is frequent. Besides cardiac surgery, these patients often present for umbilical and/or inguinal hernia repair. Recurrent infections (upper respiratory tract, pneumonia, otitis media) are an ongoing issue in these patients. In a subset of patients, recurrent hypoglycemic attacks, gastric outlet obstruction, intestinal malrotation, and intussusception have been described.

Precautions before anesthesia: Obtain a full developmental history. Assess the upper airway (choanal atresia), examine for evidence of recent respiratory tract infection and for signs of difficult airway management. Obtain a chest radiograph if evidence of recurrent pneumonia is present. Specifically exclude cardiac anomalies by clinical examination, electrocardiogram, and echocardiography as indicated. Check serum levels of electrolytes and glucose and assess renal function in the presence of renal abnormalities. Assess spine anatomy (spina bifida occulta) if central neuraxial blockade is considered.

Anesthetic considerations: Because the facial appearance of patients has been described as being similar to that of ☞Hurler Syndrome, be prepared for difficult airway management. Spontaneous ventilation should be maintained until the airway has been secured. Alternative airway management techniques (e.g., fiberoptic bronchoscope, laryngeal mask airway) should be ready. There are reports indicating that airway management becomes more difficult with age. Premedication may be needed, as some children demonstrate aggressive behavior. However, severe hypotonia and/or respiratory insufficiency may be a contraindication for preoperative sedation. The presence of cardiac disease dictates the anesthetic technique. Regional or local anesthesia rather than opioid-based analgesia may be preferable for some patients. Prolonged postoperative mechanical ventilation may be required because the upper airway tends to be obstructed already preoperatively (macroglossia, hypotonia) in some patients. Regular perioperative control of serum glucose is recommended. Vascular access may be difficult. Careful intraoperative positioning is needed.

Pharmacological implications: In the presence of generalized hypotonia, succinylcholine is relatively contraindicated. Avoid neuromuscular blockers until the airway has been secured. Subacute bacterial endocarditis prophylaxis may be required.

Other condition to be considered:

☞**BRACHMANN-DE LANGE SYNDROME:** A characteristic syndrome of craniofacial malformations associated with neurologic impairment.

REFERENCES:

Dimaculangan D, Lokhandwala B, Wlody D, Gross R: Difficult airway in a patient with Coffin-Siris syndrome. *Anesth Analg* 92:554, 2001.

Fleck BJ, Pandya A, Vanner L, et al: Coffin-Siris syndrome: Review and presentation of new cases from a questionnaire study. *Am J Med Genet* 99:1, 2001.

Silvani P, Camperesi A, Zoia E, et al: Anesthetic management of a child with Coffin-Siris syndrome. *Paediatr Anaesth* 14:698, 2004.

Cohen Syndrome

At a glance: An inherited disorder characterized by hypotonia, obesity, prominent incisors, and nonprogressive psychomotor retardation.

Synonyms: Norio Syndrome; Pepper Syndrome; Hypotonia-Obesity-Prominent Incisors Syndrome; Obesity-Hypotonia Syndrome.

Incidence: Approximately 100 cases have been described. An increased frequency has been reported in Finland and in the Ashkenazi Jewish population. Consanguinity is a known, but not constant risk factor. No sexual predilection.

Genetic inheritance: Autosomal recessive. The mutation has been mapped to 8q22-q23.

Diagnosis: The wide clinical variability of this disorder makes the diagnosis difficult, which is primarily based on the clinical findings of nonprogressive psychomotor retardation, microcephaly with characteristic facial appearance, early hypotonia, joint hyperextensibility, clumsiness, truncal obesity, mottled retina, and myopia in patients with isolated and intermittent neutropenia ($< 2 \times 10^9$/mm^3). Because of the highly variable features, the diagnosis often is not made until late infancy or even childhood.

Clinical aspects: Pregnancy most often is uneventful and birth occurs at term, however, poor fetal movement and growth and oligohydramnios have been described in some patients. Poor feeding in the first year of life is common. The disease involves the head and neck (microcephaly, thick scalp hair, eyebrows and eyelashes, prominent nasal bridge and beak-shaped nose, maxillary hypoplasia, prominent incisors [more the result of short and thin upper lip, which becomes even more pronounced on smiling], micrognathia [usually mild], short, upturned philtrum, high narrow palate, open mouth appearance), the heart (mitral valve prolapse is common, but rarely of clinical significance, progressive left ventricular dysfunction may occur with increasing age), the eyes (wave-shaped, downward slanting palpebral fissures, progressive pigmentary retinopathy, chorioretinal dystrophy, optic atrophy, early myopia, strabismus, vision deteriorates with age and patients are severely handicapped by the fourth to fifth decade of life), the central nervous system (mental retardation, delayed motor milestones, seizures, generalized hypotonia), and the skeleton (short stature secondary to growth hormone deficiency, kyphoscoliosis often starting after puberty, joint hyperextensibility [particularly hands, feet, knees], cubiti valgi, genua valga, narrow hands and feet with slender fingers and toes, camptodactyly, shortened metatarsals). Other features may include low birth weight, transverse palmar creases, obesity (although less common than initially thought), generally cheerful, socially interactive and cooperative personality, delayed puberty, and mild-to-moderate neutropenia (78% of patients), which does not appear to predispose the patients to infection. Stridor occurs in about one fourth of patients and most often is a result of laryngomalacia. Vocal cord paralysis was responsible for tracheostomy for more than 1 year in one patient. Lifespan appears to be normal.

Precautions before anesthesia: A detailed cardiovascular evaluation should be performed (clinically, electrocardiography, echocardiography). Evaluate head and neck anatomy with regard to airway management because of craniofacial anomalies and prominent teeth (radiographs may be required). Evaluate neurologic status (clinically, computed tomography scans or magnetic resonance imaging, electroencephalography). Obtain a complete blood count with white cell differentiation (neutropenia).

Anesthetic considerations: The combination of prominent incisors, maxillary hypoplasia, and micrognathia suggests direct laryngoscopy and tracheal intubation may be difficult. Spontaneous ventilation should be maintained until the airway has been secured. Appropriate preoxygenation is recommended secondary to obesity and possible difficult airway management. Regional anesthesia is not contraindicated, but should be expected to be difficult because of obesity and orthopedic features (e.g., kyphoscoliosis). Careful in-traoperative positioning must be performed. Strict asepsis is needed because of neutropenia. Vascular access can be difficult secondary to obesity.

Pharmacological implications: Subacute bacterial endocarditis prophylaxis may be required. Muscle relaxants should not be used until the airway has been secured. Consider the interaction of anesthetic drugs and antiepileptic treatment in patients with seizures.

Other conditions to be considered:

☞**ALSTRÖM SYNDROME:** Inherited syndrome with diabetes mellitus, cardiac, hepatic, and renal involvement, and progressive visual and hearing loss.

☞**BARDET-BIEDL SYNDROME:** Mental retardation, pigmentary retinopathy, polydactyly, obesity, renal anomalies, and hypogenitalism.

REFERENCES:

Chandler KE, Kidd A, Al-Gazali L, et al: Diagnostic criteria, clinical characteristics, and natural history of Cohen syndrome. *J Med Genet* 40:233, 2003.

Hurmerinta K, Pirinen S, Kovero O, et al: Craniofacial features in Cohen syndrome: An anthropometric and cephalometric analysis of 14 patients. *Clin Genet* 62:157, 2002.

Kivitie-Kallio S, Norio R: Cohen syndrome: Essential features, natural history, and heterogeneity. *Am J Med Genet* 102:125 2001.

Cold Agglutinin Syndrome

At a glance: A disorder that is idiopathic or secondary to a malignancy, resulting in immune-hemolytic anemia with exacerbation upon exposure to cold.

Synonyms: Cold Agglutinin Disease; Cold Hemagglutinin Disease.

History: First described in 1903 by Karl Landsteiner, an Austrian pathologist and immunologist, who is considered the father of modern transfusion medicine, since he also discovered the ABO system, for which he was awarded the Nobel Prize in 1930.

Incidence: It has been estimated that approximately 5 to 20% of all autoimmune hemolytic anemias are caused by cold agglutinins (approximately 1:300,000). No ethnic predilection has been reported, however, females are affected slightly more often than males (1.5:1). All age groups can be affected, although it most often occurs in patients in the seventh decade of life or older and rarely in children. Even in otherwise healthy persons, low cold agglutinin titers (1:64 or less) are common. Significantly higher titers may be associated with infections by *Mycoplasma pneumoniae*, cytomegalovirus, human immunodeficiency virus, influenza virus, Epstein-Barr virus, mumps virus, with malaria, listeriosis, and trypanosomiasis, but these increased levels are transient and the development of cold agglutinin syndrome is relatively uncommon, at least in the classic chronic form.

Genetic inheritance: Trisomy 3 has been found in some patients with this disorder. However, cold agglutinin syndrome is acquired and not inherited.

Pathophysiology: Cold agglutinin syndrome as a secondary disease usually is associated with a hematologic malignancy (e.g., Waldenström macroglobulinemia [production of monoclonal IgM paraprotein], multiple myeloma, lymphomas, Kaposi sarcoma) and infections. Activated B lymphocytes produce pathogenic antibodies (most commonly monoclonal IgM, rarely IgA or IgG, directed against the I antigen of the erythrocyte membrane in adults; rarely the antibodies are targeted against the fetal i antigen). When the blood cools below the "thermal threshold" (approximately 32°C, i.e., in acral areas), these autoantibodies cause red cell agglutination, slugging, and complement binding in peripheral vessels. Upon returning to the central circulation (warmer areas), the IgM antibodies dissociate, leaving complement on the cell surface. In severe cases, the red cell–antibody complexes activate the complement system, which may result in intravascular hemolysis. Sequestration of opsonized red cells occurs, mainly by the Kupffer cells in the liver.

Diagnosis: Based on the clinical picture with exacerbation on exposure to cold (finger pain and paresthesias). Anemia, spherocytosis, reticulocytosis, and in vitro agglutination of blood that resolves upon rewarming are characteristic.

Clinical aspects: Usually mild chronic anemia is present. Red blood cell agglutination may result in a Raynaud-like phenomenon upon exposure to cold (acrocyanosis, livedo reticularis). Purpura, acral gangrene, and immune complex nephritis are rare complications, but have been described. Hemolysis may lead to worsening of anemia, hemoglobinuria, and renal failure, mild hepatomegaly, jaundice, and/or splenomegaly. The presence of circulating inhibitors of specific coagulation factors has been reported and must be considered because they may be associated with hemorrhage.

Precautions before anesthesia: Prevention of hemagglutination by keeping the patient warm is paramount. Check for anemia, which most often is mild. Rule out hematologic diseases or active infections. Cyclophosphamide, steroids, interferon, and plasmapheresis have all been used to reduce the severity of the disease. Crossmatching must be performed carefully at 37°C to minimize the effects of cold agglutinins.

Anesthetic considerations: Exposure to a cold environment in the perioperative period may precipitate an attack. In the event of hemolysis, circulating complement may hemolyze transfused red cells. Preoperative plasmapheresis may be effective in preventing an attack by reducing the IgM load. Temperature regulation, with special attention being paid to maintain peripheral temperature, is the most important task. With regard to cardiopulmonary bypass, severe-to-moderate hypothermic cardiopulmonary bypass and cold cardioplegia should be avoided. Careful evaluation of arterial flow and collateral flow prior to insertion of an arterial catheter is recommended in the presence of Raynaud phenomenon or acral lesions. Strict asepsis is mandatory for any invasive procedure.

Pharmacological implications: High-dose steroid regimens have been used with variable success. Steroid stress dose supplements should be used in case of prolonged preoperative treatment.

Other condition to be considered:

☞**COLD HYPERSENSITIVITY SYNDROME:** A familial form of urticaria with systemic reactions that occurs as a result of cold exposure.

REFERENCES:

Beebe DS, Bergen L, Palahniuk RJ: Anesthetic management of a patient with severe cold agglutinin hemolytic anemia utilizing forced air warming. *Anesth Analg* 76:1144, 1993.

Neff AT: Autoimmune hemolytic anemias, in: Greer JP, Foerster J, Lukens JN, et al. (eds.): *Wintrobe's Clinical Hematology,* 11th ed. Philadelphia, Lippincott Williams & Wilkins, 2004, p 1163.

van Spronsen DJ, Oosting JD, Hoffmann JJ, et al: Factor V inhibitor associated with cold agglutinin disease. *Ann Hematol* 76:49, 1998.

Cold Hypersensitivity Syndrome

At a glance: A familial form of urticaria with systemic reactions that occurs as a result of cold exposure.

Synonyms: Familial Cold Urticaria; Familial Cold-Induced Autoinflammatory Syndrome; Familial Cold Autoinflammatory Syndrome; Familial Polymorphous Cold Eruption Syndrome.

Incidence and genetic inheritance: Approximately 1:1,000,000 of the general population is affected. Autosomal dominant inheritance, although sporadic cases (de novo mutations) have also been described. The responsible gene (CAS1) has been mapped to 1q44 and encodes for cryopyrin, a protein that is expressed on peripheral leukocytes and chondrocytes and appears to be involved in apoptosis and caspase-1 activation.

Clinical aspects: The diagnosis is based on the clinical findings and the family history and is confirmed by sequencing analysis of the CAS1 gene (although CAS1 mutations also occur in other syndromes, e.g., ☞Muckle-Wells Syndrome). Usually the onset of symptoms occurs hours after birth or as soon as the baby is exposed to a cold environment. Delayed presentation is possible, but the maximal age at onset is believed to be less than 6 months. Urticarial eruptions are triggered by exposure to cold, damp air, and/or wind (air conditioning), generally occur 1 to 2 hours after exposure, and initially present as macules and papules on exposed skin areas, which then spread to covered sites. The distinctive lesions have a purple cyanotic color and are surrounded by a white halo, causing a burning pain rather than itch. Intense cold exposure not only is associated with eruptions lasting for up to 48 hours, but potentially also with a systemic reaction of fever, sweating, arthralgia, myalgia, headache, conjunctivitis, and leukocytosis, which usually follow 4 to 6 hours after exposure. Systemic amyloidosis has been suspected in some cases, but the diagnosis in these cases was questioned and reevaluation found the diagnosis of Muckle-Wells syndrome more likely. Nevertheless, a small percentage of patients with cold hypersensitivity syndrome suffers from renal amyloidosis. Although the disorder is a lifelong issue, it does not affect life expectancy. Treatment is primarily preventive. Medications used to treat the disease are nonsteroidal antiinflammatory drugs, steroids, and gold. Some patients have also been treated with interleukin-1 antagonists and stanozolol.

Anesthetic considerations: Avoid cold exposure. Arterial hypotension and cardiovascular collapse may occur. Increasing the temperature in the operating room and warming the operating room table before patients are brought into the room are recommended. The use of warming mattresses or better forced-air convective warming devices and warmed infusions should be considered. Hypothermic cardiopulmonary bypass and cold cardioplegia should be avoided although they have been used successfully in one patient with prebypass and on-bypass antiinflammatory treatment. Because some patients are on gold therapy, a complete blood count (to rule out thrombocytopenia, leukopenia, agranulocytosis, or aplastic anemia) should be obtained, and renal function (because of possible renal amyloidosis; creatinine, blood urea nitrogen) and hepatic function (transaminases, bilirubin, coagulation profile, serum albumin) should be assessed. Patients may be on steroid therapy and, depending on the procedure, perioperative steroid stress coverage may be required.

Other conditions to be considered:

☞**MUCKLE-WELLS SYNDROME:** A very rare genetic disorder diagnosed in infancy and characterized by deafness (adolescence), nonpruritic urticaria, and renal amyloidosis type AA. Other features include arthralgias and/or conjunctivitis.

☞**Cold Agglutinin Syndrome:** A disorder that is idiopathic or secondary to a malignancy, resulting in immune-hemolytic anemia with exacerbation upon exposure to cold.

REFERENCES:

Dode C, Le Du N, Cuisset L, et al: New mutations of CIAS1 that are responsible for Muckle-Wells syndrome and familial cold urticaria: A novel mutation underlies both syndromes. *Am J Hum Genet* 70:1498, 2002.

Lancey RA, Schaefer OP, McCormick MJ: Coronary artery bypass grafting and aortic valve replacement with cold cardioplegia in a patient with cold-induced urticaria. *Ann Allergy Asthma Immunol* 92:273, 2004.

Ormerod AD, Smart L, Reid TM, et al: Familial cold urticaria. Investigation of a family and response to stanozolol. *Arch Dermatol* 129:343, 1993.

Cole-Carpenter Syndrome

At a glance: A disorder associated with craniosynostosis, exophthalmia, and palpebral ptosis. Radiography shows an osteogenesis imperfecta-like aspect of the skeleton.

Incidence and genetic inheritance: Four cases have been described. Autosomal dominant inheritance was suspected. The disorder may be caused by a defect in the collagen synthesis or structure.

Clinical aspects: Patients appear normal at birth, but multiple compression fractures of the long bones are noted soon thereafter, followed by extensive demineralization with recurrent diaphyseal fractures of the weight-bearing bones before the first birthday. Short stature, kyphosis, and scoliosis are other skeletal features. Facial abnormalities may include facial structural asymmetry, development of marked frontal and temporal bossing, hypertelorism, short midface, micrognathia, depressed premaxillary region, shallow orbits with ocular proptosis, blue sclerae, dental anomalies, and craniosynostosis of the coronal and frontal sutures with rapidly progressive hydrocephalus. Normal neurologic development has been reported, but anomalies of crying, voice, and gait and generalized hypotonia are common. Osteopenia and hypercalcemia is frequent. Hydrops fetalis has been described in one case.

Anesthetic considerations: Preoperative blood work should include a complete blood count and serum levels of electrolytes including calcium. With the aforementioned craniofacial anomalies, airway management should be expected to be difficult. Preservation of spontaneous ventilation until the airway has been secured is recommended. However, intracranial pressure may already be raised at the time of presentation for cranial surgery (secondary to craniosynostosis), requiring a rapid-sequence induction. Succinylcholine is best avoided because of its associated risk of fractures (fasciculations) and its negative impact on intracranial pressure. However, only a thorough clinical examination and review of the radiologic examinations can help in the decision regarding which induction technique (maintenance of spontaneous ventilation vs. rapid-sequence induction) is best suited for the patient. Careful protection of the eyes must be provided since they are at high risk for corneal damage because of proptosis. Careful intraoperative positioning is mandatory, secondary to multiple deformations and bone fragility. Central neuraxial anesthesia techniques are not contraindicated, but can be difficult to achieve. Local anesthetics should be titrated because of modifications of the perimedullar space as a result of vertebral compression fractures. Hypercalcemia should be evaluated to avoid arrhythmias.

Other condition to be considered:

☞**Osteogenesis Imperfecta:** A group of rare disorders affecting the connective tissue characterized by extremely fragile bones that fracture easily during the antenatal and postnatal period (brittle bones).

REFERENCES:

Amor DJ, Savarirayan R, Schneider AS, et al: A case of Cole-Carpenter syndrome. *Am J Med Genet* 92:273, 2000.

Cole DEC, Carpenter TO: Bone fragility, craniosynostosis, ocular proptosis, hydrocephalus, and distinctive facial features: A newly recognized type of osteogenesis imperfecta. *J Pediatr* 110:76, 1987.

MacDermot KD, Buckley B, Van Someren V: Osteopenia, abnormal dentition, hydrops fetalis and communicating hydrocephalus. *Clin Genet* 48:217, 1995.

Coleman-Randall Syndrome

At a glance: A disorder associated with irregular pili torti, deafness and hypogonadism with luteinizing hormone and growth hormone deficiency.

Synonym: Seizures, Mental Retardation, Hair Dysplasia Syndrome.

Incidence and genetic inheritance: Extremely rare disorder (one case report) with probably autosomal recessive transmission.

Clinical aspects: Features include coarse hair with abnormal texture, low-set ears, epicanthic folds, broad nasal root, long philtrum, thin lips, short neck, hypoplastic/absent nipples, irregularly shaped fingers, and overlapping toes. Hypotonia, mental retardation, and seizures (any type) can be observed.

Anesthetic considerations: Anesthesia associated with this disorder has not been described. Anticipate difficult airway management and maintain spontaneous ventilation until the airway has been secured. Consider interactions between antiepileptic treatment and anesthetic drugs. Mental retardation may affect patient cooperation. Hypnotic and/or anxiolytic premedication and the presence of the primary caregiver during induction may be helpful.

REFERENCE:

Coleman M, Randall J; Seizure disorder, mental retardation, unusual facies, and abnormal hair. *J Clin Dysmorphol* 1:28, 1983.

Collins-Dennis-Clarke-Pope Syndrome

At a glance: A familial disorder characterized by hip dislocation, flat facial aspect and congenital heart defect.

Synonym: Congenital Dislocation of the Hip with Hyperextensibility of Fingers and Facial Dysmorphism.

Incidence and genetic inheritance: An extremely rare disorder with three cases in one family described. Most likely autosomal dominant inheritance. The mother was tall (90th percentile) in the original report and the height of the father was below the 3rd percentile.

Clinical aspects: The disease involves the head and face (flat face, ear anomalies, epicanthic folds, hypertelorism, periorbital puffiness, broad, flattened nose with anteverted nares, microstoma [carp-shaped], high arched, narrow palate). Skeletal anomalies may include short stature, flat cheek bones, hyperextensible joints, clinodactyly, and hip and knee dislocations. All three sisters had an atrial septal defect, but tricuspid valve prolapse and patent ductus arteriosus were inconstant. Inguinal hernia and urinary tract anomalies occurred in one patient. Results of studies of collagen from skin and ligaments were normal.

Anesthetic considerations: Anesthesia in this disorder has not been described. Tracheal intubation should be expected to be difficult secondary to microstoma. Careful intraoperative positioning is mandatory to prevent dislocations of the large joints. Congenital heart defects require an adapted anesthetic management, and subacute bacterial endocarditis prophylaxis may be required.

REFERENCE:

Collins AL, Dennis NR, Clarke N, et al: A mother and three daughters with congenital dislocation of the hip and a characteristic facial appearance: A new syndrome? *Clin Dysmorphol* 4:277, 1995.

Collodion Baby

At a glance: An inherited syndrome apparent at birth and present throughout life. The newborn is born encased in a collodion-like membrane that sheds within the next 12 weeks, revealing generalized scaling with variable redness of the skin. Frequent consequences are life-threatening sepsis and dehydration by protein and electrolyte loss.

Synonyms: Ichthyosis Congenita; Lamellar Exfoliation of Newborn; Desquamation of Newborn; Collodion Fetus.

History: The term was first used by Arnold M. Seligman, an American biochemist, in 1841. It is a descriptive term for infants born encased in a membrane-like thick scale rather than a disease entity on its own. Among this group of keratinizing disorders are several heterogeneous conditions including nonbullous congenital ichthyosiform erythroderma and lamellar ichthyosis.

Incidence: Estimated 1:300,000 live births. Approximately 300 cases have been described in the literature.

Genetic inheritance: Autosomal recessive inheritance. The gene is located on 14q11.2.

Pathophysiology: The pathogenesis of "collodion baby" has not been clarified, but there is increased epidermal germinal cell activity and a failure of stratum corneum cells to separate.

Diagnosis: Characteristic clinical picture. Histopathologic examination of skin biopsies shows a compact, hyperkeratotic stratum

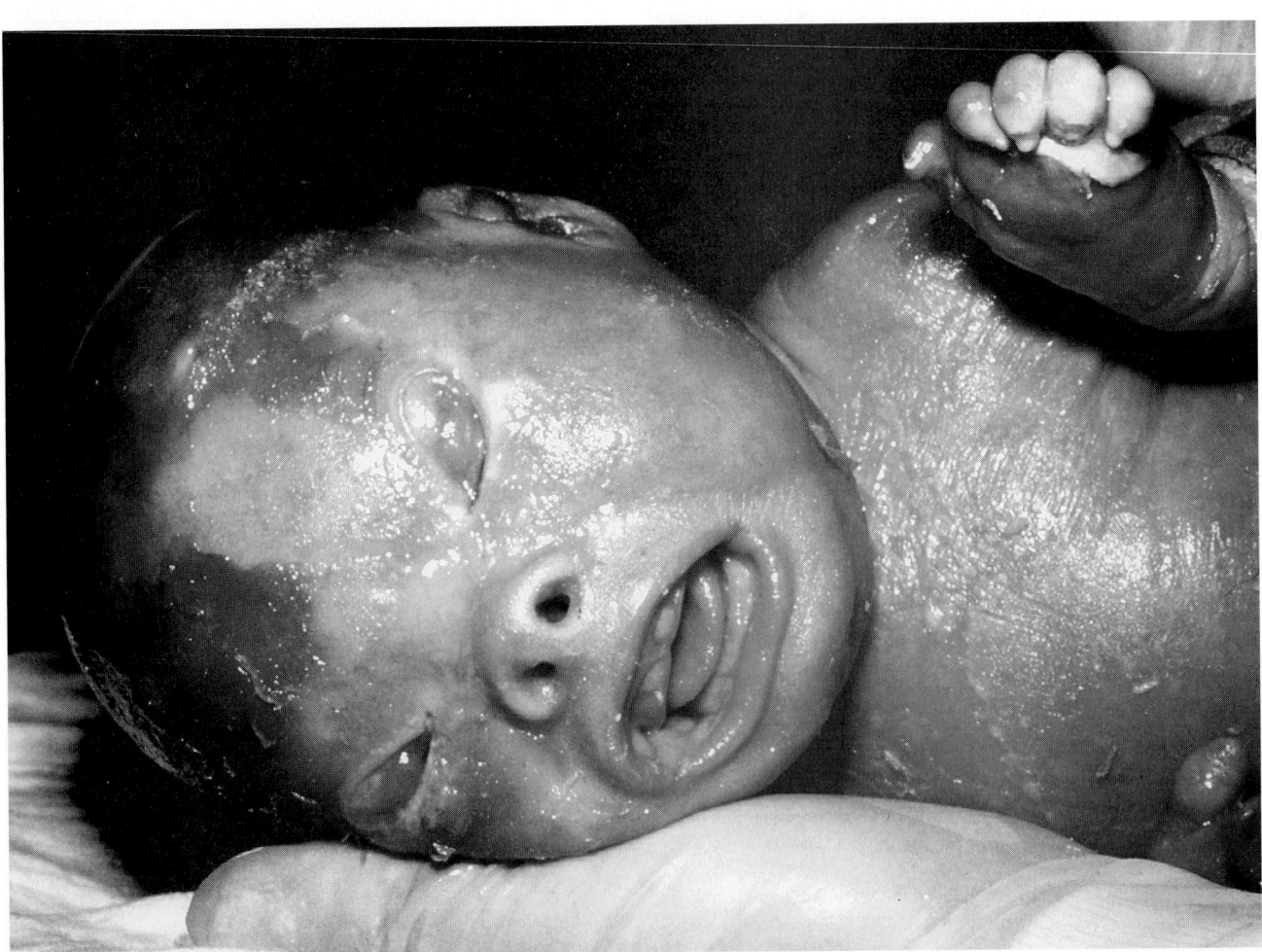

Collodion Baby   Newborn with the most severe form of collodion baby. See color plates.

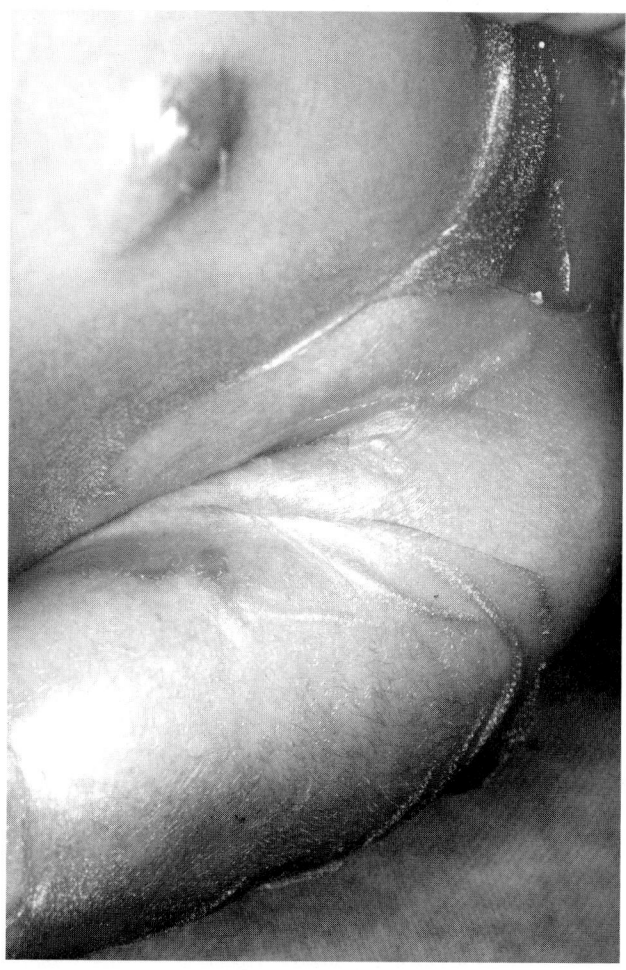

Collodion Baby Generalized scaling of the skin (shoulder area shown) leads to the collodion-like aspect in a collodion baby. The underlying skin is red but otherwise normal.

corneum and normal underlying epidermis. In the second stage of the disease (i.e., after shedding of the collodion membrane), the etiologic diagnostic approach should consist of a thorough family history (including parental consanguinity), a complete clinical examination (inspection of the skin, other associated findings), histology of the skin and hair (e.g., trichothiodystrophy, trichorrhexis invaginata), and finally laboratory tests (biochemical/metabolic screening, mutation screening).

Clinical aspects: Collodion babies are frequently born premature. The condition may be self-limiting with shedding of the parchment-like membrane within the first 1 to 4 weeks (maximally 12 weeks) of life, however, the majority of children eventually progress to a form of ichthyosis (i.e., congenital erythrodermic ichthyosis in 48%, lamellar ichthyosis in 12%, and dominant ichthyosis vulgaris in 10%), whereas only 10% of the patients eventually develop normal skin. Often the clinical course is complicated by fungal and bacterial skin infections, that may result in sepsis. Hands, feet, and the conjunctivae are the favorite sites of infections. High humidity and application of nonocclusive lubricants may facilitate shedding of the membranes. Other complications in the neonatal period include severe hypothermia, dehydration, and hypernatremia. Ectropion and/or eclabium, flattened ears and nose, and characteristic fixation of the lips in an O-shaped form are additional clinical find-

ings. Respiratory distress frequently occurs. Mortality now is below 10%, but the condition remains serious.

Precautions before anesthesia: Assess hydration state: Transepidermal water loss may be significant and lead to severe hypernatremic dehydration and hypoproteinemia (which may be masked by hypovolemia). Intravenous fluid therapy and maintenance of a temperature-regulated environment (incubator) to prevent hypovolemia and hyperthermia or hypothermia may be necessary. An up to sevenfold increase in fluid losses has been reported when compared to healthy infants. Assess for signs of infection/sepsis, commonly involving the lungs. Preoperative laboratory investigations should include a complete blood count with white cell differentiation, serum levels of urea, creatinine, and electrolytes. A chest radiograph should be obtained.

Anesthetic considerations: These patients have an increased morbidity (and mortality) as a result of impaired barrier function of the skin. Thermoregulation is impaired. On the one hand, hyperthermia commonly occurs if the ambient temperature is set too high. On the other hand, hypothermia may occur with excessive transcutaneous water losses. Venous access often is difficult in the presence of the skin changes. Fixation of the endotracheal tube probably is best done with a band of gauze than with adhesive tape. Ectropion requires careful protection and lubrication of the eyes. A poor nutritional status is often present with negative nitrogen balance and lower serum protein and albumin levels. Strict perioperative asepsis is mandatory because intravenous catheters are a well-known risk factor for severe infections in these children.

Pharmacological implications: Hypovolemia, hypoalbuminemia, and a reduction in renal blood flow may affect the pharmacokinetics and pharmacodynamics of drugs.

Other condition to be considered:

☞**HARLEQUIN SYNDROME:** Congenital skin disease in which the skin builds up and scales ("fish skin disease"). Associated with a very poor prognosis, with death generally occurring in the first week of life.

REFERENCES:

Buyse L, Graves C, Marks R, et al: Collodion baby dehydration: The danger of high transepidermal water loss. *Br J Dermatol* 129:86, 1993.

Vabres P, Larregue M: Collodion baby syndrome. *Ann Dermatol Venereol* 128:265, 2001.

Van Gysel D, Lijnen RL, Moekti SS, et al: Collodion baby: A follow-up study of 17 cases. *J Eur Acad Dermatol Venereol* 16:472, 2002.

Colpocephaly

At a glance: Disproportionate enlargement of the occipital horns of the lateral ventricles in association with partial or complete agenesis of the corpus callosum.

Synonym: Vesiculocephaly.

History: First described in 1946 by P.I. Yakovlev and R.C. Wadsworth.

Incidence and genetic inheritance: Approximately 40 cases have been described. Some cases are thought to be X-linked or autosomal dominant inherited with incomplete penetrance. Colpocephaly has been associated with trisomy 8 mosaicism and trisomy 9 mosaicism, *Toxoplasma gondii* infection during pregnancy, and maternal ingestion of ethanol, oral contraceptive medications, and other medications during pregnancy.

Clinical aspects: The main feature is an enlargement of the occipital horns of the lateral ventricles with partial or complete agenesis of the corpus callosum. Normally, the densely packed axons of the corpus callosum help stabilize the lateral ventricles. In partial or complete agenesis of the corpus callosum, this support for the lateral ventricles is missing, particularly in the posterior areas, where enlargement of the dorsal horns is characteristic. This finding is pronounced if the cingulum is hypoplastic or aplastic, which is typically the case in colpocephaly. Common symptoms include learning disabilities, seizures, and motor and visual abnormalities. It may be associated with other anomalies, such as microcephaly, micrognathia, lissencephaly, cerebellar atrophy, pachygyria, microgyria and macrogyria, ☞Pierre-Robin Syndrome, neurofibromatosis, optic nerve hypoplasia, chorioretinal coloboma, cleft palate, and myelomeningocele. Mental retardation, seizures, and motor and visual abnormalities may be present.

Anesthetic considerations: Considerations should mainly focus on associated disorders because colpocephaly per se should not significantly affect the anesthetic management. The main concern is airway management. Chronic antiepileptic treatment may interfere with the metabolism and elimination of anesthetic drugs.

REFERENCES:

Cerullo A, Marini C, Cevoli S, et al: Colpocephaly in two siblings: Further evidence of a genetic transmission. *Dev Med Child Neurol* 42:280, 2000.

Yakovlev PI, Wadsworth RC: Schizencephalies: A study of the congenital clefts in the cerebral mantle. I. Clefts with fused lips. *J Neuropathol Exp Neurol* 5:116, 1946.

Complete Androgen Insensitivity Syndrome

At a glance: An inherited disorder caused by androgen insensitivity with affected males having a female phenotype with normal female external genitalia but abnormal or absent internal female organs. Testes are often intraabdominal, in the inguina, or in the labia. Normal male (46,XY) karyotype.

Synonyms: Testicular Feminization; Androgen Receptor Deficiency; Dihydrotestosterone Receptor Deficiency; Male Pseudohermaphroditism as a Result of Androgen Insensitivity; Hairless Women Syndrome.

Incidence: Estimates vary from 1:7,000–20,000 male live births. No racial predilection has been reported.

Genetic inheritance: X-linked recessive with the responsible gene encoding for the androgen receptor being located on Xq11-q12. More than 200 different mutations have been described.

Pathophysiology: The basic etiology of androgen insensitivity syndrome (AIS) is a mutation in the androgen receptor gene that results in the gene's loss of function. The functional defects can range from complete absence of receptors on the cell surface to decreased substrate binding affinity with loss of signal transmission. Despite normal or elevated levels of androgen, functional loss of the androgen receptor is clinically equivalent to a lack of androgen and results in prenatal undervirilization of external genitalia, and absence of pubic and axillary hair, lack of acne, and absence of voice changes at puberty. Leydig cell stimulation to estrogen production occurs probably because of a failure in feedback repression of the pituitary gland, which shares the unresponsiveness to androgen. Peripheral conversion of testosterone and androstenedione to estradiol finally results in elevated estrogen serum levels. This on the one hand explains the absence of (androgen mediated) axillary and pubic hair, acne, and voice changes and on the other hand the development of normal breasts in these patients.

Diagnosis: The clinical findings of inguinal hernia with a labial mass in infancy and primary amenorrhea despite typical female secondary sex characteristics, but scant or absent pubic and axillary hair in puberty should raise suspicion for AIS. Affected males have female external genitalia associated with normal or high testosterone serum levels. In infancy, plasma luteinizing hormone (LH) and testosterone levels and the response to luteinizing hormone-releasing hormone (LHRH) are higher than in age-matched controls. In puberty, the androgen insensitivity, which also affects the hypothalamic-pituitary area, results in elevated testicular androgen and estradiol synthesis.

Clinical aspects: These genotypic male patients are phenotypic females. Anatomically, they have normal female external genitalia but a blind-ending vaginal pouch and absent uterus and fallopian tubes. The testes usually are located intraabdominally, in the inguinal canal, or in the labia. Leydig cells appear hyperplastic and form adenomatous clumps. Primary amenorrhea and scant pubic and axillary hair contrast with well developed female personality and body shape (including breasts). Patients often appear tall for females, and the clinical signs result from high estrogen levels. Other features include inguinal hernia and an increased risk of testicular malignancies (Sertoli cell adenomas, seminomas, malignant sex-cord stromal tumor) after 25 years of age. Patients often present for orchiectomy and vaginal lengthening procedures, both now often done at the end of the second or at the beginning of the third decade of life so that the patient is mature enough to participate actively in the treatment decisions. Patients are mentally absolutely normal. Gender identity is that of a normal female.

Precautions before anesthesia: Bear in mind that some patients may not know the exact details of their genetic status, anatomy, or endocrinology.

Anesthetic considerations: The larynx may be smaller and the trachea shorter than expected. Otherwise no specific anesthetic consideration should arise from this disorder.

Pharmacological implications: An increased tolerance to steroidal neuromuscular blocking agents has been described. After orchiectomy, hormone replacement therapy with estrogens is standard for patients with AIS.

Other conditions to be considered:

☞**REIFENSTEIN SYNDROME:** A condition characterized by partial androgen receptor deficiency resulting in hypogonadism or male pseudohermaphroditism.

☞**MAYER-VON ROKITANSKY-KÜSTER-HAUSER SYNDROME:** A syndrome characterized by congenital absence of the vagina, rudimentary cornua uteri, and morphologically normal ovaries and fallopian tubes situated on the pelvic sidewall. Primary amenorrhea with normal ovulation, breast development, body, and hair. Affected women are infertile. Frequently associated with urinary tract anomalies, skeletal abnormalities, congenital heart conditions, and inguinal hernia.

REFERENCES:

Boehmer AL, Brinkmann O, Bruggenwirth H, et al: Genotype versus phenotype in families with androgen insensitivity syndrome. *J Clin Endocrinol Metab* 86:4151, 2001.

Lee HT, Appel MI: Increased tolerance to vecuronium in a patient with testicular feminization. *J Clin Anesth* 10:156,1998.

Pollard BJ: Anaesthesia in the testicular feminisation syndrome. *Anaesthesia* 44:169, 1989.

Complex Disease/Deficiency (Overview)

At a glance: The mitochondrial myopathies are a rare group of conditions affecting the respiratory chain and oxidative phosphorylation. A total of five protein complexes make up the mitochondrial electron transport chain. The clinical consequences of a deficiency in their normal physiology is associated with numerous syndromes as described in this section and presented in this book. Because of the complexity of this group of diseases, an overview is presented here, followed by a short description of the five individual deficiencies. On page 186, the reader will find a table listing the names of the associated medical disorders that are described as specific syndromes in this book.

Historical note: "Mitochondrial medicine" was defined by Luft and Moyan-Hughes in the late 1980s and became the subject of numerous investigations of the metabolic disorders affecting the muscles and the brain. Mitochondria were first recognized in 1898 by Bend. The term comes from the Greek *mitos* (thread) and *chondros* (grain). The concept of cellular respiration was defined and studied in the 1920s.

Biochemical features: In the 1970s and mid-1980s, the standard classification of respiratory chain disorders rested on the biochemical phenotype; however, this approach for mitochondrial DNA (mtDNA) mutations leading to respiratory inefficiencies is now less clear. It is accepted that most mtDNA mutations affect the subunit synthesis either through a mutation in a key tRNA (transfer RNA) gene or through deletion of a series of tRNA genes. The presence of tRNA mutations may, among other mechanisms, lead to amino acid dysfunction most probably within larger subunits.

Classification: See Table C-2.

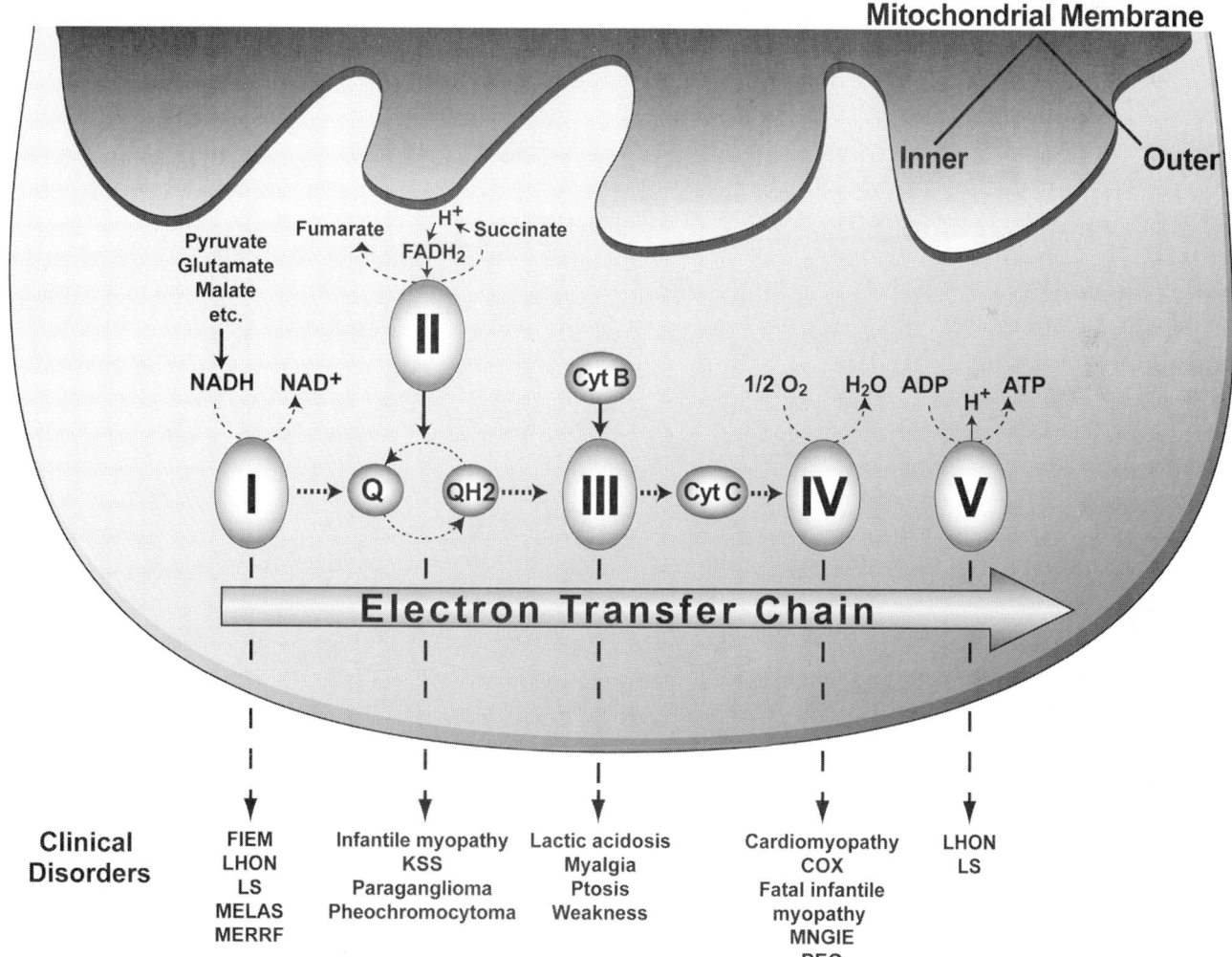

Complex Deficiency Graphic illustration of the electron transfer chain within the mitochondrium and corresponding clinical disorders. COX, cytochrome C oxidase deficiency; FIEM, fatal infantile encephalomyopathy; LHON, Leber hereditary optic atrophy; LS, Leigh syndrome; MELAS, mitochondrial encephalomyopathy-lactic acidosis-stroke syndrome; MERRF, myoclonus epilepsy ragged-red fibers; MNGIE, mitochondrial neurogastrointestinal encephalopathy syndrome; KSS, Kearns-Sayre syndrome; PEO, progressive external ophthalmoplegia.

Table C-2 *Mitochondrial Respiratory Chain Composition by Complex*

Complex	I	II	III	IV	V
Enzyme	NADH-CoQ reductase	Succinate-CoQ reductase	CoQ-cytochrome C reductase	Cytochrome C oxidase	ATP synthase
Inhibitor	Rotenone, Amytal	TTFA malonate	Antimycin A	Cyanide carbon, monoxide azide	Oligomycin
Nuclear DNA subunits	39	4	10	10	$\approx$14
Mitochondrial DNA subunits	7 ND1-6, ND4L	0	1 Cytochrome b	3 Cytochrome oxidase I, II, III	2 ATPase 6, ATPase 8
Flavoprotein	Flavin mononucleotide	FAD (SDAH)			
Iron protein	Iron sulfur (FeS) protein	FeS protein, SDHB	Rieke FeS, cytochrome (heme) b, c1	Cytochrome (heme) a, a3	
Other features		Membrane proteins, Cytochrome b560, SDHC, SDHD		Copper protein	
Associated disorders	Alzheimer, parkinsonism, cardiomyopathy, Barth syndrome, lethal infantile encephalopathy, Infantile Crigler-Najjar syndrome, LHON, Leigh, MELAS, MERRF, Myopathy $\pm$ Crigler-Najjar syndrome, PEO	KSS, Leigh, Myopathy during infancy $\pm$ Crigler-Najjar syndrome, paraganglioma, pheochromocytoma	Cardiomyopathy, fatal infantile myopathy, Leber myopathy $\pm$ Crigler-Najjar syndrome, PEO 6 Fragile syndrome	Alpers ataxia; deafness; Leber atrophy; Leigh; myopathy, infantile; myopathy, benign; myopathy, fatal; adult rhabdomyolysis, PEO; KSS; MNGIE; MERRF; MELAS	Leber atrophy, Leigh, NARP

KSS, Kearns-Sayre syndrome; LHON, Leber hereditary optic atrophy, neuropathy; MELAS, mitochondrial encephalopathy, lactic acidosis, and stroke; MERRF, myoclonic epilepsy, ragged-red fibers; MNGIE, myopathy and external ophthalmoplegia, neuropathy, gastrointestinal, encephalopathy; NARP, neuropathy, ataxia, retinitis pigmentosa; PEO, progressive external ophthalmoplegia; TTFA malonate, thenoyltrifluoroacetone malonate.

(Adapted from Neuromuscular Disease Center. Washington University, St Louis, MO, USA. website: http://www.neuro.wustl.edu/neuromuscular/index.html)

Table C-3 General System/Organ Manifestations for All Complex Deficiencies

System/Organ	Manifestations
Central nervous system	Seizures, stroke-like episodes, dementia, sensorineural deafness, ataxia, myoclonic movements, dystonia, chorea, migraine
Skeletal muscle	Hypotonia, myopathy, ptosis, myoglobinuria
Peripheral nerves	Neuropathy
Bone marrow	Pancytopenia, sideroblastic anemia
Kidney	Renal tubular necrosis (de Toni-Debré-Fanconi syndrome)
Endocrine	Diabetes mellitus (type II), hypoparathyroidism, growth hormone deficiency
Heart	Cardiomyopathy, conduction defects
Gastrointestinal system	Pancreatic failure, hepatomegaly
Metabolic	Lactic acidosis,
Ocular	Optic nerve atrophy, retinal pigmentary degeneration

Modified from Thyagarajan D, Byrne E: Mitochondrial disorders of the nervous system: Clinical, b ochemical, and molecular genetic features. *Int Rev Neurobiol* 53:93, 2002.

Complex I Deficiency

At a glance: This is the most common type of respiratory chain disease. Complex I is the largest respiratory chain complex and involved in numerous clinical conditions (see Table C-2 on page 186). Forty-six polypeptide subunits form Complex I, of which 7 are encoded by mitochondrial DNA (mtDNA) and the residual 39 by nuclear DNA (nDNA). The major subunits are flavoprotein, iron-sulphur protein, and hydrophobic fraction. Complex I is involved in the electron transport from NADH to ubiquinone, from where the electrons are transported to the next respiratory chain complex. This is the most commonly identified respiratory chain disease phenotype, which is most likely related to the large number of subunits encoded by both, nuclear and mitochondrial DNA and the size of the complex subunit. Complex I deficiency is often part of a combined deficiency because deficiencies in other complexes may result in a loss of Complex I function. It is the result of a number of situa-

tions where mtDNA point mutations are associated with deletions. In the absence of known mtDNA abnormalities, it may be associated with fatal infantile encephalomyopathy. As an isolated deficit, the clinical presentation occurs at the age of 4 to 5 months and in about 70% of patients death occurs within 2 years. Severe lactic acidosis occurs in 85% of patients. Most infants also present with severe cardiomyopathy, childhood encephalopathy, macrocephaly with progressive leukodystrophy, hepatomegaly and real tubulopathy. The most frequent myopathy is known as ☞MELAS syndrome.

Synonyms: NADH-Coenzyme Q Reductase Deficiency; NADH-Ubiquinone Oxido–reductase Deficiency.

Incidence: The estimated incidence for all forms of respiratory chain diseases combined is approximately 1 in 10,000 live births. The male-to-female ratio is approximately 3.5:1.

Genetic inheritance: Inheritance is usually autosomal recessive. It can also be caused, as with all mitochondrial encephalopathies, by mutations in multiple different genes. Complex I deficiency presents both nuclear-encoded and mitochondrial-encoded mutations. Human complex I (NADH-ubiquinone reductase) consists of at least 36 nuclear-encoded and 7 mitochondrial-encoded subunits. Mutations in any of these subunits can cause the disorder, which explains the complexity of this disorder.

REFERENCE:
Cheam EW, Critchley LA: Anesthesia for a child with complex I respiratory chain enzyme deficiency *J Clin Anesth* 10:524, 1998.

Complex II Deficiency

At a glance: Complex II is, as in Complex I, caused by mutations in nDNA. This mutation is defined as a "direct hit" in the genes that encode subunits of respiratory chains complexes. It affects the enzyme succinate CoQ reductase which is responsible for the transfer of electrons by the reduction of succinate to fumarate in the electron chain pathway (see Table C-2 on page 186). Deficiency of complex II is characterized by highly variable phenotypic expression. The clinical features include encephalomyopathy, failure to thrive, severe developmental delay, muscle hypotonia, lethargy, respiratory failure, ataxia, and myoclonic seizures. The presence of lactic acidosis is common. The most frequent clinical condition is ☞Leigh syndrome.

Synonyms: Succinate CoQ Reductase Deficiency; Succinate Dehydrogenase.

Incidence: If we consider only cases with documented mutations, complex II deficiency appears to be a rare cause of mitochondrial disorders.

Genetic inheritance: Inheritance is usually autosomal recessive. Deficiency of complex II is characterized by highly variable phenotypic expression. It can be caused by mutation in the nuclear-encoded SDHA gene on chromosome 5p.

REFERENCE:
Cheam EW, Critchley LA. Anesthesia for a child with complex I respiratory chain enzyme deficiency. *J Clin Anesth* 10:524, 1998.

Table C-4   Summary of Mitochondrial Syndromes and Common Clinical Manifestations

Syndrome	Common Clinical Manifestations
Coenzyme Q deficiency	Familial mitochondrial encephalomyopathy, ataxia, seizures, mental retardation, proximal muscle weakness, pyramidal signs, exertional fatigue with lactic acidosis (ATT: administration of coenzyme Q10 may contribute to control of seizure activities)
MELAS	Short stature, sensorineural deafness, stroke-like episodes that most often are occipital and not conforming to metabolic territories), seizures, exercise intolerance, asthenia, severe muscle weakness, diabetes mellitus, cerebral atrophy
NARP	Neuropathy, ataxia, retinitis pigmentosa
MNGIE	Gastric hypomotility, PEO, muscle wasting and weakness, deafness
KSS	PEO with onset before 30 years of age, retinal pigmentary degeneration, high cerebrospinal fluid protein, heart block (always present before 50 years of age), identification of white matter abnormalities on magnetic resonance imaging, intracranial calcification, often raised intracranial pressure
PEO	Ptosis and progressive complex external ophthalmoplegia, limb muscle weakness and wasting, exercise intolerance, intracerebral calcification, white matter abnormalities
LS	Psychomotor retardation, reduced ability to suck and swallow in infancy leading to failure to thrive, signs of brainstem dysfunction (respiratory abnormalities, sudden death in infancy, eye movement disturbance, nystagmus), peripheral neuropathy, dystonia, other movement disorders
LHON	Subacute visual failure (particularly in males; male-to-female ratio 9:1), dystonia

NARP, Neuropathy, ataxia, retinitis pigmentosa; MELAS, mitochondrial encephalopathy, lactic acidosis, and stroke; MERRF, myoclonic epilepsy, ragged-red fibers; MNGIE, myopathy and external ophthalmoplegia, neuropathy, gastrointestinal, encephalopathy; LHON, Leber hereditary optic atrophy, neuropathy; KSS, Kearns-Sayre syndrome; PEO, progressive external ophthalmoplegia; LS, Leigh syndrome.

Modified from Thyagarajan D, Byrne E; Mitochondrial disorders of the nervous system: Clinical, biochemical, and molecular genetic features. *Int Rev Neurobiol* 53:93, 2002.

Complex III Deficiency

At a glance: Complex III is located within the inner membrane of the mitochondria and is the second enzyme in the electron transport chain of the oxidative phosphorylation process. The ubiquinol cytochrome c reductase catalyses the electron transfer from succinate and nicotinamide adenine dinucleotide-linked dehydrogenases to cytochrome c within the respiratory chain located within the inner membrane of the mitochondria. The clinical features usually include progressive ataxia, predominantly proximal muscle weakness, areflexia, extensor plantar responses, dementia, and concomitant nonspecific myopathic and neuropathic changes in muscle. External ophthalmoplegia, ptosis and cardiomyopathy are often present. The most frequent clinical condition is ☞Leber Myopathy.

Synonyms: Ubiquinone-cytochrome Oxidoreductase; Coenzyme Q-Cytochrome C Reductase Deficiency.

Incidence: The incidence for Complex III deficiency remains unknown.

Genetic inheritance: Inheritance is usually autosomal recessive, however, an autosomal dominant inheritance has also been suggested. Mutations in the BCS1L gene on chromosome 2q33 or the UQCRB gene on chromosome 8 have been demonstrated. The BCS1L gene are associated with tubulopathy, encephalopathy, and liver failure. GRACILE syndrome, which belongs to the Finnish disease heritage, is also caused by mutation in the BCS1L gene, but displays a different phenotype.

REFERENCES:

Seijo-Martinez M, Castro del Rio M, Campos Y, et al: Unusual clinical findings and Complex III deficiency in a family with myotonic dystrophy. *J Neurol Sci* 208:87, 2003.

Thyagarajan D, Byrne E; Mitochondrial disorders of the nervous system: Clinical, biochemical, and molecular genetic features. *Int Rev Neurobiol* 53:93, 2002.

Complex IV Deficiency

At a glance: Complex IV deficiency, also known as cytochrome c oxidase (COX) deficiency, is a very rare inherited metabolic disorder characterized by the absence of this enzyme. Several medical conditions have been associated with the cytochrome c oxidase deficiency (see Table C-2 on page 186). Clinical features vary according to the type of skeletal muscles affected by the COX deficiency. Two major forms exist and are determined by the organ involvement: encephalopathic or myopathic. Affected infants with the benign infantile mitochondrial myopathy present similar clinical features than infants affected with the more severe infantile form of the disease, without either cardiac (hypertrophic cardiomyopathy) or kidney dysfunction. In Leigh's Disease (Subacute Necrotizing Encephalomyelopathy), a progressive degeneration of the brain is associated with significant dysfunction of the heart, kidneys, skeletal muscles, and the liver. The COX Deficiency French-Canadian Type affects skeletal muscles, connective tissue, and the liver. As observed in Leigh's Disease, the brain can be involved in this form of COX deficiency. Renal Fanconi Syndrome can be the first manisfestation of Complex IV deficiency (intermittent lactic acidosis). Complex IV is the terminal enzyme of the respiratory chain and consists of 13 polypeptide subunits. Three of these proteins are encoded by the mitochondrial DNA and the responsible catalytic subunits that carry out the electron transport function.

Synonyms: Cytochrome C Oxidase Deficiency; COX Deficiency.

Incidence: Complex IV or cytochrome c oxidase (COX) deficiency is the most common disorder involving complexes of the respiratory chain in the pediatric age. Cytochrome c oxidase deficiency is clinically heterogeneous, ranging from isolated myopathy to severe multisystem disease, with onset from infancy to adulthood. In the French-Canadian population of the Saguenay-Lac St. Jean region of the province of Quebec, the estimated prevalence at birth for cytochrome c oxidase deficiency is believed to be 1 in 2,473, giving a carrier frequency of 1 in 28.

Genetic inheritance: Many cases of COX deficiency are inherited as an autosomal recessive genetic trait. However, it is possible that other cases may be inherited due to abnormal changes in genetic material (mutations in genes needed for the assembly of their subunits) found within mitochondria (mtDNA).

REFERENCES:

Kuwertz-Broking E, Koch HG, Marquardt T, et al: Renal Fanconi syndrome: First sign of partial respiratory chain complex IV deficiency. *Pediatr Nephrol* 14:495, 2000.

Thyagarajan D, Byrne E; Mitochondrial disorders of the nervous system: Clinical, biochemical, and molecular genetic features. *Int Rev Neurobiol* 53:93, 2002.

Complex V Deficiency

At a glance: Complex V (Adenosine triphosphate (ATP) synthase or ATPase) couples proton flow from the inter-membrane space back to the matrix by the conversion of ADP and inorganic phosphate to ATP. Mitochondrial ATPase is a multisubunit enzyme that catalyzes ATP synthesis during oxidative phosphorylation. The complete loss of the ATP synthase enzyme activity is probably not compatible with life. However, partial loss or complex V deficiency, reflected by a lower amount of functional ATP synthase, causes a medical condition characterized by progressive myopathy, hypertrophic cardiomyopathy, seizures, and severe lactic acidosis. It is often associated with evidence of brainstem degeneration leading to coma. The presence of methyl glutaconic aciduria can be a major clue in the diagnosis of Complex V deficiency in an infant. Only few cases have been described in the literature. The clinical features included craniofacial dysmorphism, micrognathia, and hypospadias. Progressive muscle hypotonia, severe lactic acidosis, hypertrophic cardiomyopathy, and hepatomegaly were also present. Heart failure is reported as the cause of death within the first week of life.

Synonyms: ATPase Deficiency; TPAF2 Deficiency; ATP Synthase Deficiency.

Incidence: The incidence is unknown.

Genetic inheritance: It has been suggested that a mutation in the encoded assembly gene for the development of ATPase enzyme might be responsible for Complex V deficiency.

REFERENCES:

Kuwertz-Broking E, Koch HG, Marquardt T, et al: Renal Fanconi syndrome: First sign of partial respiratory chain complex IV deficiency. *Pediatr Nephrol* 14:495, 2000.

Thyagarajan D, Byrne E; Mitochondrial disorders of the nervous system: Clinical, biochemical, and molecular genetic features. *Int Rev Neurobiol* 53:93, 2002.

Cone-Rod Retinal Dystrophies

At a glance: Inherited dystrophy of retinal photoreceptors and pigment epithelium characterized by simultaneous abiotrophic degeneration of rods and cones.

Incidence and genetic inheritance: The incidence is unknown. Autosomal dominant inheritance is more frequent, but autosomal recessive and X-linked transmission and sporadic cases have also been described. Cone Rod Retinal Dystrophy (CRD) Type I refers to an autosomal dominant inherited form of CRD that has been described in one patient only and is caused by a deletion of the 18q21.1-qter segment. CRD Type II is more common, also autosomal dominant inherited and caused by mutations in the CRX gene (Cone-rod homeo box-containing gene) located on 19q13.3. However, genetic heterogeneity may exist.

Clinical aspects: The diagnosis of CRD II is based on a positive family history in association with the clinical findings (visual field defects and abnormal electroretinography). The clinical signs are limited to the eyes with initial loss of color vision (cone-mediated; most often red-green or blue-yellow defects) and visual acuity, then followed by nyctalopia (night blindness; rod-mediated) and peripheral visual field loss and early blindness. Severe photophobia and a fine nystagmus are common and chorioretinal atrophy may occur in severe cases. Examination shows cone-rod retinal dystrophy, "Bull's eye" macular lesions, widespread retinal pigmentation, and chorioretinal atrophy. The onset of decreased central vision with progredient shrinkage of the peripheral visual field and loss of visual acuity usually manifests before the age of 10 years. Onset of nyctalopia occurs in the third decade of life, and after the fifth decade of life, visual function is severely reduced. Unfortunately, progression to complete lack of light perception in CRD is inexorable. CRD II is not associated with extraocular findings.

Beside the typical eye features described above, the patient with CRD I also suffered from hypogonadism and impaired hearing.

Anesthetic considerations: No specific anesthetic considerations should arise from this disorder. Dealing with a blind patient unable to see what is happening requires more explicit explanations in general and clear warnings before painful procedures in particular.

Other conditions to be considered:

☞LEBER CONGENITAL AMAUROSIS (Do not confuse with Leber Hereditary Optic Neuropathy): This is an inherited degenerative disease of the retina characterized by severely decreased vision manifesting already at birth or shortly thereafter. Other ocular anomalies may include sensory (wandering) nystagmus, amaurotic pupils, and deep-set eyes. Central nervous system anomalies have been described in some of these patients.

☞**STARGARDT SYNDROME:** This is the most common form of inherited juvenile macular degeneration. It is characterized by a reduction of central vision with a preservation of peripheral vision. Onset is usually before the age of 20 years. The macula presents with yellow-white spots of irregular shapes.

REFERENCES:

Evans K, Duvall-Young J, Fitzke FW, et al.: Chromosome 19q cone-rod retinal dystrophy: ocular phenotype. *Arch Ophthal* 113:195, 1995.

Evans K, Fryer A, Inglehearn C, et al.: Linkage of cone-rod retinal dystrophy to chromosome 19q and evidence for segregation distortion. *Nature Genet* 6:210, 1994.

Moore AT: Cone and cone-rod dystrophies. *J Med Genet* 29:289, 1992.

Congenital Afibrinogenemia

At a glance: An inherited bleeding syndrome resulting from an absence of fibrinogen.

Synonyms: Familial Afibrinogenemia; Familial Dysfibrinogenemia; Familial Hypofibrinogenemia.

Incidence: Approximately 150 cases have been described in the medical literature. The incidence is estimated to be 1–2:1,000,000 live births. No racial or sexual predilection has been reported.

Genetic inheritance: Autosomal recessive. A high rate of consanguinity in the parents of affected children has been reported. The mutations have been mapped to 4q28.

Pathophysiology: The fibrinogen molecule is a hexamer consisting of three polypeptide chain pairs (α, β, γ). Each chain is controlled by a different gene, with all genes located on chromosome 4. Congenital afibrinogenemia results from a defective fibrinogen synthesis in the liver. It can be caused by mutations in any of the three genes, but the most common mutation affects the fibrinogen α-gene. The genetic defect leads to errors in the assembly of the hexamer and problems with its secretion from the hepatocytes. Complete (homozygous type) or partial (heterozygous type) absence of fibrinogen results in mild-to-severe bleeding.

Diagnosis: The homozygous form often is lethal and is diagnosed at birth secondary to severe bleeding from the umbilical stump. Other common presentations include splenic rupture, osseous hemorrhages, and hepatic hemorrhage. Surprisingly, some affected persons have only minor bleeding troubles. Diagnosed by partial or complete afibrinogenemia in blood samples, and prolonged bleeding time, prothrombin time (PT), and activated partial thromboplastin time (PTT).

Clinical aspects: Bleeding may be mild to severe and affect the gastrointestinal tract, the cranial vault and central nervous system, the joints (hemarthros), the bones (osseous hemorrhages), the liver (hepatic hemorrhage), and the spleen (rupture). Death is most often attributable to postoperative bleeding and intracranial hemorrhage. Recurrent spontaneous abortions (most commonly between 6 and 8 weeks of gestation if no fibrinogen replacement therapy is used) and heavy menstrual bleeding have been described in women with congenital afibrinogenemia. During pregnancy where fibrinogen is also involved in maintaining the integrity of placental implantation, fibrinogen levels of at least 0.6 g/liter (better 1.0 g/liter) have been recommended and should be started before 5 weeks of gestation. For delivery (spontaneous or cesarean section), the fibrinogen level should be maintained at 1.5 g/liter (better 2.0 g/liter) with a continuous infusion of fibrinogen.

Precautions before anesthesia: Obtain bleeding history, serum fibrinogen levels, PT, PTT, bleeding time, and a complete blood count with differentiation. Consider hematology consultation. Since these patients are exposed to recurrent transfusions, they have a higher risk for transfusion related diseases (e.g., hepatitis, HIV).

Anesthetic considerations: Patients are at high risk for severe hemorrhage in the perioperative period because of partial or complete incoagulability of the blood. Regional anesthesia in general and central neuraxial blockade in particular should be avoided. Fibrinogen serum levels usually are less than 0.1 g/liter, and increasing it perioperatively to at least 0.5 g/liter (better 1.0 g/liter) is recommended. Either fibrinogen concentrate or cryoprecipitate can be used to achieve this level. Fresh-frozen plasma also can be used, but significant amounts are required to bring the fibrinogen level in the desired range. The half-life of fibrinogen is approximately 4 to 7 days.

Pharmacological implications: Fibrinogen replacement therapy in the form of fresh-frozen plasma, cryoprecipitate, or fibrinogen concentrate prior to surgery usually is required.

REFERENCES:

Kobayashi T, Kanayama N, Tokunaga N, et al: Prenatal and peripartum management of congenital afibrinogenaemia. *Br J Haematol* 109:364, 2000.

Neerman-Arbez M, de Moerloose P, Bridel C, et al: Mutations in the fibrinogen A-alpha gene account for the majority of cases of congenital afibrinogenemia. *Blood* 96:149, 2000.

Neerman-Arbez M, de Moerloose P, Honsberger A, et al: Molecular analysis of the fibrinogen gene cluster in 16 patients with congenital afibrinogenemia: Novel truncating mutations in the FGA and FGG genes. *Hum Genet* 108:237, 2001.

Congenital Atresia of Larynx

At a glance: A very rare developmental abnormality of the larynx.

Incidence and genetic inheritance: The exact incidence remains to be determined. Approximately 50 cases with no sexual predilection have been reported. Inheritance is most likely autosomal dominant with the responsible gene located on chromosome 5.

Clinical aspects: Laryngeal atresia is defined as a complete absence of the laryngeal lumen and results from an arrest in the embryonic development of the larynx at different stages. Depending on the localization of the atresia, three types of laryngeal atresia can be distinguished: atresia is both supraglottic and infraglottic in type I, infraglottic in type II, and glottic in type III. Partial laryngeal atresia may result from congenital webs, which may be localized between the cords, or from supraglottic and/or infraglottic stenoses leading to a laryngeal lumen with reduced size at birth. Clinical signs of complete atresia at birth may include stridor, laryngeal obstruction or absent cry, and require tracheostomy within minutes after birth. Partial atresia of the larynx may be revealed by direct laryngoscopy. A common finding in complete laryngeal atresia (but not in partial atresia) is pulmonary hyperplasia with dilatation of the tracheobronchial tree. Approximately half of the patients described in the literature also suffer from other anomalies, some of which are potentially life-threatening. These anomalies may affect the central nervous system (hydrocephalus), the heart (single ventricle, cardiac failure secondary to venous obstruction), the respiratory and gastrointestinal tracts (tracheal atresia, tracheoesophageal fistula, esophageal atresia, duodenal atresia), the urogenital tract (aplastic/hypoplastic kidneys, hydroureter, urethral atresia, hypospadias), and the musculoskeletal system (craniofacial anomalies, cervical vertebral anomalies, pes varus). Because complete atresia requires immediate therapy (tracheostomy/tracheotomy) after birth, most children born with this condition will die unless the condition is diagnosed prenatally (minority of cases), which is possible only in complete, but not in partial atresia (polyhydramnios, pulmonary hyperplasia, hydrops fetalis, ascites). However, survival also depends on other concomitant anomalies. Although survival in general is rare, the lifespan of a few patients with immediate and successful therapy of isolated laryngeal atresia reportedly is normal.

Anesthetic considerations: These patients present immediately after birth. As mentioned earlier, immediate action in the form of a tracheo(s)tomy is required for complete laryngeal atresia. Preserve spontaneous ventilation in partial atresia until the airway has been secured. Anesthesia for this procedure must mainly rely on local anesthesia. Ex utero intrapartum treatment (so-called EXIT procedure) has been used successfully in a fetus at 35 weeks of gestation just prior to delivery via cesarean section.

Other conditions to be considered:

☞**FRASER SYNDROME:** A polymalformative condition characterized by the association of cryptophthalmos with a wide range of abnormalities (orofacial defects, syndactyly, decreased number of digits, urogenital and renal malformations), easily recognized at birth by the evident absence of eyelids.

☞**CAT CRY SYNDROME:** A syndrome clinically characterized by microcephaly, round face, macrostomia and micrognathia, scoliosis, muscular hypotonia, severe mental retardation and often congenital heart defects. One of the most important signs in the newborn is a high-pitched cat-like cry that usually is considered diagnostic.

REFERENCES:

Bui TH, Grunewald C, Frenckner B, et al: Successful EXIT (ex utero intrapartum treatment) procedure in a fetus diagnosed prenatally with congenital high-airway obstruction syndrome due to laryngeal atresia. *Eur J Pediatr Surg* 10:328, 2000.

Okada T, Ohnuma N, Tanabe M, et al: Long-term survival in a patient with congenital laryngeal atresia and multiple malformations. *Pediatr Surg Int* 13:521, 1998.

Wiatrak BJ: Congenital anomalies of the larynx and trachea. *Otolaryngol Clin North Am* 33:91, 2000.

Congenital Dyserythropoietic Anemias

At a glance: This is a group of inherited disorders characterized by quantitatively and qualitatively altered erythropoiesis resulting in usually mild-to-moderate anemia. Premature destruction of erythroblasts in the bone marrow reduces the number of them reaching maturity. In addition, there is peripheral destruction of these dysplastic erythroblasts. Three main types of congenital dyserythropoietic anemia (CDA; types I, II, and III) and four other extremely rare types have been described.

Synonyms: *For CDA III:* Anemia with Multinucleated Erythroblasts; Hereditary Benign Erythroreticulosis.

Incidence and genetic inheritance:

CDA I: Almost 200 cases of this autosomal recessive inherited disorder have been described. Most cases originate from Europe, and consanguinity is a known risk factor. The defect has been mapped to 15q15.1-q15.3.

CDA II: More than 120 cases have been reported. Inheritance is also autosomal recessive, but the mutations have been mapped to

20q11.2. Consanguinity is present in a few families. Both sexes are equally affected.

CDA III: The rarest of the three well-defined forms of CDA. Most of the knowledge about this type of CDA derives from the Swedish Västerbotten family. Inheritance is autosomal dominant (although sporadic cases have been reported), and the genetic defect has been mapped to 15q21-q25.

Diagnosis: Based on the clinical findings, examination of peripheral blood smear and bone marrow biopsy, laboratory results (bilirubin, ferritin, transferrin, haptoglobin), and genealogic tree.

Clinical aspects:

CDA I: Clinically, the spectrum ranges from mild to severe. In approximately half of the cases, the diagnosis is made in the neonatal period secondary to significant anemia. In the other half, the diagnosis is commonly made later in childhood or adolescence secondary to mild anemia with intermittent jaundice, splenomegaly, and sometimes hepatomegaly. The hemoglobin level typically stays at around 90 g/liter (range 66–116 g/liter), so transfusions are rarely required. Macrocytosis may be present, and the reticulocyte count is normal or low. The peripheral blood smear shows anisocytosis (elliptocytosis) and poikilocytosis with dacryocytosis. Serum concentration of bilirubin is elevated, while haptoglobin is decreased. Iron overload (even without transfusions) may result in hepatic cirrhosis and skin and endocrine changes. Biliary complications (e.g., bile duct obstruction, pancreatitis, bile peritonitis) may lead to sepsis. Bone marrow aspirate reveals erythroid hyperplasia with significantly dysplastic nuclei (irregular, karyorrhectic, binucleate, trinucleate appearance). Long chromatin strands surrounded by microtubules forming intercellular bridges and connecting the nuclei of two otherwise almost separated cells are considered typical for CDA I (although it may be seen in other forms of CDA). Erroneously, a β-thalassemia trait can be mimicked by increased percentage of hemoglobin A_2 and the α/non–α-globin chain synthesis ratio. Severe forms, usually occurring before or at birth with hemoglobin levels as low as 30 g/liter requiring regular transfusions, have been described. Occasionally, the presenting features are dysmorphic body signs rather than anemia related and may include short stature, platyspondyly, hypoplastic ribs, hearing loss, hypertelorism, micrognathia, large mouth, thick lips, large ears, syndactyly, aplasia/hypoplasia of distal phalanges, onychodysplasia, and brown skin patches. These patients may be on interferon-α therapy.

CDA II: The main clinical features are anemia (which can be absent, mild or severe), jaundice, splenomegaly, and occasionally hepatomegaly. Rarely, frontal and parietal bossing, mental retardation, and posterior mediastinal tumors (extramedullary hemopoietic tissue) may occur. Like in CDA I, iron overload and biliary complications determine the course of this disorder. If CDA II is severe, often other conditions are associated. The combination of CDA II with ☞Gilbert Syndrome results in an almost fivefold increased risk for gallstones compared to patients with isolated CDA II. Hemoglobin levels are usually above the transfusion threshold with normal or decreased reticulocyte count, but occasional drops related to acute infections are common. The peripheral blood cells show normocytosis, anisocytosis, and a varying degree of anisochromasia and poikilocytosis including teardrop poikilocytes. Many erythroblasts are binucleated; less commonly they are multinucleated. Erythroid hyperplasia dominates the bone marrow with an up to 10-fold increase in erythroblasts. Lipid-laden macrophages in the bone marrow lead to a pseudo-Gaucher appearance. The typical feature of CDA II can be detected only with electron microscopy: erythroblasts containing peripheral cisternae with a more or less interrupted double membrane running parallel to the erythroblast cell membrane in a distance of 40 to 60 nm. These cisternae appear to be derived from smooth endoplasmic reticulum and fail to be cleared away as a consequence of dyserythropoiesis. Their persistence can be shown even in circulating red cells. In CDA II, red cells are preferentially destroyed in the spleen, which seems to support the benefit of splenectomy.

CDA III: Clinical features are variable but usually well tolerated, with some fatigue and mild jaundice. Splenomegaly may be present. Hemoglobin levels are commonly above the transfusion threshold with a normal or low reticulocyte count. Peripheral blood smears show anisocytosis and basophilic stippling. Bone marrow examination reveals erythroid hyperplasia with sometimes impressive giant, multinucleated erythroblasts. The haptoglobin concentration is decreased, while serum bilirubin and lactic dehydrogenase (LDH) concentrations are elevated. Iron overload is rarely an issue in these patients. Hemosiderinuria may be present and partially explain the absence of iron overload. There seems to be an increased prevalence of lymphoproliferative disorders (Hodgkin lymphoma, T-cell lymphoma, monoclonal gammopathy, multiple myeloma). Other rare clinical features may include mental retardation, visual problems with macular degeneration and angioid streaks, mongoloid facial appearance, "hair-on-end" skull phenomenon on radiographs (expansion of the diploetic portion of the calvarium), and elevated serum thymidine kinase levels.

CDA IV: Severe, transfusion-dependent, autosomal recessive inherited form with nonspecific, moderately megaloblastic erythroid dysplasia and mild-to-moderate splenomegaly.

CDA V: Extremely rare, autosomal dominant inherited form with mild anemia and jaundice, unconjugated hyperbilirubinemia, and normoblastic erythroid hyperplasia without evidence of dyserythropoiesis.

CDA VI: Extremely rare form of CDA (only five cases have been described) characterized by vitamin B_{12}- and folate-independent megaloblastic and dysplastic erythropoiesis. Anemia is usually mild with marked macrocytosis, slight hyperbilirubinemia, and absent splenomegaly.

CDA VII: Extremely rare form of CDA presenting with severe, transfusion-dependent anemia and prominent erythroid hyperplasia, anomalies of the erythroblast nuclei, and characteristic inclusions in polychromatophilic erythroblasts.

Precautions before anesthesia: Obtain a complete blood count with differentiation. Check for signs of secondary hemochromatosis (as a result of iron overload). Assess cardiac function (clinically, echocardiography, electrocardiogram) and liver function (serum concentrations of bilirubin, transaminases, albumin, and clotting factors). Evaluate for endocrinopathies. Correct anemia if necessary prior to surgery. Check for dysmorphic features that sometimes are associated with this disorder (e.g., micrognathia, short stature, vertebral anomalies) and may have an impact on the anesthetic management.

Anesthetic considerations: Airway management may be challenging in the presence of micrognathia. Central neuraxial anesthesia techniques are not contraindicated but should be expected to be difficult in patients with vertebral anomalies. However, if hepatic function appears to be compromised, coagulation status should be checked beforehand. Depending on the procedure, ensure that blood is easily available for transfusion because patients with repeated transfusions may have antibodies that may delay the availability of matching blood units.

Pharmacological implications: There are no specific implications for these conditions.

Other conditions to be considered:

☞**BLACKFAN-DIAMOND SYNDROME:** Congenital hypoplastic anemia manifesting in the first year of life with an increased risk for leukemia.

☞**FANCONI ANEMIA:** Spontaneous chromosomal aberrations associated with hypocellular marrow, pancytopenia, and constitutional aplastic anemia presenting in the first years of life associated with growth retardation. In older patients, a variety of cancers (head and neck, esophageal, gastrointestinal, vulvar, anal) have been described.

REFERENCES:

Delaunay J, Iolascon A: The congenital dyserythropoietic anaemias. *Baillieres Best Pract Res Clin Haematol* 12:691, 1999.

Heimpel H: Congenital dyserythropoietic anemias: Epidemiology, clinical significance, and progress in understanding their pathogenesis. *Ann Hematol* 83:613, 2004.

Wickramasinghe SN: Dyserythropoiesis and congenital dyserythropoietic anaemias. *Br J Haematol* 98:785, 1997.

Congenital Factor VII Deficiency

At a glance: A rare coagulation factor deficit with poor correlation between serum levels and clinical manifestations.

Synonyms: Hypoproconvertinemia; Congenital Proconvertin Deficiency.

Incidence: Not precisely known, but estimates range between 1:500,000–1,000,000 live births. Approximately 250 cases have been described in the medical literature.

Genetic inheritance: Autosomal recessive inheritance. Parental consanguinity is a known risk factor. Heterozygous patients are asymptomatic. No sexual predilection. The factor VII (FVII) gene is located on chromosome 13q34, and more than 120 different mutations have been described.

Pathophysiology: FVII is a vitamin K-dependent clotting factor synthesized in the liver. It is part of the extrinsic clotting cascade and has a half-life of approximately 3 to 4 hours. Specifically, FVII becomes activated (FVIIa) by binding to tissue factor at sites of vascular injury or inflammation. After binding to tissue factor, FVIIa further promotes coagulation by activating FIX and FX. Thus, FVII deficiency prevents initiation of coagulation by the extrinsic pathway and results in a highly variable degree of clinical bleeding, which often does not correlate with plasma levels of FVII, which may be influenced by individual (weight, age, gender), dietary, environmental, and genetic factors. However, generally FVII levels less than 2% of normal values are associated with a significantly increased risk of bleeding.

Diagnosis: FVII deficiency is the only hereditary clotting factor deficiency with a prolonged prothrombin time (PT) and a normal activated partial thromboplastin time (aPTT), although confirmation of the diagnosis requires a specific FVII assay.

Clinical aspects: Depending on the presence of FVII antigen (FVII:Ag) in the plasma, congenital FVII deficiency can be divided in type I or type II. In type I, FVII:Ag deficiency results from either decreased biosynthesis or accelerated clearance, whereas a dysfunctional FVII:Ag characterizes type II. Generally, features may include hemarthros, menorrhagia, hematuria, epistaxis, gingival bleeding, gastrointestinal bleeding, retroperitoneal hematomas, and fatal cerebral hemorrhages or hematomas. Clinically, the disease has been divided in four forms: (1) severe life-threatening form (15%

of patients) manifesting with neonatal intracranial bleeding and often lethal course in infancy; (2) severe hemorrhagic form (20%) with recurrent hemarthros and consequently chronic arthropathy; (3) mild, late-onset form (60%) with postoperative cutaneous or mucosal bleeding; and (4) asymptomatic form. Exclude acquired FVII deficiency secondary to liver disease, vitamin K deficiency (warfarin therapy, malabsorption), and, rarely, severe infections. Paradoxically, a few patients develop thrombotic complications such as pulmonary embolus and/or myocardial infarction.

Precautions before anesthesia: Consult a hematologist for recommendations regarding the use of plasma-derived FVII, a heated-vapor treated product safe from viral transmission. However, because of the delay associated with obtaining FVII concentrate, emergency surgery requires use of prothrombin complex concentrates (FII, FVII, FIX, FX), recombinant FVIIa (rFVIIa), or fresh-frozen plasma (FFP). Because the half-life of FVII is only approximately 3 to 4 hours, repeated replacement therapy quite possibly will be necessary (which, in case of FFP, results in huge amounts of volume required). On very rare occasion, patients develop antibodies against rFVIIa, so patients receiving FVII replacement therapy should be monitored for FVII antibodies. Major surgery has been performed with FVII levels as low as 10%; however, maintenance of FVII levels of at least 15 to 25% are recommended for surgical procedures to be performed safely (some sources even recommend 50%).

Anesthetic considerations: Obtain a complete blood count and measure PT, PTT, and activity of FVII. Regional anesthesia in general and central neuraxial blockade in particular are best considered contraindicated in these patients. Avoid nasal intubation and nasopharyngeal airways and temperature probes if possible. Also avoid intramuscular injections. Chronic arthropathy in patients with recurrent hemarthros may make positioning difficult. Ensure that appropriate replacement therapy is available before starting surgery or other invasive procedures. Ideally, replacement therapy starts prior to surgery so that therapeutic FVII levels are achieved on time and can be checked before surgery starts.

Pharmacological implications: Vitamin K therapy is of minimal value. Avoid aspirin and nonsteroidal antiinflammatory drugs.

Other conditions to be considered:

☞**HEMOPHILIA A:** Most severe hereditary coagulation disorder resulting from defective synthesis of plasma protein FVIII.

☞**HEMOPHILIA B:** A coagulation disorder resulting from defective synthesis of plasma protein FIX.

REFERENCES:

Blanot S, Hivert P, Lienhart A: Anesthesia and coagulation factor VII deficiency. *Ann Fr Anesth Reanim* 10:91, 1991.

Hunault M, Bauer KA: Recombinant factor VIIa for the treatment of congenital factor VII deficiency. *Semin Thromb Hemost* 26:401, 2000.

Perry DJ: Related factor VII deficiency. *Br J Haematol* 118:689, 2002.

Congenital Hypothyroidism

At a glance: This syndrome results from inadequate thyroid hormone (TH) levels during pregnancy or in the neonatal period and during infancy. Characterized in newborns by failure to thrive and physical and mental retardation.

Synonym: Cretinism.

Incidence: :3000–4000. Eighty-five percent of cases are sporadic, with wide ethnic variations (1:4000 in Caucasians, 1:2000 in Hispanics, 1:32,000 in Blacks). Females are affected twice as often as men.

Genetic inheritance: Varying etiology. Thyroid dysgenesis is occasionally autosomal recessive inherited but mostly is nonhereditary. Inborn errors of TH biosynthesis are most often autosomal recessive transmitted, except for defects in TH receptor actions that are autosomal dominant inherited.

Pathophysiology: Congenital hypothyroidism can be classified into two groups: endemic cretinism and sporadic cretinism. Endemic cretinism is caused by intrauterine and/or neonatal iodine deficiency frequently occurring in certain areas (e.g., alpine regions of Europe), whereas sporadic cretinism may be the result of basically three different mechanisms:

Thyroid dysgenesis (85% of all cases): Thyroid dysgenesis includes thyroid (hemi-)agenesis, ectopic thyroid tissue, cysts of the thyroglossal duct, and thyroid hypoplasia. In the vast majority of cases, thyroid dysgenesis is sporadic, but is familial in about 2%. The pathogenesis is largely unknown, but suggested mechanisms include mutations in the genes coding for thyroid transcription factor-1 (TTF-1), thyroid transcription factor-2 (TTF-2, which is important for thyroid morphogenesis and differentiation), and paired box 8 transcription factor (PAX-8, involved in the regulation of TH production), and mutations resulting in dysfunction of the thyrotropin (thyroid-stimulating hormone [TSH]) receptor (important for thyroid growth and function).

Inborn errors of TH biosynthesis (dyshormogenesis) (10% of patients): They are the result of a defect in any step of TH synthesis, secretion, and/or action, including mutations in the sodium/iodide symporter, defects in thyroid peroxidase, thyroglobulin, and deiodinase. In fewer than 1% of patients the cause is hypothalamic and/or pituitary failure.

Transplacental transfer of maternal antibodies (5% of patients): Maternal autoimmune thyroid disease (Graves disease, Hashimoto autoimmune thyroiditis) with transplacental passage of thyrotropin receptor-blocking antibodies (TRB Abs).

Diagnosis: Based on the clinical findings and laboratory investigations: low levels of total and free thyroxine (T_4 and fT_4) and triiodothyronine (T_3), altered TSH levels (depending on the etiology may be either decreased or increased), and low serum thyroglobulin concentrations can be seen. Serum, salivary, and urine iodine studies are required to confirm errors of biosynthesis, the presence of maternal and neonatal serum TRB-Abs, or low urinary iodine excretion in iodine deficiency. Imaging studies (e.g., nuclear medicine) can be used to determine the location and size of the gland, and to assess skeletal maturation (e.g., conventional radiography of the distal femur epiphysis).

Clinical aspects: Signs of hypothyroidism usually are difficult to diagnose at or immediately after birth. In severe cases, it may take a few weeks until symptoms become apparent. In milder cases, diagnosis may be delayed for months or even longer. Screening programs with measurement of TSH and T_4 are important because congenital hypothyroidism is one of the most common preventable causes of mental retardation. Early signs may include an abnormally high birth weight, delayed passage of meconium, constipation, and a large abdomen. Later symptoms include persistent neonatal icterus, feeding difficulties with little appetite, failure to thrive, choking spells, respiratory distress and apneas (partly as a result of macroglossia and nasal obstruction), wide anterior and posterior fontanelles (an important and common sign), hoarse voice, umbilical hernia, and disturbances in thermoregulation with temperatures often below 35°C, leading to cold and mottled skin. Somnolence and lethargy, bradycardia (despite frequently present anemia) and cardiomegaly, pericardial and pleural effusions, and genital and peripheral edemas are frequent findings. Physical and psychomotor development are delayed and become more obvious at 3 to 6 months of age in severe cases. The changes are more subtle in milder cases and therefore are more difficult to detect. Dysmorphic features may include coarse, brittle hair with low anterior hairline, hypertelorism, depressed nasal bridge, constantly open mouth with protruding tongue secondary to macroglossia, short and thick neck, short stature, wide hands with brachydactyly, and generalized muscular hypotonia with a clumsy gait. The skin often appears dry and scaly. In endemic cretinism, the above described findings are often accompanied by deaf-mutism and motor dysfunction with spasticity.

Precautions before anesthesia: Evaluate thyroid function (clinically, and serum levels of T_3, free T_4, and TSH), and obtain a chest radiograph to exclude pleural effusions. Given the possible anomalies mentioned, the airway should be assessed carefully with regard to difficult airway management. Frequent apneas in the neonatal period and in infancy require appropriate postoperative monitoring and care. In addition, anemia, hyponatremia, and hypoglycemia have been described in these patients, so a complete blood count and serum levels of electrolytes and glucose should be checked. Mental retardation may affect patient compliance. Preoperative mild sedation (mild to preserve airway patency) and the presence of the primary caregiver during induction of anesthesia may be helpful.

Anesthetic considerations: Difficult airway management is common. Spontaneous ventilation should be maintained until the airway has been secured. However, gastric emptying may be delayed and, depending on the clinical findings, a rapid-sequence induction may be preferred. There is an increased risk of perioperative bradycardia and cardiac failure in these patients. The patients appear to be sensitive to the sedative and respiratory depressing effects of opioids and other anesthetic drugs. Depending on the extent of respiratory symptoms and the planned surgery, prolonged postoperative mechanical ventilation may be necessary or favored. Hypothyroidism and hypothermia result in delayed metabolism and elimination of drugs, so reduced doses may be necessary. Hypoglycemia may occur, hence regular perioperative control is recommended. Because thermoregulation is altered, every effort should be made to keep the patients warm (e.g., forced-air convective warmer, heating blanket). Peripheral venous access may be difficult because of edema and skin changes.

Pharmacological implications: Avoid neuromuscular blockers in patients with suspected difficult airway management until the airway has been secured. Delayed clearance of drugs has been reported (partly because of delayed maturation of glucuronide conjugation).

Other condition to be considered:

AKESSON SYNDROME (**Cutis Verticis Gyrata with Thyroid Aplasia and Mental Retardation Syndrome**)**:** Characterized by the presence of cutis vertices gyrata, hypothyroidism, mental retardation, skull abnormality, shagreen patch, short stature (occasionally considered dwarfism). The thyroid gland is either ectopic, absent (aplastic), or hypoplastic. Although an X-linked inheritance seems likely, most other cases of cutis verticis gyrata and mental retardation present with an autosomal dominant inheritance. It is important to evaluate the thyroid function (serum T4, T3, T3RU, TSH) and ensure proper therapeutic replacement of thyroid hormones before anesthesia. Impairment of thermoregulatory responses requires proper care to minimize heat loss intraoperatively.

REFERENCES:

de Vijlder JJ: Primary congenital hypothyroidism: Defects in iodine pathways. *Eur J Endocrinol* 149:247, 2003.

Kopp P: Perspective: Genetic defects in the etiology of congenital hypothyroidism. *Endocrinology* 143:2019, 2002.

LaFranchi S: Congenital hypothyroidism: Etiologies, diagnosis, and management. *Thyroid* 9:735, 1999.

Congenital Muscular Dystrophy: An Overview

See chart (below) indicating the two different pathophysiological conditions and clinical presentation for congenital muscular dystrophy.

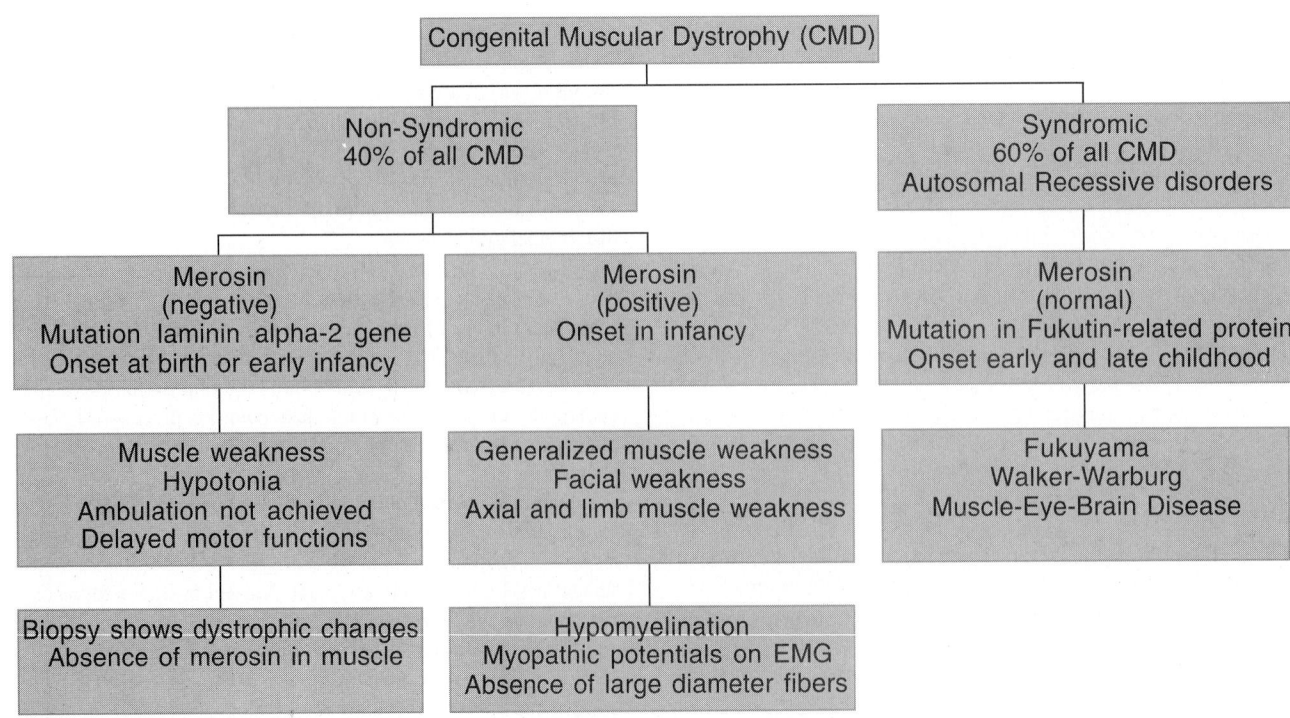

Congenital Myopathy with Fiber-Type Disproportion

At a glance: A rare genetic myopathy presenting at birth with hypotonia and muscle weakness. Findings occurring later in life include short stature, progressive scoliosis, hip dislocation, and deformities of the feet.

Synonym: Congenital Fiber-type Disproportion Myopathy.

Incidence and genetic inheritance: The exact incidence of congenital myopathies is unknown, however, congenital myopathy with fiber-type disproportion (CMFTD) seems to account for approximately 20% of cases. Autosomal recessive transmission is the most common form; however, autosomal dominant inheritance and sporadic cases have been described. Genetic heterogeneity is probable.

Clinical aspects: CMFTD can be found in other forms of congenital myopathy and other diseases (e.g., ☞Duchenne Muscular Dystrophy, ☞Spinal Muscular Atrophy, metabolic myopathies, central nervous system diseases such as leukodystrophies, ☞Lowe Syndrome, and ☞Moebius Syndrome); however, it also exists as a distinct diagnostic entity. Generalized hypotonia and weakness are noticeable at birth, and failure to thrive is common. The prognosis is often good because the disease is usually not progressive. In some cases, improvement with age has been reported. However, in approximately 25% of patients, the course is severe, with death resulting from respiratory failure in approximately 10% of patients. Skeletal involvement is common and may present with short stature, (kypho)scoliosis, contractures, joint laxity, and congenital hip dislocation. Bulbar palsy and ophthalmoplegia are less common and associated with a poor prognosis. Cardiac involvement (dilated cardiomyopathy, arrhythmias) is rare, but can be significant and require medical treatment or even heart transplant. In a minority of these patients, facial anomalies (e.g., high arched palate) and insulin-resistant diabetes mellitus have been reported. The diagnosis is confirmed by muscle biopsy, which commonly shows small, atrophic type I fibers and compensatory hypertrophic type II fibers. In CMFTD, type I fiber mean diameter should be at least 12% smaller than that of type II fibers, although some groups consider a difference of 25% more appropriate. Rarely, a small number of type I fibers shows signs of hypertrophy.

Anesthetic considerations: This disease requires a complete workup, including assessment of neurologic and motor milestones, family history, and past medical history. Respiratory function should be checked preoperatively (e.g., chest radiographs, arterial blood gas analysis, pulmonary function tests), and preoperative physiotherapy likely will be beneficial. Nevertheless, one should be prepared for prolonged postoperative mechanical ventilation. Regular and close monitoring of blood glucose in the perioperative period is recommended. Scoliosis not only may make airway management more difficult but also may lead to restrictive lung disease and cor pulmonale. A rapid-sequence induction technique should be considered in the presence of bulbar symptoms. Patient positioning may be difficult but must be done with great care because joint laxity with dislocation (hip) is a common problem in these patients. Because cardiac problems have been described in some of these patients, the threshold for a cardiac consult and/or echocardiography should be low. In case of cardiac anomalies, invasive monitoring is recommended. Regional anesthesia per se is not contraindicated, however, positioning problems and scoliosis can affect the success rate negatively (particularly for central neuraxial blockade).

Pharmacological implications: The use of succinylcholine and volatile anesthetics has not been described in this disease. However, it seems prudent to avoid succinylcholine in muscular disorders. Maintain spontaneous ventilation until the airway has been secured.

Other conditions to be considered:

☞**CENTRAL CORE DISEASE:** Congenital myopathy with a specific histologic pattern and high susceptibility to malignant hyperthermia.

☞**MYOTUBULAR MYOPATHY:** Congenital muscle disease characterized by generalized hypotonia, muscle weakness, and central nuclei on muscle biopsy (myotube-like aspect).

☞**NEMALINE ROD MYOPATHY:** A rare congenital and slowly progressive inherited neuromuscular disease usually apparent at birth and characterized by extreme hypotonia.

REFERENCES:

Banwell BL, Becker LE, Jay V, et al: Cardiac manifestations of congenital fiber-type disproportion myopathy. *J Child Neurol* 14:83, 1999.

Clarke NF, North KN: Congenital fiber type disproportion—30 years on. *J Neuropathol Exp Neurol* 62:977, 2003.

Vestergaard H, Klein HH, Hansen T, et al: Severe insulin-resistant diabetes mellitus in patients with congenital muscle fiber type disproportion myopathy. *J Clin Invest* 95:1925, 1995.

Congenital Pancreatic Agenesis

At a glance: This extremely rare condition results in early-onset insulin-dependent diabetes mellitus (IDDM) and exocrine pancreatic insufficiency.

Synonym: Congenital Pancreatic Hypoplasia.

Incidence: Approximately 10 cases of pancreatic agenesis have been reported.

Genetic inheritance: Autosomal recessive transmission. The genetic defect results from a mutation of the human insulin promoter factor-1 (IPF1) gene, which is located on 13q12.1.

Pathophysiology: The homeodomain protein IPF1 is critical for the development of the pancreas and is a key factor in the regulation of the insulin gene in the beta cells of the endocrine pancreas. Targeted disruption of the gene encoding IPF1 results in failure of the pancreas to develop (pancreatic agenesis). Intrauterine growth retardation appears to be related to the fact that insulin is a major intrauterine growth factor.

Diagnosis: Exclude ☞Mucoviscidosis, which is the most common cause of exocrine pancreatic insufficiency in childhood. The findings of intrauterine growth retardation (insulin is a known prenatal growth factor that does not cross the placenta in clinically significant amounts) and early-onset IDDM combined with clinical and biochemical evidence of pancreatic exocrine insufficiency may fit the diagnosis of congenital pancreatic aplasia/hypoplasia. In contrast to cases with absence of islets of Langerhans or complete pancreatic aplasia, serum levels of C peptide and glucagon may be measurable in partial aplasia. The diagnosis of pancreatic agenesis is difficult to establish in the newborn period. The size of the infant makes use of endoscopic retrograde cholangiopancreatography hazardous, and normal newborn comparisons are not well established for radiologic examinations. Clues pointing to the diagnosis include intrauterine growth retardation, failure to thrive, persistent hyperglycemia, polyuria, glycosuria, and steatorrhea.

Clinical aspects: Intrauterine growth retardation with early-onset IDDM is typical. Affected infants may develop profound polydipsia and polyuria because of increased osmotic load resulting in rapidly progressing dehydration. Hyperglycemia in newborns can be associated with an increased incidence of intraventricular hemorrhage. Overly aggressive insulin therapy can result in hypoglycemia with adverse neurologic sequelae. Ketoacidosis is a rare finding in these patients, and some researchers hypothesized this finding results from the lack of hyperglucagonemia. Despite appropriate insulin and exocrine pancreas hormone replacement therapy, some patients fail to gain weight. Serum insulin levels may be very low or undetectable. Limited joint mobility has been reported in some patients.

Precautions before anesthesia: Admit the patient 24 to 48 hours preoperatively to optimize insulin therapy and try to keep the blood glucose levels slightly higher (i.e., 5–12 mmol/liter) than generally accepted for older children. These patients should be booked at the beginning of the operating list. Different treatment options are available for the management of IDDM. We recommend the treatment you commonly use and with which you are familiar. One regimen consists of omitting the morning dose of insulin, starting an intravenous glucose-insulin infusion (either separately or mixed), and adding potassium as required. Preoperative laboratory investigations should include a 24-hour serum glucose profile, glycosylated hemoglobin or fructosamine, fasting blood glucose level, complete blood count, and serum concentrations of electrolytes, creatinine, and urea. Limited joint mobility may affect the head and neck, and the "prayer sign" (attempt to press the two palms as flat as possible against each other without leaving a gap in between) can be helpful in determining the degree of joint involvement, which can be important for the anticipation of difficult airway management.

Anesthetic considerations: Check blood glucose levels at least hourly intraoperatively because symptoms of hypoglycemia are masked under anesthesia and every 2 hours postoperatively until normal oral intake has been established. Serum potassium levels should be monitored at least every 4 hours if clinically indicated. The glucose-insulin infusion is continued until the patient has resumed a normal calorie intake. Regional anesthesia techniques are preferable to general anesthesia because they usually allow for better control of clinical signs of hypoglycemia and an earlier return to normal dietary patterns.

Pharmacological implications: Consider compatibility of solutions and drugs with insulin.

Other conditions to be considered:

☞**Mucoviscidosis:** Congenital multiorgan disease affecting mainly the lungs, liver, and pancreas. Frequent lung infections, hemoptysis, intolerance to exercise, presence of finger clubbing suggesting pulmonary hypertension, rectal prolapse, and nasal polyps.

☞**Johanson-Blizzard Syndrome:** An inherited syndrome characterized by nasal alar hypoplasia (beak-shaped nose), scalp defects, hypothyroidism, pancreatic achylia, and congenital deafness.

☞**Shwachman Syndrome:** A rare congenital defect characterized by pancreatic insufficiency with neutropenia (60% of cases) and growth retardation. Other features may include recurrent and fatal infections, aplastic anemia, leukemia, skeletal abnormalities (metaphyseal dysostosis, thoracic dystrophy), hepatic failure, and ichthyotic skin changes.

REFERENCES:

Schwitzgebel VM, Mamin A, Brun T, et al: Agenesis of human pancreas due to decreased half-life of insulin promoter factor 1. *J Clin Endocrinol Metab* 88:4398, 2003.

Stoffers DA, Zinkin NT, Stanojevic V: Pancreatic agenesis attributable to a single nucleotide deletion in the human IPF1 gene coding sequence. *Nat Genet* 15:106, 1997.

Winter WE, Maclaren NK, Riley, et al: Congenital pancreatic hypoplasia: A syndrome of exocrine and endocrine pancreatic insufficiency. *J Pediatr* 109:465, 1986.

Congenital Pseudarthrosis of Clavicle

At a glance: A rare syndrome with most often right-sided clavicular pseudarthrosis.

Incidence and genetic inheritance: More than 200 cases have been reported worldwide. Most likely autosomal dominant inheritance, although the majority of cases (approximately two thirds) seem to occur sporadically.

Clinical aspects: Commonly, the disorder is characterized by a painless, prominent lump or spike under the skin causing some discomfort with activity combined with short stature, high arched palate, and irregular upper teeth. Vascular thoracic outlet syndrome has been described in a small number of patients. Radiography shows a pseudoarthrosis in the middle third of the clavicle, closer to the junction with the lateral third. The two segments are not in continuity, the ends are enlarged, and no callus or reactive bone formation can be seen. The lesion manifests almost always on the right side (fewer than 10 left-sided cases have been reported, almost all of which were associated with dextrocardia; in 10% the lesion occurs bilaterally), leading to speculations that excessive pressure from the right subclavian artery, normally at a higher level on the right, causes the pathology. Other researchers hypothesized that the anomaly results from failed coalescence of the two primary ossification centers of the clavicle. Differential diagnosis includes ☞Cleidocranial Dysostosis and posttraumatic pseudarthrosis. Treatment is either conservative or surgical.

Anesthetic considerations: The airway should be assessed for difficult management because of the maxillary anomalies. In cases with suspected or known difficult intubation, spontaneous ventilation should be maintained until the airway has been secured. Central venous access via the subclavian route on the affected side probably should be avoided because access may be distorted and therefore difficult.

Other conditions to be considered:

☞**Cleidocranial Dysplasia:** Generalized skeletal dysplasia resulting in defects in the development of the skull, clavicles and pelvis, and dental abnormalities.

☞**Craniofrontonasal Dysplasia:** An X-linked syndrome, strangely more severe in females, combining frontonasal dysplasia, coronal craniosynastosis, various other skeletal and soft tissue abnormalities (including clavicular pseudarthrosis) and mental retardation.

REFERENCES:

Ahmadi B, Steel HH: Congenital pseudarthrosis of the clavicle. *Clin Orthop* 126:130, 1977.

Eltl V, Wild A, Krauspe R, Raab P: Surgical treatment of congenital pseudarthrosis of the clavicle: a report of three cases and a review of the literature. *Eur J Pediatr Surg* 15:56, 2005.

Schnall SB, King JD, Marrero G: Congenital pseudarthrosis of the clavicle: A review of the literature and surgical results of six cases. *J Pediatr Orthop* 8:316. 1988.

Congenital Pulmonary Hypoplasia

At a glance: A congenital or acquired syndrome with underdevelopment of one or both lungs.

Incidence and genetic inheritance: Congenital pulmonary hypoplasia (CPH) is considered autosomal recessive inherited. However, it more often may be secondary to other intrauterine anomalies.

Clinical aspects: The hypoplastic lung has all the normal anatomical components, but fails to develop to normal size. CPH is extremely rare. More commonly, pulmonary hypoplasia occurs secondary to other anomalies, such as intrauterine compression of the developing lungs (diaphragmatic hernia, tumor, pleural effusion, skeletal anomalies, tracheobronchial stenoses), oligohydramnios, and impaired fetal breathing movements secondary to phrenic nerve agenesis or neuromuscular diseases. The compressive lesions may lead to unilateral hypoplasia, while systemic causes and CPH most often result in bilateral hypoplasia, which is generally lethal shortly after birth. Respiratory distress usually manifests within the first 5 minutes after birth, which reflects on the Apgar scores. Mechanical ventilation with highest oxygen concentrations and ventilator pressures is required to initially maintain reasonable arterial saturations. Nevertheless, most infants deteriorate further and die of respiratory failure (on average 9 hours after birth). Only a few infants survive and are discharged home from the hospital. Small clear lungs, pneumothoraces, and bilaterally raised diaphragms are considered diagnostic radiologic features for CPH. Most often, the ratio of lung weight to body weight is decreased, although secondary (ventilator-induced) lung changes may result in increased lung weight.

Anesthetic considerations: Unilateral hypoplasia may cause recurrent pneumonia and/or hypoxemia. Patients may require pulmonary lobectomy or pneumonectomy and are at risk for pulmonary barotrauma, pneumothorax, pneumomediastinum, or interstitial emphysema on either side. Persistent pulmonary hypertension of the newborn may be present and lead to right-to-left shunting through a persistent ductus arteriosus or patent foramen ovale with hypoxemia. Treatment with nitric oxide has been used successfully in some patients. It is obvious that these patients are at extremely high risk and should not be brought to the operating room until they have been stabilized, which probably is possible only in patients with milder forms of this disease.

REFERENCES:

Frey B, Fleischhauer A, Gersbach M: Familial isolated pulmonary hypoplasia: A case report, suggesting autosomal recessive inheritance. *Eur J Pediatr* 153:460, 1994.

Langer R, Kaufmann HJ: Primary (isolated) bilateral pulmonary hypoplasia: A comparative study of radiologic findings and autopsy results. *Pediatr Radiol* 16:175, 1986.

Tanigaki S, Miyakoshi K, Tanaka M, et al: Pulmonary hypoplasia: Prediction with use of ratio of MR imaging-measured fetal lung volume to US-estimated fetal body weight. *Radiology* 232:767, 2004.

Congenital Shortness of the Costocoracoid Ligament

At a glance: A very rare syndrome characterized by costocoracoid ligament shortness resulting in cosmetic deformity with limitation of the rotation movements of the shoulder.

Incidence and genetic inheritance: Described in one large Canadian kindred. Autosomal dominant transmission with variable expression.

Clinical aspects: The scapula is fixed to the first rib by a congenitally short costocoracoid ligament. The rib cage may be narrow and the shoulders sloping. The contour of the anterior clavicle is lost, the shoulders rounded, and the scapular motion limited. Movements depending on rotation or retraction of the scapula are limited, but usually do not interfere with normal activities. Surgical excision of the costocoracoid ligament results in some correction of the cosmetic deformity.

Anesthetic considerations: No literature regarding anesthesia in these patients is available. Careful intraoperative positioning is needed, particularly in the prone position because of limited shoulder mobility. The subclavian approach for central venous line insertion or axillary plexus blockade probably should be avoided because of altered landmarks (loss of anterior clavicle contour). Chest narrowing theoretically can result in decreased chest wall compliance, but this problem has not been reported.

REFERENCE:

Bamforth JS, Bell MH, Hall JG, et al: Congenital shortness of the costocoracoid ligament. *Am J Med Genet* 33:444, 1989.

Congenital Stridor

At a glance: A symptom characterized by noisy breathing because of turbulent flow in the narrowed airways indicating partial obstruction of the upper airway, glottis, or trachea. Congenital stridor is a symptom rather than a syndrome.

Genetic inheritance: Depends on the underlying cause.

Pathophysiology: Fixed or variable partial obstruction of the upper airway, glottis, or trachea may change the air flow pattern from laminar to turbulent, which results in noisy breathing or stridor. Extrathoracic obstructions usually are associated with inspiratory stridor, whereas intrathoracic lesions usually result in expiratory stridor, and (sub)glottic stenoses may result in biphasic (inspiratory and expiratory) stridor. Causes of congenital stridor are variable and can be divided into four categories: supralaryngeal, laryngeal, tracheal, and nonanatomical. They may include tracheoesophageal fistula, laryngomalacia, narrowing of the mainstem bronchus, Pierre-Robin syndrome, dysfunction of cranial nerves IX to XII, curled epiglottis, congenital subglottic stenosis, laryngotracheal cleft, epipharyngeal fibroma, vascular rings, and bronchogenic cysts. In severe cases, gastroesophageal reflux may lead to stridor.

Diagnosis: Patients usually present with stridor starting just after birth or shortly thereafter (first 4–6 weeks of life), feeding difficulties, frequent coughing, and recurrent aspirations. The diagnosis is based on the clinical finding of the characteristic breath sounds. Clinical circumstances may give an idea about the etiology (association with position and feeding, persistent versus intermittent, abnormal phonation, foreign body exposure, presence of other congenital abnormalities). Laryngo-broncho-esophageal examination usually reveals the exact cause of the symptom. Check the percentiles for weight and height because increased respiratory work may lead to increased energy requirements with growth retardation.

Clinical aspects: Congenital stridor is a symptom rather than a syndrome, so the cause of the stridor must be explored. The most common cause of inspiratory stridor in the neonatal period is laryngomalacia, which accounts for approximately three fourths of all cases. Stridor generally improves in the prone position with the head up. Laryngomalacia usually requires no therapy and disappears spontaneously around 1 year of age. Rarely, in patients with severe obstruction, supraglottoplasty may be required. Unilateral vocal cord paralysis is probably the second most common cause of stridor in the neonatal period. It is either congenital or acquired (related to cardiothoracic surgery or birth trauma). Incomplete canalization of the subglottic area and cricoid rings is the anatomical correlate in congenital subglottic stenosis, while acquired subglottic stenosis is most often caused by prolonged intubation (often related to an endotracheal tube with a diameter that is too big). Severe episodes of airway obstruction may require resuscitation with intubation and/or tracheo(s)tomy. Ask about associated features such as cyanosis, increased respiratory efforts (indrawings), tachypnea, and apnea to determine the severity of the stridor. The most common cause of expiratory stridor in the neonatal period is tracheomalacia, which is caused by a loss of the stability of the tracheal ring cartilages and results in persistent stridor. However, tracheal collapse also can be caused by external compression (double aortic arch, vascular rings, slings). An increased risk of obstructive sleep apnea has been reported in children with congenital stridor.

Precautions before anesthesia: Assess the airway for evidence of stridor when the patient is awake, during sleep, and during activity. Also assess the airway for potentially difficult management. Evaluate the respiratory status for evidence of aspiration with a detailed history and examination, chest radiographs, and arterial blood gas analysis if indicated. Special attention should be paid to craniofacial anomalies, presence of choanal atresia/stenosis, and cutaneous hemangiomas. Try to pinpoint the precise localization of stridor by auscultation of the nose, oropharynx, neck, and chest. Check the risk of pulmonary aspiration.

Anesthetic considerations: Anesthesia of a patient with stridor requires a clear protocol. All equipment, including emergency tracheostomy instruments and resuscitation drugs, must be present in the operating room. In severe cases, a surgeon experienced in emergency airway procedures should be present. Tracheobronchoscopy can be performed under ventilation through the bronchoscope, through a laryngeal mask airway, or with jet ventilation under total intravenous anesthesia. In all other cases, preserving spontaneous ventilation and obtaining venous access prior to tracheal intubation are necessary. Therefore, inhalational induction is often preferred. Direct laryngoscopy requires a sufficiently deep level of anesthesia, and topicalization of the airway with lidocaine can be helpful. Moderate continuous positive airway pressure can prevent expiratory collapse of the airway during spontaneous breathing. Extubation of the trachea is performed under the same safety conditions and can require adrenaline nebulization or nasal jet continuous positive airway pressure.

Pharmacological implications: Muscle relaxants should be avoided until the airway has been secured and the level of the stridor been assessed. Antisialogues can be useful; atropine is indicated. Halothane is often preferred to sevoflurane because of its longer action.

REFERENCES:

Holzki J, Laschat M, Stratmann C: Stridor in the neonate and infant. Implications for the paediatric anesthetist. Prospective description of 155 patients with congenital and acquired stridor in early infancy. *Paediatr Anaesth* 8:221, 1998.

Phelan P, Stocks J, Williams H, et al: Familial occurrence of congenital laryngeal clefts. *Arch Dis Child* 48:275, 1973.

Congenital Varicella Syndrome

At a glance: A rare congenital nongenetic disorder resulting from maternal transmission of varicella in the first and second trimesters of pregnancy manifesting with cutaneous, neurologic, and limb involvement.

Synonyms: Fetal Varicella Syndrome; Varicella Virus Antenatal Infection; Varicella Embryopathy; Varicella Fetopathy.

Incidence: Because most women of child-bearing age (>90%) have antibodies (IgG) against the varicella-zoster virus, infection during pregnancy is rare. Approximately 2% of babies suffer from the syndrome following maternal varicella infection in the first 20 weeks of pregnancy (greatest risk between weeks 8 to 20). In industrialized countries, approximately 0.5–3:1000 pregnancies are affected. However, a significantly higher rate is expected in developing countries. Approximately 100 cases have been described in the medical literature. Two thirds of affected neonates are females.

Genetic inheritance: Not a genetic disorder.

Pathophysiology: The route of infection most likely is transplacental and leads to fetal viremia, although ascending infection from the cervix uteri is possible. Organ injuries reflect the neurotropic nature of the varicella virus.

Diagnosis: Based on the history of maternal chickenpox in the first or second trimester of pregnancy and clinical and serologic (IgM-specific antibodies, persistence of IgG antibodies beyond the first 6 months of life) findings in the neonate with low birth weight and multiple, characteristic abnormalities (see *Clinical Aspects*).

Clinical aspects: At any stage of pregnancy, severe maternal chickenpox may result in fetal death. The features of the disorder may involve the skin (cicatricial lesions associated with underlying tissue hypoplasia; the lesions appear depressed and hyperpigmented and often have an irregular border; certain skin areas [mainly arms and legs in dermatomal distribution] may exhibit thickened and hypertrophic scars with induration, redness, and inflammation of the surrounding skin), the eyes (microphthalmia, microcornea, anisocoria, chorioretinitis, optic nerve atrophy and hypoplastic optic disc, cataract, corneal opacities, enophthalmia, strabismus, and nystagmus), the central nervous system (cortical and spinal cord atrophy, cerebellar aplasia, seizures, encephalitis, deafness, generalized hypotonia, hyperreflexia, intermittent myoclonic seizures, Horner syndrome, developmental delay, limb paresis), the musculoskeletal system (signs of hypoplasia and/or reduction deformities of the limbs including fingers and toes, hypoplastic mandible, clavicle, scapula, ribs, muscles), the gastrointestinal tract (hepatic calcifications, gastroesophageal reflux, duodenal stenosis, jejunal dilatation, chronic constipation, microcolon, colonic atresia, anal sphincter dysfunction), the urogenital tract (vesicoureteral reflux, neurogenic bladder), and the cardiovascular system. Intrauterine growth retardation is common. Almost one third of these patients die in the first months of life.

Precautions before anesthesia: The patient is infectious, so avoid contact with medical personnel who is at risk for contracting varicella or whose immune status is unknown. Isolation from other patients is required because varicella is highly contagious. Evaluate the patient for less common manifestations, such as cardiovascular abnormalities (in 8% of patients) and maintain a low threshold for echocardiography. Obtain a full medical history and evaluate neurologic development, seizure control, and extent of paresis. Laboratory investigations should include a complete blood count, serum concentrations of electrolytes, creatinine, and urea (because vesicoureteral reflux may affect kidney function), and hepatic function tests (e.g., serum concentrations of transaminases, albumin, bilirubin, and coagulation parameters) in case of hepatic lesions. Treating secondary bacterial infections prior to surgery seems appropriate. Facial anomalies (e.g., micrognathia) may be present, so careful assessment of the airway with regard to airway management is recommended.

Anesthetic considerations: Vascular access may be challenging in the presence of multiple skin lesions and reduction anomalies of the limbs. Maintain spontaneous ventilation until the airway has been secured in patients at risk for difficult airway management. However, if intestinal atresias are suspected or proven, a rapid-sequence technique may be indicated. Given that these patients often show signs of muscular hypoplasia, the requirements for neuromuscular blockers most likely are reduced. Monitoring of their effect with a peripheral nerve stimulator is recommended.

Pharmacological implications: Consider interaction between anesthetic drugs and antiepileptic treatment. Avoid neuromuscular blockers until the airway has been secured in patients with suspected difficult airway management.

Other condition to be considered:

☞**TORCH SYNDROME:** A syndrome referring to a group of fetal infectious malformations (TORCH is an acronym for *t*oxoplasma, *r*ubella, *c*ytomegalovirus and *h*erpes). Common signs involve essentially intracranial anomalies that must be considered for anesthetic management.

REFERENCES:

Harger JH, Ernest JM, Thurnau GR, et al: Frequency of congenital varicella syndrome in a prospective cohort of 347 pregnant women. *Obstet Gynecol* 100:260, 2002.

Mirlesse V, Lebon P: [Chickenpox during pregnancy]. *Arch Pediatr* 10:1113, 2003.

Sauerbrei A, Wutzler P: The congenital varicella syndrome. *J Perinatol* 20:548, 2000.

Conn Syndrome

At a glance: An endocrine disorder caused by hyperaldosteronism presenting with symptoms associated with hypertension and hypokalemia.

Synonyms: Primary Hyperaldosteronism; Aldosteronoma.

Incidence: Previously thought to be rare; however, the detection rate has increased tremendously with more sensitive screening options now available. Prevalence rates in hypertensive patients now vary between 3 and 32%, depending on the patient selection and the diagnostic criteria used.

Genetic inheritance: Most cases are sporadic; however, a genetic basis for the disorder has been identified in some patients. An au-

tosomal dominant inherited form is known as familial hyperaldosteronism, which is caused by an abnormal hybrid gene encoding an enzyme that has 11-β-hydroxylase and aldosterone synthase activity and is regulated by adrenocorticotropic hormone instead of angiotensin II.

Pathophysiology: Primary hyperaldosteronism results from adrenal cortical hyperplasia (diffuse or nodular), adrenal adenoma, or rarely adrenal carcinoma. This results not only in excessive sodium reabsorption in the distal nephron with hypertension and suppression of the renin–angiotensin II system, but also in increased urinary losses of potassium and hydrogen ions (in exchange with sodium) leading to hypokalemia and metabolic alkalosis.

Diagnosis: Based on clinical findings (hypertension, polyuria, polydipsia, fatigue, tinnitus, paresthesia, paralysis of variable duration, failure to thrive, muscle loss). Hypokalemia (<3.5 mmol/liter; present in approximately 20% of patients), metabolic alkalosis associated with inappropriate kaliuresis, increased plasma levels of aldosterone (>40 ng/dl), decreased plasma renin activity (<0.3 ng/ml/hour), nonsuppressible aldosterone response to ambulation, and a pathologic fludrocortisone suppression test confirm the diagnosis. Dexamethasone does not suppress aldosterone levels (except in familial hyperaldosteronism, where small doses of dexamethasone are used therapeutically). Magnetic resonance imaging is the diagnostic imaging tool of choice. It shows that the adrenal gland on the left side is involved four times more often than the gland on the right.

Clinical aspects: Morbidity in Conn syndrome results mainly from hypertension, which can range from mild to severe and be associated with significant headache. Increasing evidence indicates aldosterone in excess can trigger adverse cardiovascular sequelae (myocardial remodeling and fibrosis) independent of hypertension. Hypervolemia and hyperglycemia may occur. Renal failure as a result of acute rhabdomyolysis because of severe hypokalemia has been reported, as well as a lumbar plexopathy. Visual disturbances are less frequent. Severe growth retardation has been reported as a result of severe potassium depletion.

Precautions before anesthesia: Evaluate serum electrolyte status and correct hypokalemia. Restrict sodium intake. Administer spironolactone and stop captopril or enalapril (if used) 24 hours before general anesthesia. Check cardiovascular status. Check for signs of long-standing arterial hypertension (left ventricular hypertrophy, peripheral arterial and coronary artery sclerosis, heart failure). Obtain a chest radiograph, an electrocardiogram, and potentially an echocardiogram. Check renal function (creatinine, urea, serum electrolytes).

Anesthetic considerations: If hypokalemia is not corrected prior to anesthesia, hyperventilation could be very dangerous by further decreasing potassium plasma levels. In young children, regional anesthesia techniques may be preferred because of the absence of hemodynamic effects. In older patients, however, significant drops in arterial blood pressure can occur in combination with spinal anesthesia. No specific anesthetic agents can be recommended or are contraindicated considering the risk of acute hypotension. Depending on the procedure, invasive arterial blood pressure and central venous pressure monitoring should be considered. Hypokalemia may prolong the action of neuromuscular blockers, so reduced doses should be used and monitoring with a peripheral nerve stimulator is recommended.

Pharmacological implications: Close attention should be paid to the possible interaction between the antihypertensive drugs that are used in these patients (e.g., captopril, enalapril, spironolactone) and the risk of hyperkalemia. Clonidine should be avoided because it decreases plasma renin activity. The use of enflurane may be questionable if signs of nephropathy exist preoperatively. Supplementation with exogenous cortisol is indicated only in patients with excision of multiple adenomas with bilateral mobilization of adrenal glands.

Other condition to be considered:

☞**LIDDLE SYNDROME:** Renal tubular defect causing severe hypertension with hypokalemia and metabolic alkalosis.

REFERENCES:

Stowasser M, Gordon RD: Primary aldosteronism. *Best Pract Res Clin Endocrinol Metab* 17:591, 2003.

Wheeler MH, Harris DA: Diagnosis and management of primary aldosteronism. *World J Surg* 27:627, 2003.

Winship SM, Winstanley JH, Hunter JM: Anaesthesia for Conn's syndrome. *Anaesthesia* 54:569, 1999.

Cooks Syndrome

At a glance: A disorder involving nail dysplasia and bone abnormalities.

Synonym: Anonychia-Onychodystrophy with Hypoplasia/Absence of Distal Phalanges.

Incidence and genetic inheritance: Extremely rare disorder described in a total of 11 members from only two families. Autosomal dominant inheritance.

Clinical aspects: The diagnosis is made based on family history and the characteristic clinical features of hand and nails, which include onychodystrophy that can progress to complete loss of nails, digitalization of the thumbs, fifth finger brachydactyly, and absent or hypoplastic distal phalanges of hands and feet.

Anesthetic considerations: Because the findings are limited to the hands, no specific anesthetic concerns are expected to arise from this disorder.

Other condition to be considered:

☞**COFFIN-SIRIS SYNDROME:** A congenital syndrome with growth and mental retardation, coarse facies, nail dysplasia and skeletal anomalies.

REFERENCES:

Cooks RG, Hertz M, Katznelson MB, et al: A new nail dysplasia syndrome with onychonychia and absence and /or hypoplasia of distal phalanges. *Clin Genet* 27:85, 1985.

Nevin NC, Thomas PS, Eedy DJ, et al: Anonychia and absence/hypoplasia of distal phalanges (Cooks syndrome): Report of a second family. *J Med Genet* 32:638, 1995.

Corneal Cerebellar Syndrome

At a glance: An inherited syndrome combining ataxia, corneal dystrophy, and orthopedic anomalies.

Synonyms: Der Kaloustian Jarudi Khoury Syndrome; Spinocerebellar Degeneration and Corneal Dystrophy; Corneal-Cerebellar Syndrome; Corneal Dystrophy with Spinocerebellar Degeneration.

Incidence and genetic inheritance: Extremely rare genetic autosomal recessive disorder. It has been described in only two sisters of healthy, but consanguineous parents. Autosomal recessive inheritance has been suggested.

Clinical aspects: Onset is in the second year of life, when bilateral corneal opacifications of the corneas (which eventually result in severe visual impairment) and slowly progressive cerebellar anomalies with variable spinocerebellar involvement begin. Patients may be mentally delayed. In addition to the ocular findings (ptosis, corneal edema, pannus and dystrophy with clouding and visual loss requiring penetrating keratoplasty), the disorder may involve the face (triangular shape, micrognathia, low-set ears with posterior angulation), the nervous system (abnormal electroencephalogram, spinocerebellar degeneration, ataxia, muscular hypertonia and spasticity, hemiparesis), and the musculoskeletal system (lordosis, scoliosis, dislocation of the hips). Histologic anomalies of nerves and muscles exist.

Anesthetic considerations: Airway management may be difficult because of the facial features. Spontaneous ventilation should be maintained until the airway has been secured. Careful intraoperative positioning is needed to prevent dislocations and pressure sores. Regional anesthesia is not contraindicated per se but should be expected to be difficult to perform secondary to vertebral deformities. Spinocerebellar degeneration likely precludes most anesthetists from giving a central neuraxial blockade. Because of upper motor neuron involvement, hyperkalemia can result from succinylcholine, so succinylcholine should be avoided. Perioperative eye protection should include ointment and tape to keep the eyes shut.

REFERENCE:

Der Kaloustian VM, Jarudi NI, Khoury MJ, et al: Familial spinocerebellar degeneration with corneal dystrophy. *Am J Med Genet* 20:325, 1985.

Corneodermatoosseous Syndrome

At a glance: A syndrome characterized by the association of corneal changes with diffuse, palmoplantar hyperkeratosis, short stature, and premature birth.

Synonym: Stern-Lubinsky-Durrie Syndrome.

Incidence and genetic inheritance: Extremely rare syndrome (probably fewer than 15 cases have been described) with autosomal dominant inheritance.

Clinical aspects: Premature birth is frequent. Patients have a mild degree of short stature. Clinical features involve the eyes (astigmatism, abnormal corneal structure with mild dysplastic changes in the corneal epithelium, photophobia with burning/blurring of the eyes), the teeth (early dental decay and fragility secondary to abnormal softness), the skin (erythematous scaly skin, onychodysplasia and/or onycholysis, palmoplantar acanthosis, hyperkeratosis), and the limbs (brachydactyly, terminal hypoplasia of the fingers, shortening of the fourth metacarpal and anomalies of the metacarpal heads, medullary narrowing of the hand bones).

Anesthetic considerations: Anesthesia in this condition has not been described. Initially, problems may arise from prematurity. Otherwise, careful protection of the eyes (lubrication and taping) is recommended to prevent corneal injuries. Skin and nail lesions could make difficult placement and removal of skin electrodes for electrocardiography and (particularly self-adhesive) sensors for pulse oximetry.

Other conditions to be considered:

☞**TYROSINEMIA TYPE II:** A form of tyrosinemia characterized by herpetiform corneal ulcers and hyperkeratotic lesions of the tongue, digits, palms and soles, and mental retardation. Most patients are photophobic in bright light. These patients may fail to thrive and develop liver cirrhosis, renal tubular dysfunction, and vitamin D-resistant rickets. For other disorders associated with Hyperkeratosis Palmaris et Plantaris, please refer to:

☞**KERATOSIS PALMARIS ET PLANTARIS** (Overview).

REFERENCE:

Stern JK, Lubinsky MS, Durrie DS, et al: Corneal changes, hyperkeratosis, short stature, brachydactyly, and premature birth: A new autosomal dominant syndrome. *Am J Med Genet* 18:67, 1984.

Corpus Callosum Agenesis

At a glance: A disorder of neuronal migration characterized by partial or complete agenesis of the corpus callosum.

Incidence: Corpus callosum agenesis (CCA) is the most common cerebral malformation. It has been estimated that 0.05 to 0.7% of the general population and 2.3% of children with developmental disabilities are affected.

Genetic inheritance: Agenesis of the corpus callosum has been associated with several chromosomal rearrangements. These include autosomal dominant, autosomal recessive, and X-linked inherited syndromes.

Pathophysiology: Unknown. An insult to the commissural plate during embryogenesis interferes with migration of the cells that form the corpus callosum. This insult can be a result of chromosomal abnormalities, be part of a syndrome, a migration, or a metabolic disorder. CCA may be an isolated anomaly or part of a syndrome with other, more extensive malformations or metabolic or genetic disorders. The corpus callosum is formed between the gestational weeks 7 and 20. Consequently, partial or complete CCA may occur if this process is disrupted. Because major parts of the cortex and cerebellum develop at the same time, associated anomalies must always be excluded. As a rule, formation of the corpus callosum starts in the front and continues to the back (holoprosencephaly is the main exception to this rule), which explains why partial callosal agenesis usually involves the posterior portion of the corpus callosum.

Diagnosis: Based on the clinical findings in children undergoing extensive examination for epilepsy, cognitive impairment, or, less often, behavioral problems. Computed tomography or magnetic resonance imaging confirms the absence of the corpus callosum. Frequently, there is also upward displacement and enlargement of the third ventricle (because the corpus callosum normally forms the roof of the third ventricle), widely spaced dorsal horns, and possible evidence of other migration disorders.

Clinical aspects: Clinically and prognostically, CCA can be divided into two types. *Type I* is not associated with other disorders. Patients may have mild-to-moderate mental retardation and no or only mild neurologic manifestations, which may include seizure disorders and impaired visual, motor, and coordination skills. A peculiar facies with prominent forehead, macrocephaly or microcephaly, deep-set eyes, and preauricular skin tags is common. However, some patients have no clinical signs, which makes parental counseling difficult in the absence of radiologic and genetic markers allowing determination of future asymptomatic from symptomatic disease. *Type II* is associated with other migration, genetic, and chromosomal abnormalities, usually resulting in severe neurologic

manifestations, which may include severe mental retardation, microcephaly, hemiparesis, spasticity, seizure disorder, and failure to thrive. This condition often is accompanied by recurrent bronchopneumonia and, in the severest cases, early death in infancy.

Precautions before anesthesia: Check for associated abnormalities, particularly metabolic disorders. Assess for complications such as seizures, paralysis, and bronchopneumonia. Preoperative investigations should include a chest radiograph, pulmonary function tests (if possible), and arterial blood gas analysis. Assess for difficult airway management in case of microcephaly. Mental retardation may affect patient cooperation. Sedative and/or anxiolytic premedication and/or the presence of the primary caregiver during induction of anesthesia may be helpful.

Anesthetic considerations: Associated syndromes and abnormalities may result in extra considerations, such as preoperative fasting time and metabolic monitoring intraoperatively. Perioperative chest physiotherapy can be useful in case of recurrent bronchopneumonias. A rapid-sequence induction technique may be considered in the presence of recurrent aspiration pneumonias. Prolonged postoperative mechanical ventilation may be required.

Pharmacological implications: Ketamine may not provide adequate analgesia because of abnormal pathways between the cortex and limbic system. Succinylcholine may be relatively contraindicated in the presence of spinal neurologic abnormalities. Other drug implications may occur, depending on the presence of other associated anomalies. Consider interaction between anesthetic drugs and antiseizure medication.

Other conditions to be considered: Numerous syndromes are associated with agenesis of the corpus callosum. The following list represents the most important ones.

☞**AICARDI SYNDROME:** The combination of myoclonic seizures with a characteristic electroencephalographic pattern, lacunar chorioretinopathy, and (complete or partial) agenesis of the corpus callosum is characteristic for this X-linked dominant inherited syndrome.

☞**ARNOLD-CHIARI SYNDROME:** Depending on the type, it can be associated with hydrocephalus, raised intracranial pressure, and respiratory and cardiac center dysfunction. Infants may exhibit vomiting, weakness, and mental impairment.

☞**CEREBRO-RENO-DIGITAL SYNDROME:** Autosomal recessive inherited syndrome with corpus callosum agenesis, Dandy-Walker malformation, mental retardation, paraparesis or quadriparesis.

☞**DANDY-WALKER MALFORMATION:** Congenital anomaly of the cerebellum and fourth ventricle characterized by hypoplasia of the cerebellum and hydrocephalus because of cystic expansion of the fourth ventricle into the posterior fossa.

☞**DONNAI-BARROW SYNDROME:** Genetic disorder responsible for diaphragmatic hernia, exomphalos, absent corpus callosum, hypertelorism, eye anomalies, and sensorineural deafness.

☞**FG SYNDROME:** X-linked form of mental retardation associated with complete or partial agenesis of the corpus callosum and minor facial, skeletal, and gastrointestinal anomalies.

☞**HARD SYNDROME:** A very rare and severe autosomal recessive, quickly lethal acronymic syndrome with major neurologic impairment. Common features include *h*ydrocephalus, *a*gyria, and *r*etinal *d*ysplasia. It is characterized by type II lissencephaly in association with retinal dysplasia, obstructive hydrocephalus, and agenesis of the corpus callosum. Affected infants typically have severe growth failure, severe microcephaly, seizures, microphthalmia, and cataracts. Some affected infants have an occipital encephalocele.

☞**OPITZ-FRIAS SYNDROME:** A genetic disorder characterized by craniofacial anomalies, ocular hypertelorism, cleft lip and palate, epicanthal folds, and a wide, flat nasal bridge. Affected males present with cryptorchidism, bifid scrotum, and/or hypospadias. The most significant anomalies are the presence of clefts in the larynx and trachea, pulmonary hypoplasia, dysphagia, and respiratory obstruction. Hypoplasia or agenesis of the corpus callosum, kidney abnormalities, cardiac defects, and mental retardation have been reported.

☞**PSAUME SYNDROME:** A congenital X-linked syndrome lethal for males characterized by orofacial and digital defects associated with renal failure.

☞**RUBINSTEIN-TAYBI SYNDROME:** A rare syndrome with craniofacial anomalies and complex multiple malformations including cardiac, digestive, and respiratory. High rate of anesthetic implications concerning intubation, aspiration risk, and cardiorespiratory function.

☞**SCHINZEL ACROCALLOSAL SYNDROME:** Very rare autosomal recessive, complex disease with predominant neurologic and skeletal anomalies.

☞**TORIELLO-CAREY SYNDROME:** Multiple congenital anomalies consisting of agenesis of corpus callosum, telecanthus, short palpebral fissures, small nose with anteverted nares, Pierre-Robin sequence, malformed ears, redundant neck skin, macrocephaly, micrognathia, laryngeal and sublaryngeal abnormalities, heart defect, muscular hypotonia, occasional Hirschsprung disease, and moderate-to-severe developmental delay.

REFERENCES:

Inbar D, Halpern GJ, Weitz R, et al: Agenesis of the corpus callosum in a mother and son. *Am J Med Genet* 69:152, 1997.

Rummeny C, Ertl-Wagner B, Reiser MF: [Kongenitale Malformationen des Grosshirns. Teil 2: Entwicklungsstörungen des Balkens und Holoprosencephalien]. *Radiologe* 43:925, 2003.

Russell IF: Ketamine and agenesis of the corpus callosum. *Br J Anaesth* 51:983, 1979.

Costello Syndrome

At a glance: A syndrome characterized by postnatal growth deficiency, coarse facies, redundant skin on the neck, acanthosis nigricans, developmental delay, and papillomata.

Synonyms: Fasciocutaneoskeletal Syndrome; Mental Retardation Papillomata Syndrome.

Incidence: Approximately 50 cases have been described in the literature.

Genetic inheritance: Most likely autosomal dominant.

Pathophysiology: The abnormalities stem from abnormal development of ectodermal tissue, the mechanism of which is not understood. The responsible gene is located on 22q13.1. The etiology of Costello syndrome is unclear. Fibroblasts show increased proliferation, normal elastin gene expression, produce normal amounts of tropoelastin, and properly deposit an extracellular microfibrillar scaffold; however, the assembly of elastic fibers is defective secondary to rapid shedding of elastin binding proteins. This finding has been suggested to result from accumulation of chondroitin sulfate moieties, a phenomenon also found in ☞Mucopolysaccharidosis.

Diagnosis: Clinical recognition of the peculiar course of the disease, typical facies, and ectodermal involvement (loose and hyperpigmented skin).

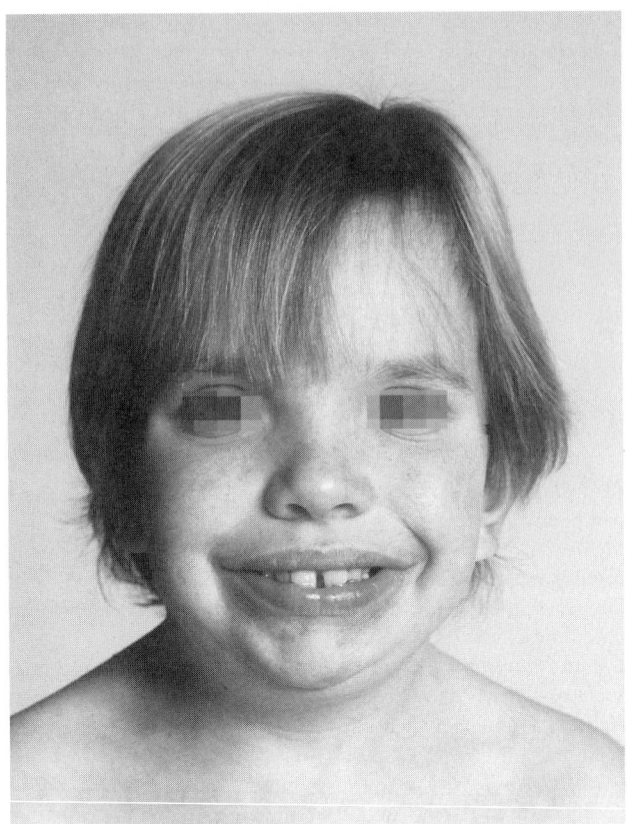

Costello Syndrome The coarse face with depressed nasal bridge, hypertelorism, large mouth, and short neck in this boy is caused by Costello syndrome.

Clinical aspects: Pregnancy is frequently complicated by polyhydramnios. Respiratory distress immediately after birth has been reported in a few patients. Characteristically, patients are born with increased birth weight and macrocephaly, which is followed by postnatal growth retardation and failure to thrive. Patients often require an enteral feeding tube because of oral motor apraxia and swallowing problems. This period is called the *marasmic phase*, which is followed by the *pseudo-thesaurismotic phase* that is characterized by a storage disease-like picture with macrocephaly, full cheeks, large mouth with thick lips, macroglossia, and gingival hyperplasia. The disease involves the head and neck (macrocephaly, coarse facies, strabismus, keratoconus, chorioretinal dystrophy, hypertelorism, epicanthal folds, downslanting palpebral fissures, low-set ears with fleshy earlobes and helices, depressed nasal bridge with bulbous nose and anteverted nostrils, full cheeks, micrognathia, retrognathia, large mouth with macroglossia, high arched palate, bifid uvula, abnormal teeth, short neck), the skeleton (short stature with adult height between 118 and 148 cm, barrel chest, pectus excavatum/carinatum, scoliosis, broad hands and feet, limited extension in elbow and wrist, pes equinovarus, subluxation of hip and elbow, osteoporosis), the skin (redundant skin on hands and feet leading to deep palmar and plantar creases and ridges, acanthosis nigricans, hyperkeratosis, fine hair, papillomata [facial, laryngeal, axillary, abdominal, cubital, popliteal, anal], multiple pigmented nevi, capillary hemangiomata on the forehead), the central nervous system (developmental delay with an IQ between 47 and 85, speech development delay, seizures, mild brain atrophy, cerebellar atrophy, generalized ventricular dilatation [occasionally requiring ventriculoperitoneal shunting], muscular hypotonia or hypertonia), and the genital region (cryptorchidism, inguinal hernia). Cardiac abnormalities including hypertrophic cardiomyopathy, pulmonary stenosis, atrial and ventricular septal defects, and dysrhythmias have been described. Hepatosplenomegaly and umbilical hernias have been described in some patients. These patients have an increased risk for malignant solid tumors (up to 17% of patients), including neuroblastoma, rhabdomyosarcoma, and bladder carcinoma. Laryngeal web, crumpled vocal cords, and tracheoesophageal fistula have been described in one patient each. Abnormal glucose metabolism occurs occasionally. A study found low levels of growth hormone and reported good response to growth hormone therapy. Cardiac problems, failure to thrive, and pneumonia are the main reasons for early death.

Precautions before anesthesia: Assess cardiac function and obtain an echocardiogram to exclude cardiac anomalies. Anticipate difficult airway management secondary to macroglossia, abnormal teeth, laryngeal anomalies, and short neck. Regular checks of perioperative glucose levels are recommended. Because these patients should undergo regular tumor screening, check the date and results of the last follow-up.

Anesthetic considerations: In one published case report, preoperative multiple atrial ectopic beats, gastrointestinal reflux, and thickened arytenoid folds were encountered. On the one hand, a rapid-sequence induction may be indicated because of gastroesophageal reflux. On the other hand, airway management may be difficult, so spontaneous ventilation should be maintained until the airway has been secured. It will therefore depend on the clinical situation, which problem will receive preference. Tracheobronchial secretions appear to be abundant and require repeated suctioning. Careful intraoperative positioning is needed because of limb deformities, osteoporosis, and a tendency to subluxations.

Pharmacological implications: Subacute bacterial endocarditis prophylaxis may be required. Avoid neuromuscular blockers until the airway has been secured (except for rapid sequence induction).

Other conditions to be considered:

☞**Cantu Syndrome:** A congenital multisystem syndrome involving neonatal macrosomia, cardiomegaly, osteodysplasia, and hypertrichosis.

☞**Noonan Syndrome:** A rare genetic disorder present at birth. Characterized by distinctive facial appearance, a broad or webbed neck, a low posterior hairline, and short stature. Micrognathia, kyphosis and/or scoliosis, and cardiac defects are present. Other features include coagulation disorders, platelet deficiencies, mild mental retardation, and cryptorchidism.

☞**Reynolds-Neri-Hermann Syndrome:** A rare syndrome characterized by postnatal growth retardation with cardiac defects (atrial septal defect, pulmonic stenosis) and craniofacial anomalies (facial features similar to Noonan syndrome). Other features include relative macrocephaly, micrognathia, high arched palate, splenomegaly, hypotonia or hypertonia, hydrocephalus and raised intracranial pressure, and brainstem atrophy (gait ataxia).

De Barsy Moens Diercks Syndrome (De Barsy Syndrome; Progeroid Syndrome of De Barsy; Corneal Clouding Cutis Laxa Mental Retardation Syndrome): Extremely rare disorder inherited as an autosomal recessive trait. The main characteristics are frontal bossing and large, prominent ears, athetosis, cornea clouding, hypotonia, hyperlaxity of the small joints, and/or short stature.

References:

Benni F, Leoni T, Iacobucci T, et al: Anaesthesiological considerations in Costello syndrome. *Paediatr Anaesth* 12:376, 2002.

Dearlove O, Harper N: Costello syndrome. *Paediatr Anaesth* 7:476, 1997.

Stein RI, Legault L, Daneman D, et al: Growth hormone deficiency in Costello syndrome. *Am J Med Genet* 129A:166, 2004.

Cousin-Walbaum-Cegarra Syndrome

At a glance: A syndrome of familial pelvic and scapular dysplasia, anomalies of the epiphyses, dwarfism, and dysmorphism.

Synonym: Pelviscapular Dysplasia.

Incidence and genetic inheritance: Presented in a North African brother and his sister whose parents were healthy first cousins. Most likely autosomal recessive inheritance. A total of three patients were reported.

Clinical aspects: Congenital dwarfism (rhizomelic micromelia), facial dysmorphism (macrocephaly, hypertelorism, low-set ears), short neck, agenesis of the scapular wings, and hypoplasia of the iliac and acetabular wings occurred in both patients. A high risk for hip dislocation is associated with the disorder. Moderate developmental delay, a cutaneous cervical diverticulum, and auricular anomalies were noted.

Anesthetic considerations: Anesthesia in this disorder has not been described. Expect difficult airway management depending on the degree of dysmorphism. Careful intraoperative positioning is needed to avoid dislocations of the hips. Mental retardation may affect patient cooperation. Sedative and/or anxiolytic premedication and/or the presence of the primary caregiver during induction of anesthesia may be helpful.

Other Condition to Be Considered:

Kosenow Syndrome (Scapuloiliac Dysplasia): Initially described in two unrelated girls presenting with marked hypoplasia of the scapulae, clavicles, and pelvis. Associated malformations included spina bifida and anomalies of the eyes (e.g., ectopic pupils) and ribs. It appears that the father of one of the girls had the same condition. Inheritance most likely is autosomal dominant.

References:

Cousin J, Walbaum R, Cegarra P, et al: Familial pelvi-scapulary dysplasia with anomalies of the epiphyses, dwarfism and dysmorphy: A new syndrome? *Arch Fr Pediatr* 39:173, 1982.

Elliott AM, Roeder ER, Witt DR, et al: Scapuloiliac dysostosis (Kosenow syndrome, pelvis-shoulder dysplasia) spectrum: Three additional cases. *Am J Med Genet* 95:496, 2000.

Hauser SE, Chemke JM, Bankier A: Pelvis-shoulder dysplasia. *Pediatr Radiol* 28:681, 1998.

Cowchock Syndrome

At a glance: An X-linked form of sensory and motor neuropathy characterized by atrophy of the peroneal muscle, but also involving other distal muscles of the legs and arms.

Synonyms: Cowchock Fischbeck Syndrome; Charcot-Marie-Tooth Disease with Deafness and Mental Retardation; Hereditary Motor Sensory Neuropathy (HMSN) II.

Incidence: Unknown. A few reports exist of familial series. Male offsprings are more severely affected.

Genetic inheritance: X-linked, with mapping to Xq24-q26. It may be either allelic to X-linked Charcot Marie Tooth (CMT) disease or a contiguous gene syndrome, with the features of ☞Charcot Marie Tooth Syndrome resulting from alterations in the CMTX1 gene or in one of the other two CMT genes on the X chromosome.

Pathophysiology: Consistent with hereditary motor sensory neuropathy type II. Electromyography demonstrates widespread denervation and occasional fibrillation. Motor nerve conduction velocities are normal to moderately delayed, however, sensory conduction in the median and sural nerves is markedly abnormal. Electron microscopy of sural nerve tissue reveals a paucity of myelinated axons. Audiometry shows sensorineural hearing loss.

Diagnosis: Based on the clinical findings in infants with foot drop, clawing of fingers, and progressive atrophy and weakness of peroneal and other distal foot muscles in combination with a positive family history. Electrophysiology plus microscopy show reduced conduction velocity, demyelination, and axonal degeneration.

Clinical aspects: Presentation is usually in infancy with slowly progressive distal or generalized muscle weakness and atrophy and diminished or absent deep tendon reflexes. Motor development is delayed. Other clinical features may include foot dropping (manifesting as frequent tripping), pes cavus deformity, muscle cramping, steppage or equine gait, "champagne bottle" or stork legs, hammertoes, and clawhand. Pain and temperature sensation are normal. The diaphragm, phrenic nerve, and vocal cords are occasionally involved. Frequently associated with mental retardation and deafness. Moderate disability in adulthood.

Precautions before anesthesia: Assess the patient neurologically and ask about respiratory and cardiac problems. Pulmonary function tests including a chest radiograph and arterial blood gas analysis should be performed if respiratory involvement (secondary to respiratory muscle weakness) is suspected. An electrocardiogram is recommended for all patients, and an echocardiogram may be indicated depending on the clinical findings.

Anesthetic considerations: Anesthesia may exacerbate preexisting respiratory disease, and prolonged postoperative mechanical ventilation may be required. A peripheral nerve stimulator should be used to monitor neuromuscular blockade if muscle relaxants will be used. However, care should be taken to place the electrodes on an unaffected nerve to prevent erroneous results. Regional anesthesia has been used successfully in multiple cases. Involvement of the autonomic nervous system may result in abnormal temperature regulation. Mental retardation and deafness may affect patient cooperation. Sedative and/or anxiolytic premedication and/or the presence of the primary caregiver during induction of anesthesia may be helpful.

Pharmacological implications: Specific experience is lacking, however, the literature indicates that the induction dose of thiopentone may need to be reduced in CMT disease. A small number of case reports indicate the use of succinylcholine in CMT may result in hyperkalemia or malignant hyperthermia-like reactions. However, this has not been confirmed by a larger, retrospective series of a total of 161 procedures in 86 patients, of whom 48% received succinylcholine and 90% received malignant hyperthermia triggering agents without significant adverse effects. It has been suggested, however, that individuals with acute exacerbations of the disease represent a subset of patients who have altered responses to muscle relaxants and that, in such a scenario, succinylcholine should be avoided and other muscle relaxants used in small incremental doses with neuromuscular monitoring only.

Other conditions to be considered: See ☞Hereditary Motor and Sensory Neuropathy for an overview of the different types.

☞**CHARCOT MARIE TOOTH DISEASE:** A hereditary polyneuropathy condition presenting with distal weakness and muscular atrophy (myopathy).

REFERENCES:

Cowchock FS, Duckett SW, Streletz LJ, et al: X-linked motor sensory neuropathy type-II with deafness and mental retardation: A new disorder. *Am J Med Genet* 20:307, 1985.

Priest JM, Fischbeck KH, Nouri N, et al: A locus for axonal motor-sensory neuropathy with deafness and mental retardation maps to Xq24-q26. *Genomics* 29:409, 1995.

Cowden Syndrome

At a glance: A rare syndrome characterized by multiple hamartomas (small flesh-colored nodules on the skin made up by hair follicles and small wart-like growths) and a risk of breast, thyroid, and uterine neoplasias.

Synonym: Multiple Hamartoma Syndrome.

History: Named after Rachel Cowden, the first patient described.

Incidence: More than 200 cases have been described in the medical literature. Males and females are equally affected, however, thyroid cancer is the most common cancer in males, whereas breast cancer is the most common in affected women.

Genetic inheritance: Autosomal dominant with interfamilial and intrafamilial variance.

Pathophysiology: Cowden syndrome results from a mutation in the PTEN (*p*hosphatase and *ten*sin homologue) tumor suppressor gene. (*Synonym:* MMAC1 [*m*utated in *m*ultiple *a*dvanced *c*ancers-1] gene), which has been mapped to 10q23. PTEN encodes a phosphatase involved in regulation of growth, survival, and death of cells. The lack of PTEN functionality appears to be responsible for the uncontrolled proliferation of certain cells and the formation of hamartomas (and neoplasias).

Diagnosis: Based on the clinical findings. Usually Cowden syndrome is diagnosed only after the first year of life. Mucocutaneous signs are most pathognomonic but least obvious. Signs include acral keratosis, facial trichilemmomas, oral papillomas, and scrotal tongue. The International Cowden Syndrome Consortium summarized the diagnostic features into major criteria (macrocephaly, thyroid cancer, breast cancer, and Lhermitte-Duclos disease [see Other Conditions to Be Considered]) and minor criteria (mental retardation, nonmalignant thyroid changes, nonmalignant breast tumors, gastrointestinal hamartomas, lipomas, fibromas, urogenital tumors). Mucocutaneous lesions alone can meet the criteria under certain circumstances (depending on the number and type of lesions). The diagnosis is considered very likely when one major and three minor criteria, two major criteria (but only if either macrocephaly or Lhermitte-Duclos disease is present), or four minor criteria are met.

Clinical aspects: Macrocephaly, not secondary to hydrocephalus, may be present in up to 39% of patients and usually becomes evident only after the first year of life. It is often accompanied by frontal bossing, adenoid facies, hypoplastic maxilla and mandible, and high arched palate. Mild mental retardation with seizures and cerebellar signs (tremor) is present in 12% of patients. Kyphosis, kyphoscoliosis, and anomalies of the thyroid gland are reported in approximately two thirds of patients and may include multinodular goiter, adenomas, and follicular adenocarcinoma. Patients should undergo regular checkups for signs of thyroid cancer (especially men). The most serious malignancy in females is (early-onset) breast cancer, which may affect up to one third of female patients and often occurs bilaterally. Gastrointestinal adenomas, hamartomatous and hyperplastic polyps, lymphangiomas, and ganglioneurofibromas may occur in almost three fourths of patients and can be localized anywhere between the esophagus and the anus (including gallbladder) but are most common in the colon. Malignant transformation is a possible risk. Urogenital lesions include carcinomas of the kidneys, urethra, and uterine cervix, ovarian cysts, leiomyomas, and teratomas, vaginal and vulvar cysts, and testicular hamartomas. Mucocutaneous lesions are present in more than 90% of patients and may appear in different forms. In more than three fourths of patients, small, white, oral papules representing fibromas with a diameter up to 3 mm can be detected on the lips, palate, gingiva, and tonsillar fossae. Involvement of the tongue can result in scrotal tongue (lingua scrotalis), with thickening and deep furrowing giving it the appearance of scrotal skin. Verruciform, flesh-colored papules (most often trichilemmomas) with a diameter of up to 5 mm are often located in periorificial areas and exhibit a keratin-plugged center. About two thirds of patients manifest acral keratosis characterized by verruciform papules on the dorsum of the hands and the feet, while approximately one third of patients have signs of keratosis palmoplantaris. Additional skin lesions may include subcutaneous lipomas, hemangiomas, and neuromas.

Precautions before anesthesia: Assessment of the upper airway is crucial because hypoplasia of maxilla and mandible have been described, and potential obstruction by tumors is possible. Be aware of other relevant problems, such as thyroid dysfunction (obtain laboratory results of thyroid function free T_4, T_3 and TSH). It may be wise to obtain a complete blood count preoperatively because anemia may result from intestinal polyps or malignancies. Mental retardation may affect patient cooperation. Sedative and/or anxiolytic premedication and/or the presence of the primary caregiver during induction of anesthesia may be helpful.

Anesthetic considerations: Patients may present for multiple surgical procedures because of multiple tumors. Airway management may be difficult because of macrocephaly, hypoplastic maxilla with high arched palate, hypoplastic mandible, thyroid tumors, and papillomatosis of the base of the tongue, pharynx, and larynx. In one case laryngeal and hypopharyngeal papillomas resulted in difficult airway management complicated with bleeding and acute airway obstruction requiring emergency tracheostomy. Maintenance of spontaneous ventilation until the airway has been secured and availability of alternative airway management options (e.g., fiberoptic bronchoscope, laryngeal mask airway) is recommended. However, if gastrointestinal obstruction results from tumors, a rapid-sequence technique is recommended or should at least be weighed against maintenance of spontaneous ventilation because of expected airway problems.

Pharmacological implications: Hepatic or renal involvement is unlikely unless these organs are affected by tumors. Avoid neuromuscular blockers until the airway has been secured (except for rapid sequence induction). One case of postoperative delirium was proposed to be related to abnormal metabolism of buprenorphine. Consider interactions between antiepileptic treatment and anesthetic drugs.

Other conditions to be considered:

☞**Bannayan-Zonana Syndrome:** This inherited disorder is characterized by excessive growth prenatally and postnatally, manifesting with macrocephaly and scaphocephaly with normal intelligence or mild mental retardation and multiple hamartomas (lipomas, intestinal polyps). As affected infants age, the growth rate slows down and commonly results in normal adult height.

☞**Carney Complex** consists of spotty skin pigmentation in association with multiple neoplasias (mainly cardiac and endocrine tumors).

☞**Proteus Syndrome:** A rare congenital hamartomatous disorder characterized by multiple, diverse, somatic manifestations: partial bilateral gigantism of hands and feet, nevi, hemihypertrophy, subcutaneous tumors, and macrocephaly with cranial hyperostoses It is named after the Greek god Proteus, "the polymorphous," who could change his shape at will to avoid capture.

☞**Riley-Smith Syndrome:** A rare syndrome very similar to the Bannayan-Zonana syndrome characterized by macrocephaly, pseudopapillomata, hemangiomas, and multiple lipomas. Subcutaneous hemangiomas may be present at birth or appear later in childhood.

Lhermitte-Duclos Syndrome (Dysplastic Gangliocytoma of the Cerebellum; Benign Hypertrophy of the Cerebellum; Diffuse Ganglioneuroma of the Cerebellar Cortex; Neurocystic Blastoma; Hamartoblastoma; Cerebellar Hamartoma; Cerebellar Gangliomatosis; Neurocytoma Myelinicum; Gangliocytoma Myelinicum Diffusum; Purkinjeoma): Approximately 100 cases have been described. Patients present in young adult age with symptoms of cerebellar dysfunction (absent or only minimal signs in 50%), occlusive hydrocephalus with signs of increased intracranial pressure. However, symptoms may already be present shortly after birth. In approximately 60% of patients, Lhermitte-Duclos syndrome occurs sporadically, in the remaining 40%, an association with Cowden syndrome can be diagnosed. Magnetic resonance imaging usually confirms the clinical diagnosis. Macroscopically, the cerebellar folia and cortex are enlarged. Histologic examination reveals replacement of the cerebellar internal granular cell layer by large dysplastic neuronal cell bodies resembling Purkinje cells. Prominent myelinated tracts with axonal enlargement in the outer molecular layer of the cerebellar cortex are considered typical.

References:

Omote K, Kawamata T, Imaizumi H, et al: Case of Cowden's disease that caused airway obstruction during induction of anesthesia. *Anesthesiology* 91:1537, 1999.

Pilarski R, Eng C: Will the real Cowden syndrome please stand up (again)? Expanding mutational and clinical spectra of the PTEN hamartoma tumour syndrome. *J Med Genet* 41:323, 2004.

Shiraishi N, Nakamura T, Saito H, et al: Anesthetic management of a patient with Cowden syndrome. *Masui* 44:282, 1995.

Cramer-Niederdellmann Syndrome

At a glance: An extremely rare syndrome combining gigantism, pigmented nevi, jaw cysts, and neurologic signs.
Synonym: Cerebral Gigantism with Jaw Cysts.

Incidence and genetic inheritance: Incidence unknown. Initially described in nine patients from two families. Autosomal dominant inheritance.

Clinical aspects: The disorder may affect the head and neck (macrocephaly, mandibular prognathia, frontal and biparietal bossing, odontogenic cysts of jaws, cleft lip and palate), the spine (scoliosis, kyphosis, abnormal cervical vertebrae, vertebral fusion), the central nervous system (hydrocephalus, ventricular malformation, cerebellar signs, intracranial calcifications, muscular hyptonia, hyporeflexia or areflexia, electroencephalographic anomalies, insensitivity to pain), and the skin (signs of ☞Gorlin-Goltz Syndrome). In addition, amyotrophy or muscle agenesis and limb and digit abnormalities have been reported. Disturbances in the calcium metabolism seem to be a prominent feature of this disorder. Perioperative control of calcium serum levels is recommended.

Anesthetic considerations: Given the features of this disorder, airway management is expected to be difficult. Maintenance of spontaneous ventilation is recommended until the airway has been secured. Caution with depolarizing and nondepolarizing muscle relaxants is advisable in view of hypotonia and neuromuscular abnormalities. Central neuraxial blockade may be difficult because of vertebral malformations and probably should be avoided considering the neurologic impairment.

Other conditions to be considered:

☞**SOTOS SYNDROME:** Characterized by excessively rapid growth during the first year of life, acromegalic craniocerebral features (macrocephaly, prominent forehead), and a nonprogressive cerebral disorder with mental retardation. Other features include high arched palate and prognathism with premature eruption of teeth, hypotonia, hyper- or hypothyroidism, and delayed motor and cognitive development.

☞**GORLIN-GOLTZ SYNDROME:** Autosomal dominant inherited ectodermal disorder with complete penetrance but variable expressivity, characterized by multiple basal cell nevi on the torso and shoulders with a potential of malignant degeneration.

REFERENCE:

Cramer H, Niederdellmann H: Cerebral gigantism associated with jaw cyst basal cell naevoid syndrome in two families. *Arch Psychiatr Nervenkr* 233:111, 1983.

Crane-Heise Syndrome

At a glance: A severe lethal syndrome combining disproportionately large head with peculiar facies and bilateral talipes equinovarus.

Incidence and genetic inheritance: Approximately 10 cases have been described. Most likely autosomal recessive transmission. Parental consanguinity was observed in some, but not all cases.

Clinical aspects: This complex polymalformative syndrome with severe intrauterine growth retardation may involve the head and neck (macrocephaly with disproportionate small face, deficient mineralization of the calvaria [or even absence of frontal, parietal, and occipital bones], agenesis of the corpus callosum, absence of the cingulate gyrus, increased ventricular size, severe hypertelorism, low-set and posteriorly rotated ears with hypoplasia of the helix, depressed nasal bridge, wide and upturned nares, lateral cleft lip, cleft palate, or even absence of hard and soft palate, severe micrognathia/retrognathia, short neck) and the skeleton (absent cervical vertebrae, absent or abnormal clavicles, hypoplastic scapulae, 11 rib pairs, large and small joint contractures, club foot, hypoplastic distal middle phalanges, soft tissue syndactyly of fingers and toes). Either hirsutism or absence of scalp and body hair, esophageal stenosis, redundant bowel loops, hypoplastic external genitalia, hypogonadism, and cryptorchidism have been described, but are not constant features. Cardiovascular anomalies are inconstant and may consist of thin myocardium and thick-walled ascending aorta and pulmonary artery. Intrauterine death or death in early infancy is common.

Anesthetic considerations: It is unlikely that these patients present for anesthesia. Difficult tracheal intubation should be anticipated, and maintenance of spontaneous ventilation is recommended until the airway has been secured. Subclavian central venous access should be avoided because of clavicular malformations. Careful intraoperative positioning is required, and the brain must be protected from external pressure in the absence of cranial bones.

Other condition to be considered:

☞**FETAL AMINOPTERIN SYNDROME:** A polymalformative teratogenic syndrome characterized by short stature, skull anomalies, hydrocephalus, and facial anomalies (abnormal auricles, hypertelorism, micrognathia, cleft palate).

REFERENCES:

Barnicoat AJ, Seller MJ, Bennett CP: Fetus with features of Crane-Heise syndrome and aminopterin syndrome sine aminopterin (ASSAS). *Clin Dysmorphol* 3:353, 1994.

Crane JP, Heise RL: New syndrome in three affected siblings. *Pediatrics* 68:235, 1981.

Zand DJ, Carpentieri D, Huff D, et al: Crane-Heise syndrome: A second familial case report with elaboration of phenotype. *Am J Med Genet* 118A:223, 2003.

Craniodiaphyseal Dysplasia

At a glance: A bone disorder characterized by marked hyperostosis of the craniofacial bones and diaphyseal expansion of the tubular bones resulting in significant clinical complications.

Synonym: Schäfer Stein Oshman Syndrome

Incidence and genetic inheritance: Fewer than 20 cases have been described in the literature. Both autosomal recessive and dominant forms but also sporadic cases have been described. In some cases the parents were consanguineous.

Clinical aspects: This syndrome is a metabolic bone disease resulting in progressive and massive thickening and sclerosis of the skull, mandible, maxilla, clavicles, and ribs. No surgical or medical cure is available. Metabolic therapy with Calcitrol to promote osteoclastic remodeling and restricted calcium intake to prevent hypercalcemia aimed at controlling the process usually are not successful. The diagnosis is confirmed by radiographs, which demonstrate diaphyseal expansion of tubular bones with sclerosis and minimal metaphyseal expansion of the epiphyses, and marked hyperostosis and sclerosis of the ribs, sternum, clavicles, and scapulae. The humeri may show endosteal cortical thickening. Diaphyseal undertubulation may lead to straightened humeri with cylindrical shape, resembling a "policeman's nightstick" or a "truncheon." Symptoms are usually seen by approximately 3 months of age, but may start at birth and progress with bone pain, pronounced deformities such as progressive cranial hyperostosis with obliteration of the diploic spaces and the paranasal sinuses, development of foraminal

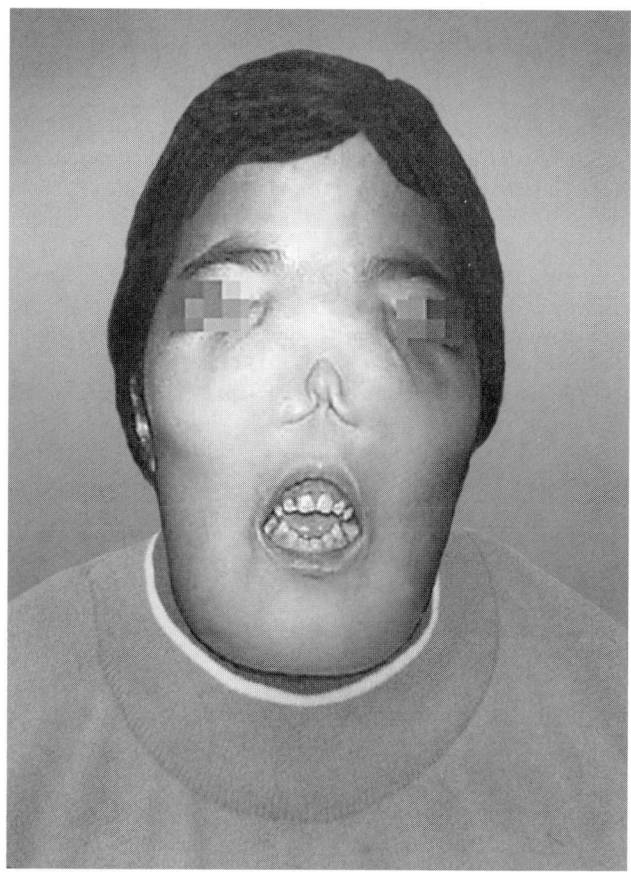

Craniodiaphyseal Dysplasia   Airway management in this adolescent boy with craniodiaphyseal dysplasia was very difficult.

encroachment leading to neuropathy with progressive deterioration of vision (nonreactive pupils have been described) and hearing, obstruction of jugular venous outflow, chronic epiphora secondary to nasolacrimal duct obstruction, chronic nasal obstruction secondary to choanal stenosis (may lead to respiratory distress in infancy), facial hyperostosis with overgrown nasal bridge, gross mandibular hyperplasia relative to the maxilla with limited mouth opening from severe immobility of the temporomandibular joints, facial muscle atrophy and weakness, mild hydrocephalus with herniation of the cerebellar tonsils through a small foramen magnum, cervical syringomyelia, mental retardation, and restricted cervical spine (especially atlantoaxial) mobility. Flexion of the neck may also be limited by the bulky mandible pressing against the chest, whereas extension of the head may be limited by the bulky occiput. Death usually occurs in childhood.

Anesthetic considerations: The combination of choanal stenosis, major mandibular hyperplasia, and significant limitation of mouth opening and cervical spine mobility puts these children at very high risk for difficult airway management. A clear backup plan must be in place prior to induction of anesthesia. An awake fiberoptic intubation is the technique of choice. An induction technique with maintenance of spontaneous ventilation may also be suitable. However, hypercapnia should be avoided because intracranial pressure may be increased. Successful tracheal intubation using a fiberoptic guided intubation through a laryngeal mask has been reported in the literature. Prolonged postoperative mechanical ventilation may be required, particularly when the surgery involves the face. Tracheal

extubation may be performed a few days later when the swelling has resolved and is best done with the patient fully awake in the operating room with all the equipment prepared for eventual need of reintubation.

Other conditions to be considered:

☞**CAMURATI-ENGELMANN SYNDROME:** Musculoskeletal syndrome leading to enhanced bone formation and hyperostosis and sclerosis of the diaphyses of the long bones.

☞**PYLE DISEASE:** An inherited bone dysplasia affecting the enchondral growth of long bones, which results in failure of metophyseal modeling and the so-called "Erlenmeyer flask deformity."

REFERENCES:

Appleby JN, Bingham RM; Craniodiaphyseal dysplasia; Another cause of difficult intubation. *Paediatr Anaesth* 6:225, 1996.

Brueton LA, Winter RM; Craniodiaphyseal dysplasia. *J Med Genet* 27:701, 1990.

Marden FA, Wippold FJ 2nd: MR imaging features of craniodiaphyseal dysplasia. *Pediatr Radiol* 34:167, 2004.

Craniofrontonasal Dysplasia

At a glance: An X-linked syndrome, strangely more severe in females, combining frontonasal dysplasia, coronal craniosynostosis, various other skeletal and soft tissue abnormalities and mild mental deficiency.

Synonyms: Frontofacionasal Dysostosis/Dysplasia.

Incidence and genetic inheritance: Incidence is not known. Females are affected approximately four to six times more often than males, with the disease being usually much more severe in females, a highly unusual feature for an X-linked (dominant) disorder. The mutation has been mapped to Xp22.

Clinical aspects: Almost all symptoms (except the urogenital findings) are either only present in females or more severe in females. Multiple malformations have been described involving the head and neck (coronal synostosis, anterior bifid cranium, brachycephaly, frontal bossing, facial asymmetry [often secondary to unicoronal craniosynostosis], downslanting palpebral fissures, hypertelorism, strabismus, nystagmus, bifid nose, high arched palate, cleft lip, cleft palate, short neck), the chest (diaphragmatic hernia, Sprengel deformity, clavicular pseudarthrosis, pectus excavatus, axillary pterygia, unilateral breast hypoplasia), and the skeleton (growth retardation, scoliosis, muscular hypotonia and joint laxity, limb abnormalities such as different leg length, brachydactyly, syndactyly of fingers and toes, broad halluces). Other features can include developmental delay, dry, thick, frizzy hair, longitudinally grooved nails, shawl scrotum, and hypospadias.

Anesthetic considerations: Airway management difficulties should be expected depending on the degree of asymmetry and palatal anomalies. Maintenance of spontaneous ventilation is recommended until the airway has been secured. Intraoperative positioning may be difficult and requires care. The subclavian approach for central venous cannulation may be difficult in the presence of clavicular pseudarthrosis. Be aware of the possibility of diaphragmatic hernias in newborns. Mental retardation and deafness may affect patient cooperation. Sedative and/or anxiolytic premedication and/or the presence of the primary caregiver during induction of anesthesia may be helpful.

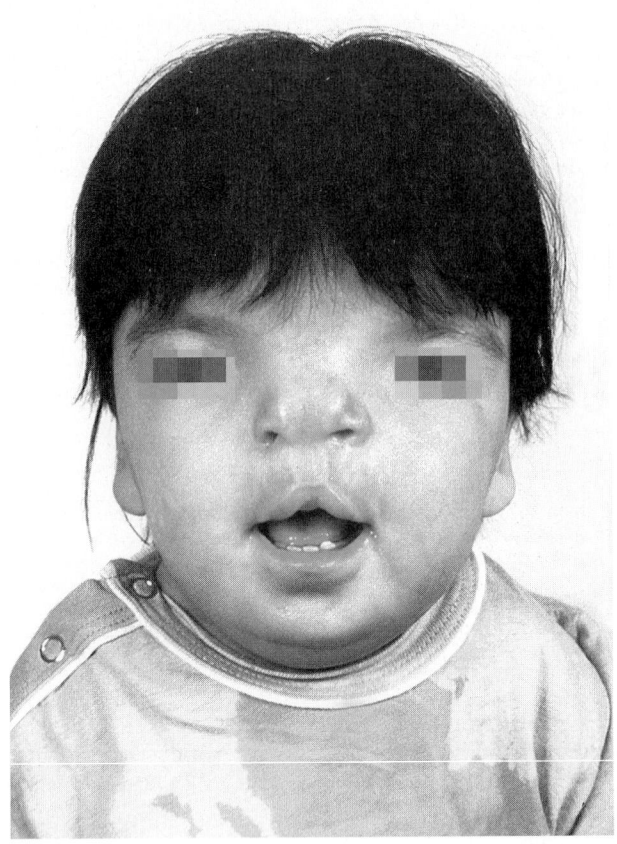

Craniofrontonasal Dysplasia Facial asymmetry, hypertelorism, bifid nose, repaired cleft lip, and short neck in a 3-year-old girl with craniofrontonasal dysplasia.

REFERENCES:

Pulleyn LJ, Winter RM, Reardon W, et al: Further evidence from two families that craniofrontonasal dysplasia maps to Xp22. *Clin Genet* 55:473, 1999.

Saavedra D, Richieri-Costa A, Guion-Almeida ML, et al: Craniofrontonasal syndrome: Study of 41 patients. *Am J Med Genet* 61:147, 1996.

Wieacker P, Wieland I: Clinical and genetic aspects of craniofrontonasal syndrome: towards resolving a genetic paradox. *Mol Genet Metab* 86:110, 2005.

Craniolacunia

At a glance: A transitory disease characterized by punched-out skull defects.

Synonyms: Lacunar Skull; Lückenschädel.

Incidence and genetic inheritance: Unknown.

Clinical aspects: Craniolacunia is considered a mesenchymal dysplasia affecting the calvarial ossification. It may be an isolated finding; however, most often it is associated with defects in neural tube closure, such as ☞Arnold-Chiari Syndrome Type II, myelomeningocele, and encephalocele. Occasionally it occurs with other cerebral lesions. The exact etiology of the defects is unknown, however, a suggestion has involved the lack of cerebral ventricular distension as a result of the open neural tube, which then results in

a lack of distension of the fetal brain, which is necessary to induce normal development of the membranous plates of the fetal calvaria. Instead, abnormally organized collagen fibers are produced and their ossification results in the defects seen in craniolacunia. The fact that the defects resolve by 6 months of age has been explained with remodeling in response to either normal expansion of cerebral tissue or development of hydrocephalus. The most commonly affected bones are the parietal and occipital bones. The lesions appear as multiple, "punched-out" skull defects with well-defined borders and bony trabecular ridges involving the inner table and the diploe (less commonly the outer table) with a diameter of up to 1 cm. Generally, craniolacunia is not associated with increased intracranial pressure and appears not to affect neurologic outcome.

Anesthetic considerations: Craniolacunia per se should not affect anesthesia. However, it seems wise to avoid any pressure on the skull, especially when handling or positioning the baby. Other anesthesia considerations are guided by the underlying disease (e.g., Arnold-Chiari Syndrome, myelomeningocele).

REFERENCES:

Wilson WG, Alford BA, Schnatterly PT: Craniolacunia as the result of compression and decompression of the fetal skull. *Am J Med Genet* 27:729, 1987.

Coley BD: Ultrasound diagnosis of luckenschadel (lacunar skull). *Pediatr Radiol* 30:82, 2000.

Craniomicromelic Syndrome

At a glance: A severe and lethal disease combining major craniofacial, cardiac, and skeletal anomalies.

Incidence and genetic inheritance: Three cases have been reported, two were sisters and one was a female fetus of 29 weeks' gestation. Most likely autosomal recessive transmission.

Clinical aspects: Numerous, severe abnormalities associated with intrauterine or neonatal death occur. The defects in these patients included intrauterine growth retardation with delayed or absent ossification, deficient skull bones, large fontanelles with wide cranial sutures, and macrocephaly. The superior portion of the parietal bones and frontal bones were deficient in one of the patients, leaving a 4-cm diameter space over the vertex. Central nervous system anomalies consisted of dilatation of the frontal horns of the lateral ventricles, "splayed" cerebellar hemispheres, irregular falx cerebri, and a posterior encephalocele containing brain tissue. Facial features consisted of low-set ears, protruding nasal spine, micrognathia, retrognathia, and cleft palate. The chest appeared narrow with normally lobulated but hypoplastic lungs and an enlarged heart. The urinary system was dilated with decreased lobulation of the kidneys. The gallbladder was absent, the intestine was short and partially distended, and the uterus was hypoplastic. Skin creases were abnormal and the fingers appeared short as a result of cutaneous syndactyly of all five fingers. Syndactyly of the toes with a bilateral sandal gap was seen.

Anesthetic considerations: It is highly unlikely that these patients will present for anesthesia. Tracheal intubation would be expected to be very difficult, as could peripheral venous access because of limb anomalies. Cardiac, pulmonary, and renal function most likely would be severely abnormal and require extensive preoperative assessment.

REFERENCES:

Baralle D, Firth H: Craniomicromelic syndrome: Report of a third case. *Am J Med Genet* 87:360, 1999.

Barr M, Heidelberger KP, Comstock CH: Craniomicromelic syndrome: A newly recognized lethal condition with craniosynostosis, distinct facial anomalies, short limbs, and intrauterine growth retardation. *Am J Med Genet* 58:348, 1995.

Craniosynostosis

At a glance: A congenital anomaly of the skull characterized by premature fusion of one or more cranial sutures.

Synonym: Craniostenosis.

Incidence: Estimated to be approximately 1:200,000 live births. Sagittal and lambdoid craniosynostosis (the most common type) are approximately four times more common in males than in females, whereas unicoronal craniosynostosis is more common in females. For the other forms, the distribution is about equal between the two genders.

Genetic inheritance: A positive family history is present in up to 40% of cases, with genetic syndromes accounting for at least 50% of those cases. The most common syndromes include ☞Apert Syndrome and ☞Crouzon Syndrome. Both autosomal dominant and autosomal recessive inheritance have been described, but sporadic occurrence also is common. Genetic mutations that may be responsible for craniosynostosis include mutations in the fibroblast growth factor receptors (FGFR1, FGFR2, FGFR3), the TWIST, and MSX2 genes.

Pathophysiology: The etiology is unknown but may involve abnormal cranial suture development resulting in failure of growth perpendicular to the affected suture and overgrowth of skull parallel to the affected suture. Environmental factors etiologically linked to craniosynostoses include rickets and hyperthyroidism. Drugs that may be involved in craniosynostosis include phenytoin, retinoids, valproic acid, aminopterin/methotrexate, fluconazole, and cyclophosphamide. In some cases, local intrauterine factors related to constraint of the fetus (e.g., abnormal positioning in utero, multiple pregnancy, oligohydramnios) have been linked to craniosynostosis. The developing brain is the driving power behind skull growth and forces the skull to compensatory growth in directions perpendicular to the fused suture along adjacent open sutures.

Diagnosis: The diagnosis may be suspected clinically if special attention is paid to the head circumference (percentiles), shape and presence of any deformities, size of the fontanelles, palpable ridges over affected sutures with absent movement of the bone on either side of the suture on palpation, neurologic behavior and development of the infant, the pupils and their reaction to light, and funduscopic evaluation for papilledema. Radiologic examinations (e.g., computed tomography scanning and/or magnetic resonance imaging) confirm the diagnosis. True craniosynostosis must be differentiated from birth molding (present at birth and resolving within days or weeks) and positional plagiocephaly without synostosis (a frequent finding resulting from local pressure on a specific area of the skull (same position), typically the occipital region leading to occipital or lambdoid plagiocephaly.

Clinical aspects: It must be differentiated between syndromic and nonsyndromic craniosynostosis. Nonsyndromic cases account for approximately 50% of all craniosynostoses and are commonly limited to synostoses of a single suture (sagittal, metopic, or

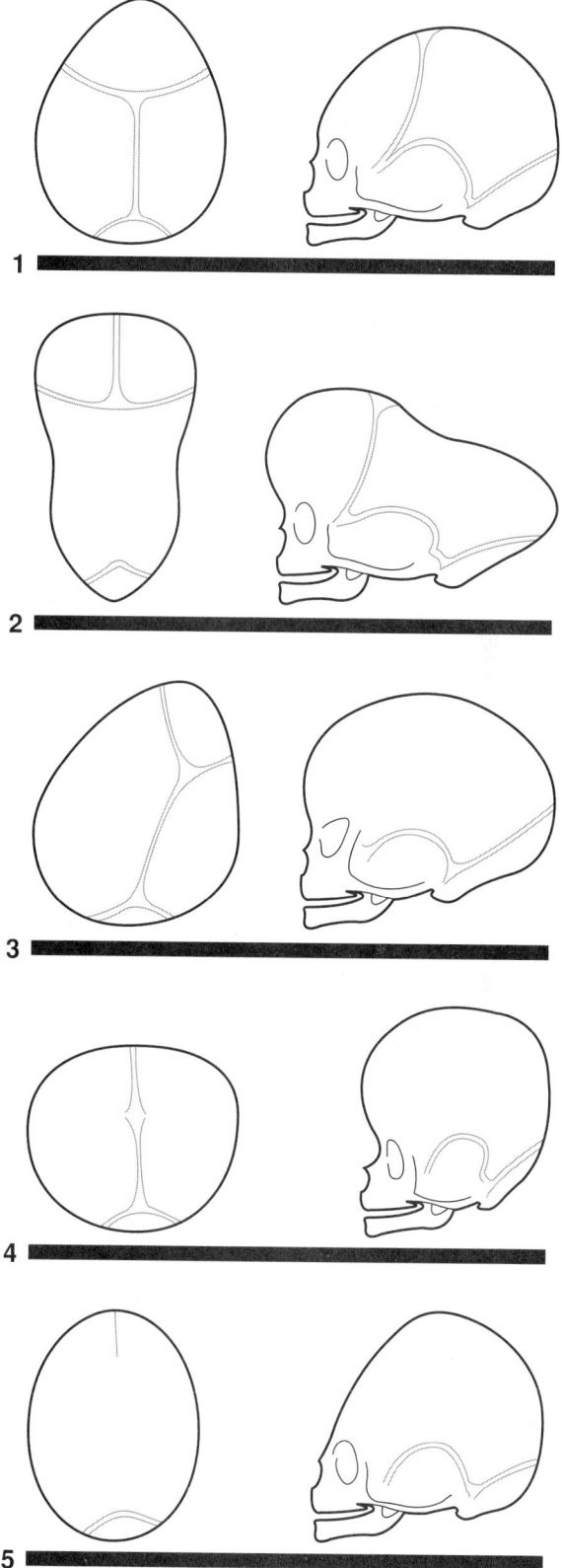

Craniosynostosis Different morphological types of craniosynostoses: 1. trigonocephaly; 2. scaphocephaly; 3. plagiocephaly; 4. brachycephaly; 5. oxycephaly. (Modified from Bissonnette B, Dalens B: *Pediatric Anesthesia,* McGraw-Hill, 2002, p. 1334, with permission).

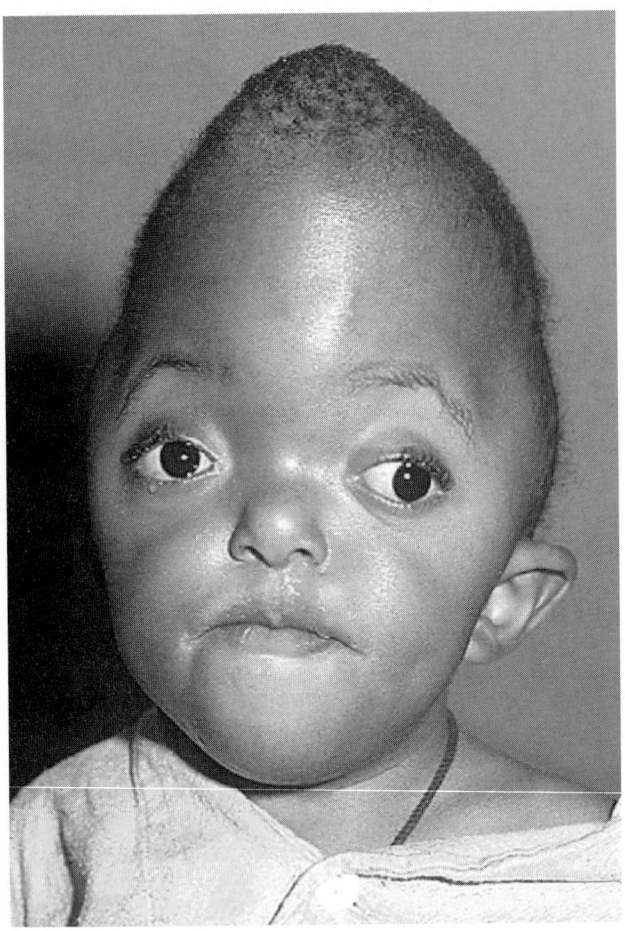

Craniosynostosis   Craniosynostosis resulting in keel-shaped forehead (trigonocephaly) in a young boy.

coronal) and usually not associated with increased intracranial pressure, whereas syndromic craniosynostosis refers (most commonly) to patients with ☞Acrocephalosyndactyly Syndromes (i.e., Apert, Crouzon, Pfeiffer, and Saethre Chotzen syndromes). Hydrocephalus, increased intracranial pressure, and developmental delay may occur secondary to craniosynostosis and are more common with bicoronal, combined coronal and sagittal, and total craniosynostosis. The anatomical classification is based on the suture(s) affected:

Sagittal craniosynostosis: Accounts for 40% of all craniosynostoses and most cases of single suture craniosynostosis. It results in dolichocephaly or scaphocephaly (decreased biparietal diameter and increased anteroposterior diameter) with frontal and occipital bossing if left untreated. The vast majority of patients are males. Increased intracranial pressure and mental retardation are rare.

Unicoronal craniosynostosis: This type of craniosynostosis is responsible for approximately 15% of all cases of craniosynostosis and is more common in females. Left uncorrected, plagiocephaly with marked craniofacial asymmetry develops with flattening of the forehead and the cheeks on the affected side, proptosis, ipsilateral elevated supraorbital ridge, and malalignment of the eyes. The orbital asymmetry may cause amblyopia. Frontal bossing occurs on the unaffected side. Increased intracranial pressure is not common.

Bicoronal craniosynostosis: 20% of all craniosynostoses leading to brachycephaly (decreased anteroposterior diameter) with a flattened, wide forehead and characteristic deformities of the orbits

(shallow) leading to eye (proptosis) and nasolacrimal duct complications. Associated anomalies include choanal atresia, hypoplasia of the maxilla (and midface), high arched palate, increased intracranial pressure, and developmental delay. This type of craniosynostosis typically is found in Apert and Crouzon syndromes.

Lambdoid craniosynostosis: Responsible for up to 3% of craniosynostoses and affects males about four times more often than females. This form of craniosynostosis has to be carefully distinguished from deformational, nonsynostotic plagiocephaly, which is much more common than previously thought and explains why older studies report a significantly higher overall percentage for lambdoid craniosynostosis. Bilateral involvement results in brachycephaly with anterior and inferior displacement of the ears, while in unilateral cases flattening of the occiput and ipsilateral forehead bulging result in rhomboid skull and the same ear displacement as in bilateral craniosynostosis.

Metopic craniosynostosis: Approximately 4% of all craniosynostoses. The metopic suture is the first suture to close, which normally occurs soon after birth. Premature closure leads to trigonocephaly (keel shaped, pointed forehead). Hypotelorism may occur if the frontonasal suture also is affected. In severe cases, the forehead appears narrow with compensatory widening of the skull posterior to the coronal sutures. This is occasionally associated with mental retardation secondary to cerebral malformations, such as arrhinencephaly or even holoprosencephaly.

Coronal and sagittal craniosynostosis: Approximately 10% of all craniosynostoses. Typically, acrocephaly (cone-shaped head) develops.

Lambdoid and sagittal craniosynostosis: Approximately 1% of all craniosynostoses. Occipital plagiocephaly typically results.

Multisuture craniosynostosis: Results in oxycephaly (short and narrow head) with underdeveloped paranasal sinuses, shallow orbits, increased intracranial pressure, and mental retardation. Most often, the sagittal and coronal sutures are affected. Involvement of all sutures except the metopic suture leads to ☞Cloverleaf Skull (Kleeblattschädel). In all these cases, increased intracranial pressure and mental retardation are common.

Total craniosynostosis: May be responsible for up to 10% of all craniosynostoses and lead to microcephaly and increased intracranial pressure.

Precautions before anesthesia: It is important to identify associated syndromes and risks related to them preoperatively. Raised intracranial pressure is not uncommon and often underestimated and should be taken into consideration for the anesthetic plan. Upper airway obstruction is a common feature, and careful evaluation of the airway is required with regard to airway management. Obtain a complete blood count, serum levels of electrolytes, and coagulation parameters preoperatively. If craniosynostosis repair is planned, ensure packed red cells are available in the operating room before skin incision is made.

Anesthetic considerations: Surgical treatment of craniosynostosis can be an anesthetic challenge with a high complication rate. Mental retardation may lead to poor cooperation upon separation from the parents or during induction of anesthesia. Difficult airway management should be expected. Maintaining spontaneous ventilation and oxygenation during attempts to control the airway is strongly recommended. Be prepared to use alternative techniques to manage the airway (e.g., laryngeal mask, fiberoptic intubation). A surgeon familiar with surgical airway management and the necessary equipment should always be present in the operating room. Specific anesthetic measures are required in case of increased intracranial pressure. Careful protection of the eyes must be provided in case of proptosis because of the high risk for corneal damage. Current surgical technique for craniosynostosis consists of total cranial vault reconstruction, which carries a high risk of major blood loss (often significantly more than one circulating blood volume). Large-bore intravenous access with the possibility for rapid transfusion is mandatory. However, vascular access in these patients often is challenging. Accurate evaluation of blood loss usually is difficult. Invasive hemodynamic monitoring with the possibility of regular intraoperative blood work sampling (complete blood count, blood gas analysis, serum electrolytes, and coagulation parameters) is required. Depending on the patient's positioning, the risk of venous air embolism should be kept in mind and the need for central venous access considered. For this reason, nitrous oxide should not be used in these patients. To reduce the amount of homologous blood transfusions, preoperative hemodilution, intraoperative cell saver techniques, and induced arterial hypotension have been used. However, arterial hypotension should not be tolerated in patients with increased intracranial pressure in order to maintain cerebral perfusion pressure. Ventilation should aim at normocapnia or mild hypocapnia. Hypothermia in these usually small patients is not uncommon because of massive transfusion and the prolonged operative time. Although mild hypothermia might offer some degree of cerebral protection, moderate hypothermia must be avoided. Postoperative ventilation may be necessary in the presence of significant facial edema associated with the surgical procedure. Securing the endotracheal tube with a suture rather than a tape is preferable because accidental extubation could be fatal (facial edema!).

Pharmacological implications: Sedative premedication in patients with increased intracranial pressure should be used with caution and under supervision of trained personnel only. Hypotensive anesthesia is most often achieved by using volatile anesthetics, opioids, and/or sympathodrenergic receptor blocking drugs. Avoid nitrous oxide secondary to the risk of venous air embolism. Avoid muscle relaxants until the airway has been secured. Avoid ketamine and succinylcholine in case of increased intracranial pressure.

REFERENCES:

Orliaguet G, Meyer P, Blanot S: Anesthetic management for craniosynostosis. *Ann Fr Anesth Reanim* 21:111, 2002.

Ridgway EB, Weiner HL: Skull deformities. *Pediatr Clin North Am* 51:359, 2004.

Scholtes JL, Thauvoy C, Moulin D, et al: Craniofaciosynostosis: Anaesthetic and preoperative management. Report of 71 operations. *Acta Anaesthesiol Belg* 36:176, 1985.

CREST Syndrome

At a glance: An autoimmune connective tissue disorder associated with anticentromere antibodies. A form of scleroderma associated with esophageal dysmotility. CREST is an acronym for *c*alcinosis, *R*aynaud phenomenon, *e*sophageal dysmotility, *s*clerodactyly, *t*elangiectasis.

Synonyms: Limited Scleroderma; Thibièrge-Weissenbach Syndrome (some authors use Thibièrge Weissenbach Syndrome to describe the calcinosis of the hand in combination with ischemia in the context of scleroderma).

History: First described in 1910 by G. Thibièrge and R.J.E. Weissenbach, two French physicians.

Incidence: The incidence of CREST syndrome is not known. The incidence of systemic sclerosis in the general population is in the range of approximately 2–7:1,000,000 (with geographical differences). All ethnicities can be affected. Females are affected two to four times more often than males.

Genetic inheritance: Although a few cases with an inheritance pattern have been described, in most cases autoimmune processes appear to be involved in the pathogenesis of this disorder. A genetic predisposition may be present.

Pathophysiology: The three primary pathologic processes of scleroderma are initially perivascular infiltration with predominantly lymphocytes and macrophages, followed by collagen (including fibronectin and proteoglycans) deposition with tissue thickening and fibrosis secondary to chronic activation of skin fibroblasts, and vascular changes mainly affecting the small arteries and presenting with endothelial injury, intima proliferation, vasospasms, and significantly decreased neovascularization. It has been suggested that several cytokines are involved in the pathogenesis of this disorder, particularly transforming growth factor β and interleukin-4, which are both present in increased concentrations in this disorder, while the level of interferon-γ, which acts as an inhibitor of collagen synthesis, is decreased.

Diagnosis: The minimal diagnostic criteria for scleroderma required by the American College of Rheumatology include either the major criterion of proximal cutaneous scleroderma (defined as symmetric thickening, tightening, and induration of the skin of the fingers and the skin proximal to the metacarpophalangeal or metatarsophalangeal joints. The changes may affect the entire limb or spread to head, neck, and trunk) or two of the three minor criteria (i.e., sclerodactyly [aforementioned findings, but strictly limited to the fingers], digital [finger pad] pitting scars, or bilateral pulmonary fibrosis with reticular or reticulonodular pattern on the chest radiograph). The presence of anticentromere antibodies in the serum may be helpful for the diagnosis (positive in approximately 50% of patients with CREST syndrome), while only approximately 20% test positive for scleroderma antibody (SCL-70/topoisomerase I). However, overall the sensitivity and specificity of these antibodies are limited.

Clinical aspects: Two different forms of scleroderma have been recognized. The localized form includes morphea and linear scleroderma ("sclérodermie en coup de sabre" if located in the facial area) and does not result in visceral organ involvement. The two types of systemic scleroderma are limited scleroderma (80% of patients) and diffuse scleroderma (20%). In limited scleroderma, the disease usually progresses slowly (over several years) and, by definition, the skin involvement remains distal to elbows and knees (however, involvement of the face and neck may occur). In more than two thirds of patients, Raynaud phenomenon is the first sign of the disease, with the characteristic triphasic color changes starting with pallor (white; vasoconstriction), changing to cyanosis (blue; low blood flow), and finally erythema (red; postischemic hyperperfusion). Over the following years, the skin of the fingers becomes thicker as the disease progresses. Calcinosis of the skin is often located periarticular in the extremities and may initially be subclinical, but later becomes painful and exulcerates with perifocal inflammation. The calcinosis is clearly visible as white, crumbly deposits on the bottom of the ulcers. Acroosteolysis may occur. Paraspinal calcifications are uncommon, but may cause pain and neurologic symptoms. The majority of patients have some degree of intestinal dysmotility, which is clinically most noticeable in the esophagus and characterized by a decrease or loss of peristalsis in the distal part of the esophagus. In many of these patients, erosive esophagitis and gastroesophageal reflux (often associated with silent aspiration) and strictures are present. Complications such as Barrett esophagus and adenocarcinoma of the esophagus have been described. Other gastrointestinal problems include autonomic dysfunction, ileal, jejunal, and colonic diverticula (also called *sacculations,* in the colon typically located along the antimesenteric border), malabsorption, and bacterial overgrowth. The patient may complain of dyspepsia and diarrhea alternating with constipation. Hyperpigmentation and hypopigmentation of the skin and pruritus are common. Telangiectases are typically located on the face, chest, and hands, but also may be seen on the mucosa in the oral cavity and throughout the entire gastrointestinal tract, where they may cause recurrent bleeding. Approximately one fourth of patients develop pulmonary hypertension with dyspnea and chronic cough. Cardiac involvement can present with arrhythmias and conduction abnormalities, patchy areas of myocardial fibrosis, pericardial effusions, and right heart failure secondary to pulmonary hypertension. The vast majority of patients have generalized, but unspecific arthralgias with morning stiffness. Clinically apparent synovitis and erosive arthritis are uncommon. Tendon friction rubs can commonly be felt and/or heard in the area of the big joints. Flexion contractures may lead to reduced joint mobility. Muscle weakness (particularly proximal) may be explained by myositis with muscle atrophy, resulting in increased serum creatine phosphokinase levels. One third of patients suffer from sicca syndrome with xerostomia and xerophthalmia. The 10-year survival rate of scleroderma depends on the extent of the disease. In isolated sclerodactyly, the rate is approximately 70%, in skin involvement also proximal to the metacarpophalangeal joints but absent trunk involvement the rate is almost 60%, while in patients with diffuse skin involvement the rate is only approximately 20%. Renal failure (secondary to vascular changes and/or glomerulonephritis) accounts for approximately 50% of all scleroderma-related deaths in patients with widespread skin involvement, whereas patients with limited skin involvement commonly die of cardiac, pulmonary, or gastrointestinal complications.

Precautions before anesthesia: Patients present with several risk factors for anesthesia. A thorough examination is recommended. The skin changes may result in microstomia with limited mouth opening (although much more common in diffuse scleroderma than in CREST syndrome), making tracheal intubation difficult. Pulmonary hypertension is a well-known and reported problem in these patients, and investigations should include auscultation (accentuated pulmonic component of the second heart sound) and pulmonary function tests (abnormal in the majority of patients) including measurement of the carbon monoxide diffusion capacity. High-resolution computed tomography scanning has proved to be a highly sensitive diagnostic tool for pulmonary fibrosis. Pulmonary venoocclusive disease has been described. Cardiac examination should include an electrocardiogram (24-hour electrocardiography if arrhythmias are suspected), and an echocardiogram to assess the extent of myocardial fibrosis and overall heart function (cor pulmonale secondary to pulmonary hypertension) and to exclude pericardial effusions. Arterial hypertension may result from renal disease. Primary biliary cirrhosis has been reported in a number of mainly female patients with CREST syndrome. Autoimmune hepatitis is considered rare. Preoperative laboratory investigations should include a complete blood count (microangiopathic hemolytic anemia secondary to small vessel disease and intestinal bleeding from telangiectases), serum concentrations of electrolytes, creatinine, urea, total protein, bilirubin, transaminases, and alkaline phosphatase, coagulation tests, and an arterial blood gas analysis in case

of pulmonary disease. Hypergammaglobulinemia and elevated erythrocyte sedimentation rate are common, and renal involvement may result in proteinuria.

Anesthetic considerations: As mentioned, CREST syndrome has a milder course than diffuse scleroderma, so clinical findings usually are less severe. Pulmonary hypertension is a frequent finding, so drugs that increase pulmonary vascular resistance (e.g., nitrous oxide) should be avoided. For the same reason, acidosis and hypercapnia must be avoided. Hypoxemia is not well tolerated by these patients; induction and emergence of anesthesia in particular pose the highest risk for pulmonary hypertensive crisis. If a spontaneous breathing induction technique is preferred secondary to expected airway management difficulties, ventilation may require assistance to prevent hypercapnia. However, esophageal dysmotility and gastroesophageal reflux may predispose to regurgitation/aspiration, and a rapid-sequence induction technique is recommended. The thickened skin can make peripheral vascular access difficult. The femoral artery probably is preferred over the radial artery for invasive pressure monitoring in the presence of significant Raynaud symptomatology and calcinosis of the fingers. Depending on the degree of muscle weakness and pulmonary disease, prolonged postoperative mechanical ventilation may be required. Careful intraoperative positioning and padding as a result of limited joint mobility are required.

Pharmacological implications: Dysproteinemia may result in altered protein binding of drugs and thus affect the efficacy (particularly for highly protein-bound drugs). Avoid vasoconstrictive drugs in the presence of Raynaud phenomenon. Use reduced doses of predominantly renally excreted drugs in the presence of renal failure and for drugs with mainly hepatic elimination in case of liver failure. Steroids usually are not effective in CREST syndrome, so a perioperative stress dose should not to be indicated.

Other conditions to be considered:

☞**PARRY-ROMBERG SYNDROME:** Progressive facial hemiatrophy characterized by unilateral atrophy of the skin including the subcutaneous tissue and underlying bone or cartilage. In contrast to "sclérodermie en coup de sabre," this form more often affects the lower half of the face (but is not limited to it) with cutaneous sclerosis and possible involvement of the tongue, developing teeth, lips, and salivary glands.

☞**RAYNAUD SYNDROME:** A disorder characterized by short-lasting vasospasms of the small arteries of the arms and legs, hands, and feet. Usually diagnosed before 40 years of age .

REFERENCES:

Marie I, Levesque H, Tranvouez JL, et al: Autoimmune hepatitis and systemic sclerosis: A new overlap syndrome? *Rheumatology (Oxford)* 40:102, 2001.

Meyer O: CREST syndrome. *Ann Med Intern (Paris)* 153:183, 2002.

Zamost BJ, Hirschberg J, Ippoliti AF, et al: Esophagitis in scleroderma. Prevalence and risk factors. *Gastroenterology* 92:421, 1987.

Creutzfeldt-Jakob Disease

At a glance: A form of neurodegenerative human prion (acronym for "proteinaceous infectious particles") disorder, which belongs to a group of diseases known as *transmissible spongiform encephalopathies.*

Incidence: Worldwide, the incidence of Creutzfeldt-Jakob disease (CJD) in the general population is approximately 1:1,000,000 per year. A variant of CJD (vCJD) has been associated with bovine spongiform encephalopathy (BSE) and has the highest occurrence in the United Kingdom. As of November 2005, the total number of definite or probable vCJD cases (dead and alive) in the United Kingdom was 158 (in 108 cases with neuropathologic confirmation). A causal association between vCJD and BSE is supported by epidemiologic and laboratory evidence in areas with high prevalence of BSE and the lack thereof in basically BSE-free regions.

Genetic inheritance: The occurrence of CJD, like other forms of prion diseases, is familial (5–10% of cases, with autosomal dominant inheritance caused by mutations in the PRNP [prion protein] gene, which has been mapped to 20pter-p12), sporadic (approximately 90% of patients with noninherited mutation of the prion protein), or infectious (iatrogenic with the first reported case of vCJD in 1974). The infectious agent in prion disease consists almost entirely of a host-encoded protease-resistant, neuronal cell surface sialoglycoprotein termed *prion protein.*

Pathophysiology: The cause is not fully understood but is believed to be related to misfolding of the normal endogenous cellular prion protein PrP^C into a new pathogenic conformation PrP^{Sc} encoded by PRNP. Prion protein is necessary for normal synaptic function. Iatrogenic and infectious transmission has occurred via tissue transplants (e.g., corneal transplants and no longer used dura mater grafts), cadaveric pituitary gland extracts (e.g., for human growth hormone [hGH] and gonadotropin production, now replaced by synthetic hormones), and contamination by neurosurgical instruments and stereotactic electroencephalography electrodes. Currently, blood is considered to pose a theoretical risk only, and no cases related to blood transmission have been reported. Accumulation of PrP^{Sc} in the central nervous system of affected individuals is responsible for the typical degenerative changes, such as loss of neurons, vacuolization, and finally death.

Diagnosis: There is no definitive clinical diagnostic test apart from the neuropathologic investigation. Patients have variable clinical and pathologic pictures. Pathology findings include diffuse nerve cell degeneration, status spongiosus, and glial proliferation. The electroencephalogram may show characteristic periodic complex changes.

Clinical aspects: The vast majority of patients are between 50 and 70 years old at the onset of the disease, although significantly younger affected patients have been reported. The onset of familial cases is significantly earlier than in other forms. The course of the illness may last from a few weeks to several years, although in general it is rapidly progressive. It is uniformly fatal, with the average length of survival from onset of the disease being approximately 6 months. Affected patients present with signs of dementia that often are accompanied by behavioral changes and psychiatric anomalies. Characteristic electroencephalographic changes can be detected (a slow background rhythm with superimposed periodic biphasic or triphasic synchronous sharp-wave complexes), which are clinically often accompanied by myoclonus and progressive motor dysfunction. Numerous other neurologic symptoms such as pyramidal and extrapyramidal signs (muscular rigidity), seizures, nystagmus, autonomic dysfunction, and signs of cerebellar dysfunction (unsteady or atactic gait), may occur. Forgetfulness or nervousness, supranuclear gaze paralysis, and loss of facial expression may occur. Some neurologic features may subside in the terminal phase of the disease. Autopsy reveals generalized brain atrophy; however, if the course of the disease is rapid (i.e., death in less than 6 months), the macroscopic changes may only be subtle. CJD is a spongiform encephalopathy resulting in diffuse loss of neurons,

reactive astrocytosis, and widespread vacuolization of the neuropil. Electron microscopy locates the round vacuoles within the neuroplasma and neuropil of the cortical gray matter. The vacuoles vary in diameter from 1 to 50 μm and appear to contain membranous particles.

In contrast to the classic form of CJD, vCJD predominantly affects young persons and presents initially with atypical features such as prominent psychiatric and sensory symptoms, whereas onset of neurologic symptoms is delayed and the electroencephalogram is unspecific. The course of the disease lasts longer than in the classic form (at least 6 months), and the median age at death is approximately 30 years. Spongiform encephalopathy is more pronounced and a higher number of Kuru-type amyloid plaques surrounded by prion protein accumulations and vacuoles can be detected, which may be, at least in part, a reflection of the prolonged course of vCJD.

Precautions before anesthesia: Except for the cerebral changes, these patients are otherwise healthy. However, in advanced stages of the disease, a chest radiograph may be necessary because recurrent aspirations may occur. Cooperation may be limited secondary to dementia. Sedative premedication may be helpful.

Anesthetic considerations: Not different from other forms of dementia. The main issue is preventing infections among staff. Special attention must be paid to the sterilization of medical equipment. Extensive prion infection of lymphoreticular tissues has been detected during the asymptomatic incubation period of vCJD. Medical instruments exposed to these infected tissues (e.g., Waldeyer ring of lymphoid tissue in the pharynx for the laryngoscope blade) of preclinically infected individuals might represent a potential risk of iatrogenic transmission of vCJD if reused after routine sterilization. In a recent study, lymphocytes were detected on 30% of used (and uncleaned) laryngoscope blades. Since prions are resistant to routine sterilization processes, it was concluded, that this might pose a potential risk of transmission of vCJD from patient to patient. Although the blades in that study were not sterilized before sampling them, it seems wise to use disposable equipment whenever possible in patients with known or suspected infection.

Pharmacological implications: These patients may be taking antiseizure medications, which may interact with the metabolism and elimination of anesthetic drugs.

REFERENCES:

Hirsch N, Beckett A, Collinge J, et al: Lymphocyte contamination of laryngoscope blades—a possible vector for transmission of variant Creutzfeld-Jakob disease. *Anaesthesia* 60:664, 2005.

Hernandez-Palazon J, Martinez-Lage JF, Tortosa JA, et al: Anaesthetic management in patients suspected of, or at risk of having Creutzfeldt-Jakob disease. *Br J Anaesth* 80:516, 1998.

Web site of the Department of Health of the United Kingdom, Section "Policy and Guidance", "Health and social care topics". http://www.health.gov.uk/PolicyAndGuidance/HealthAndSocialCareTopics/GJD/fs/en

Crigler-Najjar Syndrome

At a glance: A congenital disorder characterized by unconjugated hyperbilirubinemia.

Synonyms and classification: Bilirubin Uridine-Diphosphate Glucuronyltransferase Deficiency; Hereditary Unconjugated Hyperbilirubinemia.

Type I: Bilirubin Glucuronyltransferase Deficiency; Congenital Hyperbilirubinemia; Congenital Familial Nonhemolytic Jaundice.

Type II: Arias Syndrome.

Incidence: Not precisely known but estimated to be approximately 1:1,000,000 live births, with approximately 120 cases with Crigler-Najjar syndrome type I described in the literature. No racial or sexual predilection has been reported.

Genetic inheritance: Crigler-Najjar syndrome type I is an autosomal recessive inherited disorder with a mutation in the uridine diphosphate glucuronyltransferase (UGT)-1 gene located on 2q37. Crigler-Najjar syndrome type II, which is much more frequent than type I, is autosomal recessive inherited with a mutation mapping to the UGT-2 gene also on 2q37. Autosomal dominant forms have also been reported.

Pathophysiology: This enzymopathy affects the conjugation of bilirubin with glucuronic acid. Unconjugated bilirubin has the ability to penetrate into the neonatal brain and cause neurologic damage and encephalopathy (kernicterus). Uridine diphosphate glucuronyltransferases (UGT) are enzymes that detoxify numerous compounds by conjugating them with glucuronic acid and rendering them water soluble and harmless at the same time (glucuronidation). Crigler-Najjar syndrome type I is characterized by complete absence of bilirubin UGT, which leads to unconjugated hyperbilirubinemia with total serum bilirubin levels greater than 340 μmol/liter (20 mg/dl). In Crigler-Najjar syndrome type II, a partial deficiency of bilirubin UGT occurs with total serum bilirubin concentrations in the range from 100 to 340 μmol/liter (6–20 mg/dl). Because of residual enzyme activity in type II, phenobarbital treatment can be used to induce the enzyme and lower serum bilirubin concentration significantly.

Diagnosis: In Crigler-Najjar syndrome type I, biliary bilirubin concentration is decreased and bilirubin glucuronide is absent. The diagnosis is confirmed by decreased glucuronyltransferase activity on the liver biopsy specimen. In contrast to Crigler-Najjar syndrome type II, there is no response to treatment with phenobarbital. Neonatal jaundice presenting soon after birth and lasting longer than 13 days in the absence of hemolysis may point to the diagnosis. The stool color often is pale yellow. Untreated, survival past the neonatal period is uncommon. Persistent jaundice during the neonatal period occurs in Crigler-Najjar syndrome type II, however, the levels of total bilirubin are significantly lower and generally neurologic symptoms do not appear. Confirmation of the diagnosis also requires a liver biopsy specimen to measure enzyme activity. Biliary bilirubin is (sub)normal, and stool color is normal.

Clinical aspects: *Crigler-Najjar syndrome type I.* Severe unconjugated hyperbilirubinemia with intense jaundice appears in the first 3 days of life and persists through the neonatal period. Diffusion of unconjugated (lipid-soluble) bilirubin into the brain may be favored by a damaged blood-brain barrier (e.g., hypoxia, hyperosmolality), but also by prematurity and the presence of hypoalbuminemia or highly protein-bound drugs (e.g., sulfonamides). Kernicterus usually presents in the first week of life (although it may occur at any time, especially during the neonatal period, but is not limited to this period) with lethargy, loss of the Moro reflex, and poor feeding. Left untreated, it may progress to opisthotonus, signs of increased intracranial pressure (e.g., bulging fontanelle, high-pitched crying), seizures, and stiffness. Affected infants often die in the first weeks or months of life secondary to kernicterus, others survive with little or no neurologic sequelae. In survivors, these neurologic signs often do not resolve or recur after an ini-

tial improvement and may finally result in bilateral choreoathetosis, seizures, mental retardation, hearing loss, speech anomalies, and extrapyramidal signs. The neurologic sequelae reflects injury to basal ganglia, corpus subthalamicum, thalamus, globus pallidus, putamen, cerebellar and cranial nerve nuclei, and hippocampal structures. Phototherapy (450-nm wavelength light) and emergent exchange transfusion often are required in the first days of life. The only treatment for Crigler-Najjar syndrome type I is liver transplantation.

Crigler-Najjar syndrome type II is most often benign, presenting with unconjugated hyperbilirubinemia in the first 3 days of life. It sometimes mimics physiologic neonatal icterus, however, persistence for more than 2 weeks should raise suspicion for Crigler-Najjar syndrome type II. Very rarely, kernicterus with bilirubin encephalopathy occurs in these patients (again, not confined to the neonatal period). Acute exacerbations can be associated with trauma, infection, anesthesia, or drugs, and plasmapheresis and/or exchange transfusion have been used successfully for treatment. Clinical signs of neurologic involvement may include mental retardation, seizures, and movement disorders.

Precautions before anesthesia: Evaluate hepatic function (no coagulation disorders have been reported in this syndrome). Exclude a possible association with hemolysis. Correction of hypoalbuminemia should help reduce the concentration of free bilirubin. Evaluate plasma levels of bilirubin and glucuronyl transferase activity. Review electroencephalograms to evaluate preoperative brain function (seizures). If the patient is on phototherapy (some patients are on lifelong daily phototherapy for up to 20 hours per day), it should be continued as long as possible preoperatively and restarted postoperatively as soon as possible. In some cases, phototherapy has been used intraoperatively, particularly for longer procedures.

Anesthetic considerations: Keep fasting times as short as possible because it can increase bilirubin serum concentration. Acute exacerbations may be triggered by infections, so elective procedures should be postponed until the infection has been cured. Severe hypertension, hypercarbia, hyperosmolality, and acidosis should all be avoided because they may favor the passage of albumin-bound bilirubin through the blood-brain barrier. It is important to avoid hepatotoxic drugs and drugs that may displace bilirubin from its binding to serum proteins, thus increasing the risk of brain damage. Regional anesthesia is a safe alternative.

Pharmacological implications: Thiopental can be used in both types of the disease, even in type I, although it does not decrease bilirubin levels. Midazolam is best avoided because of its linkage to plasma proteins and its possible interaction with bilirubin transport. For neuromuscular blockade, succinylcholine, atracurium, and cisatracurium are the drugs of choice. If possible, halogenated inhalational agents should be avoided, although desflurane, sevoflurane, and isoflurane are considered acceptable. Some cephalosporins and contrast media for radiologic procedures are contraindicated because of their extensive albumin binding with displacement of bilirubin from albumin. Morphine can be used because it is metabolized by a different glucuronyl transferase system.

Other condition to be considered:

☞**GILBERT SYNDROME:** A benign inherited disorder characterized by chronic intermittent jaundice (unconjugated hyperbilirubinemia) that does not lead to particular complications and is not progressive (normal life expectancy; may even prolong life by preventing heart attacks).

REFERENCES:

Jansen PL: Diagnosis and management of Crigler-Najjar syndrome. *Eur J Pediatr* 158(suppl 2):S89, 1999.

Prager MC, Johnson KL, Ascher NL; Anesthetic care of patients with Crigler Najjar syndrome. *Anesth Analg* 74:162, 1992.

Shevell MI, Majnemer A, Schiff D: Neurologic perspectives of Crigler-Najjar syndrome type I. *J Child Neurol* 13:265, 1998.

Cumming Syndrome

At a glance: A disorder combining anomalies of the face, limbs, and multiple internal organs. Stillbirth occurs frequently, or death commonly occurs shortly after birth.

Synonyms: Camptomelia Cumming type; Cervical Lymphocele with Long Bowed Bones Syndrome.

Incidence and genetic inheritance: Seven cases have been described (6 females, 1 male). Autosomal recessive inheritance with parental consanguinity is a significant risk factor.

Clinical aspects: The disorder may affect the head (cloverleaf skull, dolichocephaly or scaphocephaly, marked deformation of the face, cervical cystic hygroma or lymphocele, redundant subcutaneous tissue, severe cervical edema, microphthalmos, cleft palate), the limbs (tetramelic camptomelia with bowed diaphyses, micromelia, and brachydactyly talipes equinovarus), the heart (dextrocardia, total anomalous pulmonary venous drainage, left-sided superior vena cava, aortic arch anomalies), the lungs (hypoplasia and/or abnormal lobation in a short, bell-shaped chest), the kidneys (polycystic kidney disease), the liver (hepatomegaly, multiple liver cysts), and other organs (multiple pancreatic cysts and anatomical anomalies, polysplenia, short bowel, ectopic or undescended testes, absent uterus and Fallopion tubes). Lymph edema may be generalized. Some researchers consider heterotaxia to be part of this syndrome.

Anesthetic considerations: It is unlikely that these patients come to the operating room. Cardiac anatomy and function should be determined preoperatively. Respiratory, renal, and hepatic function and blood glucose levels should be assessed. Difficult airway management should be anticipated secondary to the described head and neck features. Vascular access may be difficult because of lymph edema. Medication selection may be altered in the presence of concomitant hepatic and/or renal dysfunction.

Other condition to be considered:

☞ **GRANT SYNDROME:** A form of osteogenesis imperfecta with persistent wormian bones, blue sclerae, mandibular hypoplasia, shallow glenoid fossae, and camptomelia.

REFERENCES:

Bedeschi MF, Spaccini L, Rizzuti T, et al: Cumming syndrome with heterotaxia, campomelia and absent uterus/fallopian tubes. *Am J Med Genet A* 132:329, 2005.

Ming JE, McDonald-McGinn DM, Markowitz RI: Heterotaxia in a fetus with camptomelia, cervical lymphocele, polysplenia, and multicystic dysplastic kidneys: Expanding the phenotype of Cumming syndrome. *Am J Med Genet* 73:419, 1997.

Perez del Rio MJ, Fernandez-Toral J, Madrigal B, et al: A Two new cases of Cumming syndrome confirming autosomal recessive inheritance. *Am J Med Genet* 82:340, 1999.

Curatolo-Cilio Syndrome

At a glance: A congenital syndrome characterized by mental retardation, white matter hypoplasia, agenesis or extreme hypoplasia of the corpus callosum, and failure to thrive.

Incidence and genetic inheritance: Fewer than 10 cases have been described in the literature. The genetic inheritance pattern has not been determined, yet.

Diagnosis: Based on the clinical findings associated with neuroimaging features of cortical atrophy, ventricular dilatation, cerebellar agenesis/hypoplasia, and agenesis/hypoplasia of the corpus callosum and the septum pellucidum.

Clinical aspects: Patients present with short stature, generalized hypotonia, and hyperreflexia. Mental retardation (of varying severity), microcephaly, frontal bossing, hypertelorism, broad nasal root, micrognathia or retrognathia, and failure to thrive appear to be common findings. Magnetic resonance imaging of the brain reveals severe white matter hypoplasia, extreme hypoplasia or even agenesis of the cerebellum and the corpus callosum, and minor midline facial abnormalities.

Precautions before anesthesia: Anesthetic management in this syndrome has not been described. Obtain a history of the seizures and their response to treatment. Check for possible difficult airway management. Mental retardation may affect patient compliance. Preoperative sedation and/or the presence of the primary caregiver during induction may be helpful.

Anesthetic considerations: Difficult airway management should be expected, and spontaneous ventilation maintained until the airway has been secured. Alternative airway management techniques such as laryngeal mask or fiberoptic bronchoscope should be easily available.

Pharmacological implications: The metabolism of some anesthetic agents may be altered by long-term use of antiepileptic drugs. Avoid medications that lower the seizure threshold. Avoid neuromuscular blockers until the airway has been secured.

REFERENCES:

Curatolo P, Cilio MR, Del Giudice E, et al: Familial white matter hypoplasia, agenesis of the corpus callosum, mental retardation and growth deficiency: A new distinctive syndrome. *Neuropediatrics* 24:77, 1993.

Septien L, Gras P, Giroud M, et al: Agenesis of the corpus callosum and epilepsy. 26 cases. *Rev Neurol* 149:257, 1993.

Cutis Laxa

At a glance: Cutis laxa is a rare autosomal recessive or sporadic connective tissue disorder characterized by the lack of elasticity manifesting mostly by hanging or wrinkled skin. Clinically, the affected skin normally is thickened and dark.

Synonyms: Generalized Chalazodermia; Generalized Dermatochalasia; Generalized Elastorrhexis.

Important Notice: Numerous medical conditions are associated with similar skin conditions as observed in cutis laxa, but most of these disorders have specific findings, such as characteristic facial features, joint hypermobility, and age of onset, that are so distinctive that they should typically not be confused with cutis laxa. These include Turner syndrome, neurofibromatosis, systemic lupus erythematous, complement deficiencies, and pseudoxanthoma elasticum.

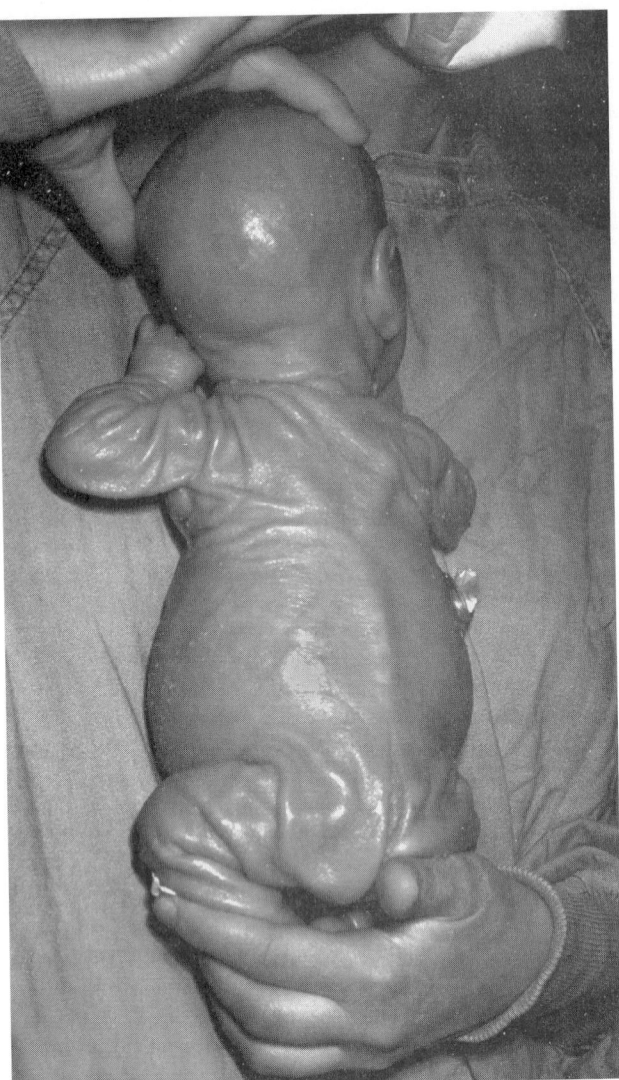

Cutis Laxa This newborn child suffers from congenital cutis laxa characterized by a lack of elasticity manifesting mainly by skin hanging and wrinkling on arms and legs. The affected skin appears thickened and edematous.

Incidence and genetic inheritance: Cutis laxa is a rare skin disorder that affects males and females in equal numbers. Approximately 50 cases have been reported in the medical literature. Most cases of cutis laxa are inherited as an autosomal recessive trait. It has been suggested that cutis laxa in some cases is inherited as an autosomal dominant transmission; in this situation, the skin manifestations can be minimal but systemic effects (lungs) may still occur. An X-linked form of cutis laxa has been classified as Ehlers-Danlos type IX. The acquired form of cutis laxa may develop following a severe illness involving fever, polyserositis, or erythema multiforme. It has been suggested that acquired cutis laxa results from an autoimmune process.

Pathophysiology: Reduced levels of elastin mRNA and elastic fibers throughout the dermis are associated with abnormal elastin components noted by electron microscopy.

Clinical aspects: Congenital cutis laxa typically is diagnosed at birth or early infancy. Transient edema, especially of the arms and legs, often is perceived as the first manifestation. During infancy, the skin lacks elasticity that may be most apparent on the face. The symptoms of cutis laxa progress during infancy, but usually become less noticeable after puberty. Patients may present with emphysema and occasionally flaccid trachea. Diverticula in the esophagus, duodenum and bladder are common findings. Cardiovascular anomalies may include cor pulmonale, supravalvular aortic stenosis, arterial aneurysms, arterial tortuosity, multiple pulmonary artery stenoses, and fibromuscular renal artery dysplasia. Joint laxity and potential hip dislocation are characteristic. The association of cutis laxa and diaphragmatic hernia has been suggested. The presence of a large fontanelle with delayed closure has been reported. The symptoms of the acquired form of cutis laxa develop slowly and may not appear until puberty or later during early adulthood. Episodes of transient angioedema, especially in the face and neck, and inflammation are frequently the first signs of the acquired form of the disease. Skin changes develop slowly and may be widespread or limited to the face, trunk, and/or neck. Small blood vessels under the skin in the affected area may rupture easily and result in purpura-like spots on the skin. It is important to notice that life-threatening complications have been reported in congenital and acquired cutis laxa, including rupture of the aorta and severe emphysema.

Precautions before anesthesia: Proper preoperative evaluation of pulmonary and cardiovascular function is necessary. The presence of emphysema usually is an indicator of the severity of the disease. Cutis laxa patients can bruise easily because of vascular fragility, however, this does not suggest patients have coagulation problems or prolonged bleeding time. The presence of major vessel aneurysms should be evaluated, especially of the aorta. The patient may be receiving chronic steroid therapy, and supplementation may be required for the perioperative period.

Anesthetic considerations: The presence of abnormal skin may make vascular access difficult. The possibility of prolonged mechanical ventilation postoperatively must be kept in mind for patients with significant pulmonary manifestations. Cor pulmonale and pulmonary arterial hypertension have been reported in some of these patients. Avoid further increases in pulmonary artery pressures (avoid acidosis, hypercapnia and hypoxia) and maintain inotropy.

Pharmacological implications: Avoid nitrous oxide in patients with severe emphysema and/or pulmonary arterial hypertension.

Other conditions to be considered:

De Barsy Moens Diercks Syndrome is inherited as an autosomal recessive trait. It is characterized by degeneration of the elastic tissue in the skin (cutis laxa), athetosis, loss of muscle tone, unusual flexibility of the small joints, clouding of the corneas, large prominent ears, frontal bossing, and short stature. Other clinical features may include mental retardation, dislocated joints at birth, sparse hair, and thin lips.

☞**Ehlers-Danlos Syndrome** is a group of inherited systemic connective tissue disorders characterized by a wide variety of joint and skin problems. Eleven types have been described. Clinically, this entity is characterized by fragile, soft, velvety, elastic skin and hyperextensibility of joints causing frequent dislocations. When the skin is pulled, it normally returns to its original position. Vascular fragility has been suggested because most patients bruise and bleed easily.

REFERENCES:

Armstrong L, Jimenez C, Hunter AGW: A boy with developmental delay, malformations, and evidence of a connective tissue disorder: Possibly a new type of cutis laxa. *Am J Med Genet* 119A:57, 2003.

Loeys B, van Maldergem L, Mortier G, et al: Homozygosity for a missense mutation in fibulin-5 (FBLN5) results in a severe form of cutis laxa. *Hum Mol Genet* 11:2113, 2002.

Urban Z, Gao J, Pope FM, Davis EC: Autosomal dominant cutis laxa with severe lung disease synthesis and matrix deposition of mutant tropoelastin. *J Invest Dermatol* 124:193, 2005.

Cutis Marmorata Telangiectatica Congenita

At a glance: A congenital cutaneous condition with persistent cutis marmorata, telangiectasia, and phlebectasia. It is often reported in association with a variety of other congenital anomalies.

Synonyms: Van Lohuizen Syndrome; Congenital (Generalized) Phlebectasia; Nevus Vascularis Reticularis; Livedo Telangiectatica; Congenital Livedo Reticularis.

History: First described by C.H.J. Van Lohuizen in 1922.

Incidence: More than 100 cases have been published worldwide.

Genetic inheritance: Unclear. Autosomal recessive and autosomal dominant trait with low penetrance have been discussed, although most cases seem to be sporadic.

Pathophysiology: The role of external factors, including viral infections, have been discussed, as several cases of cutis marmorata telangiectatica congenita (CMTC) occurred in the same geographic area. Histologic examination shows an increased number and size of capillaries and veins, perivascular lymphocytic infiltrates, occasional areas of microthrombosis and cutaneous atrophy or ulceration. An underlying connective tissue abnormality has been postulated.

Diagnosis: Generally, the lesions are present at birth or shortly thereafter. They may be localized (most often on the legs) or generalized. A skin biopsy may confirm the diagnosis.

Clinical aspects: Consists of cutis marmorata, which is a marbled or mottled skin appearance caused by prominent capillaries and veins; vascular lesions present as telangiectasias that look like spider angiomas, venous dilatation or phlebectasias, and superficial ulceration. Major vessel stenosis resulting in claudication or gangrene have been described. There is a high incidence of abnormalities associated with CMTC, some studies estimated in up to almost 90% of patients. These other abnormalities may include mental retardation, macrocephaly, cerebrovascular malformations, glaucoma, micrognathia, cleft palate, dystrophic teeth, cardiac malformations (e.g., double aortic arch, patent ductus arteriosus), congenital hypothyroidism, multicystic kidney disease, hemihypertrophy, hemiatrophy, syndactyly, and nevi flammei. Some researchers suggested CMTC belongs to a group of vascular diseases (e.g., ☞Sturge-Weber Syndrome, ☞Klippel-Trénaunay Syndrome) associated with other mesodermal defects occurring during embryogenesis.

Precautions before anesthesia: Perform a thorough search for other associated abnormalities in particular heart (clinical, echocardiography, electrocardiography) and kidneys (complete blood count, serum electrolytes, creatinine and blood urea nitrogen). Check thyroid function and correct hypothyroidism if necessary. Assess the airway with regard to difficult airway management.

Anesthetic considerations: Maintain spontaneous ventilation until the airway has been secured in patients with suspected or have difficult airway management. Watch out for dysotropic teeth. Venous access may be difficult because of numerous fragile branching

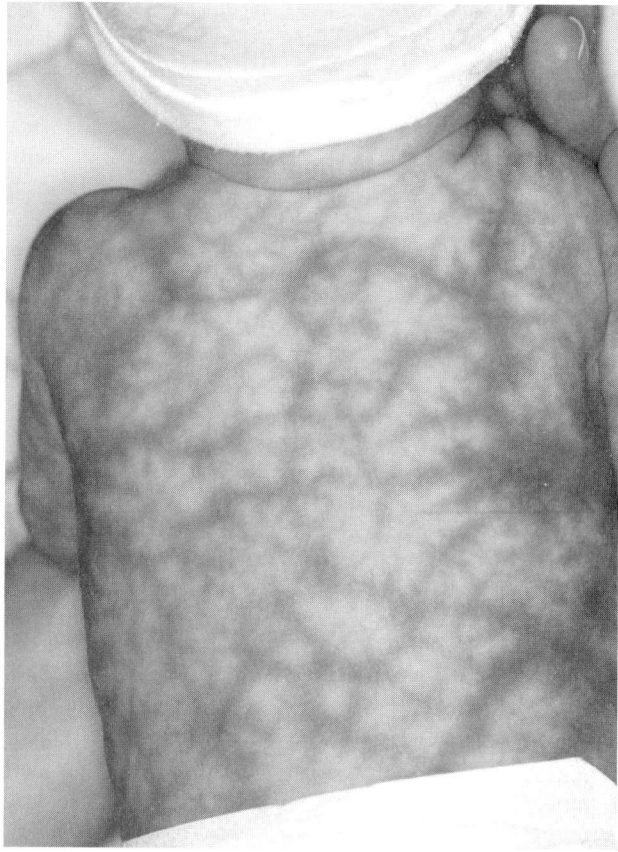

Cutis marmorata telangiectatica congenita in a newborn See color plates.

veins. Areas of skin ulceration are a potential entry site for infections and should be kept clean and covered. Avoid sudden increases in blood pressure in patients with known cardiovascular malformations. Careful positioning and padding are necessary to prevent damage to the already delicate skin.

Pharmacological implications: Avoid neuromuscular blocker until the airway has been secured. Avoid succinylcholine and atropine in the presence of glaucoma. Reduce the dose of anesthetic agents in the presence of uncorrected hypothyroidism.

Other conditions to be considered:

☞**ADAMS-OLIVER SYNDROME:** A very rare inherited disorder characterized by defects of the scalp associated with multiple scarred and hairless areas that usually have dilated blood vessels directly under the skin. Scalp defects are present at birth. The extremities are either short (hypoplastic fingers and toes) or characterized by absent hands and lower legs. Congenital heart defects must be ruled out.

☞**APLASIA CUTIS CONGENITA:** A most often inherited disorder with circumscribed or more extensive skin lesions that may involve underlying tissues. Neurologic and cardiac anomalies have been described in these patients.

☞**KLIPPEL-TRÉNAUNAY SYNDROME:** Congenital malformation of unknown origin characterized by the association of soft tissue and osseous hypertrophy, venous malformations, lymphatic abnormalities, and cutaneous capillary malformations.

☞**STURGE-WEBER SYNDROME:** A neurocutaneous syndrome characterized by the presence of vascular tumors of the face (facial hemangioma capillary (nevus flammeus) usually called "port wine stain"), ipsilateral vascular anomalies (most often of meningeal and choroidal vessels), and intracranial calcifications. Other features may include contralateral hemiparesis, hemianopia, and seizures.

MEGALENCEPHALY-CUTIS MARMORATA TELANGIECTATICA CONGENITA: Distinct phenotype of CMTC associated with macrocephaly and frontal bossing, macrosomia, and neurologic abnormalities (e.g., hydrocephalus, mental retardation). Joint and skin laxity, facial and limb asymmetry, generalized hypotonia, and venous malformations (venous "aneurysms") may occur.

REFERENCES:

Enjolras O: Cutis marmorata telangiectatica congenita. *Ann Dermatol Venereol* 128:161, 2001.

Garzon MC, Schweiger E: Cutis marmorata teleangiectatica congenita. *Semin Cuton Med Surg* 23:99, 2004.

Vogel AM, Paltiel HJ, Kozakewich HP, et al: Iliac artery stenosis in a child with cutis marmorata teleangiectatica congenita. *J Pediatr Surg* 40:89, 2005.

Cystic Hygroma

At a glance: Cystic hygroma is a benign, multiloculated cystic structure. Cystic hygromas form as a result of budding lymphatics. They may occur anywhere in the body, although they are most frequently encountered in the neck and axilla. Cystic hygromas frequently abut and/or encompass neurovascular structures. Surgical excision remains the therapy of choice.

Synonyms: Cystic Lymphangioma; Familial Nuchal Bleb; Fetal Cystic Hygroma; Hygroma Colli.

Incidence: Approximately 1:6,000 live births suffers from cystic hygroma.

Genetic inheritance: Cystic hygroma with a normal karyotype may be inherited as an autosomal recessive trait.

Pathophysiology: Cystic hygromas can range from increased nuchal translucency to thin-walled cystic masses that can become larger than the fetal head. The cysts may result from a lymphatic abnormality, possibly because of absent or inefficient connections between the lymphatic and venous systems. The concept that correct communications between these two systems develop later during gestation in some fetuses may account for cystic areas that resolve with merely a residual of redundant skin (pterygium colli). Other theories for the development of cystic hygromas include possible abnormal sequestration of embryonic lymphatic tissue that does not communicate with normal lymph flow channels and budding of lymphatics that canalize to form lymph-filled cysts.

Diagnosis: Prenatal diagnosis is often possible (ultrasound). Approximately two thirds of children present at birth or within the first year of life and in 90% within 2 years of age. Most often, the lesion is a cosmetic problem, however, compression of the airway, esophagus, and/or great vessels may occur as the hygroma invades the deeper structures of the neck or the mediastinum. The clinical course is characterized by intermittent or progressive growth, spontaneous regression, hemorrhage, and infection.

Clinical aspects: Cystic hygromas, most often occurring in the neck (75%) and axilla (20%), belong to a group of diseases that now are considered lymphatic malformations. Occasionally, cystic hygromas become very large and extend into the mediastinum, axillae, mouth, and chest. Occasionally, they occur exclusively in those

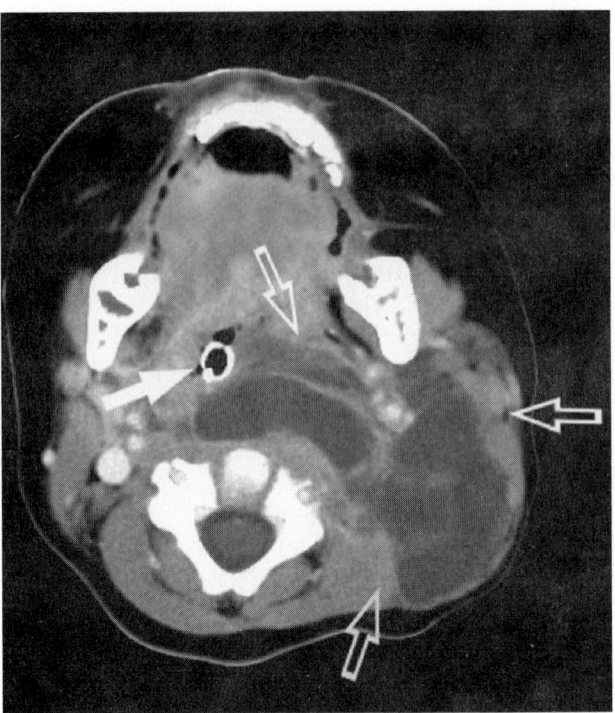

Cystic Hygroma   Cystic hygroma of the neck *(outlined arrows)* resulting in deviation of the trachea *(solid arrow)* to the contralateral side.

areas. Cystic hygromas are often associated with lymphedema, congenital cardiac defects, and chromosomal anomalies. Other features may include cleft lip/palate, single umbilical artery, and horseshoe, fused, or ectopic kidneys. Umbilical hernia, thymic aplasia, and holoprosencephaly/arrhinencephaly have also been described. The risk of infection of a cystic hygroma is approximately 16% and may result in additional swelling, pain, fever, and localized erythema. The risk of hemorrhage is approximately 13%. Consider this complication with an enlarging and painful cystic hygroma in a patient with evidence of acute blood loss. In up to half of patients, fetal cystic hygromas are associated with chromosomal anomalies such as ☞Turner Syndrome (most frequent), ☞Trisomy 21, ☞Trisomy 18, and ☞Noonan Syndrome. Although surgical therapy remains the treatment of choice for large cystic hygromas, smaller lesions may be treated with laser therapy or repeated injections of alcohol to induce sclerosis.

Precautions before anesthesia: Closely evaluate children who present with cystic hygroma of the neck for tracheal deviation or other evidence of impending airway obstruction (e.g., stridor, coughing, feeding difficulties). Closely evaluate the tongue, oral cavity, hypopharynx, and larynx because any involvement of these structures may lead to airway obstruction and difficult airway management upon induction of anesthesia. Chest radiography or better computed tomography scanning or magnetic resonance imaging to evaluate the neck, mediastinum, and chest for assessment of the anatomical structures and the degree of their involvement by the cystic hygroma is recommended. Because chromosomal anomalies are common and may be associated with numerous other features, it is recommended that a complete blood count (also because of possible hemorrhage into the cystic hygroma) and serum concentrations of electrolytes, creatinine, and urea be obtained preoperatively.

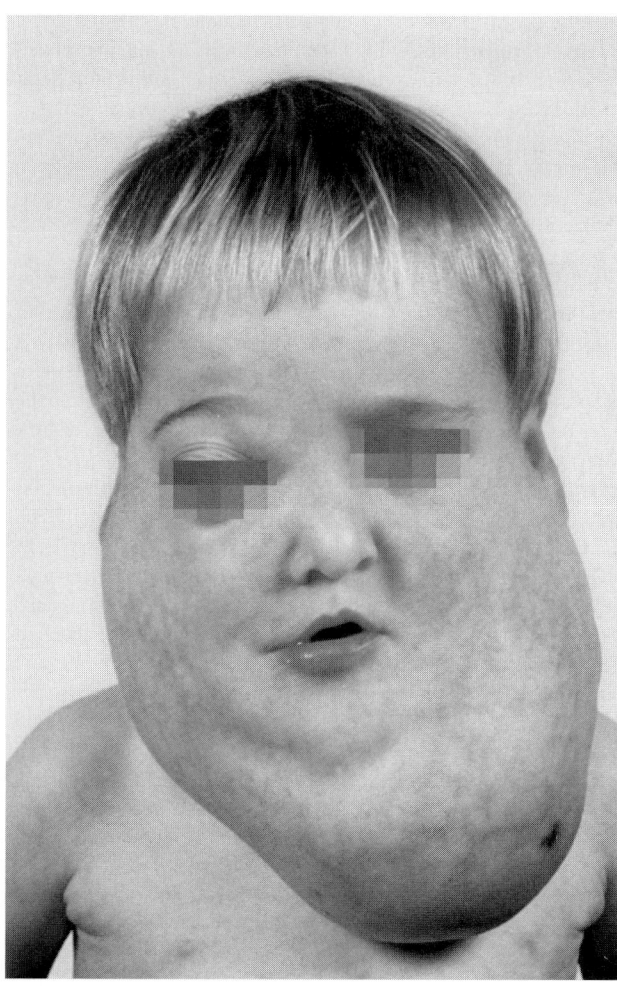

Cystic Hygroma Facial asymmetry as a result of a big cystic hygroma in an infant boy.

Anesthetic considerations: Airway obstruction is the most significant complication of cystic hygroma involving the neck and mediastinum. To assess the risk of airway obstruction, carefully evaluate the child with cystic hygroma of the head and neck for any signs of tracheal deviation and for involvement of the oropharynx, hypopharynx, and infraglottic area. Airway involvement is often accompanied by involvement of the tongue, its base and the supraglottic part of the larynx. Awake fiberoptic intubation is the technique of choice for cystic hygromas with oral or pharyngeal extension. Maintain spontaneous ventilation in the presence of airway infiltration/compression at least until the airway has been secured. Although rare in patients with cystic hygroma, airway collapse is possible after administration of neuromuscular blockers, therefore, they should be avoided if airway compression is suspected. In the presence of chromosomal aberrations, the anesthetic management is also guided by the underlying disease. Surgical therapy most likely results in neck swelling, and prolonged postoperative mechanical ventilation may be required until the swelling in and around the neck has subsided.

Pharmacological implications: Avoid muscle relaxant until the airway has been secured or better at all in the presence of airway compression/infiltration.

Other condition to be considered:

COWCHOCK WAPNER KURTZ SYNDROME: An exceptional, often lethal congenital genetic disorder combining nuchal cystic hygroma, cleft palate, and lymphedema.

REFERENCES:

Bryan Y, Chwals W, Ovassapian A: Sedation and fiberoptic intubation of a neonate with cystic hygroma. *Acta Anaesthesiol Scand* 49:122, 2005.

Chervenak FA, Isaacson G, Blakemore KJ, et al: Fetal cystic hygroma. Cause and natural history. *N Engl J Med* 309:822, 1983.

Gershanik JJ, Lacassie Y, Sargent W: Exit procedure: A case report. *J La State Med Soc* 155:46, 2003.

Cystinosis

At a glance: Cystinosis is an inherited metabolic disease resulting in the accumulation of cystine in various organs of the body (e.g., kidneys, eyes, liver, muscles, pancreas, brain, leukocytes). Untreated, the infantile nephropathic form will result in end-stage renal failure before the age of 10 years.

Incidence: Estimated to be in the range of 1:100,00–200,000 live births, although a wide geographic variability has been reported. Males are slightly more often affected (M:F = 1.5:1). Cystinosis is the most common inherited cause of ☞De Toni-Debré-Fanconi syndrome (renal Fanconi syndrome).

Genetic inheritance: All types of cystinosis are transmitted in an autosomal recessive manner. The defect affects the cystinosin gene (CTNS) that has been mapped to 17p13. Hitherto, more than 50 different CTNS mutations have been described.

Pathophysiology: Cystine is a degradation product of cysteine, which originates from ingested and in lysosome hydrolyzed proteins. Cystinosis is a lysosomal storage disease caused by impaired transport of cystine out of the lysosomes into the cytoplasm. This energy-dependent transport relies on cystinosin, an integral membrane protein that acts as the lysosomal cystine transporter. In the nephropathic form of cystinosis (see "Diagnosis" and "Clinical aspects"), this results in cystine depositions within the cells of various organs where they affect the cellular energy metabolism. Cystine crystal deposits in the proximal tubule cells of the kidney result in early renal involvement and eventually renal Fanconi syndrome. It is characterized by a generalized transport defect in the proximal tubules of the kidneys with renal losses of glucose, phosphate, calcium, uric acid, amino acids, and bicarbonates eventually leading to short stature, osteomalacia, and renal failure.

Diagnosis: *Infantile nephropathic cystinosis* (Synonyms: Classic or early onset cystinosis): The diagnosis is based on growth retardation manifesting after the first six months of life and the features of renal Fanconi syndrome before one year of age with progressive deterioration of renal function to end-stage renal disease usually before the age of 10 years. Measurement of leukocyte cystine content is used to confirm the diagnosis. Cystine crystals can be detected in the cornea and conjunctiva and in biopsies from brain, bone marrow, kidneys, liver, spleen, pancreas, intestinal mucosa, thyroid, lymph nodes, and muscles.

Intermediate nephropathic cystinosis (Synonyms: Juvenile, adolescent, or late onset cystinosis): This form of cystinosis is basically characterized by the same renal pathology, however the onset is delayed and the severity (initially) less pronounced. In the beginning, the symptoms of renal Fanconi syndrome in these patients can be so subtle that they diagnosis may be missed for a while. However, eventually renal function also decreases in these patients and end-stage renal failure develops between the age of 15 and 25 years.

Non-nephropathic cystinosis (Synonyms: Benign, adult or ocular cystinosis): These patients present with photophobia and ocular discomfort (burning, pruritus) secondary to cystine crystal accumulation in the corneae (and conjunctivae), which can easily be detected on slit lamp examination. Crystalline deposits are also detected in bone marrow and leukocytes (but not in the retina or kidneys), however, they seem not to affect the function clinically.

Clinical aspects: *Infantile nephropathic cystinosis:* Initially, these patients present with polydipsia, polyuria, vomiting, constipation, and inappetence leading to failure to thrive. Most often, the disease is diagnosed during an acute exacerbation with dehydration, metabolic acidosis and electrolyte imbalance frequently triggered by an intercurrent (gastrointestinal) infection. Poor growth (typically below the third percentile for height and weight) and renal Fanconi syndrome characterize the clinical course. Renal Fanconi syndrome may lead to painful hypophosphatemic rickets, hypocalcemia with tetany, and hypokalemia with arrhythmias. Hyponatremia and hypomagnesemia have also been described. Photophobia usually presents at approximately 8 years of age and can be severe. Corneal erosions and ulcers can occur. Defective sweat production may result in heat intolerance in some patients. These patients also salivate and tear abnormally. Delayed puberty (males and females) and primary hypogonadism in untreated males is common. Hypothyroidism develops at about the same time as end-stage renal failure presents. Renal damage becomes irreversible already after one year of age. However, early replacement therapy of renal losses and a cystine-depleting therapy may not only prevent the laboratory anomalies, but also attenuate renal Fanconi syndrome, rickets, and tetany, and allow for a normal growth rate. Although these patients may have behavioral issues, intelligence is usually normal. Idiopathic intracranial hypertension (pseudotumor cerebri) with cerebrospinal fluid (CSF) opening pressures over 20 cm of H_2O and papilledema have been described in some patients. Drugs (e.g., steroids, cyclosporine, cysteamine), hypercoagulability with increased risk for thrombosis (as a result of renal disease), or decreased CSF reabsorption in the arachnoid villi secondary to cystine deposition have been discussed as possible risk factors. Renal transplantation is the treatment of choice and has been very successful, however cystine accumulation in other tissues continues, which explains some of the late complications. One of the main complications from an anesthetic point of view occurs usually in the third to fourth decade of life and consists of a distal vacuolar myopathy resulting in (initially) distal weakness, muscle wasting, restrictive lung disease, and dysphagia. Other, even earlier presenting complications may include insulin-dependent diabetes mellitus, retinal blindness, and central nervous system dysfunction (personality and cognitive changes, progressive dementia, hemiparesis, pseudobulbar, pyramidal and extrapyramidal dysfunction).

Intermediate nephropathic cystinosis: The patients show basically the same symptoms (growth retardation, renal Fanconi syndrome, photophobia) as in infantile nephropathic cystinosis, although they occur delayed and are initially less severe.

Precautions before anesthesia: Review the past medical history and check for signs of potentially involved organ systems. Anemia is a common problem in these patients (renal anemia, decreased hematopoiesis secondary to bone marrow affection), hence a complete blood count should be obtained. In addition, blood glucose, serum electrolytes (including calcium, magnesium and phosphate), creatinine, blood urea nitrogen, acid-base status and volume status should be assessed and corrected if indicated. Assessment of hepatic function may be indicated in older patients (transaminases, albumin, coagulation status, bilirubin). Since these patients may have polyuria and isosthenuria, ask about daily drink and urine volume. Keep the preoperative fasting time as short as possible and consider intravenous fluid replacement during this time. Depending on the age of the patient, thyroid function tests may be added. Clinical assessment of muscle function is important (weakness, muscle wasting) since this may result in prolonged postoperative mechanical ventilation. Also assess for signs of increased intracranial pressure in older patients. Admission to an intensive care unit postoperatively to closely monitor vital signs, electrolytes, acid-base, and volume status is recommended.

Anesthetic considerations: Upon arrival of the patient in the operating room, the lights should be dimmed to avoid photophobia, and direct light into the patient's face should be avoided (also applies for emergence of anesthesia). The threshold for an arterial line should be kept low in these patients to allow for frequent perioperative blood work (including blood glucose levels, electrolytes, and acid-base status). Perioperative replacement of sodium bicarbonate and potassium decreases the risk for significant electrolyte disturbances. Urine output in these patients does not reliably reflect the volume status and invasive monitoring (central venous line) is recommended for procedures with significant fluid shifts or of longer duration (alternatively, blood can then be sampled from the central venous line). Due to involvement of the intestinal mucosa, diabetes mellitus or increased intracranial pressure, these patients may be at risk for gastroesophageal reflux and aspiration during induction of (and emergence from) anesthesia. A rapid sequence induction is therefore recommended. If signs of increased intracranial pressure exist, elective surgery should be postponed, otherwise standard anesthesia implications for management of patients with raised intracranial pressure apply. Strict aseptic technique for all invasive procedures is mandatory in patients under immunosuppressive therapy (after kidney transplant). Keep the eyes taped shut and use lubricants during surgery. Careful monitoring of body temperature is required to avoid hyperthermia.

Pharmacological implications: Potentially nephrotoxic drugs should be avoided and drugs with predominantly renal elimination may require adapted dosage. Repeated doses of morphine or meperidine (pethidine) should be avoided. (Cis-)atracurium and mivacurium are the neuromuscular blockers of choice. Titration under the control of a peripheral nerve stimulator is recommended. Succinylcholine is best avoided once signs of myopathy are detected or suspected to avoid the consequences of exaggerated hyperkalemia due to rhabdomyolysis. A patient with a malignant hyperthermia-like reaction has been described, but this was most likely caused by abnormal (decreased) sweating function. Since atropine affects sweating, it should be used with strict indications only.

Other conditions to be considered:

☞**DE TONI-DEBRÉ-FANCONI SYNDROME:** A rare acquired or inherited condition involving a generalized transport defect in the proximal tubules with renal losses of glucose, phosphate, calcium, uric acid, amino acids, and bicarbonates leading to short stature, osteomalacia, and renal failure.

☞**GALACTOSEMIA:** An inborn error of metabolism with the inability to metabolize galactose appropriately. This results in toxic effects on brain, liver, kidney, and eyes. Early diagnosis and galactose free diet are key.

☞**LOWE SYNDROME:** A genetically transmitted syndrome mainly affecting males and characterized by the association of ocular problems with renal dysfunction and mental retardation.

☞**WILSON DISEASE:** An inherited, potentially fatal disease of copper metabolism characterized by liver cirrhosis and central nervous system findings.

REFERENCES:

Anikster Y, Lacbawan F, Brantly M, et al: Pulmonary dysfunction in adults with nephropathic cystinosis. *Chest* 119:394, 2001.

Dogulu CF, Tsilou E, Rubin B, et al: Idiopathic intracranial hypertension in cystinosis. *J Pediatr* 145:673, 2004.

Gahl WA, Thoene JG, Schneider JA: Cystinosis. *N Engl J Med* 347:111, 2002.

Ray TL, Tobias JD: Perioperative care of the patient with nephropathic cystinosis. *Paediatr Anaesth* 14:878, 2004.

D

D-2-Hydroxyglutaric Aciduria

At a glance: Metabolic disease resulting in abnormal MRI findings and psychomotor retardation, hypotonia, and nonneurologic signs.

Incidence and genetic inheritance: Incidence is unknown, but approximately 30 cases have been reported. Inheritance is autosomal recessive.

Clinical aspects: The enzymatic defect causing this progressive neurometabolic disorder has not been found. D-2-Hydroxyglutaric acid is a stereoisomer of L-2-hydroxyglutaric acid and an intermediate in glutamate, 5-aminolevulinic acid, and gamma-aminobutyric acid (GABA) metabolism. Elevated levels of GABA were found in the cerebrospinal fluid of some patients with D-2-hydroxyglutaric aciduria. A mild and a severe phenotype have been reported, with a more variable clinical picture and less consistency seen on MRI findings of the mild phenotype. Regardless of the phenotype, progressive psychomotor degeneration with macrocephaly, epilepsy (hypsarrhythmia), hypotonia, cerebral and/or cerebellar atrophy with cerebellar ataxia, and mental and motor developmental delay can be found. The most consistent MRI findings are enlargement of the lateral ventricles, subependymal cysts, and signs of delayed cerebral maturation. Nonneurologic manifestations include prenatal and postnatal growth retardation, cardiomyopathy, facial anomalies, and episodic vomiting. Inspiratory stridor and apnea were the reasons for tracheotomy in one patient at age 4 months.

Anesthetic considerations: Facial anomalies, which may affect the airway management, have been reported in a minority of cases. Anomalies include macrocephaly and microcephaly, micrognathia, prognathia, and midface hypoplasia. Hypertrophic cardiomyopathy and aortic insufficiency have been reported and warrant preoperative investigation. Check serum electrolytes and volemia in case of recurrent vomiting, and perform a rapid-sequence induction if general anesthesia is required.

Other condition to be considered:

☞L-2-HYDROXYGLUTARIC ACIDURIA: Inborn error of metabolism manifesting as progressive neurodegenerative disorder with psychomotor retardation.

REFERENCES:

Amiel J, de Lonlay P, Francannet C, et al: Facial anomalies in D-2-hydroxyglutaric aciduria. *Am J Med Genet* 86:124, 1999.

Nyhan WL, Shelton D, Jakobs C, et al: D-2-hydroxyglutaric aciduria. *J Child Neurol* 10:137, 1995.

Van der Knaap MS, Jakobs C, Hoffmann GF, et al: D-2-hydroxyglutaric aciduria: Further clinical delineation. *J Inherit Metab Dis* 22:404, 1999.

Da Silva Syndrome

At a glance: Mental retardation with hypoplastic corpus callosum and preauricular tag.

Incidence and genetic inheritance: Extremely rare disorder with autosomal recessive transmission.

Clinical aspects: The most consistent features of this syndrome are microcephaly, hypoplastic corpus callosum, aqueductal stenosis with enlarged ventricles, severe mental retardation, large ears with preauricular skin tags, profound growth retardation, camptodactyly, and recurrent bronchopneumonias. Electroencephalographs reportedly are normal; however, hypertonicity and hyperreflexia of all limbs have been described as a common symptom. Mild micrognathia and high arched palate were additional signs. Death in the three patients initially described occurred between age 10 and 32 months, most likely as a consequence of bronchopneumonia. One patient who was alive at age 7 years suffered from recurrent pneumonias and persistent esophagitis secondary to gastroesophageal reflux.

Anesthetic considerations: No references to anesthesia exist. However, intracranial pressure can be elevated, and an anesthetic technique tailored accordingly should be provided. Micrognathia usually is mild, and airway management should not be affected. Because of gastroesophageal reflux, a rapid-sequence induction is strongly suggested. Depending on the procedure, patients may need postoperative mechanical ventilation. A preoperative chest radiograph is recommended. Elective surgery should be postponed until bronchopneumonia and other airway infections are resolved. Recurrent bronchopneumonias may affect pulmonary gas exchange, and increased secretions in the acute phase (for emergency surgery) may result in obstruction of the endotracheal tube (particularly in small patients).

Other conditions to be considered:

☞ZELLWEGER SYNDROME: Characterized by the congenital absence of functioning peroxisomes resulting in a cerebrohepatorenal syndrome.

☞AICARDI SYNDROME: Combination of myoclonic seizures with a characteristic EEG pattern, lacunar chorioretinopathy, and complete or partial agenesis of the corpus callosum is characteristic for this X-linked dominant inherited syndrome.

☞SCHINZEL ACROCALLOSAL SYNDROME: Very rare autosomal recessive, complex, polymalformative disease with prominent neurologic and skeletal anomalies. Anesthetic procedure must consider craniofacial malformations (intubation).

☞FG SYNDROME: X-linked form of mental retardation associated with complete or partial agenesis of the corpus callosum and minor facial, skeletal, and gastrointestinal anomalies.

☞ANDERMANN SYNDROME: Inherited neurodegenerative disorder with progressive sensorimotor neuropathy.

☞CEREBRO-RENO-DIGITAL SYNDROME: Autosomal recessive inherited syndrome with corpus callosum agenesis, Dandy-Walker malformation, mental retardation, and paraparesis or quadriparesis. Succinylcholine should be used with caution.

REFERENCES:

da-Silva EO: Callosal defect, microcephaly, severe mental retardation, and other anomalies in three sibs. *Am J Med Genet* 29:837, 1988.

Naritomi K, Tohma T, Goya Y, et al: Delineation of the da-Silva syndrome. *Am J Med Genet* 49:313, 1994.

Danbolt-Closs Syndrome

At a glance: Inherited vesiculobullous disorder characterized by intermittent simultaneous occurrence of diarrhea and bullous dermatitis (dry lesions surrounding the mouth, ears, nose, and eyes, but also affecting the fingers, feet, and knees) and failure to thrive in premature babies. In children, periorificial lesions of the face and anogenital region. Alopecia and absence of eyebrows, eyelashes, and thymus are common.

Synonyms: Acrodermatitis Enteropathica; Zinc-Deficiency Syndrome; Periorificial Dermatitis.

History: Named after Niels C.G. Danbolt and Karl P. Closs, two Norwegian physicians who described the disease in 1942, although the first description was given by Thore E. Brandt, a Swedish dermatologist, in 1936.

Genetic inheritance: Exact incidence is not known, but estimates are about 2:1,000,000 live births. No racial or sexual predilection has been reported.

Pathophysiology: Results in decreased synthesis of picolinic acid that causes an impaired ability to utilize zinc from common food. The metabolic defect appears to be related to a cellular defect in zinc metabolism rather than in zinc absorption. However, oral or intravenous administration of zinc rapidly improves the condition. Fibroblasts of these patients contain 60% less zinc than in normal subjects. The immune system also is affected by zinc deficiency, which not only may result in decreased cellular and humoral immune response with increased susceptibility to infections but also may be involved in the association with connective tissue disorders. Zinc concentrations are decreased in the mucosa of the small intestine.

Diagnosis: Vesiculobullous and/or pustular disorder caused by a disturbance of intraepidermal or dermal-epidermal adherence with subsequent accumulation of serous fluid within the cavities formed by tissue separation. The disorder develops during the first year of life as periorificial and acral vesiculobullous eruptions, which are followed by alopecia, ungual dystrophy, severe diarrhea, failure to thrive, cachexia, and psychological symptoms such as irritability or apathy. Laboratory tests reveal a significant decrease in zinc serum and tissue levels (*caveat:* special laboratory tubes may be required because many may contain zinc in the rubber cap or other parts) and a low level of alkaline phosphatases (because it is a zinc metalloenzyme). Be aware that hypoalbuminemia can result in falsely low zinc serum concentrations.

Clinical aspects: In addition to the inherited form of zinc deficiency, several clinical conditions may result in zinc deficiency, particularly during total parenteral nutrition (TPN) without zinc supplementation. In babies, the symptoms usually appear during the third month of life. Symptoms consist of dry skin lesions surrounding the mouth, ears, nose, and eyes, and the fingers, feet, and knees. In older children, the clinical aspect is that of periorificial lesions of the face and the anogenital region. Sacral lesions and vesiculobullous mucosal lesions are constant findings. Failure to thrive, anorexia, alopecia, nail dystrophy, and recurrent infections are almost always present. Bullous dermatitis, alopecia, absence of eyebrows and eyelashes, pallor, delayed wound healing, pancreatic islet hyperplasia, absent or hypoplastic thymus, and hypogonadism are common findings. Children may have neurologic and behavioral changes (intellectual capacity is most often normal) and be nutritionally deprived, hypovolemic, anemic, and weak (because of muscle loss). Other manifestations include photophobia, glossitis,

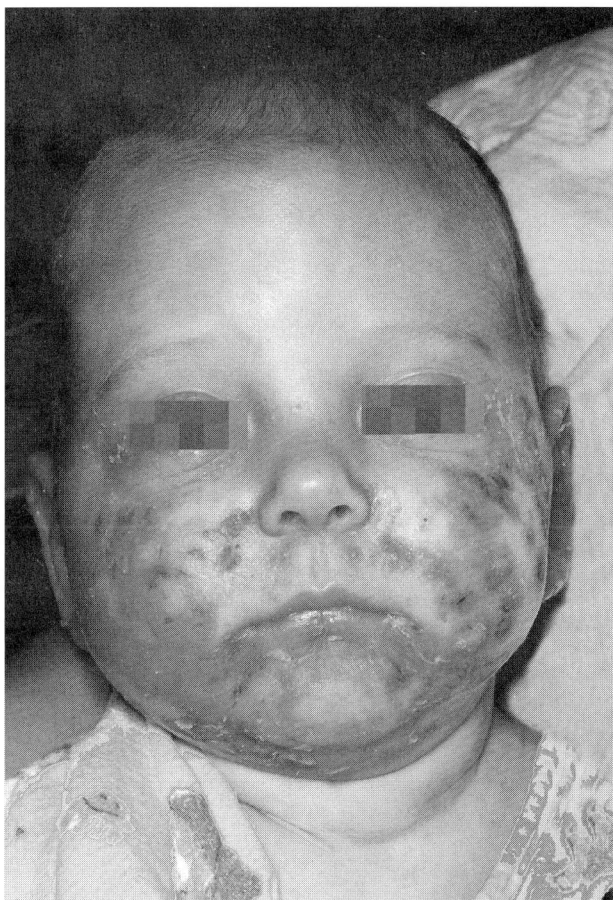

Danbolt-Closs Syndrome   Periorificial skin lesions in the face of a toddler. See color plates.

stomatitis, and bacterial and fungal (candida) infections. A possible association with Crohn disease, ulcerative colitis, malabsorption syndromes (acquired or congenital), intestinal lymphangiectasia, cow milk protein intolerance, ataxia telangiectatica, immune deficiency, cystic fibrosis, or hypersudation has been reported. The condition has been reported in exclusively breast-fed premature babies whose mothers present with a zinc transfer defect from blood to breast milk. Left untreated, patients suffer from severe growth retardation and recurrent bacterial and fungal infections, which finally result in death within the first few years of life. Treated properly, the condition should not affect life expectancy. Acute exacerbations may be fatal. Lifelong zinc supplementation is required.

Precautions before anesthesia: Preoperative blood work should include a complete blood count (anemia) and electrolytes (diarrhea). Because these patients reportedly tolerate inhalational anesthetics poorly, careful assessment of the volume status is recommended. The zinc deficit requires approximately 2 to 3 weeks to be corrected, but most symptoms (except cutaneous lesions) disappear within the first week of treatment. Awaiting preoperative correction of treatable parameters (anemia, infections, cachexia) is strongly recommended if possible or actively treated if necessary. In patients with long-term disease, mouth opening should be checked because perioral scarring may limit mouth opening. A preoperative chest radiograph may be indicated to rule out any bronchopulmonary fungal or bacterial infections.

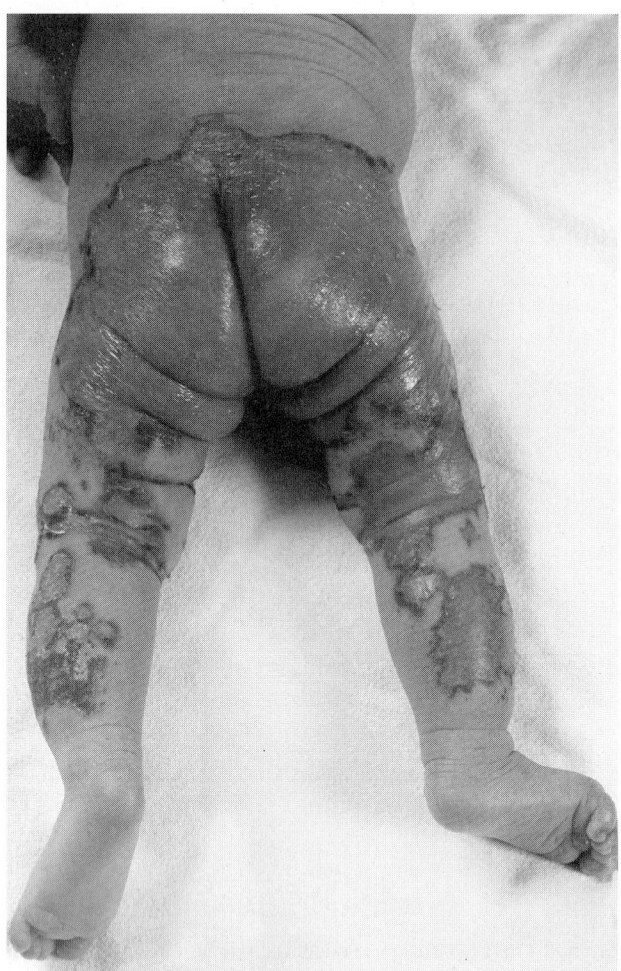

Danbolt-Closs Syndrome Extended periorificial dermatitis affecting the anal region and the legs in a small infant.

Anesthetic considerations: Strict aseptic technique is recommended to prevent infections. Behavior changes may affect patient cooperation. A sedative and/or anxiolytic premedication and the presence of the primary caregiver during induction of anesthesia may be helpful. Careful positioning is required to prevent further

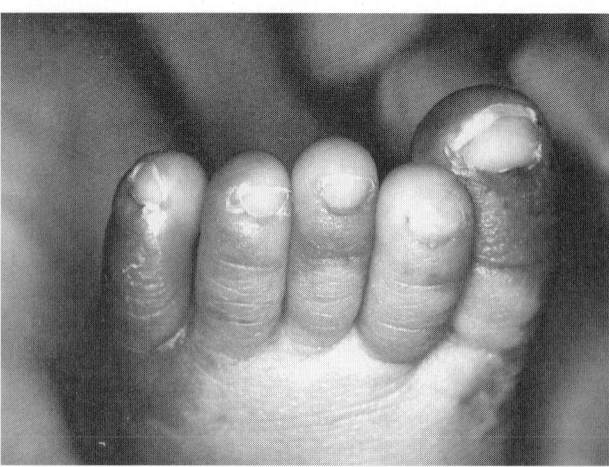

Danbolt-Closs Syndrome Acral skin lesions on the toes of a small child.

exacerbation of the skin lesions, which may affect the positioning of the intravenous cannula and pulse oximetry. Because taping of the endotracheal tube may be difficult, use of a sterile gauze to hold the tube in place is recommended. To prevent further exacerbation, skin lesions should be covered with Vaseline and gauze. The eyes should be well lubricated and then taped to prevent (further) lesions. No literature regarding anesthesia in these patients exists. Depending on the severity of the symptoms, the dosage of anesthetic drugs should be on the lower side because anemia, hypovolemia, hypalbuminemia, and reduced muscle mass (failure to thrive) may render patients susceptible to the adverse effects of these drugs.

Pharmacological implications: Careful titration of anesthetic drugs and use of a peripheral nerve stimulator to assess the degree of neuromuscular blockade are recommended. Reduction of the dose is required for highly protein-bound medications in the presence of hypalbuminemia.

Other conditions to be considered:

☞**EPIDERMOLYSIS BULLOSA:** Genetic disorder characterized by cutaneous blistering and scarring following minor trauma. More than 20 different subtypes of the disease have been grouped into three main categories: epidermolysis bullosa simplex, dystrophic epidermolysis bullosa, and junctional epidermolysis bullosa.

☞**ERYTHEMA MULTIFORME:** Acute mucocutaneous hypersensitivity reaction of variable severity characterized by symmetrical skin eruptions, with or without mucous membrane lesions.

☞**KWASHIORKOR:** Acquired disorder resulting from malnutrition secondary to insufficient protein intake leading to multisystemic chronic failure with generalized edemas.

REFERENCES:

Prasad AS: Zinc: An overview. *Nutrition* 11(suppl):93, 1996.

Sandström B, Cederblad A, Lindblad BS, et al: Acrodermatitis enteropathica, zinc metabolism, copper status, and immune function. *Arch Pediatr Adolesc Med* 148:980, 1994.

Dandy-Walker Malformation

At a glance: Congenital anomaly of the cerebellum and fourth ventricle characterized by hypoplasia of the cerebellum and hydrocephalus caused by cystic expansion of the fourth ventricle in the posterior fossa.

Incidence: Approximately 1:25,000 newborns is affected. Accounts for less than 5% of hydrocephalus patients. Frequency is higher in females than in males.

Genetic inheritance: Heterogenous. Some autosomal recessive cases with a possible genetic defect on the long arm of chromosome 9. Recurrence risk is considered low (1–5%) if it is not associated with a mendelian disorder. Exposure to isotretinoin in the first trimester was associated with the malformation but now is uncommon.

Pathophysiology: Unknown. Syndrome initially thought to result from atresia of the fourth ventricle's foramina during embryologic differentiation, resulting in cystic transformation of the roof of the fourth ventricle. Cerebellar malformation now is considered to be independent of this atresia. The cyst arises from compromised cerebrospinal fluid absorption.

Diagnosis: In approximately 80% of cases, the diagnosis is made in the first year of life, and in approximately 25% of cases it is made in the neonatal period. Affected children present with hydrocephalus associated with bulging fontanelles and occiput. Transillumination of the skull is positive. MRI or CT scans confirm enlargement of the posterior fossa, fourth ventricle (grossly), aqueduct of Sylvius, and third and lateral ventricles. The posterior fossa cyst may extend through the foramen magnum into the spinal canal. Partial or complete absence of the cerebellar vermis and elevated imprints of the transverse sinuses are additional features. The bones forming the posterior fossa are thinned. This malformation has been reported to occur in combination with other genetic syndromes.

Clinical aspects: Obstructive hydrocephalus is present in approximately 90% of patients and is often associated with cranial nerve palsies. Most children have cerebellar signs (ataxia, nystagmus) and evidence of long-tract signs (spasticity). Signs of raised intracranial pressure (irritability, vomiting, convulsions), infantile hypotonia, developmental delay, and mental retardation (in up to 70%). Associated anomalies occur in almost 50% of cases. Agenesis of the corpus callosum with associated mental retardation and interference with medullary control of respiration leads to medullary failure. Pontine lesions involving the apneustic center result in abnormal respiratory control (e.g.: apneas). The clinical picture in older children involves delayed motor development with poor coordination and gait control. Intellectual development is delayed, and learning problems are frequently reported. Seizures have been reported in up to 30% of patients. Extracerebral anomalies are present in approximately one third of patients and include cleft palate, micrognathia, eye abnormalities (increased intraocular pressure), skeletal abnormalities of lumbar vertebrae, and polydactyly. Congenital cardiac defects have been reported in approximately 15% (ventriculoseptal defect) of patients. Renal abnormalities have been reported. Infundibular hematomas, posterior fossa lymphomas, and syringomyelia are reported features that complicate Dandy-Walker syndrome. The reported mortality rates vary from 26 to 50%.

Precautions before anesthesia: Assess the airway for associated abnormalities such as cleft palate or micrognathia and be prepared for difficult laryngoscopy and tracheal intubation. Positioning of the head with the enlarged posterior fossa may be difficult. Obtain history regarding apneas or other respiratory abnormalities such as aspiration pneumonia. Look for signs of raised intracranial pressure and provide anesthesia accordingly if positive. Check for other associated abnormalities (kidney and cardiac defects).

Anesthetic considerations: Direct laryngoscopy and tracheal intubation may be difficult because of anatomical abnormalities. Preexisting laryngeal incompetence is possible. Consideration must be given to problems associated with raised intracranial pressure, such as the presence of a full stomach (rapid-sequence induction is recommended), respiratory depression, and bradycardias. Intraoperative measures to reduce intracranial pressure, such as mild hyperventilation, mannitol, and diuretics, should be considered. Postoperatively, patients should be monitored in the intensive care unit because recurrent apneas are likely. Depending on preoperative breathing abnormalities, a period of postoperative mechanical ventilation may be required.

Pharmacological implications: Although succinylcholine is not contraindicated, it should be used carefully in a potentially difficult airway. The dosage of narcotics must be reduced if there is a history of respiratory control abnormalities. Tracheal extubation must be planned at the end of the case.

Other conditions to be considered:

☞**JOUBERT SYNDROME:** Autosomal recessive transmitted syndrome with agenesis of the cerebellar vermis, cystic dilatation of the fourth ventricle, and poor respiratory control. Variable combina-

tion of central nervous system (CNS), eye, and renal abnormalities exists.

☞**MECKEL-GRUBER SYNDROME:** Genetic disorder with main features of encephalocele, polydactyly, and polycystic kidneys but a wide phenotypic variation.

☞**CEREBRO-RENO-DIGITAL SYNDROME:** Autosomal recessive inherited syndrome with corpus callosum agenesis, Dandy-Walker malformation, mental retardation, and paraparesis or quadriparesis. Succinylcholine should be used with caution.

REFERENCES:

Ewart M, Oh TE: The Dandy-Walker syndrome. Relevance to anaesthesia and intensive care. *Anaesthesia* 45:646, 1990.

Hart MN, Malamud N, Ellis WG: The Dandy-Walker syndrome: A clinicopathological study based on 28 cases. *Neurology* 22:771, 1972.

Darier-White Disease

At a glance: Autosomal dominant, slowly progressive disorder of keratinization. Lesions usually coalesce and result in crusted papillomatous lesions.

Synonyms: Keratosis Follicularis; Dyskeratosis Follicularis.

Incidence: Four new cases per million per 10 years. Gene map locus is 12q23-q24.1

Genetic inheritance: Autosomal dominant.

Pathophysiology: Results from an abnormal desmosome–keratin filament complex that leads to disruption of cell adhesion.

Diagnosis: Diagnosis is made by family history and clinical aspect. Histological studies of the skin are diagnostic and characterized by hyperkeratosis, dyskeratotic epidermal cells, suprabasal separation of the spinal layer with formation of clefts and lacunae containing acantholytic cells, dermal villi extending in the epidermis, and mild nonspecific perivascular dermal infiltration.

Clinical aspects: Age of onset is usually between 6 and 20 years, with peak onset around puberty. Keratotic papules appear predominantly on the upper trunk and may involve the face, scalp, neck, hands (palms), feet (soles), and limb flexures (axillae, groins). The papillomatous masses may become malodorous. Nail dystrophy manifests as subungual hyperkeratosis, fragility, longitudinal ridging and splitting, and longitudinal red and white lines. Mucous membranes, such as lips, buccal mucosa, hard palate, alveolar ridges, uvula, pharynx, larynx, and vulva, are rarely involved. However, if involved, papules, fissures, crusts, and ulcers may result. Secondary cutaneous infection (herpes virus, bacterial) is a frequent complication. The disease is exacerbated by sunlight or sunburn. Occasionally, patients suffer from a seizure disorder and mild mental retardation.

Precautions before anesthesia: Inquire about dermatologic treatment. Adverse effects of oral retinoid derivatives include increased intracranial pressure, pseudotumor cerebri, hypoplastic anemia, leukopenia, optic neuropathy, hypercalcemia, bone demineralization, increased alkaline phosphatase level, hepatomegaly, splenomegaly, dermatotoxicity, carcinogenicity, photosensitization, and teratogenicity. A newer generation of more selective topical retinoids seems almost devoid of toxic side effects. Topical steroids are of little use in Darier disease. In the presence of oral retinoid treatment, obtain a complete blood count, hemoglobin level, liver function tests, and calcium level, and evaluate for the presence of increased intracranial pressure. If necessary, obtain a neurologic consultation.

Anesthetic considerations: Involvement of the mucous membranes is extremely rare and does not compromise airway management. In the presence of retinoic acid toxicity, correction of anemia and hypercalcemia may be necessary. In the rare cases of increased intracranial pressure, precautions to prevent further elevation should be taken. In cases with an associated seizure disorder, patients on anticonvulsant treatment should receive their medication perioperatively.

Pharmacological implications: In the presence of a seizure disorder, avoid potentially epileptogenic drugs such as methohexital, ketamine, enflurane, atracurium, *cis*-atracurium, and meperidine (the last three only if given in large quantities because of their metabolites laudanosine and normeperidine, respectively).

REFERENCES:
Burge SM, Wilkinson JD: Darier-White disease: A review of the clinical features in 163 patients. *J Am Acad Dermatol* 27:40, 1992.

Weinstein GD: Safety, efficacy and duration of therapeutic effect of tazarotene used in the treatment of plaque psoriasis. *Br J Dermatol* 135(suppl 49):32, 1996.

De Die Smulders Vles Fryns Syndrome

At a glance: Genetic disorder characterized by a characteristic facies, marfanoid habitus, and mental delay.

Synonym: Arachnodactyly Mental Retardation Dysmorphism Syndrome.

Incidence: Approximately 10 cases have been described.

Genetic inheritance: Postulated to be autosomal recessive.

Pathophysiology: Unknown.

Diagnosis: Symptoms of the syndrome are apparent at birth. Diagnosis is based on physical signs of arachnodactyly and the characteristic facies associated with mental retardation.

Clinical aspects: Facies is long, narrow, and triangular in shape, with a large forehead and brachycephalic skull. Other facial characteristics are hypertelorism, microstomia with thin lips and flat philtrum, and an underdeveloped maxilla. Moderate-to-severe mental retardation with or without seizures is found. Patients present with long slender extremities, arachnodactyly comparable to Marfan syndrome, and, in some cases, hyperextensible joints. Finger and toe anomalies, such as clinodactyly of the fourth and fifth fingers, triphalangeal thumbs, and hammer-shaped toes, can be present. Patients may be hypotonic with increased reflexes and underdeveloped musculature. Development of the external genitalia is delayed. Mitral regurgitation has been described in one case.

Precautions before anesthesia: Evaluate the airway carefully. If a cardiac lesion is suspected, obtain an ECG and an echocardiogram.

Anesthetic considerations: Direct laryngoscopy and tracheal intubation may be challenging. An inhalation induction while the child is kept spontaneously breathing probably is the best choice, considering the child is mentally delayed and can hardly cooperate with an awake fiberoptic intubation. In the presence of a cardiac lesion, antibiotic prophylaxis for subacute bacterial endocarditis should be given.

Pharmacological implications: Secondary to the generalized hypotonia and poorly developed musculature, neuromuscular blocking agents may not be needed at all or only in a reduced dosage.

If the patient is on anticonvulsant medication, liver enzymes may be induced and hasten the metabolism of drugs with predominantly hepatic metabolism.

Other conditions to be considered:

☞**LUJAN FRYNS SYNDROME:** Inherited syndrome with marfanoid features and X-linked mental retardation.

☞**MARFAN SYNDROME:** Autosomal dominant inherited disorder with generalized connective tissue abnormalities. Aortic regurgitation and dissection are responsible for premature death in the third to fifth decade.

REFERENCES:
de Die-Smulders C, Vles H, Fryns JP: Characteristic facial dysmorphism, arachnodactyly and mental handicap in two unrelated girls: A distinct MCA/MR syndrome? *Genet Couns* 4:165, 1993.

Mégarbané A, Chammas C: Severe mental retardation with marfanoid habitus in a young Lebanese male. A diagnostic challenge. *Genet Couns* 8:195, 1997.

Van Buggenhout GJCM, Akkermans-Scholten ACM, Hamel BCJ: Characteristic facial dysmorphism, arachnodactyly and mental retardation: Another case. *Genet Counsel* 6:61, 1995.

De Morsier Syndrome

At a glance: Genetic disease that causes the triad of optic nerve hypoplasia, structural brain abnormalities, and hypothalamic/pituitary deficiencies.

Synonyms: Septo-Optic Dysplasia; Optic Nerve Hypoplasia; Dwarfism-Septo-Optic-Dysplasia.

Incidence: Unknown.

Genetic inheritance: Some cases are sporadic, whereas other cases seem to indicate autosomal dominant and recessive patterns of inheritance.

Pathophysiology: Caused by mutation in the homeobox gene HESX1. The typical picture includes optic hypoplasia, pituitary hypofunction, and midline defects of the prosencephalon. Milder forms exist in individuals with heterozygous mutations of the gene.

Diagnosis: Clinical picture, family history, brain imaging, and cytogenetic identification of mutations of the HESX1 gene.

Clinical aspects: Wide variability in the clinical picture. The syndrome is characterized by hypoplasia of the optic disk and nerve, hypothalamic–pituitary axis defects, and agenesis of the septum pellucidum. Agenesis of the corpus callosum, hypoplastic cerebellar changes similar to Dandy-Walker malformation, hemiparesis or hemiplegia, spasticity, and mental retardation (mild-to-severe) have been described as optional signs. The extent of pituitary involvement ranges from growth hormone deficiency only to panhypopituitarism. The clinical picture of decreased hormone levels may result not only in short stature but also in hypoglycemia (decreased levels of adrenocorticotropic hormone), diabetes insipidus, and precocious puberty. Visual impairment is usually noted at birth, ranging from decreased vision in one eye to no vision in both eyes secondary to optic disc atrophy and corneal opacification. Variable pupillary dilatation and searching nystagmus can often be found. Facial features include a flat face and midline cleft lip. Abnormal external genitalia (cryptorchidism, micropenis) have been reported. Patients are prone to intercurrent infections.

Precautions before anesthesia: The hazards of anesthetizing a patient in whom the syndrome has not been recognized have been documented. Bear the diagnosis in mind in a patient with visual impairment and small stature. Ideally, the patient is under the care of an endocrinologist. Ask about episodes of hypoglycemia. The patient may be on chronic hormone replacement therapy, requiring additional hydrocortisone stress coverage in the perioperative period. Preoperative assessment should include evaluation of hydration and electrolytes in view of possible diabetes insipidus. Check seizure control.

Anesthetic considerations: Sudden unexpected death has been described in these patients, probably as a consequence of intercurrent viral illness and consecutive adrenal crisis. Specific attention must be paid to prevent hypoglycemia. Maintaining hydration, if diabetes insipidus is present, is crucial, and extra doses of hydrocortisone to cover for perioperative stress are required. Temperature control is important because patients may suffer from thermoregulatory disturbances.

Pharmacological implications: Be aware of interactions between anticonvulsants and anesthetic drugs. Hormone replacement therapy must be maintained.

REFERENCES:

Brodsky MC, Conte FA, Taylor D, et al: Sudden death in septo-optic dysplasia: Report of 5 cases. *Arch Ophthalmol* 115:66, 1997.

Sherlock DA, McNicol LR: Anaesthesia and septo-optic dysplasia. Implications of missed diagnosis in the peri-operative period. *Anaesthesia* 42:1302, 1987.

Thomas PQ, Dattani MT, Brickman JM, et al: Heterozygous HESX1 mutations associated with isolated congenital pituitary hypoplasia and septo-optic dysplasia. *Hum Mol Genet* 10:39, 2001.

De Sanctis Cacchione Syndrome

At a glance: Genetic disorder with xeroderma pigmentosum and progressive neurologic degeneration.

Synonym: Xerodermic Idiocy of De Sanctis and Cacchione.

Incidence: Not known for De Sanctis Cacchione syndrome; however, the incidence of xeroderma pigmentosum is estimated to be 1:250,000 in general population, and the percentage of patients with associated neurologic changes is 15 to 20%. Both genders are equally affected. Seems to occur in all ethnic groups.

Genetic inheritance: Autosomal recessive.

Pathophysiology: Xeroderma pigmentosum causes pigmentary and atrophic skin changes as a result of a defective ability to repair normally occurring DNA changes (cross-linkage of thymidine nucleotides, called *dimers)* following exposure to ultraviolet (UV) light. The nucleotide excision repair mechanism, responsible in healthy individuals for elimination of these dimers, fails to excise and replace them by normal nucleotides. Early and diffuse neuronal death occurs in correlation with the degree of inability to repair DNA, which may account for the neurologic changes in this subgroup of xeroderma pigmentosum. Polyneuropathy has been attributed to diffuse axonal loss in peripheral nerves in affected patients.

Diagnosis: Clinical and family history. Cytogenetic testing can be used to elucidate the complementation subtype of xeroderma pigmentosum. The De Sanctis Cacchione syndrome usually is associated with subtypes A (subgroup with the most profound defect and basically absent DNA repair function) and D (subgroup with the highest rate [about half of patients] of neurologic involvement) but may occur with any of the seven subtypes (A through G).

Clinical aspects: Skin changes include atrophy, photosensitivity, and hyperpigmentation and hypopigmentation. Skin cancer is the major cause of morbidity in these patients, with basal cell and squamous cell carcinoma being the most common tumors, presenting at a median age of approximately 8 years. The risk of developing a malignant melanoma is up to 2000-fold higher than in a healthy person. Commonly, these skin tumors are multiple and do not spare the eye. Interestingly, and sadly enough, patients also suffer from a significantly higher incidence of other tumors. The most common neurologic symptoms are mental retardation, spasticity, ataxia, microcephaly, epilepsy, deafness, areflexia, and choreoathetosis. Other signs include the eye abnormalities (photophobia, keratitis, impaired vision), dwarfism, and gonadal hypoplasia.

Anesthetic considerations: Communication will be difficult because of mental impairment, possible deafness, and impaired vision. Careful positioning and padding are required because of the vulnerability of the skin. Mouth opening may be restricted as a result of skin atrophy and scarring. According to a case report, volatile anesthetic agents should be avoided in patients with xeroderma pigmentosum because of in vitro evidence that the defective DNA repair may be further worsened by exposure to halothane. Vascular access can be challenging in the presence of extensive skin changes. Be careful when applying adhesive tapes and strips and even more so when removing them.

Pharmacological implications: Secondary to liver enzyme induction, chronic anticonvulsant medication may affect the metabolism of predominantly hepatic eliminated drugs.

Other conditions to be considered:

☞**XERODERMA PIGMENTOSUM:** Rare autosomal recessive inherited defect affecting the DNA repair mechanisms for damages induced by UV radiation. Characterized by severe sensitivity to all sources of UV radiation (especially sunlight), resulting in chronic skin changes and a high frequency of skin malignancies similar to De Sanctis Cacchione syndrome.

☞**BLOOM SYNDROME:** Autosomal recessive inherited disorder characterized by prenatal and postnatal growth retardation, photosensitivity, telangiectasias, skin pigment anomalies, and increased risk of malignancies most likely caused by chromosomal instability.

☞**COCKAYNE SYNDROME:** Characteristics of this autosomal-recessive inherited disease are dwarfism, precociously senile appearance, pigmentary retinal degeneration, optic atrophy, progressive sensorineural deafness, sensitivity to sunlight, and mental retardation. Disproportionately long limbs with large hands and feet and flexion contractures of joints are the usual skeletal features.

☞**ROTHMUND-THOMSON SYNDROME:** Poikiloderma, alopecia or sparse hair, dystrophic teeth and nails, saddle nose, short stature, skeletal defects, juvenile cataract, premature aging, and a high incidence of cutaneous and noncutaneous malignancies characterize this disorder.

☞**WERNER SYNDROME:** Rare genetic disease characterized by premature aging. Development of endocrine disturbance with diabetes, early atherosclerosis, and potentially difficult airway management are known features.

REFERENCES:

Butler MG, Hayes BG, Hathaway MM, et al: Specific genetic diseases at risk for sedation/anesthesia complications. *Anesth Analg* 91:837, 2000.

Kraemer KH, Lee MM, Scotto J: Xeroderma pigmentosum. Cutaneous, ocular, and neurologic abnormalities in 830 published cases. *Arch Dermatol* 123:241, 1987.

Masuda Y, Imaizumi H, Okanuma M, et al: Anesthesia for a patient with xeroderma pigmentosum. *Masui* 51:169, 2002.

De Toni Debré Fanconi Syndrome

At a glance: Rare acquired or inherited condition involving a generalized transport defect in the proximal tubules with renal losses of glucose, phosphate, calcium, uric acid, amino acids, and bicarbonates, leading to short stature, osteomalacia, and renal failure.

Synonyms: Lignac De Toni Debré Syndrome; Fanconi Syndrome; Renal Fanconi Syndrome; Fanconi Renal-Tubular Syndrome.

Nature: Genetic disorder but also can be caused by inborn errors of metabolism, Wilson disease, Lowe syndrome, cystinosis, glycogenoses, hereditary fructose intolerance, mitochondrial diseases, heavy-metal poisoning, glue sniffing, and toxicity from some chemotherapeutic drugs.

Incidence: Inherited form is estimated to occur in approximately 1:40,000 live births.

Genetic inheritance: Autosomal dominant, but autosomal recessive and X-linked transmission have been reported. Gene located on 15q15.3.

Pathophysiology: Syndrome may be inherited (idiopathic familial), secondary to other genetic diseases or secondary to exposure to certain toxins. Cystinosis is the most common genetic cause in childhood. Others are galactosemia, Wilson disease, tyrosinemia, and glycogen storage diseases. Toxins include heavy metals such as cadmium, lead, and mercury, ifosfamide, gentamicin, expired tetracycline, and various solvents. The disease causes failure of proximal renal tubular reabsorption.

Diagnosis: Diagnosis is mainly clinical and biochemical. The presenting symptoms are polyuria, polydipsia, and dehydration. The biochemical findings are glucosuria with normal glycemia, hypophosphatemia, hyperaminoaciduria, acidosis, uricosuria, proteinemia, progressive renal insufficiency, and renal sodium and potassium wasting. Following the diagnosis of renal tubular acidosis, an underlying cause should be sought with appropriate investigations for inborn metabolic disease or environmental exposure.

Clinical aspects: Excessive renal loss of glucose, amino acids, potassium, bicarbonate, phosphate, calcium, water, and magnesium lead to growth retardation/dwarfism, polyuria, polydipsia, metabolic acidosis, muscle weakness, and rickets or osteomalacia (depending on age of onset). De Toni Debré Fanconi syndrome can be the first manifestation of complex IV deficiency.

Precautions before anesthesia: Assess for dehydration and treat accordingly. Detailed assessment of acid-base and serum electrolyte status is mandatory.

Anesthetic considerations: Patients are said to be particularly anxious; consequently, sedative premedication is recommended. Patients have ongoing polyuria and losses of bicarbonate, potassium, phosphate, calcium, and magnesium, which require regular assessment and replacement. It may be appropriate to monitor circulatory volume status during important surgical procedures with the aid of central venous pressure monitoring or monitoring of left ventricular filling. Careful positioning and handling are required because of rickets/osteomalacia.

Pharmacological implications: A case of hyperthermia under general anesthesia in a patient with this syndrome secondary to cystinosis has been reported. After the event, malignant hyperthermia was considered unlikely and pyrexia, which developed during a subsequent nonmalignant hyperthermia-triggering anesthetic, was treated successfully with acetaminophen. Avoid drugs eliminated mainly by the renal system. Remember that some drugs, such as certain antibiotics or neuromuscular relaxant drugs, may require dosage adjustment. Succinylcholine is not contraindicated except in the presence of hyperkaliemia. Uremic patients may be more sensitive to the central depressant effect of benzodiazepines and opioids.

Other conditions to be considered: Those associated with renal tubular acidosis:

☞**PERIODIC PARALYSIS:** Congenital abnormality in membrane electrolyte conductance leading to episodic muscle weakness.

☞**LIGHTWOOD SYNDROME:** Nonhereditary form of primary tubular acidosis presenting with hypercalcemia, hypercalciuria, and nephrocalcinosis.

☞**ALBRIGHT BUTLER SYNDROME:** Patients present with renal tubular acidosis, nephrocalcinosis, and renal failure. Hypokalemia with muscle weakness and periodic paralysis is frequent. Polyuria, vomiting, and dehydration lead to fluid and electrolyte imbalances.

☞**ADENOSINE DEAMINASE DEFICIENCY:** Heterogeneous systemic disorder caused by deficiency of adenosine deaminase resulting primarily in severe combined (cellular and humoral) immunodeficiency but also systemic abnormalities.

☞**GITELMAN SYNDROME:** Inherited renal tubular defect resulting in urinary loss of magnesium, sodium, potassium, and chloride with otherwise normal kidneys.

☞**LOWE SYNDROME:** Genetically transmitted polymalformative syndrome characterized by the association of ocular problems with renal dysfunction and mental retardation.

☞**PHOSPHOENOLPYRUVATE CARBOXYKINASE DEFICIENCY:** Congenital metabolic disease leading to a defect in gluconeogenesis.

☞**PROPIONIC ACIDEMIA:** Inborn error of metabolism affecting the mitochondrial catabolism of valine and isoleucine; untreated resulting in ketoacidosis, lethargy, coma, and finally death.

☞**PYRUVATE CARBOXYLASE DEFICIENCY:** Mitochondrial disease impairing synthetic pathways and leading to hypoglycemia and severe lactic acidosis.

☞**TYROSINEMIA:** Elevated blood tyrosine levels are present in several clinical entities. The term *tyrosinemia* is used to describe several syndromes. In general, the association of liver and renal failure, marked edema, epistaxis, and distinctive cabbage-like odor are characteristic of the disease.

REFERENCES:

Izzedine H, Launay-Vacher V, Isnard-Bagnis C, et al: Drug-induced Fanconi's syndrome. *Am J Kidney Dis* 41:292, 2003.

Joel M, Rosales JK: Fanconi syndrome and anesthesia. *Anesthesiology* 55:455, 1981.

Lichter-Konecki U, Broman KW, Blau EB, et al: Genetic and physical mapping of the locus for autosomal dominant renal Fanconi syndrome on chromosome 15q15.3. *Am J Hum Genet* 68:264, 2001.

Deafness-Optic Atrophy Syndrome

At a glance: Genetic disorder with congenital deafness and progressive visual loss.

Genetic inheritance: Autosomal dominant.

Clinical aspects: Hearing loss is sensorineural and severe at birth. Although many patients do not develop any speech, some still have residual hearing in the lower frequencies, allowing amplification and development of speech if treated in early childhood. Bilateral optic nerve atrophy begins at an early age but is very slowly progressive, with visual loss noticeable by the patient by age 24 to 30 years. This syndrome has no other associated findings.

Anesthetic considerations: In the presence of hearing loss without significant visual loss, optimize communication by remaining in the visual field of the patient. Writing and drawing, when appropriate, are useful tools. When sign language is used, a qualified translator available preoperatively and postoperatively is an ideal helper. If the patient uses an amplifying hearing device, keeping it available during induction and emergence of anesthesia helps to reduce anxiety.

Other conditions to be considered:

SYLVESTER SYNDROME: Autosomal dominant inherited form of Friedreich ataxia described in 6 of 9 children of one family. Combined findings of Friedreich ataxia with optic atrophy and progressive sensorineural hearing loss.

☞NYSSEN-VAN BOGAERT SYNDROME: Rare genetic disorder with blindness, deafness, developmental delay, and spasticity.

☞ALSTRÖM SYNDROME: Inherited syndrome with progressive visual and hearing loss, diabetes mellitus, and cardiac, hepatic, and renal involvement.

☞COCKAYNE SYNDROME: Characteristics of this autosomal-recessive inherited disease are dwarfism, precociously senile appearance, pigmentary retinal degeneration, optic atrophy, progressive sensorineural deafness, sensitivity to sunlight, and mental retardation. Disproportionately long limbs with large hands and feet and flexion contractures of joints are usual skeletal features.

☞BALLINGER-WALLACE SYNDROME: Maternally transmitted diabetes mellitus, neurosensory deafness, and ophthalmic abnormalities.

☞WOLFRAM SYNDROME: Genetic syndrome sometimes referred to as DIDMOAD (diabetes insipidus, diabetes mellitus, optic atrophy, and deafness).

☞ROGERS SYNDROME: Rare syndrome caused by a defect in a transporter of thiamine, which results in anemia, diabetes, puffiness, and deafness. Situs inversus viscerum totalis is characteristic.

☞CAPOS SYNDROME: Congenital neurologic syndrome with presentation in infancy.

☞ROSENBERG-CHUTORIAN SYNDROME: Inherited neurodegenerative disorder with polyneuropathy, optic atrophy, and deafness. Features resemble those of Charcot-Marie-Tooth disease combined with deafness.

☞USHER SYNDROME: Autosomal recessive disease associated with retinitis pigmentosa and sensorineural deafness.

☞REFSUM DISEASE: Syndrome caused by accumulation of nicotinic acid that leads to polyneuropathy, cutaneous ichthyosis, cardiac failure, deafness, and visual anomalies.

REFERENCES:

Konigsmark BW, Knox DL, Hussels IE, et al: Dominant congenital deafness and progressive optic nerve atrophy. Occurrence in four generations of a family. *Arch Ophthalmol* 91:99, 1974.

Kollarits CR, Pinheiro ML, Swann ER, et al: The autosomal dominant syndrome of progressive optic atrophy and congenital deafness. *Am J Ophthalmol* 87:789, 1979.

Sylvester PE: Some unusual findings in a family with Friedreich's ataxia. *Arch Dis Child* 33:217, 1958.

Degos Syndrome

At a glance: Rare form of systemic occlusive arteriopathy of small- and medium-size arteries with a typical two-stage evolution. Disease affects vessels of the dermis with an aspect of erythematous, dome-shaped papules that develop a central area of necrosis and leave a porcelain-like scar. Gastrointestinal tract and CNS can be affected. Can be fatal.

Synonyms: Malignant Atrophic Papulosis; Papulosis, Malignant Atrophic; Degos Disease; Degos-Kohlmeier Disease; Kohlmeier-Degos Disease.

History: Disease was first described in 1941 by W. Kohlmeier, a German radiologist, and first individualized in 1942 by Robert Degos, a French dermatologist.

Genetic inheritance: Autosomal dominant inheritance is observed in familial cases.

Pathophysiology: Unknown. Familial cases have been described. Immunologic, infectious, or thrombotic factors have been evocated.

Diagnosis: Clinically evocated onset usually in young adults between 20 and 40 years old, probably with male predominance. Characteristic skin lesions (pink, asymptomatic, diffuse papules with a telangiectatic border followed by umbilication and a porcelain-white center) appear. Histologic appearance is typically characterized by a wedge-shaped area of necrosis from the epidermis through the dermis.

Clinical aspects: Skin lesions can be followed by systemic manifestations, sometimes a few years later. Features can involve the eyes (avascular patches), CNS (20% cerebrovascular or medullar accident), and GI system (40–60%, particularly small bowel with abdominal pain, bleeding, and diarrhea; intestinal perforations and peritonitis are the leading causes of death). Pleural and pericardial effusion can be observed.

Precautions before anesthesia: Obtain full history. Evaluate neurologic lesions (clinical, CT/MRI). Pleural and pericardial effusion must be searched and treated before anesthesia if necessary (clinical, ECG, chest radiographs, echography). Full blood count is necessary.

Anesthetic considerations: Eye protection is needed. Spinal and perimedullar blockades probably should be avoided because of the frequency of medullar accidents. Should obtain a bleeding time and coagulation profile.

Pharmacological implications: Aspirin is often used to treat patients. Heparin substitution should be considered.

REFERENCES:

Degos R, Delort J, Triscot R: Dermatite papulo squameuse atrophiante. *Bull Soc Franc Derm Syph* 49:148, 1942.

Ojeda Cuchillero RM, Sanchez Regana M, Umbert Millet P: Benign cutaneous Degos' disease. *Clin Exp Dermatol* 28:145, 2003.

Torrelo A, Sevilla J, Mediero IG, et al: Malignant atrophic papulosis in an infant. *Br J Dermatol* 146:916, 2002.

Dejerine-Sottas Syndrome

At a glance: Hereditary degenerative disorder that primarily involves peripheral motor nerves but also involves sensitive and autonomic components.

Synonyms: Hypertrophic Neuropathy of Dejerine Sottas; Hereditary Motor and Sensory Neuropathy type III; HMSN III; Dejerine-Sottas Neuropathy.

Incidence: Rare disorder.

Genetic inheritance: Autosomal dominant. Gene possibly located on chromosome 8.

Pathophysiology: Interstitial hypertrophic neuropathy with abnormal myelin.

Diagnosis: Usually, the nerve enlargements lead to palpable nerves by age 3 to 5 years. Cranial nerve or spinal nerve root enlargement may be seen on MRI or myelography. Elevated levels of cerebrospinal fluid protein are common. Ultimately, genetic mapping and nerve biopsy confirm the diagnosis. The histology shows onion-bulb aspects of nerve sheets.

Clinical aspects: Clinical manifestations begin in early infancy and are rapidly progressive. The course is characterized by exacerbations and remissions. They begin with distal muscular weakness, followed by gait disturbances, deformities of feet, kyphoscoliosis, and fasciculations. There is a distal sensory loss of all four extremities with incoordination of the arms and areflexia. Pupillary reflex is often blunted. Clinical differentiation between the different types of Dejerine-Sottas syndrome is sometimes difficult.

Precautions before anesthesia: Often, children are scheduled for orthopedic procedures of the lower limbs (clubfoot or ulcers of the feet). Assess respiratory function with at least a chest radiograph to assess kyphoscoliosis and complete spirometry including voluntary maximal ventilation.

Anesthetic considerations: Poor airway control and poor pharyngeal tone place patients at high risk for aspiration. Autonomic nervous system involvement may jeopardize cardiovascular stability.

Pharmacological implications: Peripheral denervation with excessive potassium response to succinylcholine. Nondepolarizing neuromuscular blocking agent may be used, and there is no prolonged response to these agents. However, because of poor respiratory reserve, extubate only when neuromuscular blocking agents are fully reversed and patient is fully awake.

REFERENCES:

Beisty JC, Alloza C, Alvarez J, et al: General anesthesia in a patient with Dejerine-Sottas disease. *Rev Esp Anesthesiol Reanim* 40:99, 1993.

Murakami T, Garcia CA, Reiter LT, et al: Charcot-Marie-Tooth disease and related inherited neuropathies. *Medicine* 75:233, 1996.

Delleman Oorthuys Syndrome

At a glance: Multiple congenital anomaly syndrome mainly affecting the central nervous system (CNS), eyes, and skin.

Synonyms: Delleman Syndrome; Oculocerebrocutaneous (OCC) Syndrome; Orbital Cyst with Cerebral and Focal Dermal Malformations.

Incidence: Approximately 30 cases have been described. Males are affected approximately 2.5 times more often than females.

Genetic inheritance: Most cases are sporadic and may result from mutation of a lethal gene compatible with survival only in the mosaic state. In a few cases, transmission may be autosomal dominant with variable penetrance.

Pathophysiology: Mechanism causing the anomalies is poorly understood. Abnormal development in week 5 or 6 of gestation could explain most of the symptoms. Several authors agree that, independent of the causal factor, the pathogenetic mechanism most likely is a disruption of the anterior neuroectodermal plate leading to neurocristopathy with primary craniofacial dysmorphogenesis.

Diagnosis: The most common features of Delleman syndrome are orbital cysts, microphthalmia/anophthalmia, focal hypoplastic skin defects, skin appendages, and cerebral malformations. The triad of ocular, cutaneous, and cerebral features is considered characteristic for the syndrome, with the ocular findings being the most typical and consistent. However, the minimal diagnostic criteria for Delleman syndrome include CNS cysts or hydrocephalus, orbital cysts or microphthalmia, and focal skin defects. To differentiate this syndrome from encephalocraniocutaneous lipomatosis, orbital cysts and agenesis of the corpus callosum are the most reliable signs.

Clinical aspects: CNS anomalies may include agenesis/hypoplasia of the corpus callosum, hydrocephalus, porencephaly, Dandy-Walker malformation, cerebral atrophy, arachnoid cysts, encephalocele, and meningocele. Pathologic changes affecting the eye are anophthalmia/microphthalmia and colobomata of eyelids and iris. Skin anomalies include auricular tags, periorbital cysts, pedunculated, hamartomatous (most often periorbital) skin appendages, café au lait spots, and focal dermal hypoplasia. Psychomotor retardation and seizures have been reported in most patients. Midline cleft lip/palate and bifid/fused ribs can be seen occasionally.

Precautions before anesthesia: Syndrome may go unrecognized, so silent neuroectodermal abnormalities may be present. Therefore consider CNS imaging in patients with facial skin tags and orbital cysts. Assess neurodevelopment and seizure control. Ask about previous episodes suggestive of aspiration pneumonia and obtain a chest radiograph if in doubt.

Anesthetic considerations: Airway management will be difficult in the presence of severe hydrocephalus and other anomalies, such as a high arched palate. Watch for seizure activity under anesthesia, which may manifest as unexpected autonomic changes. Muscle relaxants may mask seizure activity. Seizures may be the cause of slow emergence from anesthesia and predispose the patient to pulmonary aspiration. Postoperative apneic episodes may be a sign of seizures, and apnea monitoring might be useful. In a case report of anesthesia in a 2-month-old child with the syndrome, no perioperative problems other than a suboptimal view on direct laryngoscopy were reported.

Pharmacological implications: Be aware of interactions with anticonvulsant drugs. Avoid potentially epileptogenic drugs.

Other conditions to be considered:

ENCEPHALOCRANIOCUTANEOUS LIPOMATOSIS: This disease is now considered to be a variant of Proteus syndrome, which is a congenital hamartomatous disorder characterized by partial gigantism (hands and feet, macrodactyly), hemihypertrophy, macrocephaly, scoliosis, exostoses, and nevi.

There is phenotypic overlap in terms of eye and skin signs with

☞GOLDENHAR SYNDROME: Common birth defect of vascular origin involving first and second branchial arch derivatives resulting mainly in facial and vertebral anomalies.

☞ADAMS-OLIVER SYNDROME: Very rare inherited disorder characterized by defects of the scalp associated with multiple scarred and hairless areas that usually have dilated blood vessel directly under the skin. Scalp defects are present at birth. The extremities are either short (hypoplastic fingers and toes) or characterized by absent hands and lower legs. Congenital heart defect must be ruled out.

☞APLASIA CUTIS CONGENITA: Most often inherited disorder with circumscribed or more extensive skin lesions that may also involve underlying tissues. Neurologic and cardiac anomalies have been described in these patients.

☞CUTIS MARMORATA TELANGIECTATICA CONGENITA: Congenital cutaneous disorder with persistent cutis marmorata, telangiectasia, and phlebectasia. Often reported in association with a variety of other congenital anomalies.

☞**EPIDERMAL NEVUS SYNDROME:** Genetically transmitted neurodermatosis characterized by epidermal nevi, odontodysplasia, mental retardation, and various malformations.

☞**EPIDERMOLYSIS BULLOSA:** Group of inherited bullous disorders characterized by blister formation in response to mechanical trauma.

☞**JOHANSON-BLIZZARD SYNDROME:** Polymalformative syndrome characterized by nasal alar hypoplasia (beak-shaped), scalp defects, hypothyroidism, pancreatic achylia, and congenital deafness.

☞**GOLTZ SYNDROME:** Complex mesoectodermal hereditary disorder characterized by focal dermal atrophy with herniation of fat producing multiple papillomas, in association with a skeletal, dental, ocular, and other anomalies.

☞**SETLEIS SYNDROME:** Puckered periorbital skin, absent or multiple rows of eyelashes.

☞**STREETER ANOMALY:** Constricting amniotic bands leading to amputation with scarring, distal syndactyly, cleft lip/palate, anencephaly, encephalocele, hydrocephaly, omphalocele, and gastroschisis. Other internal anomalies involve the heart, lungs, diaphragm, kidneys, and gonads.

REFERENCES:

McCandless SE, Robin NH: Severe oculocerebrocutaneous (Delleman) syndrome: Overlap with Goldenhar anomaly. *Am J Med Genet* 78:282, 1998.

Moog U, de Die-Smulders C, Systermans JM, et al: Oculocerebrocutaneous syndrome: Report of three additional cases and aetiological considerations. *Clin Genet* 52:219, 1997.

Sadhasivam S, Subramaniam R: Delleman syndrome: Anesthetic implications. *Anesth Analg* 87:553, 1998.

Dent Disease

At a glance: Very rare, X-linked, inherited disorder characterized by onset in childhood or adulthood, tubular proteinuria hypercalciuria, calcium nephrolithiasis, nephrocalcinosis, and chronic renal failure.

Synonyms: Renal Fanconi Syndrome with Nephrocalcinosis and Renal Stones; Nephrolithiasis, X-Linked Recessive, Type II; Nephrolithiasis II.

History: Genetic disorder first described by C.E. Dent and M. Friedman in 1964.

Genetic inheritance: X-linked recessive inheritance.

Pathophysiology: Generalized transport dysfunction of the proximal renal tubule caused by mutation in the CLCN5 chloride channel gene (gene map locus at Xp11.22), leading to impaired reabsorption of amino acids, glucose, calcium, phosphate, bicarbonate, magnesium, sodium, potassium, water, uric acid, and low-molecular-weight proteins. Urinary losses can lead to polyuria, polydipsia, dehydration, hypokalemia, metabolic acidosis, and hypophosphatemia. The second component of the syndrome is a vitamin D-resistant metabolic bone disease that is responsible for rickets in children and osteomalacia in adults.

Diagnosis: Clinically evocated in males presenting with Fanconi syndrome and nephrocalcinosis or renal stones.

Clinical aspects: Clinical manifestations are related to the underlying disease. In the pediatric population, failure to thrive results from chronic acidosis, dehydration, hypokalemia, hypophosphatemia, and vitamin D-resistant rickets. Urinalysis reveals hypercalciuria, phosphaturia, microglobulinuria, particularly β_2-microglobulin, α_1-microglobulin, and retinol-binding protein. Microglobulinuria is seen in asymptomatic female heterozygotes. Plasma amino acids levels are normal because urinary losses are minimal compared to amino acid intake. Hyperchloremic metabolic acidosis with normal anion gap is usually moderate. When it increases in severity, urinary pH decreases. Hyponatremia, hypophosphatemia, and occasionally hypouricemia may occur. Renal biopsy reveals a "swan-neck" deformity of the proximal convoluted tubule.

Precautions before anesthesia: Obtain renal function tests (sodium, potassium, calcium, phosphate blood levels); urinalysis; creatinine clearance test if creatinine blood level is increased; request nephrology consultation if necessary. Obtain arterial blood gases (hyperchloremic nonanion gap metabolic acidosis), blood cell count, and hemoglobin level (anemia). Evaluate cardiac function by ECG for arrhythmias resulting from electrolyte abnormalities. Further testing, such as echocardiography, and radionuclide imaging, when necessary, may reveal decreased cardiac function secondary to uremia. Elective surgery should not be performed before optimization of acid–base and fluid-electrolyte status.

Anesthetic considerations: Metabolic acidosis with bicarbonate loss and sodium/potassium wasting is treated with administration of intravenous fluids having bicarbonate and electrolyte supplements. Under general anesthesia, mild intraoperative hyperventilation contributes to improvement of acid–base status. In cases where large volume shifts are expected, a central venous pressure line, a pulmonary arterial catheter in the presence of end-stage renal failure with cardiac dysfunction, or transesophageal echocardiography may facilitate volume management and assessment of ventricular function. An arterial line is required for close follow-up of blood gases, electrolytes, and blood pressure variations. Monitor urine output. Patients with rickets or osteomalacia should be carefully positioned and padded. Although renal Fanconi syndrome is different from Fanconi pancytopenia, anemia and coagulopathy may result as a consequence of end-stage renal failure.

Pharmacological implications: Avoid nephrotoxic drugs (e.g.: tetracyclines, aminoglycosides). When renal function is decreased, titrate carefully all anesthetic agents eliminated by the kidney.

REFERENCES:

Bergeron M, Gougoux A, Vinay P: The renal Fanconi syndrome, in Scriver CR, Beaudet AL, Sly WS, et al. (eds): *The Metabolic and Molecular Bases of Inherited Disease.* 7th ed. New York, McGraw-Hill, 1995, p 3691.

Fisher SE, Van Bakel I, Lloyd SE, et al: Cloning and characterization of CLCN5, the human kidney chloride channel gene implicated in Dent disease (an X-linked hereditary nephrolithiasis). *Genomics* 29:598, 1995.

Joel M, Rosales JK: Fanconi syndrome and anesthesia. *Anesthesiology* 55:455, 1981.

Denys-Drash Syndrome

At a glance: Denys-Drash syndrome (DDS) manifests in small children and consists of the triad of congenital nephropathy, Wilms tumor, and ambiguous genitalia.

Synonym: Drash Syndrome.

Incidence: Unknown. Approximately 150 cases have been reported. No racial predilection.

Genetic inheritance: Probably arises as a spontaneous mutation. The mutation is usually not present in parents; however, affected sibling pairs have been reported. DDS is the result of a so-called heterozygous dominant-negative mutation in the Wilms tumor suppressor gene 1 (WT1), with the gene locus mapping to 11p13. The same mutation has been reported in patients with isolated Wilms tumor. Most patients are pseudohermaphrodites with a 46,XY karyotype.

Pathophysiology: The dominant-negative mutation results in cellular WT1 levels less than 50% of normal in these patients. Diffuse mesangial fibrosis of the kidney results in progressive nephropathy and subsequent renal failure and associated hypertension. Wilms tumor is present in 74% and gonadal malignancies (gonadoblastoma) in 4% of patients.

Diagnosis: The majority of patients have an ambiguous genitalia or appear phenotypically female. The combination of ambiguous genitalia with typical renal involvement and arterial hypertension is suggestive of the disease. Kidney biopsy shows diffuse mesangial sclerosis with expansion of the mesangial matrix and subcapsular atrophy. Intracytoplasmic deposits of fibrillary material results in mesangial cell expansion.

Clinical aspects: Although pure gonadal dysgenesis with male pseudohermaphroditism is typical, the clinical variability of the external genitalia ranges from bifid scrotum with micropenis and palpable gonads to penoscrotal hypospadias with cryptorchidism or clitoral hypertrophy with labial fusion. Gonadal dysgenesis presents as streak ovaries and dysgenetic testes, respectively. Usually, patients present in their first year of life with the typical symptoms of nephrotic syndrome (marked proteinuria with hypoproteinemia [hypalbuminemia] resulting in recurrent infections, marked edema, abdominal distension secondary to ascites, hyperlipidemia, and hypercholesterolemia). Patients may have varying degrees of renal dysfunction/failure, but glomerular filtration rate usually declines quickly and results in end-stage renal disease requiring either dialysis or renal transplantation at approximately age 3 years. Hypertension, failure to thrive, and delayed psychomotor milestones may develop as a result of renal failure. Wilms tumor is usually detected at approximately age 2 years and is most often unilateral (80%). However, bilateral nephrectomy may be prudent management for unilateral nephropathy to reduce the high likelihood of developing a Wilms tumor in the contralateral kidney. Elective gonadectomy can be performed because of the difficulty in screening for gonadal malignancies. Most associated findings probably are incidental.

Precautions before anesthesia: Expect chronic renal anemia and evaluate renal function with serum electrolytes, creatinine, and urea preoperatively. Ask about the date of last hemodialysis, daily urine output, and maximal allowable daily fluid intake. Depending on the laboratory results and the clinical status (hypervolemia), hemodialysis may be necessary. Consider end-organ involvement related to arterial hypertension, hyperlipidemia, and/or hypercholesterolemia and whether chemotherapeutic agents were used preoperatively for treatment of Wilms tumor. The patient may have undergone renal transplantation requiring immunosuppressant drugs (corticosteroids) and manifest related adverse effects.

Anesthetic considerations: Avoid hypovolemia and nephrotoxic agents in patients undergoing unilateral nephrectomy, and avoid renally excreted drugs in patients with renal failure or who are undergoing bilateral nephrectomy. Postoperative pain management may take the form of regional anesthesia or parenteral narcotics. Both must be viewed in the light of reduced or absent renal function.

Pharmacological implications: Avoid drugs that depend on renal excretion or are nephrotoxic. Consider perioperative corticosteroid coverage for postrenal transplant patients.

Other conditions to be considered:

FRASIER SYNDROME: Similarly to DDS, the mutation responsible for this disorder is on the WT1 gene, located on 11p13. However, this syndrome is caused by mutations of the alternative splice donor site of exon 9 and therefore is different from DDS. Patients present with complete gonadal dysgenesis (streak gonads) and pseudohermaphroditism. The nephrotic syndrome is caused by focal glomerular sclerosis, which progresses to end-stage renal disease between the ages of 10 and 20 years and requires either hemodialysis or kidney transplantation. Gonadoblastoma, but not Wilms tumor, is a frequent complication of Frasier syndrome and occurs later in life than does Wilms tumor in DDS. Nevertheless, clinical differentiation between the two syndromes may be difficult. Basically the same precautions before anesthesia, anesthetic considerations, and pharmacological implications apply as for DDS, except that the malignancy is gonadoblastoma instead of Wilms tumor.

☞ANIRIDIA: It is estimated that approximately one third of patients with sporadic aniridia will develop a Wilms tumor, whereas approximately half of patients with aniridia, genitourinary anomalies (e.g., hypospadias), and mental retardation will develop a Wilms tumor. The association of *W*ilms tumor with *a*niridia, *g*enitourinary anomalies, and mental *r*etardation is known as the WAGR syndrome. Most patients have prominent lips and macrognathia. Other features may include congenital cataracts, nystagmus, ptosis, and blindness. The presence of ptosis and generalized hypotonia in a subgroup of patients suggests a susceptibility to malignant hyperthermia.

☞WAGR SYNDROME: Characterized by congenital developmental abnormalities such as aniridia, genitourinary abnormalities, and mental retardation. With a probability of 30%, the risk of developing a Wilms tumor in patients with this syndrome is very high.

☞BECKWITH-WIEDEMANN SYNDROME: Most often sporadic occurring syndrome with exomphalos, macroglossia, gigantism, and hypoglycemia resulting from hyperinsulinism.

REFERENCES:

McTaggart SJ, Algar E, Chow CW, et al: Clinical spectrum of Denys-Drash and Frasier syndrome. *Pediatr Nephrol* 16:335, 2001.

Mueller RF: The Denys-Drash syndrome. *J Med Genet* 31:471, 1994.

Poulat F, Morin D, König A, et al: Distinct molecular origins for Denys-Drash and Frasier syndrome. *Hum Genet* 91:285, 1993.

Dermatomyositis and Polymyositis

At a glance: Both diseases belong to a group of connective tissue disorders known as idiopathic inflammatory myopathies. They are a multisystem disease characterized by necrotizing inflammatory myopathy of striated muscles and a skin rash, both of unknown etiology.

Incidence: Approximately 5–10:100,000 in the general population. Female preponderance (male-to-female ratio = 1:2) but no racial predisposition.

Genetic inheritance: Both are autoimmune-mediated diseases, but the mechanisms are different and the exact etiology is unknown.

Classification:

- Primary idiopathic polymyositis (adult)
- Primary idiopathic dermatomyositis (adult)
- Childhood dermatomyositis or polymyositis with necrotizing vasculitis
- Polymyositis associated with connective tissue disorder (i.e., overlap syndrome, mixed connective tissue syndrome)
- Polymyositis or dermatomyositis associated with malignant tumors

Pathophysiology: Whether the pathophysiologies for dermatomyositis and polymyositis are different or the same is controversial. For some authors, these two diseases differ from each other mainly by the presence of dermatologic features (dermatomyositis) or the lack thereof (polymyositis). In the opinion of the proponents of a different pathophysiology, the two diseases differ as follows:

- *Dermatomyositis:* Activation of the *humoral* part of the immune system with antibodies directed against small arterioles and capillaries of the muscles seems to be the main culprit. Deposition of the complement factors C5b–9 (so-called membrane attack factor) results in antibody-mediated cell death. As the inflammatory process continues, capillary destruction results in atrophy, necrosis of muscle fibers, and, finally, muscle weakness and muscle tenderness.
- *Polymyositis:* Abnormal *cellular* immune response is considered responsible for the symptoms of this disease. Some evidence exists for a cytotoxic, T-cell–mediated attack directed toward muscular components. The factors triggering this cascade are unknown, but viruses could play a role (picornavirus-like structures have been found in affected muscle cells). Electron microscopy revealed tubular inclusions in endothelial cells of affected skin and muscle vessels and in surrounding monocytes, similar to those seen in other viral infections. Other viruses that have been blamed include retroviruses (HIV, HTLV-1) and coxsackievirus B.

Diagnosis: Pathognomonic features are heliotrope rash (violaceous erythema and edema) of the periorbital region and the eyelids, a reddish rash on the face and upper torso, and Gottron papules (violaceous-colored papules found on metacarpophalangeal and distal interphalangeal joints [knuckles] and the extensor aspects of knees and elbows). Sun exposure can exacerbate the skin lesions. Dilated cuticular telangiectasias at the base of the fingernails also are characteristic for dermatomyositis. Muscle biopsy, if obtained, detects degeneration and necrosis of muscle fibers that cause them to lose their staining characteristics so that the cytoplasm appears empty, resulting in the term *ghost fibers.* These changes combined with inflammatory cell infiltrates around blood vessels enforce the diagnosis of dermatomyositis. Four of the five following diagnostic criteria must be present for definite diagnosis: (1) cutaneous lesions typical for dermatomyositis; (2) elevated muscle enzyme levels (creatine kinase, transaminases, aldolase, lactate dehydrogenase); (3) progressive, proximal, symmetrical muscle weakness (shoulder and hip) developing over weeks to months; (4) pathologic electromyography (EMG), and (5) typical findings on muscle biopsy.

Clinical aspects: Childhood onset usually occurs between 5 and 15 years of age. Dermatomyositis in children is similar to the adult form. However, healing of affected muscles by fibrosis, which may result in incapacitating contracture deformities (flexion contractures of the ankles often result in a tiptoe gait), gastrointestinal ulcers, and infections, seem to be more common in children. Anemia is common as a result of gastrointestinal ulcerations and hemorrhages. In addition to these ulcerations with melena and/or hematemesis, extensive bowel infarctions caused by necrotizing arteritis can complicate the course of the disease. Progressive weakness of proximal muscles is present, usually in combination with elevated serum levels of creatinine phosphokinase (not mandatory), transaminases (aspartate aminotransferase [ASAT], alanine aminotransferase [ALAT]), lactate dehydrogenase, and aldolase. Results of EMG are abnormal. The degree of weakness can range from mild to severe, and even quadriparesis has been reported. Weakness of swallowing musculature (dysphagia), intercostal muscles, and the diaphragm may lead to problems with airway protection and respiration (10% of cases). Myocardial fibrosis can cause arrhythmias (heart block), ventricular dysfunction (dilated cardiomyopathy), and heart failure. Interstitial lung disease may be present and usually is mild (these patients often are anti–Jo-1 antibody [a myositis-specific antibody] positive). Use of steroids has improved mortality but with the expense of inherent problems of steroid therapy. Additional immunosuppressive drugs may be needed. A negative nitrogen balance is present when the disease is active. Sensation is not altered, and tendon reflexes are preserved unless the muscle strength is severely compromised by the inflammatory process. Death usually results from respiratory failure, heart failure, or a complicating infection. Up to 20% of adult cases (especially when the rash is present and the age of onset is late) are associated with occult neoplasms (lung, breast, ovary, stomach, prostate, nonmelanoma skin cancer), and dermatomyositis is considered a paraneoplastic syndrome in these patients. Steroids, salicylates, and immunosuppressives (azathioprine, cyclophosphamide, intravenous immunoglobulins) are used to suppress the inflammatory process. Subcutaneous calcifications can cause skin ulcerations and infections when they protrude through the skin.

Precautions before anesthesia: Obtain a full history of motor milestones and of complications following previous surgeries. Evaluate pulmonary function (forced vital capacity [FVC], peak expiratory flow rate, forced expiratory volume in 1 second [FEV_1], FEV_1:FVC ratio, arterial blood gas analysis). Evaluate cardiac function (ECG, echocardiography, radionuclide imaging when necessary). Preoperative laboratory investigations should include hemoglobin level, arterial blood gas analysis, and serum levels of total protein and albumin. Calculate the nitrogen balance if active disease is present. Serum creatinine phosphokinase and serum myoglobin levels are said to be the most sensitive indicators of disease activity. Perform a systemic assessment for other associated autoimmune disorders. Review drug therapy and possible complications. Continue steroid coverage and give additional perioperative stress prophylaxis.

Anesthetic considerations: A high complication rate is expected in the presence of muscle weakness, respiratory insufficiency, and cardiac dysfunction. Mechanical ventilation may be necessary following major surgery. Endotracheal intubation should be performed to minimize the risk of pulmonary aspiration in view of difficulties with swallowing and the resulting pooling of oral secretions. A rapid-sequence induction should be used if pharyngeal, esophageal, or gastric symptoms are present. Some papers have recommended avoiding malignant-hyperthermia triggering agents in the presence of muscle pathology. Avoid intramuscular injections. Extubation and termination of assisted ventilation should follow measurement of lung volumes (e.g., tidal volume, minute volume). Because of the risk of aspiration, tracheal extubation may be performed with the patient in the lateral position. If preoperative pulmonary function was significantly reduced, short-term postoperative ventilatory support following major surgery should be anticipated. Postoperative chest physiotherapy should be provided when necessary to minimize pulmonary complications.

Pharmacological implications: In the presence of muscle weakness, small incremental doses of neuromuscular blockers should be used and the effects monitored by a peripheral nerve stimulator. Normal response to neuromuscular blockers has been reported. Both normal and increased sensitivity to nondepolarizing neuromuscular blockers have been reported. Acute inflammation of muscles is present in the acute form of the disease, so suxamethonium should be avoided because of the possibility of hyperkalemia. Titrate opioids to avoid respiratory depression.

Other conditions to be considered:

☞**AMYOTROPHIC LATERAL SCLEROSIS:** Degenerative motor neuron disease evolving to progressive muscle weakness resulting in paralysis.

☞**MYASTHENIA GRAVIS:** Neuromuscular disorder characterized by muscle weakness and rapid muscle fatigue. Usually apparent during adulthood, but onset may occur at any age. Most individuals present eyelid ptosis, diplopia, and excessive muscle fatigue following exercise. Other features commonly include dysarthria, dysphagia, and proximal limb weakness. Approximately 10% may develop potentially life-threatening complications as a result of severe respiratory depression (myasthenic crisis).

REFERENCES:

Bohan A, Peter JB: Polymyositis and dermatomyositis (first of two parts). *N Engl J Med* 292:344, 1975.

Ganta R, Campbell IT, Mostafa SM: Anesthesia and acute dermatomyositis/polymyositis. *Br J Anaesth* 60:854, 1988.

Rockelein S, Gebert M, Baar H, et al: [Neuromuscular blockade with atracurium in dermatomyositis]. *Anaesthesist* 44:442, 1995.

Desbuquois Syndrome

At a glance: Autosomal recessive osteochondrodysplastic disease with typical skeletal anomalies and high mortality in the first year of life.

Synonyms: Desbuquois Dysplasia; Desbuquois Grenier Michel Syndrome; Micromelic Dwarfism with Vertebral and Metaphyseal Abnormalities and Advanced Carpotarsal Ossification.

Incidence: Exact incidence is unknown. Approximately 40 cases have been described in the literature.

Genetic inheritance: Autosomal recessive. The gene has not been identified.

Pathophysiology: Cause of dwarfism is not understood. Because of a strong radiologic similarity with diastrophic dysplasia, abnormalities in the diastrophic dysplasia sulfate transporter gene have been sought but were not found in Desbuquois syndrome.

Diagnosis: Made by the clinical picture plus distinct radiologic findings at the femoral neck ("monkey wrench" or "Swedish key" appearance), advanced carpal bone age, and a supernumerary ossicle at the base of the second phalanx in some patients.

Clinical aspects: High variability in the expression of the syndrome. Facial features consist of microcephaly with a round, flat profiled face, early closure of the fontanelles, micrognathia, cleft palate, depressed nasal bridge, short neck, glaucoma, proptosis, and blue sclerae. Orthopedic anomalies are micromelic dwarfism, scoliosis, and abnormal joint laxity resulting in recurrent luxations of hip and patella. Infants may show some distinctive additional skeletal signs, which may disappear after the first year of life and include coronal clefts in thoracolumbar vertebrae, and extra ossification centers, most often in the area of the metacarpophalangeal joint of the index finger, resulting in supernumerary phalanges and deviation of the fingers. The chest appears narrow and "funnel" shaped, and the abdominal wall is hypoplastic. These children are mentally retarded and approximately one third of them die in early infancy, most commonly as a result of respiratory infections. Some also suffer from obstructive sleep apnea syndrome. Ventricular septal defect, tracheomalacia, and laryngomalacia have been reported, with the latter two findings requiring tracheotomy in at least one patient. Long-term problems of these children include worsening joint problems, chest and spine deformities, recurrent aspiration pneumonias, and progressive psychomotor developmental delay.

Precautions before anesthesia: Careful assessment of the respiratory status is required. Inquire about sleep apnea, examine clinically and radiologically for chest infection and atelectasis, and treat as necessary. Consider assessment of arterial blood gases. Echocardiography may be necessary to exclude congenital cardiac lesions.

Anesthetic considerations: No literature on anesthesia for these patients was found. Patients may present most often for surgery of glaucoma and joint dislocations. Airway management may be challenging in some patients because of short neck and facial anomalies. Pulmonary ventilation and oxygenation may be difficult as a result of the restrictive nature of the chest deformity and preexisting collapse and consolidation. Neuraxial blockade not only may be difficult but also dangerous if vertebral abnormalities are present. Radiologic examination of the spine may be helpful. Careful positioning is required to prevent luxation of the joints (especially hip). Because of the high mortality associated with this syndrome in the first year of life (33%), some authors suggest routine use of apnea, bradycardia, and oxygen saturation monitoring of these patients. This is especially true in the postoperative period when prolonged observation may be required. Nasal continuous positive airway pressure may be helpful in milder cases of tracheomalacia and laryngomalacia.

Pharmacological implications: Careful use of opioids in view of obstructive sleep apnea syndrome is required. Antibioprophylaxis in case of cardiac defect.

Other conditions to be considered:

☞**DIASTROPHIC DYSPLASIA:** Autosomal recessive inherited form of short-limb dwarfism associated with spine anomalies.

☞**LARSEN SYNDROME:** Congenital dysmorphic syndrome associated with characteristic anomalies of face, hand, and feet, and multiple congenital dislocations. Spine, airway, and cardiac abnormalities.

CATEL-MANZKE SYNDROME (HYPERPHALANGY-CLINODACTYLY OF INDEX FINGER WITH PIERRE ROBIN SYNDROME; INDEX FINGER ANOMALY WITH PIERRE ROBIN SYNDROME; PALATODIGITAL SYNDROME): X-linked recessive disorder characterized by micrognathia, high arched palate, cleft palate/lip, Robin anomaly, glossoptosis, malformed ears, and short neck. Other features include cardiovascular anomalies (ventricular septal defect, aortic coarctation, dextrocardia), pectus carinatum or excavatum, seizures, joint laxity and dislocations, hyperphalangy of index finger, fifth finger clinodactyly, single transverse palmar crease, and talipes equinovarus.

REFERENCES:

Desbuquois G, Grenier B, Michel J, et al: Nanisme chondrodystrophique avec ossification anarchique et polymalformations chez deux soeurs. *Arch Fr Pediatr* 23:573, 1966.

Hall BD: Lethality in Desbuquois dysplasia: Three new cases. *Pediatr Radiol* 31:43, 2001.

Shohat M, Lachman R, Gruber HE, et al: Desbuquois syndrome: Clinical, radiographic, and morphologic characterization. *Am J Med Genet* 52:9, 1994.

Devriendt Legius Fryns Syndrome

At a glance: Syndrome characterized by hypogonadism, alopecia, and progressive neurologic and intellectual symptoms.

Incidence and genetic inheritance: Has been suggested to be a newly discovered autosomal recessive disorder based on its presence in two children (a boy and a girl) of consanguineous parents.

Clinical aspects: The boy's childhood was described as uneventful. First symptoms were noted at about age 12 years, when speech difficulties and learning problems and gait abnormalities were noted. Fine motor skills started to decline thereafter, mainly as a consequence of reduced muscle strength and neurologic control. Absence of puberty (prepubertal penis and testes) and nondevelopment of secondary male sex characteristics were diagnosed at age 17 years. Neurologic examination at that time showed dystonia and dysarthria that, by age 47 years, had progressed to almost complete inability to walk (as a consequence of dystonic and choreoathetotic movements) and speak, combined with eating and drinking difficulties. Alopecia was noted in early adulthood. The sister was affected earlier than her brother, with learning problems noted in primary school, requiring special education. Her motor skills declined faster, and she was wheelchair-bound by the time she was in her early 20s. She also showed signs of primary hypogonadism and no development of secondary female sex characteristics. Dysarthria and alopecia occurred at age 14 years and were slowly progressive.

Anesthetic considerations: None reported. However, depending on the age and severity of neurologic symptoms, recurrent pulmonary aspirations are possible, and a preoperative chest radiograph might be helpful. Long-term muscle inactivity (wheelchair-bound) precludes the use of succinylcholine because of the risk of a hyperkalemic response.

REFERENCE:

Devriendt K, Legius E, Fryns JP: Progressive extrapyramidal disorder with primary hypogonadism and alopecia in sibs: A new syndrome? *Am J Med Genet* 62:54, 1996.

D-Glyceric Acidemia

At a glance: Inborn error of metabolism resulting in D-glyceric acidemia, developmental delay, and seizures.

Synonym: D-Glycerate Kinase Deficiency.

Incidence and genetic inheritance: Extremely rare disorder (fewer than 10 cases have been reported) with autosomal recessive transmission.

Clinical aspects: Initially described case of a mentally retarded boy of nonconsanguineous Serbian parents suffered clinically from nonketotic hyperglycinemia. Extremely high concentrations of

D-glyceric acid were found in both serum and urine. Enzyme assays of D-glyceric dehydrogenase (glyoxylate reductase) on blood leukocytes demonstrated significantly lower activity in the patient compared to five normal children. Further measurements of glycine cleavage activity in autopsic liver tissue from this patient revealed only 10% of normal activity. The two compounds, 2-methylbutyryl-CoA and isobutyryl-CoA, are known inhibitors of the glycine cleavage system. Based on the findings of increased urinary excretion of both free and conjugated isobutyric acid, 2-methylbutyric acid, and isovaleric acid, it was hypothesized that decreased glycine cleavage activity might be a result of inhibition by these three substances. However, in the liver of another patient with this disease, glycerate kinase activity was less than 5% of normal, and D-glycerate dehydrogenase and triokinase activities were not deficient. Therefore D-glycerate kinase deficiency was suggested to be the cause of D-glyceric aciduria. However, a primary defect in the catabolism of L-serine catabolism cannot be excluded. An oral fructose loading dose resulted in a sharp increase of D-glycerate excretion. Subjective clinical improvement was reported after a diet moderately restricted in fructose. Clinical symptoms of this disease are global developmental delay and seizures. Severe metabolic acidosis and failure to thrive are common and may require chronic therapy with bicarbonate.

Anesthetic considerations: No references to anesthesia were found. However, the presence of severe acidemia, seizures, and developmental delay are considerations individually associated with their manifestations. Anticonvulsant medication should be continued.

REFERENCES:

Duran M, Beemer FA, Bruinvis L, et al: D-Glyceric acidemia: An inborn error associated with fructose metabolism. *Pediatr Res* 21:502, 1987.

Kolvraa S, Christensen E, Brandt NJ: Studies of the glycine metabolism in a patient with D-glyceric acidemia and hyperglycinemia. *Pediatr Res* 14:1029, 1980.

Kolvraa S, Rasmussen K, Brandt NJ: D-Glyceric acidemia: Biochemical studies of a new syndrome. *Pediatr Res* 10:825, 1976.

Diaminopentanuria

At a glance: Genetic disorder with increased renal clearance of cystine, lysine, arginine, and ornithine caused by a dysfunction of the reabsorptive capacity of the renal tubules. In addition, defective intestinal absorption results in increased degradation of these amino acids by bacteria in the intestine.

Synonyms: Cystine-Lysinuria; Cystinuria.

Incidence and genetic inheritance: Fewer than five patients reported in the literature. Genetic inheritance is unknown.

Pathophysiology: Increased renal clearance of cystine and the dibasic amino acids lysine, arginine, and ornithine, in the presence of normal or low plasma levels of these compounds, is secondary to dysfunction of the reabsorptive capacity of the renal tubule. Defective intestinal absorption of cystine, lysine, arginine, and ornithine results in increased degradation of these amino acids by bacteria in the intestinal tract. Alternate intestinal transport routes may protect cystinuric patients from amino acid malnutrition because they respond to a large oral dose of lysine with a normal increase of its plasma concentration. Although cystinuria may be associated with CNS abnormalities, the precise mechanism of action remains to be determined. In cystine-lysinuria, production of cadaverine (1,5-diaminopentane) and putrescine by bacterial conversion of lysine and ornithine may play a role in the pathophysiology.

Diagnosis: Diagnosis made by the clinical course, microscopic examination of the urinary sediment (cystine crystals), screening for crystalluria by cyanide-nitroprusside urine test, urinary amino acids measurements by ion exchange chromatography, or liquid chromatography mass spectrometry. Cystine-lysinuria also can be diagnosed by an oral lysine loading test: urinary excretion of cystine and lysine is increased and, in case of associated neurologic abnormalities, the EEG reveals mild background slowing following lysine loading.

Clinical aspects: Peak times for clinical expression of cystinuria are usually during the second and third decades of life (the disease may appear as early as in the first year or as late as in the ninth decade of life). Renal cholics with hematuria as a consequence of nephrolithiasis, urinary tract infections, and obstructive uropathies are common manifestations. Hypertension and renal failure occur occasionally. Onset of neurologic symptoms, such as progressive loss of motor and cognitive milestones, seizures, spasticity, and ataxia, have been reported to occur in early childhood. Further deterioration of neurologic status often coincides with urinary tract infections. Alteration of intestinal flora by neomycin and *Lactobacillus acidophilus* may lessen the neurologic injury. Maintaining good hydration can help reduce the risk of nephrolithiasis.

Precautions before anesthesia: Assess renal function. If serum creatinine levels are increased, obtain a creatinine clearance test and request, if necessary, urology/nephrology consultation. Check serum electrolytes, hemoglobin, and blood cell counts (frequent urinary tract infections and hematuria). Leukopenia, agranulocytosis, or even aplastic anemia are possible adverse effects of D-penicillamine treatment. Severe allergic reactions, nephrotic syndrome with membranous glomerulonephritis, bronchoalveolitis with respiratory distress, myasthenia gravis, and dermatologic affections (e.g., pemphigoid, lupus erythematosus, dermatomyositis) have been reported as a consequence of D-penicillamine treatment. In the presence of an associated seizure disorder (rare), ask about anticonvulsant therapy (efficacy and toxicity) and check for treatment and potential adverse effects. Captopril and neomycin are other therapeutic options.

Anesthetic considerations: Chronic renal failure occurs occasionally, and its potential consequences, such as chronic anemia, coagulopathy, altered hydration, electrolyte imbalance, acidosis, and systemic hypertension, must be considered in the perioperative management.

Pharmacological implications: In the presence of depressed renal function, carefully titrate all anesthetic agents with predominantly renal elimination and avoid nephrotoxic drugs (e.g., tetracyclines, aminoglycosides). In case of nephrotic syndrome (a potential adverse effect of treatment), hypoalbuminemia is present and mandates cautious dosage of highly protein-bound drugs. Potentially epileptogenic drugs (e.g., ketamine, methohexital, enflurane, meperidine, atracurium *cis*-atracurium) should be avoided in patients with an associated seizure disorder.

Other conditions to be considered:

☞**BLUE DIAPER SYNDROME:** Genetic disorder with defective transport for L-tryptophan resulting in blue urine.

☞**HARTNUP SYNDROME/DISEASE:** Autosomal recessive disorder caused by defective transport of tryptophan and other neutral (i.e., monoamino-monocarboxylic) amino acids in the small intestine and kidney. Patients may present with a pellagra-like skin condition, cerebellar ataxia, and gross aminoaciduria.

☞**HYPERPROLINEMIA:** Autosomal recessive inherited disorder with decreased renal tubular reabsorption of glycine and the imino acids proline and hydroxyproline. Patients with type II of the disease may be taking antiseizure medication, and epileptogenic drugs should be avoided.

☞**LYSINURIC PROTEIN INTOLERANCE:** Autosomal recessive disease characterized by defective transport of the dibasic amino acids.

REFERENCES:

Berry HK, Norman EJ, Oppenheimer SG, Steiner JS, Denton MD: A new defect of lysine metabolism: 1,5-Diaminopentanuria. *Am J Hum Genet* 31:38A, 1979.

Ross DL, Berry HK, Norman EJ, Oppenheimer S: A new treatment for neurologic deterioration in patients with cystine-lysinuria. *Neurology* 31:87A, 1981.

Segal S, Their SO: Cystinuria, in Scriver CR, Beaudet AL, Sly WS, et al. (eds): *The Metabolic and Molecular Bases of Inherited Disease.* 7th ed. New York, McGraw Hill, 1995, p 3581.

Diastematomyelia

At a glance: Disorder of spinal dysraphism resulting in division of the spinal cord into two parts by a fibrocartilaginous or bony posterior projection of the posterior vertebral body.

Synonym: Split Cord Syndrome.

Incidence: Unknown, but girls are affected more often than boys.

Genetic inheritance: There are a few reports of autosomal recessive cases in the literature.

Pathophysiology: Differentiation of the neural ectoderm from the epithelial ectoderm occurs between weeks 3 and 5 of gestation. Diastematomyelia is a result of a defect in neural tube fusion with persistence of the mesodermal tube from the developing neurenteric canal, which acts as a septum. Neurologic signs are thought to result from traction and trauma with extension and flexion of the cord.

Diagnosis: Neurologic presentation and confirmation by imaging of the spinal cord by either CT or MRI scanning. Approximately 50% of cases involve the first three lumbar vertebrae. The symptoms usually are not obvious until the child starts to walk. Most often, however, patients present at preschool age. The spinal cord is (often asymmetrically) split into two hemicords (with a separate central canal and a spinal anterior artery supplying each half), which reunite caudally of the defect, or, if the lesion extends very low down the lumbar spine, extends in two separate coni medullares and fila terminales.

- *Type I:* Affects 55% of patients. The two spinal hemicords are surrounded by one dural-arachnoid sleeve. This form often is asymptomatic initially, unless tethering or hydromelia occurs.
- *Type II:* Affects 45% of patients. Each spinal hemicord has its own dural-arachnoid sleeve, separated by a bony, cartilaginous, or fibrous septum. By fixing the spinal cord to the vertebral bodies on the affected level, this sagittal septum precludes the normal cephalad shift of the spinal cord during growth, resulting in the symptoms described below.

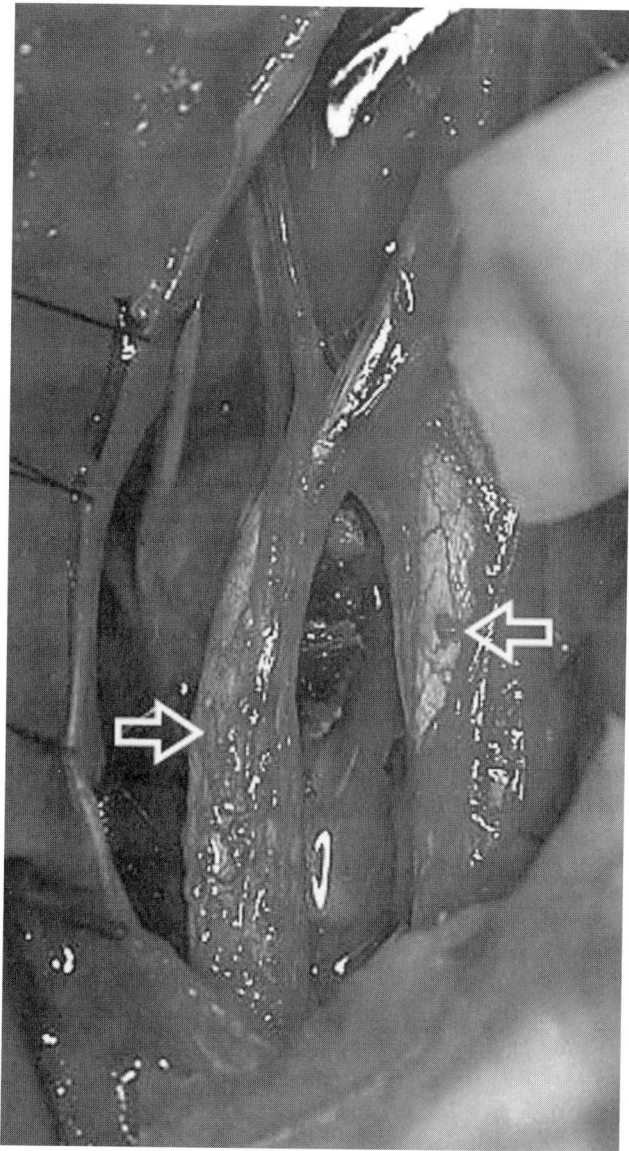

Diastematomyelia   Asymmetrical splitting of the spinal cord into two hemicords *(arrows)* in a patient. See color plates.

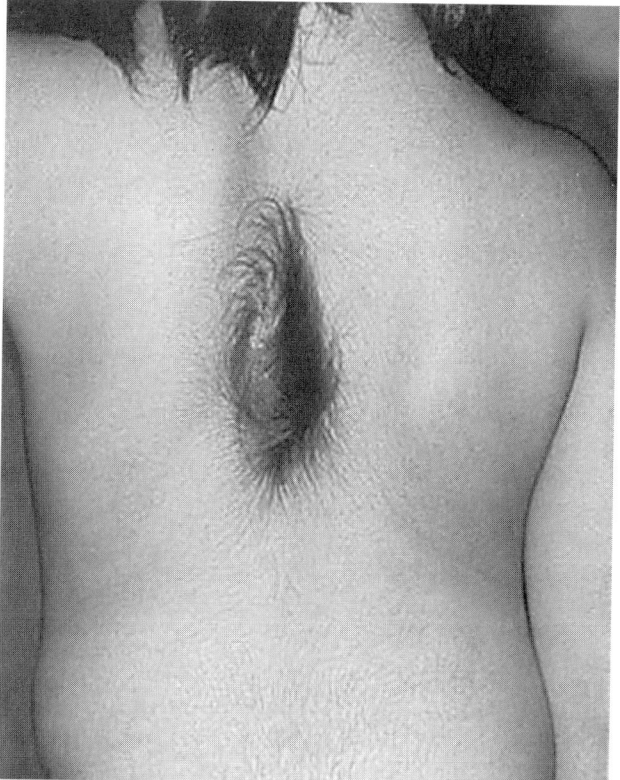

Diastematomyelia   Localized hypertrichosis along the spine is often an indicator of an underlying pathology in that area, as seen in this patient with diastematomyelia.

Clinical aspects: In more than 70% of patients, a localized area of hyperpigmentation and/or hypertrichosis can be found in the skin area directly overlying the defect. The symptomatology varies from asymptomatic to significant neurologic and skeletal abnormalities. Unilateral changes may include foot abnormalities (talipes equinovarus), loss of pain and temperature sensation, and atrophy of the gastrocnemius muscle. Bilateral abnormalities present with sensory and motor changes (gait disturbances) and lead to muscle atrophy, absent ankle jerks, urinary incontinence, and back pain. Neurologic symptoms arise from flexion–extension movements of the spine, resulting in traction and potential trauma. In most of these patients, the conus medullaris is located below the L2 level, and thickening of the filum terminale has been reported in more than half of these patients. Associated anomalies may include vertebral fusion defects, hemivertebrae, butterfly vertebrae, kyphoscoliosis, spina bifida, myelomeningocele, tethered cord, intraspinal neuroenteric cysts, dermoid cysts, lipomas, hemangiomas, and teratomas.

Precautions before anesthesia: Routine preoperative assessment. In addition, check and document the extent of neurologic dysfunction, especially if regional anesthesia is considered.

Anesthetic considerations: Central neuraxial blockade is not recommended because the anatomy may be distorted (scoliosis, hamartomas) and the conus medullaris most often extends further caudal than usual.

Pharmacological implications: Depending on the degree of neurologic involvement, succinylcholine could elicit a hyperkalemic response and therefore is probably best avoided.

Other conditions to be considered: Other syndromes are associated with spina bifida, such as the following:

☞**ARNOLD-CHIARI SYNDROME:** Collection of anatomical abnormalities caused by a bony defect in the posterior fossa and upper cervical spine. This results in herniation of the cerebellar vermis and choroid plexus through the foramen magnum, with elongation of the medulla and fourth ventricle and noncommunicating hydrocephalus.

☞**ALAGILLE SYNDROME:** Congenital disorder with abnormalities of the liver, heart, eye, skeleton, and kidneys, and characteristic facial features.

☞**INCONTINENTIA PIGMENTI:** Ectodermal disorder characterized by dermatologic, dental, and ocular features.

☞**KOUSSEFF SYNDROME:** Genetic disorder with sacral meningocele, conotruncal heart malformations, and anomalies of the head and neck.

☞**NAIL-PATELLA SYNDROME:** Inherited connective tissue disorder with the cardinal features of nail dysplasia and absent or hypoplastic patellae.

☞**KRAUSE-KIVLIN SYNDROME:** Introduced to describe the association of Peters anomaly with cleft lip/palate, short stature, abnormal ears, and mental retardation. Has been reported in conjunction with short-limb dwarfism.

☞**TETHERED SPINAL CORD SYNDROME:** Syndrome resulting from abnormal development of the filum terminale resulting in persistent anchoring of the spinal cord conus medullaris at or below the L2 level.

☞**THREE-M SYNDROME:** Congenital disorder with low birth weight, short stature, and dysmorphic features.

REFERENCES:

Drolet BA: Cutaneous signs of neural tube dysraphism. *Pediatr Clin North Am* 47:813, 2000.

Northrup H, Volcik KA: Spina bifida and other neural tube defects. *Curr Probl Pediatr* 30:313, 2000.

Scatliff JH, Kendall BE, Kingsley DP, et al: Closed spinal dysraphism: Analysis of clinical, radiological, and surgical findings in 104 consecutive patients. *Am J Roentgenol* 152:1049, 1989.

Diastrophic Dysplasia

At a glance: Autosomal recessive inherited form of short-limb dwarfism associated with spine anomalies.

Synonyms: Diastrophic Dwarfism; Diastrophic Nanism Syndrome.

Incidence: 1:100,000 live births, with an approximately three times higher incidence in Finland.

Genetic inheritance: Transmission is autosomal recessive, with a broad phenotypical range. The responsible gene maps to 5q32-q33.1 (also called SLC26A2).

Pathophysiology: The defect on chromosome 5 affects the diastrophic dysplasia sulfate transporter (DTDST) and leads to depletion of intracellular sulfate and insufficient sulfation of sulfated macromolecules such as cartilage matrix proteoglycans, which results in abnormally soft cartilage with decreased resistance to stress.

Diagnosis: Made by the clinical findings and molecular genetic testing.

Clinical aspects: This form of rhizomelic (short-limb) dwarfism is characterized by a proportionate shortening of the tubular bones, which are approximately 50% of the normal length. Abduction of the thumbs results from a short and oval-shaped first metacarpal bone, which gives it the aspect of a "hitchhiker thumb." Severe clubfoot deformity with luxation of the big toes and ulnar deviation of the hands are typical. These findings, which are present in prenatal ultrasonographs, make very likely the diagnosis of diastrophic dysplasia. A patient may suffer from hyperlaxity with recurrent dislocations of some joints, while other joints show stiffness and contractures. During the first 2 to 5 weeks of life, more than 80% of patients suffer from swelling and inflammation of the ear cups with subsequent calcification and "cauliflower"-like ears. The palate is high arched and broad, and cleft palate (complete, partial or submucous, double or bifid uvula) may occur in up to 25% of patients. The abnormally soft cartilage is responsible for laryngotracheobronchomalacia and often causes respiratory distress. Spinal deformities, such as mid-cervical kyphosis with potential compression of the medulla, cervical spina bifida occulta, and scoliosis (with lung volumes inversely correlated to the angle of scoliosis) with decreased chest mobility, contribute to the respiratory problems. In fact, respiratory failure is responsible for the increased mortality in the first months of life. Although

cervical kyphosis resolves spontaneously in more than 90% of patients, progression to quadriplegia and death has been reported. The median adult height in a Finnish study of 121 affected men and women was 135 cm (53.1 in) and 129 cm (50.8 in), respectively. Most of the patients are mentally normal, but as a consequence of the orthopedic problems, motor skills are delayed and their exercise tolerance is reduced secondary to respiratory problems.

Precautions before anesthesia: The pulmonary situation should be optimized as much as possible before surgery, and the need for postoperative mechanical ventilation should be anticipated. A chest radiograph should be obtained. Cervical spine anomalies are frequent and require a thorough clinical and radiologic evaluation. Lateral flexion and extension radiograph and/or MRI of the neck may be necessary to evaluate the grade of spinal compression.

Anesthetic considerations: Death as a result of anesthetic complications has been described. If tracheal intubation is required, either inline cervical stabilization or fiberoptic intubation is recommended. Careful handling and positioning of these patients are mandatory in the presence of cervical instability, contractures, and skeletal deformities. Depending on the type of surgery, somatosensory evoked potential during induction, but especially for positioning, has been recommended in patients with cervical instability to monitor for signs of cord compression. If tracheal intubation is not mandatory, a face mask or alternatively a laryngeal mask may be a good alternative, avoiding not only tracheal but also cervical spine manipulations. However, continuous positive airway pressure may be required secondary to laryngotracheobronchomalacia. Abnormalities of tracheal, laryngeal, and bronchial cartilage resulting in airway collapse and death have been described.

Pharmacological implications: Cervical instability may result in spinal cord compression and consecutive weakness of distal muscles. Consequently, succinylcholine could lead to a hyperkalemic response.

Other conditions to be considered:

☞**DESBUQUOIS SYNDROME:** Autosomal recessive osteochondrodysplastic disease with typical skeletal anomalies and high mortality in the first year of life.

☞**LARSEN SYNDROME:** Congenital dysmorphic syndrome associated with characteristic anomalies of face, hands, and feet, and multiple congenital dislocations. Spine, airway, and cardiac abnormalities are associated.

☞**CHONDRODYSPLASIA: GIANT CELL TYPE:** Lethal form of chondrodysplasia characterized by rhizomelic limb shortening with giant cell chondrodysplasia.

☞**THANATOPHORIC DWARFISM:** Severe form of micromelic dwarfism with narrow thorax. Death generally occurs in the first hours of life.

REFERENCES:

Makitie O, Kaitila I: Growth in diastrophic dysplasia. *J Pediatr* 130:641, 1997.

Remes VM, Helenius I, Peltonen J, et al: Lung function in diastrophic dysplasia. *Pediatr Pulmonol* 33:277, 2002.

Diencephalic Syndrome

At a glance: Very rare neurologic disorder characterized by failure to thrive, emaciation, amnesia, intense sleepiness, unusual eye position, and sometimes blindness. It is normally seen in infancy or early childhood but some cases in older children and even adults have been reported. Diencephalic syndrome usually is caused by a brain tumor such as a low-grade glioma or astrocytoma.

Synonyms: Russell Diencephalic Cachexia Syndrome; Russell Syndrome

Incidence and genetic inheritance: Very rare disorder that affects males and females equally. Onset age of presentation usually is the young infant or child between the ages of 18 months and 3 years. However, it also can develop during adolescence and even adulthood. The syndrome occurs worldwide. Childhood brain tumors arise in 2.5–3.5:100,000 children per year.

Pathophysiology: Results from the development of a brain tumor in the hypothalamic region, often a low-grade glioma or astrocytoma. The tumor may invade the anterior portion of the third ventricle and affect the optic nerve or optic chiasm. The presence of this expanding intracerebral mass leads to raised intracranial pressure. The cause of the weight loss is unknown, but excessive growth hormone secretion, activation of proteins produced by the pituitary gland that break down fat, or secretion of a fat mobilizing compound have been implicated. There is no known genetic predisposition for diencephalic syndrome.

Clinical aspects: Very rare disorder that usually affects infants and young children. It is characterized by a failure to thrive, emaciation, and normal linear growth. A history of normal development and weight gain is normally followed by either a prolonged period of failure to gain weight or weight loss. The individual may have anorexia or bulimia. Over time, loss of body fat occurs and leads to an emaciated appearance. The child may have a relatively large head compared with body weight. Overall development is often slowed, but results of neurologic testing are normal. The eyes are often affected, and the infant or child may present a strabismus, nystagmus, papilledema, or blindness. The child may be unusually sleepy. The patient usually behaves in a normal, alert, happy manner that is not in keeping with the physical appearance. Growth hormone plasma level is usually higher than normal.

Anesthetic considerations: Presence of emaciation must be assessed preoperatively for electrolytes and glucose imbalances. Intraoperative thermoregulatory heat loss must be carefully managed. Presence of elevated intracranial pressure must be ruled out. If present, proper anesthesia management for raised intracranial pressure must be ensured. The anesthetic considerations for brain tumour are not specific to this syndrome and are reviewed in the textbook entitled *Pediatric Anesthesia: Principles and Practice* by the same author.

Other condition to be considered:

☞**TOLOSA-HUNT SYNDROME:** Rare disorder that includes headaches, fever, and vision impairment. There may be eye muscle paralysis, swelling and protrusion of the eye, drooping eyelid, and diminished vision.

REFERENCE:
Menzes AH, Bell WE, Perret GC: Hypothalmic tumors in children: Their diagnosis and management. *Child Brain* 3:265, 1977.

Diferrante Syndrome

At a glance: Mucopolysaccharidosis with questionable glucosamine-6-sulfate sulfatase deficiency. Scientific fraud in Diferrante's laboratory is suspected, and this syndrome has been retained here only for historical reasons.

Synonyms: Glucose-6-Sulfate Sulfatase Deficiency; Mucopolysaccharidosis Type VIII.

Incidence: Only one patient has been described.

Genetic inheritance: Autosomal recessive.

Pathophysiology: Mucopolysaccharidoses represent a group of hereditary disorders involving lysosomal enzymatic defects affecting the degradation of mucopolysaccharides present in connective tissue. Nearly every organ of the body shows an accumulation of incompletely metabolized mucopolysaccharides.

Diagnosis: The patient excreted keratan and heparan sulfate in the urine. Lymphocytes stained with toluidine blue show a peculiar ring-shaped metachromasia underlying the cell membrane.

Clinical aspects: The syndrome combines clinical and biochemical features of the Morquio and Sanfilippo syndromes. The affected patient had a short stature with mild dysostosis multiplex and hypoplasia of the odontoid. He was mentally retarded and presented with hepatomegaly and hirsutism. He had no ocular involvement.

Precautions before anesthesia: Obtain radiographs of the cervical spine to document atlantoaxial instability. Pulmonary function testing should be obtained in view of a probable restrictive pulmonary syndrome in relation with the short stature. Baseline liver function should be obtained.

Anesthetic considerations: Difficult tracheal intubation is the rule and fiberoptic intubation should be considered. In spite of the atlantoaxial instability, mucopolysaccharides may accumulate in the tongue and nasopharyngeal tissues, making visualization of the glottic opening difficult during direct laryngoscopy. Hence, patients may also present with obstructive apnea and increased sensitivity to the ventilatory depressant effect of narcotics, so regional anesthesia for postoperative pain control is recommended, as well as observation in the intensive care unit for 24 to 48 hours. Finally, the heart may be affected by mucopolysaccharide accumulation in different ways, so the dose of anesthetics should be adjusted accordingly.

Pharmacological implications: If liver function is decreased, then certain medications, such as muscle relaxants, should be given in a reduced dose.

REFERENCE:
Stoelting RK, Dierdorf SF: Metabolic and nutritional disorders, in Stoelting RK (ed): *Anesthesia and Coexisting Disease.* 3d ed. New-York, Churchill Livingstone, 1993, p 383.

DiGeorge Syndrome

At a glance: Genetic defect leading to a wide range of phenotypic presentations, mainly developmental defects in the outflow tract of the heart, hypoparathyroidism with hypocalcemia, and thymic hypoplasia/aplasia with immune defects.

Synonyms: Pharyngeal Pouch Syndrome; Thymic Aplasia.

Incidence: Both sexes are equally affected. Deletion of 22q11 is estimated to occur in approximately 1:3000–5000 live births. It is more frequent in children with congenital cardiac defects (up to 25% of these patients) and with cleft lip/palate (up to 8% of children with a cleft reportedly have this deletion).

Genetic inheritance: Autosomal dominant; possibly a contiguous gene syndrome. Only 25% of 22q deletions are inherited, and most cases of DiGeorge Syndrome are isolated. In 90% of cases, DiGeorge syndrome is related to a monoallelic microdeletion of 22q11.2 (so-called DiGeorge syndrome critical region [DGCR]). This is the most frequent human gene deletion and, after trisomy 21, the second most common genetic cause of congenital heart defect. A few patients with DiGeorge syndrome have defects in other chromosomes (10p13, 18q21.33, 4q21.3-q25). In noninherited cases, maternal alcohol abuse, isotretinoin exposure, and uncontrolled diabetes mellitus during pregnancy have been considered risk factors.

Pathophysiology: The chromosomal deletion leads to an abnormal migration of the cephalic and cardiac neural crest cells in the fourth week of embryogenesis, causing a developmental field defect that involves the third and fourth pharyngeal pouches. The developmental field defect theory is used to explain the narrow range of clinical expression of the different causes of DiGeorge syndrome. The principal basic defect leads to thymic aplasia or hypoplasia, heart defects, and hypoparathyroidism.

Diagnosis: The finding of thymic aplasia or hypoplasia radiologically, intraoperatively (for correction of congenital cardiac defect), or on autopsy, combined with the clinical features, confirms the diagnosis. However, immune function correlates poorly with thymus size. Measurement of the CD4+ subset of white cells, standard karyotype to exclude major rearrangements, and fluorescent in situ hybridization using probes from within the deletion segment (close to translocation breakpoint site preferably) finalize the diagnosis. Although CD3+, CD4+, and CD8+ T-lymphocyte counts are abnormally low, the number of natural killer cells and B lymphocytes is normal.

Clinical aspects: Severe cases present with neonatal hypocalcemia (caused by hypoplasia of the parathyroid glands), which may result in tetany or seizures (presenting symptom in approximately 10% of patients) and susceptibility to infection as a consequence of a deficit of T cells (hypoplasia or aplasia of the thymus gland). Several cardiac malformations (tetralogy of Fallot, type B interrupted aortic arch [typical], persistent truncus arteriosus, double-outlet right ventricle, transposition of the great arteries, ventriculoseptal defect, pulmonary stenosis, right infundibular stenosis, right aortic arch, aberrant right subclavian artery) are common and the main cause of death during the first weeks of life. Recurrent infections start in the first 6 months of life. Cases with delayed diagnosis (late childhood) present usually with a milder spectrum of cardiac defects (mainly membranous ventricular septal defect), absence of, hypocalcemia and nearly normal immune function. Facial abnormalities are present in up to 60% of patients and may include small dysplastic ears; hypertelorism with lateral displacement of the inner canthi; short and downward-slanted palpebral fissures; anteverted nostrils and short philtrum; a cupid-bow mouth (fish mouth); midface hypoplasia; retrognathia; micrognathia; high arched palate; and bifid uvula. Other common, but inconstant, features are short stature, variable learning difficulties, mild psychomotor retardation (holoprosencephaly and arrhinencephaly have been reported), and various psychiatric disorders (most often paranoid schizophrenia). Airway anomalies have been recognized in a number of patients and include tracheoesophageal fistula, short trachea with a reduced number of tracheal rings, abnormal thyroid cartilage, and laryngomalacia, tracheomalacia, and bronchomalacia. Esophageal muscle dysfunction, hydronephrosis, nephrocalcinosis, and limb anomalies may occur. DiGeorge syndrome can be associated with autoimmune disorders (e.g., Graves disease, immune thrombocytopenic purpura, juvenile rheumatoid arthritis-like polyarthritis).

Precautions before anesthesia: Assess cardiovascular function with ECG, request echocardiography, and, if necessary, request cardiac catheterization. Evaluate for difficult tracheal intubation. The

aforementioned airway anomalies can cause significant morbidity and mortality. Make sure pulmonary function is optimized as much as possible, although airway infections are already very common in otherwise healthy children and even more so in these patients. Prophylaxis of *Pneumocystis carinii* pneumonia with trimethoprim and sulfamethoxazole or pentamidine isocyanate should be considered. Laboratory examination should include a complete blood count (including lymphocyte count) and serum levels of potassium, calcium, blood urea nitrogen, and creatinine. Keep in mind that these patients are immunoincompetent. Blood transfusions have to be cytomegalovirus-negative and irradiated, as fatal graft-versus-host disease from transfusion has been described. The immunocompromised recipient is unable to eliminate the transfused, but viable, T lymphocytes, which, by proliferation and attack of the host, lead to graft-versus-host disease. Irradiation prevents this proliferation of transfused, immunocompetent T lymphocytes. Check for infections and hypothyroidism.

Anesthetic considerations: Anticipate difficult airway management and risk of gastric aspiration. Strict asepsis is mandatory to prevent infection. Intravenous catheters should be inserted as distal as possible to the forearm veins protecting them for future use of arteriovenous shunt in case of renal impairment. The degree of hemodynamic surveillance must be a compromise among heart function, renal function, and risk for infection, but mainly depends on the type of surgical procedure. Special anesthetic care is required for management of preexisting cardiac lesions. Anomalies of the carotid arteries have been reported and require special attention during insertion of an internal jugular venous catheter. Beware of hypocalcemia (repeated checks intraoperatively are required) and risk of cardiac arrest. Anticipate admission to the critical care unit and prolonged postoperative mechanical ventilation, and keep in mind the danger of nosocomial infections.

Pharmacological implications: Cardiodepressive drugs are contraindicated. Avoid drugs with predominantly renal excretion in the presence of associated renal impairment. Antibiotic prophylaxis may be indicated.

Other conditions to be considered: The velocardiofacial syndrome and the conotruncal anomaly-face syndrome are considered phenotypical variants of one genetic entity. The term "chromosome 22q11 deletion syndrome" has been suggested to name this group.

☞**VELOCARDIOFACIAL SYNDROME:** Includes typical facies and cardiac anomalies. Various other malformations can be associated (including endocrine and ophthalmic structures). Anesthetic implications are frequent (intubation, cardiac, infectious).

CONOTRUNCAL ANOMALY-FACE SYNDROME: Autosomal recessive congenital disorder characterized by facial and cardiac abnormalities. It is part of the spectrum of clinical manifestations of the 22q11.2 deletion syndrome. It is considered a variant of DiGeorge syndrome. This is the most frequent known microdeletion syndrome found in humans, with an incidence of 1:4000 live births. Clinical features include ocular hypertelorism, short palpebral fissures, microglossia, cleft lip/palate, bifid uvula, strabismus, bloated eyelids, and conductive deafness. A variety of cardiac defects have been described, including tetralogy of Fallot, pulmonary atresia, double-outlet right ventricle, truncus arteriosus communis, and aortic arch anomalies. Mental retardation and brain atrophy (occasional), short stature, hypoplasia of thymus and parathyroid glands, susceptibility to infection, neonatal hypocalcemia, anal atresia, abdominal hernias, and thrombocytopenia (occasional) have been described.

☞**CHARGE SYNDROME:** Life-threatening, congenital syndrome of multiple abnormalities, consisting of coloboma, heart disease, choanal atresia, mental and growth retardation, genital and urinary anomalies, and ear anomalies with deafness. The prognosis worsens if the disorder is associated with concomitant cyanotic congenital heart disease, CNS anomalies, and esophageal atresia.

☞**PIERRE ROBIN SYNDROME:** Frequent syndrome with multiple etiologies resulting in mandibular aplasia. Characterized by association of cleft palate, glossoptosis, and micrognathia with significant anesthetic implications, particularly for airway management. These problems decrease with age.

☞**OPITZ FRIAS SYNDROME:** Genetic disorder characterized by hypertelorism, hypospadia, and other midline defects. In particular, congenital heart defects are frequent.

GENITOPALATOCARDIAC SYNDROME (GARDNER-SILENGO-WATCHEL SYNDROME; SMITH-LEMLI-OPITZ SYNDROME TYPE III): Autosomal recessive or X-linked disorder with distinct dysmorphic features predominant and male pseudohermaphrodism. It is associated with poor survival outcome. Multiple malformations include micrognathia, cleft palate, complex heart defect (double-outlet right ventricle, ventricular septal defect, transposition of the great vessels, right-sided aortic arch), polycystic kidneys, and hypospadias. Oral contraceptives have been suggested as a probable causative agent.

☞**KOUSSEFF SYNDROME:** Severe polymalformative syndrome involving the nervous system (sacral meningocele), heart (conotruncal heart defect), unilateral renal agenesis, low-set and posteriorly angulated ears, retrognathia, and short neck with low posterior hairline. Significant craniofacial deformities.

REFERENCES:

Emanuel BS, McDonald-McGinn D, Saitta SC, et al: The 22q11.2 deletion syndrome. *Adv Pediatr* 48:39, 2001.

Huang RY, Shapiro N: Structural airway anomalies in patients with DiGeorge syndrome: A current review. *Am J Otolaryngol* 21:326, 2000.

Leana-Cox-J, Pangkanon S, Eanet KR, et al: Familial DiGeorge/velocardiofacial syndrome with deletions of chromosome area 22q11.2. Report of five families with a review of the literature. *Am J Med Genet* 65:309, 1996.

Digitotalar Dysmorphism

At a glance: Genetic disorder consisting of hand and foot deformities.

Synonyms: Hereditary Ulnar Drift; Deviation de la main en Coup de Vent; Windblown Hand Deformity.

Incidence and genetic inheritance: Unknown, but described only in a few kindreds. Autosomal dominant with varying clinical expression.

Pathophysiology: The deformities of the hand may, in part, be a result of the abnormal flexor and extensor mechanisms and the absence of the lateral portion of the extensor tendons expansions. This abnormality could explain the soft tissue deficiency over the middle phalanges and the flexion deformity of the terminal phalanges. The intrinsic muscles may either be shortened or tight, atrophic, or even absent. The extensor tendons are often subluxed into the ulnar valleys between the metacarpal heads. In some individuals, the joint capsules may be involved. When present, the vertical talus is responsible for the "rocker bottom" aspect of the foot.

Clinical aspects: For some authors, this is a forme fruste of arthrogryposis multiplex congenita. However, the affection limited to hands and feet and its pattern of inheritance allow for differentiation from arthrogryposis multiplex congenita. Deformities of the hands and feet are present at birth and may progress over time. Constant features are flexion contractures of the metacarpophalangeal joints, ulnar deviation, and narrowing of the fingers. Adduction contraction of the thumb with soft tissue webbing to the palm limits the range of motion and is the most limiting disability of this disorder. In some cases, the other digits are flexed in all joints. Metacarpal synostosis is not uncommon. The palms are described as having only a single palmar crease and a very soft and shiny skin. The muscles of the shoulder girdle and the entire upper extremity may be underdeveloped with a limited range of motion. Although some patients have normal feet, bilateral vertical talus with "rocker bottom" feet is a frequent finding and could result in minor gait anomalies ("waddling").

Anesthetic considerations: Careful positioning and padding of the hands are the only specific anesthetic considerations for this syndrome.

Other condition to be considered: Many other syndromes show the same or similar deformities of the hands and feet. However, digitotalar dysmorphism, in its original description, is limited to the features above and does not include any facial stigmata. Freeman-Sheldon syndrome is one of the most important of these syndromes.

☞**FREEMAN-SHELDON SYNDROME:** Genetic disorder characterized by a flat face with a small, pinched mouth mimicking whistling, clubfeet, and contracted muscles of the joints of fingers and hands. The hand deformities may resemble those of digitotalar dysmorphism.

REFERENCES:

Dhaliwal AS, Myers TL. Digitotalar dysmorphism. *Orthop Rev* 14:90, 1985.

Sallis JG, Beighton P: Dominantly inherited digitotalar dysmorphism. *J Bone Joint Surg Br* 54:509, 1972.

Wood VE, Biondi J: Treatment of the windblown hand. *J Hand Surg [Am]* 15:431, 1990.

Dihydropyrimidinase Deficiency

At a glance: Very rare metabolic disease with highly variable clinical expression, including seizures, mental retardation, and craniofacial anomalies.

Synonym: Dihydropyrimidinuria.

Incidence: Approximately 10 cases have been reported worldwide.

Genetic inheritance: Autosomal recessive with variable clinical phenotype.

Pathophysiology: Dihydropyrimidinase (DHP) catalyzes the degradation of 5,6-dihydrouracil and 5,6-dihydrothymine to N-carbamyl-β-alanine and N-carbamyl-β-aminoisobutyric acid, respectively. In the absence of DHP, large quantities of dihydrouracil and dihydrothymine and moderate amounts of uracil and thymine are excreted in the urine. The absence of DHP is responsible for a variety of clinical features.

Diagnosis: Clinical aspects and urinary metabolite profile (increased excretion of dihydrouracil, dihydrothymine, uracil, and thymine). Liver biopsy for measurements of DHP activity confirms the diagnosis.

Clinical aspects: The small number of patients limits the experience with the clinical picture. However, a wide range of inconstant clinical features has been reported, including seizures, extrapyramidal dyskinesia and pyramidal signs, mental retardation, plagiocephaly (oblique skull), and facial dysmorphism. Metabolic acidosis may occur.

Precautions before anesthesia: Obtain a full history of the seizures and anticonvulsant therapy (efficacy and toxicity). Consider neurologic consultation in cases with associated extrapyramidal involvement. Sedative premedication may be helpful in the presence of mental retardation. Check arterial blood gases and postpone elective surgery until metabolic acidosis (rare) is corrected. Check for difficult airway management in the presence of facial dysmorphism.

Anesthetic considerations: No literature is available. However, difficult airway management should be expected to be difficult. Depending on the kind of the procedure, intraoperative arterial or venous blood gas analysis is recommended.

Pharmacological implications: Avoid potentially epileptogenic drugs (e.g., methohexital, ketamine, enflurane, atracurium, cisatracurium, meperidine). In cases with associated extrapyramidal manifestations, avoid drugs with antidopaminergic effects (e.g., droperidol, domperidone, metoclopramide). Consider interaction between antiepileptic treatment and anesthetic drugs. Muscle relaxants should be avoided until airway is secured.

Other condition to be considered:

☞**DIHYDROPYRIMIDINE DEHYDROGENASE DEFICIENCY:** Genetic disorder with a high phenotypic variability, ranging from asymptomatic to developmental delay and seizures. Increased toxicity of 5-fluorouracil.

REFERENCES:

Duran M, Rovers P, De Bree PK, et al: Dihydropyrimidinuria: A new inborn error of pyrimidine metabolism. *J Inherit Metab Dis* 14:367, 1991.

Hamajima N, Kouwaki M, Vreken P, et al: Dihydropyrimidinase deficiency: Structural organization, chromosomal localization, and mutation analysis of the human dihydropyrimidinase gene. *Am J Hum Genet* 63:717, 1998.

Van Gennip AH, De Abreu RA, Van Lenthe H, et al: Dihydropyrimidinase deficiency: Confirmation of the enzyme defect in dihydropyrimidinuria. *J Inherit Metab Dis* 20:339, 1997.

Dihydropyrimidine Dehydrogenase Deficiency

At a glance: Genetic disorder with a high phenotypic variability ranging from asymptomatic to developmental delay and seizures. Increased toxicity of 5-fluorouracil.

Synonym: DPD Deficiency,

Incidence: Only approximately 50 cases have been described, with the majority reported from the Netherlands. Whether the prevalence is higher in the Netherlands, or whether this is finding is related only to a more extensive screening program, is not clear; 1:10,000 live births in Japan has been suggested.

Genetic inheritance: Autosomal recessive transmission. The defect has been mapped to chromosome 1p22.

Pathophysiology: The rate-limiting step in the degradation of uracil and thymine is catalyzed by the nicotinamide adenine dinucleotide phosphate (NADPH)-dependent enzyme dihydropyrimidine dehydrogenase (DPD) and results in the formation of 5,6-dihydrouracil and 5,6-dihydrothymine, respectively (also dihydropyrimidinuria). Although this enzyme is found in many organs throughout the body, the highest concentrations are found in the liver and leukocytes (monocytes and lymphocytes). Increased toxicity (neurotoxicity more pronounced than cardiotoxicity) has been reported for 5-fluorouracil (5-FU) administered in regular doses to these patients. Covalent binding of a metabolite of 5-FU to thymidylate synthase (the enzyme catalyzing the conversion of desoxyuridine monophosphate [dUMP] to desoxy-thymidine monophosphate [dTMP]) results in a complex that blocks the formation of thymidylate from uracil, thereby interfering with DNA synthesis. Approximately 80% of the administered 5-FU dose is metabolized by DPD.

Diagnosis: High urinary concentrations of uracil and thymine and low concentrations of N-carbamyl-β-alanine and N-carbamyl-β-aminoisobutyric acid (because of a lack of 5,6-dihydrouracil and 5,6-dihydrothymine, respectively) are usually the first findings in the search for an inborn error of metabolism in these patients. The diagnosis is finally confirmed by measuring DPD activity in liver cells, fibroblasts, or leukocytes.

Clinical aspects: The range of phenotypic variability is considerable. Whereas some patients are diagnosed only after they undergo 5-FU therapy, which resulted in increased toxicity, others (approximately 50%) present with seizures and delayed psychomotor development, usually starting in the first years of life. Other signs are less frequent and may include growth retardation, microcephaly, and other forms of dysmorphism.

Precautions before anesthesia: Obtain a full history of the seizures and anticonvulsant therapy (efficacy and toxicity).

Anesthetic considerations: No literature available about this disorder in association with anesthesia is available. No specific anesthesia-related problems should arise. However, sedative premedication may be helpful in the management of patients with signs of developmental delay.

Pharmacological implications: To our knowledge, increased toxicity of 5-FU is the only, but a potentially fatal, adverse drug effect specific to this population. Avoid potentially epileptogenic drugs in patients with a history of seizures (e.g., methohexital, ketamine, enflurane, atracurium, cisatracurium, meperidine). Chronic antiepileptic therapy may induce hepatic enzymes and therefore change the metabolism of drugs with predominately hepatic elimination.

Other conditions to be considered:

☞**DIHYDROPYRIMIDINASE DEFICIENCY:** Very rare metabolic disease with a highly variable clinical expression, including seizures, mental retardation, and craniofacial anomalies.

HEREDITARY THYMINE-URACILURIA: Allelic variant of DPD first described by van Gennip et al. in 1994. This condition features include microphthalmia, coloboma of the iris, choroid, nystagmus, and a gradually increasing psychomotor retardation, with no growth retardation or neurologic abnormalities.

5-FLUOROURACIL TOXICITY: Condition is an allelic condition.

REFERENCES:

Diasio RB, Beavers TL, Carpenter JT: Familial deficiency of dihydropyrimidine dehydrogenase: Biochemical basis for familial pyrimidinemia and severe 5-fluorouracil-induced toxicity. *J Clin Invest* 81:47, 1988.

Van Kuilenburg ABP, Vreken P, Abeling NGG, et al: Genotype and phenotype in patients with dihydropyrimidine dehydrogenase deficiency. *Hum Genet* 104:1, 1999.

Vreken P, Van Kuilenburg ABP, Meinsma R, et al: Identification of a four-base deletion (delTCAT296-299) in the dihydropyrimidine dehydrogenase gene with variable clinical expression. *Hum Genet* 100:263, 1997.

Dionisi Vici Sabetta Gambarara Syndrome

At a glance: Genetic disorder characterized by developmental delay, immunodeficiency, cleft lip/palate, cataract, hypopigmentation, and absent corpus callosum.

Incidence: Fewer than 10 cases have been reported in the literature.

Genetic inheritance: Autosomal recessive.

Pathophysiology: Unknown. There is speculation about a defect involving the embryogenic organization of both the CNS and the immune system such as regulating gene products.

Diagnosis: Clinical findings and combined immunodeficiency with reduced IgG levels (particularly IgG2 subclass), normal IgA and IgM levels, and low number of circulating T lymphocytes, mainly T$_4$.

Clinical aspects: Patients present with profound developmental delay associated with agenesis of the corpus callosum, microcephaly, hypotonia, seizures, and, occasionally, severe hypoplasia of the cerebellar vermis. Cortical dysplasia and schizencephaly have been described. One of the main features of this syndrome is a combined immunodeficiency with decreased levels of T$_4$ lymphocytes and serum IgG. This is a result of profound hypoplasia of the thymus and the peripheral lymphoid tissue. Activity of the natural killer cells, however, was reported to be normal. Recurrent infections, particularly pulmonary infections (partially also related to recurrent aspirations) and chronic mucocutaneous candidiasis, are a consequence of this immunodeficiency. The disease is also characterized by hypopigmentation of skin, hair, and retina. Cataract, nystagmus, unilateral or bilateral cleft lip/palate, micrognathia, and postnatal growth retardation are other, but inconstant, features. Cardiac involvement can occur in the form of endocardial fibroelastosis and/or progressive cardiomyopathy with dilatation or hypertrophy of the left ventricle. None of the reported patients has survived beyond age 3 years. Death from cardiac failure has been described, but most often death is the result of bronchopneumonia.

Precautions before anesthesia: Patients are most often booked for percutaneous gastric tube insertion secondary to failure to thrive. Request a chest radiograph to rule out respiratory tract infection. Obtain an ECG and an echocardiogram if cardiomyopathy is suspected. Continue antiseizure medication up to the morning of surgery.

Anesthetic considerations: Airway management may be more difficult than usual because of the micrognathia and cleft lip/palate. Sterile precautions are mandatory for all line insertions because of immunodeficiency. If cardiomyopathy is present, then medical therapy to improve left ventricular function should be optimized before the patient presents for an elective procedure.

Pharmacological implications: Avoid drugs with negative inotropic effect. Avoid or decrease the dose of muscle relaxants in the context of hypotonia. In the presence of a seizure disorder, potentially epileptogenic drugs such as methohexital, ketamine, enflurane, atracurium, *cis*-atracurium, and meperidine (applies to the latter three only if given in large quantities, because of their metabolites, laudanosine and normeperidine, respectively) should be avoided. Chronic antiseizure medication can lead to induction of hepatic en-

zymes and therefore accelerate the metabolism of predominantly hepatically eliminated drugs. Antibioprophylaxis should be adapted because of the immunodeficiency.

Other conditions to be considered:

☞**AICARDI SYNDROME:** Rare disorder characterized by partial or complete agenesis of the corpus callosum, infantile spasms (spasm-like epilepsy), mental retardation, and an ocular abnormality called lacunae of the retina. Often associated with other features such as microcephaly and porencephalic cysts. Age at onset is generally between 3 and 5 months.

☞**CHEDIAK HIGASHI SYNDROME:** Frequently fatal disease of childhood characterized by albinism, photophobia, hypopigmentation, loss of binocular vision, and marked susceptibility to infections.

☞**GRISCELLI SYNDROME:** Albinism with immunodeficiency characterized by partial pigmentary dilution of the skin and hair (silvery gray hair), frequent infections, neurologic abnormalities, and fatal outcome caused by uncontrolled T-lymphocyte and macrophage activation syndrome. Clinical features include the presence of large clumps of pigment in hair shafts and an accumulation of melanosomes in melanocytes.

REFERENCES:

Del Campo M, Hall BD, Aeby A, et al: Albinism and agenesis of the corpus callosum with profound developmental delay: Vici syndrome, evidence for autosomal recessive inheritance. *Am J Med Genet* 85:479, 1999.

Dionisi Vici C, Sabetta G, Gambarara M, et al: Agenesis of the corpus callosum, combined immunodeficiency, bilateral cataract, and hypopigmentation in two brothers. *Am J Med Genet* 29:1, 1988.

Disaccharide Intolerance Type I

At a glance: Congenital enzyme defect resulting in chronic diarrhea and failure to thrive.

Synonym: Congenital Sucrase-Isomaltase Deficiency; Disacchardase Deficiency Type I.

Incidence: Varies with ethnic group (whites: 1:2500, native Alaskans: 1:33, native Canadians: 4–7:100).

Genetic inheritance: Autosomal recessive. The gene encoding for sucrase-isomaltase deficiency is localized on the long arm of chromosome 3.

Pathophysiology: The absence or severe reduction in sucrase and isomaltase activity in the brush-border membrane of the small intestine is responsible for malabsorption of dietary disaccharides and starch. When these carbohydrates are introduced into the diet, they generate an osmotic pressure gradient in the intestinal lumen, attracting large volumes of isotonic fluid with normal sodium concentration. The capacity for colonic bacteria to ferment malabsorbed carbohydrates is rapidly overwhelmed, and osmotic diarrhea ensues.

Diagnosis: Starch is a mixture of the two polysaccharides amylopectin and amylose. Hydrolysis of amylopectin and amylose yields mainly maltose, maltotriose, and glucose. Clinical presentation, oral tolerance test with the corresponding disaccharides, sucrose breath hydrogen test, differential urinary disaccharide excretion, and measurement of intestinal disaccharidase activity in a small intestine biopsy lead to the diagnosis. Disaccharidase deficiency is defined as an enzyme activity of at least two standard deviations below the normal mean value. A jejunal biopsy is the gold standard for the diagnosis because the disaccharidase levels are normally the highest here; however, the specimen is difficult to obtain. Furthermore, the circadian rhythm of enzyme activity must be considered.

Clinical aspects: The clinical presentation varies and depends on the introduction of sucrose and starch to the diet. Once the diet ceases to consist exclusively of breast milk and lactose-free formulas, the introduction of sucrose-containing juices, solid food, or even medications causes chronic osmotic-fermentative diarrhea and, occasionally, failure to thrive. Decreased duodenal-ileal transit time may compromise fat absorption. Empiric avoidance of dietary sucrose load may delay the diagnosis up to the toddler age (children show relatively normal growth but suffer from intermittent diarrhea with meteorism and abdominal cramps). A minority of patients requires hospitalization for severe dehydration, malnutrition, and muscle wasting. Lifelong elimination of sucrose and reduction of starch content in the diet leads to complete recovery.

Precautions before anesthesia: Obtain a full history of gastrointestinal symptoms (severity of diarrhea and degree of malnutrition) causing failure to thrive. In rare cases, TPN is required. Evaluate volume status clinically and check electrolytes, blood urea nitrogen, and creatinine. If the patient is on TPN, also check serum concentrations of albumin, glucose, phosphate, calcium, magnesium, transaminases, alkaline phosphatase, and bilirubin. Optimize volume status preoperatively by intravenous rehydration.

Anesthetic considerations: Consider repeated intraoperative blood glucose monitoring if the patient is on TPN.

Pharmacological implications: In the presence of severe malnutrition (rare) or depressed renal and/or hepatic function secondary to complications from TPN, highly protein-bound drugs must be titrated carefully secondary to low protein levels (in particular α_1-acid glycoprotein and albumin), which may result in decreased drug binding and increased free drug levels.

Other condition to be considered:

☞**DISACCHARIDE INTOLERANCE TYPE II:** Congenital enzyme defect resulting in chronic diarrhea, dehydration, and failure to thrive.

REFERENCES:

Newton T, Murphy MS, Booth IW: Glucose polymer as a cause of protracted diarrhea in infants with unsuspected congenital sucrase-isomaltase deficiency. *J Pediatr* 128:753, 1996.

Treem WR: Congenital sucrase-isomaltase deficiency. *J Pediatr Gastroenterol Nutr* 21:1, 1995.

Disaccharide Intolerance Type II

At a glance: Congenital enzyme defect resulting in chronic diarrhea, dehydration, and failure to thrive.

Synonyms: Congenital Lactase Deficiency; Disaccharidase Deficiency Type II.

Nature: Genetic disorder manifested by chronic diarrhea.

Incidence: Fewer than 100 cases have been reported worldwide, with the majority in Finland.

Genetic inheritance: Autosomal recessive. The congenital lactase deficiency gene is localized on the long arm of chromosome 2.

Pathophysiology: Lactose, the main carbohydrate in milk and dairy products, is a disaccharide composed of glucose and galactose. In congenital lactase deficiency, the enzyme is present only at trace levels in the small intestine brush-border membrane. As a consequence of lactase deficiency, high concentrations of unabsorbed lactose remain in the intestinal lumen and generate an osmotic diarrhea.

Diagnosis: Clinical presentation, a trial of lactose-free diet, breath hydrogen test, and assay of lactase activity in a jejunal biopsy specimen.

Clinical aspects: Onset is very early in life (in the first hours or days of life), with watery diarrhea upon introduction of lactose-containing milks. Diarrhea is severe and results in rapid dehydration, malnutrition, failure to thrive, and high lactose concentration in the feces. Total remission with normal growth and psychomotor development occurs with a lactose-free diet.

Precautions before anesthesia: Evaluate volume status clinically and check serum electrolytes, blood urea nitrogen, and creatinine. Pay special attention to renal function and serum calcium levels because hypercalcemia and nephrocalcinosis have been described. Delay elective surgery until the patient is well rehydrated and acid–base status is corrected. If the patient is on TPN, also obtain serum concentrations of albumin, glucose, phosphate, magnesium, transaminases, alkaline phosphatase, and bilirubin. Optimize volume status preoperatively by intravenous rehydration.

Anesthetic considerations: Consider repeated intraoperative blood glucose monitoring if the patient is on TPN.

Pharmacological implications: In the presence of severe malnutrition (rare) or depressed renal and/or hepatic function secondary to complications from TPN, highly protein-bound drugs have to be titrated carefully, secondary to low protein levels (particularly α_1-acid glycoprotein and albumin), which may result in decreased drug binding and increased free drug levels.

Other conditions to be considered:

☞**DISACCHARIDE INTOLERANCE TYPE I:** Congenital enzyme defect resulting in chronic diarrhea and failure to thrive.

SEVERE INFANTILE LACTOSE INTOLERANCE: On a lactate-containing diet, affected children become severely ill and present with vomiting, acidosis, lactosuria, aminoaciduria, and failure to thrive. Cataract occurs occasionally. The cause of this disorder has not been fully elucidated, but it seems that jejunal lactase activity is normal and that the defect is caused by an abnormal permeability of the intestinal mucosa.

REFERENCES:

Jarvela I, Sabri Enattah N, Kokkonen J, et al: Assignment of the locus for congenital lactase deficiency to 2q21, in the vicinity of but separate from the lactase-phlorizin hydrolase gene. *Am J Hum Genet* 63:1078, 1998.

Semenza G, Auricchio S, Mantei N: Small-intestinal disaccharidases, in Scriver CR, Beaudet AL, Sly WS, et al. (eds): *The Metabolic and Molecular Bases of Inherited Disease.* 8th ed. New York, McGraw Hill, 2001, p 1623.

Donnai-Barrow Syndrome

At a glance: Genetic disorder responsible for diaphragmatic hernia, exomphalos, absent corpus callosum, hypertelorism, eye anomalies, and sensorineural deafness.

Incidence: Six cases have been reported since its first description by Donnai and Barrow in 1993. Some researchers believe that Donnai-Barrow Syndrome and facio-oculo-acoustico-renal (FOAR) syndrome belong to the same entity.

Genetic inheritance: Autosomal recessive.

Pathophysiology: The precise mechanism resulting in the findings of this syndrome remains to be determined.

Diagnosis: Pregnancy may be complicated by polyhydramnios, and prenatal diagnosis can be made by ultrasonography.

Clinical aspects: Patients are born with bilateral absence of the diaphragm (some die shortly after birth as a result of severe pulmonary hypoplasia). Congenital heart disease may coexist (double-outlet right ventricle, ventricular septal defect, patent foramen ovale, persistent ductus arteriosus). Omphalocele (exomphalos), intestinal malrotation, absent corpus callosum, severe myopia (15–20 diopters), iris coloboma, retinal detachment, sensorineural deafness, and variable degree of developmental delay are characteristic of this syndrome. Other distinct features include facial dysmorphism with enlargement of both fontanels, hypertelorism with down-slanting palpebral fissures, broad nose, angulated ears, and mild micrognathia.

Precautions before anesthesia: Evaluate the degree of the newborn's illness. Depending on the amount of abdominal contents in the chest and the severity of pulmonary hypoplasia, the neonate may require immediate tracheal intubation and controlled ventilation or even extracorporeal membrane oxygenation (ECMO). In the presence of severe pulmonary hypoplasia with pulmonary hypertension, an attempt at inhalation of nitric oxide to reduce pulmonary vascular resistance may be worthwhile, before ECMO is considered. ECMO is the ultimate bridging management for refractory cases; however, the prognosis is unfavorable for patients with severely hypoplastic lungs and pulmonary vasculature. The size of the omphalocele is usually moderate. Obtain a chest radiograph and echocardiography to rule out possible congenital cardiac lesions. Laboratory investigations should include serum electrolytes and glucose, hemoglobin, blood type, cross-match, and arterial blood gas analysis. Later in life, consider administration of an anxiolytic premedication for elective surgery if mental retardation is present.

Anesthetic considerations: Any surgery should be preceded by optimization of the infant's volume and electrolyte status, intensive respiratory care, and prevention of further intrathoracic distension of bowel loops by permanent low suction through a gastric tube. Avoid high airway pressures (>25 mmHg) and accept permissive hypercapnia instead. If the patient is on ECMO, care should be taken to avoid kinking the cannulas when positioning the patient for surgery. Hypothermia increases morbidity significantly. Invasive monitoring, such as arterial (preferentially preductal) and central venous line, is required. The upper extremities are preferred for peripheral venous access because reduction of the diaphragmatic hernia and/or the omphalocele increases the intraabdominal pressure and may obstruct the inferior vena cava. Preductal and postductal pulse oximetry allow for early detection of right-to-left shunting. Nitrous oxide should be avoided as it distends gas-filled intestinal loops and worsens the pulmonary situation. Pulmonary mechanics change rapidly intraoperatively, and any acute deterioration in lung compliance, oxygenation, and/or hemodynamic parameters suggests a pneumothorax. When reducing an omphalocele, intragastric pressures higher than 20 mmHg usually are poorly tolerated. Postoperatively, an intensive care unit bed is required for continued respiratory and hemodynamic management.

Pharmacological implications: No specific considerations for this condition.

Other condition to be considered:

☞**Facio-Oculo-Acoustico-Renal (FOAR) Syndrome:** Genetic disorder affecting the eyes (blindness), ears (deafness), face, kidneys, and the bones.

References:

Donnai D, Barrow M: Diaphragmatic hernia, exomphalos, absent corpus callosum, hypertelorism, myopia, and sensorineural deafness: A newly recognized autosomal recessive disorder? *Am J Med Genet* 47:679, 1993.

Gripp KW, Donnai D, Clericuzio CL, et al: Diaphragmatic hernia-exomphalos-hypertelorism syndrome: A new case and further evidence of autosomal recessive inheritance. *Am J Med Genet* 68:441, 1997.

Donohue Syndrome

At a glance: Rare inherited condition caused by resistance to insulin with growth deficiency and characterized by dysmorphic facies ("elfin-like"), severe growth retardation, hirsutism, and multiple endocrine disorders.

Synonym: Leprechaunism.

Nature: Endocrine disorder characterized by resistance to insulin caused by abnormal insulin receptors. First described by W.L. Donohue and I.A. Uchida in 1954.

Incidence: Approximately 50 cases have been reported in the literature, but the incidence is estimated to be approximately 1:4,000,000 live births.

Genetic inheritance: Autosomal recessive. The defective gene, which is responsible for encoding of the insulin receptor, has been mapped to 19p13.2. Parental consanguinity is likely for this disorder.

Pathophysiology: The primary defect in leprechaunism is located in the insulin receptor, but a secondary associated defect probably is responsible for growth failure because of an impaired response to endogenous growth hormone. This finding may be explained by the fact that the cytoplasmic subunit of the insulin receptor shares similarities with other receptors that have tyrosine kinase activity (e.g., insulin-like growth factor-1, epidermal and platelet-derived growth factor, and certain protooncogenes).

Diagnosis: Clinical aspect and measurement of blood glucose and insulin levels. Prenatal diagnosis is available.

Clinical aspects: The synonym for this syndrome, leprechaunism, is derived from "leprechaun," the name of a mythical little hairy elf originating from the Irish folklore. Patients have an elfin or gnome-like face with microcephaly, protuberant and low-set ears, large, wide-set eyes, high arched palate, thickened lips, and severely diminished subcutaneous fat (general lipodystrophy) and muscle mass. Skin abnormalities include hypertrichosis (also reflected in the name leprechaun), acanthosis nigricans, and pachyderma. Insulin resistance characterizes the metabolic abnormalities, such as severe hyperinsulinemia, postprandial hyperglycemia, and paradoxical fasting hypoglycemia. Intrauterine and postnatal growth retardation seem to result from a diminished response to growth hormone, at least partially because of downregulation of growth hormone receptors by high insulin levels. The genitalia are enlarged, and cystic changes in the gonads occur frequently in girls. The abdomen often is distended, and the presence of umbilical and/or inguinal hernias is not uncommon. Some patients have cardiac involvement, such as atrial septal defect or, more commonly, myocardial hypertrophy, which may be severe. Although some patients survived for several years, most die of severe failure to thrive with recurrent infections in the first year of life. Rare cases of survival beyond infancy have been attributed to the presence of residual insulin receptor function.

Precautions before anesthesia: Obtain a blood sugar level prior to going to the operating room. If cardiac disease is suspected, obtain an ECG and an echocardiogram.

Anesthetic considerations: General and regional anesthesia, in the same newborn, for two different surgeries have been reported with no major complications related to the type of anesthesia. Except for very short surgeries, regular blood glucose measurements should be performed and a dextrose-containing intravenous solution administered to detect and prevent hypoglycemia, respectively. In the presence of hypertrophic cardiomyopathy, tachycardia, hypotension, hypovolemia, and an increase in contractility must be avoided.

Pharmacological implications: Depending on the congenital cardiac defect and the type of procedure, subacute bacterial endocarditis prophylaxis may be necessary.

Other conditions to be considered: Other progeroid syndromes including the following:

☞**PROGERIA:** Premature aging with increased urinary excretion of hyaluronic acid caused by a sporadic dominant mutation.

☞**BERARDINELLI-SEIP SYNDROME:** Inherited disorder with hyperinsulinemia as a consequence of insulin resistance combined with lipodystrophy and acromegaloid features (enlarged external genitalia, increased skeletal growth with acromegaloid appearance, diabetes mellitus with generalized loss of body fat, hepatomegaly, and acanthosis nigricans).

DE BARSY MOENS DIERCKS SYNDROME: Autosomal recessive disorder featuring cutis laxa, frontal bossing and prominent ears, athetosis, cloudy cornea, hypotonia and hyperlaxity of joints, and/or short stature.

☞**COCKAYNE SYNDROME:** DNA repair syndrome characterized by short stature, premature aging, and photophobia, which is aggravated by UV exposure but has no link to cancer development.

☞**HALLERMAN-STREIFF SYNDROME:** Sporadic malformation syndrome characterized by short stature, microphthalmia, brittle teeth, growth retardation, upper respiratory tract obstruction, and scoliosis.

☞**CONGENITAL DISORDERS OF GLYCOSYLATION:** Group of multisystemic disorders characterized by dysmorphism, coagulation disorders, and psychomotor retardation. Multiple subtypes exist, of which type Ia is by far the most common.

☞**RABSON-MENDENHALL SYNDROME:** Genetic disorder with pineal hyperplasia, insulin-resistant diabetes mellitus, and somatic abnormalities.

☞**ALSTRÖM SYNDROME:** Inherited syndrome with progressive visual and hearing loss, diabetes mellitus, and cardiac, hepatic, and renal involvement.

REFERENCES:

Desbois-Mouthon C, Girodon E, Ghanem N, et al: Molecular analysis of the insulin receptor gene for prenatal diagnosis of leprechaunism in two families. *Prenat Diagn* 17:657, 1997.

Longo N, Wang Y, Smith SA, et al: Genotype-phenotype correlation in inherited severe insulin resistance. *Hum Mol Genet* 11:1465, 2002.

DOOR Syndrome

At a glance: DOOR is an acronym standing for sensorineural *d*eafness, *o*nychodystrophy, *o*steodystrophy, microcephaly, and global developmental *r*etardation. The disorder is characterized by sensorineural deafness, progressive blindness, onychodystrophy, triphalangeal thumbs, mental retardation, and seizures.

Incidence: Approximately 20 cases have been reported in the literature.

Genetic inheritance: There are two forms of this syndrome, one being inherited autosomal dominantly (without mental retardation), the other inherited autosomal recessively. Parental consanguinity is a risk factor.

Pathophysiology: Unknown.

Diagnosis: Diagnosis is mainly clinical. However, patients with the recessive type and a more severe phenotype, who are classified as DOOR syndrome type I (with early onset of seizures, i.e., within the first 6 months of life, and a progressive course with blindness, deafness, and early death), show increased plasma and urinary concentrations of 2-oxoglutarate and its metabolite α-hydroxyglutarate. (2-Oxoglutarate, a precursor of glutamate, is involved in the regulation of gluconeogenesis in liver and kidney and of ammoniagenesis in the kidney). DOOR syndrome type II is not associated with increased concentrations of organic acids and shows a less severe clinical course.

Clinical aspects: Main clinical characteristics of this syndrome are the presence of congenital sensorineural deafness, mental retardation, and onychoosteodystrophy, which consists of hypoplasia of the terminal phalanges, triphalangeal thumbs, dysplastic or absent fingernails and toenails, and pathologic (arch pattern) dermatoglyphics. Affected patients usually develop seizures early in life, which may be difficult to control and can cause death. Other, but less frequent, anomalies include microcephaly, plagiocephaly, low-set ears, hypertelorism, broad nose with large nostrils, thin upper lip with long philtrum, micrognathia, retrognathia, and high arched palate. Cardiac defects and urinary tract anomalies have been described. Mental retardation is not a feature of the autosomal dominant transmitted form of the DOOR syndrome.

Precautions before anesthesia: Ensure that seizure control is optimized. Administer the patient's medication up to the morning of surgery. Check kidney function because urinary tract abnormalities are common in DOOR syndrome type I. If cardiac disease is suspected, an ECG and echocardiogram should be obtained.

Anesthetic considerations: In the presence of mental retardation, deafness, and progressive blindness, the patient coming to the unknown environment of the operating room may be anxious and agitated. Sedative and anxiolytic premedication and the presence of the primary caregiver during induction of anesthesia may be helpful. If the patient presents with micrognathia or retrognathia, airway management should be expected to be more challenging.

Pharmacological implications: With anticonvulsive medication, the hepatic enzyme system may be induced and the metabolism of other drugs with predominantly hepatic elimination altered, requiring dose adjustment.

Other conditions to be considered:

☞**ERONEN SYNDROME:** Genetic disorder characterized by severe digital, renal, and cerebral malformations.

☞**COFFIN-SIRIS SYNDROME:** Probably an autosomal dominant transmitted syndrome. Characteristics of the syndrome include developmental delay, hypoplasia of the fifth digit nails and phalanges, sparse scalp hair, bushy eyebrows, wide mouth, hirsutism, and prominent or hypertrophied lips.

REFERENCES:

Hess RO, Pecotte JK: Additional case report of the DOOR syndrome. *Am J Med Genet* 19:401, 1984.

Nevin NC, Thomas PS, Calvert J, et al: Deafness, onychodystrophy, mental retardation (DOOR) syndrome. *Am J Med Genet* 13:325, 1982.

Rajab A, Riaz A, Paul G, et al: Further delineation of the DOOR syndrome. *Clin Dysmorphol* 9:247, 2000.

Drachtman Weinblatt Sitarz Syndrome

At a glance: Disease characterized by the combination of congenital neurologic anomalies and late-onset bone marrow hypoplasia.

Incidence and genetic inheritance: Only two cases have been described. Inheritance could be autosomal recessive. Chromosome studies were normal and did not show increased fragility.

Diagnosis: Diagnosis is clinical based on the presence of neurologic anomalies combined with easy bruising. Diagnosis is confirmed by CT or MRI scans of the brain, complete blood count (nonmegaloblastic macrocytosis), and bone marrow biopsy that reveals hypocellular bone marrow with erythroid hyperplasia, reduced granulopoiesis, and quasi-absence of megakaryocytes.

Clinical aspects: The main feature of this syndrome is the late appearance (around age 4 years) of easy bruising with purpuric lesions and scattered petechiae as a result of a low platelet count. In addition, patients may present with acute bleeding as a consequence of minor trauma, which, in turn, leads to anemia. The other characteristic of this syndrome is the presence of neurologic anomalies, which seem to be quite variable (hemiparesis with dilated left ventricle and asymmetry of the peduncles, partial agenesis of the corpus callosum, hydrocephalus, Dandy-Walker syndrome, developmental delay, and seizures). Congenital ocular anomalies include strabismus, optic nerve hypoplasia, and rotary nystagmus. No skeletal anomalies have been described in association with this syndrome. The disorder usually is not responsive to steroid therapy. Bone marrow transplant seems to be the only therapeutic solution.

Precautions before anesthesia: Obtain a complete blood count and consult a hematologist if necessary. Ensure that blood products are readily available before going to the operating room.

Anesthetic considerations: In the presence of bone marrow aplasia, it may be wise to avoid neuraxial anesthesia and the placement of central lines via the subclavian route. Good padding for positioning is advised. To decrease the formation of petechiae or bruises, less-frequent cycling of the blood pressure cuff is recommended if the patient is stable or when an arterial line is in place. Use sterile technique for catheter insertion because these patients may also be neutropenic.

Pharmacological implications: In order to not further compromise hemostasis, drugs that inhibit thromboxane A_2 synthesis (e.g., acetylsalicylate, nonsteroidal antiinflammatory drugs) or otherwise interfere with hemostasis should be avoided or used with caution only. Acetaminophen, although less potent, should be preferred instead.

Other conditions to be considered:

☞**BLACKFAN-DIAMOND SYNDROME:** Congenital hypoplastic anemia that manifests in the first year of life and has an increased risk for leukemia.

☞**FANCONI ANEMIA:** Inherited anemia leading to bone marrow failure, myelogenous leukemia, and, in older patients, many cancers (head and neck, esophageal, gastrointestinal, vulvar, and anal).

REFERENCE:

Drachtman R, Weinblatt M, Sitarz A, et al: Marrow hypoplasia associated with congenital neurologic anomalies in two siblings. *Acta Paediatr Scand* 79:990, 1990.

Du Pan Syndrome

At a glance: Genetic disorder characterized by complex brachydactyly and fibular hypoplasia.

Incidence: Approximately 20 cases have been described in the literature.

Genetic inheritance: Autosomal recessive. The responsible gene has been mapped to 20q11.2. Parental consanguinity is a risk factor.

Pathophysiology: The cartilage-derived morphogenetic protein-1 (CDMP1) is crucial in the patterning of chondrogenesis, longitudinal bone growth, and appendicular skeleton. The genetic defect results in a missense substitution in the active domain of CDMP1, which leads to a change in the conformation and finally in the activity of CDMP1.

Diagnosis: Mainly clinical, based on the combination of short stature and limb malformations.

Clinical aspects: Patients affected with this syndrome present with short stature as a result of symmetrical limb malformations. In the upper limbs, the main findings are short metacarpal bones (especially the first metacarpals), short phalangeal bones (particularly the middle ones), and hypoplasia of the carpal bones. The thumbs are button-like, and all fingers tend to have radial deviation. In the lower limbs, the fibulas are either absent or severely hypoplastic, and the knees may be dislocated with hypoplastic and displaced patellae. The feet usually have an equinovalgus deformation associated with tibiotarsal dislocation of the ankle. The metatarsals are hypoplastic, as are the phalanges of all toes, which resemble ball-like remnants with hypoplastic nails. Intelligence and craniofacial features are normal.

Precautions before anesthesia: No particular precautions for this syndrome.

Anesthetic considerations: Careful padding and positioning are required to prevent dislocations of the joints. Because of the malformations, peripheral vascular access may be challenging.

Pharmacological implications: No specific implications for this condition.

Other condition to be considered:

☞**ACROMESOMELIC DYSPLASIA TYPES II (HUNTER-THOMPSON) AND III (GREBE):** Extremely short stature as a result of acromesomelic dysplasia of the limbs (forearms, forelegs, hands, feet). In general, patients have normal intelligence. Joint dislocations may occur. Normal craniofacial and axial skeleton.

REFERENCES:

Ahmad M, Abbas H, Wahab A, et al: Fibular hypoplasia and complex brachydactyly (Du Pan syndrome) in an inbred Pakistani kindred. *Am J Med Genet* 36:292, 1990.

Faiyaz-Ul-Haque M, Ahmad W, Zaidi SH, et al: Mutation in the cartilage-derived morphogenetic protein-1 (CDMP1) gene in a kindred affected with fibular hypoplasia and complex brachydactyly (Du Pan syndrome). *Clin Genet* 61:454, 2002.

Duane Retraction Syndrome

At a glance: Neurophthalmologic condition associated with abnormal ocular movement, usually not accompanied by other congenital anomalies.

Synonym: Stilling Turk Duane Syndrome.

Incidence: Duane retraction syndrome (DRS) is an unusual form of congenital strabismus and accounts for 1 to 4% of children with strabismus. It is slightly more common in females than in males (about 60:40), often is bilateral (20−57%), and is significantly more frequent in the left eye (about 3−4:1). Reported frequencies vary widely.

Genetic inheritance: Approximately 56 to 90% are sporadic cases. In the residual cases, a positive family history with autosomal dominant transmission has been suggested, although some cases with most likely autosomal recessive inheritance have been reported. Several gene defects can account for hypoplastic or absent brainstem motor neurons and aberrant innervation and therefore have been linked to DRS. Defects have been mapped to loci 2q31, 4q27-31, 8q12.2-q21.1, and 22pter-22q11.2, to mention a few.

Pathophysiology: Innervation of the lateral rectus muscle emanates from axons of oculomotor nuclei, which supposedly supply the medial rectus muscle. The abducens nucleus may be hypoplastic or even absent. Attempted adduction of the eye basically results in simultaneous contractions of the lateral and the medial rectus muscle, with the net effect being retraction of the globe. At the same time, the palpebral fissure narrows and horizontal eye movement is limited (depending on the type of DRS, abduction is severely compromised). A teratogenic event (e.g., thalidomide exposure) between days 20 and 35 of gestation has been held responsible for the genetic defect.

Diagnosis: Severe limitation of horizontal eye movement accompanied by narrowing of the palpebral fissure and eyeball retraction with attempted adduction leads to the diagnosis of DRS.

Clinical aspects: Different classifications have been suggested for DRS. The following classification is based on EMG findings:

- *Type I:* Abduction is more compromised than adduction, which results in globe retraction and narrowing of the palpebral fissure, whereas abduction results in widening of the palpebral fissure. Adduction, but not abduction, shows EMG activity in the lateral rectus muscle. This type accounts for 70 to 90% of cases.
- *Type II:* Adduction is absent or limited with exotropia of the affected eye. Attempted adduction results in globe retraction. Adduction and abduction result in EMG activity in the lateral rectus muscle.
- *Type III:* Both adduction and abduction are severely limited. Attempted adduction results in globe retraction and narrowing of the palpebral fissure. EMG activity can be recorded for the lateral and the medial rectus muscles during attempted adduction and abduction.

In addition to the described horizontal restrictions of eye movement, vertical eye movement anomalies are possible.

A few other anomalies have been reported in conjunction with DRS, including other ocular anomalies such as anisometropia, amblyopia (both in approximately 15% of DRS patients), anisocoria, ptosis, and nystagmus. Conductive hearing loss and sensorineural hearing loss (each in approximately 5% of cases) have been reported. Furthermore, DRS has been described in patients with Arnold-Chiari I Syndrome, cerebro-oculofacioskeletal syndrome, Goldenhar syndrome, Holt-Oram syndrome, or Rubinstein-Taybi syndrome. DRS can be associated with intracerebral vascular malformations.

Precautions before anesthesia: No specific anesthetic problems with DRS. However, the frequent association of this disorder with other anomalies or syndromes indicates the need for thorough and careful examination of the patient to exclude more anesthesia relevant findings.

Anesthetic considerations: Dictated by the syndrome associated with DRS. Isolated DRS should not affect anesthetic management and outcome.

Pharmacological implications: Isolated DRS is not expected to have any pharmacological implications.

Other conditions to be considered: The following syndromes must be considered in a patient with DRS.

☞**ARNOLD-CHIARI I SYNDROME:** Defect in the formation of the lower portion of the medulla (posterior fossa). Can be associated, according to the type, with hydrocephalus, raised intracranial pressure, and respiratory and cardiac center dysfunction. Infants may present with vomiting, mental impairment, and weakness. Limb paralysis is possible. The presence in adolescents usually is milder. Dizziness, weakness of the legs, headaches, double vision, or deafness may be present. Raised intracranial pressure. In type I, cerebellar displacement into the spinal canal occurs; however, hydrocephalus and syringomyelia are variable.

☞**PENA-SHOECKER SYNDROME TYPE II:** Rapidly progressive congenital neurologic disorder.

☞**GOLDENHAR SYNDROME:** Common birth defect of vascular origin involving first and second branchial arch derivatives resulting mainly in facial and vertebral anomalies with potentially severe anesthetic implications (both caused by reconstructive surgery and difficult intubation).

☞**HOLT-ORAM SYNDROME:** Inherited malformation syndrome characterized by the association of a congenital heart disease (septal defect) and upper limb malformation (underdevelopment of bones and/or extra bones).

☞**RUBINSTEIN-TAYBI SYNDROME:** Rare syndrome with craniofacial anomalies and complex and multiple malformations of the cardiac, digestive, and respiratory systems.

REFERENCES:

Gutowski NJ: Duane's syndrome. *Eur J Neurol* 7:145, 2000.

Marshman WE, Schalit G, Jones RB, et al: Congenital anomalies in patients with Duane retraction syndrome and their relatives. *J AAPOS* 4:106, 2000.

Yamanouchi H, Iwasaki Y, Sugai K et al: Duane retraction syndrome associated with Chiari I malformation. *Paediatr Neurol* 9:327, 1993.

Dubin-Johnson Syndrome

At a glance: Benign disease characterized by familial idiopathic jaundice presenting with chronic intermittent conjugated hyperbilirubinemia.

Synonym: Dubin-Johnson-Sprinz Nelson Syndrome.

Incidence: Occurs in both sexes (although males are affected about 1.5 times more often than females) and in all nationalities and races. The highest prevalence in the general population (1:1300) is found in Iranian Jews.

Genetic inheritance: Autosomal recessive, with a reduced penetrance in females. The gene encoding for the human canalicular multispecific organic anion transporter (cMOAT) protein has been mapped to 10q24.

Pathophysiology: The cMOAT protein is involved in the energy-dependent transport of certain bilirubin glucuronides and organic acids (except bile acids) against a concentration gradient across the canalicular membrane of the hepatocyte. The cMOAT protein defect in Dubin-Johnson syndrome (DJS) leads to decreased hepatobiliary transport and seems to be responsible for the predominantly conjugated hyperbilirubinemia and the intralysosomal accumulation of pigment in hepatocytes.

Diagnosis: In healthy people, the total daily biliary coproporphyrinogen (CPG) excretion (a by-product of the heme synthesis) is about three times higher than urinary CPG excretion, and urinary CPG III concentration is about three times higher than CPG I concentration. In DJS, the total amount of urinary CPG is normal, but CPG isomer I accounts for 80% of total CPG. Hence, the diagnosis is based on increased levels of CPG I in the urine, whereas the CPG III level is below normal. Furthermore, the rise in the sulfobromophthalein sodium test is delayed, and the liver appears macroscopically dark blue or even black. Histologically, the cytoplasm of hepatocytes (especially in zone III) contains big lysosomes packed with a lipochromic pigment, which is responsible for the brown-black color. This pigment has many similarities to melanin but is not melanin. It has been theorized that the pigment may be composed of polymers of epinephrine metabolites. The amount of pigment is variable; for example, it can disappear almost completely during an acute viral hepatitis but then reappear slowly after recovery.

Clinical aspects: Main findings of the disease are hepatomegaly associated with abdominal pain and jaundice. Although cases in neonates have been described, onset usually is in early adulthood, presenting with a nonpruritic jaundice that is caused by increased conjugated hyperbilirubinemia. Liver function is otherwise normal. However, in up to two thirds of DJS patients (especially those of Iranian Jewish descent), a prolonged prothrombin time secondary to reduced activity of factor VII has been reported.

Precautions before anesthesia: Ensure the liver anomalies truly result from DJS and that no other intercurrent disease is causing the liver dysfunction. Ask about prolonged bleeding; if in doubt or before major surgery, check for coagulation disorder.

Anesthetic considerations: If blood loss is significant, check coagulation and treat accordingly.

Pharmacological implications: Jaundice may transiently increase postoperatively. Consequently, it seems prudent to avoid halothane to prevent its implication in the development of postoperative jaundice. Pregnancy, exogenous administration of hormones (e.g., oral contraceptives), and stress can trigger or exacerbate an existing jaundice. Factor VII concentrate is available, but its use likely is not indicated in DJS.

Other conditions to be considered:

☞**GILBERT SYNDROME:** Genetic disorder resulting in mild jaundice, which tends to fluctuate in severity and results from a mutation in the uridyl diphosphate-glucuronosyltransferase gene, thus being allelic to the mutation for the Crigler-Najjar syndrome.

☞**CRIGLER-NAJJAR SYNDROME:** Genetic disorder leading to severe neonatal jaundice (typically with kernicterus).

☞**ROTOR SYNDROME:** Rare autosomal recessive disease characterized by a chronic, predominantly conjugated hyperbilirubinemia. It has many similarities to DJS, but total urinary CPG is elevated, as is the CPG I concentration; however, CPG I accounts for less than 80% of total urinary CPG. The liver is a normal color on biopsy, unlike DJS.

REFERENCES:

Chowdry J, Wolkoff A, Chowdry N, et al: Hereditary jaundice and disorders of bilirubin metabolism, in Scriver C, Beaudet A, Valle D, et al. (eds): *The Metabolic and Molecular Bases of Inherited Disease.* 8th ed. New York, McGraw-Hill, 2000, p 3085.

Kartenbeck J, Leuschner U, Mayer R, et al: Absence of the canalicular isoform of the MRP gene-encoded conjugate export pump from the hepatocytes in Dubin-Johnson syndrome. *Hepatology* 23:1061, 1996.

Sherlock S, Dooley J: Dubin Johnson syndrome, in Sherlock S, Dooley J: *Diseases of the Liver and Biliary System.* 11th ed. Blackwell Science, 2002, p 243.

Dubowitz Syndrome

At a glance: Genetic disorder with craniofacial (craniosynostosis), neurologic, orthopedic and dermatologic anomalies.

Incidence: Approximately 150 cases have been reported in the literature since the first description of the syndrome by V. Dubowitz in 1965.

Genetic inheritance: Autosomal recessive.

Pathophysiology: The precise mechanisms leading to the very wide phenotypic presentations of the syndrome remain to be determined.

Diagnosis: No biochemical characterization to confirm Dubowitz syndrome is available. Diagnosis is based on clinical features (mainly facial appearance), which show a high variability and may result in underdiagnosis of the disorder.

Clinical aspects: Very high variety of combinations of multiple anomalies may be present, which is at least in part responsible for the difficulties in confirming the diagnosis. Intrauterine and postnatal growth retardation and delayed osseous maturation lead to (proportionate) short stature in approximately 80% of patients. Mental retardation ranges from mild (common) to severe (rare), but average intelligence has been reported. Patients are often described as hyperactive with a short attention span (67%), stubborn, and shy. Muscular hypotonia is common (40%). Seizures are rare. Craniofacial anomalies may include microcephaly (with head circumference below the third percentile), premature craniosynostosis, distinctive, small face with high forehead, flat supraorbital ridge, short palpebral fissures, scanty or absent lateral part of the eyebrows, lateral telecanthus, hypertelorism, epicanthal folds, ptosis, blepharophimosis, and other ocular anomalies (e.g., strabismus, microphthalmia, iris hypoplasia, coloboma, and ocular albinism). The nasal tip is broad, and the ears are prominent or dysplastic. Micrognathia (may be severe) and retrognathia (rare), submucous cleft palate (44%), occasional velopharyngeal insufficiency, multiple dental problems (delayed eruption, missing teeth, extensive caries), and a high-pitched and hoarse voice (68%) have been described. Cardiovascular anomalies are rare but can occur in the form of coarctation of the aorta, aberrant subclavian artery (dysphagia lusoria), occlusion of the internal carotid artery, persistent ductus arteriosus, ventricular septal defect, and mitral valve prolapse. Patients often suffer from eczema (58%), which tends to improve with age; sparse hair; and pilonidal dimples. Brachyclinodactyly of the fifth finger is a constant feature, the joints are hyperextensible, and, patients occasionally present with scoliosis or spina bifida occulta. Genital abnormalities, such as cryptorchidism, hypospadias, and inguinal hernia, are common.

Gastroesophageal reflux disease, vomiting, chronic diarrhea, or chronic obstipation may be present. Bone marrow hypoplasia may occur in up to 6% of patients, and case reports of fatal aplastic anemia exist. On the one hand, patients have increased susceptibility to recurrent infections (of upper airway, ears, and urinary tract, most likely secondary to IgA, IgG, and/or IgM deficiencies) and malignancies (leukemia, lymphoma, neuroblastoma, rhabdomyosarcoma). On the other hand, allergies are very frequent findings.

Precautions before anesthesia: Obtain a full medical history and clinical assessment of the airway and the degree of muscular hypotonia. Request a pulmonary function test if any doubt about respiratory compromise exists. Ask about previous anesthesias and any related complications. Blood examination should include a complete blood count and a hemoglobin level (because of possible bone marrow hypoplasia, immunodeficiency). Check electrolyte levels (hypoparathyroidism has been described). In the rare case of seizure disorder, inquire about anticonvulsant therapy, and its efficacy and toxicity. Depending on the degree of mental retardation, sedative and anxiolytic premedication and the presence of the primary caregiver during induction may be helpful.

Anesthetic considerations: Micrognathia and submucous cleft rarely make tracheal intubation difficult. In the presence of retrognathia (infrequent) or any type of anticipated difficult airway, spontaneous respiration should be maintained while securing the airway by fiberoptic intubation. In cases of gastroesophageal reflux or recurrent vomiting, a rapid-sequence intubation is recommended. However, keep in mind that almost half of patients show signs of muscular hypotonia. Correction of anemia and thrombocytopenia may be necessary in cases of bone marrow hypoplasia, and good vascular access is recommended. Allergies are frequent, and the anesthetist should be prepared to treat them should they occur.

Pharmacological implications: Succinylcholine is contraindicated because of the risk of hyperkalemia. Nondepolarizing muscle relaxants are often unnecessary or should be titrated under the control of a peripheral nerve stimulator because increased sensitivity has been reported. If a seizure disorder is present, potentially epileptogenic drugs (methohexital, ketamine, enflurane, meperidine, atracurium, and *cis*-atracurium) should be avoided. Some antiseizure drugs induce the hepatic enzyme system, which may result in altered metabolism of predominantly hepatically eliminated drugs. Subacute bacterial endocarditis prophylaxis may be required, depending on the presence of cardiac lesions and the kind of procedure.

REFERENCES:

Kuster W, Majewski F: The Dubowitz syndrome. *Eur J Pediatr* 144:574, 1986.

Lerman-Sagie T, Merlob P, Shuper A, et al: New findings in a patient with Dubowitz syndrome: Velopharyngeal insufficiency and hypoparathyroidism. *Am J Med Genet* 37:241, 1990.

Tsukahara M, Opitz JM: Dubowitz syndrome: Review of 141 cases including 36 previously unreported patients. *Am J Med Genet* 63:277, 1996.

Duchenne Muscular Dystrophy

At a glance: Inherited and progressive myopathy affecting boys. Presents with muscular, respiratory, and cardiac disease.

Synonyms: DMD; Pseudohypertrophic Muscular Dystrophy; Duchenne Type of Progressive Muscular Dystrophy; Progressive Muscular Dystrophy Type I.

Incidence: Approximately 1:3500 boys is affected, which makes it the most common form of muscular dystrophy. No preferences in race or nationality have been reported. The disease affects almost exclusively males, although females rarely can be affected, for example, when they have a translocation between autosomal chromosomes and the X chromosome, uniparental disomy (i.e., when the chromosome pair or specific segments of a chromosome pair are inherited from one parent only), or suffer from Turner syndrome.

Genetic inheritance: About one third results from spontaneous mutation (negative family history does not exclude DMD); the rest is inherited in an X-gonosomal recessive way. Simplified, in DMD a frameshift mutation results in the absence of dystrophin, whereas in Becker muscular dystrophy a non-frameshift mutation results in decreased levels of dystrophin. The responsible gene (with 2400 kbp, one of the largest known human genes) has been mapped to the short arm of the X chromosome at position 21 (Xp21).

Pathophysiology: The DMD gene product, a protein called dystrophin, is absent or nonfunctional in patients with DMD. Dystrophin, an important structural part of a large sarcolemmal glycoprotein complex, stabilizes the sarcolemma and plays an important role in the interaction between sarcoplasm and extracellular matrix. Dystrophin is expressed in skeletal and cardiac muscle and in the brain. In the absence of dystrophin (or its function), the entire function of this sarcolemmal complex appears to be disrupted (dystrophin links the actin filaments to the glycoprotein complex in the sarcolemma). This defect may result in either decreased sarcolemmal stability to the mechanical stress of contraction-relaxation or disturbed calcium homeostasis with excessive calcium influx into the muscle cell and pathologic activation of intracellular enzymes. Finally, this results in destruction and necrosis of muscle fibers, which are eliminated by macrophages (myophagocytosis) and later replaced by scar and fat tissue with endomysial and perimysial fibrosis. Although some muscle fibers may show a compensatory hypertrophy, most often the fibers are atrophic, split, or even missing in later stages of the disease. The clinically diagnosed pseudohypertrophy of muscles (particularly the calves) refers to this phenomenon and is, in fact, the result of scarring and fatty degeneration of the muscles, which is muscle wasting.

Diagnosis: The clinical course, elevated plasma levels of creatine phosphokinase and other enzymes (e.g., troponin I, lactate dehydrogenase, and transaminases), and muscle biopsy (fatty degeneration and scarring and immunostaining confirm the lack of dystrophin) lead to the diagnosis. Molecular biology allows for intrauterine diagnosis. Age at diagnosis is before birth (familial context), otherwise between 2 and 5 years (occasionally later). Female carriers of the disease may have increased creatine phosphokinase levels, but most often they are clinically asymptomatic.

Clinical aspects: Progressive and symmetrical wasting of muscles of the legs and pelvis and later of the thorax and upper limbs. Muscle weakness appears insidiously between 2 and 5 years of age, producing a waddling gait and lordosis. Soon thereafter, the calf muscles become enlarged (pseudohypertrophy). These boys have difficulty standing up (Gowers sign) and climbing stairs, develop contractures, and become wheelchair-bound by age 10 to 12 years (sometimes earlier). Joint deformities, muscle retractions, and degenerations are common. Collapse of the spine results in severe scoliosis and restrictive pulmonary disease. Often these patients are obese (secondary to lack of physical activity and fatty degeneration of the muscles), show mild mental retardation (with an average IQ in the mid-80s), and hypertrophy of the tongue. Clinically apparent dilated cardiomyopathy (which initially may have been hypertrophic), often with persistent sinus tachycardia and conduction system abnormalities (ECG changes, most often consisting of signs of right ventricular hypertrophy and/or right bundle branch block, occur in 40–90% of patients), is a common feature in adolescents with DMD. Occasionally, left-sided endocardial thickening (left atrial and left ventricular) occurs. Echocardiography may reveal normal systolic but pathologic diastolic left ventricular function (i.e., decreased diastolic relaxation). Mitral valve prolapse has been reported in about one fourth of patients and may be secondary to fatty degeneration of the papillary muscles. Weakness of the diaphragm is an ominous sign that usually occurs in the second decade of life and may result in hypoventilation and hypoxia. Death most often occurs late in the second decade from respiratory complications (>90%) and/or cardiac complications (10%).

Precautions before anesthesia: Obtain a full history of motor milestones, previous complications (especially following surgeries), and familial related disorders. Evaluate pulmonary function test (forced vital capacity [FVC], peak expiratory flow rate, forced expiratory volume (1 sec) [FEV_1], FEV_2: FRC [functional residual capacity] ratio, arterial blood gas analysis, and chest radiograph). Evaluate cardiac function with ECG, echocardiography, and, if necessary, radionuclide imaging. Blood work should include a complete blood count, serum levels of creatine phosphokinase and electrolytes, and arterial blood gas analysis. Elective surgery under general anesthesia is contraindicated when respiratory and/or cardiac function is severely reduced.

Anesthetic considerations: Serious complications, including death associated with anesthesia, have repeatedly been reported. The high complication rate is a result of muscle weakness with respiratory insufficiency, metabolic changes (hyperkalemia and hyperthermia), and cardiomyopathy (late onset). Expect difficult airway management in patients with enlarged tongue and/or ankylosis of the temporomandibular joints. Cervical lordosis may result in tracheal and bronchial compression in the prone position and may not be relieved by tracheal intubation. Hazards of severe hyperthermia have been described (which may be different from malignant hyperthermia unless succinylcholine has been used) with hyperkalemia and myoglobinuria (dark discoloration of urine) secondary to rhabdomyolysis. Renal impairment and acute renal failure can occur as a result of myoglobinuria. Arrhythmias (tachycardia, ventricular fibrillation) and cardiac arrest have been reported. They are mainly, but not exclusively, associated with succinylcholine use and most often occur shortly after succinylcholine administration. However, late and sudden cardiac arrest in the postoperative period following recovery of consciousness is possible. Furthermore, it seems that hyperkalemia can be precipitated by halogenated inhalational anesthetics alone (most often halothane but also isoflurane). Joint deformities and contractures make difficult not only patient positioning on the operating room table (with danger of pressure necrosis) but also vascular access, which is further complicated by obesity and thickening of subcutaneous tissues. Mechanical ventilatory support is almost mandatory following major surgery (spinal fusion). Patient compliance occasionally is reduced because of anxiety and mild mental retardation.

Pharmacological implications: Whether patients are at increased risk to experience a malignant hyperthermia reaction is controversial. For clinical purposes, however, this is not of fundamental importance because both reactions (malignant hyperthermia and nonmalignant hyperthermia) are triggered by the same agents. Succinylcholine (absolute contraindication) and halogenated agents (halothane, particularly if creatine phosphokinase levels are elevated) must be avoided because of a possible and potentially fatal hyperkalemic response. Dantrolene should be easily available. Persisting metabolic acidosis (despite adequate volume status) and hypercapnia in the presence of signs of rhabdomyolysis should always raise concerns about the possibility of a malignant hyperthermia or malignant hyperthermia-like reaction. Calcium-induced hypermetabolism seems to be the common denominator in both situations, and dantrolene has the potential to interrupt the vicious cycle. Muscle relaxants (preferably *cis*-atracurium) can be used (under control of a peripheral nerve stimulator), but recovery may be significantly prolonged. However, they often are unnecessary because of preexistent muscle weakness. Opioids are not contraindicated but should be used with caution in patients with already compromised respiratory function. If possible, a regional anesthetic technique should be used for postoperative pain therapy. Because of the muscle relaxing effects, benzodiazepines for premedication should be used with caution in these patients.

Other conditions to be considered:

BECKER MUSCULAR DYSTROPHY (BMD; ADULT PSEUDO-HYPERTROPHIC MUSCULAR ATROPHY; BENIGN X-LINKED RECESSIVE MUSCULAR HYPERTROPHY; BECKER TYPE OF PROGRESSIVE MUSCULAR DYSTROPHY; PROGRESSIVE MUSCULAR DYSTROPHY TYPE II): Allelic disorder of DMD affecting approximately 1:30,000 males. However, in contrast to DMD, dystrophin in BMD is partially functional, which results in less severe symptoms. Its onset is usually during the second decade of life, with slow progression and normal life expectancy in most cases. However, the same clinical features as in DMD can be observed. As such, cases of BMD with isolated cardiomyopathy and unexpected deaths from a malignant hyperthermia or a malignant hyperthermia-like reaction during anesthesia in undiagnosed cases have been described. Therefore, for anesthetic purposes, the same precautions and considerations apply as in DMD. Unfortunately, generalized myotonia, which is a congenital anomaly of the muscular chloride channels resulting in prolonged contraction of skeletal muscles and significant anesthetic implications, is also called myotonia congenita Becker type or just Becker disease. Do not mix them up.

☞**BETHLEM MYOPATHY:** Genetic disorder consisting of a benign congenital myopathy and contractures. Significant anesthetic implications.

☞**LIMB-GIRDLE TYPE OF MUSCULAR DYSTROPHY:** Inherited symmetrical muscular weakness, initially of the lower limbs, with slow progression and associated cardiac anomalies.

☞**EMERY-DREIFUSS MUSCULAR DYSTROPHY:** Relatively benign congenital muscular dystrophy usually beginning in childhood or adolescence and characterized by early muscle contractures (mainly shoulders and upper arms) and cardiac conduction disorders.

☞**SCHWARTZ-JAMPEL SYNDROME:** Progressive congenital disorder characterized by hypertrophic myotonic myopathy, dwarfism, chondrodystrophy, and ocular and facial abnormalities. Contractures are most severe by mid-adolescence.

☞**MYOTONIC DYSTROPHY:** Genetic multisystem disorder affecting skeletal and smooth muscles, heart, and CNS with a wide range of clinical expression.

☞**MYOTONIA CONGENITA:** Rare genetic disorder characterized by myotonia, muscle stiffness, and abnormal muscle hypertrophy giving the impression of a "Herculean" or "bodybuilder-like" appearance. Two main forms of myotonia congenita have been described: Thomsen disease and Becker disease. In Thomsen disease, symptoms and findings usually are apparent from infancy to approximately 2 to 3 years of age. In many cases, muscles of the eyelids, hands, and legs may be most affected. In Becker disease, symptoms most commonly become apparent between the ages of 4 and 12 years. Affected individuals develop progressive myotonia. Muscle rigidity and hypertrophy tend to be more severe.

REFERENCES:

Chalkiadis GA, Branch KG: Cardiac arrest after isoflurane anaesthesia in a patient with Duchenne's muscular dystrophy. *Anaesthesia* 45:22, 1990.

Kleopa KA, Rosenberg H, Heiman-Patterson T: Malignant hyperthermia-like episode in Becker muscular dystrophy. *Anesthesiology* 93:1535, 2000.

Morris P: Duchenne muscular dystrophy: A challenge for the anaesthetist. *Paediatr Anaesth* 7:1, 1997.

Duker Weiss Siber Syndrome

At a glance: Genetic disorder mainly characterized in affected males by ocular anomalies (e.g., microphthalmos), microencephaly, mental retardation, agenesis of the corpus callosum, and urogenital anomalies. Lethal in infancy.

Synonym: Cerebro-Oculo-Genital Syndrome.

Incidence and genetic inheritance: The first report described four related males in 1985. Transmission is X-linked recessive.

Clinical aspects: Diagnosis is clinical, based mostly on the ocular findings and on imaging studies confirming absence of the corpus callosum. Affected male patients present with complicated ocular anomalies such as microphthalmos, corneal hypoplasia and pannus, cataracts, uveal and optic nerve hypoplasia, retinal dysplasia, and congenital blepharoptosis and swollen eyelids. Other consistent findings are microcephaly, agenesis of the corpus callosum, mental retardation, hypospadias, and cryptorchidism. The condition is lethal in infancy or early childhood.

Anesthetic considerations: Because patients with this syndrome are mentally delayed and almost blind, obtaining their cooperation may be difficult. Sedative and anxiolytic premedication and the presence of the primary caregiver during induction of the anesthesia may be helpful.

Other condition to be considered:

☞**LENZ SYNDROME:** Very rare disorder with multiple anomalies, such as neurologic, craniofacial, ocular, skeletal, and urogenital findings.

REFERENCE:

Duker JS, Weiss JS, Siber M, et al: Ocular findings in a new heritable syndrome of brain, eye, and urogenital abnormalities. *Am J Ophthalmol* 99:51, 1985.

Dyggve-Melchior-Clausen Syndrome

At a glance: Short-spine–type dwarfism associated with mental retardation and skeletal abnormalities.

Incidence: Only 58 cases have been reported in the literature. Seems to occur more frequently in Lebanon.

Genetic inheritance: Autosomal recessive. Linkage studies localized the responsible genes to chromosome 18q12-21.1. This gene seems to be involved in normal skeletal development and brain function.

Pathophysiology: Electron microscopy of chondrocytes shows dilated cisternae of rough endoplasmic reticulum, containing fine granular or amorphous material. Protein accumulation within the rough endoplasmic reticulum has been hypothesized to be secondary to an enzyme defect that has not been characterized.

Diagnosis: Clinically, thoracic deformities in the form of barrel chest become visible in the first 18 months of life. Radiographs of the iliac crests show a characteristic, lace-like appearance, which is caused by an irregular pattern in the bone tissue deposits at the osteochondral junction. Abnormal enchondral ossification and absent columnarization of chondrocytes are found in the growth plates. The vertebral bodies are characteristic, presenting with double-hump endplates associated with a central constriction (platyspondyly). These signs usually are present by age 4 years and become more prominent with increasing age.

Clinical aspects: Phenotypically, patients share some features of Morquio and Hurler syndromes. In fact, the disorder initially was named Morquio-Ullrich disease. Affected patients present with dwarfism because of both short trunk and short limbs. The mean adult height is approximately 130 cm (51.2 in). They also have a coarse facies, although the degree is highly variable, ranging from almost normal to very severe, where the bulky jaws and microcephaly are striking. The neck is short. Patients have a variable degree of odontoid hypoplasia, which may lead to atlantoaxial instability and place them at risk for complications related to spinal cord compression. The chest is barrel shaped, and malalignment of the spine with kyphoscoliosis is common. The hands and feet are broad, and the fingers might be clawed. Dislocation of hips and shoulders are common (secondary to dysplastic joints). Although mental retardation is present, general health is otherwise good and survival into adulthood is the rule.

Precautions before anesthesia: Short stature in association with the spine deformity leads to restrictive lung disease so pulmonary function tests are recommended, although cooperation may be limited. Blood gas analysis and echocardiography (cor pulmonale) may be warranted, depending on the results of the lung function tests. Obtain flexion and extension radiographs or CT scans of the cervical spine to rule out atlantoaxial instability. Anxiolytic or sedative premedication may be helpful in the presence of mental retardation.

Anesthetic considerations: Difficult tracheal intubation is likely (even without atlantoaxial instability) because of the presence of a short neck, prominent, big jaws, macroglossia, and limited mouth opening. Tracheal intubation should be performed either fiberoptically or, if possible, conventionally with inline stabilization of the cervical spine. Restrictive lung disease may render ventilation and oxygenation more challenging and may preclude the use of neuraxial regional anesthesia. Proper patient positioning is difficult because of atlantoaxial instability, dislocations (hip, shoulder), deformities, and contractures affecting the musculoskeletal system.

Pharmacological implications: Titrate sedation carefully to avoid respiratory depression in the presence of restrictive lung disease.

Other condition to be considered:

SMITH-MCCORT DYSPLASIA/DWARFISM: Allelic disorder similar to the Dyggve Melchior Clausen syndrome, with the only significant difference being the absence of mental retardation.

REFERENCES:

Beighton P: Dyggve-Melchior-Clausen syndrome. *J Med Genet* 27:512, 1990.

Cohn DH, Ehtesham N, Krakow D, et al: Mental retardation and abnormal skeletal development (Dyggve-Melchior-Clausen dysplasia) due to mutations in a novel, evolutionarily conserved gene. *Am J Hum Genet* 72:419, 2003.

Kandziora F, Neumann L, Schnake KJ, et al: Atlantoaxial instability in Dyggve-Melchior-Clausen syndrome: Case report and review of the literature. *J Neurosurg* 96:112, 2002.

Dyke-Davidoff-Masson Syndrome

At a glance: Syndrome characterized by cerebral hemiatrophy with marked asymmetry of the cerebral hemispheres and characteristic changes on skull radiograph. These changes usually are associated with facial asymmetry, mental retardation, seizures, and contralateral hemiplegia.

Synonym: Cerebral Hemiatrophy Syndrome.

Incidence: Unknown. Only a small series of case reports has been published since the first description in 1933.

Genetic inheritance: Unknown. Normal chromosomal karyotypes and amino acid excretion patterns on testing. Males and females are equally affected.

Pathophysiology: Condition results from two different etiologies.

- *Primary:* Caused by perinatal asphyxia with symptoms apparent soon after birth and often resulting in severe white matter lesions and marked asymmetry of the pyramidal tracts.

- *Secondary:* Caused by loss of cortical neurons with symptoms presenting later in childhood after a generally normal early development. Syndrome may be postictal, particularly if there is a history of early childhood febrile seizures (multifocal neuronal loss) following a vascular insult such as middle cerebral artery stroke or trauma (more focal abnormality).

Diagnosis: Clinical suspicion is confirmed by the classic changes on skull radiograph showing ipsilateral osseous hypertrophy of the calvaria and hyperpneumatization of the paranasal sinuses and mastoid cells. This is a result of the failure of brain growth leading to inward growth of bony structures, resulting in increased size of the frontal sinus and elevation of the greater wing of sphenoid and petrous ridge on the affected side. CT and MRI scans are used to assess the etiology and extent of cerebral parenchymal involvement. They usually reveal dilation of the ventricles and low density of the involved cortical side. Thickening of the calvaria and midline shift are seen in about half of cases. Temporal sclerosis is frequent if there is a history of febrile convulsions.

Clinical aspects: Asymmetry of the face and calvaria and contralateral hemiplegia are the main characteristics. Moderate-to-severe mental retardation is often associated with cerebral palsy, visual perception problems, language (slurred or immature) or speech problems (repetitive speech patterns, simple jargon), and seizures. Patients may present with symptoms of schizophrenia without neurologic abnormalities. Coarctation of the midthoracic aorta has been reported.

Precautions before anesthesia: General clinical assessment including the ability to cooperate. Obtain a full history of seizures and the medication and its efficacy. Look for signs of adverse effects of antiseizure medication. Antiepileptics should be continued preoperatively.

Anesthetic considerations: Separation from parents may be difficult, so sedative and anxiolytic premedication may be helpful. Neuroaxial blockade is relatively contraindicated.

Pharmacological implications: If a seizure disorder is present, potentially epileptogenic drugs (methohexital, ketamine, enflurane, meperidine, atracurium, and *cis*-atracurium) should be avoided. Some antiseizure drugs induce the hepatic enzyme system, which may result in altered metabolism of predominantly hepatically eliminated drugs. Emergence seizures on emergence are not uncommon.

Other condition to be considered:

☞**RUSSELL-SILVER SYNDROME:** Very rare genetic disorder characterized by intrauterine growth retardation, hemihypertrophy, and asymmetry of the head, trunk, arms, and/or legs. The extent and severity of asymmetry vary greatly among affected children. Characteristic facial features may include a triangular-shaped face with a small, pointed chin, frontal bossing, blue sclera, an unusually small and wide mouth, down-turned corners of the mouth, and micrognathia.

REFERENCES:

Dix JE, Cail WS: Cerebral hemiatrophy: Classification on the basis of MR imaging findings of mesial temporal sclerosis and childhood febrile seizures. *Radiology* 203:269, 1997.

Parker CE, Harris N, Mavalwala J: Dyke-Davidoff-Masson syndrome: Five case studies and deductions from dermatoglyphics. *Clin Pediatr (Phila)* 11:288, 1972.

Vosskamper M, Schachenmayr W: Cerebral hemiatrophy: A clinico-pathological report of two cases with a contribution to pathogenesis and differential diagnosis. *Clin Neuropathol* 9:244, 1990.

Dyskeratosis Congenita

At a glance: Dyskeratosis congenita is a genodermatosis characterized by hyperpigmentation of the skin, dystrophy of the nails, leukoplakia of mucous membranes, and progressive pancytopenia.

Synonyms: Zinsser-Cole-Engman Syndrome; Dyskeratosis Congenita Scoggins type.

Incidence: Unknown, but approximately 200 cases have been described.

Genetic inheritance: X-linked recessive disorder that affects almost exclusively males (male-to-female ratio = 10:1). However, there are rare case reports of autosomal recessive and autosomal dominant inheritance. The mutant gene has been mapped to Xq28 and encodes for a 514-amino-acid protein called dyskerin.

Pathophysiology: Dyskerin seems to have a major role in the regulation of cell proliferation (biogenesis of ribosomes and pseudouridylation of recombinant RNA messengers) and therefore primarily affects rapidly proliferating tissues (e.g., skin, gastrointestinal mucosa, and bone marrow).

Diagnosis: The phenotype is highly variable; however, bone marrow failure and the triad of reticulated hypopigmentation and hyperpigmentation of the skin, nail dystrophy, and mucocutaneous leukoplakia is typical for dyskeratosis congenita. The onset of skin and nail changes usually is around age 10 years and precedes epiphora and mucocutaneous changes. Although signs of bone marrow failure and malignancy begin to develop in the early to mid-teens, manifestation before age 10 years is not uncommon.

Clinical aspects: Changes in skin pigmentation (reticulated hypopigmentation and hyperpigmentation) often in combination with telangiectases are more pronounced on the flexures of the big joints, neck, and axillae, and along the inner thigh. Nail dystrophy is progressive and initially may result in longitudinal ridges and finally in complete loss of nails. The hair may be affected, leading to baldness. Leukoplakia most often occurs in the mouth but also may affect other mucosal sites (e.g., esophagus, vagina, anus, urethral meatus, and lacrimal duct resulting in strictures with dysphagia, dyspareunia, dysuria, and epiphora) and is associated with an increased risk for malignancies (most often squamous cell carcinoma). In male patients, testes often are undescended and hypoplastic. Dental abnormalities (extensive cavities, premature loss) and increased fragility of the bones caused by abnormal metaphyseal trabeculation and osteoporosis have been reported. Lacrimal duct stenosis or atresia is present in up to 80% of patients and leads to continuous epiphora. Up to 90% of patients suffer from bone marrow failure; rarely the diagnosis of aplastic anemia precedes the diagnosis of dyskeratosis congenita. Some patients develop myelodysplasia and acute myeloid leukemia. Pancytopenia or complications related to bone marrow transplant (high rate of pulmonary complications) are responsible for approximately 70% of the premature deaths in this population. Approximately 20% of these patients show pulmonary changes with progressive pulmonary fibrosis and restrictive lung disease, arteriovenous shunting with microvascular changes, and reduced diffusion capacity. It has been hypothesized that these underlying changes are, at least in part, responsible for the high rate of pulmonary complications in association with bone marrow transplant. Liver cirrhosis with a nutmeg aspect may be present, and mucosal ulcerations may cause gastrointestinal hemorrhage. Elevated immunoglobulin levels and increased risk of opportunistic infections have been reported. Additional findings (each in approximately 15–20% of patients) include prenatal and postnatal growth retardation and mild-to-moderate mental retardation (intracerebral calcifications) associated with mainly deafness-related learning difficulties. In general, female patients tend to have a milder course of the disease; nevertheless, bone marrow failure with death has been reported.

Precautions before anesthesia: Obtain a complete blood count because of possible bone marrow failure and gastrointestinal hemorrhage. Perioperative prophylaxis with H_2 antagonists or proton pump inhibitors should be considered. A chest radiograph, lung function tests, and arterial blood gas analysis are recommended preoperatively because the incidence of pulmonary disease is high. Depending on the results and the planned procedure, arrangements should be made for postoperative mechanical ventilation. The presence of obstructive sleep apnea, which has been reported in some patients, requires the possibility for close postoperative monitoring and judicious use of opioids. Liver function and coagulation tests may be indicated for possible cirrhosis.

Anesthetic considerations: Strictly aseptic technique is required to prevent iatrogenic infections. Anemia is often a major concern. Patients may have undergone bone marrow transplant, and special attention must be paid to the type of blood given (irradiated). As a consequence of extensive cavities and premature loss of teeth, careful direct laryngoscopy is mandatory in order to prevent further damage. Careful positioning is required because of increased bone fragility. Esophageal strictures may be present, and, in case of liver cirrhosis, esophageal varices should be expected, so nasogastric tube insertion should be done very carefully or avoided. Because a significant number of patients received chemotherapy and/or radiation therapy, the inspired oxygen concentration should be kept as low as safely possible. Intraoperative monitoring of arterial and/or mixed venous oxygen partial pressures helps in finding this lowest safe level.

Pharmacological implications: Drugs with pulmonary toxicity (e.g., antimetabolites, alkylating agents, bleomycin, mitomycin, amiodarone) should be avoided in these patients. In the presence of liver cirrhosis, drugs with predominantly hepatic metabolism and elimination should be given in reduced doses and if possible titrated to the desired effect. Hypalbuminemia may increase the effect of highly protein-bound drugs, requiring a dose reduction.

Other conditions to be considered:

☞**BLOOM SYNDROME:** Autosomal recessive inherited disorder characterized by prenatal and postnatal growth retardation, photosensitivity, telangiectasias, skin pigment anomalies, and increased risk of malignancies most likely caused by chromosomal instability.

☞**FANCONI ANEMIA:** Inherited anemia leading to bone marrow failure, myelogenous leukemia, and, in older patients, many cancers (head and neck, esophageal, gastrointestinal, vulvar, and anal).

☞**KINDLER SYNDROME:** Polymalformative syndrome of unknown inheritance pattern characterized by neonatal skin blistering on the extremities appearing spontaneously and after minor trauma. Other features include limb hyperkeratosis, mucous membrane fragility with esophageal and urethral strictures, and webbing of the fingers and the toes.

☞**ROTHMUND-THOMSON SYNDROME:** Rare genetic syndrome with extensive bullous skin anomalies, juvenile cataract, skeletal disorders, and predisposition to malignancy.

HOYERAAL-HREIDARSSON SYNDROME (CEREBELLAR HYPOPLASIA WITH PANCYTOPENIA; PRENATAL GROWTH RETARDATION WITH PROGRESSIVE PANCYTOPENIA AND CEREBELLAR HYPOPLASIA): Considered to be a severe variant of X-linked dyskeratosis congenita. In addition to many of the features found in dyskeratosis congenita (although skin and nail changes are uncommon), patients present with microcephaly and cerebellar hypoplasia with reduced cellularity of the molecular and granular layers, but only minimal gliosis and relative preservation of Purkinje cells. Clinically, developmental delay, spastic paresis, and ataxia may develop. In addition, growth retardation, facial dysmorphism, and recurrent infections caused by lymphopenia (B-cell depletion and T-cell dysfunction) and low or abnormal levels of IgG and IgM can occur. The average age at the onset of aplastic anemia, which is approximately 22 months, is significantly lower than in dyskeratosis congenita. The prognosis is dismal, with the most patients dying at about age 3.5 years. Death is most often caused by infection and sepsis.

REFERENCES:

Drachtman RA, Alter BP: Dyskeratosis congenita [review]. *Dermatol Clin* 13:33, 1995.

Knight SW, Heiss NS, Vulliamy TJ, et al: Unexplained aplastic anaemia, immunodeficiency, and cerebellar hypoplasia (Hoyeraal-Hreidarsson syndrome) due to mutations in the dyskeratosis congenita gene, DKC1. *Br J Haematol* 107:335, 1999.

Knight S, Vulliamy T, Copplestone A, et al: Dyskeratosis congenita (DC) registry: Identification of new features of DC. *Br J Haematol* 103:990, 1998.

Langston AA, Sanders JE, Deeg HJ, et al: Allogenic marrow transplantation for aplastic anaemia associated with dyskeratosis congenita. *Br J Haematol* 92:758, 1996.

Dysosteosclerosis

At a glance: Genetic disorder with unfavorable prognosis manifesting as blindness, mental retardation, and characteristic skeletal changes.

Incidence: Unknown. Approximately 15 cases have been reported.

Genetic inheritance: Both autosomal recessive (common) and X-linked recessive transmission (rare) have been reported. Parental consanguinity is considered a risk factor.

Pathophysiology: Dysplasia of the bone with areas of thickening and areas of sclerosis is responsible for this very distinctive osseous disease. However, the underlying mechanism is unknown.

Diagnosis: Made by clinical course and findings of the disorder in combination with the typical radiologic features.

Clinical aspects: Most typical radiologic finding is platyspondyly (flattening of the vertebral bodies), especially of the thoracic spine with irregular endplates and wide intervertebral spaces. As in osteopetrosis, vertebral bodies and the ribs show a diffusely increased density. Sclerosis is found in the diaphyses and epiphyses of the long bones. The metaphyses are splayed and osteoporotic as a result of cortical thinning, particularly in the lower extremities. Metaphyseal widening extends progressively with time. There is an increased risk of fractures even after trivial trauma. Thickening and sclerosis of the skull base result in macrocephaly and impingement of the basal foramina but particularly of the optic nerve canal, causing optic atrophy with severe visual impairment or blindness, which probably is the most important clinical finding. The electroretinogram and visual evoked potentials confirm the gross loss of function of visual pathways. Other radiologic findings include thickening and sclerosis of the clavicles and scapulae and absent pneumatization of the paranasal sinuses and the mastoids. Less commonly, hearing impairment or deafness may occur. Growth hormone levels are abnormally low, resulting in progressive growth retardation. Occasionally, hydrocephalus, hypertelorism, and micrognathia with a high arched palate and excessive drooling are found. Progressive mental retardation with loss of acquired milestones, sometimes associated with seizures, is another important clinical finding. Dental hypoplasia with delayed eruption of the first teeth and failure of the permanent teeth to erupt are frequent findings. The teeth themselves are of diminished quality, fall out prematurely, and show significant cavities. Macular, violet, or dark rose areas of skin atrophy, which are caused by discrete fragmentation and rarefaction of the elastic layer in the middle and deep sections of the dermis, and flattening of the fingernails may occur.

Precautions before anesthesia: Evaluate the degree of micrognathia. If drooling is excessive, consider anticholinergic premedication. Assess the severity and locations of skeletal lesions. If an epidural or spinal anesthesia is planned, consider obtaining radiographs of the spine.

Anesthetic considerations: If micrognathia is significant enough to generate any doubt about airway management, consider fiberoptic tracheal intubation while maintaining spontaneous ventilation. Apply the standard measures for management of increased intracranial pressure in the presence of hydrocephalus. The tendency for bones to fracture easily and the skin changes warrant careful positioning and padding. Regional anesthesia (e.g., epidural or spinal) may be challenging because of the dysplastic vertebrae. Mental retardation and blindness can make cooperation difficult. Careful sedative and anxiolytic sedation (beware of oversedation if difficult airway management is expected) and the presence of the primary caregiver during induction of anesthesia may be helpful.

Pharmacological implications: No known specific implications for this syndrome.

Other condition to be considered:

☞**OSTEOPETROSIS:** Heterogenous genetic disorder resulting in increased bone mass as a result of defective bone resorption. Depending on the mode of inheritance, its course can be either uniformly fatal with pancytopenia, recurrent pathologic fractures, blindness, and other neurologic symptoms or a much milder form with later manifestation and favorable prognosis.

REFERENCES:

Elcioglu NH, Vellodi A, Hall CM: Dysosteosclerosis: A report of three new cases and evolution of the radiological findings. *J Med Genet* 39:603, 2002.

Maheshwari A, Rao KM, Kohli N: Case report: Dysosteosclerosis: A unique entity. *Clin Radiol* 51:224, 1996.

Pascual-Castroviejo I, Casas-Fernandez C, Lopez-Martin V, et al: X-linked dysosteosclerosis. Four familial cases. *Eur J Pediatr* 126:127, 1977.

Dysplasia Epiphysealis Hemimelica

At a glance: Uncommon skeletal developmental disorder affecting the epiphysis in the form of aberrant cartilage growth in children.

Synonyms: Trevor Disease; Tarsomegaly; Tarsoepiphyseal Aclasis.

Incidence: Estimated to be approximately 1:1,000,000 live births. More than 120 cases have been reported in the literature since the first description in 1926. Male-to-female ratio is 3:1.

Pathophysiology: Etiology is unknown, but the pathogenesis and histology are identical to osteochondromas. In fact, this disease is considered to be a variant of osteochondroma occurring in the joint. Abnormal cartilage proliferation in the epiphysis is associated with enchondral ossification before ossification is complete. A cartilage cleavage zone can be found between the ossification centers of the lesion and the epiphysis.

Clinical aspects: Age at onset is usually between 2 and 14 years. Patients usually present with unilateral, most often painless, asymmetrical swelling on one side of a lower limb joint, most often the knee or ankle (talus, tarsonavicular, or first cuneiform joints). Other anatomical sites affected by the disease are the upper limbs, sacroiliac joint, and acetabulum. Multiples of these chondromas may be present. Deformity of the limb, differences in length, or a limp may be the initial symptoms. In suspected cases, the diagnosis is confirmed by imaging studies of the affected limb. Most often, the medial portion of the epiphysis is involved. Treatment is surgical, but recurrence is common.

Anesthetic considerations: No specific considerations for this condition.

Other condition to be considered:

☞**MAFUCCI SYNDROME:** Association of skeletal lesions (enchondromatosis) and soft tissue hemangiomas, often involving the head and neck. Major anesthetic implications.

REFERENCES:

Keret D, Spatz DK, Caro PA, et al: Dysplasia epiphysealis hemimelica: Diagnosis and treatment. *J Pediatr Orthop* 12:365, 1992.

Segal LS, Vrahas MS, Schwentker EP: Dysplasia epiphysealis hemimelica of the sacroiliac joint, a case report. *Clin Orthop* 333:202, 1996.

E

Eastman-Bixler Syndrome

At a glance: This disorder is characterized by a classic facies (malar hypoplasia, prominent antegonial notch of the mandible), horseshoe kidney, congenital heart defects, muscular hypoplasia, mental retardation, and delayed physical development.

Synonyms: Faciocardiorenal Syndrome.

Incidence: Unknown. Few scientific papers published in the medical literature since 1977.

Genetic inheritance: Autosomal recessive.

Pathophysiology: Unknown.

Diagnosis: Based on the association of mental retardation with a characteristic facies and the presence of horseshoe kidney confirmed by imaging studies.

Clinical aspects: Patients present with characteristic facial features consisting of mild plagiocephaly, relatively stiff, prominent and low-set ears, malar hypoplasia, broad nasal bridge and upturned nares, hypoplastic nasal alae, a poorly developed philtrum with a vermillion border, microstomia, cleft palate, and hypodontia. Microtia has been described. Other major manifestations are the presence of a horseshoe kidney, severe mental retardation, microsomia, and congenital heart defects such as conduction anomalies, atrial septal defects (ASDs), tricuspid valve prolapse, enlarged left ventricle, and endocardial fibroelastosis. The nipples are hypoplastic, the testes undescended, and the dermatoglyphics abnormal. The musculature is poorly developed, with a higher risk of pulmonary infection because of ineffective cough. Isolated growth hormone deficiency with good response to treatment has been reported in one patient.

Precautions before anesthesia: Check the airway anatomy for difficult airway management. If a heart defect is suspected, obtain an echocardiogram preoperatively. Also obtain baseline renal function tests (creatinine, urea). Mental retardation may limit patient compliance. Sedative and/or anxiolytic premedication and the presence of the primary caregiver during induction of anesthesia may be helpful.

Anesthetic considerations: Direct laryngoscopy and tracheal intubation may be difficult in the presence of a microstomia with restricted mouth opening. In a 2-year-old patient, the mouth was barely big enough to allow the insertion of an index finger. Spontaneous ventilation should be maintained until the airway has been secured. The electrocardiogram should be constantly monitored for evidence of abnormal cardiac conduction. Muscle hypoplasia may be associated with prolonged muscle paralysis. Prolonged postoperative mechanical ventilation may be required due to poorly developed muscles, weak cough, and frequent respiratory infections.

Pharmacological implications: Subacute bacterial endocarditis prophylaxis may be required. Maintain spontaneous respiration. Avoid neuromuscular blockers before the airway has been secured. If renal function is decreased, the dose and choice of drugs and amounts of fluids should be adjusted accordingly.

Other condition to be considered:

☞**OPITZ-FRIAS SYNDROME (G SYNDROME):** Genetic disorder characterized by craniofacial anomalies, ocular hypertelorism, cleft lip/palate, epicanthal folds, and a wide, flat nasal bridge. Affected males present cryptorchidism, bifid scrotum, and/or hypospadias. The most significant anomalies are the presence of cleft in the larynx and trachea, pulmonary hypoplasia, dysphagia, and respiratory obstruction. Hypoplasia or agenesis of the corpus callosum, kidney abnormalities, cardiac defects, and mental retardation have been reported.

REFERENCES:

Eastman JR, Bixler D: Facio-cardio-renal syndrome: A newly delineated recessive disorder. *Clin Genet* 11:424, 1977.

Nevin NC, Hill AE, Carson DJ: Facio-cardio-renal (Eastman-Bixler) syndrome. *Am J Med Genet* 40:31, 1991.

Ebstein Syndrome

At a glance: Congenital tricuspid valve anomaly (deformation and improper placement between the right atrium and right ventricle) resulting in tricuspid insufficiency, which may present in the neonatal period as a cyanotic heart disease but also may remain asymptomatic throughout life.

Synonyms: Congenital Tricuspid Dysplasia; Ebstein Anomaly; Ebstein Malformation. (Do not confuse with Epstein Syndrome.)

History: First described in 1866 by the German physician Wilhelm Ebstein.

Incidence: Accounts for approximately 0.5% of all congenital heart defects (1:20,000–50,000 live births). No sexual predilection has been reported.

Genetic inheritance: Sporadic in most cases. Lithium ingestion during pregnancy has been strongly related to Ebstein syndrome. A few familial cases with a possible autosomal recessive transmission have been reported.

Pathophysiology: The tricuspid annulus is displaced downward into the right ventricle such that part of the right ventricle becomes "atrialized" (i.e., lies above the valve). The anterior and septal valve leaflets are affected the most and may be severely dysplastic, resulting in tricuspid regurgitation. The distal ends of the valve leaflets may be fused, resulting in a variant degree of tricuspid stenosis. The anterior leaflet may obstruct the right ventricular outflow tract. Atrial septal defect (ASD) or enlarged patent foramen ovale (PFO) is present in almost all cases. Most often, the tricuspid lesion results in tricuspid insufficiency, but stenosis also is possible. Tricuspid regurgitation causes distention of the atrium and the atrialized ventricular portion, which is usually thin-walled with paradoxical movement during ventricular systole. Even distention may be seen during atrial systole. Because part of the right ventricle is atrialized, the functional right ventricle is smaller than normal, and secondary dilatation may result in thinning of the wall, predisposing to right ventricular failure. Forward flow of blood is also affected by the fact that, during atrial contraction, part of the blood from the right atrium is pumped into the atrialized portion of the right ventricle causing its dilatation, whereas during ventricular contraction the blood in the atrialized part is pushed back into the (dilated) atrium. Right-to-left shunting occurs across the ASD or PFO, leading to a variable degree of cyanosis. Cyanosis is thus a common feature of this anomaly occurring in more than 50% of patients.

Diagnosis: Based on the clinical findings of cyanosis associated with signs of tricuspid regurgitation. The chest radiograph shows cardiomegaly with diminished pulmonary markings. A history of paroxysmal supraventricular tachycardia is possible. The final diagnosis is confirmed by echocardiography or magnetic resonance imaging.

Clinical aspects: Neonates may often present with cyanosis, heart failure, tricuspid regurgitation (with cannon v waves and pulsatile liver), and right ventricular failure. These symptoms may improve once the initially high pulmonary vascular resistance (PVR) decreases. Not uncommonly, cyanosis recurs or exacerbates later in childhood secondary to right heart failure with dilatation of the right heart. The clinical findings may include episodic cyanosis, decreased exercise tolerance, and dysrhythmias in combination with signs of tricuspid regurgitation. Electrocardiographic findings include right bundle branch block, Wolff-Parkinson-White syndrome–like pattern (up to 20% of patients may have an accessory pathway), and supraventricular tachycardia secondary to atrial distention. Tachydysrhythmias worsen cardiac function and result in decreased cardiac output and increased right atrial pressure and right-to-left shunting with marked cyanosis.

Precautions before anesthesia: Obtain an electrocardiogram in presence of a history of dysrhythmias. Effectiveness of the current treatment must be assessed. A preoperative echocardiogram should be obtained to define right and left ventricular function, degree of tricuspid regurgitation and/or stenosis, and extent of right-to-left shunting. Also assess cardiac function clinically. Check preoperative saturation or better consider obtaining arterial blood gas analysis.

Anesthetic considerations: The goals during anesthesia are to avoid tachyarrhythmias (decrease the time for ventricular filling), maintain (or re-establish) appropriate filling pressures and myocardial contractility, minimize PVR (avoid acidosis, hypercapnia, and hypoxemia) in order to reduce regurgitation and support forward flow, and reduce right-to-left shunting. Appropriate premedication assists in controlling preoperative heart rate increases; however, deep sedation may result in increased PVR and should be avoided. Careful placement of central venous catheters is required to avoid triggering tachydysrhythmias. Treat intraoperative supraventricular tachycardias aggressively (e.g., adenosine, cardioversion) because they may start a vicious circle. Massive atrial enlargement has been reported and may prolong the onset of action of intravenous drugs. Paradoxical emboli may occur because of right-to-left shunting, so special attention should be paid to prevent air bubbles or clots from entering the circulation.

Pharmacological implications: Continue antidysrhythmic medication perioperatively. Minimize use of anesthetic agents with myocardial depressant effects. Avoid drugs that may induce tachycardia and trigger tachydysrhythmia (e.g., atropine).

REFERENCES:

Frescura C, Angelini A, Daliento L, et al: Morphological aspects of Ebstein's anomaly in adults. *Thorac Cardiovasc Surg* 48:203, 2000.

Huang CJ, Chiu IS, Lin FY, et al: Role of electrophysiological studies and arrhythmia intervention in repairing Ebstein's anomaly. *Thorac Cardiovasc Surg* 48:347, 2000.

Knott-Craig CJ, Overholt ED, Ward KE, et al: Repair of Ebstein's anomaly in the symptomatic neonate: An evolution of technique with 7-year follow-up. *Ann Thorac Surg* 73:1786, 2002.

Ectodermal Dysplasia

Ectodermal dysplasia is a rare group of inherited disorders. It was first described by Charles Darwin in 1875. The disorders arise from disturbances in one or more ectodermal structures and their accessory appendages. The absence, or deficient function, of at least two derivatives of the ectoderm constitutes a form of ectodermal dysplasia. Each combination of defects represents another type of ectodermal dysplasia and has a specific name. At least 150 different forms of ectodermal dysplasia have been identified; some of the most common are presented here.

Individuals affected with ectodermal dysplasia have at least two of the following manifestations:

- Absent or malfunctioning sweat glands. Temperature regulation can be dysfunctional and lead to hyperthermia.
- Dental anomalies, including missing or underdeveloped teeth.
- Varying degrees of alopecia resulting from defective hair follicles.
- Malformed or missing fingers or toes.
- Malformed fingernails and toenails.
- Cleft lip/palate, deficient saliva, hearing and visual defects, and inadequate eye fluids and tears.
- Neurologic and respiratory abnormalities may be present.

CLOUSTON SYNDROME

At a glance: Autosomal dominant ectodermal dysplasia characterized by the triad of palmoplantar hyperkeratosis, nail dystrophy, and alopecia. Facial appearance, teeth, and sweating are normal.

Synonyms: Fischer-Jacobsen-Clouston Syndrome; Hidrotic Ectodermal Dysplasia.

Incidence: Unknown. A higher incidence has been reported in the French Canadian population, but it occurs in all ethnicities.

Genetic inheritance: Autosomal dominant. The defect has been linked to 13q11-q12.1.

Pathophysiology: Abnormality in the molecular structure of keratin seems to be responsible for the disease.

Diagnosis: Based on the typical clinical features and family history.

Clinical aspects: In contrast to the X-linked form of ectodermal dysplasia (anhidrotic ectodermal dysplasia), most of the affected patients have normal sweat and sebaceous glands, and the teeth are usually only mildly affected (in contrast to the first description by Clouston). However, as in other forms of ectodermal dysplasia, the patients suffer from severe dystrophy of nails (thickened, striated, very slow growing, often discolored) and hair (resulting in total alopecia, sometimes in infancy but usually after puberty). Ultrastructural analysis of the hair shows an altered organization of hair fibrils with loss of the cuticular cortex suggesting a biochemical defect in the keratin of the integumentary system. Skin changes include palmoplantar hyperkeratosis, which can involve the periungual area and result in thickening of the fingertips with the aspect of clubbing. Skin hyperpigmentation is common over the joints.

Precautions before anesthesia: Although no specific reports for this disease exist, because of mild depression of the immune system and hypoplasia/absence of the respiratory mucus glands, other forms of ectodermal dysplasia are often associated with a predisposition to respiratory tract infections, which can be life-threatening. Although no such reports exist specifically for this syndrome, it should be kept in mind when assessing the patient.

Anesthetic considerations: Altered heat regulation does not seem to be a problem in these patients because sweat glands are functional. Direct laryngoscopy and tracheal intubation may be difficult because of maxillary and/or mandibular abnormalities. Because of

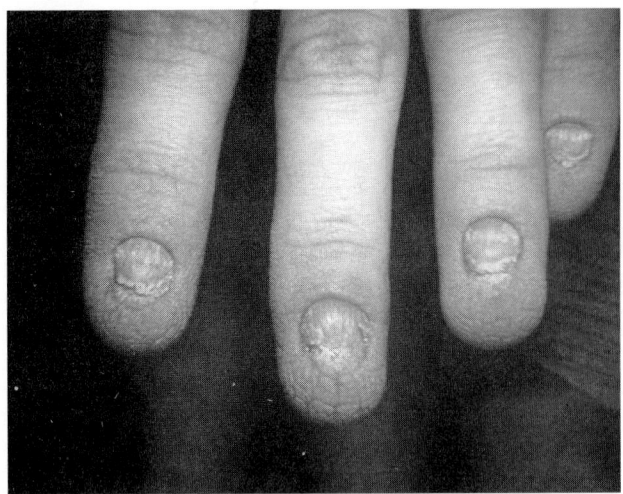

Ectodermal Dysplasia Nail dystrophy and hyperkeratotic skin changes in a patient with Clouston syndrome.

hypoplasia/absence of mucous glands in the respiratory tract, humidified air should be used for general anesthesia and in the postanesthesia care unit.

Pharmacological implications: No adverse drug reactions specific for this disease have been reported.

Other conditions to be considered:

☞**INCONTINENTIA PIGMENTI:** X-linked, dominant genodermatosis with skin pigmentation changes that are often associated with ocular, dental, and central nervous abnormalities and with malignancies (Wilms tumor, retinoblastoma, myeloid leukemia, rhabdomyosarcoma).

☞**EEC SYNDROME (Ectrodactyly-Ectodermal Dysplasia-Cleft Lip/Palate Syndrome):** Autosomal dominant inherited anomaly complex characterized by ectrodactyly of hands and feet, ectodermal dysplasia, and cleft lip/palate.

☞**GORLIN-GOLTZ SYNDROME:** Autosomal dominant transmitted neurocutaneous syndrome characterized by facial, skin, and skeletal abnormalities and later (usually after puberty) occurrence of multiple basal cell carcinomas.

☞**SETLEIS SYNDROME:** Characterized by an aged leonine face with absent or multiple rows of eyelashes, redundant facial soft tissue, and rubbery feel to facial skin. Characteristic bitemporal skin marks and association with imperforate anus.

☞**CHANDS:** Autosomal recessive inherited form of ectodermal dysplasia associated with ankyloblepharon.

☞**CHRIST-SIEMENS-TOURAINE SYNDROME:** Heterogeneous genetic disorder caused by abnormal development of the ectodermal tissue and characterized by the association of hypohidrosis, hypotrichosis, defective dentition, peculiar facies, abnormal thermoregulation, and exocrine gland insufficiency.

☞**OCULODENTODIGITAL SYNDROME:** Ectodermal dysplasia with autosomal dominant inheritance characterized by mental retardation, microcephaly, microphthalmia, glaucoma, enamel hypoplasia, syndactyly and camptodactyly, and hypotrichosis.

PACHYONYCHIA CONGENITA (Jadassohn-Lewandowsky Syndrome; Jackson-Lawler Type of Pachyonychia Congenita; Schaffer-Brunauer Syndrome (with steatocystoma multiplex); Nonepidermolytic Palmoplantar Keratoderma): Onychogryposis, hyperkeratosis of the palms, soles, knees, and elbows. Tiny cutaneous horns in many areas and leukoplakia of the oral mucosa.

☞**CRANIODIAPHYSEAL DYSPLASIA:** Bone disorder characterized by marked hyperostosis of the craniofacial bones and diaphyseal expansion of the tubular bones resulting in significant clinical complications.

☞**SCHOPF-SCHULTZ-PASSARGE SYNDROME:** Autosomal recessive inherited keratosis palmoplantaris with cystic eyelids, hypodontia, and hypotrichosis. Increased frequency of tumors of exocrine glands.

☞**CARNEVALE HERNANDEZ CASTILLO SYNDROME:** Extremely rare syndrome characterized by triphalangeal thumbs, brachy (syn)dactyly, and occasionally ectrodactyly of the feet and hands.

☞**TRICHODENTO-OSSEOUS SYNDROME:** Autosomal dominant inherited disorder featuring enamel hypoplasia and hypocalcification, combined with curly, dry hair.

AMELOGENESIS IMPERFECTA, HYPOMATURATION-HYPOPLASIA-TYPE WITH TAURODONTISM SYNDROME: Clinically very similar to the trichodento-osseous syndrome. The dental changes are identical to those found in trichodento-osseous syndrome but without hair changes and osteosclerosis; however, it is reported to be genetically different.

☞**XERODERMA, TALIPES, AND ENAMEL DEFECT SYNDROME:** Extremely rare, autosomal dominant inherited form of ectodermal dysplasia is characterized by xeroderma, talipes, and tooth enamel defects. Further signs include growth and mild mental retardation, congenital mitral stenosis, cleft palate, absent eyelashes of the lower lid, short-lasting skin vesicles, reduced number of sweat glands associated with hypohidrosis. and increased photosensitivity.

ONYCHOTRICHODYSPLASIA WITH NEUTROPENIA: Clinical signs of this extremely rare disorder, which is caused by an autosomal recessive mutation, include onychotrichodysplasia, chronic neutropenia, and mild mental retardation. However, patients with normal intelligence have been reported. Trichorrhexis nodosa with bamboo-like appearance of the hair results in brittle hair. Chronic neutropenia may be part of the so-called lazy leukocyte syndrome. No case reports related to anesthesia have been found, but strict asepsis seems mandatory in the perioperative care to prevent infections.

☞**ODONTOTRICHOMELIC SYNDROME:** Autosomal recessive inherited, extremely rare syndrome presents most often with severe absence deformities of all four extremities, abnormal teeth, hypoplastic nipples, malformation of the ears, absent or decreased eyelashes and eyebrows, and hypotrichosis. Other less frequent signs include nail anomalies, hypogonadism, thyroid enlargement and dysfunction, cleft lip, ECG and EEG abnormalities, and growth and mental retardation. Increased concentrations of tyrosine and/or tryptophane in the urine were reported.

☞**TOOTH AND NAIL SYNDROME:** Rare autosomal dominant ectodermal dysplasia characterized by defects of the nail plates of the fingers (onychorrhexis) and toes (koilonychia). Familial hypodontia with normal hair and sweat gland function.

NAEGELI ECTODERMAL DYSPLASIA (Naegeli Franceschetti Jadassohn Syndrome): Autosomal dominant inherited disease, which is limited to the ectoderm (hypohidrosis, palmoplantar keratoderma, lack of dermatoglyphics [fingerprint lines], characteristic reticular hyperpigmentation on neck, chest, and abdomen, onychodystrophy and yellowish spots on their enamel). Other organ systems have not been reported to be affected; mental retardation particularly is not a feature of this disease.

☞**TRICHORHINOPHALANGEAL SYNDROME:** Most often autosomal dominant inherited syndrome with mental retardation, microencephaly, multiple exostoses, musculoskeletal dysplasia, and redundant skin.

☞**MONILETHRIX:** Although the symptoms of these syndromes may resemble ectodermal dysplasia, it is suggested that monilethrix does not belong to this group. It is an autosomal dominant disorder characterized by a beaded appearance (because of periodic narrowing of the shaft) of the scalp hair as a result of periodic thinning of the shaft. The cause of this disease seems to be a mutation in the genes responsible for the hair keratin, which has been mapped to 12q13. Phenotypically, this results in breakage of the hair (brittle, dry, lusterless look) and patchy alopecia. Onset usually is in infancy, and symptoms may ameliorate to a certain degree after puberty and during pregnancy.

REFERENCES:

Clouston HR: A hereditary ectodermal dystrophy. *Can Med Assoc J* 21:18, 1929.

Lamartine J, Essenfelder GM, Kibar Z, et al: Mutations in GJB6 cause hidrotic ectodermal dysplasia. *Nat Genet* 26:142, 2000.

Radhakrishna U, Blouin JL, Mehenni H, et al: The gene for autosomal dominant hidrotic ectodermal dysplasia (Clouston syndrome) in a large Indian family maps to the 13q11-q12.1 pericentromeric region. *Am J Med Genet* 71:80, 1997.

Ectodermal Dysplasia, Ectrodactyly, and Macular Dystrophy (EEM) Syndrome

At a glance: EEM is an acronym that stands for *e*ctodermal dysplasia; *e*ctrodactyly, and *m*acular dystrophy syndrome. This genetic disorder affects ectoderm derivatives, upper and lower extremities, and retina.

Synonyms: EEM-Albrectsen Syndrome.

Incidence: Unknown, but approximately 13 cases have been described.

Genetic inheritance: Autosomal recessive with parental consanguinity as a risk factor. Variable expression or genetic heterogeneity has been suspected.

Pathophysiology: Remains to be determined.

Diagnosis: Based on family history, specific clinical features, radiologic studies, and ophthalmologic examination.

Clinical aspects: Ectodermal dysplasia may present with sparse and thin scalp hair, eyebrows and eyelashes, partial anodontia, and small, widely spaced teeth. Ectrodactyly of the upper and lower extremities can be associated with syndactyly and/or clefting of hand and feet. Hypoplastic distal phalanx of the index finger with onychodysplasia has been described. Ocular fundus examination reveals presumably progressive macular dystrophy and optic nerve changes. Sweating seems to be unaffected. Mild developmental delay may occur.

Precautions before anesthesia: No specific precautions are required.

Anesthetic considerations: Peripheral intravenous access can be challenging because of deformities of hands and feet. For the same reasons, careful positioning and padding are required. If indicated for postoperative pain management, use of a PCA device can be facilitated by replacing the PCA button by a wide pad.

Pharmacological implications: No specific considerations should arise from this syndrome.

Other condition to be considered:

☞**KUSTER MAJEWSKI HAMMERSTEIN SYNDROME:** Extremely rare condition combining growth retardation, repeated

hair loss, and ring-shaped degeneration of the retinal pigmentary epithelium.

REFERENCES:

Hayakawa M, Yanashima K, Kato K, et al: Association of ectodermal dysplasia, ectrodactyly and macular dystrophy: EEM syndrome (case report). *Ophthalmic Paediatr Genet* 10:287, 1989.

Ohdo S, Hirayama K, Terawaki T: Association of ectodermal dysplasia, ectrodactyly, and macular dystrophy: The EEM syndrome. *J Med Genet* 20:52, 1983.

Senecky Y, Halpern GJ, Inbar D, et al: Ectodermal dysplasia, ectrodactyly and macular dystrophy (EEM syndrome) in siblings. *Am J Med Genet* 101:195, 2001.

Ectrodactyly

At a glance: Congenital limb malformation involving the central rays of the hands or feet. Ectrodactyly (derived from Greek *ektroma* [abortion] and *daktylos* [finger]) refers to a situation where at least one entire digit (both metacarpal/metatarsal and phalanges) is missing. It is a nonspecific term applied to a variety of malformations.

Synonym: Absent Finger Syndrome.

Incidence: 1:90,000 live births (typical split hand); 1:150,000 live births (atypical split hand).

Genetic inheritance: Atypical forms are usually sporadic. Typical cases (absence of central rays or deficiency of radial rays with no cleft) are usually inherited as an autosomal dominant trait with complete penetrance and variable expression. Autosomal recessive forms have been reported. Five loci for split-hand/foot malformation have been mapped (7q21, Xq26, 10q24, 3q27, and 2q31).

Pathophysiology: Unknown.

Diagnosis and clinical aspects: This "split-hand/foot" malformation with absence of multiple fingers varies from monodactyly to syndactyly. Multiple metacarpal anomalies, radioulnar synostosis, and tarsal/toe hypoplasia are associated. Other syndromes may coexist with ectrodactyly, such as the ☞Ectrodactyly, Ectodermal Dysplasia, and Clefting (EEC) Syndrome.

Precautions before anesthesia: If ectrodactyly is associated with EEC syndrome, renal function should be assessed (serum concentrations of electrolytes, creatinine, urea). Check for signs of central diabetes insipidus and, if present, evaluate the response to vasopressin treatment. Optimize intravenous hydration prior to surgery.

Anesthetic considerations: Placement of intravenous and arterial lines and pulse oximeter on the extremities may be challenging. Pay particular attention to positioning and padding. Because of the hand deformities, triggering the button of a patient-controlled analgesia (PCA) device by the patient could be difficult. However, this is not a big problem for most patients because they encounter similar difficulties on a regular basis.

Pharmacological implications: No special considerations for isolated ectrodactyly are required.

Other conditions to be considered: Because ectrodactyly is a descriptive term, it may be part of several syndromes.

ANONYCHIA-ECTRODACTYLY: Absent fingers or oligodactyly, absent nails and phalanges, osseous and cutaneous syndactyly of fingers.

☞**ECTRODACTYLY-ECTODERMAL DYSPLASIA-CLEFTING SYNDROME:** Autosomal dominant inherited syndrome with maxillary hypoplasia, mild malar hypoplasia, cleft lip/palate, choanal atresia, hearing loss, photophobia and blepharophimosis, dacryocystitis, cryptorchidism, hypogonadotropic hypogonadism renal agenesis or dysplasia, hydronephrosis, occasionally mental retardation, central diabetes insipidus.

RÜDIGER SYNDROME: Extremely rare disorder with prominent forehead, flat nasal bridge, stubby nose, and protuberant upper lip. Low-pitched and hoarse voice, short digits, and palmar flexion contractures. Patients may present for inguinal hernia repair.

SAAL BULAS SYNDROME: Extremely rare syndrome characterized by diaphragmatic hernia, agenesis of the corpus callosum, and ectrodactyly. Other features include ventricular septal defect and frequent respiratory distress.

VAN DEN ENDE BRUNNER SYNDROME: Extremely rare disorder presenting with microcephaly, microphthalmia, ectrodactyly of the lower limbs, premature aging of the skin, and prognathism. Other findings may include cardiomyopathy, ventricular septal defect, and dysmorphism.

☞**CLEFT HAND AND ABSENT TIBIA SYNDROME:** Syndrome characterized by cleft hand and tibial aplasia with ectrodactyly.

REFERENCE:

Sifakis S, Bael D, Ianakiev P, et al: Distal limb malformations: Underlying mechanisms and clinical associations. *Clin Genet* 60:165, 2001.

Ectrodactyly, Ectodermal Dysplasia, and Clefting (EEC) Syndrome

At a glance: Autosomal dominant inherited syndrome with maxillary hypoplasia, mild malar hypoplasia, cleft lip/palate, choanal atresia, hearing loss, photophobia and blepharophimosis, dacryocystitis, cryptorchidism, hypogonadotropic hypogonadism renal agenesis or dysplasia, hydronephrosis, occasionally mental retardation, central diabetes insipidus.

Synonyms: EEC Syndrome; Cleft Lip/Cleft Palate–Lobster-Claw Deformity Syndrome; Ectrodactyly-Cleft Lip/Palate Syndrome; Ectrodactyly-Ectodermal Dysplasia-Cleft Lip/Palate Syndrome; Ectrodactyly-Ectodermal Dysplasia-Cleft Lip/Palate Syndrome; Split Hand-Cleft Lip/Palate and Ectodermal (SCE) Dysplasia; Walker-Clodius Syndrome.

Incidence: More than 250 cases have been published in the medical literature.

Genetic inheritance: Autosomal dominant inheritance with variable phenotypic expression. The gene locus has been mapped to 7p11.2-q21.3 (EEC1). The chromosome 19-linked variety is referred to as EEC2. EEC3 has been mapped to 3q27, which is also the location for the limb-mammary and the ☞ADULT Syndrome. A number of sporadic cases have been described.

Diagnosis: Cardinal features are ectrodactyly of hands and feet, ectodermal dysplasia with severe keratitis, and cleft lip/palate. There are variable manifestations, and no sign is obligatory for the diagnosis.

Clinical aspects: Facial features included cleft lip with or without cleft palate (72% of patients), maxillary hypoplasia, mild malar hypoplasia, partial anodontia, microdontia, and choanal atresia. Mental retardation (7%), growth hormone deficiency, hypopituitarism, and central diabetes insipidus (rare) are additional features. Genitourinary malformations (50% of patients) include renal dysplasia and agenesis. Conductive hearing loss is present in approximately 14% of patients. Lacrimal duct anomalies result in repeated infections of the eyes. Ectodermal dysplasia consists of complete/partial adon-

tia, microdontia, oligodontia, enamel hypoplasia, dental caries, and slow-growing, dysplastic nails. Feeding difficulties in the presence of the cleft predispose to pulmonary aspiration and subsequent chest infections. Malnutrition and anemia are major problems resulting from poor oral intake and loss of proteins from skin ulcers. Hypohidrosis secondary to hypoplastic sweat glands may result in abnormal body temperature regulation. Abnormal bleeding tendency has been reported.

Precautions before anesthesia: Perform a thorough examination to exclude active infections commonly involving the chest, urinary system, or eyes. Chest physiotherapy may be required to help clear retained copious secretions (recurrent aspirations). Assess airway for difficult intubation that may be related to clefting. Because an abnormal bleeding tendency may occur, the patient's blood should be crossed and typed, and blood should be readily available for transfusion. Chest radiograph, complete blood count with white cell differentiation, coagulation screen, and urinalysis should be obtained prior to anesthesia. Cooperation may be limited in patients with mental retardation and hearing impairment (approximately 10% of patients). Sedative and/or anxiolytic premedication and/or the presence of the primary caregiver during induction of anesthesia may be helpful.

Anesthetic considerations: Difficult laryngoscopy and tracheal intubation may be associated with cleft lip/palate and maxillary hypoplasia. Avoid trauma to the cleft with the laryngoscope blade. Tracheal intubation and controlled ventilation with humidification are essential to cope with the often thick and copious secretions. Wide fluctuations of body temperature secondary to impaired thermoregulation may require close monitoring and facilities to maintain normothermia. The fragile skin condition secondary to malnutrition requires extreme care to prevent further perioperative damage (careful while removing electrocardiogram electrodes!). Intraoperative eye protection is mandatory in the presence of blepharitis, conjunctivitis, and keratitis to prevent further ocular injuries.

Pharmacological implications: Avoid atropine to prevent exacerbation of hypohidrosis and heat retention. Avoid deep sedative premedication if the airway is compromised.

Other conditions to be considered:

ECTRODACTYLY-MANDIBULO-FACIAL DYSOSTOSIS SYNDROME: Extremely rare disorder with monomelic to tetramelic ectrodactyly, cleft uvula, and mandibulofacial dysostosis. The phenotype overlaps in part with the EEC syndrome.

PATTERSON-STEVENSON-FONTAINE SYNDROME: Extremely rare syndrome characterized by malar hypoplasia and microretrognathia and complete or occult posterior cleft palate and bifid uvula.

RÜDIGER SYNDROME: Extremely rare disorder with prominent forehead, flat nasal bridge, stubby nose, and protuberant upper lip. Low-pitched and hoarse voice, short digits, and palmar flexion contractures. Patients may present for inguinal hernia repair.

SAAL BULAS SYNDROME: Extremely rare disorder characterized by diaphragmatic hernia, agenesis of the corpus callosum, and ectrodactyly. Other features include ventricular septal defect and frequent respiratory distress.

VAN DEN ENDE BRUNNER SYNDROME: Extremely rare disorder presenting with microcephaly, microphthalmia, ectrodactyly of the lower limbs, premature aging of the skin, and prognathism. Other findings may include cardiomyopathy, ventricular septal defect, and dysmorphism.

☞**ADULT SYNDROME:** Main findings are hypodontia, very brittle and/or premature loss of permanent teeth, and ectrodactyly (split hands and feet). There is no evident impairment of general health in patients with ADULT syndrome.

☞**ANKYLOBLEPHARON FILIFORME ADNATUM AND CLEFT PALATE:** Form of ectodermal dysplasia associated with cleft lip/palate. It is most often associated with congenital filiform fusion of the eyelids.

LIMB MAMMARY SYNDROME: Very rare syndrome characterized by severe anomalies of the hands and feet in combination with hypoplasia or aplasia of the mammary gland and nipple. As in ADULT syndrome, the lacrimal duct can be atretic or obstructed and the nails thickened and dystrophic. Hypodontia and cleft palate have been described. A newer study placed the ADULT syndrome gene locus in the same chromosome region as the LMS locus, thereby suggesting these two conditions are allelic.

☞**CLEFT HAND AND ABSENT TIBIA SYNDROME:** Syndrome characterized by cleft hand and tibial aplasia with ectrodactyly.

REFERENCES:

Maas SM, de Jong TP, Buss P, Hennekam RC: EEC syndrome and genitourinary anomalies: An update. *Am J Med Genet* 63:472, 1996.

Mizushima A, Satoyoshi M: Anaesthetic problems in a child with ectrodactyly, ectodermal dysplasia and cleft lip/palate. *Anaesthesia* 47:137, 1992.

Roelfsema NM, Cobben JM: The EEC syndrome: A literature study. *Clin Dysmorphol* 5:115, 1996.

Ehlers-Danlos Syndrome (EDS): An Overview

See table, p. 262.

Ehlers-Danlos Syndrome (EDS)

At a glance: Heterogeneous group (six major types) of inherited connective tissue disorders characterized by joint hyperlaxity, skin hyperextensibility, and tissue fragility.

Synonyms: Ehlers-Danlos Disease; Chernogubov Syndrome; Cutis Elastica; Danlos Syndrome; Meekeren-Ehlers-Danlos Syndrome; Van Meekeren Syndrome I; Sack Syndrome; Sack-Barabas Syndrome; Indian Rubber Man.

History: First described by the Dutch surgeon J.J. van Meekeren in 1668, when he described a young Spanish sailor man who was able to pull the skin of his chin up to the eyes and down to the chest. In 1892, the Russian dermatologist Nikolai A. Chernogubov described this syndrome in a 17-year-old boy, but this description went unnoticed in Western medicine. In 1899, Edvard L. Ehlers, a Danish dermatologist, presented a patient with this disorder at a meeting in Paris, France, before his findings were published in 1901. Seven years later, Henri A. Danlos, a French dermatologist, published his view of the syndrome. The Italian composer Niccolo Paganini (1782–1840) was one of the famous persons suffering from this disorder.

Incidence: Incidence of EDS ranges from 1: 150,000–300,000 and the prevalence ranges from 1:5000–10,000. The disorder affects males and females of all racial and ethnic backgrounds. EDS types I and III account for 90% of all cases (each approximately 30%).

Genetic inheritance: The classic, hypermobility, vascular, and arthrochalasis types are autosomal dominant inherited, whereas the kyphoscoliosis and dermatosparaxis types are autosomal recessive transmitted. In a few cases, X-linked inheritance has been described.

Pathophysiology: Depends on the type of EDS. Generally, collagen synthesis is abnormal, resulting in reduced strength of the collagen in numerous tissues.

Diagnosis: Prenatal diagnosis is possible by detection of abnormally low lysyl hydroxylase enzyme activity in cultured amniotic fluid cells. The soft, hyperextensible, velvety skin (so-called marshmallow skin), joint hypermobility, scoliosis, and ocular fragility (severe myopia), all features of ☞Marfan Syndrome, are also features of EDS. Instability is a result of the marked joint laxity and leads to delayed motor development in affected children.

Clinical aspects: The clinical picture is highly variable and depends on the type of EDS. The skin is generally hyperelastic and hyperextensible (difficult to assess in neonates and infants) but most often is thin and highly vulnerable with a tendency to hematomas associated with already minor trauma. Patients often have impaired wound healing with inappropriate (either hypertrophic or atrophic) scarring, particularly affecting the most exposed body areas (knee, shin bone). The occurrence of knuckle pads on hands and feet, molluscoid pseudotumors from scars on elbows and knees, subcutaneous calcifications, spheroids (small, mobile, hard nodules on forearms and lower legs), and acrogeria are common findings. Easy bruising is noticed in infancy, commonly occurring in exposed body areas and often presenting as spontaneous ecchymoses that later change into areas of brownish discoloration. This is explained by increased tissue fragility. The laxity of the ligaments not only leads to hyperextensibility of the joints, which is most pronounced in (but not limited to) shoulder, elbow, ankle, and temporomandibular joint and may result in recurrent (sub)luxations, but also to skeletal anomalies (e.g., kyphoscoliosis, clubfoot). The Beighton Score is used to assess the degree of joint hyperextensibility and the criteria include (1) passive dorsiflexion of the little fingers beyond 90 degrees, (2) passive apposition of the thumb to flexor aspect of the forearm, (3) hyperextension of the elbow beyond 10 degrees, (4) hyperextension of the knees beyond 10 degrees (genua recurvatum), and (5) forward flexion of the trunk with the knees fully extended so that the palms of the hand rest flat on the floor. Chronic joint and musculoskeletal pain is a common problem in EDS patients. Cardiovascular anomalies include multiple aneurysms (rarely of the aorta) and rupture and dissection of arteries, varicosis, mitral valve prolapse (common), orthostatic hypotension, and acrocyanosis. Although dilatation of the aortic root is rare, it should be kept in mind and checked on a regular basis (echocardiography) because sudden cardiac death secondary to aortic rupture has been described. Facial appearance is often (but not always) typical in vascular type of EDS, presenting with a slender face, sunken cheeks, thin or pinched nose, thin (upper) lips, prominent eyes with periorbital pigmentation, and firm, lobeless ears. Vascular type of EDS is the most severe form, with arterial rupture occurring in 25% of these patients before age 20 years and in 80% before age 40 years. This complication is the most common cause of death in these patients, whose average life expectancy is 48 years. Arterial rupture may present with acute abdominal or flank pain, which should prompt urgent investigations in these patients. Because of the increased tissue fragility, which also involves the arteries, the repair is often very difficult or even impossible. Ophthalmologic features may include strabismus, ptosis, keratoconus, blue sclerae, glaucoma, photophobia, (sub)luxation of the lens, rupture of the globe, and blindness from recurrent retinal hemorrhages. Gastroesophageal, inguinal, and umbilical hernias, anal prolapse, and spontaneous ruptures of intestinal organs have been reported.

Table E-1

EDS Type	Former Type	Inheritance	Major Criteria	Minor Criteria	Pathogenesis
Classic	Gravis type (EDS type I) Mitis type (EDS type II)	Autosomal dominant	Skin hyperextensibility Wide, atrophic scars Joint hypermobility	Smooth, velvety skin Subcutaneous spheroids Molluscoid pseudotumors Easy bruising Manifestations/complications of joint hypermobility (dislocations/subluxations), tissue hyperextensibility, and fragility (hiatal hernia, anal prolapse) Surgical complications (postoperative hernias) Muscle hypotonia with delayed motor development Positive family history	Abnormal electrophoretic mobility of the proα1(V) or proα2(V) chains of collagen type V Mutations on COL5A1 and COL5A2 Abnormal electron microscopic findings in the collagen fibril structure ("cauliflower" deformity of collagen fibrils)
Hypermobility	Hypermobile type (EDS type III)	Autosomal dominant	Hyperextensible, smooth, velvety skin Generalized joint hypermobility	Recurring joint dislocations Chronic joint/limb pain Positive family history	Unknown In some cases anomalies of collagen V have been described
Vascular	Arterial-ecchymotic type (EDS type IV)	Autosomal dominant	Thin, translucent skin Arterial/intestinal (colon)/uterine fragility or rupture Extensive bruising Typical facial appearance	Acrogeria Hypermobility of small joints Tendon and muscle rupture Talipes equinovarus Early-onset varicosis Arteriovenous, carotid-cavernous sinus fistulas Pneumo(hemato)thorax Gingival recession Positive family history Sudden death in close relative(s)	Structural anomalies in the proα1(III) chain of collagen type III encoded by the COL3A1 gene
Kyphoscoliosis	Ocular-scoliotic type (EDS type VI)	Autosomal recessive	Generalized joint laxity Severe muscle hypotonia and progressive scoliosis at birth Scleral fragility and rupture of the ocular globe after minor trauma	Tissue fragility, including atrophic scars Easy bruising Arterial rupture Marfanoid habitus Microcornea Radiologically osteopenia Positive family history	Lysyl hydroxylase deficiency
Arthrochalasia	Arthrochalasis multiplex congenital type (EDS types VIIA and VIIB)	Autosomal dominant	Severe joint hypermobility with recurrent subluxations Congenital bilateral hip dislocation	Skin hyperextensibility Tissue fragility and atrophic scars Easy bruising Muscle hypotonia Kyphoscoliosis Mild osteopenia	Mutations of COL1A1 or COL1A2 result in defects of proα1(I) (type A) or proα2(I) (type B) chains of collagen
Dermatosparaxis	Human dermatosparaxis type (EDS type VIIC)	Autosomal recessive	Severe skin fragility Sagging, redundant skin	Soft, doughy skin texture Easy bruising Premature rupture of fetal membranes Large hernias (umbilical, inguinal)	Procollagen I N-terminal peptidase deficiency

Ehlers-Danlos Syndrome   Cutis laxa at the knee in a patient with Ehlers-Danlos syndrome.

Precautions before anesthesia: The heterogeneous nature of EDS results in a mixed picture in many cases. Obtain a thorough history of complications with previous surgeries and ask about excessive bleeding after minor trauma. The clinical examination should also determine the degree of cardiorespiratory compromise associated with kyphoscoliosis (restrictive lung disease, cor pulmonale). Lung function tests (including arterial blood gas analysis) and echocardiography should be considered. Aortic and mitral insufficiency may be associated with the classic and vascular types and should be graded by echocardiography. Right bundle branch block and left anterior hemiblock have been described, so a preoperative electrocardiogram is recommended. Excessive bleeding is a feature of the classic and vascular types of EDS and may manifest as increased bleeding time rather than abnormal coagulation tests. The patient's blood should be cross-matched prior to surgery, and adequate amounts of blood products should be easily available. Check

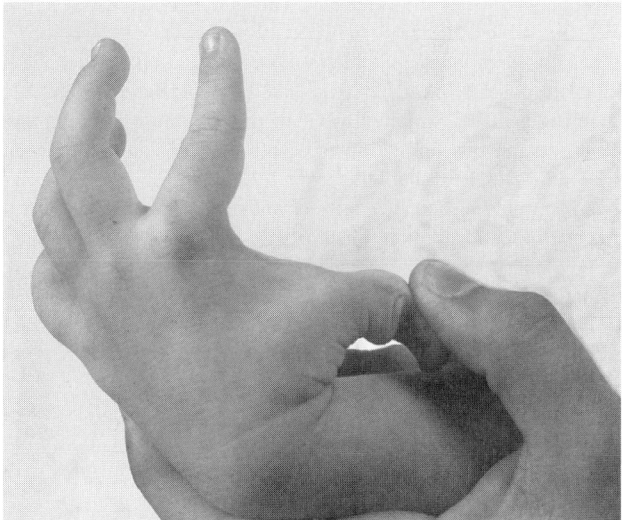

Ehlers-Danlos Syndrome   Joint hyperlaxity in patient with Ehlers-Danlos syndrome. However, this finding can be demonstrated in 10 to 15% of normal people without Ehlers-Danlos syndrome.

for difficult airway management because mandibular hypoplasia, recurrent temporomandibular joint dislocations, and gingival anomalies have been described. Atlantoaxial instability has been described as a feature of the vascular type of EDS.

Anesthetic considerations: Care with positioning of the surgical patient is needed to prevent damage to the delicate skin and to avoid joint dislocations. Venous access must be adequate to cope with potential heavy blood loss, which often results from delicate skin. Central venous access may be complicated by mediastinal or pleural hematomas. Arterial cannulation may be complicated by aneurysm formation or excessive hematoma formation. Both central venous and arterial monitoring should be used only when essential to patient management. Regional techniques have been described, but central blocks are associated with a higher risk of hematoma formation. These should be kept in mind and checked accordingly if regional anesthesia has been performed. Local anesthesia may have an insufficient effect in many patients with the hypermobility type of EDS. General anesthesia should be accomplished using minimal airway trauma. Mask anesthesia is probably the management of choice, but when appropriate, airway intubation and extubation should be accomplished as gently as possible to minimize airway bruising. Avoid temporomandibular joint dislocation or subluxation and cervical spine subluxation. Peak airway pressure must be kept as low as possible to reduce the risk of pneumothorax. Avoid wide swings in blood pressure to reduce the risk of hemorrhage and aneurysm rupture. The risk of cerebral hemorrhage from intracranial aneurysms is considered low but should be kept in mind for patients with the vascular type of EDS. The same type of EDS also has a high risk of uterine rupture in parturients, with pregnancy-related mortality of up to 25% reported (secondary to uterine, aortic, pulmonary artery, or vena cava rupture). However, severe hemorrhage may also occur in the early postpartum period. Epidural anesthesia has been used successfully in some of these patients. Large-bore intravenous access (although sometimes difficult to establish in these patients) and availability of blood products are recommended for these women. Despite normal parameters, prolonged bleeding has been described in EDS patients.

Pharmacological implications: There are no strict contraindications, but agents interfering with blood coagulation and hemostasis should be used with considerable care. Subacute bacterial endocarditis prophylaxis usually is recommended if mitral valve prolapse is associated with thickened leaflets and/or mitral regurgitation.

Other condition to be considered:

☞**Marfan Syndrome:** Familial disorder of generalized connective tissue abnormalities leading to connective tissue weakness with hyperextensible joints, eye anomalies (dislocation of the lens), increased risk of valvular/aortic disease, and spontaneous pneumothorax.

References:

Beighton P, De Paepe A, Steinmann B, et al: Ehlers-Danlos syndromes: Revised nosology, Villefranche, 1997. *Am J Med Genet* 77:31, 1998.

Germain DP: Clinical and genetic features of vascular Ehlers-Danlos syndrome. *Ann Vasc Surg* 16:391, 2002.

Halko GJ, Cobb R, Abeles M: Patients with type IV Ehlers-Danlos syndrome may be predisposed to atlantoaxial subluxation. *J Rheumatol* 22:2152, 1995

North KN, Whiteman DA, Pepin MG, et al: Cerebrovascular complications in Ehlers-Danlos syndrome type IV. *Ann Neurol* 38:960, 1995.

Eisenmenger Reaction

At a glance: Cyanotic condition in which patients with an initially intracardiac (or surgically created extracardiac) left-to-right shunt show shunt reversal (i.e., now right-to-left shunting) secondary to significantly increased pulmonary vascular resistance (PVR).

Synonym: Eisenmenger Disease.

History: The Austrian physician Viktor E. Eisenmenger was the first to describe in 1897 severe pulmonary vascular disease in a 32-year-old man with cyanosis and dyspnea since infancy secondary to an unrestricted ventricular septal defect, who died of massive pulmonary hemorrhage.

Incidence: Approximately 8% of patients with congenital heart disease and 11% of those with left-to-right intracardiac shunting develop Eisenmenger reaction.

Genetic inheritance: Eisenmenger reaction per se is not inherited; it is an acquired complication of a congenital cardiac lesion. No sexual predilection has been reported.

Pathophysiology: In congenital cardiac lesions with intracardiac shunting, blood initially shunts from the high-pressure systemic circulation to the low-pressure pulmonary circulation. If the defect is unrestricted and sustained, exposure of the pulmonary vascular bed to systemic arterial pressure initially results in increased pulmonary blood flow and pressure that over time triggers progressive adaptation processes in the microvasculature, including arteriolar intima proliferation, media hypertrophy, and finally capillary and/or arteriolar occlusion. Obliteration of pulmonary arterioles and capillaries may result from necrotizing arteritis. Decreased endothelium-dependent pulmonary arteriolar dilatation and increased pulmonary endothelin and plasma thromboxane B_2 levels (both pulmonary vasoconstrictors) have been described; all of these factors ultimately lead to increased PVR. Once systemic and pulmonary vascular resistances and pressures approach each other, a process called *shunt reversal* occurs, where the blood now shunts bidirectionally or from the right (pulmonary) side to the left (systemic) side. Reduced pulmonary blood flow and right-to-left shunting explain the arterial hypoxemia. Endothelium-dependent pulmonary arteriolar relaxation is impaired, pulmonary endothelin production is increased, and plasma thromboxane B_2 concentrations are elevated in patients with the Eisenmenger reaction, suggesting that endothelial dysfunction or platelet activation plays a causative role in this condition.

Diagnosis: Dyspnea, chest pain (right ventricular ischemia), and new cyanosis in the presence of congenital heart disease. Echocardiography or cardiac catheterization (*Caveat:* radiographic contrast material may cause systemic arterial vasodilatation) can be used to determine the degree of pulmonary hypertension and demonstrate and quantify the shunting.

Clinical aspects: The term *Eisenmenger reaction* describes cyanosis secondary to severe pulmonary hypertension in the systemic range as a result of significantly increased PVR with reversed or bidirectional shunting resulting from a connection between systemic and pulmonary circulation (such as septal defects, atrioventricular canal, patent ductus arteriosus, or aortopulmonary windows). Obtain a history of cyanotic episodes, syncopes, fatigue, dyspnea, check for finger clubbing, plethora, and polycythemia, which may be associated with hyperviscosity. Exercise tolerance is significantly reduced because of the inability to increase pulmonary blood flow. Hemoptysis is a common finding and often caused by pulmonary infarction, rupture of a pulmonary artery aneurysm, or a thin-walled pulmonary arteriole. There is an increased risk of hyperuricemia (increased production and reduced renal clearance of urate), cholelithiasis, hypertrophic osteoarthropathy, cerebral abscesses, and thromboembolic events (cerebrovascular insults). Renal function may be decreased, with evidence of glomerulopathy (hematuria, proteinuria, increased serum creatinine levels) reported in these patients. Syncope, increased right-sided filling pressures, and severe hypoxemia (i.e., systemic SpO_2 <85%) are associated with a poor prognosis. Sudden death as a result of arrhythmia and hypoxemia, but also pulmonary artery rupture, has been reported. Death as a result of Eisenmenger reaction usually occurs in the third decade of life. Patients with sleep apnea in association with congenital heart disease may demonstrate accelerated development of the disorder (e.g., patients with ☞Trisomy 21).

Precautions before anesthesia: Some studies reported a high perioperative mortality in these patients undergoing noncardiac surgery. Full clinical cardiac assessment (right parasternal heave, palpable pulmonary valve closure, right-sided fourth heart sound, and a loud pulmonic component of the second heart sound are constant findings) in combination with electrocardiography, echocardiography, chest radiograph is strongly recommended to define the degree of lesion and cardiac function. Arterial blood gas analysis may be considered. Obtain a complete blood count and consider iron replacement therapy for iron deficiency anemia. Check renal function (serum concentrations of creatinine, urea and electrolytes, and urine analysis for proteinuria and hematuria). Antiarrhythmic management for atrial arrhythmias and prophylaxis against thromboembolism should be considered. Isovolumetric hemodilution has been used to decrease the hematocrit in these patients, which not only increases cardiac output and systemic oxygen delivery but also decreases systemic vascular resistance (SVR) and improves the patient's symptoms. Avoid prolonged preoperative fasting, which may result in hypovolemia and hyperviscosity. It is recommended to start an intravenous infusion with maintenance fluid replacement at the beginning of the fasting period.

Anesthetic considerations: Consider suitability for local anesthesia because general anesthesia may cause systemic vasodilation aggravating the right-to-left shunt. Anesthesia should be administered by an experienced cardiac anesthetist, with the possibility of postoperative care in an intensive care unit setting. Avoid hypovolemia, which may lead to hypotension, hypoxemia, and sometimes hemoconcentration and thromboembolic events (volume expansion should be provided immediately). Avoid decreases in SVR in relation to PVR, which results in increased right-to-left shunting. Both spontaneous ventilation and controlled ventilation have been used; however, care should be taken to avoid hypercarbia, alveolar hypoxia, acidosis, and atelectasis. Avoid high airway pressures during controlled ventilation. There is a risk of paradoxical embolism throughout surgery, so careful deaeration of syringes and stop cocks is mandatory. Epidural analgesia (bupivacaine 0.125% with fentanyl 5 μg/ml) has been used successfully for laparotomy without adverse effects. Patients with Eisenmenger reaction can be eligible for heart and heart-lung transplantation.

Pharmacological implications: Ketamine 1 to 2 mg/kg IV reportedly has minimal effects on PVR and SVR as long as ventilation is controlled and has been used successfully in patients with Eisenmenger reaction. Both thiopental and propofol, but also inhalational anesthetics, decrease SVR and should be used with caution and in low doses only. Prophylactic use of vasopressors (methoxamine, phenylephrine) has resulted in reflex bradycardia and increased right-to-left shunt. Vasopressors are probably best used only if increased right-to-left shunting develops. Nitrous oxide is contraindicated because it may increase PVR. Avoid nonsteroidal antiinflammatory drugs in the presence of renal failure.

Other condition to be considered: Avoid confusion with **Eisenmenger Complex (Eisenmenger Syndrome):** Congenital cardiac lesion presenting with ventricular septal defect and overriding aorta, pulmonary hypertension with right-to-left shunt, and right ventricular hypertrophy. However, the terms Eisenmenger disease, Eisenmenger complex, and Eisenmenger syndrome are all used interchangeably in the literature and a consensus seems to be missing. In the editors' opinion, only the term "Eisenmenger reaction" clearly refers to the pathologic process of shunt reversal, which explains why we have chosen it as the title of this section.

REFERENCES:

Berman EB, Barst RJ: Eisenmenger's syndrome: Current management. *Prog Cardiovasc Dis* 45:129, 2002.

Lyons B, Motherway C, Casey W, et al: The anaesthetic management of the child with Eisenmenger's syndrome. *Can J Anaesth* 42:904, 1995.

O'Kelly S, Hayden-Smith J: Eisenmenger's syndrome: Surgical perspectives and anaesthetic implications. *Br J Hosp Med* 51:250, 1994.

Elejalde Syndrome

At a glance: Rare inherited disorder characterized by silvery hair, pigment abnormalities of the skin, and early-onset central nervous system dysfunction.

Synonym: Melanolysosomal Neurocutaneous Syndrome. (*Caveat:* The name Elejalde syndrome has also been used synonymously for ☞Acrocephalopolysyndactylous Dysplasia. To avoid confusion, we recommend reserving this name for the syndrome described here.)

Incidence: Approximately 11 cases have been reported.

Genetic inheritance: Autosomal recessive. Candidate genes for Elejalde syndrome have been sought in a variety of genes involved in organellogenesis and intracellular trafficking. These genes are directly or indirectly involved in pigmentation disorders throughout the expression of adaptor-like protein complex(AP)-3 factor, which is involved in the budding of coated vesicles from the Golgi system.

Pathophysiology: Abnormal melanocytes, melanosomes, and inclusion bodies in fibroblasts may be present. There are speculations that myosin V protein may be affected and probably responsible for the severe generalized hypotonia. The molecular basis of the disease remains to be elucidated.

Diagnosis: Light microscopy of the hair is characterized by the presence of small and large melanin clumps irregularly distributed along the hair shaft but predominantly in the medulla. Skin biopsy specimens may reveal a normal number of melanocytes but irregular distribution and irregular size of melanin granules in the basal layer. Electron microscopy of the skin reveals melanocytes with melanosomes of various sizes and at various developmental stages. Because of a maturation defect, melanization of the melanosomes is incomplete; however, in contrast to ☞Griscelli and ☞Chediak-Higashi Syndrome (the two other "Silvery Hair Syndromes"), both humoral and cellular immunity are normal.

Clinical aspects: Scalp hair, eyelashes, and eyebrows are silver. Sun exposure leads to pronounced and long-lasting skin tanning. The age at onset of neurologic signs can range from 1 month to 11 years and include severe muscular hypotonia, ataxia, seizures, hyperreflexia or hyporeflexia, spastic or flaccid hemiplegia or quadriplegia, and ocular features (e.g., congenital amaurosis, nystagmus, diplopia, pupillary areflexia). Mental retardation with delayed psychomotor development usually is obvious in the first month of life. Magnetic resonance imaging can demonstrate cerebellar hypoplasia/atrophy.

Precautions before anesthesia: No data regarding anesthetic management or pharmacological implications in this disorder have been published. Seizure control, assessment of muscular hypotonia, and the potential presence of recurrent pulmonary aspirations are the main focus points in the preoperative evaluation. A chest radiograph might be indicated. Failure to thrive may be present secondary to poor feeding and results in electrolyte and fluid imbalances. Blood work should include serum levels of electrolytes. Depending on the type and extent of surgery, prolonged postoperative mechanical ventilation may be required. Mental retardation may limit patient cooperation. Sedative premedication and/or the presence of the primary caregiver during induction of anesthesia may be helpful.

Anesthetic considerations: Recurrent aspiration is a described complication in this syndrome. A rapid-sequence induction technique is recommended. Severe hypotonia may require reduced amounts or no neuromuscular blocking agents. Positioning may be difficult in the presence of spastic paraplegia or tetraplegia.

Pharmacological implications: In the presence of severe hypotonia, use of depolarizing neuromuscular relaxants may result in exaggerated hyperkalemia. The sensitivity to nondepolarizing blocking agents can be increased and should be properly monitored with a peripheral nerve stimulator.

Other conditions to be considered:

☞**GRISCELLI SYNDROME:** Albinism with immunodeficiency characterized by partial pigmentary dilution of the skin and hair (silvery-gray hair), frequent infections, neurologic abnormalities, and fatal outcome caused by uncontrolled T-lymphocyte and macrophage activation syndrome. The clinical features include the presence of large clumps of pigment in hair shafts and an accumulation of melanosomes in melanocytes.

☞**CHEDIAK-HIGASHI SYNDROME:** Frequently fatal disease of childhood characterized by the association of immune deficiency, partial oculocutaneous albinism, easy bruisability, bleeding, and recurrent infections.

☞**HERMANSKY-PUDLAK SYNDROME:** Autosomal recessive disorder presenting with oculocutaneous albinism, visual impairment, platelet dysfunction, severe bleeding disorder, and progressive symptoms including pulmonary fibrosis, inflammatory bowel, and kidney disease. The severity of this syndrome ranges from very mild with few symptoms to severe and disabling.

☞**OCULOCEREBRAL WITH HYPOPIGMENTATION SYNDROME:** Extremely rare autosomal recessive inherited syndrome (fewer than 20 cases have been described). Most symptoms are present at birth or develop shortly thereafter and may include very light skin color and silvery hair in combination with ophthalmologic (microphthalmia, corneal clouding, cataract, ectropion) and central nervous system anomalies (dolichocephaly, mental retardation, athetosis, ataxia, spastic paraplegia or tetraplegia). Gingival fibromatosis may develop at the age of emergence of the first teeth and may result in complete coverage of the teeth and become so significant that ventilation is impaired. Ventilation can be decreased further by a dysfunctional diaphragm.

REFERENCES:

Cahali JB, Fernandez SA, Oliveira ZN, et al: Elejalde syndrome: Report of a case and review of the literature. *Pediatr Dermatol* 21:479, 2004.

Thornton CM, Stewart F: Elejalde syndrome: A case report. *Am J Med Genet* 69:406, 1997.

Ellis-Van Creveld Syndrome

At a glance: Inherited form of short-limbed dwarfism often seen among the Old Order Amish community in Lancaster County, Pennsylvania (USA).

Synonyms: Chondroectodermal Dysplasia; Mesoectodermal Dysplasia Syndrome.

History: Genetic skeletal dysplasia first described by Richard W.B. Ellis (1902–1966) from Edinburgh and Simon van Creveld (1895–1971) from Amsterdam. Together with ☞Jeune Syndrome, it is grouped into the nonlethal short rib-polydactyly syndromes.

Incidence: Approximately 250 cases have been described. No sexual predilection has been reported.

Genetic inheritance: Autosomal recessive with linkage of the Ellis-van Creveld (EVC) phenotype to genetic markers on the short arm of chromosome 4p16.

Pathophysiology: Unknown; however, the cartilage of long bones and vertebrae of fetuses with EVC syndrome shows disorganization of the chondrocytes in the physeal growth zone and retardation of the short columellar arrangements in the physis.

Diagnosis: Dwarfism with profound shortening of the distal parts of the extremities (mesomelic shortening), already identifiable at birth. Skeletal histopathology via fetoscopy and ultrasound can be used for prenatal diagnosis.

Clinical aspects: Features may include micrognathia, polydactyly, and abnormalities of the ectoderm (onychodystrophy, anomalies in the upper lip variously called "partial hare lip" or "lip tie," and cleft lip/palate), and dysodontiasis (congenital teeth, partial anodontia, malpositioned teeth). Of particular importance are the presence of cardiac malformations in 60% of affected patients (commonly a septal defect or single atrium). Respiratory distress is frequent in neonates as a result of hypoplastic lungs within a narrow dysplastic thorax with extremely short ribs. Hypoplasia of the tracheobronchial cartilage tends to result in collapse of the tracheobronchial tree causing tension lobar emphysema and may further exacerbate any respiratory compromise. ☞Dandy-Walker malformation, hydrocephalus, and mental retardation occur occasionally. Genital anomalies are common (epispadias and hypospadias, cryptorchism, megaureter, hydronephrosis, renal agenesis). Management consists of dental care, plastic surgery for treatment of polydactyly, and correction of cardiac defects.

Precautions before anesthesia: Assess the airway for difficult management secondary to the presence of cleft lip/palate and micrognathia. Check for cardiac lesions including cor pulmonale (clinical examination, electrocardiography, and echocardiography). Evaluate for signs of airway collapse (stridor) and assess pulmonary function (clinical examination, chest radiographs, arterial blood gas analysis, and pulmonary function tests). Assess renal function (serum concentrations of electrolytes, creatinine, and urea). Check for signs of increased intracranial pressure.

Anesthetic considerations: Intravenous access can be difficult secondary to excessive lax skin and subcutaneous tissue. If difficult airway management is suspected, spontaneous ventilation should be maintained until the airway has been secured. In patients with pulmonary hypertension, anesthetic management should aim to avoid any further increase in pulmonary artery pressure (avoid acidosis, hypercarbia, and hypoxia). Ventilation may require assistance to some degree during an induction with maintained spontaneous ventilation to prevent significant hypercapnia with consequently increased pulmonary vascular resistance (PVR). The patient's weight rather than the age best predicts endotracheal tube size. Airway collapse as a result of bronchial cartilage hypoplasia may complicate general anesthesia. Avoid high airway pressures during controlled ventilation to minimize barotrauma and further gas trapping in the presence of lobar emphysema. Repeated arterial blood gas analyses are strongly recommended for patients with respiratory impairment (arterial catheter may be considered). Prolonged postoperative mechanical ventilation may be required in patients with dysplastic thorax.

Pharmacological implications: Anticholinergic agents may be useful in patients with suspected airway management problems. Restrictive lung disease prolongs inhalational induction. Neuromuscular blockers should be avoided until the airway has been secured. Subacute bacterial endocarditis prophylaxis may be required. Kidney dysfunction may affect elimination of (predominantly renally excreted) drugs.

OTHER CONDITIONS TO BE CONSIDERED:

☞**JEUNE SYNDROME:** Very rare form of chondrodysplasia often leading to death in infancy from respiratory insufficiency as a result of severe thoracic restrictive deformation. Commonly associated with multiple skeletal malformations and liver, renal, and retinal dysfunction.

SALDINO-NOONAN SYNDROME (☞SHORT-RIB POLYDACTYLY SYNDROME): Lethal, autosomal recessive inherited skeletal dysplasia characterized by a hypoplastic thorax, short ribs and limbs, polydactyly, and visceral abnormalities (e.g., transposition of the great arteries, polycystic kidneys, atretic lesions of the gastrointestinal and genitourinary systems). The pelvis resembles that in the Ellis-van Creveld syndrome and Jeune syndrome.

MAJEWSKI SYNDROME (☞SHORT-RIB POLYDACTYLY SYNDROME): Autosomal recessive inherited disorder characterized by short stature with extremely short limbs, preaxial and postaxial polysyndactyly of hands and feet, short ribs, premature ossification of the proximal humerus and femur epiphyses and the lateral cuboids, malformed ears, short and flat nose, median cleft lip/palate, genital abnormalities (ambiguous genitalia), anomalies of the epiglottis and larynx (malformed larynx with hypoplastic epiglottis), pulmonary hypoplasia, and glomerular and renal tubular cysts leading to renal failure. Sometimes associated with polyhydramnios and hydrops fetalis.

VERMA-NAUMOFF SYNDROME (☞SHORT-RIB POLYDACTYLY SYNDROME): Autosomal recessive inherited disorder characterized by polydactyly, short ribs, and narrow chest with neonatal asphyxia, often resulting in early death. Craniofacial anomalies include frontal bossing, flat occiput, and depressed nasal bridge. Genitourinary anomalies are common.

☞**BEEMER LANGER SYNDROME:** Genetic disorder characterized by multiple skeletal (and other) anomalies and death either in utero or in the early neonatal period as a result of respiratory failure.

☞**WEYERS SYNDROME II:** Recognized phenotype of the Ellisvan Creveld syndrome, also presenting with heart defects (atrial or ventricular septal defects in >70% of patients) and postaxial polydactyly of the hands and feet, hexadactyly, fusion of the fifth and sixth metatarsals and metacarpals, and bony clefts of the mandibular symphysis. Other features may include short stature, micrognathia, small mouth, orodental anomalies, hypoplasia of the larynx, and hypoplastic and dysplastic nails.

REFERENCES:

Sergi C, Voigtlander T, Zoubaa S, et al: Ellis-van Creveld syndrome: A generalized dysplasia of enchondral ossification. *Pediatr Radiol* 31:289, 2001

McKusick VA: Ellis-van Creveld syndrome and the Amish. *Nat Genet* 24:203, 2000.

Wu CL, Litman RS: Anesthetic management for a child with the Ellis-van Creveld syndrome: A case report. *Paediatr Anaesth* 4:335, 1994.

Emery-Dreifuss Muscular Dystrophy (EDMD)

At a glance: Relatively benign congenital muscular dystrophy usually beginning in childhood or adolescence and characterized by early muscle contractures (mainly shoulders and upper arms) and cardiac conduction disorders.

Synonym: Scapuloilioperoneal Atrophy with Cardiomyopathy.

Incidence: No precise data are available. The X-linked form (males only) is more frequent and has been reported in more than 70 families. The estimated prevalence is approximately 1:100,000 in the general population. The autosomal dominant form is much less frequent.

Genetic inheritance: Two forms of EDMD exist: (1) X-linked, resulting from a mutation in the emerin gene (>100 mutations have been reported and mapped to X28q) that usually results in complete absence of emerin from the muscles, and (2) autosomal dominant, resulting from a mutation in the lamin A/C gene on 1q21. Lamins A/C are part of the nuclear lamina, a fibrous layer on the nucleoplasmic side of the inner nuclear membrane, where they interact with chromatin and other proteins of the inner nuclear membrane (lamina-associated proteins and emerin) through various binding sites. Significant intrafamilial and interfamilial variability have been described. Sporadic cases have been described.

Pathophysiology: Almost all known mutations result in a complete absence of emerin, an inner nuclear membrane protein not limited to muscle cells but mostly expressed in skeletal and cardiac muscles. It is believed to interact with the nuclear lamins (components of the nuclear lamina), chromatin, and nuclear actin. Its exact role is unknown, but it seems to protect the nuclear membrane from mechanical lesions during muscle contraction. It also may favor reassembly of the nuclear membrane at the end of mitosis. Lamins A/C is also an inner nuclear membrane protein with properties similar to emerin, which would account for the similarity in phenotype between X-linked and autosomal dominant EDMD. For emerin (and presumably lamins A/C) to function properly, the protein must be correctly positioned on the nuclear membrane. Any defect in the nuclear membrane could interfere with skeletal muscle regeneration because emerin seems to play an important role in the organization of the nuclear membrane during cell division. Emerin seems to be associated with cardiac desmosomes and fasciae adherentes, which not only suggests a physiologic role for the protein in cardiac function but also explains the cardiac involvement.

Diagnosis: Mainly based on the clinical findings. It is easier to diagnose if a relative has the disease. Serum creatinine kinase levels are moderately increased. Electromyography and nerve conduction studies confirm the myopathic nature of the disease. Muscle biopsy using antibodies to emerin can help confirm the diagnosis in the X-linked form.

Clinical aspects: The two forms of the disorder are clinically similar. Onset of the clinical manifestations usually occurs in the second or third decade of life. The following triad characterizes the disorder. (1) Early contractures affecting the Achilles tendons (resulting in toe walking), elbows (biceps and triceps), and posterior cervical muscles (initially resulting in limited cervical flexion, which later extends to the whole spine) often occur before any muscle weakness is apparent. (2) Early in the course of the disease, a slowly progressive muscle wasting and weakness (which is rarely severe) with a distinctive humeroperoneal distribution (i.e., proximal in the upper limbs and distal in the lower limbs) can be detected. As the disease progresses, weakness extends to the proximal limb girdle musculature. (3) Cardiac conduction defects may range from sinus bradycardia to prolongation of the PR interval and complete heart block. Atrial paralysis is almost considered pathognomonic of EDMD. A dilated right atrium on echocardiography and isolated atrial standstill and absent P waves on the electrocardiogram should prompt exclusion of EDMD. A generalized cardiomyopathy has been described, resulting in progressive cardiac failure or sudden cardiac death from heart block (which occurs in up to 40% of affected patients). Cardiac involvement is by far the most serious and important feature of this disorder, occurring almost exclusively after muscle weakness has become obvious. Almost all patients show some degree of cardiac involvement by age 30 years. Early diagnosis is crucial, allowing pacemaker implantation before fatal arrhythmias occur. Some patients develop a scoliosis. These patients are mentally normal.

Precautions before anesthesia: Obtain an electrocardiogram (consider 24-hour Holter ECG), an echocardiogram to assess cardiac function, and a cardiac consultation if the patient has a pacemaker. In the presence of significantly decreased muscle weakness and/or scoliosis, pulmonary function tests should be obtained prior to any major surgery. Prolonged postoperative mechanical ventilation may be required. Check neck mobility, particularly neck extension.

Anesthetic considerations: Be prepared for difficult airway management because of patient's neck stiffness. Maintain spontaneous ventilation until the airway has been secured. In the presence of scoliosis, there may be a restrictive pulmonary disease or even cardiac involvement. The presence of contractures makes patient positioning more difficult. Good padding is required. Regional anesthesia per se is not contraindicated; however, proper positioning for central neuraxial blockade may be difficult. The requirement for muscle relaxants will be minimal in patients with muscle weakness. Finally, cardiac involvement is frequent with conduction anomalies, so a defibrillator, resuscitation drugs, and a magnet if the patient has a pacemaker should be available immediately. No association with malignant hyperthermia has been reported.

Pharmacological implications: Succinylcholine should not be used in these patients because of an increased risk of exaggerated hyperkalemia. In the presence of significant cardiomyopathy, myocardial depressant drugs should be avoided. Avoid neuromuscular blockers in suspected difficult airway management until the airway has been secured.

Other conditions to be considered:

SCAPULOPERONEAL MUSCULAR DYSTROPHY AND SCAPULOPERONEAL NEUROPATHY have a distribution of weakness similar to that of EDMD but are not genetically defined.

References:

Emery AEH: Emery Dreifuss muscular dystrophy—A 40 year retrospective. *Neuromuscul Disord* 10;228, 2000.

Shende D, Agarwal R: Anaesthetic management of a patient with Emery-Dreifuss muscular dystrophy. *Anaesth Intensive Care* 30:372, 2002.

Wehnert MS, Bonne G: The nuclear muscular dystrophies. *Semin Pediatr Neurol* 9:100, 2002.

Encephalocele

At a glance: Malformation characterized by cerebral anomalies and a median skull gap originating from the nasal root, orbits, or forehead (sincipital encephalocele), or the skull base or occiput (occipital encephalocele), allowing cerebrospinal fluid and/or brain to herniate. The encephalocele itself is defined as a herniation of part of the cranial contents through this skull defect. It may contain meninges (meningocele), meninges and brain (meningoencephalocele), or meninges, brain, and ventricle (meningoencephalocystocele).

Synonyms: Cephalocele; Craniocele; Cranial Meningoencephalocele.

Definition: Defect of neural tube development resulting in a osseous defect in the midline of the skull that allows herniation of the meninges and portions of the brain.

Incidence: 1:5000–10,000 live births. No sexual predilection.

Genetic inheritance: Multifactorial inheritance pattern.

Pathophysiology: Dysraphism of the skull with a defect that may occur anywhere from the nasal cavity to the foramen magnum. Herniation of cerebral structures with (encephalocystocele) or without ventricular components (cenencephalocele) are distinguished. If meningeal structures are involved in the herniation, the terms encephalomenigocele and meningoencephalocele have been used. Another classification distinguishes just between meningocele or encephalocele. The herniated brain is often abnormal, and there are frequently associated structural and functional abnormalities that also affect the nonherniated brain areas.

Diagnosis: Based on the obvious clinical findings and confirmation by computed tomography scanning or magnetic resonance imaging. In utero diagnosis can be made by ultrasound, elevated maternal (and patient) alpha-fetoprotein, and amniocentesis.

Clinical aspects: The clinical picture depends on the type of encephalocele: *Sincipital encephaloceles* (25% of all encephaloceles) most often originate from the orbits, nose, or forehead and occur most commonly in Asians. (1) *Anterior sincipital encephaloceles* present as a mass in the nasopharynx. They are often diagnosed late and may present because of persistent nasal discharge or recurrent meningitis. (2) *Basal sincipital encephaloceles* may extend into the upper pharynx and present with feeding difficulties and/or upper airway obstruction. The content of the encephalocele may include hypothalamus or pituitary gland, which may result in neuroendocrine disturbances and preclude resection. The associated mortality is high.

Notencephaloceles (75% of all encephaloceles) extend from the occipital region aspect of the skull. Portions of the brain found in the herniated sac may include abnormal cerebral cortex, cerebellum, brainstem, and ventricles. There are often extensive malformations throughout the neuraxis with involvement of the midbrain, optic pathways, venous drainage, and skull. There may be a disturbance of the central autonomic control with abnormalities in temperature

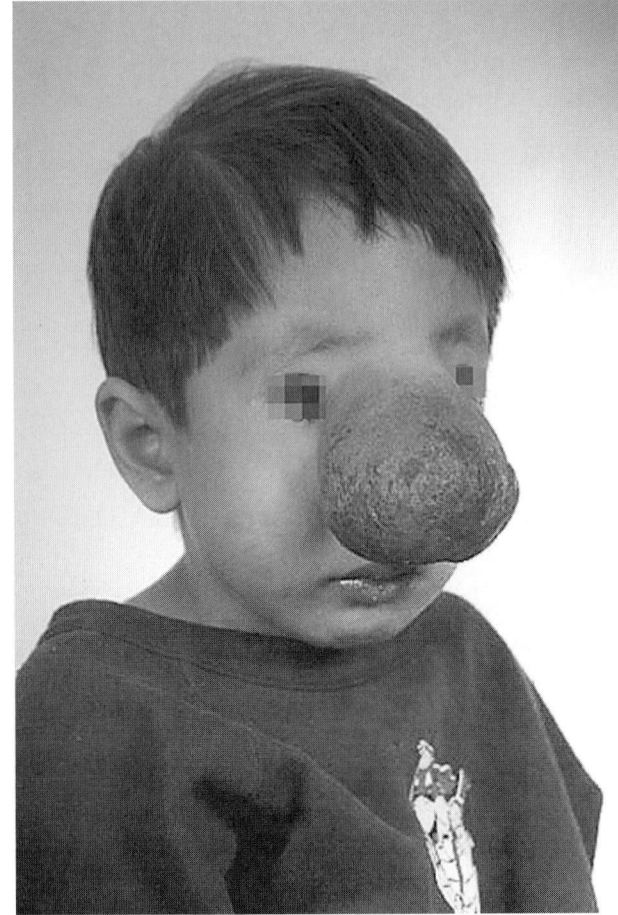

Encephalocele   Sincipital encephalocele in a 6-year-old boy.

regulation. Seizures are common, and mental retardation is associated with extensive brain involvement. The hernia is usually covered with skin or membrane and may be pulsatile. The size may vary from a small sac to a cyst-like structure greater than the size of the head. Complications at presentation may include rupture of the sac with infection or necrosis. Associated neural abnormalities may include developmental delay, microcephaly, seizures, and mental retardation. Occipital encephaloceles may be associated with ☞Arnold-Chiari Syndrome and hydrocephalus.

Several malformations have been identified to often coexist with encephaloceles, such as hydrocephalus, ☞Klippel-Feil Syndrome (cervical vertebral synostosis and neck webbing), ☞ Arnold-Chiari Syndrome, porencephaly, agenesis of the corpus callosum, myelodysplasia, optic nerve dysplasia, and cleft lip/palate.

Precautions before anesthesia: Coexisting syndromes and their associated anesthetic risks should be identified prior to anesthesia. Surgery may occur within the first 24 hours of life or may be delayed until after age 6 months depending on the location, size, and type of the encephalocele. Early complete surgical treatment is indicated to allow the developing brain and eyes to remodel the facial deformity. The goals of surgery include urgent closure of open skin defects to prevent infections and desiccation of brain tissue, removal or invagination of nonfunctional tissue, watertight closure of the dura, and total craniofacial reconstruction, particularly avoiding the "long-nose deformity." To correct the deformity caused by hypertelorism and a long midface, Holmes et al. lower the supraorbital bar by

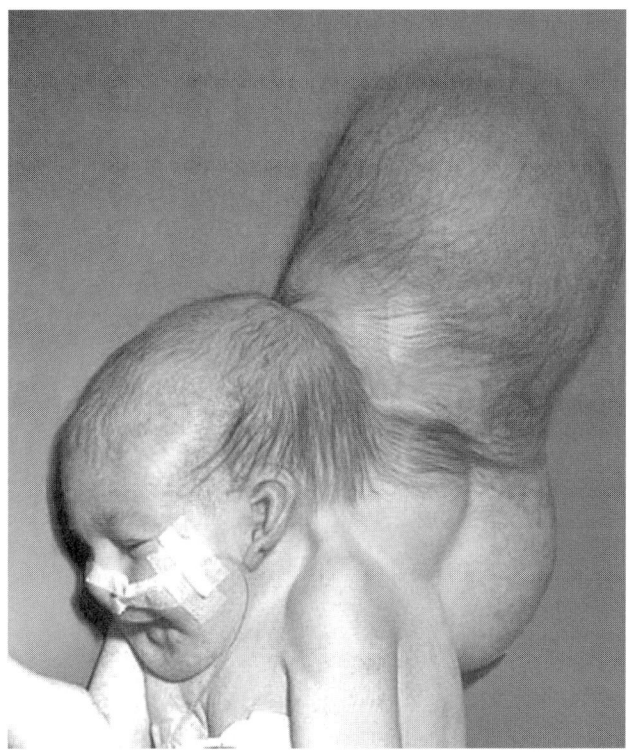

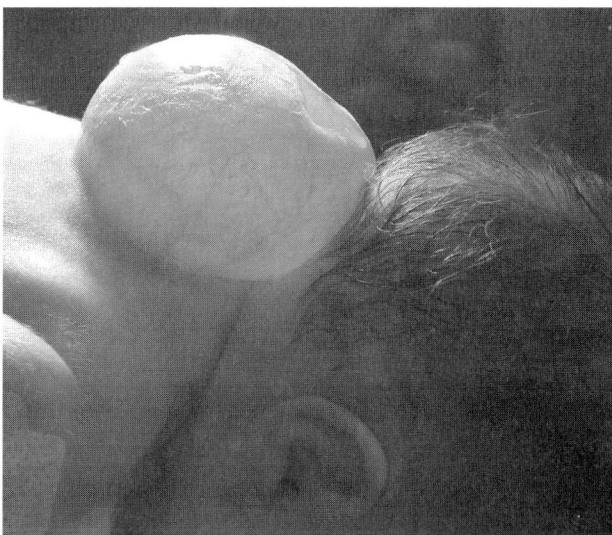

Encephalocele Transilluminated nuchal encephalocele in a new-born baby positioned in the prone position for surgery. See color plates.

Encephalocele Huge occipital meningoencephalocystocele in an infant.

rotating it medially, posteriorly, and downward in the midline, with lateral widening to correct the trigonocephalic deformity. Review computed tomography scans and/or magnetic resonance images if available before anesthesia.

Anesthetic Implications: These children may have difficult airway management secondary to the position of the encephalocele

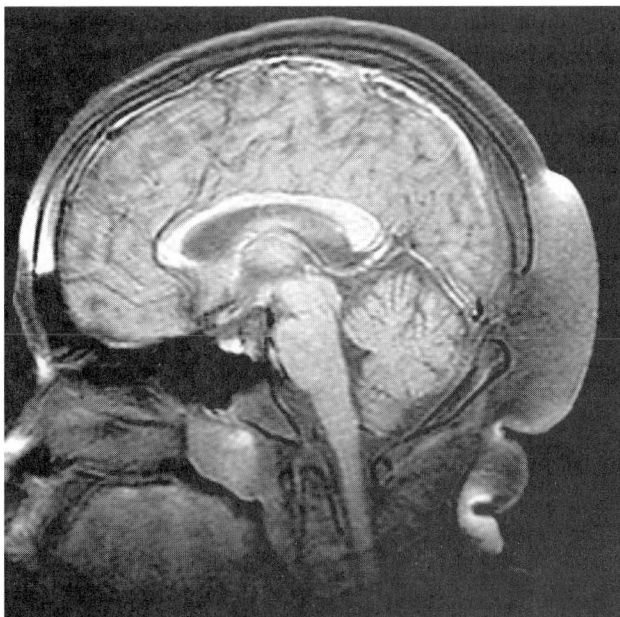

Encephalocele Three-dimensional MRI reconstruction of the head of a patient with a large occipital encephalocele revealing the impressive underlying bone lesion associated with the encephalocele.

and associated abnormalities. Because subglottic stenosis has been reported in some patients, an endotracheal tube one size smaller than expected should be prepared as well. An anterior encephalocele may be associated with a large mass in the nasopharynx, so nasal tracheal intubation should be avoided. Supine positioning with a posterior encephalocele may be difficult even in the presence of bolsters to prevent external pressure on the encephalocele, so tracheal intubation should be performed in the (left) lateral position. Neonates have had their tracheas intubated awake in some cases. Maintenance of spontaneous ventilation is recommended until the airway has been secured if airway problems are expected. If there are any concerns regarding aspiration in combination with difficult airway management, a fiberoptic awake tracheal intubation is probably the technique of choice. Posterior encephaloceles are positioned prone, and nasal intubation using armored endotracheal tubes has been recommended as there are case reports of kinking or dislocation of the endotracheal tube that resulted in cardiac arrest. Changes in heart rate and/or rhythm may indicate brainstem compromise. Correct positioning of bolsters allows normal abdominal movement and venous flow in the inferior vena cava to reduce bleeding from the cerebral vessels and the vertebral venous plexus. Preparation for significant blood loss should be made because of potential bleeding from the suboccipital bone and dural sinus. Large-bore intravenous access is recommended, and invasive blood pressure monitoring with the possibility of drawing arterial blood gas samples (including complete blood count, hemoglobin, and coagulation parameters) should be considered. Maintenance of normal body temperature may be a problem because of brain exposure and significant volume replacement and may be complicated further by decreased central autonomic control. Use of forced-air warmers, heating blankets, warmed infusions, and other standard heating methods is recommended.

Pharmacological Considerations: Use of atropine (0.02 mg/kg) prior to laryngoscopy and tracheal intubation has been recommended for all patients. Lumbar intrathecal morphine has been used for repair of frontal encephalocele via single-shot technique and provided effective analgesia for up to 24 hours.

Others conditions to be considered: Encephaloceles can be an isolated finding, but they may also be part of numerous syndromes, such as Acrocephalosyndactyly Syndromes, Median Cleft Facial Syndrome, Aplasia Cutis Congenita, Morning Glory Syndrome, Catlin Marks, MURCS Association, Cerebrorenodigital Syndrome, Pallister Hall Syndrome, Chondrodysplasia (giant cell type), Pentalogy of Cantrell, COACH Syndrome, Roberts Syndrome, Craniomicromelic Syndrome, Rolland Desbuqois Syndrome, HARD Syndrome, Smith-Lemli-Opitz Syndrome, Knobloch Syndrome, Streeter Anomaly, Krause Reese Syndrome, VACTERL Association (with hydrocephalus).

REFERENCES:

Hunt JA, Hobar PC: Common craniofacial anomalies: Facial clefts and encephaloceles. *Plast Reconstr Surg* 112: 606, 2003.

Mahapatra AK, Suri A: Anterior encephaloceles: A study of 92 cases. *Pediatr Neurosurg* 36:113, 2002.

Tobias JD, Mateo C, Ferrer MJ, et al: Intrathecal morphine for postoperative analgesia following repair of frontal encephalocoele in children: Comparison with intermittent, on-demand dosing of nalbuphine. *J Clin Anaesth* 9:280, 1997.

Tubbs RS, Wellons JC 3rd, Oakes WJ: Occipital encephalocele, lipomeningomyelocele, and Chiari I malformation: Case report and review of the literature. *Childs Nerv Syst* 19:50, 2003.

Eosinophilic Endomyocardial Disease

At a glance: Progressive and restrictive cardiomyopathy associated with a hypereosinophilic state and endocarditis resulting in impaired ventricular filling with normal or decreased diastolic volume of either or both ventricles, associated with multiple organ involvement.

Synonyms: Löffler Endocarditis; Fibroplastic Parietal Endocarditis with Eosinophilia; Nontropical Eosinophilic Endomyocardial Fibrosis.

History: Named after the Swiss Physician W. Löffler, who described this disorder in 1936.

Incidence: Rare disorder that primarily occurs in people living in the rain forest in the tropical and subtropical areas of Africa, Asia, and South America. Males are affected more often than females.

Genetic inheritance: The condition has a predilection for African populations, especially in tribes from Rwanda, which may or may not be caused by genetic factors (yet unknown epidemiology of underlying environmental factors may play the major role).

Pathophysiology: Pathophysiology remains unclear, but many hypotheses have been discussed. The basis of the cardiac injury seems to involve eosinophil granule proteins that produce muscular and vascular injury that in turn leads to endomyocardial fibrosis. How eosinophilic infiltration and degranulation occur are unknown. Studies have shown that interleukin-5 is produced by eosinophils and could have a role in chemotaxis and degranulation.

Diagnosis: Based on clinical and biochemical findings such as a high eosinophil blood count, but confirmation requires endocardial and/or myocardial biopsy. The echocardiogram is not useful as a diagnostic tool in the early stages of the disease. In the later stages, echocardiography may show a markedly thickened endocardium and the chest radiograph a widespread shadowing of both lung fields. Widespread T-wave inversions may be seen on the electrocardiogram.

Clinical aspects: Eosinophilic endomyocardial disease may be the result of numerous disorders, including the idiopathic hypereosinophilic syndrome, which mainly affects young men. Idiopathic hypereosinophilic syndrome is a heterogeneous group of disorders characterized by an absolute eosinophil count of more than 1500/mm^3 that lasts for more than 6 months in the absence of any known cause of hypereosinophilia and with signs of organ involvement. Cardiac involvement occurs in more than half of patients and is the major cause of morbidity and mortality. However, eosinophilic endomyocardial disease may also be associated with bronchial carcinomas, medullary carcinoma of the thyroid, malignant fibrous histiocytoma, eosinophilic leukemia, sarcoma, and several other disorders (parasites, adverse drug reactions) associated with hypereosinophilia. Patients with the disease initially may be asymptomatic or present with tachypnea, shortness of breath, elevated central venous pressure, ascites, and pulmonary edema as a consequence of global heart failure. The endomyocarditis progresses in three different stages. The early necrotic stage presents in up to one third of patients with systemic disease and hypereosinophilia (unspecific signs such as fever, lymphadenopathy, splenomegaly) and in up to half of the patients with signs of acute endomyocarditis with inappetence, pulmonary infiltrates, cough, mitral and tricuspid regurgitation, and global heart failure. Thromboembolic complications may follow and can be found in up to 20% of patients. They originate from mural thrombi over endomyocardial lesions and may lead to anemic infarctions of brain, spleen, kidneys, bowel, and heart. Progressive scarring characterizes the late stage of the disease with endomyocardial fibrosis and restrictive cardiomyopathy and right and/or left ventricular failure.

Precautions before anesthesia: Check for concomitant disorders (e.g., cancer). Obtain a chest radiograph, electrocardiogram, echocardiogram, complete blood count with white cell differentiation, and serum electrolyte levels. Carefully assess intravascular volume and treat any signs of heart failure (pulmonary edema) before the patient goes to the operating room.

Anesthetic considerations: The anesthesiologist must consider, until proven otherwise, the patient as having a failing heart. Thus, for general anesthesia, high-dose opioids are recommended because volatile anesthetics may cause cardiac depression in a dose-dependent fashion; halothane is the worst. Ketamine and etomidate may be useful as induction agents. Inotropic support may be required, and invasive monitoring (i.e., arterial line, central venous catheter, or even pulmonary artery catheter) is advised for any type of major surgery to help optimize fluid status and hemodynamics. If the patient is treated with digoxin, hyperventilation should be avoided because it may lower the potassium level and potentiate digitalis toxicity. Regional anesthesia is not contraindicated per se, but be careful with the decrease in systemic vascular resistance (SVR) resulting from central neuraxial techniques because a slight decrease in afterload may improve cardiac output, whereas significant peripheral vasodilatation can negatively affect cardiac output.

Pharmacological implications: If the patient is taking a loop diuretic, potassium serum concentration should be monitored, especially if the patient is also taking digoxin.

REFERENCES:

Corradi D, Vaglio A, Maestri R, et al: Eosinophilic myocarditis in a patient with idiopathic hypereosinophilic syndrome: Insights into mechanisms of myocardial cell death. *Hum Pathol* 35: 1160, 2004.

Galiuto L, Enriquez-Sarano M, Reeder GS, et al: Eosinophilic myocarditis manifesting as myocardial infarction: Early diagnosis and successful treatment. *Mayo Clin Proc* 72:603, 1997.

Horenstein MS, Humes R, Epstein ML, et al: Loffler's endocarditis presenting in 2 children as fever with eosinophilia. *Pediatrics* 110:1014, 2002.

Epidermal Nevus Syndrome

At a glance: Genetically transmitted group of neurocutaneous disorders characterized by epidermal nevi, odontodysplasia, mental retardation, and various other malformations (including skeleton, heart, kidneys, and eyes).

Synonyms: Jadassohn Nevus Phakomatosis; Solomon Syndrome; (Inflammatory) Linear Nevus Sebaceous Syndrome; Nevus Sebaceous of Jadassohn. The terms Porcupine Man, Ichthyosis Hystrix Gravior, and Lambert type Ichthyosis are considered by some authors as synonyms.

Incidence: Approximately 500 cases have been described in the medical literature.

Genetic inheritance: Most cases appear to be sporadic, but a few seem to be familial with autosomal dominant transmission.

Pathophysiology: Unknown.

Diagnosis: Based on the clinical findings. The Epidermal Nevus Syndromes are a group of five different syndromes:

1) Schimmelpenning Syndrome (sebaceous nevus associated with cerebral anomalies, coloboma, and lipodermoid of the conjunctiva)
2) Nevus Comedonicus Syndrome (with cataracts as a distinguishing feature)
3) Pigmented Hairy Epidermal Nevus Syndrome (with Becker Nevus and skeletal defects [e.g., scoliosis], and ipsilateral breast hypoplasia)
4) ☞CHILD (*c*ongenital *h*emidysplasia with *i*chthyosiform erythroderma and *l*imb *d*efects) syndrome
5) ☞Proteus Syndrome

The latter two syndromes are described separately; the first three are described together. The majority of epidermal nevi either are present at birth or occur within the first year of life (later onset is possible but unusual). Typically, the distribution of nevi follows the lines of Blaschko. Verrucous plaques of the scalp usually extend to the cheeks and other facial structures. The distribution, surface characteristics, and histology of the lesions are variable. Smaller lesions tend to be limited to the face, scalp, and neck, whereas larger lesions may affect any part of the body. In newborns, the nevi appear in a linear distribution as ovoid, flat, velvety plaques. During adolescence, the lesions often become more raised, verrucous, and hyperpigmented. Orbital hypoplasia, frontal bossing, asymmetry of the skull, facial hemihypertrophy, and premature closing of the sphenofrontal suture are the principal craniofacial defects. Hypoplasia of the teeth and odontodysplasia ("ghost teeth") are the main dental disorders. Facial nevi may extend to the oral mucosa and cause friable, papillomatous, bleeding masses. Cleft or highly arched palate and bifid uvula occur in some cases. Rib defects and abnormal clavicles, kyphosis, scoliosis, lordosis, and vertebral anomalies, short limbs, hemihypertrophy (or localized gigantism), spontaneous fractures, hypoplasia of the talar bone, genua valga, luxation of the ankle, pes equinovarus, and camptodactyly, clinodactyly, and brachydactyly are all features that have been described. Vitamin D-resistant rickets and cystic changes in the long bones and mandible have been described.

Clinical aspects: Epidermal nevi of the face and neck seem to be associated with a higher rate of cerebral anomalies when compared to epidermal nevi limited to the trunk. Seizures (that may be difficult to treat) and mental retardation (mild to very severe) complicate the neurologic abnormalities and occur in approximately two thirds of patients. Seizures typically start by the end of the first year of life and may include apneic, myoclonic, psychomotor, Jacksonian, and grand mal types of seizures. Cranial nerve disorders usually involve palsy of the sixth, seven, and eighth cranial nerve. Occasional cortical atrophy, hydrocephalus, cerebral hemangiomas or vascular malformations, hemimegalencephaly (typically ipsilateral to the skin lesions), agenesis of the corpus callosum and/or the cerebellar vermis, cysts continuous with the fourth ventricle of the brain, porencephaly, macrocephaly, hypotonia, hyperkinesia, hemiparesis or hemiplegia, cerebral calcifications, and cerebral tumors may be associated. ☞Dandy-Walker Syndrome (absence of the cerebellar vermis, hydrocephalus, and posterior fossa cyst continuing with the fourth ventricle) occurs in some cases. Neurogenic tumors may occur along the spinal cord. The skin shows epidermal nevi associated with nevus flammeus, sebaceous hypertrophy, hypopigmentation, café au lait spots, acanthosis nigricans, and mixed verrucous lesions. Blindness (retinal changes similar to those in ☞Coats Disease have been reported) is not an uncommon finding, and additional ocular features may include colobomas of the eyelid, iris, and retina, subconjunctival lipodermoids, corneal clouding and vascularization, ptosis, ectopic displacement of the pupils, exotropia/ esotropia tear duct stenosis, macrophthalmia/microphthalmia, and nystagmus.

The sebaceous epidermal nevus is associated with an increased risk of secondary tumors, both benign and malignant. Basal cell carcinoma is the most common cutaneous malignancy in these patients (up to 22% of patients). Generally, it does not occur until after puberty, although prepubertal manifestation has been reported. Squamous cell carcinoma has been described but is a rare complication of sebaceous nevus. Other tumors that have a higher incidence in these patients are hemangioma, keratoacanthoma, Wilms tumor, rhabdomyosarcoma, and various adenocarcinomas. Cardiovascular complications may include ventricular septal defect, coarctation of the aorta, pulmonary stenosis, dilated pulmonary artery, tetralogy of Fallot, patent ductus arteriosus, and hypoplastic left heart. Urogenital anomalies may include renal hypoplasia, hydronephrosis, hydroureter, ureteropelvic junction obstruction, vesicoureteral reflux, Wilms tumor, horseshoe kidney, cystic kidney, and cryptorchidism and hypospadia in males.

Precautions before anesthesia: There does not appear to be any literature about anesthesia associated with this condition, but certain considerations are be made. The disease requires a complete workup, including neurologic and motor milestones, family history, and problems with previous anesthetics. Assess the airway for difficult management and check for enoral lesions. Exercise tolerance and full cardiac workup including echocardiography to quantify heart function are essential because various cardiac diseases are associated with the disease. A history of seizures and effectiveness of treatment should be obtained, and antiseizure medications should be continued until day of surgery. Respiratory function should be checked by chest radiographs and arterial blood gas analysis. Preoperative chest physiotherapy likely will be of benefit. A complete blood count and serum concentrations of electrolytes, creatinine, and urea should be obtained.

Anesthetic considerations: Patients may have raised intracranial pressure as a result of hydrocephalus. They may have a large head with prominent occiput and facial abnormalities that may make airway management difficult, as does the increased likelihood of bleeding from lesions of the oral mucosa. The threshold for invasive monitoring should be low in the presence of congenital cardiac lesions. Ventilation could be problematic because of kyphoscoliosis (decreased chest compliance) and other bony abnormalities and may be of particular significance if intracranial pressure is increased. Regular perioperative arterial blood gas analyses are recommended. The choice of anesthetic agents should take into account the patient's epileptic status.

Pharmacological implications: Chronic treatment with antiseizure medications may interact with the metabolism and elimination of certain anesthetic drugs. Chronic administration of phenytoin increases requirements for nondepolarizing neuromuscular blocker, produces gingival hyperplasia and bleeding, and may cause hepatic dysfunction. Ketamine, enflurane, and methohexital are relatively contraindicated. Subacute bacterial endocarditis prophylaxis may be required.

Others conditions to be considered:

☞**ADAMS-OLIVER SYNDROME:** Very rare inherited disorder characterized by defects of the scalp associated with multiple scarred and hairless areas that usually have dilated blood vessels directly under the skin. Scalp defects are present at birth. The extremities are either short (hypoplastic fingers and toes) or characterized by absent hands and lower legs. Congenital heart defect must be ruled out.

☞**APLASIA CUTIS CONGENITA:** Most often inherited disorder with circumscribed or more extensive skin lesions that may also involve underlying tissues. Neurologic and cardiac anomalies have been described in these patients.

☞**CHILD SYNDROME:** Inherited syndrome characterized by unilateral inflammatory nevus with strict midline demarcation, sparing the face, and ipsilateral defects involving all skeletal structures and internal organs.

☞**CUTIS MARMORATA TELANGIECTATICA:** Congenital cutaneous disorder with persistent cutis marmorata, telangiectasia, and phlebectasia. Often reported in association with a variety of other congenital anomalies.

☞**DELLEMAN OORTHUYS SYNDROME:** Multiple congenital anomaly syndrome mainly affecting the central nervous system, eyes, and skin.

☞**EPIDERMOLYSIS BULLOSA:** Group of inherited bullous disorders characterized by blister formation in response to mechanical trauma.

☞**JOHANSON-BLIZZARD SYNDROME:** Polymalformative syndrome characterized by nasal alar hypoplasia (beak shaped), scalp defects, hypothyroidism, pancreatic achylia, and congenital deafness.

☞**GOLTZ SYNDROME:** Complex mesoectodermal hereditary disorder characterized by focal dermal atrophy with herniation of fat producing multiple papillomas, in association with skeletal, dental, ocular, and other anomalies.

☞**PROTEUS SYNDROME:** Rare congenital hamartomatous disorder characterized by multiple, diverse, somatic manifestations: partial bilateral gigantism of hands and feet, nevi, hemihypertrophy, subcutaneous tumors, and macrocephaly with cranial hyperostoses. It is named after the Greek god Proteus, "the polymorphous," who could change his shape at will to avoid capture.

☞**SETLEIS SYNDROME:** Puckered periorbital skin, absent or multiple rows of eyelashes.

☞**STREETER ANOMALY:** Constricting amniotic bands leading to amputation with scarring, distal syndactyly, cleft lip/palate, anencephaly, encephalocele, hydrocephaly, omphalocele, and gastroschisis. Other internal anomalies involve the heart, lungs, diaphragm, kidneys, and gonads.

REFERENCES:

Baker RS, Ross PA, Baumann RJ: Neurologic complications of the epidermal nevus syndrome. *Arch Neurol* 44:227, 1987.

Grebe TA, Rimsza ME, Richter SF, et al: Further delineation of the epidermal nevus syndrome: Two cases with new findings and literature review. *Am J Med Genet* 47:24, 1993.

Vujevich JJ, Mancini AJ: The epidermal nevus syndromes: Multisystem disorders. *J Am Acad Dermatol* 50: 957, 2004

Epidermolysis Bullosa

At a glance: Genetic disorder characterized by cutaneous blistering and scarring following minor trauma.

Classification: More than 20 different subtypes of the disease are grouped into three main categories: epidermolysis bullosa simplex (EBS), dystrophic epidermolysis bullosa (DEB), and junctional epidermolysis bullosa (JEB).

Junctional	Herlitz type (lethal type)
epidermolysis	Non-Herlitz type
bullosa	JEB with pyloric atresia
	(☞**Carmi syndrome**)
Epidermolysis bullosa	Weber-Cockayne type
simplex	Dowling-Mara type (EBS herpetiformis)
	Koebner type
Dystrophic	
epidermolysis	
bullosa	

Incidence: Seems to vary widely, depending on the country, from as high as 1:12,500 in the United States and 1:17,000 in the United Kingdom to 1:300,000 in Canada. The incidence of DEB and EBS is approximately 2 in 100,000, for each of them.

Genetic inheritance: DEB has two modes of transmission that are autosomal dominant and more frequently autosomal recessive. EBS is inherited as an autosomal dominant trait. JEB form is an autosomal recessive trait.

Pathophysiology: In *EBS*, skin separation occurs at the level of mid basal cells and is most commonly associated with mutations affecting the genes responsible for keratins 5 and 14. The molecular background of *JEB* is highly variable and most likely represents a collection of different diseases. The separation of the skin layers with blister formation occurs in the lamina lucida. The responsible mutations have been assigned to the genes coding for the laminin 5 subunits, collagen XVII, and α_6 and β_4 integrin. *DEB* is associated with mutations in the gene coding for collagen type VII (COL7A1), which is a protein that anchors the lamina densa within the superficial dermis.

Diagnosis: Based on the clinical features of blisters and scarring associated with minor trauma of the skin, oropharynx, and esophagus.

Clinical aspects: In general, patients are very sensitive to touch because frictional or shearing forces damage their skin and lead to blistering and scarring. These blisters can be very painful (and sometimes itchy) and often are present at birth or shortly thereafter. Application of direct pressure (without shearing forces), such as related to blood pressure measurement, is not as damaging. Affected patients may present with severe syndactyly of their fingers and toes (so-called "pseudosyndactyly" or "mitten deformity") and contractures of their limbs caused by scarring as a consequence of the disease. Depending on the type of epidermolysis bullosa, onychodystrophy and repeated loss of fingernails and toenails are common. At later stages, mutilation of the extremities may occur. Involvement of the oral mucosa leads to microstomia, narrowed nasal apertures, and esophageal strictures with poor oral feeding. Constipation may result from poor feeding but also from anal blister and fissure formation associated with painful and therefore retained defecations. Eyelid retraction (entropium and symblepharon) can lead to corneal abrasion. Skin bullae render patients more prone to infection and anemia secondary to bleeding from the lesions.

JUNCTIONAL EPIDERMOLYSIS BULLOSA: *Herlitz Type (Lethal Type):* This most common form of JEB is caused by the absence or a defect in the anchoring filament glycoprotein laminin 5 in the skin. It is also the most severe form commonly affecting the mouth and pharynx, including the larynx, resulting not only in feeding difficulties and hoarse voice but also in potentially life-threatening respiratory distress. Death as a result of respiratory distress and/or sepsis (favored by poor nutritional state) originating from skin infections often occurs before age 2 years. Scalp involvement is characteristic for this type of JEB, as is onychodystrophy with excessive granulation leading to bulbous enlargement of the finger tips ("drumstick fingers"). Anemia is a frequent finding.

Non-Herlitz Type: Initially similar to Herlitz type of JEB; however, the frequency and severity of blister formation decrease with increasing age.

JEB with Pyloric Atresia: This rarest from of JEB is associated with a poor prognosis. Death often occurs in the first year of life.

EPIDERMOLYSIS BULLOSA SIMPLEX: *Weber-Cockayne Type:* Milder variant of EBS that usually starts in early childhood and most often is limited to hands and feet. The lesions tend to heal quickly, although infections are a common complication often resulting in delayed wound healing. The nails are unaffected.

Dowling-Mara Type: This form has an extremely wide range of clinical appearance, ranging from only mild symptoms to early neonatal death. The blisters are often hemorrhagic. In contrast to the Weber-Cockayne type, this type is not limited to hands and feet, although they are the most commonly affected sites and later result in keratoderma palmoplantaris. Enoral and laryngeal involvement interfering with feeding and/or breathing is frequently seen in these patients.

Koebner Type: Blister formation most often starts in the first months of life. The blisters usually heal quickly, and secondary infections are less common than in other forms of EB. The frequency of blisters seems to decrease as the children become older and onychodystrophy is not a feature of this type.

DYSTROPHIC EPIDERMOLYSIS BULLOSA: Probably the type most common in patients presenting for surgery. Chronic poststreptococcal glomerulonephritis secondary to skin infections and

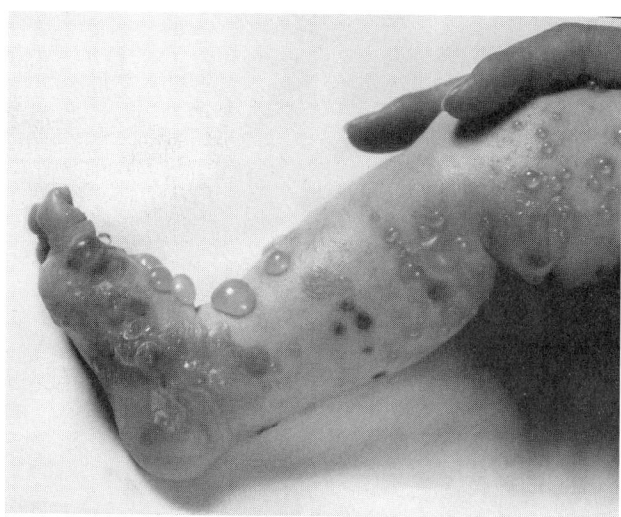

Epidermolysis Bullosa Different stages of epidermolysis bullosa on the leg of an infant. See color plates.

nephrotic syndrome secondary to renal amyloidosis have been described in these patients. Some of the lesions may turn into squamous cell carcinomas later in the evolution of the disease (usually in the third and fourth decades of life) and are the main cause of death in DEB patients surviving into adulthood.

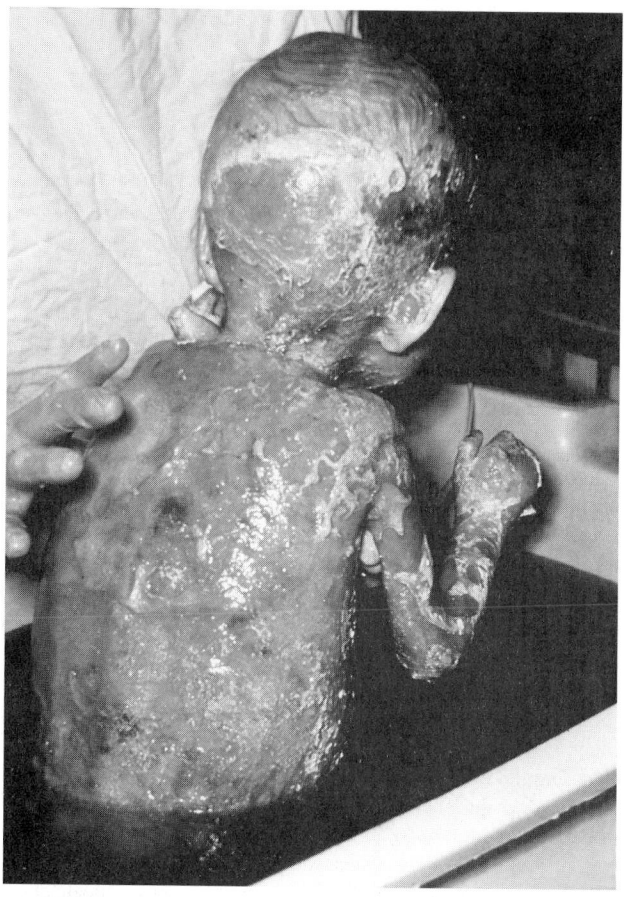

Epidermolysis Bullosa Severe, autosomal recessive form of epidermolysis bullosa.

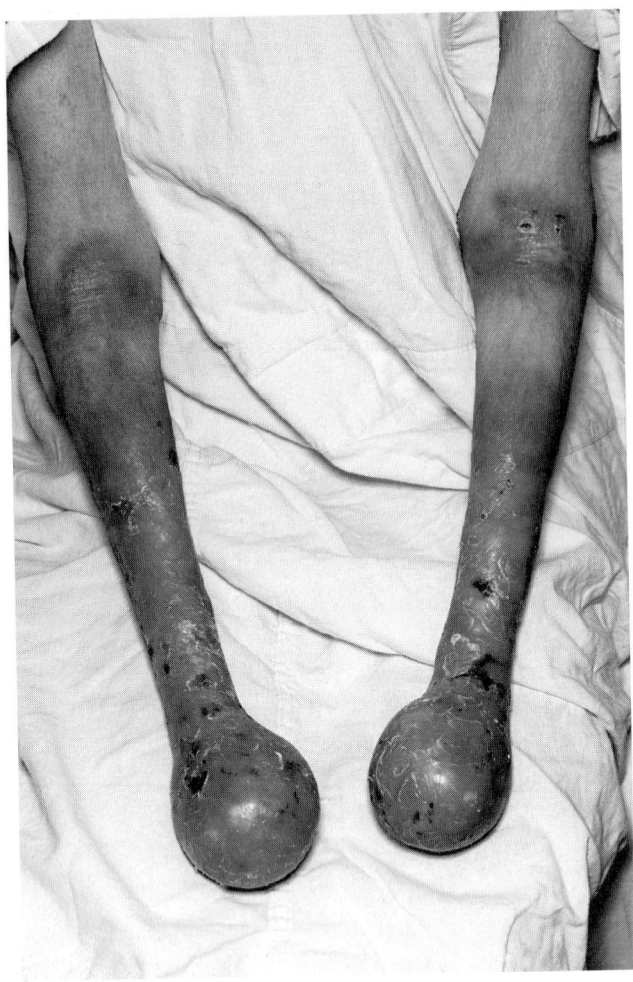

Epidermolysis Bullosa Epidermolysis bullosa results in painful mutilations of the arms. Similar findings are found on the legs. Vascular access may be very challenging in these patients.

Precautions before anesthesia: Obtain a complete blood count because many of the patients are anemic as a result of poor nutrition and frequent trauma. Renal function should be evaluated if there are any concerns about renal involvement. Assess mouth opening (microstomia), check tongue (scarring), neck mobility (contractures), and status of the teeth (pain associated with tooth brushing may result in poor dental hygiene). Peripheral vascular access can be extremely difficult because of scarring and/or mutilation. Rarely, epidermolysis bullosa is associated with muscular dystrophy, characterized by progressive muscle weakness or ☞Myasthenia Gravis. A possible association with cutaneous ☞Porphyria has been reported.

Anesthetic considerations: The main anesthetic management point to remember is to use a nontouch technique to prevent induction of blisters. Venous access can be difficult to obtain, and securing the intravenous cannula is an issue because dressing can cause blistering. Therefore use of Vaseline gauzes over and around the cannula followed by a light bandage around the insertion site is recommended. Monitoring can cause new bullae, and care must be taken to avoid adhesive electrode pads directly on the skin whenever possible and to wrap the underlying skin with Vaseline gauze before applying the blood pressure cuff. Needle electrodes for the electrocardiogram have been used successfully instead. Airway man-

agement can be difficult because of scarring around the mouth (microstomia) and of the tongue, so a padded (air-cushion type, if possible) and well-lubricated (Vaseline) face mask and laryngoscope blade must be used. Difficult airway management is associated with a higher risk of new bullae formation. In severe cases, fiberoptic intubation is needed because of restricted mouth opening. Oral intubation is preferred, and an endotracheal tube half to one size smaller than predicted should be used. Hoarse voice may be an indicator for laryngeal bullae/scarring, also potentially requiring a smaller endotracheal tube. Again, endotracheal tube securing may be complicated, and suturing it in place is often the best choice. The lips should be well lubricated too, especially where they come in contact with the endotracheal tube. Laryngeal mask airway use with few complications from new bullae formation has been reported. In addition, tracheal lesions do not appear to occur frequently after intubation (may be explained by respiratory columnar epithelium instead of squamous epithelium). Oropharyngeal suctioning should be avoided or done under direct vision only (also to check for new bullae before extubation) because it can easily cause bullae formation. Regional anesthesia is not contraindicated if the skin over the region is unaffected, but use of a sterile technique is imperative because these patients are prone to infections. Avoid rubbing the skin for disinfection; use a spray such as aqueous chlorhexidine instead. Finally, because of esophageal scarring, affected patients are at higher risk for regurgitation and aspiration, so antacid prophylaxis is recommended prior to surgery. Esophageal involvement also leads to malnutrition as a result of poor feeding and sometimes requires correction prior to elective surgery. Infections are more common because of the broken epidermal barrier and should be treated prior to the patient going to the operating room. Blood for transfusion should be easily available in the operating room, particularly if the hemoglobin level already is borderline. Administering a sedative premedication prior to taking young children to the operating room may be wise to prevent them from struggling during induction, which may lead to new bullae formation. Be very careful while positioning these patients because inappropriate handling may cause new bullae formation. Ideally, the patient should position him/herself on a well-padded operating table. Corneal abrasions are common among affected patients secondary to scarring of the eyelids with poor coverage of the cornea, so lubricant eye ointment and Vaseline gauzes should be applied. However, in small children, eye ointment resulting in blurred vision may trigger eye rubbing with new blister formation postoperatively. Avoid nasopharyngeal, esophageal, or rectal temperature probes. These patients are often already in significant pain preoperatively, which will be even worse postoperatively. Adequate pain relief is mandatory. Regional anesthesia is an elegant and effective way to achieve this goal; however, not all procedures are suitable for this approach. The oral and rectal routes may not be options in these patients (dysphagia and anal blisters/fissures, respectively), leaving the intravenous route as the only option. Patient-, parent-, or nurse-controlled analgesia has been used successfully in these cases.

Pharmacological implications: Avoid using succinylcholine in patients with associated muscular dystrophy. Some patients seem to be very sensitive to nondepolarizing muscle relaxants, so titration under the control of a peripheral nerve stimulator (*Caveat:* use needle electrodes instead of self-adhesive) is recommended. Perioperative steroid stress coverage may be necessary for patients on long-term oral steroids. Atropine preoperatively has been recommended to reduce oral secretions, particularly in sedated and spontaneously breathing patients. Drugs to be avoided in the presence of porphyria are given under ☞Porphyria.

Other conditions to be considered:

☞**ADAMS-OLIVER SYNDROME:** Very rare inherited disorder characterized by defects of the scalp associated with multiple scarred and hairless areas that usually have dilated blood vessels directly under the skin. Scalp defects are present at birth. The extremities are either short (hypoplastic fingers and toes) or characterized by absent hands and lower legs. Congenital heart defect must be ruled out.

☞**APLASIA CUTIS CONGENITA:** Most often inherited disorder with circumscribed or more extensive skin lesions that may also involve underlying tissues. Neurologic and cardiac anomalies have been described in these patients.

☞**ERYTHEMA MULTIFORME:** Acute mucocutaneous hypersensitivity reaction of variable severity characterized by symmetrical skin eruptions, with or without mucous membrane lesions.

☞**DANBOLT-CLOSS SYNDROME:** Inherited vesiculobullous disorder characterized by intermittent simultaneous occurrence of diarrhea and bullous dermatitis (dry lesions surrounding the mouth, ears, nose and eyes, but also affecting the fingers, feet, and knees) and failure to thrive in premature babies. In children, periorificial lesions of the face and anogenital region. Alopecia and absence of eyebrows, eyelashes, and thymus are common.

☞**PEMPHIGUS:** Rare autoimmune blistering disease that affects the skin and mucous membranes. Patients have circulating antibodies to an intercellular cement substance of the basal membrane.

REFERENCES:

Herod J, Denyer J, Goldman A, et al: Epidermolysis bullosa in children: Pathophysiology, anesthesia and pain management. *Paediatr Anaesth* 12:388, 2002.

Iohom G, Lyons B: Anaesthesia for children with epidermolysis bullosa: A review of 20 years' experience. *Eur J Anaesth* 18:745, 2001.

Yonker-Sell AE, Connolly LA: Twelve-hour anaesthesia in a patient with epidermolysis bullosa. *Can J Anaesth* 42:735, 1995.

Epstein Syndrome

At a glance: Genetic disorder characterized by platelet disorder, renal failure, and sensorineural deafness.

Synonyms: Alport Syndrome with Macrothrombocytopenia; Alport Syndrome Type V; Macrothrombocytopathy, Nephritis, and Deafness.

> Epstein Syndrome can also refer to a disorder associated with splenomegaly, high platelet count, and prolonged bleeding time. This disorder has also been termed Di Guglielmo Disease II or Di Guglielmo Syndrome, Epstein-Goedel Syndrome, Mortensen Disease/Syndrome, or Revol Disease/Syndrome.

History: First reported in two families by C.J. Epstein in 1972.
Incidence: Unknown; however, more than 30 families have been reported. No sexual predilection has been reported.
Genetic inheritance: Autosomal dominant with the genetic defect mapping to 22q11.2.
Pathophysiology: The bleeding tendency is a result of thrombocytopenia and the presence of a majority of giant spheroid platelets with a disorganized microtubular system and a lesser number of normal-size discoid platelets. Renal dysfunction occurs secondary to proliferative and sclerosing glomerulonephritis with interstitial nephritis and fibrosis. Hearing loss is gradual and of sensorineural etiology.

Diagnosis: Based on family history, clinical features, hematologic and nephrologic studies, and auditory examination. Hematologic studies reveal thrombocytopenia, prolonged bleeding time, and the above described giant platelets with abnormal ultrastructure, impaired platelet aggregation response to collagen and epinephrine, defective platelet adherence to glass, and impaired release of platelet factor III. The renal abnormality mainly manifests as proteinuria, which remains stable with normal renal function, although deterioration as a result of episodes of acute glomerulonephritis has been described.

Clinical aspects: Patients may develop multiple ecchymoses when they start walking and recurrent episodes of epistaxis beginning in early childhood. Bleeding from other sites is rare and usually not significant. High-frequency sensorineural hearing loss becomes noticeable by approximately 5 to 8 years of age, and progression to almost complete deafness may occur around the middle of the second decade of life. Proteinuria begins in childhood, usually without impairment of renal excretory function. In rare cases, episodes similar to acute glomerulonephritis occur.

Precautions before anesthesia: Laboratory investigations should include a complete blood count and coagulation studies, including bleeding time, platelet count, and a blood smear (thrombocytopenia and ultrastructural and functional studies showing macrothrombocytopathy). Preoperative and intraoperative platelet transfusions are often required, and packed red blood cells should be easily available. Evaluate renal function with serum concentrations of electrolytes, creatinine, urea, and urine analysis (proteinuria is common, and hematuria or red blood cell casts suggest nephritis), and obtain a nephrology consult if necessary. If renal function is severely altered (rare), check cardiac function with electrocardiogram (arrhythmias as a result of electrolyte abnormalities), and further testing such as echocardiography (with or without dobutamine-stress test) may be necessary to detect decreased cardiac function secondary to long-standing uremia.

Anesthetic considerations: Platelets transfusions should be available in the operating room before any invasive procedure. Avoid regional anesthesia. In case of renal failure (rare), attempt to optimize the patient's preoperative and intraoperative fluid and acid–base status. If large volume shifts and/or blood loss are expected, consider invasive monitoring with arterial line and central venous catheter.

Pharmacological implications: Avoid nephrotoxic drugs (e.g., tetracyclines, aminoglycosides), carefully titrate all anesthetic agents predominantly eliminated by the kidney. Despite proteinuria, the serum protein level is usually within normal limits, and adequate drug-protein binding can be expected.

Other conditions to be considered:

☞**ALPORT SYNDROME:** Familial nephritis characterized by hematuria, proteinuria, nephrotic syndrome (edema, hypoalbuminemia, hyperlipidemia), progressive renal failure, neurosensory hearing loss, and ocular abnormalities (10–15% of patients, nystagmus, cataracts). It accounts for 3% of all cases of chronic renal failure in childhood. Autosomal dominant and X-linked variants have been described.

☞**BERNARD-SOULIER SYNDROME:** Genetic disorder characterized by giant platelets, mild-to-moderate thrombocytopenia, abnormal platelet function, and bleeding out of proportion to the reduced number of platelets.

FECHTNER SYNDROME (Macrothrombocytopathy, Nephritis, Deafness, and Leukocyte Inclusion Syndrome; Alport Syndrome with Leukocyte Inclusions and Macrothrombocytopenia). Can be considered a variant of Epstein syndrome (because the features are very similar, except for the cataracts and the leukocyte inclusion bodies), characterized by a combination of nephritis (with symptoms ranging from microhematuria to end-stage renal failure), high-frequency sensorineural deafness, macrothrombocytopenia, congenital cataracts, and inclusion bodies in neutrophils and eosinophils.

REFERENCES:

Basile C, Schiavone P, Heidet L, et al: Hereditary nephritis with macrothrombocytopenia: Phenotypic variety and the genotypic defect. *J Nephrol* 15:320, 2002.

Bernheim J, Dechavanne M, Bryon PA, et al: Thrombocytopenia, macrothrombocytopathia, nephritis and deafness. *Am J Med* 61:145, 1976.

Seri M, Savino M, Bordo D, et al: Epstein syndrome: Another renal disorder with mutations in the nonmuscle myosin heavy chain 9 gene. *Hum Genet* 110:182, 2002.

Erb and Klumpke Palsy

At a glance: Neonatal brachial plexus palsy caused by obstetric trauma.

Synonyms: Applying to both: Brachial Plexus Injury from Birth Trauma; Obstetric Brachial Plexus Palsy.

For Erb Palsy: Duchenne Erb Palsy.

For Klumpke Palsy: Dejerine-Klumpke Palsy/Paralysis/Syndrome.

History: The first description of (a bilateral) obstetric brachial plexus palsy was reported by the Scottish obstetrician William Smellie (1697–1763) in 1752 in a newborn after difficult labor. In 1861, the famous French neurologist Guillaume Benjamin A. Duchenne (de Boulogne) (1806–1875) analyzed four newborns with brachial palsy and came up with the correct pathogenesis (traction injury). The German neurologist Wilhelm Heinrich Erb (1840–1921) further investigated this topic and concluded in 1875 that a radicular nerve lesion at the level C5 and C6 was responsible for the palsy. At the same time, the American-born neurologist Augusta Marie Dejerine-Klumpke (1859–1927) described lower trunk lesions of the brachial plexus associated with palsy and Horner Syndrome resulting from C8 and T1 lesions.

Incidence: The incidence of obstetric brachial plexus palsy is estimated at 1–3 cases per 1000 live births in industrial countries. Males are more commonly affected than females. The right side is more often affected than the left. In countries with lower average birth weights, it is most likely less frequent.

Genetic inheritance: No genetic component (traumatic brachial plexus injury). However, a history of a previous child with brachial plexus injury carries a high risk of repetition in the next child (no genetic background).

Diagnosis: Clinical findings and history of difficult vaginal delivery (shoulder dystocia or breech presentation). MRI or CT-myelography are used to visualize the lesions.

Four types of brachial plexus injuries are known: *avulsion* is the most severe form where the nerve is torn from the spinal cord. *Rupture* denotes the state where the nerve is torn, but not at the spinal cord level. *Neuroma* describes the state where the nerve has been torn and healed, but scar tissue affects proper signal conduction in the affected nerve. *Neurapraxia*, the most common form of brachial plexus injury, is caused by the damaged, but not torn nerve.

Clinical aspects: The brachial plexus is made up of the nerves exiting the spinal cord from root C5–T1. They form the three trunks: upper (formed by C5 and C6), middle (formed by C7), and lower trunk (formed by C8–T1). Each trunk then divides further to form the cords and finally subdivide further to form radial, median, and ulnar nerve. The injury to the brachial plexus may range from mild palsy to flaccid paralysis.

Four different types of brachial plexus palsy have been defined:

- Erb (-Duchenne) palsy is caused by nerves arising from C5 and C6.
- (Dejerine-) Klumpke palsy results from injury to the nerve fibers at the levels C8 and T1 (although it is controversial if pure C8/T1 lesions are possible). This lesion is rare.
- Lesions affecting C5, C6, and C7 result in upper and middle trunk brachial plexus injury.
- If all levels of the brachial plexus are affected, a total plexus paralysis is diagnosed.

The injury occurs at the time of delivery as a result of excessive stretch of the brachial plexus. This results in palsy or paralysis of muscles supplied by these nerve roots, such as triceps and intrinsic muscles of the hand. Sensory deficits in the corresponding dermatomes do exist, but are difficult to verify in the neonate. Phrenic nerve palsy may be present. Damage to the sympathetic fibers of the first thoracic root results in Horner Syndrome (enophthalmos, ptosis, miosis, and anhydrosis).

Anesthetic considerations: Neurologic deficits should be carefully documented prior to anesthesia. Intravenous access may be challenging, since these babies are often big and only the healthy arm can be used for vascular access (both legs are usually used for the nerve harvesting). Assess for signs of phrenic nerve palsy. The repair of the brachial plexus injury takes several hours. Fixation of the nasal endotracheal tube is crucial to avoid accidental extubation. Appropriate measures should be in place to avoid hypothermia (e.g., convective forced-air warmers, fluid warmers). Blood loss is usually minimal. Fluid overload is a common problem in these patients. Reducing the amount of fluids to 60–70% of the calculated maintenance dose intraoperatively helps to avoid pulmonary edema. Urinary output during this procedure is usually low, but chasing it with repeated fluid boluses may again result in fluid overload. Hypoglycemia is not a common intraoperative problem, however some clinicians prefer to mix a 2.5–5% dextrose containing lactated Ringer's solution.

Pharmacological implications: Succinylcholine, if necessary, is safe to use.

REFERENCES:

Marcus JR, Clarke HM: Management of obstetrical brachial plexus palsy evaluation, prognosis, and primary surgical treatment. *Clin Plast Surg* 30:289, 2003.

Piatt JH Jr: Birth injuries of the brachial plexus. *Clin Perinatol* 32:39, 2005.

Shenaq SM, Bullocks JM, Dhillon G, et al: Management of infant brachial plexus injuries. *Clin Plast Surg* 32:79, 2005.

Erdheim-Chester Disease (ECD)

At a glance: Systemic non-Langerhans cell histiocytic disorder characterized by development of lipoid granulomas in many organs and tissues of the body. Clinical manifestations range from asymptomatic to fatal multisystem involvement.

Synonyms: Lipid Granulomatosis; Polyostotic Sclerosing Histiocytosis.

History: First described by the American pathologist William Chester in 1930. Credit was later also given to Chester's mentor during his time in Vienna, the Austrian pathologist Jakob Erdheim, although he was not an author on the paper.

Incidence: Fewer than 100 cases have been described in the medical literature. Erdheim-Chester disease (ECD) has a male predilection and most often affects adults older than 40 years, although the reported age range is wide.

Genetic inheritance: Etiology is unknown. No genetic basis has been described.

Pathophysiology: ECD results from infiltration of the bones and other tissues by foamy histiocytes. These histiocytes are derived from monocytes/macrophages, lack intracytoplasmic granules (Birbeck granules), and do not stain positive for S-100 protein, which makes them histologically distinguishable from histiocytes derived from Langerhans cells. (However, researchers now have found extensive S-100–positive staining in some ECD histiocytes, so further evaluation seems necessary.) ECD characteristically affects the long bones symmetrically.

Diagnosis: Based on clinical and histopathologic findings. Symmetrical long bone osteosclerosis is the characteristic radiologic finding. However, histologic confirmation is required for the final diagnosis, preferentially from specimens from bone or retrobulbar tissue.

Clinical aspects: ECD is a systemic, xanthogranulomatous, proliferative, infiltrative disease with foamy (lipid-laden) macrophages/histiocytes of unknown etiology. The signs and symptoms are unspecific and mainly result from the histiocytic infiltration of different tissues. The bones most often affected are the femora, tibiae, and fibulae; humeri, ulnae, and radius are less often involved. The axial skeleton is usually spared. The diaphyses and metaphyses of the long bones are characterized by a diffuse or patchy increase in density, coarsening of the trabecular pattern, medullary sclerosis, and cortical thickening. The epiphyses usually are not affected. The most common presenting features include lower limb pain (knees, ankles), exophthalmos, diabetes insipidus, and general symptoms such as fever and weight loss. Retroperitoneal involvement with paraaortic and perirenal infiltration may cause postrenal obstructive uropathy. Pulmonary interstitial involvement is seen in approximately 35% of cases, with the upper parts of the lungs usually being more severely affected. Pulmonary lesions are characterized by interstitial accumulations of histiocytes and fibrosis in a mainly perilymphangitic and subpleural pattern. Computed tomographic scanning may demonstrate centrilobular nodularity and thickening of the interlobular septa and the visceral pleura. Other nonbony sites affected may include skin (pruritic rash, xanthelasma, periorbital xanthomata), retroorbital tissue (resulting in exophthalmos and rarely blindness), and central nervous system (dural and falcine masses possibly compressing the brain, seizures, dysarthria, cerebellar symptoms such as nystagmus, hypermetric saccades, negative suppression of the vestibuloocular reflex, dysmetria and ataxia, and diabetes insipidus with polyuria and polydipsia from infiltration of the pituitary gland). Pericardial effusion and hepatosplenomegaly have been described. Jaw infiltration (mandibula and maxilla) resulting in periodontitis and loss of teeth has been reported in a small number of patients. The clinical course is quite variable. Steroids, chemotherapy (vincristine, vinblastine, cy-

clophosphamide, doxorubicin), radiotherapy, immunotherapy (cyclosporin, interferon-α-2A), and surgery have all been used with various success in the treatment of this disease. Reports about response to therapy and overall survival are limited and highly variable; however, survival after diagnosis in the largest study was approximately 32 months, with pulmonary fibrosis, respiratory distress, and/or heart failure the most common causes of death.

Precautions before anesthesia: Pulmonary involvement must be assessed by clinical examination, chest radiograph, and pulmonary function tests (including arterial blood gas analysis) often revealing moderate restrictive lung disease and reduced carbon monoxide diffusion capacity. Cardiac/pericardial involvement should be evaluated by echocardiography. Look for cor pulmonale in patients with significant pulmonary symptoms. Urine analysis and serum levels of electrolytes, creatinine, and urea should be checked in the presence of suspected renal disease. In addition, plasma and urine osmolality should be checked preoperatively to exclude diabetes insipidus, because it may cause electrolyte abnormalities and water depletion, if left untreated. Therapy with vasopressin is usually successful. A complete blood count is recommended, because medullary sclerosis could theoretically affect hemopoiesis. Assess dental status for vulnerability during direct laryngoscopy.

Anesthetic considerations: The choice of anesthetic technique is guided by the degree of organ compromise from the disease. A urinary catheter may be helpful to diagnose diabetes insipidus and follow-up of the effect of vasopressin. Attention should be paid to protecting the eyes in the presence of exophthalmos. Depending on the chemotherapy drugs that have been used, high oxygen concentrations may not be appropriate (in order to prevent pulmonary oxygen toxicity).

Pharmacological implications: These patients may be on oral steroid therapy, and perioperative stress coverage may be required. Careful dosage (titration) of predominantly renally excreted drugs in the presence of decreased kidney function is recommended.

Other conditions to be considered:

☞**HISTIOCYTOSIS:** Group of disorders characterized by infiltration and accumulation of histiocytes in various tissues, such as the skin, bones, brain, lungs, spleen, and liver. Despite nonmalignant growth, the prognosis is poor.

☞**GAUCHER DISEASE:** Most common inherited lipid storage disease, particularly common in Ashkenazi Jewish people (Eastern European ancestry). Accumulation of glucocerebrosides (derived from red blood cells) in many tissues, especially the macrophages in the bone marrow (the normal functions of which are impaired). Significant-to-major anesthetic implications.

☞**NIEMANN-PICK DISEASE:** Group of rare inherited disorders of fat metabolism. Lysosomal storage disorder caused by a defect in sphingolipid metabolism and involving brain and/or viscera. Clinical features include jaundice, progressive loss of motor skills, feeding difficulties, learning disabilities, and hepatosplenomegaly.

REFERENCES:

Shamburek RD, Brewer HB Jr, Gochuico BR: Erdheim-Chester disease: A rare multisystem histiocytic disorder associated with interstitial lung disease. *Am J Med Sci* 321:66, 2001.

Wright RA, Hermann R, Parisi J: Neurological manifestations of Erdheim-Chester disease. *J Neurol Neurosurg Psychiatry* 66:72, 1999.

Eronen Syndrome

At a glance: Very rare disorder characterized by severe digital, renal, and cerebral malformations.

Synonyms: Eronen Somer Gustafsson Syndrome; Digitorenocerebral (DRC) Syndrome.

Incidence: Unknown. Fewer than a dozen case reports since its first description by Eronen in 1985.

Genetic inheritance: Autosomal recessive with variable clinical expression.

Pathophysiology: Unknown.

Diagnosis: Mainly based on clinical features, neurologic studies (CT and/or MRI scan of the brain, electroencephalogram, auditory and brainstem evoked potentials), urologic imaging (ultrasonography examination, intravenous pyelogram), and radiographs of the hands and feet.

Clinical aspects: Absent distal phalanges with dysplastic or absent nails of all fingers and toes are a constant feature of this syndrome and result in brachydactyly. Renal manifestations are variable and may include unilateral agenesis, cystic dysplasia, or double kidney with two ureters and two renal arteries. Facial features are a high and sloping forehead, wide nasal bridge, short nose with full tip and wide base, low-set ears, high arched palate, and gingival hyperplasia. Neurologic manifestations are variable but always severe: microcephaly, cerebral atrophy, dilated cerebral ventricles, Dandy-Walker malformation, severe seizures, muscular hypotonia, and blindness with optic nerve atrophy. Respiratory distress, heart murmurs, and cyanosis have been described in some patients, with further examination leading to the diagnosis of atelectases, patent ductus arteriosus, small ventriculoseptal defect, or open foramen ovale. Profound mental retardation is a permanent feature. The majority of patients die in infancy, with very few surviving beyond age 2 years. Increased levels of plasma and urinary 2-oxoglutarate are common findings.

Precautions before anesthesia: Obtain full assessment of the neurologic status and check for the presence of increased intracranial pressure. Evaluate the efficacy and eventual toxicity of antiepileptic treatment and the degree of muscular hypotonia. Renal function is usually adequate, but blood electrolytes and creatinine levels should be obtained.

Anesthetic considerations: Because of the high arched palate and gingival hypertrophy, intubation may be challenging. The increased risk of aspiration warrants a rapid-sequence induction. In the presence of hypotonia, avoidance of succinylcholine (because of potential severe hyperkalemia) is recommended. Instead, use of a nondepolarizing muscle relaxant with a rapid onset of action is preferred (e.g., rocuronium). In the presence of increased intracranial pressure, intravenous lidocaine on induction may help decrease systemic hypertension associated with laryngoscopy. Mild hyperventilation lowers the intracranial pressure, and a 10- to 30-degree head-up position improves cerebral venous drainage.

Pharmacological implications: In the presence of a seizure disorder, avoid potentially epileptogenic drugs such as methohexital, ketamine, enflurane, atracurium, *cis*-atracurium, and meperidine (applies to the latter three only if given in large quantities because of their metabolites, laudanosine and normeperidine, respectively). Cautious titration of nondepolarizing muscle relaxants (under control of nerve stimulator) is required in the presence of muscular hypotonia (increased sensitivity to their effects). If renal function is decreased, adjustment of drugs with predominantly renal elimination (e.g., some muscle relaxants and antibiotics) may be required.

Other conditions to be considered:

☞**Brachymorphism-Onychodysplasia-Dysphalangism Syndrome:** Presumed genetic disorder causing short stature, hand abnormalities, and mild intellectual impairment.

☞**Coffin-Siris Syndrome:** Probably autosomal dominant transmitted syndrome with developmental delay. Hypoplasia of the nails and phalanges is confined to toes and the fifth digit. Sparse scalp hair, bushy eyebrows, wide mouth, hirsutism, prominent or hypertrophied lips. Mental retardation is less severe than in Eronen syndrome.

☞**DOOR Syndrome:** Characterized by onychodystrophy, triphalangeal thumbs, mental retardation, seizures, sensorineural deafness, and progressive blindness. In contrast to the Eronen syndrome, urine organic acid analysis shows an up to 10-fold increase of 2-oxoglutarate excretion. Some authors assume this is the same as Eronen syndrome.

REFERENCES:

Eronen M, Somer M, Gustafsson B, et al: New syndrome: A digito-reno-cerebral syndrome. *Am J Med Genet* 22:281, 1985.

Le Merrer M, David A, Goutieres F, et al: Digito-reno-cerebral syndrome: Confirmation of Eronen syndrome. *Clin Genet* 42:196, 1992.

Winter RM: Eronen syndrome identical with DOOR syndrome? *Clin Genet* 43:167, 1993.

Erythema Multiforme (EM)

At a glance: Acute mucocutaneous hypersensitivity reaction of variable severity characterized by symmetrical skin eruptions, with or without mucous membrane lesions.

Synonyms: Erythema Polyforme (French appellation); EM.

Classification: EM minor form or EM major form (Stevens-Johnson syndrome).

History: The terminology of the disorder is confusing, and the many names represent the spectrum of one disease that is part of mucocutaneous syndromes. Historically, erythemas were first described by Willan in 1808, but the fact that they are different clinical presentations of the same entity was first noted by Hebra in 1860. Then, in 1916 Rendu described mucosal lesions with or without skin lesions, which were later named "ectodermosis erosiva pluriorificialis" by Fiessinger in 1923. Meanwhile, in 1922 the American and English literature reported the association of skin and mucosal lesions with a systemic reaction, the Stevens-Johnson syndrome. The common nature of all these conditions was noticed in 1965 by Ströhm, who gave them the term "mucocutaneous fever." Currently, this entity is considered an immunologic disease that may be linked to the presence of HLA-B15.

Incidence: The reported incidence of EM is 0.03 to 0.1% in the general population. Males are affected more often than females (ratio of 3:1). The majority of cases occur in individuals younger than 20 years. The disease is almost nonexistent in those younger than 3 years and older than 50 years. The disease is recurrent in approximately 30% of cases. The incidence of drug-related cases of EM major is equal in males and females.

Genetic inheritance: Not a genetic disorder, although a genetic predisposition has been discussed.

Pathophysiology: Can be caused by drugs (nonsteroidal antiinflammatory drugs (e.g., ibuprofen, naproxen, valdecoxib, oxaprozin), sulfonamides, penicillins, cephalosporins, erythromycin, tuberculostatics, salicylates, pyrazolones, carbamazepine, phenobarbital, phenytoin), viral (e.g., adenovirus, herpes simplex virus, Epstein-Barr virus, cytomegalovirus, hepatitis A and B virus, measles virus, varicella virus, mumps virus, influenza virus, coxsackie virus B5), bacterial (e.g., *Proteus* species, *Salmonella* species, *Mycobacterium* species, *Brucella* species, *Corynebacterium diphtheriae*), fungal (e.g., histoplasmosis), parasitic (e.g., coccidiosis) or mycoplasma infections, endocrine factors, neoplasms, collagen diseases, sarcoidosis, and physical factors. However, of all the possible causative factors, only drugs, herpes simplex, and mycoplasma have been implicated without doubt. The disease is speculated to be caused mainly by a cell-mediated hypersensitivity reaction to a drug or another type of antigen. Humoral involvement with the presence of IgM and C3 are part of the immunologic reaction. These immune complexes are found in the vasculature and at the dermal-epidermal junction and cause vasculitis and skin lesions.

Diagnosis: Results of laboratory tests are nonspecific and may show leukocytosis and an elevated erythrocyte sedimentation rate. The diagnosis is clinical, based on the presence of typical skin and mucosal lesions, with or without systemic involvement. Drug history and possible recent infections should be taken into account.

Clinical aspects: In its *minor form,* the disease is characterized by a self-limited course with a duration of 1 to 4 weeks. The prodromal symptoms are compatible with an upper respiratory tract infection, and the skin lesions usually appear after 7 to 10 days. The typical cutaneous manifestations are the target or iris lesions, which are symmetrical and present mostly on the dorsum of the hands and feet, palms, and soles, and finally on the extensor surfaces of the limb. After a few days, the center of the lesion changes to a cyanotic reddish color surrounded by a lighter peripheral ring. Blisters may form in the center. In the end, the lesions retract and leave a transient hyperpigmentation. Symptoms are mild and consist mainly of a burning sensation. Mucosal involvement is present in only 25% of cases and usually limited to modest oral erosions of short duration. In all cases, complete healing takes approximately 2 weeks.

In the *majus* or *major* or *Stevens-Johnson form,* the disease is characterized by a more important prodromal episode with high fever, asthenia, malaise, muscular pain associated with migrant arthralgia, diarrhea, vomiting, and pharyngitis. After a few days, skin and mostly mucosal lesions, which are always present in this form of the disease, appear. The mucosal involvement is severe and usually involves two or more mucosal sites simultaneously (minimum of two sites is required for the diagnosis). In the worst cases, the pharynx, larynx, bronchial mucosa, and esophagus are involved. The mucosal lesions rapidly change to blisters, which in turn ulcerate and produce painful erosions resulting in significant swallowing problems. The eyes can be affected by the disease in the form of purulent conjunctivitis and permanent visual loss in up to 10%. The skin lesions are also more extensive in this form, and massive denudation of the skin can be seen with transudation of proteins. Of note, the skin manifestations are asymmetrical in the Stevens-Johnson form. In the majus form, healing is complete in the great majority of cases, but the course of the disease is longer, lasting for up to 6 weeks. Death is rare but has been reported. Corticosteroids and cyclosporin A can be used for treatment of severe forms.

Precautions before anesthesia: No patient should undergo an elective surgical procedure during the acute episode, especially with Stevens-Johnson syndrome. However, anesthesia may be required

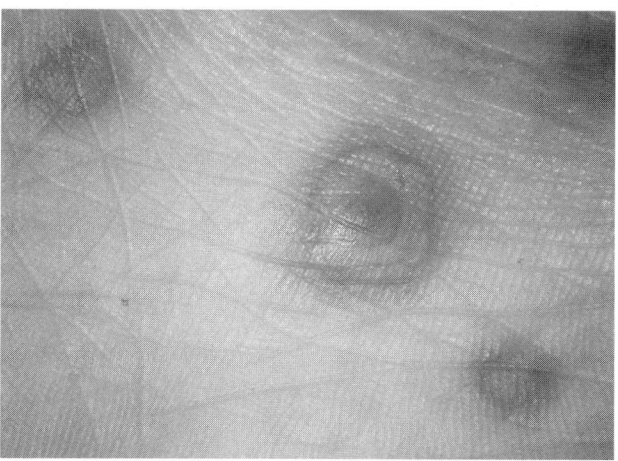

Erythema Multiforme Typical iris or target lesions and a central blister on the palm of a patient with erythema multiforme.

for dressing changes and skin debridement. A complete blood count and serum concentrations of electrolytes and albumin should be obtained. Because fluid losses through the skin defects may be significant, adequate volume status should be ensured before induction of anesthesia. A chest radiograph should be obtained.

Anesthetic considerations: Affected patients should be considered like ☞ Epidermolysis Bullosa patients. The presence of lesions in the respiratory tract can result in pulmonary blebs and increase the risk of pneumothorax. Vascular access may be challenging in the presence of extensive skin lesions.

Pharmacological implications: Many drugs are involved in the development of EM (see *Pathophysiology).* In the severe forms, hypalbuminemia results in an increased free fraction and efficacy of drugs with high protein binding.

Other conditions to be considered:

☞**Epidermolysis Bullosa:** Genetic disorder characterized by cutaneous blistering and scarring following already minor trauma. More than 20 different subtypes of the disease have been grouped into three main categories: epidermolysis bullosa simplex, dystrophic epidermolysis bullosa, and junctional epidermolysis bullosa.

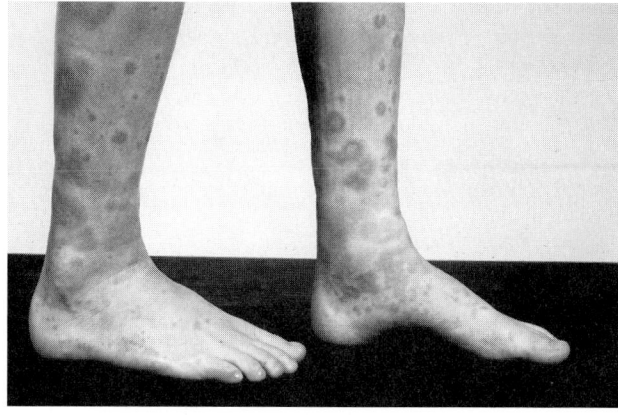

Erythema Multiforme More extensive form of erythema multiforme affecting both legs in a patient who received sulfonamides for treatment of a urinary tract infection.

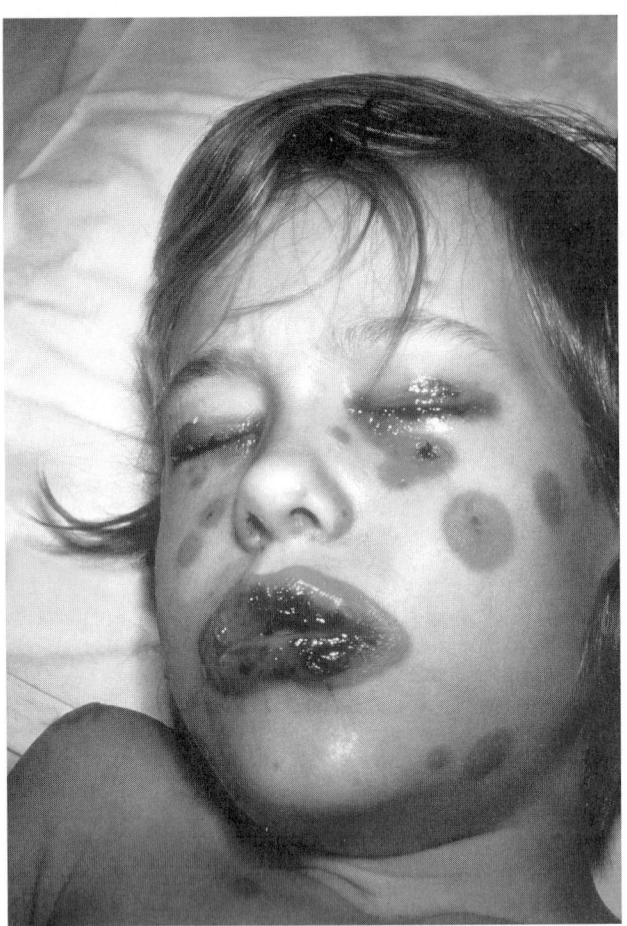

Stevens-Johnson Syndrome Facial manifestation of Stevens-Johnson syndrome in a 9-year-old boy.

☞**LYELL SYNDROME:** Severe allergic syndrome characterized by extensive bullous eruptions of the skin and mucous membranes, fever, malaise, conjunctivitis, and diffuse erythema. Often lethal in children.

☞**DANBOLT-CLOSS SYNDROME:** Inherited vesiculobullous disorder characterized by intermittent simultaneous occurrence of

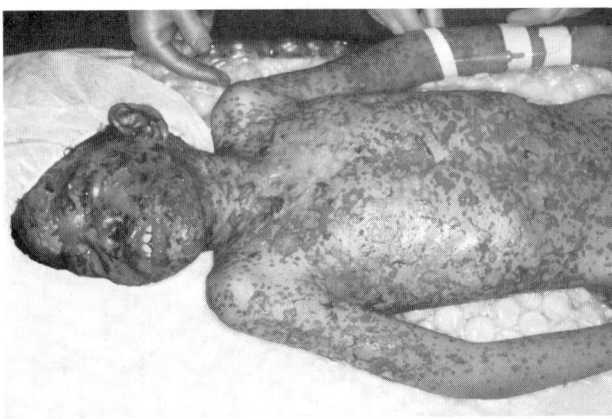

Stevens-Johnson Syndrome Severest form of Stevens-Johnson syndrome, with generalized skin involvement, in a 10-year-old girl.

diarrhea and bullous dermatitis (dry lesions surrounding the mouth, ears, nose, and eyes, but also affecting the fingers, feet, and knees) and failure to thrive in premature babies. In children, periorificial lesions of the face and anogenital region. Alopecia and absence of eyebrows, eyelashes, and thymus are common.

REFERENCES:

Auquier-Dunant A, Mockenhaupt M, Naldi L, et al: Correlations between clinical patterns and causes of erythema multiforme majus, Stevens-Johnson syndrome, and toxic epidermal necrolysis: Results of an international prospective study. *Arch Dermatol* 138:1019, 2002.

Ayangco L, Rogers RS: Oral manifestations of erythema multiforme. *Dermatol Clin* 21:195, 2003.

Forman R, Koren G, Shear NH: Erythema multiforme, Stevens-Johnson syndrome and toxic epidermal necrolysis in children: A review of 10 years' experience. *Drug Saf* 25:965, 2002.

Erythromelalgia

At a glance: Disorder characterized by vasodilatation associated with paroxysmal, intense burning pain and episodic reddening of the extremities (mainly feet). The symptoms of redness, heat, pain, and swelling, when not associated with an organic disease, constitute the primary form, which has also been termed "erythermalgia" because of the significance of the heat. The secondary or acquired form is related to underlying medical conditions.

Synonyms: Acromelalgia; Erythermalgia; Gerhardt Disease; Weir-Mitchell Disease.

History: The first case was reported by the Irish physician Richard James Graves in 1834. The American physician Silas Weir Mitchell suggested the term "Erythromelalgia" in 1878, and the German physician Carl Jakob Gerhardt provided further insights into erythromelalgia in 1892.

Incidence: Approximately 0.25:100,000 in the general population.

Genetic inheritance: Autosomal dominant inheritance for primary erythromelalgia susceptibility, with the responsible gene located on chromosome 2q31-32.

Pathophysiology: Pathogenesis unknown. Proposed mechanisms involve abnormalities in platelet aggregation, with contributing factors such as vessel wall damage, changes in blood flow patterns, and disturbances in prostaglandin metabolism. Intravascular platelet aggregation appears to play a major role. Endothelial cells in affected areas appear swollen with enlarged nuclei. Smooth muscle cell proliferation and vacuolization of the cytoplasm in the tunica media of the vessels and deposition of interstitial collagen lead to narrowing of the vessels lumen. The internal elastic lamina seems to be split between the proliferated smooth muscle cells resulting in a picture of fibromuscular intimal proliferation, which is (with or without occlusive intravascular thrombosis) a specific erythromelalgia finding. Arterioles are frequently occluded by thrombi rich in platelets or which become completely fibrotic in the presence of peripheral necrosis. Immunofluorescence findings have failed to indicate a specific inflammatory process. It seems therefore that erythromelalgia is not a separate disease entity but rather a pathophysiologic response (microvascular arteriovenous shunting) of the skin microcirculation, with shunting induced by opening of anatomical arteriovenous anastomosis normally present in hands, feet, nose, and ears, or by angioneogenesis.

Diagnosis: Primary and secondary/acquired types occurred. The primary type occurs in children, especially boys, whereas the secondary form is found almost entirely in adults who have an underlying disease (typically polycythemia vera, essential thrombocythemia, chronic myelogenous leukemia, and idiopathic myelofibrosis and other forms of myeloproliferative disorders) but may also include connective tissue disorders, autoimmune collagen vascular diseases (e.g., rheumatoid arthritis, ☞Systemic Lupus Erythematosus), infectious diseases (e.g., AIDS), neurologic diseases (e.g., multiple sclerosis, neuropathies), cardiovascular disorders (e.g., arterial hypertension, arteriosclerosis), diabetes mellitus, and drugs (e.g., iodine contrast injection, vaccinations, calcium antagonists). The clinical appearance of both primary and secondary forms is basically identical. The pathognomonic diagnostic criterion of secondary erythromelalgia is rapid pain relief that lasts a few days after one low dose of aspirin, which irreversibly inhibits platelet cyclooxygenase activity. Heat intolerance (and aggravation of symptoms with standing or exercise) and relief of symptoms with cooling (and elevation of the affected body part and rest) are hallmarks of erythromelalgia, whereas warmth exposure not only triggers flaring but also increases the severity of the episode. Pain relief from immersing the affected body parts in ice water is considered almost pathognomonic for the disease (similarly, immersing a limb in warm water may trigger an attack). In all cases of newly diagnosed erythromelalgia, polycythemia, thrombocythemia, and other diseases (neuropathies) must be excluded by appropriate laboratory and diagnostic studies. Regular followups are recommended.

Clinical aspects: Onset of erythromelalgia may be gradual, with some cases remaining mild and unchanged for decades but in other cases beginning acutely and spreading or becoming disabling within a few weeks. Episodes of erythromelalgia may occur spontaneously or are more commonly provoked by heat (in most patients, distress is triggered by ambient temperatures from 29–32°C), exercise, or dependency of limbs. A dusky red or cyanotic color change in the hands or feet is accompanied by intense pain and a sensation of heat. The episodes may be brief initially but with time may last longer. In primary erythromelalgia, the feet and lower legs are affected, with relative sparing of the toes. In contrast, in the secondary form, the burning pain and red congestion preferentially involve one or more toes or fingers or the sole of the forefoot. Typically the episodes are bilateral; however, unilateral occurrence has been described, particularly in secondary cases. In severe forms of erythromelalgia, the vasodilatation may be bilateral and spread proximally up the legs or arms, from the lower to upper limbs or vice versa, or to the face or ears. Some patients describe a diurnal cycle in their symptoms, which are most often worse in the evening or at night. The therapy is directed at reversal of the precipitating causes, applications of cold packs, and administration of indomethacin. Erythromelalgia vanishes with lowering of the platelet count to normal levels with chemotherapy in myeloproliferative disorders. A number of drugs have been used for treatment of erythromelalgia with varying success (e.g., vasoactive drugs [ephedrine, propranolol, calcium antagonists, α_2-agonists], aspirin, serotonin-reuptake inhibitors [fluoxetine, sertraline], anticonvulsants [gabapentin], misoprostol). The same applies for epidural anesthetics and other forms of sympathetic blockade. Allodynia and paresthesias have been described by some patients.

Precautions before anesthesia: Ask about precipitating causes of attacks and drug therapy. If secondary/acquired erythromelalgia is present, take steps to account for the primary disease process, such as phlebotomy and isovolemic hemodilution for polycythemia vera.

Obtain a complete blood count and coagulation status, including bleeding time.

Anesthetic considerations: Avoid factors that precipitate an attack (e.g., aggressive warming techniques). In this instance, mild perioperative hypothermia is preferred. Careful positioning of the limbs to avoid dependency is recommended. Expose feet and hands outside of blankets or covers and try to maintain the patient below the critical temperature that triggers symptoms. When present, erythromelalgia pain is often resistant to a wide range of analgesic therapies, including high-dose narcotics.

Pharmacological implications: Patients are often taking a number of different medications, so interactions with anesthetic drugs are possible.

Other conditions to be considered:

☞**Raynaud Syndrome:** Disorder characterized by shortlasting vasospasms of the small arteries of the arms and legs, hands, and feet. Usually diagnosed before age 40 years.

Reflex Sympathetic Dystrophy Syndrome: Also known as CRPS. Progressive disease of the autonomic nervous system that can follow a simple trauma, heart problems, infections, surgery, spinal cord injuries, or major trauma.

Shoulder-Hand Syndrome: Variant of the reflex sympathetic dystrophy syndrome that affects the feet and the hands after an injury.

References:

Cohen JS: Erythromelalgia: New theories and new therapies. *J Am Acad Dermatol* 43:841, 2000.

Kalgaard OM, Seem E, Kvernebo K: Erythromelalgia: A clinical study of 87 cases. *J Intern Med* 242:191, 1997.

Sandroni P, Davis MDP, Low PA et al: Neurophysiologic characteristics of patients with erythromelalgia. A retrospective study. *Neurology* 48: 130, 1997.

Tarach JS, Nowicka-Tarach BM, Matuszek B, et al: Erythromelalgia— A thrombotic complication in chronic myeloproliferative disorders. *Med Sci Monit* 6:204, 2000.

Erythropoietic Protoporphyria

At a glance: Rare genetically transmitted disorder of the porphyrin-heme in which reduced activity of the enzyme ferrochelatase leads to accumulation of protoporphyrins in erythrocytes with cutaneous and systemic manifestations.

Synonyms: Congenital Erythropoietic Protoporphyria; Erythrohepatic Protoporphyria; Heme Synthetase Deficiency; Protoporphyria.

Genetic inheritance: Mode of inheritance in erythropoietic protoporphyria (EPP) is complex and can be either autosomal dominant with low clinical penetrance, as is in most cases, or autosomal recessive. The gene for human ferrochelatase (FECH) has been mapped to 18q21.3.

Pathophysiology: The basic defect affects the mitochondrial enzyme ferrochelatase. The nature of the defect on the molecular level is uncertain. Protoporphyrin diffuses from the erythrocytes into the plasma to be bound to albumin and the heme-binding protein hemopexin. Protoporphyrin deposits in the skin are responsible for the extreme photosensitivity. The excess porphyrin comes from both erythropoietic and hepatic tissues. Ultraviolet light photoactivates protoporphyrins that then cause tissue damage by release of free oxygen radicals, which manifests as photosensitivity.

Diagnosis: Fluorescence of a significant proportion of red blood cells is detectable by ultraviolet microscopy because of the presence of free erythrocyte protoporphyrin. A reduction in the activity of the enzyme ferrochelatase (also called heme synthase, a mitochondrial enzyme responsible for the final step in the heme synthesis pathway, which is the incorporation of ferrous iron into protoporphyrin) to 10 to 25% of normal levels has been demonstrated. This is unlike the other dominantly inherited forms of porphyria, in which only a 50% reduction of activity of the specific enzyme is observed.

Clinical aspects: Stinging or burning of the skin may result within 1 hour of sun exposure. This is followed by edema and erythema. Solar urticaria, petechiae, vesicles, purpura, and crustification may develop and last for several days. Late skin changes include thickening of the skin with a waxy appearance, shallow pits, and linear creases on the face (particularly cheeks and nose). Artificial lights, particularly operating room lamps, may cause photosensitivity. Cholelithiasis is fairly common (in approximately 30% of patients) and may present at an unusually early age. Hepatic cholestasis is rare (1–4% of patients) but often has a severe course. Rarely, hemolytic or mild hypochromic anemia is present, and mild (nonhemolytic) anemia has been described in up to 25% of cases. Polyneuropathy and quadriparesis may occur. Excessive protoporphyrin is excreted in bile, and hence in feces, but not in urine because protoporphyrin is only poorly water-soluble. It may be deposited in the liver, resulting in progressive and even fatal liver damage. Management includes avoidance of exposure to sunlight (ensure that the chosen sunscreen also protects in the 400-nm range, as common commercial sunscreens often only effectively block light with a wavelength of approximately 300 nm) and/or skin protection by parenteral administration of beta-carotene. Liver disease may be ameliorated by treatment with cholestyramine (to prevent enterohepatic recirculation of protoporphyrin), activated charcoal, and bile salts.

Precautions before anesthesia: In general, EPP is considered a benign disorder with clinical symptoms mainly affecting the skin. Although it should not be confused with hepatic porphyrias, abnormalities of the liver and biliary tract are not uncommon. Even rapidly progressive liver disease and cirrhosis have been described, so the presence and severity of hepatic involvement must be evaluated. Laboratory investigations should include a complete blood count, serum concentrations of electrolytes, urea, and creatinine, and liver function tests (including coagulation test in jaundiced patients). Hepatobiliary ultrasound may be indicated if symptoms of cholelithiasis are present. Avoid intramuscular premedication in patients with coagulopathy.

Anesthetic considerations: Anemia may require treatment prior to surgery. Perioperative maintenance of appropriate hemoglobin levels is desirable because it may reduce hemoglobin synthesis and therefore minimize protoporphyrin levels. In patients without significant hepatic involvement, the anesthetic technique is dictated by the planned procedure and the surgical requirements. Patients with significant hepatic impairment should be managed according to the severity of the dysfunction. Operating room lamp filters should be used (yellow acrylate) to prevent exposure of the patient to light with wavelengths near 400 nm. Recovery should be conducted in a dimly lit room or in a room with light filters if possible.

Pharmacological implications: Morphine may induce or exacerbate spasms of the sphincter of Oddi. The action of succinylcholine may be prolonged in patients with severe hepatic impairment. Pan-curonium and vecuronium actions may be prolonged in such patients, and atracurium or cisatracurium may be preferred. Succinylcholine should be avoided in the quadriplegic patient. Attacks in EPP are not triggered by drugs.

REFERENCES:

Asokumar B, Kierney C, James TW, et al: Anaesthetic management of a patient with erythropoietic protoporphyria for ventricular septal defect closure. *Paediatr Anaesth* 9:356, 1999.

Jensen NF, Fiddler DS, Striepe V: Anesthetic considerations in porphyrias. *Anesth Analg* 80:591, 1995.

Sarkany RP: Erythropoietic protoporphyria (EPP) at 40. Where are we now? *Photodermatol Photoimmunol Photomed* 18:147, 2002.

Torrance JM: Anaesthetic management of erythropoietic protoporphyria. *Paediatr Anaesth* 10:571, 2000.

Essential Thrombocythemia

At a glance: Chronic myeloproliferative disorder caused by a clonal increase in platelets resulting in thromboembolic and hemorrhagic complications.

Synonyms: Primary Thrombocytosis; Idiopathic Thrombocytosis; Hemorrhagic Thrombocytosis.

Incidence: Estimated at 1.4–2.5:100,000 per year. Overall, both genders are approximately equally affected; however, there is a predilection for females at younger ages. Although the majority of patients at presentation are approximately 60 years old, approximately 20% of the patients are younger than 40 years. Only rarely has essential thrombocytosis (ET) been described in children.

Genetic inheritance: Rare familial form with autosomal dominant transmission has been described. However, in the vast majority of patients, no genetic background is detectable.

Pathophysiology: Not fully elucidated yet. ET is caused by proliferation of megakaryocytes, of which the exact pathogenesis remains to be elucidated. However, evidence now indicates that a mutation of the thrombopoietin gene (located on 3q26.3-q27) may play a major role. Thrombopoietin is the key hormone in the regulation of megakaryocyte differentiation and proliferation. The mechanisms by which ET leads to thromboembolic and hemorrhagic complications remain unclear, although different laboratory findings have been used to explain them (intrinsic abnormality of the platelets resulting in hypoaggregation and hyperaggregation of platelets, anomalies or decreased concentrations of "von Willebrand factor," or deficiencies of proteins C and S and/or antithrombin III).

Diagnosis: Based on the clinical findings of a sustained, not otherwise explained platelet count greater than 600×10^9/liter, a hematocrit less than 40 (mild erythrocytosis is present in approximately one third of patients, while others have a mild hypochromic, microcytic anemia), and normal or increased leukocyte count. The mean platelet volume usually is increased, but microcytosis has also been described. Giant platelets can be found in the peripheral blood smear. A bone marrow aspirate and biopsy are needed and show an increased cellularity with megalokaryocytic predominance (often in clumps or sheets). Increased red and white cell hyperplasia are common. The stainable iron in the bone marrow, serum ferritin levels, and mean corpuscular erythrocyte volume are normal. Bone marrow fibrosis is either absent or affects less than one third of the biopsy area. No cytogenetic or morphologic evidence of a myelodysplastic syndrome can be found. No cause for reactive thrombocytosis. Essential thrombocythemia is diagnosed once reactive thrombocytosis has been excluded.

Clinical aspects: Up to 50% of patients present with microvascular occlusions (e.g., fingers and toes with risk of gangrene if left untreated, priapism), whereas major vessel occlusions (e.g., coronary, renal and femoral arteries, or hepatic-vein thrombosis [☞Budd-Chiari Syndrome], portal vein, splenic, or femoral vein thrombosis) are less common. Cerebrovascular infarction, transient ischemic attacks, and myocardial infarction, although common in elderly patients, are less common in young patients. Pulmonary embolism is a common finding and may result in chronic pulmonary artery hypertension. Hemorrhage can be a presenting feature, is generally not severe, and often is associated with platelet counts greater than 1000×10^9/liter, with the gastrointestinal tract (duodenum) the most common site of bleeding. Other sites of bleeding may include the urogenital tract, skin, gums, eyes, and central nervous system. Results of screening tests of coagulation usually are normal, but bleeding time may be prolonged. Splenomegaly and hepatomegaly (less common) are present in a significant number of patients. B symptoms (weight loss, fever, sweating) but also pruritus have been described in up to one third of patients. The risk of transformation into an acute leukemia reported in the literature varies between 2% and 20%. Death is usually the result of thromboembolic complications. Ten-year survival may be as high as 80%. Aspirin is the mainstay of management against recurrent thrombotic events (and places these patients at high risk for bleeding). Hydroxyurea, busulphan, and pipobroman have been used to lower very high platelet counts, although they may increase the rate of conversion to acute leukemia (leukemogenicity). This has suggested use of a conservative approach to management in younger patients. Anagrelide (an imidazoquinazoline compound that not only inhibits platelet aggregation but also results in suppression of megakaryocyte maturation with a decreased platelet count) has been used successfully to reduce the platelet count, while α-interferon currently is being investigated for use in ET. Plateletpheresis is used for patients with acute cerebrovascular complications or digital ischemia, for which rapid reduction of the platelet count is required.

Precautions before anesthesia: A full examination for past or recent vascular occlusions, especially affecting the central nervous and/or cardiovascular systems but also kidneys and liver, is mandatory. A 12-lead electrocardiogram can help diagnose recent or old infarctions, major pulmonary embolism, or pulmonary hypertension. Echocardiography may be required to assess myocardial function and detect myocardial wall-motion abnormalities, myocardial scars from infarction and/or cor pulmonale, and signs of pulmonary hypertension. Laboratory investigations should include a complete blood count, coagulation studies (including bleeding time), serum concentrations of electrolytes (pseudohyperkalemia resulting from thrombocytosis), phosphate, urea, creatinine, and urate, and renal function. Pseudohypoxemia has been described in some patients, which is explained by the increased oxygen consumption in stored blood samples (so transport on ice and rapid processing of blood samples is recommended). Ensure appropriate fluid resuscitation and consider prophylaxis against thromboembolism. In approximately one third of patients, anagrelide may cause vasodilatory and positive inotropic effects, fluid retention, palpitations, arrhythmias, heart failure, and headache. Another side effect of this treatment may be a progressive anemia.

Anesthetic considerations: Ensure normovolemia throughout the perioperative period to minimize the risk of vascular occlusions and thromboembolic events. Avoid or limit the use of tourniquets when possible. Regional anesthesia has been used successfully; however, careful timing with thromboembolism prophylaxis and assessment of bleeding time is mandatory preoperatively, particularly for central neuraxial blockade.

Pharmacological implications: No known specific implications for this condition.

Other condition to be considered:

☞**ERYTHROMELALGIA:** Disorder characterized by vasodilatation associated with paroxysmal, intense burning pain and episodic reddening of the extremities (mainly feet). The symptoms of redness, heat, pain, and swelling, when not associated with an organic disease, constitute the primary form, which has also been termed "erythermalgia" because of the significance of the heat. The secondary or acquired form is related to underlying medical conditions.

REFERENCES:

Bazzan M, Tamponi G, Schinco P, et al: Thrombosis-free survival and life expectancy in 187 consecutive patients with essential thrombocythemia. *Ann Hematol* 78: 539, 1999.

Mesa R, Silverstein M, Jacobsen S, et al: Population based incidence and survival figures in essential thrombocythemia and agnogenic myeloid metaplasia: An Olmsted County Study, 1976–1995. *Am J Hematol* 61:10, 1999.

Murphy S, Peterson P, Lland H, et al: Experience of the Polycythemia Vera Study Group with essential thrombocythemia: A final report on diagnostic criteria, survival, and leukaemic transition by treatment. *Semin Hematol* 34:29, 1997.

Michiels JJ, Thiele J: Clinical and pathological criteria for the diagnosis of essential thrombocythemia, polycythemia vera, and idiopathic myelofibrosis (agnogenic myeloid metaplasia). *Int J Hematol* 76:133, 2002.

F Syndrome

At a glance: Skeletal dysplasia, broad short thumbs, and pectoral and sternal deformities. Assess vertebral anomalies by radiologic examination of spine. Spina bifida occulta may be present.

Synonyms: Acropectorovertebral Dysplasia; Opitz F Syndrome.

Incidence and genetic inheritance: Autosomal dominant. Fewer than 15 cases reported in the literature.

Clinical aspects: Skeletal dysplasia, broad short thumbs, distal thumb phalanx duplication, thumb and index finger syndactyly, fused capitate and hamate, syndactyly of toes, malformed toes. Pectoral and sternal deformities. Vertebral anomalies and spina bifida occulta at L5 or S1.

Anesthetic considerations: Assess vertebral anomalies by radiologic examination of spine. Because spina bifida occulta may be present, there is an increased risk of dural puncture with lumbar extradural block.

Pharmacological implications: No specific pharmacological implications.

Other condition to be considered:

GROSSE SYNDROME (Cranioacrofacial Syndrome): Autosomal dominant condition characterized by cardiac anomalies (ventricular septal defect, pulmonic stenosis), narrow head and face, minor head anomalies, and Dupuytren contractures.

REFERENCES:

Grosse F, Herrmann J, Opitz JM: The F-form of acropectorovertebral dysplasia: The F-syndrome. *Birth Defects Orig Artic Ser* 3:48, 1969.

Dundar M, Gordon TM, Ozyasgan I, et al: A novel acropectoral syndrome maps to chromosome 7q36. *J Med Genet* 38: 304, 2001.

Camera G, Camera A, Pozzolo S, et al: F-Syndrome (F-form of acropectoro-vertebral dysplasia): Report on a second family. *Am J Med Genet* 57:472, 1995.

Fabry Disease

At a glance: Genetically transmitted lysosomal storage disorder caused by a deficiency in α-galactosidase and characterized by an accumulation of substrate in many organs and tissue resulting in progressive neurologic and vascular degeneration.

Synonyms: Angiokeratoma Corporis Diffusum; Anderson-Fabry Disease; Alpha-Galactosidase A Deficiency.

Incidence: Second most prevalent metabolic storage disorder. ☞Gaucher disease being the most prevalent. Incidence is 1:117,000 live births.

Genetic inheritance: Transmission is recessive and X-linked. Men are affected, but women carriers can present symptoms of the disease.

Pathophysiology: Lack of α-galactosidase A leads to intracellular accumulation of its substrate globotriaosylceramide. This defect leads to severe painful neuropathy with progressive renal, cardiovascular, and cerebrovascular dysfunction and finally death.

Diagnosis: Diagnosis is clinical and biochemical. The clinical signs indicating Fabry disease are the presence of angiokeratomas in the skin and mucous membrane and benign corneal abnormalities.

Diagnosis is confirmed by white blood cells or cultured skin fibroblasts showing a decreased α-galactosidase A activity. Treatment is symptomatic.

Clinical aspects: The main features of the disease are caused by the deposit of the glycolipid (Gb^3) in the vascular endothelium, smooth muscle cells, renal epithelium, myocardium, dorsal root ganglia, autonomic nervous system, and brain. Clinically, it translates into stroke, progressive renal failure with proteinuria, cardiac hypertrophy, arrhythmias, valvular insufficiency, and myocardial infarction. Other manifestations of the disease are progressive sensorineural hearing loss, vertigo, postprandial abdominal cramps, and achalasia. Pain in the hands and feet as a result of neuropathy is common. Skeletal involvement translates to arthralgia, articular erosion, avascular necrosis, and limitation of the temporomandibular joint. As the disease evolves, the lungs become involved and pulmonary function tests show an obstructive disease. Finally, they present characteristics of angiokeratomas in the skin and mucous membranes, corneal abnormalities, and a lack of sweating.

Precautions before anesthesia: Because it is a multisystemic disease, all major systems must be evaluated thoroughly. The patient should undergo a cardiac evaluation with an ECG and echocardiogram, pulmonary function tests, and renal function tests. If the patient has symptoms of achalasia, he/she should be given sodium citrate as a gastric prophylaxis before undergoing a general anesthetic.

Anesthetic considerations: Because of the disseminated vascular involvement in the major organs, aim at preventing important shifts in blood pressure, particularly hypotension, and ensure phenylephrine is available. The ECG should be monitored for the presence of arrhythmias. Signs of cardiac involvement because of the disease should be managed accordingly. Direct laryngoscopy may be more difficult because of limited mouth opening as a consequence of temporomandibular joint stiffness.

Pharmacological implications: In the presence of arrhythmias, avoid using halothane; however, halothane is the drug of choice in the presence of cardiac hypertrophy. Anticholinergic drugs can worsen the hypohidrosis and are best avoided. If renal function is decreased, drugs eliminated by this route, such as neuromuscular relaxants and antibiotics, should be avoided or their dosage adjusted.

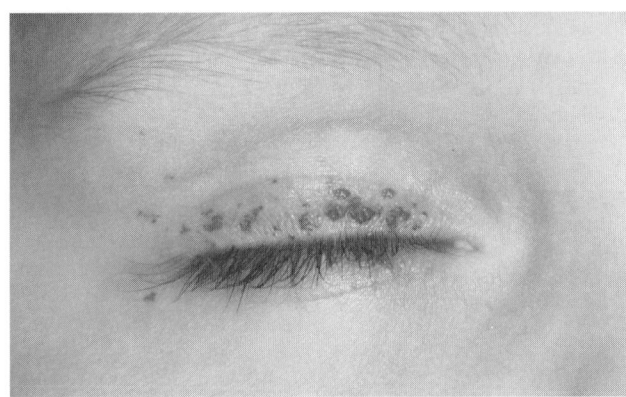

Fabry Disease Angiokeratomata on the eyelids in a patient with Fabry disease. See color plates.

REFERENCES:

Brady RO, Schiffmann R: Clinical features of and recent advances in therapy for Fabry disease. *JAMA* 284:2771, 2000.

Luciano CA, Russell JW, Banerjee TK, et al: Physiological characterization of neuropathy in Fabry's disease. *Muscle Nerve* 26:622, 2002.

Perrot A, Osterziel KJ, Beck M, et al: Fabry disease: Focus on cardiac manifestations and molecular mechanisms. *Herz* 27:699, 2002.

Facio-Oculo-Acoustico-Renal (FOAR) Syndrome

At a glance: Genetic disorder affecting the eyes (blindness), ears (deafness), face, kidneys, and bones.

Synonym: FOAR Syndrome.

Incidence and genetic inheritance: Very rare syndrome (fewer than 10 cases have been reported), which most likely is transmitted as an autosomal recessive trait. FOAR syndrome and Donnai-Barrow syndrome are believed to be the same entity.

Clinical aspects: Characterized by anomalies of the eye (high myopia, iris coloboma, retinal detachment, chorioretinal atrophy, poorly differentiated maculae, cataract, glaucoma), the face (macrocephaly, flat nasal bridge, true hypertelorism, telecanthus, antimongoloid slanting of the palpebral fissures, prominent eyebrows), the ears (moderate-to-severe sensorineural deafness), the skeleton (epiphyseal dysplasia of the femoral heads), and the kidneys (structural abnormalities, proteinuria, hematuria, aminoaciduria). Psychomotor development may range from moderately delayed to normal.

Precautions before anesthesia: No special precautions other than the usual patient preparation for a general anesthesia.

Anesthetic considerations: Patients often present for eye surgery (retinal detachment). No anesthetic complications have been reported. Airway management is not expected to be difficult. Check renal function (creatinine, blood urea nitrogen) and serum concentrations of protein, electrolytes, and hemoglobin (renal anemia) preoperatively. Patients are blind and deaf; consequently, their cooperation may be reduced. Sedative and anxiolytic premedication and the presence of the primary caregiver during induction of anesthesia may be helpful.

Pharmacological implications: Ketamine and succinylcholine should not be used in the presence of increased intraocular pressure. Avoid using drugs with predominantly renal elimination in patients with decreased kidney function. Carefully titrate highly protein-bound drugs because hypoproteinemia may result from proteinuria and lead to increased concentrations of the free drug.

Other conditions to be considered:

☞**DONNAI-BARROW SYNDROME:** Genetic disorder responsible for diaphragmatic hernia, exomphalos, absent corpus callosum, hypertelorism, eye anomalies, and sensorineural deafness.

☞**WAARDENBURG SYNDROME, TYPE I:** Characterized by a wide bridge of the nose resulting from lateral displacement of the inner canthus of each eye, pigmentary disturbance (frontal white blaze of hair, heterochromia iridis, white eye lashes, leukoderma), and cochlear deafness. Severity varies widely; some affected persons escape deafness. Confusion between FOAR syndrome and Waardenburg syndrome is frequent.

REFERENCES:

Devriendt K, Standaert L, Van Hole C, et al: Proteinuria in a patient with the diaphragmatic hernia-hypertelorism-myopia-deafness

syndrome: Further evidence that the facio-oculo-acoustico-renal syndrome represents the same entity. *J Med Genet* 35:70, 1998.

Schowalter DB, Pagon RA, Kalina RE, et al: Facio-oculo-acoustico-renal (FOAR) syndrome. *Am J Med Genet* 69:45, 1997.

Facio-Thoraco-Genital Syndrome

At a glance: Congenital malformation that mainly involved the face, thorax, and genitalia.

Incidence: Only two cases reported in the literature. The first case was described by R. Wilf-Miron and R.M. Goodman in 1987.

Genetic inheritance: Believed to be transmitted as an autosomal recessive trait.

Diagnosis and clinical aspects: Diagnosis is clinical based on the dysmorphic findings. This syndrome has some characteristics similar to the Smith-Lemli-Opitz syndrome and the Aarskog-Scott syndrome. Affected patients present with facies characterized by the presence of microphthalmia, asymmetrical ears, anteverted nares, long flat philtrum associated with a thin upper lip, and micrognathia. The thorax features an important pectus excavatum and widely spaced nipples. The genitalia defect includes a "saddlebag" configuration of the scrotum associated with a prominent raphe and hypospadias. Other minor anomalies include the widening of the thumbs and great toes with hypoplastic nails and the presence of a prominent crease on the ventral aspect of the feet. No skeletal, renal, or cardiac anomalies noted.

Anesthetic considerations: Craniofacial features suggest a potential for difficult laryngoscopy and tracheal intubation. Proper evaluation of the airway must be conducted prior to induction of anesthesia. Maintenance of spontaneous ventilation until the airway has been secured and ventilation confirmed is highly recommended.

Other conditions to be considered:

☞**AARSKOG SYNDROME:** X-linked disorder characterized by ocular hypertelorism, anteverted nostrils, broad upper lip, and peculiar penoscrotal relations ("saddlebag " or "shawl" scrotum). Occurrence of ligamentous laxity manifested by hyperextensibility of the fingers, genu recurvatum, and flat feet. A very important characteristic is the presence of cervical hypermobility with anomaly of the odontoid that may result in neurologic deficit during extension. Believed to be transmitted as a sex-influenced autosomal dominant inheritance.

☞**SMITH-LEMLI-OPITZ SYNDROME TYPE I:** Characterized by severe growth retardation, developmental delay, severe dysphagia, microcephaly, micrognathia, cleft palate, cataracts, ptosis, polysyndactyly and syndactyly of the second and third toes, and congenital heart defects (transposition of the great vessels frequent). Congestive heart failure and liver failure are not uncommon.

MULTIPLE OSTEOCHONDRITIS DISSECANS: Characterized by hypertelorism, cryptorchidism, digital contractures, sternal deformity, and osteochondritis dissecans at multiple sites. Early fusion of the manubrium and corpus sterni occurred. Transmitted most probably as an autosomal dominant inheritance (with sex influence).

REFERENCE:

Wilf-Miron R, Goodman RM: Facio-thoraco-genital syndrome: A newly recognized birth defect syndrome. *J Craniofac Genet Dev Biol* 7:19, 1987.

Fahr Syndrome

At a glance: Very rare degenerative neurologic syndrome characterized by microcephaly, mental and growth retardation, seizures and dystonic movements, and athetosis with evidence of multiple intracranial calcifications in parts of the gray and dentate nuclei, particularly of smaller brain vessels.

Synonyms: Cerebral Nonarteriosclerotic Calcification; Idiopathic Basal Ganglia Calcification; Fahr Intracerebral Calcinosis; Fahr Disease; Morbus Fahr Ferrocalcinosis; Nonarteriosclerotic Cerebral Calcifications; Striopallidodentate (SPD) Calcinosis.

Nature: Presence of idiopathic intracranial calcifications has been recognized for many years. The initial report by Fahr was about an adult. The heterogeneous nature of the disease was later recognized and genetic conditions occurring in infants were included.

Genetic inheritance: Autosomal recessive and autosomal dominant transmission have been reported. In some cases, the condition appears to be sporadic and may result from an unidentified infection during pregnancy affecting the developing fetus.

Pathophysiology: Pathogenesis is unclear, but a few hypotheses have been stated, such as the possible role of abnormal iron transport, fetal viral infection, and hypoparathyroidism.

Diagnosis: Diagnosis of exclusion after ruling out common causes of microcephaly with intracranial calcifications, such as TORCH (toxoplasmosis, other agents, rubella, cytomegalovirus, herpes simplex) infection, varicella virus, and cytomegalovirus infections.

Clinical aspects: Children affected with the disease are normal at birth but then show poor psychomotor developmental progress. Seizures appear early in life and are of variable nature. Affected patients present with severe microcephaly, hypotonia, spasticity, and growth retardation. Some children also have thrombocytopenia and hepatosplenomegaly manifesting shortly after birth but lasting for only a few weeks and then resolving spontaneously. CT scan of the brain may show cerebral atrophy, dilated ventricles, calcifications, and a lower density of white matter consistent with dysmyelination. Hypoparathyroidism may be associated with this disorder. Clinical course and outcome are highly variable.

Precautions before anesthesia: If the child needs surgery in the first few weeks of life, obtain a complete blood count (CBC) to rule out anemia and thrombocytopenia. Blood calcium should be checked to rule out hypocalcemia caused by hypoparathyroidism.

Anesthetic considerations: Locoregional anesthesia should be avoided in case of thrombopenia.

Pharmacological implications: Presence of undetermined cause for hepatomegaly should limit the use of inhalational agent likely to affect the liver (e.g., halothane). Hepatic enzyme induction may occur in the presence of anticonvulsant, so the dose of some drugs, such as neuromuscular relaxants, may require adjustment. It is best to avoid succinylcholine if the patient has severe spastic paraplegia.

REFERENCES:

Hempel A, Henze M, Berghoff C, et al: PET findings and neuropsychological deficits in a case of Fahr's disease. *Psychiatry Res* 108:133, 2001.

Morgante L, Trimarchi F, Benvenga S: Fahr's disease. *Lancet* 359:759, 2002.

Reardon W, Hockey A, Silberstein P, et al: Autosomal recessive congenital intrauterine infection-like syndrome of microcephaly, intracranial calcification, and CNS disease. *Am J Med Genet* 52;58, 1994.

Familial Amyotrophic Dystonic Paraplegia

At a glance: Very rare syndrome characterized by progressive amyotrophy, mental retardation, nystagmus, and incontinence of bowel and bladder in association with spastic paraplegia.

Incidence and genetic inheritance: Twelve patients have been described in the literature. Autosomal dominant.

Clinical aspects: Because the disease has a variable expression, the degree of symptoms ranges from an asymptomatic condition to a severe disease. Features include dystonia, spastic paraplegia, amyotrophy, mental retardation, bowel incontinence, bladder incontinence, and nystagmus.

Anesthetic considerations: Assess airway reflexes and history of gastroesophageal reflux (recurrent pulmonary aspiration). Because patient may be prone to frequent chest infections, assess respiratory function, including chest radiography, arterial blood gas analysis, and pulmonary function tests, if possible. In presence of severe pulmonary dysfunction, postoperative mechanical ventilatory support may be necessary and should be planned accordingly. Mental retardation may complicate communication and preoperative assessment. May suffer from gastroesophageal reflux (regurgitation) and poor swallowing (rapid-sequence induction). Care with positioning of patient with spastic paraplegia. Use of neuromuscular blocking agents should be done with titration considering muscle atrophy and under control of nerve stimulator.

REFERENCE:

Gilman S, Horenstein S: Familial amyotrophic dystonic paraplegia. *Brain* 87:51, 1964.

Familial Atrial Myxoma

At a glance: Atrial myxoma is the most common primary heart tumor. It usually is nonmalignant and sporadic, but 10% are familial.

Synonyms: Atrial Myxoma; Intracardiac Myxoma.

Incidence: Cardiac myxomas account for 40 to 50% of primary cardiac tumors. They are solitary and pedunculated and usually involve only the left atrium in the nonfamilial form (90% of cases) and both sides of the heart in the familial form (10% of atrial myxomas). In the sporadic cases, the female-to-male ratio is 3:1, whereas both sexes are equally involved in the familial cases. The overall prevalence of primary cardiac tumors is approximately 0.02% (200 tumors per one million autopsies); approximately 37.5% of them are myxomas (75 cases of myxoma per one million autopsies).

Genetic inheritance: In cases of familial occurrence (10% of atrial myxomas), the transmission is autosomal dominant.

Pathophysiology: The tumor is benign but can be lethal if it obstructs a valve or causes major embolic events. It arises from the epithelium and acts as a space-occupying lesion. A left atrial lesion behaves as a mitral valve stenosis and leads to pulmonary edema, whereas a right atrial lesion acts as a tricuspid valve stenosis and manifests with dyspnea and hypoxemia. These tumors are friable, resulting in tumor embolism that occurs in approximately 30 to 40% of patients. Symptomatology depends on the location of the tumor (left or right atrium) and the presence of an intracardiac shunt.

Diagnosis: Confirmed by an echocardiogram in suspected cases.

Clinical aspects: Symptoms are produced by mechanical interference with cardiac function or embolization. It seems that familial disease involves younger patients with more frequent lesions on the right side of the heart and more recurrences over the years. Complications associated with the disease, such as vascular aneurysms, are not more common in the familial cases.

Precautions before anesthesia: An echocardiogram and ECG are needed preoperatively to document the extent and number of lesions and their effect on the hemodynamics of the heart. An angiogram should be part of the workup to rule out the presence of vascular aneurysms in the cerebral, coronary, and pulmonary vasculature. If the syndrome form is suspected, rule out involvement of the adrenals.

Anesthetic considerations: Affected patients present with lesions that can obstruct cardiac valves and thus decrease cardiac output considerably. Consider avoiding use of medication with the potential to depress myocardial function (especially contractility), prevent tachycardia, and maintain adequate preload. In the case of right-sided lesions, use of a central line in the superior vena cava should be assessed carefully.

Pharmacological implications: No specific implications reported for this condition.

Other condition to be considered: In familial cases, atrial myxoma can be isolated or occasionally is associated with other disorders, constituting distinct entities.

☞**CARNEY COMPLEX TYPE I:** Multiple neoplasia syndrome characterized by spotty skin pigmentation, cardiac and other myxomas organs (e.g., breast, skin, thyroid gland, neural tissue), endocrine tumors, and psammomatous melanotic schwannomas. Clinical features include lentigines (brown discoloration of skin) and pigmented nevi, pituitary overactivity (Cushing syndrome), ventricular myxoma, subcutaneous myxoid neurofibromata, and mammary fibroadenosis. Hirsutism and spotty facial and labial (female) pigmentation are characteristics of this medical condition. Severe atherosclerotic narrowing of the left anterior descending coronary artery has been reported as the cause of death in a 44-year-old man following surgical hernioplasty. NAME (nevi, atrial myxoma, myxoid neurofibroma, and ephelides [tanned skin macules]) syndrome and LAMB (lentigines, atrial myxoma, and blue nevi) syndrome now are considered under the group of Carney complex.

REFERENCES:

Casey M, Vaughan CJ, He J, et al: Mutations in the protein kinase A R1alpha regulatory subunit cause familial cardiac myxomas and Carney complex. *J Clin Invest* 106:R31, 2000.

Farah MG: Familial cardiac myxoma: A study of relatives of patients with myxoma. *Chest* 105:65, 1994.

van Gelder HM, O'Brien DJ, Staples ED, et al: Familial cardiac myxoma. *Ann Thorac Surg* 53:419, 1992.

Familial Benign Copper Deficiency

At a glance: Infant presenting with seizures as a result of low serum copper with normal ceruloplasmin levels and normal copper urinary excretion. Improvement of the physical status can be observed following oral supplementation. Postulated to result from a defect in copper absorption.

Incidence: One case with two affected relatives has been described in the literature.

Genetic inheritance: Autosomal dominant or X-linked dominant.

Clinical aspects: Other causes of copper deficiency (e.g., low intake, prolonged parenteral nutrition, alkali medication for renal acidosis, long-term zinc therapy) must be excluded to make the diagnosis. Development of seizures responsive to dietary copper supplementation and recurring on withdrawal. Failure to thrive. Iron-deficient anemia. Very curly hair. Radiology shows spurring of femora and tibiae.

Anesthetic considerations: Check complete blood count. Consider whether preoperative transfusion is needed. Avoid substances that reduce the seizure threshold and could lead to intraoperative seizure activities.

Other condition to be considered:

☞**MENKES SYNDROME:** Differentiated by severe neurologic deterioration leading to death by age 3 to 4 years, pili torti, tortuosity of arteries, and decreased ceruloplasmin levels.

REFERENCES:

Llanos RM, Mercer JF: The molecular basis of copper homeostasis copper-related disorders. *DNA Cell Biol* 21:259, 2002.

Mehes K, Petrovicz E: Familial benign copper deficiency. *Arch Dis Child* 57:716, 1986.

Mehes K, Petrovicz E: Familial benign copper deficiency: An old case re-examined. *Acta Paediatr Hung* 89;29:313, 1988.

Familial Generalized Anhidrosis

At a glance: Familial disorder characterized by anhidrosis present at birth and resulting in heat intolerance. Muscarinic stimulation results in significantly reduced sweat production (10–50% of normal).

Incidence: Extremely rare; only a few cases reported.

Genetic inheritance: X-linked inheritance as the disorder in mothers appears to be less severe than observed in their sons.

Pathophysiology: Reduced reaction to muscarinic stimulation of sweat glands.

Diagnosis: Three types of generalized anhidrosis:

1. Ectodermal dysplasia with anomalies of hair, sweat glands, and teeth, with or without additional congenital defects.
2. Ectodermal dysplasia with no other defects except for morphologically and functionally abnormal sweat glands.
3. Isolated ectodermal dysplasia with no other anomalies. The clinical history of heat intolerance and the markedly reduced response to muscarinic stimulation of the sweat glands (10% in males and approximately 50% of normal in affected females) are characteristic. However, the sweat glands appear to be morphologically normal on biopsy, and autonomic cardiovascular response is normal. A postganglionic defect has been suggested.

Clinical aspects: Reduced sweating capability results in heat intolerance.

Precaution before anesthesia: Check the teeth for damage (and document them clearly); otherwise routine preoperative assessment.

Anesthetic considerations: Careful perioperative temperature monitoring is necessary to prevent intraoperative hyperthermia. Careful direct laryngoscopy is required in the presence of preexisting dental defects.

Pharmacological implications: Muscarinic antagonists (e.g., atropine) should be avoided in the presence of an already reduced sweat function.

Other conditions to be considered:

☞**HEREDITARY SENSORY AND AUTONOMIC NEUROPATHY IV:** Genetic neurodegenerative disorder (peripheral nerve degeneration involving small fiber) characterized by congenital insensitivity to pain (resulting in painless injuries), episodic fever (hot weather) resulting from anhidrosis, autonomic disorders, mental retardation, short stature, self-mutilation, and joint deformities.

VAN DEN BOSCH SYNDROME: Transmitted as an X-linked recessive trait. Associated with mental deficiency, choroideremia, acrokeratosis verruciformis, and skeletal deformities. The syndrome is extremely rare and has been described in only a single kindred.

HELWEG-LARSEN SYNDROME (Anhidrosis–Congenital Neurolabyrinthitis; Anhidrosis–Neurolabyrinthitis Syndrome): Anhidrosis is present from birth. Ectodermal dysplasia and neurolabyrinthian deafness developing in the fourth or fifth decade of life.

REFERENCES:

Dann EJ, Epstein Y, Sohar E: Familial generalized anhidrosis. *Isr J Med Sci* 26:451, 1990.

Ingber A: Familial generalized anhidrosis. *Israel J Med Sci* 26: 457, 1990.

Familial Hyperaldosteronism

At a glance: Genetically inherited endocrine disorder entity that is clinically characterized by fatigue, ileus (from hypokalemia), hypertension, strokes, and other significant cardiovascular events in young persons because of overproduction of aldosterone.

Classification and synonyms: ACTH-Dependent Hyperaldosteronism Syndrome.

Type I: Aldosteronism Sensitive to Dexamethasone; Glucocorticoid-Suppressible Hyperaldosteronism; Glucocorticoid-Remediable Aldosteronism.

Type II: Aldosteronism Insensitive to Dexamethasone; Glucocorticoid Nonsuppressible Hyperaldosteronism; Glucocorticoid Nonremediable Aldosteronism.

Incidence: Fewer than 150 validated cases reported in the literature.

Genetic inheritance: Autosomal dominant. The glucocorticoid-sensitive form (type I) of familial hyperaldosteronism is related to a chimeric gene product combining (by crossover) the promoter of the 11β-hydroxylase gene with the coding region of the aldosterone synthetase gene on chromosome 8q21 (anti-Lepore–type fusion of Cyp11B1 and Cyp11B2). Type II is caused by a mutation in chromosome 7p22.

Pathophysiology: Hyperaldosteronism is a consequence of aldosterone-producing adenoma. The effects of aldosterone are mediated through activation of the epithelial sodium channel, and activating mutations of this channel lead to signs of mineralocorticoid excess.

Diagnosis: Hypertension, polyuria, polydipsia, fatigue, tinnitus, paresthesia, and paralysis of variable duration (from 1 hour to weeks), failure to thrive, and muscle loss. Laboratory investigations include hypokalemia (<3.5 mmol/liter), metabolic alkalosis associated with inappropriate kaliuresis, increased plasma levels of aldosterone (>40 ng/dl), decreased plasma renin activity (<0.3 ng/ml/hour), and nonsuppressible aldosterone response to ambulation. Dexamethasone test did not suppress aldosterone level. Magnetic resonance imaging is better for locating the adenoma than is CT. The left gland is four times more frequently involved than the right gland. In Conn syndrome, the ratio of deoxycorticosterone to corticosterone is unaffected by adrenocorticotropic hormone.

Clinical aspects: The clinical presentation of familial hyperaldosteronism is not distinctive, and diagnosis requires expertise on the part of the physician. Familial hyperaldosteronism patients usually have a long history of fatigue, muscle loss, paresthesia (even paralysis), tinnitus, and headache (caused by hypertension). Polyuria and polydipsia are common features. The main physical symptom is hypertension. It is not unusual for the diagnosis to be established when a severe complication of hypertension occurs (stroke, cardiac problem). Laboratory examinations reveal hypokalemia (often severe), metabolic alkalosis, inappropriate kaliuresis, decreased plasma rennin activity, and high basal plasma levels of aldosterone. Imaging reveals either diffuse adrenocortical hyperplasia or multiple adrenocortical adenomas. Depending on the efficacy of glucocorticoid given to correct the symptomatology, two types of this familial disease exist: *type I,* which is glucocorticoid sensitive and caused by multiple adrenocortical adenomas, and *type II,* which is caused by adrenal hyperplasia and is not glucocorticoid remediable. Otherwise the two forms are clinically similar.

Precaution before anesthesia: Evaluate electrolytes status and correct hypokalemia. Restrict sodium intake. Administrate spironolactone (5–10 mg/kg/d) . Stop captopril or enalapril 24 hours before general anesthesia. Evaluate immune status because of treatment by agents that inhibit angiotensin-converting enzyme.

Anesthetic considerations: If hypokalemia has not been corrected prior to anesthesia, hyperventilation could be dangerous by decreasing further potassium plasma levels. Regional anesthesia technique such as epidural anesthesia can be used safety in children, especially in patients less than 8 years of age, because of the absence of induced hemodynamic effects in this age group. No specific anesthetic agents can be recommended or contraindicated considering the risk of acute hypotension. Monitoring of arterial blood pressure as well as central venous pressure is recommended perioperatively.

Pharmacological implications: Pay close attention to the possible interaction between hypotensive drugs that can be used, such as captopril or enalapril and spironolactone, and the risk of hyperkalemia. Clonidine must be avoided because it decreases plasma renin activity. Enflurane may be questionable if a nephropathy exists preoperatively. Supplementation with exogenous cortisol (cortisone hemisuccinate) is indicated only in cases of excision of multiple adenomas with bilateral mobilization of adrenal glands.

Other conditions to be considered:

☞**BARTTER SYNDROME:** Family of disorders characterized by hypokalemic, hypochloremic, metabolic alkalosis, and normotensive, hyperreninemic hyperaldosteronism.

☞**CONN SYNDROME:** Rare and potentially curable endocrine disorder caused by hyperaldosteronism. Presenting symptoms associate hypertension to severe hypokalemia.

☞**GITELMAN SYNDROME:** Inherited renal tubular defect resulting in urinary loss of magnesium, sodium, potassium, and chloride with otherwise normal kidneys.

REFERENCES:

Pascoe L, Jeunemaitre X, Lebrethon MC, et al: Glucocorticoid-suppressible hyperaldosteronism and adrenal tumors occurring in a single French pedigree. *J Clin Invest* 96:2236, 1995.

Stowasser M, Gunasekera TG, Gordon RD: Familial varieties of primary aldosteronism. *Clin Exp Pharmacol Physiol* 28:1087, 2001.

Familial Hyperlysinemia

At a glance: The enzyme deficiencies of α-aminoadipic semialdehyde dehydrogenase and the saccharopine dehydrogenases have been associated with increased serum levels of L-lysine. The clinical presentation is very variable and may include developmental delay, hypotonia, lethargy recurrent emesis, and diarrhea.

Synonyms: Alpha-Aminoadipic Semialdehyde Synthase Deficiency; Lysine Intolerance; Lysine:Alpha-Ketoglutarate Reductase Deficiency; L-Lysine:NAD-Oxido-Reductase Deficiency.

Incidence: Extremely rare.

Genetic inheritance: Inherited in a autosomal recessive way. Parental consanguinity has been reported in some cases and is considered a risk factor. The defect has been related to a mutation in the α-aminoadipic semialdehyde synthase (AASS) gene, which maps to gene locus 7q31.3.

Pathophysiology: The enzyme AASS has both lysine ketoglutarate reductase and saccharopine dehydrogenase activity and therefore is bifunctional. It is involved in the first two steps of the lysine degradation pathway in humans. Lysine-ketoglutarate reductase catalyzes the metabolism of L-lysine to saccharopine, which is cleaved to α-aminoadipic semialdehyde and glutamic acid by saccharopine dehydrogenase. A defect either in one or both of these enzymes results in familial hyperlysinemia, lysinuria, and saccharopinuria of variable degree. An alternative metabolism, the so-called "pipecolic acid pathway," functions only as an overflow pathway and is not suited to handle the relatively large amounts of L-lysine from oral intake.

Diagnosis: Most often, the disease is diagnosed by a general screening for metabolic disease initiated by clinical signs. The enzyme AASS is present in almost all body cells, with the highest concentration found in the liver. However, skin fibroblast can be used to perform the standard test (incubation of the fibroblast with radioactive/labeled L-lysine and measurement of the carbon dioxide production) and confirm the diagnosis. In most cases, the enzyme activity is less than 10% of normal.

Clinical aspects: Clinical manifestation is highly variable. The descriptions range from symptom-free to severe developmental delay, spastic diplegia, seizures, rigidity, coma, episodic vomiting, and diarrhea. In one case, coma and hyperammonia resolved with a low-protein diet. However, it now seems that hyperlysinemia is not associated with an ill effect in the majority of cases. A special diet seems not indicated, but some physicians prefer to limit protein intake in their patients.

Precautions before anesthesia: Evaluate antiseizure medication, frequency of emesis, and diarrhea. Electrolyte and volume status should be watched carefully in the presence of vomiting and diarrhea. Patients with mental retardation may benefit from sedative and anxiolytic premedication and/or presence of the primary caregiver during induction of anesthesia.

Anesthetic considerations: With a history of vomiting, rapid-sequence induction and endotracheal intubation are recommended. Check blood gases and electrolytes at least once intraoperatively (or better preoperatively) in association with recent or ongoing vomiting/diarrhea.

Pharmacological implications: Patients on chronic antiseizure medication may show altered hepatic drug metabolism.

Other conditions to be considered: Hyperlysinemia can also be found in the following disorders:

☞**PYRUVATE CARBOXYLASE DEFICIENCY:** Mitochondrial disease impairing synthetic pathways and leading to hypoglycemia and severe lactic acidosis.

☞**D-2-HYDROXYGLUTARIC ACIDURIA:** Metabolic disease resulting in abnormal MRI findings and psychomotor retardation, hypotonia, and nonneurologic signs.

☞**L-2-HYDROXYGLUTARIC ACIDURIA:** Inborn error of metabolism manifesting as progressive neurodegenerative disorder with psychomotor retardation.

☞**PROPIONIC ACIDEMIA:** Inborn error of metabolism affecting the mitochondrial catabolism of valine and isoleucine. Left untreated it results in ketoacidosis, lethargy, coma, and eventually death.

REFERENCES:

Cox RP: Errors of lysine metabolism, in Scriver CR, Beaudet AL, Sly WS, et al. (eds.): *The Metabolic and Molecular Bases of Inherited Disease.* 8th ed. New York, McGraw Hill, 2001, p 1965.

Sacksteder KA, Biery BJ, Morrell JC, et al: Identification of the alpha-aminoadipic semialdehyde synthase gene, which is defective in familial hyperlysinemia. *Am J Hum Genet* 66:1736, 2000.

Familial Hypogonadotrophic Eunuchoidism

At a glance: Genetically transmitted pituitary gonadotropin deficiency with hypothalamic–pituitary–prolactin dysfunction, absence of secondary sex characteristics, and long limbs.

Synonym: Familial Idiopathic Gonadotropin Deficiency (FIGD).

Genetic inheritance: Mostly autosomal recessive, although autosomal dominant and X-linked (rare) transmissions have been reported. Most cases are sporadic and thus could represent new mutations.

Pathophysiology: Hypothalamic deficiency of gonadotropin-releasing hormone (GnRH) is responsible for decreased pituitary gonadotropin secretion. Associated hypothalamic–pituitary–prolactin dysfunction may be present. Hypogonadotropic hypogonadism occurs as a consequence of these hormonal deficiencies.

Diagnosis and Clinical Aspects: Diagnosis is suggested by familial history, clinical features such as delayed puberty (menarche after age 15 years age in females, onset of pubic hair development after age 16 years in males), relatively long limbs, and need for hormonal treatment for appearance of secondary sexual characteristics. Serum hormonal levels are in the hypogonadal range: estradiol less than 20 pg/ml in women, testosterone less than 100 ng/dl in men, follicle-stimulating hormone and luteinizing hormone levels decreased with absence of normal adult pattern of pulsatile gonadotrophin secretion during a baseline evaluation of serum gonadotrophins with frequent (every 20 minutes) blood sampling. Testing of anterior pituitary hormone secretion during insulin tolerance and thyroid-stimulating hormone-releasing factor stimulation testing are within normal limits. No anomalies are seen on radiologic imaging of the hypothalamic and pituitary areas. Treatment consists of administration of synthetic luteinizing hormone-releasing hormone (GnRH).

Precautions before anesthesia: No specific precautions before anesthesia.

Anesthetic considerations: Other than the usual anesthetic considerations and preoperative evaluation for anesthesia, no known specific complications with this medical condition are reported in the literature.

Pharmacological implications: No pharmacological implications.

Other conditions to be considered:

☞**KALLMANN SYNDROME:** Congenital syndrome characterized by the association of hypogonadotropic hypogonadism with anosmia (or hyposmia).

☞**KLINEFELTER SYNDROME:** Chromosomal disorder consisting of supernumerary X chromosome(s) in male subjects associated with infertility and hypogonadism.

REFERENCES:

Toledo SPA, Luthold W, Mattar E: Familial idiopathic gonadotropin deficiency: A hypothalamic form of hypogonadism. *Am J Med Genet* 15:405, 1983.

Waldstreicher J, Seminara SB, Jameson JL, et al: The genetic and clinical heterogeneity of gonadotrophin-releasing hormone deficiency in the human. *J Clin Endocrinol Metab* 81:4388, 1996.

Familial Inverted Choreoathetosis

At a glance: Extremely rare form of familial choreoathetosis with infantile onset.

Synonym: Infantile Choreoathetosis of Fisher.

Incidence and genetic inheritance: Described in only one family, affecting four generations. Autosomal dominant inheritance.

Clinical aspects: Distinguishing features were infantile onset with exclusive neurologic impairment including progressive choreoathetosis predominantly affecting the legs and consequently impairing gait. Occasionally, pyramidal tract signs can occur. Patients do not show any signs of dementia, seizures, or rigidity.

Anesthetic considerations: No specific anesthetic considerations are expected to arise.

REFERENCE:

Fisher M, Sargent, J, Drachman D: Familial inverted choreoathetosis. *Neurology* 29:1627, 1979.

Familial Juvenile Nephronophthisis (NPH)

At a glance: Inherited disorder characterized by progressive polyuria preceding the decline of renal function and leading to end-stage renal disease during childhood or adolescence.

Synonyms: Nephronophthisis.

History: First reported in the literature in 1945 by Smith and Graham, but the first description is attributed to Guido Fanconi, a Swiss pediatrician, in 1951.

Incidence: Most frequent genetic cause of end-stage renal disease in childhood. Represents approximately 10 to 15% of end-stage renal disease in children.

Classification: Four types of nephronophthisis (NPH), often determined by the age at onset of end-stage renal failure. Terminal renal failure develops at median ages of 1 year, 13 years, and 19 years in NPH II, NPH I, and NPH III, respectively. Type IV is variable.

Type I (Familial Juvenile Nephronophthisis; NPH I): Characterized by anemia, polyuria, polydipsia, isosthenuria, and death in uremia. It represent 80% of all NPH cases.

Type II (Infantile Nephronophthisis; NPH II): Characterized by hypertension, respiratory failure, pulmonary hypoplasia, renal failure by age 3 years, hyperkalemic metabolic acidosis, hyperkalemia, oligohydramnios, and neonatal death secondary to pulmonary insufficiency.

Type III (Adolescent Nephronophthisis; NPH III): Adolescent nephronophthisis is considered clearly distinct by clinical and genetic findings than the other types. Most patients suffered from anemia, and onset of terminal renal failure occurred significantly later than in juvenile nephronophthisis.

Type IV (NPH IV): Characterized by a triad of interstitial cell infiltrates, renal tubular cell atrophy with cysts arising from the corticomedullary junction of the kidneys, and renal interstitial fibrosis. Chromosomal localization is reported on a fourth gene locus NPHP4. End-stage renal disease commenced within a wider age range of 11 to 34 years. It usually is considered type III.

☞Loken-Senior Syndrome is characterized by nephronophthisis in association with retinitis pigmentosa or retinal aplasia, which is consistent with Leber Congenital Amaurosis. The association of ☞Leber Congenital Amaurosis is present in 15% of all cases affected with nephronophthisis. It is often considered a type III with retinal dysplasia.

Genetic inheritance: Depends on the clinical form. NPH I (80% of cases) is inherited as a recessive trait (linkage for 2q13; possible second locus 9q22-31). NPH II has recessive inheritance (unknown gene localization). NPH III has no linkage for chromosome 2. NPH IV (medullary cystic disease) is transmitted as an autosomal trait (gene map locus 1q21).

Pathophysiology: Changes are characteristic and include the presence of atrophic tubules, irregularly thickened tubular basement membrane, and focal interstitial fibrosis. As the disease progresses, diffuse tubulointerstitial changes and medullary cysts are found. The biochemical defect underlying the production of the defective tubular basement membrane is unknown.

Diagnosis: Confirmed by pathologic renal findings obtained from biopsy.

Clinical aspects: Patients will complain of polyuria caused by decreased renal concentrating ability. Progressive renal function deterioration follows. Other features of the disease are growth retardation, cerebellar dysfunction, liver involvement, and bone anomalies. Ocular involvement is common. Patients require dialysis or renal transplant; otherwise death occurs in early adulthood.

Precautions before anesthesia: The hydration status of the patients should be carefully evaluated. Assess all the other characteristic changes associated with chronic renal failure: anemia, thrombocytopenia, electrolyte balance, metabolic acidosis, blood pressure, and susceptibility to infection. In presence of uremia, the coagulation system might be affected and should be checked.

Anesthetic considerations: Patients are managed as chronic renal failure patients. Maintain renal function intraoperatively by preventing overt dehydration and cardiovascular depression. According to the type of surgical procedure, invasive monitoring can be helpful for assessing intravascular volume. Patients with arteriovenous shunt for the purpose of dialysis should receive special attention to prevent thrombosis as a result of extrinsic compression. The patency of the shunt should be monitored intraoperatively with a Doppler examination, and the shunt should never be used as intravenous access.

Pharmacological implications: Avoid or reduce the administration of sevoflurane in these patients given the potential production of fluoride anions compound A and their effects on the kidney. The muscular relaxant of choice in the presence of renal failure is *cis*-atracurium or atracurium. However, other muscular relaxants can be used but in reduced dosage because renal clearance is decreased.

Other condition to be considered:

☞**LOKEN-SENIOR SYNDROME:** Autosomal recessive disorder characterized by progressive nephronophthisis, with or without medullary cystic disease. Other features include progressive eye disease (retinitis pigmentosa) and ataxia. Apparent during the first year of life. Blindness develops within the first 2 years of life. It is most often associated with tubulointestinal nephropathy and renal cystic disease.

REFERENCES:

Antignac C, Arduy CH, Beckmann JS, et al: A gene for familial juvenile nephronophthisis (recessive medullary cystic kidney disease) maps to chromosome 2p. *Nat Genet* 3:342, 1993.

Cohn DH, Shohat T, Yahav M, et al: A locus for an autosomal dominant form of progressive renal failure and hypertension at chromosome 1q21. *Am J Hum Genet* 67:647, 2000.

Saunier S, Calado J, Benessy F, et al: Characterization of the NPHP1 locus: Mutational mechanism involved in deletions in familial juvenile nephronophthisis. *Am J Hum Genet* 66:778, 2000.

Familial Mediterranean Fever

At a glance: Genetically transmitted disorder characterized by recurrent episodes of fever with abdominal pain, arthritis, or pleurisy.

Synonym: Recurrent Polyserositis.

Incidence: Incidence is higher in the Mediterranean population. Carrier state can be as high as 1:5 in at-risk population (Sephardic Jews, Armenians, Arabs, Turks).

Genetic inheritance: Autosomal recessive. The syndrome is caused by missense mutations in the MEFV gene located on chromosome 16 leading to alteration in the shape of the pyrin (or marenostrin) protein, exclusively found in granulocytes, which is thought to activate the biosynthesis of a chemotactic-factor inactivator.

Pathophysiology: Affected patients lack a specific protease that is usually present in serosal fluids and that normally inactivates interleukin-8 and the chemotactic complement factor 5a inhibitor. It is believed that it accumulates and causes exaggerated inflammatory response.

Diagnosis: Based on the clinical course and the presence of elevated C-reactive protein, erythrocyte sedimentation rate, fibrinogen, serum amyloid A, and leukocyte count during an acute episode but are nonspecific. Usually there is no increase in platelets. The diagnosis usually is made at age approximately 5 years and almost always before age 20 years.

Clinical aspects: Familial Mediterranean fever (FMF) is characterized by recurrent episode of fever, serositis, oligoarticular arthritis, and rash, beginning between the ages of 5 and 15 years and tending to occur every 2 to 4 weeks. Abdominal pain of short duration is present in 90% of patients and represents acute peritonitis. Peritoneal adhesions may form and cause small-bowel obstruction. Acute scrotal pain may be a manifestation of FMF and should be distinguished from testicular torsion. Pleuritis occurs in approximately 30% of cases and can lead to recurrent atelectasis. Monoarticular arthritis involving large joints is present in up to 70% of patients. The most serious complication of FMF is amyloidosis of the AA type,

which can lead to renal failure and death. Splenomegaly is a common complication of amyloidosis; other organs are rarely involved. Amyloidosis is mostly prevalent among Sephardic Jews. Symptoms of an acute attack appear suddenly and last from a few hours up to 96 hours. The disease has a variable and unpredictable course in each patient. Prophylactic therapy with colchicine prevents inflammatory attacks and the development of amyloidosis. The therapy should be continued throughout pregnancy and during lactation as long-term follow-up does not reveal any adverse effect on the children. The association of FMF with seronegative spondyloarthropathies remains controversial.

Precautions before anesthesia: Laparotomy during an acute episode should be avoided because it might cause a flare-up of the disease. Evaluate renal function and test for the presence of proteinuria. Test electrolytes and acid–base status if severe renal failure is diagnosed. If patient has presented pleuritis with atelectasis, a chest radiograph should be obtained.

Anesthetic considerations: If possible, avoid any type of anesthesia during an acute episode. If surgery is mandatory during an attack, avoid regional anesthesia in the context of fever and acute inflammatory response. Keep in mind that in the presence of pleuritis and atelectasis, ventilation and oxygenation may be more of a challenge. Avoid overhydration in the presence of renal failure.

Pharmacological implications: In the presence of renal failure, the muscle relaxants of choice are atracurium and *cis*-atracurium. A lower dose of other muscle relaxants should be given if chosen. Certain antibiotics require dose adjustment in case of renal failure.

REFERENCES:

Arav-Boger R, Spirer Z: Periodic syndromes of childhood. *Adv Pediatr* 44;389, 1997.

Direskeneli H, Ozdogan H, Yazici H: First international conference on familial Mediterranean fever. *J Rheumatol* 25:2236, 1998.

Drenth JPH, Van Der Meer JWM: Hereditary periodic fever. *N Engl J Med* 345:1748, 2001.

Familial Nonchromaffin Paragangliomas

At a glance: Genetically transmitted disorder characterized by the development of highly vascularized tumors derived from neuroectodermal cells, preferentially localized in the carotid body (80% of cases) and in the glomus jugulare (20% of cases).

Synonyms: Carotid Body Tumors; Chemodectomas; Glomus Jugulare Tumors; Hereditary Paraganglioma.

Nature: Familial paragangliomas, or glomus tumors, are slow growing, highly vascular, generally benign neoplasms, usually of the head and neck, that arise from neural crest cells outside of the adrenal medulla. Tumors arising in chemoreceptor structures include carotid body tumors and glomus jugulare tumors.

Incidence: Glomus tumors accounts for only 0.03% of all neoplasms and 0.6% of head and neck tumors. They are sometimes familial, bilateral, and associated with other neoplasms. They can be malignant, although this is rare.

Genetic inheritance: Inheritance is autosomal dominant. The paraganglioma gene PGL1 has been mapped to 11q22.3-q23. Germline missense mutations in the gene encoding succinate dehydrogenase subunit D (SDHD) gene have been identified. The disease is subject to age-dependent penetrance and imprinting.

Pathophysiology: Tumors may be bilateral or unilateral. The most common sites are the carotid body, the vagal body, and the jugulotympanic site. It is postulated that the tumor starts secondary to stimulus of hypercarbia or hypoxemia (the carotid bodies are the peripheral chemoreceptors that act as sensors for both hypoxia and hydrogen ion concentration). Others postulate that there is a connection between living at high altitude, emphysema, and carotid body tumors. There may be an association between paraganglioma and pheochromocytoma. The tumors have a tendency to reproduce the microscopic structure of the normal carotid body. These carotid body tumors are referred to as nonfunctional with regards to the nonchromaffin nature of the tumor, but chemoreceptor function is still present.

Diagnosis: Most patients present for evaluation of an anterior neck mass discovered on clinical examination or self-examination or detected during duplex scanning for carotid artery disease. In patients with tympanic chemodectomas, the condition may be suspected because of tinnitus aurium and a transtympanic reddish image by otoscopy. Arteriography remains the gold standard for diagnosis. Doppler color flow imaging, dynamic angioscintigraphy, CT, and MRI contribute additional information about tumor extension.

Clinical aspects: Age at onset of symptoms was significantly different between fathers and children (affected children have earlier age of onset). Clinical manifestations depend on tumor location and are often related to the middle ear (pulsatile tinnitus, conductive hearing loss, aural fullness, discharge or bleeding, and a bluish mass behind the tympanic membrane are characteristic). Cranial nerve dysfunction (facial paralysis, dysphonia, marked hearing loss, pain). The most common complaint was swelling in the anterolateral region of the neck. Familial carotid body tumors tend to be multiple. All paragangliomas are capable of catecholamine production. Of the paragangliomas of the head and neck, 1 to 4% can secrete sufficient amounts of catecholamines to mimic a pheochromocytoma. Patients with glomus tumors have a higher incidence of developing a pheochromocytoma, especially those with familial glomus tumor disease. Many authors believe that nonoperative treatment is preferred in many cases because of the benign course of the tumors and the considerable risks of the surgery, but others recommend early surgery to minimize major risks associated with resection of a larger tumor and advocate selective embolization to enable safer surgery with less bleeding. Triplex scanning and CT are helpful for postoperative follow-up.

Precautions before anesthesia: Secretory activity of the tumors (e.g., catecholamines and serotonin) should be investigated before surgery and treated appropriately. Carotid arteriography (and ball occlusion) is useful for assessing vascularization of the tumor and determining the need to clamp the carotid artery during the procedure. Multisystem preoperative assessment is necessary, with special emphasis on the cardiovascular system of those patients with secretory tumors. In addition, there may be an association between glomus tumor and deficiency of factors VII and X. Patients may have altered response to O_2 and CO_2, so a reference baseline blood gas may be useful.

Anesthetic considerations: Surgical treatment of glomus jugulare tumors yields high rates of perioperative morbidity and mortality for several reasons, including neuroendocrine secretory activity, high degree of vascularization, intracranial extension, long duration of surgery, and cranial nerve lesion. During surgery, monitor for potential complications, such as hemodynamic alterations (bleeding or endocrine response), pulmonary embolism (air or thrombotic), hypothermia, and facial nerve lesions. After surgery, cranial nerve

involvement, which can lead to dysphagia and pulmonary aspiration, must be ruled out. The risk of cerebrospinal fluid fistula is high. After surgery, oral intake is delayed until intestinal function is established and glottic sphincter competence is verified by fiberoptic laryngoscopy. For tumors that are catecholamine secretory, appropriate preoperative pharmacologic blockade is essential (alphablockade using phenoxybenzamine or prazosin with concomitant beta-blockade). Full invasive cardiovascular monitoring is mandatory in such cases to detect and guide therapy of sudden hemodynamic changes during the perioperative period.

Pharmacological implications: Administration of a normal dose of opioid has been reported to cause severe postoperative respiratory depression following excision of both unilateral and bilateral carotid body tumors by abolishment of the peripheral chemoreceptor function. Potent inhalational anesthetics may exacerbate the attenuation of hypoxic drive at a concentration as low as 0.1 minimum alveolar concentration (MAC). Surgical excision of carotid body tumors, whether unilateral or bilateral, can be followed by severe postoperative respiratory depression. The complication may be attributed to opioid administration in the absence of peripheral chemoreceptor drive.

REFERENCES:

Jensen NF: Glomus tumors of the head and neck: Anesthetic considerations. *Anesth Analg* 78:112, 1994.

Leonetti JP, Donzelli JJ, Littooy FN, et al: Perioperative strategies in the management of carotid body tumors. *Otolaryngol Head Neck Surg* 117:111, 1997.

Patetsios P, Gable DR, Garrett WV, et al: Management of carotid body paragangliomas and review of a 30-year experience. *Ann Vasc Surg* 16:331, 2002.

Familial Osteodysplasia

At a glance: Inherited disorder believed to be an autosomal recessive trait. Characterized by midface hypoplasia, malformation of the mandible, hypoplastic zygomatic bones, and abnormally pointed chin.

Synonym: Anderson Syndrome.

Incidence and genetic inheritance: Seems to be extremely rare. Transmission appears to be autosomal recessive. Consanguinity in the parents of the first described patients was noted.

Clinical aspects: The typical facies has prominent eyebrows and ear lobes and a broad, flat nose with a flat nasal bridge. The forehead is usually quite prominent. The face showed a V-shaped configuration with midface hypoplasia, straightening of the gonial angle (the angle between the ramus and the body of the mandible), flattening of the malar eminences, hypoplastic zygomatic bones, and abnormally pointed chin. The opening of the gonial angle leads to overclosure of the mandible with functional prognathism. Alveolar and sutural bone growth in the face is decreased and associated with partial dental agenesis. Craniosynostosis can occur. Skull radiographs show a striking thinning of the calvaria and brachycephaly. The morphology of the cervical vertebrae may be abnormal, and some degree of thoracic scoliosis seems to be common. The lumbosacral spine, however, was described as normal. Cortical thickening of the bone appears to be a prominent feature, most commonly found in the long bones, which can result in encroachment of the medullary cavity. The ribs and the superior pubic ramus are often thin. Minor changes were found in the bones of clavicles, hand, and feet. In one of the patients, thinning of the mandible led to recurrent mandibular fractures (only in one case with a trauma appropriate enough to explain the fracture). All patients in the initially described family were hyperuricemic but not hyperuricosuric, and no other metabolic abnormalities could be detected. However, increased erythrocyte sedimentation rate (30–40 mm/hour) and C3 complement levels have been reported. The plasma fibrinogen level was low in all family members. Diastolic hypertension was present in three of the four initially described patients. The patients are mentally normal.

Precautions before anesthesia: Obtain personal medical history for (spontaneous) fractures. Laboratory examinations should include a complete blood cell count (hematopoiesis may be affected by bone marrow encroachment), electrolytes, creatinine, uric acid, and coagulation tests. Ask about spontaneous or prolonged bleeding. Check for difficult airway management (face-mask and tracheal intubation), which should include examination of neck mobility (abnormal cervical vertebrae). If scoliosis is significant, a preoperative lung function test and an echocardiography may be indicated. Assess treatment and efficacy of antihypertensive medication. Check for elevated intracranial pressure in the presence of craniosynostosis.

Anesthetic considerations: Expect airway management to be difficult because of the described anomalies. Furthermore, the teeth may be loose and the bone of the mandible fragile, resulting in fracture during overly vigorous laryngoscopy attempts for tracheal intubation. Depending on the degree and extension of scoliosis, central neuraxial blockade may be difficult, although the lumbosacral spine was described as normal. In the presence of craniosynostosis, an anesthetic technique should be used to avoid a further increase in intracranial pressure. Careful positioning and padding are recommended to prevent (the overall probably low risk of) spontaneous fractures.

Pharmacological implications: The patient may be on antihypertensive therapy, so depending on the type of drug and the planned procedure, decide whether the medication needs to be stopped or continued on the day of surgery.

Other conditions to be considered:

☞**DESBUQUOIS SYNDROME:** Autosomal recessive osteochondrodysplastic disease with typical skeletal anomalies and high mortality in the first year of life.

☞**HAJDU-CHENEY SYNDROME:** Very rare diffuse connective tissue disorder with osteolysis involving mainly head and musculoskeletal system.

☞**NAIL-PATELLA SYNDROME:** Rare genetic disorder usually apparent at birth or during infancy. Characterized by dysplasia of the fingernails and toenails, aplasia or hypoplasia of the patellae, webbing of skin at the elbow(s), and abnormal bilateral projections of the iliac superior crest. Other features include glaucoma (open-angle glaucoma) and "cloverleaf iris-shaped" (Lester iris). Approximately 30 to 40% may develop nephropathy that usually is apparent during childhood or later in life.

☞**PYLE DISEASE:** Inherited bone dysplasia affecting the enchondral growth of long bones, which results in failure of modeling and causes increased circumference of the ends of the shafts.

☞**CLEIDOCRANIAL DYSPLASIA:** Generalized skeletal dysplasia resulting in defects in the development of skull, clavicles, pelvis, and dental abnormalities in particular.

REFERENCES:

Anderson LG, Cook AJ, Coccaro PJ, et al: Familial osteodysplasia. *JAMA* 220:1687, 1972.

Buchignani JS, Cook AJ, Anderson LG: Roentgenographic findings in familial osteodysplasia. *AJR Am J Roentgenol* 116:602, 1972.

Schendel SA, Delaire J: Familial osteodysplasia. *Head Neck Surg* 4:335, 1982.

Familial Porencephaly

At a glance: Heterogenous group of extremely rare familial malformative disorders characterized by intracerebral cerebrospinal fluid (CSF)-filled cavitations associated with various malformations and neurologic impairments.

Synonym: Infantile Hemiplegia with Porencephaly.

Classification: Type I: encephaloclastic porencephaly; Type II: schizencephalic porencephaly.

History: A developmental defect of the brain, porencephaly is defined as any cavitation or CSF-filled cyst in the brain that communicates directly with the ventricular system. It may occur prenatally or postnatally. Berg et al. provided the first description of familial porencephaly in 1983.

Incidence: An autopsy review showed an incidence of 22:1000 infants with intracerebral injuries.

Genetic inheritance: Infantile hemiplegia with porencephaly is transmitted as an autosomal dominant trait.

Pathophysiology: *Type I*, or *encephaloclastic porencephaly*, is an acquired and usually unilateral condition thought to occur in the third trimester. It can result from fetal vascular occlusion, birth trauma, ventricular puncture, inflammatory processes, coxsackie virus infection, hemorrhage, or embolism. *Type II*, or *schizencephalic porencephaly*, usually is symmetrical, is thought to occur during the second trimester, and represents a primary defect in morphogenesis of the neuroectoderm. Later findings indicate that deficiencies in the protein C anticoagulant pathway have an important role in the etiology of congenital porencephaly.

Diagnosis: Prenatal and postnatal ultrasonography and MRI can demonstrate characteristic images of porencephaly. Cranial transillumination may be positive. Types I and II are distinguishable both anatomically and histopathologically. Type I usually presents as a unilateral cyst, whereas type II usually is bilateral, located around the sylvian fissure, and often communicating with the lateral ventricles. Angiographically, type I porencephaly shows preexisting vessels, which cross the cavitation, whereas type II is noted for the continuity between the cortical vessels and the subependymal vessels. Histologic findings in type I reveal that the cavity is lined by a cicatricial glial membrane, whereas the type II cavity is lined by ependymal tissue.

Clinical aspects: Patients with infantile hemiplegia and porencephaly usually present with permanent neurologic disabilities. Prognosis generally depends on the extent of the lesion. In most patients, symptoms begin in the first decade of life. A few patients develop only minor neurologic signs and have normal intelligence. The character and etiology of porencephaly, congenital or acquired, is diversiform and often difficult to recognize. Classically, those with type I lesions have severe impairment, ranging from mental retardation and seizures to spastic hemiparesis or tetraplegia and blindness. Infants with type I cysts have a more variable course. The use of cocaine during pregnancy is associated with a higher risk (four times normal) of porencephaly. Progressive hydrocephalus may require a shunt procedure.

Precautions before anesthesia: Detailed neurologic assessment, documenting any raised intracranial pressure and the presence of other neurologic deficits. Look for seizures, the presence of bulbar involvement, feeding difficulties, and recurrent pulmonary aspiration syndrome. Evaluate the respiratory system, especially in tetraplegic patients. Investigations include complete blood count, serum electrolytes, arterial blood gas, and chest radiography. Avoid sedative premedications in patients with raised intracranial pressure because any respiratory depression further compromises cerebral perfusion.

Anesthetic considerations: Carefully position the hemiplegic or tetraplegic patient to prevent trauma to the spastic limbs. Neuromuscular junction monitoring should be performed on the unanalyzed limb, to prevent administration of excessive doses of muscle relaxants. In spastic tetraplegic patients with respiratory muscle involvement, problems of weaning from artificial ventilation postoperatively may occur. The anesthetic technique for patients with raised intracranial pressure should consider a smooth induction with total control of the hemodynamic changes. Rapid reversibility of the effects of anesthetics must be considered so that an adequate neurologic assessment may be performed at the end of the operation. In addition, perioperative institution of cerebral protective maneuvers (such as mannitol and hyperventilation) must be evaluated.

Pharmacological implications: Hemiplegia has been associated with resistance to nondepolarizing muscle relaxants and hyperkalemia following the administration of succinylcholine. Tetraplegia, on the other hand, is known to have increased sensitivity to nondepolarizing muscle relaxants in the affected muscles. The intravenous induction anesthetic agents decrease intracranial pressure via a reduction in the cerebral metabolic rate and blood flow. Ketamine remains the exception because it increases both cerebral blood flow and cerebral oxygen consumption. Volatile inhalational agents are potent cerebrovasodilators and cause uncoupling of the relationship between cerebral blood flow and cerebral metabolic rate. Narcotics should be administered with care because they result in some degree of respiratory depression and increase CSF production, which may have significant effects on intracranial pressure. Succinylcholine is contraindicated in the presence of hemiparesis or quadriparesis.

Other condition to be considered:

BONNEMANN MEINECKE SYNDROME (Porencephaly-Cerebellar Hypoplasia-Internal Malformations Syndrome): Autosomal recessive disorder characterized by bilateral porencephaly, cerebellar hypoplasia (including absence of the vermis), and internal malformations, including severe congenital heart anomalies (e.g., tetralogy of Fallot, total situs inversus, atrial septal defect). In cases of extensive bilateral porencephaly, the term "basket brain" has been coined, referring to the remaining parasagittal tissue that gives the brain the appearance of a basket with a handle.

REFERENCES:

Berg RA, Aleck KA, Kaplan AM: Familial porencephaly. *Arch Neurol* 40:567, 1983.

Bonnemann CG, Meinecke P: Bilateral porencephaly, cerebellar hypoplasia, and internal malformations: Two siblings representing a probably new autosomal recessive entity. *Am J Med Genet* 63:428, 1996.

Eller KM, Kuller JA: Fetal porencephaly: A review of etiology, diagnosis, and prognosis. *Obstet Gynecol Surv* 50:684, 1995.

Familial Progressive Scleroderma

At a glance: Disorder characterized by progressive systemic sclerosis (scleroderma), calcium deposits (calcinosis) usually in the fingers, Raynaud syndrome, loss of muscle control of the esophagus (difficult swallowing), osseous deformity of the fingers (sclerodactyly), and small red spots (telangiectasia) on the skin (fingers, face) or inside the mouth.

Synonym: Calcinosis.

Incidence: 5:10,000,000 in adults; only 3% of total cases affect children.

Genetic inheritance: Unknown, but female-to-male ratio is 3:1. Dominant form described.

Pathophysiology: Collagen (types I and III), fibronectin, and proteoglycans are deposited in the interstitium and the intima of small arteries. Fibrosis (involving several cytokines, especially interleukin-4) is found in clinically affected and unaffected tissue. Calcinosis is caused by deposits of carbonated apatite B. Autoimmune mechanism is suspected (increased chromosomal breakage rate is predominantly observed in linkage disequilibrium with HLA haplotype A1, Cw7, B8, C4AQ0B1, DR3, which is frequently observed in autoimmune diseases). A linkage between the fibrillin-1 gene locus and the scleroderma phenotype is suspected. Because of the similarity of scleroderma to chronic graft-versus-host disease, microchimerism is suspected in the pathogenesis of the disorder.

Diagnosis: Multisystemic disorder of connective tissue affecting the skin, which becomes hardened. Visceral involvement may be severe and affects the heart (myocardial fibrosis and secondary conduction defects, pericardial effusions), lung, kidneys (renal failure), intestinal tract (gastroesophageal reflux and strictures), and synovium. Whitish creamy discharge from the fingertips is observed occasionally. The deposit consists of carbonated apatite type B. The mineral substance seems to be less reactive and more stable than normal calcium pyrophosphate deposit in bone, explaining the total lack of effectiveness of calcium chelating agents.

Clinical aspects: Because of the numerous combinations of potential signs of the disorder, many clinical aspects are observed. Calcinosis (subcutaneous calcareous concretions), telangiectasia, and scleroderma (systemic sclerosis) are constant. Raynaud syndrome is very common. Scleroderma often results in esophageal motility disorders (with permanent strictures occasionally) and sclerodactyly. Calcinosis can involve many joints (elbows, shoulders), periarticular areas (flank), and viscera (heart). Clinically, the disorder is divided into *two groups:* (1) "pure" CREST (calcinosis cutis, Raynaud phenomenon, esophageal motility disorder, sclerodactyly, and telangiectasia), which occurs when patients have two or more symptoms of CREST but do not meet the criteria for either limited or diffuse scleroderma (no tight skin above their wrists, no pitting digital ulcers, no lung fibrosis; and (2) "plus CREST," when CREST symptoms appear with another form of scleroderma (e.g., limited scleroderma plus CREST, diffuse scleroderma plus CREST, any other autoimmune disease plus CREST).

Precautions before anesthesia: These patients are often treated with a systemic corticosteroid therapy; consequently, salt and water balance must be evaluated. Patients taking acetylsalicylic acid must be evaluated for bleeding. Evaluate mouth opening because of contracted perioral skin. Fiberoptic tracheal intubation should be available for induction of anesthesia. Pulmonary function tests prior to major procedures. Evaluation of cardiac, hepatic, and renal function is needed. Evaluation of venous access because of possible difficulties as a result of affected skin. Administration of antacid and cimetidine as premedication.

Anesthetic considerations: Regional anesthesia, particularly peripheral nerves blocks, must be used as often as possible. Depending on the type of surgery, regional anesthesia has proved to be very successful in adults and can be safely proposed in children. If general anesthesia is chosen, difficult tracheal intubation should be anticipated because of the association of limited mouth opening. The use of a rapid-sequence intubation technique because of gastric reflux must be evaluated in light of the mouth opening limitation. Inhalational induction using sevoflurane associated with cricoid pressure (even under fiberscope) seems to be the safest technique. Tracheal extubation should be performed only when the patient is completely awake and displays fully competent laryngeal reflexes.

Pharmacological implications: Only depends on the multisystemic involvement and medication taken. Intraoperative corticosteroid supplementation must be considered.

Other conditions to be considered:

☞**HEREDITARY TELANGIECTASIA:** Autosomal dominant mucocutaneous and visceral fibrovascular dysplasia in which telangiectasia, arteriovenous malformations, and aneurysms may be widely distributed throughout the cardiovascular system. It is usually recognized as a "triad" of telangiectasia, recurrent epistaxis, and a family history of the disorder.

MORPHEA (Morphoea; Localized Scleroderma): Localized form of scleroderma characterized by thickening and induration of the skin and subcutaneous tissue as a consequence of excessive collagen deposition. Morphea subtypes are classified according to clinical presentation and depth of tissue involvement. They include plaque-like, generalized, linear, and deep varieties. Morphea lacks features such as sclerodactyly, Raynaud phenomenon, and internal organ involvement. Because of overproduction of collagen by lesional fibroblast, probably as a result of endothelial cell injury, inflammation and immunologic responses occur. The incidence rate is estimated to be 27 new cases per one million general population per year.

SCLERODERMA EN COUP DE SABRE (Proliferative Retinopathy): Bilateral linear scleroderma en coup de sabre is associated with facial hemiatrophy and neurologic dysfunctions. Affects usually one side of the face and head in the frontoparietal area with band-like indurated skin lesions. "En coup de sabre" is defined by a localized patch of scleroderma in the frontal region of the scalp, causing a cicatricial alopecia (resembles the scar of a wound made by a sabre).

☞**PARRY ROMBERG SYNDROME:** Rare disorder characterized by progressive atrophy of one side of the face occasionally extending to other parts of the body. The process may, however, be bilateral in 5 to 10% of cases. Tissues involved include the skin, tongue (difficult intubation), gingiva, soft palate, nose, subcutaneous fat, larynx, muscle, and bone.

☞**CREST SYNDROME:** One of the three divisions of scleroderma, which are morphea, linear scleroderma, and CREST syndrome.

REFERENCES:

Akiyama Y, Tanaka M, Takeishi M, et al: Clinical, serological and genetic study in patients with CREST syndrome. *Intern Med* 39:451, 2000.

Hussmann J, Russell RC, Kucan JO, et al: Soft tissue calcifications: Differential diagnosis and therapeutic approaches. *Ann Plast Surg* 34:138, 1995.

Fanconi Anemia

At a glance: Inherited anemia leading to bone marrow failure, myelogenous leukemia, and, in older patients, many cancers (head and neck, esophageal, gastrointestinal, vulvar, anal).

Synonym: Type I Fanconi Pancytopenia.

History: Genetically inherited anemia. Named after the Swiss pediatrician, Guido Fanconi.

Incidence: Rare, with carrier frequency of 1:300 in the general population (1:89 in the Ashkenazi Jewish population). Occurs equally in males and females and is found in all ethnic groups. The International Fanconi Anemia Registry (Rockefeller University, New York, NY) maintains case data on more than 3000 patients.

Genetic inheritance: Fanconi anemia (FA) comprises a group of monogenic autosomal recessive disorders resulting from mutations in one of eight Fanconi anemia genes (A, B, C, D1, D2, E, F, G). Although caused by rather simple mutations, the disorder shows a complex phenotype with many features, including developmental abnormalities, severe anemia, and/or eventually leukemia and various cancers. Many patients die during their mid-teen years. Mutations in FA-A and FA-C account for 76% of patients worldwide.

Pathophysiology: Spontaneous chromosomal aberrations associated with hypocellular marrow, pancytopenia, and constitutional aplastic anemia.

Diagnosis: Usually diagnosed by age 6 years, after onset of hematologic abnormalities. It may be diagnosed as early as the neonatal period while investigated for other associated anomalies. Diepoxybutane, a DNA cross-linking agent, is a unique marker for Fanconi anemia cells. Currently, the definitive diagnostic test is a chromosome breakage test with a chemical, either diepoxybutane or mitomycin C, that cross-links DNA. Normal cells are able to correct most of the damage caused by these agents, whereas Fanconi anemia cells show marked chromosome breakage. These tests can be performed prenatally on cells from chorionic villi or from the amniotic fluid.

Clinical aspects: Pancytopenia, with mean survival of 5 years after diagnosis, low birth weight, skeletal anomalies (hips, spine, ribs), short stature, microcephaly, microphthalmia, microstomia, radial ray/thumb abnormalities, polydactyly, syndactyly, misplaced radial artery, renal abnormalities, cardiac defects, and developmental delay.

Precautions before anesthesia: Check a complete blood cell count (CBC) for anemia and thrombocytopenia. Check electrolytes in presence of renal defects. Complete physical evaluation must be obtained to eliminate the presence of cardiac defects.

Anesthetic considerations: Maintain oxygen carrying capacity with red blood cell transfusion. Anticipate need for platelet transfusion. Avoid central neuraxial anesthesia techniques in presence of coagulopathy. Direct laryngoscopy and tracheal intubation can be difficult in the presence of macrostomia.

Pharmacological implications: Prophylactic antibiotic must be considered in case of cardiac defect.

Other conditions to be considered:

☞**BLOOM SYNDROME:** Autosomal recessive inherited disorder characterized by prenatal and postnatal growth retardation, photosensitivity, telangiectasias, skin pigment anomalies, and increased risk of malignancies most likely caused by chromosomal instability. Most interchanges occur between homologous chromosomes, not between nonhomologous chromosomes as in Fanconi anemia.

☞**BLACKFAN-DIAMOND SYNDROME:** Congenital hypoplastic anemia manifesting in the first year of life, with increased risk for leukemia. High adenosine deaminase activity in the blood.

☞**TAR SYNDROME:** Rare condition associated with thrombocytopenia and bilateral radial aplasia first described in 1951. The frequency is 0.42:100,000 live births in Spain. Autosomal recessive inheritance, also presenting abnormalities in skeletal, gastrointestinal, hematologic, and cardiac systems. Pancytopenia similar to Fanconi anemia. The major cause of mortality is hemorrhage. The incidence of hemorrhage is limited to the first 14 months of life. Male and females are affected equally.

☞**CONGENITAL DYSERYTHROPOIETIC ANEMIAS:** Group of inherited disorders characterized by quantitatively and qualitatively altered erythropoiesis resulting in usually mild-to-moderate anemia. Premature destruction of erythroblasts in the bone marrow reduces the number of them reaching maturity. In addition, there is also peripheral destruction of these dysplastic erythroblasts.

HEXOKINASE-DEFICIENCY HEMOLYTIC ANEMIA, CHRONIC: Autosomal recessive pattern characterized by chronic hemolytic anemia associated with severe deficiency of red cell glucose phosphate isomerase. Some cases of autosomal dominant transmission have been reported. Like the phosphofructokinase and pyruvate kinase, the hexokinase enzyme is a rate-limiting factor in the metabolism of glucose in the Embden-Meyerhof pathway. Because glycolysis is the only source of energy for the red cells, deficiency in hexokinase results in chronic hemolytic anemia. A few *allelic variants* have been described for this chronic form: *Fukuoka:* Reported in the Japanese literature as the association of chronic glucose phosphate deficiency and a history of prolonged neonatal jaundice. *Iwate:* Chronic form of hemolytic anemia most often homozygous in pattern and detected early in life. *Homburg:* Association of chronic hemolytic anemia and neurologic deficits. Anesthetic considerations must include a proper evaluation of the hematocrit and the possibility of intraoperative transfusion. Administration of glucose solution can exaggerate the hemolytic reactions.

REFERENCES:

Ahmad SI, Hanaoka F, Kirk SH: Molecular biology of Fanconi anaemia—An old problem, a new insight. *Bioessays* 24:439, 2002.

Giampietro PF: The need for more accurate and timely diagnosis in Fanconi anemia: A report from the International Fanconi Anemia Registry. *Pediatrics* 91:1116, 1993.

Fanconi-Bickel Syndrome (FBS)

At a glance: Genetically transmitted metabolic disorder of carbohydrates characterized by accumulation of glycogen in the liver with hepatomegaly, proximal tubular nephropathy, fasting hypoglycemia, glucose (and galactose) intolerance, and dwarfism.

Synonyms: Hepatorenal Glycogenosis with Renal Fanconi Syndrome; Hepatic Glycogenosis with Fanconi Nephropathy; Hepatic Glycogenosis with Aminoaciduria and Glucosuria; Fanconi Syndrome with Intestinal Malabsorption and Galactose Intolerance; Pseudo-Phlorizin Diabetes; Glycogenosis, Fanconi type; Glycogen Storage Disease IX; Bickel-Fanconi Syndrome.

History: Inborn error of carbohydrate metabolism with tubular nephropathy. First reported in 1949 by Guido Fanconi, a Swiss pediatrician, and Horst Bickel, a German physician.

Incidence: Approximately 100 cases reported in the literature.

Genetic inheritance: Autosomal recessive inheritance. Caused by mutations in the glucose transporter protein 2 (GLUT2 gene) that is expressed in liver, pancreas, intestine, and kidney. Gene map locus is 3q26.1-q26.3.

Pathophysiology: Primary defect of monosaccharide transport across the membranes. Hyperglycemia (and hypergalactosemia) in the fed state could be explained by (1) a decreased monosaccharide uptake by the liver or (2) an inappropriately low insulin secretion caused by impairment of the glucose-sensing mechanism of the beta cells. Hypoglycemia during fasting may result from (1) an altered glucose transport out of the liver, resulting in an increased intracellular glucose level that, in turn, may inhibit glycogen degradation, leading to glycogen storage and hepatomegaly, or (2) exacerbation of hypoglycemia due to an increased renal loss of glucose caused by a transport defect for glucose and galactose across the basolateral membranes of the proximal tubular cells. As a consequence, renal glycogen accumulation may occur, with impairment of other functions of the proximal tubular cells and the characteristic clinical picture of Fanconi nephropathy with disproportionately severe glucosuria. As a consequence of a transport defect for glucose and galactose at the basolateral membrane, intestinal monosaccharide transport also is affected, resulting in malabsorption and diarrhea.

Diagnosis: Characterized by hepatomegaly. It is caused by hepatorenal glycogen accumulation, proximal renal tubular dysfunction, and impaired utilization of glucose and galactose. Glucosuria is considered a most prominent finding.

Clinical aspects: Present in infancy (fever, vomiting, growth failure, and rickets). Later patients present with dwarfism, protuberant abdomen, hepatomegaly, moon-shaped face, and fat deposition about the shoulders and abdomen. Emergence of the teeth and development of puberty are retarded. Fractures and pancreatitis are complications. Rickets and osteoporosis later in life are constant features. Glomerular filtration rate is normal or low normal, and there is no progression to glomerular insufficiency or deterioration of tubular defects. Polyuria, probably a result of osmotic diuresis, is a constant finding. Clinical management by symptomatic replacement treatment (water, electrolytes, and vitamin D, restriction of galactose, a diabetes mellitus-like diet presented in frequent small meals with adequate caloric intake). Administration of uncooked cornstarch has been reported to be beneficial for promoting growth. Few patients reported still alive in their 50s.

Precautions before anesthesia: Preoperative fasting should be kept as brief as possible and intravenous glucose started to minimize the possibility of hypoglycemia. Frequent measurement of blood glucose concentrations is mandatory. Detailed assessment of hepatic functions in view of glycogen accumulation. Blood work should include serum concentrations of urea, creatinine, and electrolytes and liver function tests.

Anesthetic considerations: Anesthetic management depends on the severity of the disease. Intraoperative hypoglycemia may be difficult to recognize because the signs and symptoms are masked by general anesthesia. Consequently, regular blood glucose level monitoring is mandatory. Adequate intravascular fluid replacement in the presence of osmotic diuresis. Sympathetic blockade induced by spinal or epidural anesthesia may abolish any homeostatic adrenergic responses to hypoglycemia.

Pharmacological implications: Sedative premedications are not recommended because they may mask hypoglycemic symptoms. Similarly, postoperative analgesia and sedation must be administered in guarded doses. Avoid any drug that is a potential threat to hepatocellular integrity. Sevoflurane is not associated with an increased risk of renal toxicity when compared with other commonly used volatile anesthetics. However, prolonged low-flow administration of sevoflurane must be done with caution because of the significant increase in compound A. Avoid nephrotoxic agents. Avoid drugs that are dependent upon the liver or kidneys for metabolism and elimination (e.g., gallamine, pancuronium).

REFERENCES:

Brown GK: Glucose transporters: Structure, function and consequences of deficiency. *J Inherit Metab Dis* 23:237, 2000.

Santer R, Groth S, Kinner M, et al: The mutation spectrum of the facilitative glucose transporter gene SLC2A2 (GLUT2) in patients with Fanconi-Bickel syndrome. *Hum Genet* 110:21, 2002.

Santer R, Steinmann B, Schaub J: Fanconi-Bickel syndrome—A congenital defect of facilitative glucose transport. *Curr Mol Med* 2:213, 2002.

Farber Uzman Syndrome

At a glance: Inborn error of the fatty metabolism caused by a lysosomal enzyme deficiency and resulting in the accumulation of ceramide in body tissues with multiple organ failure and death in infancy (but mildly affected patients can reach adulthood). Severe motor and mental retardation is evident.

Synonyms: Acid Ceramidase Deficiency; Farber Lipogranulomatosis; Farber Disease.

Incidence: Approximately 50 cases have been reported in the literature. Equally represented in males and females.

Genetic inheritance: Autosomal recessive.

Pathophysiology: Accumulation of ceramide in tissue as a result of a deficiency of lysosomal acid ceramidase. This accumulation causes cell damage with an inflammatory response resulting in the formation of nodules or granules (not involving the CNS).

Diagnosis: Suspected based on the classic triad of symptoms: synovial thickening associated with joint stiffness, subcutaneous granulomas, and hoarseness as a consequence of laryngeal involvement. It is established by the deficiency of ceramidase activity in lymphocytes or cultured skin fibroblasts and the identification of Farber bodies on biopsy of nodules (characteristic inclusions). Prenatal diagnosis is available (deficiency of ceramidase activity in cultured chorionic villi or amniocytes).

Clinical aspects: Characterized by progressive hoarseness, noisy respiration, nutritional failure associated with poor growth and development, multiple subcutaneous and periarticular nodules, and progressive arthropathies. Accumulation of ceramide in the nervous system causes psychomotor retardation, peripheral neuropathy, and muscle denervation. The heart can be involved in the disease process, with the presence of granulomas on cardiac valves. This clinical picture mainly fits the classic type I disease. Some other subtypes, which are even more unusual, may present with ocular, neurologic, and bone marrow involvement.

Precautions before anesthesia: If bone marrow involvement is suspected, a CBC is recommended. An ECG and echocardiogram are recommended if valvular involvement caused by the disease is suspected.

Anesthetic considerations: Because of the presence of granulomas in the oral cavity, direct laryngoscopy and tracheal intubation may be difficult as a consequence of diminished space and poor visualization. Also, nutritional failure decreases albumin level and so

increases the unbound fraction of many drugs. Cardiac disease, if present, should be managed appropriately. Antibioprophylaxis may be required. Finally, joint contractures require proper positioning of the patient on the operating room table.

Pharmacological implications: Increased level of unbound drug because of decreased albumin level. Lower threshold for local anesthetic toxicity. Use of succinylcholine is not recommended if there is a severe denervation myopathy and the overall need for muscular relaxant will be minimal.

Other condition to be considered:

☞**ERDHEIM-CHESTER DISEASE:** Rare histiocytic disorder characterized by non-Langerhans cell histiocytosis resulting in extensive lipoid granulomas in various parts of the body and organs. Clinical manifestations range from asymptomatic to fatal multisystem involvement, typically bones, kidneys, hearts, and lungs.

REFERENCES:

Bar J, Linke T, Ferlinz K, et al: Molecular analysis of acid ceramidase deficiency in patients with Farber disease. *Hum Mutat* 17:199, 2001.

Haraoka G, Muraoka M, Yoshioka N, et al: First case of surgical treatment of Farber's disease. *Ann Plast Surg* 39:405, 1997.

Salo MK, Karikoski R, Hallstrom M, et al: Farber disease diagnosed after liver transplantation. *J Pediatr Gastroenterol Nutr* 36:274, 2003.

Faulk Epstein Jones Syndrome

At a glance: Polymalformative syndrome characterized by the association of congenital blepharoptosis of the eyelid and lumbosacral vertebral fusion.

Synonyms: Posterior Lumbosacral Vertebral Fusion-Blepharoptosis Syndrome; Familial Posterior Lumbosacral Vertebral Fusion and Eyelid Ptosis Syndrome.

Genetic inheritance: Autosomal dominant.

Diagnosis Based on clinical findings and radiologic findings of vertebral fusions, especially in the lumbosacral region.

Clinical aspects: Patients have eye and musculoskeletal involvement. They present with a congenital and bilateral ptosis and elevator palsy. Other clinical features consist of contractures at the hip and knee, Achilles tendon tightness, and fusion of the posterior elements of the lumbosacral spine.

Anesthetic considerations: Limited movement of the hips, knees, and lumbosacral region may complicate patient positioning and increase risk of nerve compression and skin damage. However, the main concern is that neuraxial regional anesthesia in the lumbar and lower thoracic region is not recommended because of the posterior fusion.

REFERENCE:

Faulk WP, Epstein CJ, Jones MD: Familial posterior lumbosacral vertebral fusion and eyelids ptosis. *Am J Dis Child* 119:510, 1970.

Feigenbaum Bergeron Richardson Syndrome

At a glance: Neurodegenerative disorder with progressive atherosclerosis, diabetes mellitus, and nephropathy.

Incidence: The syndrome was originally described in two brothers. Few cases have been reported in the literature.

Genetic inheritance: Uncertain; either X-linked or autosomal recessive.

Pathophysiology: The pathologic findings led the authors to conclude that the syndrome probably is caused by a mitochondrial defect in the respiratory chain and that it was the cause of the neuronal damage and of the premature atherosclerosis.

Diagnosis: Based mainly on the clinical findings. If this syndrome is suspected, skin fibroblast culture may show a partial deficiency of the mitochondrial enzymes of complexes III and IV.

Clinical aspects: The disease is slowly progressive, and the patients often die of complications in their third decade of life. Patients first present with sensorineural deafness at a young age and later present with other neurologic symptoms, such as deterioration in cognitive function, shuffling gait, incoordination, tremor, dysmetria, dysdiadokinesis, slurred speech, and finally photomyoclonic seizures. They may have increased spasticity mainly in the lower limb. Affected patients also present with diabetes mellitus type I beginning in their 20s and nephropathy in the form of a nephritic syndrome. The other remarkable finding is the presence of severe atherosclerosis affecting mainly the coronary, renal, and cerebral vessels.

Precautions before anesthesia: In the presence of renal disease, hemoglobin level may be reduced, thus a CBC is recommended. Also, because of the associated diabetes, patients will have delayed gastric emptying, so gastric prophylaxis is recommended prior to operation. Proper cardiac evaluation for signs of ischemia must be performed.

Anesthetic considerations: Keep in mind that gastric emptying is delayed and that a rapid sequence may be warranted, especially in the absence of a prophylaxis. However, with the combination of diabetes and atherosclerosis, patients are more prone to cardiac ischemia and renal and cerebral hypoperfusion. The recommendation is to prevent significant changes in blood pressure and to have a vasopressor, such as phenylephrine, readily available.

Pharmacological implications: Drugs used for seizure control can cause induction of liver enzymes, so the dose of certain medications, such as neuromuscular agents, may need to be increased.

REFERENCE:

Feigenbaum A, Bergeron C, Richardson R, et al: Premature atherosclerosis with photomyoclonic epilepsy, deafness, diabetes mellitus, nephropathy, and neurodegenerative disorder in two brothers: A new syndrome? *Am J Med Genet* 49:118, 1994.

Feingold Syndrome

At a glance: Polymalformative condition characterized by esophageal/duodenal atresia, limb abnormalities (hand/foot), short palpebral fissures, microcephaly and learning disabilities.

Synonyms: Microcephaly-Oculo-Digito-Esophago-Duodenal Syndrome; MODED Syndrome; Brunner-Winter Syndrome; Oculodigitoesophagoduodenal Syndrome.

Incidence and genetic inheritance: Incidence unknown. Autosomal dominant with gene map locus at 2p24.

Clinical aspects: Most common clinical features are microcephaly with prominent occiput, mental retardation, narrow palpebral fissures, telecanthus, retrognathia and low-set ears. The presence of a laryngeal cleft/vocal cord palsy gives an abnormal cry and voice. The gastrointestinal defects include esophageal atresia (EA) [with or without tracheoesophageal fistula (TEF) or duodenal atresia (DA)],

occurs in 30% of patients. Other features include a patent ductus arteriosus, sacral spine anomalies (sagittal cleft), and blockage of C5-C6 vertebrae. Neural arch fusion at C6-C7 has been reported. Short stature, syndactyly of toes, brachydactyly type A, clinodactyly, slender thumbs with limited flexion in the distal interphalangeal joint.

Precautions before anesthesia: Evaluate the airway due to facial malformations. Mental retardation may limit patient cooperation. Sedative premedication and/or the presence of the primary caregiver may be helpful.

Anesthetic considerations: Airway management should be expected to be difficult due to microretrognathia and potential cervical motility problems. Patients with DA and/or TEF are at increased risk for aspiration. The association of EA and TEF requires that the tracheal tube be positioned below the level of the fistula to avoid gastric distention during positive pressure ventilation. Venous access may be difficult. Regional anesthesia is not contraindicated, but caudal anesthesia may be difficult in presence of sacral anomalies.

Pharmacological implications: Avoid neuromuscular blockers until the airway has been secured.

REFERENCES:

Celli J, van Bokhoven H, Brunner HG: Feingold syndrome: clinical review and genetic mapping. *Am J Med Genet* 122:294, 2003.

Felty Syndrome

At a glance: Late immunologic complication of seropositive (rheumatic factor–positive) rheumatoid arthritis (RA) characterized by splenomegaly and granulocytopenia.

History: Immunologic disorder complicating RA first described in 1924 by Augustus Roi Felty, an American physician.

Incidence: Only three reported cases of Felty Syndrome complicating juvenile RA versus an incidence of approximately 1% in adults with RA. Predominance in whites (rare in blacks) and predominantly in females (3:1).

Genetic inheritance: The human leukocyte antigen DR4 (HLA-DR4) genotype is strongly associated with Felty syndrome.

Pathophysiology: Laboratory studies show a lower granulocyte count in the splenic vein compared to the splenic artery, the presence of immune complexes coating the granulocytes, low granulocyte growth factor levels, and numerous circulating autoantibodies (especially those against granulocyte surface antigens).

Diagnosis: Development of splenomegaly and granulocytopenia ($<2000/mm^3$) in patients with severe RA; confirmed by immunologic studies. Cryoglobulins may be present.

Clinical aspects: Felty syndrome usually develops after many years of destructive RA with extraarticular manifestations (rheumatoid nodules, vasculitis, pleuropericarditis, peripheral neuropathy, ocular complications, Sjögren syndrome, adenopathy, skin ulcers). Patient frequently present with bacterial infections (possibly life-threatening) and pain in the upper quadrant of the abdomen (splenic infarct, capsular distention). Immunosuppressive therapy for RA often improves granulocytopenia and splenomegaly, confirming the immune-mediated nature of the disease. Recombinant granulopoietic growth factors quickly raise the granulocyte count and improve the physical condition of the patient in case of life-threatening infections. Splenectomy is only a last-chance therapy; granulocytopenia recurs in approximately 25% of splenectomized patients.

Precautions before anesthesia: In presence of severe RA, complete evaluation of cardiac and renal function is highly recommended. Chronic corticosteroid therapy and potential side effects must be evaluated. Use of gold salt must be confirmed and their effect on the kidneys assessed. Obtain a CBC. Obtain full history (infection, Sjögren syndrome)

Anesthetic considerations: Patients are more prone to infection, so intravenous access or invasive monitoring should be done under sterile conditions. Regional technique should be avoided in the presence of a thrombocytopenic patient. Other considerations are those related to RA, such as joint stiffness and deformations and temporomandibular involvement, which can complicate tracheal intubation.

Pharmacological implications: Methotrexate can induce hepatorenal dysfunction; if it is a concern, appropriate blood tests and management are warranted. Patients receiving gold salt medication must be carefully assessed for renal dysfunction. If so, anesthetic medications must be selected appropriately. Consider these patients to be immunodeficient.

REFERENCES:
Bloom BJ, Smith P, Alario AJ: Felty syndrome complicating juvenile rheumatoid arthritis. *J Pediatr Hematol Oncol* 20;511, 1998.

Bowman SJ: Hematological manifestations of rheumatoid arthritis. *Scand J Rheumatol* 31:251, 2002.

Hellmich B, Csernok E, Schatz H, et al: Autoantibodies against granulocyte colony-stimulating factor in Felty's syndrome and neutropenic systemic lupus erythematosus. *Arthritis Rheum* 46:2384, 2002.

Femoral-Facial Syndrome

At a glance: Osteoarticular disorder characterized by the presence of a typical facial appearance, cleft palate, and underdeveloped bowed femurs.

Synonyms: Bilateral Femoral Dysgenesis; Femoral Dysgenesis-Robin Anomaly; Femoral Hypoplasia-Unusual Facies Syndrome.

Genetic inheritance: Mostly sporadic but autosomal dominant forms with incomplete penetrance have been reported.

Pathophysiology: Unknown.

Diagnosis: Mainly clinical and usually can be suspected antenatally during routine ultrasonogram.

Clinical aspects: Affected patient presents with a facies characterized by up-slanted palpebral fissures. Micrognathia associated with a small, pointed chin, short nose, thin upper lip, long philtrum, and cleft palate is found in some cases. The musculoskeletal findings show mainly short, bowed femora and acetabular and sacral anomalies, resulting in a short stature. All other bone lengths are within normal. Some of the other features are hypoplasia of the penis, testes, and labia major and possible renal abnormalities.

Precautions before anesthesia: No special precautions required before administration of anesthesia except for careful evaluation of the airway in the presence of micrognathia. Evaluate renal function.

Anesthetic considerations: The potential for difficult direct laryngoscopy and tracheal intubation cannot be eliminated. Because of musculoskeletal involvement, special attention to intraoperative position must be given.

Pharmacological implications: No specific implications with this condition. Limit use of prolong neuromuscular relaxants once the trachea has been secured.

REFERENCES:
Burn J, Winter RM, Baraitser M, et al: The femoral hypoplasia-unusual facies syndrome. *J Med Genet* 21:331, 1984.

Leal E, Macias-Gomez N, Rodriguez L, et al: Femoral-facial syndrome with malformations in the central nervous system. *Clin Imaging* 27:23, 2003.

Robinow M, Sonek J, Buttino L, et al: Femoral-facial syndrome—Prenatal diagnosis—Autosomal dominant inheritance. *Am J Med Genet* 57:397, 1995.

Femur-Fibula-Ulna Syndrome

At a glance: Polymalformative syndrome characterized by multiple osteoarticular anomalies of long bones of upper and lower extremities. The upper limbs and the right side are usually affected more often.

Synonyms: FFU Syndrome; Proximal Focal Femoral Deficiency.

Incidence and genetic inheritance: Male-to-female ratio is 9:1. Mostly sporadic but possible autosomal recessive inheritance in some cases.

Clinical aspects: Based on clinical presentation and radiologic confirmation of the characteristic malformed limbs. The affection is asymmetrical and highly variable in its clinical expression. Males are affected more often, and usually the upper limb and the right side are more commonly malformed. Some of the more common malformations encountered are amelia of the arm, peromelia of the upper arm, humeroradial synostosis, peromelia of the femur, missing fingers, defect of the ulna or ulnar rays, and hypoplasia of the fibula.

Anesthetic considerations: Venous access may be difficult because of the limb anomalies. Installation of monitoring devices also can be affected by the limb abnormalities. Considerations for invasive monitoring may be justified only on the basis of inability to ensure proper placement and functioning of noninvasive devices. No specific pharmacological implications with this condition.

REFERENCE:
Lenz W, Zygulska M, Horst J: FFU complex: An analysis of 491 ceases. *Hum Genet* 91:347, 1993.

Fenton Wilkinson Toselano Syndrome

At a glance: Caused by an inborn error of tryptophan metabolism. Ataxia with photosensitivity, short stature, and a high-vaulted, narrow palate.

Genetic inheritance: Unsure but could be autosomal recessive.

Pathophysiology: Unknown.

Diagnosis: Diagnosis is clinical and biochemical. Low serum tryptophan levels with normal 5-hydroxytryptophan pathways, low urinary N-methyl nicotinamide levels, and absent 5-hydroxyanthrilic acid are observed. The response to tryptophan loading is abnormal, with low-to-absent level of 3-hydroxyanthranilic acid. Monochromator studies show abnormal photosensitivity.

Clinical aspects: The main features of the disease are a short stature, cerebellar-like ataxia associated with intention tremor of the upper limb, photosensitivity of the face and trunk, and mental retardation. Other common findings are clinodactyly, high arched palate, pseudohypertrophy of the calf, and bicuspid aortic valve malformation.

Precautions before anesthesia: Obtain an ECG and an echocardiogram if a cardiac valve lesion is suspected.

Anesthetic considerations: Because of the high arched palate and small maxilla, insertion of a laryngoscope with a curve blade may be more difficult. Spontaneous respiration may have to be maintained until the airway is secured.

Pharmacological implications: In the presence of a valve lesion, antibioprophylaxis may be recommended, and the management should be made accordingly.

Other condition to be considered:

☞**COCKAYNE SYNDROME:** Complex congenital genetic disorder characterized by the association of dwarfism, deafness, microcephaly, facies similar to progeria syndrome, ataxia, photosensitivity and eye malformations, retinal atrophy, and renal insufficiency with premature aging and atherosclerosis.

REFERENCE:
Fenton DA, Wilkinson JD, Toseland PA: Family exhibiting cerebellar-like ataxia, photosensitivity and shortness of stature—A new inborn error of tryptophan metabolism. *J R Soc Med* 76:736, 1983.

Fetal Alcohol Syndrome (FAS)

At a glance: Syndrome characterized by a series of physical, mental, and neurobehavioral birth defects resulting from chronic alcohol consumption during pregnancy.

Synonyms: Alcohol Antenatal Exposition; Alcoholic Embryopathy.

History: First described in France by J. Lemoine in 1968 and in the United States by Jones and Smith in 1973. The literature is prominent because FAS is considered the leading known cause of mental retardation affecting all socioeconomic groups and races.

Incidence: Between 0.5 and 5 per 1000 live births, making fetal FAS the leading cause of mental retardation and birth defects. More frequent in infants born to black mothers, especially those with ADH2-1/3 phenotype (an unusual phenotype in white women). The incidence among children born to heavy drinkers is 4%.

Genetic inheritance: Not a genetic condition; rather it is a toxic syndrome. However, women with the alcohol dehydrogenase 2 genotype 1/3 (ADH2-1/3) seem to be at greater risk for having an affected infant, but this may be the result of greater ingestion of alcohol.

Pathophysiology: Unknown, but the teratogenic effect of alcohol on the fetus is suspected to result from the formation of free radicals causing cellular damage on the developing tissues of the fetus. Exposure early in pregnancy is responsible for the defective organogenesis and abnormal craniofacial development, whereas continuing alcohol exposure throughout pregnancy causes growth deficiency. Neurodevelopmental effects caused by alcohol are present during the three trimesters because the brain undergoes development at all stages of pregnancy.

Diagnosis: Diagnosis is clinical based on the physical findings in the infant and the history of alcohol consumption during early pregnancy. Diagnosis criteria have been established by the Institute of Medicine and the National Academy of Sciences.

Clinical aspects: FAS is an ensemble of findings found in children exposed to alcohol in utero. They include prenatal and postnatal

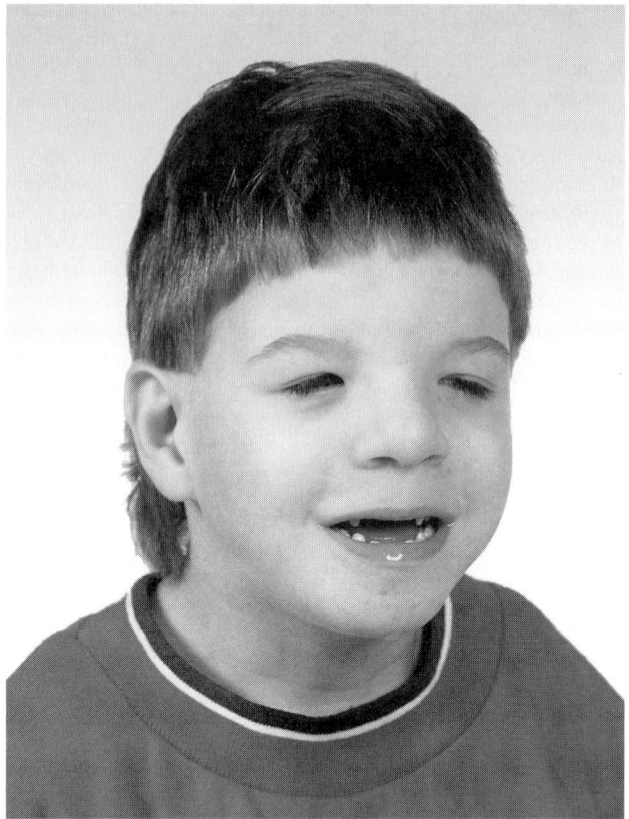

Fetal Alcohol Syndrome Five-year-old boy with fetal alcohol syndrome shows short palpebral fissures, ptosis, and a smooth, long philtrum with a thin upper lip.

growth deficiency, short palpebral fissures, ptosis, flat midface, upturned nose, smooth philtrum with thin upper lip, microcephaly, learning disabilities associated with mild-to-moderate mental retardation, fine motor dysfunction, hyperactivity, ventriculoseptal defect, atrial septal defect, and minor musculoskeletal findings.

Precautions before anesthesia: Clinically suspected cardiac defects should be ruled out with an echocardiogram.

Anesthetic considerations: Cooperation may be absent in some children with behavioral dysfunction, so premedication is advisable. Rarely patients have micrognathia and/or a short, webbed neck that may make direct laryngoscopy and tracheal intubation more difficult.

Pharmacological implications: In the presence of a cardiac defect, antibioprophylaxis may be required.

REFERENCES:
Rovasio RA, Battiato NL: Ethanol induces morphological and dynamic changes on in vivo and in vitro neural crest cells. *Alcohol Clin Exp Res* 26:1286, 2002.

Stoler JM, Ryan LM, Holmes LB: Alcohol dehydrogenase 2 genotypes, maternal alcohol use, and infant outcome. *J Pediatr* 141:780, 2002.

Thackray HM, Tifft C: Fetal alcohol syndrome. *Pediatr Rev* 22:47, 2001.

Fetal Aminopterin Syndrome

At a glance: Polymalformative teratogenic syndrome characterized by short stature, skull anomalies, hydrocephalus, and facial anomalies (abnormal auricles, hypertelorism, micrognathia, cleft palate).

Synonym: Aminopterin Antenatal Infection.

Pathophysiology: Aminopterin is a folic acid antagonist that was used both as an antineoplastic and an abortive agent in the 1950s and 1960s. It is teratogenic when absorbed during the first trimester of pregnancy (affecting the morphogenesis of 50% of embryos and fetuses). Methotrexate, which is the methyl derivative of aminopterin, can have the same effect in dosages greater than 10 mg/wk.

Diagnosis: Diagnosis is clinical based on the drug ingestion history and the dysmorphism of the fetus.

Clinical aspects: Drug ingestion causes fetal and early postnatal death, but some infants survive beyond the first year. The main feature is growth deficiency that usually has a prenatal onset and continues postnatally. They are born with microcephaly and hypoplasia of most of the cranial bones. Other facial feature findings are the presence of a broad nasal bridge, shallow supraorbital ridges, prominent eyes, low-set ears, epicanthal folds, micrognathia, and maxillary hypoplasia. Intelligence and motor development are normal. Musculoskeletal findings are a relative shortness of the limbs, mostly of the forearm, and talipes equinovarus. Other occasional abnormalities, such as cleft palate, neural tube defect, dextroposition of the heart, and hypotonia, are observed.

Precautions before anesthesia: Carefully evaluate the airway.

Anesthetic considerations: Tracheal intubation may be difficult because of the micrognathia and the maxillary hypoplasia, so have an alternate intubation tool readily available.

Pharmacological implications: Avoid long-acting muscular relaxants until the airway is secured.

Other conditions to be considered: This syndrome can be compared to other toxic antenatal expositions, such as fetal methotrexate syndrome, fetal aminopterin-like syndrome (exposure to antifolate drugs other than aminopterin).

RETINOIC ACID EMBRYOPATHY: Syndrome characterized by significant anomalies in response to the teratogenic effects of retinoic acid (isotretinoin, 1,3-*cis*-retinoic acid [Accutane]). The risk to the fetus is usually present when maternal ingestion of Accutane occurs after day 15 of pregnancy. The patient presents with microcephaly, facial asymmetry, facial nerve palsy, micrognathia, and cleft palate. The cardiovascular system includes conotruncal anomalies. Mental retardation and hydrocephalus have been reported. There is an association with ☞DiGeorge syndrome. Anesthetic considerations include difficult airway management, hypocalcemia (because of parathyroid gland dysfunction), and the potential for congenital heart defects.

☞**FETAL RETINOID SYNDROME:** Characteristic pattern of mental and physical birth defects resulting from maternal use of retinoids, the synthetic derivatives of vitamin A, during pregnancy. Affects males and females equally. Exact incidence is unknown, and because many cases of fetal retinoid syndrome often go unrecognized, the disorder is underdiagnosed. The most well-known retinoid is isotretinoin (Accutane®), a drug used for treatment of severe cystic acne. The range and severity of associated abnormalities vary greatly from case to case. Characteristic features may include prenatal and postnatal growth retardation, craniofacial malformations, and central nervous system abnormalities. The cardiovascular system is generally affected with congenital defects such as tetralogy of Fallot, ventricular septal defect, and transposition of the great vessels. Some infants may develop hydrocephalus and present with posterior fossa cysts. Learning disabilities and motor developmental delays are reported. Thymus gland dysfunction has been reported, and calcium problems caused by dysfunctional

parathyroid glands are known. Additional features include polysyndactyly, skeletal malformations affecting the legs and spines, and hypotonia.

☞**DIGEORGE SYNDROME:** Rare immunodeficiency disorder characterized by various congenital abnormalities that develop because of defects that occur during early fetal development. These defects occur in areas known as the third and fourth pharyngeal pouches, which later develop into the thymus and parathyroid glands. The symptoms vary greatly, depending upon the extent of the missing thymus and parathyroid tissue. The primary problem caused is the repeated occurrence of various infections as a result of a diminished immune system.

☞**CHARGE SYNDROME:** Life-threatening, congenital syndrome of multiple abnormalities, consisting of coloboma, heart disease, choanal atresia, mental and growth retardation, genital and urinary anomalies, and ear anomalies with deafness. The prognosis worsens if the disorder is associated with concomitant cyanotic congenital heart disease, central nervous system anomalies, and esophageal atresia.

☞**GOLDENHAR SYNDROME:** Rare disorder apparent at birth. Characterized by developmental abnormalities involving craniofacial anatomical structures, usually in a unilateral pattern. Malar hypoplasia, maxillary and mandibular hypoplasia, temporal hypoplasia, macrostomia, and cleft palate are present. In most cases, Goldenhar syndrome appears to occur randomly, with no apparent cause. Vertebral malformations may include vertebral hypoplasia, fusion, and/or absence of certain vertebrae. Many affected individuals may have additional skeletal, neurological, cardiac, pulmonary, renal, and/or gastrointestinal abnormalities.

☞**CRANE HEISE SYNDROME:** Severe lethal syndrome combining disproportionately large head with peculiar facies and bilateral talipes equinovarus.

REFERENCES:
Bawle EV, Conard JV, Weiss L: Adult and two children with fetal methotrexate syndrome. *Teratology* 57:51, 1998.

Del Campo M, Kosaki K, Bennett FC, et al: Developmental delay in fetal aminopterin/methotrexate syndrome. *Teratology* 60:10, 1999.

Wheeler M, O'Meara P, Stanford M: Fetal methotrexate and misoprostol exposure: The past revisited. *Teratology* 66:73, 2002.

Fetal Cocaine Syndrome

At a glance: Polymalformative teratogenic syndrome characterized by growth disturbances, abnormalities of the fingers and toes, gastrointestinal and/or genitourinary tract, irritability, and arrhythmia with a danger of heart attack or stroke.

Synonym: Cocaine Antenatal Infection.

Nature: This "syndrome" has been challenged because even though cocaine is a known teratogen, there is no specific set of malformations associated with it, unlike the fetal alcohol syndrome.

Incidence: Cocaine is used by approximately 1% of pregnant women in the United States.

Genetic inheritance: The condition is not genetic; rather it is a toxic syndrome therefore acquired.

Pathophysiology: The main effects of cocaine are mediated via dopamine and norepinephrine, the former being responsible for the euphoria and the latter for the harmful effects. Cocaine inhibits norepinephrine reuptake; thus it accumulates at the synaptic level and causes sympathetic activation, which translates to tachycardia, vasoconstriction, hypertension, and arrhythmias. During pregnancy, cocaine use can lead to decreased uteroplacental blood flow, vasoconstriction of the uterine vasculature, and subsequently hypoperfusion of the placenta. Finally, it also crosses the placenta and affects the fetus directly.

Diagnosis: In most of the studies, cocaine use was obtained through history or positive urine testing from the mother. However, if cocaine is not used for a few days (approximately 3 days), no metabolites will be detected in the urine.

Clinical aspects: Initially more preterm labor, precipitous labor, abruptio placentae, and small-for-gestational-age babies in women taking cocaine were reported, but some studies concluded that these occurrences were not related to cocaine use per se but to the absence of adequate prenatal care. Many malformations and behavioral effects caused by cocaine have been reported in the fetus, but with no specific pattern. Consequently, it is thought that the abnormalities are related to the timing and amount of drug used during the pregnancy and to the fact that abusers often use more than one type of drug. Some of the anomalies reported are skull malformations, cerebral infarcts, congenital cardiac defects (atrial septal defect, ventriculoseptal defect, valve stenosis, tetralogy of Fallot, hypoplastic left heart syndrome), neonatal arrhythmias and tachycardia, intestinal atresia, necrotizing enterocolitis, genitourinary malformations, limb defects, microcephaly, hypoplasia of the optic nerve, hypotonia, irritability, and seizures. Behavioral problems associated with attention deficit disorder are controversial. The association with an increased risk for sudden infant death syndrome has been suggested but not confirmed.

Precautions before anesthesia: Perform a complete physical examination to rule out the more obvious anomalies and then obtain an ECG, echocardiogram, and abdominal ultrasonogram based on the clinical findings.

Anesthetic considerations: The acute cardiovascular effects of cocaine on the fetus last for approximately 2 days, so surgery should be postponed to allow for elimination of the drug. If this waiting period is not possible, a narcotic-based anesthesia, but not halothane and desflurane because of their effects on the cardiovascular and sympathetic nervous systems, respectively, is recommended. Continuous ECG monitoring and postoperative stay in the neonatal intensive care unit are mandatory.

Pharmacological implications: Indirect-acting vasopressor drugs should be avoided because catecholamine stores are already depleted. Avoid direct sympathetic activation with agents such as ketamine. Antibioprophylaxis in case of cardiac defect.

REFERENCES:

Birnbach DJ: Substance abuse, in Chestnut DH: *Obstetric Anesthesia Principles and Practice.* 2nd ed. St. Louis, Mosby, 1999, p 1027.

Chiriboga CA, Brust JC, Bateman D, et al: Dose–response effect of fetal cocaine exposure on newborn neurologic function. *Pediatrics* 103:79, 1999.

Plessinger MA, Woods JR: Cocaine in pregnancy: Recent data on maternal and fetal risks. *Obstet Gynecol North Am* 25;99, 1998.

FG Syndrome

At a glance: Genetically transmitted polymalformative syndrome characterized by short stature with a disproportionately large head, imperforate anus, hypotonia, and agenesia of corpus callosum.

Synonyms: FGS I Syndrome; Keller Syndrome; Opitz-Kaveggia Syndrome; Megalocornea-Mental Retardation Syndrome.

Incidence: Approximately 50 cases have been documented since the syndrome was first described in 1974.

Genetic inheritance: X-linked recessive inheritance (affects males). The severity of symptoms varies from patient to patient. Some females ("carriers") present with some characteristics of FG syndrome, but they are not affected by the disorder itself. Gene map loci are Xq28, Xq12-q21.31, and Xp22.3.

Pathophysiology: Neuropathology findings are suggestive of a diffuse defect of neuronal cell migration.

Diagnosis: Mainly clinical. The presence of subtle facial anomalies and the characteristic behavior in mid-childhood facilitate the diagnosis, as does the presence of other affected male relatives in the maternal family. Usually, the child presenting with the disease has a friendly, loquacious hyperactive behavior, with occasional aggressive outbursts.

Clinical aspects: Patients present with severe mental deficiency, seizures, and delayed motor development associated with hypotonia. The hypotonia eventually evolves in spasticity and joint contractures. Some of the major features are the presence of macrocephaly, a high, broad forehead, frontal cowlick, and long philtrum. They also have ocular hypertelorism with epicanthal folds and down-slanting of the palpebral fissures. Many have some form of anal anomaly, such as stenosis or imperforation, and complain of chronic constipation. There are reports of patients with FG syndrome and associated sensorineural deafness. Affected individuals may present with minor skeletal anomalies involving fingers, toes, vertebrae, and sternum. Occasionally, patients may have a fatal cardiac defect, with death prior to age 2 years occurring in approximately one third of patients, mainly because of bronchopulmonary and cardiac complications.

Precautions before anesthesia: If a cardiac defect is suspected, obtain an ECG and an echocardiogram before surgery. Ensure the patient does not have a respiratory infection that tends to be recurrent in these patients as a result of the hypotonia.

Anesthetic considerations: Neuromuscular relaxants are probably best avoided or used in a reduced dose because of the presence of hypotonia. Some patients have a narrow palate and mild micrognathia, making direct laryngoscopy and tracheal intubation difficult. Joint contractures require a careful positioning in the operating room.

Pharmacological implications: In the presence of a cardiac defect, antibioprophylaxis may be required.

REFERENCES:

Graham JM Jr, Superneau D, Rogers RC, et al: Clinical and behavioral characteristics in FG syndrome. *Am J Med Genet* 85:470, 1999.

Graham JM Jr, Tackels D, Dibbern K, et al: FG syndrome: Report of three new families with linkage to Xq12-q22.1. *Am J Med Genet* 80:145, 1998.

Ozonoff S, Williams BJ, Rauch AM, et al: Behavior phenotype of FG syndrome: Cognition, personality, and behavior in eleven affected boys. *Am J Med Genet* 97:112-8, 2000.

Fibrin Stabilizing Factor (Factor XIII) Deficiency

At a glance: Inherited coagulation disorder resulting in life-long bleeding tendency in homozygotes with poor wound healing and easy bruising.

Synonym: Congenital Factor XIII Deficiency.

History: Coagulation disorder first described by François Henri Duckert, a Swiss hematologist, in 1960 (before factor XIII [FXIII], the "forgotten coagulation factor" was considered a clotting factor). Factor XIII was determined to be a coagulation factor in the coagulation cascade in 1963.

Incidence: Approximately 1:2–5,000,000 population.

Genetic inheritance: Autosomal recessive, often with consanguinity. Caused by mutations (>40) in the gene encoding the catalytic α subunit on chromosome 6. Whereas the concentration of β subunits is relatively normal, the α subunit is absent in plasma, platelets, and monocytes and results in severe bleeding diathesis.

Pathophysiology: FXIII is a transglutaminase enzyme that forges covalent bonds between adjacent strands of monomeric fibrin after thrombin activation, thereby converting fibrin monomers into fibrin polymer. Deficiency leads to clot instability, bleeding, and poor wound healing. This disease has a high incidence of intracranial bleeding ($>25\%$) and is commonly diagnosed in the neonatal period, when bleeding is noted at the umbilical stump.

Diagnosis: Umbilical stump bleeding is pathognomonic. Laboratory diagnosis requires a clot solubility test with 5M urea or 1% monochloroacetic acid, or FXIII assay.

Clinical aspects: Umbilical stump bleeding ($>90\%$), intracranial bleeding ($>25\%$), superficial bleeding/subcutaneous hematomas ($>50\%$), hemarthrosis (25%), normal prothrombin time, partial thromboplastin time, and platelet count. Treatment usually entails fresh-frozen plasma 5 ml/kg at monthly intervals as prophylaxis. Treatment with cryoprecipitate is effective. Virally inactivated FXIII concentrates exist but are reportedly not commercially available everywhere.

Precautions before anesthesia: Suspect FXIII deficiency when bleeding exists in the presence of normal coagulation parameters and platelet count. Consult hematologist for treatment recommendations and availability of FXIII concentrates. Treat patients emergently with fresh-frozen plasma 5 ml/kg.

Anesthetic considerations: Avoid regional anesthesia. Ensure blood bank support. Avoid IM injections.

Pharmacological implications: Avoid aspirin and nonsteroidal antiinflammatory drugs.

Other conditions to be considered:

ACQUIRED FXIII DEFICIENCY: Caused by liver disease, inflammatory bowel disease, and disseminated intravascular coagulation but has no clinically relevant bleeding.

OTHER CONGENITAL COAGULATION FACTOR DEFICIENCIES (Dysfibrinogenemia, Decreased Fibrinogen Levels): Differential diagnosis is obtained following proper laboratory examinations.

REFERENCES:

Anwar R, Miloszewski KJ: Factor XIII deficiency. *Br J Haematol* 107:468, 1999.

Gerlach R, Tolle F, Raabe A, et al: Increased risk for postoperative hemorrhage after intracranial surgery in patients with decreased factor XIII activity: Implications of a prospective study. Stroke 33:1618, 2002.

Pernod G, Barro C, Arnutti B, et al: Surgery in severe factor XIII deficiency: Report of a case of epilepsy neurosurgery and review. *Haemophilia* 9:121, 2003.

Fibrocystic Pulmonary Dysplasia

At a glance: Genetically transmitted respiratory disease characterized by rapidly progressive dyspnea and cyanosis, digital clubbing, polycythemia, pulmonary hypertension, and diffuse pulmonary fibrosis (fatal within months of onset).

Synonyms: Corrigan Cirrhosis; Cryptogenetic Fibrosing Alveolitis; Familial Interstitial Lung Disease; Hamman Rich Disease; Idiopathic Pulmonary Fibrosis; Liebow Pneumonia; Usual Interstitial Pneumonia of Liebow.

History: First described by Sir Dominic John Corrigan in 1838. Respiratory disorder characterized by chronic nonproductive cough and dyspnea with changes in the diffusion capacity of the lung. The disease evolves toward respiratory failure and death.

Incidence: Prevalence: 1.34:1,000,000 population in the United Kingdom. Occurs more frequently in males than in females.

Genetic inheritance: Autosomal dominant.

Pathophysiology: Could result from an inherited anomaly in the immune system, but it is yet to be confirmed.

Diagnosis: Based on clinical, radiologic, and respiratory function tests and lung biopsy if necessary. Radiologic changes show a nodular ground-glass appearance, predominantly in the bases. Respiratory function tests indicate a diffusion defect that is associated with a decrease in arterial oxygen saturation made worse by exercise. Usually, there is no restrictive pulmonary disorder until very late in the disease. Biopsy demonstrates the presence of interstitial fibrosis and cysts.

Clinical aspects: Affected patients present with a nonproductive cough that is associated with dyspnea, chest pain, and cyanosis. The disease evolves over many years toward hypoxemia, respiratory failure, and right heart failure. It can be exacerbated by spontaneous pneumothorax and recurrent infections. Clubbing and pulmonary osteoarthropathy are usually present. Patients become very disabled in the third or fourth decade, and death usually occurs in their 50s or earlier if they are victims of complications.

Precautions before anesthesia: Before going to the operating room, the patient should be evaluated by a pneumologist for respiratory function testing, arterial blood gas, recurrent infections, and exacerbation of symptoms. Also obtain a chest radiograph and an ECG. If right heart failure is suspected, an echocardiogram is recommended. An anesthesiology consultation is highly recommended for elective surgery.

Anesthetic considerations: Because patients are "respiratory cripples," tracheal intubation should be avoided as much as possible to prevent serious postoperative complications, including prolonged mechanical ventilation. Regional anesthesia may be preferable.

Pharmacological implications: Be careful when using opioids alone or in combination with benzodiazepines because patients may be sensitive to the respiratory depressant effect of the medication.

REFERENCES:

Green FH: Overview of pulmonary fibrosis. *Chest* 122(6 suppl):334S, 2002.

Verleden GM, du Bois RM, Bouros D, et al: Genetic predisposition and pathogenetic mechanisms of interstitial lung diseases of unknown origin. *Eur Respir J Suppl* 32:17s, 2001.

Whitsett JA: Genetic basis of familial interstitial lung disease: Misfolding or function of surfactant protein C? *Am J Respir Crit Care Med* 165:1201, 2002.

Fibrodysplasia Ossificans Progressiva

At a glance: Genetically transmitted malformative syndrome affecting the connective tissue system. It is characterized by malformed big toes that are often monophalangic, mild mental retardation, and intermittently progressive ectopic ossification.

Synonyms: Myositis Ossificans; Münchmeyer Disease.

Incidence: Incidence is 1:2,000,000 live births and seems to affect both genders equally.

Genetic inheritance: Autosomal dominant. Gene map locus is 4q27-q31.

Pathophysiology: Results from overexpression of a potent bone-inducing morphogen (bone morphogenetic protein 4) in lymphocytes that is responsible for ectopic osteogenesis.

Diagnosis: Mainly clinical, based on the presence of new bone formation in the soft tissue. There is also an increase in alkaline phosphatase during active phase of the disease. Diagnosis established by molecular biology studies (increased levels of bone morphogenetic protein 4 and its mRNA).

Clinical aspects: Symptoms usually appear around 6 years of age and consist of cartilaginous and osteoid transformation of connective tissue. This ectopic bone formation leads to skeletal muscle mass displacement and serious limitation of joint movement, mainly in the elbow, hip, and knee. There is a characteristic hallux deformity, which consists of shortened and angulated halluces with associated brachymesodactyly. Cervical spine involvement is common, with varying degrees of cervical fusion and the possibility of atlantoaxial subluxation. Temporomandibular joint involvement may occur. Muscles of the face, larynx, eyes, anterior abdominal wall, diaphragm, and heart usually escape involvement. Finally, limitation of rib movement may lead to a restrictive, shallow type of breathing but rarely to respiratory failure, although pneumonia is a common complication. ST-segment changes and right bundle branch block are however often seen.

Precautions before anesthesia: Obtain an ECG and pulmonary function testing. Also obtain baseline alkaline phosphatase level. Cervical spine radiography to rule out atlantoaxial subluxation should be done preoperatively.

Anesthetic considerations: Because of the temporomandibular and atlantoaxial involvement, direct laryngoscopy may be difficult and fiberoptic tracheal intubation may be wise. Positioning of the patient on the operating room table might be more problematic because of the joint limitations. Successful execution of regional techniques may be impossible because of the ectopic bone formation. Also, local trauma may induce more ectopic bone formation. General anesthesia is recommended.

Pharmacological implications: A few patients might be taking corticosteroids and/or warfarin, so steroid coverage may be warranted or vitamin K for reversal of warfarin in major surgery.

REFERENCES:

Mahboubi S, Glaser DL, Shore EM, et al: Fibrodysplasia ossificans progressiva. *Pediatr Radiol* 31:307, 2001.

Shafritz AB, Shore EM, Gannon FH: Overexpression of an osteogenic morphogen in fibrodysplasia ossificans progressiva. *Lancet* 335:555, 1996.

Semonin O, Fontaine K, Daviaud C, et al: Identification of three novel mutations of the noggin gene in patients with fibrodysplasia ossificans progressiva. *Am J Med Genet* 102:314, 2001.

Fibromatoses

At a glance: Group of disorders characterized by expanding benign fibrous tissue that are more aggressive than benign isolated fibromas and less aggressive than fibrosarcoma.

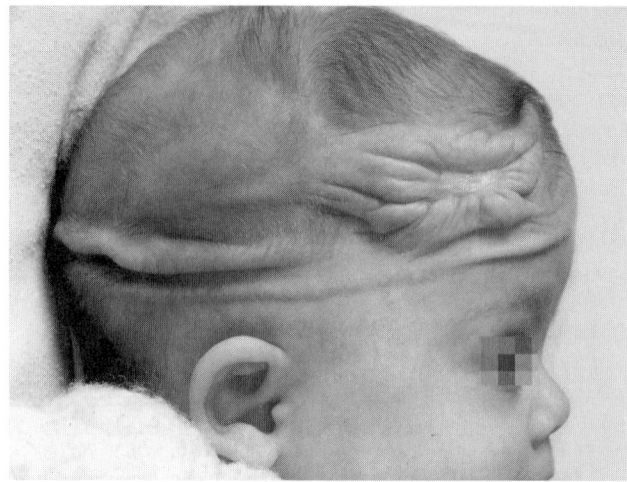

Fibromatosis   Congenital fibromatosis affecting the scalp in an infant.

Classification: Fibromatoses can be divided in three syndromes:

1.   Hereditary desmoid disease
2.   Congenital generalized fibromatosis
3.   Jaffe Campanacci syndrome

HEREDITARY DESMOID DISEASE

At a glance: Autosomal dominant disorder characterized by infiltrative fibromatosis of the mesentery without colonic polyps, osteomas and sebaceous cysts. It is known to predispose to desmoid tumor but its association with colon cancer is unknown.

Incidence and genetic inheritance: Incidence unknown. Autosomal dominant inheritance.

Clinical aspects: These are fibroproliferative disorders in which histologically benign tumors of musculoaponeurotic tissue arise and are often locally invasive. They occur more commonly in patients with familial adenomatous polyposis. The fibromatosis may be intraabdominal (mesenteric) or extraabdominal, such as paraspinal, limb, buttock, flank, head, and neck.

Anesthetic considerations: Patients receive multidisciplinary treatment, so they may present for surgery after having received chemotherapy or radiotherapy. Patients with tumors of the head and neck may require careful airway management planning according to the site of the tumor(s).

REFERENCE:

Dormans JP, Spiegel D, Meyer J, et al: Fibromatoses in childhood: The desmoid/fibromatosis complex. *Med Pediatr Oncol* 37:126, 2001.

CONGENITAL GENERALIZED FIBROMATOSIS

At a glance: Characterized by multiple fibroblastic tumors involving skin, striated muscles, bones, and viscera. Tumors are present at birth or develop during the first weeks of life.

Synonym: Juvenile Myofibromatosis.

Incidence and genetic inheritance: Incidence is unknown. Autosomal recessive transmission is suggested, but there are also cases of autosomal dominance.

Clinical aspects: Solitary or multicentric fibroblastic tumors of skin, striated muscle, bone, and viscera, which are congenital or develop in the first weeks of postnatal life. The multicentric type may be visceral or nonvisceral. The former has a higher mortality and may involve lungs, myocardium, gastrointestinal tract, and rarely the central nervous system. Nonvisceral tumors tend to regress spontaneously.

Anesthetic considerations: Patients may present for surgery for removal of locally aggressive tumors. Very rarely patients with central nervous system involvement present with extrinsic cord compression or with an intracranial space-occupying lesion. One third of solitary lesions affect head and neck structures.

REFERENCE:

Netscher DT, Eladoumikdachi F, Popek EJ: Infantile myofibromatosis: Case report of a solitary hand lesion with emphasis on differential diagnosis and management. *Ann Plast Surg* 46:62, 2001.

JAFFE CAMPANACCI SYNDROME

At a glance: Syndrome of unknown etiology with variable expression characterized mainly by nonossifying fibromata, extraskeletal congenital anomalies such as café au lait spots, mental retardation, hypogonadism or cryptorchidism, and ocular and cardiovascular malformations. Other clinical features include chylothorax, stenosis of aortic isthmus, mitral insufficiency, chylopericardium, mental retardation, and precocious puberty.

Synonym: Multiple Nonossifying Fibromatosis.

Incidence and genetic inheritance: Incidence is unknown. Genetics are not understood. Males and females appear to be equally affected. There usually is no family history of the syndrome or of neurofibromatosis, which has similar characteristics.

Clinical aspects: Usually presents between the ages of 10 and 15 years, typically with a pathologic fracture. Smooth-bordered café-au-lait spots, axillary freckling, and multiple nonossifying fibromas are present without soft tissue neurofibromas.

Anesthetic considerations: Be careful with handling and movement in view of the predisposition to pathologic fractures.

REFERENCE:

Hau MA, Fox EJ, Cates JM, et al: Jaffe-Campanacci syndrome. A case report and review of the literature. *J Bone Joint Surg Am* 84A:634, 2002.

Floating-Harbor Syndrome (FHS)

At a glance: Rare, autosomal dominant syndrome associated with short stature, delayed bone age, and characteristic triangular face with a prominent nose and deep-set eyes. Language delay is frequent (usually in the presence of normal motor development).

Synonyms: Leisti Hollister Rimoin Syndrome; Pelletier-Leisti Syndrome.

History: The unusual name of this syndrome is derived from the Boston Floating Hospital and the Harbor General Hospital, where the first cases were described.

Clinical aspects: Features include *characteristic facies* (dolichocephaly/scaphocephaly, short neck, prominent occiput, triangular face, short midface, low-set ears, broad nasal root, bulbous nose, long eyelashes, enophthalmos, thickened gingivae, narrow palate), *limbs anomalies* (brachydactyly, delayed bone age, joint dislocation, restricted joint mobility, clinodactyly of toes, clinodactyly of fifth finger), *genitourinary signs* (micropenis, urethral anomalies), and short stature. Difficult feeding in infancy, mental retardation,

and speech defect are common. Cardiac septal defect and celiac disease may be associated.

Anesthetic considerations: Tracheal intubation can be difficult because of skull and neck abnormalities and may require adapted anesthetic management. Avoid using muscle relaxants until airway is secured. Careful intraoperative positioning is needed. Prophylactic antibiotics in case of cardiopathy as indicated.

REFERENCES:

Patton MA, Hurst J, Donnai D, et al: Floating-Harbor syndrome. *J Med Genet* 28:201, 1991.

Penaloza JM, Garcia-Cruz D, Davalos IP, et al: A variant example of familial Floating-Harbor syndrome? *Genet Couns* 14:31, 2003.

Foix Alajouanine Syndrome

At a glance: Rare entity presenting with onset of age of approximately 50 years and characterized by a subacute myelopathy evolving over 1 to 5 years. It is caused by an arteriovenous malformation of the spinal cord predominantly affecting the lower thoracic and/or lumbosacral levels.

Synonyms: Foix-Alajouanine Disease; Spinal Dural Arteriovenous Fistula; Varicositas Medullae Spinalis.

Incidence: Rare (no specific statistics). Male-to-female ratio of 4:1. No racial predilection.

Genetic inheritance: Uncertain. Spinal dural arteriovenous malformations may be acquired, although the specificity for the spinal cord is not easily explained.

Pathophysiology: Not well understood. In most cases there is an arteriovenous fistula in the lower thoracic dura, resulting in increasing the pressure within the dura, compromising perfusion, and leading to iterative infarction of the spinal cord parenchyma. Thrombosis may occur, but venous stasis is probably the primary cause of infarction. Proliferation of intramedullary blood vessels is frequently observed and may be accompanied by fibrinoid degeneration of the vessel walls. Another proposed mechanism is that remittent leakage of blood from the arteriovenous malformation promotes progressive adhesive arachnoiditis resulting in iterative "chokes" of the spinal cord. The same mechanism has been evocated to be possible when blood patches are realized.

Diagnosis: On MRI, T1-weighted images show decreased signal intensity within the affected spinal cord segments; the lesions are hyperintense on T2-weighted images. Contrast administration usually produces serpentine areas of enhancement. Spinal angiography is the definitive diagnostic procedure for evaluation of this disease.

Clinical aspects: Onset between 20 and 60 years of age (usually a male who is older than 50 years). Progressive paraplegia (manifested as increasing weakness and numbness or tingling in the lower extremities, frequent falls), urinary and fecal incontinence, and nonradiating lower back pain. Affected patients initially are spastic but eventually develop flaccid paralysis of the limbs and may become wheelchair bound. Four different types of arteriovenous malformation have been described: dural arteriovenous fistulas, glomus malformations, juvenile type arteriovenous malformations, and intradural extramedullary arteriovenous fistulas.

Precautions before anesthesia: Corticotherapy is often prescribed: evaluate sodium and potassium status. If angiographic evidence of thrombosis exists, anticoagulation with heparin is indicated. Evaluate neurologic function (history, clinical, CT, MRI).

Anesthetic considerations: Avoid central block procedures that can break a preexisting delicate neurologic balance. Somatosensory evoked potential intraoperative monitoring could be impossible because of coronal lesion. Padding and positioning are critical, as it is for any paraplegic patient.

Pharmacological implications: As with other lower motor neuron diseases, avoid succinylcholine (hyperkalemic cardiac arrests). The sensitivity and duration of action of nondepolarizing drugs is markedly increased. Must reduce the dose and monitor the neuromuscular junction. Consider antibioprophylaxis and anticoagulant therapy. Steroid stress dose if necessary. There are no indications that malignant hyperthermia occurs; however, avoiding trigger anesthetic agents during the acute phase of neuromuscular degeneration is recommended.

Other condition to be considered:

CAUDA EQUINA SYNDROME: Defined as low back pain, bladder and bowel dysfunction, and variable lower extremity motor and sensory loss. Not a genetic disorder but rather an acquired complication from extrinsic mass compression, local anesthetic complication, or trauma.

REFERENCES:

Foix C, Alajouanine T: La myélite nécrotique subaiguë (Myélite centrale angiohypertrophique à évolution progressive). Paraplégie amyotrophique lentement ascendante d'abord spasmodique, puis flasque. *Rev Neurol (Paris)* 2:1, 1926.

Saraf-Lavi E, Bowen BC, Quencer RM, et al: Detection of spinal dural arteriovenous fistulae with MR imaging and contrast-enhanced MR angiography: Sensitivity, specificity, and prediction of vertebral level. *AJNR Am J Neuroradiol* 23:858, 2002.

Van Dijk JM, TerBrugge KG, Willinsky RA, et al: Multidisciplinary management of spinal dural arteriovenous fistulas: Clinical presentation and long-term follow-up in 49 patients. *Stroke* 33:1578, 2002.

Folic Acid Deficiency

At a glance: Megaloblastic anemia resulting from folic acid deficiency secondary either to dietary deficiency or malabsorption syndrome. A genetically transmitted disorder with poor prognosis unless folinic acid is regularly administered.

Synonyms: Congenital Folate Malabsorption; Hereditary Folate Malabsorption; Transport Defect Involving Folic Acid.

Genetic inheritance: Not well identified. Twelve cases of this rare disorder have been reported, mostly in females (but males can be affected).

Pathophysiology: Folic acid is reduced by dihydrofolate reductase to form tetrahydrofolate. Tetrahydrofolate is important in one carbon transfer reaction and essential in the methylation of deoxyuridylate to thymidylate during DNA synthesis. This leads to megaloblastic anemia, although the mechanism is poorly understood in nutritional diseases. Folic acid deficiency is caused by dietary deficiency, impaired absorption, or increased requirements. Nutritional deficiency is seen in the elderly, alcoholics, premature infants, infants raised on goat's milk and in hemodialysis, hyperalimentation, and gastrectomy patients. Impaired absorption occurs in sprue, regional enteritis, after extensive small bowel resections, in Whipple disease, and in leukemic infiltration of the intestine. Increased requirements are seen in pregnancy and in diseases with increased cell turnover, such as hemolytic anemia.

Diagnosis: Clinical signs and symptoms are those of chronic anemia. Onset is insidious and associated with weakness, palpitation, fatigue, light-headedness, and dyspnea. Pallor and jaundice are common. Leukocyte and platelet counts may be depressed. Laboratory features include low serum and red cell folate, low reticulocyte count, macrocytic anemia, and hypersegmented neutrophils. Bone marrow examination reveals erythroid megaloblastic changes.

Clinical aspects: Hereditary form manifests as recurrent megaloblastic anemia, mental retardation, convulsions, movement disorder (ataxia), diarrhea, susceptibility to infections, and calcification of basal ganglia. Most patients die within the first few months of life as a consequence of diarrhea, vomiting, drowsiness, pallor, and glossitis.

Precautions before anesthesia: Check hematocrit. Elective surgery is contraindicated until anemia resolves with treatment. In hereditary forms, avoid anesthesia unless there is a life-threatening surgical indication. Most infants are in very poor physical status with malnutrition and chronic dehydration. Check carefully fluid losses and avoid both underinflation and overinflation of fluids (intraoperatively and postoperatively). Provide IV folic acid and consider prophylactic antibiotics. Check acid balance status and plasma protein levels.

Anesthetic considerations: No specific anesthetic consideration with this condition except for potential severe anemia and epilepsy in the hereditary form. Transfuse with packed red blood cells as needed.

Pharmacological implications: In hereditary form, reduce doses in patients with clinical and biologic signs of dehydration.

Other conditions to be considered:

DIHYDROPTERIDINE REDUCTASE DEFICIENCY: Same calcification of basal ganglia and same efficiency of folinic acid therapy.

☞PHENYLKETONURIA TYPE II: Inborn error of phenylalanine metabolism. Results in severe irreversible mental retardation at thrive of infancy.

REFERENCES:

Geller J, Kronn D, Jayabose S, et al: Hereditary folate malabsorption: Family report and review of the literature. *Medicine (Baltimore)* 81:51, 2002.

Jebnoun S, Kacem S, Mokrani C, et al: A family study of congenital malabsorption of folate. *J Inherit Metab Dis* 24:749, 2001.

Steinschneider M, Sherbany A, Pavlakis S, et al: Congenital folate malabsorption: Reversible clinical and neurophysiologic abnormalities. *Neurology* 40:1315, 1990.

Forsius-Ericksson Syndrome

At a glance: Congenital form of albinism characterized by retinal disorder with marked vision impairment and color blindness. Patients should be considered as muscular dystrophic patients unless proven otherwise.

Synonyms: Aland Island Eye Disease (ACE); Ocular Albinism Type II; OA II.

Genetic inheritance: X-chromosome recessive ocular albinism.

Pathophysiology: Results from a mutation at Xp21.3-Xp212.2 leading to decreased dystrophin production and congenital stationary night blindness.

Diagnosis: Ophthalmic symptoms and signs include iris transillumination, fundus hypopigmentation, congenital nystagmus, and typical electroretinogram appearance.

Clinical aspects: Aland Island eye disease is an ophthalmic diagnosis and is not associated with any other abnormalities. However, the gene locus is in close proximity to that coding for Duchenne muscular dystrophy. The coexistence of these two pathologies is well documented and should be suspected in a child with congenital night blindness who fails to reach motor milestones.

Precautions before anesthesia: Careful history and examination should reveal symptoms and signs of coexisting pathology such as muscular dystrophy.

Anesthetic considerations: Patients with confirmed Aland Island eye disease should probably be treated as if they had muscular dystrophy unless there is overwhelming evidence to the contrary.

Pharmacological implications: The usual pharmacological precautions for patients with Duchenne muscular dystrophy should be observed.

REFERENCE:

Forsius H, Eriksson AW: Ein neues Augensyndrom mit X-chromosomaler Transmission: eine Sippe mit Fundusalbinismus, Foveahypoplasie, Nystagmus, Myopie, Astigmatismus und Dyschromatopsie. *Klin Monatsbl Augenheilkd* 144:447-57, 1964.

Fragile X Syndrome

At a glance: Most common form of X-linked mental retardation. Affects males more often and more severely than females. Only subtle dysmorphic features. Behavioral issues may be more pronounced.

Synonyms: FRAXA Syndrome; Martin Bell Syndrome; X-linked Mental Retardation with Macroorchidism.

Incidence: The incidence for boys is estimated to be 1:1000–5000 live births, making it the most common chromosomal cause of mental retardation second only to trisomy 21. The clinical picture can vary significantly.

Genetic inheritance: Inheritance is X-gonosomal dominant. The genetic defect has been mapped to Xq27.3. Advanced maternal age seems to be a risk factor for this disorder.

Diagnosis: The clinical picture may be suggestive of the disease, although the dysmorphic features are rather subtle. The diagnosis can be confirmed using molecular genetic testing (Southern blot) and relies on the detection of an altered *f*ragile X *m*ental *r*etardation-1 (FMR1) gene. In almost all patients, the mutation is caused by a significantly increased number of CGG (C = cytosine, G = guanosine) trinucleotide repetitions, which is also associated with abnormal methylation of the FMR1 gene. The absence of or mutation in the fragile mental retardation protein (FMRP) is responsible for the Fragile X syndrome. FMRP is an RNA binding protein that shuttles between the nucleus and the cytoplasm. It seems that FMRP is located at synapses, where it is involved in signal transduction and encoding of cytoskeletal proteins. It also appears that lack of FMRP affects synaptic plasticity. Prenatal diagnostic is possible.

Clinical aspects: This progressive X-linked mental retardation affects boys (moderate mental retardation) more often and more severely than girls (mild mental retardation). The main neurologic symptoms include delayed language skills, delayed motor development, autism or autistic-like behavior, behavioral problems (attention deficit hyperactivity disorder, oppositional defiant disorder, enuresis, encopresis), and poor sensory skills. Anatomical features may include macrocephaly, a long face with prognathism (which in fact is often just a prominent symphysis of the mandibula rather than real prognathism), strabismus, prominent large ears, high arched palate, and a high-pitched voice. The external male genitalia show pronounced growth during puberty, which results in macroorchidism. Overall, muscle tone is low with generalized joint laxity (particularly of the fingers). Pectus excavatum, flat feet, shortening of the tubular bones of the hands, and hyperlordosis may be present. Heart defects (e.g., mitral valve prolapse), dilatation of the aortic root, and seizures have been described. Researchers found that the hippocampus often shows an age-related increase in size, whereas the superior temporal gyrus and the posterior cerebellar vermis are diminished in size. After age 50 years, patients show an increased rate of progressive parkinsonism, cognitive decline, and generalized brain atrophy.

Precautions before anesthesia: The cardiovascular findings may prompt the anesthetist to request an echocardiography. If pectus excavatum is present and significant, a chest radiograph should be obtained. Because these patients are mentally retarded and may have some additional behavior issues, preoperative sedation is most often helpful and therefore recommended.

Anesthetic considerations: Careful positioning and padding are needed in the presence of joint laxity to prevent luxations. Facial anomalies are not expected to be severe enough to cause airway management problems. The dose of neuromuscular blockers can probably be reduced in the face of generalized muscular hypotonia. Depending on the procedure, postoperative mechanical ventilation may be indicated.

Pharmacological implications: If mitral valve prolapse is present and associated with mitral regurgitation, subacute bacterial endocarditis prophylaxis is indicated.

Other conditions to be considered:

☞**ALLAN-HERNDON SYNDROME:** Although most neonates and infants with this disorder appear to develop normally in the first few months of life, the presence of poor muscle tone is most often present at birth. By age 6 months, hypotonia, inability to hold the head, and severe muscle atrophy are detectable. Severe mental retardation is associated with multiple congenital anomalies.

☞**JUBERG-MARSIDI SYNDROME:** X-linked recessive inherited syndrome characterized by severe mental retardation, deafness, failure to thrive, microgenitalism, and early death.

☞**HAPPY PUPPET SYNDROME:** Rare disorder characterized by developmental delay, ataxia, dysmorphic facial features, and seizures associated with a happy, sociable disposition.

☞**MASA SYNDROME:** Extremely rare inherited disorder that is one of several disorders known as X-linked mental retardation (XLMR) syndromes.

RENPENNING SYNDROME (Escalante Syndrome): Extremely rare form of X-linked (moderate-to-severe) mental retardation. It has been linked to Xp11.2-p11.4. Other findings may include short stature, moderate microcephaly, prognathism, and small testes. Affected patients may use repetitive speech and show an aggressive behavior. Longevity seems not to be impaired, and female carriers do not show any heterozygous signs.

SUTHERLAND-HAAN SYNDROME (Sutherland-Haan X-Linked Mental Retardation Syndrome; X-Linked Mental Retardation With Spastic Diplegia): Extremely rare form of X-linked severe mental retardation. Features include short stature, spastic diplegia, significant congenital heart defects, and craniofacial abnormalities (microcephaly, cleft palate or high arched palate, abnormal ears, bulbous nose, broad nasal bridge, malar hypoplasia, micrognathia, and a small mouth. No reports exist about anesthesia in these patients; however, difficult airway management seems likely.

REFERENCES:

Hessl D, Rivera SM, Reiss AL: The neuroanatomy and neuroendocrinology of fragile X syndrome. *Ment Retard Dev Disabil Res Rev* 10:17, 2004.

Mandel JL, Biancalana V: Fragile X mental retardation syndrome: From pathogenesis to diagnostic issues. *Growth Horm IGF Res* 14(suppl A):158, 2004.

Zalfa F, Bagni C: Molecular insights into mental retardation: Multiple functions for the Fragile X mental retardation protein? *Curr Issues Mol Biol* 6:73, 2004.

Fraser Syndrome

At a glance: Malformative condition present at birth and characterized by the association of cryptophthalmos with a wide range of abnormalities (orofacial defects, syndactyly, decreased number of digits, urogenital and renal malformations).

Synonyms: Fraser-François Syndrome; Cryptophthalmos Syndrome; Cryptophthalmos Syndactyly Syndrome; Cryptophthalmos Syndactyly Cyclopism Syndrome; Meyer-Schwickerath Syndrome.

Incidence: 0.043:10,000 liveborn infants and 1.1:10,000 stillbirths.

Genetic inheritance: Autosomal recessive.

Pathophysiology: Pathogenesis is unclear. However, embryologically, it has been suggested that the neural ectodermal optic vesicle is responsible for induction of lens development. Abnormal lack of lens development prevents adequate migration of anterior neural crest structures leading to deficiency in the development of the eyelids, cornea, lens, and anterior chamber. A defect of apoptosis has been suggested, as several of the anomalies result from failure of programmed cell death (fusion of the eyelids, digits, larynx, and vagina).

Diagnosis: The diagnosis should be considered in patients with a combination of acrofacial and urogenital malformations with or without cryptophthalmos. The occurrence of the cryptophthalmos syndrome without cryptophthalmos is an argument for using the eponym Fraser syndrome rather than cryptophthalmos-syndactyly syndrome. The most characteristic malformations of the Fraser syndrome are temporarily fused eyelids in utero, digits, and the vagina. Pulmonary hyperplasia, laryngeal stenosis, and renal agenesis have been associated. Markedly enlarged echogenic lungs can be observed at 16 and 17 weeks of gestation. The reported frequency of cryptophthalmos is 93% and syndactyly 54%. The major diagnostic criteria are cryptophthalmos, syndactyly, and abnormal genitalia. Minor criteria are congenital malformation of the nose, ears, larynx, cleft lip/palate, skeletal defects, umbilical hernia, renal agenesis, and mental retardation. The presence of two major and one minor criteria or one major and four minor criteria are necessary for diagnosis.

Clinical aspects: Clinical features include bilateral cryptophthalmos, absent or malformed lacrimal ducts, middle and outer ear malformations, high arched palate, cleavage along the midplane of nares and tongue, hypertelorism, laryngeal stenosis, syndactyly, wide separation of symphysis pubis, displacement of umbilicus and nipples, primitive mesentery of small bowel, maldeveloped kidneys; fusion

of labia and enlargement of clitoris, and bicornuate uterus. In the male infant, undescended testes and small penis with hypospadias are characteristic when associated with bilateral cryptophthalmos. Death or serious morbidity is common in the first year of life. This is related to upper respiratory tract infection associated with the abnormal anatomy of the airway. Renal abnormalities (including renal agenesis) contribute to mortality and morbidity in early life. Very few patients are reported to have light perception, and they are considered clinically or profoundly blind.

Precautions before anesthesia: The airway is of primary concern to the anesthesiologist. Often, the airway difficulty is noticed at delivery of the newborn and may be associated with bad outcome. In elective surgery, in addition to concerns regarding the airway, renal agenesis or impairment must be considered.

Anesthetic considerations: The pattern of airway abnormalities causes significant problems with airway management, and most of these children require tracheostomies early in life. Orotracheal intubation has been very challenging in several case reports. Anesthesiologists must be prepared for difficulty in endotracheal intubation with all the usual means of securing difficult pediatric airways.

Pharmacological implications: No specific pharmacological implications, although renal agenesis, if present, limits the choice of anesthetic agent.

Other conditions to be considered:

☞**OCULODENTODIGITAL (ODD) SYNDROME:** Craniofacial and ocular abnormalities, dental and skeletal defects, hand and foot malformations, and delayed mental development. Ocular features include microcorneas with or without microphthalmos, secondary glaucoma, optic nerve atrophy, hypertelorism or hypotelorism, and Adie-Holmes syndrome. Digital anomalies include clinodactyly, camptodactyly, and occasional syndactyly of the fourth and fifth fingers. Autosomal dominant inheritance pattern. Weyers type III or ODD type III is defined by the type of syndactyly present. Syndactyly of fingers 4 and 5 must be present. The ODD syndrome type II presents rather than syndactyly of fingers 4 and 5 with unilateral preaxial polydactyly of the hand, fifth finger camptodactyly, and absent terminal phalanges of fingers 2 and 5.

☞**ULLRICH-FEICHTIGER SYNDROME:** Comparable to Weyers syndrome type III, including micrognathia, polydactyly, and genital anomalies triad. Blepharoptosis and cleft palate are present in this disorder.

REFERENCES:

Martinez-Frias ML, Bermejo Sanchez E, et al: Fraser syndrome: Frequency in our environment and clinical-epidemiological aspects of a consecutive series of cases. *An Esp Pediatr* 48:634, 1998.

Sarman G, Speer ME, Rudolph AJ: Fraser syndrome. *J Perinatol* 15:503, 1995.

Freeman-Sheldon Syndrome (FSS)

At a glance: Genetic malformative disorder characterized by a microstomia; flat midface with a small, pinched mouth mimicking whistling; clubfeet; and contracted muscles of the joints of the fingers and hands malformations.

Synonyms: Craniocarpotarsal Disease or Dystrophy; Distal Arthrogryposis Type IIA; Whistling Face Syndrome; Whistling Face-Windmill Vane Hand Syndrome; "Whistler" Syndrome.

Incidence: Unknown. More than 50 cases have been reported in the literature.

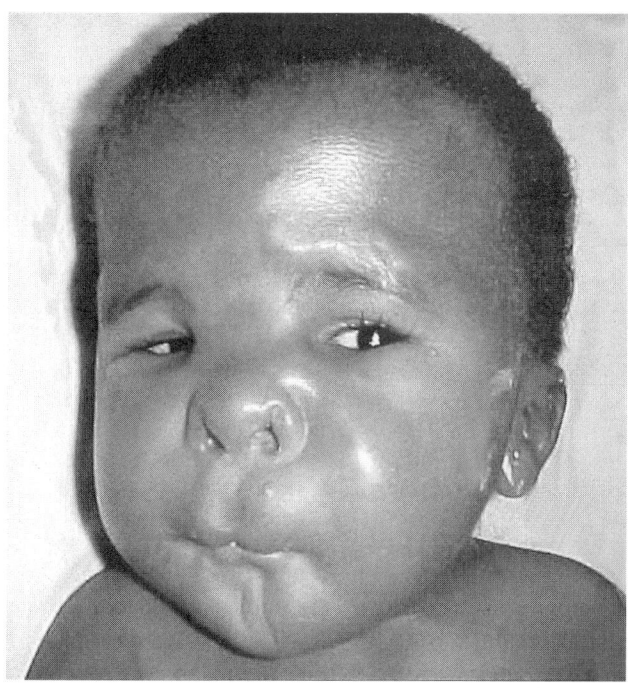

Freeman-Sheldon Syndrome Infant with Freeman-Sheldon syndrome showing the typical whistling face, long philtrum, and flat face.

Genetic inheritance: Autosomal dominant inheritance with variable expressivity. No gene has been identified for this condition. No prenatal diagnosis available.

Pathophysiology: Unknown, but it is thought to involve fibrous replacement of muscles fibers.

Diagnosis: Facial features and malformations of limbs are typical. Radiographs of the skull show abnormal appearance of the floor of the anterior cranial fossa. Biopsy of the buccinator muscle reveals fibrous connective tissue. Electromyographic studies show a reduced activity most pronounced in the muscles involved in facial expression.

Clinical aspects: The facies looks immobile with a flat midface, long philtrum, and puckered mouth with whistling shape to lips. The palate is highly arched; mandible and tongue tend to be small; there is an H or V groove on the chin and deeply set eyes with hypertelorism. Patients present with ulnar deviation (90%) and flexion contracture of fingers (88%) accompanied with adduction of the thumb giving the "windmill vane" appearance. Kyphoscoliosis is present in 85% of cases. Talipes equinovarus is common (60%). Intelligence and lifespan are normal.

Precautions before anesthesia: Evaluate the airway for difficult tracheal intubation (microstomia). Use of fiberoptic laryngoscope may be required. Evaluate physical status: failure to thrive is common as a result of vomiting and swallowing difficulties. Muscle rigidity following halothane anesthesia has been reported, suggesting the presence of an underlying myopathy. Laboratory data should include blood chemistries, blood group, hemoglobin, and coagulation studies.

Anesthetic considerations: Several anesthetic challenges include difficult airway, intravenous cannulation, and the use of regional technique. The presence of facial anomalies is highly suggestive of the potential for difficult airway management. Direct laryngoscopy and tracheal intubation may be difficult, and alternatives (e.g., fiberoptic intubation, Bullard laryngoscope, laryngeal mask) should be considered. Use of a laryngeal mask for a short anesthesia procedure was reported as successful. The suspected underlying myopathy (never proven physiopathologically but suggested following rigidity after halothane anesthesia in a few cases) must not be ignored. The potential for malignant hyperthermia is present because of the myopathic anomaly. Tachycardia, hyperpyrexia, and severe masseter spasm have all been reported. In a few cases, the administration of dantrolene was needed to stop the process. Use of halothane and succinylcholine, as well as other inhalational agents, should not be automatically assumed to be safe in patients with FSS. Individuals presenting with FSS are believed to be at risk for postoperative pulmonary complications (pneumonia, empyema, respiratory insufficiency, recurrent infections from aspirations). Regional anesthesia should always be considered in the anesthetic plan reducing the risk of respiratory problems subsequent to systemic use of narcotics for pain management, although some difficulties may be encountered.

Pharmacological implications: No pharmacological implications with this condition.

Other conditions to be considered:

DISTAL ARTHROGRYPOSIS (TYPE I): Camptodactyly and hammertoes; cleft palate; clubfeet; joint contractures; overlapping fingers (trisomy 18-like); ptosis of the eyes; and thick, broad neck, usually webbed.

ILLUM SYNDROME (Arthrogryposis Multiplex Congenita with Central Nervous System [CNS] Calcifications/Whistling Face; Freeman-Sheldon Syndrome Variant): Same clinical features as described for FSS except that this is a genetic variant inherited as an autosomal recessive pattern.

☞**HECHT SYNDROME:** Characterized by the inability to open the mouth (partially or completely). Associated with short muscle-tendon units in the fingers, causing camptodactyly. Believed to be an autosomal dominant inheritance pattern.

☞**ADDUCTED THUMBS SYNDROME:** Stiff myopathic facies, open mouth, high arched palate with cleft. Craniostenosis and microcephaly. Swallowing difficulties and generalized myopathic hypotonia. Respiratory insufficiency that generally leads to death in early infancy.

SIMOSA CRANIOFACIAL SYNDROME (Simosa Penchaszadeh Bustos Syndrome): Characterized by high forehead, elongated and flattened face, arched and sparse eyebrows, short palpebral fissures, telecanthus, long nose and hypoplastic nostrils, long philtrum, microstomia, high and narrow palate, nasal speech, chin dimples, and a highly unusual bilateral auricular malformation. The individual presents usually with normal intelligence and hearing. Although to some extent the facies suggested the "whistling face" syndrome, the entity appeared to be distinct.

REFERENCES:

Bamshad M, Jorde LB, Carey JC: A revised and extended classification of the distal arthrogryposes. *Am J Med Genet* 65:277, 1996.

Cruickshanks GF, Brown S, Chitayat D: Anaesthesia for Freeman-Sheldon syndrome using a laryngeal mask airway. *Can J Anaesth* 46:783, 1999.

Vas L, Naregal P: Anaesthetic management of a patient with Freeman Sheldon syndrome. *Paediatr Anaesth* 8:175, 1998.

Friedreich Ataxia (FRDA)

At a glance: Genetic disorder characterized by progressive dysfunction of the posterior spinal cord, cerebellum (ataxia, nystagmus), and peripheral nerves. It typically becomes apparent before adolescence. Clinical features include unsteady posture, frequent falling, progressive ataxia, characteristic foot deformities, increasing incoordination of the arms and hands, dysarthria, and nystagmus. It may be associated with cardiomyopathy, chest pain, arrhythmias, and diabetes mellitus. All patients have normal intelligence.

Synonyms: FRDA I; Spinocerebellar Degeneration; Hereditofamilial Spinal Ataxia; Friedreich Tabes.

History: First described in 1863 by the German neurologist Nicholaus Friedreich.

Nature: Degeneration of the posterior spinal column, corticospinal, spinocerebellar, and pyramidal tracts. Mixed upper and lower motor neuron disease. Loss of ambulation typically occurs 15 years after disease onset. More than 95% of patients are wheelchair bound by age 45 years.

Incidence: Estimated 1:30,000–50,000 in the general population. Carrier frequency is 1:60–110 with a disease prevalence of 1:29,000. Incidence is low in Africans and Asians.

Genetic inheritance: Autosomal recessive. Gene map locus is 9q13. FRDA is associated with a mutation that consists of unstable expansion of GAA repeats on chromosome 9. FRDA alleles are found in approximately 11.4% of apparently recessive patients and 5.2% of apparently sporadic patients.

Pathophysiology: Spinocerebellar degeneration involving the spinocerebellar tracts, dorsal columns, pyramidal tracts, and, to a lesser extent, the cerebellum and medulla. Frataxin, the protein produced by the FRDA gene, which is part of the cellular energy of mitochondria, is severely reduced in the nervous system, heart, and pancreas of patients with FRDA. Patients have abnormally high levels of iron in their heart tissue and it is believed that the nervous system, heart, and pancreas may be particularly susceptible to damage from the free radicals produced when the excess iron reacts with oxygen. Many enzymatic activities are defective, but reduced activity of FE-S cluster-containing subunits (located in mitochondrial complexes I, II, and III and in aconitase) play a major role in disease progression.

Diagnosis: Neurologic examination, EMG, muscle biopsies, and measurement of nerve conduction. Direct molecular test of GAA expansion is useful for the diagnosis, prognosis (size of GAA expansion is associated with the frequency of cardiomyopathy and loss of reflexes in the upper limbs), and genetic counseling. Prenatal diagnosis is available.

Clinical aspects: Symptoms usually begin between the ages of 5 and 15 years but can appear earlier. The first sign is usually difficulty in walking. The ataxia gradually worsens and slowly spreads to the arms and trunk. Foot deformities, such as clubfoot, flexion of the toes, hammertoes, or foot inversion, may be early signs. Rapid, rhythmic, involuntary movements of the eyeball are common. Most people with FRDA develop scoliosis, which may be extremely severe. Hypertrophic cardiomyopathy and congestive heart failure (often a cause of death) are usual. Of patients with FRDA, 25% have diabetes mellitus; diabetic ketosis is not infrequent.

Precautions before anesthesia: For elective surgery, an anesthesiology consultation is highly recommended. Evaluate neurologic status (preferably with the help of an independent neurologist), cardiac status (ECG tracings, echocardiography aimed at grading the severity of cardiomyopathy and risks of cardiac failure), and metabolic status (diabetes). Check for scoliosis, possible associated difficult airway, and restrictive lung disease. Plan adequate postoperative analgesia and postoperative ECG monitoring. Depending on the physical status of the patient and the severity of surgery, postoperative transfer to the intensive care unit may be mandatory. Neurologic signs may be enhanced during the postoperative period, with spasticity that may become a sustained tetanus. Consider preoperative treatment with vitamin E and idebenone (antioxidants to decrease sensitivity to catecholamines, limit the cardiomegaly, and probably improve myocardial function).

Anesthetic considerations: Regional anesthetic techniques have long been denied in these patients, even though no scientific data are available. As for all demyelinating disorders, as the disease progresses, nerve stimulation becomes technically more difficult, thus making nerve location more unreliable, and less concentrated local anesthetic solutions are sufficient. Epidural and spinal anesthesias have been performed without adverse effects in many patients. FRDA patients have a marked sensitivity to depolarizing muscle relaxants, which induces hyperkalemia. The sensitivity to nondepolarizing muscle relaxants is increased, and proper neuromuscular monitoring is essential. However, monitoring of muscle relaxation may be difficult, depending on the progress of the disease. If general anesthesia is used, transesophageal echocardiographic monitoring is helpful to maintain continuous evaluation of cardiac contraction. As with any hypertrophic cardiomyopathy, maintain adequate volume status and avoid tachycardia, vasoplegia, and adrenergic stimulation during the intraoperative and postoperative periods. Postoperative supervision must emphasize hemodynamic and cardiac rhythm monitoring, adequate analgesia, and careful clinical muscular monitoring, especially of the pharyngeal and respiratory muscle. Postoperative mechanical ventilation must be considered to ensure adequate ventilation and facilitates adequate pain management.

Pharmacological implications: Marked sensitivity but also normal response to nondepolarizing muscle relaxants have been reported. Succinylcholine can induce hyperkalemia in these patients and result in cardiac arrhythmias. Because of the potential risk of cardiac arrhythmias, halothane should be used with caution and combined with adequate analgesia, limiting the potential for sympathomimetic responses. Propofol, fentanyl, and low doses of *cis*-atracurium is probably a good anesthetic regimen. Short-acting beta-blockers (esmolol, atenolol) may be useful to blunt adrenergic responses on the heart.

Other conditions to be considered:

☞SPINOCEREBELLAR ATAXIA: Characterized by degeneration of the cerebellum and its afferent and efferent connections. Clinical features include ataxia, cerebellar dysarthria, oculomotor disturbances, retinopathy, optic nerve atrophy, spasticity, extrapyramidal movement disorders, peripheral neuropathy, sphincter disturbances, and epilepsy. More than 25 variants of the spinocerebellar ataxia exist, and an overview is available under *Spinocerebellar Ataxia.*

FRIEDREICH ATAXIA TYPE II (FRDA II): Clinical features similar to Friedreich ataxia type I but with frataxin gene mutations (at a different locus than in FRDA1). Slow progression of the degeneration.

FAMILIAL EPISODIC CEREBELLAR ATAXIA (Episodic Ataxia Type II): Characterized by episodic cerebellar ataxia, particularly in children, followed by amelioration of symptoms later in life with no permanent or progressive cerebellar abnormalities. Autosomal dominant pattern of inheritance. It is believed to be a variant of episodic ataxia syndrome, called EA1 (resulting from mutations of the potassium channel gene KCNA1 on 12p13) and EA2 (resulting from mutations of the calcium channel gene CACNL1A4 on 19p, which is highly expressed in the cerebellum).

PERIODIC VESTIBULOCEREBELLAR ATAXIA (Episodic Ataxia Type III): Characterized by recurrent attacks of vertigo, diplopia, and ataxia beginning in early adulthood. Slowly progressive cerebellar ataxia occurred in some patients. Assumed to be an autosomal dominant ataxia.

☞**ROUSSY-LÉVY SYNDROME:** Hereditary disease inherited as autosomal dominant characterized by spinocerebellar degeneration. Not usually associated with motor ataxia and gait problems. Other features include lower limb muscular atrophy, bilateral pes cavus, and loss of deep reflexes. Severe scoliosis, camptodactyly, and clubfeet have been associated. Distinguished from FRDA by the absence of cerebellar and pyramidal signs and from Charcot-Marie-Tooth disease by the absence of sensory and vasomotor changes.

☞**FOIX-ALAJOUANINE SYNDROME:** Rare entity presenting as a subacute myelopathy evolving over 1 to 5 years as a result of an arteriovenous malformation of the spinal cord predominantly affecting the lower thoracic and/or lumbosacral levels.

☞**GORDON-HOLMES SYNDROME:** Characterized by late-onset cerebellar ataxia and hypogonadotropic hypogonadism. Hypogonadotropism was reflected in failure of secondary sexual characteristics, eunuchoidism, absence of libido, and infertility.

MARIE ATAXIA: Characterized by progressive degeneration of spinal nerves causing tremors and severe muscle atrophy in the arms, legs, head, and neck. It can appear in either early adulthood or middle age. Clinical features include abnormal reflexes, muscle contractions, and decreased pain or touch perception.

☞**CHARCOT-MARIE-TOOTH DISEASE:** Characterized by muscle weakness and atrophy, primarily in the legs. *Type I Charcot-Marie-Tooth disease* usually begins in middle childhood or teenage years and is associated with a deformity of the foot often referred to as gampsodactyly or clawfoot, which produces a "stork leg" deformity. With time, it spreads to the upper extremities and produces a "stocking-glove" pattern of diminished sensitivity. There is decreased sensitivity to vibration, pain, and temperature. There are several other types of this genetic condition.

☞**LOUIS-BAR SYNDROME:** Progressive cerebellar ataxia characterized by the loss of motor coordination in the limbs and head. The onset of disease is usually in infancy. Impaired muscle coordination is an early sign of the disease that becomes most evident when walking. At age 3 to 6 years, telangiectasias appear in the eyes and on the face and palate. Other clinical features include an increased risk of sinus and respiratory infections, neoplasms, and premature aging. It has been associated with an immune deficiency (IgA or IgE). Mental development may be normal in the early stages, but loss of intellectual capacities may occur during the second decade of life. It is often misdiagnosed as FRDA until the telangiectasias appear.

HEREDITARY OLIVOPONTOCEREBELLAR ATROPHY (OPCA): Rare group of disorders characterized by a progressive sense of disequilibrium, cerebellar ataxia, and dysarthria. There are at least five distinct forms of hereditary OPCA. Most forms of hereditary OPCA are inherited as autosomal dominant traits.

REFERENCES:

Finley GA, Campbell AM: Spinal anesthesia and Friedreich's ataxia. *Anesth Analg* 74:311, 1992.

Lynch DR, Farmer JM, Balcer LJ, et al: Friedreich ataxia: Effects of genetic understanding on clinical evaluation and therapy. *Arch Neurol* 59:743, 2002.

Mouloudi H, Katsanoulas, Frantzeskos G: Requirement for muscle relaxation in Friedreich's ataxia. *Anesthesia* 53;177, 1998.

Fronto-Metaphyseal Dysplasia of Gorlin (FMD)

At a glance: Congenital syndrome involving multiple abnormalities of the face and airway, poorly developed musculature, and limited joint mobility.

Synonyms: Gorlin Syndrome I; Gorlin-Cohen Frontometaphyseal Dysplasia; Gorlin-Holt Syndrome.

History: First described in 1969 by Robert James Gorlin, an American pathologist and geneticist.

Incidence: Rare; only 20 to 30 cases are known.

Genetic inheritance: Probable X-linked inheritance, with severe manifestations in males and variable manifestations in females.

Pathophysiology: Unknown.

Diagnosis: Usually asymptomatic at birth and then gradually progressive, particularly contractures. Radiography shows bony changes of dysplasia and osteosclerosis. Metachromatic fibroblasts on blood work.

Clinical aspects: Prominent supraorbital ridges, incomplete sinus development, micrognathia with decreased angle, high palate, and delayed eruption of teeth. Defective vision and hearing (conductive and sensorineural). Congenital stridor, subglottic stenosis, laryngomalacia, vocal cord paralysis, tracheal web, recurrent respiratory infection, restrictive lung disease, and pulmonary hypertension secondary to scoliosis. Scoliosis, cervical vertebral abnormalities and limited movement, and winged scapula. Flexion contracture of joints (particularly fingers), poorly developed musculature. Cardiac murmurs are common, but often no abnormalities are found. However, mitral valve prolapse has been reported. Bradycardia. Prognosis depends on the progression of ankylosis and thoracic restriction (respiratory failure). Genitourinary tract obstructive anomalies and hydrocephaly are not unusual.

Precautions before anesthesia: Assessment of associated abnormalities, particularly the airway. A congenital stridor, if present, may be the presenting complaint for diagnosis under anesthesia, and imaging of the airway may be available for assessment. If scoliosis is present, the patient should be assessed for the degree of restrictive lung disease (spirometry) and the presence of pulmonary hypertension (chest radiographs, MRI, blood gases, ECG, and echocardiography). If cardiac murmur is noted, an ECG and echocardiographic evaluation should be performed to rule out arrhythmia and structural abnormality.

Anesthetic considerations: Abnormality of the airway is usual in these patients, so the potential for a difficult tracheal intubation should always be considered. If stridor is present, a sedative premedication may not be appropriate and narcotic premedication certainly is contraindicated. Atropine should be considered at induction to reduce the risk of bradycardia and to decrease oral secretions. Induction should be performed after placement of all routine monitoring devices. Inhalational induction in 100% O_2 is the preferred technique so that spontaneous ventilation can be maintained and the airway can be fully assessed. Preparation should be made for use of a smaller tube than expected, aiming for a moderate leak. Atropine should be available to treat intraoperative bradycardia. Patient positioning should be done carefully in view of strictures. Intravenous access in the hands may be difficult. Postoperatively, these children may require a period of mechanical ventilation allowing for complete recovery and decreasing the possibility of an increased incidence of tracheal damage and severe stridor after reintubation. Postoperative continuous positive airway pressure has been recommended as an alternative.

Pharmacological implications: Avoid using neuromuscular blocking agents until tracheal intubation and proper lung ventilation are achieved. Care is necessary because of the tendency toward bradycardia and possible sensitivity in these children. Postoperative respiratory problems occur, so narcotics should be titrated carefully or avoided where possible.

Other conditions to be considered:

☞**OTOPALATODIGITAL SYNDROME, TYPES I AND II:** Congenital association of coarse facies, posterior cleft palate, conduction deafness, clinodactyly on the fifth fingers, and broad big toes. The skull and limb are most often abnormal. Possibly a variant of FMD.

☞**MELNICK-NEEDLES SYNDROME:** X-linked dominant; lethal in boys. Abnormal facial anomalies (prominent forehead, bulging eyes, full cheeks, small chin with dental malalignment), short stature, orthopedic anomalies, and small chest. Possibly a variant of FMD.

☞**SERPENTINE FIBULA–POLYCYSTIC KIDNEY SYNDROME:** Elongated serpentine fibulas, bowed lower legs and forearms, bowed radii, polycystic kidneys, small stature, unusual facial appearance, large skull and occipital depression, severe pectus excavatum, hirsutism, and deafness but normal intelligence.

ATELOSTEOGENESIS TYPE III: Characterized by the absence of metatarsals, bowed femur, tibia, and radius, camptodactyly and hammertoes, hydrocephalus, cleft lip/palate, short stature, and microstomia.

☞**BOOMERANG DYSPLASIA:** Dwarfism associated with an unusual shape of the long bones of the legs. Few cases have been reported, and all of the patients died in the neonatal period. All patients had characteristic facies, large nose, and severe hypoplasia of the nares and septum.

REFERENCES:

Mehta Y, Schou H: The anaesthetic management of an infant with frontometaphyseal dysplasia (Gorlin-Cohen syndrome). *Acta Anaesthesiol Scand* 32:505, 1988.

Morava E, Illes T, Weisenbach J, et al: Clinical and genetic heterogeneity in frontometaphyseal dysplasia: Severe progressive scoliosis in two families. *Am J Med Genet* 116:272, 2003.

Verloes A, Lesenfants S, Barr M, et al: Fronto-otopalatodigital osteodysplasia: Clinical evidence for a single entity encompassing Melnick-Needles syndrome, otopalatodigital syndrome types 1 and 2, and frontometaphyseal dysplasia. *Am J Med Genet* 28;90:407, 2000.

Frydman Cohen Karmon Syndrome

At a glance: Inherited syndrome with blepharophimosis, ptosis, short stature, and syndactyly.

Synonym: Blepharophimosis with Ptosis, Syndactyly, and Short Stature.

Incidence: Extremely rare syndrome with unknown incidence.

Genetic inheritance: No genetic background or molecular data concerning this syndrome are available. The mode of inheritance is autosomal recessive, which distinguishes this syndrome from other blepharophimosis-ptosis syndromes.

Pathophysiology: Weakness of extraocular and frontal muscles.

Diagnosis: Diagnosis is made by the typical facial appearance (combination of blepharophimosis, ptosis, orbital asymmetry), short stature, syndactyly of toes 2 and 3, and camptodactyly of the fingers.

Clinical aspects: In addition to the aforementioned stigmata, the patient may have plagiocephaly, a broad nasal bridge, prognathism, and thick eyebrows with synophrys. In one case, borderline mental retardation and anosmia were reported.

Precautions before anesthesia: No specific considerations concerning this syndrome, and no description of evident impairment of general health is available.

Anesthetic considerations: In general, patients are not different from healthy children undergoing the same procedure. However, depending on the degree of prognathism, airway management could be difficult. Oculocardiac reflex with profound bradycardia should be expected, especially in younger patients undergoing ophthalmic examination with general anesthesia. Treatment is twofold and includes firstly; stopping the stimulation and secondly; if still necessary, the administration of anticholinergic drugs. No other specific precautions are required.

Pharmacological implications: No known implications with this condition.

Other conditions to be considered: Other blepharophimosis-ptosis syndromes, including the following:

☞**BLEPHAROPHIMOSIS, EPICANTHUS INVERSUS, AND PTOSIS SYNDROME (BPES):** Hereditary autosomal dominant syndrome affecting the eyelids, with the clinical symptom triad of blepharophimosis, ptosis, and epicanthus inversus (fold curving in the mediolateral direction inferior to the inner canthus).

☞**BLEPHAROPTOSIS WITH MYOPIA AND ECTOPIA LENTIS:** Extremely rare autosomal dominant genetic disease with features limited to the eye and its appendices.

BLEPHAROPTOSIS, PTOSIS, SYNDACTYLY, AND MENTAL RETARDATION (CAMERA-MARUGO-COHEN SYNDROME): Characterized by blepharoptosis, truncal obesity, syndactyly, camptodactyly, retrognathia, mental retardation, body asymmetry, and muscle weakness. It has been found that one of these patients showed diploid/triploid mixoploidy (69,XXY/46,XY) on cytogenetic analysis of skin fibroblasts. Karyotyping of skin fibroblasts should be performed when the diagnosis of Camera-Marugo-Cohen syndrome is considered.

DE DIE SMULDERS DROOG VAN DIJK SYNDROME: Blepharophimosis, nasal groove, and growth retardation.

JORGENSON LENZ SYNDROME: Mild short stature, microcephaly, ptosis-blepharophimosis, facial asymmetry, prognathism, restricted joint mobility, and radioulnar synostosis. The name of this syndrome is based on a single paper.

OHDO MADOKORO SONODA SYNDROME (Blepharophimosis Syndrome, Ohdo Type): Blepharophimosis, ptosis, mental retardation, congenital heart disease, and hypoplastic teeth.

SIMOSA PENCHASZADEH BUSTOS SYNDROME (Simosa Craniofacial Syndrome; Blepharophimosis Telecanthus Microstomia Syndrome): High forehead, elongated and flattened face, arched and sparse eyebrows, short palpebral fissures, microstomia, and high and narrow palate. Intelligence is normal. Facies has similarities with the whistling face syndrome (Freeman-Sheldon syndrome).

REFERENCE:

Frydman M, Cohen HA, Karmon G, et al: Autosomal recessive blepharophimosis, ptosis V-esotropia, syndactyly, and short stature. *Clin Genet* 41:57, 1992.

Fryns Syndrome

At a glance: Very rare polymalformative syndrome characterized by diaphragmatic hernia and unusual facies. The proportion of patients who survive the neonatal period represents only 14% of reported cases. The majority are stillborn or die in early neonatal period.

Synonyms: Diaphragmatic Hernia, Abnormal Face, and Distal Limb Anomalies; FRNS.

History: First reported in two female siblings by J.P. Fryns in 1979.

Genetic inheritance: Autosomal recessive.

Clinical aspects: The features are extremely numerous but dominated by diaphragmatic hernia. Patients have *characteristic facies* (thin lips, macrostomia or microstoma, microretrognathia, short neck, coarse face, broad forehead, anteverted nares, broad nasal root, down-slanted fissures, decreased lashes and eyebrows, microphthalmia, narrow or cleft palate, cleft lip). Other features involve *viscera* (hypoplastic lungs, polycystic kidneys, polysplenia, malrotation or duplication of the gut, esophageal atresia, Meckel diverticulum, duodenal atresia), *heart* (cardiac septal defect, tetralogy of Fallot, patent ductus arteriosus), *limb* (brachydactyly, small fingernails, clinodactyly of fifth finger, syndactyly of toes), and *central nervous system* (*CNS*) (hydrocephaly, Dandy-Walker anomaly, cranial nerve anomalies, holoprosencephaly, corpus callosum agenesis). Absent or abnormally placed nipples, excess nuchal skin, tracheoesophageal fistula, and uterine anomalies have been described.

Anesthetic considerations: High rate of anesthetic implications. Main risks concern direct laryngoscopy and tracheal intubation, pulmonary aspiration, respiratory distress, and cardiac and renal function. Full preoperative assessment is needed and should include chest radiographs, renal and cardiac echography, CT, and laboratory analysis. Anesthetic management may conciliate imperative requirement of the associate defects. Postoperative stay in an intensive care unit with mechanical ventilatory support may be anticipated.

REFERENCES:

Fryns JP, Moerman F, Goddeeris P, et al: A new lethal syndrome with cloudy corneae, diaphragmatic defects, and distal limb deformities. *Hum Genet* 50:65, 1979.

Veldman A, Schlosser R, Allendorf A, et al: Bilateral congenital diaphragmatic hernia: Differentiation between Pallister-Killian and Fryns syndromes [letter]. *Am J Med Genet* 111:86, 2002.

Ramsing M, Gillesen-Kaesbach G, Holzgreve W, et al: Variability in the phenotypic expression of Fryns Syndrome: a report of two sibships. *Am J Med Genet* 95:415, 2000.

Fucosidosis

At a glance: Lysosomal storage disease resulting from nearly complete deficiency of alpha-L-fucosidase enzyme activity characterized by accumulation of lipids (glycosphingolipids) in the central nervous system (CNS) and peripheral tissues.

Synonyms: Alpha-l-Fucosidase Deficiency; Mucopolysaccharidosis F; Mucopolysaccharidosis Storage Disease F; FUCA Deficiency; Glycoproteinoses.

Classification: Many researchers believe there are two types of fucosidosis (types I and II), which are determined by the severity of symptoms. Others theorize there are three types, with the age at onset and disease severity the determining factors.

Fucosidosis type I is the most severe form of the disease. The age at onset is the infancy period, and it may become apparent as early as age 6 months. Clinical symptoms include progressive deterioration of the brain and spinal cord, mental retardation, loss of previously acquired intellectual skills, and growth retardation leading to short stature. Dysostosis multiplex, coarse facial features, cardiomegaly, hepatosplenomegaly, and seizures complete the clinical picture.

Fucosidosis type II is characterized by age at onset within the first few years of life and clinical symptoms that progress more slowly than in type I. Other symptoms may be similar to type I but are milder. The most noticeable feature distinguishing the two types is the appearance of angiokeratomas on the skin of individuals with type II.

Incidence: Fewer than 100 cases have been reported. Equally distributed in males and females. Pan-ethnic, but frequency is increased in populations of Italian and Spanish descent.

Genetic inheritance: Autosomal recessive. The gene (alpha-L-fucosidase) is mapped to chromosome 1p34 with a homologous site on chromosome 2. Seventeen mutation types have been reported.

Pathophysiology: Deficiency of alpha-L-fucosidase (a lysosomal enzyme that catalyzes removal of fucose residues from glycosphingolipids) results in accumulation and excretion of oligosaccharides and glycoproteins (mainly H antigen glycolipid).

Diagnosis: Based on history and physical findings. Increased sweat sodium chloride (infantile form) and urinary fucose-rich oligosaccharides, sphingolipids, and glycopeptides (about 22 glycopeptides) detected by thin-layer chromatography (no mucopolysaccharides). Enzyme assay of alpha-L-fucosidase in white blood cells or cultured fibroblasts. Prenatal diagnosis available (deficiency of alpha-L-fucosidase activity in cultured chorionic villi or amniocytes).

Clinical aspects: More severe cases (type I or infantile form) are affected in the first year of life with mental and growth retardation, dysostosis multiplex, and coarse faces. Hepatosplenomegaly, cardiomegaly, seizures, and infections are variable. Death occurs around age 5 years. The milder form (type II or juvenile form) has similar but less severe features, longer survival (early adulthood), and is distinguished from the infantile form with the presence of angiokeratoma.

Anesthetic considerations: The potential for difficult direct laryngoscopy and tracheal intubation must be reviewed in view of the unstable cervical spine. Proper preoperative evaluation of the cervical spine motion must be achieved. Gingival hyperplasia may be present and occasionally can be significant enough to affect the airway management. Neuraxial regional blockade may be difficult because of skeletal dysplasia. In patients affected with fucosidosis type I, the implications of cardiomegaly, hepatosplenomegaly, and severe seizure disease are important to the management of anesthesia. Postoperative mechanical ventilation may be required. The presence of severe seizure activities must be evaluated, and an intraoperative intravenous anticonvulsant medication must be administered as a relay to the oral form of therapy. Electrolyte measurements are important because of the presence of atrophic adrenal glands.

Other conditions to be considered:

☞**FABRY DISEASE:** Characterized by a deficiency of the enzyme alpha-galactosidase A leading to abnormal accumulation of glycolipids (glycosphingolipid) in various organs of the body, particularly blood vessels and the eyes. Clinical features include angiokeratomas, abdominal pain, and visual impairment. Later in the course of the disease, kidney failure, heart problems, and progressive neurologic abnormalities are serious complications. Inherited as an X-linked recessive trait; primarily affects males. A milder form of the disease has been identified in females.

☞**SIALIDOSIS TYPE II:** Caused by a deficiency of the enzyme alpha-neuraminidase leading to accumulation of mucopolysaccharides and mucolipids in many tissues of the body. The age at onset of symptoms may vary; congenital, infantile, and juvenile forms have been identified. Characterized by sudden myoclonic activities, ocular problems causing visual impairment, mild coarse facial features, dysostosis multiplex, hepatosplenomegaly, and mild mental retardation. Muscle hypotonia and atrophy, choreoathetosis, inguinal hernia, and dyspnea are common symptoms. Inherited as an autosomal recessive genetic trait.

☞**MANNOSIDOSIS:** Characterized by age at onset during the first year of life. Results from abnormally low levels of the enzyme alpha-D-mannosidase. Clinical features include rapid progression of mental retardation, hepatosplenomegaly, skeletal abnormalities, and coarse facial features. A milder form of mannosidosis is characterized by mild-to-moderate mental retardation during childhood or adolescence. Impaired immune system response may result in increased risk of respiratory infections. Inherited as an autosomal recessive trait.

☞**MUCOPOLYSACCHARIDOSES:** Group of hereditary lysosomal storage diseases characterized by abnormal accumulations of mucopolysaccharides in the arteries, skeleton, eyes, joints, ears, skin, and teeth. They may be found in the respiratory system, liver, spleen, central nervous system, blood, and bone marrow. Symptoms are progressive and typically begin around age 1 year, at which time signs of both growth and mental retardation may become apparent. After age 3 or 4 years, significant delay in growth is observed. Stiff joints, hirsutism, dwarfism, hepatosplenomegaly, breathing irregularities, and heart abnormalities are common features. These disorders, except for the mucopolysaccharidosis type II (Hunter Syndrome), are inherited as autosomal recessive genetic traits.

REFERENCES:

Ismail EA, Rudwan M, Shafik MH: Fucosidosis: Immunological studies and chronological neuroradiological changes. *Acta Paediatr* 88:224, 1999.

Michalski JC, Klein A: Glycoprotein lysosomal storage disorders: alpha- and beta-mannosidosis, fucosidosis and alpha-*N*-acetylgalactosaminidase deficiency. *Biochim Biophys Acta* 1455:69, 1999.

Willems PJ, Seo HC, Coucke P, et al: Spectrum of mutations in fucosidosis. *Eur J Hum Genet* 7:60, 1999.

G

Galactosemia

At a glance: Inborn error of metabolism with the inability to metabolize galactose appropriately. This results in toxic effects on brain, liver, kidney, and eyes. Early diagnosis and galactose-free diet are key.

Synonyms: Galactose-1-Phosphate Uridyltransferase Deficiency; GALT Deficiency.

Incidence: The incidence in the general population is estimated between 1:30,000 and 1:70,000, with the highest incidence in Ireland. It occurs in all races, but the incidence is lower among Asian people. Both genders are equally affected.

Genetic inheritance: Transmission is autosomal recessive. The responsible gene encoding galactose-1-phosphate uridyltransferase (GALT) has been mapped to 9p13.

Pathophysiology: Lactose is a disaccharide consisting of galactose and glucose that is metabolized to glucose-6-phosphate via uridine diphosphate (UDP)-glucose in the Leloir pathway. Three different enzyme defects within the Leloir pathway can lead to galactosemia. Classic galactosemia, the most common form, is caused by GALT deficiency. The inability to metabolize galactose-1-phosphate to UDP-galactose results in accumulation of the former in brain, kidney, and liver, where it exerts a toxic effect. Galactosemia also can be caused by a deficiency in galactokinase, the enzyme responsible for the initial phosphorylation of galactose to galactose-1-phosphate. Erythrocytic galactokinase activity (used for diagnostic purposes) is significantly diminished in homozygous patients, whereas intermediate activities are measured in heterozygous children. Increased galactose levels are found in blood and urine samples after ingestion of lactose. In general, the prognosis is better than observed for the classic form. Finally, UDP-galactose-4-epimerase is necessary for the conversion of UDP-galactose to UDP-glucose. The deficiency of this enzyme comes in two different clinical forms. The benign form usually is detected during newborn screening tests with increased levels of erythrocytic galactose-1-phosphate concentrations, whereas galactokinase and uridyltransferase activities are normal. In this benign form, the defect affects only blood cells, so no treatment is required. In the generalized form, however, the clinical course is indistinguishable from classic galactosemia. In patients with black ethnic background, the most frequent mutation (S135L, which was previously called "Negro" or "African American" variant) accounts for approximately 45% of the mutant alleles. Homozygosity for the S135L allele and for two other mutant alleles (Duarte and Los Angeles variants) results in approximately 50% of normal GALT activity and a mild clinical course. A certain amount of free galactose may be reduced to galactitol through aldose reductase; however, this is a dead-end pathway and the poorly diffusable galactitol accumulates in the cells. It is partly responsible for the toxic effects seen in galactosemia.

Diagnosis: Most often galactosemia is detected by standard newborn screening tests for inborn errors of metabolism. The test requires that the child be fed with human or cow's milk or a lactose-containing formula. A galactose breath test with orally administered stable isotope-labeled galactose can be used to determine whole-body galactose oxidation to CO_2. The absence of a marked CO_2 peak after 2 to 5 hours is found in patients with a severe clinical course or in affected neonates exposed to galactose.

Clinical aspects: Upon being fed with milk, newborns develop a variable combination of the following symptoms: lethargy, irritability, hypotonia, vomiting, hypoglycemia, seizures, failure to thrive, jaundice, hepatomegaly, liver dysfunction (including coagulopathy with bleeding), ascites, and splenomegaly. Cataracts are typical and already present in the neonatal period. It is essential to diagnose galactosemia early, otherwise hardly reversible or even irreversible and severe damage to brain (mental retardation), liver (macronodular cirrhosis, portal hypertension, hypersplenism), and eyes (cataract) may be established. Transfer of galactose from maternal into fetal circulation can lead to toxic changes in utero. Although not common on a normal diet, hypoglycemic episodes can occur after ingestion of galactose and are caused by either elevated levels of galactose-1-phosphate, which can inhibit the conversion of glycogen to glucose, or increased insulin release. A higher risk of *Escherichia coli* sepsis in galactosemia patients has been reported. In fact, galactosemia should be ruled out in neonates with sepsis from this pathogen. Renal tubular dysfunction and albuminuria with later transition into generalized amino aciduria has been described. Hypergonadotropic hypogonadism is a common finding. The condition should be suspected in males presenting with small testes. Females with primary ovarian failure and primary (or secondary) amenorrhea but normal development and even uncomplicated pregnancy have been described. Short stature, ataxia, tremor, EEG abnormalities, and difficulties with learning and speech (verbal dyspraxia) are other features of galactosemia. Treatment consists of elimination of galactose from the diet as soon as the diagnosis is made. No specific drug therapy exists. Although a galactose-free diet protects the body from the severe toxic effects of galactose-1-phosphate, it cannot prevent all the long-term complications (e.g., hypogonadism, cerebellar signs). These long-term complications have been suggested to be caused by "self-intoxication" of the body with galactose, because UDP-galactose can be synthesized from glucose through the enzymes UDP-glucose-pyrophosphorylase and UDP-galactose-4-epimerase, which both are part of the Leloir pathway. Other researchers believe that cerebral complications are the result of in utero exposition to high levels of galactose-1-phosphate.

Precautions before anesthesia: Obtain a complete blood count (renal anemia, thrombocytopenia), check electrolytes (hypokalemia) and glucose levels, and assess renal and hepatic function (coagulation). Sedative or anxiolytic premedication may be helpful in the presence of mental retardation.

Anesthetic considerations: Blood glucose should be monitored perioperatively, depending on the degree of renal dysfunction and the nature of the procedure. An arterial line for a close followup of acid-base changes is recommended.

Pharmacological implications: Depending on the degree of renal and hepatic dysfunction, drugs with predominantly renal and hepatic elimination, respectively, should be titrated carefully. In the presence of known seizures, avoid potentially epileptogenic drugs such as methohexital, ketamine, enflurane, atracurium, *cis*-atracurium, and meperidine (the last three only if given in large quantities because of their metabolites, laudanosine and normeperidine, respectively). The potential association of seizure activity during induction of anesthesia with high concentration of sevoflurane should be considered. Lactulose and voriconazole contain lactose and should not be used in these patients.

Other condition to be considered:

FRUCTOSE 1-PHOSPHATE ALDOLASE DEFICIENCY (Fructose Intolerance): Severe autosomal recessive inborn error affecting the metabolism of glucides caused by a deficiency of hepatic fructose 1-aldolase becomes clinically apparent only when fructose is ingested. Characterized by vomiting, hypoglycemia, severe metabolic acidosis, coma, growth retardation (even cachexia), hepatomegaly, jaundice, coagulopathy, and renal Fanconi syndrome. The responsible gene has been mapped to 9q22.3.

REFERENCES:

Forges T, Monnier-Barbarino P: [Premature ovarian failure in galactosemia: pathophysiology and clinical management.] *Pathol Biol (Paris)* 51:47, 2003.

Leslie ND: Insights into the pathogenesis of galactosemia. *Annu Rev Nutr* 23:59-80, 2003

Galactosialidosis

At a glance: Neurodegenerative disorder characterized by dwarfism, gargoyle facies, myoclonic seizures, progressive neurologic dysfunction (dementia and ataxia), and macular cherry-red spots.

Synonyms: Deficiency of Cathepsin; Goldberg Syndrome; Neuraminidase Deficiency with Beta-Galactosidase Deficiency; Neuraminidase/Beta-Galactosidase Expression (NGBE); PPCA Deficiency; Beta-Galactosidase Protective Protein Deficiency.

Nature: Inborn error of metabolism. Lysosomal storage disease belonging to the group of progressive myoclonus epilepsies.

Incidence: Approximately 70 cases have been described worldwide. The majority of patients are of Japanese origin.

Genetic inheritance: Autosomal recessive. The gene is mapped to chromosome 20q13.1. Predominance in populations of Japanese origin. Equal distribution between males and females.

Pathophysiology: Lysosomal storage disease associated with combined deficiency of beta-galactosidase and neuraminidase. Deficiency of a protein (cathepsin) that is essential for the catalytic activity of alpha-N-acetyl-neuraminidase and normally protects beta-galactosidase from degradation. Accumulation of sialyloligosaccharides and sialylglycopeptides in lymphocytes, fibroblasts, bone marrow cells, Kupffer cells, and Schwann cells.

Diagnosis: Combined enzyme deficiency demonstrable in lymphocytes or cultured skin fibroblasts. Sialyloligosaccharides/sialylglycopeptides are detected by (1) light microscopy as periodic acid–Schiff-positive inclusions (vacuolations) within cells throughout the body and (2) thin layer chromatography in urine. Prenatal diagnosis is available (deficiency of alpha-N-acetylneuraminidase and beta-galactosidase activities in cultured chorionic villi or amniocytes).

Clinical aspects: In all forms, coarsened facial features, vertebral anomalies, and often bilateral macular cherry-red spots result in progressive loss of vision. Infantile form presents with fetal hydrops, or with death from renal and cardiac failure in infancy. Late infantile form has better prognosis. Hepatosplenomegaly and valvular heart disease are common in this form. The majority of patients have juvenile/adult form of galactosialidosis. Features include spinal deformities, myoclonus, ataxia, seizures, mental retardation, and hearing loss.

Precautions before anesthesia: Assess neurologic status (myoclonus and seizures), cardiac status (may have cardiac failure or valvular heart disease), airway (potentially difficult tracheal intubation), and renal function.

Anesthetic considerations: Anesthetic management has not been described but depends upon systemic manifestations of the disease. In the more common juvenile/adult form, attention should be directed toward potential airway anomalies and skeletal deformities. The presence of renal or cardiac dysfunction requires appropriate precautions in infantile forms. The association with myoclonic seizures and anesthetic medications potentially able to trigger seizure must be avoided.

Pharmacological implications: Agents that might precipitate seizures, such as ketamine, enflurane, and methohexital, should be avoided. Seizure medications should be continued until the day of surgery when an intravenous anticonvulsant should be administered. Antibiotic prophylaxis as indicated in case of cardiopathy.

Other conditions to be considered:

☞SIALIDOSIS: Lysosomal storage disease caused by a deficiency of the enzyme alpha-neuraminidase resulting in tissue accumulation of mucopolysaccharides and mucolipids, resulting in the development (usually in the second decade) of red macules in the eyes, myoclonus, mild seizures, Hurler-like facies, skeletal dysplasia, psychomotor retardation, and normal excretion of urinary mucopolysaccharides. Autosomal recessive; gene map locus is 6p21.

☞G_{M1}-GANGLIOSIDOSIS, TYPE I: Autosomal recessive lysosomal storage disease characterized by coarse facies and progressive neurodegeneration caused by accumulation of G_{M1} ganglioside, oligosaccharides, and the mucopolysaccharide keratan because of deficient activity of lysosomal enzyme beta-galactosidase. Gene map locus is 3p21.33.

REFERENCES:

Achyuthan KE, Achyuthan AM: Comparative enzymology, biochemistry and pathophysiology of human exo-alpha-sialidases (neuraminidases). *Comp Biochem Physiol B Biochem Mol Biol* 129:29, 2001.

Claeys M, Van der Hoeven M, de Die-Smulders C, et al: Early-infantile type of galactosialidosis as a cause of heart failure and neonatal ascites. *J Inherit Metab Dis* 22:666, 1999.

Gangliosidosis (G_{M1}) Type I

At a glance: Lysosomal storage disease. Affected patients have clinical features resembling those of mucopolysaccharidoses types I and VI but without mucopolysacchariduria. Clinical features include joint stiffness, scoliosis, and skeletal dystrophy. Valvular heart diseases are present, of which aortic insufficiency is the most common. Obstructive sleep apnea is frequent, and 50% of reported cases have mild mental retardation.

Synonyms: Caffey Pseudo-Hurler Syndrome; Caffey Syndrome; Hurler-Like Syndrome; Landing Syndrome; Norman-Landing Syndrome; Beta-Galactosidase-1 (GLB 1) Deficiency; Cerebral G_{M1} Gangliosidosis; Familial Neurovisceral Lipidosis; Generalized Gangliosidosis G_{M1}, Type I; Generalized Infantile Gangliosidosis.

Classification: Three forms of gangliosidosis have been described:

- *Infantile form:* Classic infantile subtype combines the features of a neurolipidosis (i.e., neurodegeneration, macular cherry-red spots) with those of a mucopolysaccharidosis (i.e., visceromegaly, dysostosis multiplex, coarsened facial features). It most frequently presents in early infancy and may be evident at birth.
- *Juvenile form:* Juvenile subtype is marked by a slightly later age of onset and clinical variability in the classic physical features.
- *Adult form:* Adult subtype is marked by normal early neurologic development with no physical stigmata and subsequent development of a slowly progressive dementia with parkinsonian features, extrapyramidal disease, and dystonia.

Incidence: Incidence is estimated at 1:3700 live births in the population of Malta. The incidence in the international general population is unknown.

Genetic inheritance: Autosomal recessive, the gene has been mapped to chromosome 3p21-33.

Pathophysiology: Ganglioside storage disorder caused by beta-galactosidase deficiency resulting in abnormal accumulation of G_{M1} ganglioside in the lysosomes of neurons and of oligosaccharides in hepatic, splenic, and other histiocytes and in renal glomerular cells.

Diagnosis: Vacuolated lymphocytes in peripheral blood and foam cells in bone marrow; Hurler-like radiographic bone anomalies in infantile form; measurement of enzymatic activity in peripheral leukocytes or fibroblasts.

Clinical aspects: *Infantile form:* Symptoms appear shortly after birth and include hypotonia, slow psychomotor development, failure to thrive, feeding difficulty, startle reaction to sounds, and hepatosplenomegaly. Coarse facies with macrocephaly, frontal bossing, full cheeks, and mandibular prognathism. Puffy eyelids, cherry-red macular spots in 50% of patients and occasional corneal opacity. Depressed nasal bridge and prominent philtrum. Macroglossia and enlarged alveolar process. Wide ribs. Hypoplastic ilia and pelvic trabeculation. Short and stubby hands with bullet-shaped phalanges. Flexion contractures of joints and faulty tubulation of long bones. Kyphoscoliosis and short vertebrae in their anteroposterior diameter with convex endplates and hook-like deformities at the thoracolumbar junctions. Cardiomyopathy and paroxysmal supraventricular tachycardia have been described. Severe cerebral degeneration follows, with death in the first 2 years of life, usually as a result of bronchopneumonia. Affected infants often are blind, deaf, and quadriplegic.

Juvenile form: Onset during the second year of life; progressive loss of skills, autistic behavior, ataxia, epilepsy, and spastic paresis develop progressively. Dysostosis multiplex on bone radiograph. Death by around 10 years of age.

Adult-onset form: Onset during childhood or adolescence. Presents as an extrapyramidal disorder with dystonia, dysarthria, and ataxia. No ocular or skeletal anomalies. Dementia may be severe.

Precautions before anesthesia: Cardiac function should be assessed in light of cardiomyopathic potential. Epileptic history and control factors, including seizure termination, should be ascertained and medications continued where possible. Respiratory function should be checked by chest radiographs and preoperative physiotherapy. Blood tests are necessary because of bone marrow and histiocyte involvement.

Anesthetic considerations: Vascular access will likely be difficult because of short, misshapen limbs and contractures with/

without spasticity. In the infantile form, airway management likely will be difficult as in Hurler syndrome: have laryngeal mask airway and nasopharyngeal airway ready for use. Expect face-mask ventilation, direct laryngoscopy, and tracheal intubation to be very difficult; odontoid hypoplasia with possibility of an unstable neck; thickened tracheal wall, necessitating a smaller endotracheal tube than predicted; valvular heart disease. Obstructive sleep apnea. Ventilation could be problematic because of kyphoscoliosis (causing a stiff ribcage), visceromegaly, and bronchopneumonia. The child may be blind, deaf, quadriplegic, and profoundly mentally handicapped, making handling of a difficult anesthetic case even more of a challenge. Choice of anesthetic agents should take the patient's epileptic status into account.

Pharmacological implications: High probability of interaction with epilepsy medications. Avoid anesthetic agents with intrinsic ability to trigger seizure activity.

REFERENCES:

Barth PG: Disorders of sphingolipid metabolism, in Fernandes J, Saudubray J-M, Van den Bergh G (eds): *Inborn Metabolic Diseases.* 3rd ed. Berlin, Springer, 2000, p 400.

Caffey J: Gargoylism (Hurler-Hunter disease, dysostosis multiplex, lipochondrodystrophy): Prenatal and neonatal bone lesions and their early postnatal evolution. *Bull Hosp Joint Dis* 12:38, 1951.

Landing BH, Silverman FN, Craig JM, et al: Familial neurovisceral lipidosis. An analysis of eight cases of a syndrome previously reported as "Hurler-variant," "pseudo-Hurler disease" and "Tay-Sachs disease with visceral involvement." *Am J Dis Child* 108:503, 1964.

Gangliosidosis (G~M2~) Type II

At a glance: Heritable lysosomal storage disorder with ganglioside accumulation leading to severe neurologic impairment with premature death. Tay-Sachs disease (TSD) and its variants are caused by absence or defects of the alpha subunit of hexosaminidase A.

Synonyms and Classification:

- *G_{M2} Gangliosidosis B Variant: Tay-Sachs Disease* (TSD; Hexosaminidase A Deficiency [Hex A deficiency]; Pseudo AB variant): Three types of TSD are described (infantile, juvenile, and adult, which is characterized by a pseudodeficiency mutation in one or both *HEXA* alleles).
- *G_{M2} Gangliosidosis B1 variant.*
- *G_{M2} Gangliosidosis AB Variant* (Hexosaminidase Activator Deficiency) is caused by absence or defects of the hexosaminidase activator. It represents a deficiency of sphingolipid activator protein G_{M2} required for in vivo degradation of G_{M2} ganglioside by beta-hexosaminidase A.
- *G_{M2} Gangliosidosis O Variant: Sandhoff disease* and its variants are caused by absence or defects of the beta subunit of hexosaminidase A and the subunits of hexosaminidase B. It is also known as SD (Sandhoff Disease), Hex A and Hex B deficiency, or G_{M2} gangliosidosis, O variant, and it includes the juvenile subacute type.

Incidence: Incidence in the general US population is 1:320,000 live births, and only 1 in 283 persons is a heterozygous unaffected carrier of a *HEXA* mutation. However, in the Ashkenazi Jewish population, the incidence of affected individuals is 1:2500–3600 newborns. The carrier of the *HEXA* mutations in this subgroup of population is 1 in 30 individuals. In certain isolated populations, such as Louisiana Cajuns and Pennsylvania Dutch, the incidence of this disease appears even higher than in individuals of Ashkenazi Jewish descent. The incidence of Sandhoff disease in the United States is estimated to be 1:309,000 non-Jewish newborns. One in 278 persons of non-Jewish descent is a heterozygous unaffected carrier of a *HEXB* mutation. Approximately 1:1,000,000 Jewish newborns is affected. Individuals affected with the hexosaminidase activator deficiency are very rare. Internationally, the incidence for TSD is estimated at 1:360,000 live births in the general population, and 1:300 individuals is a carrier of the *HEXA* mutation. Increased frequencies have been reported in Moroccan Jews and some isolated populations in Switzerland and Japan. The incidence in French Canadians living along the border of the eastern St. Lawrence River in the Province of Quebec is similar to the incidence reported for those of Ashkenazi Jewish descent. The international incidence for Sandhoff disease is approximately 1:310,000 non-Jewish newborns. Increased incidences have been suggested in Creoles of northern Argentina, Metis Indians of northern Saskatchewan in Canada, Lebanese, and Hispanics of Mexican or Central American heritage. The mortality associated with this medical condition depends on the type. The classic infantile form usually is fatal by 2 to 4 years of age. In the late infantile subacute, B1 variant form, disease progression is particularly aggressive, leading to death within 2 to 4 years of disease onset. In the juvenile subacute form, death occurs by 10 to 15 years of age. It usually is caused by infection and most often is preceded by several years of vegetative state with decerebrate rigidity. In the adult chronic form, most patients survive to 60 to 80 years of age. Death in Sandhoff disease occurs by approximately 4 years of age.

Genetic inheritance: Autosomal recessive inheritance. The gene for *HEXA* has been mapped to 15q23, while *HEXB* is located on 5q13.

Pathophysiology: As mentioned earlier, G$_{M2}$ gangliosidosis comprises a group of lysosomal lipid storage disorders caused by mutations affecting at least three enzymes: the alpha subunit of β-hexosaminidase A (*HEXA*), the beta subunit of hexosaminidase A (*HEXB*), and the G$_{M2}$ activator protein (G$_{M2}$A). A normal catabolism of G$_{M2}$ ganglioside requires all three enzymes to function properly. A deficient activity of one or more of these enzymes leads to accumulation of the substrate inside neuronal lysosomes. This accumulation of G$_{M2}$ ganglioside in lysosomes results in the formation of so-called membranous cytoplasmic bodies in neuronal cells and ultimately cell death, which is responsible for the clinical symptoms of developmental delay and progressive neurodegeneration.

Diagnosis: Clinically evocated in patients with progressive developmental retardation, followed by paralysis, dementia, and blindness.

Clinical aspects: Features can include hearing loss, optic disc atrophy with visual loss, neurologic regression with dementia, mental retardation, seizures, and hyperreflexia. Quadriparesis, myotonia, hypotonia or hypertonia, and spasticity are frequent.

Three variants have been described according to age of onset: In *type I* (classic infantile acute form with hexosaminidase A extremely low or absent), onset is between 2 and 6 months of age and death occurs in a few months. In *type II* (juvenile subacute form, hexosaminidase A is decreased but not absent), onset is between 2 and 6 years. *Type III* is an adult or chronic form with diagnosis generally at the adult age.

Precautions before anesthesia: Evaluate neurologic function (clinical, EEG, CT) and seizure activities.

Anesthetic considerations: Aspiration risk can exist as a consequence of neurologic dysfunction and may require rapid-sequence induction. Visual and neurologic impairment may make cooperation of the patient difficult. Postoperative mechanical ventilation must be planned in children with severe neurologic dysfunction (e.g., quadriparesis).

Pharmacological implications: Consider interaction between antiepileptic treatment and anesthetic drugs. Avoid medications that might precipitate seizures (e.g. ketamine, enflurane, methohexital) Succinylcholine should be avoided because of the potential risk of hyperkalemia.

Other conditions to be considered:

☞**ALPERS DISEASE:** Very rare and progressive neurologic disorder, predominantly involving the gray matter, characterized by spasticity, myoclonus, and dementia in combination with hepatic cirrhosis. Poor prognosis with death usually within a few months after onset.

☞**NEURONAL CEROID LIPOFUSCINOSES:** Hereditary progressive neurodegenerative disorders with mental retardation, visual loss, and seizures. The neuronal ceroid lipofuscinoses probably are the most common class of neurodegenerative disease in children.

☞**LEIGH SYNDROME:** Severe progressive necrotizing encephalopathy caused by a mitochondrial disorder impeding oxidative phosphorylation.

REFERENCES:

Mark BL, Mahuran DJ, Cherney MM, et al: Crystal Structure of human beta-hexosaminidase B: Understanding the molecular basis of Sandhoff and Tay-Sachs disease. *J Mol Biol* 327:1093, 2003.

Myerowitz R, Lawson D, Mizukami H, et al: Abstract molecular pathophysiology in Tay-Sachs and Sandhoff diseases as revealed by gene expression profiling. *Hum Mol Genet* 11:1343, 2002.

Garcia-Lurie Syndrome

At a glance: Anomalies of the prosencephalic structures, atelencephaly and microcephaly in association with congenital heart defects (ventricular and atrial septal defects, patent ductus arteriosus, coarctation of the aorta), preaxial limb malformations, eye (cyclopia), and genital abnormalities. Micrognathia and craniofacial disproportion.

Synonyms: Aprosencephaly Syndrome; Aprosencephaly-Atelencephaly Syndrome; XK Syndrome; XK-Aprosencephaly Syndrome.

Nature: Aprosencephaly is a lethal malformation of the central nervous system.

Incidence: Very rare malformation of unknown incidence.

Genetic inheritance: Autosomal recessive inheritance suggested. Chromosome 13 has been implicated, with suspicion of a deletion of the long arm of chromosome 13.

Pathophysiology: Aprosencephaly has been attributed to a post-neurulation encephaloclastic process. Cause of aprosencephaly syndrome is unknown.

Diagnosis: Diagnosis of a severe brain malformation can already be made antenatally by ultrasonography. Reported cases describe autopsy finding in fetuses and postnatally dead infants.

Clinical aspects: Aprosencephaly is characterized by a midline oculofacial defect in association with limb and genital anomalies. Anencephaly has been described. Other findings include congenital heart defects (ventricular and atrial septal defects, patent ductus arteriosus, coarctation of the aorta), preaxial limb malformations (humerus-radial fusion, hip dislocation), eye (cyclopia, hypertelorism), and genital abnormalities. Furthermore, micrognathia and craniofacial disproportion, high arched palate, and adrenal hypoplasia have also been described.

Precautions before anesthesia: Complete evaluation of all systems is mandatory, especially cardiac and pulmonary. Adrenal function should be evaluated and corticosteroid supplementation considered, if necessary. Laboratory reports must include electrolytes, acid-base status, coagulation profile, renal function, and CBC.

Anesthetic considerations: Difficult direct laryngoscopy and tracheal intubation should be expected. The presence of congenital heart defects must be considered in the preparation of the anesthetic. Cortisol supplement may be necessary in the presence of adrenal insufficiency.

Pharmacological implications: Indicated by the complexity of the associated conditions. Subacute bacterial endocarditis prophylaxis may be required. No specific known implications with this condition.

REFERENCE:

Adkins WN, Kaveggia EG: Sporadic case of apparent aprosencephaly. *Am J Med Genet* 3:311, 1979.

Gaucher Disease

At a glance: Most common inherited lipid storage disease. It is particularly common in Ashkenazi Jewish people. Accumulation of glucocerebrosides (derived from red blood cells) in many tissues, especially the macrophages in the bone marrow.

Synonyms and Classification: Sphingolipidosis I.

- *Gaucher Disease Type I* (Noncerebral Juvenile Gaucher Disease; Glucocerebrosidase Deficiency; Acid Beta Glucosidase Deficiency; GBA Deficiency) is characterized by hematologic abnormalities with hypersplenism, bone lesions, skin pigmentation, and pingueculae (brown spots of Gaucher cells at corneoscleral limbus). The disorder is particularly frequent in Ashkenazi Jews. The disease has been diagnosed as early as in the first week of life and as late as 86 years of age.

- *Gaucher Disease Type II* (Infantile Cerebral Gaucher Disease; Acute Neuropathic Gaucher Disease) is characterized by enlargement of the abdomen from hepatosplenomegaly and neurologic signs such as retroflexion of the head, strabismus, dysphagia, choking spells, and hypertonicity. Death usually occurs before the end of the second year of life.

- *Gaucher Disease Type III* (Juvenile and Adult Cerebral Gaucher Disease; Chronic Neuronopathic Gaucher Disease; Subacute Neuronopathic Gaucher Disease; Norrbottnian Type Gaucher Disease) is characterized by hepatosplenomegaly that usually precedes neurologic abnormalities, which include ataxia, spastic paraplegia, grand mal and/or psychomotor seizures, supranuclear ophthalmoplegia, and dementia. Supranuclear gaze palsies (ocular motor apraxia) are characteristic of type III Gaucher disease. Age of onset is variable.

- *Perinatal Lethal Gaucher Disease* is characterized by nonimmune hydrops fetalis. When hydrops is absent, neurologic involvement begins in the first week of life and leads to death

within 3 months. Hepatosplenomegaly is a major sign and is associated with ichthyosis, arthrogryposis, and facial dysmorphism in 35 to 43% of cases.

History: Genetic disorder first described in 1882 by the French physician Philippe Charles Ernest Gaucher. At least 34 mutations are known to cause Gaucher disease, but only four (N370S, L444P, 84gg, IVS2[+1]) account for 95% of cases in the Ashkenazi Jewish population, and 50% of cases in the general population. Enzyme replacement therapy is available (mainly for type I). A clinical trial of gene therapy is under progress.

Incidence: Estimated at 1:60,000 live births (all forms considered). The carrier rate for the mutations may be as high as 1 in 14 Ashkenazi Jews and 1 in 100 of the general population. Males and females are equally affected. Incidence approximates up to 1:250 live births for type I (in Ashkenazi Jews), 1:100,000 live births for type II and 1:50,000 for type III.

Genetic inheritance: Autosomal recessive; locus is the long arm of chromosome 1 at position 21 (1q21). Gene is 7 kb in length with 11 exons. Missense mutation is the most common form.

Pathophysiology: In lysosomes, glucosylceramide is broken down by acid beta-glucosidase (glucocerebrosidase) into ceramide and glucose. A reduction in the catalytic function of acid beta-glucosidase leads to glucosylceramide accumulation in monocytes and macrophages, which become Gaucher cells. These engorged cells can be found in varying degrees throughout the body and cause cell necrosis, mainly through its pressure effects.

Diagnosis: Clinical course, radiology (Erlenmeyer flask deformity of distal femur), bone marrow (Gaucher cells have wrinkled tissue paper appearance on light microscopy), quantitative measurement of glucocerebrosidase activity (in blood, leukocytes, urine), and molecular biology. Age at diagnosis is first year of life to late adulthood. Prenatal diagnosis is available (low glucocerebrosidase activity in chorionic villi).

Clinical aspects: Most common symptoms are enlargement of the liver and spleen, anemia, reduced platelet count (resulting in prolonged bleeding time), coagulation disorders, painful bone infarctions ("bone crises") often leading to deterioration of joint mobility (shoulder, hip), and osteoporosis (with spontaneous fractures). The course of the disease is variable, depending on the type.

Type I which accounts for the vast majority of cases presents with hepatosplenomegaly (anemia, thrombocytopenia, low factor XI concentration), raised intramedullary pressure (bone ischemia/infarction or fractures), and hypermetabolism. Spleen may account for 15 to 20% of body weight; if it infarcts, it can present as acute abdomen. Vertebral collapse may cause spinal cord compression, especially during pubertal growth. Gaucher cell infiltration can result in pulmonary hypertension/failure, with right-to-left intrapulmonary shunt.

Type II is characterized by muscular hypertonia resulting in neck retroflexion and limb rigidity. Bulbar signs and seizures occur. Death usually occurs within 2 years.

Type III presents with mainly visceral involvement and ataxia. Treatment options have included alglucerase (a modified glucocerebrosidase from human placental tissue) and bone marrow transplantation, with variable success.

Treatment of Gaucher disease consists mainly of replacement therapy for the enzyme glucocerebrosidase. Miglustat has been approved for therapy of Gaucher disease type I. Its mechanism of action is reduction of glucocerebroside synthesis by inhibition of the enzyme glucosylceramide synthase. However, it seems to have a slow onset, requires therapy over a long period to be effective, and has significant (mainly gastrointestinal) side effects.

Precautions before anesthesia: Evaluate neurologic status, especially the status of seizure activity and treatment. Spinal cord compression should be ruled out. Evaluate degree of respiratory involvement: SpO_2, forced expiratory volume at 1 second/forced vital capacity (FEV_1/FVC) (restrictive pattern from limited diaphragmatic movement), and arterial blood gases. Possible upper airway obstruction from glycolipid deposition. Blood examination should include liver function tests, electrolytes, CBC, and coagulation screen. Increased opioid requirements may occur if patient has chronic bone pain.

Anesthetic considerations: General anesthesia with rapid-sequence induction, and intermittent positive pressure ventilation are recommended. The presence of raised intraabdominal pressure may reduce lung compliance and increase the risk of pulmonary aspiration. Muscular hypertonia may interfere with respiratory movements. Coagulation disorders are common. Anesthetic requirements may be higher because of hypermetabolism (analogous to hyperthyroidism). Patient handling and positioning during the operation must be meticulous because of extremely thin bones and delicate pressure points because of fragile skin.

Pharmacological implications: Succinylcholine should be avoided if there is spinal cord compression. Atracurium or *cis*-atracurium should be used if liver function is reduced. Meperidine is relatively contraindicated if seizures are present.

Other conditions to be considered:

   GAUCHER-LIKE DISEASE (Pseudo-Gaucher): Glucocerebrosidase deficiency, but none of the common mutations in the glucocerebrosidase gene are found. Characterized by communicating hydrocephalus, corneal opacities, deafness, valvular heart disease, and deformed toes, associated with deficiency of the enzyme involved in Gaucher disease (i.e., glucosylceramide-(glc-cer)-beta-glucosidase). However, the usual manifestations of Gaucher disease are not present. Supranuclear gaze palsies, which are characteristic of type III Gaucher disease, can be detected from early childhood on, although the major signs are not present until early adult life. Individuals affected with this condition present on autopsy with thickened leptomeninges having perivascular fibrosis, nonrheumatic calcified aortic and mitral stenosis, and mild infiltration of Gaucher cells in the reticuloendothelial organs. None of the common mutations in the glucocerebrosidase gene can be demonstrated. Corneal opacities and cardiac valve involvement are manifestations of other lysosomal storage diseases, particularly the mucopolysaccharidoses, but are virtually unknown in Gaucher disease.

   ☞NIEMANN-PICK DISEASE: Lysosomal storage disorder involving brain and/or viscera. Similar clinical features except that the enzyme defect affects the sphingomyelinase.

REFERENCES:

Beutler E, Grabowski GA: Gaucher Disease, in Scriver CR, Beaudet AL, Valle D, et al. (eds.): *The Metabolic and Molecular Bases of Inherited Disease*, 8th ed, New York, McGraw Hill, 2001; p 3635.

Charrow J, Andersson HC, Kaplan P, et al: The Gaucher registry. Demographics and disease characteristics of 1698 patients with Gaucher disease. *Arch Intern Med* 160:2835, 2000.

Tobias JD, Atwood R, Lowe S, et al: Anesthetic considerations in the child with Gaucher disease. *J Clin Anaesth* 5:150, 1993.

Geleophysic Dysplasia

At a glance: Very rare disorder characterized by a child with happy face (*gelios* = happy, and *physis* = nature). This condition is believed to be a "focal" mucopolysaccharidosis. The presence of dysostosis-multiplex-like changes, predominantly in the hands and feet, associated with cardio- and hepatomegaly has been reported. Right ventricular hypertrophy, severe mitral valve stenosis and aortic regurgitation as the patient ages has been observed.

Incidence and genetic inheritance: This rare syndrome is inherited as an autosomal recessive genetic trait.

Pathophysiology: This form of "focal" mucopolysaccharidosis is defined by specific organ lysosomal storage affecting especially the trachea, liver, cartilage, and heart.

Clinical aspects: The most important characteristic of children affected with geleophysic dysplasia is the presence of a pleasant, happy-looking, round, full face and a high-pitched voice. However, the facial characteristic has been suggested to not always be associated with a "geleophysic" behavior. The short stature is associated with a normal head circumference. The cardiovascular system is affected with cardiomegaly and right ventricular hypertrophy leading to cardiac failure. The valvular system presents with mitral and tricuspid valve stenosis, aortic valve regurgitation, and/or stenosis. The respiratory system can be affected with tracheal and bronchial stenosis. Usually, a significant pectus excavatum is noted. The liver is highly affected by storage of mucopolysaccharides, and hepatomegaly develops at an early age. The skeletal system shows osteopenia, coxa valga, shortened long tubular bones, short hands, wrist contractures, short metacarpals with rounded proximal ends, and short feet. The skin is thickened and tight. The neurologic system may present important developmental delay and seizure activity. Radiologically, the shape of the sella turcica shows a characteristic J-form.

Anesthetic considerations: The most important considerations affect the pulmonary and cardiovascular systems. The presence of tracheal stenosis or main bronchi stenosis may have a considerable effect on tracheal intubation and mechanical ventilation. Maintenance of spontaneous ventilation is highly recommended until proper ventilatory support is confirmed. A smaller than expected tracheal tube should be used. The association of valvular disease (most probably stenosis, but also possible association with regurgitation) and heart muscle disease should direct the administration of anesthesia accordingly. Intraoperative positioning could be difficult because of joint contractures or reduced mobility.

Other conditions to be considered:

   ☞ACROMICRIC DYSPLASIA: Characterized by severe growth retardation, mild facial anomalies, and markedly shortened hands and feet secondary to short and stubby metacarpals and phalanges.

   ☞MOORE-FEDERMAN SYNDROME: Dwarfism with disproportionately short legs. Reduced joint mobility (or stiffness) and ocular anomalies (hyperopia, glaucoma, cataract and retinal detachment).

REFERENCES:

Lipson AH, Kan AE, Kozlowski K: Geleophysic dysplasia: Acromicric dysplasia with evidence of glycoprotein storage. *Am J Med Genet Suppl* 3:181, 1987.

Santolaya JM, Groninga LC, Delgado A, et al: Patients with geleophysic dysplasia are not always geleophysic. *Am J Med Genet* 72:85, 1997.

Generalized Arterial Calcification of Infancy

At a glance: Very rare metabolic disorder characterized by deposition of calcium salts in the intima of the aorta, coronary, iliac, and carotid arteries. Coronary artery disease occurs in early infancy with heart failure and myocardial infarction. Death usually occurs before 6 months of age.

Synonyms: Idiopathic Infantile Arterial Calcification; Idiopathic Arterial Calcification in Infancy; Infantile Arterial Calcifications; Infantile Occlusive Arteriopathy; Medial Coronary Sclerosis of Infancy; Occlusive Infantile Arteriopathy.

Genetic inheritance: Autosomal recessive.

Pathophysiology: Calcification of the internal elastic lamina of arteries leading to rupture of the lamina and occlusive changes in the affected artery. Altered iron metabolism may play a role in the pathogenesis. Deficient extracellular inorganic pyrophosphate and a deficiency of plasma cell membrane glycoprotein-1 (PC-1) nucleoside triphosphate pyrophosphohydrolase activity can be associated with or is responsible for the disease.

Diagnosis: ECG changes of occlusive coronary artery disease, calcification in peripheral arteries demonstrable by ultrasound or CT scan. Periarticular calcification may be present. Prenatal ultrasound diagnosis is possible.

Clinical aspects: Respiratory difficulties and coronary artery disease occur in early infancy with heart failure and myocardial infarction. Vomiting, abdominal distension, ileus, joint swelling, and hypertension may coexist. Death usually occurs before the age of 6 months. Treatment with diphosphonate resolved the calcification in one reported case.

Precautions before anesthesia: Full assessment of cardiovascular system with ECG, echocardiography, and angiography. Treatment of hypertension and cardiac failure should be optimized. Correct anemia or any preoperative electrolyte disturbances.

Anesthetic considerations: Very poor long-term outlook. Anesthetic technique should be chosen to ensure cardiovascular stability; prevent hypertension/hypotension and maintain diastolic pressure to ensure coronary perfusion. Maintain heart rate; prevent excessive tachycardias. Prevent hypoxia and acidosis. Ensure adequate analgesia. Postoperative oxygen therapy and monitoring in an intensive care unit may be required.

Pharmacological implications: Avoid drugs that cause tachycardias or hypotension to ensure diastolic coronary perfusion is maintained.

REFERENCES:

Levine JC, Campbell J, Nadel A: Prenatal diagnosis of idiopathic infantile arterial calcification. *Circulation* 103:325, 2001.

Rutsch F, Vaingankar S, Johnson K, et al: PC-1 nucleoside triphosphate pyrophosphohydrolase deficiency in idiopathic infantile arterial calcification. *Am J Pathol* 158:543, 2001.

Genoa Syndrome

At a glance: Extremely rare syndrome with primary craniosynostosis and holoprosencephaly.

Synonyms: Camera Lituania Cohen Syndrome; Holoprosencephaly Craniosynostosis Syndrome.

Incidence and genetic inheritance: The disorder has been described in only two sisters. The parents were healthy and nonconsanguineous. Transmission seems to be autosomal recessive.

Clinical aspects: Body length and weight were below the third percentile at birth. Craniofacial signs included facial asymmetry with brachioplagiocephaly, upslanted palpebral fissures, hypertelorism, blepharophimosis, and epicanthal folds. Magnetic resonance imaging of the brain showed a semilobar type of holoprosencephaly. Primary craniosynostosis involving the coronal and lambdoid sutures was present at birth. The hands and feet were small with clinodactyly of the fifth finger. Generalized hypotonia may result at least in part from significantly reduced muscle mass. Severe growth retardation continued to be an issue in infancy, with body weight and length still below the third percentile. Reexamination at 3 years of age showed persistent skull asymmetry, slender long bones, small vertebral bodies, coxa valga, hypoplastic terminal phalanges, and cone-shaped epiphyses of the fingers. The second phalanx of both fifth fingers were hypoplastic. At 3 years of age, speech was absent, the gait was unsteady, and the electroencephalogram was normal. The second patient was diagnosed in utero, and the pregnancy was electively terminated at 21 weeks of gestation. Basically, the same morphologic findings were found in the fetus.

Anesthetic considerations: Craniosynostosis may be associated with raised intracranial pressure. Perioperative poikilothermia, convulsions, airway obstruction, and bradycardia have been described in the perioperative course of patients with holoprosencephaly and must be taken into consideration for the anesthetic management.

Other conditions to be considered: Disorders associated with holoprosencephaly.

☞**AGNATHIA-HOLOPROSENCEPHALY:** Infant presents with agnathia associated with cleft lip/palate, hypertelorism, and dysregulation of the sympathetic nervous system. The holoprosencephaly is associated with agenesis of the corpus callosum.

☞**FRYNS SYNDROME:** Very rare polymalformative syndrome characterized by diaphragmatic hernia and unusual facies. The proportion of patients who survive the neonatal period represents 14% of reported cases. Majority are stillborn or die in the early neonatal period.

☞**TRISOMY 13:** Chromosomal disorder characterized by specific midline dysmorphic features and organ malformations. Usually leads to death before the age of 6 months.

☞**TRISOMY 3P:** Duplication of the short arm of chromosome 3 with severe delay in mental development, craniofacial dysmorphism, urogenital maldevelopment, and various occasional anomalies, including cardiac defects, cleft lip/palate, holoprosencephaly, dermatoglyphic findings, and other malformations.

REFERENCE:

Camera G, Lituania M, Cohen MM: Holoprosencephaly and primary craniosynostosis: The Genoa syndrome. *Am J Med Genet* 47:1161, 1993.

Geroderma Osteodysplastica Syndrome

At a glance: Connective tissue disease resulting in early aging processes of the skin and generalized osteopenia with predisposition to fractures. Other features include joint hyperlaxity, bone fragility, muscle hypotonia, hip dislocation, sunken eyes, microcorneas, and failure to thrive.

Synonyms: Bamatter Syndrome; Bamatter-Franceschetti-Klein-Sierro Syndrome; Geroderma Osteodysplastica Hereditaria; Hereditary Geroderma Osteoplastica; Osteoplastic Geroderma; Premature Senility Syndrome; Walt Disney Dwarfism Syndrome ("Snow White and the Seven Dwarfs").

History: Familial connective tissue disorder first described in 1950 in a Swiss family by Frederic Bamatter, a Swiss pediatrician.

Incidence: Rare; approximately 50 cases reported in the literature, mainly in endogamous Mennonite religious population.

Genetic inheritance: Inheritance is X-linked recessive with occasional manifestations in females. Less severe in female heterozygotes.

Pathophysiology: Unknown. Altered activity of the activator protein-1 (AP-1) in fibroblasts may lead to relevant changes in the extracellular matrix composition, which could explain the possible correlation between some of the defects shown in these patients.

Diagnosis: Characteristic skin changes suggesting precocious aging and osseous changes, including osteoporosis and multiple lines similar to growth rings of trees. Facies shows a "droopy, jowled, prematurely aged appearance"—linked to the dwarfs in Walt Disney's "Snow White and the Seven Dwarfs"—hence the synonym. Metaphyseal pegs indenting the epiphyses of long bones may represent a primary, age-dependent (only visible at 4 to 5 years of age) alteration of bone shape which could be used as a new bone marker specific to the condition.

Clinical aspects: Premature skin aging of the face and dorsum of hands and feet is recognizable from birth. The skin appears thin and creased with reduced turgidity and elasticity, more marked over the hands and feet. Generalized joint hyperextensibility and severe osteoporosis usually are present. Intelligence is normal. Presentation with hypotonia in childhood is possible. Bones are osteoporotic and susceptible to fracture, particularly the vertebrae, which may show compression with anterior wedging and biconcavity. Dental and facial abnormalities, including maxillary hypoplasia and mandibular prognathism, have been described.

Precautions before anesthesia: No known reports in the anesthetic literature. Obtain full history of motor milestones, previous complications (especially following surgeries), and familial-related disorders. Assess potential airway difficulties because of dental, maxillary, and mandibular abnormalities.

Anesthetic considerations: Vascular access may be difficult because of laxity of the subcutaneous tissues. Careful positioning of patients is required because of osteoporotic bones (danger of fractures, particularly the vertebrae). Spontaneous breathing should be maintained until the airway has been secured.

Pharmacological implications: No known implications with this condition.

Other conditions to be considered:

DE BARSY MOENS DIERCKS SYNDROME (De Barsy Syndrome; Progeroid Syndrome of De Barsy; Corneal Clouding Cutis Laxa Mental Retardation Syndrome): Rare disorder inherited as an autosomal recessive trait. The main characteristics are degeneration of the elastic tissue in the skin (cutis laxa), involuntary movement of the arms and legs (athetosis), cloudy cornea of the eye, large prominent ears, generalized hypotonia, hyperlaxity of small joints, frontal bossing, and short stature.

☞**EHLERS-DANLOS SYNDROME:** A heterogenous group of inherited connective tissue disorders characterized by joint hyperlaxity, skin hyperextensibility and tissue fragility.

REFERENCES:
Eich GF, Steinmann B, Hodler J, et al: Metaphyseal peg in geroderma osteodysplasticum: A new genetic bone marker and a specific finding? *Am J Med Genet* 63:62, 1996.

Gherzi R, Bellini C, Bonioli E: Altered response to stimuli of the AP-1/DNA binding activity in a syndrome of precocious ageing (geroderma osteodysplastica hereditaria). *Mech Ageing Dev* 100:169, 1998.

Hunter AGW: Is geroderma osteodysplastica underdiagnosed? *J Med Genet* 25:854, 1988.

Gerstmann-Sträussler Disease

At a glance: Rare familial form of subacute spongiform encephalopathy resulting in widespread degeneration of the nervous system, usually beginning in the fourth or fifth decade of life. Special consideration must be given to potential contamination of the attending personnel, other patients, and medical materials.

Synonyms: Amyloid Dependent Subacute Spongiform Encephalopathy; Cerebellar Ataxia-Progressive Dementia Syndrome; Cerebellar Ataxia with Progressive Dementia and Amyloid Deposits in CNS; Cerebral Amyloidosis with Spongiform Encephalopathy Syndrome; Gerstmann Syndrome I; Gerstmann-Sträussler-Scheinker Disease (or Syndrome); Prion Dementia; Sträussler Disease (or Syndrome); Subacute Spongiform Encephalopathy, Gerstmann-Sträussler Type.

Incidence: Rare; incidence estimated to be 1–10:100,000,000 in the general population.

Genetic inheritance: Autosomal dominant with point mutation of the prion protein gene (20 different mutations of the human PrP gene are reported). Gene map locus is 20pter-p12.

Pathophysiology: Evidence indicates this disorder is caused by mutation in the prion protein gene (PRNP). PrPC is a normal glycoprotein that seems to have a central role in the pathogenesis of transmissible subacute spongiform encephalopathies. The isoform, which is associated with the disease, is the result of a conformational change of PrPC and designated PrPSc. Mutations in the 102nd codon of the PrP gene can produce neurodegeneration, which is the main feature of the prion diseases.

Diagnosis: Classified with other transmissible spongiform encephalopathies that represent a group of neurodegenerative diseases with lethal outcome. The differential diagnosis between Creutzfeldt-Jakob disease (CJD) and Gerstmann-Sträussler disease (GSD) has proved to be difficult because of the clinical similarities. However, it differs histologically from CJD by the presence of Kuru-type amyloid plaques and numerous multicentric, floccular plaques in the cerebral and cerebellar cortex, basal ganglia, and white matter. Whereas only 5 to 15% of CJD cases are familial, most cases of GSD are familial. In addition to spinocerebellar and corticospinal tract degeneration, extensive amyloid plaques are found throughout the CNS, and in many cases spongiform degeneration is found. An abnormal isoform of prion protein (PrP) in the brain can be detected by Western blotting and immunohistochemistry.

Clinical aspects: Characterized by cerebellar ataxia, progressive dementia, and absent reflexes in the legs. Onset is usually in the fifth decade of life. In the early phase, ataxia is predominant. Dementia develops later. Atactic symptoms, dysarthria, and personality changes characterize the clinical course of this disorder. Pyramidal, pseudobulbar, or cerebellar symptoms (usually preceding dementia), age of onset, course, and familial character of the disorder distinguish it among presenile dementias. The disease course ranges from 2 to 10 years. There is a progressive decline of physical and intellectual function until death.

Precautions before anesthesia: Prions are highly resistant to traditional disinfection and sterilization processes. Patients known to have, or suspected of having, transmissible prion diseases, such as CJD and GSD, should be managed in the hospital ward with precautionary measures similar to those used for patients with hepatitis B or acquired immune deficiency syndrome.

Anesthetic considerations: Unlike iatrogenic CJD, there have been no cases of GSD as a result of iatrogenic spread. Disposable items should be used and then incinerated. Personnel should use gloves, masks, and eye protection. The laryngoscope can be sterilized by immersion in a 5% sodium hypochlorite solution for 1 hour. Surgery in these patients should be performed at the end of the operating list to allow for thorough cleaning and disinfection of equipment and operating room. General anesthesia may precipitate mental decline; regional block procedures are preferable when applicable.

Pharmacological implications: Benzodiazepines may worsen memory tests in the elderly. Anesthesia with isoflurane may induce more vegetative symptoms than will propofol.

Other conditions to be considered:

☞CREUTZFELDT-JAKOB DISEASE: Characterized by the loss of facial expression, diminished visual activity, supranuclear gaze paralysis, gait ataxia, extrapyramidal muscular rigidity, myoclonus, and dementia. The cerebrospinal fluid examination is normal, but occasionally protein content is slightly elevated. The three forms of CJD are determined by the mode of transmission: infectious (prion contamination), sporadic, and inherited (autosomal dominant). Fifteen percent of cases are familial, and most are sporadic. Neuropathology includes spongiform changes, diffuse nerve cell degeneration, and glial proliferation. Characteristic periodic EEG complexes.

KURU DISEASE: Largely restricted to the Fore linguistic group of the Papua New Guinea Highlands. This medical entity is a neurodegenerative disorder caused by a "slow virus." Whether significant genetic factors are also involved is uncertain. "Scrapie" is a chronic neurologic disease of sheep also believed to be caused by a "slow virus"; however, genetic factors may also be involved. In Kuru disease, the virus is transmitted during endocannibalistic feasts. Heterozygosity for a common polymorphism in the human prion protein gene may confer relative resistance to prion diseases. Elderly survivors of the kuru epidemic, who had multiple exposures to cannibalistic feasts, are, in marked contrast to younger unexposed Fore, predominantly PRNP 129 heterozygotes. Evidence suggests that cannibalism was widespread in many prehistoric populations and may have provided the setting for selection pressure as protection against prion disease.

FATAL FAMILIAL INSOMNIA: Characterized by progressive insomnia and dysautonomia (pyrexia, diaphoresis, myosis, sphincter disturbances), diplopia, dysarthria, tremor, myoclonus, ataxia, dementia, and dreamlike status leading to coma and death within 1 year. It is a neurodegenerative disorder with reactive astrocytosis limited to the anterior and dorsomedial thalamic nuclei and without spongiosis or vascular or inflammatory changes. Inheritance is autosomal dominant.

REFERENCES:

Collins S, McLean CA, Masters CL: Gerstmann-Sträussler-Scheinker syndrome, fatal familial insomnia, and kuru: A review of these less common human transmissible spongiform encephalopathies. *J Clin Neurosci* 8:387, 2001.

Hernandez-Palazon J, Martinez-Lage JF, Tortosa JA, et al: Anaesthetic management in patients suspected of, or at risk of having Creutzfeldt-Jakob disease. *Br J Anaesth* 80:516, 1998.

Hsiao K, Baker HF, Crow TJ, et al: Linkage of a prion protein missense variant to Gerstmann-Sträussler syndrome. *Nature* 338:342, 1989.

Gianotti-Crosti Syndrome

At a glance: Childhood exanthem with a characteristic distribution. Cases often are associated with viral infections. Systemic features are rare.

Synonyms: Acrodermatitis Papulosa Infantum; Gianotti Disease.

History: First case was described by C. Gianotti, an Italian pediatrician, in 1955. All originally described patients were affected with hepatitis B virus infection (although nowadays other viral infections account for the majority of cases).

Incidence: Affects children of both sexes, 80% of patients are between 2 and 6 years of age. Well known in Italy, where more than 300 cases were examined between 1955 and 1990. Worldwide distribution of the disease.

Genetic inheritance: None, although the incidence is higher in children with Down syndrome.

Pathophysiology: Specific and self-limited response to cutaneous or mucosal contamination, opposite to the classic parenteral contamination. The disorder seems related to the presence of immune complexes in the vascular wall. Existence of immune cellular deficiency can explain the higher incidence of the disease in children with trisomy 21.

Diagnosis: Based on the clinical dermatological findings associated with a viral or streptococcal infection.

Clinical aspects: Historically, hepatitis B surface antigen-positive (HBsAg-positive) papular acrodermatitis of childhood (named Gianotti Disease) was first described and distinguished from HBsAg-negative papulovesicular, acral syndrome (called Gianotti-Crosti Syndrome), which was reported after contamination with different infectious agents (Ebstein-Barr virus, Coxsackie virus, Cytomegalovirus, Herpes virus 6, HIV, human Parvovirus B19). The affected children present with sometimes asymmetric, papulous or papulovesiculous, asymptomatic skin eruptions of up to 1 cm in diameter that usually develop over 3 to 4 days, starting on the thighs or the buttocks and later spreading to the extensor surfaces of the extremities, and finally the face. The trunk is usually spared. Typically, these eruptions last at least 10 to 14 days, however in more than half of the patients the course is longer than 6 weeks. Secondary to leakage of blood from the capillaries, these lesions may turn into purple spots later in the course of the disease. Fluid-filled blisters may also occur. Pruritus is present only in about one quarter of the children and is particularly uncommon in patients where hepatitis B is responsible for the skin lesions. Other symptoms are mainly related to the underlying viral illness and may include malaise, a low-grade fever and other flulike symptoms. The classic form associated with hepatitis B (HB$_s$Ag-positive) typically presents with an acute, nonicteric hepatitis.

Precautions before anesthesia: Assess liver function (e.g., transaminases, coagulation) and the degree of cytolysis in patients with underlying hepatitis. Exclude fever and respiratory tract infections. A complete blood count is recommended to assess transient lymphoblastosis, lymphocytosis, and thrombocytopenia.

Anesthetic considerations: Take the usual precautions for patients with hepatitis B.

Pharmacological implications: Agents undergoing hepatic metabolism probably should be avoided.

REFERENCES:

Caputo R, Gelmetti C, Ermacora E: Gianotti-Crosti syndrome: A retrospective analysis of 308 cases. *J Am Acad Dermatol* 26:207, 1992.

Chuh AA, Chan HH, Chiu SS, et al: A prospective case control study of the association of Gianotti-Crosti syndrome with human herpesvirus 6 and human herpesvirus 7 infections. *Pediatr Dermatol* 19:492, 2002.

Gilbert Syndrome

At a glance: Benign inherited disorder characterized by chronic intermittent jaundice (unconjugated hyperbilirubinemia) that does not lead to particular complications and is not a progressive disorder (normal life expectancy; may even prolong life by preventing heart attacks).

Synonyms: Constitutional Hepatic (or Liver) Dysfunction; Familial Cholemia; Familial Nonhemolytic Jaundice; Hyperbilirubinemia I; Icterus Intermittens Juvenilis; Gilbert-Lereboullet Syndrome; Gilbert-Meulengracht Syndrome; Low-Grade Chronic Hyperbilirubinemia; Meulengracht Disease; Unconjugated Benign Bilirubinemia.

History: Gilbert syndrome was first described in 1900 by Nicolas Augustin Gilbert, a French gastroenterologist.

Incidence: Affects 5 to 7% of the population; male-to-female ratio is 2–7:1.

Genetic inheritance: Transmission is autosomal recessive. Mutation was identified as affecting the promoter gene of the enzyme UDP-glucuronosyltransferase, whereas the gene coding for the protein itself is normal. Prevalence of the mutation is 40%, but only 16% are homozygous. Most homozygous patients have normal levels of bilirubin.

Pathophysiology: Reduced hepatic UDP-glucuronosyltransferase (30%) activity toward bilirubin is observed in all cases. Some patients also have defective hepatic uptake of bilirubin and other organic anions from serum, resulting in a chronic, nonhemolytic, intermittent, unconjugated hyperbilirubinemia.

Diagnosis: Unconjugated hyperbilirubinemia without overt hemolysis is suspicious for the diagnosis. Serum transaminases, phosphatases, bile salt concentration, hepatic function, and liver biopsy are normal. Elevation of unconjugated bilirubinemia often occurs after reduced caloric intake.

Clinical aspects: Gilbert syndrome appears often by 10 to 12 years of age. The patient is frequently asymptomatic or has intermittent nonhemolytic jaundice. Fatigue and abdominal discomfort are frequent complaints that can lead to multiple diagnostic investigations and even exploratory laparotomy. The syndrome can be associated with perioperative jaundice in children with malnutrition and in those who received halothane or morphine. Clinical signs are increased by fasting or infections and decreased by phenobarbital treatment.

Precautions before anesthesia: Obtain full history of familial-related disorders. Blood work should include a CBC (to exclude hemolytic anemia) and assessment of liver function. Avoid unconjugated hyperbilirubinemia by close followup on preoperative fasting.

Anesthetic considerations: Regional anesthesia can be used. Phenobarbital induces hepatic microsomal enzyme activation and reduces bilirubin levels; however, the anesthesiologist should be aware of the implications of enzyme induction with regard to anesthetic drugs in patients receiving phenobarbital therapy. The halogenated agents halothane and enflurane should be avoided because they both decrease hepatic blood flow; isoflurane and sevoflurane appear to be acceptable agents. Concerning muscle relaxants, drugs eliminated by the Hoffmann elimination pathway (atracurium, *cis*-atracurium) or by esterases (succinylcholine, mivacurium) should be preferred. Narcotics are metabolized in the liver, and prolonged effects of morphine have been reported in patients with the disorder.

Pharmacological implications: Inhalational anesthetics of choice are desflurane, sevoflurane or isoflurane. Muscle relaxants such as *cis*-atracurium, mivacurium or succinylcholine should be preferred. Propofol and thiopental are equally suited for induction of anesthesia. Despite the enzyme defect, opioids can be safely used in regular doses, although prolonged effects have been described. Remifentanil can be used without any specific adverse effects. Patients with Gilbert Syndrome are heterogeneous in terms of acetaminophen/paracetamol metabolism and a subgroup of them may exhibit a higher sensitivity to liver damage.

Other condition to be considered:

☞**CRIGLER-NAJJAR SYNDROME:** Familial form of inherited error of bilirubin metabolism leading to hyperbilirubinemia and severe central nervous system disorder (degeneration of the basal ganglia). Caused by an enzyme deficiency in the liver in which bilirubin cannot be converted into water-soluble bilirubin glucuronide because of a defect in glucuronyl transferase.

REFERENCES:

Green DW, Fisher M, Sockalingham I: Mivacurium compared with succinylcholine in children with liver disease. *Br J Anaesth* 81:463, 1998.

Mendoza-Hernandez JL, Garcia-Paredes I, Larrubia-Marfil JR: Diagnosis of Gilbert syndrome: Current status of the fasting test. *An Med Interna* 14:2:57, 1997.

Vitek L, Jirsa M, Brodanova M, et al: Gilbert syndrome and ischemic heart disease: A protective effect of elevated bilirubin levels. *Atherosclerosis* 160:449, 2002.

Gilles De La Tourette Syndrome

At a glance: Neurologic syndrome characterized by repeated and involuntary, stereotype motor movement or vocalization (tics).

Synonyms: Tourette Syndrome; Brissaud Syndrome; Maladie des Tics; Tic Impulsif; Chronic Motor Tics.

History: Georges Albert Édouard Brutus Gilles de la Tourette was a French neurologist (1857–1904) who described this rare psychoneurologic disorder with onset in childhood, usually at 7 to 10 years of age, characterized by echolalia, palilalia and coprolalia, stuttering and a craving to touch. Gilles de la Tourette became Doctor in Paris in 1879.

Incidence: Common; estimates range from 0.05 to 1% in the general population. Up to 20% of schoolchildren may have a transient tic disorder at some point.

Genetic inheritance: Controversial; probably autosomal dominant with incomplete penetrance and variable expression. Environmental factors seem to influence the risk, severity, and course of the disorder.

Pathophysiology: Postulated to be a result of dopamine excess or supersensitivity of the postsynaptic dopamine receptors in the basal ganglia and frontal cortex. Another hypothesis is a neurophysiologic deficit secondary to neurotransmitter abnormalities, resulting in failed inhibition of frontal-subcortical motor circuits.

Diagnosis: Diagnostic criteria for Gilles de la Tourette syndrome recommended by the American Psychiatric Association include both multiple motor and vocal tics over a period of more than 1 year, voluntary suppression of symptoms, a waxing and waning course, and onset between 2 and 15 years of age.

Clinical aspects: Initial symptoms usually are involuntary, tic-like movements. The disorder progresses with development of echolalia (repeating another's words or phrases), grunting, and coprolalia (use of obscene words). Most cases are mild and do not come to medical attention. Waxing and waning course, with one tic appearing and typically being replaced by another. Long-term outcome is generally favorable. Commonly associated with attention deficit hyperactivity disorder, obsessive-compulsive disorder, behavior problems, and learning disabilities. Management includes behavior or pharmacologic therapies (neuroleptic medications and dopamine D_2 antagonist agents).

Precautions before anesthesia: Tics should be differentiated from other movement disorders, such as chorea, stereotypy, and dystonia. Urine drug screening for cocaine and stimulants should be considered in a teenager with sudden onset of tics and inappropriate behavior symptoms. Every patient with a family history of liver disease associated with hyperkinetic movement disorder should be investigated to rule out ☞Wilson disease (hepatolenticular degeneration). Details of current drug therapy are essential to prevent unwanted drug interactions.

Anesthetic considerations: Anxiety, stress, and fatigue often intensify tics. Behavioral disorders may limit cooperation during induction and emergence.

Pharmacological implications: Psychoactive drugs, particularly cocaine and other stimulants, have a tendency to worsen tics. Drug interactions may arise from existing pharmacologic therapy: neuroleptic agents (haloperidol), atypical neuroleptic agents (risperidone), α_2-adrenergic presynaptic agonists (clonidine), benzodiazepines (clonazepam), and CNS stimulants (pemoline, used for attention deficit hyperactivity disorder). Benzodiazepines may result in hypnotic synergism on induction of anesthesia, and a lower dose of induction agent may be required. Recovery may be delayed. Pemoline-sevoflurane interaction reportedly may cause severe intraoperative hypotension.

Other condition to be considered:

☞**JUMPING FRENCHMAN OF MAINE SYNDROME:** Neurologic disease characterized by exaggerated startle reflexes produced by the slightest stimulus, echolalia, and echopraxia.

REFERENCES:

American Psychiatric Association. *Diagnostic and Statistical Manual,* fourth edition text revision (DSM-IVTR). Washington DC: American Psychiatric Association Press, 2000, p 108.

Bagheri MM, Kerbeshian JK, Burd L: Recognition and management of Tourette's syndrome and tic disorders. *Am Fam Physician* 59:2263, 1999.

Leckman JF: Tourette's syndrome. *Lancet* 360:1577, 2002.

Gillespie Syndrome

At a glance: Inherited polymalformative, nonprogressive disorder characterized by aniridia, mental deficiency, cerebellar ataxia, and gross incoordination. Characteristic appearance of the eyes in the first month is crucial in making the diagnosis.

Synonyms: Aniridia-Cerebellar Ataxia-Mental Retardation Syndrome; Aniridia, Partial-Cerebellar Ataxia-Oligophrenia; Gillespie Syndrome II. [*NB:* Avoid confusing Gillespie syndrome II with Gillespie Syndrome I, which is more commonly referred to as ☞Oculo-Dento-Digital (ODD) Syndrome (also Meyer-Schwickerath-Weyers Syndrome, or Weyers Syndrome III)].

Incidence: 1:61,000 newborns in the United States, 1:96,000 live births worldwide. No racial or sex predilection.

Genetic inheritance: Typically transmitted as an autosomal recessive trait, but one case report suggests autosomal dominant transmission (from mother to daughter).

Pathophysiology: Unknown. No mutation in the *PAX6* gene on chromosome 11, which usually is responsible for familial aniridia. No development of Wilms tumor as in ☞WAGR syndrome [Wilms tumor, aniridia, genitourinary abnormalities, and mental retardation] or ☞Monosomy 11p, another inherited disorder with aniridia.

Diagnosis: Diagnosis rests on the presence of partial or complete aniridia, cerebellar ataxia, and mental retardation. Common presentation is fixed and dilated pupils in a hypotonic infant.

Clinical aspects: Neurologic involvement can be demonstrated by white matter loss on MRI and is manifested as severe motor delay, hypotonia, disabling ataxia, and mental retardation. There may be fusion of cervical vertebrae with neck rigidity. Congenital pulmonary stenosis may be present.

Precautions before anesthesia: Thorough assessment of mental state and neurologic state is necessary. Assessment must be made regarding airway and neck manipulation. Cervical vertebral fusion may result in difficulties instrumenting and maintaining the airway. Obtain a cardiac ultrasound in the presence of a heart murmur.

Anesthetic considerations: In the presence of even moderate mental retardation, regional anesthetic techniques will be challenging. Difficulties in endotracheal intubation may make these patients significant challenges to the anesthetist. Thorough preoperative assessment of motor function enhances monitoring of recovery from anesthesia.

Pharmacological implications: No specific implications or contraindications to specific anesthetic agents. Subacute bacterial endocarditis prophylaxis may be required in the presence of pulmonary stenosis.

Other conditions to be considered:

OTHER SYNDROMES ASSOCIATED WITH ANIRIDIA: ☞Aniridia type I (AN 1); Aniridia type II (AN 2); ☞WAGR syndrome.

☞**Marinesco-Sjögren Syndrome:** Cataracts, cerebellar ataxia, mental retardation, muscle weakness, short stature, and hypergonadotropic hypogonadism. Autosomal recessive.

References:

Kieslich M, Vanselow K, Wildhardt G, et al.: [Present limitations of molecular biological diagnostics in Gillespie syndrome] *Klin Pädiatr* 213;47, 2001.

Nelson J, Flaherty M, Grattan-Smith P: Gillespie syndrome: A report of two further cases. *Am J Med Genet* 71:134, 1997.

Gitelman Syndrome

At a glance: Inherited renal tubular defect resulting in urinary loss of magnesium, sodium, potassium, and chloride with otherwise normal kidneys.

Synonym: Primary Renotubular Hypomagnesemia-Hypokalemia with Hypocalciuria.

Genetic inheritance: Autosomal recessive; caused by mutation in the thiazide-sensitive sodium-chloride cotransporter gene (*SLC12A3* gene). More than 100 different mutations distributed throughout the whole protein have been reported. Gene locus is 16q13.

Pathophysiology: Alteration of the thiazide-sensitive sodium chloride transporter impairs sodium and chloride reabsorption and stimulates renin and aldosterone secretion, resulting in hypokalemia and metabolic alkalosis. Reasons for renal magnesium wasting are unknown.

Diagnosis: Made by biochemical changes (alkalosis, hypokalemia, hypomagnesemia, hypocalciuria). Although some features overlap with ☞Bartter syndrome, in contrast to Bartter syndrome, Gitelman syndrome patients present later in life with hypomagnesemia, high fractional excretion of magnesium, and low calcium excretion, but no overt hypovolemia.

Clinical aspects: Late childhood presentation with hypokalemic metabolic alkalosis and hypomagnesemia. Either asymptomatic or occasional mild episodes of muscle weakness. Symptoms are precipitated by nonspecific illness and may consist of tetany. Patients are neither polyuric nor polydipsic, but they have hypocalciuria, renal magnesium wasting, and absence of nephrocalcinosis. Chronic dermatitis, skeletal problems with growth retardation (as a consequence of rickets), and chondrocalcinosis; rarely rhabdomyolysis (secondary to severe hypokalemia) can be observed in some patients. Long-term prognosis is rather good, especially when potassium losses are corrected. Treatment with oral magnesium corrects the magnesium deficit but not the metabolic alkalosis. The relationship of these skeletal abnormalities to magnesium wasting and hypomagnesemia is not clear.

Precautions before anesthesia: Obtain history of frequency and severity of tetany and muscle weakness as an indicator of disease severity. Obtain electrolyte levels (potassium, magnesium, calcium) and arterial blood gas analysis. Correct electrolyte abnormalities preoperatively.

Anesthetic considerations: The catecholamine stress response associated with direct laryngoscopy and tracheal intubation further exacerbates hypokalemia (intracellular entry). The arrhythmogenic potential of hypokalemia is thought to result from electrical inhomogeneity, alterations in conduction, changes in automaticity, and disturbances in sodium pump kinetics. Hypomagnesemia favors atrial dysrhythmias. Use of a nerve stimulator is mandatory if general anesthesia with muscle relaxants is considered. Postanesthetic care should be in a high-dependency area for 24 to 48 hours or until the patient is stable with normal potassium and magnesium levels. Should cardiac dysrhythmias occur, determination of serum potassium, calcium, and magnesium concentrations are essential in guiding the therapy.

Pharmacological implications: Muscle relaxants (preferably atracurium or *cis*-atracurium) can be used (under the monitoring of peripheral nerve stimulator). Use of catecholamines and other vasoactive drugs may exacerbate preexisting hypokalemia because of the intracellular shift of potassium. Careful administration of glucose-based intravenous solution may contribute to exaggeration of the hypokalemia.

Other conditions to be considered:

☞**Bartter Syndrome:** Family of disorders characterized by hypokalemic, hypochloremic, hypomagnesemic variants with hypocalciuria, metabolic alkalosis, and normotensive hyperreninemic hyperaldosteronism linked to the gene encoding the thiazide-sensitive Na/Cl-cotransporter (TSC). The responsible gene here is located on chromosome 1p 36.

☞**Gullner Syndrome:** Findings differ from those of Bartter syndrome in which hyperaldosteronism and juxtaglomerular hyperplasia are important features and sodium conservation occurs. It is associated with hyperreninemia, high urinary prostaglandin E_2, normal blood pressure, and resistance of blood pressure to the pressor effect of angiotensin II. Hypokalemia is corrected by magnesium repletion. Abnormal magnesium metabolism may be responsible for the hypokalemia in this syndrome. Magnesium treatment does not affect renin levels but causes an increase in plasma aldosterone concentration in both the supine and upright positions.

☞**Liddle Syndrome:** Autosomal dominant disorder characterized by early, and frequently severe, hypertension associated with hypokalemic metabolic alkalosis, low plasma renin activity, and suppressed aldosterone secretion, another disorder with hypokalemia. It is differentiated from the Gitelman syndrome, Gullner syndrome, and Bartter syndrome by the presence of hypertension.

☞**De Toni Debré Fanconi Syndrome:** Rare acquired or inherited condition involving a generalized transport defect in the proximal tubules with renal losses of glucose, phosphate, calcium, uric acid, amino acids, and bicarbonates leading to short stature, osteomalacia, and renal failure.

☞**Periodic Paralysis:** Congenital abnormality in membrane electrolyte conductance leading to episodic muscle weakness.

☞**Lightwood Syndrome:** Nonhereditary form of primary tubular acidosis presenting with hypercalcemia, hypercalciuria, and nephrocalcinosis.

☞**Albright Butler Syndrome:** Patients present with renal tubular acidosis, nephrocalcinosis, and renal failure. Hypokalemia with muscle weakness and periodic paralysis is frequent. Polyuria, vomiting, and dehydration lead to fluid and electrolyte imbalances.

☞**Adenosine Deaminase Deficiency:** Heterogeneous systemic disorder caused by the deficiency of adenosine deaminase resulting primarily in severe combined (cellular and humoral) immunodeficiency but also systemic abnormalities.

☞**Lowe Syndrome:** Genetically transmitted polymalformative syndrome characterized by the association of ocular problems with renal dysfunction and mental retardation.

☞**Phosphoenolpyruvate Carboxykinase Deficiency:** Congenital metabolic disease leading to a defect in gluconeogenesis.

☞**Propionic Acidemia:** Inborn error of metabolism affecting the mitochondrial catabolism of valine and isoleucine that, left untreated, results in ketoacidosis, lethargy, coma, and finally death.

☞**PYRUVATE CARBOXYLASE DEFICIENCY:** Mitochondrial disease impairing synthetic pathways, leading to hypoglycemia and severe lactic acidosis.

☞**TYROSINEMIA:** Elevated blood tyrosine levels are present in several clinical entities. The term *tyrosinemia* is used to describe several syndromes. In general, the association of liver and renal failure, marked edema, epistaxis, and distinctive cabbage-like odor are characteristic of the disease.

REFERENCES:

Ring T, Knoers N, Oh MS, et al: Reevaluation of the criteria for the clinical diagnosis of Gitelman syndrome. *Pediatr Nephrol* 17:612, 2002.

Shaer AJ: Inherited primary renal tubular hypokalemic alkalosis: A review of Gitelman and Bartter syndromes. *Am J Med Sci* 322:316, 2001.

Zelikovic I, Szargel R, Hawash A, et al: A novel mutation in the chloride channel gene, CLCNKB as a cause of Gitelman and Bartter syndromes. *Kidney Int* 63:24, 2003.

Glanzmann Thrombasthenia

At a glance: Genetic platelet disorder resulting in blood clotting disorder and hemorrhage. Life-threatening condition under stress (e.g., surgery, anesthesia).

Synonyms: Athrombocytopenic Purpura; Congenital Hemorrhagic Thrombocytic Dystrophy; Glanzmann Syndrome; Glanzmann-Nägeli Syndrome; Glycoprotein IIb (GPIIb/III) Complex Deficiency; Hemorrhagic Thrombasthenia; Hereditary Thrombasthenia; Hereditary Thrombocytopenic Purpura; Nägeli Syndrome II; Platelet Fibrinogen Receptor Deficiency; Platelet Glycoprotein IIb/III Deficiency; Révol Syndrome; Thrombasthenia; Thrombocytasthenia; Thrombocytopathic Purpura.

History: Eduard Glanzmann (1887–1959) was a Swiss pediatrician, Otto Nägeli (1871–1938) was a Swiss hematologist.

Incidence: Rare. Approximately 200 cases reported.

Genetic inheritance: Autosomal recessive disorder in one of two genes of chromosome 17, either GPIIb (or integrin αIIb) or GPIIa (or integrin αIIbβ3), where GP indicates glycoprotein. Genetic mutations split equally between GPIIb and GPIIIa. Some cases are suspected to be transmitted as an autosomal dominant trait.

Pathophysiology: In platelets, GPIIb and GPIIIa are joined together as a dimer (referred to as GPIIb/IIIa). Once activated, GPIIb/IIIa binds to one end of fibrinogen (and/or von Willebrand factor), while another platelet, with its own GPIIb/IIIa, can bind to the other extremity of the fibrinogen, thus leading to a large aggregation of bound platelets (so-called white blood clot). In patients with Glanzmann thrombasthenia, GPIIb/IIIa is defective and platelets cannot aggregate; no blood clot is formed and bleeding does not stop.

Diagnosis: Normal to increased platelet count, giant platelets, absent platelet surface thrombosthenin, prolonged bleeding time, poor clot retraction, and absent platelet aggregation. Adenosine diphosphate-induced platelet aggregation does not occur.

Clinical aspects: Bleeding diathesis, petechiae, anemia. Two forms described: type I (severely affected patients, especially girls at time of menarche) and type II (mild form).

Precautions before anesthesia: Check CBC. Ensure platelet availability. Check for platelet antibodies.

Anesthetic considerations: Avoid central neuraxial anesthetics. Anticipate need for platelet transfusion. Platelet transfusions must be restricted to serious bleeding because antibodies against platelets can develop (and would compromise the vital prognosis in case of further bleeding). Postoperative bleeding may be severe. Perioperative treatment with recombinant FVIIa supplements has proven to be safe and efficient.

Pharmacological implications: Avoid use of antiplatelet drugs such as acetylsalicylic acid.

Other conditions to be considered:

☞**BERNARD-SOULIER SYNDROME:** Autosomal recessive bleeding disorder with low platelet count and bleeding out of proportion to the reduced platelet count.

☞**WISKOTT-ALDRICH SYNDROME:** X-linked recessive disorder with altered platelets, bleeding disorder, and susceptibility to infections as a consequence of B- and T-cell immunodeficiencies.

REFERENCES:

Marchant W, Mallet S: Platelet function assessment in Glanzmann's thrombasthenia. *Br J Anaesth* 89:525, 2002.

Poon MC, D'Oiron R, von Depka M, et al: Prophylactic and therapeutic recombinant factor VIIa administration to patients with Glanzmann's thrombasthenia: results of an international survey. *J Thromb Haemost* 2;1096, 2004.

Tomiyama Y: Glanzmann thrombasthenia: Integrin alpha IIb beta 3 deficiency. *Int J Hematol* 72:448, 2000.

Glucose-6-Phosphate Dehydrogenase Deficiency

At a glance: Most common human enzyme deficiency in the world. Clinically characterized by an acute red cell hemolysis resulting from intake of oxidative agents. Glucose-6-phosphate dehydrogenase (G6PD)-deficient individuals are more resistant to *Plasmodium falciparum* (malaria-causing parasite).

Synonyms: Baghdad Anemia; Broad Bean Syndrome; Favism (usually in persons of Mediterranean area descent).

Nature: Genetic enzyme deficiency (>400 variant alleles, or different forms of the same gene). Favism has been known to exist since antiquity; Pythagoras had warned his disciples against the dangers of eating fava beans.

Incidence: Most of the affected individuals reside in Africa, the Middle East, tropical, subtropical Asia, some areas of the Mediterranean, Papua New Guinea, and Southeast Asia (areas where malaria is common); 100 million people worldwide are believed to be affected.

Genetic inheritance: X-linked (thus predominantly a male syndrome). Most of the variants arise from a single point mutation (amino acid substitution) in the structural gene encoding for G6PD, which is located at the Xq28 region on the tip of the long arm of the X chromosome.

Pathophysiology: G6PD catalyzes the first step in the hexose monophosphate pathway, producing nicotinamide adenine dinucleotide phosphate (NADPH). This pathway is the only source of NADPH in the erythrocyte. NADPH is required to reduce oxidized glutathione. Reduced glutathione is the substrate for peroxide removal from the red blood cells. When G6PD-deficient patients are given drugs that form peroxides in contact with oxyhemoglobin, the lack of glutathione peroxide removal leads to hemolysis and formation of Heinz bodies. There exist at least five variants of this syndrome: the rare class 1, or hereditary nonspherocytic hemolytic anemia (associated with chronic hemolysis); class 2, or severe deficiency (<10%); class 3, or moderate-to-mild deficiency; class 4, or very mild-to-no enzyme deficiency (60%); and class 5, an increase in enzyme activity. The degree of hemolysis also may be related to other non–G6PD-related issues, such as acetylator status (i.e., a rapid acetylator will metabolize drug quicker than a slow or nonacetylator, and the lack of drug accumulation prevents hemolysis).

Diagnosis: A variety of laboratory tests are available for patients who have not hemolyzed, including the dye reduction test and the fluorescent spot test. Oxidant stress causes hemoglobin denaturation and the formation of Heinz bodies. For patients who have hemolyzed, the most powerful diagnostic technique is genomic DNA analysis.

Clinical aspects: *Class 1:* Chronic hemolysis without exposure to "classic" trigger agents (Table G-1), often beginning at birth (neonatal jaundice potentially leading to kernicterus). *Classes 2* and *3 :* Variable degrees of hemolysis, depending on pharmacologic exposure. Hemolysis usually occurs 1 to 2 days after drug exposure and may be associated with back pain and dark urine. Numerous bacterial, viral, and rickettsial infections have been reported as precipitants.

Precautions before anesthesia: Evaluate for anemia and chronic hemolysis (bilirubin, red blood cell and reticulocyte count).

Anesthetic considerations: Avoid triggering agents.

Pharmacological implications: All known antimalarial drugs are contraindicated for G6PD-deficient individuals. (See also Tables G-1 and G-2.)

Other conditions to be considered:

☞**HEREDITARY SPHEROCYTOSIS:** Autosomal dominant (occasionally recessive) mild hemolytic anemia in people of Mediterranean descent; caused by spectrin deficiency; no acute hemolytic episodes after drug intake.

Table G-1   Drugs to Avoid in All Class 1 Variant Patients

Acetaminophen	Phenylbutazone
Acetophenetidin	Phenytoin
Acetylsalicylic acid	Probenecid
Actazoline	Procainamide hydrochloride
Aminopyrine	Pyrimethamine
Antipyrine	Quinine
Ascorbic acid	Quinidine
Benzhexol	Streptomycin
Chloramphenicol	Sulfacytine
Chlorguanidine	Sulfadiazine
Chloroquine	Sulfaguanidine
Colchicine	Sulfamerazine
Diphenylhydramine	Sulfamethoxypyridazine
Isoniazid	Sulfisoxazole
L-Dopa	Tiaprofenic acid
Menadione sodium	Trimethoprim
bisulfite	Tripelennamine
Menaphthone	Vitamin K
p-Aminobenzoic acid	

Table G-2   Drugs to Avoid in All G6PD-Deficient Patients

Acetanilid	Nitrofurantoin	Sulfanilamide
Furazolidone	Phenazopyridine	Sulfapyridine
Isobutyl nitrite	Phenylhydrazine	Thiazolsulfone
Methylene blue	Primaquine	Toluidine blue
Nalidixic acid	Sulfacetamide	Trinitrotoluene
Naphthalene	Sulfamethoxazole	Urate oxidase
Niridazole		

HOMOZYGOUS BETA THALASSEMIA MAJOR (☞THALASSEMIA): Severe autosomal recessive hemoglobinopathy characterized by an abnormal rate of synthesis of the hemoglobin chains resulting in faulty erythropoiesis with severe anemia, bone marrow hyperplasia, and hepatosplenomegaly; death often occurs before puberty.

☞**SICKLE CELL ANEMIA:** Severe autosomal recessive hemoglobinopathy caused by an alteration of the two beta chains in which a valine amino acid is substituted for glutamic acid, resulting in sudden change of the shape of the molecule of hemoglobin under certain conditions (low oxygen concentration, dehydration) resulting in acute hemolysis and thrombosis (vasoocclusive episodes in many organs) termed "sickle cell crisis".

REFERENCES:
Beutler E: Glucose-6-phosphate-dehydrogenase deficiency. *Blood* 84:3613, 1994.

Kwok CJ, Martin AC, Au SW, et al: G6PDdb, an integrated database of glucose-6-phosphate dehydrogenase (G6PD) mutations. *Hum Mutat* 19:217, 2002.

Martin LD, Casella ES: Anesthesia and glucose-6-phosphate dehydrogenase deficiency in a child with congenital heart disease. *J Cardiothorac Vasc Anesth* 5:596, 1991.

Glucose Phosphate Isomerase Deficiency

At a glance: Autosomal recessive disease caused by a deficiency in the enzyme glucose phosphate isomerase and clinically characterized by nonspherotic hemolytic anemia and spontaneous hemolytic crises.

Synonyms: Glucose Phosphate Isomerase Deficiency; Phosphohexose Isomerase Deficiency; Autocrine Motility Factor Deficiency.

Incidence: Glucose Phosphate Isomerase deficiency is the third most common enzymopathy (after Glucose-6-Phosphate Dehydrogenase Deficiency and Pyruvate Kinase Deficiency) that results in hemolysis.

Genetic inheritance: This autosomal dominant disorder (19cen-q12) is most symptomatic in cases presenting homozygous or compound heterozygous pattern.

Pathophysiology: The enzyme glucose phosphate isomerase catalyzes the interconversion of the second step of the Embden-Myerhof (glucose metabolism) pathway into fructose-6-phosphate. This enzyme is known as the rate-limiting factor in the mitochondrial energy pathway.

Clinical aspects: Patients present with nonspherocytic hemolytic anemia, most often as spontaneously occuring crises. Jaundice, splenomegaly, and cholecystitis are often associated. Muscle weakness is reported. The cardiovascular system is not affected. Neurologically, the presence of mental retardation and mixed sensory and cerebellar ataxia is noted.

Anesthetic considerations: Preoperatively, a complete laboratory assessment should be conducted to confirm the presence of phosphohexose isomerase deficiency (essential to the risk of spontaneous hemolytic crises) and evaluate the level of red cell osmotic fragility. The patient's hematocrit should be obtained. The presence of reduced leukocyte superoxide anion production should raise the concern of infection because of reduced leukocyte bactericidal activity. Patients appear to respond positively to splenectomy.

Other conditions to be considered:

CHRONIC HEXOKINASE DEFICIENCY HEMOLYTIC ANEMIA: Autosomal recessive inherited disease characterized by chronic hemolytic anemia associated with severe deficiency of red cell glucose phosphate isomerase. Some cases of autosomal dominant transmission have been reported. Like phosphofructokinase and pyruvate kinase, the hexokinase enzyme is a rate-limiting factor in the metabolism of glucose in the Embden-Meyerhof pathway. Because glycolysis is the only source of energy for the red cells, deficiency in hexokinase results in chronic hemolytic anemia. Few allelic variants have been described of the chronic form. *Fukuoka variant:* Reported in the Japanese literature as the association of chronic glucose phosphate deficiency and a history of prolonged neonatal jaundice. *Iwate variant:* Chronic form of hemolytic anemia most often homozygous in pattern and detected early in life. *Homburg variant:* Association of chronic hemolytic anemia and neurologic deficits.

☞**PYRUVATE KINASE DEFICIENCY:** Blood disorder characterized by a deficiency of the enzyme pyruvate kinase. Physical findings include hemolytic anemia, hyperbilirubinemia, splenomegaly, and/or other abnormalities. Inherited as an autosomal recessive genetic trait.

TRIOSE PHOSPHATE ISOMERASE DEFICIENCY: Inherited autosomal dominant disease presents with several alleles. Triose phosphate isomerase catalyzes the interconversion of dihydroxyacetone phosphate and glyceraldehyde-3-phosphate (Embden-Meyerhof glycolytic pathway). Clinically, the entity is characterized by moderate hemolytic anemia (nonspherocytic; called Dacie type II), cardiac failure, and sudden cardiac arrest most probably related to dysrhythmias, developmental retardation, severe myopathy and hypotonia, jaundice, splenomegaly, cholelithiasis, and recurrent systemic infection. Patients may have normal intelligence. The spasticity is the result of a neurologic degenerative process involving the lower motor neurons and manifests as pyramidal tract signs, tremor, dystonia, and dyskinesia. Anesthetic considerations should include preoperative evaluation of the hematocrit. Administration of medications with antidopaminergic effects, such as phenothiazines, butyrophenones, and metoclopramide (because of extrapyramidal effects) should be avoided. Ondansetron is considered safe as an antiemetic because it does not have antidopaminergic effects. Succinylcholine should not be used because of central neuron degeneration and the risk of triggering a hyperkalemic response.

FRUCTOSE 1,6-DIPHOSPHATE ISOMERASE DEFICIENCY (Hereditary Fructose-1,6-Biphosphatase Deficiency): There are three inherited disorders of fructose metabolism. *Essential fructosuria* is a mild disorder not requiring treatment; *hereditary fructose intolerance* (HFI) and *hereditary fructose-1,6-biphosphatase deficiency* (HFBP) are treatable and controllable, however, must be treated seriously. Hereditary fructose intolerance is an inherited inability to digest fructose or its precursor sorbitol. This condition is caused by a deficiency of the enzyme fructose-1-phosphate aldolase, resulting in accumulation of fructose-1-phosphate in the liver, kidneys, and small intestine. The disorder can be life-threatening in infants and ranges from mild to severe in older children and adults. People affected with HFBP usually develop a strong dislike for sweets and fruits. After eating foods containing fructose, symptoms of severe abdominal pain, vomiting, and hypoglycemia often occur. Early diagnosis is important because most people who have HFI can live normal lives if they adopt a fructose-free diet. Left untreated, patients present signs of serious liver and kidney damage. Clinical manifestations are characterized by prolonged vomiting, failure to thrive, jaundice, and growth retardation. Hepatomegaly and cirrhosis are often present. Spontaneous gastrointestinal bleeding is often associated because of deficiency of clotting factors. There are decreased levels of glucose and phosphate in the blood and increased levels of fructose in the blood and urine. The pattern of inheritance is autosomal recessive, and the gene locus has been mapped to 9q22.3. Anesthetic considerations must include complete assessment of the hepatic, renal, and hematologic functions. Spontaneous bleeding must be noted. Administration of glucose containing solutions should be guided only by the periodic measurement of plasma glucose level.

REFERENCE:

Kugler W, Breme K, Laspe P, et al: Molecular basis of neurological dysfunction coupled with haemolytic anaemia in human glucose-6-phosphate isomerase (GPI) deficiency. *Hum Genet* 103:450, 1998.

Glutaric Acidemia Type I (GA-I)

At a glance: Progressive neurologic disorder caused by a genetically transmitted inborn error of metabolism of glutaric acid.

Synonyms: Glutaric Aciduria; Glutaryl-CoA Dehydrogenase Deficiency.

Incidence: May be more prevalent in Sweden and in Amish Pennsylvania. Affects males and females equally.

Genetic inheritance: Autosomal recessive. Defective gene coding for glutaryl-CoA dehydrogenase located on chromosome 19. Forty-five mutations have been identified.

Pathophysiology: Deficiency of glutaryl-CoA dehydrogenase, a mitochondrial flavin adenine dinucleotide (FAD)-dependent enzyme of the liver and kidney. This enzyme normally catalyzes the conversion of glutaryl-CoA to glutaconyl-CoA, which is an intermediate in the catabolism of lysine, hydroxylysine, and tryptophan. Deficiency of glutaryl-CoA dehydrogenase results in accumulation of glutaric acid in the body, which leads to progressive neurologic damage (degeneration of the basal ganglia of the brain) with acute episodes often triggered by stress such as infections or surgery.

Diagnosis: During acute episodes, high concentrations of glutaric acid are found in blood and urine. Enzyme activity may be assayed in leukocytes or fibroblasts. Prenatal diagnosis is available (deficiency of glutaryl-CoA dehydrogenase activity in cultured chorionic villi/amniocytes; inconstantly, elevated glutaric acid levels in the amniotic fluid).

Clinical aspects: Early development may be normal. The pediatric patient develops progressive dystonia and choreoathetosis. Acute encephalopathy often develops between 6 to 18 months of age, causing striatal damage with severe neuronal loss. Spongiform changes restricted to brainstem white matter and mild lymphocytic infiltrates have been described. Acute exacerbation may occur after a minor infection, presenting with vomiting, ketosis, seizures, and coma. Death commonly occurs during one of these episodes. A low-protein diet and high doses of riboflavin may result in clinical improvement in some patients.

Precautions before anesthesia: Maintain adequate hydration. Check acid-base status. Assess neurologic status.

Anesthetic considerations: Periods of stress, such as surgery, may precipitate acute deterioration. Adequate hydration should be ensured perioperatively and acid-base status monitored during major surgery. Severity of neurologic abnormalities may dictate changes in anesthetic technique, for example, children with bulbar involvement may be at risk for pulmonary aspiration.

Pharmacological implications: No agents specifically contraindicated. Neurologic status may warrant avoidance of drugs that can precipitate seizures, such as enflurane and meperidine.

Other condition to be considered:

☞**Glutaric Acidemia Type II:** Progressive neurologic disorder caused by a genetically transmitted inborn error of metabolism in which the body cannot oxidize fatty acids. Typical clinical features include respiratory distress, muscular hypotonia, sweaty odorous feet, and death often occuring in the neonatal period.

REFERENCES:

Bjugstad KB, Goodman SI, Freed CR: Age at symptom onset predicts severity of motor impairment and clinical outcome of glutaric acidemia type 1. *J Pediatr* 137:681, 2000.

Funk CB, Prasad AN, Frosk P, et al: Neuropathological, biochemical and molecular findings in a glutaric acidemia type I cohort. *Brain* 128;711, 2005.

Glutaric Acidemia Type II (GA-II)

At a glance: Progressive neurologic disorder caused by a genetically transmitted inborn error of metabolism in which the body cannot oxidize fatty acids. Typical clinical features include respiratory distress, muscular hypotonia, sweaty odorous feet, and death often in the neonatal period.

Synonyms: Glutaric Aciduria II; Multiple Acyl-CoA Dehydrogenase Deficiency (MADD); Electron Transfer Flavoprotein (ETF) Deficiency; ETF-Ubiquinone Oxidoreductase (ETF:QO) Deficiency

Classification:

- *Glutaric Aciduria Type IIA:* Neonatal form of glutaric aciduria II
- *Glutaric Aciduria Type IIB:* Adult form of glutaric aciduria II. Also known as the late onset form of glutaric aciduria
- *Glutaric Aciduria Type IIC:* Ethylamonic adipicaciduria

Genetic inheritance: X-linked (neonatal form) or autosomal recessive (mild or "adult" form). Affects males and females equally.

Pathophysiology: Two enzyme deficiencies may be associated with this disorder: electron transfer flavoprotein (ETF) and ETF-ubiquinone oxidoreductase (ETF:QO), which play major roles in the catabolism of fatty acids and proteins.

Diagnosis: Typical abnormal pattern of organic acids in the urine of neonates with GA-II (far less typical in milder forms).

Clinical aspects: *Neonatal GA-II* is characterized by severe hypoglycemia, metabolic acidosis, hypotonia, heart disease, hepatomegaly, and, frequently, an odor of "sweaty feet." Often fatal dur-

ing the first week of life. *Milder forms* (late-onset glutaric acidemia type II) do not display congenital anomalies, and symptoms usually consist of intermittent episodes of nausea and vomiting, lethargy, weakness, and liver enlargement. Acute episodes of hypoglycemia may be extremely severe, often after infection, exercise, or any form of stress (including surgery). The *ethylamonic adipicaciduria form* is characterized by distinctive congenital malformations (e.g., pulmonary hypoplasia, facial dysmorphism) and severe hypoglycemia. Vascular lesions of the skin (petechiae, ecchymoses), acrocyanosis and retinal lesions have been described. Prolonged diarrhea may occur. Respiratory failure may precede death.

Precautions before anesthesia: Maintain adequate hydration and avoid fasting whenever possible (diet high in carbohydrates, low in protein and fat). Prevent hypoglycemia (glucose infusion). Check acid-base status. Assess neurologic status. Consider prophylactic antibiotics.

Anesthetic considerations: Periods of stress, such as surgery, may precipitate acute deterioration. Adequate hydration and prevention of hypoglycemia should be ensured perioperatively and acid-base status monitored during major surgery. In patients with pulmonary hypoplasia, ventilation may be difficult and pulmonary arterial pressure increased.

Pharmacological implications: No agents specifically contraindicated. Neurologic status may warrant avoidance of drugs that can precipitate seizures, such as enflurane and meperidine.

Other condition to be considered:

☞**Glutaric Acidemia Type I:** Progressive neurologic disorder caused by a genetically transmitted inborn error of metabolism of glutaric acid.

REFERENCES:

Ozand PT, Rashed M, Millington DS, et al: Ethylmalonic aciduria: an organic acidemia with CNS involvement and vasculopathy. *Brain Dev* 16 (Suppl);12, 1994.

Slukvin II, Salamat MS, Chandra S: Morphologic studies of the placenta and autopsy findings in neonatal-onset glutaric acidemia type II. *Pediatr Dev Pathol* 5:315, 2002.

Glycogen Storage Diseases (GSD): An Overview

Table G-3 Glycogen Storage Disease (GSD): An Overview

GSD no.	Deficient Enzymatic Activity	Eponym
I	Glucose-6-phosphatase I	Von Gierke disease
II	Alpha 1,4-glucosidase (acid maltase)	Pompe disease
III	Debrancher (amylo-1,6 glucosidase)	Cori disease
IV	Brancher	Andersen disease
V	Muscle phosphorylase	McArdle disease
VI	Liver phosphorylase	Hers disease
VII	Phosphofructokinase	Tarui disease
VIII	Phosphorylase kinase of liver	

Glycogen Storage Disease Type 0

At a glance: Inborn error of metabolism of glucose caused by decreased glycogen synthetase activity and characterized by fasting hypoglycemia with ketosis beginning in early infancy. Unlike other GSDs, GSD 0 does not result in tissue accumulation of normal or abnormal glycogen.

Synonym: Glycogen Synthetase Deficiency.

Incidence: Less than 1:250,000 live births.

Genetic inheritance: Autosomal recessive trait. Male-to-female ratio is 1:1. Disease is caused by a defect in the gene coding for liver glycogen synthetase (*GYS2*), which is located on chromosome band 12p12.2.

Pathophysiology: A decrease or absence of hepatic glycogen synthetase, which is the rate-limiting enzyme for glycogen synthesis, by transferring glucose units from UDP-glucose to a glycogen primer. This action depends on phosphorylation/dephosphorylation mechanisms and is regulated by several hormones, including insulin, epinephrine, and glucagon. Secondary to a lack of storage of glycogen, GSD 0 patients develop hypoglycemia in the early stages of fasting, when the main source of glucose is provided by glycogenolysis, while gluconeogenesis is not able to maintain normoglycemia. On the other hand, feeding results in postprandial hyperglycemia and increased blood lactate levels because glycogen synthesis is very limited; excess glucose mainly undergoes lactate conversion through the glycolytic pathway. Muscle glycogen synthetase is coded by a different gene and is not affected in patients with GSD 0.

Diagnosis: After 5 to 7 hours of fasting, patients demonstrate hypoglycemia and ketosis (and ketonuria), while lactate and alanine levels remain normal. Injection of glucagon fails to elicit a rise in plasma glucose in fasted patients, whereas after a meal, it elicits hyperglycemia and decreased levels of plasma lactate and alanine. Oral intake of glucose, fructose, or galactose elicits a consistent rise in blood lactate. Definitive diagnosis of GSD 0 requires a liver biopsy for enzyme assay (defective glycogen synthetase activity) and microscopic analysis (decreased amounts of normal glycogen stores, increased fat accumulation).

Clinical aspects: Early-onset symptomatic hypoglycemia in infancy, commonly presenting as seizures, disorientation, abnormal eye movements, and/or coma occurring in the morning before breakfast or after inadvertent fasting. Mild forms may display less suggestive signs, such as drowsiness, lethargy, mental confusion, sweating, pallor, attention deficit, and headache. Evolution is characterized by growth retardation. Physical examination may reveal mild hepatomegaly.

Precaution before anesthesia: Preoperative examination of a child with GSD 0 must document the presence or absence of hepatomegaly, lactic acidosis, hyperketosis or hypoketosis, and associated signs of hepatic insufficiency. The characteristic schedule of hypoglycemia following fasting (delay, intensity, predictability, precipitating factors) should be closely evaluated; this can be achieved only by monitored assessment of fasting adaptation in an inpatient setting. Outpatient surgery is contraindicated in GSD 0 patients. Evaluate serum electrolytes to calculate the anion gap, thus determining the existence of metabolic acidosis (which is absent in typical GSD 0 patients). Evaluate liver enzymes; mild elevations of aspartate aminotransferase and alanine aminotransferase are consistent with mild hepatocellular damage.

Anesthetic considerations: Aim to maintain normal intake of carbohydrate by intravenous glucose infusion during the perioperative period (including preoperative fasting period). Main risk is the development of severe perioperative hypoglycemia. Establish infusion of dextrose preoperatively to maintain normal carbohydrate intake (may require 20% dextrose). Maintain good hydration status. Avoid fasting, even short fasting, with early establishment of enteral feeding postoperatively if possible. Monitor blood glucose and blood gases; place arterial catheter for longer cases.

Pharmacological implications: No agents specifically contraindicated.

Other conditions to be considered:

FRUCTOSE 1-PHOSPHATE ALDOLASE DEFICIENCY (Fructose Intolerance): Severe autosomal recessive inherited inborn error of metabolism of glucides as a result of a deficiency of hepatic fructose 1-aldolase. Becomes apparent only when fructose is ingested and is characterized by vomiting, hypoglycemia, severe metabolic acidosis, coma, growth retardation (even cachexia), hepatomegaly, jaundice, coagulopathy, and renal Fanconi syndrome. Gene map locus is 9q22.3.

☞GLYCOGEN STORAGE DISEASE TYPE I: Severe inborn liver dysfunction caused by an almost total deficiency of hepatic glucose-6-phosphatase (type Ia) or defect in intracellular transport of the enzyme substrate (type Ib), resulting in severe hypoglycemia and its consequences (seizures, cyanosis, apnea).

REFERENCE:

Bachrach BE, Weinstein DA, Orho-Melander M, et al: Glycogen synthase deficiency (glycogen storage disease type 0) presenting with hyperglycemia and glucosuria: Report of three new mutations. *J Pediatr* 140:781, 2002.

Glycogen Storage Disease Type I (GSD I)

At a glance: Severe inborn liver dysfunction caused by an almost total deficiency of hepatic glucose-6-phosphatase (type Ia) or a defect in intracellular transport of the enzyme substrate (type Ib), resulting in severe hypoglycemia and its consequences (seizures, cyanosis, apnea).

Synonyms: ☞von Gierke Disease; Hepatorenal Glycogenosis Disease; Glycogenosis Type I.

Classification:

- *Type Ia: Glucose-6-Phosphate Deficiency:* Characterized by a deficiency in the enzyme glucose-6-phosphatase.

- *Type Ib: Glucose-6-Phosphate Translocase Deficiency:* Characterized by a deficiency of the specific translocase T1. The clinical consequences are related to the result of altered neutrophil functions predisposing them to Gram-positive bacterial infections.

- *Type Ic: Glucose-6-Phosphate Translocase T2 Deficiency:* Characterized by a deficiency of translocase T2, which carries anorganic phosphates from microsomes into the cytosol and pyrophosphates from the cytosol into microsomes

- *Type Id: Glucose-6-Phosphate Transporter Deficiency:* Characterized by a deficiency in the transporter that translocates free glucose molecules from microsomes into the cytosol.

History: First described by Edgar Otto C. von Gierke, a German pathologist (1877–1945), in 1929 under the name *hepatonephromegalia glycogenica*. In 1952, Cori and Cori demonstrated that glucose-6-phosphatase deficiency was a cause of GSD type I. In 1978, Narisawa proposed that a transport defect of glucose-6-phosphate into the microsomal compartment may be present in some patients with GSD type I. Following this observation, GSD type I was divided into GSD Ia resulting from deficiency in glucose-6-phosphatase and GSD type Ib resulting from deficiency of a specific translocase T1. Apart from the substrate translocation defect, patients with GSD type Ib have altered neutrophil functions predisposing them to Gram-positive bacterial infections.

Incidence: Type I glycogenosis is unlikely to occur more frequently than 1:50,000 infants.

Genetic inheritance: Autosomal recessive. Two main types described:

- *Type Ia:* Deficient activity of glucose-6-phosphatase enzyme as a result of mutations (at least 14 allelic variants described) at locus 17q21.
- *Type Ib:* Deficient activity of glucose-6-phosphate translocase as a result of mutations at locus 11q23.

Two other types, *Ic* and *Id,* have been reported and correspond to unusual mutations in the translocase gene at locus 11q23.

Pathophysiology: Inability of the liver to release free glucose and accumulation of glycogen in the liver. Hypoglycemia elicits a flood of glucose-6-phosphate that cannot be released from the cell. Glucose-6-phosphate is also the substrate for glycolysis and produces lactate, which exits the hepatocyte, thus producing lactic acidosis with a large anion gap. At the same time, accumulated phosphorylated intermediate compounds of glycolysis inhibit rephosphorylation of adenine nucleotides, thus activating the nucleic acid degradation pathway and increasing the production of uric acid (danger of nephrolithiasis). Hypoglycemia stimulates the release of epinephrine, thus activating lipoprotein lipase and secretion of free fatty acids, which are used for triglyceride synthesis and exported as very-low-density lipoproteins (VLDLs, which are increased in GSD I patients). GSD I patients do not develop significant ketosis because the abundance of acetyl-coenzyme A (derived from glycolysis) activates the acetyl-CoA carboxylase that produces malonyl-CoA (first step of fatty acid synthesis). However, malonyl-CoA inhibits fatty acid transport into mitochondria; therefore fatty acids cannot be used for energy production to support hypoglycemic cells, which causes a continuing decrease in glycemia and explains the absence of ketone bodies.

Diagnosis: Hypoglycemia without significant ketosis, high VLDLs, increased blood lactate, acidosis with large anion gap, chronic leukopenia (type Ib only). Glucagon administration produces no hyperglycemic response, although it causes a marked increase in plasma lactic acid level. Oral administration of galactose causes no change in blood glucose but results in increased lactic acid level in plasma. Liver biopsy (fresh specimen for enzymatic evaluation): considerable glycogen and, to a lesser extent, lipid storage, and absent glucose-6-phosphatase activity.

Clinical aspects: Main clinical signs are (1) severe hypoglycemia, beginning at birth, with its complications of twitching, seizures, cyanosis, apathy, hypotonia, hypothermia, apnea, and coma (either secondary to convulsive disorders or to cerebral edema), and (2) massive liver enlargement (without splenomegaly). Long-term con-

sequences of glycogen storage disease type I consist of short stature, hepatic adenomas and carcinomas, hyperuricemic nephrocalcinosis with progressive renal insufficiency, and hyperlipidemic xanthomas. Young children with type Ia glycogenosis may experience frequent epistaxis. In type Ib glycogenosis, patients are susceptible to Gram-positive infections because of significantly impaired respiratory-burst response of neutrophils to stimuli. Neutropenia is common, and GSD Ib patients often experience recurrent infections, otitis, gingivitis with compromised dentition, brain abscess, and pseudocolitis. In middle childhood, GSD patients often manifest evidence of rickets and anemia.

Precautions before anesthesia: Check history for dietary management, abnormal bleeding, and recurrent infections. Obtain a complete blood cell count. Check levels of blood glucose, electrolytes, and creatinine, urate, blood gases, and liver function. Hyperuricemia may require treatment and postponing of surgery until normal levels are reached. Treat intercurrent infections. Control adequacy of iron intake and ascertain that weekly administration of granulocyte colony-stimulating factor (G-CSF) is really given in type 1b patients.

Anesthetic considerations: Aim to maintain normal intake of carbohydrate by intravenous glucose-containing solutions during the perioperative period. Main risk is development of hypoglycemia and lactic acidosis perioperatively. Establish infusion of dextrose preoperatively to maintain normal carbohydrate intake (may require 20% dextrose). Maintain good hydration status. Avoid prolonged fasting with early establishment of enteral feeding postoperatively, if possible. Monitor blood glucose level and blood gases; place an arterial catheter for longer cases. Avoid regional techniques (bleeding tendency). Hepatomegaly may be sufficient to cause respiratory compromise during mask anesthesia. Careful attention should be paid to aseptic technique.

Pharmacological implications: *cis*-Atracurium is the muscle relaxant of choice (renal dysfunction). Avoid lactate-containing intravenous fluids (e.g., Ringer's lactate). No agents are specifically contraindicated.

Other conditions to be considered: Other glycogen storage diseases (however, GSD I is the only form responsible for severe neonatal hypoglycemia).

REFERENCES:

Chou GY: The molecular basis of type 1 glycogen storage diseases. *Curr Mol Med* 1:25, 2001.

Shenkman Z, Golub Y, Meretyk S, et al: Anaesthetic management of a patient with glycogen storage disease type 1b. *Can J Anaesth* 43:467, 1996.

Veiga-da-Cunha M, Gerin I, Van Schaftingen E: How many forms of glycogen storage disease type I? *Eur J Pediatr* 159:314, 2000.

Glycogen Storage Disease Type II

At a glance: Inborn error of metabolism that results from the deficiency of acid alpha-glucosidase, a lysosomal hydrolase. The three variants are infantile, juvenile, and adult onset. In the classic infantile form (Pompe disease), cardiomyopathy and muscular hypotonia are the cardinal features. In the juvenile and adult forms, involvement of skeletal muscles dominates the clinical presentation.

Synonyms: Acid Maltase Deficiency; Pompe Syndrome; Pompe Disease; Cardiomegalia Glycogenica Diffusa; Cardiac form of

Generalized Glycogenosis; GAA Deficiency; Alpha-1, 4-Glucosidase Deficiency; Glycogenosis type II.

History: First described by the Dutch pathologist Joannes Cassianus Pompe (1901–1945) in 1932, when he reported a 7-month-old girl who died after developing idiopathic hypertrophic cardiomyopathy.

Incidence: In the United States, the frequency is estimated at 1:40,000 live births for all three variants of GSD II. Internationally, the frequency in Taiwan and southern China is estimated at 1:50,000 individuals. In the Dutch population, the frequency is 1:40,000 (1:138,000 for the infantile category). In this population, 63% carry at least one of the three common mutations.

Genetic inheritance: Autosomal recessive. The gene for the affected enzyme has been mapped to 17q25.2-q25.3.

Pathophysiology: Absent acid alpha-1,4-glucosidase (acid maltase), a lysosomal enzyme, in muscle and liver. The enzyme degrades alpha-1,4 and alpha-1,6 linkages in glycogen, maltose, and isomaltose. Deficiency of the enzyme results in accumulation of glycogen within lysosomes and in the cytoplasm, eventually leading to tissue destruction.

Diagnosis: Neonates appear normal at birth but develop hypotonia and poor feeding within a few weeks. Specific enzyme assay in muscle cells, leukocytes, or amniocytes confirms the diagnosis. Creatine kinase elevation, muscle biopsy, demonstration of massive glycogen deposits in lymphocytes in peripheral blood, measurement of acid alpha-1,4-glucosidase activity in leukocytes.

Clinical aspects: There are three major forms of the disorder.

- *Infantile Form:* Infants may appear normal at birth but after a few weeks they begin to develop cardiomyopathy and generalized hypotonia and muscle weakness, which are the cardinal features of the disease. Biventricular hypertrophy and either congestive or obstructive cardiomyopathy result from the accumulation of glycogen, which leads to progressive cardiac failure. Poor swallowing reflexes and decreased muscle tone contribute to feeding difficulties and aspiration. An enlarged tongue (macroglossia) and diminished airway reflexes may cause upper airway obstruction. Characteristic facial appearance with open mouth and protruding tongue. The ECG classically shows signs of biventricular hypertrophy with a short PR interval. The chest radiograph confirms the presence of cardiomegaly and may show evidence of atelectasis and aspiration. The liver is not affected, although it may be enlarged as a result of cardiac failure. Normal mental development. Normal blood glucose concentration. No effective treatment. Death usually results from respiratory failure, which is often complicated by aspiration pneumonia and/or congestive cardiac failure. The disease is rapidly progressive, and few children survive beyond the age of 1 year. Death usually results from respiratory failure and/or end-stage cardiomyopathy. Two different recombinant human α-glucosidase enzymes are now available, which showed an improved outcome for the infantile form of GSD II.
- *Juvenile Form:* These infants and children (onset after 6 months of age) present with delayed motor milestones, weakness, and hypotonia, but no cardiac involvement. Intelligence is normal. Other features include respiratory distress, hypotonia, macroglossia, and hepatomegaly (typically present), but no cardiomegaly or cardiomyopathy.
- *Adult-Onset Form:* Slowly progressive disease in which the heart is not affected. Usually the presentation is by complaints related to proximal muscle weakness, such as difficulty climbing stairs. Respiratory problems are significant in 33% of cases. Other features include exercise intolerance, orthopnea, somnolence, nighttime headache, and diminished deep tendon reflexes.

Precautions before anesthesia: Ensure baseline ECG to establish rhythm and evidence of biventricular hypertrophy. Evaluate cardiac function; echocardiography to assess ventricular function, degree of myocardial hypertrophy and whether any cardiomyopathy is congestive or obstructive. Perform chest radiography and evaluate respiratory function. Blood examination: sodium, potassium, and creatine kinase levels, and arterial blood gas analysis. Full assessment of airway. Macroglossia may be present. Treat intercurrent respiratory infections.

Anesthetic considerations: Indications for surgery should be reviewed. Cardiac arrest during induction of anesthesia with halothane, but also with sevoflurane/propofol, has been reported. Monitoring and intravenous access should be established before induction of anesthesia. Direct measurement of arterial blood pressure may be useful. Hypotonic infants with macroglossia may require awake fiberoptic intubation. Maintenance of airway patency may be difficult because of macroglossia. Anesthetic agents should be selected to avoid myocardial depression; high concentrations of inhaled agents should be avoided. Muscle relaxants may not be required in hypotonic infants and may complicate postoperative recovery. Postoperative mechanical ventilation may be necessary, and weaning may be difficult with profound muscle weakness and cardiopulmonary insufficiency. Pulmonary aspiration may increase oxygen requirements. Intermittent positive pressure ventilation is mandatory in the presence of severe hypotonia. With congestive cardiomyopathy, care should be taken to maintain adequate filling pressures, increase myocardial contractility, and reduce afterload. Obstructive cardiomyopathy requires maintenance of appropriate (high normal) cardiac filling pressures and avoidance of inotropes, chronotropes, and peripheral vasodilatation which may worsen obstruction. Invasive monitoring is indicated. Watch for signs of myocardial ischemia. Spinal and epidural anesthesia may be contraindicated.

Pharmacological implications: Extreme caution with myocardial depressant drugs. Conversely, myocardial hypertrophy may relatively contraindicate drugs with positive inotropic actions, such as ketamine. If muscle relaxants are required, rocuronium or *cis*-atracurium are the agents of choice. Select agents that allow rapid recovery postoperatively. Myocardial depressant drugs, such as barbiturates, propofol, halothane, enflurane, and nitrous oxide, should be used with extreme care. Ketamine is contraindicated in obstructive cardiomyopathy because of its inotropic and chronotropic effects, but has been successfully used in congestive (non-obstructive) cardiomyopathy. Its effect of increasing secretions may also be undesirable. Nondepolarizing muscle relaxants should be used with extreme care and only once the airway has been secured. Suxamethonium is contraindicated because of risk of hyperkalemia and rhabdomyolysis. Opioids should be used with caution because of their effects on respiratory function.

Other conditions to be considered: Other glycogen storage diseases.

REFERENCES:

Ausems MG, Lochman P, van Diggelen OP, et al: A diagnostic protocol for adult-onset glycogen storage disease type II. *Neurology* 52:851, 1999.

Ing RJ, Cook DR, Bengur RA, et al: Anaesthetic management of infants with glycogen storage disease type II: A physiological approach. *Paediatr Anaesth* 14:514, 2004.

McFarlane HJ, Soni N: Pompe's disease and anesthesia. *Anesthesia* 41:1219, 1986.

Glycogen Storage Disease Type III (GSD III)

At a glance: Inherited metabolic disease resulting in accumulation of abnormal glycogen in different tissues of the body.

Synonyms: Cori Disease; Forbes Disease; Illingworth-Cori-Forbes Disease; Amylo-1,6-Glucosidase Debrancher Deficiency; Glycogenosis III; Debranching Enzyme Deficiency; Limit Dextrinosis.

Incidence: Incidence of GSD type III in the United States and other countries is estimated to make up for 24% of all patients affected with GSD.

Genetic inheritance: Autosomal recessive. The responsible defect has been mapped to 1p21.

Pathophysiology: Deficiency of amylo-1,6-debrancher enzyme, an enzyme found in all tissues, that converts glycogen to glucose-1,6-phosphate, resulting in accumulation of dextrin. The site of glycogen accumulation is primarily cytoplasmic. Disease results from generalized liver and muscle (GSD IIIa) or isolated (liver only) deficiency of glycogen debranching enzyme (GSD IIIb).

Diagnosis: Low blood glucose levels, elevated glycogen content in red blood cells, and elevated levels of fat. Uric acid and lactic acid levels are usually normal. Liver biopsy shows inflammatory changes, significantly abnormally structured glycogen content, and deficiency of the debrancher enzyme. Biopsy of muscle shows an accumulation of abnormally structured glycogen in type IIIa.

Clinical aspects: Affected organs vary. Moderate-to-marked hepatomegaly. May have moderate hypotonia and cardiomegaly. Hypoglycemia is rare (but can be profound), occurring mainly after fasting periods. Hepatic or cardiac failure is rare. Normal mental development. May have recurrent pneumonia. Muscle weakness is commonly present in childhood and occasionally is severe. Often the liver returns to a normal size at puberty, although the enzyme defect persists and transition into hepatic cirrhosis and later hepatocellular carcinoma is a known complication. Survival to adulthood however is common.

Precautions before anesthesia: Assess extent of cardiac or hepatic involvement. Assess extent of muscle weakness, which can become a prominant feature after puberty in GSD IIIa. Treat intercurrent infections.

Anesthetic considerations: No specific difficulties with anesthesia have been described. A bleeding tendency may be present, which contraindicates regional anesthesia (central block procedures). Although hypoglycemia is rarely a clinical problem, blood glucose concentrations should be measured in the perioperative period and intravenous dextrose-containing solutions given if required. Depending on the operation, prolonged mechanical ventilation may be required postoperatively in patients with predominant muscle weakness.

Pharmacological implications: Muscle relaxants and drugs with prolonged sedative properties should be used cautiously in children with marked hypotonia. If cardiac function is reduced, agents should be selected to avoid further myocardial depression.

Other conditions to be considered: Other glycogen storage diseases.

REFERENCES:

Cox JM: Anesthesia and glycogen-storage disease. *Anesthesiology* 29:1221, 1968.

Kiechl S, Kohlendorfer U, Thaler C, et al: Different clinical aspects of debrancher deficiency myopathy. *J Neurol Neurosurg Psychiatry* 67:364, 1999.

Glycogen Storage Disease Type IV (GSD IV)

At a glance: Inherited metabolic disorder characterized by hepatosplenomegaly and failure to thrive during the first year of life, followed by progressive liver cirrhosis with portal hypertension and death by 5 years of age.

Synonyms: Amylopectinosis; Andersen Disease; Brancher Deficiency; Glycogenosis type IV.

History: Also named Anderson Disease after the American pathologist and pediatrician Dorothy Hansine Anderson (1901–1963) who described the disease in 1938.

Incidence: GSD IV accounts for only 3% of all glycogen storage diseases, which translates to an incidence of about 1:800,000–1,200,000 neonates.

Genetic inheritance: Autosomal recessive. Both sexes are affected. The disease is caused by defects in the gene coding for the glycogen-branching enzyme located on chromosome 3p12.

Pathophysiology: Deficiency of amylo-1,4 to 1,6-transglucosidase (glycogen-branching enzyme), which results in production of abnormal glycogen with long, unbranched outer chains and decreased solubility (amylopectin-like). Tissue glycogen concentration is usually not increased, but the presence of insoluble glycogen induces foreign-body reactions, leading to cellular injury and organ dysfunction. Ultimately, patients develop terminal hepatic cirrhosis. In skeletal muscles, the presence of abnormal glycogen leads to weakness, exercise intolerance, and muscle atrophy. Cardiac involvement yields to dilated cardiomyopathy and progressive heart failure. In the nervous system, the presence of abnormal glycogen results in cognition disorders and both neuromuscular and neurovisceral dysfunction.

Diagnosis: Clinical features. Diagnosis of GSD IV relies on demonstration of deficient glycogen-branching enzyme activity (1–10% of normal values) by an indirect enzyme assay. Heterozygotes display an intermediate reduction in enzyme activity. Definitive diagnosis may involve biopsy of the liver or other affected organs for microscopic examination and enzyme assay. Antenatal diagnosis consists of measuring the levels of glycogen-branching enzyme activity in cultured amniocytes and chorionic villi. Molecular diagnosis may be performed in selected cases.

Clinical aspects: Clinical heterogeneity with variable age of onset, specific organ involvement, and degree of accumulation of abnormal glycogen in different tissues. Typically, GSD IV patients present with hepatosplenomegaly and progressive development of cirrhosis and portal hypertension. Death commonly occurs before 5 years of age from hepatic failure. Liver transplant may stop disease progression in some patients. Liver disease may be associated with hypoalbuminemia, coagulopathy, and thrombocytopenia. Esophageal varices, ascites, splenomegaly, renal failure and hepatic encephalopathy may complicate the clinical course. Associated features described in some patients include cardiomyopathy with congestive cardiac failure, peripheral neuropathy, and hypoglycemia. Prolongation of the QT interval on the ECG has been described and may predispose to arrhythmias. Several neuromuscular forms of GSD IV have been identified. A common variant consists of the development of myopathy or cardiomyopathy during childhood. A perinatal form is distinguished by severe neuromuscular involvement and death. Some patients with clinically diagnosed adult polyglucosan body disease have deficient glycogen-branching enzyme activity and diffuse neurologic (central and peripheral nervous system) dysfunction. After liver transplantation, some patients continue to have progressive accumulation of abnormal glycogen in other organs, ultimately leading to death.

Precautions before anesthesia: Assess for signs and symptoms of cardiac failure. Obtain chest radiograph, ECG, and echocardiogram if indicated. Assess history for muscle weakness, perhaps periodic in nature. Assess for history of neuropathy. Check liver function, coagulation profile (major alterations are frequent), platelet count, and serum electrolytes and blood glucose levels. Ultrasonography may reveal the existence of portal hypertension, esophageal varices, and altered liver echogenicity; it allows determination of the portal vein diameter and blood flow directionality (important data when hepatic transplantation is considered).

Anesthetic considerations: Anesthetic management depends upon the severity of liver dysfunction and other manifestations of the disease. If heart failure is present, further depression of cardiac output by anesthetic agents should be avoided. Monitor ECG for arrhythmias. Regional techniques are contraindicated secondary to coagulopathy or neuropathy. Monitor serum potassium and blood glucose levels in perioperative period and administer intravenous fluids to maintain normal values. Naso- or orogastric tubes should be well lubricated and inserted very carefully in the presence of esophageal varices.

Pharmacological implications: Avoid succinylcholine and reduce doses of nondepolarizing muscle relaxants if myopathy is present; *cis*-atracurium is the muscle relaxant of choice. Reduce doses of highly protein-bound drugs (e.g., thiopentone) if hypoalbuminemic. Liver failure may prolong the action of drugs eliminated by hepatic metabolism, for example, morphine. Preexisting renal failure and thrombocytopenia should preclude the use of nonsteroidal antiinflammatory drugs.

Other conditions to be considered: Other glycogen storage diseases.

REFERENCES:

Bao Y, Kishnani P, Wu JY, et al: Hepatic and neuromuscular forms of glycogen storage disease type IV caused by mutations in the same glycogen-branching enzyme gene. *J Clin Invest* 97:941, 1996.

Sahoo S, Blumberg AK, Sengupta E, et al: Type IV glycogen storage disease. *Arch Pathol Lab Med* 126:630, 2002.

Glycogen Storage Disease Type V (GSD V)

At a glance: Autosomal recessive inherited inborn error of metabolism, probably underdiagnosed, characterized by muscle fatigue, myalgia, and cramping following exercise.

Synonyms: McArdle Disease (or Syndrome, or Myopathy); Muscle Glycogen Phosphorylase Deficiency; Myophosphorylase Deficiency; Glycogenosis type V.

History: This inborn error of metabolism was first described in 1951 by Brian McArdle (1911–2002), a British pediatrician, in a 30-year-old man who complained of pain followed by weakness and stiffness after exercise.

Incidence: GSD V accounts for approximately 2.5% of all patients affected with GSD worldwide.

Genetic inheritance: Autosomal recessive. Although males and females should be equally affected, more males than females have been reported. The gene encoding the muscular isoform of phosphorylase is located on band 11q13. Nonsense, deletion, missense, and splice-junction mutations usually result in almost complete absence of myophosphorylase in skeletal muscle. Three common mutations in the gene (R49X, G204S, K542T) account for approximately 90% of the mutant alleles in the white population.

Pathophysiology: Deficiency of muscle phosphorylase (myophosphorylase or alpha-1,4-glucan orthophosphate glycosyl transferase), which initiates glycogenolysis by removing 1,4-glucosyl groups with release of glucose-1-phosphate. Myophosphorylase is the only isoform present in skeletal muscle (but also in the heart and the brain). Patients are unable to release glucose from glycogen in muscle. The production of adenosine triphosphate via the Krebs cycle is compromised and the exercising muscle derives its energy from blood glucose and free fatty acids, which might account for the second-wind phenomenon experienced by these patients, (i.e., progressive fatigue and muscle weakness develops after 10 to 15 min of exercise. Following a rapid recovery, exercise can be resumed without difficulties for a prolonged time period.)

Diagnosis: Painful muscle cramps following exercise. No rise in serum lactate following ischemic exercise. Phosphorus-31 nuclear magnetic resonance (^{31}P-NMR) shows a lack of cytoplasmic acidification following exercise. DNA diagnosis possible. No electrical activity may be observed on EMG during cramps. The disease may be asymptomatic during childhood.

Clinical aspects: Clinical heterogeneity. Onset often in adolescence or early adulthood. Weakness and cramping of skeletal muscles after exercise. May have episodes of rhabdomyolysis and myoglobinuria after vigorous exercise (half of patients develop acute renal failure). Muscle wasting develops later. Heart muscle unaffected. Prognosis generally good with avoidance of excessive exercise. Seizures have been described in 4% of patients. A rare fatal infantile form is described (hypotonia, diminished tendon reflexes); death results from respiratory failure as a consequence of severe muscular weakness. A late-onset form, also very rare, has been reported.

Precautions before anesthesia: Assess history for episodes of myoglobinuria and severity of episodes of muscle weakness. Check renal function, which may be impaired by myoglobinuria. Patients with GSD V may be depleted in pyridoxine, which is normally bound to myophosphorylase.

Anesthetic considerations: Tourniquets may lead to prolonged muscle cramping, even compartment syndrome, and should be avoided. Maintain normothermia to prevent shivering in the postoperative period. Dextrose-containing solutions should be infused perioperatively.

Pharmacological implications: Succinylcholine should be avoided because of the risk of severe myoglobinuria. Nondepolarizing muscle relaxants have been used without problems, although reduced doses may be required (nerve stimulator).

Other conditions to be considered: Other glycogen storage diseases.

REFERENCES:

Kubisch C, Wicklein EM, Jentsch TJ: Molecular diagnosis of McArdle disease: Revised genomic structure of the myophosphorylase gene and identification of a novel mutation. *Hum Mutat* 12:27, 1998.

Lindner A, Reichert N, Eichhorn M, et al: Acute compartment syndrome after forearm ischemic work test in a patient with McArdle's disease. *Neurology* 56:1779, 2001.

Martin MA, Rubio JC, Buchbinder J, et al: Molecular heterogeneity of myophosphorylase deficiency (McArdle's disease): A genotype-phenotype correlation study. *Ann Neurol* 50:574, 2001.

Glycogen Storage Disease Type VI (GSD VI)

At a glance: Autosomal recessive inborn error of metabolism of glycogen producing a heterogeneous group of hepatic glycogenoses with mild clinical manifestations and benign course.

Synonyms: Glycogen Phosphorylase Deficiency; Hepatic Phosphorylase Kinase Deficiency; Hers Syndrome; Liver Phosphorylase Deficiency; X-Linked Liver Glycogenosis; Glycogenosis type VI; Phosphorylase b Kinase Deficiency.

Nature: Inborn error of metabolism consisting of a deficiency of liver phosphorylase (classic form) or other enzyme defects of the phosphorylase cascade system such as phosphorylase b kinase deficiency (formerly GSD IX, GSD VIII by McKusick) and adenosine 3',5'-cyclic monophosphate (cyclic AMP)-dependent protein kinase deficiency (formerly GSD X).

Incidence: Accounts for about 30% of all GSD, of which approximately 75% result from the X-linked recessive form of phosphorylase kinase deficiency. Incidence up to 0.1% in the Mennonite population (3% incidence of specific splice-site mutation in the liver phosphorylase gene of this religious group).

Genetic inheritance: Autosomal recessive (classic form; accounts for about 25% of cases) and X-linked recessive form (phosphorylase kinase deficiency). Phosphorylase b kinase genes are multimeric (four different subunits, each coded by a unique gene located on different chromosomes). Different isoforms of each enzyme with differential tissue expression exist.

Pathophysiology: Deficiency of liver phosphorylase, the rate-limiting enzyme of glycogenolysis, is activated by an enzyme cascade by a succession of enzymes resulting in insufficient liberation of glucose from the glycogen molecule. Neoglycogenesis is not affected. Even though the enzyme deficiency is usually incomplete, mild fasting hypoglycemia and associated hyperketosis with ketonuria are frequent.

Diagnosis: Enzyme deficiency demonstrated on liver biopsy. Associated biologic disorders include mild hyperlipidemia, hypercholesterolemia, and, to a lesser extent, hypertriglyceridemia. Elevated serum transaminases with no other evidence of liver dysfunction is frequent. Molecular diagnostic testing is used to identify carriers and affected children.

Clinical aspects: Typically, symptomatology becomes apparent in children at the age of 1 to 5 years, who present with a protuberant abdomen, growth and mild motor retardation, mild fasting hypoglycemia, and hypotonia. Some patients are asymptomatic, but physical abdominal examination reveals hepatomegaly, which may be massive. Severe hypoglycemia is rare. Mild cardiomyopathy may occur in some patients.

Precautions before anesthesia: Check blood glucose level, liver function and cardiac function. Assess degree of hypotonia.

Anesthetic considerations: Anesthetic management in this condition has not been described, but no particular problems would be predicted except for the potential for severe hypotonia. Dextrose-containing fluid may be used in patients at risk for hypoglycemia. If hypotonia is present, neuromuscular blocking agents should be titrated to effect (nerve stimulator) and depending on the planned procedure, postoperative mechanical ventilation may be required.

Pharmacological implications: No agents specifically contraindicated. *Cis*-atracurium should be preferred in patients with altered liver function.

Other conditions to be considered: Other glycogen storage diseases.

REFERENCES:

Burwinkel B, Bakker HD, Herschkovitz E, et al: Mutations in the liver glycogen phosphorylase gene (PYGL) underlying glycogenosis type VI. *Am J Hum Genet* 62:785, 1998.

Cox JM: Anesthesia and glycogen-storage disease. *Anesthesiology* 29:1221, 1968.

Wolfsdorf JI, Holm IA, Weinstein DA: Glycogen storage diseases. Phenotypic, genetic, and biochemical characteristics, and therapy. *Endocrinol Metab Clin North Am* 28:801, 1999.

Glycogen Storage Disease Type VII (GSD VII)

At a glance: One of the four glycogen storage diseases characterized by phosphofructokinase deficiency in the muscles and associated with abnormal deposition of glycogen in muscle tissues, exercise intolerance, and anemia.

Synonyms: Muscle Phosphofructokinase Deficiency; Tarui Disease; Glycogenosis type VII.

History: Also named Tarui disease after the Japanese physician Seiichiro Tarui (born in 1927) who first described the disease in 1965.

Incidence: Less than 50 cases reported (<10 for the infantile lethal form). This condition is mainly observed in the Ashkenazi Jewish people.

Genetic inheritance: Autosomal recessive; however, more males than females have been reported. The gene causing GSD VII (M subunit gene) has been mapped to chromosome 1.

Pathophysiology: Deficiency of muscle phosphofructokinase, which catalyzes the irreversible conversion of fructose-6-phosphate to fructose-1,6-bisphosphate in glycolysis. As a consequence, free or glycogen-derived glucose cannot be used as a source of energy and glycogen accumulates because of impaired degradation and/or excess synthesis. Increased levels of glucose-6-phosphate activate the hexose monophosphate shunt, thus enhancing nucleotide formation and uric acid production. The enzymatic block also causes a decrease in 2,3-diphosphoglycerate (DPG). Oxygen affinity of hemoglobin is therefore increased, as is the production of new erythrocytes, resulting in compensated anemia.

Diagnosis: Based on the clinical findings in patients with muscular exercise intolerance exacerbated by glucose infusion prior to exercise, fatigue, vomiting, muscle weakness, myalgia, cramps, and myoglobinuria. Phosphofructokinase deficient in skeletal muscle, but not in the liver. No rise in blood lactate concentration after ischemic exercise. Plasma creatine phosphokinase is increased. ^{31}P-NMR spectroscopy reveals a specific peak of phosphorylated monoesters (accumulation of glycolytic intermediates resulting from the enzymatic block). A severe *infantile form* with arthrogryposis, cardiomyopathy, and frequent respiratory failure has been described. Death occurs early. Antenatal detection possible in families with identifiable mutations.

Clinical aspects: Clinical features similar to GSD type V. Temporary weakness and painful muscle cramps occur after exercise. Myoglobinuria may occur with extreme exertion. Patients tend to develop hemolytic anemia (with jaundice as a result of partial erythrocyte phosphofructokinase deficiency) and myogenic hyperuricemia.

Three clinical forms have been described: classic, infantile onset, and late onset type. The *classic form* includes exercise intolerance, fatigue, and myoglobinuria. The *infantile form* may include myopathy, mental retardation, cataracts, joint contractures, and death during childhood. The *late-onset form* consists of progressive muscle weakness developing in adults.

Precautions before anesthesia: Assess history of muscle weakness. Monitor hemoglobin and reticulocyte count and renal function in cases of myoglobinuria. Perform ultrasonography to evaluate the presence of gallstones in case of hyperbilirubinemia. Evaluate cardiac and respiratory function if necessary, particularly in the infantile form (clinical aspects, radiographs, echocardiography, pulmonary function tests). Check renal function in the presence of myoglobinuria.

Anesthetic considerations: Tourniquets may precipitate painful muscle cramps. Maintain normothermia to prevent shivering in the postoperative period, which could trigger severe muscle cramps and myoglobinuria. Careful intraoperative positioning is needed in patients with myalgia and weakness. Postoperative ventilatory support can be necessary in severe forms.

Pharmacological implications: Avoid succinylcholine. Use of nondepolarizing muscle relaxants should not cause problems, but should be administered with proper monitoring. Due to its metabolism, *cis*-atracurium seems to be the relaxant of choice. Propofol increases uric acid excretion and should probably be avoided for long-term infusion (total intravenous anesthesia, sedation). Effect of perioperative glucose infusion is unknown.

Other conditions to be considered: Other glycogen storage diseases.

REFERENCES:

Nakajima H, Raben N, Hamaguchi T, et al: Phosphofructokinase deficiency: Past, present and future. *Curr Mol Med* 2:197, 2002.

Vorgerd M, Karitzky J, Ristow M, et al: Muscle phosphofructokinase deficiency in two generations. *J Neurol Sci* 141:95, 1996.

Glycogen Storage Disease Type VIII (GSD VIII)

At a glance: One of the mildest form of the glycogenoses. It is characterized by hepatomegaly, growth retardation, elevation of glutamate-pyruvate transaminase and glutamate-oxaloacetate transaminase, hypercholesterolemia, hypertriglyceridemia, and fasting hyperketosis.

Synonyms: Hepatic (or Liver) Phosphorylase Kinase Deficiency; Phosphorylase Kinase Deficiency of Liver; Phosphorylase Kinase-Deficient Liver Glycogenosis; Glycogenosis type VIII. [*NB:* Also classified as GSD type VIa. GSD type IX is a variant of the recessive form of defective enzyme without brain involvement.]

Incidence: Fewer than 10 cases have been reported, but it may be underdiagnosed because it is often asymptomatic and, when symptomatic, often classified as GSD VI.

Genetic inheritance: X-linked recessive (GSD VIII) and autosomal recessive (GSD IX) types described. Gene map loci are Xp22.2-p22.1 (GSD VIII) and 16q12-q13 (GSD IX).

Pathophysiology: Deficiency of liver phosphorylase kinase, which is required to activate liver phosphorylase. Protein phosphorylation is a major mechanism of signal transduction.

Diagnosis: Clinical finding of hepatomegaly. Enzyme deficiency on liver biopsy.

Clinical aspects: Massive hepatomegaly in infancy that may regress later in life. Otherwise, children are normal and prognosis is good.

Precautions before anesthesia: Check liver function.

Anesthetic considerations: Anesthetic management has not been described. If hepatomegaly is significant, functional residual capacity of the lungs may be reduced. Proper preoxygenation would be recommended. Case reports exist where hepatomegaly finally progressed to liver cirrhosis and formation of a hepatocellular adenoma.

Pharmacological implications: No agents specifically contraindicated.

Other conditions to be considered: Other glycogen storage diseases.

REFERENCES:

Burwinkel B, Tanner MS, Kilimann MW: Phosphorylase kinase deficient liver glycogenosis: Progression to cirrhosis in infancy associated with PHKG2 mutations (H144Y and L225R). *J Med Genet* 37:376, 2000.

Shiomi S, Saeki J, Kim K, et al: A female case of type VIII glycogenosis who developed cirrhosis of the liver and hepatocellular tumor. *Gastroenterol Jpn* 24:711, 1989.

Goldenhar Syndrome

At a glance: Common birth defect of vascular origin involving first and second branchial arch derivatives, resulting mainly in hemifacial microsomia with anomalies of the ear, eye, and vertebral bodies. Usually associated with cardiovascular anomalies including ventriculoseptal defect, atrial septal defect, patent ductus arteriosus, tetralogy of Fallot, and coarctation of the aorta. Arnold-Chiari syndrome and hydrocephalus are reported. Airway problems (unilateral hypoplasia of the facial bones and muscles). Epibulbar dermoids. Limited mouth opening, micrognathia, cleft palate.

Synonyms: Facio-Auriculo-Vertebral Sequence (or Spectrum) (FAV Sequence); Goldenhar-Gorlin Syndrome; Hemifacial Microsomia; Oculo-Auriculo-Vertebral Dysplasia (OAV Dysplasia); Oculo-Auriculo-Vertebral Anomaly (or Spectrum).

History: Described by Maurice Goldenhar, an American physician (1924–2002) who attended medical school in Geneva and in 1940 emigrated from Belgium to the United States. He was a general practitioner. The "Maurice Goldenhar Family Medicine Update," Stony Brook University Hospital, State University of New York, is named in his honor.

Incidence: Frequency ranges from 1:3000–26,500 live births. Male-to-female ratio is 3:2. Infants born to Gulf War veterans displayed a higher rate of Goldenhar syndrome, probably secondary to toxic exposures.

Genetic inheritance: Most cases are sporadic; familial cases are consistent with autosomal recessive, autosomal dominant, and multifactorial patterns of transmission. Gene location has not been identified.

Pathophysiology: Vascular disruption in the blood supply to the first and second branchial arches, especially at the time of switching from stapedial to external carotid artery supply, is believed to be the cause in many cases of the Goldenhar anomaly; this disruption could be genetically linked. Another hypothesis suggests that a defect of blastogenesis results from deficiency in migration of neural crest cells, deficiency of mesodermal formation, or defective interaction between neural crest cells and mesoderm. A transgenic mouse line model with autosomal dominant hemifacial microsomia suggested the anomaly consisted of a mutational deletion (23 kb at least) on the locus Hfm (hemifacial microsomia-associated locus) on chromosome 10 (in the mouse). The disorder may be present in monozygotic twins, with only one twin being affected.

Diagnosis: Based on the clinical features. Radiographic studies of the vertebral column and the malformations of the mandible and its annexes may be a useful diagnostic aid. Muscular lesions (hypotrophic and hypoplastic muscles) are associated with these skeletal malformations.

Clinical aspects: Variable phenotypic expression, ranging from mild to severe cases even within the same affected family. The presence of a scleral dermolipoma on the lateral aspect of the eyeball is a condition sine qua non for Goldenhar syndrome. Associated malformations include facial asymmetry (right side in 60% of cases), mandibular hypoplasia, macrostomia, unilateral hypoplastic palate, unilateral hypoplasia of tongue muscles, parotid agenesis, epibulbar dermolipomas, upper eyelid coloboma, blepharophimosis, microphthalmia (even anophthalmia), anomalies of the ear (external and middle ear are frequently involved, inner ear may be involved, hearing loss may be conductive or mixed, preauricular cartilaginous tags or sinuses, external auditory canal atresia), scalp hemangiomas, vertebral dysplasia, and acroosteolysis of terminal phalanges. Other manifestations include microcephaly or hydrocephaly with mental retardation in 5 to 15% of patients, Arnold-Chiari malformation, encephalocele, spina bifida, and cardiac malformations. Cervical subluxation at the level C1 and C2 has been described in some patients. Patients often have feeding difficulties, and they are prone to develop obstructive sleep apnea. Normal lifespan is usual.

Precautions before anesthesia: Physical examination. Sparing techniques of blood loss (autotransfusion program is recommended if extensive reconstructive surgery is planned). Evaluation for difficult intubation due to mandibular hypoplasia. Standard preoperative laboratory examinations are appropriate in most patients (blood chemistry, blood group, complete blood cell count, coagulation). Echocardiography to exclude associated cardiac defects (atrial and ventricular septal defects, patent ductus arteriosus, tetralogy of Fallot, coarctation of the aorta).

Anesthetic considerations: Must be prepared for difficult laryngoscopy and tracheal intubation. Some patients have subluxation of C1-C2. Plastic and/or maxillofacial surgery are often required for correction of malocclusion and cleft palate. Blood loss may be significant and require invasive monitoring of hemodynamic parameters, estimation of blood loss, and repeated blood gas and electrolyte analyses. Postoperative care often requires transfer to an intensive

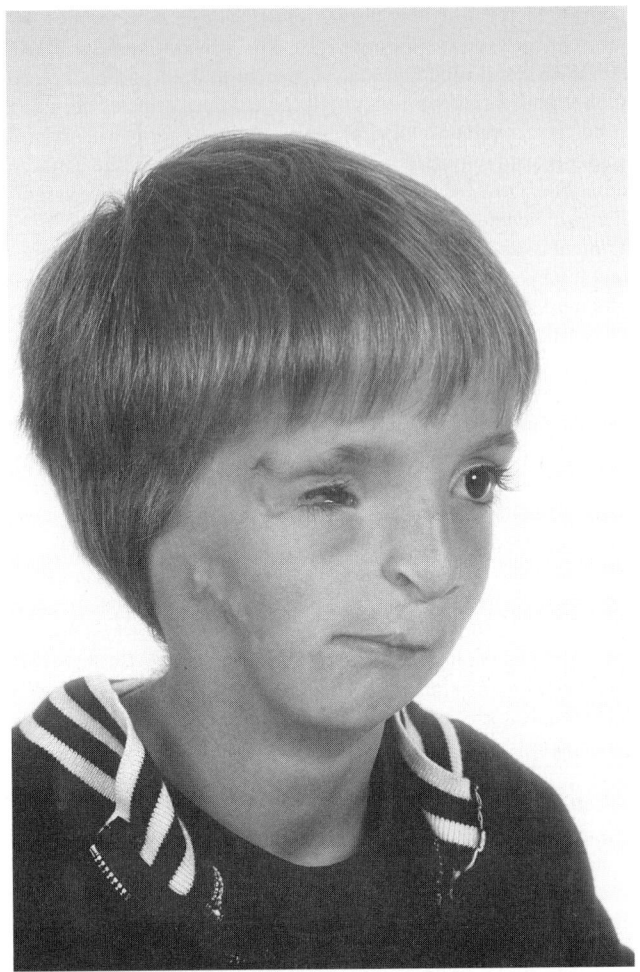

Goldenhar Syndrome Facial asymmetry with mandibular hypoplasia, agenesis of the parotid gland, eyelid coloboma, blepharophimosis, microphthalmia, and anomalies of the ear with atresia of the external auditory canal characterize Goldenhar syndrome in a 9-year-old boy.

care unit and prolonged mechanical ventilation until the facial swelling (in the case of reconstructive surgery) has decreased to a level safe enough for extubation.

Pharmacological implications: None currently identified that are specific to this condition. Muscle relaxants should be avoided until the airway has been secured. The only pharmacological implications are those associated with the cardiovascular anomalies. Subacute bacterial endocarditis prophylaxis may be necessary.

Other conditions to be considered:

AKSU STOCKHAUSEN SYNDROME: This autosomal dominant medical condition is defined by the association of brachial arch defects. Characterized by the presence of anotia/microtia, microstomia, preauricular pits, respiratory distress, pharyngeal abnormality, hearing loss, sacral sinus/dimple, hypertonia, spasticity, and muscle rigidity. A proper evaluation of the airway must be done to eliminate problems related to difficult airway management during face-mask ventilation and tracheal intubation. The potential for hyperkalemia following the administration of succinylcholine must be considered if hypertonia is present.

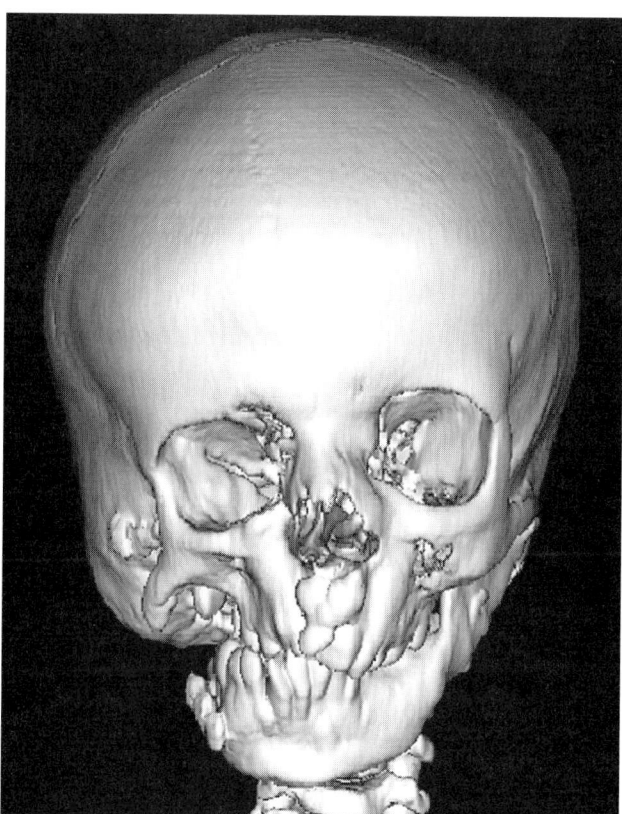

Goldenhar Syndrome Frontal three-dimensional reconstruction of the CT scan (of a different patient) confirms the findings.

☞**CHARGE SYNDROME:** A life-threatening, congenital syndrome with multiple anomalies consisting of choanal atresia, coloboma, heart defects, mental and growth retardation, genital and urinary anomalies, and ear anomalies with deafness. Prognosis worsens if concomitant cyanotic heart lesions, esophageal atresia or central nervous system anomalies are present.

☞**TREACHER COLLINS SYNDROME:** Autosomal dominant polymalformative syndrome characterized by craniofacial malformations, including hypoplastic zygomatic arches and supraorbital rims, mandibular hypoplasia, micrognathia, macrostomia, palatal malformation, palpebral fissures, and coloboma.

FRANCESCHETTI KLEIN SYNDROME: Mandibulofacial dysostosis presenting less severe micrognathia than observed in ☞Pierre Robin syndrome. The facial appearance is characterized by palpebral fissures sloping downward the outer canthi, colobomas (lower eyelids), large mouth but receding chin. Although similar to Treacher Collins syndrome, in this situation the mandible is not as hypoplastic; however, the undersurface is profoundly concave.

☞**PIERRE ROBIN SYNDROME:** Micrognathia with associated pseudomacroglossia, glossoptosis, and high arched or cleft palate. The posterior displacement of the genioglossus muscle contributes to the abnormal tongue position. Severe micrognathia and small mouth opening.

TRISOMY 22: The complete form is usually lethal; mosaicism, however, has a good survival rate. Intrauterine growth retardation, microcephaly, facial malformations (hypertelorism, epicanthal folds, midface hypoplasia, low-set ears), digital malformations, and genitourinary malformations in males; cleft palate, cardiac and anal malformations are common features.

REFERENCES:

Chen PP, Cheng CK, Abdullah V, et al: Tracheal intubation using suspension laryngoscopy in an infant with Goldenhar's syndrome. *Anaesth Intensive Care* 29:548, 2001.

Lam CH: A theory on the embryogenesis of oculo-auriculo-vertebral (Goldenhar) syndrome. *J Craniofac Surg* 11:547, 2000.

Van Meter TD, Weaver DD: Oculo-auriculo-vertebral spectrum and the CHARGE association: Clinical evidence for a common pathogenetic mechanism. *Clin Dysmorphol* 5:187, 1996.

Goldston Syndrome

At a glance: Very rare congenital genetic disorder with hepato-reno-pancreatic involvement combined with Dandy-Walker malformation.

Synonym: Renal-Hepatic-Pancreatic Dysplasia with Dandy-Walker Cyst.

Incidence and genetic inheritance: Very rare syndrome (<10 cases worldwide) with probably autosomal recessive inheritance.

Clinical aspects: Main features are dysplastic kidneys, pancreas and liver anomalies, and presence of ☞Dandy-Walker malformation. Other features can include oligoamnios, polyhydramnios, hypoplastic lungs, and duplication of the gut.

Precautions before anesthesia: Assess liver, renal and pancreatic function. Obtain a complete blood cell count (renal anemia) and check blood glucose. Check for history of apnea (Dandy-Walker malformation) and signs of increased intracranial pressure. Assess for signs of difficult airway management.

Anesthetic considerations: High rate of anesthetic implications. Hepatic, renal, neurologic, respiratory, and liver function should be assessed and their influence on anesthetic drug metabolism and perioperative fluid regimen should be considered. Avoid hypotension, hypercapnia and increased body temperature in the presence of increased intracranial pressure.

Pharmacological implications: In the presence of hepatic and/or renal anomalies, *cis*-atracurium is the neuromuscular blocker of choice, and isoflurane and desflurane are the inhalational anesthetics of choice, although sevoflurane is expected not to cause any harm if used for a short period of time (e.g., induction of anesthesia).

REFERENCES:

Goldston AS, Burke EC, D'Agostino A, et al: Neonatal polycystic kidney with brain defect. *Am J Dis Child* 106:484, 1963.

Gulcan H, Duman N, Kumral A, et al: Goldston syndrome: Report of a case. *Genet Couns* 12:263, 2001.

Moerman P, Pauwels P, Vandenberghe K, et al: Goldston syndrome reconsidered. *Genet Couns* 4:97, 1993.

Goltz Syndrome

At a glance: Complex mesoectodermal hereditary disorder characterized by focal dermal atrophy, with herniation of fat-producing multiple papillomas, in association with skeletal, dental, ocular, and other anomalies.

Synonym: Focal Dermal Hypoplasia (FDH). [*NB:* Avoid confusion with Goltz-Gorlin syndrome (inheritable disease characterized by multiple cutaneous nodules with a tendency to become malignant).]

Incidence: Frequency is approximately 2:100,000 newborns.

Genetic inheritance: 95% sporadic. X-linked dominant with in utero lethality in males or by a sex-limited dominant gene of variable expressivity. Gene is located on Xp22.31. Only 10% of cases occur in males (possibly the result of half-chromatid mutations).

Pathophysiology: The underlying molecular defect in FDH is not clear. Based on the common findings of syndactyly, oligodactyly, and polydactyly, the fetal expression of FDH is postulated to occur before week 8 of gestation because the hands and feet have differentiated and developed separate and elongated digits by the eighth week. Because skin and bone lesions generally follow the lines of Blaschko, mosaicism with random X-chromosome inactivation is probable. Clinical abnormalities indicate a profound dysplasia of ectodermal, neuroectodermal, endodermal, and mesodermal elements. Various in vitro observations of fibroblasts from lesional skin reveal abnormal growth kinetics of fibroblasts (increase in the fibroblast doubling time), abnormal glycosaminoglycan metabolism (decreased accumulation of hyaluronic acid), and absence of basement membrane type IV collagen. A hypothesis that aberrant dermal fibroblast growth and altered collagen fibers may be the basis of the skin defects in FDH has been suggested.

Diagnosis: Usually female gender. Characteristic skin findings are present at birth (streaky areas of hyperpigmentation, atrophy, and telangiectasia and groups of soft, yellow-red nodules). Radiologic examination shows longitudinal striation of the long bones with crossing of the epiphyses (osteopathia striata). The combination of split-hand with syndactyly and absence of rays, the so-called lobster-claw hand, is a striking feature of the disorder.

Clinical aspects: Patients with areas of total absence of skin at birth have been reported. More commonly, skin changes are usually present at birth or develop shortly thereafter from erythematous areas. Papillomas usually develop later, involving the mucous membranes or skin. Lesions of the oropharynx and peritonsillar regions have been described. Laryngeal papillomas requiring tracheostomy in one case and esophageal papillomas associated with strictures have been described. In addition, anomalies involving the *hands* (syndactyly, polydactyly, camptodactyly, missing digits or entire hand), *skeleton* (hypoplasia or aplasia or the truncal skeleton), *mouth* (lip papillomas, hypoplastic teeth), and *eyes* (coloboma of iris and choroid, strabismus, microphthalmia) have been present in some cases. Gastroesophageal reflux, short stature, and mental retardation occur in many patients. Course and prognosis dependent upon the type and severity of noncutaneous involvement. Treatment is symptomatic. One case report describes a stillborn girl with Goltz syndrome who had truncus arteriosus II with hypoplastic pulmonary vasculature (arteries and veins) and lungs, massive diaphragmatic hernia and absence of one kidney.

Precautions before anesthesia: Look for stridor and signs of increased work of breathing. Fiberoptic examination may be required to determine whether verrucous lesions in the hypopharynx and supraglottic larynx are obstructing visualization of the vocal cords during direct laryngoscopy and tracheal intubation. Evaluate the respiratory system in the presence of kyphoscoliosis (arterial blood gas analysis, chest radiographs, pulmonary function tests). If kyphoscoliosis is significant, echocardiography may be indicated (cor pulmonale).

Anesthetic considerations: Difficult cooperation in the presence of mental retardation should be expected and sedative/hypnotic premedication as well as the presence of the primary caregiver for induction of anesthesia may be helpful. Careful positioning is needed to protect the atrophic or absent skin areas. Thermoregulation may be impaired in patients with large areas of involvement. Monitoring of the body temperature and precautions to prevent hypothermia are necessary. General anesthesia with spontaneous respiration may be complicated by persistent partial upper airway obstruction secondary to supraglottic lesions. Tracheal intubation may be difficult as a result of these growths and the presence of facial abnormalities. Hypoplastic, anomalous teeth may be more prone to damage during direct laryngoscopy. Spinal and epidural anesthesia might be difficult because of spinal abnormalities (kyphoscoliosis). Frequent gastroesophageal reflux may require rapid-sequence induction. Secondary to the skin and anatomical anomalies, vascular access may be difficult.

Pharmacological implications: Muscle relaxants should be avoided until the airway has been secured.

Other conditions to be considered:

Microphthalmia with Linear Skin Defects (MLS) Syndrome: Some similar features, but associated with a deletion of the tip of the X chromosome; all main features are confined to the neck and head.

Osteopathia Striata with Cranial Sclerosis: Severe bone dysplasia in which osteopathia striata is associated with cranial sclerosis, dysmorphic facies, cleft palate, deafness, heart defects, and vertebral anomalies with variable expression. Neurologic findings range from normal development to psychomotor retardation and hydrocephalus.

☞**Adams-Oliver Syndrome:** Very rare inherited disorder characterized by defects of the scalp associated with multiple scarred and hairless areas that usually have dilated blood vessels directly under the skin. Scalp defects are present at birth. The extremities are either short (hypoplastic fingers and toes) or characterized by absent hands and lower legs. Congenital heart defects must be ruled out.

☞**Aplasia Cutis Congenita:** Most often inherited disorder with circumscribed or more extensive skin lesions that may also

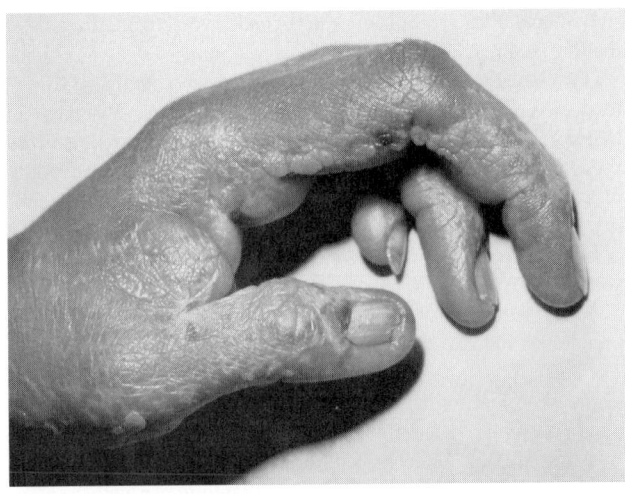

Goltz Syndrome Multiple papillomata and areas of hyperpigmentation in an adult with Goltz syndrome.

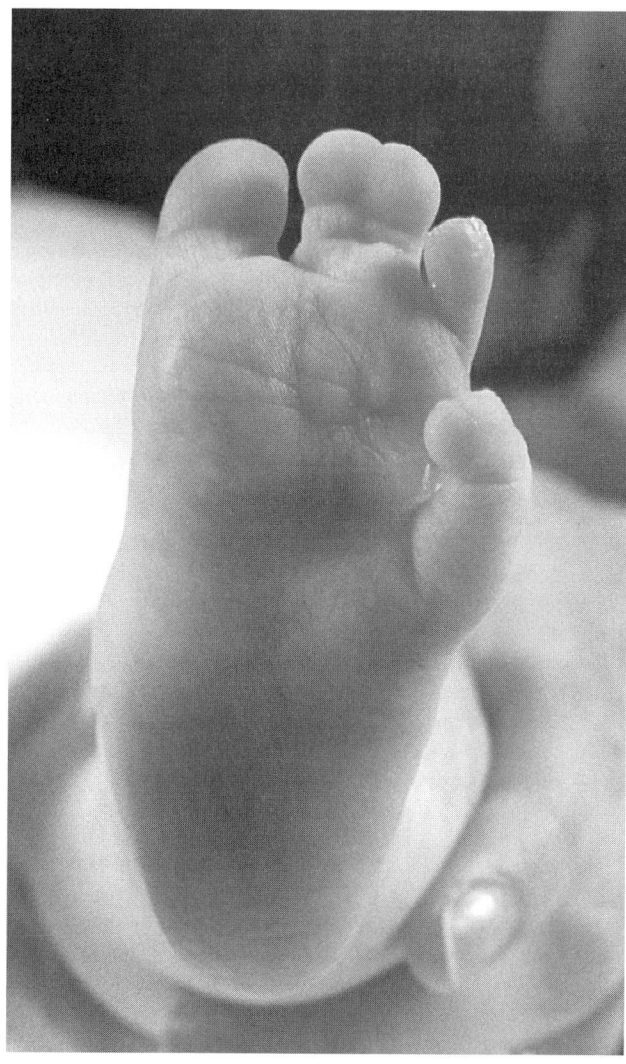

Goltz Syndrome   Split foot and syndactyly in a neonate with Goltz syndrome.

involve underlying tissues. Neurologic and cardiac anomalies have been described in these patients.

☞**DELLEMAN-OORTHUYS SYNDROME:** Multiple congenital anomaly syndrome mainly affecting the central nervous system, eyes and skin.

☞**EPIDERMOLYSIS BULLOSA:** Group of inherited bullous disorders characterized by blister formation in response to mechanical trauma.

☞**JOHANSON-BLIZZARD SYNDROME:** Polymalformative syndrome characterized by nasal alar hypoplasia (beak-shaped), scalp defects, hypothyroidism, pancreatic achylia, and congenital deafness.

☞**SETLEIS SYNDROME:** Puckered periorbital skin, absent or multiple rows of eyelashes.

REFERENCES:

Han XY, Wu SS, Conway DH, et al: Truncus arteriosus and other lethal internal anomalies in Goltz syndrome. *Am J Med Genet* 90:45, 2000.

Holzman RS: Airway involvement and anesthetic management in Goltz syndrome. *J Clin Anesth* 3:422, 1991.

Goodman Camptodactyly

At a glance: Mental retardation associated with cardiac and limb anomalies.

Synonym: Camptodactyly Fibrous Tissue Hyperplasia Skeletal Dysplasia.

Incidence and genetic inheritance: Extremely rare (two sisters and a brother); autosomal recessive.

Clinical aspects: Features include expressionless face with broad nose and flared nares, limb anomalies (camptodactyly, arachnodactyly of fingers and toes, clawhand, hammertoes, large hands), mental retardation, fibrous tissue hyperplasia, and scoliosis. Patent ductus arteriosus was present in the boy.

Anesthetic considerations: Involvement warrants thorough cardiovascular evaluation. Vascular access may be difficult due to the anatomical anomalies.

REFERENCE:

Goodman RM, Katznelson MB, Manor E: Camptodactyly: Occurrence in two new genetic syndromes and its relationship to other syndromes. *J Med Genet* 9:203, 1972.

Goodpasture Syndrome

At a glance: Time-limited (2 to 48 months) autoimmune disease with circulating antiglomerular basement membrane (anti-GBM) antibodies affecting the lungs and the kidneys of unknown cause (viral and streptococcal infections and exposure to hydrocarbon fumes have been suggested as causes). Often lethal during the acute phase; most patients who survive progress to end-stage renal disease.

Synonym: Antiglomerular Basement Membrane Disease.

Nature: Autoimmune disease, the major antigen target is the carboxyl terminus of the noncollagenous (NC-1) domain of the α_3-chain in type IV (basement membrane) collagen. The antibodies are directed against a 28-kDa monomeric subunit present within the noncollagenous domain. The disease may also occur in the transplanted kidneys of patients with Alport syndrome. There is an inherited predisposition to this syndrome (HLA-DRw2 is associated with anti-GBM disease).

Incidence: 1:100,000 people, most often males approximately 20 years old. White people are more affected than black people, as are certain ethnic groups (e.g., Maoris of New Zealand). A bimodal distribution has been reported (young men presenting with a pulmonary-renal syndrome and elderly women presenting mainly with glomerulitis).

Genetic inheritance: Genetic predisposition depends on genes localized on chromosomes 2 and 6.

Pathophysiology: The primary cause of the syndrome is the presence of antibodies directed against specific collagen chains, which are present in the glomerular and the pulmonary alveolar capillary basement membrane. Following an initiating event, for example infection or toxin exposure, an autoimmune response is set in motion, resulting in crescentic glomerulonephritis and progressive deterioration in renal function and leakage of blood from alveolar capillaries into the air spaces.

Diagnosis: The presence of bound anti-GBM antibodies in renal glomeruli is diagnostic. The antibodies are usually IgG, but may be IgA or IgM. Circulating anti-GBM antibodies are present in 90% of patients. Radioimmunoassays are more specific and sensitive than anti-GBM analysis. These findings, in addition to the presence of pulmonary hemorrhage, are pathognomonic of Goodpasture syndrome.

Clinical aspects: Hemoptysis ranging from blood-streaked sputum to massive hemorrhage is commonly the presenting feature. Patients may complain of dyspnea and cough. Pulmonary hemorrhage may be associated with severe hypoxemia and death. Intubation, assisted ventilation, and hemodialysis are often required in the acute phase. Renal function can range from normal to severe insufficiency, and the deterioration in renal function can occur rapidly. Some proteinuria is common, but nephrotic syndrome is rare. Hypertension is an unusual finding. Renal ultrasonography is usually normal. Pulmonary hemorrhage is often responsive to pulse methylprednisolone therapy, whereas renal involvement rarely is. Cyclophosphamide has also been used in the management. Plasmapheresis is frequently useful in the management of renal manifestations; however, many patients develop renal failure and require dialysis or renal transplantation. Transplanted kidneys may develop glomerulonephritis if anti-GBM antibodies are still present at the time of transplantation.

Precautions before anesthesia: Evaluate renal function: urea, creatinine, and electrolytes, and optimize K^+ if necessary. Evaluate pulmonary function: pulse oximetry, chest radiograph, and pulmonary function tests if indicated clinically. Consider perioperative corticosteroid coverage and plasmapheresis in the most severe cases.

Anesthetic considerations: The presence of renal failure must be considered when selecting anesthetic technique and agents. Patients may be dialyzed. The presence of pulmonary hemorrhage may affect the ability to oxygenate the patient adequately. Most patients are treated with corticosteroids and/or immunosuppressive agents, which may interfere with anesthesia care and make patients more prone to intraoperative and postoperative infections (consider nonnephrotoxic antimicrobial therapy).

Pharmacological implications: Agents requiring renal clearance must be used with care.

Other conditions to be considered:

WEGENER GRANULOMATOSIS: Autoimmune inflammatory vasculitis of unknown origin usually beginning as a localized granulomatous inflammation of the nasal and bronchial mucosa, progressing into generalized necrotizing granulomatous inflammation of the blood vessels and ultimately leading to general sepsis and multiorgan failure.

ACUTE COLLAGEN DISEASES: These diseases can temporarily mimic Goodpasture syndrome, especially systemic lupus erythematosus (positive antinuclear antibodies, positive antibodies to double-stranded DNA, presence of rheumatic factor, and extractable nuclear antigen antibodies).

REFERENCES:

Bolton WK: Goodpasture's syndrome. *Kidney Int* 50:1753, 1996.

Gallagher H, Kwan JT, Jayne DR: Pulmonary renal syndrome: A 4-year, single-center experience. *Am J Kidney Dis* 39:42, 2002.

Salama AD, Levy JB, Lightstone L, et al: Goodpasture's disease. *Lancet* 358:917, 2001.

Gordon-Holmes Syndrome

At a glance: Genetic disorder with hypogonadism and progressive cerebellar ataxia.

Synonyms: Cerebellar Ataxia and Hypogonadotropic Hypogonadism; Deficiency of Luteinizing Hormone-Releasing Hormone with Ataxia.

History: Gordon Holmes (1876–1966), an English neurologist, described this autosomal-recessive transmitted syndrome almost 100 years ago.

Incidence and genetic inheritance: Only a few case reports exist, and the underlying pathophysiology is not completely clear.

Clinical aspects: The first symptoms are that of hypogonadotropic hypogonadism, although there seems to be a broad clinical spectrum of this disease as patients with hypergonadotropic hypogonadism have been described as well. A defect in the production or the release of gonadotropins in the pituitary gland is responsible for the hypogonadotropic state. Most often, plasma concentrations of luteinizing hormone and follicle-stimulating hormone fail to rise after repetitive stimulation with gonadotropin-releasing hormone, which is consistent with a primary pituitary defect. However, a small number of patients do respond to exogenous gonadotropin-releasing hormone, suggesting a primary hypothalamic disturbance. Usually, in the third to fourth decade of life, progressive cerebellar ataxia and profound dementia develop, resulting in patients who are bedridden with no purposeful movements and finally death secondary to aspiration pneumonia. CT and/or MRI scans may reveal marked cerebellar and, to a lesser degree, cortical atrophy, as well as hypodensities in the cerebral white matter. Spasticity and nystagmus are not features of this disorder.

Anesthetic considerations: Although no case reports on this disease in association with anesthesia exist, it is probably best to apply the same precautions as in ☞Friedreich ataxia with regard to muscle relaxants (however, cardiomyopathy has not been described in Gordon Holmes syndrome). The use of a peripheral nerve stimulator during induction is essential to titrate the relaxants to effect and to closely monitor recovery. Because different muscle groups may be affected differently by the disease, it might be necessary to monitor (residual) paralysis in more than one site.

Pharmacological implications: Succinylcholine may elicit a hyperkalemic response, and the sensitivity to nondepolarizing drugs may be altered.

REFERENCES:

Holmes G: A form of familial degeneration of the cerebellum. *Brain* 30:466, 1907.

Seminara SB, Acierno JS Jr, Abdulwahid NA, et al: Hypogonadotropic hypogonadism and cerebellar ataxia: Detailed phenotypic characterization of a large, extended kindred. *J Clin Endocrinol Metab* 87:1607, 2002.

Gordon Hyperkalemia-Hypertension Syndrome

At a glance: Rare form of familial hypertension. Syndrome is characterized by hyperkalemia, metabolic acidosis, suppressed plasma renin activity, and hyperchloremia, but no renal failure. Positive effects of thiazide diuretics are associated.

Synonyms: Hypertensive Hyperkalemia; Familial Hyperpotassemia and Hypertension Pseudohypoaldosteronism Type II; PHA II.

History: Genetic disorder first described by Paver and Pauline in 1964 and singularized by Gordon in 1970.

Genetic inheritance: Transmitted as an autosomal dominant trait, but genetically heterogeneous.

Pathophysiology: Caused by mutations in WNK4 (a serine-threonine protein kinase) (17q21) or WNK1 (a lysine deficient protein kinase) (12p). An additional locus is probably located on 1q. A resistance to aldosterone regarding potassium, but not sodium transport, and a generalized cellular defect in transmembrane potassium transport, has been evocated to explain this disease.

Diagnosis: Based on the clinical findings (hyperkalemia, metabolic acidosis, absent plasma renin activity, hyperchloremia) in a patient with hypertension, already presenting in childhood.

Clinical aspects: Besides the main features, muscular weakness and periodic paralysis have been described.

Precautions before anesthesia: Evaluate renal function and electrolytes. Arterial blood gas analysis can be useful. Evaluate cardiac function because of hypertension and hyperkalemia (clinical, ECG, echocardiography). Check for signs of muscle weakness.

Anesthetic considerations: Perioperative cardiac monitoring (including invasive arterial blood pressure measurement if necessary) has to be considered. Hyperkalemia has to be corrected before surgery. Central regional anesthesia should be considered.

Pharmacological implications: Both insulin and bicarbonates have no effect on hyperkalemia. Thiazide diuretics can treat main features. Potassium-free intravenous solutions with reduced sodium concentration might be preferable.

REFERENCES:

Gereda JE, Bonilla-Felix M, Kalil B, et al: Neonatal presentation of Gordon syndrome. *J Pediatr* 129:615, 1996.

Mansfield TA, Simon DB, Farfel Z, et al: Multilocus linkage of familial hyperkalaemia and hypertension, pseudohypoaldosteronism type II, to chromosomes 1q31-42 and 17p11-q21. *Nat Genet* 16:202, 1997.

Gorham-Stout Disease

At a glance: Rare syndrome affecting bones and characterized by osteolysis; often associated with swelling or diffuse cystic angiomatous proliferation. Associated with massive resorption of bone matrix, often called the *vanishing bone disease*. Can affect only one bone or may have extension to nearby soft tissue and adjacent bones.

Synonyms: Diffuse Cystic Angiomatosis of Bone; Massive Gorham Osteolysis; Vanishing Bone Disease.

Incidence: More than 175 cases have been reported in the literature. Both genders seem to be equally affected.

Genetic inheritance: Autosomal dominant.

Clinical aspects: The monofocal osteolytic lesion may occur at any age, but is more common in the first three decades of life. While the lesion may affect any part of the skeleton, the skull, shoulders and the pelvis are the most frequently affected areas. Spontaneous fractures with absent fracture healing are common. The lesions may be painful to touch and temperature during the acute phase. Small intramedullary lesions of the bones later coalesce to form extensive areas of destruction with involvement of the cortical bone. The affected areas show sclerosis and significant proliferation of vessels (angiomatosis). Severe complications including death have been described, mainly resulting from spinal cord compression and severe chest wall involvement. Progressive deformations and contractures may occur. Laboratory investigations are usually normal. The disease seems to be the result of an in-

creased sensitivity of osteoclast precursors to humoral factors, which promote osteoclast formation and activity and hence bone resorption. Biphosphonates have resulted in clinical improvement in some patients.

Anesthetic considerations: They are related to the affected area. If the lesion affects the cervical spine, careful intubation with inline stabilization of the spine is recommended and since neck movement is expected to be limited in these patients, fiberoptic intubation may be the technique of choice. Careful positioning and padding are required to avoid spontaneous fractures.

Pharmacological implications: Succinylcholine should be used only after precurarization to avoid fasciulations that may result in spontaneous fractures.

REFERENCES:

Bruch-Gerharz D, Gerharz CD, Stege H, et al: Cutaneous vascular malformations in disappearing bone (Gorham-Stout) disease. *JAMA* 289:1479, 2003.

Hirayama T, Sabokbar A, Itonaga I, et al: Cellular and humoral mechanisms of osteoclast formation and bone resorption in Gorham-Stout disease. *J Pathol* 195:624, 2001.

Gorlin-Chaudry-Moss Syndrome

At a glance: Very rare syndrome characterized by craniosynostosis, midfacial hypoplasia, hypertrichosis, and anomalies of the heart, eyes, teeth, and external genitalia.

Synonyms: Craniofacial Dysostosis, Genital, Dental, Cardiac Syndrome; Craniofacial Dysostosis, Hypertrichosis, Hypoplasia of Labia Majora Syndrome.

Incidence: Less than 10 cases have been reported in the literature.

Genetic inheritance: Autosomal recessive.

Pathophysiology: Unknown.

Diagnosis: Characteristic features include dental anomalies, multiple eye malformations, and craniofacial dysostosis with genital and cardiac anomalies.

Clinical aspects: Patients present with either normal intelligence or mild mental retardation and short stature. This complex polymalformative syndrome associates facial anomalies that involve eyes (microphthalmos, down-slanted fissures, coloboma of the eyelid, defect of lacrimal system), mouth (anodontia or oligodontia, high-vaulted, narrow palate, cleft soft palate), ear (hypoplastic lobe and deafness), and skull (midface hypoplasia, brachycephaly, premature synostosis of the coronal sutures, hypertelorism, low hairline, and elevation of the lesser sphenoid wings). Other features include skeletal abnormalities (syndactyly of fingers, hypoplastic distal phalanges of hands and feet, and pectus excavatum), external female genitalia anomalies (hypoplasia of the labia majora, short vagina, and malformed uterus), umbilical hernia, hypertrichosis, and patent ductus arteriosus.

Precautions before anesthesia: Assess for signs of difficult intubation (clinical, radiographs) and evaluate cardiac function (clinical, echography, radiographs), particularly to determine size of the patent ductus arteriosus and the pulmonary artery pressure.

Anesthetic considerations: Careful intraoperative positioning is needed because of skeletal malformations. Face-mask ventilation and direct laryngoscopy can be difficult because of craniofacial anomalies. Venous access and pulse oximetry can be a challenge because of limb deformations and dermatoglyph modifications.

Pharmacological implications: Anesthetic drug choice must consider the existence of a patent ductus arteriosus with potentially increased pulmonary arterial pressures.

REFERENCES:

Gorlin RJ, Chaudry AP, Moss ML: Craniofacial dysostosis, patent ductus arteriosus, hypertrichosis, hypoplasia of labia majora, dental and eye anomalies: A new syndrome? *J Pediatr* 56:778, 1960.

Ippel PF, Gorlin RJ, Lenz W, et al: Craniofacial dysostosis, hypertrichosis, genital hypoplasia, ocular, dental, and digital defects: Confirmation of the Gorlin-Chaudry-Moss syndrome. *Am J Med Genet* 44:518, 1992.

Gorlin-Goltz Syndrome

At a glance: Autosomal dominant inherited ectodermal disorder characterized by basal cell nevi on the torso and shoulders with a potential of malignant degeneration.

Synonyms: Basal Cell Nevus Syndrome; Gorlin Syndrome. *[NB: Avoid confusion with focal dermal hypoplasia syndrome, which is also termed Goltz-Gorlin syndrome (or Goltz syndrome, Goltz-Peterson-Gorlin-Ravits syndrome, Jessner-Cole syndrome, or Liebermann-Cole syndrome).]*

History: Neurocutaneous syndrome first reported by the Hungarian dermatologist Moritz Kaposi in 1874 and 20 years later by Adolf Jarisch, an Austrian dermatologist. Further description by Robert James Gorlin, an American pathologist and geneticist, and the American dermatologist Robert William Goltz in 1960.

Incidence: Minimum estimated prevalence is 1:57,000 in the general population; 1:200 patients with basal cell carcinomas (one or more) had the syndrome, but the proportion is much higher (1:5) among those in whom a basal cell carcinoma develops before 19 years of age.

Genetic inheritance: Autosomal dominant inheritance with variable expressivity and high penetrance that appears to follow a similar course within single families. Evidence indicates the disorder results from mutations in PTCH, the human homologue of the *Drosophila* "patched" gene. Approximately 40% of cases represent a new mutation. Gene map locus is 9q22.3.

Pathophysiology: The causative gene probably functions as a tumor suppressor. This is based on the findings that deletion of the relevant region of chromosome 9q is found in many neoplasms occurring in the syndrome.

Diagnosis: Characterized by multiple basal cell nevi of the skin. The rib anomalies described below may be helpful for the early diagnosis. Molecular identification of the gene markers can be used in risk estimation and presymptomatic surveillance.

Clinical aspects: The main clinical characteristic is an enlarged head (macrocephaly) with facial abnormalities such as hypertelorism, keratocysts of the maxilla and mandible, dental dysplasia, skeletal abnormalities, calcified falx cerebri, and typical alterations at the sole and palm "pits" that are already obvious during infancy. The basal cell nevi occur in enormous numbers, most often increasing in numbers around the time of puberty. Basal cell carcinomas developed in approximately 85% of affected persons. Radiation treatment can result in fresh crops of aggressive basal cell carcinomas. Lip and/or palatal clefts are present in approximately 5% of cases, and mental retardation occurs at about the same frequency. Associated congenital lung cysts have been reported. Other skeletal abnormalities include bifid, splayed or fused ribs, kyphoscoliosis, and

spina bifida. There is also a predisposition to other tumor formations (medulloblastomas, ovarian tumors, and, rarely, cardiac tumors).

Precautions before anesthesia: Examine the airway for possible difficult intubation (facial asymmetry, dental defects, cleft lip/palate); endoscopic examination may be required to exclude verrucous lesions in the hypopharynx and supraglottic larynx obstructing visualization of the vocal cords. Evaluate pulmonary function tests (chest radiograph, arterial blood gas, forced vital capacity (FVC), peak expiratory flow rate (PEFR), (FEV_1) forced exspiratory volume in the first second, FEV_1/FRC (functional residual capacity). Elective surgery under general anesthesia is contraindicated when respiratory function is severely reduced (FVC <25%, PEFR <30%). A previous series of 36 patients with this syndrome reported three patients who developed severe bradycardia, hypotension, and bronchospasm with general anesthesia. The cause is unknown. Assess the effects of any associated hormone-secreting tumors.

Anesthetic considerations: General anesthesia with spontaneous respiration may be complicated by persistent partial upper airway obstruction secondary to supraglottic lesions. Tracheal intubation may be difficult as a result of these lesions and the presence of mandibular abnormalities. Scoliosis or kyphoscoliosis may compromise ventilation, and cardiac function (cor pulmonale) requiring postoperative mechanical ventilation.

Pharmacological implications: Nitrous oxide should be avoided in the presence of lung cysts. The presence of cleft palate, maxillary and mandibular cysts, and dental dysplasia may result in intubation problems; muscle relaxants should therefore not be used until the airway has been secured.

REFERENCES:

Bitar GJ, Herman CK, Dahman MI, et al: Basal cell nevus syndrome: Guidelines for early detection. *Am Fam Physician* 65:2501, 2002.

Gorlin RJ: Nevoid basal-cell carcinoma syndrome. *Medicine (Baltimore)* 66:98, 1987.

Veenstra-Knol HE, Scheewe JH, van der Vliest GJ, et al: Early recognition of basal cell nevus syndrome. *Eur J Pediatr* 164;126, 2005.

Gottron Syndrome

At a glance: A familial form of progeria in which premature aging of the skin and growth retardation predominantly affects the hands and feet. Small stature and micrognathia may be present. Cardiac assessment to rule out ischemic heart disease and/or congestive heart failure.

Synonyms: Familial Acrogeria; Familial Acromicria; Metageria; Acrometageria.

History: Described by Heinrich Adolf Gottron (1890–1974), a German dermatologist.

Incidence: Approximately 40 cases have been reported in the literature.

Genetic inheritance: Probably an autosomal dominant, sporadic, spontaneous gene mutation.

Pathophysiology: Underlying mutation of collagen gene leading to abnormality of collagen metabolism.

Diagnosis: Clinical course and features, raised urinary hyaluronic acid levels.

Clinical aspects: A premature aging syndrome where patients present with aged facies, wrinkled skin of feet and hands, joint hypermobility, and learning difficulties. Small stature and micrognathia may be present. Prominent vessels on the skin over the torso have been described. Premature aging syndromes may be associated with premature atherosclerosis, myocardial infarction, and congestive heart failure.

Precaution before anesthesia: Full cardiac assessment to rule out premature ischemic heart disease and/or congestive heart failure is recommended.

Anesthetic considerations: Mental retardation may be a feature, so the patient may require a sedative premedication prior to anesthesia. Possibility of difficult tracheal intubation in patients with micrognathia. Careful attention to patient positioning and pressure areas is mandatory since the skin may be thin and atrophic and the bone osteoporotic. The distal skin areas of the extremities may be bruised and ulcerated, making vascular access potentially difficult.

Pharmacological implications: All those associated with the potential presence of ischemic heart diseases and congestive heart failure.

Other conditions to be considered:

☞**PROGERIA SYNDROME (Hutchinson-Gilford Syndrome):** Severe form of progeria. The clinical characteristics include rapid aging, dwarfism, large head, small face, beak-like nose, exophthalmos, blue sclerae, and a receding chin. Other symptoms include dry, thin, and wrinkled skin that appears aged. Patients affected with this condition present with usually normal intelligence, but their life expectancy is significantly shorter than normal.

DE BARSY-MOENS-DIERCKS SYNDROME (De Barsy Syndrome; Progeroid Syndrome of De Barsy; Corneal Clouding-Cutis Laxa-Mental Retardation Syndrome; Cutis Laxa-Growth Deficiency Syndrome): Extremely rare, autosomal recessive disorder characterized by progeria, corneal clouding, dwarfism, and mental retardation. Other clinical features include ocular, facial, skeletal, dermatologic, and neurologic abnormalities.

☞**GRANDDAD SYNDROME:** Premature aging of the face combined with generalized growth retardation.

REFERENCES:

Blaszczyk M, Depaepe A, Nuytinck L, et al: Acrogeria of the Gottron type in mother and son. *Eur J Derm* 10:36, 2000.

Greally JM, Boone L, Lenkey SG, et al: Acrometageria: A spectrum of "premature aging" syndromes. *Am J Med Genet* 44:334, 1992.

Gradenigo Syndrome

At a glance: Now rare postinfectious syndrome caused by the extension of a middle ear infection to the petrous apex with abducens palsy.

Synonyms: Gradenigo Petrosum Syndrome; Gradenigo Triad; Gradenigo-Lannois Syndrome; Abducens Nerve Palsy-Petrous Osteomyelitis Syndrome; Petrous Osteomyelitis-Abducens Nerve Palsy Syndrome.

History: Guiseppe Conte Gradenigo, an Italian Otolaryngologist (1859–1926), described this syndrome in 1904.

Incidence: Incidence has widely decreased since the development of antibiotics.

Genetic inheritance: No genetic inheritance.

Pathophysiology: Caused by extension of an infection of the middle ear, mastoid sinus, or both to the petrous apex that occurs because of extensive pneumatization and the presence of bone marrow. The proximity of the venous sinuses to the petrous apex is the reason for the historically high incidence of venous sinus thrombosis as-

sociated with petrous apicitis. Petrous apicitis is believed to result when organisms, typically pseudomonas, become trapped within the complex air cell system of the petrous apex. Blockage of this air cell system may result from acute or chronic inflammation or from mechanical blockage by an obstructing lesion. The inflammation may extend into the Dorello canal, which contains cranial nerve (CN) VI and the Gasserian ganglion (CN V). Inflammation of the canal produces the triad of symptoms recognized by Gradenigo: lateral rectus (CN VI) palsy, retroorbital pain, and otorrhea.

Diagnosis: Based on the clinical findings of a coexisting ear infection and ipsilateral paralysis of the abducens nerve and otorrhea. Severe pain in the area supplied by the ophthalmic branch of the trigeminal nerve is generally associated. The MRI can show focal enhancement of the meninges over the petrous apex and extension of the infection into Meckel cave (the cavity that harbors the trigeminal ganglion).

Clinical aspects: Pain is typically severe, centered within the ear, burning or throbbing, worse at night, aggravated by jaw movement, pressure over the tragus, and traction upon the auricle. Pain can be observed simultaneously in the frontal and parietal regions. In the largest series of patients with petrous apicitis, the most common presenting symptoms were hearing loss in 60% of patients, deep pain (50%), CN VIII involvement (50%), CN VI involvement and meningitis (25%), facial paralysis (25%), CN IX palsy (15%), and CN X palsy (15%). Other features include excessive lacrimation, fever, and reduced corneal sensitivity. Extension of the inflammatory process can involve palsy of CN II through X, Horner syndrome. Thrombosis of the venous sinuses, hemorrhage of the carotid artery, and meningoencephalitis are the most serious complications. Before the introduction of antibiotics, mortality rate was greater than 50%.

Precautions before anesthesia: Evaluate neurologic function and review history (clinical, history, CT, MRI).

Anesthetic considerations: Avoid all intranasal probes because of infection. Since jaw movement may exacerbate pain, mouth opening may be limited in the awake state, but is expected to normalize once anesthesia has been induced.

Pharmacological implications: Avoid nitrous oxide because of its effect on pneumatized spaces that may result in increased pain.

REFERENCES:

Chole RA, Donald PJ: Petrous apicitis. Clinical considerations. *Ann Otol Rhinol Laryngol* 92:544, 1983.

De Graf J, Cats H, De Jager AE: Gradenigo's syndrome—A rare complication of otitis media. *Clin Neurol Neurosurg* 90:237, 1998.

Sherman SC, Buchanan A: Gradenigo syndrome: A case report and review of a rare complication of otitis media. *J Emerg Med* 27:253, 2004.

Graham-Boyle-Troxell Syndrome

At a glance: Very rare, non-malignant syndrome characterized by abnormal morphogenesis affecting both kidneys and lungs.

Synonym: Cystic Hamartoma of Lung and Kidney.

Incidence and genetic inheritance: Three cases have been reported worldwide. Inheritance unknown.

Clinical aspects: Clinical features involve the lungs (hamartomatous pulmonary cysts, lung fibrosis respiratory distress, chronic inflammatory lung disease) and the genitourinary system (bilateral multilocular cysts of the kidney, abdominal masses, renovascular hypertension, cellular mesoblastic nephroma, and possible markedly hyperplastic renomegaly with medullary dysplasia).

Anesthetic considerations: No literature available. Evaluate renal function (clinical, ultrasound, laboratory) and adapt intraoperative fluid regimen and drug choice (avoid nephrotoxic drugs and prefer those with nonrenal elimination). Evaluate respiratory function (clinical, chest radiographs, CT, pulmonary function tests, arterial blood gas analysis). Postoperative ventilatory support might be necessary. Perioperative chest physiotherapy can be useful. Avoid excessive airway pressures that could lead to rupture of pulmonary malformations. Intraoperative invasive blood pressure monitoring may be justified.

REFERENCE:
Graham JM Jr, Boyle W, Troxell J, et al: Cystic hamartomata of lung and kidney: A spectrum of developmental abnormalities. *Am J Med Genet* 27:45, 1987.

Grand-Kaine-Fulling Syndrome

At a glance: Rare form of cerebroretinal vasculopathy with characteristic subcortical degenerative lesions.
Synonyms: Retinal Vasculopathy with Cerebral Leukodystrophy; Cerebroretinal Vasculopathy.
History: Genetic disorder first described by M.G. Grand et al. in 1988.
Incidence: No known international incidence.
Genetic inheritance: Autosomal dominant inheritance. The responsible gene has been mapped to 3p21.3-p21.1.
Pathophysiology: Histopathologic analysis of brain tissue in affected persons demonstrated white matter "necrosis" without vasculitis.
Diagnosis: Based on the clinical findings of visual impairment and neurologic signs. Disease is characterized by progressive subcortical contrast-enhancing lesions with surrounding edema, mimicking tumors and often leading to biopsies in numerous patients. The association of retinopathy, ☞Raynaud syndrome, migraine, and kidney involvement should raise suspicion of this condition.
Clinical aspects: Features involve the eyes (retinal changes such as vasculopathy, exudates, or hemorrhage, visual loss, cataract, glaucoma, buphthalmos) and central nervous system (structural anomalies, speech defect, hemiparesis, seizures). Leg pain and weakness are frequent. Punctate vasculitic skin lesions can be observed.
Precautions before anesthesia: Evaluate neurologic function (clinical, CT, MRI, EEG, epilepsy control). Evaluate visual impairment (clinical, ophthalmologic consult).
Anesthetic considerations: Visual impairment and speech difficulties may make the operating area a scary environment for these patients. Sedative and/or anxiolytic premedication may therefore be helpful. Lubrication and protection of the eyes are required for patients with buphthalmos.
Pharmacological implications: Consider interaction between antiepileptic treatment and anesthetic drugs. Avoid drugs that can increase intraocular pressure or those that may trigger seizures.
Other condition to be considered:

VASCULAR RETINOPATHY WITH CEREBRAL AND RENAL INVOLVEMENT, RAYNAUD AND MIGRAINE PHENOMENA SYNDROME: Allelic to Grand Kaine Fulling syndrome.

REFERENCE:
Grand MG, Kaine J, Fulling K, et al: Cerebroretinal vasculopathy. A new hereditary syndrome. *Ophthalmology* 95:649, 1988.

Granddad Syndrome

At a glance: Very rare syndrome of premature aging facies combined with growth retardation.
Synonym: Growth Retardation, Aged Facies, Normal Development, Decreased Subcutaneous Fat Syndrome.
Incidence and genetic inheritance: Seven cases have been described worldwide. Probably autosomal dominant inheritance.
Clinical aspects: Patients present with intrauterine growth retardation and postnatal growth delay with normal mental development. There is decreased subcutaneous fat and thin or absent scalp hair. Main features involve the face, which seems prematurely aged with a triangular facies, prominent forehead, deep-set eyes, midfacial hypoplasia, prominent nasal septum, hypoplastic alar nasae, prominent ears, and thin lips.
Anesthetic considerations: Tracheal intubation and face-mask ventilation may be difficult because of anatomical abnormalities. Nasal intubation should be avoided secondary to small nares.

REFERENCE:
Marion RW, Goldberg RB, Young RS, et al: The GRANDDAD syndrome: A disorder combining growth delay, "aged facies," normal development, and deficiency of subcutaneous fat. *Am J Hum Genet* 45(suppl):A53, 1989.

Grant Syndrome

At a glance: Form of osteogenesis imperfecta with persistent wormian bones, blue sclerae, mandibular hypoplasia, shallow glenoid fossae, and camptomelia.
History: This disease is considered part of the large osteogenesis imperfecta family. However, because it could not be precisely categorized, Maclean called it by the family name of the first patient described.
Incidence and genetic inheritance: Only three cases of the same family that gave the name to this syndrome have been described. Probably autosomal dominant inheritance.
Clinical aspects: Patients present with short stature. Features involve head (blue sclera, frontal bossing, large fontanels with delayed closure, wormian bones, brachycephaly, poorly ossified skull, facial structural asymmetry with flat large face, depressed nasal bridge, high vaulted and narrow palate, micrognathia/retrognathia, and malocclusion) and skeleton (cortical hyperostosis, joint dislocation with hyperextensible knees, shoulder and wrist dislocation, bowed femur, tibia and clavicles, clubfoot, talipes-varus, narrow rib cage, sloping shoulders with scapula anomaly, pelvis anomaly). Hypotonia can occur.
Anesthetic considerations: Evaluate tracheal intubation that could be difficult because of facial malformations and may require adapted anesthetic techniques. Careful intraoperative positioning is required to avoid dislocations. Evaluate respiratory function (clinical, chest radiographs, CT, pulmonary function tests, and arterial blood gas analysis). Postoperative ventilatory support should be available.
Other condition to be considered:

☞OSTEOGENESIS IMPERFECTA: Group of disorders affecting the connective tissue, characterized by brittle bones, often fracturing without apparent cause. Four main types of osteogenesis imperfecta (OI) have been identified. *OI type I* is the most common and the mildest form of the disorder. *OI type II* is the most severe form. In most cases, the various forms of osteogenesis imperfecta are inherited as autosomal dominant traits.

REFERENCE:

Maclean JR, Lowry RB, Wood BJ: The Grant syndrome: Persistent wormian bones, blue sclerae, mandibular hypoplasia, shallow glenoid fossae and camptomelia—An autosomal dominant trait. *Clin Genet* 29:523, 1986.

Graves Disease

At a glance: Autoimmune disease resulting in nonsuppressible overproduction of thyroid hormone characterized by hyperthyroidism, goiter, and exophthalmos. There is often a family history of both Graves disease and autoimmune thyroiditis.

Synonyms: Basedow Disease; Begbie Disease; Diffuse Thyrotoxic Goiter; Flajani Disease; Flajani-Basedow Syndrome; Graves-Basedow Disease; Marsh Disease; Parry Disease.

History: First reported 800 years ago by the Persian physician Sayyid Ismail Al-Jurjani (in *Thesaurus of the Shah of Khwarazm*); Robert James Graves (1797–1853) was an Irish physician who described the disease including exophthalmos in 1835. The German physician Karl Adolph von Basedow (1799–1854) described the disease in 1840.

Nature: Autoimmune disease involving thyroidal and orbital tissue resulting in a goiter with thyrotoxicosis and ophthalmic abnormalities.

Incidence: 1% of the population suffers from Graves disease, with a female predominance (female-to-male ratio 4:1). Peak onset is in the third and fourth decades of life; only 5% of cases arise in childhood and adolescence. It is extremely rare in neonates (1:50,000 live births).

Genetic inheritance: Etiology is unknown, but there is a genetic predisposition to the disease. Both autosomal dominant and autosomal recessive inheritance have been suggested. May be multifactorial.

Pathophysiology: Production of thyroid-stimulating IgG immunoglobulins (TSI), which are antibodies to the thyroid stimulating hormone (TSH)-receptors of the thyroid follicular cell. TSI activate TSH receptors, which induces the intracellular production of cyclic AMP via adenylate cyclase, leading to excessive thyroid hormone secretion. In approximately 40% of cases, lymphocytic infiltration and deposition of glucosaminoglycans into the exterior eye muscles leads to Basedow ophthalmopathy. In neonates, the most common source of TSI is active transplacental transfer of IgG immunoglobulin from mothers with Graves disease and is therefore self-limited (4 to 8 weeks) and resolves with the disappearance of these TSI from the neonatal serum. Secondary to pituitary suppression of TSH production by the elevated levels of TSI, a transient period of hypothyroidism may follow.

Diagnosis: Clinical features; biochemical (high circulating levels of T_4 and T_3, low serum TSH, presence of TSI); imaging studies (diffuse and increased ^{123}I uptake).

Clinical aspects:

- *Antenatal:* Intrauterine growth retardation, fetal tachycardia, premature birth, and intrauterine death.
- *Neonatal:* Arrhythmias, systemic and pulmonary hypertension, heart failure, hepatosplenomegaly, prolonged neonatal jaundice, flushing, fever, diaphoresis, diarrhea, vomiting, failure to thrive (with sometimes profound weight loss), goiter that

may cause airway obstruction, and eye signs (lid lag, exophthalmos, and stare).

- *Childhood:* Marked weight loss despite enormous appetite, enlarged thyroid gland with bruit, tachycardia, hypertension, high output cardiac failure, tremors, nervousness, sweating, heat intolerance, diarrhea, hyperactivity, fatigue, behavior disturbances, poor concentration, hyperreflexia, and ophthalmic manifestations that are less severe than in adults; pretibial myxedema is rare in children.

Precautions before anesthesia: Thyroid function must be well controlled prior to anesthesia to avoid thyrotoxic crisis, which can be triggered by any form of stress including surgery, but also by iodine-based contrast agents. Baseline therapy consists of antithyroid drugs, such as methimazole, carbimazole, and propylthiouracil. However, it is important to realize that, in order to be effective, either of these drugs must be given 6 to 8 weeks before anesthesia. For more emergent interventions, potassium iodide and beta-blockers (e.g., propranolol or atenolol) for 7 to 10 days are effective in controlling the symptoms. A complete blood count with differentiation should be ordered, especially for patients on antithyroid drugs, which rarely can cause agranulocytosis, aplastic anemia, liver problems, and lupus-like syndromes. Cardiac function should be assessed by appropriate means. Adequate anxiolysis should be provided.

Anesthetic considerations: Difficult tracheal intubation should always be expected because neck imaging studies might not reliably indicate airway distortion or compression. Of significant concern in strumectomy patients is the risk of perioperative hematoma formation, which makes meticulous hemostasis adamant, and postoperative care personnel must be aware of this potentially serious complication. Expect respiratory compromise after extubation because of postoperative vocal cord pareses or tracheomalacia, although both complications are rare. Some patients might develop hypocalcemia, usually 24 to 48 hours after surgery. Treatment for thyroid crisis consists of antithyroid drugs, iodine, and supportive measures such as beta-blockers, fluid resuscitation, cooling, and inotropes if necessary. Steroids are often used to treat relative adrenal insufficiency during thyroid crisis. A few reports describe the successful application of dantrolene in refractory cases of thyroid crisis.

Pharmacological implications: For acute perioperative symptoms of hyperthyroidism, beta-blockers such as propranolol or esmolol are recommended. Unless there is evidence of congestive heart failure, propofol is safe and increased dosages might be needed in hyperthyroid patients.

Other conditions to be considered:

    ☞MCCUNE-ALBRIGHT SYNDROME: Characterized by polyostotic fibrous dysplasia, café-au-lait skin pigmentation, and autonomous endocrine hyperfunction, including hyperthyroidism.

    THYROIDITIS: Inflammatory acute (bacterial) or subacute (viral) infection, more common in patients with the human leukocyte antigen [HLA]-Bw35 antigen disease of the thyroid gland that can produce hyperthyroidism at the beginning of the evolution, thus mimicking Basedow disease.

REFERENCES:

Aust G, Sittig D, Steinert M, et al: Graves' disease is associated with an altered CXCR3 and CCR5 expression in thyroid-derived compared to peripheral blood lymphocytes. *Clin Exp Immunol* 127:479, 2002.

Chistyakov DA, Savost'anov KV, Turakulov RI, et al: Genetic determinants of Graves disease. *Mol Genet Metab* 71:66, 2000.

Hollingsworth DR, Mabry CC, Eckerd JM: Hereditary aspects of Graves' disease in infancy and childhood. *J Pediatr* 81:446, 1972.

Greig Cephalopolysyndactyly Syndrome

At a glance: Inherited polymalformative syndrome characterized by supernumerary digits, webbing or fusion of digits, large and unusually shaped skull, frontal bossing, and hypertelorism.

Synonyms: Polysyndactyly with Peculiar Skull Shape; Polysyndactyly-Dysmorphic Craniofacies, Greig type; Frontodigital Syndrome; Hootnik-Holmes Syndrome.

Incidence: Unknown; more than 100 cases have been described. First reported in 1926.

Genetic inheritance: Autosomal dominant. There is evidence that this disorder is caused by a mutation in the zinc finger domain of the GL13 gene (gene map locus 7p13). There is phenotypic overlap with the ☞Schinzel Acrocallosal syndrome.

Diagnosis: Based on clinical findings, family history, and genetic testing.

Clinical aspects: The range and severity of symptoms is quite variable. Macro- and scaphocephaly, a high forehead with frontal bossing and a broad nasal root with hypertelorism result in craniofacial dysmorphism, which however can be subtle in some cases. Although the gene for craniosynostosis is also located on chromosome 7, craniosynostosis is not a common feature of this disease. Intelligence is most often normal, but a few cases (less than 10%) have been described with agenesis of the corpus callosum, seizures and mild mental retardation. Broad thumbs and halluces, syndactyly (mainly of the fingers 3 and 4 and the toes 1–3), postaxial polydactyly of the hands, and preaxial polydactyly of the feet are typical. Hip dislocations have been reported.

Precautions before anesthesia: Although rare, signs of craniosynostosis associated with increased intracranial pressure should be ruled out. Cooperation may be limited in patients with mental retardation and sedative and/or anxiolytic premedication as well as the presence of the primary caregiver for induction of anesthesia may be helpful.

Anesthetic considerations: Peripheral vascular access may be a bit more challenging given the anatomical features of the disease. Careful positioning is recommended to avoid dislocation of the hips. Avoid arterial hypotension, hypoxia, hypercapnia, and hyperthermia in the presence of increased intracranial pressure (ICP).

Pharmacological implications: Avoid drugs that could result in a further increase in ICP and avoid premedication in this patient group (risk of hypercapnia and arterial hypotension).

Other conditions to be considered:

☞**Schinzel Acrocallosal Syndrome:** Polymalformative syndrome characterized by polydactyly and/or syndactyly, macrocephaly, mental retardation, ocular hypertelorism, agenesis of the corpus callosum, small nose and dysplastic ears; mostly sporadic but autosomal recessive forms have been reported.

☞**Acrocephalopolysyndactyly Type II:** Very similar clinical features but dwarfism is constant and genetic transmission is autosomal recessive.

☞**Pallister-Hall Syndrome:** Polymalformative syndrome characterized by craniofacial anomalies, polydactyly, cardiac and renal malformations, hypothalamic hamartoblastoma and endocrine disorders, and mild mental retardation; mostly sporadic but autosomal dominant mutations in chromosomes 3 and 7 have been reported in some cases.

Meckel-Gruber Syndrome: Autosomal recessive lethal polymalformative syndrome characterized by occipital encephalocele, polycystic kidneys, polydactyly, and pulmonary hypoplasia (leading cause of death); mapped to chromosome 17.

☞**Short Rib-Polydactyly Syndrome:** Congenital dwarfism with micromelia and narrowed thorax, polydactyly, and respiratory manifestations; constantly lethal.

☞**Ellis-van Creveld Syndrome:** Autosomal recessive disorder with short-limb dwarfism, polydactyly, dystrophic fingernails, cleft lip, cardiac malformations, and often prenatal eruption of the teeth; mapped to chromosome 4.

☞**McKusick-Kaufman Syndrome:** Autosomal recessive polymalformative syndrome characterized by congenital hydrometrocolpos, cardiac malformation, postaxial polydactyly, and respiratory, urinary, intestinal, and circulatory disorders.

☞**Psaume Syndrome:** Polymalformative syndrome characterized by oral (macroglossia, cleft palate, hypodontia), facial (hypertelorism, cleft lip, hypoplasia of the alae nasi, and micrognathia), digital (polydactyly, syndactyly, clinodactyly of fifth digit), and additional malformations (agenesis of corpus callosum, cerebral/cerebellar atrophy, Dandy-Walker malformation, polycystic kidney disease, mental retardation); caused by a mutation in the OFD1 gene (Xp22.3-p22.2).

☞**Mohr Syndrome:** Polymalformative syndrome characterized by cleft palate, facial deformities, short limbs with malformations of hands and feet, episodic neuromuscular disturbances, and mental retardation.

☞**Biemond Syndrome Type I:** Rare autosomal dominant polymalformative syndrome with cerebellar ataxia, mental retardation, nystagmus, strabismus, and short metacarpal and metatarsal bones.

References:

Jones KL: *Smith's Recognizable Patterns of Human Malformations.* 5th ed. Philadelphia, WB Saunders, 1997.

Kroisel PM, Petek E, Wagner K: Phenotype of five patients with Greig syndrome and microdeletion of 7p13. *Am J Med Genet* 102:243, 2001.

Griscelli Syndrome

At a glance: Albinism with immunodeficiency characterized by partial pigmentary dilution of the skin and hair (silvery gray hair), frequent infections, neurologic abnormalities, and fatal outcome caused by uncontrolled T lymphocyte and macrophage activation. Clinical features include the presence of large clumps of pigment in hair shafts and a pathological accumulation of melanosomes in melanocytes. Two types are described: type I with severe neurologic impairment and type II with immunologic deficiency.

Classification and synonyms:

- *Type I:* Griscelli Syndrome with Neurologic Impairment; Partial Albinism and Primary Neurologic Disease without Hemophagocytic Syndrome; Cutaneous and Neurologic type of Griscelli Syndrome.
- *Type II:* Chediak-Higashi–Like Syndrome; Partial Albinism Immunodeficiency Syndrome; PAID Syndrome.

Incidence: Approximately 60 cases have been described; most reported cases are from Turkish and other Mediterranean populations. The age at diagnosis ranged from 1 month to 8 years, with a median of 17.5 months (in 20 patients).

Genetic inheritance: Autosomal recessive disorder. The responsible gene is located on 15q21.

Pathophysiology: Histopathology of Griscelli syndrome (GS) involves prominent, mature melanosomes in skin and hair follicle melanocytes, but sparse pigmentation of adjacent keratinocytes. This leads to large, clumped melanosomes in hair shafts, resulting in hair that has a silvery-gray sheen. *Type I* is caused by mutation in the MyoVa (Myo5a)-gene, which is involved in melanocytic and neuronal cell vesicle transport. *Type II* is caused by mutations in the RAB27A gene, which encodes for a membrane-bound protein that is involved in signal transduction and similar to, or in combination with MyoVa, in the melanosome transport. Immunodeficiency often involves impaired natural killer cell activity, absent delayed-type hypersensitivity, and a poor cell proliferation response to antigenic challenges. The two genes encode for proteins, which are key effectors of intracellular vesicular transport. RAB27A seems also to be involved in the cytotoxic granule exocytosis.

Diagnosis: The single most consistent dermatological expression of albinism is the presence of silvery-gray hair. GS must be considered for any child with combined hypopigmentation and neurologic abnormalities (type I) or what is called hemophagocytic lymphohistiocytosis, (the acute phase of severe infections may be characterized by an uncontrolled activation of macrophages and lymphocytes, which is also called the accelerated phase) (type II). Microscopy examination of the hair shaft provides strong support for the diagnosis of Griscelli syndrome. The characteristic neurologic symptoms and analysis of lymphocyte cytotoxic activity of patients tend to incriminate one of the two molecular causes. Confirmation by DNA analysis.

Clinical aspects: Features include partial pigmentary dilution or albinism with silvery-gray hair, and down-slanted palpebral fissures. *Type I* is characterized by severe neurologic impairment (hypotonia, absence of coordinated voluntary movements and severely retarded psychomotor development, isolated congenital cerebellar atrophy) presenting early in life. *Type II* is characterized by frequent infections, cellular immune deficiency, and fatal outcome caused by an uncontrolled T-lymphocyte and macrophage activation syndrome. This is the accelerated phase (fever, jaundice, hepatosplenomegaly, lymphadenopathy, pancytopenia, and generalized lymphohistiocytic infiltrates of various organs, including the central nervous system) called hemophagocytic lymphohistiocytosis or hemophagocytic syndrome, which leads to death in the absence of bone marrow transplantation. It seems to be associated with viral or bacterial infection. When remission is obtained, recurrent accelerated phases with increasing severity will be observed. Neurologic signs (hyperreflexia, seizures, signs of intracranial hypertension, regression of developmental milestones, generalized hypertonia, nystagmus, and ataxia) appear during the accelerated phase and may regress with remission.

Precautions before anesthesia: Evaluate immunologic status (history, clinical, laboratory findings including a complete blood cell count). Evaluate respiratory function (because of frequent infections) and neurologic status (clinical, EEG, CT). During the accelerated phase, also assess renal and hepatic, function.

Anesthetic considerations: Strict asepsis is required. Severe anemia and/or thrombocytopenia should be corrected preoperatively and may need to be continued intra- and postoperatively. Increased intracranial pressure may exist and requires proper anesthesia technique according to standard neuroanesthetic guidelines. Avoid central neuraxial anesthesia techniques in patients with pancytopenia (bleeding, infection).

Pharmacological implications: Prophylactic antibiotics may be required in these immunodeficient patients. Consider interaction between antiepileptic treatment and anesthetic drugs. Appropriate choice of drugs according to hepatic and renal function.

Other conditions to be considered:

☞**CHEDIAK-HIGASHI SYNDROME:** Syndrome different from the Griscelli syndrome, which also associates partial albinism with immunodeficiency, but without giant organelle inclusion bodies in virtually all granulated cells, which is a hallmark of Griscelli syndrome.

☞**ELEJALDE SYNDROME:** GS Type I seems to be very similar to the Elejalde Syndrome, which features silvery hair and severe dysfunction of the central nervous system (neuroectodermal melanolysosomal disease). Clinical features include silver-leaden hair, bronze skin after sun exposure, and neurologic involvement (seizures, severe hypotonia, and mental retardation).

☞**HERMANSKY-PUDLAK SYNDROME:** Autosomal recessive inherited disorder associated with cardiomyopathy, restrictive lung disease, frequent abdominal pain, and severe coagulation disorder. Nystagmus and reduced visual acuity.

☞**OCULOCEREBRAL SYNDROME WITH HYPOPIGMENTATION:** Extremely rare autosomal recessive inherited syndrome (<20 cases have been described). Most symptoms are present at birth or develop shortly thereafter and may include very light skin color and silvery hair in combination with ophthalmologic (microphthalmia, corneal clouding, cataract, ectropion) and central nervous system anomalies (dolichocephaly, mental retardation, athetosis, ataxia, spastic paraplegia or tetraplegia). Gingival fibromatosis may develop at the age of eruption of the first teeth and may result in complete coverage of the teeth and become so significant that ventilation may be impaired. Ventilation can be further decreased by a dysfunctional diaphragm.

REFERENCES:

Griscelli C, Durandy A, Guy-Grand D, et al: A syndrome associating partial albinism and immunodeficiency. *Am J Med* 65:691, 1978.

Habermehl P, Althoff S, Knuf M, et al: Griscelli syndrome. *Klin Padiatr* 215:82, 2003.

Menasche G, Fischer A, de Saint Basile G: Griscelli syndrome types 1 and 2. *Am J Hum Genet* 71:1237, 2002.

Grisel Syndrome

At a glance: Subluxation of the atlantoaxial joint secondary to inflammatory processes (pharyngitis and pharyngeal abscess) and head and neck surgery. Major anesthetic implications (danger of quadriplegia, especially during laryngoscopy and tracheal intubation; massive bacterial pulmonary contamination if there is a rupture of a pharyngeal abscess).

Synonym: Nontraumatic Atlanto-Axial Subluxation.

History: Although first described in 1830 by the Scottish physician Charles Bell, it is named after the French otorhinolaryngologist P. Grisel who described the features in 1930.

Incidence: Rare. Literature suggests approximately 1:100,000,000 per year. Males and females are affected equally. Usually affects children, but may be diagnosed late into adulthood.

Genetic inheritance: Not inherited disorder.

Pathophysiology: Infection in the head and neck area spreads toward the upper cervical vertebrae. The inflammation causes laxity of the atlantoaxial ligament complex, leading to anterior subluxation of the atlas on the axis. This probably follows rupture of the transverse ligament and may result in spinal cord compression. The cause of infection may be (1) *postsurgery:* mastoidectomy, tonsillectomy, adenoidectomy, removal of tumors, or choanal atresia repair, (2) *contiguous infection:* rhinopharyngitis, tonsillitis, abscess (retropharyngeal to alveolar), or ear infections, or (3) *other more rare associations,* such as acute rheumatic fever or inflammatory bowel disease.

Diagnosis: Usually clinical and it may be missed for months until significant symptoms occur. Radiographs are of minimal value in the first 4 weeks, although flexion-extension views may be suggestive. CT- and MRI scans usually confirm the presence of rotational dislocation or anterior subluxation. Flexible nasopharyngoscopy is useful.

Clinical aspects: Usually presents with progressive unrelenting throat and neck pain followed by torticollis and subluxation. There is often little systemic reaction. The torticollis is usually acute and often occurs with sleep or minimal motion. Neurologic complications occur in approximately 15% of cases and range from radiculopathy to myelopathy, transient or permanent paraplegia, and even death. This can occur if the atlas becomes dislocated and can occur following only minimal trauma. Treatment includes antibiotics, surgical drainage of pus collections, bony stabilization and neurologic protection. In the acute phase of the disease, spinal protection often involves spinal traction treatment. Chronic disease may require fixation, which is commonly performed by an anterior approach.

Precautions before anesthesia: Once the diagnosis is made, the major concerns are spinal stability and the degree of neurologic compromise. This is usually well established by clinical examination and scan results. Assessment of the cause is important and may involve consideration of a retropharyngeal or other upper airway abscess. Full assessment of the neck is required because movement is usually severely restricted regardless of stability.

Anesthetic considerations: Tracheal intubation may be extremely difficult for several reasons: (1) unstable upper cervical spine with increased risk for any movements, such as jaw support for face mask; (2) high risk of complications if neurologic abnormalities are present; (3) causal abscess or other airway inflammation/infection; (4) limited neck movement and mouth opening because patient may be in traction; and (5) positioning is best performed awake when neurologic assessment is optimal. The position may be prone, although outcome is often better via an oral approach, in which case a nasal armored tube is preferred. Awake intubation using a fiberoptic scope is the technique of choice but often is impractical in children. This may be possible, however, under a spontaneously ventilating gas or intravenous general anesthetic technique; and spinal cord monitoring can be used to assess cord integrity. Once intubated and positioned, a wake-up test is used by some to establish cord function; but again, this is difficult and may be unpredictable in children. Maintenance of spontaneous ventilation is a way to ensure clinical upper cord function monitoring. Shared airway may lead to surgical and anesthetic problems, such as endotracheal tube compression and accidental extubation/disconnection.

Pharmacological implications: Use of neuromuscular blockade is best avoided because of loss of spinal cord integrity monitoring via respiration and response to motor and/or sensory stimulations (if unable to perform wake-up test). If succinylcholine is deemed necessary, fasciculations should be avoided (precurarization), since they may pose a serious risk to spinal stability. Induction with inhalational general anesthesia, intravenous propofol infusion, or ketamine may be considered.

Other conditions to be considered: Congenital causes of atlantoaxial instability may include the following disorders:

- Os odontoideum (absent, hypoplastic, or incompletely fused dens to body of C2). Atlantoaxial instability, as seen in ☞Morquio syndrome (mucopolysaccharidosis IV), ☞Osteogenesis imperfecta, and ☞Trisomy 21.

REFERENCES:

Baker LL, Bower CM, Glasier CM: Atlantoaxial subluxation and cervical osteomyelitis: two unusual complications of adenotonsillectomy. *Ann Otol Rhinol Laryngol* 105:295, 1996.

Guleryuz A, Bagdatoglu C, Duce MN, et al: Grisel's syndrome. *J Clin Neurosci* 9:81, 2002.

Mathern WM, Batzdorf U: Grisel's syndrome: Cervical spine clinical, pathological, and neurological manifestations. *Clin Orthop* 244:131, 1989.

Grix-Blankenship-Peterson Syndrome

At a glance: Very rare syndrome characterized by craniofacial malformations associated with osseous signs, mental retardation, and seizures.

Synonym: Craniofacial and Osseous Defects with Mental Retardation.

Incidence: unknown, but extremely rare.

Genetic inheritance: Autosomal recessive inheritance.

Clinical aspects: Features involve head (microcephaly, puffy eyelids (defect of lacrimal system), thick eyebrows, high nasal bridge, long bulbous nose, long philtrum, micrognathia, retrognathia, cleft tongue, cleft palate, thickened gingivae), abdomen (inguinal hernia, ectopic testes), and skeleton (bifid thumbs and toes, overlapping fingers, abnormal soles, sacrococcyx and rib anomalies). Dry skin, osteosclerosis, hypertonia and spasticity, mental retardation, seizures, and short stature are associated. Ventricular septal defects have been observed.

Anesthetic considerations: Evaluate cardiac function (clinical, echography, ECG). Anesthetic technique should be adapted in case of ventricular septal defect. Facial malformations may require tracheal intubation evaluation and adequate anesthetic management (fiberoptic intubation if necessary). Neurologic function and history of seizures and their control should be assessed.

Pharmacological implications: Subacute bacterial endocarditis prophylaxis is required in the presence of a ventricular septal defect. Avoid muscle relaxants until the airway has been secured. Consider interactions of anesthetic drugs with chronic antiseizure medications.

REFERENCE:

Grix A, Blankenship W, Peterson R, et al: A new familial syndrome with craniofacial abnormalities, osseous defects, and mental retardation. *Birth Defects Orig Artic Ser* 11:107, 1975.

Groenblad-Strandberg Syndrome

At a glance: Inherited connective tissue disorder characterized by progressive calcification and fragmentation of elastic fibers in skin, retina, and cardiovascular system leading to multiple vascular lesions caused by medial calcification of medium-sized and major arteries. Severe cardiovascular complications must be expected.

Synonyms: Pseudoxanthoma Elasticum; PXE.

History: First described by Ester Elizabeth Groenblad, a Swedish ophthalmologist, and James Victor Strandberg, a Swedish dermatologist, in 1929.

Incidence: Incidence in the general population is estimated at 1:100,000. Male-to-female ratio is 2:1.

Genetic inheritance: Various patterns: two autosomal dominant forms (type II, characterized by isolated skin manifestations) and two autosomal recessive forms (type I, represents 95% of patients), caused by mutations in the ABCC6 gene (adenosine triphosphate-binding cassette, subfamily C, member 6) probably mapped on 16p13.1. Sporadic cases have also been observed.

Pathophysiology: Unknown; An abnormal secretion of glycosaminoglycans by fibroblasts may result in coating of the elastic fibers. Another hypothesis is the presence of an abnormal protease that renders elastic fibers prone to calcification.

Diagnosis: Based on the clinical findings of skin lesions, which are almost always present, and start in the teen years at the neck, progressing to armpits, elbows, and groins and consisting of yellow papules, followed by visual impairment at approximately 25 years of age, but never leading to blindness (peripheral vision is preserved).

Clinical aspects: Features involve skin (small, yellow papules in mouth, neck, axilla, elbow, groin, and periumbilical region; orange peel appearance, elastosis perforans serpiginosa), eyes (angioid streaks of the retina in Bruch membrane, macular degeneration, decreased visual acuity, myopia, blue sclerae, retinal hemorrhages), heart and vessels (mitral valve prolapse, angina pectoris from premature occlusive vascular disease, arteriosclerosis, medial calcification of medium-sized and major arteries, diminished or absent peripheral pulses, claudication, congestive heart failure, restrictive cardiomyopathy myocardial infarction), gastrointestinal system (gastrointestinal hemorrhage, gastric and duodenal microaneurysms, arteriovenous malformations), skeleton (pectus deformities, kyphosis, scoliosis), and central nervous system (stroke, cerebral hemorrhage calcification of falx cerebri).

Precautions before anesthesia: Assess for occult blood loss (red blood cell count, fecal test, urine analysis). Evaluate cardiovascular function (clinical, ECG, Doppler ultrasonography, echocardiography). Evaluate ophthalmologic lesions (clinical, ophthalmologic examination).

Anesthetic considerations: Vascular risk is major and requires appropriate perioperative cardiac monitoring. Arterial blood pressure should be strictly controlled, but invasive monitoring is often difficult because of frequent loss of peripheral pulses and calcifications of the arteries. Avoid arterial hypotension. Regional anesthesia is not contraindicated, but vascular resistance response to sympathetic blockade is unpredictable. Renal failure may occur, so kidney function should be assessed.

Pharmacological implications: When choosing an anesthetic drug, consider these patients as suffering from coronary and arteriosclerosis. Postoperative hypocoagulation should be considered. Subacute bacterial endocarditis prophylaxis may be required if mitral valve prolapse is associated with mitral regurgitation or mitral stenosis is present.

Other conditions to be considered:

☞**EHLERS-DANLOS SYNDROME:** Characterized by joint hypermobility, hyperelasticity of the skin, and generalized tissue fragility including blood vessels and skin. The blood vessels may rupture even when exposed to minor trauma.

☞**MARFAN SYNDROME:** Inherited disorder that affects the connective tissues of the cardiovascular system. The musculoskeletal system is also affected, especially with scoliosis. Clinical features include anomalies of the lungs and the eyes.

REFERENCES:

Chassaing N, Martin L, Calvas P, et al: Pseudoxanthoma elasticum: A clinical, pathophysiological and genetic update including III novel ABCC6 mutations. *J Med Genet* 42:881, 2005.

Krechel SL, Ramirez-Inawat RC, Fabian LW: Anesthetic considerations in pseudoxanthoma elasticum. *Anaesth Analg* 60:344, 1981.

Levitt MW, Collison JM: Difficult endotracheal intubation in a patient with pseudoxanthoma elasticum. *Anaesth Intensive Care* 10:62, 1982.

Groll-Hirschowitz Syndrome

At a glance: Inherited syndrome characterized by progressive deafness, neuropathy, digestive and potential cardiac involvement.

Synonym: Deafness, Mesenteric Diverticula of Small Bowel, and Neuropathy Syndrome.

Incidence: Fewer than 10 cases reported in the literature.

Genetic inheritance: Autosomal recessive.

Clinical aspects: Features include *digestive signs* (small bowel diverticula, gastric motility loss, jejunoileal ulcerations, fat malabsorption, chronic diarrhea), progressive neuropathy, hemiplegia, and progressive sensorineural deafness (possibly due to cochleosaccular degeneration). Unexplained tachycardia and loss of the carotid sinus reflex may occur.

Anesthetic considerations: Evaluate neurologic function, particularly the severity of the neuropathy. Evaluate nutritional status and hydration (clinical, laboratory, including albumin, electrolytes, creatinine serum level, and urea). Perioperative cardiac monitoring (including invasive blood pressure monitoring if necessary) may be considered. A rapid sequence induction is recommended because of a high risk of aspiration secondary to abnormal gastric motility. Avoid succinylcholine in case of neuropathy.

REFERENCES:

Groll A, Hirschowitz BI: Steatorrhea and familial deafness in two siblings. *Clin Res* 14:47, 1966.

Potasman I, Stermer E, Levy N, et al: The Groll-Hirschowitz syndrome. *Clin Genet* 28:76, 1985.

Gsell-Erdheim Syndrome

At a glance: Aneurysms and dissections of the aorta usually result from degenerative changes in the aortic wall. Thoracic aortic aneurysms and dissections are primarily associated with a characteristic histologic appearance known as "medial necrosis" or "Erdheim cystic medial necrosis" which is characterized by degeneration and fragmentation of elastic fibers, loss of smooth muscle cells, and accumulation of basophilic ground substance. The association between congenital bicuspid aortic valve and medial necrosis of the aorta has been suggested. Ectopia of the pigment layer of the iris onto the anterior surface of the iris has been associated with this medical condition.

Synonyms: Annuloaortic Ectasia; Cystic Medial Necrosis of Aorta; Erdheim Disease; Erdheim-Gsell Cystic Medial Necrosis; Familial

Aortic Dissection; Erdheim Cystic Medial Necrosis of Aorta; Medionecrosis Cystica Erdheim-Gsell.

History: The first comprehensive description was published by Robert Otto Gsell, a Swiss physician in 1928, while the Austrian pathologist Jakob Erdheim contributed the pathoanatomical findings in 1929. King George II of England died of this condition while straining on a commode.

Incidence: The true incidence is difficult to estimate. However, based on autopsy results, the prevalence is approximately six new aneurysms per 100,000 persons per year. Evidence of aortic dissection is found in 1 to 3% of all autopsies.

Genetic inheritance: Autosomal dominant.

Pathophysiology: Loss of elastic fibers, deposits of mucopolysaccharide-like substances, and cystic medial changes in the aortic wall predispose to dilatation and dissection/rupture.

Diagnosis: Familial history (aortic dissecting aneurysms over generations), clinical features, chest radiographs revealing prominent ascending aorta, confirmed by echocardiography, and on arteriogram demonstrating dilatation of aortic root and sinuses of Valsalva. Left ventricular hypertrophy and bicuspid aortic valve may be present, as well as dilatation of the aorta more distally and dilatation of some of the major aortic branches. Histologic examination reveals the cystic medial necrosis of the aorta and deposits of mucopolysaccharide-like material (mucoid degeneration). Differential diagnosis includes ☞Marfan or ☞Ehlers-Danlos syndrome (patients with Gsell-Erdheim Syndrome are usually not tall and do not have hyperextensible joints and skin, or lens subluxation, or collagen and skin fibroblast anomalies).

Clinical aspects: A majority of affected patients are normotensive throughout life. A systolic ejection click is often heard on the left parasternal border. If not followed up and treated early, patients may die from ruptured or dissecting aortic aneurysm at a young age (teen years and early adulthood). Occasionally, coloboma and/or ectopia of the iris pigment layer on the anterior surface of the iris are observed.

Precautions before anesthesia: Cardiovascular evaluation: echocardiography (visualization of aortic valve and degree of dilatation of aorta, estimation of ventricular function); arterial angiogram if any doubt about involvement of distal aorta and its major branches. Inquire about beta-blocker treatment.

Anesthetic considerations: Prophylactic administration of beta-blockers to patients with documented aortic dilatation decreases myocardial contractility and the rate of rise of aortic pressure. Because left ventricular ejection velocity may be increased with vasodilators alone, the concomitant use of beta-blockers is recommended. Beat-to-beat blood pressure monitoring via an arterial line is indicated. In cases of severe ventricular dysfunction (very rare), further monitoring, such as intraoperative transesophageal echocardiography or pulmonary arterial catheter, may be considered. Any form of stress associated with tachycardia and high blood pressure should be avoided.

Pharmacological implications: The principal anesthetic goal consists of avoidance of sudden increases in myocardial contractility producing aortic wall stress. Anesthetic medications associated with sympathetic nervous system stimulation (e.g., ketamine, pancuronium) should be avoided.

Other conditions to be considered:

☞**Ehlers-Danlos Syndrome:** Heterogeneous group of heritable connective tissue disorders, characterized by joint hyperlaxity, skin extensibility, and tissue fragility.

☞**Marfan Syndrome:** Generalized connective tissue weakness with hyperextensible joints, increased risk of valvular/aortic disease, and pneumothorax.

References:

Burri H, Dielbold-Berger S, Didier D: Erdheim-Gsell cystic medial necrosis as a cause of giant aneurysm of the ascending aorta. *Heart* 87:22, 2002.

Leu HJ: Erdheim-Gsell medial necrosis and mucoid degeneration of the media as a cause of aortoarterial aneurysms. Pathologico-anatomical analysis of 150 excised vessels. *Schweiz Med Wochenschr* 118, 687, 1988.

Wells DG, Podolakin W: Anesthesia and Marfan syndrome: Case report. *Can J Anaesth* 34:311, 1987.

Guizar-Vasquez-Luengas Syndrome

At a glance: Inherited syndrome characterized by dermoids of cornea associated with short stature.

Synonym: Corneal Epithelial Dystrophy Short Stature syndrome.

Incidence and genetic inheritance: Two cases reported in the literature; autosomal recessive.

Clinical aspects: Features include skin tumors, short stature, corneal opacity (caused by corneal dermoids), and pupillary anomalies. The condition is distinct from other corneal dermoids by its inheritance mode.

Anesthetic considerations: Consider ocular protections. Careful intraoperative positioning is needed.

Reference:

Guizar-Vasquez J, Luengas-Munoz F, Antillon F: Corneal dermoids and short stature in brother and sister—A new syndrome? *Am J Med Genet* 8:229, 1981.

Gullner Syndrome

At a glance: Inherited syndrome that is similar to ☞Bartter syndrome, but with normal juxtaglomerular apparatus and abnormalities in the proximal renal tubule.

Synonym: Familial Hypokalemic Alkalosis with Specific Renal Tubulopathy.

History: First described by H.G. Gullner in 1979.

Incidence: Less than 10 cases have been described.

Genetic inheritance: Autosomal recessive.

Pathophysiology: Unknown. Hypokalemia is corrected by magnesium repletion, suggesting an interrelationship of magnesium and potassium metabolism.

Diagnosis: Clinically evocated by signs of hypokalemia and confirmed by biologic studies.

Clinical aspects: Fatigue and muscle cramps are the main features; they are associated with nausea and intermittent vomiting. Laboratory findings include hypokalemic alkalosis, abnormal magnesium metabolism, resistance of blood vessels to angiotensin II, sodium wasting by proximal tubular defect, elevated plasma renin, and elevated prostaglandin E_2 levels.

Precautions before anesthesia: Evaluate hypokalemia and hydration (clinical, electrolytes, creatinine and urea serum levels).

Anesthetic considerations: Hypokalemia and dehydration should be corrected before anesthesia is performed. Central venous catheterization may lead to cardiac rhythm disorder by direct endocavitary stimulation. Avoid advancement of the guidewire into the heart during central venous catheter insertion since endocavitary mechanical stimulation of the heart may easily trigger cardiac arrhythmias in these patients. Close perioperative monitoring of heart rhythm and hemodynamics is recommended.

Pharmacological implications: Care with use of bicarbonate, insulin, β_2-agonists or other drugs that could lower potassium serum levels. Try to avoid drugs that primarily rely on renal function for elimination or dose appropriately.

Other conditions to be considered:

☞**BARTTER SYNDROME:** Characterized by failure to thrive, growth deficiency, dwarfism, muscle weakness and cramps, and hypokalemia as a result of a renal potassium wasting syndrome. Mental retardation has been observed in some patients. An acid-base imbalance associated with hypokalemic alkalosis is pathognomonic of the condition. Low potassium levels may result from hyperaldosteronism. The exact cause is not known, but inheritance as an autosomal recessive trait has been suggested.

☞**GITELMAN SYNDROME:** Inherited renal tubular defect resulting in urinary loss of magnesium, sodium, potassium, and chloride with otherwise normal kidneys.

REFERENCES:

Gullner HG, Gill JR Jr, Bartter FC, et al: A familial disorder with hypokalemic alkalosis, hyperreninemia, aldosteronism, high urinary prostaglandins and normal pressure that is not Bartter's syndrome. *Trans Assoc Am Physicians* 92:175, 1979.

Gullner HG, Tiwari JL, Terasaki PI, et al: Genetic linkage between histocompatibility antigens (HLA) and a new syndrome of familial hypokalemia. *IRCS Med Sci* 8:369, 1980.

Gunn Syndrome

At a glance: Physical phenomenon that involves jaw movements and upper eyelid. Controversies exist about sensibility to malignant hyperthermia.

Synonyms: Jaw-Winking Syndrome; Marcus Gunn Syndrome; Trigemino Oculomotor Synkinesis Syndrome.

Incidence: Gunn syndrome is estimated to account for approximately 5% of all congenital cases of blepharophimosis.

Genetic inheritance: Several presentations have been suggested: sporadic cases, and autosomal dominant transmissions.

Pathophysiology: Caused by an aberrant connection between the motor branches of the trigeminal nerve (innervating the external pterygoid muscle) and the fibers of the superior division of the oculomotor nerve that innervate the levator superioris muscle of the upper eyelid.

Diagnosis: Generally possible to evocate at birth or after a few weeks when facing a child with unilateral congenital ptosis and rapid, exaggerated elevation of the ptotic lid on moving of the lower jaw.

Clinical aspects: Principal features are ophthalmic with strabismus (50–60% of cases), anisometropia (5–25% of cases), and amblyopia (30–50% of cases). Superior rectus palsy is found in 25% of cases and double elevator palsy in another 25% of cases.

Precautions before anesthesia: Obtain full personal and familial history with regard to malignant hyperthermia reaction in the past. Laboratory investigations may include preoperative creatine phosphokinase level because of the potential for malignant hyperthermia, although normal levels do not exclude a predisposition to malignant hyperthermia.

Anesthetic considerations: Relation with malignant hyperthermia susceptibility has been evocated on the findings of rare cases of histologic muscle anomalies. Close monitoring for signs of beginning malignant hyperthermia is therefore recommended, although to the best of our knowledge, no such care has been reported in connection with this disorder.

Pharmacological implications: Avoid halogenated agents and succinylcholine if possible.

REFERENCES:

Bullock JD: Marcus-Gunn jaw-winking ptosis: Classification and surgical management. *J Pediatr Ophthalmol Strabismus* 17:375, 1980.

Pratt SG, Beyer CK, Johnson CC: The Marcus Gunn phenomenon. A review of 71 cases. *Ophthalmology* 91:27, 1984.

Hageman Factor (Factor XII) Deficiency

At a glance: Inherited coagulation disorder caused by a deficiency in plasma protein factor XII (FXII) characterized by in vitro delayed blood clotting without a clinical bleeding tendency. The condition may also be acquired and temporary.

Synonyms: Factor XII Deficiency; HAF Deficiency; Hageman Trait.

History: Coagulation disorder first described in 1955 after routine preoperative laboratory examination of a patient named John Hageman.

Incidence: From 1955 to 2002, only a few hundred reported cases. Incidence is greater in patients of Asian origin.

Genetic inheritance: Autosomal recessive. Location of the Hageman factor gene was difficult; it was successively assigned to chromosome 6 and then 7, and now the gene map locus has been established as 5q33-ter.

Pathophysiology: FXII is a contact factor belonging to the kallikrein-kinin system or plasma. Patients affected with a deficiency in FXII do not experience abnormal bleeding because there is activation by other contact factors. The diagnosis is usually serendipitous. Partial thromboplastin time is elevated.

Diagnosis: Prolonged partial thromboplastin time; considerably decreased FXII assay. Condition usually discovered during routine laboratory examination.

Clinical aspects: Elevated partial thromboplastin time, no clinical bleeding in normal conditions. Occasionally, mild blood loss has been reported, mainly following trauma or surgery. Severe liver disease may lead to reduced production of FXII, worsening the (biologic) condition. FXII deficiency was reported to be a risk factor for thromboembolism as a result of inactivation of fibrinolysis. The disorder may be a risk factor for early gestational losses.

Precautions before anesthesia: Evaluate the coagulation profile and specific dosage of clotting factors. Even when partial thromboplastin time is considerably prolonged, there is no indication for fresh-frozen plasma, and common surgical procedures should not be contraindicated. These patients are not prone to develop a bleeding tendency but, on the contrary, might be at risk for thromboembolism (spontaneously and perioperatively).

Anesthetic considerations: Classically, there are no specific contraindications to anesthesia. However, bleeding problems may arise in procedures requiring use of anticoagulants (cardiac surgery), requiring close followup of both global coagulation tests and individual dosages of clotting factors. Despite contradictory statements in the literature, these patients might be at increased risk for thromboembolism. Close monitoring of coagulation status and clinical and Doppler ultrasonography evaluation for suspected thromboembolism are highly recommended.

Pharmacological implications: Administration of heparin may result in FXII deficiency; its use should be avoided in affected patients unless absolutely necessary (cardiac surgery, thromboembolism). Similarly, use of all anticoagulant agents is questionable and, basically, should be avoided.

REFERENCES:

Hasegawa T, Uematsu M, Tsukube T, et al: Huge left atrial thrombus with mitral stenosis in congenital factor XII deficiency. *Ann Thorac Surg* 73:286, 2002.

Roberts HR, Hoffman M: Hemophilia and related conditions—Inherited deficiencies of prothrombin (factor II), factor V, and factors VII to XII, in Beutler E, Lichtman MA, Coller BS (eds): *Hematology.* 5th ed. New York, McGraw-Hill, 1995, p 1434.

Zeerleder S, Schloesser M, Redondo M, et al: Reevaluation of the incidence of thromboembolic complications in congenital factor XII deficiency—A study on 73 subjects from 14 Swiss families. *Thromb Haemost* 82:1240, 1999.

Haim Munk Syndrome

At a glance: Rare syndrome characterized by the development of palmoplantar hyperkeratosis, pyogenic skin lesions, onychogryposis, and degeneration of the periodontosis.

Synonyms: Keratosis Palmoplantaris with Periodontopathia and Onychogryposis; Cochin Jewish Disorder.

History: Genetic disorder first described by S. Haim and J. Munk in 1965.

Incidence: Rare syndrome; only reported in a small community of Jews from Cochin, India.

Genetic inheritance: Autosomal recessive.

Pathophysiology: Caused by mutations in the gene encoding cathepsin C (CTSC). Gene mapped on 11q14.1-q14. Allelic with Papillon-Lefèvre syndrome.

Diagnosis: Evocated in patients combining hyperkeratosis, skin lesions, onychogryposis, and periodontodysplasia, particularly if patients come from the Cochin area.

Clinical aspects: Features involve *skin* (congenital keratosis palmoplantaris, onychogryposis), *teeth* (periodontosis, anodontia, oligodontia), and *skeleton* (pes planus, arachnodactyly, acroosteolysis). Frequent skin infections.

Precautions before anesthesia: Evaluate skeletal involvement (history, clinical, radiographs), teeth lesions (clinical, radiographs), and skin lesions. The investigation must include electrolytes and calcium levels.

Anesthetic considerations: Care with tracheal intubation because of possibility of teeth lesions. Strict asepsis is needed because of skin infections.

Pharmacological implications: Prophylactic antibiotics may be adapted to infectious status.

Other conditions to be considered:

☞**PAPILLON-LEFEVRE SYNDROME:** Characterized by the presence of palmar-plantar hyperkeratosis, periodontium, and periodontoclasia. Additional clinical features may include pyogenic skin infections, nail dystrophy, and hyperhidrosis. It is inherited as an autosomal recessive trait. There is some evidence that Papillon-Lefevre syndrome may result from certain mutations of the same gene responsible for Cochin-Jewish disorder.

☞**SCHOPF-SCHULZ-PASSARGE SYNDROME:** Characterized by the presence of palmar-plantar hyperkeratosis, fragile nails, hypodontia, hypotrichosis, and development of cysts on the eyelids. It is thought to be inherited as an autosomal dominant trait.

PACHYONYCHIA CONGENITA (Jadassohn-Lewandowsky Syndrome): Characterized by palmar-plantar hyperkeratosis and onychogryposis. Other clinical features include neonatal dentition, hypotrichosis, hyperhidrosis of the hands and feet, hoarseness, and potential for respiratory distress. Mental retardation may be present. It is thought to be inherited as an autosomal dominant trait.

MAL DE MELEDA: Characterized by palmar-plantar hyperkeratosis with unusually red skin that becomes abnormally thick. Affected children may present with abnormal nails, hyperhidrosis associated with an unpleasant odor (bromhidrosis), and lichenoid plaques. It is thought to be inherited as an autosomal recessive trait.

REFERENCES:

Haim S, Munk J: Keratosis palmo-plantaris congenita, with periodontosis, arachnodactyly and peculiar deformity of the terminal phalanges. *Br J Dermatol* 77:42, 1965.

Hart TC, Hart PS, Michalec MD, et al: Haim-Munk syndrome and Papillon-Lefèvre syndrome are allelic mutations in cathepsin C. *J Med Genet* 37:88, 2000.

Hajdu Cheney Syndrome

At a glance: Very rare diffuse connective tissue disorder with osteolysis involving mainly head and musculoskeletal system.

Synonyms: Cheney Syndrome; Arthrodentoosteodysplasia; Osteopathia Dysplastica Familiaris; Familial Osteodysplasia; Cranioskeletal Dysplasia with Acroosteolysis.

History: First described by N. Hajdu and R. Kauntze in 1948 and later by W.D. Cheney in 1965.

Incidence: Approximately 60 cases have been described.

Genetic inheritance: Autosomal dominant. Sporadic cases apparently represent new mutations.

Pathophysiology: Unknown. The disorder probably results from defective development of bone rather than destruction of bone already formed.

Diagnosis: Based on the clinical findings of short stature, hand pain, weakness, pathologic fractures, and distal osteolytic lesions.

Clinical aspects: The clinical phenotype is variable, and none of the patients have all the signs mentioned in the following description. At birth, many of these patients look normal or only show mild and unspecific dysmorphic signs, such as downslanted palpebral fissures, flat and broad nasal bridge, long philtrum, low-set ears, or hypertelorism. However, the facial appearance changes over time, that is, they become coarser, not starting before early or middle childhood. The diagnosis may be delayed until the patient is in the second or even third decade, when they typically present with swelling and pain of the fingers. The features of this disorder may involve the *head and neck* (normal intelligence, although mild developmental delay has been described in some cases), progressive hearing loss (one third of patients), speech abnormalities, bathrocephaly (a form of posterior sagittal synostosis), platybasia (basilar invagination, a developmental deformity resulting from seemingly upward pushing of the cervical spine and consecutive bulging of the occipital bone), multiple wormian bones, enlarged pituitary fossa without endocrine abnormalities, open cranial sutures, absent or hypoplastic frontal sinuses, low-set ears, midfacial flattening, mi-

crognathia or retrognathia (>50% of patients), cleft lip, high arched or cleft palate, early loss of teeth, hypertelorism, limited neck movement) and the *musculoskeletal system* (with short stature in >50% of patients), generalized osteoporosis predisposing to multiple fractures, terminal phalangeal acroosteolysis, cervical spine instability, vertebral anomalies (collapsed "fishbone" vertebrae), kyphosis, scoliosis, and joint hyperextensibility and dislocations). Other features are associated with the *respiratory system* (upper airway obstruction, vocal cord paralysis, deep voice), the *nervous system* [☞Arnold Chiari Malformation, hydrocephalus and cranial nerve damage (both possibly caused by platybasia), mental retardation, sensory changes such as pain and paresthesias may accompany the acroosteolytic lesions], the *cardiovascular system* (atrial and ventricular septal defects, patent ductus arteriosus, mitral and aortic valve disease, arterial hypertension), the *genitourinary tract* (cystic kidney disease in 14% of patients), hypoplastic kidneys, glomerulonephritis, reflux nephropathy, hypogonadism), the *abdomen* (intestinal malrotation, umbilical and inguinal hernias, hepatosplenomegaly), and the *skin* (hirsutism in childhood, dry and coarse skin, thick scalp hair). Although life expectancy reportedly has been normal in these patients, the literature supporting this statement is insufficient.

Precautions before anesthesia: The stability of the cervical spine should be assessed clinically and radiologically. Echocardiography should be obtained if cardiac lesions are suspected. The presence of hydrocephalus with increased intracranial pressure should be determined. Check renal function (creatinine, blood urea nitrogen), respiratory function, and airway (clinically, chest radiographs or computed tomography scanning, pulmonary function tests, arterial blood gas analysis).

Anesthetic considerations: The facial features in association with limited neck mobility and possible cervical instability suggest that airway management may be difficult. Maintain spontaneous respiration until the trachea is intubated and proper lung ventilation confirmed. Have a laryngeal mask available. Controlled ventilation with normocapnia or mild hypocapnia is recommended in the presence of increased intracranial pressure. Particular care is required for patient handling and positioning because of the predisposition to fractures and joint dislocations. Central neuraxial blockade is not contraindicated but should be expected to be difficult because of spinal deformities.

Pharmacological implications: Reduced dosage of predominantly renally excreted drugs in the presence of kidney failure. Subacute bacterial endocarditis prophylaxis may be required in the presence of cardiac lesions.

Other conditions to be considered:

☞**MELNICK-NEEDLES SYNDROME:** Genetic disorder characterized by abnormal bone development. Bowing of the bones in the arms and legs is characteristic. Particular facial appearance includes hypertelorism, full cheeks, small facial bones, and severe micrognathia. Other features include a relatively small chest cavity with irregular ribbon-like ribs, short clavicles, short stature, and narrow shoulders. Pectus excavatum is often present. Occasionally, dislocation of the hip may occur. Hydronephrosis caused by urinary retention as a result of small ureters may be present.

☞**SERPENTINE FIBULA-POLYCYSTIC KIDNEY SYNDROME (SFPKS):** Probably X-linked dominant inherited disorder with normal intelligence characterized by S-shaped (serpentine-shaped) elongation of the fibulas, bowed long bones of forearms and lower legs. Patients present with proportionate short stature, short neck, shield thorax with pectus excavatum and increased intermamillary distance. Other features include polycystic kidneys, large head with low-set ears, full cheeks, prominent eyes with megalocornea and ptosis, and micrognathia. Sensorineural deafness is not uncommon. Other characteristics may include congenital cardiac defects (e.g., atrial and/or ventricular septal defects, persistent ductus arteriosus), intestinal malrotation, joint laxity, and hirsutism. It has been suggested that SFPKS and ☞Melnick-Needles Syndrome are allelic disorders.

REFERENCES:

Ades LC, Morris LL, Haan EA: Hydrocephalus in Hajdu-Cheney syndrome. *J Med Genet* 30:175; 1993.

Brennan AM, Pauli RM: Hajdu-Cheney syndrome: Evolution of phenotype and clinical problems. *Am J Med Genet* 100:292, 2001.

Crifasi PA, Patterson MC, Bonde D, et al: Severe Hajdu-Cheney syndrome with upper airway obstruction. *Am J Med Genet* 70:261, 1997.

Hakim-Adams Syndrome

At a glance: Syndrome characterized (in adults) by the clinical triad of dementia (memory loss, bradyphrenia), gait ataxia (mimicking Parkinson disease), and urinary incontinence, caused by progressive hydrocephalus (without increase in CSF pressure) following previous trauma, subarachnoid hemorrhage, neoplasm, and infection. Children may present with at least two elements of the triad. Can be idiopathic with genetic predisposition.

Synonyms: Hakim Syndrome; Normal-Pressure Hydrocephalus; Normotensive Hydrocephalus; Occult Hydrocephalus.

History: Syndrome characterized by the presence of slowly developing normal-pressure hydrocephalus. Hydrocephalus was first described by Hippocrates.

Incidence: Internationally, the estimate in the general population is 1:25,000 cases and as many as 6% of patients affected with dementia. No gender proclivity. Increasing in the premature neonatal population as a result of periventricular/intraventricular hemorrhage. The likelihood of developing hydrocephalus is related to the severity of hemorrhagic lesions. The most common progression is to normal-pressure hydrocephalus.

Genetic inheritance: Not defined in the literature.

Pathophysiology: Following intraventricular/periventricular bleed in the newborn, the condition may result from obliterative arachnoiditis affecting mainly the posterior fossa or, less commonly, obstruction of cerebrospinal fluid (CSF) flow within the ventricular system by clots or other debris. The precise relationship between this and the genesis of brain injury in the newborn is unknown. In older children, there is usually clearly identifiable etiology or previous shunt surgery. Clinical symptoms result from stretching of the corona radiata by the distended ventricles. Dementia is attributed to distension of the fornix by the third ventricle, and incontinence is attributed to the involvement of sacral motor fibers. There seems to be an association between Hakim syndrome and either generalized vascular disease or deep white matter infarctions in adults.

Diagnosis: Usually clinical, initially with progressive dilation of the ventricles that may take days to weeks to reach the classic signs of hydrocephalus (head enlargement in infants, sun-setting eyes, irritability, lethargy, nausea, vomiting, weakness, cognitive difficulties, incontinence, headache). The older child may show signs of subtle psychomotor deterioration. Diagnosis of hydrocephalus is confirmed by ultrasonography through the anterior fontanelle (in infants) and by computerized tomography or magnetic resonance imaging when the fontanelle is closed. Nuclear medicine cisternogram reveals absent (or delayed) passage of tracer over convexities. Most patients undergo ventriculoperitoneal shunt derivation without prior assessment of CSF pressure, so the term *chronic hydrocephalus* has been proposed as an alternative title.

Clinical aspects: Neurologic examination usually reveals the presence of normal-pressure hydrocephalus, such as bulging fontanelle and inappropriate increase in head circumference. Most children also have at least two elements of the adult triad, consisting of psychomotor retardation, gait disturbance psychotic-like behavior, mild dementia, and urinary or fecal incontinence.

Precautions before anesthesia: Assessment of general considerations in the premature neonate. Assessment of previous medical or surgical management; if the hydrocephalus developed slowly, it may have been treated conservatively as many spontaneously resolve with time. Other therapies, such as use of drugs to reduce formation of CSF or repeated lumbar punctures to remove CSF, may have been given. If so, these treatments, plus complications such as the presence of infection, must be considered. Also assess for other abnormalities, especially Arnold-Chiari malformation.

Anesthetic considerations: Intracranial pressure by definition should be normal. However, a patient presenting for insertion of a ventriculoperitoneal shunt is usually in a worsening state, and general measures for increased intracranial pressure may be indicated, including use of cricoid pressure during laryngoscopy for tracheal intubation after a modified rapid-sequence induction and use of mild hypocapnia. Patients affected with psychotic-like behavior may present a significant challenge at induction of anesthesia. The use of sedative medication should be balanced against the risk of slight hypoventilation in the presence of raised intracranial pressure.

Pharmacological implications: Tracheal intubation following succinylcholine or rocuronium is preferable if progressive hydrocephalus has been confirmed.

Other conditions to be considered:

SYNDROMES WITH HYDROCEPHALUS: Aqueductal stenosis (can be inherited as an X-linked trait; gene map location is Xq28), myelomeningocele, Arnold-Chiari malformation, intraventricular hemorrhage, meningitis, tumor (including X-linked hydrocephalus).

☞DANDY-WALKER MALFORMATION: Congenital hydrocephalus syndrome caused by blockage of foramina of the fourth ventricle. This condition is associated with agenesis of the cerebellar vermis.

REFERENCES:

Bret P, Chazal J: Chronic ("normal pressure") hydrocephalus in childhood and adolescence. A review of 16 cases and reappraisal of the syndrome. *Childs Nerv Syst* 11:687, 1995.

Hakim CA, Hakim R, Hakim S: Normal-pressure hydrocephalus. *Neurosurg Clin N Am* 12:761, 2001.

Hill A: Ventricular dilation following intraventricular haemorrhage in the premature infant. *Can J Neurol Sci* 10:81, 1983.

Hall Riggs Syndrome

At a glance: Progressive disorder characterized by a flat nasal bridge, microcephaly, severe mental retardation, short stature, and metaphyseal–epiphyseal abnormalities.

Synonym: Hall Riggs Mental Retardation Syndrome.

Incidence and genetic inheritance: Very rare (described in two families with consanguinity); autosomal recessive.

Clinical aspects: Patients present with growth, motor, speech, and mental retardation. Features involve *head* (microcephaly, prominent forehead, depressed nasal bridge, anteverted nostrils, epicanthal folds, large lip, malformed teeth), *skeleton* (prominent sternum, brachydactyly and clinodactyly, clubbed fingers, short arms, joint hypermotility, scoliosis, bullet-shaped vertebrae, delayed bone age, epiphyseal and metaphyseal defects). Recurrent pneumonia and unexplained vomiting may occur.

Anesthetic considerations: Careful preoperative evaluation must include neurologic function [clinical computed tomography (CT), electroencephalogram (EEG)], tracheal intubation (clinical, radiographs) because of microcephaly, and respiratory because of recurrent infections (chest radiographs, pulmonary function tests if necessary). Direct laryngoscopy and tracheal intubation can be difficult. Prophylactic antibiotics may be considered to prevent pulmonary infections. Careful intraoperative positioning is needed. Postoperative mechanical ventilation must always be considered in presence of decreased respiratory functions.

REFERENCES:

Hall BD, Riggs FD: A new familial metabolic disorder with progressive osseous changes, microcephaly, coarse facies, flat nasal bridge and severe mental retardation. *Birth Defects Orig Artic Ser* 9:79, 1975.

Silengo M, Rigardetto R: Hall-Riggs syndrome: A possible second affected family? *J Med Genet* 37:886, 2000.

Hallerman-Streiff Syndrome

At a glance: Genetic polymalformative dysostotic syndrome characterized by distinctive craniofacial malformations including brachycephaly, bird-like facies with "parrot-beaked" nose, hypoplastic mandible, hypotrichosis, ocular abnormalities (congenital cataracts, microphthalmia), dental defects, skin atrophy (scalp and nasal area), severe tracheomalacia, and dwarfism.

Synonyms: Hallerman-Streiff-François Syndrome; François Dyscephalic (or dyscephaly) Syndrome; François Syndrome; Oculomandibulofacial Syndrome; Oculo-Mandibulo-Dyscephaly-Hypotrichosis Syndrome; Ullrich-Fremerey-Dohna Syndrome.

Incidence: Rare; 70 cases reported in the literature.

Genetic inheritance: Most cases have been sporadic (but with high frequency of parental consanguinity) with no sex predilection. Autosomal recessive and dominant forms have been reported.

Diagnosis: Based on clinical features and clinical course. Radiographic examination of the temporomandibular joints shows a characteristic change.

Clinical aspects: The syndrome associates a bird-like facies with hypoplastic mandible (in all dimensions) and "parrot-beaked" nose, microphthalmia, and congenital cataract. The cornea is small (diameter <11 mm) and coloboma is common, confirming the early disturbance of eye development. Hypoplastic mandible, high arched palate, microstomia, glossoptosis, natal teeth (inconstant), and hypodontia with malformed teeth contribute to the recognizable facial features of the patients. Proportionate dwarfism, hypotrichosis, skin atrophy, hypoplastic clavicles and ribs, and daytime hypersomnolence are usual. Mental retardation is observed in 15% of patients. Because of a narrow upper airway and most often associated tra-

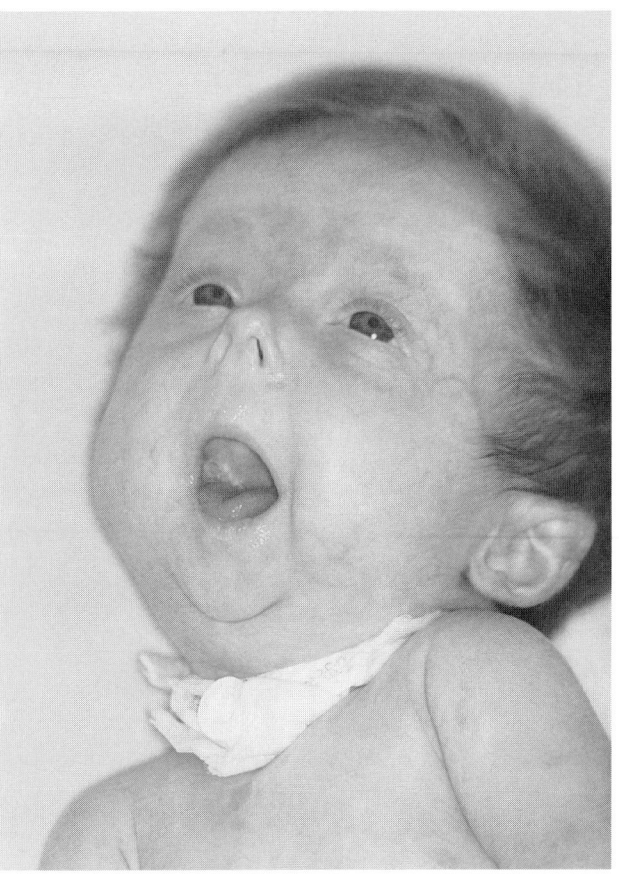

Hallermann-Streiff syndrome Airway obstruction secondary to small nares, glossoptosis, hypoplastic mandible, and tracheomalacia resulted in chronic respiratory failure, which required tracheotomy in this infant with Hallermann-Streiff syndrome.

cheomalacia, there is a danger of upper airway obstruction, particularly during the neonatal period and infancy. Obstruction may be a result of small nares and glossoptosis secondary to micrognathia, which may result in cor pulmonale. Tracheomalacia is a frequent complication that can lead to chronic respiratory insufficiency (subsequent biventricular cardiac failure and death has been reported in a 6-month-old infant). Sleep apnea is common in these patients.

Precautions before anesthesia: Anesthesia consultation is highly recommended prior to elective surgical procedures. Evaluation for difficult direct laryngoscopy and tracheal intubation because of hypoplasia of the mandible (use of fiberscope may be required, and nasotracheal intubation may be difficult because of the small nares). Management of the airway is expected to be difficult because of anatomical factors. Physical examination is directed primarily toward the central nervous system, cardiovascular system (cor pulmonale), lungs, and upper airway (tracheomalacia). Echocardiography is indicated. Standard preoperative laboratory examinations are appropriate in most patients (blood chemistries, blood group, hemoglobin, and coagulation).

Anesthetic considerations: Airway management represents the most significant anesthetic consideration. Maintenance of spontaneous respiration is highly recommended until the airway has been secured. Alternative airway management technique (e.g., fiberoptic,

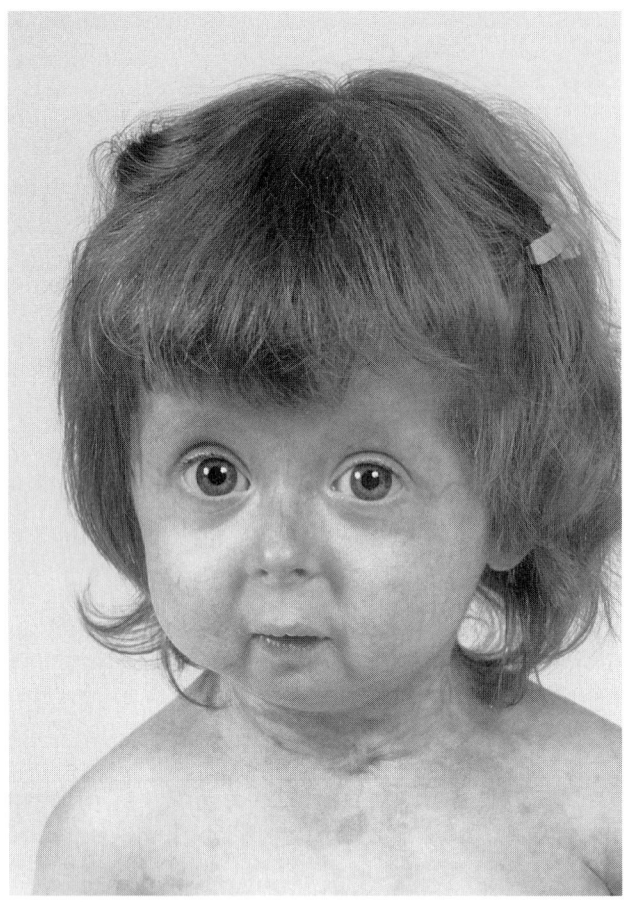

Hallermann-Streiff syndrome Toddler with Hallermann-Streiff syndrome had undergone a previous tracheotomy (scar) which, with increasing age and growth, was no longer required. However, this does not imply that airway management now is easy (note the small mouth and hypoplastic mandible).

retrograde intubating technique, etc.) must be available. A laryngeal mask might be useful but the presence of severe microstomia may prevent its insertion. The potential for cardiovascular involvement and pulmonary hypertension must be accounted. Postoperative mechanical ventilation may be required.

Pharmacological implications: All pharmacological considerations are not specific but rather determined by associated condition.

Other condition to be considered:

☞OCULODENTODIGITAL SYNDROME: Characterized by ocular abnormalities (microcorneas, microphthalmos, glaucoma, optic atrophy, short palpebral fissures), dental defects, craniofacial dysmorphism, many skeletal anomalies (including hand and foot malformations), and mild mental retardation.

REFERENCES:

Cohen MM Jr: Hallermann-Streiff syndrome: A review. *Am J Med Genet* 41:488, 1991.

Malde AD, Jagtap SR, Pantvaidya SH: Hallermann-Streiff syndrome: Airway problems during anaesthesia. *J Postgrad Med* 40:216, 1994.

Hallervorden-Spatz Disease

At a glance: Inherited disorder characterized by progressive degeneration of the nervous system caused by iron deposition in basal ganglia. Most commonly begins in childhood as a dystonic syndrome. Other clinical features include distorting muscle contractions of the face, limbs, and trunk, choreoathetosis, muscle rigidity, spasticity, seizures, and dementia. Less common symptoms include painful muscle spasms, mental retardation, and visual impairment.

Synonyms: Neurodegeneration Brain Iron Accumulation Syndrome; Late Infantile Neuroaxonal Dystrophy; Pantothenate Kinase-Associated Neurodegeneration.

Incidence: Very rare condition. Fewer than 100 cases described. No racial or sex predominance.

Genetic inheritance: The disease can be familial or sporadic. When familial, it is an autosomal recessive trait linked to chromosome 20 (gene map locus is 20p13-p12.3).

Pathophysiology: Not clearly established. The key factors seem to be an abnormal peroxidation of lipofuscin to neuromelanin and deficient cysteine dioxygenase, which result in iron accumulation in the brain. Whether the deposition of iron in basal ganglia in Hallervorden-Spatz disease is the cause or the consequence of neuronal loss and gliosis is not clear. A mutation in the *PANK2* gene (20p13) resulting in deficiency of pantothenate kinase may cause accumulation of cysteine, which can cause chelation of iron in the globus pallidus and produce neurotoxic free radicals.

Diagnosis: No biochemical markers yet found. Presence of abnormal cytosomes, including fingerprint, granular, and multilaminated bodies (suggesting the presence of ceroid lipofuscin), in bone marrow histiocytes and peripheral lymphocytes. Currently, the diagnosis can be ascertained only by histologic findings (postmortem).

Clinical aspects: Progressive rigidity, first in the lower and then in the upper limbs. Equinovarus deformity of the feet with walking difficulties. Involuntary choreoathetoid movements. Cranial nerves involved with chewing and swallowing difficulties. Torticollis and scoliosis. Oromandibular rigidity makes airway assessment difficult. Followed by dysarthria, epilepsy, and dementia. Onset occurs at 5 to 15 years of age, with death within 10 years following the diagnosis. At autopsy, brown coloration of the substantia nigra is seen.

Precautions before anesthesia: Proper evaluation of the airways and pulmonary function must be obtained, when feasible. Patients affected with this condition often receive chronic myorelaxant medication, which must be continued until the day of the operation. The use of an antisialagogue agent must also be considered.

Anesthetic considerations: Because of unpredictable and potentially difficult airway management, a spontaneous ventilation technique is recommended (however, because of choreoathetoid movements and muscle rigidity, neuromuscular blockade may often be needed, thus requiring tracheal intubation with assisted face-mask ventilation). However, before administration of neuromuscular blocking agents, ensure that lung ventilation can be supported by face-mask ventilation. With deepening of anesthesia, the torticollis, scoliosis, and oromandibular muscular rigidity disappear. However, following a long course of dystonic attacks and muscle rigidity, musculoskeletal deformations become fixed. Usual treatment should not be discontinued and should be resumed during the immediate postoperative period through a nasogastric tube. Signs of basal ganglias dysfunction (chorea, athetosis, and rigidity) reappear on emergence. Aspiration pneumonitis occurs easily. In the most severe situation, maintenance of postoperative mechanical ventilation might be indicated for better pain control management.

Pharmacological implications: Because of diffuse axonal changes and muscular denervation, hyperkalemic cardiac arrest following succinylcholine is a possibility. No problems related to inhalational anesthetics. Patients often receive antiparkinson agents and/or anticholinergics and benzodiazepines, which often interact with anesthetic agents. These interactions should be carefully considered throughout the perioperative period.

Other conditions to be considered:

HARP SYNDROME: Hypoprebetalipoproteinemia, acanthocytosis, retinitis pigmentosa, and pallidal degeneration (could be a variant of Hallervorden-Spatz disease).

☞HUNTINGTON CHOREA: Autosomal dominant neurodegenerative disorder characterized by involuntary (choreiform) movements and slowly progressive dementia, leading to death 15 to 20 years after the first clinical symptoms.

NEUROACANTHOCYTOSIS: Progressive neurodegenerative disease characterized by abnormal movements, seizures, cognitive deterioration, personality changes, and axonal neuropathy. At some point during the course of the disease, patients have acanthocytosis on peripheral blood smear.

☞NEURONAL CEROID LIPOFUSCINOSES: Group of neurogenetic (lysosomal) storage diseases characterized by seizures, progressive dementia, visual loss, and cerebral atrophy.

REFERENCES:

Hayflick SJ, Penzien JM, Michl W, et al: Cranial MRI changes may precede symptoms in Hallervorden-Spatz syndrome. *Pediatr Neurol* 25:166, 2001.

Roy RC, McLain S, Wise A, et al: Anesthetic management of a patient with Hallervorden-Spatz disease. *Anesthesiology* 58:382, 1983.

Swaiman KF: Hallervorden-Spatz syndrome and brain iron metabolism. *Arch Neurol* 48:1285, 1991.

Haltia-Santavuori Syndrome

At a glance: Neurodegenerative disorder caused by cricoid lipofuscinosis and characterized by onset at 6 to 18 months of age with rapid psychomotor deterioration, hypotonia, microcephaly, blindness, loss of speech, seizures, and ataxia.

Synonyms: Acute Infantile Neuronal Ceroid-Lipofuscinosis; CLN Type I; Hagberg-Santavuori Disease; Infantile Finnish Type of Neuronal Ceroid-Lipofuscinosis; Infantile Neuronal Ceroid-Lipofuscinosis (INCL); Neuronal Ceroid Lipofuscinosis Type I (early infantile); Santavuori-Haltia Disease; Polyunsaturated Fatty Acid Lipidosis.

Nature: Inherited neurometabolic disorder characterized by abnormal storage of the autofluorescent proteolipopigments in neuronal and other structures as a consequence of low or absent activity of palmitoyl-protein thioesterase 1.

Incidence: Average incidence of all lipofuscinoses is estimated at 1.5:100,000 live births. Haltia-Santavuori syndrome is one of the least frequent and affects mainly Finnish people.

Genetic inheritance: Autosomal recessive. Disorder caused by a defective gene (CLN1) coding for the palmitoyl-protein thioesterase, which is mapped to chromosome 1p32.

Pathophysiology: Palmitoyl-protein thioesterase is a small glycoprotein that removes palmitate groups from cysteine residues in lipid-modified proteins. It is thought to be involved in the catabolism of lipid-modified proteins and is involved in neuronal maturation processes.

Diagnosis: Deposition of lipofuscin in neural perikaryon, hepatocytes, heart muscle, retina, conjunctiva, skin, and lymphocytes.

Clinical aspects: Haltia-Santavuori syndrome is the infantile form of neuronal ceroid lipofuscinosis, which becomes clinically apparent between 6 and 18 months of age and presents as a rapidly progressive mental and psychomotor deterioration with hypotonia, microcephaly, convulsive disorders, blindness, and ataxia.

Precautions before anesthesia: Carefully evaluate neurologic status and seizure disorders [electroencephalography (EEG) recommended if not yet performed]. Consider visual and somatosensory evoked potentials and electroretinogram to identify eye conditions. The presence of abnormal dark retinal patches are common at eye examinations.

Anesthetic considerations: Not reported. Same anesthetic management as described for other neuronal ceroid lipofuscinoses.

Pharmacological implications: Antiepileptic drugs should be continued until day of surgery. Consider interaction between antiepileptic drugs and anesthesia. Cystagon might be a potential therapy for the disease.

Other conditions to be considered:

JANSKY-BIELSCHOWSKY DISEASE (☞Neuronal Ceroid Lipofuscinoses): Late infantile form of neuronal ceroid lipofuscinosis (NCF). It has an onset between 2 and 4 years of age. Until that time, children appear normal or may exhibit slight delays in psychomotor development. Clinical features include seizure episodes characterized by sudden breaks in action or thought, twitching of certain facial muscles, and petit mal seizures and/or grand mal seizures. Myoclonic seizures, ataxia, muscle hypotonia, gradual intellectual deterioration, and progressive blindness may be present. A variant has been identified in individuals of Finnish descent in whom the symptoms tend to appear later, at approximately 5 to 7 years of age and progress more slowly. It is inherited as autosomal recessive traits.

VOGT-SPIELMEYER DISEASE (☞Neuronal Ceroid Lipofuscinoses): Characterized by symptoms similar to the other two forms (infantile and late infantile forms) but with an onset later in life, at approximately 5 to 13 years of age. The clinical manifestations include gradual intellectual deterioration, seizure episodes, progressive motor impairment, and, particularly, progressive visual impairment.

KUFS DISEASE (☞Neuronal Ceroid Lipofuscinoses): Characterized by an onset during adulthood (third or fourth decade). The clinical symptomatology includes gradual intellectual deterioration, seizure episodes, progressive motor impairment, and progressive visual impairment.

☞ALPERS DISEASE: Characterized by an onset of symptoms during early childhood. The clinical features include progressive mental deterioration and motor impairment, intractable epilepsy, and impaired liver function. Most of the neurologic symptoms disappear because of degeneration of nerve cells of the brain.

☞RETT SYNDROME: Neurologic disorder that occurs only in females. Affected children appear to develop normally until approximately 6 to 18 months of age, at which time their psychomotor development stops and signs of developmental regression occur. Although the head circumference is normal at birth, infants show microcephaly by 1 year of age. Stereotypical hand movements, hyperventilation, retractable seizures, and loss of psychomotor development have been observed.

REFERENCES:

Goebel HH: The neuronal ceroid-lipofuscinoses. *J Child Neurol* 10:424, 1995.

Weimer JM, Kriscenski-Perry E, Elshatory Y, et al: The neuronal ceroid lipofuscinoses: Mutations in different proteins result in similar disease. *Neuromolecular Med* 1:111, 2002.

Young EP, Worthington VC, Jackson M, et al: Pre- and postnatal diagnosis of patients with CLN1 and CLN2 by assay of palmitoyl-protein thioesterase and tripeptidyl-peptidase I activities. *Eur J Paediatr Neurol* 5(suppl A):193, 2001.

Hanot-Chauffard Syndrome

At a glance: Very rare syndrome combining diabetes mellitus and hemochromatosis.

Synonyms: Troisier-Hanot-Chauffard Syndrome; Leschke Syndrome; Recklinghausen Applebaum Syndrome; Troisier Syndrome.

Incidence and genetic inheritance: Greatest frequency in men between 40 and 60 years old. The hereditary type is transmitted as an autosomal recessive trait first described by Troisier in 1871 and by Hanot and Chauffard in 1882.

Clinical aspects: Diabetes mellitus associated with hypertrophic cirrhosis of the liver and dark brownish skin pigmentation caused by deposition of excess of melanin, iron pigment, or both in tissues. Lassitude, weakness, weight loss, upper right abdominal quadrant sharp pain, dyspnea, and loss of libido occur. Occasionally, specific progressive polyarthropathy appears.

Anesthetic considerations: Assess diabetes and adapt intraoperative fluid regimen. The insulin management should be based on perioperative glucose level monitoring. Assess liver function (clinical, echography, CT, laboratory, including coagulation) and adapt anesthetic technique and choice of agents in consideration for the potential presence of hepatic toxicity.

REFERENCES:

Hanot VC, Chauffard AME: Cirrhose hypertrophique pigmentaire dans le diabète sucré. *Rev Med (Paris)* 2:385, 1882.

Troisier CE: Diabète sucré. *Bull Soc Anat (Paris)* 16:231, 1871.

Happy Puppet Syndrome

At a glance: Rare disorder characterized by developmental delay, ataxia, dysmorphic facial features, and seizures associated with a happy, sociable disposition.

Synonyms: Angelman Syndrome; Puppet Children; Puppet-Like Syndrome; Syndrome du Pantin Hilare (French).

History: Genetic or sporadic disease first described by Harry Angelman in 1965.

Incidence: 1:12,000–20,000 live births.

Genetic inheritance: Some cases are transmitted as an autosomal dominant trait.

Pathophysiology: Caused by a gene encoding ubiquitin-protein ligase (UBE3A) located on 15q11-13.

Diagnosis: Onset between 3 and 7 years of age. The affected children have a happy disposition and laugh frequently for almost any reason. Movements are jerky, like those of a marionette or puppet. Seizures are present in 96% of cases with a characteristic EEG.

Clinical aspects: Features include *neurologic disorders* (jerky movements caused by ataxia associated with hypertonia, brisk tendon reflexes, hyperreflexia, hyperkinesia, hypsarrhythmia, epilepsy, cerebral atrophy/myelin abnormality at MRI), *craniofacial malformations* (brachycephaly with occipital flattening, microcephaly, prognathism, macrostomia, oligodontia, protruding tongue, open mouth, widely spaced teeth, deficient pigmentation of the choroid with optic pallor and characteristic blue irides and Brushfield spots), and *skin* (hypopigmentation, blond hair). Associated with happy disposition, children present with hyperactivity, restlessness, absent speech, sleeping disorders, feeding problems, and drooling. Thoracic scoliosis can be observed.

Precautions before anesthesia: Evaluate tracheal intubation because of skull anomalies (clinical, radiographs). Evaluate neurologic function (clinical, CT, MRI, EEG, epileptic treatment efficiency).

Anesthetic considerations: Cooperation is impossible to obtain and often makes anesthetic induction difficult. Tracheal intubation can be difficult and may require adapted anesthetic management.

Pharmacological implications: Consider interaction between antiepileptic treatment and anesthetic drugs. Muscle relaxants should be avoided until airway is secure.

Other conditions to be considered:

☞**ALLAN-HERNDON SYNDROME:** Although most neonates and infants with this disorder appear to develop normally in the first few months of life, the presence of poor muscle tone is most often already present at birth. By 6 months of age, hypotonia, inability to hold up the head, and severe muscle atrophy are detectable. Severe mental retardation is associated with multiple congenital anomalies.

☞**FRAGILE X SYNDROME:** Most common form of X-linked mental retardation that affects males more often and more severely than females. Only subtle dysmorphic features, but behavioral issues may be more pronounced.

☞ **JUBERG-MARSIDI SYNDROME:** X-linked recessive inherited syndrome characterized by severe mental retardation, deafness, failure to thrive, microgenitalism, and early death.

☞ **MASA SYNDROME (Mental retardation, Aphasia, Shuffling gait, Adducted Thumbs Syndrome):** Extremely rare inherited disorder that is one of several disorders known as X-linked mental retardation syndrome.

RENPENNING SYNDROME: Extremely rare form of X-linked (moderate-to-severe) mental retardation. It has been linked to Xp11.2-p11.4. Other findings may include short stature, moderate microcephaly, prognathism, and small testes. Affected patients may use repetitive speech and show aggressive behavior. Longevity seems not to be impaired, and female carriers do not show any heterozygous signs.

SUTHERLAND-HAAN SYNDROME (Sutherland-Haan X-Linked Mental Retardation Syndrome; X-Linked Mental Retardation with Spastic Diplegia): Extremely rare form of X-linked severe mental retardation. Features of this disorder include short stature, spastic diplegia, significant congenital heart defects, and craniofacial abnormalities (microcephaly, cleft palate or high arched palate, abnormal ears, bulbous nose, broad nasal bridge, malar hypoplasia, micrognathia, and a small mouth). No reports exist about anesthesia in these patients; however, difficult airway management seems to be likely.

REFERENCES:

Angelman H: "Puppet children." A report of three cases. *Dev Med Child Neurol* 7:681, 1965.

Clayton-Smith J, Laan L: Angelman syndrome: A review of the clinical and genetic aspects. *J Med Genet* 40:87, 2003.

Williams CA, Lossie A, Driscoll D R, et al: Angelman syndrome: Mimicking conditions and phenotypes. *Am J Med Genet* 101:59, 2001.

Harboyan Syndrome

At a glance: Very rare condition characterized by corneal opacities present at birth and later-onset deafness.

Synonym: Corneal Dystrophy Perceptive Deafness.

Incidence and genetic inheritance: Very rare; autosomal recessive inheritance. Gene located on 20p13.

Clinical aspects: Features involve *eyes* (corneal clouding or opacity, abnormal corneal structure, severe visual loss, glaucoma, buphthalmos). Sensory neural *deafness* also occurs but later in age.

Anesthetic considerations: Avoid ototoxic drugs. Eye care protection is necessary because of buphthalmos. Medications that might increase eye pressure, such as atropine, succinylcholine, and ketamine, should be avoided.

REFERENCES:

Abramowicz MJ, Albuquerque-Silva J, Zanen A: Corneal dystrophy and perceptive deafness (Harboyan syndrome): CDPD1 maps to 20p13. *J Med Genet* 39:110, 2002.

Harboyan G, Mamo J, Der Kaloustian VM, et al: Congenital corneal dystrophy, progressive sensorineural deafness in a family. *Arch Ophthamol* 85:27, 1971.

HARD Syndrome

At a glance: HARD is an acronym for *h*ydrocephalus, *a*gyria, and *r*etinal *d*ysplasia. Very rare and severe autosomal recessive syndrome quickly lethal, with major neurologic impairment. It is characterized by type II lissencephaly in association with retinal dysplasia, obstructive hydrocephalus, and agenesis of the corpus callosum. Affected infants typically have severe growth failure, severe microcephaly, seizures, microphthalmia, and cataracts.

Synonyms: Walker-Walburg Syndrome; Warburg Syndrome; Chemke Syndrome; Pagon Syndrome (different from Pagon Bird Detter Syndrome); Cerebroocular Dysgenesis (COD); Cerebroocular Dysplasia Muscular Dystrophy Syndrome (COD MD).

Genetic inheritance: Autosomal recessive.

Pathophysiology: Caused by mutation in the gene encoding protein O-mannosyl transferase. Could be related to a primitive meningeal pathology (neurocristopathy).

Diagnosis: Clinical features. Prenatal diagnosis is possible.

Clinical aspects: Present at birth with polyhydramnios, decreased fetal movement and growth retardation. It is usually lethal within the first few months of life. This complex polymalformative disease involves the *head* with neurologic malformations (microcephaly, microtia, agyria, hydrocephalus type II, lissencephaly, corpus callosum and pellucidum agenesis, disorganized brain cytoarchitecture,

cerebellar malformation, ventriculomegaly and polymicrogyria), *ear* (absent auditory canals, low-set and bat ears), *eyes* (retinal detachment, cataract, microphthalmia, retinal pigmentary changes, anterior chamber malformation, hyperplastic primary vitreous, optic nerve hypoplasia, coloboma, glaucoma, and corneal clouding), and *mouth* (cleft lip/palate). Profound mental retardation and seizures are constant. Other features can include imperforate anus, genital abnormalities (cryptorchidism, small penis and testes), renal dysplasia, congenital contractures, and muscular dystrophy.

Precautions before anesthesia: Evaluate neurologic function (clinical, history, CT, MRI, EEG), renal function (clinical, echography laboratory investigations including urea, creatinine, electrolytes), and muscular function (clinical, serum creatine kinase level).

Anesthetic considerations: Careful intraoperative positioning is needed because of contractures and muscular anomalies. Avoid procedures that can increase intracranial or intraocular pressure, considering the neurologic and ocular malformations. Ocular signs for measurement of the depth of anesthesia cannot be used in these patients.

Pharmacological implications: Atropine must be avoided because of ocular lesions. Consider interaction between antiepileptic treatment and anesthetic drugs. Succinylcholine use is not recommended because of muscular dystrophy and risk of hyperkalemic response. Ketamine probably should be avoided because of its effect on intracranial and intraocular pressure.

Other conditions to be considered:

HARDE SYNDROME (Walker-Walburg Harrod Doman Keele Syndrome): Presents all the characteristics of the HARD syndrome plus encephalocele. Lissencephaly, malformation of the cerebellum, mental impairment, seizures, hypotonia, and eventually spastic quadriplegia accompany the clinical presentation. Dandy-Walker malformation, cleft lip/palate, microcephaly, and microphthalmia occasionally present.

HARROD SYNDROME: Autosomal recessive condition characterized by mental retardation, unusual facial appearance, hypotelorism, high arched palate, numerous genitourinary anomalies, hydrocephalus, and pyloric stenosis.

REFERENCES:

Dobyns WB, Pagon RA, Armstrong D, et al: Diagnostic criteria for Walker-Warburg syndrome. *Am J Med Genet* 32:195, 1989.

Karadeniz N, Zenciroglu A, Yavuz Gurer YK, et al: De novo translocation t(5;6)(q35;q21) in an infant with Walker-Warburg syndrome [letter]. *Am J Med Genet* 109:67, 2002.

Walker AE: Lissencephaly. *Arch Neurol Psychiatry* 48:13, 1942.

Hardcastle Syndrome

At a glance: Genetic disorder with dysplasia of the long bones associated with a high risk for transition in malignant histiocytoma.

Synonyms: Diaphyseal Medullary Stenosis with Malignant Fibrous Histiocytoma; Bone Dysplasia with Medullary Fibrosarcoma; Hereditary Bone Dysplasia with Malignant Fibrous Histiocytoma.

Incidence: Unknown but rare. Only four families with this syndrome have been reported in the literature since its first recognition by Arnold in 1973.

Genetic inheritance: Autosomal dominant pattern of inheritance with probable variable penetration of the gene. Gene linkage studies have isolated the syndrome to 9p22-p21.

Pathophysiology: Precise pathophysiology is unknown, but the region of chromosome 9 has been linked to the syndrome. It contains a number of genes whose protein products are involved in growth regulation, protein synthesis, and breakdown. At a cellular level, abnormal fibroblast function is the most likely cause of dysplasia.

Diagnosis: Made by clinical features and characteristic radiologic findings, which include diffuse diaphyseal medullary stenosis with overlying endosteal cortical bone thickening, scalloping, metaphyseal striations, infarctions, scattered sclerotic bone areas, and decrease of metaphyseal bone density with sparing of the epiphysis. Family members at risk are advised to have yearly radiographs of the lower limbs after puberty, and those with abnormalities on plain radiographs should have yearly bone scintigraphy scans thereafter (scintigraphy scanning will detect tumors within areas of dysplasia). Biochemical and parathyroid screening are normal.

Clinical aspects: Characterized by bone dysplasia with cortical growth abnormalities, which symmetrically affects the long tubular bones of the extremities. Spine and pelvis are unaffected. Radiographic evidence of the bone dysplasia has been reported from puberty onward, with a peak between the second and fifth decade of life. Of affected individuals, 35% develop malignant fibrous histiocytoma, a highly malignant bone sarcoma. Survival following diagnosis of malignant fibrous histiocytoma is very poor (usually less than 2 years). Morbidity results from pathologic fractures (prolonged healing and nonunion occur), bowing of the limbs, wasting of affected limbs, and painful debilitation. An association with presenile cataracts has been reported. Death is most often caused by multiple metastases (brain, lung, liver, kidney, heart, and bone). Current treatment is directed toward early diagnosis of malignant changes in dysplastic areas followed by amputation with or without chemotherapy.

Precautions before anesthesia: Detailed clinical history and examination to determine the extent of bone dysplasia and evidence of malignant changes and tumor metastases. If indicated (metastatic disease), assess cardiac function (ECG, echocardiography), pulmonary function (chest radiograph, spirometry, arterial blood gases), liver function, and renal function (blood urea nitrogen, electrolytes). CT or MRI scans (brain, lungs, heart, liver, kidney, bones) and hematologic screening (complete blood count and clotting screen) may be required.

Anesthetic considerations: Anesthetic technique is influenced by the metastatic disease and depends on the affected organs. Care with patient positioning must be taken because even minimal trauma may cause bone fracture.

Pharmacological implications: All routine medications should be continued preoperatively unless contraindicated. No other specific pharmacological considerations except for patients receiving chemotherapy and/or corticosteroids.

REFERENCES:

Arnold WH: Hereditary bone dysplasia with sarcomatous degeneration. Study of a family. *Ann Intern Med* 78:902, 1973.

Hardcastle P, Nade S, Arnold W: Hereditary bone dysplasia with malignant change. Report of three families. *J Bone Joint Surg Am* 68:1079, 1986.

Martignetti JA, Desnick RJ, Aliprandis E, et al: Diaphyseal medullary stenosis with malignant fibrous histiocytoma: A hereditary bone dysplasia/cancer syndrome maps to 9p21-22. *Am J Hum Genet* 64: 801, 1999.

Harlequin Syndrome

At a glance: Congenital skin disease in which the skin builds up and scales ("fish skin disease"). Associated with a very poor prognosis (usually death if infant is younger than 1 week).

Synonyms: Harlequin Fetus; Harlequin-Type Ichthyosis.

History: First reported in the diary of the Reverend O. Hart in 1750. Inheritable disorder of keratinization caused by a structural defect of tonofibrils (abnormal alpha-protein structure of keratin). This lesion is distinct from the lamellar exfoliative type of congenital ichthyosis, the prognosis of which is better.

Incidence: Rare (three cases per year in the United Kingdom). Harlequin syndrome is one of the four reported genetic disorders of keratinization displaying a structural defect of tonofibrils; the other three are bullous (or congenital) ichthyosiform erythroderma, Curth-Macklin form of ichthyosis hystrix, and ichthyosis hystrix gravior.

Genetic inheritance: Autosomal recessive. Chromosome 18 might carry the gene responsible for the disorder (transglutaminase 1 [TGM1]). Prenatal diagnosis is available (skin biopsies of the fetus).

Pathophysiology: In the harlequin fetus, an abnormal radiographic diffraction pattern of the horn material points to a cross–beta-protein structure instead of the normal alpha-protein structure of keratin. A suggested cause for this finding is an abnormality of keratinization.

Diagnosis: Characteristic clinical picture. Skin biopsy demonstrating severe cornification. Mutations in TGM1 are identified by sequence analysis of complementary DNA isolated from a fresh 2-mm skin punch biopsy.

Clinical aspects: Many are stillborn. Others are of low birth weight for dates and, as a rule, die in less than 1 week as a consequence of severe restriction of chest movement and abdomen incompatible with respiration and feeding. Thermoregulation disorders. Plaques, measuring up to 4 or 5 cm per side, have a diamond-like configuration resembling the suit of a harlequin clown. One patient survived 6 years with considerable failure to thrive, probably related to the enormous losses of protein in desquamated skin.

Precautions before anesthesia: In practice, because of the severity of the disease, harlequin syndrome patients are not eligible for surgery and anesthesia. Assess the severity of the disease, particularly in regard to the thoracic and abdominal involvement. Limit skin desiccation by providing continuous warm humidification of the baby. Assess nutritional state. Exclude the presence of hypovolemia caused by poor feeding. Check core temperature since hypothermia is often present. Investigations: hemoglobin, arterial blood gas analysis, serum protein, and albumin levels.

Anesthetic considerations: Venous access is often difficult. Strict aseptic measures must be taken for venous cannulation because the impaired skin barrier is predisposed to infection. Secure the venous cannulas with petroleum jelly gauze and tie or suture down. Adhesive tape likely will denude the skin and cause bleeding. ECG monitoring may require needle electrodes or pads without adhesive for the same reason. Semiflexed rigid limbs require careful positioning to prevent pressure sores. Severe ectropion and bulging eyes require ointment and careful taping to prevent ocular injury. Measures to maintain normothermia should be instituted. Involvement of the chest and abdomen that interferes with respiration may necessitate mandatory postoperative ventilatory support.

Pharmacological implications: Dehydration and hypoalbuminemia may affect the kinetics of drug distribution and excretion.

Other conditions to be considered:

BULLOUS ICHTHYOSIFORM ERYTHRODERMA (Epidermolytical Hyperkeratosis): Autosomal dominant disorder present at birth. It is characterized by thick warty scales on most of the body, especially in the creases of skin surfaces involved mostly with flexures. Blisters may occur. It is believed to result from an abnormal arrangement of tonofibrils.

CURTH-MACKLIN TYPE of ICHTHYOSIS HYSTRIX: Characterized by ichthyosis ranging from mild to severe. Severe palmoplantar keratoderma may occur with no other symptoms, or the whole body surface may be covered with scales. It is caused by concentric unbroken shells of abnormal tonofilaments around the nucleus.

ICHTHYOSIS HYSTRIX GRAVIOR (Porcupine Man; Lambert type Ichthyosis): Part of a group of epidermal nevus syndrome characterized by distinctive nevi on the skin apparent at birth that form in a line and usually are excessively pigmented. Often associated with neurologic and skeletal abnormalities (e.g., excessive bone growth, scoliosis, and clubfeet). Mental retardation, brain atrophy, brain cysts, seizures, and eye abnormalities may occur. Transmission is suggested to be an autosomal dominant trait that occurs in approximately two thirds of cases. Singular or multiple forms of the five major types of epidermal nevi have been described: raised wart-like streaks, polyp-like masses forming in lines, dark velvety spots, scaly streaks, or an orange, hairless, velvety patch covering part of the face, nose, eyes and scalp.

ICHTHYOSIS LAMELLAR: Serious skin disorder characterized by cornification that is the conversion of the upper layer of the skin into scaly or plate-like (squamous) skin. In serious cases, the ectropion of the eyelids and lips may be present. Erythroderma and palmoplantar keratoderma are present in the newborn. Lipid analysis from the stratum corneum of the skin shows increased free sterols and ceramides but normal hydrocarbon (alkane) content. Autosomal recessive and dominant forms have been reported.

☞**KERATOSIS ICHTHYOSIS DEAFNESS SYNDROME:** Present at birth and characterized by corneal keratitis, skin plaques on the extremities and face, palmar-plantar keratosis, and deafness. It is genetically transmitted as autosomal recessive and autosomal dominant forms.

RECESSIVE X-LINKED ICHTHYOSIS: X-linked ichthyosis occurs only in males and usually is present at birth or during infancy. It is characterized by large, dark, sometimes fine scales that are prominent on the neck and trunk. Skin on the palms and soles is normal. Opacities in the cornea of the eye occur. It is believed to result from an inborn error of metabolism and a steroid sulfatase deficiency.

☞**NETHERTON SYNDROME:** Hereditary polymalformative syndrome characterized by abnormal hair, ichthyosis, abnormal finger- and toenails, loss of subcutaneous fat resulting in a prematurely aged-looking face, mild mental retardation, and various neurologic disorders.

REFERENCES:

Akiyama M: The pathogenesis of severe congenital ichthyosis of the neonate. *J Dermatol Sci* 21:96, 1999.

Prasad RS, Pejaver RK, Hassan A, et al: Management and follow-up of harlequin siblings. *Br J Dermatol* 130:650, 1994.

Smith GB: Disorders of epidermal cell kinetics and differentiation, in Goldstone JC, Pollard BJ (eds): *Handbook of Clinical Anesthesia.* Churchill Livingston, New York, 1996, p 213.

Hartnup Disease

At a glance: Inherited metabolic disorder characterized by a pellagra-like skin eruption, cerebellar ataxia, and gross aminoaciduria. Most children are asymptomatic.

Synonyms: H Disease; Hart Syndrome; Hartnup Disorder or Syndrome; Pellagra-Cerebellar Ataxia-Renal Aminoaciduria Syndrome; Tryptophan Pyrrolase Deficiency.

History: Metabolic disorder of amino acids named after the first family in which the disorder was found (Hartnup family of London).

Incidence: Approximately 1:15,000 live births in the United States (similar to phenylketonuria); 1:18,000–42,000 live births in the rest of the world. No racial or sex predilection.

Genetic inheritance: Autosomal recessive (probably a monogenic defect that interacts with polygenic and environmental factors, giving a wide clinical spectrum). Gene located on 5p15.

Pathophysiology: Defect of transport of neutral alpha-amino acids (mainly tryptophan) across the intestinal mucosa and renal tubules as a result of defective tryptophan pyrrolase. Retained amino acids are converted by intestinal bacteria to indolic compounds, which have a cerebral toxicity.

Diagnosis: Amino aciduria limited to neutral alpha-amino acids, indicanuria (excludes nutritional pellagra). Oral tryptophan load causes urinary excretion of 5-hydroxyindoleacetic acid. Jejunal and skin biopsies may be required in selected patients.

Clinical aspects: Routine neonatal urine screening has indicated that many individuals with this defect are asymptomatic. Affected patients develop a photosensitive skin rash, usually beginning in children 3 to 9 years old (but may present during the neonatal period). Typically, after sunlight exposure, the skin reddens. A dry, scaly, well-marginated eruption may develop on the face and other light-exposed areas. With time, pigmentation changes may become definitive. More rarely, episodes of cerebellar ataxia, emotional lability, encephalopathy, and ocular manifestations occur. The episodes are reversible with treatment, which consists of nicotinic acid supplementation with a high-protein diet (in addition to use of creams for protection from sunlight). Exacerbations occur most often in spring or early summer after exposure to sunlight. They may be favored by febrile illness, poor nutrition, treatment with sulfonamides, and emotional stress.

Precautions before anesthesia: Assess extent of skin and neurologic involvement.

Anesthetic considerations: No particular difficulties with anesthesia have been reported. Periods of induced stress may be associated with acute exacerbation in some patients.

Pharmacological implications: Administration of sulfonamides should be avoided because they may exacerbate the disease.

Other conditions to be considered:

HYDROA VACCINIFORME (Bazin Hydroa Vacciniforme): Rare, chronic photodermatosis of unknown etiology. Recurrent vesicles on sun-exposed skin that heal with vacciniform or varioliform scarring. The histopathology is distinctive with intraepidermal reticular degeneration and cellular necrosis. May be accompanied by mild keratoconjunctivitis and photophobia.

PITYRIASIS ALBA: Common hypopigmented dermatitis that occurs primarily in school-age children (3–16 years of age). Occasionally occurs in adults. In the United States, the incidence is believed to be 33% of school-age children; the condition is more obvious during sun exposure. Approximately 40% of Egyptian children are affected. Nonspecific dermatitis of unknown etiology.

☞**XERODERMA PIGMENTOSUM:** Syndrome characterized by a defect in ultraviolet radiation-induced DNA repair mechanisms. It is characterized by severe sensitivity to all sources of UV radiation (especially sunlight). Xeroderma pigmentosum is categorized into seven complementation groups according to the capacity of the body to repair DNA. It is a life-threatening disorder. DNA damage is cumulative and irreversible. Often lethal in infancy or childhood.

REFERENCE:

Nozaki J, Dakeishi M, Ohura T, et al: Homozygosity mapping to chromosome 5p15 of a gene responsible for Hartnup disorder. *Biochem Biophys Res Commun* 284:255, 2001.

HDR Syndrome

At a glance: HDR is an acronym for *h*ypoparathyroidism, *d*eafness, and *r*enal dysplasia. DiGeorge-like syndrome characterized by hypoparathyroidism, heart defects, immune deficiency, deafness, and renal malformations caused by a haplo-insufficiency of the zinc-finger transcription factor GATA3.

Synonyms: Baraka Syndrome; Nephrosis Nerve Deafness Hypoparathyroidism Syndrome.

Incidence: Approximately 40 cases described in the literature worldwide.

Genetic inheritance: Autosomal dominant disorder caused by mutations in the GATA3 gene on chromosome 10. Gene map location is 10p15.

Pathophysiology: The GATA3 gene is part of the family of zinc-finger transcription factors; it is involved in vertebrate embryonic development and in the development of the parathyroids, inner ear, and kidneys.

Diagnosis: Diagnosis is based on clinical and laboratory stigmata, genetic testing, and family history.

Clinical aspects: The typical triad of HDR—sensorineural deafness, hypocalcemia and/or hypoparathyroidism, and nephropathy—is present in almost all patients. The manifestation of renal involvement is variable and may range from vesicoureteral reflux to kidney aplasia. Developmental delay, seizure disorder, and a high incidence of cerebral infarcts have been described. Mild dysmorphic features may be present and may include hypertelorism, flat nose, proptosis, high arched palate, micrognathia, and limb anomalies.

Precautions before anesthesia: Clinical examination with emphasis on facial malformations and routine blood work, including complete blood count, electrolytes, calcium, glucose, and kidney function test are required. Hematologic or biochemical disturbances, especially hypocalcemia, must be corrected prior to anesthesia. A complete medical history and current medication, for example, antiseizure drugs with the potential for drug interactions with anesthetic agents, must be documented. Anxiolysis is particularly important with deafness and mental retardation.

Anesthetic considerations: Calcium levels should be monitored regularly during blood transfusions or albumin infusions and corrected if necessary. Tracheal extubation can be difficult in patients with severe mental retardation because of the presence of chronic lung disease from recurrent aspirations and reduced ability to cough. In these more severely affected patients, the potential for postoperative mechanical ventilation must be considered and intensive care admission planned ahead.

Pharmacological implications: Negative inotropic effects of anesthetic agents and response to neuromuscular blockade might be enhanced in the presence of hypocalcemia. Drugs with predominantly renal elimination should be used with caution in the presence of impaired kidney function. Consider antibioprophylaxis because these patients have potentially severe impairment of immune function.

Other conditions to be considered:

☞**DIGEORGE SYNDROME:** Developmental field defect with facial dysmorphism, congenital heart defect, hypocalcemia, hypoparathyroidism, thymus hypoplasia, and increased susceptibility to infections. The hallmarks include conotruncal absence or hypoplasia of thymus and parathyroid glands. Mostly caused by a microdeletion in chromosome 22q11.2.

☞**VELOCARDIOFACIAL SYNDROME:** Unusual face syndrome. Seems associated with a defect of chromosome 22 (deletion 22q11). The most common features are cleft palate, congenital heart defects (interrupted aortic arch, truncus arteriosus, tetralogy of Fallot with pulmonary atresia, absent pulmonary valve syndrome, simple tetralogy of Fallot, ventriculoseptal defect, and D-transposition of the great arteries), hypoparathyroidism, seizures, muscular hypotonia, short stature, and scoliosis. The incidence of velocardiofacial syndrome is 8% of all children born with cleft palate.

CONOTRUNCAL ANOMALY FACE SYNDROME (Takao Syndrome): Overlaps with DiGeorge syndrome with the phenotypic spectrum of a deletion of chromosome 22q11. Presents with congenital heart defects (tetralogy of Fallot, transposition of the great arteries, double-outlet right ventricle, ventriculoseptal defect), microstomia, cleft palate, mental retardation, strabismus, hypertelorism.

REFERENCES:

Hameed R, Raafat F, Ramani P, et al: Mitochondrial cytopathy presenting with focal segmental glomerulosclerosis, hypoparathyroidism, sensorineural deafness, and progressive neurological disease. *Postgrad Med J* 77:523, 2001.

Muroya K, Hasegawa T, Ito Y, et al: GATA3 abnormalities and the phenotypic spectrum of HDR syndrome. *J Med Genet* 38:374, 2001.

Van Esch H, Devriendt K: Transcription factor GATA3 and the human HDR syndrome. *Cell Mol Life Sci* 58:1296, 2001.

Hecht Syndrome

At a glance: Rare, inherited disorder, characterized by trismus and pseudocamptodactyly. Patients cannot open completely their mouth.

Synonyms: Trismus Pseudocamptodactyly Syndrome; Camptodactyly Limited Jaw Excursion; Hecht-Beals-Wilson Syndrome; Dutch-Kentucky Syndrome.

History: Genetic disorder first described in 1969 by Frederik Hecht, an American pediatrician, and Rodney Kenneth Beals, an American surgeon.

Incidence: Rare syndrome; possible same familial origin for all cases has been evocated.

Genetic inheritance: Autosomal dominant; more common in females.

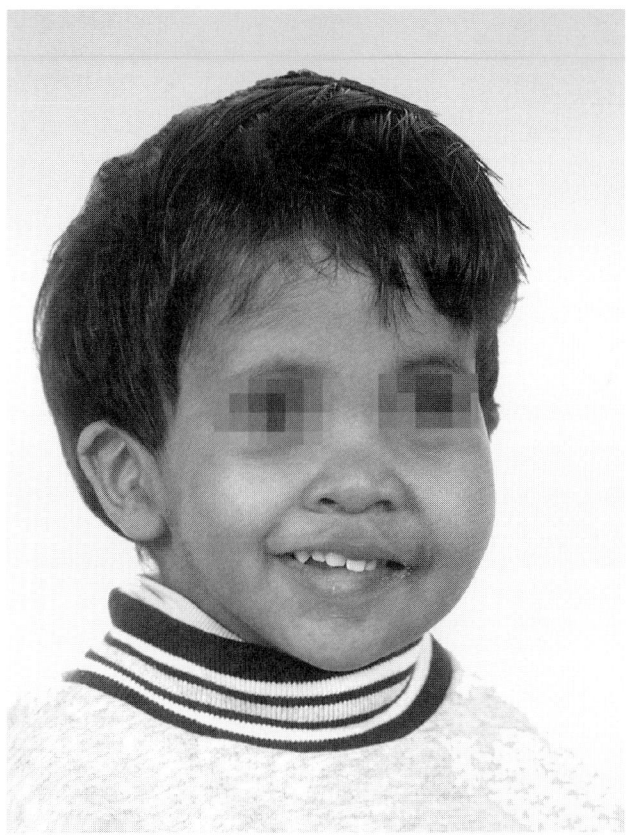

Hemifacial hyperplasia   Almost 3-year-old child with left hemifacial hypertrophy. No visual or otologic impairment was noted.

Diagnosis: Clinically evocated in patients presenting with an inability to open their mouth completely, combined with abnormally short muscle-tendon units in the fingers, causing the fingers to curve or bend with wrist dorsiflexion.

Clinical aspects: Features involve *mouth* (trismus), *muscle,* and *bones* (short stature, symphalangy, muscle anomalies, restricted joint mobility, pseudocamptodactyly). Ptosis, prognathism, dislocated hip and foot anomalies (metatarsus adductus, down-turning or hammer toes, talipes equinovarus), and heart malformations (mitral valve prolapse, aortic root dilatation) may occur. Feeding difficulties are frequent.

Precautions before anesthesia: An anesthetic consultation is highly recommended. Evaluate the airway for potential difficulty during direct laryngoscopy and tracheal intubation (clinical, radiographs) and orthopedic function (clinical).

Anesthetic considerations: Direct laryngoscopy and tracheal intubation can be difficult because of trismus and may require adapted anesthetic techniques such as fiberoptic intubation. Careful intraoperative positioning is needed because of skeletal malformations but can be difficult to realize.

Pharmacological implications: Avoid muscle relaxant until airway is secured and lung ventilation confirmed. Trismus is not related to a structural muscle anomaly, and the administration of succinylcholine and volatile anesthetic agents does not have to be avoided. Prophylactic antibiotics in case of cardiopathy may be indicated.

References:

Hecht F, Beals RK: Inability to open the mouth fully: An autosomal dominant phenotype with facultative camptodactyly and short stature. Preliminary note. *Birth Defects Orig Artic Ser* 5:96, 1969.

Mabry CC, Barnett IS, Hutcheson MW, et al: Trismus pseudocamptodactyly syndrome; Dutch-Kentucky syndrome. *J Pediatr* 85:503, 1974.

Vaghadia H, Blackstock D: Anaesthetic implications of the trismus pseudocamptodactyly (Dutch-Kentucky or Hecht Beals) syndrome. *Can J Anaesth* 35:80, 1988.

Hemochromatosis

At a glance: Hereditary hemochromatosis is a disorder in which iron is significantly absorbed by the digestive tract and accumulates in body tissues, which progressively causes diabetes, joint disorders, cardiac arrhythmia then heart failure, hepatic cirrhosis, skin color change, and increased risk of cancer.

Synonyms: Adult Hemochromatosis; Hereditary Hemochromatosis; Idiopathic Hemochromatosis.

History: Genetic disorder of iron metabolism described in 1865 by Trousseau and named from the Greek words *heme* ("of the blood") and *chroma* ("color").

Incidence: Fewer than 1:250,000 per year in the general population but approximately 1:200 people in the United States is believed to have a mutation necessary for iron overload.

Genetic inheritance: Autosomal recessive. Males are affected more severely with an earlier onset. Two mutations in the HFE gene

Table H-1   Hemochromatosis: Genetic Mutations

Combination Mutations	Patients with Hemochromatosis	Patients without Symptoms	Clinical Features
C282Y/C282Y	60–90%	7–50%	Severe form
C282Y/H63D	3%	98–99.5%	Moderate form
H63D/H63D	1%	>99%	Mild form
C282Y/Normal	Should not have symptoms and should be healthy carriers	>99%	Some patients may have mildly increased iron levels and a 1.5–2-fold increased risk for cardiac disorders

can cause hereditary hemochromatosis: H63D (less severe and later onset form) and C282Y. HLA-A3 is found in 78.4% of cases (27% of controls) and HLA-B14 in 25.5% of cases (3.4% of controls). Gene located on 6p21.3, close to HLA-A locus.

Pathophysiology: The HFE protein is normally expressed in crypt enterocytes of the duodenum (and the placenta) where it has a predominantly intracellular localization and forms a stable association with the transferrin receptor. The HFE protein is believed to modulate the uptake of transferrin-bound iron from plasma by crypt enterocytes. Impairment of this function could result in a paradoxical signal in crypt enterocytes, which causes them to absorb more dietary iron when they mature into villus enterocytes.

Diagnosis: Usually delayed until adulthood after onset of clinical symptoms, although screening of family members may lead to early, asymptomatic diagnosis. Orientation tests include serum ferritin, sideremia, and liver biopsy for iron staining, which are all consistent with iron accumulation. Diagnosis established by molecular biology on blood samples (presence of HFE mutation).

Clinical aspects: Symptomatology usually begins at middle age but may be detected earlier. Early symptoms are nonspecific: weakness, joint and digestive pains, palpitations, and loss of menstrual periods. Abnormal liver function tests can be detected earlier, in the absence of other symptoms. Left untreated, late symptoms appear: bronze skin pigmentation, liver cirrhosis, or hepatocellular carcinoma, diabetes mellitus, panhypopituitarism, dysrhythmias, and cardiac failure, joint disorders, chronic abdominal pain, extreme weakness, and tendency to recurrent infections.

Precautions before anesthesia: Ascertain that ferritin is at the low end of normal values; if not, postpone surgery (if possible) until this is achieved. Check ECG for conduction abnormalities; rule out cardiomyopathy by clinical findings and/or echocardiogram. Evaluate liver function: liver function test, prothrombin time, partial thromboplastin time for signs of liver dysfunction. Prepare to treat the presence of coagulopathy.

Anesthetic considerations: Avoid myocardial depressants. Titrate hepatic metabolized drugs to effect in patients with liver dysfunction. Avoid regional anesthesia in presence of coagulopathy.

Pharmacological implications: Avoid any iron and vitamin C supplementation. Avoid any medication or nutriment that can cause hepatic toxicity.

Other conditions to be considered:

JUVENILE HEMOCHROMATOSIS: Not caused by an *HFE* defect; more severe with earlier clinical course but otherwise very similar.

NEONATAL HEMOCHROMATOSIS: Not caused by an *HFE* defect; lethal.

☞**PORPHYRIA VARIEGATA:** Autosomal dominant disease of porphyrin-heme metabolism characterized by cutaneous photosensitivity, acute episodes of abdominal pain and vomiting, central nervous system (CNS) disorders, peripheral and autosomal neuropathy; caused by a defective protoporphyrinogen oxidase mapped to chromosome 14.

☞**CERULOPLASMIN DEFICIENCY:** Group of genetic disorders affecting expression of the ceruloplasmin gene leading to an iron storage disorder with hepatic failure and progressive dementia.

REFERENCES:

Bacon BR: Diagnosis and management of hemochromatosis. *Gastroenterology* 113:995, 1997.

Powell LW: Diagnosis of hemochromatosis. *Semin Gastrointest Dis* 13:80, 2002.

Turlin B, Deugnier Y: Iron overload disorders. *Clin Liver Dis* 6:481, 2002.

Hemoglobin Disorders: Overview

Hemoglobinopathy is a genetic defect that causes abnormal structure of one of the globin chains of the hemoglobin molecule. *Thalassemia* is a genetic defect resulting in the production of an abnormally low quantity of a given hemoglobin chain or chains.

HEMOGLOBIN C DISEASE

At a glance: Genetically inherited hemolytic anemia, usually mild and often inapparent until adulthood. Mainly encountered in populations of African descent but also in populations of Sicilian and Hispanic descent.

Synonyms: CC Disease; Hemoglobinopathy C.

Nature: Hemolytic anemia with moderate reduction in red cell lifespan. In the oxyhemoglobin state, hemoglobin C is less soluble than normal hemoglobin, thus forming intraerythrocytic crystals

Table H-2 Hemoglobin Disorders: An Overview

Classification	Diseases
Hemoglobinopathies	
Sickle cell syndromes	Sickle cell trait (Hb S heterozygotes)
	Sickle cell anemia (Hb S homozygotes)
	Combination disorders Sickle B thalassemia Sickle cell C disease (hemoglobin C disease) Sickle cell SC disease Sickle cell D disease Sickle cell SD disease
No sickling and crystallization	Hemoglobin E disease
Unstable Hemoglobins	Congenital Heinz body hemolytic anemia
	Köln hemoglobin
	Methemoglobinemia
Thalassemias (Cooley Anemias)	α-Thalassemia
	β-Thalassemia (minor, major)
Hemoglobin Variants	Fetal hemoglobin (F)
	Hemoglobin A_2, G, D, J, H
	Hemoglobin Bart

(tactoids); deoxygenation further reduces solubility and increases blood viscosity. Patients with hemoglobin C disease have a survival advantage in areas of endemic *Plasmodium falciparum* malaria.

Incidence: Prevalence in the general population is 0.017% in African Americans but approximately 0.03% in Northern Africa. No sex prevalence.

Genetic inheritance: Autosomal codominant (biparental inheritance). The beta gene cluster is on chromosome 11.

Pathophysiology: The double helix of hemoglobin C is composed of two normal alpha-chains and two variant beta-chains, in which glutamic acid is replaced by lysine at position 6. Hemoglobin C is unstable and tends to precipitate in erythrocytes where it crystallizes. This changes the physical properties of the erythrocytic membrane (decreased deformability and increased viscosity of blood). These crystal-containing red blood cells are removed by the spleen, which becomes enlarged with time (splenomegaly).

Diagnosis: Examination of the erythrocytes (blood smear) reveals several morphologic disorders (caused by crystallization of hemoglobin): target cells mainly, but also appearance of an off-center target, occasional pyknotic spherocytes, and polychromasia. Diagnosis is established by hemoglobin electrophoresis (100% hemoglobin C in homozygotes, up to 35% in heterozygotes). Reticulocyte count and lactic acid dehydrogenase levels determine the extent of hemolysis.

Clinical aspects: Except for mild-to-moderate hemolytic anemia, most patients remain asymptomatic until adulthood. Symptoms usually consist of joint and musculoskeletal pain, visual disorders (retinopathy as a result of iron deposition in the Bruch membrane causing angioid streaks), cholelithiasis, and radiographic anomalies of the maxilla and mandible (overgrowth of erythrocyte-forming marrow). Physical examination reveals splenomegaly but is otherwise normal.

Precautions before anesthesia: Check hematocrit, reticulocyte count, and lactic acid dehydrogenase levels to determine the extent of hemolysis.

Anesthetic considerations: Maintain oxygen-carrying capacity. Avoid oxygen desaturation of blood and all conditions favoring desaturation, including use of tourniquets and hypotensive techniques of anesthesia.

Pharmacological implications: No known specific implications for this condition.

Other conditions to be considered:

    Sᴵᴄᴋʟᴇ Cᴇʟʟ/Hᴇᴍᴏɢʟᴏʙɪɴ C Dɪsᴇᴀsᴇ (SC): Intermediate symptomatology between sickle cell disease and hemoglobin C disease caused by genetic transmission of both autosomal traits.

    Hᴇᴍᴏɢʟᴏʙɪɴ C β-Tʜᴀʟᴀssᴇᴍɪᴀ Dɪsᴇᴀsᴇ: Clinically similar to typical hemoglobin C disease but caused by genetic transmission of a hemoglobin C gene from one parent and a β-thalassemia gene from the other parent.

REFERENCES:

Almeida AM, Henthorn JS, Davies SC: Neonatal screening for haemoglobinopathies: The results of a 10-year programme in an English Health Region. *Br J Haematol* 112:32, 2001.

Bernaudin F, Verlhac S, Freard F, et al: Multicenter prospective study of children with sickle cell disease: Radiographic and psychometric correlation. *J Child Neurol* 15:333, 2000.

Weatherall DJ: The thalassemias, in Beutler E, Marshall A, Lichtman MD (eds): *Hematology*. 5th ed. New York, McGraw-Hill, 1995, p 607.

HEMOGLOBIN E DISEASE

At a glance: Genetically inherited minor anomaly of hemoglobin resulting in mild anemia and slight anomalies of size and shape of red blood cell.

Incidence: Most commonly found in Southeast Asia, where the incidence varies from approximately 0 to 0.2% of the population.

Genetic inheritance: Autosomal dominant. Homozygotes have hemoglobin E disease, whereas heterozygotes have hemoglobin E trait.

Pathophysiology: Substitution of glutamic acid at the 26th position of the beta-globin chain where lysine is substituted for glutamic acid. This compound is unstable under oxidative stress.

Diagnosis: Hemoglobin electrophoresis demonstrates approximately 98% hemoglobin E (HbE) and 2% HbF (no HbA) in homozygotes versus approximately 30% (no more than 45%) in heterozygotes (the remaining being normal HbA). Peripheral blood smear reveals numerous target forms (up to 75%) and bone marrow smear usually reveals mild erythroid hyperplasia. Patients with combined HbE/β-thalassemia have a predominance of HbE (up to 75%), with increased HbF (7–40%) and variable HbA (1–30%).

Clinical aspects: *Homozygotes* (HbE disease) have marked microcytosis and hypochromia but usually are not anemic. Red blood cells have a normal lifespan. Splenomegaly is absent. The clinical picture is similar to thalassemia trait.

    Hemoglobin E carriers (HbE trait) are asymptomatic, although 30 to 35% (no more than 45%) of the hemoglobin is HbE. Peripheral blood smear demonstrates microcytosis without anemia. Patients with both *hemoglobin E and β-thalassemia* (double heterozygotes) have significant-to-severe microcytic anemia, increased reticulocyte count and splenomegaly, and usually require chronic transfusion by 6 years of age. Peripheral blood smear reveals the existence of target cells (typical of HbE) and the basophilic stippling typical of β-thalassemia.

Precautions before anesthesia: Check hematocrit. Standard preoperative management of patient.

Anesthetic considerations: No specific considerations except for patients with combined HbE/β-thalassemia (see *Thalassemia*). Maintain oxygen-carrying capacity.

Pharmacological implications: No specific pharmacological implications with this condition. Hemoglobin E disease offers possible protective effects against malaria.

REFERENCES:

Chotivanich K, Udomsangpetch R, Pattanapanyasat K, et al: Hemoglobin E: A balanced polymorphism protective against high parasitemias and thus severe *P. falciparum* malaria. *Blood* 100:1172, 2002.

Lubin BH: Laboratory diagnosis of hemoglobinopathies. *Clin Biochem* 24:363, 1991.

Hemolytic Anemia, Congenital, with Emphysema and Cutis Laxa

At a glance: Very rare syndrome characterized by hemolytic anemia of unknown origin associated with early-onset emphysema and cutis laxa. Poor prognosis.

Synonym: Cutis Laxa, Emphysema, and Hemolytic Anemia; Emphysema Hemolytic Anemia Syndrome.

Incidence and genetic inheritance: Extremely rare (three cases described in consanguineous family); autosomal recessive.

Clinical aspects: Features include severe congenital hemolytic anemia, early-onset pulmonary emphysema, diffuse pulmonary giant cell infiltration, hemorrhagic adrenal necrosis, cutis laxa. Two of the three cases described died of septic shock before 7 years of age.

Anesthetic considerations: Evaluate severity of anemia (clinical, full blood count), and respiratory function (clinical, chest radiographs, CT, pulmonary function test, arterial blood gas analysis).

REFERENCE:

Anderson CE, Finklestein JZ, Nussbaum E, et al: Association of hemolytic anemia and early onset pulmonary emphysema in three siblings. *J Pediatr*105:247, 1984.

Hemophagocytotic Lymphohistiocytosis (HLH)

At a glance: Genetic disorder associated with failure to establish an effective immune response to infection. Caused by normal but overactive histiocytes. Clinical features include fever, hepatomegaly, cytopenia, and neurologic abnormalities. Lethal if not treated.

Synonyms: HPLH 1; HLH 1

Incidence: 1:50,000 live births. Two forms are described: (1) primary or familial hemophagocytic lymphohistiocytosis (FHL), a heterogeneous autosomal recessive disorder, and (2) secondary or acquired HLH (related to systemic infection, immunodeficiency, or underlying malignancy).

Genetic inheritance: Heterogeneous autosomal recessive inheritance for FLH.

Pathophysiology: Proliferation of activated macrophages and histiocytes, which phagocytose other cells (red and white blood cells, platelets), leading to the clinical symptoms. Spleen, lymph nodes, bone marrow, liver, and central nervous system are preferential sites of involvement. The role of perforin and NK cells has been evocated in familial forms.

Diagnosis: Evocated by the association of fever, hepatosplenomegaly, cytopenia, hypofibrinogenemia, hypertriglyceridemia, and hemophagocytosis. Rash may occur. Frequently affects infants from birth to 18 months.

Clinical aspects: Patients can present with coagulopathy with an increased partial thromboplastin time. Jaundice is often present as a consequence of hyperbilirubinemia. Lymphadenopathy, malaise, anorexia with weight loss, and failure to thrive can occur. Neurologic abnormalities including seizures have been observed. The skin can be involved in a variety of ways; clinically best characterized as erythroderma, generalized purpuric macules and papules, or morbilliform eruptions.

Precautions before anesthesia: Preoperative evaluation must concern localization of infection and identification of the causal agent. Preoperative laboratory investigations should include full blood count, liver function (bilirubinemia, albuminemia, aspartate aminotransferase, alanine aminotransferase), and triglyceride.

Anesthetic considerations: Strict asepsis is needed. Coagulopathy and thrombopenia should be corrected if necessary and may require more transfusions than expected. Regional anesthesia is not contraindicated but should be avoided in case of infection or severe thrombopenia.

Pharmacological implications: Repeated nitrous oxide administration should be avoided. Hepatotoxic drugs or drugs with hepatic metabolism should be avoided. Prophylactic antibiotics may consider immunologic status.

REFERENCES:

Arico M, Allen M, Brusa S: Haemophagocytic lymphohistiocytosis: Proposal of a diagnostic algorithm based on perforin expression. *Br J Haematol* 119:180, 2002.

Dufourcq-Lagelouse R, Pastural E, Barrat FJ, et al: Genetic basis of hemophagocytic lymphohistiocytosis syndrome [review]. *Int J Mol Med* 4:127, 1999.

Hemophilia A

At a glance: Most severe hereditary coagulation disorder. It is caused by defective synthesis of plasma protein factor VIII.

Synonyms: Classical Hemophilia; F-VIII Deficiency.

Incidence: 1:5000–10,000 live male births; 30% of cases are the result of new mutations.

Genetic inheritance: X-linked recessive with expression in male children only. Gene locus is Xq28.

Pathophysiology: Defective factor VIII gene produces low levels of functional factor VIII. Factor VIII is required in the intrinsic coagulation cascade and, when activated and in the presence of factor XIa, leads to activation of factor X. Affected patients are classified as mild, moderate, or severe. Mildly afflicted patients have factor VIII levels 6 to 30% of normal activity and experience hemorrhage secondary to trauma or surgery, but rarely spontaneously. Patients moderately afflicted have factor VIII levels of 1 to 5% of normal activity and experience hemorrhage secondary to trauma or surgery with occasional spontaneous hemarthroses. Severely afflicted patients have less than 1% of normal factor VIII activity and experience frequent spontaneous hemorrhages from early infancy requiring replacement therapy. Although carriers usually have 50% normal activity and experience no bleeding difficulties, levels should be obtained, as those with less than 50% activity can experience significant hemorrhage after trauma.

Diagnosis: Elevation of the partial thromboplastin time with normal prothrombin time and normal bleeding time. Diagnosis is established by dosage of factor VIII antigen and factor VIII serum factor activity. Prenatal and carrier detection are possible with restriction fragment length polymorphism DNA analysis but are contingent upon parental analysis.

Clinical aspects: Soft tissue hematomas, including retroperitoneal/pharyngeal hemarthroses (75%), most often of the same target joint, pseudotumor of bone, with rare erosion into viscera, hematuria, intracranial hemorrhage, cord compression secondary to epidural bleeding, nerve compression secondary to hematoma, mucous membrane hemorrhage (epistaxis, hemoptysis), peptic ulcer disease, and excessive postsurgical bleeding.

Precautions before anesthesia: Hematology and anesthesiology consultation are highly recommended before elective surgical procedures. Schedule procedures early in the week to avoid weekend pharmaceutical delays. Ensure supply of virally inactivated or recombinant factor VIII concentrate, which does not have the infectious risks of fresh-frozen plasma or cryoprecipitate. Dose calculations are based on the following formula: *1 unit factor VIII /kg increases factor VIII activity by 2%.* Half-life is 8 to 12 hours. Consider desmopressin acetate (DDAVP 0.3 μg/kg) in mild-to-moderate disease because it increases factor VIII levels up to threefold by an unknown mechanism. Consider antifibrinolytic therapy (ε-aminocaproic acid [EACA] or tranexamic acid), as these agents may be useful adjuvants for mucosal and dental bleeding although they are contraindicated with hematuria. Raise factor VIII to normal levels before major surgical procedures.

Anesthetic considerations: In conjunction with a hematologist consultation, maintain factor VIII levels postoperatively because factor replacement may be required for 7 to 10 days, with twice-daily factor VIII assays. Avoid regional anesthesia and intramuscular (IM) injections.

Pharmacological implications: Avoid aspirin and NSAIDs.

Other conditions to be considered:

☞**HEMOPHILIA B:** Hereditary coagulation disorder caused by defective synthesis of plasma protein factor IX.

☞**VON WILLEBRAND DISEASE:** Inherited coagulation disorder characterized by frequent nosebleeds, easy/spontaneous bruising, prolonged bleeding after injury/surgery. Caused by a lack of production (types I and III) or by nonfunctional (type II) von Willebrand coagulation factor.

REFERENCES:

Baujard C, Gouyet L, Murat I : Diagnosis and anaesthesia management of haemophilia during the neonatal period. *Paediatr Anaesth* 8:245, 1998.

Donmez A, Turker H, Sekerci S, et al: Dealing with a hemophilia—A patient undergoing cerebral aneurysm surgery. *J Neurosurg Anesthesiol* 11:214, 1999.

Roberts HR, Hoffman M: Hemophilia and related conditions—Inherited deficiencies of prothrombin (factor II), factor V, and factors VII to XII, in Beutler E, Marshall A, Lichtman MD (eds): *Hematology.* 5th ed. New York, McGraw-Hill, 1995, p 1413.

Hemophilia B

At a glance: Hereditary coagulation disorder caused by defective synthesis of plasma protein factor IX.

Synonyms: Christmas Disease; F-IX Deficiency.

History: Also called *Christmas disease* after Steven Christmas, who was first diagnosed with the disease at 5 years of age in 1952 (and who died of AIDS at age 46 in 1993). Sir Jonathan Hutchinson was responsible for naming clinical disorders after patients and has become familiar for serologic research.

Incidence: 1:40,000 males (15–20% of hemophiliacs).

Genetic inheritance: X-linked. Defective coagulation factor IX. Gene map location is Xq27.1-q27.2.

Pathophysiology: Factor IX is a vitamin K-dependent clotting factor. It is activated by either factor XIa or factor VIIa-tissue factor complex. Once activated, it activates factor X in the presence of calcium, phospholipid, and factor VIIIa. Because deficiency of factor VIII or factor IX decreases factor X activity, hemophilia B is clinically indistinguishable from hemophilia A. Affected patients are classified as mild, moderate, or severe. Mildly afflicted patients have factor IX levels 5 to 40% of normal activity, moderately af-

flicted patients have levels 1 to 5% of normal activity, and severely afflicted patients have less than 1% of normal activity.

Diagnosis: Based on assays of factor IX antigen and factor IX activity. According to the residual factor IX activity, the disorder is classified as severe (<1%), moderate (1 to 5%), or mild (5–20% of normal value). Prenatal and carrier detection are possible with restriction fragment length polymorphism DNA analysis but are contingent upon parental analysis. Elevation of the partial thromboplastin time with normal prothrombin time and bleeding times are found.

Clinical aspects: Early onset of symptoms: increased tendency to bleeding becomes evident in 90% of affected patients by 1 year of age. Clinical picture very similar to hemophilia A, namely, soft tissue hematomas, including retroperitoneal/pharyngeal hemarthroses (75%), often at the same target joint, pseudotumor of bone, with rare erosion into viscera, hematuria, intracranial hemorrhage, cord compression secondary to epidural bleeding, nerve compression secondary to hematoma, mucous membrane hemorrhage (epistaxis, hemoptysis), peptic ulcer disease, and excessive postsurgical bleeding. Hepatitis infection from previous transfusions is common.

Precautions before anesthesia: Hematology and anesthesiology consultation are highly recommended before elective surgical procedures. Schedule surgical procedures early in the week to avoid pharmaceutical delays. Ensure supply of virally inactivated factor IX concentrate, which does not have the infectious risks of fresh-frozen plasma. Dose calculations are based on the following formula: *1 unit factor IX/kg increases factor IX activity by 1%.* Half-life is 18 to 24 hours. Consider antifibrinolytic therapy [epsilon-aminocaproic acid (EACA), tranexamic acid or aprotinin] because these agents may be useful adjuvants for dental bleeding. Raise factor IX to normal levels before major surgical procedures.

Anesthetic considerations: In conjunction with a hematologist consultation, maintain factor IX levels peri- and postoperatively. Avoid regional anesthesia and intramuscular injections.

Pharmacological implications: Avoid aspirin and NSAIDs.

Other conditions to be considered:

☞**HEMOPHILIA A:** More severe hereditary coagulation disorder but otherwise a clinically similar syndrome caused by defective synthesis of plasma protein factor VIII.

HEMOPHILIA B LEYDEN: Variant of hemophilia B in which the mutation affects the adjacent promoter region of the gene instead of the functional region of the factor IX gene. The prevalence is unknown (this variant accounts for a small percentage of hemophilia B). The disease is characterized by a gradual increase in factor IX levels that begins at puberty. The patients progressively eliminate their hemophilia because the promoter gene is sensitive to hormonal changes. Hemophilia B Leyden was first described in families of Dutch ancestry.

REFERENCES:

Bowen DJ: Haemophilia A and haemophilia B: Molecular insights. *Mol Pathol* 55:127, 2002.

Koren JP, Klein RL, Kavic MS, et al: Management of splenic trauma in the pediatric hemophiliac patient: Case series and review of the literature. *J Pediatr Surg* 37:568, 2002.

Roberts HR, Hoffman M: Hemophilia and related conditions—Inherited deficiencies of prothrombin (factor II), factor V, and factors VII to XII, in Beutler E. (ed): *Hematology.* 5th ed. New York, McGraw-Hill, 1995, p 1423.

Hennekam Syndrome

At a glance: Rare, severe syndrome combining intestinal lymphangiectasia and lymphedema of the limbs, genital, and face, with a dysmorphic facial appearance and severe mental retardation.

Synonym: Intestinal Lymphangiectasia-Lymphedema-Mental Retardation Syndrome.

History: First described by Hennekam in 1989.

Genetic inheritance: Autosomal recessive.

Diagnosis: Clinical. The patient presents with severe lymphedema of limbs, genitalia, and face. Also associated with intestinal lymphangiectasis, facial anomalies, and progressive neurologic involvement. The intestinal lymphangiectasia is accompanied by hypoproteinemia, hypogammaglobulinemia, and lymphocytopenia, which help confirm the diagnosis.

Clinical aspects: Features include *head* (lymphedematous flat facies, retrognathia, atresia of ear canal, low-set ears, hearing loss, hypertelorism, flat nasal bridge, epicanthal folds, glaucoma, small mouth, narrow palate, flat upper lip, oligodontia, conical crowns, delayed eruptions), *skeleton* (horizontal clavicles, pectus excavatum, coronal craniosynostosis, scoliosis, syndactyly, camptodactyly, small hands and feet, talipes equinovarus), *extremities* (lymphedema), *skin* (alopecia, frontal upsweep, heavy eyebrows, hirsutism), *gastrointestinal* (*GI*) *tract* (lymphangiectasia of the small intestine, rectal prolapse, umbilical hernia), *urogenital system* (genital lymphedema, ectopic or horseshoe kidney, vesicoureteral reflux, cryptorchism), *central nervous system* (*CNS*) (seizures, conductive hearing loss, mental retardation, focal parietal pachygyria, hyperactivity), and *heart* (ventricular or atrial septal defect, pericardial lymphangiectasia, pericardial effusions). Lymphangiectasia may affect pleura and thyroid. Infection of oozing lymph may cause erysipelas.

Precautions before anesthesia: Evaluate the airway for potential difficulties with tracheal intubation because of facial malformations (clinical, radiographs), the neurologic function (clinical, EEG, CT, MRI, seizure control), cardiac function (clinical, echography, ECG), and respiratory function because of skeletal deformation and lung lymphangiectasia (clinical, history, pulmonary function test, chest radiographs, CT, arterial blood gas analysis) must also be evaluated. Look for existence and severity of glaucoma (clinical, ophthalmologic examination). Evaluate protein loss (clinical, laboratory including proteinemia, albuminemia, agammaglobulinemia). The intravascular volume and oncotic pressure must be corrected before elective surgical procedures.

Anesthetic considerations: High rate of risk for anesthetic implications. Direct laryngoscopy and tracheal intubation can be difficult and require adapted anesthetic techniques including fiberoptic intubation. Venous access can be difficult because of lymphedema. Subclavian venous access can be difficult and probably should be avoided because of clavicle and rib anomalies. Postoperative cardiac monitoring is recommended; ventilatory support can be necessary. If pericardiocentesis because of pericarditis is scheduled, an adapted anesthetic technique must be defined based on the amount of fluid present and how it affects cardiac performance.

Pharmacological implications: Muscle relaxants should be avoided until airway is secured. Avoid drugs that increase intraocular pressure or that are contraindicated in case of glaucoma (atropine, succinylcholine, ketamine). Consider interaction between antiepileptic treatment and anesthetic drugs. The presence in plasma level of albumin (hypoalbuminemia) could influence the pharmacodynamics of anesthetic agents administered. The proportion of active medication between the bound and free portion of the drug used will be modified. It is recommended to reduce the dose administered until albumin level is confirmed. Prophylactic antibiotics in case of cardiopathy as indicated.

REFERENCES:

Hennekam RCM, Geerdink RA, Hamel BCJ, et al: Autosomal recessive intestinal lymphangiectasia and lymphedema, with facial anomalies and mental retardation. *Am J Med Genet* 34:593, 1989.

Van Balkom ID, Alders M, Allanson J, et al: Lymphedema-lymphangiectasia-mental retardation (Hennekam) syndrome: A review. *Am J Med Genet* 112:412, 2002.

Hereditary Acromelalgia

At a glance: Neurologic movement disorder characterized by an unpleasant sensation in the lower extremities, eliciting intolerable restlessness with twitching and jumping of the legs when the patient is at rest, especially at night.

Synonyms: Restless Legs Syndrome; Acromelalgia-Painful Legs-Moving Toes Syndrome; Anxietas Tibialis Syndrome; Asthenia Crurum Dolorosa; Asthenia Crurum Paresthetica Syndrome; Ekbom Syndrome; Leg Jitters Syndrome; Moving Toe Syndrome; Painful Leg Syndrome, Wittmaack-Ekbom Sequence.

History: First described by the English anatomist Thomas Willis in 1672, then by Theodor Wittmaack, a German clinician, in 1861. Restless legs syndrome may occur as a primary condition (idiopathic) or may be a result of other conditions (secondary or symptomatic restless legs syndrome).

Incidence: Prevalence is evaluated at 5.5% of the general population, with a female predominance. Prevalence increases with age.

Genetic inheritance: The disorder is usually familial and inherited as an autosomal dominant trait. Candidate gene map locus is 12-q21.

Pathophysiology: Unknown. Idiopathic myoclonic jerks occur just prior to sleep and severely affect it. However, it disappears with the onset of stage 1 REM (rapid eye movement) sleep. It is associated with a variety of conditions, including iron deficiency, folic acid anemia, B vitamin deficiency, drug intake (phenothiazine), barbiturate withdrawal, diabetes, renal insufficiency, neuropathy, stroke, and chronic respiratory illness. It is common during pregnancy and is precipitated by fatigue, anxiety, and stress.

Diagnosis: History of repeated, asymmetric flexion jerks of the legs occurring at night just before and interfering with sleep. Acromelalgia, myoclonus, and paresthesia are characteristic.

Clinical aspects: Symptoms worsen with age. Hereditary acromelalgia is a lifelong condition with no cure. Opioids are effective for relieving pain, and correction of iron deficiency may improve symptoms for some patients. Sleep deprivation may become severe with increasing age.

Precautions before anesthesia: Check usual medication (affected patients often take either neuroleptic and/or sedative medications). Ensure that regular medications are continued until the morning of surgery. Check red blood cell count and evaluate for iron deficiency.

Anesthetic considerations: No specific considerations with this condition.

Pharmacological implications: None reported. Most affected patients take medications such as temazepam, levodopa/carbidopa, bromocriptine, pergolide mesylate, oxycodone, propoxyphene, and codeine, which are effective in relieving symptoms but may interfere with anesthetic techniques and requirements for postoperative pain relief.

Other condition to be considered:

☞ERYTHROMELALGIA: Characterized by repeated episodes of paroxysmal vasodilation with burning pain in the hands and feet. Diminished sensitivity to temperature changes, especially with cold acting as pain depressor and heat as stimulator. Affects middle-aged patients of both sexes. Unknown etiology but may occasionally be inherited as an autosomal dominant trait.

REFERENCES:

Odin P, Mrowka M, Shing M: Restless legs syndrome. *Eur J Neurol* 9(suppl 3):59, 2002.

Ohayon MM, Roth T: Prevalence of restless legs syndrome and periodic limb movement disorder in the general population. *J Psychosom Res* 53:547, 2002.

Stiasny K, Oertel WH, Trenkwalder C: Clinical symptomatology and treatment of restless legs syndrome and periodic limb movement disorder. *Sleep Med Rev* 6:253, 2002.

Hereditary Desmoid Disease (HDD)

At a glance: Variant of familial adenomatous polyposis (FAP) characterized by benign growths of fibrous tissue (hyperproliferation of epithelial mesenchymal tissues) that form either spontaneously or after surgery. These tumors can become large and aggressive, compressing abdominal organs.

Synonyms: Aggressive Fibromatosis; Familial Infiltrative Fibromatosis (FIF).

Incidence: Up to 13% of patients with FAP have associated desmoid disease (FAP affects 1:8000 individuals). The incidence of HDD occurring alone remains to be determined.

Genetic inheritance: Autosomal dominant with 100% penetrance. The majority of mutations affect the adenomatous polyposis coli (APC) gene (a tumor suppressor) on chromosome 5 distal to the beta-catenin–binding domain (5q15-22). New mutations account for 20 to 30% of families affected with this condition (direct mutation testing is required to establish diagnosis).

Pathophysiology: The *APC* gene is a tumor suppressor. The APC protein seems to act like a cell-signaling protein. Mutations in the *APC* gene are responsible for generating slowly growing fibrous masses consisting of bundles of spindle cells with variable amounts of collagen. Hereditary desmoid disease occurs with or without colonic polyposis and consists of infiltrative fibromatosis of connective tissues invading multiple parts of the body. Desmoid tumors may also present as extracolonic manifestations in some patients with FAP.

Diagnosis: Based on clinical aspect, familial history, genetic studies, and tissue biopsy.

Clinical aspects: HDD patients develop multifocal fibromatosis: arms, breast, paraspinal muscles, occiput, lower ribs, abdominal wall, and mesentery. Desmoid tumors may proliferate in various areas: arms, ribs, breasts, occiput, mesentery, abdominal wall, and paraspinal muscles. Epidermal cysts and osteomata of the skull and mandible, as well as scoliosis caused by desmoid disease, have been described. Desmoid tumors are not considered malignant per se, but their local aggressiveness and recurrence after surgical removal are frequent. Although some families with HDD are predisposed to colonic carcinoma, colonic polyposis is rare. Up to 90% of FAP patients have congenital hypertrophy of the retinal pigment epithelium (<40% of control patients).

Precautions before anesthesia: Inquire about associated familial colonic polyposis (anemia). Inquire about the location of the lesions to be excised (some locally invasive desmoid tumors may be close to major blood vessels). Obtain hemoglobin level and blood cell count.

Anesthetic considerations: Careful positioning and padding are required to avoid trauma to superficial lesions. Although very rare, mandibular osteomata have not been known to make tracheal intubation difficult. Should mandibular lesions become such that they interfere with laryngoscopy, fiberoptic intubation should be considered by either oral or nasal route. Depending on the location and degree of invasion of the tumor, significant blood loss is possible.

Pharmacological implications: No known specific implications with this condition.

Other conditions to be considered: Other mutations within the *APC* gene, including the following:

FAMILIAL ADENOMATOUS POLYPOSIS (FAP): Most severe autosomal dominant variant of mutation in the *APC* gene (tumor suppressor gene). FAP is characterized clinically by the development of a considerable number of adenomatous polyps within the colon that become cancerous if they are not treated.

GARDNER SYNDROME: Another autosomal dominant variant of FAP characterized by congenital hypertrophy of the retinal pigment epithelium, gastrointestinal polyps, multiple osteomas, and skin and soft tissue tumors.

☞ PEUTZ-JEGHERS SYNDROME: Autosomal dominant inherited disorder characterized by intestinal hamartomatous polyps in association with mucocutaneous melanocytic macules. In most cases, it is caused by a germline mutation of the *STK11* (serine threonine kinase 11) gene (gene map locus is 19p13.3).

☞ TURCOT SYNDROME: Autosomal recessive syndrome characterized by the association of a primary brain tumor and multiple colorectal adenomas (could be a variant of Gardner syndrome).

REFERENCES:

Abraham SC, Reynolds C, Lee JH, et al: Fibromatosis of the breast and mutations involving the APC/beta-catenin pathway. *Hum Pathol* 33:39, 2002.

Eccles DM, Van der Luijt R, Breukel C, et al: Hereditary desmoid disease due to a frameshift mutation at codon 1924 of the APC gene. *Am J Hum Genet* 59:1193, 1996.

Maher ER, Morson B, Beach R, et al: Phenotypic variation in hereditary nonpolyposis colon cancer syndrome. Association with infiltrative fibromatosis (desmoid tumor). *Cancer* 69:2049, 1992.

Hereditary Keratitis

At a glance: Inherited condition characterized by recurrent stromal keratitis and vascularization.

Genetic inheritance: Autosomal dominant. Probably caused by a mutation in the PAX6 gene, which is also involved in the development of aniridia and Peters anomaly (anterior segment malformations of the eye). Gene map locus is 11p13.

Pathophysiology: Characterized by the presence of a circumferential band of opacification and vascularization at the level of Bowman membrane adjacent to the limbus. Histopathologic studies confirm the inflammatory nature and the anterior stomal localization of the keratitis.

Clinical aspects: Hereditary childhood corneal clouding. Recurrent episodes of "keratoendothelitis" associated with mild iritis and stromal edema. Propensity for early recurrence after keratoplasty.

Precautions before anesthesia: No specific precautions associated with this medical condition. Only the presence of underlying medical problems affects preparation for anesthesia.

Table H-3　Hereditary Motor Sensory Neuropathies (HMSN): An Overview

Type	Inheritance	Eponym/Synonym	Characteristics
HMSN I (classic CMT I)	Autosomal dominant	☞*Charcot-Marie-Tooth Disease*	Onset during late childhood or adolescence Variable degree of nerve hypertrophy Myelin sheath degeneration At least three subtypes (IA, IB, IC)
HMSN I variant	Autosomal dominant	☞*Roussy-Lévy Syndrome*	Combination of HMSN type I and Friedrich's ataxia
HMSN II	Autosomal dominant	☞*Cowchock Syndrome*	Onset usually later than type I Known as neuronal type No nerve hypertrophy
HMSN III	Autosomal recessive	*Dejerine Sottas Syndrome*	Onset in infancy or childhood Delayed motor development Often severe nerve hypertrophy
HMSN IV	Autosomal recessive	☞*Refsum Syndrome*	Slow motor nerve conduction velocity Retinitis pigmentosa Cerebellar signs
HMSN V	Mainly autosomal dominant (recessive forms exist)	*Strümpell-Lorrain Disease*	Neuropathy with spastic paraplegia with peroneal muscular atrophy and sensory loss
HMSN VI	Mitochondrial DNA transmission (from mother only)	☞*Leber Hereditary Optic Atrophy*	Neuropathy with optic atrophy
HMSN VII		*Often Included in Refsum Syndrome*	Neuropathy with retinitis pigmentosa
X-Linked HMSN	X-Linked		Similar to HMSN I but limited to males Females can be mildly affected
HMSNL	Autosomal recessive	*Hereditary Motor and Sensory Neuropathy-Lom Type*	Peripheral neuropathy Tendon areflexia Sensory loss

Anesthetic considerations: No specific anesthesia considerations.

Pharmacological implications: No known pharmacological implications with this syndrome. However, some patients may be on chronic corticosteroid treatment, which indicates administration of intravenous steroids preoperatively might be necessary according to the surgical stress.

Other condition to be considered: Other hereditary syndromes with keratitis, especially the following:

☞**KERATITIS ICHTHYOSIS DEAFNESS SYNDROME:** Polymalformative syndrome characterized by inflammation of the corneas (keratitis), skin scales, and deafness; both autosomal dominant and autosomal recessive forms have been reported.

REFERENCES:

Pearce WG, Mielke BW, et al: Autosomal dominant keratitis: A possible aniridia variant. *Can J Ophthalmol* 30:131, 1995.

Prosser J, van Heyningen V: PAX6 mutations reviewed. *Hum Mutat* 11:93, 1998.

Hereditary Motor Sensory Neuropathies (HMSN): Overview

See Table H-3.

Table H-4   Hereditary Neurocutaneous Angiomatoses: An Overview

Syndrome	Features
☞**Louis Bar Syndrome** (ataxia–telangiectasia)	Progressive ataxia with degeneration of Purkinje cells, loss of myelinated fibers in peripheral nerves, multiple cutaneous telangiectasia, specific immunologic abnormalities, hypersensitivity to irradiation. Ataxia-telangiectasia cells divide before DNA repair can occur, leading to an increased number of observed chromosomal breaks
☞**Sturge-Weber Syndrome** (encephalotrigeminal angiomatosis)	Unilateral facial angioma in the dermatomes of the first or second division of the trigeminal nerve (V), ipsilateral leptomeningeal venous angiomatosis, and cortical atrophy with calcifications, cystic choroid plexus; somatic mutation rather than germ cell mutation (sporadic rather than inherited)
☞**Klippel-Trenaunay Syndrome** (spinal cutaneous angiomatosis)	Spinal variant of Sturge-Weber syndrome; extensive skin hemangiomas following dermatomal pattern with associated hemangiomas of the spinal cord
☞**Hereditary Telangiectasis** (Rendu-Osler-Weber syndrome)	Multiple red or purple angiomas, arteriovenous malformations of the skin, viscera, and central nervous system that may cause intracranial bleeding with seizures or localized dysfunction; autosomal dominant
☞**Fabry Disease** (angiokeratoma, corporis diffusum)	Acroparesthesias in the extremities with acute episodes (Fabry crises), development of angiokeratoma, heat intolerance, progressive accumulation of glycosphingolipids in tissues resulting in progressive degeneration and major organ failure; X-linked disease caused by a deficiency of the lysosomal enzyme α-galactosidase
☞**Wyburn Mason Syndrome**	Arteriovenous malformations in the CNS and retina; congenital but nonhereditary disorder, without sex or race predilection

Hereditary Neurocutaneous Angiomatoses: Overview

See Table H-4.

Hereditary Neurocutaneous Angioma

At a glance: Phakomatoses characterized by multiple arteriovenous malformations that may cause intracranial or spinal hemorrhage with neurologic sequelae.

Synonyms: Angioma Hereditary Neurocutaneous; Disseminated Hemangiomatosis; Spinal Arterial Venous Malformations with Cutaneous Hemangiomas.

Genetic inheritance: Autosomal dominant.

Pathophysiology: Multiple arteriovenous malformations affecting the central nervous system and other organs, which have a marked tendency to bleed.

Diagnosis: Family history, clinical features, larger hemangiomas on the skin. MRI examination of central nervous system, cerebral angiography.

Clinical aspects: Multiple angiomas within the brain and spinal cord have a marked tendency to bleed, leading to paralysis, cerebral hemorrhage, epilepsy. Angiomas elsewhere can lead to gastrointestinal hemorrhage, hematuria. Large flat hemangiomas on the skin.

Precautions before anesthesia: History of cerebral or spinal hemorrhage, full neurologic examination to define any preexisting deficit, radiologic examination of central nervous system to define presence of hemangiomas. History of seizures and bleeding from other systems (GI hemorrhage, hematuria). Obtain complete blood count, clotting screen ECG, chest radiograph. Cross-matched blood must be available.

Anesthetic considerations: *Neurologic surgery:* May present with cerebral hemorrhage and raised intracranial pressure or sudden paralysis. More than one cerebral or spinal arteriovenous malformation may be present, thereby increasing chance of major hemorrhage. Postoperative focal seizures. *Nonneurologic surgery:* Careful control of blood pressure to reduce risk of cerebral hemorrhage. Spinal hemangiomas may be present, so central nerve blockade should be used with great caution. Careful positioning of the patient with large cutaneous hemangiomas is necessary.

Pharmacological implications: No known specific implications with this condition.

Other conditions to be considered:

☞**VON HIPPEL-LINDAU SYNDROME:** Hereditary phakomatosis characterized by multiple angiomas. Autosomal dominant; gene map locus is 3p25-26.

☞**HEREDITARY TELANGIECTASIA:** Autosomal dominant syndrome characterized by the presence of spinal hemangioma and multiple telangiectasias of the skin and the oral, nasal, and gastrointestinal mucous membranes.

☞**KLIPPEL-TRENAUNAY-WEBER SYNDROME:** Congenital malformation of unknown origin characterized by the presence of spinal hemangiomas and the association of soft tissue and bony hypertrophy, venous malformations, lymphatic abnormalities, and cutaneous capillary malformations.

REFERENCE:

Leblanc R, Melanson D, Wilkinson RD: Hereditary neurocutaneous hemangiomatosis. Report of four cases. *J Neurosurg* 85:1135, 1996.

Hereditary Pancreatitis

At a glance: Genetic condition characterized by recurrent episodes of painful pancreatic attacks, which can progress to chronic pancreatitis.

History: Inherited disorder characterized by relapsing chronic pancreatitis. First described by Comfort and Steinberg in 1952.

Incidence: It is the most common form of chronic relapsing pancreatitis in childhood. May account for approximately 25% of adult cases with chronic idiopathic pancreatitis. Equal sex predilection. At least 1000 individuals in the United States are affected with hereditary pancreatitis.

Genetic inheritance: Autosomal dominant disorder with incomplete penetrance. Hereditary pancreatitis is mainly caused by a mutation of exon 3 of the cationic trypsinogen gene (protease-serine 1 gene, PRSS-1), resulting in an arginine to histidine substitution. Gene map locus is 7q35.

Pathophysiology: Inherited condition characterized by typical symptomatology and laboratory features of pancreatitis. Pancreatitis results from inappropriate activation of pancreatic proenzymes. Active trypsin is normally inhibited by a limited supply of trypsin inhibitor. If trypsin activity exceeds the inhibitory capacity of pancreatic secretory trypsin inhibitor, then proenzymes, including mesotrypsin and enzyme Y, are activated. The activation of these enzymes is postulated to be part of a feedback mechanism for inactivating wild-type trypsinogen, trypsin, and other zymogens. When the Arg117 cleavage site for mesotrypsin, enzyme Y, and trypsin is replaced by histidine, trypsin continues to activate trypsinogen and other zymogens unabated, leading to autodigestion of the pancreas and pancreatitis. Congenital anomalies of the pancreatic duct or biliary duct system may play a role. The histopathologic findings of pancreatitis are related to the release of activated proteolytic and lipolytic enzyme. Interstitial edema and blood vessel disruption (thrombosis in the portal or splenic vein occurs with an inflammatory response) may appear early. As pancreatitis progresses, necrosis may appear, leading to hemorrhage hereditary pancreatitis with hyperparathyroidism in the multiple endocrine adenomatosis syndrome.

Diagnosis: Based on a positive family history of pancreatitis and early onset of symptoms. Characterized by the presence of calculi in pancreatic ducts. Serum amylase (measured up to 4 days) is elevated and lipase activity may be elevated for 8 to 14 days. A puzzling feature is the urinary excretion of lysine and cystine by about half the members of affected kindred (with or without pancreatitis). Endoscopic retrograde cholangiopancreatography is diagnostic for chronic pancreatitis and shows a distorted duct with multiple strictures and dilatations similar to a "chain of lakes" pattern. Children may have complications seen in pancreatitis—pseudocysts, diabetes mellitus, thrombosis of portal or splenic veins, coagulopathy, pleural effusions, and pulmonary edema.

Clinical aspects: May present with symptoms of pancreatitis late in the first decade. Typical recurrent abdominal pain starting in childhood. Diagnosis confirmed by laboratory studies. Children may be well during attacks. The attacks were characterized by severe abdominal pains, fever, and marked elevation of serum amylase. Pancreatic insufficiency (5.5%), diabetes mellitus (12.5%), pseudocysts (5.5%), and hemorrhagic pleural effusion were observed in a review of 72 patients. Portal vein thrombosis occurred in two patients and was suspected in three other patients. Patients seemed to improve later in life. Attacks were precipitated by emotional upset, alcohol, or high fat intake. The link with adenocarcinoma is unclear. Treatment is conservative, but treatment of complications must be individualized.

Precautions before anesthesia: Assess pancreatic exocrine and endocrine functions. Evaluate the severity of diabetes mellitus and its sequelae, particularly the presence of cardiovascular, renal, and autonomic impairment. Optimize diabetic control. Patients with stable, well-controlled diabetes undergoing relatively minor surgery may be admitted as "day admit" cases, whereas patients with brittle diabetes may require preoperative admission for stabilization and optimal preparation. Derangement in intravascular volume status is not uncommon during an acute attack of pancreatitis and should be corrected. Chronic exocrine pancreatic insufficiency may result in malnutrition and fat-soluble vitamin deficiencies. Electrolyte abnormalities are common, particularly calcium and potassium homeostasis, and any abnormalities should be corrected preoperatively. Many of these patients with chronic pancreatitis are opioid dependent and alcoholics. Investigations include complete blood count, serum electrolytes, urea and creatinine levels, serum albumin and proteins, coagulation studies, urine ketones, and chest radiography (pleural effusion or pulmonary edema). Anxiety and stress result in an increased sympathetic discharge with its sequelae on substrate metabolism and cardiovascular system; a sedative premedication is advocated. Consider insulin-dependent diabetes mellitus precautions if diabetes mellitus is established. Consider antithrombotic prophylaxis if history of venous thrombosis.

Anesthetic considerations: Drainage of pseudocysts is now mainly done percutaneously. Thus patients are presenting increasingly less often for surgery of the pancreas, which usually is very tedious, technically difficult, and fraught with potential complications of hypothermia, significant fluid shifts and electrolyte imbalances, massive blood loss, and hyperglycemia. In addition, systemic complications may arise from the release of multiple cytokines and other toxic factors from the pancreatitis process or during manipulation of the pancreas, because renal failure, hepatic failure, neurologic dysfunction, and cardiorespiratory failure are possible. Although an epidural technique may offer excellent postoperative analgesia and avoid prolonged ventilatory support because of inadequate pain control, the presence of preoperative clotting studies and the potential for postoperative coagulation derangements may be relative contraindications to the wider use of this option. One of the primary goals is preventing hypoglycemia and hyperglycemia with ketosis.

Pharmacological implications: No particular anesthetic agents are specifically beneficial or contraindicated for diabetes. Avoid alcohol and alcohol-containing solutions.

REFERENCES:

Charnley RM: Hereditary pancreatitis. *World J Gastroenterol* 9:1, 2003.

Whitcomb DC: Hereditary pancreatitis: A model for understanding the genetic basis of acute and chronic pancreatitis. *Pancreatology* 1:565, 2001.

Whitcomb DC, Gorry MC, Preston RA, et al: Hereditary pancreatitis is caused by a mutation in the cationic trypsinogen gene. *Nat Genet* 14:141, 1996.

Hereditary Sensory and Autonomic Neuropathies (HSAN): Overview

See Table H-5.

HEREDITARY SENSORY AND AUTONOMIC NEUROPATHY TYPE I (HSAN I)

At a glance: Genetic neurodegenerative disorder characterized by a loss of sensations, especially in the lower extremities, leading to perforating skin ulceration and bone destruction as a result of abnormal functioning of the autonomic nervous system.

Synonyms: Acrodystrophic Neuropathy; Burning Feet Syndrome; Denny-Brown Syndrome I; Hereditary Sensory Neuropathy type I (HSN I); Hereditary Sensory Radicular Neuropathy; Hick Syndrome; Lumbosacral Syringomyelia; Mutilating Acropathy; Sensory Radicular Neuropathy, type I; Smith-Thévenard Syndrome; Thévenard Disease II; Thévenard Syndrome; Ulcerative and Mutilating Acropathy.

History: First reported by Auguste Nélaton, a French physician and surgeon, in 1852.

Genetic inheritance: Autosomal dominant, chromosome 9q22.

Pathophysiology: Shorter lifespan of ganglion cells in sacral and lumbar dorsal root ganglia.

Diagnosis: Ganglia biopsy showing loss of neuronal cells with sometimes amyloid deposits, mainly around the capillaries. At the beginning, Meissner corpuscles count in skin biopsies are normal. With disease progression, loss of these sensory corpuscles occurs. Sometimes associated with brain atrophy.

Clinical aspects: Onset is between 15 and 40 years of age. Loss of sensitivity in the feet, with painless ulcers, occurs first, followed by shooting pain and lightning pain in the lower legs. Ulcers require years to heal. There is thermal sensory loss of the lower extremities, often extending to the thigh, sometimes thermal loss in the hands, and restless legs and burning sensations in the feet. Shortly thereafter, the patient complains of bilateral neurosensory deafness. Normal sweating. The other cranial nerves are not involved. Normal ocular motility, normal pupils and pupillary reactions, no nystagmus. Disappearance of ankle jerks and knee jerks. Secondary Charcot-type neurotrophic arthropathy and mutilating acropathy. Upper extremities seldom affected. No motor involvement. Deafness is a common feature of the syndrome.

Precautions before anesthesia: Usually patients present with painless cutaneous ulcers for orthopedic procedures. For medicolegal reasons, it is advisable to obtain a neurologic evaluation before and after the procedure. Search for signs of autonomic dysfunction before induction.

Anesthetic considerations: General anesthesia is often preferred, even though regional anesthesia cannot be contraindicated on scientific grounds. However, the undetected preoperative presence of nerve dysfunction may be a source of confusion after the use of regional anesthesia. Proper positioning on the operating table and

Table H-5 Hereditary Sensory and Autonomic Neuropathies (HSAN)

Type	Inheritance	Eponym/Synonym
HSAN type I	Autosomal dominant	***Hick Syndrome*** ***Denny-Brown Syndrome*** ***Thévenard Syndrome*** ***Hereditary Sensory Radicular Neuropathy***
HSAN type II	Autosomal recessive	***Neurogenic Acroosteolysis*** ***Giaccai Syndrome***
HSAN type III	Autosomal recessive	***Familial Dysautonomia*** ***Riley-Day Syndrome***
HSAN type IV	Autosomal recessive	***Familial Dysautonomia Type II*** ***Swanson Syndrome*** ***Congenital Sensory Neuropathy with Anhidrosis***
HSAN type V	Autosomal recessive	***Strümpell-Lorrain Syndrome*** ***Familial Spastic Paraplegia***
Posterior column ataxia	Autosomal dominant	***Biemond Congenital Anesthesia***
Ataxic neuropathy	Autosomal dominant	***Sensory Ataxic Neuropathy***

after the procedure. No particular airway involvement. Check blood pressure carefully during procedure. Usually uneventful recovery.

Pharmacological implications: No specific implications with this condition.

REFERENCES:

Stogbauer F, Young P, Kuhlenbaumer G, et al: Autosomal dominant burning feet syndrome. *J Neurol Neurosurg Psychiatry* 67:78, 1999.

Thomas PK: Hereditary sensory neuropathies. *Brain Pathol* 3:157, 1993.

Hereditary Sensory and Autonomic Neuropathy Type II (HSAN II)

At a glance: Genetic neurodegenerative disorder characterized by inflammation of the fingers and/or toes with paronychia and whitlows, multiple ulcers (fingers, soles of the feet), and sensory loss in both arms and legs.

Synonyms: Giaccai (often misspelled Giacci) Familial Neurogenic Acrosteolysis; Giaccai Syndrome; Hereditary Sensory Radicular Neuropathy, Recessive form; Hereditary Sensory Neuropathy Type II (HSN II); Neurogenic Acrosteolysis.

Incidence: Very rare (fewer than 50 cases reported).

Genetic inheritance: Autosomal recessive.

Pathophysiology: Peripheral nerve degeneration of unknown cause. A high urinary excretion of sphingomyelin and lecithin in three sibs of a Turkish family suggested that the pathogenetic mechanism was a disorder of phospholipid metabolism. Several authors believe the disease is nonprogressive.

Diagnosis: Nerve biopsy shows wallerian degeneration of the axons, with reduction of the number of myelinated fibers. Unmyelinated fibers also were involved but to a lesser degree.

Clinical aspects: Age of onset usually is between 5 and 15 years, which is earlier than the dominant type. There is a loss of all modalities of cutaneous sensation in the lower extremities. It is associated with joint and leg swelling that leads to cylinder-shaped limbs. Proximal sensation is preserved and tendon reflexes are lost. There is no deafness or other cranial nerve involvement. No nystagmus or ocular involvement. There is generalized neurogenic osteoporosis, with acrosteolysis and collapse of the distal phalanges, leading to digital clubbing.

Precautions before anesthesia: Patients are often scheduled for amputations secondary to osteomyelitis. Usually no specific cardiovascular or respiratory involvement. No central nervous system problem. No airway problems related to the syndrome.

Anesthetic considerations: Difficult venous access as a result of pachydermoperiostosis and soft tissue swelling. Enhanced body temperature loss caused by hyperhydrosis. Airways usually are not involved by soft tissue swelling, but special attention must be given to this possibility. Proper positioning on the operation table and in the postoperative period to prevent pressure sores. Use of regional anesthesia is controversial.

Pharmacological implications: Effect of local anesthetics remains unclear. Normal response to neuromuscular blockers.

Other conditions to be considered:

☞**Hereditary Sensory and Autonomic Neuropathy Type I:** Characterized by a loss of sensation usually affecting the feet and legs more severely than the hands and forearms. Other clinical features include open sores on the feet and anomalies of pain and temperature sensations that are affected more than touch-pressure sensation.

☞**Charcot-Marie-Tooth Disease:** Neurologic disorder characterized by muscle atrophy and weakness most prominent in the legs and the small muscles of the hands. A decrease in vibration, pain, and thermal sensation in the hand, foot, and lower part of the leg may occur. Stretch reflexes are usually absent.

Peripheral Neuropathy: Produced by disease of a single nerve (mononeuropathy, mononeuritis), several nerves in asymmetrical areas of the body (mononeuritis multiplex), or many nerves simultaneously (polyneuropathy, polyneuritis, multiple peripheral neuritis). These symptoms may involve sensory, motor, reflex, or blood vessel (vasomotor) function.

☞**Syringomyelia:** Caused by the development of a syrinx within the spinal cord destroying the fascicle of Lissauer. Clinically, it is characterized by loss of pain and temperature sensations first noticed in the fingers, hands, arms, and upper chest. In the early stages, a sense of touch is still present. As the disease evolves, a loss of feeling may spread over the shoulders and back. Chronic progressive degeneration of the stress-bearing part of a bone joint (Charcot joint) is another symptom. Other clinical features include loss of tendon reflexes in the upper extremities, spasticity, muscle weakness, muscular incoordination in the lower extremities, and paralysis of the bladder.

☞**Roussy-Lévy Syndrome:** Motor sensory disorder characterized by a foot deformity in the shape of a claw (clawfoot), muscle weakness, atrophy of the leg muscles, and tremor in the hands.

References:

Basu S, Paul DK, Basu S: Four siblings with type II hereditary sensory and autonomic neuropathy. *Indian Pediatr* 39:870, 2002.

Jedrzejowska H, Milczarek H: Recessive hereditary sensory neuropathy. *J Neurol Sci* 29:371, 1976.

Hereditary Sensory and Autonomic Neuropathy III (HSAN III)

At a glance: Genetically transmitted neurodegenerative disorder characterized by the absence of overflow tears with emotional crying in infants, hypotonia, difficult feeding, inappropriate reactions to stress, speech, and motor incoordination, progressive loss of thermal and pain perceptions, and absence of fungiform papillae on the tongue.

Synonyms: Familial Dysautonomia; Riley-Day Syndrome; Hereditary Sensory Neuropathy Type III (HSN III).

History: Peripheral nerve degeneration involving unmyelinated fibers. First reported in 1949 by Conrad Milton Riley and Richard Lawrence Day, American pediatricians.

Incidence: Incidence is 1:3800 in Eastern European Jews. Only reported in individuals of Ashkenazi Jewish descent (classified as one of the Jewish genetic diseases). The familial dysautonomia gene is carried by 1:30 individuals of Eastern European Jewish ancestry.

Genetic inheritance: Autosomal recessive with complete penetrance. Chromosome 9 (9q31). Two mutations of the familial dysautonomia gene (IKBKAP) can cause the disease: (1) a mutation in intron 20 (99% of cases) in which the gene product IKAP is not expressed in the brain (but is in lymphoblasts), and (2) a missense mutation in exon 19 that causes a disruption of a phosphorylation site of IKAP, which decreases its activity.

Pathophysiology: Loss of small unmyelinated nerve fibers carrying pain, temperature, and central autonomic nervous control.

Diagnosis: Nerve biopsy shows a loss of unmyelinated fibers. Muscle biopsies shows loss of Golgi tendon organs. Tongue has few or no papillae. Urinary catecholamines and metabolites excretion are decreased. Definitive diagnosis established by molecular biology (DNA analysis by genetic linkage testing). Prenatal diagnosis and carrier genetic testing (when there is a family history) is available.

Clinical aspects: In early infancy, there is poor swallowing with pharyngeal dyscoordination and aspiration. Poor sucking. Swallowing difficulties remain the main problem, leading to significant failure to thrive. Sweating during meals. Delayed and ataxic walking. Ataxia is secondary to loss of feedback by muscle spindles.

Progressively, pain and thermal sensation are lost. When children are 2 to 6 years old, painless corneal ulcerations and numerous painless traumatic injuries occur frequently. Tendon stretch reflexes are absent. Skeletal deformity and scoliosis are often present. Generalized convulsions can be observed in 40% of these patients. Autonomic crises begin between 3 and 6 years. They include cyclic vomiting every 20 minutes, with hypertension, sweating, mottled skin, and irritability. Prognosis is poor, with patients dying of aspiration or respiratory failure, unopposed vagal stimulation, or sleep abnormality. Prior to 1960, 50% of patients died before 5 years of age; currently, approximately 50% of patients reach 30 years of age.

Precautions before anesthesia: An anesthesia consultation is highly recommended for elective surgery. Patients often require anesthesia care for trauma, burns, or eye surgery. Spinal correction procedure is frequent. Nissen fundoplication is indicated to prevent chronic pulmonary aspiration. There are no airway problems directly related to the syndrome. Check for scoliosis and respiratory restrictive syndrome. Check and correct electrolyte imbalances and intravascular volemia before induction. Invasive arterial pressure monitoring is recommended.

Anesthetic considerations: In the absence of cardiovascular hemodynamic stability and poor thermoregulatory control, the anesthetic management must specifically account for these potential complications. All measures to prevent hypothermia must be implemented. In the absence of corneal protection reflexes, use artificial tears and careful eye closure during anesthesia to prevent corneal desiccation. Regional anesthesia has been safely used in several reported cases. Postoperative nausea and vomiting frequently occur. Protection from injuries is important in the postoperative period because of irritability and loss of pain sensation. Depending on pulmonary status, patients may require postoperative mechanical ventilation.

Pharmacological implications: Because of the possibility of an excessive response to vasopressors, doses should be titrated to effect. Normal response to neuromuscular blockers, opiates, and local anesthetics. Increased cardiovascular depression (bradycardia and hypotension) following hypnotics.

REFERENCES:

Axelrod FB, Donenfeld RF, Danziger F, et al: Anesthesia in familial dysautonomia. *Anesthesiology* 68:631, 1988.

Challands JF, Facer EK: Epidural anesthesia and familial dysautonomia (Riley-Day syndrome). Three case reports. *Paediatr Anaesth* 8:83, 1998.

Kaplan L, Margulies JY, Kadari A, et al: Aspects of spinal deformity in familial dysautonomia (Riley-Day syndrome). *Eur Spine J* 6:33, 1997.

HEREDITARY SENSORY AND AUTONOMIC NEUROPATHY IV (HSAN IV)

At a glance: Genetic neurodegenerative disorder (peripheral nerve degeneration involving small fibers) characterized by congenital insensitivity to pain (resulting in painless injuries), episodic fever (hot weather) as a consequence of anhidrosis, autonomic disorders, mental retardation, short stature, self-mutilation, and joint deformities.

Synonyms: Congenital Sensory Neuropathy with Anhidrosis; Familial Dysautonomia Type II; Congenital Insensitivity to Pain with Anhydrosis (CIPA) of Swanson; Swanson Syndrome.

Incidence: Very rare disease. High prevalence in Israeli-Bedouin Arabs.

Genetic inheritance: Autosomal recessive. Gene map location is chromosome 1q21-q22. Mutations in the same gene are associated with familial medullary thyroid carcinoma. The protein has a single extracellular domain (nerve growth factor binding) that acts as a signal peptide and a single intracellular domain (tyrosine kinase).

Pathophysiology: Nociceptive neurons in the dorsal root ganglia derive from the neural crest, and they can survive only if they are stimulated by the nerve growth factor through the TrkA receptor. Mutations in the TrkA gene have shown a correlation with the defective development of the nociceptive neurons. It results in the loss of small "C" nerve fibers responsible for carrying pain, temperature and autonomic control. HSAN IV is a result of a defect of the high-affinity tyrosine kinase (TrkA) receptor (neurotrophin signal transduction system) for nerve growth factor. Consequently, there is a defect in neural crest differentiation and the system responsible for pain and temperature sensation, the first-order afferent system, is lost. The Lissauer spinothalamic tract is absent. Temperature regulation and sensation are inexistent, which may represent a life-threatening condition. Nerve growth factor modulates synaptic plasticity and nervous transmission and plays a modulating role among the nervous, immune, and endocrine systems. It may interfere with the skeletal cell metabolism.

Diagnosis: Clinically evocated by progressive insensitivity to pain, associated with anhydrosis. Nerve biopsy shows a loss of unmyelinated fibers. Small myelinated and unmyelinated axons are almost absent (0–5% of normal); large myelinated axons are mildly reduced (45–65% of normal). Absence of innervation of sweat glands. Provocative sweating tests are negative. Normal sweat glands in the skin, with absence of sweating.

Clinical aspects: Symptoms present from birth. There is a progressive insensitivity to pain, associated with anhydrosis. HSAN IV shares some clinical similarities with HSAN III, but instead of profuse sweating there is complete anhydrosis. Children present with unexplained fever up to 43°C (109.4°F) because of loss of thermal regulation. Self-mutilating behavior, with numerous trauma, tongue bites, and burns. Mental retardation with IQ in the 60s is often observed. Other features include fingernail dystrophy and various neurogenic joint disorders. Prognosis is poor; 30% of children die before 3 years of age uncontrolled fever and/or massive infection.

Precautions before anesthesia: Patients often require anesthesia care for trauma, burn, or eye surgery. No airway problems should be expected directly related to the syndrome. The absence of central autonomic response must be evaluated, especially for the cardiovascular hemodynamic stability.

Anesthetic considerations: Poor cardiovascular stability, poor temperature control, no corneal protection reflexes. Perioperatively, it is mainly a temperature-control problem. The presence of self-mutilating behavior and severe mental retardation make be a challenge during induction of anesthesia. The use of preoperative sedation must be evaluated. Protection from injuries is important in the postoperative period because of irritability and loss of pain sensation. All measures must be taken preoperatively to prevent hypothermia or hyperthermia responses.

Pharmacological implications: Because of an excessive response to vasopressors, doses must be titrated to effect. Normal response to neuromuscular blockers, opiates, and local anesthetics is expected.

Other condition to be considered:

☞**FAMILIAL GENERALIZED ANHIDROSIS:** Familial disorder characterized by anhidrosis already present at birth and resulting in heat intolerance. Muscarinic stimulation results in significantly reduced sweat production (10–50% of normal).

REFERENCES:

Axelrod FB, Donenfeld RF, Danziger F, et al: Anesthesia in familial dysautonomia. *Anesthesiology* 68:631, 1988.

Okuda K, Toshimi A, Miwa T, et al: Anaesthetic management of children with congenital insensitivity to pain with anhidrosis. *Paediatr Anaesth* 10:543–8, 2000.

Rozentsveig V, Katz A, Weksler N, et al: The anaesthetic management of patients with congenital insensitivity to pain with anhidrosis. *Paediatr Anaesth* 14:344, 2004.

HEREDITARY SENSORY AND AUTONOMIC NEUROPATHY TYPE V (HSAN V)

At a glance: Group of genetically inherited disorders that share the primary feature of progressive, generally severe, lower extremity spasticity. Also termed *congenital absence of pain without anhidrosis.*

Synonyms: Diplegia Spinalis Progressive; Familial Spastic Paraplegia (or Paraparesis) (FSP); French Settlement Disease (FSD); Hereditary Charcot Disease; Hereditary Progressive Spastic Paraplegia; Hereditary Sensory Neuropathies type V; Spastic Paraplegia (SPG); Spastic Spinal Paralysis (SSP); Strümpell-Lorrain Syndrome; Strümpell Disease.

History: First described by Ernst Adolf Gustav Gottfried von Strümpell, a German neurologist, in 1880. Subclassified into *pure* (or uncomplicated) and *complicated* forms based on the presence of additional neurologic or nonneurologic features.

Incidence: Pure hereditary spastic paraplegia is the most common form of hereditary spastic paraplegia, with a prevalence of 9.6:100,000 in the general population of Spain.

Genetic inheritance: Autosomal dominant inheritance accounts for 70 to 80% of cases, with autosomal recessive inheritance responsible for most of the remainder. X-linked recessive inheritance is very rare. Three autosomal dominant genes causing pure hereditary spastic paraplegia have been mapped on chromosomes 2p, 14q, and 15q. A new locus for HSP gene has been mapped to chromosome 13q12.3 (encoding spartin); it is responsible for a recessive form of complicated HSP (Troyer syndrome) that is found mainly in patients of Old Order Amish descent.

Pathophysiology: Axonal degeneration involving the terminal ends of the longest fibers of the corticospinal tracts and dorsal columns. The spinocerebellar tracts are less affected. The cell bodies of the involved fibers are normal.

Diagnosis: Magnetic resonance imaging (MRI) scans may show spinal cord atrophy, especially in the cervical region. Sensory polyneuropathy on electrophysiologic studies. Normal motor nerve conduction velocities. Severe loss of large diameter fibers and relative preservation of small myelinated and nonmyelinated fibers on sural nerve biopsy. Prenatal testing is possible in families with SPG2 with an identified *PLP* gene (chromosomal locus Xq28) mutation only.

Clinical aspects: Progressive spastic paraplegia manifests as insidious onset of an abnormal gait. The age of onset ranges from childhood (as delayed motor milestones) to adulthood. Considerable variation with regard to onset of symptoms and severity of disease. Affected subjects range from entirely asymptomatic (10–20% of cases) to chair bound (10–15% of cases). Urinary symp-

toms (frequency, urgency, or hesitancy) are common (50% of cases). Hypertonicity of the lower limbs is often disproportionate to weakness and is the most disabling feature. Mild upper limb incoordination may occur. Subclinical sensory abnormalities are present in most cases. No therapy that slows the disease process is available. Treatment is aimed at maximizing functional ability and preventing contractures.

Precautions before anesthesia: Document all existing neurologic involvement, with emphasis on the level of cord involvement. The presence of autonomic hyperreflexia should be excluded. The suitability of a regional anesthetic technique should be discussed, taking into account the presence of any existing anticoagulation therapy. Investigations include urinalysis, complete blood count, electrolytes, urea and creatinine levels, chest radiography, and electrocardiogram.

Anesthetic considerations: Although there is no reported anesthetic experience in these patients, the considerations should be similar to those involving patients with chronic spinal cord injury. However, because the involvement in these patients is limited mainly to the lower limbs, the degree of cardiopulmonary involvement is minimal. Chair-bound patients are prone to thromboembolic disease, and appropriate perioperative measures should be taken (stockings, anticoagulation, or pneumatic compressive devices for long operations). Osteoporosis and hypercalcemia may be present in these non–weight-bearing patients, and careful positioning is required to prevent fractures and pressure areas. Although a regional anesthetic technique may be useful, difficulty in testing sensory levels after a spinal or epidural block and use of anticoagulation often preclude the use of these routes.

Pharmacological implications: Thromboembolic prophylaxis should be continued into the perioperative period.

Other conditions to be considered:

☞**AMYOTROPHIC LATERAL SCLEROSIS:** Adult-onset idiopathic, progressive degeneration of anterior horn cells involving both upper and lower motor neurons characterized by progressive muscle weakness with fasciculations and atrophy; sporadic in most cases, but autosomal dominant transmission has been reported.

MULTIPLE SCLEROSIS: Most common disease of the central nervous system (brain and spinal cord), which presents as a progressive immune-mediated inflammatory neurodegenerative disease resulting in myelin loss, destruction of oligodendrocytes, and astrogliosis affecting multiple body systems.

☞**HEREDITARY SENSORY AND AUTONOMIC NEUROPATHY TYPE IV:** Characterized by congenital pain insensitivity and severe temperature sensation defect and anhidrosis. Patients present with severe mental retardation and self-mutilating behavior. Other clinical features include absent corneal sensation, corneal opacities, and ulceration because of very poor corneal healing. Unexplained high fever is often associated with episodic hyperpnea. Most individuals affected with HSAN type IV present with repeated traumatic and thermal injuries. Laboratory investigation confirms the presence of normal-appearing sweat glands on skin biopsy, absent afferent system for pain and temperature, absent small myelinated and unmyelinated fibers, and no sweat response to thermal, painful, emotional, or chemical stimuli. There are no histamine-evoked axonflare and no tearing with methacholine (Mecholyl) or neostigmine. The inheritance mode is believed to be autosomal recessive.

TROYER SYNDROME (Autosomal Recessive Spastic Paraplegia; Childhood-Onset Spastic Paraplegia with Distal Muscle

Wasting; designated Troyer Syndrome for the surname of many of the affected persons in the Amish population): Clinical presentation includes onset in early childhood with dysarthria and distal muscle wasting. Lower limb spasticity and contractures usually make walking impossible by the third or fourth decade. Drooling and mild cerebellar signs may occur. All have weakness and atrophy of thenar, hypothenar, and dorsal interosseous muscles.

REFERENCES:

Fink JK, Hedera P: Hereditary spastic paraplegia: Genetic heterogeneity and genotype-phenotype correlation. *Semin Neurol* 19:301, 1999.

Reid E: Pure hereditary spastic paraplegia. *J Med Genet* 34:499, 1997.

Tallaksen CM, Durr A, Brice A: Recent advances in hereditary spastic paraplegia. *Curr Opin Neurol* 14:457, 2001.

Hereditary Spherocytosis

At a glance: Hereditary spherocytosis is characterized by a membrane defect within red blood cells resulting in a shortened survival time. The red cells have low amounts of lipid within the bilayer membrane that lead to an abnormally small amount of surface area. Because the red blood cells are spherocytic, flow through the spleen is difficult, resulting in hemolysis. It is caused by an inherited metabolic defect.

Synonyms: Congenital Spherocytic Anemia; Minkowski-Chauffard Syndrome; Spherocytosis.

Nature: Hemolytic anemia caused by red blood cell membrane defect. Although a spectrin deficiency is seen in most hereditary spherocytosis patients, the principal defect is an abnormality of the RBC membrane protein ankyrin.

Incidence: 1:5000 in the general population; mainly in white populations originating from areas around the Mediterranean sea.

Genetic inheritance: Autosomal dominant in most cases, but autosomal recessive forms exist (spectrin deficiency). Four subsets can be defined by the protein defect: (1) partial spectrin deficiency (mutations of alpha-spectrin are associated with recessive forms, whereas mutations of beta-spectrin produce autosomal dominant forms); (2) combined partial spectrin/ankyrin deficiency; (3) partial band 3 protein deficiency; and (4) protein 4.2 deficiency.

Pathophysiology: The protein abnormality causes defects in vertical stabilization of the phospholipid bilayer of the red cell membrane, which causes a separation of the spectrin-phospholipid bilayer. As a consequence, portions of the phospholipid bilayer form vesicles and thus are lost from the red blood cell (RBC) surface—the surface area is decreased and spherocytes are formed. These abnormal RBCs are retained in the spleen and destroyed, leading to anemia.

Diagnosis: Based on clinical signs of anemia, analysis of the peripheral smear (numerous spherocytes), moderate anemia with reticulocyte count greater than 10%, and osmotic fragility test (which reflects the decreased surface-to-volume ratio of red blood cells). Erythrocytes also have increased autohemolysis, increased metabolic depletion of glucose, and increased mechanical fragility.

Clinical aspects: Symptoms can be quite variable. The erythrocytic fragility and hepatic enzyme immaturity may cause significant neonatal jaundice. Whether or not occasional acute aplastic crises (especially after parvovirus infection) is revealing; the clinical picture is mainly that of an anemia that may vary from mild to severe.

Hyperbilirubinemia, predisposing to cholelithiasis, elevated plasma lactate dehydrogenase, splenomegaly, endocrine dysfunctions, and acute renal failure following hemolytic crisis, is not unusual. Splenectomy markedly improves anemia.

Precautions before anesthesia: Obtain a complete cell blood count (CBC) and coagulation profile. In case of severe anemia, elective surgical procedures should be delayed until hemoglobin level has been corrected. For surgical procedures with the potential for large blood loss and fluid shift, preoperative blood cross-match must be obtained.

Anesthetic considerations: Oxygen-carrying capacity is the most important consideration associated with this medical condition. It is essential to prevent red cell hemolysis often caused by hyperdynamic cardiovascular responses. The prevention of hypothermia is also important to limit venous stasis, red cells fragility, and hemolysis. Glucose intravenous solutions must be administered to maintain red cells energy across the membrane and limit the possibility of spherocytosis.

Pharmacological implications: No specific pharmacological implications associated with this medical condition.

Other conditions to be considered:

HEREDITARY ELLIPTOCYTOSIS: Autosomal dominant hemolytic disease in which erythrocytes are elongated into either an oval or a bizarre poikilocytic shape as a consequence of mutation disrupting the formation of spectrin tetramers; at least four loci are implicated.

☞**HEREDITARY STOMATOCYTOSIS:** Series of inherited red blood cell disorders in which the outer membrane of the cell "leaks" sodium and potassium.

HEREDITARY PYROPOIKILOCYTOSIS: Autosomal dominant hemolytic medical condition in which erythrocytes have a bizarre morphology similar to that seen in thermal burns. It is probably the result of co-inheritance of a mutation impairing spectrin association (and causing hereditary elliptocytosis) and a second mutation that results in quantitative spectrin deficiency.

REFERENCES:

Brandenberg JB, Demarmels Biasiutti F, Lutz HU, et al: Hereditary spherocytosis and hemochromatosis. *Ann Hematol* 81:202, 2002.

Nakao M: New insights into regulation of erythrocyte shape. *Curr Opin Hematol* 9:127, 2002.

Palek J: Hereditary spherocytosis, elliptocytosis, and related disorders, in Beutler E (ed): *Hematology.* 5th ed. New York, McGraw-Hill, 1995, p 596.

Hereditary Stomatocytosis

At a glance: Series of inherited forms of hemolytic anemia caused by alterations in the red cell membrane, resulting in leakage of sodium and potassium. After resaturation of normal permeability, red cell membrane rigidity, morphology, water content, and cell cation return to normal. Low potassium is dominant to high potassium.

Synonyms: Cryohydrocytosis; Overhydrated Hereditary Stomatocytosis.

Incidence: Unknown. Approximately 1:10,000 kindreds in France and the United Kingdom have hereditary xerocytosis. Familial pseudohyperkalemia does not seem to occur in the United States.

Genetic inheritance: Autosomal dominant. Mutation located on chromosome 16, but the gene is not yet identified. Except for hereditary xerocytosis, the red blood cell membrane of stomatocytoses is defective for the stomatin protein (or "erythrocyte membrane protein 7.2b").

Pathophysiology: The red blood cells have a membrane abnormality with increased permeability to cations, with a greater efflux of potassium than sodium. Consequently, these red cells lose potassium in excess of the sodium gained, with a decrease in total cation content.

Diagnosis: Laboratory findings include hemoglobinuria, reticulocytosis, increased red cell hemolysis by shear stress, increased mean corpuscular volume, and increased mean corpuscular hemoglobin concentration. The visual aspect of red blood cells varies depending on the variant: very stomatocytic for the rather common overhydrated hereditary stomatocytosis, xerocytic for the rarer dehydrated hereditary stomatocytosis, and no anemia in familial pseudohyperkalemia.

Clinical aspects: Patients generally have few symptoms but may have exercise-induced episodes of fatigue, associated with jaundice, pallor, or darkened urine. Splenomegaly and cholelithiasis may occur. Hemoglobin levels are often normal or near-normal, despite clinical and laboratory evidence of mild-to-moderate hemolysis (except for familial pseudohyperkalemia). Blood transfusions are generally not required, and the benefit of splenectomy is slight. Furthermore, if the spleen is removed, problems with excessive blood clotting may arise later in life. Iron overload may develop later in life.

Precautions before anesthesia: Check hemoglobin level and reticulocyte count.

Anesthetic considerations: Potential reduction in oxygen delivery because of decreased levels of 2,3-diphosphoglycerate.

Pharmacological implications: No known specific implications for this condition.

Other conditions to be considered:

☞**Hereditary Spherocytosis:** Genetically transmitted hemolytic anemia as a result of mutations in the spectrin gene in people of circum-Mediterranean descent; autosomal dominant and recessive forms are described.

Hereditary Pyropoikilocytosis: Autosomal dominant hemolytic medical condition in which erythrocytes have a bizarre morphology similar to that seen in thermal burns. It is probably the result of coinheritance of a mutation impairing spectrin association (and causing hereditary elliptocytosis) and a second mutation that results in quantitative spectrin deficiency.

☞ **Hereditary Xerocytosis:** Characterized by red cell membrane abnormality with increased permeability to cations causing a greater efflux of potassium than sodium. Consequently these red cells lose potassium in excess of sodium gained, with a decrease in total cation content. Osmotically resistant xerocytes result. Clinically, the patient may present with episodes of fatigue, jaundice, pallor, and darkened urine, especially during intense physical activity. At the other end of the spectrum from xerocytosis is hereditary stomatocytosis (or hydrocytosis), in which the red cells are overhydrated and sodium loaded.

References:

Chetty MC, Stewart GW: Pseudohyperkalaemia and pseudomacrocytosis caused by inherited red-cell disorders of the "hereditary stomatocytosis" group. *Br J Biomed Sci* 58:48, 2001.

Delaunay J: Molecular basis of red cell membrane disorders. *Acta Haematol* 108:210, 2002.

Grootenboer S, Barro C, Cynober T, et al: Dehydrated hereditary stomatocytosis: A cause of prenatal ascites. *Prenat Diagn* 21:1114, 2001.

Hereditary Telangiectasia

At a glance: Autosomal dominant mucocutaneous and visceral fibrovascular dysplasia in which telangiectasia, arteriovenous malformations, and vascular aneurysms may be widely distributed throughout the cardiovascular system. It is usually recognized as a "triad" of telangiectasia, recurrent epistaxis, and a family history of the disorder.

Synonym: Osler-Rendu-Weber (ORW) Disease.

Classification: The different types of Osler-Rendu-Weber disease are classified according to either the gene map locus or, clinically, the presence or absence of pulmonary arteriovenous malformations.

- *ORW I:* Presence of pulmonary malformation with polycythemia and clubbing; mutation on the long arm of chromosome 9.
- *ORW II:* Absence of pulmonary malformation; gene map location is 12q11-q14.
- *ORW III:* Unlinked to either chromosome 9 or 12, in which the frequency of pulmonary arteriovenous fistulas is intermediate between the two first types. Patients seem to be more prone to have liver vascular malformations.

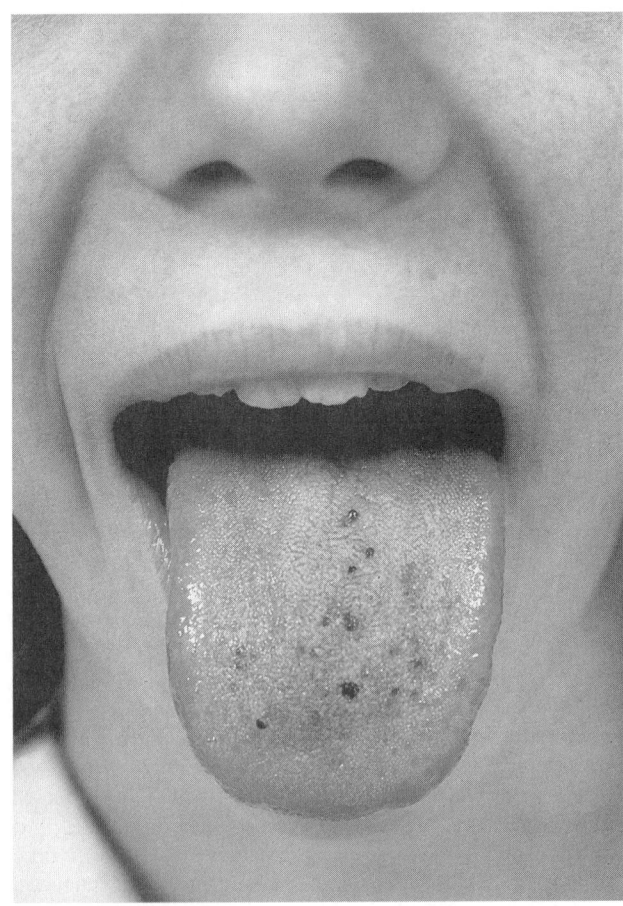

Hereditary telangiectasia Pinpoint and nodular telangiectasias on the tongue of a patient with hereditary telangiectasia. See color plates.

Incidence: Incidence is estimated at 1:100,000 in the general population, but in some areas of the world the estimate is 1:40,000, and in Vermont, U.S., the estimate is 1:16,500. The difference in incidence observed probably is a result of the different subtypes.

Genetic inheritance: All types of hereditary telangiectasia are autosomal dominant with some genetic heterogeneity but highly penetrant. The candidate genes are the genes for endoglin, CLO5A1 (type V collagen), and ZNF79, which all map to the long arm of chromosome 9.

Pathophysiology: The disease seems to result from the combination of defective perivascular connective tissue, insufficient smooth muscle contractile element, endothelial cell junction defects, and increased endothelial tissue plasminogen activator impairing thrombus formation in case of vascular damage.

Diagnosis: Hereditary telangiectasia is a vascular dysplasia leading to telangiectasias and arteriovenous malformations of skin, mucosa, and viscera (especially tongue, lips, face, ears, and fingers), with a jaundiced appearance to the skin. Epistaxis and gastrointestinal bleeding are frequent complications of mucosal involvement. Visceral involvement includes that of the lung, liver, and brain. It may be difficult to differentiate from the ☞CREST (calcinosis cutis, Raynaud phenomenon, esophageal motility disorder, sclerodactyly, and telangiectasia) syndrome. It is often associated with von Willebrand disease. The angiographic methods can demonstrate various types of visceral angiodysplasia, including arterial aneurysm, arteriovenous communication, including direct arteriovenous fistulas, conglomerate masses of angiectasia, phlebectasia, and angiomas. Pulmonary arteriovenous malformations may be life-threatening. Some are large enough to cause heart failure, polycythemia, and clubbing. Paradoxical emboli may cause abscess and infarction in the brain. Cirrhosis of the liver may occur with hepatic portocaval shunts of sufficient magnitude to cause repeated episodes of encephalopathy and esophageal varices. The arteriovenous malformations are also renal with episodic hematuria from mucosal telangiectasias and renal colic caused by clots. Migraine headaches are very common. The eyes are involved by conjunctival telangiectasia and retinal vascular malformations, but visual loss is rare. Danazol, a weak synthetic androgen, may be a good treatment for immobilization of the major arteriovenous malformations.

Precautions before anesthesia: An anesthesiology consultation is indicated before elective surgery. Check pulmonary and cardiac function to exclude high-output cardiac insufficiency and pulmonary arteriovenous malformations (clubbing). Check cell blood count (CBC) for anemia from bleeding or polycythemia from pulmonary shunt. Obtain a careful history of bleeding tendency. In case of doubt, test platelet function (often associated with the von Willebrand disease). Check renal and liver function. Perform a neurologic assessment to exclude previous paradoxical emboli and severe brain and medulla arteriovenous malformations leading to neurologic symptoms.

Anesthetic considerations: The condition may appear in the neonatal period. If the patient is treated with danazol, continue the medication until the morning of surgery. Pay special attention with use of locoregional anesthesia involving the neuraxial region because of the possibility of arteriovenous shunt, although no case in the literature describes a complication.

Pharmacological implications: No specific implications with this condition other than those associated with the underlying medical problem (e.g., liver dysfunction, cardiac, and von Willebrand

association). In case of von Willebrand association, consider administration of an octreopeptide.

Other conditions to be considered:

☞**CREST SYNDROME:** Scleroderma variant characterized by telangiectasia (morphologically indistinguishable from those of hereditary telangiectasia), sclerodactyly, Raynaud phenomenon, calcinosis, and esophageal motor dysfunction. Mucosal hemorrhage is not a main feature of CREST syndrome, whereas the presence of anticentromere antibodies is typical of CREST syndrome.

☞**LOUIS BAR SYNDROME:** Complex genetic neurodegenerative disorder that becomes apparent during infancy or early childhood. Characterized by progressive ataxia, telangiectasia, and impaired functioning of the immune system (i.e., cellular and humoral immunodeficiency), resulting in increased susceptibility to upper and lower respiratory tract infections (sinopulmonary infections). Other features include an increased risk of developing lymphomas, leukemia, and brain tumors. Progressive ataxia typically develops during infancy and usually is characterized by abnormal swaying of the head and trunk, dysarthria, drooling, and oculomotor apraxia and fixation nystagmus. Affected children may present with choreoathetosis movements. Telangiectasias may develop by midchildhood, often appearing on sun-exposed areas of the skin, such as the bridge of the nose, the ears, and certain regions of the extremities and conjunctiva. Inherited as an autosomal recessive trait.

☞**VON WILLEBRAND DISEASE:** Inherited blood clotting disorder characterized as deficiency of the von Willebrand factor protein and factor VIII protein (the factor VIII complex). Platelet adhesion is not functional, causing excessively slow clotting time and increased risk of excessive bleeding. von Willebrand disease has occurred in individuals who also have hereditary hemorrhagic telangiectasia.

REFERENCES:

Guttmacher AE, Marchuk DA, White RJ: Hereditary hemorrhagic telangiectasia. *N Engl J Med* 333:918, 1995.

Mitchell RO, Austin EH: Pulmonary arteriovenous malformations in the neonate. *Pediatr Surg* 28:1536, 1993.

Radu C, Reich DL, Tamman R: Anesthetic considerations in a cardiac surgical patient with Osler-Rendu-Weber disease. *J Cardiothorac Vasc Anesth* 6:461, 1992.

Hereditary Vitamin D-Resistant Rickets (HVDRR)

At a glance: Defect in the vitamin D receptor results in hypocalcemia, tetanic seizures, and rickets.

Synonyms: Rickets-Alopecia Syndrome; Hypocalcemic Vitamin D-Resistant Rickets; Pseudo-Vitamin D Deficiency Type II.

Incidence: Fewer than 50 kindreds are known.

Genetic inheritance: Autosomal recessive transmission, with parental consanguinity as a risk factor. It seems to be more common in people of Mediterranean origin. The defect has been mapped to 12q12-q14.

Pathophysiology: Vitamin D is well known to have biologic effects that extend far beyond the control of mineral metabolism. This is supported by the fact that vitamin D receptors are present in a wide variety of cells and can be induced by increased cell proliferation, the ontogenetic state, or exposure to calcitriol. The name *vitamin D* refers to a group of steroid molecules whose intake is possible in two forms: as vitamin D_2 (ergocalciferol), which is derived from plants, and as vitamin D_3 (cholecalciferol), which is produced in humans (skin) and animals. However, neither vitamin D_2 nor D_3 has significant biologic activity. Therefore, a two-step activation in the body is necessary. The first step takes place in the liver and results in hydroxylation of cholecalciferol, resulting in 25-hydroxycholecalciferol (or calcidiol). Passing through the enterohepatic circulation, this molecule is reabsorbed and then transported to the kidneys, where further hydroxylation results in 1,25-dihydroxycholecalciferol (calcitriol), which is the biologically active form of vitamin D. Although hydroxylation in the liver is not under very tight control, control of the enzyme 1-α-hydroxylase in the kidney (responsible for the hydroxylation on carbon molecule 1 of cholecalciferol) is regulated within very narrow limits and represents the key control point in the production of the active vitamin D_3. The main activator of 1-α-hydroxylase is parathormone, which stimulates the enzyme in the proximal tubules of the kidney. Calcitonin also results in an activation of 1-α-hydroxylase, but further distally in the proximal tubule. Inhibitors of 1-α-hydroxylase are calcium, phosphate, and calcitriol. The main function of activated vitamin D is to increase calcium serum concentration. This is achieved in three ways:

1. Increased intestinal absorption of dietary vitamin D_3 and calcium by activation of a specific calcium-binding protein (calbindin, cholecalcin, or vitamin D-dependent calcium-binding protein) in the duodenal mucosa
2. Increased release of calcium from the bone into the bloodstream by (indirect) activation of osteoclasts
3. Increased renal reabsorption of calcium

Steps 2 and 3 require the simultaneous action of parathormone.

The specific physiologic effects of calcitriol are mediated by the vitamin D receptor (VDR), a 50-kDa phosphoprotein member of the steroid/thyroid/retinoid receptor gene superfamily of transcription factors that regulates gene expression. Calcitriol enters the target-cell nucleus to form a complex with the VDR. This complex further combines with the so-called retinoic acid X receptor, forming a heterodimer. This heterodimer then regulates the biosynthesis of vitamin D-dependent calcium transport proteins in the small bowel and in osteoblasts. Mutations in the VDR results in target organ resistance to calcitriol and causes HVDRR.

Diagnosis: Hypocalcemia unresponsive to calcitriol treatment is the key symptom. Serum levels of calcidiol (25-hydroxycholecalciferol) are normal and calcitriol levels are high. About half of patients also suffer from alopecia, which usually characterizes the severe form of HVDRR. The exact relation between hair loss and HVDRR is not known; however, VDRs have been found in the basal layers of the epidermis and in epidermal keratinocytes. Resistance to calcitriol leads to diminished intestinal calcium absorption with hypocalcemia. Hypocalcemia results in secondary hyperparathyroidism. Parathormone increases renal phosphate and bicarbonate excretion, leading to hypophosphatemia, hyperchloremic acidosis, and aminoaciduria. Alkaline phosphatase serum concentration is increased.

Clinical aspects: The course of the disease may show unexplained fluctuations in the severity. HVDRR may result in profound muscular weakness and generalized hypotonia. Tetany is not common, as hypocalcemia is mild to moderate and its onset is usually slow. The most rapidly growing bones show the most striking malformation. In the first year of life, the most rapidly growing bones are the cranium, ribs, and wrist, resulting in widened cranial sutures, frontal bossing, occipital flattening, bulging costochondral junctions, and

enlarged wrists. The deformities of the ribs may, in combination with the generalized muscle weakness, result in respiratory failure. Once the child starts walking, the most affected bones are the long bones of the legs secondary to their weight-bearing function. Bone pain is a common complaint. Radiographs show a thinned bone cortex and sparse trabeculae. The growth plates are widened and distorted. Body length is often reduced. Approximately 50% of patients suffer from complete or partial alopecia, which often starts at 2 to 12 months of age and indicates the most severe form of HVDRR. Other ectodermal defects have been reported and include oligodontia, delayed dental eruption and hypoplastic enamel, and unspecific skin rashes. Supplements with high supraphysiologic doses of calcitriol and/or oral calcium can be successful in some patients. However, the more severe forms of HVDRR require more aggressive therapy, including long-term high-dose oral or intravenous infusion of calcium to restore serum calcium levels and reverse the rickets. Serum phosphate levels may decrease under this therapy, necessitating phosphate supplementation at the same time.

Depending on the treatment response, three different severities of HVDRR can be distinguished:

1. Successful treatment with calciferol analogues
2. Successful treatment with calcium in combination with high doses of calcitriol (can bypass the step catalyzed by 1-α-hydroxylase)
3. Successful treatment with extremely high doses of oral or intravenous calcium supplements

Precautions before anesthesia: Electrolytes including calcium, phosphate, and acid-base status should be checked preoperatively. If muscle hypotonia and chest wall deformity are present, preoperative lung function tests and a chest radiograph are recommended when possible. Evaluate personal medical history for spontaneous fractures. Depending on the extent of surgery, postoperative mechanical ventilation may be required and should be arranged with the intensive care unit beforehand.

Anesthetic considerations: Careful positioning and padding is recommended. Medications that decrease calcium levels should be avoided or their effects treated with additional doses of intravenous calcium. Monitor for calcemia regularly. Albumin and fresh-frozen plasma reduce serum calcium levels. Teeth anomalies require careful laryngoscopy to prevent any damage. Muscle relaxants probably are not required for most procedures in the presence of generalized muscle hypotonia.

Pharmacological implications: Antiseizure drugs such as phenytoin and phenobarbital may affect the hepatic hydroxylation of vitamin D, resulting in reduced calcidiol serum levels. Oral antifungal medications, (miconazole, ketoconazole, other imidazole derivatives) reduce serum calcitriol levels. Antihyperlipidemic drugs (e.g., cholestyramine, colestipol, orlistat) may reduce intestinal vitamin D absorption. Corticosteroids, glucagon, heparin, loop diuretics, sodium nitroprusside, and angiographic contrast media (which may contain calcium chelating agents) may lower serum calcium levels. Hypercalcemia (iatrogenic as a result of high-dose calcium supplements) may precipitate cardiac arrhythmias in patients being treated with digoxin or verapamil. Hypocalcemia and hypercalcemia affect the duration of neuromuscular blockade. Although the effects are variable, most often hypocalcemia prolongs the duration of the block. The use of a peripheral nerve stimulator is therefore recommended.

Other conditions to be considered: Rickets may also be found in the following disorders:

☞**X-LINKED HYPOPHOSPHATEMIA:** Characterized by impaired renal phosphate reabsorption and diminished vitamin D metabolism. Intestinal calcium and phosphate absorption is impaired.

PSEUDO-VITAMIN D DEFICIENCY TYPE I: Inherited in an autosomal recessive way and characterized by severe rickets, low or normal serum calcium, normal calcidiol and subnormal calcitriol plasma levels, hypophosphatemia, and generalized aminoaciduria. The disease is caused by a defect in the renal 1-α-hydroxylase. Patients respond to the administration of physiologic doses of calcitriol.

☞**ALBRIGHT HEREDITARY OSTEODYSTROPHY:** Round face, short stature and neck, significant obesity are present. Intracranial and subcutaneous calcification, neuromuscular problems such as fatigue and muscle cramps may also be present. Seizures. Pseudohypoparathyroidism and hypocalcemia. Hypertension. Correction of chronic hypocalcemia is treated by oral calcium and vitamin D. Evaluate for difficult tracheal intubation and venous access because of the deformities. Surgery should be postponed until serum calcium concentration reaches normal levels. Prevent respiratory or metabolic alkalosis. If surgery cannot be delayed, intravenous calcium therapy must be given with continuous ECG monitoring.

☞**DE TONI DEBRÉ FANCONI SYNDROME:** Rare, acquired or inherited condition involving a generalized transport defect in the proximal tubules with renal losses of glucose, phosphate, calcium, uric acid, amino acids, and bicarbonates leading to short stature, osteomalacia, and renal failure.

☞**CELIAC DISEASE:** Chronic disease of the digestive tract resulting from intolerance to gluten.

☞**DENT DISEASE:** Very rare X-linked inherited disorder characterized by onset in childhood or in adulthood of tubular proteinuria hypercalciuria, calcium nephrolithiasis, nephrocalcinosis, and chronic renal failure.

☞ **EPIDERMAL NEVUS SYNDROME:** Genetically transmitted neurodermatosis characterized by epidermal nevi, odontodysplasia, mental retardation, and various malformations.

☞**HYPOPHOSPHATASIA:** Inherited inborn error of metabolism characterized by severe bone disease (similar to vitamin D-resistant rickets), failure to thrive, movement disorders, and low plasma levels of alkaline phosphatase.

☞**LOWE SYNDROME:** Genetically transmitted polymalformative syndrome characterized by the association of ocular problems with renal dysfunction and mental retardation. Significant anesthetic implications in case of renal failure.

☞**PROGRESSIVE FAMILIAL INTRAHEPATIC CHOLESTASIS:** Rare and severe type of cholestasis liver disease, beginning in infancy and progressing to cirrhosis before adolescence.

☞ **PSEUDOHYPOPARATHYROIDISM:** Very rare disorder characterized by renal and/or bony anomalies caused by their insensitivity to parathyroid hormone.

☞**TYROSINEMIA:** Elevated blood tyrosine levels are present in several clinical entities. The term *tyrosinemia* is used to describe several syndromes. In general, the association of liver and renal failure, marked edema, epistaxis, and distinctive cabbage-like odor is characteristic of the disease. Four types of tyrosinemia-related syndromes are described under tyrosinemia. Type II, the **Richner Hanhart syndrome,** is considered a syndrome related to HVDRR.

REFERENCES:

Gardezi SA, Nguyen C, Malloy PJ, et al: A rationale for treatment of hereditary vitamin D-resistant rickets with analogs of 1 alpha, 25-dihydroxyvitamin D(3). *J Biol Chem* 276:29148, 2001.

Liberman UA, Marx SJ: Vitamin D and other calciferols, in Scriver CR, Beaudet AL, Sly WS, et al. (eds): *The Metabolic and Molecular Bases of Inherited Disease.* 8thed. New York, McGraw-Hill, 2001, p 4223.

Malloy PJ, Eccleshall TR, Gross C, et al: Hereditary vitamin D resistant rickets caused by a novel mutation in the vitamin D receptor that results in decreased affinity for hormone and cellular hyporesponsiveness. *J Clin Invest* 99:297, 1997.

Hereditary Xerocytosis

At a glance: Hereditary xerocytosis is characterized by red cell membrane abnormality with increased permeability to cations and a greater efflux of potassium than of sodium. Consequently, these red cells lose potassium in excess of sodium gained, with a decrease in total cation content. Osmotically resistant xerocytes result. Clinically, the patient may present with episodes of fatigue, jaundice, pallor, and darkened urine, especially during intense physical activity. At the other end of the spectrum from xerocytosis is hereditary stomatocytosis (or hydrocytosis), in which the red cells are overhydrated and sodium loaded.

Synonym: Hereditary Hyperphosphatidylcholine Hemolytic Anemia; Dehydrated Hereditary Stomatocytosis; Hereditary Desiccytosis.

Incidence: Approximately 1:10,000 kindreds in France and the United Kingdom.

Genetic inheritance: Autosomal dominant. Mutation located on chromosome 16, but the gene is not yet identified. Hereditary xerocytosis differs from other stomatocytoses in that the stomatin protein (or "erythrocyte membrane protein 7.2b") is not missing from the red cell membrane.

Pathophysiology: The red blood cells have a membrane abnormality with increased permeability to cations, with a greater efflux of potassium than of sodium. Consequently, these red cells lose potassium in excess of sodium gained, with a decrease in total cation content. Osmotically resistant xerocytes result.

Diagnosis: Laboratory findings include hemoglobinuria, increased red cell hemolysis by shear stress, increased mean corpuscular volume, and increased mean corpuscular hemoglobin concentration.

Clinical aspects: Patients generally have few symptoms but may have exercise-induced episodes of fatigue, associated with jaundice, pallor, or darkened urine. Splenomegaly and cholelithiasis may occur. Hemoglobin levels are often normal or near-normal, despite clinical and laboratory evidence of mild-to-moderate hemolysis. Transfusions are generally not required, and the benefit of splenectomy is slight. Iron overload may develop later in life.

Precautions before anesthesia: Check hemoglobin level and reticulocyte count.

Anesthetic considerations: Potential reduction in oxygen delivery as a consequence of decreased levels of 2,3-diphosphoglycerate.

Pharmacological implications: No known specific implications with this condition.

Other conditions to be considered:

☞**HEREDITARY SPHEROCYTOSIS:** Genetically transmitted hemolytic anemia caused by mutations in the spectrin gene in people of circum-Mediterranean descent. Autosomal dominant and recessive forms are described.

☞**HEREDITARY STOMATOCYTOSIS:** Series of inherited red blood cell disorders in which the outer membrane of the cell "leaks" sodium and potassium.

HEREDITARY PYROPOIKILOCYTOSIS: Autosomal dominant hemolytic medical condition in which erythrocytes have a bizarre morphology similar to that seen in thermal burns. Probably caused by coinheritance of a mutation impairing spectrin association (and causing hereditary elliptocytosis) and a second mutation that results in quantitative spectrin deficiency.

REFERENCES:

Carella M, Stewart G, Ajetunmobi J, et al: Genomewide search for dehydrated hereditary stomatocytosis (hereditary xerocytosis): Mapping of locus to chromosome 16 (q23-qter). *Am J Hum Genet* 63:8106, 1998.

Entazami M, Becker R, Mensen H, et al: Xerocytosis with concomitant intrauterine ascites: First description and therapeutic approach. *Blood* 90:5392, 1996.

Hermansky-Pudlak Syndrome (HPS)

At a glance: Genetically transmitted metabolic disorder causing albinism, visual impairment, platelet pool storage deficiency resulting in bleeding diathesis, and lysosomal accumulation of ceroid lipofuscin resulting in pulmonary fibrosis, inflammatory bowel disease, and renal insufficiency.

NB: "Hermansky" is often misspelled as "Hermanski."

Synonyms: Albinism with Hemorrhagic Diathesis; Oculocutaneous Albinism type VIA; Platelet Delta Storage Pool Disease; Albinism Hemorrhagic Diathesis; Albinism-Thrombocytopathy; Oculocutaneous Albinism-Hemorrhagic Diathesis Syndrome.

History: Inherited disorder of metabolism of ceroid lipofuscin first reported in 1959 by the Czech internist Frantisek Hermansky and P. Pudlak. They described two patients with oculocutaneous albinism and bleeding diathesis.

Incidence: The third most common type of albinism affecting diverse ethnic populations, mainly in Puerto Rico and the Swiss Alps. The highest incidence is in the Puerto Rican general population, with a prevalence of at least 1:1000. In Puerto Rico, approximately 1:21 persons carry the gene encoding HPS. Also, five of six Puerto Ricans with oculocutaneous albinism have HPS. However, the disease is by no means restricted to this population, and clusters exist in most populations internationally.

Genetic inheritance: This autosomal recessive disorder is caused by a mutation within the gene HPS1 consisting of a 16-bp duplication and localized on chromosome 10q23. It encodes a transmembrane protein locus that is likely to be a component of multiple cytoplasmic organelles, the granular fraction of melanocytes, and the cytoplasm of nonmelanotic cells.

Pathophysiology: In addition to the photophobia and hypopigmentation of eyes, skin, and hair exhibited by other albinos, patients with HPS demonstrate a mild bleeding diathesis. This is a result of a combination of impaired platelet function caused by storage pool deficiency and of accumulation of ceroid in tissues.

As well as impairing coagulation, ceroid accumulation results in fibrosis in various sites, resulting in organ damage.

Diagnosis: The combination of albinism with ceroid deposition and bleeding diathesis defines HPS. For proper diagnosis the platelets must be examined by electron microscopy, which reveals the absence of dense bodies.

Clinical aspects: Wide variety of phenotypic appearances. Bleeding disorders and ocular anomalies, including blindness, nystagmus, iris transillumination, foveal hypoplasia, and albinotic retinal mid-periphery, are often revealing symptoms. Albinism is tyrosinase positive, which means that patients present with varied amounts of pigmentation. A light skin color associated with numerous freckles, hypertrichosis of the eyelashes, and trichomegaly on the arms and legs are found in 36% of affected individuals. Acanthosis nigricans-like lesions (without pigmentation) are found in 29% of HPS1-positive patients. Bruising is normally observed in more than 90% of patients. In later childhood and adult life, the fibrosis caused by ceroid deposition causes considerable physical limitation because of development of fibrotic restrictive lung disease. Gingivitis is complicated by dental problems, and the resulting surgery is complicated by bleeding. Granulomatous colitis is a frequent complaint and has led to lower gastrointestinal hemorrhage. Renal infiltration causes gradual onset of renal failure. Cardiac deposition of ceroid causes a cardiomyopathy. Seventy percent of patients affected with HPS die of causes directly related to this syndrome. Pulmonary fibrosis leads to early mortality in 50% of patients. Hemorrhagic episodes lead to death in 10% of patients.

Precautions before anesthesia: Complete evaluation of the coagulation system, bleeding time, and platelet count are essential. Most often the platelet count is in the normal range, but the platelets' ability to adhere is nonexistent. Pulmonary function should be checked. Chest radiography is mandatory to eliminate or assess the importance of the fibrosis. Renal impairment should be assessed by urea and electrolyte estimations. Cardiac function must be carefully assessed, especially in individuals in whom restrictive lung disease limits exercise. If myocardial function is hard to assess, echocardiography should be performed. In any event, 12-lead electrocardiogram (ECG) is mandatory, and a 24-hour ECG may demonstrate arrhythmias in patients with significant myocardial dysfunction. The possibility of postoperative ventilatory support should always be kept in mind, and proper arrangements with the intensive care unit should be made before the day of surgery.

Anesthetic considerations: Excessive blood loss during surgery. Bleeding time should be determined prior to any minor or major surgery. Regional anesthesia is relatively contraindicated. Central regional anesthesia block should be considered a major contraindication. The risk of potential bleeding (even in presence of minor surgery and normally consider low) should not be overestimated. Proper blood cross-match should be obtained. Some patients may be on a steroid regimen for gastrointestinal problems. Be prepared to support ventilation postoperatively if pulmonary fibrosis is severe and the pulmonary function test suggests limitations.

Pharmacological implications: Because the bleeding tendency is considerably increased after ingestion of aspirin, surgery should be delayed if possible. No specific pharmacological considerations.

Other conditions to be considered: Other congenital hypopigmentary diseases resulting from a defect in the production of melanin in the skin, eyes, and/or ears.

OCULOCUTANEOUS ☞**ALBINISM:** Group of autosomal recessive inherited diseases divided into three different types. *OCA type I*

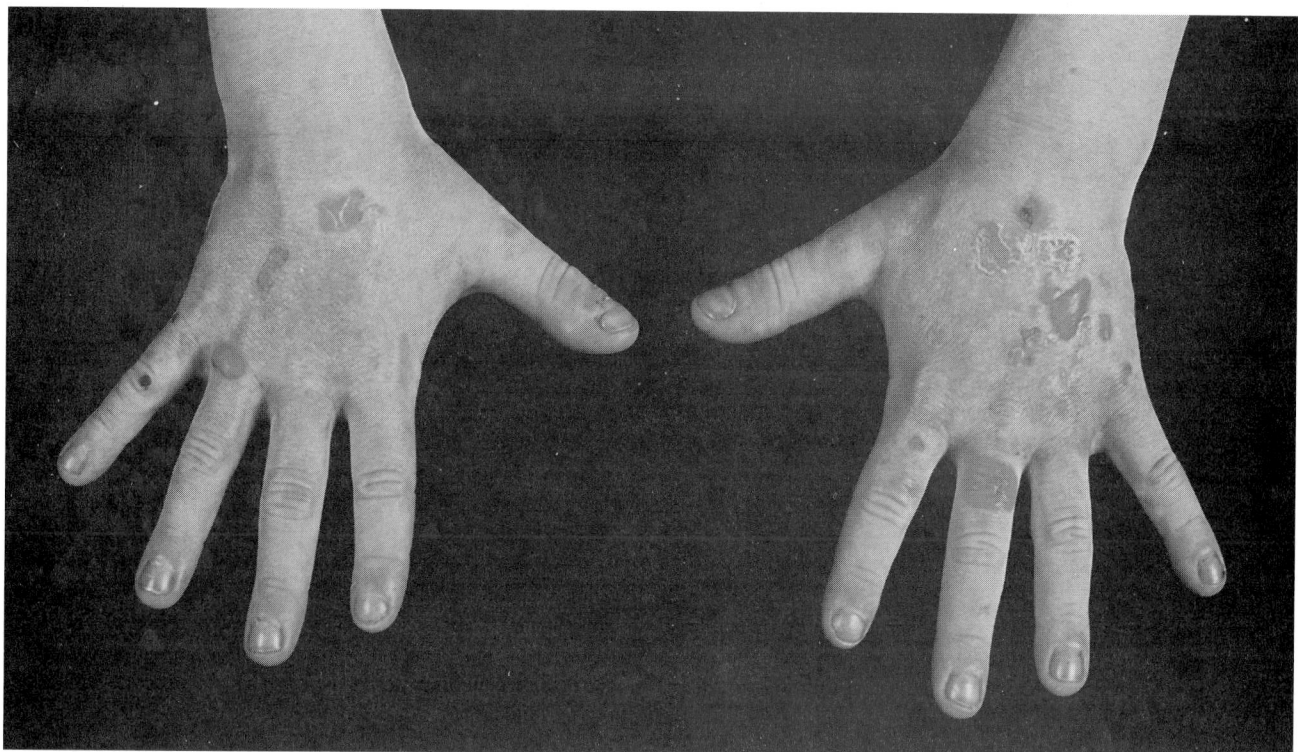

Hermansky-Pudlak syndrome Skin bleeding secondary to thrombocytopenia in a patient with Hermansky-Pudlak syndrome.

primarily presents with complete absence of pigment in the skin, the hair, and the eyes. All forms of OCA type I present with photophobia, moderate-to-severe reduced visual acuity, and nystagmus. The incidence in the general population is estimated at 1:40,000. *OCA type II* presents with incomplete absence of skin, hair, and eye pigmentation. Many patients have pigmented freckles, lentigines, and/or nevi with age. The ocular presentations are similar to those in OCA type I. *OCA type III* presents with minimal pigment reduction in the skin, hair, and eyes. It has been genetically confirmed only in dark-skinned individuals of African descent. The ocular presentations are similar to those in OCA type I, but they are not as severe. The incidence in the general population is unknown.

OCULO ☞ALBINISM: X-linked recessive ocular depigmentation and iris translucency, congenital nystagmus, reduced visual acuity, refractive errors, and strabismus. Gene map locus is Xp22.3-22.2.

☞**CHEDIAK-HIGASHI SYNDROME:** Autosomal recessive disorder characterized by immunodeficiency, partial oculocutaneous albinism (partial or complete hypopigmentation of the skin, eyes, and hair, which are silvery), bleeding disorder as a result of platelet dysfunction, and neutropenia (recurrent infections, impaired chemotaxis and bactericidal activity, and abnormal natural killer cell functions).

☞**GRISCELLI SYNDROME:** Albinism with immunodeficiency characterized by partial pigmentary dilution of the skin and hair (silvery gray hair), frequent infections, neurologic abnormalities, and fatal outcome caused by uncontrolled T lymphocyte and macrophage activation syndrome. Clinical features include the presence of large clumps of pigment in hair shafts and accumulation of melanosomes in melanocytes. Two types are described: *type 1* with severe neurologic impairment and *type II* with immunologic deficiency.

☞**ELEJALDE SYNDROME:** Silver hair and severe dysfunction of the central nervous system (neuroectodermal melanolysosomal disease). Clinical features include silver-leaden hair, bronze skin after sun exposure, and neurologic involvement (seizures, severe hypotonia, mental retardation).

☞**OCULOCEREBRAL WITH HYPOPIGMENTATION SYNDROME:** Extremely rare autosomal recessive inherited syndrome (<20 cases have been described). Most symptoms are present at birth or develop shortly thereafter and may include very light skin color and silvery hair in combination with ophthalmologic (microphthalmia, corneal clouding, cataract, ectropion) and central nervous system anomalies (dolichocephaly, mental retardation, athetosis, ataxia, spastic paraplegia or tetraplegia). Gingival fibromatosis may develop at the age of emergence of the first teeth and may result in complete coverage of the teeth and become so significant that ventilation may be impaired. Ventilation can be decreased further by a dysfunctional diaphragm.

REFERENCES:

Depinho RA, Kaplan KL: The Hermansky-Pudlak syndrome: Report of three cases and review of pathophysiology and management considerations. *Medicine (Baltimore)* 64:192, 1985.

Hermansky F, Pudlak P: Albinism associated with hemorrhagic diathesis and unusual pigmented reticular cells in the bone marrow: Report of two cases with histochemical studies. *Blood* 14:162, 1959.

Huizing M, Gahl WA: Disorders of vesicles of lysosomal lineage: The Hermansky-Pudlak syndromes. *Curr Mol Med* 2:451, 2002.

HHH Syndrome

At a glance: HHH is an acronym for *h*yperornithinemia-*h*yperammonemia-*h*omocitrullinuria. It is a genetically transmitted inborn error of metabolism caused by a defect in the transport of ornithine into the mitochondrial matrix characterized clinically by early growth retardation, learning disabilities, periodic confusion, and ataxia.

Incidence: Approximately 50 cases reported worldwide, mostly in French-Canadian populations of Quebec, Canada.

Genetic inheritance: Autosomal recessive; gene map locus is 13q14.

Pathophysiology: Defect of ornithine transport into mitochondria leads to accumulation of ornithine in cytosol and deficiency of ornithine inside mitochondria, thus altering the urea cycle. This results in hyperornithinemia and hyperammonemia.

Diagnosis: High plasma levels of ornithine and homocitrulline.

Clinical aspects: Clinical findings in these patients are the result of neurologic toxicity. There is failure to thrive, spastic paraparesis, mental retardation, myoclonus, and seizures. There may be retinal depigmentation and chorioretinal thinning. Protein restriction is beneficial. Four clinical types are described:

- *Neonatal-Onset Type:* Vomiting and lethargy following feeding of high-protein formula leading to severe hyperammonemia with rapidly progressive deterioration (asymptomatic in breast-fed infants)
- *Infant-Onset Type:* Choreoathetosis episodes, seizures, hypotonia, and developmental and growth retardation (often coinciding with introduction of high-protein solid food)
- *Childhood-Onset Type:* Mental retardation, seizures, refusal of milk, fish, and meat, behavioral disorders, and growth retardation
- *Adult-Onset Type:* Learning disabilities, avoidance of high-protein content food, confusion, and ataxia

Precautions before anesthesia: Provide adequate hydration and calories in the perioperative period.

Anesthetic considerations: Problems with anesthesia have not been described in this condition. The stress of surgery may result in acute metabolic decompensation. The severity of the neurologic abnormalities determine the anesthetic management. Adequate hydration and supply of calories from dextrose-containing intravenous fluid should be ensured perioperatively and intraoperatively. Plasma glucose concentration must be monitored regularly.

Pharmacological implications: Agents that may precipitate seizures, such as methohexitone and enflurane, should be avoided. The use of sevoflurane in these patients must be done judiciously by monitoring carefully the depth of anesthesia, preferably with an EEG monitor.

Other conditions to be considered:

☞**ORNITHINE CARBAMOYLTRANSFERASE DEFICIENCY:** X-linked inborn error of metabolism of the urea cycle caused by a mutation in the OCT gene, resulting in impairment of the reaction, allowing condensation of carbamyl phosphate with ornithine to form citrulline, resulting in hyperornithinemia and hyperammonemia.

CARBAMOYLPHOSPHATE SYNTHETASE I (CPS) DEFICIENCY: Autosomal recessive inborn error of the urea cycle characterized by hyperammonemia (but low plasma levels of citrulline and arginine), resulting in persistent vomiting and mental confusion/coma. Gene located on 2p.

☞**CITRULLINEMIA:** Inborn error of metabolism of the urea cycle caused by deficiency of argininosuccinic acid synthetase, leading to accumulation of citrulline and hyperammonemia. Gene map locus is 9q34 (20 mutations reported).

☞**ARGININEMIA:** Urea cycle disorders that lead to hyperammonemia and neurologic symptoms, which are less severe than in other forms of urea cycle abnormalities.

☞**METHYLMALONIC ACIDEMIA:** Heterogeneous inborn error of metabolism leading to metabolic acidosis and accumulation of methylmalonic acid and its byproducts.

☞**N-ACETYLGLUTAMATE SYNTHETASE DEFICIENCY:** Congenital mitochondrial disorder affecting the metabolism of ammonium and results in hyperammonemia.

☞**PROPIONIC ACIDEMIA:** Inborn error of metabolism affecting the mitochondrial catabolism of valine and isoleucine. Untreated, the result in ketoacidosis, lethargy, coma, and finally death.

REFERENCES:
Camacho JA, Obie C, Biery B: Hyperornithinaemia-hyperammonaemia-homocitrullinuria syndrome is caused by mutations in a gene encoding a mitochondrial ornithine transporter. *Nat Genet* 22:151, 1999.

Muhling J, Dehne MG, Fuchs M, et al: Conscientious metabolic monitoring on a patient with hyperornithinemia-hyperammonemia-homocitrullinuria (HHH) syndrome undergoing anaesthesia. *Amino Acids* 21:303, 2001.

HHHH Syndrome

At a glance: HHHH stands for *h*ereditary *h*emihypotrophy, *h*emiparesis, and *h*emiathetosis. Characterized by congenital unilateral (left or right) hemiparesis with subsequent development of hemihypoplasia and athetoid posturing of the left hand. Other clinical features include hemiatrophy, involuntary movements, and seizures. It has been suggested that either an autosomal dominant or X-linked inheritance is likely.

Incidence and genetic inheritance: Very rare disease. X-linked or autosomal dominant (variable expression in heterozygous females); autosomal recessive inheritance also has been evocated.

Clinical aspects: Congenital unilateral (left or right) progressive hemiparesis followed by hemihypotrophy with particular athetoid posturing of the hand. Seizures are frequent.

Anesthetic considerations: Evaluate neurologic function (clinical, history, CT, EEG). Careful intraoperative positioning is needed. Consider interaction between antiepileptic treatment and anesthetic drugs.

REFERENCE:
Haar F, Dyken P: Hereditary nonprogressive athetotic hemiplegia: A new syndrome. *Neurology* 27:849, 1977.

Hirschsprung Syndrome

At a glance: Congenital disorder characterized by absence of enteric ganglia along a variable length of the intestine leading to chronic constipation, abdominal distension, and fecal impaction in infancy, with growth retardation.

Synonyms: Hirschsprung Disease; Hirschsprung-Galant Infantilism; Mya Disease; Ruysch Disease; Aganglionic Megacolon; Colonic Agangliosis; Congenital Megacolon; Megacolon Congenitum.

History: Congenital disorder first described in 1888 by Harald Hirschsprung, a Danish pediatrician. Can be associated with various syndromes, such as Down syndrome or Waardenburg-Shah syndrome.

Incidence: Approximately 1:5000 live births. Prevalent in males.

Genetic inheritance: Sporadic cases; 10% of familial cases (autosomal dominant).

Pathophysiology: Hirschsprung disease results from the absence of parasympathetic ganglion cells in the myenteric and submucosal plexus of the rectum and/or colon. Ganglion cells, which are derived from the neural crest, migrate caudally with the vagal nerve fibers along the intestine. Arrest in migration leads to an aganglionic segment. The transition zone is seen most frequently in the rectosigmoid region in 70% of cases, but it can be seen in the small bowel. Five to 10% of cases involve the entire colon and are called total colonic Hirschsprung disease. Can result from mutation in any one of several different genes operating either alone or in combination.

Diagnosis: Diagnosis is clinical at birth in case of failure to pass meconium (cause of 15–20% of newborns presenting with intestinal obstructions) or later in children with constipation. Barium enema shows transition zone between aganglionic contracted segment and dilated proximal bowel. The definitive diagnosis rests on histologic review of rectal tissue biopsy (absence of ganglion cells in the myenteric plexuses). Acetylcholinesterase staining reveals nerve trunk hypertrophy.

Clinical aspects: Features include only digestive signs. Of children with Hirschsprung disease, 17 to 28% develop enterocolitis.

Precautions before anesthesia: Evaluate hydration in case of occlusion (clinical, electrolytes).

Anesthetic considerations: Rapid-sequence induction should be considered in case of severe colonic occlusion.

Pharmacological implications: Prophylactic antibiotics considering translocation risk.

REFERENCES:

Gabriel SB, Salomon R, Pelet A, et al: Segregation at three loci explains familial and population risk in Hirschsprung disease. *Nat Genet* 31:89, 2002.

Hirschsprung H: Stuhlträgheit Neugeborener in Folge von Dilatation und Hypertrophie des Colons. *Jahrbuch für Kinderheilkunde und physische Erziehung* 27:1, 1888.

Passarge E: Dissecting Hirschsprung disease. *Nat Genet* 31:11, 2002.

Histidinemia

At a glance: Histidinemia is a rare hereditary metabolic disorder characterized by a deficiency of the enzyme histidase, which is necessary for the metabolism of the amino acid histidine. The majority of individuals are asymptomatic.

Synonyms: Histidase Deficiency Syndrome; Histidine Ammonia-Lyase Deficiency; HAL Deficiency; HIS Deficiency; Hyperhistidinemia.

Incidence and genetic inheritance: Histidinemia is inherited as an autosomal recessive trait and is considered one of the most common inborn errors of metabolism. It is present at birth and affects males and females in equal numbers. It is now thought to be a primarily benign disorder. In a study of more than 20 million newborns, the incidence of this disease was estimated to be 1:11,500 births. This medical condition seems to be most prevalent among people of

French Canadian or Japanese descent. In the Province of Quebec, Canada, the incidence is estimated approximately 1:8600 infants. In Japan, the incidence is reported to be 1:9500 infants in Japan.

Clinical aspects: Histidinemia is considered a benign condition. For years, it was believed that mental retardation and speech defects were associated with histidinemia; however, it has now been established that these findings are coincidental. Infants with histidinemia are asymptomatic. Individuals with histidinemia have elevated levels of the amino acid histidine in the blood and excessive amounts of histidine, imidazole pyruvic acid, and other imidazole metabolism products in the urine.

Anesthetic considerations: No specific anesthetic considerations with this medical conditions.

Other condition to be considered:

HISTIDINURIA AS A RESULT OF RENAL TUBULAR DEFECT: Disorder characterized by mild mental retardation and histidinuria despite normal blood levels. Histidine loading showed impaired intestinal absorption. Clinical findings include myoclonic seizures, sensorineural deafness, thin upper lips and long shallow philtrum, and short thick fingers and toes. Radiologically, the middle phalanges are short, rounded, and abnormally shaped. The inheritance is presumably autosomal recessive transmission.

REFERENCES:

Lam WK, Cleary MA, Wraith JE, et al: Histidinemia: A benign metabolic disorder. *Arch Dis Child* 74:343 346, 1996.

Lemieux B: Newborn urine screening experience with over one million infants in the Quebec network of genetic medicine. *J Inherit Metab Dis* 11:45,1988.

Histiocytosis

At a glance: Group of disorders that have in common, as a primary event, the accumulation and infiltration of histiocytes, monocytes, macrophages, and dendritic cells in the affected tissues. Involves mainly the skin, bones, brain, lungs, spleen, and liver. Presents as nonmalignant growths that represent accumulation of histiocytes. Poor prognosis (70% mortality).

Synonyms: Langerhans Cell Histiocytosis; LCH.

Incidence: Estimated annual incidence ranges from 0.5–5.4: 1,000,000 persons per year, but this probably is underestimated. Male-to-female ratio is 2:1.

Genetic inheritance: Consanguinity has been reported.

Pathophysiology: LCH could arise secondary to a somatic mutation of a gene with clonal proliferation of the specific cells as a consequence. LCH cells synthesize various cytokines, including *interleukin (IL)-1, tumor necrosis factor-α,* and *granulocyte-macrophage colony-stimulating factor (GM-CSF),* which can explain certain systemic signs of the disease.

Diagnosis: Clinically evocated and confirmed by laboratory investigations. Different levels of probability have been described for the diagnosis:

- *Presumed:* Light morphologic characteristics
- *Probable:* Light morphologic features plus two or more supplemental positive stains for the following: adenosinetriphosphatase, S-100, α-D-mannosidase protein, and peanut lectin
- *Definitive:* Light morphologic characteristics plus Birbeck granules in the lesional cell (electron microscopy) and/or staining positive for CD1a antigen (T6) on the lesional cell.

Clinical aspects: Because of the dissemination of the disease, clinical signs are multiple and can involve a large part of the body.

Bones (78%): Typical punched-out cavity. Lesions can be asymptomatic or revealed by pathologic fracture or regional complications (loss of teeth, pain, periosteal inflammation). Most frequently involved bones are skull (49%), innominate bone 23%, femur 17%, orbit 11%, and ribs 8%.

Skin (50%): Lesions occur during the first months of life. Rash is frequent. Bronzing of the skin can occur. Infiltrates (maculoerythematous, petechial xanthomatous, nodular papula) have a predilection for the midline of the trunk and the peripheral and flexural areas of skin. Scalp lesion can lead to alopecia. There is no pruritus.

Chest (20–40%): Interstitial syndrome (nodular images) caused by a restrictive syndrome with clinical manifestations such as cough tachypnea and dyspnea. Diagnosis is based on bronchoalveolar washing. Pulmonary fibrosis and pneumothorax can occur.

Digestive System: Relatively rare, ranging from focal intestinal infiltration without any signs to severe serous diarrhea or bleeding. Liver can be variously involved, from simple, moderate biologic signs to hepatomegaly or even sclerosing cholangitis complicated by biliary cirrhosis and, finally, hepatic failure.

Nervous System: Rare; cerebral tumor or parenchymatous infiltration (usually the cerebellum) that could lead to intracranial hypertension, localization signs, ataxia, or seizures. Pituitary gland can be involved, causing diabetes insipidus and deficit of growth hormone and/or thyroid-stimulating hormone.

Other: Features can include lymph node enlargement, hematopoiesis dysfunction (anemia, thrombopenia, rarely neutropenia), abnormalities of spleen, eye, or heart (pericarditis).

Precautions before anesthesia: Because of the great variety of lesions, preanesthetic evaluation must start by obtaining full history of the disease and meticulous clinical examination. Because of the high frequency of organ involvement, some evaluation should be systematic: evaluate pulmonary function (clinical, pulmonary function test, arterial blood gas analysis, chest radiographs, CT), liver function (clinical, echography, CT, MRI, laboratory investigations including albumin, transamidinases, bilirubin, prothrombin), and nervous function (clinical, CT, MRI, EEG). Other evaluations based on clinical signs (cardiac echography, hormonal investigations, hydration, platelet count, blood cell count).

Anesthetic considerations: The high risk rate is dependent on the clinical features. Lung ventilation with low pressure must be used because of the risk of pneumothorax. Careful intraoperative positioning is needed because of bone fragility. Regional anesthesia is not contraindicated but should be evaluated in each case, considering cutaneous lesions, nervous involvement, platelet count, and hepatic function.

Pharmacological implications: Consider interaction between anesthetic drugs and antiepileptic treatment and hepatic function. Succinylcholine should be avoided if there is a large bone defect because of the risk of fracture during fasciculation. Nitrous oxide should be avoided because of the increased frequency of pneumothorax. In case of steroid treatment, intraoperative steroid supplementation must be used. Avoid situations and drugs that can affect intracranial pressure in case of central neurologic lesions.

Other conditions to be considered: Histiocytosis X disseminated form, which includes the following:

Eosinophilic Granuloma: Mildest form with only bone involvement.

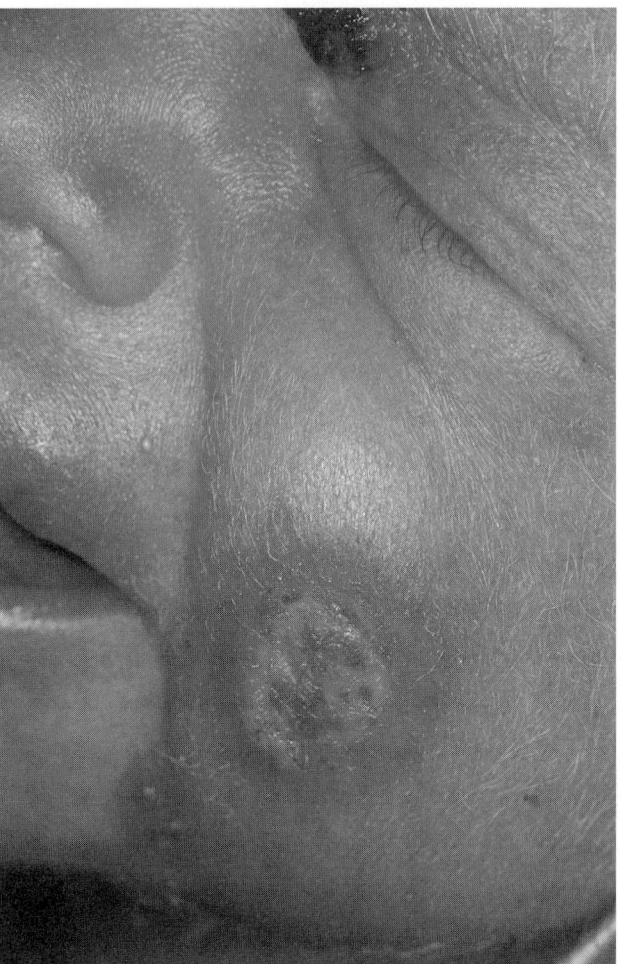

Histiocytosis Ulceration, infiltrates, and bronzing of the skin in a 3-month-old girl with congenital, self-healing histiocytosis. See color plates.

Hand-Schüller-Christian Disease: Affects children older than 2 to 3 years of age who have diabetes insipidus, cranial bone cavities, and exophthalmia.

Familial Lipochrome Histiocytosis: Autosomal recessive medical condition with immunologic involvement and susceptibility to infection.

☞**Letterer-Siwe Disease:** Childhood disorder characterized by a pathologic proliferation of histiocytes caused by the Langerhans cells. Involves mainly the skin, bones, brain, lungs, spleen, and liver. Presents as nonmalignant growths that represent accumulation of histiocytes. Poor prognosis (70% mortality).

☞**Erdheim-Chester Disease:** Systemic non-Langerhans cell histiocytic disorder characterized by development of lipoid granulomas in many organs and tissues of the body. Clinical manifestations range from asymptomatic to fatal multisystem involvement.

REFERENCES:

Egeler RM, D'Angio GJ: Langerhans cell histiocytosis. *J Pediatr* 127:1, 1995.

Kaltsas GA, Powles TB, Evanson J, et al: Hypothalamo-pituitary abnormalities in adult patients with Langerhans cell histiocytosis: Clinical, endocrinological, and radiological features and response to treatment. *J Clin Endocr Metab* 85:1370, 2000.

Holt-Oram Syndrome

At a glance: Genetically transmitted malformation syndrome characterized by congenital thenar hypoplasia and the association of a congenital heart disease (ventricular and atrial septal defect) and upper limb malformation (underdevelopment of bones and/or extra bones).

Synonyms: Atriodigital Dysplasia; Cardiac-Limb Syndrome; HOS; Heart-Hand Syndrome, Holt-Oram Type.

History: Congenital disorder of digital and/or radial dysostosis associated with congenital heart disease. First described in 1960 by Holt and Oram in a four-generation family with atrial septal defects and thumb abnormalities.

Incidence: Prevalence estimated at 0.95:100,000 live births. More than 50% of cases are caused by new mutations (no parental inheritance).

Genetic inheritance: Autosomal dominant, variable expression but strong penetrance (90–100%). Mutation of the long arm of chromosome 12 (12q24.1). No sex predilection.

Pathophysiology: Holt-Oram syndrome is caused by mutations in the transcription factor *TBX5,* which is critical for development of the heart and upper limbs. No contributory environmental factors are known. A number of syndromes phenotypically resemble Holt-Oram syndrome but arise from different mutations.

Diagnosis: Absent, bifid, hypoplastic, or triphalangeal thumb associated with cardiac septation defects, classically atrial septal defect (often with conduction defects) but also ventricular septal defect.

Clinical aspects: As well as dysostosis of the thumb, the Holt-Oram syndrome may be associated with radial dysgenesis. Clinical presentation depends on the severity of cardiac disease (atrial septal defect in 70% of cases) but may include severe endocardial cushion defects, mitral valve prolapse, and hypoplastic left heart syndrome.

Precautions before anesthesia: An anesthesiology consultation is recommended before elective surgery. Obtain a history and examine for signs and symptoms suggestive of ventricular failure and cyanosis. Perform an electrocardiogram (ECG) and echocardiography to define cardiac anatomy. Cardiac catheterization may be indicated for complex lesions.

Anesthetic considerations: The anesthetic technique is dictated by the presence of cardiac disease. Consider premedication, use measures to limit increases in pulmonary artery pressure (prevent hypercarbia, maintain PaO_2). If the pulmonary and systemic circulations are in parallel as in the hypoplastic left heart syndrome, strict attention must be paid to maintaining the balance of flow to the pulmonary and systemic vascular beds, primarily by manipulating pulmonary vascular resistance.

Pharmacological implications: No specific drug contraindications other than those dictated by individual cardiac lesions. Antibiotic prophylaxis of endocarditis is recommended.

Other conditions to be considered:

☞**AASE SYNDROME:** Autosomal recessive syndrome characterized by bilateral triphalangeal thumbs, radial hypoplasia, congenital hypoplastic anemia, joint and skeletal deformities, delayed fontanelle closures, poor peripheral vascular access, possible ventricular septal defect.

CAVANAGH SYNDROME: Rare anomaly of the upper extremities that presents with unilateral or bilateral hypoplasia of the thenar eminence. Typical clinical, radiographic, and electrophysiologic findings emphasize the diagnosis. Differentiation from carpal tunnel syndrome is important to prevent unnecessary surgical intervention. Electrophysiologic and radiographic findings are necessary tools to establish a correct diagnosis.

HAAS MALFORMATION: Congenital thenar hypoplasia associated with hand anomaly defined as complete and bilateral syndactyly, marked by six metacarpals and digits and fingers flexion. Autosomal dominant inheritance.

OKIHIRO SYNDROME (Duane-Radial Ray Syndrome): Autosomal dominant malformation characterized by radial anomalies of the upper extremities with a Duane anomaly (nerve abducens paresis of the ipsilateral lateral rectus muscle of the eye). Other features include congenital heart defects, vascular anomalies, dysplastic ears, hearing loss, and renal anomalies. Thenar hypoplasia.

☞**TAR SYNDROME (Thrombocytopenia, Absent Radius):** Characterized by severe bleeding episodes during infancy. Other features include aplasia of the thumb (radii) and hypoplasia ulnae. Congenital heart and renal defects, mental retardation secondary to brain hemorrhages. Inherited as autosomal recessive trait.

☞**VATER ASSOCIATION:** Acronym for *v*ertebral anomalies, *a*nal atresia, (cardiac defects), *t*racheo-*e*sophageal fistula, *r*enal (and limb anomalies). The name describes the most important defects of this disorder. The diagnosis usually is made based on the presence of three of the characteristic findings.

REFERENCES:

Bossert T, Walther T, Gummert J, et al: Cardiac malformations associated with the Holt-Oram syndrome—Report on a family and review of the literature. *Thorac Cardiovasc Surg* 50:312, 2002.

Huang T: Current advances in Holt-Oram syndrome. *Curr Opin Pediatr* 14:691, 2002.

Shono S, Higa K, Kumano K, et al: Holt-Oram syndrome. *Br J Anaesth* 80:856, 1998.

Homocystinuria (HCU)

At a glance: Genetically transmitted error of metabolism of the amino acid methionine characterized by severe myopia, Marfan-like stature with pectus excavatum, slight mental retardation, and tendency to develop spontaneous, generalized arterial, and venous thromboses under stress.

Synonyms: Cystathionine Beta-Synthetase (CBS) Deficiency; Homocystinemia.

Nature: Inborn error of metabolism of methionine that cannot be converted to cysteine; methionine accumulates and cysteine is lacking. Left untreated, this imbalance results in mental retardation, osteoporosis and other bone problems, dislocated lenses of the eyes, heart disease, and excessive blood clot formation.

Incidence: Incidence in the general population is estimated at between 1:50,000 and 1:200,000. Cystathionine β-synthase is a vitamin B_6-dependent enzyme; 50% of patients with homocystinuria show pyridoxine responsiveness, including 13% who can be completely controlled with pyridoxine alone.

Genetic inheritance: Autosomal recessive. Chromosome 21q22. Carrier detection possible using methionine loading tests. An abnormal gene on chromosome 1 has been proposed as the cause of reduction in methylene tetrahydrofolate reductase ([MTHFR] or homocystinuria III).

Pathophysiology: Deficiency of cystathionine synthase (homocystinuria I) leads to a failure of transsulfuration of precursors of cysteine, an important component of collagen. The weakened collagen is responsible for many of the clinical manifestations. Two other interrelated pathways of methionine metabolism can produce accumulation of homocysteine and its metabolites: defective methylcobalamin synthesis (homocystinuria II) and abnormality in MTHFR (homocystinuria III).

Diagnosis: Confirmed by findings of homocystinuria and methioninuria. P-methionine elevated in blood (up to 2 mmol/l). Homocystine, mixed disulfide, and other sulfur-containing compounds may be present (homocysteine binds to plasma proteins by disulfide bonds). Increased amounts of methionine in the cerebrospinal fluid (CSF) (homocystine may be present). Prenatal diagnosis possible by measuring enzyme activity in amniocytes.

Clinical aspects: Weakened collagen accounts for the clinical manifestations of subluxation of lens of eye, generalized osteoporosis, pectus excavatum, and marfanoid appearance (without joint hyperextensibility). Mental retardation is common but may be prevented by early dietary intervention. Breakage of collagen in blood vessel endothelium leads to a high incidence of thromboembolic events, causing cerebrovascular accident or myocardial infarction that frequently result in premature death of patients. Management consists of a low-methionine diet with supplements of cystine and betaine. Large doses of pyridoxine may control some of the clinical manifestations.

Precautions before anesthesia: Patient should be receiving appropriate diet, including pyridoxine supplements. Prolonged fasting should be avoided because of risks of dehydration leading to hypercoagulability and hypoglycemia. Dextrose-containing intravenous fluids should be started preoperatively. Assess hematocrit, platelet count, and coagulation profile (prothrombin time, partial thromboplastin time).

Anesthetic considerations: The major hazard in the perioperative period is vascular thrombosis; this has been particularly associated with angiography and the administration of nitrous oxide. The goals of anesthetic management are to maintain peripheral perfusion and prevent dehydration. Agents should be selected to avoid excessive depression of cardiac output. Fluid therapy should be started preoperatively. Generous fluid therapy should be continued intraoperatively to maintain circulating volume. Dextran-40 solutions have been advocated to reduce platelet adhesiveness. Dextrose-containing fluids should be given to prevent hypoglycemia. The patient should be positioned carefully to avoid vascular compression and venous stasis. Calf compression devices may aid in promoting venous return from the lower extremities. The anesthetic technique should allow rapid recovery with early postoperative ambulation. A significant increase in postoperative cardiac ischemic episode has been reported after administration of nitrous oxide. Regional techniques may be contraindicated: nerve blocks may be complicated by damage to adjacent blood vessels with the potential for vascular thrombosis as a result and spinal or epidural analgesia may lead to vascular stasis. Intravenous hydration should be continued postoperatively until oral intake is reestablished.

Pharmacological implications: The use of nitrous oxide is contraindicated because of its effect on homocysteine plasma concentration and thromboembolic consequences. After 48 hours of nitrous oxide administration, Badner et al. reported a significant increase in the postoperative period of cardiac ischemia in 42 patients when compared with those not receiving nitrous oxide. No other anesthetic agents are specifically contraindicated.

Other condition to be considered:

☞**MARFAN SYNDROME:** Autosomal dominant generalized connective tissue weakness with hyperextensible joints, increased risk of valvular/aortic disease, ectopia lentis, megalocornea, and pneumothorax, caused by a mutation in the fibrillin gene on chromosome 15.

REFERENCES:

Badner NH, Beattie WS, Freeman D, Spence JD. Nitrous oxide-induced increased homocysteine concentrations are associated with increased postoperative myocardial ischemia in patients undergoing carotid endarterectomy. *Anesth Analg* 5:1073–1079, 2000.

Kelly PJ, Furie KL, Kistler JP, et al: Stroke in young patients with hyperhomocysteinemia due to cystathionine beta-synthase deficiency. *Neurology* 60:275, 2003.

Teng YH, Sung CS, Liao WW, et al: General anesthesia for patient with homocystinuria—A case report. *Acta Anaesthesiol Sin* 40:153, 2002.

Yap S, Naughten E: Homocystinuria due to cystathionine beta-synthase deficiency in Ireland: 25 years' experience of a newborn screened and treated population with reference to clinical outcome and biochemical control. *J Inherit Metab Dis* 21:738, 1998.

Horton Syndrome

At a glance: Severe throbbing headache syndrome characterized by inflammation of the temporal (pulseless, enlarged superficial artery) and other cranial arteries. Patients present with anorexia, insomnia, and low-grade fever. Blindness may occur if process reaches the ophthalmic artery. Rarely presents before the sixth decade of life.

Synonyms: Arteritis Temporalis (of Horton); Horton Arteritis; Horton Disease I; Horton Giant Cell Arteritis; Horton Temporal Arteritis; Horton-Gilmour Disease; Horton-Magath-Brown Syndrome; Hutchinson-Horton Syndrome; Giant Cell Arteritis (GCA); Granulomatosis Arteritis; Senile Arteritis; Temporal Arteritis; Temporal Megacellular Arteritis.

> *NB:* Do not confuse with Bing-Horton syndrome or Horton disease II (cluster headache and erythroprosopalgia).

History: Systemic arteritis affecting major and small arteries. First described by Jonathan Hutchinson in 1890.

Incidence: More common in the northern latitudes (15–30: 100,000 persons) compared to southern latitudes (<2:100,000 persons). Rather common in northern Europe. Rare in nonwhites. Both sexes affected, but females twice as often as males.

Genetic inheritance: Not a genetic disorder even though genetic factors may predispose to the disease (three allelic variants of the HLA-DRB1*04 family are overrepresented in patients with biopsy-proven disease). Familial aggregation has been observed. People of Hispanic descent seem genetically protected against the syndrome.

Pathophysiology: The pathogenesis is not fully understood, but the underlying cause of the inflammation is an autoimmune reaction to the lining of temporal and related arteries (mainly the adventitia); however, Horton syndrome cannot be considered an autoimmune disease. Histologically, there is lymphocyte, plasma cell, and multinucleated giant cell infiltration of the vessel wall. A cell-mediated autoimmune mechanism against elastin is suggested. The cellular infiltrate predominantly consists of CD4 + T lymphocytes and monocytes. High levels of IL-1 and IL-2 have been identified in the lesions of Horton syndrome, as well as in polymyalgia rheumatica, suggesting a common pathogenesis. *Chlamydia pneumoniae* may play a significant role (data suggest the organism could be viable and undergo active vegetative growth in temporal artery tissues in affected patients). Increased endothelin-1 plasma levels have been reported, and the significance is under evaluation.

Diagnosis: Positive temporal artery biopsy. Characteristic history in the absence of biopsy.

Clinical aspects: General symptoms include weight loss, pyrexia (may have acute onset), symmetrical muscle stiffness, and pain that is worse in the morning. Cranial symptoms include paroxysmal burning pain (typically unilateral and beginning behind one eye), headache, jaw claudication, rarely scalp necrosis, or lingual ischemia secondary to arterial occlusion. Skin overlying arteries may appear inflamed in the acute phase. Ocular problems include blindness caused by anterior ischemic optic atrophy, transient visual loss, and diplopia. The vasculitis increases the risk of aortic aneurysm (usually thoracic/dissecting), coronary arteritis causing myocardial ischemia, and cerebral arteritis causing infarction, most usually in a posterior cerebral artery distribution. Vertebral arteritis may result in auditory loss and vestibular dysfunction (vertigo). Abdominal claudication and bowel necrosis are reported. Erythrocyte sedimentation rate and C-reactive protein are elevated. Treatment consists of high-dose glucocorticoid therapy in the acute phase, subsequently reduced to a lower maintenance dose for up to 6 months.

Precautions before anesthesia: Full medical history and physical examination for evidence of coronary artery disease and cerebral infarction must be obtained. History of chronic steroid use, must plan to supplement the steroid prior to anesthesia. Examine for coexisting disease. ECG mandatory; echocardiogram as clinically indicated. Chest radiograph to examine for evidence of thoracic aortic aneurysm.

Anesthetic considerations: The potential for myocardial ischemia is the major concern; therefore, avoid myocardial depression, treat hypotension aggressively, and avoid tachycardia. Consider use of invasive monitoring. Consider suitability for regional anesthesia. Some patients have reduced jaw opening (trismus) and are at risk for difficult tracheal intubation.

Pharmacological implications: Ensure adequate perioperative steroid supplementation in the presence of long-term treatment.

Other conditions to be considered:

POLYMYALGIA RHEUMATICA: Severe aching and stiffness in the neck, shoulder girdle, and pelvic girdle; unknown origin.

BING-HORTON SYNDROME (Cluster Headache; Horton Disease Type II; Paroxysmal Nocturnal Cephalalgia; Erythromelalgia of the Head; Sphenopalatine Neuralgia): Characterized by cluster headache consisting of recurrent brief attacks of sudden, severe, unilateral periorbital pain. The pathophysiology is not understood; however, typical periodicity has been attributed to hypothalamic (particularly suprachiasmatic nuclei) hormonal influences. It is thought to be generated at the level of the pericarotid/cavernous sinus complex. Immunologic and vasoregulatory factors, as well as the influence of hypoxemia and hypocapnia, have been suggested but are controversial. The incidence in the United States is estimated at 0.4% in men and 0.08% in women. It is predominant in the republic of San Marino with a prevalence of 0.7%. More common in men, with a male-to-female ratio of 5:1.

REFERENCES:

Amatucci G, Del Mastro G, Iandoli R: Horton giant cell arteritis of the legs. *J Cardiovasc Surg* 38:309, 1997.

Liu NH, LaBree LD, Feldon SE, et al: The epidemiology of giant cell arteritis: A 12-year retrospective study. *Ophthalmology* 108:1145, 2001.

Nir-Paz R, Gross A, Chajek-Shaul T: Reduction of jaw opening (trismus) in giant cell arteritis. *Ann Rheum Dis* 61:832, 2002.

Hughes Syndrome

At a glance: Coarse (acromegaloid) facies (flat and sloping forehead) with thick lips, micrognathia, overgrowth of the intraoral mucosa, blepharophimosis, bulbous nose with thick alae and prominent philtrum, cutis verticis gyrata, corneal leukoma, hyperextensible joints, and occasional mental retardation.

Synonyms: Acromegaloid Facial Appearance (AFA) Syndrome; Thick Lips and Oral Mucosa Syndrome.

Nature and incidence: Described by Helen B. Hughes, a Canadian pediatrician. Extremely rare abnormality of fetal development of unknown cause. Some familial AFA syndrome cases have been reported.

Genetic inheritance: Autosomal dominant transmission of combined phenotype. The phenotype is highly variable and appears to show complete penetrance. There is no genetic background and no molecular data concerning the syndrome.

Pathophysiology: Unknown.

Diagnosis and clinical aspects: Hughes syndrome is suspected at birth based on the clinical aspects of acromegaloid facial features, thickened lips, arched eyebrows, blepharophimosis, bulbous nose, overgrowth of the intraoral mucosa with exaggerated rugae and frenula, thickened upper lids, narrowing palpebral fissures (blepharophimosis), bulbous nose, and large and doughy hands without clubbing. Pachydermoperiostosis, Asher syndrome, and multiple neuroma syndrome must be considered in the differential diagnosis.

Precautions before anesthesia: In the Hughes syndrome, there is no evident impairment of general health. In neonates, eliminate a multiple endocrine adenomatosis syndrome (☞ MEN) and research carefully for the association of hypoglycemia. Evaluate for airway obstruction and difficult tracheal intubation related to excessive enlargement of the tongue and epiglottis, coarse facial features, and increased thickness and length of mandible.

Anesthetic considerations: Airway management may be the most important consideration with this condition. Because of the facial features suggestive of difficult direct laryngoscopy and tracheal intubation, maintain spontaneous ventilation until tracheal intubation has been secured and lung ventilation confirmed. The potential for postoperative mechanical ventilation support should be considered after major surgical procedures. This approach also allows better pain management without the consequences of respiratory depression and/or obstruction.

Pharmacological implications: No specific pharmacological considerations with this medical condition.

REFERENCES:

Dallapiccola B, Zelante L, Accadia L, et al: Acromegaloid facial appearance (AFA) syndrome: Report of a second family. *J Med Genet* 29:419, 1992.

Hughes HE, McAlpine PJ, Cox DW, et al: An autosomal dominant syndrome with "acromegaloid" features and thickened oral mucosa. *J Med Genet* 22:119, 1985.

Hunter Syndrome

At a glance: Genetically transmitted lysosomal storage disorder characterized by the accumulation of acid mucopolysaccharides (heparan and dermatan sulfates) in the central nervous system and peripheral tissues, affecting only male children and resulting in severe neurologic impairment.

Synonyms: Mucopolysaccharidosis Type II (MPS II); Hurler-Hunter Disease.

History: Inborn error of metabolism first described by Charles A. Hunter in 1917.

Incidence: 1:100,000 live births.

Genetic inheritance: X-linked (male only). Gene map location is Xq27.3-q28. Defective gene is iduronate 2-sulfatase (IDS).

Pathophysiology: Deficiency of iduronosulfate sulfatase, which catalyzes the breakdown of heparan sulfate (HS) and dermatan sulfate (DS), leading to tissue accumulation of these two mucopolysaccharides. The disease leads to severe disorders of the extracellular matrix, which is made up of several proteins and sugars including proteoglycan. The metabolism of proteoglycan yields mucopolysaccharides [also termed glycosaminoglycans (GAGs)]. Depending on the severity of the deficiency of iduronosulfate sulfatase, accumulation of HS and DS is delayed (mild forms with residual enzyme activity) or rapidly severe (MPS IIA).

Diagnosis: Typical phenotype. Increased urinary excretion of dermatan and heparan sulfates. Specific enzyme defect demonstrable (deficiency of iduronate 2-sulfatase activity in leukocytes and cultured skin fibroblasts). Prenatal diagnosis available (defective enzyme activity in cultured chorionic villi or amniocytes).

Clinical aspects: Two clinical variants—MPS IIA (severe form) and MPS IIB (mild form)—represent the two ends of a wide spectrum of clinical severity.

- *MPS IIA:* Children develop coarse facial features (not visible at birth) with thick tongue and short neck, hernias, hepatosplenomegaly and skeletal deformities (pectus excavatum, kyphosis, pes cavus, progressive joint stiffening), growth retardation (dwarfism), obstructive airway disorders, pulmonary hypertension, and development of small nodules over the skin. Severe mental retardation and hearing loss. Cardiac involvement common (myocardial thickening, valvular dysfunction, coronary artery anomalies). Progression slower than in Hurler syndrome, with survival to early adulthood common.
- *MPS IIB:* Mild form. Normal intelligence or mild mental retardation, same skeletal disorders but at a reduced rate, carpal tunnel syndrome, upper airway obstruction syndrome, corneal opacities, and progressive development of congestive heart failure and hearing loss. Life expectancy is up to the sixth decade.

Precautions before anesthesia: Assess cardiorespiratory status carefully and obtain appropriate investigations, for example, an echocardiogram. Assess airway (difficult direct laryngoscopy and tracheal intubation because of facial features, macroglossia, short neck). Check history of obstructive sleep apnea.

Anesthetic considerations: Children with Hunter syndrome most frequently present with problems with airway management. The presence of cardiomyopathy or obstructive sleep apnea further complicates anesthesia. In general, anesthetic considerations are similar to those in Hurler syndrome (see *Hurler Syndrome*). If tracheal intubation is predicted to be difficult, spontaneous ventilation should be preserved until the airway is secured and lung ventilation is confirmed. Postoperatively, the patient should be carefully monitored for episodes of airway obstruction. Opioids should be avoided and analgesia provided by NSAIDs or regional techniques may be more appropriate.

Pharmacological implications: The use of sedative medication pre- and postoperatively should be avoided.

Other condition to be considered:

☞**HURLER SYNDROME:** Characterized by high urine concentrations of mucopolysaccharides, dermatan, and heparan sulfates. It is the most severe form. Clinically, the first symptoms become evident at 6 months to 2 years of age and correspond to severe developmental delay, upper respiratory infections, noisy breathing, and persistent nasal discharge. Hydrocephalus is commonly present after 2 to 3 years of age. Other physical manifestations may include cataracts, macroglossia, teeth malformation, scoliosis, and severe arthrosis associated with claw-like hands. Mental development usually reaches a peak at approximately 2 years of age, followed by progressive mental retardation.

REFERENCES:

Busoni P, Fognani G: Failure of the laryngeal mask to secure the airway in a patient with Hunter's syndrome (mucopolysaccharidosis type II). *Paediatr Anaesth* 9:153, 1999.

Shih SL, Lee YJ, Lin SP, et al: Airway changes in children with mucopolysaccharidoses. *Acta Radiol* 43:40, 2002.

Walker RWM, Darowski M, Morris P, et al: Anesthesia and mucopolysaccharidoses. A review of airway problems in children. *Anesthesia* 49:1078, 1994.

Huntington Chorea (HC)

At a glance: Genetically transmitted progressive neurologic disease characterized by involuntary (choreiform) movements and slowly progressive dementia, leading to death 15 to 20 years after the first clinical symptoms.

Synonyms: Chorea Chronica Progressiva; Chorea Chronica Progressiva Hereditaria; Chorea Hereditaria Chronica; Chorea Progressiva Hereditaria; Chronic Degenerative Chorea; Chorea Major; Erb Vitus Dance; Hereditary Chorea; Huntington Disease (HD); Lund-Huntington Chorea (or Syndrome); Microcellular Striatal Syndrome.

History: Neurodegenerative disorder first described in 1872 by George Huntington of Ohio, U.S. as a progressive degenerative disorder of the central nervous system (CNS) of unknown etiology with involuntary movements and dementia.

Incidence: Prevalence in the general population is estimated at 4–7:100,000. No sex or racial predilection. However, localized geographic clusters of disease exist (lowest frequencies have been found in South African blacks, individuals in Japan, and North American blacks.

Genetic inheritance: Autosomal dominant with complete penetrance. New mutations are rare. The HC gene is located on the tip of the long arm of chromosome 4 (locus 4p16.3) and leads to increased length of a CAG triplet repeat at the end of the mRNA. This longer repeat [46 (range 37–86) in Huntington disease v 18 (range 9–37) in normals] leads to unstable gene and gene products. Fully autosomal dominant and homozygotes are no more severely affected than heterozygotes. Juvenile rigid early-onset form is usually paternally inherited.

Pathophysiology: The disease is characterized by premature degeneration of nerve cells. The abnormal protein product (huntingtin) of the HC gene accumulates in selective brain cells in the basal ganglia, particularly the caudate nucleus and putamen, which are severely damaged. The mutant huntingtin protein causes neurodegeneration by a direct effect on mitochondria (decrease in mitochondrial membrane potential and depolarization at lower calcium loads). There is a general reduction in the neuronal population in the cerebral cortex. Neurochemical analysis reveals a decreased gamma-aminobutyric acid and acetylcholine neuronal content. Neuropathologic changes in juvenile forms are similar to the adult-onset forms. Marked deficiency of the mitochondrial respiratory chain in the caudate nucleus of patients with HC, but not in the platelets, has been found.

Diagnosis: Usually not made until the choreic movements are recognized. Although nondiagnostic, in the late stages of the disease, CT scanning of the CNS demonstrates loss of the bulge in the wall of the lateral ventricles, which is normally caused by the head of the caudate nucleus. Mean bifrontal-to-bicaudate ratio is decreased, indicating atrophy of the caudate nucleus and putamen. An electroencephalogram (EEG) is not diagnostic. A positron-emission tomography (PET) scan shows reduced glucose uptake in the caudate nucleus preceding tissue loss and may be a valuable indication of affection in the presumed presymptomatic period. Genetic counseling is necessary.

Clinical aspects: Average age of onset is 35 to 55 years, but in 1% of cases the disease manifests during the first decade of life. Affected children develop normally until 4 to 9 years of age. Early signs include changes in behavior and personality, diminished facial expression, and slurred speech. Later presentations are progressive involuntary movements of the face, tongue, and limbs, and abnormal eye movement. Clinically, there are stiff limbs, dystonia, rigidity (more common with early onset juvenile disease), and propulsive gait with involvement of proximal muscles (patients may be mistaken for being drunk). Behavioral problems may be the first noticeable issues, with patients being argumentative, impulsive, or erratic. Later, tremor and generalized tonic–clonic seizures typically resistant to anticonvulsants may occur. Ataxia and other cerebellar signs are present in 50% of cases and oculomotor apraxia in approximately 20%. Intellectual changes range from moderate intellectual impairment to progressive dementia, and mental depression with suicidal attempts is frequent. The course of disease is more rapid in children (average of 8 years) than in adults (14–17 years). Death usually occurs from aspiration pneumonia. There is no specific treatment for Huntington disease, but drugs that relieve movement disorder are helpful. Butyrophenone and phenothiazines provide the best results in movement disorder control.

Precautions before anesthesia: With disease progression, pharyngeal muscles are involved by the disease. Check airway patency and tonus. Rule out aspiration pneumonia before induction of major surgical procedure. Check preoperative pulse rate and earlier occurrences of bradycardia. Patients affected are susceptible to body temperature changes.

Anesthetic considerations: Anesthetic experience consists of small series and case reports. No specific anesthetic regimen required, usually performed under general anesthesia. However, the safe use of locoregional anesthesia has been reported. Bradycardia following small doses of opiates respond to atropine at normal doses. There is a case report of delayed awakening with thiopental and good recovery with propofol. There is also a case report of exaggerated response to scoline and the report of an increased incidence of decreased pseudocholinesterase activity. Huntington patients may be sensitive to nondepolarizing neuromuscular blockers for an unexplained reason. Therefore, monitoring of the level of neuromuscular blockade is helpful. Proper measures to prevent hypothermia must be undertaken. Intravenous fluids must be warmed to prevent shivering postoperatively. If preoperative or postoperative sedation is needed, drugs that improve movement disorders are useful (butyrophenones, phenothiazines).

Pharmacological implications: No specific drug is either required or is to be avoided. Decrease doses of pentothal, benzodiazepines, and nondepolarizing neuromuscular blockers. Succinylcholine effect is prolonged.

Other conditions to be considered:

SYDENHAM CHOREA: Major manifestation of acute rheumatic fever; occurs most commonly between the ages of 7 and 14 years, with peak incidence at 8 years of age. Characterized by rapid, irregular, aimless, involuntary movements of the muscles of the limbs, face, and trunk. More frequent in girls than boys. Patients can be affected by severe endocarditis. The diagnosis is based on evidence of streptococcal infection leading to neuroimmune disorder.

☞**MOUNT REBACK SYNDROME:** Transmitted as an autosomal dominant trait. Characterized by repeat acute episodes of choreotathetosis and torsion without loss of consciousness. The attacks never occur during sleep, and at their height are similar to Huntington chorea. Alcoholic beverages, coffee, hunger, fatigue, tobacco, and emotional stress are precipitating factors. The presence of a Kayser-Fleischer ring (copper ocular deposition) is the principal feature.

☞ **WILSON DISEASE:** Autosomal recessive inborn error of copper metabolism in which copper initially accumulates in the liver, then in other organs of the body (brain, eyes, and kidneys). Caused by a mutation in the ATP7B gene located at 13q14.3. Characterized by cirrhosis, central nervous finding, and the presence of a Kayser-Fleischer ring in the eyes.

DENTATORUBROPALLIDOLUYSIAN ATROPHY (DRPLA): Autosomal dominant neurodegenerative disorder characterized by myoclonus, epilepsy, cerebellar ataxia, choreoathetosis, and dementia. Particularly prevalent in Japan. The age of onset varies from younger than 10 years to the seventh decade. Individuals with juvenile onset usually show rapid progression compared to late-onset cases.

HAW RIVER SYNDROME (HRS, Ataxia Chorea Seizures and Dementia): Autosomal dominant neurodegenerative disease encountered in five generations of the African American population in rural North Carolina, U.S. Resembles Huntington disease, spinocerebellar atrophy, and dentatorubropallidoluysian atrophy (DRPLA). Caused by the same expanded CTG-B37 repeat observed in the DRPLA. In comparison to DRPLA, HRS is characterized by the absence of myoclonic seizures; however, patients present with ataxia, chorea, and dementia.

REFERENCES:
Gencik M, Hammans C, Strehl H, et al: Chorea Huntington: A rare case with childhood onset. *Neuropediatrics* 33:90, 2002.

Gupta K, Leng CP: Anaesthesia and juvenile Huntington's disease. *Paediatr Anaesth* 10:107, 2000.

Panov AV, Gutekunst CA, Leavitt BR, et al: Early mitochondrial calcium defects in Huntington's disease are a direct effect of polyglutamines. *Nat Neurosci* 5:731, 2002.

Hurler Syndrome

At a glance: Genetically transmitted lysosomal storage disease resulting in accumulation of acid mucopolysaccharides in the central nervous system and peripheral tissues characterized by coarse facies (gargoyle-like), profound mental retardation, considerable hepatomegaly, hernias, enlarged tongue, skeletal disorders (kyphoscoliosis), dwarfism, and respiratory and cardiac impairment.

Synonyms: Alpha-L-Iduronidase Deficiency Syndrome; Dysostosis Multiplex; Dysostotic Idiocy; Johnie McL Disease; Hurler-Pfaundler Syndrome; Gargoylism; Lipochondrodystrophy; Mucopolysaccharidosis type IH; Pfaundler-Hurler Syndrome; Thompson Syndrome; Hurler-Scheie Syndrome.

History: Inborn error of metabolism of GAGs. First described in 1919 by Gertrud Hurler, a German pediatrician (1889–1965).

Incidence: 1:10,000–100,000 live births.

Genetic inheritance: Autosomal recessive. Defective gene responsible for the production of alpha-L-iduronidase is located at chromosome 4p16.3. No sex predilection.

Pathophysiology: Deficiency of alpha-L-iduronidase leads to tissue accumulation of dermatan and heparan sulfates. The disease leads to severe disorders within the extracellular matrix, which is made up of several proteins and sugars, including proteoglycan, the catabolism of which yields dermatan and heparin sulfates.

Diagnosis: Typical phenotype. Increased urinary excretion of dermatan and heparan sulfates. Deficiency of alpha-L-iduronidase activity in leukocytes and cultured skin fibroblasts. Prenatal diagnosis available (deficiency of enzyme activity in cultured chorionic villi or amniocytes, increased GAGs in amniotic fluid). Carrier detection possible using 4-methylumbelliferyl-α-iduronate.

Clinical aspects: Infants appear normal at birth but develop typical phenotype by the end of first year of life, including coarse facial features, large, deformed skull, short stature, kyphoscoliosis, multiple skeletal abnormalities, clouded corneas, hernias, and hepatosplenomegaly. As the disease progresses, there may be narrowing of the coronary arteries and thickening of the cardiac valves and myocardium leading to heart failure. The course of the disease is associated with a progressive deterioration with mental retardation. Death from cardiorespiratory failure commonly occurs in the early teens.

Precautions before anesthesia: Assess cardiorespiratory status carefully and obtain appropriate investigations, for example, chest radiograph, echocardiogram. Assess airway and degree of cervical spine instability. Check medical history for evidence of airway obstruction during sleep. Treat intercurrent respiratory infections.

Anesthetic considerations: Children with Hurler syndrome frequently present difficulties with airway management that increases with age. About half of direct laryngoscopy and tracheal intubations are very difficult, and securing the airway may fail in 10%. The airway is compromised by accumulation of mucopolysaccharides in the soft tissues of the head and neck. Airway obstruction may occur during induction of anesthesia, and face-mask fit may be poor. The trachea may be narrowed or flattened, necessitating the availability

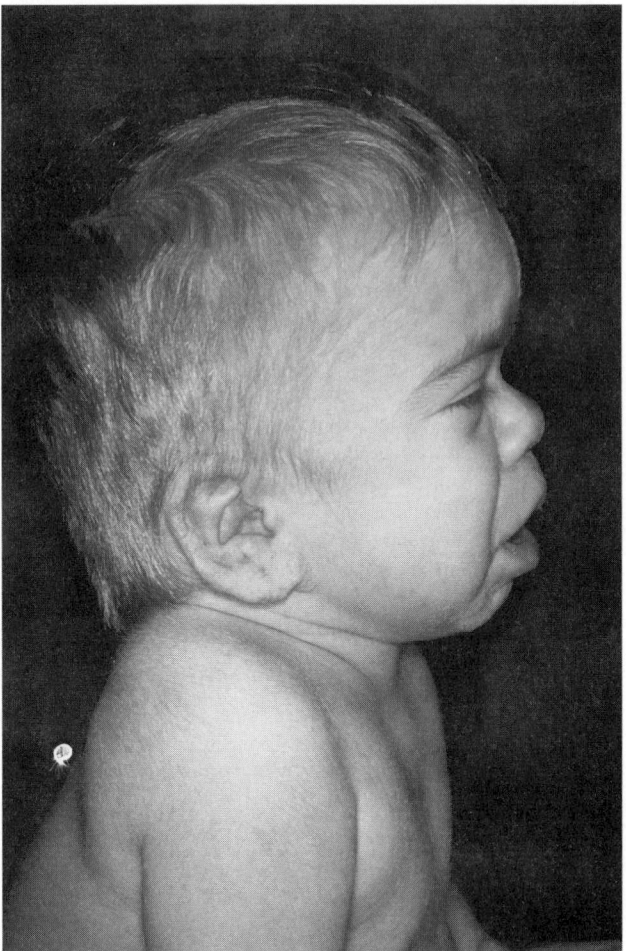

Hurler syndrome Almost 4-year-old boy shows the typical facial features of Hurler syndrome.

of a range of endotracheal tube sizes. There is frequently severe limitation of movement of the cervical spine and restrictive lung disease. Progressive cardiac failure or pulmonary hypertension occur in some patients, further complicating management. The skin is thickened, and venous cannulation may be difficult. Because of the progressive nature of the disease, previous uneventful anesthesia cannot be relied upon as reassurance. If the airway is predicted to be difficult, the aim should be to maintain spontaneous breathing during induction of anesthesia, with halothane or sevoflurane considered the agents of choice. The trachea must be secured, lung ventilation confirmed with the presence of endtidal CO_2 and by chest auscultation before any neuromuscular blockade agents is given. Antisialogogue premedication is indicated. The laryngeal mask has been useful for airway maintenance in these children and serves as a conduit for intubation, aided if necessary by a fiberoptic bronchoscope. Attempts at nasal intubation may be hindered by narrowing of the nasal airway. In some cases, emergent tracheostomy has been necessary to secure the airway. Regional anesthesia alone for surgery is often impaired by mental retardation. Postoperatively, there are risks of airway obstruction, particularly if opioids are used. Pain relief may be provided using local anesthetic techniques or nonsteroidal anti-inflammatory drugs (NSAIDs). Be prepared to support ventilation in the postoperative period, especially to facilitate proper pain management.

Pharmacological implications: Avoid sedating drugs in the postoperative period in patients where the airway is not secured. There are no specific implications with this condition; however, the underlying cardiopulmonary status may dictate each indication.

Other conditions to be considered:

☞**GANGLIOSIDOSIS G$_{M1}$ TYPE I:** Autosomal recessive lysosomal storage disease characterized by coarse facies and progressive neurodegeneration. It is caused by an accumulation of G$_{M1}$ ganglioside, oligosaccharides, and the mucopolysaccharide keratan. There is a deficient activity of lysosomal enzyme β-galactosidase. Gene map locus is 3p21.33. Pseudo-Hurler polydystrophy is milder than mucolipidosis type II or I cell disease (see *I Cell Disease*) with a later onset (2–4 years), slower progression, and possible survival into adulthood. It is caused by a mutation in the UDP-N-acetylglucosamine-1 phosphotransferase gene located on chromosome 4q21-q23. The genetics and pathophysiology is similar to that of mucolipidosis type II. Affected patients have clinical features resembling those of mucopolysaccharidoses types I and VI but without mucopolysacchariduria. Joint stiffness, scoliosis, and skeletal dystrophy are present. Cardiac valvular lesions are present, of which aortic insufficiency is most common. Although puberty is normal, approximately 50% of reported cases have mild mental retardation. Although type III is a milder illness, all the anesthetic considerations—including difficult mask ventilation, direct laryngoscopy, and tracheal intubation must be considered. The presence of odontoid hypoplasia with the possibility of an unstable neck must be taken for granted in all patients. The association of thickened trachea wall necessitating smaller endotracheal tube and the presence of obstructive sleep apnea are very important features. The clinical presentation is very similar to patients affected with I cell disease.

☞**MUCOPOLYSACCHARIDOSIS TYPE II (Hunter Syndrome):** X-linked lysosomal storage disease characterized by accumulation of acid mucopolysaccharides (heparan and dermatan sulfates) in the central nervous system and peripheral tissues, affecting only male children and resulting in severe neurologic impairment. The defective gene is iduronate-2-sulfatase (IDS). Gene map location is Xq27.3-q28.

☞**I CELL DISEASE:** Rare inherited metabolic disorder characterized by coarse facial features, skeletal abnormalities, and mental retardation. The symptoms of I cell disease are similar to, but more severe, than those of Hurler syndrome. The onset of age is during infancy (6–10 months). Craniofacial abnormalities include coarse facial features, depressed nasal bridge, long and narrow head, unusually high and narrow forehead, and/or epicanthal folds. Skeletal malformations including scoliosis, kyphosis, short neck, congenital hip dislocation, lumbar gibbus (swelling of the top portion of the spine), and limited mobility of the shoulders. Other clinical features include hypotonia, dwarfism, hepatomegaly, umbilical hernia, and inguinal hernia.

REFERENCES:

Cleary MA, Wraith JE: The presenting features of mucopolysaccharidosis type IH (Hurler syndrome). *Acta Paediatr* 84:337, 1995.

Shih SL, Lee YJ, Lin SP, et al: Airway changes in children with mucopolysaccharidoses. *Acta Radiol* 43:40, 2002.

Walker RWM, Darowski M, Morris P, et al: Anesthesia and mucopolysaccharidoses. A review of airway problems in children. *Anesthesia* 49:1078, 1994.

Hypereosinophilic Syndrome (HES)

At a glance: HES is a syndrome (i.e., a collection of similar entities), not a disease, characterized by the simultaneous existence of (1) eosinophil count greater than 1500/mm^3 for more than 6 months, (2) absence of any known cause of eosinophilia, and (3) existence of symptoms of organ involvement (benign eosinophilia is excluded).

Synonym: Idiopathic Hypereosinophilic Syndrome.

History: Leukoproliferative disorder of unknown origin characterized by overproduction of eosinophils that results in multiple organ damage. First described by Hardy and Anderson in 1968.

Incidence: Not known but rare. No racial predilection is reported, but male-to-female ratio is 9:1 (male predominance). Survival rate is 80% at 5 years and 42% at 10 years.

Genetic inheritance: None.

Pathophysiology: The etiology of this syndrome is unknown, but it is characterized by proliferation of eosinophils. These cells damage tissue, especially cardiac and neural tissue, by release of peroxidase and neurotoxin. The production of eosinophil is regulated by several cytokines (IL-3, GM-CSF, IL-5). Usually, eosinophils reach areas of inflammation and quickly undergo apoptosis after degranulation. In HES, eosinophils survive longer in the tissues, thus increasing the amount of damage they can inflict because they store (and release) toxic cationic proteins, which are the primary mediators of tissue damage. The most serious complication of HES is cardiac involvement (myocardial fibrosis and congestive heart failure); however, hypereosinophilia alone is insufficient to cause cardiac damage.

Diagnosis: Leukocytosis with eosinophilia. Bone marrow examination is required to rule out eosinophilic leukemia. Treatable parasitic infections must be sought. Some cases previously diagnosed as HES involved malignant transformation of eosinophils, but these constitute a minority and malignant evolution and are not a feature of HES.

Clinical aspects: HES is a heterogenous disease process. Multiple clinical manifestations may occur simultaneously or individually. Central nervous system (CNS) dysfunction (confusion, delirium, coma, dementia), congestive heart failure, arrhythmias, pulmonary infiltrates/effusion, nonproductive cough, hepatosplenomegaly, anemia and/or thrombocytopenia, anorexia, weight loss, fatigue, nausea, abdominal pain, diarrhea, pruritic rash, fever, night sweats, hepatosplenomegaly, peripheral neuritis, and venous thrombosis. Most commonly diagnosed between 20 and 50 years of age; rare in children.

Precautions before anesthesia: Baseline neurologic examination must be obtained. Evaluate for cardiac dysfunction and arrhythmia. Review baseline chest radiographs, ECG, cell blood count (CBC), and liver function. Echocardiography is recommended.

Anesthetic considerations: Avoid regional anesthesia if thrombocytopenia is present.

Pharmacological implications: Avoid myocardial depressants. Prophylaxis against thrombosis postoperatively.

Other conditions to be considered: Other syndromes with eosinophilia, especially the following:

CHURG-STRAUSS SYNDROME (Allergic Granulomatous Angiitis): Autoimmune disorder affecting small- to medium-sized arteries and veins, associated with antibodies to neutrophil cytoplasmic antigens; symptoms include asthma, asthenia, weight loss, fever, purpura, eosinophilia, anemia, and multivisceral disorders.

EOSINOPHILIA-MYALGIA SYNDROME: Multisystemic, chronic, autoimmune disease caused by ingestion of impure L-tryptophan (usually ingested as an amino acid dietary supplement).

KIMURA DISEASE: Chronic inflammatory disorder of unknown origin, characterized by solitary or multiple nonpainful subcutaneous nodules located on the head or neck with peripheral eosinophilia.

REFERENCES:

Bunc M, Remskar Z, Brucan A: The idiopathic hypereosinophilic syndrome. *Eur J Emerg Med* 8:325, 2001.

Samsoon G, Wood ME, Knight-George AB, et al: General anaesthesia and the hypereosinophilic syndrome: Severe postoperative complications in two patients. *Br J Anaesth* 69:653, 1992.

Watanabe K, Tournilhac O, Camilleri LF: Recurrent thrombosis of prosthetic mitral valve in idiopathic hypereosinophilic syndrome. *J Heart Valve Dis* 11:447, 2002.

Hyperlipoproteinemia: An Overview

Synonym : Familial Hyperlipoproteinemia (see Table H-6).

HYPERLIPOPROTEINEMIA TYPE IA

At a glance: Inherited inborn error of metabolism characterized by massive accumulation of chylomicrons and triglycerides in plasma resulting in recurrent abdominal pain and hepatosplenomegaly.

Synonyms: Buerger-Gruetz Syndrome; Essential Familial Hyperlipemia; Exogenous Hypertriglyceridemia; Fat-Induced Hyperlipemia; Hyperchylomicronemia; Hyperlipidemia I; Hyperlipoproteinemia Type I; Idiopathic Familial Hyperlipemia; Lipoprotein Lipase Deficiency; Familial Retention Hyperlipemia.

Incidence: Mostly prevalent among the French Canadian population.

Genetic inheritance: Autosomal recessive. Gene map locus is 8p22.

Pathophysiology: The decrease in the enzyme activity leads to an abnormally elevated accumulation of chylomicrons in the blood associated with an increase in the triglyceride level.

Diagnosis: Diagnosis is confirmed by low enzyme activity and is often first suspected by the observation of a lactescent plasma and elevated triglyceride concentration.

Clinical aspects: Patients affected with this disorder usually present in infancy or early childhood with complaint of abdominal pain often associated with recurrent pancreatitis and hepatosplenomegaly. Presenting symptoms in small children can be nonspecific, with irritability, fever, lower GI bleeding, diarrhea, and vomiting. Other features include the presence of lipemia retinalis, anemia, and xanthomas. Treatment consists of strictly restricted fat intake and avoidance of alcohol, steroids, estrogens, and isotretinoin, which increase triglyceride level. Cholesterol levels are normal, and the risk of cardiac disease is low.

Precautions before anesthesia: Obtain a cell blood count (CBC) and phosphatase alkaline and amylase levels to rule out acute pancreatitis.

Anesthetic considerations: Avoid prolonged infusion of lipidic emulsions of propofol, which increases triglyceride level.

Pharmacological implications: Avoid propofol in lipid emulsions.

REFERENCES:

Ameis D, Kobayashi J, Davis RC, et al: Familial chylomicronemia (type I hyperlipoproteinemia) due to a single missense mutation in the lipoprotein lipase gene. *J Clin Invest* 87:1165, 1991.

Holt LE, Aylward FX, Timbers HG: Idiopathic familial lipemia. *Bull Johns Hopkins Hosp* 64:279, 1939

HYPERLIPOPROTEINEMIA TYPE IIA

At a glance: Genetic disorder of lipid metabolism causing accumulation of cholesterol, thus increasing the risk of cardiovascular diseases.

Synonyms: Hypercholesterolemia; Low-Density-Lipoprotein (LDL) Receptor Disorder.

Incidence: Estimated incidence is 1:500 of general population.

Genetic inheritance: Autosomal dominant.

Pathophysiology: In most cases the patients are heterozygotes. They have a defective low-density lipoprotein (LDL) receptor that has no activity or up to only 10% of normal activity; the other allele is normal, so globally the total activity is 50 to 60%. Afterward there is an increase in plasmatic level of LDL that can infiltrate arterial vessels and cause endothelial damage, platelet aggregation, atherosclerosis and, ultimately, ischemic cardiac disease.

Diagnosis: Diagnosis is made in the presence of isolated elevation of cholesterol without concomitant elevation of triglycerides. Also, in the familial type, the total cholesterol concentration is more elevated than with other causes of elevated cholesterol. Finally, the presence of xanthomas on tendons is pathognomonic of this type of hyperlipidemia.

Clinical aspects: Patients are often detected at birth through the blood sample taken from the umbilical cord, in which LDL levels are two to three times normal for heterozygotes and six to eight times normal for homozygotes. Levels remain high throughout life, but symptoms appear around 30 to 40 years of age in the case of heterozygotes. The symptoms associated with this disease are the result of accelerated coronary atherosclerosis causing myocardial infarctions. The other major finding in this disorder is the presence of xanthomas deposition on tendon, eyelid, and cornea. In the homozygote form, the manifestations are the same but appear earlier, with ischemic lesions occurring as early as 18 months of age and death around 20 years of age. Treatment is a strict diet with low saturated fat and high polyunsaturated fat. If diet alone is insufficient, patients are placed on pharmacologic treatment.

Precautions before anesthesia: Perform a thorough cardiac evaluation before taking the patient to the operating room. If patient is on drug therapy, obtain liver function tests and glycemia and uric acid levels.

Anesthetic considerations: Consider these patients as affected with coronary artery disease until proven otherwise and thus avoid any increase in cardiac oxygen consumption pre- and postoperatively. Plan for adequate pain relief after surgery, knowing that most adverse events occur in the first 3 postoperative days. A bed in the critical care unit may be advised for closer followup during the immediate postoperative period. Invasive monitoring is warranted for surgeries with major hemodynamic fluctuations.

Pharmacological implications: Some of the drugs used for treatment of this disease may cause hepatotoxicity. so halothane should be avoided. Drugs eliminated via the kidney should be chosen, such as atracurium/*cis*-atracurium.

Table H-6

Type	Synonyms and Inclusions	Pathophysiology	Inheritance	Genetic
Lp	Apolipoprotein(a); LPA	Allelic serum lipoprotein system	Autosomal dominant	Mutations in apolipoprotein Lp(a) gene; 6q27
Ia	Familial hyperchylomicronemia	Lipoprotein lipase deficiency	Autosomal recessive	8p22
Ib	APOC2 deficiency; Apolipoprotein C-II deficiency	Apolipoprotein C-II deficiency	Autosomal recessive	19q13.2
Ic	Chylomicronemia	Lipoprotein lipase inhibitor activity	Autosomal dominant	
II	Hyperbetalipoproteinemia; familial hypercholesterolemic xanthomatosis; hyper-low-density-lipoproteinemia	Defect of the cell membrane receptor for LDL	Autosomal dominant	Mutations in LDL receptor gene; probably 19p13.2–p13.12
IIa	Familial hypercholesterolemia without hypertriglyceridemia	Defect of the cell membrane receptor for LDL	Autosomal dominant	Mutations in LDL receptor gene; probably 19p13.2–p13.12
IIb	Familial hypercholesterolemia with hypertriglyceridemia	Defect of the cell membrane receptor for LDL	Autosomal dominant	Mutations in LDL receptor gene; probably 19p13.2–p13.12
III	Apolipoprotein E deficiency; broad-betalipoproteinemia; familial hypercholesterolemia with hyperlipemia; hyperbetaproteinemia and prebetalipoproteinemia; hyperlipemia with familial floating-betalipoproteinemia; familial hypercholesterolemic xanthomatosis	Apolipoprotein E deficiency	Autosomal recessive with pseudodominance due to high gene frequency	19q13.2
IV	Carbohydrate-inducible hyperlipemia; endogenous hypertriglyceridemia; familial combined hyperlipidemia; hypercholesterolemia type IV; hyperprebetalipoproteinemia	Heterogeneous with strong influence of environmental factors	Autosomal dominant, heterogeneous	
Norum disease	Lecithin-cholesterol acyltransferase deficiency; LCAT deficiency	Lecithin-cholesterol acyltransferase deficiency	Autosomal recessive	16q22.1
Wolman disease	Lysosomal acid lipase deficiency; LAL deficiency; LIPA deficiency; cholesterol ester storage disease (CESD)	Lysosomal acid lipase deficiency (acid cholesteryl ester hydrolase deficiency)	Autosomal recessive	10q24–q25
Familial hyper-triglyceridemia		Apolipoprotein C-II deficiency	Autosomal dominant	15q11.2–q13.1
Familial hyper-cholesterolemia type B	Familial hypercholesterolemia due to ligand-defective apolipoprotein B; familial ligand-defective apolipoprotein B-100	Abnormal LDL	Autosomal dominant	2p24
Hyperalphalip-oproteinemia		Elevated levels of α-lipoprotein (as in Tangier disease)	Probably autosomal dominant	Chromosome 1? (APOA2 gene)

LDL, low-density lipoprotein.

REFERENCES:

Saint-Jore B, Varret M, Dachet C, et al: Autosomal dominant type IIa hypercholesterolemia: evaluation of the respective contributions of LDLR and APOB gene defects as well as a third major group of defects. *Eur J Hum Genet* 8:621, 2000.

Stoelting RK, Dierdorf SF: Metabolic and nutritional disorders, in Stoelting RK, Dierdorf SF: *Anesthesia and Co-existing Disease.* 3d ed. New York, Churchill Livingstone, 1993, p 378.

Hyperoxaluria, Primary

At a glance: Inherited error of metabolism of glyoxylate causing urolithiasis and progressive renal insufficiency. Two types are described, depending on the missing enzyme.

Synonyms and classification:

Type I: Oxalosis I; Glycolic aciduria; Alanine-Glyoxylate Aminotransferase Deficiency; Peroxisomal Alanine: Glyoxylate Aminotransferase Deficiency; Hepatic AGT Deficiency.

Type II: Oxalosis II; Glyceric aciduria; D-Glycerate Dehydrogenase Deficiency.

Incidence: Incidence is estimated between 1:60,000 and 1:120,000 children (United Kingdom, France, Switzerland). It may be responsible for 10 to 13% of end-stage renal failure in children in developing countries. Type II is less frequent than type I.

Genetic inheritance: Autosomal recessive inheritance. In type I, the missing enzyme is alanine-glyoxylate aminotransferase (i.e., the *AGT* gene), which is normally found only in the hepatic peroxisomes. This enzyme is necessary to detoxify glyoxylate (gene map locus 2q36-q37). In type II, the missing enzyme is D-glyceric dehydrogenase, which can be detected in leukocyte preparations.

Pathophysiology: Loss of specific enzymatic activity in glyoxylate metabolism. With the normal metabolic pathway blocked, the alternative pathway that leads to oxalate production from glycolate metabolism becomes very active and considerable amounts of oxalate are produced, leading to extremely high oxalate concentrations within the proximal tubular cells. These high oxalate levels have direct toxic effects on renal tubular cells.

Diagnosis: Family history, elevated urine oxalate excretion, high plasma levels of oxalate, progressive bilateral oxalate urolithiasis, and nephrocalcinosis. A liver biopsy can help determine which enzyme defect is present. Urinary oxalate excretion usually is more than 100 mg/day in both types of primary hyperoxaluria. Prenatal diagnosis is possible (glyoxylate metabolite analysis in amniotic fluid; linkage and mutation analysis of DNA isolated from chorionic villus samples in the first trimester; AGT enzyme assay, immunoassay, and immuno-electron microscopy of fetal liver biopsies is possible in the second trimester).

Clinical aspects: The clinical course is very similar in both types of primary hyperoxaluria (end-stage renal disease occurs slightly later and pyridoxine is usually not effective in type II). Recurrent urolithiasis and nephrocalcinosis are the main symptoms leading to progressive loss of renal function. Fifty percent of patients are affected by 5 years of age. Clinical severity is not correlated with the mutation or the degree of residual functional AGT activity. Wide variations in clinical, biochemical, and genetic heterogeneity; some patients present in infancy with renal failure, others experience only occasional passage of stones in adult life, with maintained renal function. Systemic oxalosis occurs when the critical saturation point for plasma oxalate is reached in early renal insufficiency. Clinical

manifestations of oxalate osteopathy are pain, spontaneous fractures, and erythropoietin-resistant anemia. Important sites of calcium oxalate deposits are the media of the arteries (with subsequent ischemia and gangrene), the peripheral nervous system (neuropathy), the myocardium (atrioventricular block), the thyroid gland, the skin (livedo reticularis), and the retina. Soft tissue calcifications in joints may limit mobility. Death from renal failure occurs in childhood or early adult life. Kidney transplantation is associated with a high rate of recurrence of the original disease with early graft loss.

Precautions before anesthesia: Assess cardiac function: ECG, echocardiography, and, if necessary, radionuclide imaging. Evaluate renal function: clinical (dialysis, volume restriction) and biochemistry (urea, electrolytes, creatinine clearance). Assess vascular involvement and document neurologic system involvement. Blood work should include hematocrit and electrolyte levels. For patients with chronic renal failure, control of hypertension should be optimized, as well as volume status, biochemical abnormalities, and anemia.

Anesthetic considerations: Depends on the type and severity of systemic organ involvement. Delayed gastric emptying occurs in patients affected with renal failure; rapid sequence tracheal intubation must be considered. Hypertension and cardiovascular instability may be a problem. Both fluid overload and hypovolemia readily occur. Risk of occluding the arteriovenous fistula during surgery is a serious potential complication and must be prevented at all cost. Difficult positioning of patients because of joint deformities and immobility (danger of pressure necrosis). The benefits of invasive blood pressure monitoring should be balanced with the risk of limb ischemia from existing arterial oxalate depositions.

Pharmacological implications: Avoid any potentially nephrotoxic agent (muscle relaxants such as gallamine, antibiotics such as aminoglycosides). Avoid long-acting benzodiazepines (prolonged action because of accumulation of metabolites from impaired renal function), opioids (may have increased sensitivity to morphine from decreased plasma protein binding), muscle relaxants (alcuronium, pancuronium, D-tubocurarine). Sevoflurane should be used with great caution, if at all.

REFERENCES:

Johnson SA, Rumsby G, Cregeen D, et al: Primary hyperoxaluria type 2 in children. *Pediatr Nephrol* 17:597, 2002.

Milosevic D, Rinat C, Batinic D, et al: Genetic analysis—A diagnostic tool for primary hyperoxaluria type I. *Pediatr Nephrol* 17:896, 2002.

Monico CG, Persson M, Ford GC, et al: Potential mechanisms of marked hyperoxaluria not due to primary hyperoxaluria I or II. *Kidney Int* 62:392, 2002.

Hyperprolinemia

At a glance: Inborn error of metabolism resulting from a defect in renal tubular amino acid transport leading to abnormal urinary excretion of glycine, proline, and hydroxyproline.

Synonyms and classification:

Type I: Proline oxidase deficiency

Type II: Pyrroline carboxylate dehydrogenase deficiency

Incidence: Very rare.

Genetic inheritance: Autosomal recessive; gene mapped on 22q11.2 for type I and 1p36 for type II.

Pathophysiology: Type I is a benign disorder resulting from deficiency of proline oxidase. Type II results from a deficiency of D-pyrroline-5-carboxylate (P-5-C) dehydrogenase and may be associated with neurologic manifestations. In both conditions, plasma proline levels are increased, and three amino acids (proline, hydroxyproline, glycine) are excreted in excess in urine.

Diagnosis: Excess urinary proline, hydroxyproline, and glycine levels are a normal finding in the first 6 months of life. Type I is a diagnosis of exclusion: it includes all cases of hyperprolinemia not resulting from a P-5-C dehydrogenase deficiency (type II). Plasma proline level elevated but usually less than 2000 mM (normal: 100–450 mM). Urine proline also elevated. In type II, plasma proline exceeds 2000 mM. The metabolic intermediate P-5-C is 10 to 40 times above normal in the plasma and urine.

Clinical aspects: Individuals with type I are asymptomatic. Seizures (grand mal, petit mal) and mental retardation have been associated with type II. Elevated cerebrospinal fluid (CSF) concentrations for gamma-aminobutyric acid (GABA), glutamate, and proline have been described in some patients, but their association with neurologic manifestations remains undetermined. Intestinal absorption of proline may be impaired. Heterozygotes have glycinuria only (plasma levels of amino acids are normal). Other features include dry skin, chronic inflammatory lung disease, sensorineural deafness, and ichthyosis.

Precautions before anesthesia: No specific precautions are required for type I. For type II, inquire about history of seizures, anticonvulsant therapy (efficacy, toxicity), and degree of mental retardation (possible need for sedative premedication).

Anesthetic considerations: If a seizure disorder is associated with type II, patients receiving anticonvulsants should be maintained on their medication regimen until the time of surgery, and medications should be given parenterally postoperatively until oral intake is resumed.

Pharmacological implications: Avoid potentially epileptogenic drugs: methohexital, ketamine, enflurane, atracurium, and meperidine (Demerol) (these last two, if given in large quantity, because of their respective metabolites laudanosine and normeperidine). Consider the sedation and increased drug metabolism caused by enzymatic induction effect of phenobarbital and phenytoin; the resistance to nondepolarizing muscle relaxants with phenytoin and carbamazepine; and the potential hepatic dysfunction, thrombocytopenia, and pancreatitis with valproic acid.

Other conditions to be considered:

☞**DIAMINOPENTANURIA:** Inherited metabolic disorder of amino acids (defective transport system of cystine, lysine, arginine, and ornithine) resulting in precipitation of undissolved cystine in the urine (cystinuria) and causing the formation of calculi in the urinary ducts.

☞**HARTNUP DISEASE:** Inherited disorder of basic amino acid transport resulting in urinary loss of neutral amino acids (tryptophan, alanine, asparagine, glutamine, histidine, isoleucine, leucine, phenylalanine, serine, threonine, tyrosine, valine); affected patients present with a pellagra-like rash but no evidence of dietary tryptophan insufficiency.

☞**FANCONI-BICKEL SYNDROME:** Inherited metabolic disorder of carbohydrates characterized by accumulation of glycogen in the liver with hepatomegaly, proximal tubular nephropathy, fasting hypoglycemia, glucose (and galactose) intolerance, and dwarfism.

☞**IMINOGLYCINURIA:** Benign condition in which glycine and the imino acids proline and hydroxyproline have decreased renal tubular reabsorption. Individuals are asymptomatic.

REFERENCES:

Phang, JM; Chao Yeh, G; Sciver CR: Disorders of proline and hydroxyproline metabolism, in Scriver CR, Beaudet AL, Sly WS, et al. (eds): *The Metabolic and Molecular Bases of Inherited Disease.* 7th ed. New York, McGraw-Hill, 1995, p 1125.

Gerghty MT, Vaughn D, Nicholson AJ, et al: Mutations in the Delta1-pyrroline 5-carboxylate dehydrogenase gene cause type II hyperprolinemia. *Hum Mol Genet* 7:1411, 1998.

Jacquet H, Raux G, Thibaut F, et al: PRODH mutations and hyperprolinemia in a subset of schizophrenic patients. *Hum Mol Genet* 11:2243, 2002.

Hypoglossia-Hypodactylia Syndrome

At a glance: Congenital acrofacial dysostosis obvious at birth. Characterized by an absent or incompletely developed tongue (hypoglossia), absent or partially missing fingers and/or toes (ectrodactylia), micrognathia, and malformation of arms and/or legs (peromelia).

Synonyms: Aglossia-Adactyly Syndrome; Akroteriasis Congenita; Hanhart Syndrome; Mandibular Dysostosis and Peromelia

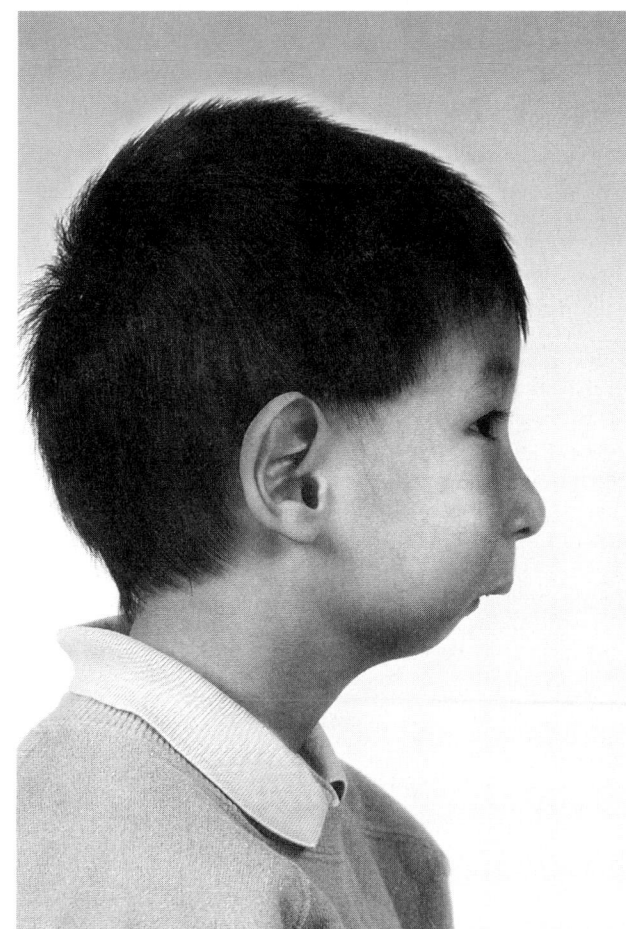

Hypoglossia-hypodactyly syndrome Marked mandibular hypoplasia in a 14-year-old boy with hypoglossia-hypodactyly syndrome.

Syndrome; Oroacral Syndrome; Oromandibular Limb Hypoplasia Syndrome; Peromelia with Micrognathism.

Incidence: Rare ("natural" incidence: 1:175,000 live births).

Genetic inheritance: Most cases are sporadic, but autosomal dominant inheritance has been reported.

Pathophysiology: Not known. Vascular disruptions at approximately the fourth embryonic week, with possible drug influence, have been hypothesized. In vivo and pathologic studies and animal models support this theory. Whether a preceding blastogenetic alteration or a disorganization mutation is an influencing factor remains unclear.

Diagnosis: Diagnosis is based only on clinical findings.

Clinical aspects: The syndrome is characterized by a small mandible, hypoglossia or aglossia, and hypodactylia. Mental retardation is reported in 10 to 15% of patients.

Precautions before anesthesia: An anesthesiology consultation is highly recommended before elective surgery. Tube feeding may be necessary in the neonatal period. Management of the airway may be difficult because of the anatomical particularities; evaluate for potential difficult tracheal intubation. Physical examination directed primarily toward the central nervous system, cardiovascular system (cor pulmonale), lungs, and upper airway (tracheomalacia). Standard preoperative laboratory examinations are appropriate in most patients (blood chemistries, blood group, hemoglobin, coagulation).

Anesthetic considerations: Anesthetic management depends on the severity of the malformations and, thus, on the surgical procedure. Special attention must be given to the airway management. All proper equipment to assist with difficult direct laryngoscopy must be available. Maintain spontaneous ventilation until the trachea is secured and lung ventilation confirmed.

Pharmacological implications: No known implications with this condition.

Other conditions to be considered:

JOHNSON HALL KROUS SYNDROME (Glossopalatine Ankylosis Cataracts Digital Syndrome): Similar condition presenting with digital anomalies and cataracts.

☞GOLDENHAR SYNDROME: Common birth defect of vascular origin involving first and second branchial arch derivatives resulting mainly with hemifacial microsomia with absent ear and eye and vertebral anomalies. Usually associated with cardiovascular anomalies, including ventriculoseptal defect, atrial septal defect, patent ductus arteriosus, tetralogy of Fallot, and coarctation of the aorta. Arnold-Chiari syndrome and hydrocephalus are reported. Severe-to-major anesthetic implications, especially the airway (unilateral hypoplasia of the facial bones and muscles). Epibulbar dermoids. Limited mouth opening, micrognathia, cleft palate.

☞MOEBIUS SYNDROME: Congenital facial diplegia as a result of underdevelopment of the sixth and seventh cranial nerves. Impaired ability to suck in the infancy period often leads to the diagnosis. Excessive drooling and crossed eyes may be present.

REFERENCES:

De Smet L, Schollen W: Hypoglossia-hypodactyly syndrome: Report of 2 patients. *Genet Couns* 12:347, 2001.

Mishima K, Sugahara T, Mori Y, et al: Case report: Hypoglossia-hypodactylia syndrome. *J Craniomaxillofac Surg* 24:36, 1996.

Hypomelanosis of Ito

At a glance: Congenital disorder characterized by hypopigmented whorls of skin along the line of Blaschko and associated with multiple other congenital defects, mostly neurologic, skeletal, hair, and dental anomalies.

Synonym: Incontinentia Pigmenti Achromians.

History: First described by the Japanese dermatologist Ito, this heterogeneous condition belongs to a group of mosaic phenotype neurodermatoses.

Incidence: Incidence was approximately 1:1000 new patients consulting a pediatric neurologic service, or 1:8000–10,000 unselected patients in a children's hospital. Females outnumber males by 2.5:1. No ethnic predilection.

Genetic inheritance: Hypomelanosis of Ito is believed to result from chromosomal mosaicism, which could explain why it is so varied in phenotype. Genes on 9q33-qter, 15q11-q13, and Xp11 have been implicated in this syndrome; however, there is no consensus in the literature.

Pathophysiology: The phenotype may result directly from the loss of specific pigmentation genes. A migration defect during central nervous system (CNS) maturation probably accounts for much of the neurologic impairment.

Diagnosis: Characterized by mental retardation, behavioral disturbances, and pigmentary anomalies. Chromosomal mosaicism in epidermal keratinocytes and confined to the hypopigmented epidermis. The normal epidermis contains only normal cells.

Clinical aspects: The disorder is characterized by unilateral or bilateral macular hypopigmented whorls, streaks, and patches that exist from birth. The lines of Blaschko are defined by a pattern determined by different nevoid on the human skin and mucosae. The cause is unknown, and their distributions do not follow nerves, vessels, or lymphatics. In 1901, Blaschko pointed out that the lines described by these conditions not only did not correspond to any known anatomical basis but were remarkably consistent both from patient to patient and even from one disease to another. Neurologic impairment (70% of cases) can be severe and present as mental retardation, seizures, neurologic syndromes, cerebellar signs, and hearing loss. Abnormalities of the eyes (strabismus, retinal changes, optic nerve hypoplasia) and the musculoskeletal system (scoliosis, syndactyly) occur in some patients. Other reported abnormalities include cleft palate, hair, nail, teeth, limb, hand and/or foot abnormalities, hemihypertrophy, hypotonia, and face and/or skull anomalies.

Precautions before anesthesia: Measurement of anticonvulsant levels and optimization of anticonvulsant therapy must be obtained. Continue morning dose of anticonvulsants until the day of surgery. Document neurologic deficits. Evaluate respiratory function in the presence of scoliosis (effort tolerance, arterial blood gas, lung function tests, chest radiograph). Assess cardiac function if there is a long-standing history of respiratory impairment.

Anesthetic considerations: In the presence of significant facial anomalies, evaluate carefully for difficulties with airway management. Triggers that potentiate occurrence of seizures are to be avoided. Preoperative intravenous seizure medication might be indicated during long surgical procedure or important fluid shift. A regional technique as the sole anesthetic may be difficult in view of the patient's mental retardation, behavioral disturbances, and deformities of the spine. No specific contraindications to regional anesthesia in patients with preexisting neurologic syndromes, but careful counseling of patients and detailed documentation of deficits should be done.

Pharmacological implications: Premedication must be avoided in presence of significant airway problem, obstruction, sleep apnea, or respiratory disease. Triggers that potentiate occurrence of seizures are to be avoided (enflurane with hypocapnia, methohexital, ketamine). Larger doses of some anesthetic medications (e.g., vecuronium) may be required on chronic phenobarbital therapy because of induction of hepatic enzymes.

Other condition to be considered:

☞**INCONTINENTIA PIGMENTI:** Genetic disease involving the skin, hair, teeth, and central nervous system. Caused by a defective NEMO gene. Gene map locus is Xq28. X-linked dominance with lethality in males.

REFERENCES:

Fritz B, Kuster W, Orstavik KH, et al: Pigmentary mosaicism in hypomelanosis of Ito. Further evidence for functional disomy of Xp. *Hum Genet* 103:441, 1998.

Ruggieri M, Magro G, Ruggieri M, et al: Tumors and hypomelanosis of Ito. *Arch Pathol Lab Med* 125:599, 2001.

Ruggieri M, Pavone L: Hypomelanosis of Ito: Clinical syndrome or just phenotype? *J Child Neurol* 15:635, 2000.

Hypoparathyroidism

At a glance: Inherited condition caused by a lack of parathyroid hormone resulting in hypocalcemia and hyperphosphatemia and their clinical manifestations.

Nature: Endocrine disorder of the parathyroid gland as a consequence of primary or secondary lack of parathormone secretion. Primary forms result from many rare diseases.

Incidence: Primary hypoparathyroidism is rare; fewer than 1000 cases of the idiopathic form, familial or not, have been reported. Rare in children.

Genetic inheritance:

- Both autosomal dominant (gene map locus 3q13) and X-linked (also related to a mutation in the parathyroid hormone gene) forms of familial idiopathic hypoparathyroidism have been reported.
- *X-Linked Agenesis of Parathyroid Gland:* Gene map locus is Xq26-q27.
- *Hypoparathyroidism-Retardation-Dysmorphism Syndrome* (HRDS): Autosomal recessive.
- *Sanjad-Sakati Syndrome* (Congenital Hypoparathyroidism with Growth Retardation, Developmental Delay, and Dysmorphism): Gene map location is 1q42-43.

Pathophysiology: Primary and secondary hypoparathyroidism are conditions in which there is a deficiency of parathyroid hormone. This deficiency induces hypocalcemia and decreases calcium resorption from bone and calcium absorption from gastrointestinal tract by preventing synthesis of vitamin D. The lack of parathyroid hormone stops the osteolytic effect of vitamin D and results in a decrease in bone metabolism. The decreased calcium concentration in the motor plate induces neuromuscular hyperexcitability. A very sensitive extracellular calcium-sensing receptor, coupled to a G protein, has been isolated from parathyroid, kidney, and brain cells. Some autosomal dominant forms of hypocalcemia result from activating mutations of this extracellular calcium-sensing receptor, which inhibits parathyroid hormone exocytosis (mechanism is unknown).

Diagnosis: In primary hyperparathyroidism, note hypocalcemia, hypomagnesemia, hyperphosphoremia, and low serum level of parathyroid hormone. Urinary excretion of calcium, phosphorus,

and cAMP is decreased. Ellsworth Howard test (infusion of 200 IU of parathyroid hormone) induces an increase of cAMP and phosphaturia. Intracerebral calcifications on CT scan.

Clinical aspects: In *neonates,* the symptoms of hyperparathyroidism are respiratory distress, cyanosis, apnea, hypertonia, agitation, and tetany. In *infants,* the symptoms are seizures and tinnitus crisis with inspiratory stridor, laryngospasm, and unexplained tachycardia. In *children,* tinnitus is the most frequent sign, with seizures that can be typical or not. Hypocalcemia may be life-threatening and can cause nephrocalcinosis and renal lithiasis.

Primary forms are related to many rare diseases, mostly genetically inherited.

Autoimmune diseases: Type I autoimmune polyglandular syndrome (or HAM syndrome) results in primary hypoparathyroidism by 10 years of age as a result of destruction of the parathyroids. Other types of autoimmune hypoparathyroidism may exist alone, in sporadic or familial forms.

Congenital diseases and syndromes with agenesis or hypoplasia of the parathyroid glands include the following:

- Isolated primary hypoparathyroidism
- X-linked primary hypoparathyroidism (band Xq26-Xq27)
- X autosomal recessive primary hypoparathyroidism
- Branchial dysgenesis (DiGeorge syndrome)
- Chromosomal defects dup(1q), del(5p), dup(8q), del(10q), del(22q)
- Monogenic hypoparathyroidism
- Isolated autosomal dominant conditions
- Isolated autosomal recessive conditions
- Velocardiofacial syndrome
- Zellweger syndrome
- Teratogenic effects
- Diabetic embryopathy
- Fetal alcohol syndrome
- Retinoid embryopathy
- CHARGE syndrome
- Kenny-Caffey syndrome
- Kearns-Sayre syndrome
- Barakat syndrome (i.e., primary hypoparathyroidism, nerve deafness, steroid-resistant nephrosis)
- Hypoparathyroidism with short stature, mental retardation, and seizures (hypoparathyroidism-retardation-dysmorphism Syndrome; Sanjad-Sakati syndrome; Kalam-Haafez syndrome)

Congenital diseases and syndromes without agenesis or hypoplasia of the parathyroid glands (functional mutations), including the following:

- Mutation of chromosome arm 3q
- Familial isolated hypoparathyroidism, which is a heterogenous mix of disorders including autosomal dominant and autosomal recessive abnormal preproparathyroid hormone allele

Secondary forms may result from several causes: ablation of parathyroid glands during thyroid or parathyroid surgery, radiotherapy, transitive neonatal hypoparathyroidism (maternal hyperparathyroidism during pregnancy), metal overload (iron overload in hemochromatosis and thalassemia, copper overload in Wilson disease, aluminum overload in hemodialyzed patients), or metal deficiency (hypomagnesemia), idiopathic.

Precautions before anesthesia: Full history and evaluation of associated syndrome. Search for neuromuscular irritability indicating chronic hypocalcemia (Chovstek or Trousseau sign); if positive, calcium levels require correction. Electromyography (EMG), EEG, CT scan, ECG (prolonged QT). Ophthalmologic examination. Skeletal radiograph. Dosages of Ca^{+2}, parathyroid hormone, cAMP. Correct calcemia: in acute hypocalcemia, calcium chloride or calcium gluconate 1 to 2 g IV; in chronic form, calcium carbonate 1 to 8 g per os with vitamin D. Correct associated electrolyte disturbances.

Anesthetic considerations: The risks are those of hypocalcemia: arrhythmia, acute hypocalcemia as a consequence of citrated blood transfusion. Monitoring of ECG preoperatively and postoperatively is highly recommended. Muscle relaxant must be controlled by nerve stimulator. Difficult tracheal intubation can occur in genetically inherited forms with associated facial malformations. For hypoparathyroidism in association with other syndromic conditions, refer to this syndrome for further information.

Pharmacological implications: Avoid agents that can prolong QT, such as local anesthetics because of their quinidine-like action. Increased efficiency of muscle relaxants because of hypocalcemia.

Other condition to be considered:

☞**ALBRIGHT HEREDITARY OSTEODYSTROPHY:** Heterogeneous group of disorders characterized by hypocalcemia, hyperphosphatemia, and increased serum concentration of parathyroid hormone. Caused by insensitivity to parathyroid hormone activity.

REFERENCES:

Goltzman D, Cole DEC: Hypoparathyroidism, in Favus MJ (ed): *Primer on the Metabolic Bone Diseases and Disorders of Mineral Metabolism.* Philadelphia, Lippincott-Raven, 1996, p 220.

Thakker RV: Genetic developments in hypoparathyroidism. *Lancet* 357:974, 2001.

Thomas BR, Bennett JD: Symptomatic hypocalcemia and hypoparathyroidism in two infants of mothers with hyperparathyroidism and familial hypercalcemia. *J Perinatol* 15:23, 1995.

Hypophosphatasia

At a glance: Inherited inborn error of metabolism characterized by severe bone disease (similar to vitamin D-resistant rickets), failure to thrive, movement disorders, and low plasma levels of alkaline phosphatase.

Synonyms and classification:

Hypophosphatasia perinatal type (neonatal hypophosphatasia)
Hypophosphatasia infantile type (phosphoethanolaminuria)
Hypophosphatasia childhood type
Hypophosphatasia adult type (mild hypophosphatasia)
Odontohypophosphatasia

History: Inborn error of metabolism initially identified by Rathbun in 1948.

Incidence: Estimated at 1:100,000 live births (and 1 carrier per 200 individuals in the United States). Some ethnic or religious groups have a higher incidence of the disease (1:2500 among Canadian Mennonites). No sex predilection.

Genetic inheritance: Autosomal recessive. However, mild adult hypophosphatasia and odontohypophosphatasia cases seem to be inherited as an autosomal dominant trait. Prenatal diagnosis is possible by measuring alkaline phosphatase activity in chorionic villus samples from amniocentesis, and the perinatal (severe) form of the disease can be detected by ultrasonography. The defective gene, called ALPL, is located at 1p36.1-34.

Pathophysiology: Deficient activity of tissue-nonspecific alkaline phosphatase, one of the four isomers of alkaline phosphatase (each of which has its own gene locus). This results in accumulation of several metabolites including phosphoethanolamine, pyridoxal-5'-phosphate (a form of vitamin B_6), and inorganic pyrophosphate, which are found in large amounts in the blood and urine. The characteristic defective calcification of bones in children (rickets) and adults (osteomalacia) is caused by the accumulation of inorganic pyrophosphate.

Diagnosis: Clinical features. Radiologic appearance: epiphyseal and metaphyseal abnormalities of long bones, vertebrae, and ribs. Elevated plasma and urine levels of phosphoethanolamine. Elevated plasma inorganic pyrophosphate and pyridoxal-5'-phosphate.

Clinical aspects: Hypophosphatasia varies widely in clinical presentation. It has been subdivided into five categories: perinatal, infantile, childhood, adult, and odontohypophosphatasia. The earlier the symptoms occur, the more severe the disease. *Perinatal form* presents with a history of poor feeding, failure to thrive, hypotonia, and skin-covered spurs extending from the forearms or legs; it is lethal in 50% of cases. *Childhood form* often presents as delayed walking, early loss of deciduous teeth, and bone pain. *Adult form* has mild symptoms (foot pain as a result of spontaneous fractures of metatarsal bones). *Odontohypophosphatasia* is limited to dental problems (premature loss of adult teeth). Severe forms are characterized by widespread failure of ossification of the skeleton and marked shortening of long bones. Multiple rib fractures may lead to flail chest and predispose to pneumonia. There may be failure of ossification of the cranial vault. Hypercalcemia may lead to nephrocalcinosis and renal failure. In milder childhood forms, the skeletal abnormalities are less severe, but frequent fractures and bone pain are typical. There is defective development of the teeth leading to premature loss. There is no effective treatment, but some spontaneous improvement may occur as the child ages.

Precautions before anesthesia: Check serum calcium level and renal function. Assess extent of skeletal abnormalities.

Anesthetic considerations: Care should be taken with positioning for surgery to avoid fracturing bones. The teeth are fragile and should be protected during direct laryngoscopy and tracheal intubation. Infants may have hypercalcemia, which leads to systemic vasoconstriction with contraction of the intravascular space. Intravenous fluid should be administered before induction of anesthesia to prevent hypotension.

Pharmacological implications: Presence of renal failure necessitates care with renally excreted drugs; *cis*-atracurium is the muscle relaxant of choice.

Other conditions to be considered:

☞**COFFIN-LOWRY SYNDROME:** X-linked polymalformative syndrome equally affecting males and females (but more severe in males). Characterized by craniofacial and skeletal abnormalities, short stature, hypotonia, and mental retardation. Caused by a mutation of RSK2 gene (Xp22.2-p22.1) that codes for a protein kinase.

☞**OSTEOGENESIS IMPERFECTA:** Disorder caused by a mutation causing abnormal type I collagen, mainly characterized by fragility of bones. Four types of osteogenesis imperfecta exist, each presenting different characteristics.

RICKETS AND ☞**HEREDITARY VITAMIN-D RESISTANT RICKETS:** Metabolic disorder of calcium and/or phosphate metabolism primarily caused by lack of vitamin D and mainly involving weakening of the bones. Hereditary forms are usually a result of kidney disorder (when kidneys are unable to retain phosphate or when renal tubular acidosis is present).

REFERENCES:

Mornet E: Hypophosphatasia: The mutations in the tissue-nonspecific alkaline phosphatase gene. *Hum Mutat* 15:309, 2000.

Zurutuza L, Muller F, Gibrat JF, et al: Correlations of genotype and phenotype in hypophosphatasia. *Hum Mol Genet* 8:1039, 1999.

Hypoplasia of the Right Ventricle

At a glance: Congenital heart disease characterized by underdevelopment of the right-sided structures of the heart, which causes inadequate blood flow to the lungs, cyanosis, and abnormal coronary supply, causing damage to the heart muscle.

Synonyms: Congenital Isolated Hypoplasia of the Right Ventricle; Hypoplastic Right Heart Syndrome; Hypoplastic Right Ventricle.

Genetic inheritance: Autosomal recessive.

Pathophysiology: In its usual form, there is attenuation of the apical trabecular zone of the right ventricle with a normal and nonobstructed pulmonary outflow tract. The tricuspid valve may be hypoplastic or frankly obstructive.

Diagnosis: Electrocardiography demonstrates sinus rhythm with right atrial enlargement. Chest radiography shows mild cardiac enlargement with an enlarged right heart border, decreased pulmonary segment, and reduced vascularity.

Clinical aspects: Significant cyanosis at birth. Signs of venous congestion with hepatomegaly may occur within the first week. Death from progressive hypoxemia is common if appropriate therapy is not commenced.

Precautions before anesthesia: Adequate treatment of hypoxemia and heart failure. Echocardiography and cardiac catheterization are recommended to assess cardiac function and degree of right ventricular inflow obstruction. Need to exclude tetralogy of Fallot, Ebstein anomaly of the tricuspid valve, pulmonary atresia with intact septum, and tricuspid atresia with pulmonary stenosis.

Anesthetic considerations: Right ventricular filling is restricted because of the small tricuspid valve and hypoplastic right ventricle. This situation necessitates unimpeded blood flow from the right atrium to the left atrium, which is commonly achieved with balloon atrioseptostomy at birth. Anesthesia may be required later for aortopulmonary shunt, Glenn anastomosis (superior vena cava to right pulmonary artery), or Fontan operation (right atrium to right ventricle anastomosis).

Pharmacological implications: Determined by cardiac function.

REFERENCES:

Joy MV, Venugopalan P, Sapru A, et al: Isolated hypoplasia of right ventricle with atrial septal defect: A rare form of cyanotic heart disease. *Indian Heart J* 51:440, 1999.

Medd, WE, Neufeld HN: Isolated hypoplasia of the right ventricle and tricuspid valve in siblings. *Br Heart J* 23:25, 1961.

Metras D, Chetaille P, Kreitmann B, et al: Pulmonary atresia with ventricular septal defect, extremely hypoplastic pulmonary arteries, major aorto-pulmonary collaterals. *Eur J Cardiothorac Surg* 20:590, 2001.

Hypoplastic Left Heart Syndrome

At a glance: Congenital heart disease characterized by underdevelopment of the left side of the heart. Lethal in 25% of infants during the first week of life.

Nature: Congenital disorder. Recurrence rate is 2% in siblings of an affected infant. Condition is fatal without palliative surgery.

Incidence: 0.1–0.27:1000 live births.

Genetic inheritance: Multifactorial; a subgroup showing autosomal recessive inheritance may exist.

Pathophysiology: Range of abnormalities, including aortic atresia/stenosis, hypoplastic left ventricle, hypoplasia of the aortic arch, and mitral atresia or hypoplasia. The left ventricle is nonfunctional; systemic perfusion is maintained by the right ventricle through a patent ductus. Coronary perfusion occurs by retrograde flow through the aortic arch. Pulmonary venous blood usually mixes with systemic venous blood through an atrial septal defect or patent foramen ovale. Most neonates have a degree of interatrial mixing, allowing sufficient pulmonary blood flow with mild pulmonary venous hypertension. Unrestricted communications cause increased pulmonary flow, pulmonary hypertension, and systemic hypoperfusion. The absence of interatrial mixing results in pulmonary hypertension and congestion and marked hypoxia as a consequence of low pulmonary blood flow. The pulmonary and systemic circulations are supplied in parallel by the right ventricle. Systemic perfusion and oxygenation are dependent on maintaining a fine balance between pulmonary and systemic flow.

Diagnosis: Neonatal cyanosis and symptoms and signs of right ventricular failure. Echocardiography is diagnostic.

Clinical aspects: Neonatal tachypnea, tachycardia, cyanosis, third heart sound, systolic murmur, and hepatomegaly. Chest radiograph may show cardiomegaly and increased pulmonary vasculature. Neonatal cardiovascular palliation is achieved by the Norwood procedure, which results in the right ventricle supplying systemic circulation. The pulmonary circulation is supplied by a systemic-to-pulmonary arterial shunt (e.g., Blalock-Taussig shunt). An atrial septectomy is performed to allow pulmonary venous blood to flow freely into the right atrium. At approximately 6 months, once pulmonary vascular resistance has fallen from the high neonatal level, a hemi-Fontan or bidirectional Glenn shunt is performed. This procedure results in the pulmonary circulation being supplied by the superior vena cava (passive process relies on superior vena cava pressure being greater than pulmonary venous pressure to maintain flow). The Fontan procedure is completed at least 6 months later to allow development of optimal right ventricular function. The completed procedure results in both superior vena cava and inferior vena cava blood being diverted to passively supply the pulmonary circulation. Heart transplantation may be required.

Precautions before anesthesia: History and examination to elicit signs and symptoms of poor ventricular function. Poor ventricular function should be considered to represent greatly increased anesthetic risk. Define stage of palliation and hence physiologic requirements for anesthesia. Cardiac function/physiology. Review recent echocardiograms and cardiac catheterization data. Assess dependence on inotropes and the need for prostaglandin E_1 in the neonatal period to maintain the patent ductus arteriosus. Measure normal SaO_2, and consider measurement of blood gases. Assess for abnormal renal function, abnormal liver function, and the presence of a lactic acidosis suggestive of poor systemic perfusion.

Anesthetic considerations: In the neonate, systemic perfusion is dependent on the patent ductus arteriosus and maintenance of prostaglandin therapy. The pulmonary and systemic circulations are supplied in parallel, to maintain the ratio of pulmonary-to-systemic flow by maintaining a raised pulmonary vascular resistance [i.e., moderate acidosis, low fraction of inspired oxygen (FiO_2), maintain preoperative $PaCO_2$]. These measures will prevent an increase in pulmonary flow and a subsequent decrease in systemic perfusion. After the Norwood procedure, pulmonary and systemic circulations are still in parallel, so careful control of the ratio of pulmonary vascular resistance to systemic vascular resistance is still required. Following hemi-Fontan and completed Fontan procedures, the pulmonary perfusion is critically dependent on a maintained high venous pressure (preload pressure) and low pulmonary venous pressure. Spontaneous respiration or controlled ventilation with low inspiratory pressures will minimize any rise in intrathoracic pressure, which would impair flow to the pulmonary circuit.

Aim to maintain a low pulmonary vascular resistance and avoid using positive end-expiratory pressure.

Pharmacological implications: Careful consideration of the effect of anesthetic agent on systemic vascular resistance and pulmonary vascular resistance. Opiate-based anesthesia with low-dose volatile agents well tolerated. Caution with inotropes that may alter the ratio of systemic vascular resistance to pulmonary vascular resistance.

REFERENCES:

Chang RK, Chen AY, Klitzner TS: Clinical management of infants with hypoplastic left heart syndrome in the United States, 1988–1997. *Pediatrics* 110:292, 2002.

Gaynor JW, Mahle WT, Cohen MI, et al: Risk factors for mortality after the Norwood procedure. *Eur J Cardiothorac Surg* 22:82, 2002.

Lake CL: *Pediatric Cardiac Anesthesia.* 3rd ed. Stamford, Connecticut, Appleton & Lange, 1998, p 337.

ICE Syndrome

At a glance: ICE is an acronym for *i*chthyosis-*c*heek-*e*yebrow. Very rare genetic disorder characterized by ichthyosis vulgaris associated with sparse lateral eyebrows.

Genetic inheritance: Autosomal dominant inheritance has been advocated.

Clinical aspects: Acronymic syndrome characterized by ichthyosis vulgaris, prominent and full cheeks, and sparse lateral eyebrows. Other features involve the *head* (brachycephaly, folded helix, large nose, high-arched palate), *thorax* and *spine* (kyphoscoliosis, pes planus, pectus excavatum or carinatum, asymmetrical rib cage with abnormally placed nipples), and *limb* (flat foot, genu valgum, arachnodactyly of toes and fingers).

Anesthetic considerations: Cutaneous lesion could make venous access difficult. Perimedullar blockade is not contraindicated however could be difficult to realize because of the presence of kyphoscoliosis and skin lesions. Careful intraoperative monitoring is needed because of skeletal deformation.

REFERENCE:

Sidransky E, Feinstein A, Goodman RM: Ichthyosis-cheek-eyebrow (ICE) syndrome: A new autosomal dominant disorder. *Clin Genet* 31:137, 1987.

I-Cell Disease

At a glance: I-cell disease stands for inclusion cell disease. It is a genetically inherited lysosomal storage disease clinically similar to Hurler syndrome (without mucopolysaccharides) and originally characterized by the presence of intracytoplasmic inclusions in fibroblasts ("inclusion cells" or "I cells").

Synonyms: GNPTA Deficiency; Inclusion Cell Disease; Leroy Disease; Mucolipidosis II (ML II); N-Acetylglucosaminyl-1-Phosphotransferase Deficiency.

Nature: Genetic disorder involving abnormal trafficking of lysosomal enzymes. The disease was classified as mucolipidosis type II because it had clinical characteristics of both the mucopolysaccharidoses and the sphingolipidoses.

Incidence: 1:640,000 live births in the Netherlands. In the French Canadian population of Saguenay Lac Saint-Jean of the province of Quebec, the estimated prevalence at birth is 1:6184, giving a carrier frequency of 1/39. No ethnic or sexual predilection. Life expectancy is reduced (first decade); patients usually die of pneumonia or congestive heart failure.

Genetic inheritance: Autosomal recessive. Caused by a deficiency of the enzyme N-acetylglucosaminyl-1-phosphotransferase, which is produced by the *GNPTA* gene located at chromosome band 4q21-q23.

Pathophysiology: The disease results from abnormal enzyme transport. The deficiency is N-acetylglucosamine-1-phosphotransferase, a membrane enzyme that catalyzes the formation of mannose-6-phosphate (Man-6-P) on nascent lysosomal enzymes (by ribosomes). This Man-6-P component is recognized by Man-6-P receptors, which direct the transfer of lysosomal enzymes into lysosomes. This failed internalization results in release of lysosome enzymes into the extracellular medium instead. Although all cells are deficient in phosphotransferase activity, not all cells are deficient in lysosomal enzyme content, indicating that some cells have Man-6-P–independent pathways. The functional deficiency of lysosomal enzymes results in abnormal cell architecture (vacuolization and formation of inclusions) in cells of mesenchymal origin, which involves several tissues of the body: skeletal system (abnormal trabeculation of bone and cartilage), heart valves (vacuolization leading to thickening of the valves), renal glomerules, and liver fibroblasts of the periportal spaces.

Diagnosis: Clinical history and physical findings. Elevated levels of lysosomal enzymes (e.g., arylsulfatase A) in serum and body fluids. Deficient enzymes can be demonstrated in cultured fibroblasts. Microscopy of fibroblasts shows numerous "inclusion bodies" for which the disease is named.

Clinical aspects: I-cell disease has many clinical and radiographic features similar to Hurler syndrome, but with earlier presentation and without mucopolysaccharides. Striking gingival hyperplasia can distinguish this disease from Hurler syndrome. Other features include kyphoscoliosis, wedging of vertebral bodies, craniofacial abnormalities, and restricted joint movements. Repeated upper respiratory infections (bronchitis and pneumonia) are frequent. Severe mucosal thickening of the epiglottis, larynx, and trachea increases with age. Macroglossia is often present. Hepatomegaly is prominent with hernias. Severe psychomotor retardation, developmental delay, myelopathy, and neonatal hypotonia are important neurologic characteristics. Mental status is variable but can present with severe progressive psychomotor retardation. The cardiovascular anomalies include hypertrophic cardiopathy, cardiomegaly, and aortic insufficiency. Death within the first decade is usually from bronchopneumonia or congestive heart failure. No specific treatment is available. Physical therapy may delay progression of joint immobility. Nasal continuous positive airway pressure has been shown to reduce respiratory infections. Successful bone marrow transplantation has been reported.

Precautions before anesthesia: Chest radiography and resting SpO_2 must be obtained in view of frequent respiratory infections/obstructive sleep apnea. Abnormal airway with macroglossia, thickened mucosal folds in oropharynx and nasopharynx and facial deformities. Evaluate cardiac function (ECG, echocardiogram). Perform liver function tests and coagulation profiles if hepatomegaly is present.

Anesthetic considerations: Airway management is a major challenge with or without tracheal intubation. Loss of muscle tone after general anesthesia induction results in rapid upper airway obstruction. Use of a laryngeal mask airway may help to provide relief. Tracheal intubation when awake or anesthetized using direct laryngoscopy or blind technique may be impossible, especially in older patients, with more thickened mucosal folds. Likewise, use of flexible fiberoptic scope or Bullard laryngoscope may be fruitless. Otolaryngology standby for tracheostomy is required, otherwise the anesthetic should be discontinued and the patient awakened. Patient positioning in the presence of contractures can be difficult. Chronic pulmonary infections and kyphoscoliosis can lead to postoperative respiratory failure.

Pharmacological implications: Avoid the use of muscle relaxants, if possible, until the trachea is intubated and proper lung ventilation confirmed. In an attempt to "break" a laryngospasm with succinylcholine, the "cannot intubate, cannot ventilate" situation may arise. Use of opioids should be prudent in the presence of sleep apnea and mental retardation.

Other conditions to be considered:

☞**SIALIDOSIS TYPE II:** Lysosomal storage disease caused by a deficiency of the enzyme alpha-neuraminidase and resulting in tissue accumulation of mucopolysaccharides and mucolipids, which results in the development (during the second decade usually) of red macules in the eyes, myoclonus, mild Hurler-like facies, skeletal dysplasia, psychomotor retardation, and normal excretion of urinary mucopolysaccharides. Autosomal recessive. Gene map locus is 6p21.

☞**HURLER SYNDROME:** Lysosomal storage disease with tissue accumulation of acid mucopolysaccharides characterized by coarse facies (gargoyle-like), severe mental retardation, considerable visceromegaly, hernias, enlarged tongue, skeletal disorders (kyphoscoliosis), dwarfism, respiratory and cardiac impairment. Gene map locus is 4p16.3.

REFERENCES:

Korneld S, Sly WS: I-cell disease and pseudo-Hurler polydystrophy: Disorders of lysosomal enzyme phosphorylation and localization, in Scriver CR, Sly WS (eds): *The Metabolic and Molecular Basis of Inherited Disease.* 8th ed. New York, McGraw-Hill, 1995, p 2495.

Lees S, Homfray T, Nicolaides KH: Prenatal ultrasound diagnosis of Leroy I cell disease. *Ultrasound Obstet Gynecol* 18:275, 2001.

Pshezhetsky AV, Ashmarina M: Lysosomal multienzyme complex: Biochemistry, genetics, and molecular pathophysiology. *Prog Nucleic Acid Res Mol Biol* 69:81, 2001.

Ichthyosis Vulgaris

At a glance: Group of cutaneous disorders of keratinization representing more than 95% of ichthyosis cases. Can be a genetic disorder that is generally present soon after birth, or it can be a nonhereditary condition associated with internal disease, such as malignancies, or it can be induced by various medications. Most patients present with asthma, eczema, and fever.

Synonym: Ichthyosis Simplex.

Incidence and genetic inheritance: Autosomal dominant inheritance.

Pathophysiology: Hereditary forms can be caused by altered profilaggrin expression leading to scaling and desquamation and is often associated with atopy. It is a retention hyperkeratosis; expression of profilaggrin is absent or reduced in the epidermis.

Diagnosis: At birth, skin is normal. It gradually becomes rough and dry in early childhood. Scaling tends to be most prominent on the extensor surfaces of the extremities and absent on the flexor surfaces. Lesions are rare in the axillae and antecubital and popliteal

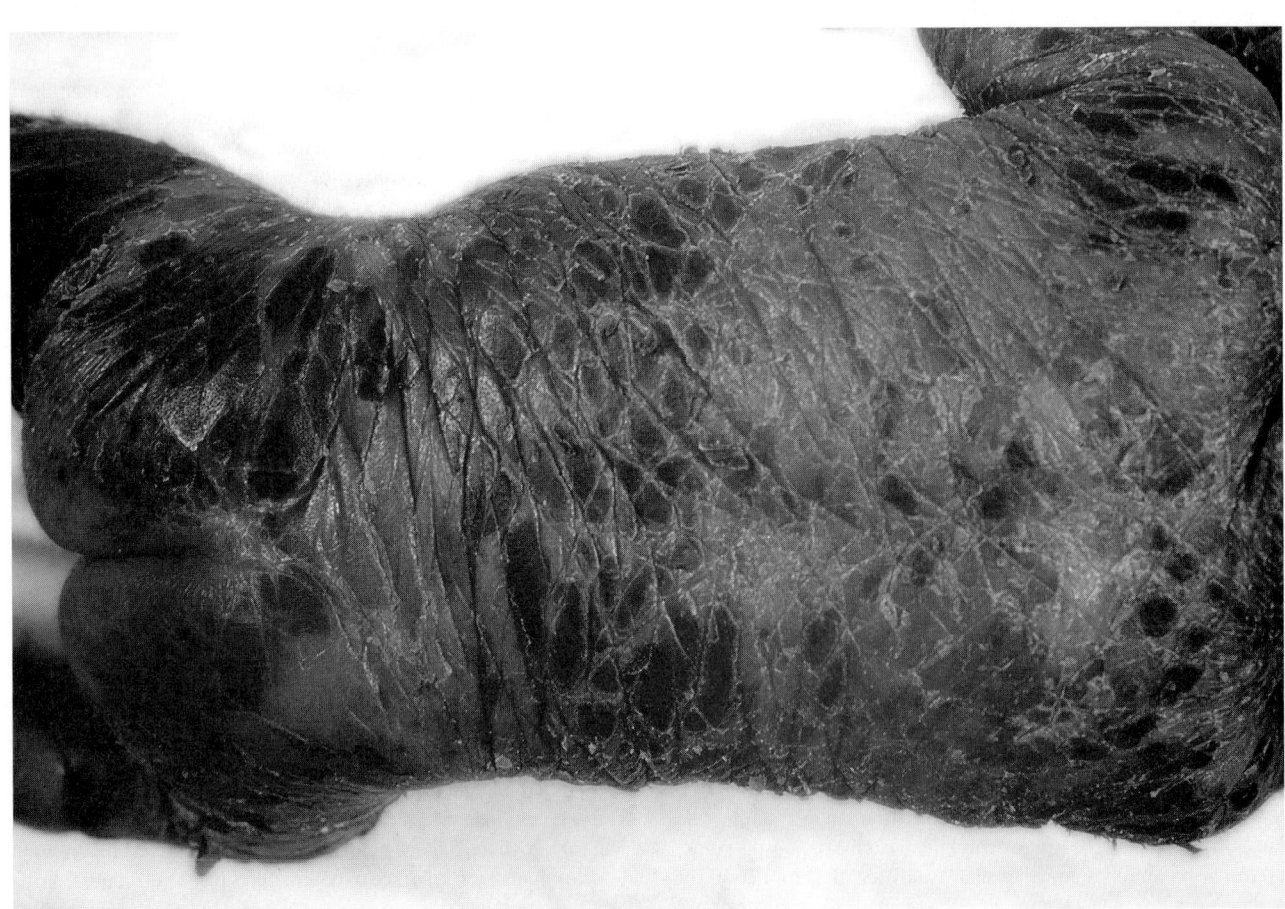

Ichthyosis lamellaris   Severe form of ichthyosis lamellaris in an infant. See color plates.

Ichthyosis lamellaris   Ichthyosis lamellaris in a teenager.

fossae. Forehead and cheeks may be involved, but lesions in these areas diminish with age. Notable amelioration in summer.

Clinical aspects: Features involve mainly skin with scales (fine, irregular, and polygonal in shape) of various sizes and colors. Lower extremities generally are more affected than the upper extremities. The face is generally spared however, hyperkeratosis of the palms and soles and follicular hyperkeratosis of the cheek and neck is often present. Pruritus is frequent. Fissures can appear with secondary infections. Inflammation is possible.

Precautions before anesthesia: Evaluate hydration status in case of extensive ichthyosis.

Anesthetic considerations: Fixation of monitoring devices and indwelling catheters on skin can be difficult. There is an increased risk of superinfection following installation of venous puncture, regional anesthesia, and any other maneuvers leading to skin damage. Patients affected are susceptible to thermoregulatory imbalance leading rapidly to severe hypothermia.

Pharmacological implications: Nicotinic acid, triparanol, butyrophenones, dixyrazine, cimetidine, and clofazimine have been implicated in acquired ichthyosis and should be avoided. Consider the administration of steroid stress doses in case of long-term treatment.

Other conditions to be considered: Multiple forms of ichthyosis.

REFERENCES:

DiGiovanna JJ, Robinson-Bostom L: Ichthyosis: Etiology, diagnosis, and management. *Am J Clin Dermatol* 4:81, 2003.

Okulicz JF, Schwartz RA: Hereditary and acquired ichthyosis vulgaris. *Int J Dermatol* 42:95, 2003.

Smart G, Bradshaw EG: Extradural analgesia and ichthyosis. *Anaesthesia* 39:161, 1984.

Idiopathic Intracranial Hypertension

At a glance: Idiopathic syndrome caused by increased intracranial pressure with papilledema of unknown origin, most often presenting with symptoms of cerebral tumor (pseudotumor cerebri) in young obese women in their childbearing years.

Synonyms: Benign Intracranial Hypertension; Pseudotumor Cerebri.

Nature: Clinical syndrome characterized by increased intracranial pressure of unknown origin with good prognosis if medical treatment (acetazolamide) is regularly taken. Severe cases (visual impairment) require neurosurgery.

Incidence: The incidence in the United States has been reported to range from 0.9–1.0:100,000 in the general population; however, this rate is estimated to be 1.6–3.5:100,000 in women and 7.9–19:100,000 in overweight women. Internationally, the incidence varies considerably among countries. However, the relationship between personal habitus such as obesity has been confirmed. In Libya, it has been demonstrated that the incidence was estimated at 2.2:100,000 in the general population, 4.3:100,000 in women, and 21.4:100,000 in obese women.

Pathophysiology: Idiopathic intracranial hypertension is a clinical syndrome characterized by an elevated intracranial pressure with normal cerebrospinal fluid (CSF) composition and no evidence of any expanding intracranial mass lesion or significant hydrocephalus. In all cases, increased vitamin A concentration is measured in the CSF of affected women. Females are more affected than males. Most often, no specific cause is found; however, multiple causes have been identified: endocrine and metabolic disorders (hypoparathyroidism, pseudohypoparathyroidism, corticosteroid therapy withdrawal, growth hormone treatment, hypervitaminosis A, Addison disease, obesity, menarche, oral contraceptives, pregnancy, galactosemia), hematologic disorders (iron deficiency and hemolytic anemia, polycythemia, Wiskott-Aldrich syndrome), infections (roseola infantum, chronic otitis media and mastoiditis, Guillain-Barré syndrome), drugs (tetracyclines, nalidixic acid), and obstruction of intracranial drainage by venous thrombosis (head injury, lateral or posterior sagittal sinus thrombosis, obstruction of superior vena cava).

Diagnosis: Clinical course; CT scan or MRI excluding any structural cause for increased intracranial pressure and showing normal ventricles; lumbar puncture revealing elevated CSF opening pressure and normal CSF composition (chemistry, cytology, bacteriology). Lumbar puncture is therapeutic, allowing CSF to escape, thereby reducing the intracranial pressure. Digital subtraction angiography may be performed if there is suspicion of venous thrombosis.

Clinical aspects: Some patients are asymptomatic. Infants may present with irritability, bulging fontanelle, and a resonant sound on skull percussion (MacEwen sign). Headache, pulsatile intracranial noises, occasional vomiting, transient visual obscuration, diplopia secondary to abducens nerve paralysis, and intermittent gait ataxia are possible findings in children and adults. Examination reveals papilledema without significant focal neurologic signs. Visual loss from optic neuropathy may occur as a long-term sequela. Treatment is aimed at controlling intracranial pressure in order to preserve the vision.

Precautions before anesthesia: Obtain a full history of any associated disorder (endocrine, hematologic, drug-related, infectious, or obstructive secondary to venous thrombosis). Inquire about the use of therapy to control the presence of benign intracranial hypertension, such as corticosteroids, diuretics (acetazolamide with/without furosemide), repeated therapeutic lumbar punctures, and surgical lumboperitoneal shunting. Obtain electrolytes and glucose levels for patients on steroid or diuretic therapy.

Anesthetic considerations: In patients receiving steroids, consider "stress-dose" supplementation and expect possible side effects from long-term steroid therapy (hypertension, hypokalemia, hyperglycemia, osteoporosis, poor wound healing, susceptibility to infections). If on diuretics, hypovolemia, electrolytes, and acid-base imbalance may require correction. Unlike patients with increased intracranial pressure caused by a space-occupying lesion in whom spinal anesthesia is contraindicated, a lumbar puncture is safe and beneficial in cases of pseudotumor cerebri. Spinal and epidural anesthesia when possible are advisable unless a lumboperitoneal shunt is present (local anesthetic injected in the subarachnoid space could escape in the peritoneum through the shunt, increasing risk of rapid absorption and toxicity). Intravenous lidocaine at induction of anesthesia decreases systemic hypertension associated with laryngoscopy. If a rapid-sequence induction is required, succinylcholine's ability to provide satisfactory intubating conditions outweighs the small increase in intracranial pressure that it may cause. Hyperventilation following induction of anesthesia lowers intracranial pressure. A 10-degree head-up position improves cerebral venous drainage and prevents kinking of the jugular veins by exaggerated rotation of the head to one side.

Pharmacological implications: Intracranial pressure reduction can be achieved with mannitol and loop diuretics; corticosteroids reduce brain edema (dexamethasone being more effective than other steroids in edema/intracranial pressure reduction). Compared to other volatile anesthetics, isoflurane below 1 minimum alveolar concentration (MAC) offers the best compromise between decreased cerebral metabolic oxygen requirement and increased intracranial pressure (as a result of an increase in cerebral blood flow). Thiopental, a potent cerebral vasoconstrictor, is the drug of choice for induction. Benzodiazepines, etomidate, and propofol are acceptable alternatives.

REFERENCES:

Haslam RHA: Pseudotumor cerebri, in Behrman RE, Kliegman RM, Arvin AM (eds): *Nelson Textbook of Pediatrics.* 16th ed. Philadelphia, WB Saunders, 1996, p 1735.

Shin RK, Balcer LJ: Idiopathic intracranial hypertension. *Curr Treat Options Neurol* 4:297, 2002.

Stanley TV: Idiopathic intracranial hypertension presenting as hemiplegic migraine. *Acta Paediatr* 91:980, 2002.

Idiopathic Thrombocytopenia Purpura

At a glance: Autoimmune disease resulting in destruction of platelets and presenting as bleeding disorders.

Synonyms: Idiopathic Thrombocytopenic Purpura; Werlhof Disease.

Incidence: *Acute*: 6:100,000 per year in the general population. No sex predilection. Peak incidence occurs between 2 and 4 years of age. *Chronic*: 1:250,000 per year in the general population. Females affected two to three times more often than males. Peak incidence occurs between 20 and 50 years of age.

Genetic inheritance: Not a genetic disorder. However, the development of antiplatelet antibodies in idiopathic thrombocytopenia purpura seems to be driven by an encounter with several platelet antigens through the clonal expansion of B cells using genetically restricted and highly specific combinations of heavy- and light-chain gene products.

Pathophysiology: The majority of patients have circulating antiplatelet antibodies, directed at glycoproteins IIb and IIIa, leading to platelet destruction in the spleen and thrombocytopenia. Although platelet production is increased, it does not prevent thrombocytopenia.

Diagnosis: Patients develop petechiae, bruising, and nosebleeds, usually after a viral illness. The remainder of the physical examination is normal. All laboratory tests are normal, with the exception of a markedly decreased platelet count and increased bleeding time. The platelet count is the only test needed to confirm the clinical diagnosis.

Clinical aspects: Petechiae, easy bruising, nosebleeds, thrombocytopenia. Typically course is benign with excellent prognosis. Treatment includes steroids, intravenous immunoglobulin, anti-D immunoglobin, chemotherapeutic agents, plasmapheresis, and splenectomy in refractory cases. Complications include intracranial hemorrhage (0.1–0.5%), usually with platelet counts below 20,000/mm^3. Fetal thrombocytopenia is secondary to transplacental crossing of antiplatelet antibodies. There are two forms of idiopathic thrombocytopenia purpura:

1. *Acute form* is encountered in children ranging in age from 2 to 6 years, often after a viral illness. It usually has a sudden onset and disappears within a few weeks (less than 6 months).
2. *Chronic form* can occur at any age but is more common in women of childbearing age. It lasts more than 6 months (often several years) and requires continual follow-up care.

Precautions before anesthesia: Consult hematologist regarding intravenous immunoglobulin and anti-D immunoglobulin. Check platelet count. Type and cross for platelets in emergency surgery (type and cross helps prevent alloimmunization in patients with frequent transfusions).

Anesthetic considerations: Bleeding usually does not occur with platelet counts greater than 50,000/mm^3. The decision to transfuse platelets should be based on clinical bleeding, not actual platelet count. Central-neuraxial anesthesia is contraindicated because of the risk of hematoma. Some patients have undergone splenectomy, which makes them more prone to develop infection. Administration of perioperative corticosteroid supplementation is highly recommended.

Pharmacological implications: Administration of pharmacological agents that affect platelet adhesion (e.g., aspirin) should be avoided. If anticoagulation is needed, extreme precautions are needed during administration (e.g., bleeding time, coagulation profile). Although some patients (e.g., children with the acute form) do not receive any treatment, most patients affected with this condition are given drugs that can affect the immune system, such as corticosteroids, infusion of immune globulin, vincristine, azathioprine, cyclophosphamide, or cyclosporine. These medications may lead to many interferences and complications both intraoperatively and postoperatively.

Other conditions to be considered:

DISSEMINATED INTRAVASCULAR COAGULATION: Acquired disorder in the context of shock.

☞THROMBOTIC THROMBOCYTOPENIC PURPURA: Severe multisystem disorder of unknown etiology associated with pregnancy, diseases such as HIV, cancer, bacterial infection, and vasculitis, bone marrow transplantation, and drugs. Hemolytic uremic syndrome is the more common pediatric variant of this syndrome, with prominent renal involvement.

REFERENCES:

Medeiros D: Current controversies in the management of idiopathic thrombocytopenic purpura during childhood. *Pediatr Clin North Am* 43:757, 1996.

Pamuk GE, Pamuk ON, Baslar Z, et al: Overview of 321 patients with idiopathic thrombocytopenic purpura. Retrospective analysis of the clinical features and response to therapy. *Ann Hematol* 81:436, 2002.

Roark JH, Bussel JB, Cines DB, et al: Genetic analysis of autoantibodies in idiopathic thrombocytopenic purpura reveals evidence of clonal expansion and somatic mutation. *Blood* 100:1388, 2002.

Imerslund Syndrome

At a glance: Inherited megaloblastic anemia caused by a constitutional malabsorption of vitamin B$_{12}$.

Synonyms: Defect of Enterocyte Intrinsic Factor Receptor; Enterocyte Cobalamin Malabsorption; Imerslund-Grasbeck Syndrome; Imerslund-Najman-Grasbeck Syndrome; Juvenile Pernicious Anemia due to Selective Intestinal Malabsorption of Vitamin B$_{12}$ with Proteinuria.

Incidence: Internationally, the incidence of megaloblastic anemia in childhood is not established; however, 29 cases have been reported in the Middle East between 1960 and 1998.

Genetic inheritance: Autosomal recessive with multiple nonallelic forms. Gene map locus is 10p12.1.

Pathophysiology: Megaloblastic anemia secondary to B$_{12}$ malabsorption, with proteinuria. The disease is caused by a selective defect between the attachment of B$_{12}$ to the ileal cell surface and binding to transcobalamin II or absence of functional receptor (cubilin); it is not influenced by the administration of intrinsic factor. Renal function studies are normal.

Diagnosis: Bone marrow exam shows megaloblastic anemia. The Schilling test, which assesses cobalamin absorption both with and without exogenous intrinsic factor, is abnormal. Urinalysis reveals proteinuria despite otherwise normal renal function studies.

Clinical aspects: Megaloblastic anemia that responds to parenteral cobalamin administration. Proteinuria. This condition has been associated with dolichocephaly, confusion, dementia, generalized paresthesias, and sensory deficits.

Precautions before anesthesia: Mandatory to obtain a complete blood cell (CBC) count, vitamin B$_{12}$ plasma level, and urinary protein level.

Anesthetic considerations: Consider postponing elective surgery in face of untreated anemia. In case of surgical emergency, complete type and crossmatch for blood must be obtained.

Pharmacological implications: Theoretically, nitrous oxide should be avoided because it reduces the activity of the vitamin B$_{12}$-dependent enzymes methionine synthetase and thymidylate synthetase.

Other conditions to be considered: Other causes of megaloblastic anemia by deficiency of either vitamin B$_{12}$ or folinic acid:

VITAMIN B$_{12}$ DEFICIENCY: Impaired absorption (insufficient release of vitamin B$_{12}$ from protein, intrinsic factor deficiency, chronic pancreatic or intestinal disorders, parasitoses) or inadequate utilization (defective enzymes, lack of transcobalamin II, chronic exposure to nitrous oxide).

☞FOLIC ACID DEFICIENCY: Prematurity, insufficient dietary intake, alcoholism, intestinal derivation, tropical sprue, treatment with sulfasalazine or folic acid antagonists such as methotrexate, hemodialysis.

REFERENCES:

Ben-Ami M: Imerslund syndrome with dolichocephaly. *Pediatr Hematol Oncol* 7:177, 1990.

Gueant JL, Chery C, Namour F, et al: Decreased affinity of urinary intrinsic factor-cobalamin receptor in a case of Grasbeck-Imerslund syndrome. *Gastroenterology* 116:1274, 1999.

Iminoglycinuria

At a glance: Benign inborn error of metabolism caused by a defect in renal tubular amino acid transport resulting in abnormal urinary excretion of glycine, proline, and hydroxyproline.

Synonyms: Familial Iminoglycinuria.

Incidence: Homozygotes: 1:15,000 live births; heterozygotes: 2:100 in the general population.

Genetic inheritance: Usually autosomal recessive, heterozygotes may be "hyperglycinuric" (incomplete recessive), or silent (completely recessive).

Pathophysiology: Benign condition in which glycine and the imino acids proline and hydroxyproline have a decreased renal tubular reabsorption. Results from a specific inborn error of metabolism involving the common membrane carrier of these amino acids in the renal tubule.

Clinical aspects: Individuals with familial iminoglycinuria are asymptomatic. Excessive urinary proline, hydroxyproline, and glycine are normal findings in the first 6 months of life. In iminoglycinuria, urinary glycine excretion exceeds 150 mg in 24 hours, or endogenous renal clearance rate exceeds 8.6 ml/min/1.73 m^2.

Anesthetic considerations: No specific precautions required for this condition.

REFERENCE:

Chesney RW: Iminoglycinuria, in Scriver CR, Beaudet AL, Sly WS, Valle D: *The Metabolic and Molecular Bases of Inherited Disease.* 7th ed. New York, McGraw-Hill, 1995, p 3643.

Immotile Cilia Syndrome

At a glance: Genetic disorder characterized by immotility of respiratory, auditory, and sperm cilia as a result of lack (or abnormality) of dynein. This anomaly is associated in approximately 50% of patients affected with situs inversus (often called Kartagener syndrome).

Synonyms: Primary Ciliary Dyskinesia; Rutland Ciliary Disorientation Syndrome (or Ciliary Dyscoordination due to Random Ciliary Orientation).

Incidence: 1:30,000–60,000 in the general population.

Genetic inheritance: Autosomal recessive with incomplete penetrance. Sporadic cases may represent new mutations with dominant expression. Identified gene map loci at 9q13.3-qter, 9p21-p13, and 5p15-p14.

Pathophysiology: Primary abnormality is absence or abnormality of dynein arms in cilia. Absence of nexin links between dynein arms is described. Dynein arms contain high levels of adenosine triphosphatase and provide the energy for ciliary beating. Absence results in akinetic or dyskinetic ciliary motion.

Diagnosis: Bronchiectasis and sinusitis or aplasia of paranasal sinuses. Clinical history, electron microscopy of cilia, ciliary motion analysis, and studies of mucociliary transport (nasal biopsy or sperm sample).

Clinical aspects: Repeated respiratory tract infections, sinusitis, persistent rhinorrhea, otitis media with hearing loss, male infertility. Bronchiectasis may develop in infancy and is common in early adult life secondary to recurrent pneumonia. Lung function shows an obstructive pattern, which may become restrictive later. Pulmonary hypertension and right ventricular dysfunction develop in later stages of the disease. Abnormal neutrophil migration has been demonstrated in vitro; however, its clinical significance is unknown.

Precautions before anesthesia: Inquire for history of recent upper airway infections, pneumonia, evidence of bronchiectasis. Cardiac assessment must include an ECG and consider an echocardiogram if there is clinical evidence of right ventricular dysfunction. Respiratory assessment including chest radiography and pulmonary function tests, especially prior to major surgery. Blood gases are mandatory prior to lung volume reduction surgery.

Anesthetic considerations: Increased risk for general anesthesia. Patients rely on forceful cough to clear secretions. The anesthetist should aim to allow early return of airway reflexes and of the ability to clear secretions. In young adults pulmonary hypertension may be present. The use of regional or local anesthesia is ideal when possible. When general anesthesia is mandatory, supplementation with regional analgesia continued postoperatively should be considered. Ensure availability of postoperative physiotherapy. The left lung may be more at risk in aspiration, and left endobronchial intubation is more likely than right. If a double-lumen endotracheal tube is used in the presence of situs inversus, a left-sided tube may occlude the left upper lung bronchus. Bronchoscopic assessment of the bronchial tree is therefore indicated.

Pharmacological implications: Chest infections should only be treated after identification of causal organism. Anticholinergics relatively contraindicated because they may prevent clearance of secretions.

Other conditions to be considered:

☞**PEUTZ-JEGHERS SYNDROME:** Same gene map locus (19p13.3) but autosomal dominant. Also considered familial in 40 to 55% of cases. Characterized by gastrointestinal polyposis (especially the small intestine) and associated with benign adenomatous (hamartous) tumors 0.5 to 0.7 cm (0.2–0.3 in) in diameter. There is a typical mucocutaneous pigmentation consisting of discrete brown to bluish-black macules about the lips, oral mucosa, and nose. Anemia caused by intestinal bleeding is frequent. Recurrent and severe abdominal pain may occur. Onset in the adolescence.

☞**KARTAGENER SYNDROME:** Association of primary ciliary dyskinesia and situs inversus. Inherited autosomal recessive disorder characterized by bronchiectasis, sinusitis, dextrocardia, and infertility.

REFERENCES:

Bartoloni L, Blouin JL, Pan Y, et al: Mutations in the DNAH11 (axonemal heavy chain dynein type 11) gene cause one form of situs inversus totalis and most likely primary ciliary dyskinesia. *Proc Natl Acad Sci U S A* 99:10282, 2002.

Bromiker R, Neeman Z, Bar-Oz B, et al: Early diagnosis of primary ciliary dyskinesia in a newborn without situs inversus. *Acta Paediatr* 91:1002, 2002.

Jaffe A, Bush A: Genetic contributions to rare childhood lung diseases. *Paediatr Respir Rev* 2:268, 2001.

Immunodeficiency Centromeric Instability and Facial Anomalies Syndrome

At a glance: Syndrome characterized by immune deficiency associated with recurrent infections and facial dysmorphism.

Synonym: ICF Syndrome.

Incidence: Approximately 50 cases have been described.

Genetic inheritance: Autosomal recessive.

Pathophysiology: The immune defect is variable. Patients tend to have a reduction in at least two immunoglobulin classes. Immunodeficiency has been suggested to be caused by the effects of an acquired viral infection in genetically predisposed individuals. Chromosomal abnormalities are multiple and affect the heterochromatic regions of chromosomes 1, 9, and 16. Chromosome 2 is occasionally affected. Chromosomal abnormalities consist of despiralization, chromosome and chromatid breaks, and pairing and interchanges between homologous and nonhomologous chromosomes. Chromosomal abnormalities are generally found only in peripheral blood lymphocytes. Low numbers of T lymphocytes and natural killer (NK) cells are noted. ICF syndrome is caused by mutations of the DNA methyl-transferase 3B (DNMT3B) gene, which has been mapped to 20q11.2.

Diagnosis: Based on the findings of severe immunodeficiency with recurrent infections, associated with a high frequency of pericentromeric decondensations and rearrangements in chromosome 1 and 16 upon karyotype analysis of blood samples. Additional clinical signs include short stature and peculiar facies. Laboratory examinations show reduced serum concentrations of immunoglobulin (Ig) A, IgG, IgE, T lymphocytes, and NK cells, whereas serum levels of IgM are increased. The diagnosis is usually made in infancy.

Clinical aspects: Patients have short stature, failure to thrive, and suffer from mental retardation. The disease affects the head and neck (hypertelorism, epicanthic folds, low-set ears, flat nasal bridge, micrognathia, macroglossia with protrusion of the tongue), gastrointestinal tract (diarrhea, malabsorption), and immune system (recurrent and prolonged respiratory tract infections, resulting in chronic bronchitis, and bronchiectases; maxillary sinusitis, otitis media, cutaneous infections). Most patients die of infections (pulmonary and/or gastrointestinal) even before they reach adolescence.

Precautions before anesthesia: Intercurrent infections should be treated. Chest radiograph, lung function tests, and arterial blood gas analysis may be helpful. Evaluate the airway for a potential difficult airway management. Mental retardation may impair cooperation.

Sedative and/or anxiolytic premedication and the presence of the primary caregiver during induction of anesthesia may be helpful.

Anesthetic considerations: Anesthesia in this condition has not been described. The described features suggest that patients may be prone to upper airway obstruction. Both direct laryngoscopy and tracheal intubation should be expected to be difficult. Alternative airway management techniques (e.g., fiberoptic bronchoscope, [intubating] laryngeal mask) should be available. Maintain spontaneous ventilation until the airway has been secured. A recent respiratory tract infection increases the incidence of perioperative complications (laryngospasm, bronchospasm, atelectases, pneumonia). Attention should be paid to strict aseptic technique for any kind of invasive procedures (intravascular catheters, regional anesthesia) in order to prevent infections. Although not described, use of irradiated blood products in these patients is advised to prevent a graft-versus-host reaction.

Pharmacological implications: Muscle relaxant should be avoided until airway has been secured.

REFERENCES:

Ehrlich M: The ICF syndrome, a DNA methyltransferase 3B deficiency and immunodeficiency disease. *Clin Immunol* 109:17, 2003.

Ehrlich M, Buchanan KL, Tsien F, et al: DNA methyltransferase 3B mutations linked to the ICF syndrome cause dysregulation of lymphogenesis genes. *Hum Mol Genet* 10:2917, 2001.

Brown DC, Grace E, Sumner AT, et al: ICF syndrome (immunodeficiency, centromeric instability and facial anomalies): Investigation of heterochromatin abnormalities and review of clinical outcome. *Hum Genet* 96:411, 1995.

Inclusion Body Myopathy

At a glance: Group of genetically transmitted muscle disorders characterized by progressive weakness of variable age onset depending on the clinical type.

Synonyms: Cytoplasmic Body Myopathy; Distal Myopathy with Rimmed Vacuoles (DMRV); Hereditary Inclusion Body Myopathy; Quadriceps-Sparing h-IBM; Nonaka Myopathy.

Genetic inheritance: Several patterns: autosomal dominant, autosomal recessive (chromosome 9, band p1-q1), and sporadic.

Pathophysiology: Cytoplasmic inclusions predominantly in type 1 fibers in the skeletal muscle. Smooth and cardiac muscles may be affected. Muscle biopsy reveals red-rimmed vacuoles, cytoplasmic or intranuclear filaments, and occasionally intracellular amyloid deposition. Progressive muscular weakness and atrophy occur as a consequence of the degenerative changes.

Diagnosis: Clinical course (symptoms appear from early to late life), tendon reflexes generally depressed, normal or elevated creatine phosphokinase, electromyogram showing predominant myopathic changes. Muscle biopsy reveals the characteristic vacuolar myopathy described. Sialuria is a characteristic feature of the quadriceps-sparing autosomal recessive myopathy.

Clinical aspects: A "malignant course" has been described in adolescents who showed a delayed onset of walking in childhood with easy fatigability. By age 14 to 15 years, they presented with scoliosis and weakness in the face, sternocleidomastoid, proximal limbs, and respiratory, spinal, and cardiac muscles. Most patients succumb from cardiorespiratory failure. Early- and late-onset adult inclusion body myopathies are characterized by distal muscle weakness of the upper and lower limbs that may progress to the girdles and result in various degrees of incapacitation. The variability of the clinical manifestations makes classification of these myopathies challenging: a quadriceps-sparing autosomal recessive myopathy of adult onset has been recognized as a distinct entity; it is caused by a defective mutation in the UDP-N-acetylglucosamine (UDP-GlcNAc) 2-epimerase/N-acetylmannosamine (ManNAc) kinase (or *GNE*) gene and was first described in Iranian Jews but it is not limited to this ethnic group.

Precautions before anesthesia: Obtain a thorough evaluation of motor function and exercise tolerance. Inquire about previous complications (cardiac, respiratory, other), especially those following surgeries. Seek any familial history of muscle weakness. Evaluate pulmonary function test (forced vital capacity [FVC], peak expiratory flow rate [PEFR], forced expiratory volume in 1 second [FEV$_1$], FEV$_1$/FVC, arterial blood gas analysis, chest radiographs) and cardiac function (ECG, echocardiography, and, if necessary, dobutamine stress echocardiography or radionuclide imaging). Plasma levels of creatine phosphokinase, serum glutamic-oxaloacetic transferase, lactate dehydrogenase, Na, and K. Avoid elective surgery if cardiac and/or respiratory function is significantly compromised (ventricular ejection fraction <0.5, FVC <25%, PEFR <30%). Inquire about corticosteroids or other immunosuppressive agents; some patients may be treated with these agents even though they are unsuccessful in controlling the disease.

Anesthetic considerations: Complications related to the various degrees of muscle weakness with the possibility of respiratory insufficiency and cardiomyopathy. If severe, spinal deformity may compress the upper respiratory tract, especially in the prone position. Careful dosing and monitoring of nondepolarizing muscle relaxants are required. Mechanical ventilatory support may be required postoperatively.

Pharmacological implications: Use of succinylcholine may trigger hyperkaliemia, arrhythmias, rhabdomyolysis, myoglobinuria, and cardiac arrest. Because of the muscle weakness, careful titration of the nondepolarizing muscle relaxants (under control of nerve stimulator) is necessary. In a spontaneously breathing patient, opioids should be given with caution, and, when possible, regional anesthesia is highly suitable.

Other condition to be considered:

SPORADIC INCLUSION BODY MYOSITIS (IBM): Acquired myopathic process of unknown origin presenting as weakness or impairment of muscle function in affected areas (predominance on knee extensor and wrist/finger flexor joints).

REFERENCES:

Eisenberg I, Grabov-Nardini G, Hochner H: Mutations spectrum of GNE in hereditary inclusion body myopathy sparing the quadriceps. *Hum Mutat* 21:99, 2003.

Sivakumar K, Dalakas MC: The spectrum of familial inclusion body myopathies in 13 families and a description of a quadriceps-sparing phenotype in non-Iranian Jews. *Neurology* 47:977, 1996.

Taratuto AL: Congenital myopathies and related disorders. *Curr Opin Neurol* 15:553, 2002.

Incontinentia Pigmenti

At a glance: Genetic disease characterized by unusual patterns of discolored skin. During the first stage, skin redness and spiral lines of blisters are encountered. Second stage includes warty skin on the arms and legs. Third stage is associated with discolorations of the skin but also hair (kinky hairs) and teeth. Other features include central nervous system dysfunction (spina bifida, skull deformity), dwarfism, club feet, cleft palate/lip, syndactyly, retinal vascular abnormalities, blindness, and congenital dislocation of the hips.

Synonyms: Bloch-Sulzberger Syndrome; Bloch-Siemens Syndrome with Incontinentia Pigmenti; Familial Incontinentia Pigmenti; Melanoblastosis Cutis Linearis; Pigmented Dermatosis, Siemens-Bloch Type.

History: Genodermatosis was first described by A.E. Garrod (1906), but the condition was defined by M. Bardach, Bruno Bloch, Swiss dermatologists, Hermann Werner Siemens, a German dermatologist, and Marion Baldur Sulzberger, an American dermatologist, during the 1920s.

Incidence: The international incidence in the general population has been estimated at 1:40,000. Up until the late 1980s, only 700 cases had been reported; however, the disease probably is not as rare as once thought because single simple cases are not usually described in the literature. Incontinentia pigmenti is a genodermatosis that can be associated with malignancies (i.e., chromosomal instability syndrome), such as acute myelogenous leukemia, Wilms tumor, malignant rhabdoid tumors, and retinoblastoma. It is more common in Caucasians than in other races. Women with incontinentia pigmenti have a 2:1 female-to-male offspring ratio. The initial skin lesions are present at birth.

Genetic inheritance: X-linked dominance with lethality in males. Gene map locus is Xq28. It affects almost only females (90–95% of cases) (Lyon effect). (Sporadic incontinentia pigmenti, usually termed hypomelanosis of Ito or incontinentia pigmenti type I, is a distinct disorder but has many features similar to those of incontinentia pigmenti; it is mapped at chromosome Xp11.21.)

Pathophysiology: Caused by a defective gene in the X chromosome, the NEMO gene (nuclear factor-κB essential modulator gene). It is an essential cellular protein allowing cells to respond to outside signals, such as growth factors. The evolution of lesions is the consequence of the death of cells bearing the mutant X chromosome and their replacement by cells with the normal X active chromosome.

Diagnosis: The cutaneous manifestations are diagnostic and present at birth. The name *incontinentia pigmenti* describes the characteristic histologic feature of incontinence of melanin from the melanocytes in the basal layer of the epidermis into the superficial dermis. Histologically, deposits of melanin pigment are seen in the corium: the designation was based on the idea that the basal layer of the epidermis is "incontinent" of melanin. The gene responsible for the disorder (NEMO gene) has been identified, thus allowing molecular testing and diagnosis.

Clinical aspects: Typically, the disease evolves in four stages that frequently overlap. The cutaneous signs are evident at or soon after birth and may be preceded by a phase suggesting inflammation in the skin. The progression is from an erythematous eruption with linear vesiculation in the newborn period (the vesicobullous stage), followed by a verrucous stage. After a few months, the verrucous growth drops off and leaves hyperpigmented areas. In the fully developed disease, the skin shows swirling patterns of melanin pigmentation, especially on the trunk, suggesting the appearance of "marble cake." The evolution of lesions can be interpreted as representing the death of cells that have the mutant-bearing X chro-

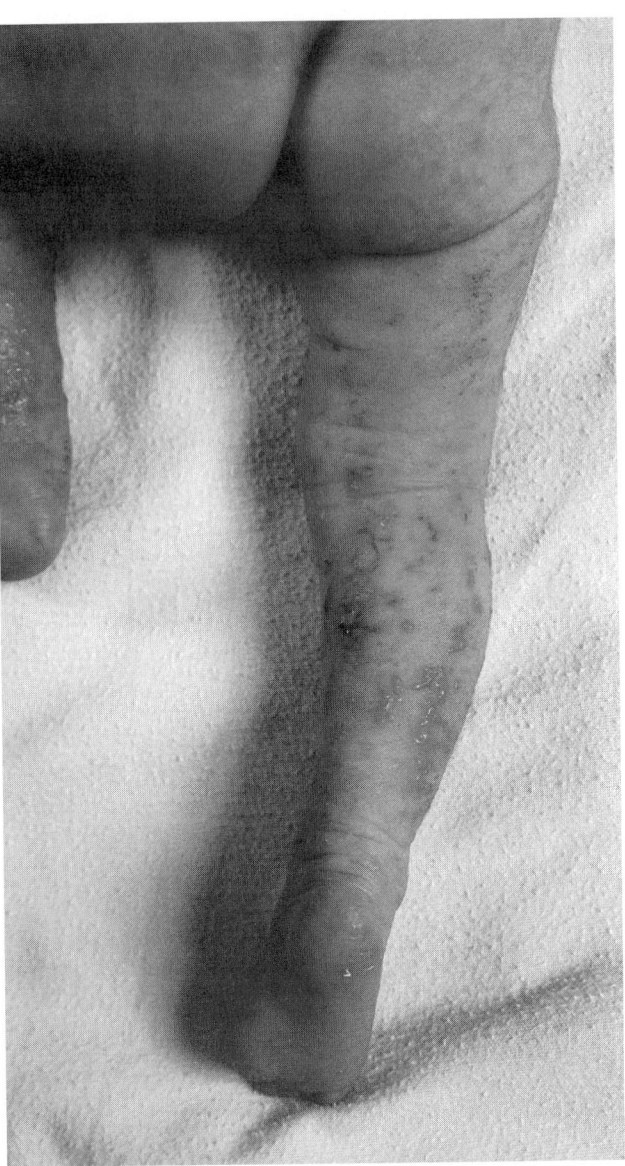

Incontinentia pigmenti First stage of incontinentia pigmenti with spiral lines and blisters on the skin of the legs in a 5-month-old infant. See color plates.

mosome as the active chromosome and replacement by cells with the normal X active. The third stage persists for several years and usually disappears at approximately age 20 years. Dental abnormalities are common (>80%), with malformation, impaction, and hypodontia. Mandibular development is normal. Neurologic features include convulsive disorders, spastic paralysis, motor and mental retardation. Ocular involvement includes retinal vascular changes, amblyopia, and strabismus. Macular ischemia is characteristic of this medical condition. It is often progressive, like typical vasculopathy. Blindness occurs in more than 15% of cases. Skeletal anomalies are less common but include spina bifida, cleft lip/palate, dwarfism, and chondrodystrophy.

Precautions before anesthesia: Missing and loose dentition should be documented. Measurement of anticonvulsant levels and optimization of anticonvulsant therapy must be achieved. Continuation of morning dose of anticonvulsants is recommended.

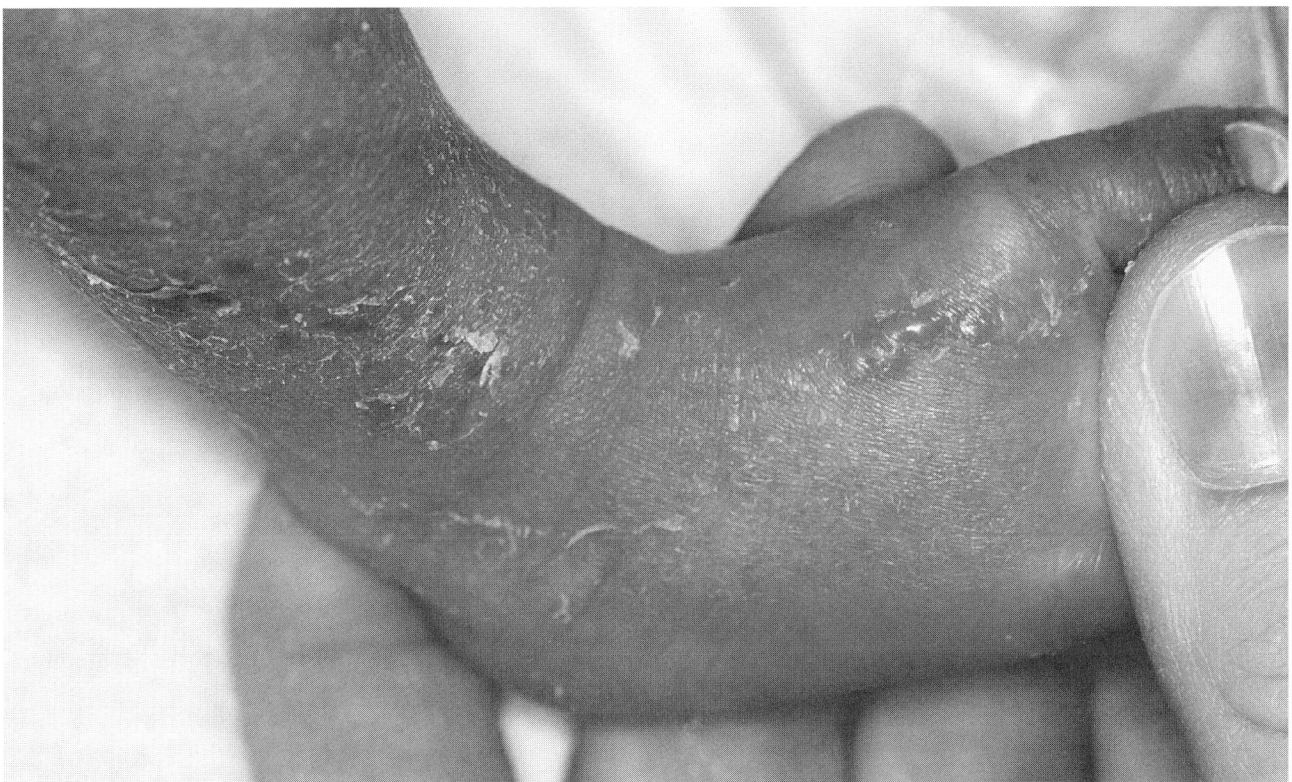

Incontinentia pigmenti Hyperpigmentation and linear vesiculation on the feet of an infant with incontinentia pigmenti.

Anesthetic considerations: No anesthetic problems have been reported. Many of the patients are blind and mentally retarded, making cooperation difficult. The room should be quiet for induction. Attention should be paid to the presence of blisters. Protection from skin trauma from the application of monitoring devices should be provided. Venous access may be difficult in the presence of widespread skin lesions. Application of the blood pressure monitor cuff may be difficult if the vesicles and bullae involve the limbs. If so, proper skin padding must be used to limit shearing forces applied to the skin during insufflation of the cuff.

Pharmacological implications: No known specific implications. However, avoiding triggers agents that potentiate occurrence of seizures (enflurane with hypocapnia, methohexital, and ketamine) is recommended.

Other condition to be considered:

☞**HYPOMELANOSIS OF ITO:** Maps to chromosome Xp11. Congenital disorder characterized by hypopigmented whorls of skin along the Blaschko lines and associated with multiple other congenital defects, mostly neurologic, skeletal, hair, and dental anomalies.

REFERENCES:

Berlin AL, Paller AS, Chan LS: Incontinentia pigmenti: A review and update on the molecular basis of pathophysiology. *J Am Acad Dermatol* 47:169, 2002.

Landy SJ, Donnai D: Incontinentia pigmenti. *J Med Genet* 30:53, 1993.

Smahi A, Courtois G, Rabia SH, et al: The NF-kappaB signalling pathway in human diseases: From incontinentia pigmenti to ectodermal dysplasias and immune-deficiency syndromes. *Hum Mol Genet* 11:2371, 2002.

Infantile Pyloric Stenosis

At a glance: Common intestinal occlusive disorder appearing during the first weeks of life typically characterized explosive vomiting following feeding, progressive dehydration, and hypochloremic alkalosis. It is a common infantile disorder characterized by enlarged pyloric musculature leading to gastric outlet obstruction.

Synonym: Infantile Hypertrophic Pyloric Stenosis

Incidence: 1:300 live births with considerable regional variation. Of the affected infants, 85% are male, with 5.7:1 male-to-female ratio. Approximately 10% are premature infants.

Genetic inheritance: Mendelian inheritance of pyloric stenosis cannot be established.

Pathophysiology: Physiopathologic mechanism is not known, but a defect in pyloric relaxation (pylorospasm) has been postulated. The pylorospasm may be the result of a lack of nitric oxide synthase in pyloric tissue.

Diagnosis: Nonbilious projectile vomiting, palpable pyloric tumor with visible peristalsis in the upper abdomen in a male infant aged 3 to 8 weeks. Confirmed diagnosis by ultrasonography. Typical laboratory finding is hypochloremic alkalosis.

Clinical aspects: Dehydration and electrolyte derangement are common (hypochloremic hypokalemic metabolic alkalosis). Full correction of the intravascular volume and of chloride and potassium deficits must be done prior to surgery and may require several days to ensure safe anesthesia and surgery. Pyloromyotomy (Ramstedt operation) remains the only satisfactory treatment, with a very low perioperative mortality rate of 0.4 to 3%. Occasional vomiting occurs postoperatively in more than half of patients, but the value of graded postoperative feeding regimen is not proven. Associated renal anomalies may occur in a small percentage of patients.

Precautions before anesthesia: This is a medical emergency, not a surgical one. Ensure that the intravascular volume and electrolyte deficits are fully corrected prior to anesthesia. Investigations include serum electrolytes, urea, creatinine, and blood sugar levels. Arterial blood gas analysis for acid-base values might be indicated in severe cases. Urine chloride concentration is indicative of the degree of hypokalemia.

Anesthetic considerations: All precautions should be taken to protect against a full stomach. The nasogastric tube should be aspirated prior to induction of anesthesia. A rapid-sequence induction with preoxygenation, cricoid pressure, thiopental, and succinylcholine is often used. Inhalation induction with cricoid pressure applied until orotracheal intubation is achieved is another alternative. Awake tracheal intubation is not superior to anesthetized, paralyzed tracheal intubation technique in maintaining adequate oxygenation and heart rate or in reducing complications. Most important for the anesthesiologist is to use the airway management technique that he/she is most comfortable with. It is not time to improvise! Blood loss usually is minimal. The infant should have his/her trachea extubated fully awake at the end of the procedure in the left lateral position. Postoperative analgesia can be provided by wound infiltration with local anesthetics and administration of acetaminophen. Postoperative hypoglycemia 2 to 3 hours after the procedure and respiratory depression have been described. Consequently, the child should be monitored closely in the immediate postoperative period.

Pharmacological implications: There are no specific implications except for a significant increase in susceptibility to opiates.

REFERENCES:

Bissonnette B, Sullivan PJ: Pyloric stenosis. *Can J Anaesth* 38:668, 1991.

Cook-Sather SD, Tulloch HV, Cnaan A, et al: A comparison of awake versus paralyzed tracheal intubation for infants with pyloric stenosis. *Anesth Analg* 86:945, 1998.

Infantile Sialic Acid Storage Disease

At a glance: Autosomal recessive inherited metabolic disorder characterized by hyperexcretion of free sialic acid in the urine and by its storage in the lysosomes of different tissues. Clinical features include coarse facial abnormalities, clear cornea, albinoid fungi, ptosis, nystagmus, anteverted nose, high-arched palate, cardiomegaly, heart failure, hepatosplenomegaly, nephrotic syndrome, hypotonia, and developmental delay. Neonatal ascites, hydrops fetalis, and early death can occur.

Classification and synonyms:

Sialuria: Rarest form of sialic acid storage disease.

Moderate Form (Salla Disease; Free Sialic Storage Disease; Sialuria Finnish Type): Adult form of sialuria mostly observed in the northeastern part of Finland. Clinical features include progressive mental and psychomotor retardation, clumsiness, onset at age 12 to 18 months with deterioration in the second decade, 4 to 15% vacuolated lymphocytes, enlarged storage lysosomes, and increased sialic acid in the urine. Ataxia, athetosis, rigidity, spasticity, impaired

speech, growth retardation, thick calvaria, and exotropia are present in more than 50% of patients. Life expectancy is reduced to the seventh decade in most patients.

Severe Form: Infantile Sialic Acid Storage Disease (ISSD; Sialuria, Infantile Form; N-Acetyl-Neuraminic Acid Storage Disease; NANA Storage Disease): Usually diagnosed in the newborn period. Unlike Salla disease, there is no ethnic prevalence. Clinically, it presents with severe visceral involvement, dysostosis multiplex, psychomotor retardation, and early death.

Genetic inheritance: Autosomal recessive.

Pathophysiology: Sialuria differs from the sialidosis in the accumulation and excretion of free sialic acid in the presence of normal or increased levels of neuraminidase activity. Sialuria occurs because of defective feedback inhibition on the enzyme UDP-GlcNAc 2-epimerase in the process of NANA synthesis. Both Salla disease and infantile sialic acid storage disease are caused by impairment of an active transport system of free sialic acid across lysosomal membrane and probably are allelic to each other, despite different clinical features. Genetic mapping of both forms is assigned to 6q14-q15 on the long arm of chromosome 6.

Diagnosis: Clinical features. Peripheral blood count may show anemia and vacuolated lymphocytes, also seen in bone marrow aspiration. Urinary free sialic acid level is increased. Cultured fibroblast presents increased free sialic acid level. Electron microscopy shows accumulation of NANA in the cytosolic fraction only in sialuria and in the lysosomal fraction only in Salla disease and infantile sialic acid storage disease, resulting in vacuole appearance. Prenatal diagnosis can be obtained by measuring free sialic acid in amniotic fluid. Normal lysosomal enzymes exclude sialidosis.

Clinical aspects: *Sialuria:* Rarest form. Clinical features include coarse facies, hepatosplenomegaly, and near-normal growth and development.

Salla Disease: Most common form. High prevalence in northern part of Finland. Presents in adulthood with growth and mental retardation, ataxia, athetosis, rigidity, spasticity, and speech impairment.

Infantile Sialic Acid Storage Disease: Most severe form. Commonly presents in infancy with early-onset psychomotor retardation, coarse facial "gargoyle-like" appearance with wispy hair, hypertelorism, prominent epicanthic folds, fluffy eyebrows, long philtrum, high-arched palate, and hepatosplenomegaly. Other presentations may include nephrotic syndrome (one case), fetal and neonatal ascites, congestive cardiac failure (one case), and esophageal atresia (one case). Other features include prematurity, failure to thrive, hypotonia, albinoid fundi, and dysostosis multiplex. Death occurs in early childhood and is commonly due to respiratory failure.

Precautions before anesthesia: The diagnosis is established by hematologic, biochemical, and genetic testing. Full cardiac evaluation including physical examination, ECG, and chest radiography; echocardiogram if cardiac failure is suspected. Assess carefully respiratory function with physical examination, chest radiography, arterial blood gas, oxygen, and ventilatory requirement because respiratory failure is the most common mode of death. Neurologic testing must include physical examination, EEG, EMG, CT scan, and MRI.

Anesthetic considerations: No reported experience despite multiple procedures performed on these patients. Anesthetic techniques should be tailored to the presence of cardiac, respiratory, and renal dysfunction. No specific consideration otherwise.

Pharmacological implications: No known specific pharmacological implications.

REFERENCES:

Cameron P, Dubowitz V, Besley G, et al: Sialic acid storage disease. *Arch Dis Child* 65:314, 1990.

Lemyre E, Russo P, Melancon SB, et al: Clinical spectrum of infantile free sialic acid storage disease. *Am J Med Genet* 82:385, 1999.

Tondeur M, Libert J, Vamos E, et al: Infantile form of sialic acid storage disorder: Clinical, ultrastructural and biochemical studies in two siblings. *Eur J Pediatr* 139:142, 1982.

Infantile-Onset Spinocerebellar Ataxia (IOSCA)

At a glance: Inherited spinocerebellar ataxia with onset usually in the first 2 years of life. Clinical features include severe muscle hypotonia and atrophy, progressive changes in sensory nerve conduction (polyneuropathy), and seizure activity.

Synonyms: OHAHA Syndrome (Ophthalmoplegia, Hypacusis, Ataxia, Hypotonia, and Athetosis Syndrome); Infantile Spinocerebellar Ataxia with Sensory Neuropathy. Some researchers also use the term Spinocerebellar Ataxia (SCA) type 8 for this disease; however, this term has not been uniformly accepted.

Incidence and genetic inheritance: Extremely rare, but more frequent in the Finnish population. The Finnish form of infantile-onset spinocerebellar ataxia (IOSCA) presents with slower progressive symptoms with clumsiness and loss of ability to walk as first manifestation. It does not share the same gene locus as OHAHA. It is an autosomal recessive inherited form of spinocerebellar ataxia with the mutation linked to 10q24.

Clinical aspects: Slowly progressive clinical symptoms appear usually between the ages of 10 and 24 months in previously healthy infants. The first symptoms are usually clumsiness and loss of the ability to walk. Ataxia, athetosis, and muscle hypotonia with loss of deep tendon reflexes, ophthalmoplegia with only convergence persisting, and hearing loss can be discovered on clinical examination. A polyneuropathy with profound decrease in sensory nerve conduction velocities and progressive loss of myelinated fibers in sural nerve biopsies may develop by adolescence. Involvement of the vestibular organ can markedly disturb the balance and may be present at the onset of symptoms. Some patients show abnormal background activity on the EEG with advancing age, and seizures (status epilepticus) have been described. Neuroradiologic investigation reveals cerebellar atrophy as the main cause of ataxia.

Precautions before anesthesia: Proper evaluation of the extent of muscle hypotonia must be obtained. Seizure medication must be maintained. An anesthesia consultation is recommended before elective surgery.

Anesthetic considerations: As the disease progresses, nerve stimulation becomes technically more difficult, on the one hand making nerve location and regional anesthesia more unreliable and on the other hand requiring reduced concentration of local anesthetic solutions to produce a sufficient nerve blockade. Depending on the progress of the disease, monitoring of muscle relaxation may be difficult secondary to polyneuropathy.

Pharmacological implications: Succinylcholine is best avoided because these patients may show increased sensitivity and hyperkalemic response. Chronic antiseizure medication can lead to hepatic enzyme induction and therefore affect the hepatic metabolism of other drugs.

Other condition to be considered:

PAGON BIRD DETTER SYNDROME: X-linked recessive condition characterized by nonprogressive cerebellar ataxia, hyperreflexia, clonus, hypochromic microcytic anemia, ringed sideroblasts on bone marrow examination, and onset in early childhood. Believed to be caused by mutations in the adenosine triphosphate–binding cassette, subfamily B, member 7 gene.

REFERENCES:

Kallio AK, Jauhiainen T: A new syndrome of ophthalmoplegia, hypoacusis, ataxia, hypotonia and athetosis (OHAHA). *Adv Audiol* 3:84, 1985.

Koskinen T, Santavuori P, Sainio K, et al: Infantile onset spinocerebellar ataxia with sensory neuropathy: A new inherited disease. *J Neurol Sci* 121:50, 1994.

Nikali K, Isosomppi J, Lonnqvist T, et al: Toward cloning of a novel ataxia gene: Refined assignment and physical map of the IOSCA locus (SCA8) on 10q24. *Genomics* 39:185, 1997.

Infertile Male Syndrome

At a glance: Azoospermia or severe oligospermia in otherwise normal men caused by androgen insensitivity.

Incidence: May account for up to 10% cases of male infertility.

Genetic inheritance: X-linked recessive but more frequently sporadic.

Pathophysiology: Androgen resistance occurs because of an abnormality of the androgen receptor of the target cells (principally the testes). A history of infertility with severe oligospermia or azoospermia in phenotypically normal individuals occurs as a consequence of the depression of the dihydrotestosterone (DHT)-binding capacity.

Diagnosis: Some affected men come from families with Reifenstein syndrome (male pseudohermaphrodism with hypospadias, hypogonadism, gynecomastia, normal XY karyotype, and pedigree consistent with X-linked recessive inheritance). The majority of patients have no family history. In the process of evaluating adolescents in a family with Reifenstein syndrome or when investigating male infertility, normal or higher plasma levels of testosterone are found with increased plasmatic levels of luteinizing hormone and markedly depressed DHT-binding capacity of cultured genital-skin fibroblasts.

Clinical aspects: Normal male external genitalia with normal wolffian duct structures, occasional gynecomastia, and sometimes minimal male beard and body hair. Infertility is a result of absence or deficiency of sperm production.

Anesthetic considerations: No anesthetic considerations specifically related to the infertile male syndrome.

Other conditions to be considered: Other forms of receptor anomalies, especially the following:

☞**COMPLETE ANDROGEN INSENSITIVITY SYNDROME:** X-linked pseudohermaphrodism caused by defective or deficient androgen receptor proteins. Usually not recognized until puberty because there is primary amenorrhea. Patients develop female secondary sex characteristics (unopposed action of adrenal estrogens), but pubic and axillary hair is scant and the vagina is atrophic. Although there is no cervix and uterus, examination finds epididymides, seminal vesicles, and prostate.

REFERENCES:

Aiman J, Griffin JE, Gazak JM, et al: Androgen insensitivity as a cause of infertility in otherwise normal men. *N Engl J Med* 300:223, 1979.

Dejager S, Bry-Gauillard H, Bruckert E, et al: A comprehensive endocrine description of Kennedy's disease revealing androgen insensitivity linked to CAG repeat length. *J Clin Endocrinol Metab* 87:3 893, 2001.

Griffin JE, Mc Phaul MJ, Russel DW, et al: The androgen resistance syndromes: Steroid 5-reductase 2 deficiency, testicular feminization and related disorders, in Scriver CR, Beaudet AL, Sly WS, Valle D (eds): *The Metabolic and Molecular Bases of Inherited Disease*. 8th ed. New York, McGraw Hill, 1995, p 2981.

Intestinal Pseudoobstruction Caused by Neuronal Disease

At a glance: Functional intestinal obstruction associated with a variety of pathologic conditions. Colonic motility disorder associated with characteristic histochemical changes of the bowel wall.

Synonyms: Chronic Idiopathic Pseudoobstruction; Deficiency of Argyrophil Myenteric Plexus; Intestinal Neuronal Dysplasia (IND) Type A; Neuronal Intestinal Dysplasia.

Incidence: Fewer than 20 patients have been reported.

Genetic inheritance: Sporadic, autosomal dominant, and autosomal recessive.

Pathophysiology: Wide spectrum of pathologic disorders: (1) neuronal intestinal dysplasia (NID) type A: hypoplasia or aplasia of the intestinal sympathetic innervation; (2) NID type B: hyperplasia of the submucosal parasympathetic plexus; and (3) other diseases: degenerative processes involving the myenteric plexus, combinations of NID B and aganglionosis (Hirschsprung), or hypoganglionosis. This group of disorders results in ineffective intestinal propulsion with various degrees of aperistalsis and clinical manifestations.

Diagnosis: Clinical course. *NID A:* Younger than 6 months with bloody stools and spastic diarrhea (in cases with immaturity of the sympathetic innervation: complete cessation of the ulcerative colitis after temporary colostomy). *NID B:* Severe constipation, subileus, sometimes attacks of or persistent malabsorption (treatment usually conservative). Although NID B appears clinically similar to Hirschsprung disease, there is no aganglionosis of intramural plexuses. NID B may be associated with intestinal malrotation, short bowel syndrome, ileal stenosis, colonic atresia, or multiple endocrine neoplasias type II (MEN IIA and IIB). Some infants with pyloric hypertrophy have an associated functional intestinal obstruction with small intestine malrotation and short bowel syndrome. Chronic neuropathic intestinal pseudoobstruction with ophthalmoplegia, ptosis, hearing loss, and severe sensory and motor peripheral neuropathy also described. Radiographic examination, electromanometry, and transit time studies do not show pathognomonic criteria for specific neuronal intestinal manifestations. Biopsies with histoimmunologic and histochemical analysis of the involved areas give the final diagnosis.

Clinical aspects: As described under *Diagnosis:* wide spectrum of recurrent episodes of intestinal obstruction in the absence of a mechanical blockage of the lumen; occasional history of prenatal oligohydramnios; and failure to thrive (some patients may be so malnourished that they require total parenteral nutrition with its potential adverse effects). Consider the possibility of associated gastrointestinal, endocrine, and neurologic manifestations.

Precautions before anesthesia: Obtain full history of gastrointestinal symptoms, failure to thrive, and associated endocrine or neurologic diseases. Evaluate patient's intravascular volume status: clinically, plasma electrolytes, coagulation profile, and hemoglobin level. If on total parenteral nutrition, obtain albumin, glucose, phosphate, calcium, and magnesium levels, liver function tests. In rare cases of associated *MEN IIA* (medullary thyroid carcinoma, parathyroid adenoma, pheochromocytoma) or *MEN IIB* (medullary thyroid carcinoma, mucosal neuromas [tongue, buccal mucosa, lips, conjunctivae, pheochromocytoma]): request endocrine consultation.

Anesthetic considerations: Optimization of fluid status most recommended prior to anesthesia. Rapid-sequence induction in the presence of intestinal obstruction or pseudoobstruction (use nondepolarizing muscle relaxants if associated myopathy); intraoperative blood glucose levels if on total parenteral nutrition. Expect prolonged postoperative mechanical ventilation if associated peripheral neuropathy affecting respiratory muscles or in presence of muscular hypotonia with MEN IIB. If MEN IIA or IIB associated with NID B: continue antihypertensive therapy, carefully monitor blood pressure (arterial indwelling catheter). One must consider the need for steroids and/or thyroid hormone supplements in patients who had a thyroidectomy (if not done, consult with endocrinologist to keep the patient as euthyroid as possible).

Pharmacological implications: Careful titration (nerve stimulator) of muscle relaxants in the presence of peripheral neuropathy or with muscular hypotonia (avoid succinylcholine). If significant degree of malnutrition or if depressed liver and renal function secondary to complications of total parenteral nutrition, cautiously titrate all anesthetic drugs (low protein: α_1-acid glycoprotein and albumin cause decreased drug binding and higher free drug level).

Other condition to be considered:

☞**HIRSCHSPRUNG DISEASE:** Congenital chronic obstruction of the colon because of complete absence of myenteric plexuses in the distal part of the gastrointestinal tract resulting in a tonically contracted aganglionic segment with a dilated segment above it (megacolon). It is caused by the absence of migration of neuroblasts into the gut epithelium from the vagal nerve trunks at the end of first trimester of intrauterine life.

REFERENCES:

Faber J, Fich A, Steinberg A, et al: Familial intestinal pseudoobstruction dominated by a progressive neurologic disease at a young age. *Gastroenterology* 92:786, 1987.

Martucciello G, Torre M, Pini Prato A, et al: Associated anomalies in intestinal neuronal dysplasia. *J Pediatr Surg* 37:219, 2002.

Oguzkurt P, Senocak ME, Akcoren Z, et al: Diagnostic difficulties in neuronal intestinal dysplasia and segmental colitis. *J Pediatr Surg* 35:519, 2000.

Iridogoniodysgenesis Syndrome

At a glance: Group of disorders characterized by malformations of the iridocorneal angle of the anterior chamber of the eye, resulting in juvenile glaucoma.

Classification and synonyms: Glaucoma Iridogoniodysgenesis; IGDA Syndrome.

Iridogoniodysgenesis type I (Autosomal Dominant Iridogoniodysgenesis Anomaly): Characterized by iris hypoplasia, goniodysgenesis, and juvenile glaucoma as a result of aberrant migration or terminal induction of the neural crest cells involved in formation of the anterior segment of the eye.

Iridogoniodysgenesis Type II (Iridogoniodysgenesis Syndrome; Autosomal Dominant Iris Hypoplasia with Early-Onset Glaucoma): Characterized by an autosomal dominant iris hypoplasia associated with early-onset glaucoma caused by maldevelopment of the trabecular meshwork and the iris. Glaucoma usually is detected in the second decade of life but may begin at any age.

Genetic inheritance: Most cases are transmitted as an autosomal dominant trait with variable expressivity and complete penetrance. Two chromosomal loci can be involved: 4q25 and 6p25, corresponding to PITX2 (or RIEG) and FKHL7, respectively. PITX2, the most studied gene, is an homeobox gene coding for a transcription factor. Different levels of expression of this gene supposedly are responsible for the phenotypic variability of the syndrome.

Pathophysiology: Abnormal differentiation of neural crest cells causes "goniodysgenesis" (abnormalities in differentiation of the iridocorneal angle tissue). The anterior iris stroma is hypoplastic and associated with increased intraocular pressure, resulting in glaucoma.

Clinical aspects: Affected individuals often have an unusual dark-gray or chocolate-brown eye color as a result of the iris epithelium showing through the hypoplastic iris stroma. All patients are at risk for developing juvenile glaucoma, which is often diagnosed in the second decade of life, although it can begin at any age. The glaucoma is often resistant to medical therapy and, in the absence of surgical intervention, blindness may occur. Nonocular features, such as maxillary hypoplasia, dental anomalies (microdontia, hypodontia), umbilical hernia, and hypospadias, may present as part of the syndrome.

Precautions before anesthesia: Inquire about severity of glaucoma and associated nonocular features. Obtain a list of topical antiglaucoma medications: echothiophate (long-acting anticholinesterase, which prolongs the effects of drugs that are metabolized by plasma cholinesterase such as succinylcholine, mivacurium, procaine, chloroprocaine, and cocaine), epinephrine (hypertension and dysrhythmias), and timolol (nonselective beta-blocker with potential for bradycardia, hypotension, bronchospasm in asthmatic patients, and decompensation of congestive heart failure). Selective beta-blockers such as betaxolol are considered safer in asthmatics.

Anesthetic considerations: The main anesthetic challenge is avoidance of intraocular pressure increases during direct laryngoscopy and tracheal intubation, as well as coughing, straining, and vomiting. In the presence of maxillary hypoplasia, intubation per se should not be technically difficult because the mandible remains normal. Intravenous lidocaine, adequate anesthetic depth, and use of a nondepolarizing muscle relaxant are the key elements in providing minimal changes in intraocular pressure during tracheal intubation. Like intracranial pressure, intraocular pressure is increased by hypercarbia and hypoxia and is reduced by hyperventilation, slight elevation of the head, osmotic diuretics, and carbonic anhydrase inhibitors.

Pharmacological implications: The majority of central nervous system depressants drugs—barbiturates, narcotics, and neuroleptics—as well as inhalational anesthetics, contribute to decreasing intraocular pressure. Both ketamine and succinylcholine increase intraocular pressure. If a rapid-sequence induction is indicated, a nondepolarizing muscle relaxant such as rocuronium can replace succinylcholine. If succinylcholine remains the only alternative, no reported method has been shown to consistently prevent the transient increases in intraocular pressure caused by the drug, although pretreatment with a nondepolarizing muscle relaxant followed by the administration of a barbiturate and then by succinylcholine may provide slightly lower changes in intraocular pressure.

Other conditions to be considered:

RIEGER ANOMALY OR SYNDROME **(Iridogoniodysgenesis with Somatic Anomalies; Rieger Syndrome Type I):** Characterized by hypodontia (partial anodontia) with malformation of the anterior chamber of the eye. The ocular features are microcornea with opacity, hypoplasia of the iris, and anterior synechiae. Myotonic dystrophy and anal stenosis are considered consistent associated features, although some authors have failed to find the presence of myotonia. Until proven otherwise, the potential association of myopathy should be considered in anesthesia. Renal malformations have been suggested.

☞CAT-EYE SYNDROME: Characterized by facies consisting of broad nasal root with telecanthus and maxillary hypoplasia with protruding lower lip. Severe developmental anomalies of the iris associated with maldevelopment of the ear and maxilla, umbilical hernia, and anal stenosis are features of this syndrome. Glaucoma is often found in association with this anomaly.

AXENFELD ANOMALY: Defects limited to the peripheral anterior segment of the eye associated with bridges of iris tissue crossing the angle to Schwalbe ring; considered a separate entity. It is one feature of Rieger syndrome. It is associated with a male-to-male transmission.

ANTERIOR SEGMENTAL OCULAR DYSGENESIS (ASOD): Characterized by the presence of iridogoniodysgenesis, glaucoma, maxillary hypoplasia, short philtrum, protruding lower lip of mild prognathism, dental anomalies (microdontia, hypodontia, and cone-shaped teeth), and failure of involution of the umbilicus (often treated surgically in the neonatal period because of confusion with umbilical hernia). Resembles Rieger syndrome.

POSTERIOR EMBRYOTOXON: Characterized by an anterior displacement and prominence of the Schwalbe line. The thickened (hypertrophied) Schwalbe's ring is visible through a clear cornea as a sharply defined, concentric white line or opacity anterior to the limbus. In the presence of posterior embryotoxon it is very important to eliminate the possibility of the Jagged syndrome.

JAGGED SYNDROME TYPE I **(Deafness, Congenital Heart Defects, and Posterior Embryotoxon Syndrome):** Characterized by multiple systemic defects with significant major development of the distal cardiac outflow tract and pulmonary artery, major arteries, portal vein, optic vesicle, otocyst, branchial arches, metanephros, pancreas, mesocardium, around the major bronchial branches, and in the neural tube. The authors conclude that the JAG1 gene is expressed in the structures affected in Alagille syndrome.

REFERENCES:

Alward WL: Axenfeld-Rieger syndrome in the age of molecular genetics. *Am J Ophthalmol* 130:107, 2000.

Héon E, Sheth BP, Kalenak JW, et al: Linkage of autosomal dominant iris hypoplasia to the region of the Rieger syndrome locus (4q25). *Hum Mol Genet* 4:1435, 1995.

Walter MA, Mirzayans F, Mears AJ, et al: Autosomal-dominant iridogoniodysgenesis and Axenfeld-Rieger syndrome are genetically distinct. *Ophthalmology* 103:1907, 1996.

Isaacs Mertens Syndrome

At a glance: Rare syndrome with peripheral nerve lesions characterized by muscle stiffness, cramps, and continuous vibrating muscle movements (myokymia).

Synonyms: Hereditary Continuous Muscle Fiber Activity; Isaacs Syndrome.

Genetic inheritance: Autosomal dominant.

Pathophysiology: Unclear; the role of autoimmunity, specifically antibodies against the potassium channel–inducing hyperexcitability of the peripheral nerve, has been advocated. Probably caused by mutations in the potassium channel gene KCNA1 located on chromosome 12p13.

Diagnosis: Characterized by muscular stiffness and cramping, particularly in the limbs with continuous fine, vibrating muscle movements (myokymia).

Clinical aspects: Neuromuscular signs dominate the disease. Progressive stiffness, cramping, weakness, and constant writhing movements of the muscles under the skin persist during sleep or under general anesthesia without muscle relaxant. Calf hypertrophy can be seen. Electromyography (EMG) shows specific anomalies (spontaneous discharges with rhythmical and continuous firing). Muscle biopsies are abnormal. Clinical examination finds hypertonia, spasticity, speech defect, ataxia, and sometimes seizures. Hyperhidrosis and tachycardia, because of autonomic nervous system involvement, are possible. Association with diaphragmatic hernia has been reported.

Precautions before anesthesia: Evaluate muscular dysfunction (clinical, EMG), neurologic function (clinical, electroencephalogram (EEG)), and autonomic nervous system involvement (clinical, heart rate variability).

Anesthetic considerations: Careful intraoperative positioning is needed. Perioperative blood pressure monitoring is necessary because of autonomic system dysregulation. Regional anesthesia is not contraindicated but probably should be avoided or the benefit must be clearly established because of peripheral nervous lesion (peripheral blocks) and autonomic nervous system involvement (perimedullar blockade).

Pharmacological implications: Consider interaction between antiepileptic treatment and anesthetic drugs. Anesthetic drugs that are suspected to induce dystonia should be used carefully (propofol). Succinylcholine probably should be avoided because of muscular lesion and potential risk of hyperkaliemic response.

Other conditions to be considered:

☞**HALLERVORDEN SPATZ DISEASE:** Characterized by dystonia (slow, steady muscle contraction distorting limbs, neck, face, mouth, or trunk into certain positions), muscular rigidity, and choreoathetosis. Muscle spasms are present in more than 33% of patients affected with this rare neurologic disorder. Other clinical features seen less often are dysarthria, mental retardation, facial grimacing, dysphasia, muscle atrophy, and seizures.

☞**HEREDITARY SPASTIC PARAPLEGIA:** Includes weakness, muscle spasms, and stiffness of the legs. Leg muscles may contract or a heel deformity may occur, making walking difficult. Dysphasia, dysphagia, exaggeration of tendon reflexes, and general muscle weakness are symptoms of this autosomal dominant or recessive transmitted disease.

STIFF MAN SYNDROME (Moersch-Woltman Syndrome): Characterized by progressive rigidity and muscles spasms of the muscles of the neck, trunk, shoulders, and proximal extremities.

Caused by abnormal nerve activity most likely in the central, rather than peripheral, nervous system. Electrical activity measured by the EMG may begin in the spinal cord rather than the peripheral nerves.

REFERENCES:

Arimura K, Sonoda Y, Watanabe O, et al: Isaacs' syndrome as a potassium channelopathy of the nerve. *Muscle Nerve Suppl* 11:S55, 2002.

Hernandez-Palazon J, Tortosa-Serrano JA, Sanchez-Ortega JL, et al: Acquired neuromyotonia (Isaacs' syndrome): Clinical characteristics and anesthesia implications. *Rev Esp Anesthesiol Reanim* 44:120, 1997.

Ischiopatellar Dysplasia

At a glance: Genetically transmitted skeletal malformation characterized by hypoplasia or aplasia of the patella, epiphyseal, and hip/pelvic girdle anomalies.

Synonyms: Coxopodo Patellar Syndrome; Small Patella Syndrome; SPS; Scott-Taor Syndrome.

Genetic inheritance: Autosomal dominant with variable penetrance (majority of patients); sporadic dominant mutation (rare).

Pathophysiology: Small patella syndrome (SPS) is a bone dysplasia affecting predominantly the pelvis, knees, and feet. The patellae are either small or absent; when present they may be laterally placed, resulting in recurrent dislocation of the patella.

Diagnosis and clinical aspects: Based on morphologic and radiologic appearances: increased space between the first and second toes, shortening and clinodactyly of the fourth and fifth toes, and flat feet are the findings in some patients. Absent or hypoplastic patellae (laterally placed or dislocated) are typical. Most patients have pelvic abnormalities: absent ischial ossification at the ischiopubic synchondrosis, infra-acetabular axe-cut notch, high iliac angles, large femoral heads with narrowed femoral necks, coxa valga or vara, and hypoplastic lesser trochanters. Patients may complain of femoropatellar pain syndrome, but symptoms referable to the pelvic girdle are very rare. Two sporadic cases of SPS associated with facial dysmorphic features have been reported: one patient had a flattened nose with prominent forehead, and the other had micrognathia, high-arched palate, and subglottic stenosis with generalized tracheomalacia; she also had bilateral talipes equinovarus (clubfeet). These facial and airway abnormalities likely are not part of the SPS itself. The differential diagnosis of SPS is either an isolated finding of displaced patellae or the "nail-patella syndrome" (iliac horns, elbow abnormalities, nail dystrophy).

Precautions before anesthesia: No specific precautions with this medical condition.

Anesthetic considerations: Obtain a "skeletal survey": SPS affects mainly pelvis, knees, and feet, but other parts of the skeleton may be abnormal. One case of minor spine involvement (mild thoracic scoliosis with normal pulmonary function, and lumbar hyperlordosis) reported. These findings should not affect anesthetic management unless scoliosis becomes significant enough to compromise breathing (pulmonary function tests are required). No anesthetic considerations specific to SPS.

Pharmacological implications: No specific pharmacological considerations.

Other conditions to be considered:

FAMILIAL RECURRENT DISLOCATION OF THE PATELLA (Congenital Dislocation of the Patella): Lateral displacement of the patella as a result of pull of the quadriceps muscle while the tibial tubercle abnormally lies lateral to the long axis of the femur. When the knee is flexed, the patella slides distally and is engaged by the trochlear groove in the femur.

☞**NAIL-PATELLA SYNDROME:** Autosomal dominant polymalformative syndrome characterized by nail dysplasia, patellar aplasia-hypoplasia, multiple joint dysplasias (elbows, iliac horns), and nephropathy.

REFERENCES:

Bongers Ernie MHF, Van Bokhoven H, Van Thienen MN, et al: The small patella syndrome: Description of five cases from three families and examination of possible allelism with familial patella aplasia-hypoplasia and nail-patella syndrome. *J Med Genet* 38:209, 2001.

Kozlowski K, Nelson J: Small patella syndrome. *Am J Med Genet* 57:558, 1995.

Isotretinoin Embryopathy-Like Syndrome

At a glance: Teratogenetic polymalformative syndrome including malformations of the head and face, heart (conotruncal defects and aortic arch anomalies), and central nervous system (hydrocephalus and posterior fossae anomalies), resulting from maternal treatment for acne with isotretinoin (vitamin A analogue).

Synonyms: Microtia-Aortic Arch Syndrome; Fetal Retinoid Syndrome; Accutane Embryopathy.

Incidence: More than 200 cases reported in the United States.

Genetic inheritance: Only a few cases of genetic inheritance, presenting as an autosomal or X-linked recessive syndrome of microtia and aortic arch anomalies resembling isotretinoin embryopathy, have been described (so-called microtia-aortic arch syndrome). This report is about a Japanese mother who did not consume any vitamin A derivative during pregnancy and who had three children with the syndrome.

Pathophysiology: Maternal use of isotretinoin for treatment of severe acne during the first trimester of pregnancy exposes the fetus to a 25-fold increased relative risk for malformations. These malformations involve ears, facial skeleton, heart, and/or central nervous system. Cellular retinoic acid–binding proteins are found in high concentration in both CNS and neural crest cells, possibly accounting for their susceptibility to isotretinoin toxicity. Isotretinoin might interfere with migration and proliferation of the neural crest cells, causing defects in branchial arch derivatives because of deficient mesenchyme.

Diagnosis: Physical appearance; history of maternal use of retinoic acid; cardiac evaluation for conotruncal heart defects and aortic arch abnormalities (echocardiogram and/or angiography); early neurologic evaluation (posterior fossa anomalies, hydrocephalus). Normal lymphocytes and calcium levels eliminate the possibility of DiGeorge syndrome.

Clinical aspects: Malformations of the head and face: prominent frontal bossing, anotia or microtia, low-set ears, telecanthus, microphthalmia, depressed nasal bridge, micrognathia, and cleft palate. Central nervous system malformations: Dandy-Walker with associated aqueductal stenosis and hydrocephalus, cerebellar vermis hypogenesis or agenesis, and mental retardation. Cardiovascular malformations: double-outlet right ventricle, ventricular septal defect, tetralogy of Fallot, patent ductus arteriosus, persistent left superior vena cava, aortic coarctation (often preductal), and occasionally lymphoid system hypoplasia (thymic aplasia with ectopic focus, generalized lymphopenia).

Precautions before anesthesia: Airway assessment: cleft palate, micrognathia. Inquire about episodes of apnea; sleep studies often reveal both central and obstructive apnea. Obtain a cardiovascular evaluation including echocardiogram/angiography. Administer prophylactic antibiotics for congenital heart defects. Obtain neurologic evaluation: CT scanner/MRI (Dandy-Walker, hydrocephalus). Inquire about thymic aplasia. If a blood transfusion is anticipated for the surgery, only irradiated blood components should be given in order to prevent graft-versus-host disease (high incidence).

Anesthetic considerations: Despite the presence of micrognathia (usually mild) and cleft palate, direct laryngoscopy and tracheal intubation in these patients usually is performed without difficulty. In case of hydrocephalus with increased intracranial pressure, rapid tracheal intubation and moderate hyperventilation should be used to lower the intracranial pressure; however, this should be weighed against the disadvantage of decreasing the pulmonary vascular resistance in the presence of congenital heart disease. Plan for prolonged postoperative monitoring because of a high frequency of apneic episodes.

Pharmacological implications: Titrate cautiously volatile anesthetics to prevent the cardiac depressant effects in the presence of congenital heart disease. An opioid-based anesthesia should be considered. In case of increased intracranial pressure, isoflurane or sevofluane offers a good compromise between decreased cerebral metabolic oxygen requirement against increase in intracranial pressure from vasodilatation. Thiopental and propofol, potent cerebral vasoconstrictors, are drugs of choice for induction in patient with increased intracranial pressure. Benzodiazepines and etomidate are acceptable alternatives.

Other conditions to be considered:

☞**DIGEORGE SYNDROME:** Characterized by neonatal hypocalcemia (parathyroid hypoplasia) causing tetany and seizures, abnormal T cells (thymic hypoplasia), and outflow tract defects of the heart (tetralogy of Fallot, truncus arteriosus, type B interrupted aortic arch, right aortic arch, aberrant right subclavian artery). In infancy, micrognathia may be present. The ears typically are low set and deficient in the vertical diameter, with abnormal folding of the pinna.

☞**VELOCARDIOFACIAL SYNDROME:** Characterized by the clinical manifestation of craniofacial anomalies, palatal abnormalities, and a rather bulbous nose and square nasal tip. Most often, patients affected with this condition have a milder spectrum of cardiac defects, with ventricular septal defect being more common than in the DiGeorge syndrome. A variety of psychiatric disorders have been described in adults affected with this condition and include paranoid schizophrenia and major depressive illness. Clinical features seen more rarely include hypothyroidism, cleft lip, and deafness.

CONOTRUNCAL ANOMALY FACE SYNDROME: Characterized by the presence of conotruncal anomaly face syndrome (often known as Takao syndrome) and clinical features similar to those reported in the DiGeorge Syndrome except for the hypocalcemia.

CATCH 22 (Cardiac Abnormality, Abnormal Facies, T Cell Deficit because of Thymic Hypoplasia, Cleft Palate,

*H*ypocalcemia because of Hypoparathyroidism): Collective acronym often used to describe these medical genetic entities.

REFERENCES:

Coberly S, Lammer E, Alashari M: Retinoic acid embryopathy: Case report and review of the literature. *Pediatr Pathol Lab Med* 16:823, 1996.

Hendrickx AG, Peterson P, Hartmann D et al: Vitamin A teratogenicity and risk assessment in the macaque retinoid model. *Reprod Toxicol* 14:311, 2000.

Isovaleric Acidemia

At a glance: Genetic disorder affecting the branched-chain organic acids, the most frequent of the leucine metabolism disorders. This inborn error of metabolism leads to body accumulation of isovaleric acid (and its metabolites) resulting in vomiting, dehydration, severe metabolic acidosis, and neurologic manifestations.

Synonym: Isovaleric Acid CoA Dehydrogenase Deficiency.

Incidence: Uncertain (lack of general population screening); more than 60 cases have been reported since the first description in 1966.

Genetic inheritance: Autosomal recessive; chromosome 15q14-q15.

Pathophysiology: Isovaleryl-CoA dehydrogenase catalyzes the first step of branched-chain organic acid metabolism of leucine. The deficiency of isovaleryl-CoA dehydrogenase activity results in accumulation of abnormal metabolites (isovaleric acid, isovalerylglycine, hydroxyisovaleric acid, isovalerylglucuronide, isovalerylglutamic acid). The build-up of these metabolites is responsible for the disease. The precise mechanism of isovaleric acid toxicity is not well known, but it is an inhibitor of succinate CoA ligase in the Krebs cycle and inhibits liver mitochondrial oxygen consumption with glutamic, 2-oxoglutaric, and succinic acids. The neutropenia often seen in the disease may be attributed to inhibition of granulopoietic progenitor cell proliferation by isovaleric acid.

Diagnosis: Clinical course; occasionally foul odor of "sweaty feet" caused by isovaleric acid in body fluids; metabolic acidosis with mild-to-moderate ketonuria and lactic acidemia; hyperammonemia. Thrombocytopenia, neutropenia, and pancytopenia may be present, as well as hypocalcemia. The "sweaty feet" odor is suggestive of, but not specific for, isovaleric acidemia because it may be present in other organic acidurias (e.g., "maple syrup" urine disease, glutaric aciduria type II). Urine analysis for nonvolatile organic acids reveals marked elevation of isovalerylglycine acid with lesser elevation of hydroxyvaleric acid and smaller, but still significant, amounts of the other abnormal metabolites. Confirmation of the diagnosis of isovaleric acidemia comes from assays on patients' fibroblasts showing deficiency of isovaleryl-CoA dehydrogenase (improved tritium release assay or fluorometric assay). Prenatal diagnosis can be made by amniocentesis by stable isotope dilution analysis of elevated isovalerylglycine in amniotic fluid or by fluorometric assay of isovaleryl-CoA dehydrogenase activity.

Clinical aspects: Two clinical categories: half of the patients present with an acute neonatal illness with poor feeding, dehydration, hypothermia, and coma, and if untreated, death secondary to severe metabolic acidosis, cerebral edema, cerebral hemorrhage, or infection. The other half of patients either are survivors of the acute

neonatal episode or later developed symptoms and suffer from a chronic intermittent form with similar episodes. The majority of patients have normal psychomotor development, but some present with various degrees of developmental delay. The recurrent episodes often follow upper respiratory infection or intake of protein-rich food to which patients frequently develop aversion. Most diagnoses of the disease are made during the first episode. Acute episodes are treated symptomatically (protein restriction, hydration, correction of acid-base disturbances, glucose infusion). Along with symptomatic treatment are more specific therapeutic approaches, such as glycine and carnitine administration. Under stable conditions of a leucine-restricted diet, the optimal regimen is 150 mg/kg/day of glycine per os or per nasogastric tube. During acute crisis, increase glycine supplements to 600 mg/kg/day. Administration of carnitine with or without glycine also decreases isovaleric acidemia, but the data are still too limited to evaluate the optimal combination for long-term management. Chronic pancreatitis may occur.

Precautions before anesthesia: Obtain full history of progression of the disease: frequency of acute crisis, nature of treatment, psychomotor development. Obtain arterial blood gases (correct metabolic acidosis preoperatively if possible); hematologic examination: pancytopenia may be significant, requiring platelets, red cells, and eventually granulocyte transfusions (consult with hematologist if necessary); pancytopenia is more frequent during infancy. Consult with competent authorities regarding leucine-restricted diet and glycine and carnitine supplements. During acute episodes, glucose infusion helps to provide calories and reduce endogenous protein catabolism.

Anesthetic considerations: Stress of surgery may precipitate acute acidosis and neurologic deterioration. In the perioperative period, the goal is maintaining adequate hydration and sufficient calorific intake to prevent catabolism. Acid-base status should be monitored during long procedures. In the presence of significant metabolic acidosis, bicarbonate infusion and mechanical ventilatory support may be necessary, including the postoperative period. Until corrected, thrombocytopenia precludes regional anesthesia. If pancytopenia is documented, platelets and red blood cells should be available before the patient enters the operating room for any type of invasive procedure.

Pharmacological implications: Salicylic acid, derived from aspirin, is a substrate for glycine N-acylase and could interfere with synthesis of isovalerylglycine, preventing the beneficial effects of glycine. Therefore it is contraindicated in isovaleric acidemia. Patients with carnitine deficiency may have a lower threshold for bupivacaine-induced cardiotoxicity, so this local anesthetic is best avoided in affected patients with carnitine deficiency.

Other condition to be considered:

☞**CARNITINE DEFICIENCY:** Disorder caused by decreased carnitine concentrations in plasma and tissues preventing mitochondria from adequate beta oxidation. Primary and secondary defects have been described. The manifestations are cardiomyopathy, encephalopathy, and myopathy.

☞**METHYLMALONIC ACIDEMIA:** Heterogeneous inborn error of metabolism affecting the amino acid metabolism, leading to metabolic acidosis and accumulation of methylmalonic acid and its by-products.

☞**PROPIONIC ACIDEMIA:** Inborn error of metabolism of branched-chain organic acids (defective propionyl-coenzyme A carboxylase) resulting in accumulation of propionic acid in the body and several toxic metabolites. Patients present with vomiting, seizures, choreoathetoid movements, lethargy, hypotonia, and encephalopathy. Autosomal recessive transmission.

REFERENCES:

Naglak M, Salvo R, Madsen K, et al: The treatment of isovaleric acidemia with glycine supplement. *Pediatr Res* 24:9, 1988.

Sweetman L, Williams JC: Branched chain organic acidurias, in Scriver CR, Beaudet AL, Sly WS, Valle D (eds): *The Metabolic and Molecular Bases of Inherited Disease.* 7th ed. New York, McGraw-Hill, 1995, p 1387.

Weinberg GL, Laurito CE, Geldner P, et al: Malignant ventricular dysrhythmias in a patient with isovaleric acidemia receiving general and local anesthesia for suction lipectomy. *J Clin Anesth* 9:668, 1997.

Ivemark Syndrome

At a glance: Polymalformative syndrome associating complex cardiac anomalies, situs inversus, absent spleen, abnormal inclusions in red blood cells, and immunocompromised state.

Synonyms: Asplenia Syndrome; Polhemus-Schafer-Ivemark Syndrome; Splenic Agenesis Syndrome.

Genetic inheritance: Autosomal recessive; a few cases transmitted as an autosomal dominant trait, but most cases are sporadic. X-linked inheritance of heterotaxy syndromes is known.

Pathophysiology: Unknown. Disorder of the laterality (i.e., heterotaxy anomaly). Trisomy 9 associated in one case. Chromosomal anomalies, intrauterine infection, and environmental/toxic factors have been suggested as etiologic factors.

Diagnosis: Asplenia (or splenic hypoplasia) associated with congenital heart disease, renal dysplasia, hepatic dysplasia, pancreatic dysplasia, and abnormal lobar development of the lungs. Could be evocated before birth by ultrasonographic examination showing asplenia and lateralization anomalies.

Clinical aspects: Asplenia is combined with bilateral right-sided organs. There are two right lungs, two right lobes of the liver, two right atria, and bilateral superior vena cava. Various abnormal localizations of single organs are observed. This syndrome cannot be qualified as situs inversus. Clinical manifestations include sensibility to infection with encapsulated germs and presence of Heinz and Howell-Jolly bodies in the blood because of asplenia. Cardiac malformations (single ventricle, transposition of great vessels, truncus arteriosus, atrioventricular defect) are frequent with their own signs; arrhythmia as a result of the presence of two sinoatrial nodes is specific. Neurologic signs could be observed in relation with anophthalmia, holoprosencephaly, hydrocephalus, or meningocele. Hepatogastrointestinal structures can be abnormal and complicate evolution of the syndrome: biliary atresia or stenosis, hiatus hernia, megaesophagus or brachyesophagus, volvulus as a result of malrotation of the gut, and malformation of the pancreas. Up to 70% of patients die within the first year of life.

Precautions before anesthesia: History and examination define the associated anomalies. Cardiac assessment. Inquire about a history of cyanosis or systemic-to-pulmonary shunt formation. Electrocardiography (ECG) and echocardiography are mandatory. Angiography and cardiac catheterization as indicated clinically. Pulmonary assessment. Chest radiography to exclude infection and pulmonary edema. Preoperative blood gases in presence of cyanosis. Laboratory tests: check electrolyte levels and renal function, liver function, coagulation status, and full blood count.

Anesthetic considerations: Cardiac and pulmonary function are the main considerations. In the presence of systemic-to-pulmonary shunts, blood pressure may vary in different limbs. Aim to maintain ratio of pulmonary flow to systemic flow and prevent large decreases in pulmonary vascular resistance or systemic vascular resistance (balanced anesthesia, minimum fraction of inspired oxygen [FiO_2], prevent hyperventilation). Maintain preoperative arterial oxyhemoglobin saturation (SpO_2). In the presence of right-to-left shunting, maneuvers to decrease pulmonary vascular resistance (hyperventilation, increased FiO_2, positive end-expiratory pressure) may be beneficial. Potential need for postoperative ventilation.

Pharmacological implications: Caution with high-dose volatile agents, myocardial depression, and decreased systemic vascular resistance. Inotropic support may be necessary. Antibiotic prophylaxis for cardiopathy as indicated.

Other conditions to be considered:

    HETEROTAXY SYNDROMES (Defects of Laterality): X-linked syndromes with laterality defects varying from situs inversus that is the complete reversal of the normal anatomical distribution of viscera to various degrees of situs ambigus (randomization of the normal organ position) that may manifest as asplenia or polysplenia syndrome.

    ☞KARTAGENER SYNDROME: Autosomal recessive polymalformative syndrome characterized by bronchiectasis, situs inversus, and chronic sinusitis. Caused by mutations in the gene encoding axonemal dynein intermediate chain (DNAI1), which maps to 9p21-p13. Can be caused by a mutation in the DNAH5 gene (5p15-p14).

    POLYSPLENIA: Some authors consider polysplenia to be a related syndrome, whereas other authors think it is the same entity. Patients with this syndrome are bilaterally left sided.

    ASPLENIA WITH CYSTIC LIVER, KIDNEY, AND PANCREAS: Autosomal recessive. Also described by Ivemark and characterized by polycystic lesions of liver, kidney, and pancreas.

REFERENCES:

Cesko I, Hajdu J, Toth T, et al: Ivemark syndrome with asplenia in siblings. *J Pediatr* 130:822, 1997.

Noack F, Sayk F, Ressel A, et al: Ivemark syndrome with agenesis of the corpus callosum: A case report with a review of the literature. *Prenat Diagn* 22:1011. 2002.

Rabakaran S, Kumaran N, Regunanthan SR, et al: Spontaneous biliary perforation in a child with features of Ivemark syndrome. *Pediatr Surg Int* 16:109, 2000.

IVIC Syndrome

At a glance: Hereditary polymalformative syndrome characterized by hearing impairment, radial ray defects and hand anomalies, internal ophthalmoplegia, thrombocytopenia, and leukocytosis.

Synonyms: Arias Syndrome; Oculo-Oto-Radial Syndrome (OO-RS).

History: IVIC is an acronym that stands for *I*nstituto *V*enezolano de *I*nvestiaciones *C*ientificas, where Sergio Arias Cazorla, a Venezuela geneticist, worked.

Incidence: This syndrome was observed in 19 living descendants of a Caucasoid family that migrated to Venezuela from the Canary Islands in the early 1800s.

Genetic inheritance: Autosomal dominant with complete penetrance and widely variable expression. Investigation on monozygotic twins indicated that modification of OORS gene expression must be environmental or epigenetic rather than genetic. It may represent an "iceberg dominant" trait because of the wide range of severity.

Pathophysiology: The gene responsible for this syndrome has variable expressivity, with the most consistent manifestation being a developmental defect of the upper limbs. A mesenchymally based defect could be implicated in the pathogenesis.

Diagnosis and clinical aspects: The radial ray is consistently involved, with degrees of severity ranging from an almost normal thumb to a hypoplastic, triphalangeal thumb attached to the radial border of the second digit. Long and slender metacarpal bones and hypoplastic carpal bones may coexist with proximally fused ulna and radius. One patient had a single forearm bone. Other findings include hearing loss (very frequent), extraocular muscle involvement in the form of strabismus (frequent), mild thrombocytopenia and leukocytosis (less frequent), and imperforated anus (10% of patients). Although very rare, incomplete right bundle branch block has been reported in both children and adults. Clinical examination, upper limb radiographs, audiograms, ophthalmologic examination, and blood cell count contribute to the diagnosis.

Precautions before anesthesia: Obtain blood cell count: possibility of mild thrombocytopenia and/or leukocytosis. Obtain an electrocardiogram (ECG): rare reported cases of incomplete right bundle branch block with occasionally increased QT interval were not associated with any significant cardiovascular dysfunction.

Anesthetic considerations: If present, thrombocytopenia is mild and usually does not necessitate platelet transfusion. Nonetheless, if locoregional anesthesia is considered, an adequate platelet level should be obtained before proceeding. The rare cardiac manifestations in the form of ECG changes mentioned under *Precautions Before Anesthesia* have been described as "benign and single cardiac sign" by the authorities on OORS.

Pharmacological implications: No known implications with this condition.

Other conditions to be considered:

☞**HOLT-ORAM SYNDROME:** Autosomal dominant polymalformative syndrome caused by defective development embryonic development of the radial ray associated with cardiac malformation (atrial septal defect). Mapped to band 12q24.1 (gene encoding the human transcription factor TBX5).

☞**TAR SYNDROME (*T*hrombocytopenia and *A*bsent *Radius*):** Autosomal recessive syndrome characterized by thrombocytopenia with potentially severe bleeding episodes, primarily during infancy, aplasia of the radius (the ulna is often involved, too), and various malformations (heart, kidneys).

REFERENCES:

Arias S, Penchaszadeh VB, Pinto-Cisternas J, et al: The IVIC syndrome: A new autosomal dominant complex pleiotropic syndrome with radial ray hypoplasia, hearing impairment, external ophthalmoplegia, and thrombocytopenia. *Am J Med Genet* 6:25, 1980.

Elcioglu N, Berry AC: Monozygotic twins discordant for the oculo-oto-radial syndrome (IVIC syndrome). *Genet Couns* 8:201, 1997.

Jacobs Syndrome

At a glance: Camptodactyly is usually present at birth or surely noticed within the first year of life. Arthropathy typically develops between 3 and 8 years of age. A noninflammatory constrictive pericarditis is often present in the first or second decade of life and may lead to pericardial effusion.

Synonyms: Arthropathy-Camptodactyly Syndrome; Congenital Familial Hypertrophic Synovitis; Familial Fibrosing Serositis; Pericarditis-Arthropathy-Camptodactyly Coxa-Vara Syndrome.

Genetic inheritance: Autosomal recessive; locus resides on chromosome 1q25-q31.

Pathophysiology: Synovial cell hyperplasia, fibrosis of pericardium.

Diagnosis: Histologic examination of synovium shows prominent fibrosis and cell infiltration. Radiologic evidence of flattened metacarpal and metatarsal heads and flattened proximal femoral ossification center. Normal erythrocyte sedimentation rate (ESR).

Clinical aspects: Childhood-onset noninflammatory arthritis. Congenital finger flexion contractures. Constrictive pericarditis and pleuritis may occur especially when associated with severe effusion. It may lead to organ function restriction. Sedimentation rate is normal. Elbow and wrist contractures may be associated.

Precautions before anesthesia: Assess temporomandibular involvement (if any), neck movements, and mouth opening. Assess presence of pericardial and pleural effusions: chest radiography, echocardiography, ECG.

Anesthetic considerations: Arthritis usually affects the large joints and hands and contractures may be present. It could be affecting patient during positioning. Pericardial and/or pleural effusion may be present. If so, the anesthetic must be tailored to avoid affecting preload and heart rate.

Pharmacological implications: Intraoperative supplementation of corticosteroids must be considered in patients receiving chronic therapy.

REFERENCE:

Verma UN, Misra R, Radhakrisnan S, et al: A syndrome of fibrosing pleuritis, pericarditis and synovitis with infantile contractures of fingers and toes in 2 sisters: "Familial fibrosing serositis." *J Rheum* 22:2349, 1995.

Jacobsen Syndrome

At a glance: Chromosome 11, partial monosomy 11q is characterized by abnormally prenatal and postnatal growth retardation, mental retardation, psychomotor retardation, craniofacial anomalies, ocular abnormalities, malformations of the hands and/or feet, and congenital heart defects (e.g., ventricular septal defect).

Synonyms: 11q- Deletion Syndrome; Partial 11q Monosomy Syndrome.

Incidence: Approximately 1:100,000 live births.

Genetic inheritance: Autosomal dominant. Parent may carry a complete but fragile 11q chromosome. Folate deficient chromosome breakage may occur in early development, leading to full Jacobsen phenotypes. The parent may not carry the syndrome despite autosomal dominant transmission. Chromosomal deletion leading to CCG repeat triplets and multiorgan involvement.

Pathophysiology: The exact cause of this chromosomal deletion and triplet expansion is unknown.

Diagnosis: Based on clinical criteria and laboratory demonstration of the deletion on the short arm of chromosome 11 (locus 11q23-24).

Clinical aspects: Present at birth with dysmorphic signs including low-set dysmorphic ears; broad, short nose with anteverted nostrils; retrognathia; U-shaped upper lip; divergent strabismus; and hammertoes and bent fingers. These children have growth and developmental retardation. Jacobsen syndrome is associated with an isoimmune thrombocytopenia.

Precautions before anesthesia: Because of the dysmorphism affecting the nose and mouth, carefully check the airway and whether difficult airway management should be anticipated. The presence of congenital heart defect must be eliminated. Check blood count for thrombocytopenia. Check for associated abnormalities, especially of the heart and lungs. An anesthesia consultation for elective surgical procedure should be obtained.

Anesthetic considerations: Use safe airway control strategy. Be prepared for difficult direct laryngoscopy and tracheal intubation. Maintain spontaneous ventilation until the trachea is intubated and lungs ventilated. A laryngeal mask should be available. Be prepared to use other means of airway management (e.g., fiberoptic, Bullard laryngoscope, retrograde intubation technique) to facilitate tracheal intubation. In most difficult cases, equipment for cricothyroidotomy should be available. Only then, if necessary, can a muscle relaxant be used. The anesthetic management also is dictated by the presence of congenital anomalies of the heart. Strict asepsis must be provided because of immune system defect.

Pharmacological implications: No specific implications with this disorder.

Other conditions to be considered:

PARIS-TROUSSEAU SYNDROME: Hematologic disorder associating low platelet count and abnormal platelet function. The intriguing fact is that all known patients with Jacobsen Syndrome have Paris-Trousseau Syndrome (which seems to be a variant of Jacobsen Syndrome, with the same gene map locus).

CHROMOSOME 11 RING: Caused by a break of the long and short arms of chromosome 11. It is characterized by failure to thrive, psychomotor retardation, craniofacial anomalies (e.g., microbrachycephaly, short nose with a low, depressed nasal bridge, microretrognathism, low-set ears), ocular abnormalities, a short neck, pancytopenia, and congenital heart defects. The exact cause of chromosome 11 ring is not fully understood.

☞**C SYNDROME:** Characterized by a "triangular-shaped" head with trigonocephaly resulting from severe craniosynostosis. Other clinical features include craniofacial anomalies, a short nose with a broad nasal bridge, epicanthus, cleft palate, and low-set, malformed ears. Joint subluxations or contractures have been observed with this condition. In some cases, congenital heart defects and mental retardation are present. It is thought to be inherited as an autosomal recessive trait.

REFERENCES:

Jones C, Mullenbach R, Grossfeld P, et al: Co-localisation of CCG repeats and chromosome deletion breakpoints in Jacobsen syndrome:

Evidence for a common mechanism of chromosome breakage. *Hum Mol Genet* 9:1201, 2000.

Michaelis RC, Velagaleti GV, Jones C, et al: Most Jacobsen syndrome deletion breakpoints occur distal to FRA11B. *Am J Med Genet* 76:222, 1998.

Jaffe-Lichtenstein Syndrome

At a glance: Very rare congenital genetic disorder characterized by bone lesions that can degenerate into sarcoma. Association with precocious puberty and other hormonal dysfunctions is possible.

Synonyms: Fibrous Bone Dysplasia; Fibrous Osteoma.

Incidence: Fewer than 100 cases reported in the literature.

Genetic inheritance: Almost sporadic; familial cases have been described.

Pathophysiology: Caused by sporadic mutation of the GNAS1 gene that encodes the alpha subunit of the stimulatory G protein (G1 medullary bone is replaced by fibrous tissue, which appears radiolu-

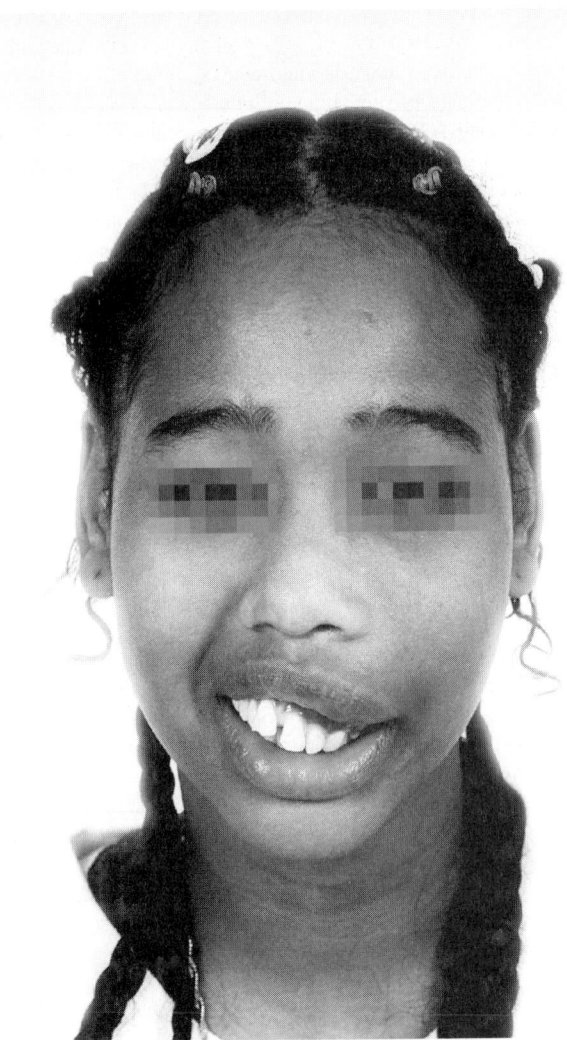

Jaffe-Lichtenstein syndrome Facial asymmetry caused by Jaffe-Lichtenstein syndrome in a 14-year-old girl.

cent on radiographs). Trabeculae of woven bone contain fluid-filled cysts that are embedded largely in collagenous fibrous matrix.

Diagnosis: Onset generally between the ages of 3 and 15 years; clinically evocated by uneven growth, pain, brittleness, and deformity of bone (particularly long bones).

Clinical aspects: May involve a single bone or multiple bones. Bone manifestations are consequences of fibrous lesions that can lead to pathologic fractures, limping, unequal limp length, chest deformity, skull asymmetry, leontiasis-like appearance, scoliosis. Sarcomatous degeneration has been described in approximately 0.5% of patients. Irregular macular dermal pigmentation can be observed. Other features can include precocious puberty, hyperthyroidism, Cushing disease, hyperparathyroidism, and hypophosphatemia.

Precautions before anesthesia: Because of the dysmorphism affecting the lower part of the face, complete evaluation of the airway must be performed. Complete evaluation of bone lesion repercussion and endocrine involvement (clinical, laboratory investigation including alkaline phosphatases, calcemia, phosphatemia, vitamin D levels, thyroid hormones, gonadotropin, and gonadosteroids).

Anesthetic considerations: Be prepared for difficult direct laryngoscopy and tracheal intubation. Spontaneous respiration may have to be maintained until the trachea is secured. Careful intraoperative positioning is needed considering bone lesions and deformities. Hormonal involvement must be stabilized before any scheduled procedure.

Pharmacological implications: Succinylcholine probably should be avoided considering risk of pathologic fractures during muscular fasciculations. Perioperative fluid regimen must be adapted to hormonal status.

Other condition to be considered:

☞**McCune-Albright Syndrome:** Defined as the triad of precocious puberty, polyostotic fibrous dysplasia, and cutaneous pigmentation.

References:

Jaffé HL, Lichtenstein L: Fibrous dysplasia of bone. A condition affecting one, several or many bones, the graver cases of which may present with abnormal pigmentation of skin, premature sexual development, hyperthyroidism or still other extraskeletal abnormalities. *Arch Pathol* 33:777, 1942.

Jarcho-Levin Syndrome

At a glance: Rare syndrome characterized by distinctive malformations of vertebrae and ribs, leading to respiratory insufficiency and death by 1 year of age.

Synonyms: Spondylocostal Dysostosis, Recessive form I; Spondylothoracic Dysplasia; Costovertebral Dysplasia; Spondylothoracic Dysostosis.

History: Genetic disorder first described by S. Jarcho and P.M. Levin in 1938.

Genetic inheritance: Autosomal recessive.

Pathophysiology: Can be caused by mutation in the DLL3 gene mapped on 19q13.

Diagnosis: Clinical, with dwarfism and multiple anomalies of bones.

Clinical aspects: Infants present with short stature. Features involve *skeleton* (scoliosis, lordosis, long limbs, short rib cage, vertebral segmentation anomaly, prominent occiput, camptodactyly, syndactyly of fingers, talipes-varus/valgus), *head* (short neck, low-set ears, anteverted nares, broad nasal root, up-slanted fissures, long philtrum, broad forehead), and *GI* (inguinal or umbilical hernia). Intrauterine growth retardation is frequent. Cleft palate, macrocephaly, microcephaly, congenital cardiac anomaly, cryptorchism, genital abnormality, and imperforate anus may occur. Respiratory deficiency caused by thoracic anomalies. Pulmonary hypertension has been described.

Precautions before anesthesia: Evaluate respiratory function (clinical, chest radiographs, pulmonary function tests, and arterial blood gas analysis). Evaluate for the possibility of difficult airway management because of the presence of a short neck and skull abnormality (clinical, radiographs).

Anesthetic considerations: Careful intraoperative positioning is needed. Tracheal intubation can be difficult and may require adapted anesthetic technique. Postoperative mechanical ventilatory support can be necessary. Regional anesthesia is not contraindicated but can be difficult to realize.

Pharmacological implications: Muscle relaxants should be avoided until airway is secured. Medication causing respiratory depression should be used carefully in the postoperative period after evaluation of the respiratory function. Prophylactic antibiotics must be considered in case of cardiopathy.

REFERENCES:

Hatakeyama K, Fuse S, Tomita H, et al: Jarcho-Levin syndrome associated with a complex congenital heart anomaly. *Pediatr Cardiol* 24:86, 2003.

Karnes PS, Day D, Berry SA, et al: Jarcho-Levin syndrome: Four new cases and classification of subtypes. *Am J Med Genet* 40:264, 1991.

Rastogi D, Rosenzweig EB, Koumbourlis A: Pulmonary hypertension in Jarcho-Levin syndrome. *Am J Med Genet* 107:250, 2002.

Jeune Syndrome

At a glance: Very rare form of chondrodysplasia often leading to death in infancy as a consequence of respiratory insufficiency caused by severe thoracic restrictive deformation. Common association with multiple skeletal malformations, liver, renal, and retinal dysfunction.

Synonyms: Asphyxiating Thoracic Dystrophy of the Newborn; Thoracic Pelvic Phalangeal Dystrophy.

History: Congenital genetic disorder first described by Jeune et al. in 1955.

Incidence: The incidence in the United States is estimated at 1:100,000–130,000 live births.

Genetic inheritance: Autosomal recessive, clinical variability.

Pathophysiology: Unknown.

Diagnosis: Clinically evocated at birth in a child with narrow thorax and pelvic anomalies confirmed by radiologic findings: short ribs and particular morphology of the pelvis (horizontal roof of the acetabulum and a trident aspect formed by a median protrusion and two lateral spurs). The term *asphyxiating thoracic dysplasia* refers to the hypoplastic thoracic cage and lungs, often resulting in respiratory distress, asphyxia, and early death in infancy.

Clinical aspects: Living patients present with short stature; disease involves *chest* (narrow thorax, short, horizontal ribs with bulbous and irregular ends) with pulmonary insufficiency (lung hypoplasia, restrictive syndrome, recurrent respiratory infections). Approximately 70% die from respiratory failure in infancy or early childhood; *skeletal* (lacunar skull, small pelvis with trident acetabular roofs, sciatic notch spur, irregular metaphyses and epiphyses, short long bones, cone-shaped epiphyses and polydactyly), *GI* (hepatic and pancreatic fibrosis, polycystic liver and pancreas disease, bile duct proliferation), and *genitourinary* (Potter type IV polycystic kidneys, chronic nephritis, and renal failure). Retinal degeneration is frequent. Hydrocephalus, cleft lip/palate, and scalp defect can be observed.

Precautions before anesthesia: Evaluate pulmonary function (clinical, chest radiographs, CT, pulmonary function test, arterial blood gases analysis) and renal, hepatic, and pancreatic function (clinical, echography, CT, and laboratory). Request complete blood count, electrolytes, creatinine, blood urea nitrogen, liver transaminases, bilirubin, and coagulation tests.

Anesthetic considerations: Careful intraoperative positioning is needed because of skeletal malformations. As a result of hypoplastic chest and lungs, high airway pressures may be required to maintain normocapnia with normal respiratory rates and tidal volumes. Hence, small tidal volumes and a higher respiratory rate are preferred to prevent pulmonary barotrauma and/or pneumothorax. Cor pulmonale and pulmonary artery hypertension must be expected, so acidosis and hypercapnia must be prevented. Both arterial and venous access can be difficult because of limb anomalies. Regional anesthesia is not contraindicated but can be difficult to realize because of skeletal deformities. Postoperative mechanical ventilation must be anticipated. If a nasogastric tube is required for surgery, be aware of the possibility of esophageal varices caused by liver cirrhosis and portal hypertension, which may render abdominal procedures prone to major blood loss [secondary to coagulopathy, thrombocytopenia (hypersplenism), venous congestion].

Pharmacological implications: Perioperative fluid regimen and the choice of anesthetic drugs should be adapted to renal and hepatic function. In case of failure of both systems, it is probably best to administer low doses of anesthetic drugs and titrate to effect.

Other conditions to be considered:

☞**SHORT RIB-POLYDACTYLY SYNDROME:** Group of four lethal skeletal dysplasias characterized by hypoplastic thorax, short ribs, short limbs, polydactyly, and multiple visceral abnormalities.

☞**BARNES SYNDROME:** Characterized by small lungs, abnormal laryngeal cartilages, and widely expanded costochondral junctions with "dystrophic" changes histologically. Respiratory failure following chest infection and cor pulmonale have been the cause of death of patients affected with this condition. In all cases, complications have occurred during anesthesia because of laryngeal stenosis and severe reduced lung volumes.

REFERENCES:

Borland LM: Anesthesia for children with Jeune's syndrome (asphyxiating thoracic dystrophy). *Anesthesiology* 66:86, 1987.

Jeune M, Beraud C, Carron R: Dystrophie thoracique asphyxiante de caractère familial. *Arch Franc Pediatr* 12:886, 1955.

Kajantie E, Andersson S, Kaitila I: Familial asphyxiating thoracic dysplasia: Clinical variability and impact of improved neonatal intensive care. *J Pediatr* 139:130, 2001.

Job Syndrome

At a glance: Genetic immunologic disorder characterized by recurrent skin and lung infections, mainly caused by *Staphylococcus* *aureus,* multiple fractures, eczematous dermatitis, coarse facies, and elevated immunoglobulin (Ig)E.

Synonyms: Hyper-IgE Syndrome; Hyperimmunoglobulin E Syndrome; HIE Syndrome; Hyperimmunoglobulin E–Recurrent Infection Syndrome; Job Buckley Syndrome

History: Genetically transmitted immunologic disorder first reported in 1966.

Incidence: Undetermined; no sex or racial prevalence.

Genetic inheritance: Autosomal recessive trait with variable penetrance.

Pathophysiology: Affected patients have an inadequate inflammatory response as a consequence of decreased chemotactic responses by neutrophils. Additionally, there is an imbalance between T-helper type 1 (Th1) cell production of interferon-gamma, which is low, and T-helper type 2 (Th2) cell production of interleukin-4, which is high. Whether these cytokine abnormalities could be consistent with increased IgE production, there is no correlation between IgE and interleukin-4 levels. These cytokine disorders cannot explain the high incidences of bone fractures, skeletal disorders, and facial features of the syndrome.

Diagnosis: Based on clinical symptoms [immunodeficiency syndrome characterized by recurrent bacterial (staphylococcal) infections and elevated IgE levels] and immunoglobulin assays.

Clinical aspects: Patients look generally well with red hair, fair skin; they have reddish-brown eyes, coarse facies, craniosynostosis and chronic eczematoid dermatitis. Infections are recurrent. Most frequent infectious agents are *S. aureus* and *C. albicans. Haemophilus influenzae, Streptococcus pneumoniae,* enteric Gram bacteria, and herpes virus can be seen. Those infections are frequent on skin (indolent staphylococcal abscesses and mucocutaneous candidiasis) and lung (abscess, empyema and pneumatocele). Laboratory investigations show mild eosinophilia, high serum IgE (not initially), neutrophil granulocyte chemotaxis defect, salivary IgA deficiency, and high serum IgD. Abnormal reactions to infectious agents are common (cutaneous hypersensitivity reactions to *S. aureus* and *C. albicans,* serum and salivary anti-*S. aureus* IgA deficiency). Recurrent bacterial infections and abscesses of skin and sinopulmonary tract, coarse facies, mucocutaneous candidiasis, recurrent otitis, frequent fractures after minor trauma, frequent pneumatoceles. and recurrent coughing. Development of malignancies such as lymphoma and squamous cell carcinoma is not infrequent.

Precautions before anesthesia: Evaluate respiratory function (clinical, history, chest x-ray films, CT, pulmonary function test, arterial blood gas analysis, bacterial). Evaluate infection sensitivity (clinical, history, laboratory). Determine location of abscesses. Query pulmonary pathology (abscess, empyema, pneumatoceles and pleural effusion).

Anesthetic considerations: Strict asepsis is needed considering immunodeficiency. Cutaneous puncture (venous access, regional anesthesia) may be realized as far as possible from any skin infection sites and/or abscesses. Regional anesthesia is not contraindicated but its benefit must be clearly established because of the potential risk of abscess.

Pharmacological implications: N_2O should be avoided because of high frequency of pneumatocele. Prophylactic antibiotics should be considered because these patients are immunodeficient.

Other conditions to be considered:

☞**CHRONIC GRANULOMATOUS DISEASE:** Inherited disorder in which phagocytic cells are unable to kill certain types of bacteria and fungi, leading to recurrent life-threatening bacterial and fungal infections.

COMMON VARIABLE IMMUNODEFICIENCY (CVID): Heterogeneous disorder characterized by failure of B-lymphocyte differentiation into plasma cells (impaired IgG and IgA antibody responses); most cases are sporadic, but various inheritance modes have been reported.

☞**OMENN SYNDROME:** Autosomal recessive immunodeficiency with erythroderma, chronic diarrhea, growth retardation, lymphadenopathy, hepatosplenomegaly, and a tendency to develop fungal, bacterial, and viral infections; elevated levels of interleukin (IL)-4 and IL-5.

☞**WISKOTT-ALDRICH SYNDROME:** X-linked immunodeficiency with thrombocytopenia leading to recurrent bacterial pulmonary infections, eczema, bleeding, autoimmune disorders, and malignancies; gene map locus is Xp11.23.

REFERENCES:

Borges WG, Augustine NH, Hill HR: Defective interleukin-12/interferon-gamma pathway in patients with hyperimmunoglobulinemia E syndrome. *J Pediatr* 136:176, 2000.

Grimbacher B, Holland SM, Gallin JI, et al: Hyper-IgE syndrome with recurrent infections—An autosomal dominant multisystem disorder. *N Engl J Med* 340:692, 1999.

Tapper JB, Giesecke AH: Spinal anaesthesia in a child with Job's syndrome, pneumatoceles and empyema. *Anaesthesia* 45:378, 1990.

Johanson-Blizzard Syndrome (JBS)

At a glance: Polymalformative syndrome characterized by nasal alar hypoplasia (beak shaped), scalp defects, hypothyroidism, pancreatic achylia, congenital heart defects, and congenital sensorineural deafness. Usually detected at birth when beak-shaped nasal defect is associated with an imperforate anus.

Synonyms: Ectodermal Dysplasia-Exocrine Pancreatic Insufficiency; Malabsorption-Ectodermal Dysplasia-Nasal Alar Hypoplasia; Nasal Alar Hypoplasia, Hypothyroidism, Pancreatic Achylia, Congenital Deafness.

Incidence: Fewer than 50 patients reported in the literature.

Genetic inheritance: Autosomal recessive. Genetic defect not yet identified.

Pathophysiology: Mainly unknown; clinically, the Johanson-Blizzard syndrome is a cluster of anomalies of preferentially midline structures formed during weeks 6 to 8 of gestation.

Diagnosis: Usually presents at birth when the nasal hypoplasia is associated with an imperforate anus. Prenatal diagnosis can be done. Usually growth retardation is only postnatal, but intrauterine growth retardation may be found in association with cardiac congenital abnormalities.

Clinical aspects: Main diagnostic features include nasal alar hypoplasia, hypothyroidism, pancreatic achylia because of acinar development disorder, and congenital neurosensorial deafness. Patients have abnormally small, malformed primary (deciduous) teeth and misshapen or absent secondary (permanent) teeth. Pancreatic achylia leads to pancreatic insufficiency with malabsorption. Growth and mental retardation are common, and imperforate anus is almost always present. Associated signs include midline ectodermal scalp defects and absent permanent teeth. Urogenital disorders include double vagina and/or uterus, rectovaginal fistula, and imperforate anus. Brain imaging may show abnormal brain gyri, and neuropathologic examinations demonstrate cortical neuronal disorganization. Congenital heart defects include situs inversus and ventricular and septal defects.

Precautions before anesthesia: Check patient development and nutritional status. Side effects of malnutrition, particularly hypoproteinemia, may lead to modified drug distribution, and infections. Thyroid status must be assessed because severe hypothyroidism may have dire consequences during anesthesia. When emergent surgery is required in severe hypothyroid patients, a suggested strategy is to draw blood for thyroid hormone dosage and immediately administer a single 25-μg thyroxin dose. Hearing loss may render communication and preoperative explanations difficult. Complete evaluation of the heart (ECG, echocardiography ultrasound) must be obtained. Check for other associated abnormalities, especially the lungs.

Anesthetic considerations: Because of the high risk of hypothermia (hypothyroidism and malnutrition), check body temperature and warm actively if necessary. Check blood glucose at regular intervals during and after intervention.

Pharmacological implications: In cases of malnutrition and decreased protein binding an increased clinical effect of protein-bound medications must be expected; therefore, doses must be reduced.

Other conditions to be considered:

☞**Mucoviscidosis:** Autosomal recessive disease of exocrine glands, involving many organs resulting in meconium ileus, chronic respiratory infections, pancreatic enzyme insufficiency with digestive malabsorption, and end-stage lung disease.

☞**Shwachman Syndrome:** Congenital disorder characterized by pancreatic insufficiency, bone marrow dysfunction, and short stature; imperforate anus and Hirschsprung disease can be associated with this syndrome.

☞**Seckel Syndrome:** Characterized by dwarfism, microcephaly, mental retardation, distinctive facial features including "beak-like" protrusion of the nose, abnormally large eyes, a narrow face, malformed ears, and micrognathism. Other clinical features include clinodactyly, hip dysplasia, and radial bone dislocation. It is inherited as an autosomal recessive trait.

☞**Trichorhinophalangeal Dysplasia (TRPS):** Types I, II, and III are extremely rare and are characterized by thin, sparse scalp hair, distinctive craniofacial abnormalities including a bulbous "pear-shaped" nose, micrognathia, brachydactyly, and dwarfism. Trichorhinophalangeal type II presents with microcephaly, multiple bone exostoses, and mental retardation. Patients affected with TRPS type III characteristically have short fingers and toes of all forms of TRPS. It is inherited as an autosomal dominant pattern.

☞**Cartilage Hair Hypoplasia Syndrome:** Characterized by progressive, short-limbed dwarfism because of abnormal development of the cartilage at the ends of long bones. Other clinical features include sparse body hairs (eyelashes, eyebrows, and scalp hair), immunologic dysfunction (abnormal T cells), intestinal malabsorption, neutropenia, lymphopenia, anemia, and dental abnormalities. It is inherited as an autosomal recessive trait.

☞**Adams-Oliver Syndrome:** Very rare inherited disorder characterized by defects of the scalp associated with multiple scarred and hairless areas that usually have dilated blood vessels directly under the skin. Scalp defects are present at birth. The extremities are either short (hypoplastic fingers and toes) or characterized by absent hands and lower legs. Congenital heart defect must be ruled out.

☞**Aplasia Cutis Congenita:** Most often inherited disorder with circumscribed or more extensive skin lesions that may also involve underlying tissues. Neurologic and cardiac anomalies have been described in these patients.

☞**Delleman Oorthuys Syndrome:** Multiple congenital anomaly syndrome mainly affecting the central nervous system, eyes, and skin.

☞**Goltz Syndrome:** Complex mesoectodermal hereditary disorder characterized by focal dermal atrophy with herniation of fat producing multiple papillomas, in association with skeletal, dental, ocular, and other anomalies.

☞**Setleis Syndrome:** Puckered periorbital skin, absent or multiple rows of eyelashes.

REFERENCES:

Alpay F, Gul D, Lenk MK, et al: Severe intrauterine growth retardation, aged facial appearance, and congenital heart disease in a newborn with Johanson-Blizzard syndrome. *Pediatr Cardiol* 21:389, 2000.

Jones NL, Hofley PM, Durie PR: Pathophysiology of the pancreatic defect in Johanson-Blizzard syndrome: A disorder of acinar development. *J Pediatr* 125:406, 1994.

Prater JF, D'Addio K: Johanson-Blizzard syndrome: A case study, behavioral manifestations, and successful treatment strategies. *Biol Psychiatry* 51:515, 2002.

Johnson Munson Syndrome

At a glance: Aphalangia of the hands and feet with hemivertebrae, including pulmonary hypoplasia, congenital heart anomalies (ventricular septal defect), and dysgenesis of the urogenital tract and rectum. Death usually occurs during the first year of life.

Synonym: Aphalangia with Hemivertebrae; Aphalangia of the Hands and Feet, Hemivertebrae, and Visceral Malformations.

Incidence and genetic inheritance: Only a few cases have been reported in the literature. Autosomal recessive.

Clinical aspects: Aphalangia of the hands and feet, hemivertebrae, pulmonary hypoplasia, ventricular septal defect, and dysgenesis of urogenital tract and rectum. May die of respiratory insufficiency in early infancy.

Anesthetic considerations: Assess respiratory function (chest radiograph, arterial blood gases) and cardiovascular system (echocardiography). May have hypoplastic lungs requiring intraoperative and postoperative ventilation. Patient may have ventricular septal defects, so endocarditis prophylaxis is required. Left-to-right intracardiac shunting leads to pulmonary hypertension. Abnormalities of the spine may make extradural and intrathecal anesthesia difficult to perform.

REFERENCE:

Johnson VP, Munson DP: A new syndrome of aphalangia, hemivertebrae, and urogenital-intestinal dysgenesis. *Clin Genet* 38:346, 1990.

Jones Syndrome

At a glance: Genetically transmitted polymalformative syndrome characterized by gingival fibromatosis and progressive sensorineural deafness.

Synonyms: Gingival Fibromatosis with Hearing Loss; Gingival Fibromatosis with Sensorineural Hearing Loss; Jones-Hartsfield Syndrome.

Incidence and genetic inheritance: Fewer than 100 cases published. Autosomal dominant.

Clinical aspects: Association of gingival fibromatosis and progressive sensorineural hearing loss.

Anesthetic considerations: Because of gingival fibromatosis, a complete evaluation of the airway, including mouth opening, must be performed to eliminate the possibility of difficult direct laryngoscopy and tracheal intubation. Difficult airway management because of gingival hypertrophy is not common but has been observed in patients affected with gingival hypertrophy caused by digitalis toxicity. Check for associated abnormalities especially of the heart and lungs.

Other conditions to be considered:

BYARS-JURKIEWICZ SYNDROME: Characterized by hypertrichosis, gingival hypertrophy, giant fibroadenomas of breast, and kyphosis.

☞**OCULOCEREBRAL WITH HYPOPIGMENTATION SYNDROME:** Extremely rare autosomal recessive inherited syndrome (<20 cases described). Most symptoms are present at birth or develop shortly thereafter. It may include very light skin color and silvery hair in combination with ophthalmologic (microphthalmia, corneal clouding, cataract, ectropion) and central nervous system anomalies (dolichocephaly, mental retardation, athetosis, ataxia, spastic paraplegia or tetraplegia). Gingival fibromatosis may develop at the age of emergence of the first teeth and may result in complete coverage of the teeth and become so significant that ventilation is impaired. Proper lung ventilation can be decreased significantly by a dysfunctional diaphragm.

GINGIVAL FIBROMATOSIS, HYPERTRICHOSIS, EPILEPSY, MENTAL RETARDATION SYNDROME: Characterized by mental retardation, epilepsy, brachymetacarpalia, hirsutism, bulbous short nose, thick floppy ears with abnormal configuration, and gingival hypertrophy. Other clinical features include congenital heart defects (e.g., tetralogy of Fallot), congenital hypothyroidism, and bilateral ureteral stenosis. Inheritance has been suggested to result from an autosomal recessive trait.

☞**LABAND SYNDROME:** Characterized by soft tissue enlargement of the nose and ears, gingival hypertrophy, skeletal abnormalities, obscure or reduced size of toenails and thumbnails, short terminal phalanges, hypermobility of several joints, and hepatosplenomegaly.

☞**JUVENILE HYALINE FIBROMATOSIS:** Autosomal recessive condition that usually presents with nodular/papular skin lesions and gingival hypertrophy during the first few years of life. The skin lesions typically occur on the hands, scalp, ears, and around the nose and require recurrent excision. Progressive joint contractures and osteopenia are characteristic and may result in severely limited mobility. Diagnosis is confirmed by demonstration of hyaline deposition in the dermis and is called *juvenile hyaline fibromatosis.*

☞**RAMON SYNDROME:** Characterized by cherubism (maxillary fibrous dysplasia), gingival fibromatosis, stunted growth, hypertrichosis, mental retardation, and epilepsy. Other clinical features may include pigmentary changes in the retina, paleness of the optic disk, Axenfeld anomaly, and giant hypertrophy of the labia minora.

RUTHERFORD SYNDROME: Characterized by gingival hypertrophy and corneal dystrophy.

REFERENCE:

Hartsfield JK Jr, Bixler D, Hazen RH. Gingival fibromatosis with sensorineural hearing loss: An autosomal dominant trait. *Am J Med Genet* 22:623, 1985.

Joubert Syndrome

At a glance: Genetic disorder characterized by cerebral malformations (vermis and brainstem) resulting in severe coordination (ataxia) and breathing (sleep apnea, hyperpnea) disorders.

Synonyms: Cerebellar Vermis Agenesis Syndrome; Cerebelloparenchymal Disorder Type IV; Chorioretinal Coloboma with Cerebellar Vermis Aplasia; Coloboma, Chorioretinal with Cerebellar Vermis Aplasia; Joubert-Boltshauser Syndrome.

History: Peroxisomal disease named after Marie Joubert, a Canadian neurologist who reported the first cases in 1989, in Montreal.

Genetic inheritance: Autosomal recessive. Gene map locus is 9q34.3.

Pathophysiology: Unknown.

Diagnosis: Typical "molar tooth" sign on axial magnetic resonance imaging (MRI) through the malformed pontomesencephalic junction. Prenatal diagnosis may be suggested by ultrasonographic features. Clinical features. Abdominal and cerebral ultrasonography diagnosis in the neonatal period.

Clinical aspects: During the neonatal period, variable combinations of central nervous system, eye, and renal abnormalities. Agenesis of the cerebellar vermix with cystic dilatation of the fourth ventricle and poor respiratory control. Episodes of tachypnea attacks alternating with apneas. Severe psychomotor retardation and ataxia. Abnormal eye movements and bilateral coloboma. Abdominal ultrasonographs reveal cortical renal cysts and interstitial renal fibrosis. Other malformations, including polydactyly (fingers and toes), cleft lip/palate, tongue malformations, and seizures, may exist. Renal function may deteriorate. Prognosis is poor.

Precautions before anesthesia: Check respiratory function, perform pulmonary function tests if patient collaboration permits [forced vital capacity (FVC), forced expiratory volume at 1 second (FEV$_1$); maximal expiratory flow rate (MEFR), residual volume (RV)]. Perform arterial blood gases in room air in all cases. Check renal function by checking electrolytes, blood urea nitrogen, and creatinine. The administration of premedication is unadvised.

Anesthetic considerations: Children with this syndrome have abnormalities of respiratory control as a consequence of neuronal changes in the brainstem and cerebellum. They are extremely sensitive to the respiratory depressant effects of anesthetic agents, including nitrous oxide. Anesthesia using inhalational induction, intermittent positive pressure ventilation, avoidance of opioids, and close postoperative monitoring are recommended.

Pharmacological implications: Opioid hypersensitivity. Respiratory depression following nitrous oxide. Children very sensitive to the depressant effects of any anesthetic agent.

Other condition to be considered:

☞**LOUIS-BAR SYNDROME:** Autosomal recessive progressive cerebellar ataxia with oculomotor apraxia, telangiectasias of the conjunctivae, choreoathetosis, immunodeficiency, recurrent infections, increased sensitivity to ionizing radiations, and tendency to develop malignancies.

REFERENCES:

Barreirinho MS, Teixeira J, Moreira NC, et al: Joubert's syndrome: Report of 12 cases. *Rev Neurol* 32:812, 2001.

Habre W, Sims C, D'Souza M: Anaesthetic management of children with Joubert syndrome. *Paediatr Anaesth* 7:251, 1997.

Zamponi N, Rossi B, Messori A, et al: Joubert syndrome with associated corpus callosum agenesis. *Eur J Paediatr Neurol* 6:63, 2002.

Juberg-Hayward Syndrome

At a glance: Very rare familial bipolar syndrome characterized by short stature resulting from growth hormone deficiency. Affected individuals have microcephaly, cleft lip/palate, and deformities of the thumbs and limbs.

Synonyms: Oro-Cranio-Digital Syndrome; Cleft Lip/Palate with Abnormal Thumbs and Microcephaly Syndrome.

Incidence and genetic inheritance: Very rare genetic disorder with probable autosomal inheritance.

Clinical aspects: Patients have short stature and mental retardation. Syndrome involves *head* (cleft lip/palate, microcephaly, hypertelorism, broad nose, bowed and upward-slanting eyebrows, and ptosis), *skeleton* (hypoplastic stiff and distally placed thumbs, brachydactyly, limited elbow extension, anomalous carpal bones, deformity of radial heads, toe anomalies, and vertebral and rib anomalies). Other features include horseshoe kidneys, micropenis, and anterior anal displacement. Laboratory investigations show growth hormone deficiency.

Anesthetic considerations: Ventilation with a face mask, direct laryngoscopy and tracheal intubation can be difficult because of facial malformations. The airway must be preoperatively assessed. Maintain spontaneous ventilation until the trachea is intubated and lung ventilated. Avoid neck extension. Careful intraoperative positioning is needed. Venous access on superior limb can be difficult.

Other conditions to be considered:

☞**FETAL AMINOPTERIN SYNDROME:** Teratogenic syndrome caused by maternal intake of aminopterin or methotrexate. Characterized by growth failure, craniofacial deformities, hydrocephalus, mental retardation, and skeletal defects.

☞**MALPUECH SYNDROME:** Malformative syndrome characterized by hypertelorism, facial clefting, urogenital abnormalities, severe growth failure, and mental retardation.

REFERENCES:

Juberg RC, Hayward JR: A new familial syndrome of oral, cranial, and digital anomalies. *J Pediatr* 74:755, 1969.

Silengo M, Tornetta L: Juberg-Hayward syndrome: Report of a case with cleft palate, distally placed thumbs and vertebral anomalies. *Clin Dysmorphol* 9:127, 2000.

Verloes A, Le Merrer M, Davin JC, et al: The orocraniodigital syndrome of Juberg and Hayward. *J Med Genet* 29:262, 1992.

Juberg-Marsidi Syndrome

At a glance: X-linked recessive syndrome characterized by severe mental retardation, seizures, deafness, failure to thrive, microgenitalism, and early death.

Synonyms: Juberg-Marsidi Mental Retardation Syndrome; X-Linked Microcephaly.

Incidence and genetic inheritance: Incidence is unknown because only a few cases have been reported in the literature. X-linked recessive at the Xq12-q21 site. The syndrome has clinical similarities with the ☞ATR-X syndrome (alpha-thalassemia, mental retardation, X-linked syndrome), which is associated with mutations of the X-linked nuclear protein (XNP) gene.

Clinical aspects: Clinical manifestations of this syndrome are apparent at birth or within the first few weeks of life. Moderate-to-severe mental retardation with developmental delay; hypotonicity; occasionally EEG abnormalities, clinical seizures, hearing loss, and microcephaly. Facial dysmorphism such as a flattened nose, high arched palate, ocular abnormalities, and telecanthus are frequent. Short stature secondary to delayed bone growth. Congenital heart disease has been reported but may not be systematically included in this condition. Genitourinary abnormalities, including undescended/atrophic testes and micropenis, are common. Other features include onychodystrophy and delayed bone age. The range and severity of symptoms vary among cases. Usually fatal in infancy or childhood.

Anesthetic considerations: Seizure control and potential interactions between anesthetic drugs and antiseizure medications (e.g., phenytoin and carbamazepine may increase nondepolarizing muscle relaxant requirements.). Antiseizure medication should be continued throughout the perioperative period. Severe muscle hypotonicity may predispose to perioperative respiratory insufficiency; consider judicious use of muscle relaxants. Consider an echocardiogram to rule out congenital heart disease. Renal function should be evaluated because of occasional incidence of hydronephrosis. Perhaps at risk for recurrent urinary tract infections.

Other conditions to be considered:

☞**ATR-X SYNDROME:** Acronym for *a*lpha-*t*halassemia, mental *r*etardation, *X*-linked syndrome. Characterized by genital abnormalities, microcephaly, midface hypoplasia, severe mental retardation, neuromotor dysfunction, seizures, and hypotonia. Occasionally the patient presents a ventricular septal defect and gastrointestinal reflux.

☞**ALLAN-HERNDON SYNDROME:** Although most neonates and infants with this disorder appear to develop normally in the first few months of life, the presence of poor muscle tone is most often present at birth. By 6 months of age, hypotonia, inability to hold up the head, and severe muscle atrophy are detectable. Severe mental retardation is associated with multiple congenital anomalies.

☞**FRAGILE X SYNDROME:** Most common form of X-linked mental retardation; affects males more often and more severely than females. Only subtle dysmorphic features, but behavioral issues may be more pronounced.

☞**HAPPY PUPPET SYNDROME:** Rare disorder characterized by developmental delay, ataxia, dysmorphic facial features, and seizures associated with a happy, sociable disposition.

☞**MASA SYNDROME:** Acronym for mental retardation, aphasia, shuffling gait and adducted thumbs. Extremely rare inherited disorder that is one of several disorders known as X-linked mental retardation (XLMR) syndromes.

RENPENNING SYNDROME: Extremely rare form of X-linked (moderate-to-severe) mental retardation. Has been linked to Xp11.2-p11.4. Other findings may include short stature, moderate microcephaly, prognathism, and small testes. Affected patients may use repetitive speech and show aggressive behavior. Longevity seems not to be impaired, and female carriers do not show any heterozygous signs.

ESCALANTE SYNDROME: Features similar to those observed in Renpenning syndrome, but associated with macroorchidism.

SUTHERLAND-HAAN SYNDROME (Sutherland-Haan X-Linked Mental Retardation Syndrome; X-Linked Mental Retardation with Spastic Diplegia): Extremely rare form of X-linked severe mental retardation. Features of this disorder include short stature, spastic diplegia, significant congenital heart defects, and craniofacial abnormalities (microcephaly, cleft/high arched palate, abnormal ears, bulbous nose, broad nasal bridge, malar hypoplasia, micrognathia, and a small mouth). No reports exist about anesthesia in these patients; however, difficult airway management seems likely.

REFERENCES:

Saugier-Veber P, Abadie V, Moncla A, et al: The Juberg-Marsidi syndrome maps to the proximal long arm of the X chromosome (Xq12-q21). *Am J Hum Genet* 52:1040, 1993.

Tsukahara M, Nasu T, Takihara H, et al: Juberg-Marsidi syndrome: Report of an additional case. *Am J Med Genet* 58:353, 1995.

Villard L, Gecz J, Mattei JF, et al: XNP mutation in a large family with Juberg-Marsidi syndrome. *Nat Genet* 12:359, 1996.

Judge Misch Wright Syndrome

At a glance: Congenital palmoplantar keratoderma and nail dystrophy. Patient presents with progressive perioral and perineal keratoderma associated with bilateral corneal epithelial dysplasia leading to severe corneal scarring and impairment of vision.

Synonym: Palmoplantar and Periorofacial Keratoderma with Corneal Epithelial Dysplasia.

Genetic inheritance: Unknown.

Clinical aspects: Dermatologic signs are very common: dry skin, palmoplantar hyperkeratosis, abnormal fingernails, and generalized absence of hair. Involvement of the corneas is common, possibly resulting in visual impairment.

Anesthetic considerations: No reports found, but possible concerns include difficulty placing and securing monitoring equipment (adhesive ECG lead pads) and indwelling lines (IV catheters, arterial lines). Hyperkeratosis, if severe, could possibly limit joint mobility, resulting in contractures, which may make positioning the patient more awkward. Care must be taken to maintain the natural position of the patient and to pad all pressure points well. Difficult airway management might be expected if mouth opening or neck mobility is limited because of contractures.

REFERENCE:

Judge MR, Misch K, Wright P, et al: Palmoplantar and periorofacial keratoderma with corneal epithelial dysplasia: A new syndrome. *Br J Dermatol* 125:186, 1991.

Jumping Frenchman of Maine Syndrome

At a glance: Neurologic disease characterized by exaggerated, and often violent, startle reflexes that are produced by the slightest stimulus. It is usually associated with echolalia and echopraxia.

Incidence and genetic inheritance: Rare. Questionable genetic component. Perhaps a psychological disease described as "operant conditioning."

Clinical aspects: Seemingly a disease isolated to French Canadians, particularly lumberjacks from the Moosehead region of Maine and the Beauce region of Quebec. The condition is often familial. Age of onset is usually between 12 and 20 years. Affected persons have an exaggerated startle reflex produced by the slightest stimulus; if given a short, sudden, quick command, they respond with the appropriate action, often echoing the words of the command (echolalia and echopraxia), even if it was expressed in a language foreign to the patient (i.e., the "parrot" response).

Anesthetic considerations: No references. Premedication prior to anesthesia may be of some value. Consider meticulous padding and immobilization.

Other condition to be considered:

☞GILLES DE LA TOURETTE SYNDROME: Repetitive compulsive involuntary stereotyped movements or vocalizations termed *tics;* for some authors, the jumping Frenchman of Maine syndrome is included in Gilles de la Tourette syndrome.

REFERENCES:

Howard R, Ford R: From the Jumping Frenchmen of Maine to post-traumatic stress disorder: The startle response in neuropsychiatry. *Psychol Med* 22:695, 1992.

Saint-Hilaire MH, Saint-Hilaire JM. Jumping Frenchmen of Maine. *Mov Disord* 16:530, 2001.

Saint-Hilaire MH, Saint-Hilaire JM, Granger L: Jumping Frenchmen of Maine. *Neurology* 36:1269, 1986.

Jung Wolff Back Stahl Syndrome

At a glance: Rare form of anterior segment dysgenesis of the eye associated with endocrine disorders, cerebral malformation, and tracheal stenosis.

Synonym: Anterior Chamber Cleavage Disorder; Cerebellar Hypoplasia, Hypothyroidism, and Tracheal Stenosis.

Incidence and genetic inheritance: Extremely rare; case report of only two patients: an unrelated boy and girl. Autosomal recessive inheritance. Questionable relationship to Peters-plus syndrome because of similar ocular abnormalities.

Clinical aspects: Both children had cerebellar hypoplasia (with Dandy-Walker malformation in the boy), hypotonia, and mental retardation. Microcephaly with a round face and broad nasal ridge, thick scalp hair with low hairline, short neck, narrow external auditory meatus, hip dysplasia, short feet, and fusion of the lower incisors were present in both patients. Tracheal stenosis was common to both; however, chronic inflammatory lung disease and abnormal vertebral shape were listed as frequent signs only; thus they probably occurred in one of the two patients. Growth hormone deficiency and congenital hypothyroidism occurred in both children. The presence of anterior chamber cleavage disorder (plus a coloboma of the right iris in the female) prompted the possible association with Peters-plus syndrome. The girl had a "shield" thorax and the boy had hypoplasia of the penis. The boy died at age 3.5 years. No mention was made of the girl's outcome.

Anesthetic considerations: No reports related to anesthetic management were found. Recommendations include screening for tracheal stenosis (stridor and/or wheeze, tachypnea, indrawing, cyanosis, chest radiograph, CT scan) and hypothyroidism (thyroid-stimulating hormone, T_3/T_4 levels). Narrow nasal passages may make nasal intubation difficult. Always consider difficulties with airway management if craniofacial abnormalities are present and tracheal stenosis. Difficulty maintaining patency of trachea if dynamic stenosis; consider maintaining spontaneous ventilation and avoiding muscle relaxants until trachea is intubated and lung ventilation confirmed. Smaller endotracheal tube may be required. May be prone to postoperative edema at site of stenosis if the endotracheal tube inserted was too tight. Correction of hypothyroidism prior to anesthesia is ideal. In case of an emergency and if suspicion of hypothyroidism is high, a suggested strategy is to draw blood for thyroid hormone dosage and administer a single 25-μg thyroxine dose. Poor muscle tone/coordination may predispose to aspiration risk and postoperative respiratory dysfunction.

Other conditions to be considered:

PETERS SYNDROME (Peters Anomaly): Anterior segment dysgenesis with abnormal cleavage of the anterior chamber of the eye secondary to mutations involving the *PAX6* gene.

☞**KRAUSE KIVLIN SYNDROME:** Same as Peters syndrome with the association of blindness, cleft lip/palate, short-limb dwarfism, delayed mental development, and cardiovascular defects (ventricular septal defect, atrial septal defect). Brain atrophy, seizures, and hydrocephalus are often present.

REFERENCE:
Jung C, Wolff G, Back E, et al: Two unrelated children with developmental delay, short stature and anterior chamber cleavage disorder, cerebellar hypoplasia, endocrine disturbances and tracheostenosis: A new entity? *Clin Dysmorphol* 4:44, 1995.

Juvenile Hyaline Fibromatosis

At a glance: Rare congenital genetic disorder characterized by papulonodular skin lesions, soft tissue masses, gingival hypertrophy, and flexion contractures of the large joints.

Synonyms: Murray Syndrome; JHF; Infantile Systemic Hyalinosis; Murray Puretic Syndrome ; Puretic Syndrome.

History: First described by J. Murray in 1873 and reported by A. Whitfield and A.H. Robinson in 1903.

Genetic inheritance: Autosomal recessive. Gene mapped on 4q21.

Pathophysiology: May be a disorder of collagen metabolism (because it is associated with abnormalities of collagen III and

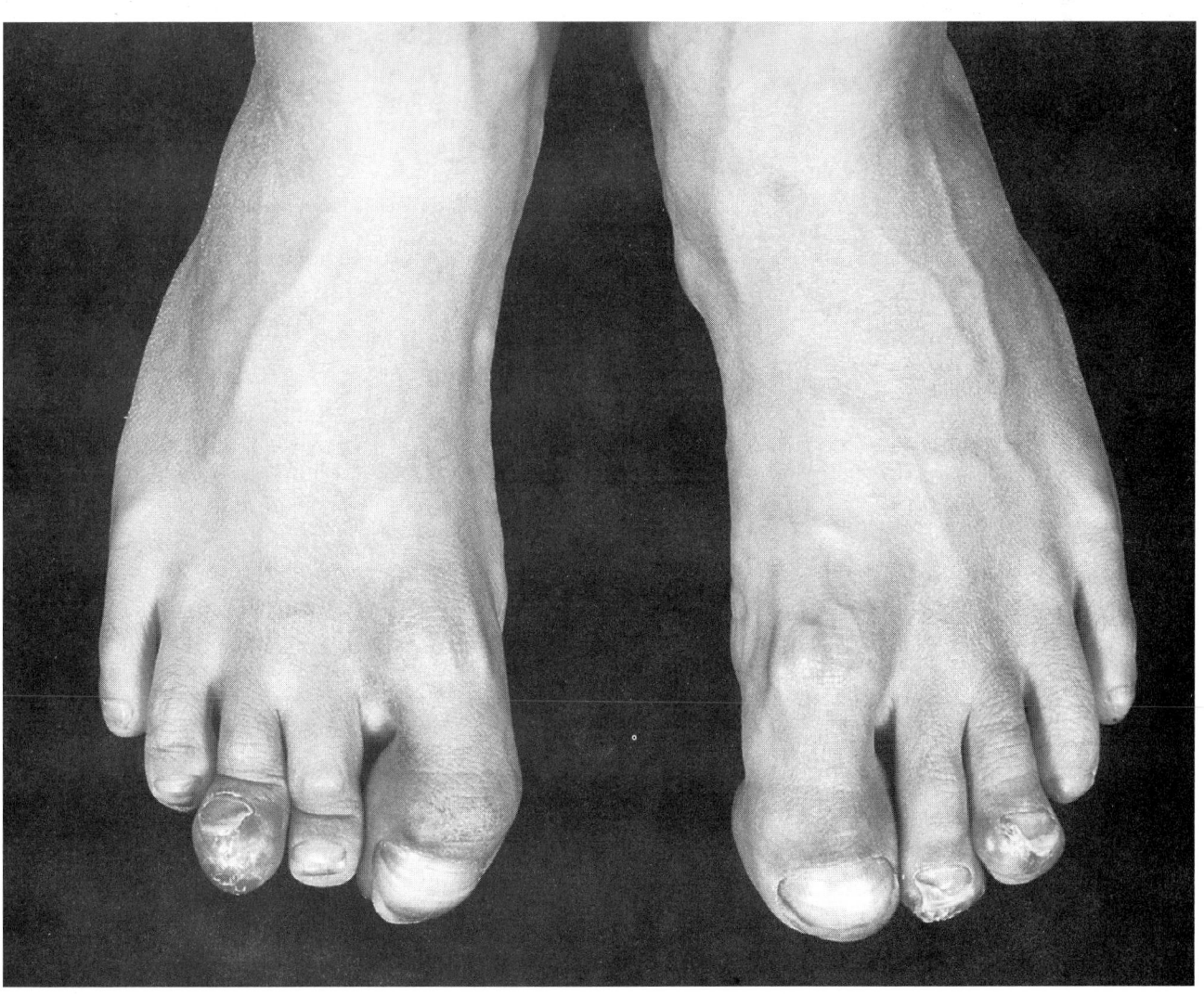

Juvenile hyaline fibromatosis Subcutaneous and subungual fibromata in an adult.

VI resulting from an underlying defect in glycosaminoglycan formation).

Clinical aspects: Onset in infancy or early childhood. Typical diagnostic criteria are multiple hyaline subcutaneous fibroma, filamentous tumors of the skin, gingival fibromatosis, muscle contractures of the extremities, and multiple osteolytic bone destruction. Features include osteolysis, diaphyseal anomaly, thickened gingivae, subcutaneous nodules, and restricted joint mobility. Deposits have been described in larynx, heart, and endocrine glands.

Anesthetic considerations: Both direct laryngoscopy and tracheal intubation can be difficult because of limited widening of the mouth and laryngeal deposits. One case of unexplained resistance to succinylcholine has been described. Preoperative cardiac function assessment can be proposed.

REFERENCES:

Murray J: On three peculiar cases of molluscum fibrosum in one family. *Med Chir Trans London* 56:235, 1873.

Norman B, Soni N, Madden N: Anesthesia and juvenile hyaline fibromatosis. *Br J Anaesth* 76:163, 1996.

Rahman N, Dunsan M, Teare ND, et al: The gene for juvenile hyaline fibromatosis maps to chromosome 4q21. *Am J Hum Genet* 71:975, 2002.

Juvenile Intestinal Polyposis

At a glance: Familial premalignant polyposis of the colon characterized by abdominal pain, rectal bleeding, and diarrhea.

Synonym: Juvenile Polyposis Syndrome.

Incidence: Solitary juvenile polyps occur in 1% of children, but juvenile polyposis is much rarer.

Genetic inheritance: There are both familial and nonfamilial polyposis. A family history of juvenile polyposis is present in 20 to 50% of patients. Autosomal dominant inheritance. There is evidence that mutations in the SMAD4/DPC4 gene located on 18q21.1 result in juvenile polyposis. Juvenile polyposis has been suggested to be caused by mutations in the PTEN gene (possible gene map location 10q23.3).

Pathophysiology: Patients have a variable number of polyps, usually between 50 and 200, distributed throughout the gastrointestinal tract, most commonly in the colon.

Diagnosis: Juvenile polyps are distinctive both macroscopically and histologically. They are usually pedunculated and spherical with a smooth surface within which are numerous large cystic spaces of variable size, filled with grayish or yellowish mucus surrounded by copious reddish stroma. In contrast to the hamartomatous polyps of Peutz-Jeghers syndrome, muscle fibers are not present in the stroma.

Clinical aspects: Usually present in childhood; less than 15% present in adulthood. Classified into three groups:

- *Juvenile polyposis of infancy* (presents with diarrhea, hemorrhage, intussusception, rectal prolapse and protein-losing enteropathy; entire gastrointestinal tract is affected, prognosis related to severity and extent of gastrointestinal involvement); usually fatal before 2 years of age.
- *Generalized juvenile polyposis*
- *Juvenile polyposis of the colon*

The latter two groups commonly present with abdominal pain, weakness, rectal bleeding, diarrhea, or rectal prolapse. Laboratory findings include anemia, hypoalbuminemia, hypokalemia, and skin test anergy. Juvenile polyposis is a premalignant condition with changes seen in children as young as 3 years of age. Patients with generalized involvement require surgical intervention. Subtotal colectomy and ileoproctostomy are the procedures of choice. Patients with a small number of polyps may choose instead to undergo periodic colonoscopy with colonoscopic polypectomy. Approximately 10 to 20% of affected patients have extracolonic abnormalities. These include finger clubbing and hypertrophic pulmonary osteoarthropathy related to pulmonary arteriovenous fistulas. Congenital cardiac defects, macrocephaly, cleft lip/palate, extra teeth, arteriovenous malformations of the skin, gut malrotation, psoriasis, and genitourinary abnormalities have been described.

Precautions before anesthesia: Correct anemia, electrolytes, and any intravascular volume deficit. Nutritional status should be assessed and metabolic deficiencies corrected prior to elective surgery. *Investigations:* complete blood count, serum electrolytes, creatinine, urea, albumin, and liver function tests. Parenteral nutrition should not be stopped suddenly, as rebound hyperglycemia may occur. Assess for any extracolonic abnormalities that may be relevant to anesthesia. Check for congenital cardiac defects. An electrocardiogram (ECG) and echocardiography may be indicated.

Anesthetic considerations: The major increase in intraoperative and postoperative complications result from the malabsorption state. Monitoring of blood sugar and electrolyte levels is mandatory. Regional anesthesia minimizes impairment of the cardiorespiratory system by general anesthetic agents. Epidural anesthesia as a perioperative adjunct provides superior pain control and has been implicated in more rapid ileus resolution after major abdominal surgery, possibly through a sympatholytic mechanism. Postoperative mechanical ventilation will be required for those with severely reduced cardiorespiratory reserves. Anemia may be significant and requires correction before surgery. Rectal bleeding may cause severe hypovolemia and must be corrected before induction of anesthesia. Diarrhea may result in electrolyte disturbances, especially hypokalemia. Cardiac defects may require specific anesthetic management or antibiotic prophylaxis.

Pharmacological implications: In severe malnutrition, there is an increased sensitivity to intravenous induction agents, succinylcholine (as pseudocholinesterase deficiency may exist), nondepolarizing neuromuscular blockers (in the presence of hypocalcemia, hypophosphatemia, and hypomagnesemia), and drugs bound to albumin (e.g., diazepam).

Other conditions to be considered:

GARDNER SYNDROME: Autosomal dominant variant of familial adenomatous polyposis characterized by intestinal polyposis, multiple osteomas, skin and soft tissue tumors. Untreated polyps spontaneously undergo malignant degeneration in 100% of cases.

☞**BANNAYAN-ZONANA SYNDROME:** Polymalformative syndrome characterized by macrocephaly, lipomas, hemangiomas, thyroid disorders, and multiple hamartomatous polyps of the small and large intestine.

☞**COWDEN SYNDROME:** Autosomal dominant disorder characterized by gastrointestinal polyps with a tendency to become malignant, mucocutaneous pigmentation, thyroiditis, and breast cysts.

☞**GORLIN GOLTZ SYNDROME:** Autosomal dominant cancer syndrome, basal cell carcinomas and medulloblastoma with sensitivity to ionizing radiation, multiple abnormalities of the skin, skeleton, and nervous system ("the fifth phakomatosis"). Gene map locus is 9q22.3-q31.

☞**PEUTZ-JEGHERS SYNDROME:** Autosomal recessive or sporadic syndrome characterized by the association of gastrointestinal polyposis with mucocutaneous pigmentation. Mutation in the *STK11* gene (at locus 19p13.3) is present in approximately 70% of familial cases and 30 to 70% of sporadic cases.

☞**TURCOT SYNDROME:** Autosomal recessive syndrome characterized by the association of a primary brain tumor and multiple colorectal adenomas. This condition could be a variant of Gardner syndrome. It has been suggested that it could result from two distinct germline defects: mutation of the APC gene or mutation of a mismatch-repair gene; candidate gene map locus 5q21-q22.

REFERENCES:

Church JM, McGannon E, Burke C, et al: Teenagers with familial adenomatous polyposis: What is their risk for colorectal cancer? *Dis Colon Rectum* 45:887, 2002.

Desai DC, Neale KF, Talbot IC, et al: Juvenile polyposis. *Br J Surg* 82:14, 1995.

Hizawa K, Sakamoto K, Akagi K, et al: Fatal colorectal cancer in juvenile polyposis syndrome. *J Gastroenterol* 37:313, 2002.

Juvenile Myoclonic Epilepsy (JME)

At a glance: Inherited epileptic disorder characterized by myoclonic jerks, generalized tonic-clonic seizures and, sometimes absence seizures shortly after awakening. Normal intelligence and onset around adolescence are characteristic.

Synonyms: Juvenile Myoclonic Epilepsy of Janz; Impulsive Petit Mal.

Incidence: 1:1000–2000 in the general population. JME represents 5 to 10% of all epileptic patients, but the condition probably is underdiagnosed. A slight prevalence among females has been reported in some (not all) studies.

Genetic inheritance: Exact mode of inheritance is not clear. One third of JME patients have a positive family history of epilepsy. Some authors reported association with human leukocyte antigen of chromosome 6 (not confirmed by other studies).

Pathophysiology: Microscopic brain alterations (dystopic neurons in stratum moleculare, white matter, hippocampus, and cerebellar cortex) have been observed. Exact cause of this disorder remains unknown.

Diagnosis: Based on clinical grounds. Video electroencephalogram (EEG) monitoring of typical seizures is the standard criterion (but not necessary to establish the diagnosis). The diagnosis should be suspected in patients with myoclonic jerks favored by reproducible precipitating factors. Sleep-deprived EEG with activation procedures (hyperventilation, photic stimulation) is the most useful test in clinical practice.

Clinical aspects: The disorder usually begins in adolescence and is characterized by absence seizures in early age. As the child ages, it is followed by myoclonic jerks in the morning (1–9 years later) and then grand mal seizures (a few years later). Patients are normally intelligent and do not lose consciousness during myoclonic jerks. Precipitating factors include sleep deprivation, psychological stress, alcohol use, and menses. Physical examination is normal.

Precautions before anesthesia: Check anticonvulsant therapy (including doses of antiepileptics) and continue normal therapy until the morning of anesthesia and surgery. Premedication, preferably with a benzodiazepine, is mandatory to reduce preoperative stress (stress is a precipitating factor of seizures in this syndrome).

Anesthetic considerations: No specific anesthetic considerations with this medical condition.

Pharmacological implications: Avoid anesthetic agents known to be associated with seizure activity or stimulation. Administration of an intravenous anticonvulsant for prolonged surgical procedures or after large blood loss must be considered.

Other condition to be considered:

FRONTAL LOBE EPILEPSY: Characterized by recurrent seizures originating in the frontal lobes, often partial with or without secondary generalization; usually symptomatic of other disorders, either congenital (cortical dysgenesis, gliosis, or vascular malformations) or acquired (neoplasms, head trauma, infections, and anoxia). One rare variant is genetically transmitted as an autosomal dominant trait.

REFERENCES:

Bai D, Alonso ME, Medina MT, et al: Juvenile myoclonic epilepsy: Linkage to chromosome 6p12 in Mexico families. *Am J Med Genet* 113:268, 2002.

Canevini MP, Mai R, Di Marco C: Juvenile myoclonic epilepsy of Janz: Clinical observations in 60 patients. *Seizure* 1:291, 1992.

Wheless JW, Kim HL: Adolescent seizures and epilepsy syndromes. *Epilepsia* 43(suppl 3):33, 2002.

Juvenile Paralysis Agitans of Hunt

At a glance: The association of progressive extrapyramidal neurologic disorder presenting in teenagers or even earlier and mild form of Parkinson disease. Characterized by tremor, bradykinesia, dysarthria, rigidity, and fixed facies. The disorder may be familial (genetically transmitted) or secondary to other heredodegenerative disorders, such as Huntington disease.

Synonyms: Corpus Striatum Syndrome; Dyssynergia Cerebellaris Myoclonica; Hunt Paralysis; Hunt Syndrome II; Juvenile Parkinson Disease of Hunt; Willige-Hunt Syndrome.

History: Degeneration of lenticular nuclei. First clinical report by Huchard in 1875.

Incidence: In Parkinson disease cases, 25% are genetically inherited, of which a small number of cases are represented by juvenile Parkinson disease.

Genetic inheritance: Familial forms may be transmitted as an autosomal dominant or autosomal recessive trait. The recessive form, called "Parkin type of juvenile Parkinson disease," is caused by mutations within the Parkin gene *PARK2,* which is located on chromosome 6q25.2-q27. The dominant form is caused by mutations in the alpha-synuclein gene *PARK1* (on chromosome 4q21); a fragment of the product of this gene is a known constituent of Alzheimer disease plaques. A few dominant forms of the disease involve other dominant loci, including ubiquitin cyclohydrolase L1 (UCHL1) on chromosome 2p12 (*PARK3*) and chromosome 4p (*PARK4*). These enzymes are part of the ubiquitin proteolytic system (UPS), which plays a central role in the regulation of many cellular processes, including removal of abnormal, misfolded, or damaged proteins.

Pathophysiology: Whatever the genetic transmission, the disease is associated with loss of dopaminergic neurons in the substantia nigra and dopamine deficiency in the striatum. There is a subsequent increase in the activity of the subthalamic nucleus and the globus pallidus, which is responsible for the extrapyramidal movements. Other nondopaminergic neurons are affected (serotonin, norepinephrine), the depletion of which causes psychological and behavioral disorders.

Diagnosis: Clinical diagnosis. An antiserum that is immunoreactive to the Parkin immunizing peptide by enzyme-linked immunoabsorbent assay (ELISA) is available.

Clinical aspects: Clinical features are very similar to the adult form of parkinsonism and begins between 5 and 15 years of age. Tremors appear first, then rigidity, dyskinesia, and unexpressive face. Disturbed gait and dysarthria. Ameliorated by L-dopa (levodopamine), monoamine oxidase (MAO) inhibitors, and anticholinergic agents.

Precautions before anesthesia: Check carefully the child's medication (L-dopa and MAO inhibitors). Do not stop medication; give the morning dose of L-dopa. L-Dopa has a short half-life and stopping it for more than 6 to 12 hours can lead to severe muscular rigidity and worsening of the ventilation.

Anesthetic considerations: Light anesthesia can favor muscular rigidity. Prevent hyperventilation (hypocarbia) which may trigger seizures. Monitor carefully the hemodynamics because of MAO inhibitors.

Pharmacological implications: There is frequent interaction between drugs commonly used to treat the condition and anesthetic agents. Drugs with antidopaminergic properties such as butyrophenones (DHBP) and phenothiazines, as well as alfentanil (dystonia), should be avoided. Ketamine is controversial because it may enhance hypertension and tachycardia. Theoretically, the association of L-dopa and halothane could predispose to cardiac arrhythmias. The use of sevoflurane must be carefully weighted against the risk of intraoperative activation of seizure activities. It may occur even at lower concentrations, and the depth of anesthesia should be monitored with intraoperative electroencephalography. Take usual precautions when patients are taking MAO inhibitors.

Other conditions to be considered:

☞**Spinocerebellar Ataxia Type 1:** Characterized by progressive cerebellar ataxia, supranuclear ophthalmoplegia, pyramidal or extrapyramidal signs, mild dementia, and peripheral neuropathy. Age at onset is in the third or fourth decade of life, most often around age 30. Involuntary choreiform movements may occur. It is believed to be an autosomal dominant spinocerebellar ataxia.

Parkin-Related Diseases: Mutation in the Parkin gene, autosomal recessive. Clinically, patients affected with Parkin gene disease present with symmetrical involvement and dystonia at onset, hyperreflexia at onset or later, a good response to levodopa therapy, and levodopa-induced dyskinesias during treatment.

Parkinson Disease: Extrapyramidal neurologic disorder resulting from progressive loss of dopaminergic neurons in the substantia nigra and nigrostriatal pathway of the midbrain, not necessarily a genetic disorder

☞**Segawa Syndrome:** Characterized by extrapyramidal symptoms, periodic neurologic episodes, generalized hypertonia with opisthotonos, and conjugate upward deviations of both eyes lasting several minutes, followed by severe hypotonia, poor contact, and excessive salivation and perspiration for several hours. Cerebrospinal fluid biochemical abnormalities are severe. Uncharacteristically, a strikingly abnormal urinary catecholamine metabolite pattern is consistently observed.

☞**Shy-Drager Syndrome:** Syndrome with mild parkinsonism, encephalomyelopathy of adult onset and consisting of orthostatic hypotension, bladder and bowel incontinence, anhidrosis,

iris atrophy, amyotrophy, ataxia, rigidity and tremor, and normal intellect.

Progressive Supranuclear Palsy (Steele-Richardson-Olszewski Syndrome): Progressive supranuclear palsy is the second most frequent cause of degenerative parkinsonism. Clinical symptoms include early postural instability and supranuclear gaze palsy. Progressive supranuclear palsy is transmitted as an autosomal dominant trait. This disorder begins with axial rigidity, slowness of movement, and gait difficulty, followed by complete vertical gaze palsy, axial dystonia, retrocollis, and severe akinesia. It is often described as a Parkinson-like syndrome without the tremor. The term "Pick complex" has been suggested to represent the overlapping with syndromes of frontotemporal dementia (FTD), primary progressive aphasia, corticobasal degeneration, progressive supranuclear palsy, and FTD with motor neuron disease.

REFERENCES:

Mason LJ, Cojocaru TT, Cole DJ: Surgical intervention and anesthetic management of the patient with Parkinson's disease. *Int Anesthesiol Clin* 34:133, 1996.

Nisipeanu P, Inzelberg R, Abo Mouch S, et al: Parkin gene causing benign autosomal recessive juvenile parkinsonism. *Neurology* 56:1573, 2001.

Severn AM: Parkinsonism and the anaesthetist. *Br J Anesthesia* 61:761, 1988.

Juvenile Sulfatidosis Syndrome

At a glance: Very rare inborn error of metabolism combining the characteristics of metachromatic leukodystrophy and mucopolysaccharidosis. Lysosomal storage disease resulting from a lack of conversion (most likely in the endoplasmic reticulum) of cysteine into formylglycine. Muscle weakness with spasticity, poor swallowing, recurrent pulmonary aspiration, and quadriplegia. Blindness and seizures (hydrocephalus) develop, eventually leading to death by the second decade of life. Aortic insufficiency and cervical cord compression have been reported.

Synonyms: Austin Disease; Mucosulfatidosis; Multiple Sulfatase Deficiency.

Genetic inheritance: Autosomal recessive.

Pathophysiology: The disease results from deficiency of at least seven different sulfatases, including arylsulfatase A, B, and C, iduronate 2-sulfate sulfatase, heparan N-sulfatase, N-acetylgalactosamine 6-sulfate sulfatase, and N-acetylglucosamine 6-sulfate sulfatase. This leads to the accumulation of a variety of sulfated compounds, including certain mucopolysaccharides, steroids, and sphingolipids. Evidence indicates the defect is a result of a disruption of the posttranslational process common to all the sulfatase enzymes, rendering them inactive.

Diagnosis: Clinical features and confirmatory laboratory results. Urinary excretion of total or individual sulfatides and glycosaminoglycans is increased. Serum and leukocytic sulfatase activity is reduced or absent. Neutrophils may show abnormal granulation. Cultured fibroblast sulfatase activity is reduced with abnormal sulfate incorporation kinetics. Cerebral fluid protein concentration is increased. Metachromic degeneration may be demonstrated in peripheral and central nerve tissue as a consequence of the accumulation of galactosphingosulfatides. Radiologic evidence of dysostosis multiplex may be present: broad ribs; narrow radial and ulnar shafts with wide and irregular metaphysis; small carpal bones; short and wide metatarsal and terminal phalanges of the great toes.

Clinical aspects: The clinical phenotypes combine the milder features of late infantile metachromic leukodystrophy and of mucopolysaccharidosis. Typically, patients have an initial period of normal development followed by the onset of motor and mental difficulty during the first or second year of life. In the later stage, most patients have developmental delay, coarse facial features ("gargoylism"), ichthyosis, hepatosplenomegaly, and skeletal abnormalities. Neurologic deterioration usually is rapid. Other reported features include seizure, deafness, hydrocephalus, chondrodysplasia calcificans, and abnormal fold of tissue between laryngeal and esophageal inlet in one case. Hemophagocytic syndrome of fever, pancytopenia, coagulopathy, liver dysfunction, and proliferation of mature histiocytes was reported in one patient.

Precautions before anesthesia: Evaluate extent of demyelination, evidence of cord compression, and bulbar palsy. Mouth opening should be checked in case of temporal mandibular ankylosis. Electrolytes and coagulation profiles must be obtained. Urine sample to exclude associated mucopolysaccharidosis. An electrocardiogram (ECG) and echocardiogram must be obtained if a cardiac lesion is suspected.

Anesthetic considerations: Potential for airway difficulty with abnormal facial features and airway anomalies, despite the lack of mention of poor mouth opening or poor neck extension in any report.

Poor cooperation because of mental retardation. Severe neurologic deterioration may predispose to lungs aspiration. Care in positioning of patients presenting with limited joint mobility.

Pharmacological implications: Succinylcholine should be avoided in the presence of cervical and thoracic spinal cord compression. Avoid drugs that rely entirely on hepatic metabolism in cases of hepatic dysfunction. Meperidine, ketamine, and enflurane are relative contraindications if seizures are present.

Other conditions to be considered:

☞**METACHROMIC LEUKODYSTROPHY:** Lysosomal storage disease caused by defective lysosomal arylsulfatase, resulting in progressive loss of white matter in the nervous system with gait disturbance, mental regression, and urinary incontinence. Gene map locus is 22q13.31-qter.

☞**MUCOPOLYSACCHARIDOSES:** Group of inherited metabolic storage disease caused by various defective lysosomal enzymes with progressive multiorgan degeneration.

REFERENCES:

Burk R, Valle D, Thomos G, et al: Early manifestations of multiple sulfatase deficiency. *J Pediatr* 104:574, 1984.

Guerra WF, Verity MA, Fluharty AL, et al: Multiple sulfatase deficiency: Clinical, neuropathological, ultrastructural and biochemical studies. *J Neuropathol Exp Neurol* 49:406, 1990.

Soong B, Casamassima A, Fink J, et al: Multiple sulfatase deficiency. *Neurology* 38:1273, 1988.

K

Kabuki Syndrome

At a glance: Congenital syndrome characterized by multiple congenital anomalies, typical facial features (regardless of ethnic origin), and mild-to-moderate mental retardation. Significant cardiac malformations have been reported.

Synonyms: Kabuki Make-up Syndrome; Niikawa-Kuroki Syndrome.

History: First described in 1980 by the two Japanese physicians N. Niikawa and Y. Kuroki. Phenotype resembles the make-up of actors in Kabuki (traditional Japanese theater). However, patients and their relatives often dislike the term "make-up."

Incidence: 1:32,000 of Japanese newborns; less in non-Japanese.

Genetic inheritance: Autosomal dominant, arising from sporadic mutations; equal male-to-female ratio. The gentetic defect has been mapped to 8p22-23.1.

Pathophysiology: Unknown. Resembles a genetic disorder; however, there is little evidence regarding the mode of inheritance.

Diagnosis: Niikawa and Kuroki described five major groups of abnormalities: (a) abnormal facies, eversion of lower lateral eyelid, arched eyebrows (sparse in the lateral third), depressed nasal tip and prominent ears; (b) skeletal anomalies; (c) dermatoglyphic anomalies; (d) mental retardation; and (e) postnatal growth deficiency.

Clinical aspects: Skeletal abnormalities include high-arched palate, cleft palate, scoliosis, sagittal cleft vertebrae, vertebral osteopenia, dysplasia of femoral acetabulum, and brachydactyly. Early breast development is seen in 23% of girls. Congenital heart disease is reported in approximately one-third of patients, including single ventricle with common atrium, ventricular septal defect, atrial septal defect, tetralogy of Fallot, coarctation of the aorta (often juxtaductal), patent ductus arteriosus, transposition of the great arteries, and right bundle branch block. Hepatic anomalies such as extrahepatic biliary atresia and neonatal sclerosing cholangitis have been described and required liver transplantation in some patients.

Kidney anomalies (fused kidneys) and ureteropelvic stenoses with hydronephrosis may result in renal failure.

Stenosis of the upper airway (main bronchus), abnormal branching pattern of the lower airways, and bronchomalacia have been reported in a few patients. Congenital diaphragmatic hernia is occasionally present. More than half of these patients have a form of hearing loss (conductive and/or sensorineural). Recurrent otitis media is a common finding. Dental anomalies (e.g., conical incisors, hypodontia) are not uncommon.

Precautions before anesthesia: Obtain a history of developmental problems. Make specific inquiries for major skeletal and cardiac abnormalities and previous cardiac surgery. Check renal and hepatic function. Airway assessment, congenital defects of spinal column, mid-face hypoplasia, high arched palate, and cleft palate may make airway management difficult. Respiratory function should be assessed carefully in the presence of scoliosis, and formal lung function tests prior to major surgery may be helpful. Assessment of the cardiac function should include a complete history and examination, ECG, and echocardiography. Cardiac catheterization as clinically indicated. Seizures are not uncommon, so assess therapy and its efficiency.

Anesthetic considerations: Prepare for a potentially difficult airway. Strictly avoid air bubbles in all intravascular lines in patients with cardiac defects and carefully maintain the ratio of pulmonary to systemic vascular resistance, depending on individual cardiac anatomy and presence of systemic to pulmonary shunts. Consider the need for postoperative intensive care unit admission after major surgery. Careful airway monitoring in the early postoperative period. Careful positioning is required to avoid joint dislocations (especially hips). Patients with Kabuki syndrome have a strong susceptibility to infections.

Pharmacological implications: No specific contraindications described. Avoid muscle relaxants until the airway has been secured. Consider interactions between anesthetic drugs and chronic antiseizure medications. Subacute bacterial endocarditis prophylaxis may be indicated. Congenital heart disease may dictate avoidance of high-dose volatile agents (decreased systemic vascular resistance resulting in increased right-to-left shunting). The potential need for vasopressors, pulmonary vasodilators, and beta blockers depends on the nature of the cardiac lesion.

Other condition to be considered:

☞**VAN DER WOUDE SYNDROME:** Autosomal dominant inherited craniofacial syndrome with cleft lip and/or palate and typical pits of the lower lip, caused by deletions in chromosome band 1q32; can occasionally be associated to Kabuki syndrome.

REFERENCES:

Niikawa N, Kuroki Y, Kajii T, et al: Kabuki make-up (Niikawa-Kuroki) syndrome: A study of 62 patients. *Am J Med Genet* 31:565, 1988.

Wessels MW, Brooks AS, Hoogeboom J, et al: Kabuki syndrome: A review study of three hundred patients. *Clin Dysmorphol* 11:95, 2002.

Kaler-Garrity-Stern Syndrome

At a glance: Inherited polymalformative syndrome originally described in two Mennonite sisters of consanguineous parents.

Synonym: Osteopenia-Mental Retardation-Sparse Hair Syndrome.

Incidence and genetic inheritance: Only two cases described, so far. Autosomal recessive inheritance.

Clinical aspects: Craniofacial dysmorphism with macrocephaly, hypertelorism, frontal bossing, bulbous nose, depressed premaxillary region, prognathism, and low-set ears. Moderate-to-severe mental retardation. Musculoskeletal abnormalities include hyperextensible joints, osteoporosis and osteosclerosis, and syndactyly of toes.

Anesthetic considerations: Craniofacial abnormalities require careful assessment of the airway for difficult face-mask ventilation or laryngoscopy. Careful positioning is mandatory to avoid fractures. Mental retardation may result in decreased patient cooperation and sedative and/or anxiolytic premedication and the presence of the primary caregiver for induction of anesthesia may be helpful.

Other condition to be considered:

☞**OSTEOGENESIS IMPERFECTA CONGENITA (TYPE II):** Severe form of osteogenesis imperfecta often fatal in early life, in contrast to Kaler-Garrity-Stern syndrome, collagen in this disorder is defective.

REFERENCE:
Kaler SG, Garrity AM, Stern HJ, et al: New autosomal recessive syndrome of sparse hair, osteopenia, and mental retardation in Mennonite sisters. *Am J Med Genet* 43:983, 1992.

Kallmann Syndrome

At a glance: Congenital syndrome characterized by the association of hypogonadotropic hypogonadism with anosmia (or hyposmia).

Synonyms: de Morsier Syndrome II; Hypogonadotropic Hypogonadism and Anosmia Syndrome; Kallmann-de Morsier Syndrome; Maestre-Kallmann-de Morsier Syndrome; Maestre de San Juan-Kallmann Syndrome; Maestre de San Juan-Kallmann-de Morsier Syndrome; Olfactogenital Dysplasia; Morsier-Gauthier Syndrome.

History: Genetic disorder first described in 1856 by the Spanish histologist Aureliano Maestre de San Juan (1828–1890). The German psychiatrist Franz Josef Kallmann in 1944 pointed out the genetic background of the disease, while the Swiss pathologist Georges de Morsier published a case series in 1954.

Incidence: 1:10,000 males, 1:50,000 females of live births.

Genetic inheritance: X-linked recessive, also present in autosomal recessive and autosomal dominant forms; locus on X chromosome at position 22.3 (Xp 22.3). In the X-linked form, there is a mutation in gene KALIG-1, which encodes for a protein with homology to neural cell-adhesive molecule (N-CAM); this form can be linked to X-linked ichthyosis, mental retardation, chondrodysplasia punctata, and short stature. Male-to-female ratio is 5:1

Pathophysiology: Interference with the migration of endogenous gonadotropin-releasing hormone (GnRH)-secreting cells arising from the nasal placode (precursor of the nose) to the hypothalamus during fetal life resulting in agenesis of the olfactory lobes and GnRH deficiency.

Diagnosis: Clinical features, biochemical (low serum levels of androgens and positive response to GnRH stimulation), and MRI/CT imaging (unilateral or bilateral absent olfactory bulbs).

Clinical aspects: Highly variable, but characterized by GnRH deficiency with hypogonadotropic hypogonadism, delayed incomplete or absent puberty, short stature, and smelling deficiencies. Neurosensory hearing loss and mild mental retardation have been reported, but the majority of these patients have normal intelligence. Choanal atresia and cleft palate and/or lip are other common features. Renal anomalies include unilateral renal agenesis and cryptorchidism in males. Infertility, erectile dysfunction, and decreased libido are common in untreated patients. Most patients have normal lifespan. Kallmann syndrome is occasionally associated with congenital heart diseases (atrial and ventricular septal defects, transposition of the great arteries, Ebstein anomaly, aortic arch anomalies, but also atrioventricular block, bundle branch blocks, and even Wolff-Parkinson-White syndrome).

Precautions before anesthesia: Assess cardiac function and rule out any anomalies and obtain further examinations (ECG, echocardiography) if required. Evaluate renal function (creatinine, urea). Examine for any indicators of difficult airway management. Sedative premedication may be helpful in patients with mild developmental delay.

Anesthetic considerations: Choanal atresia may account for respiratory distress. Difficult airway management may be encountered in patients with cleft lip and palate. Child may be uncooperative because of anxiety and mild mental retardation. Presence of congenital heart disease may require prophylactic antibiotics (endocarditis) and invasive hemodynamic monitoring.

Other conditions to be considered: Delayed puberty secondary to idiopathic hypogonadotropic hypogonadism, which is a diagnosis of exclusion, whereas anosmia and/or associated abnormalities are typical of Kallmann syndrome.

REFERENCES:
Hardelin JP: Kallmann syndrome: Towards molecular pathogenesis. *Mol Cell Endocrinol* 179:75-81, 2001.

MacColl G, Bouloux P, Quinton R: Kallmann syndrome: Adhesion, afferents, and anosmia. *Neuron* 34:675, 2002.

Kantaputra-Gorlin Syndrome

At a glance: Polymalformative syndrome characterized by dental malformations and various distal skeletal anomalies.

Synonyms: Mesomelic Dysplasia, Thai Type; Mesomelic Dysplasia with Ankle, Carpal, and Tarsal Synostosis; Mesomelic Dysplasia, Kantaputra Type; Molarization of Anterior Teeth with Deafness.

Incidence and genetic inheritance: Incidence and mode of inheritance are unknown. Only one case report of an affected female.

Clinical aspects: Molarization and premolarization of anterior teeth, possibly as a consequence of a mesenchymal defect. Histologically, tooth structure was normal; sensorineural deafness; flared nares.

Anesthetic considerations: Careful laryngoscopy is recommended to avoid dental injuries.

REFERENCE:
Kantaputra PN, Gorlin RJ: Double dens invaginatus of molarized maxillary central incisors, premolarization of maxillary lateral incisors, multituberculism of the mandibular incisors, canines and first premolar, and sensorineural hearing loss. *Clin Dysmorphol* 1:128, 1992.

Kaplowitz-Bodurtha Syndrome

At a glance: Very rare syndrome that results from a twinning abnormality with endocrine dysfunction.

Synonym: Hypopituitarism Microphthalmia Syndrome.

Incidence and genetic inheritance: Very rare syndrome that occurs in monozygotic twins by loss of an X chromosome early in embryogenesis with complete separation of 45,X and 46,XX cell lineages at the time of the twinning event.

Clinical aspects: After intrauterine growth retardation, twins present with different physical appearance. Clinical features of the syndrome combine short stature with microphthalmos and endocrine dysfunction (hypothyroid, hypoglycemia, and hypothalamo-hypophysial axis anomalies). Micropenis and ectopic testes can be associated. Mosaicism is observed in peripheral blood, but not in skin fibroblast cultures (probably by anastomoses between the placentae of the twins).

Anesthetic considerations: No literature available. Careful intraoperative monitoring is needed. Evaluate endocrine function (clinical, laboratory, CT/MRI). Fasting should include a concomitant glucose infusion and frequent blood glucose measurements. Perioperative anesthetic management may need adaptation to endocrine function, particularly concerning adrenal function that could necessitate steroid stress dose and fluid regimen adaptation.

REFERENCE:

Kaplowitz PB, Bodurtha J, Brown J, et al: Monozygotic twins discordant for Ullrich-Turner syndrome. *Am J Med Genet* 41:78, 1991.

Kaposi Sarcoma

At a glance: Cancer-like disease that can be genetically transmitted or acquired, in association with acquired immunodeficiency syndrome (AIDS).

Synonyms: Kaposi Tumor; Kaposi Malignancy; Multiple Idiopathic Pigmented Hemangiosarcoma.

History: Idiopathic multiple pigment sarcoma described initially in 1872 by the Hungarian dermatologist Moritz Kaposi (1837–1902).

Incidence: Varies dramatically according to geography. Most common AIDS-associated malignancy in the United States: 73,000-fold more frequent in homosexual HIV-infected men than in the general population; in other HIV-transmission groups, Kaposi sarcoma (KS) affects 1 to 3% of persons other than male homosexuals (however, there is a 10,000-fold increase in HIV-infected women and nonhomosexual men). Two times more frequent in white population men than in black population men.

Genetic inheritance: Rare autosomal dominant forms (rarely familial); mostly acquired (associated with herpes virus 8 infection in AIDS patients, but overexposure to nitrite might be an alternate cause).

Pathophysiology: Formed by proliferation of abnormal vascular endothelial cells. This has been established by histochemical demonstration of factor VIII-related antigen in both the cells lining the vascular channels and in the spindle-cell component of both classic and AIDS-related Kaposi sarcoma. The tumors appear in a multicentric fashion, although metastatic lesions may develop. The cutaneous distribution is occasionally symmetrical and tends to follow the path of superficial veins.

Diagnosis: Lesions have two predominant histologic features: (a) accumulation of spindle cells and (b) presence of vascular elements. The only specific vascular element is the presence of erythrocyte-containing clefts or slits, loosely outlined by tumor cells. Other vascular elements are ectatic capillaries and lymphatics and wide-lumen sinuses.

Clinical aspects: Classic KS: Multiple red or purple dermal plaques, nodules, and tumors. Lesions occur most commonly on the lower limbs, but may also occur on the upper limbs, trunk, head, neck, and genitalia. Edema is common and hemorrhage of lesions may occur. Involvement of internal organs may occur; in fact, the disease may be exclusively visceral with no cutaneous lesions. The condition is slowly progressive, with death occurring from generalized disease with cachexia, hemorrhages, or impairment of vital organ function by tumor growth.

Endemic KS: Nodular, florid, infiltrative, or lymphadenopathic lesions. The lymphadenopathic type occurs most frequently in children and young adults and may resemble lymphoma.

Epidemic KS: Associated with AIDS. Small, slowly enlarging, rounded tumors distributed over the body. Associated with lymphadenopathy.

Precautions before anesthesia: Full history of disease progression, including previous anesthesia and present medication. Check complete blood cell count, coagulation status, and serum electrolytes. Assess airway, together with cardiac and respiratory function.

Anesthetic considerations: Difficult venous access. Difficulties with tracheal intubation because of involvement of oral mucosa, tonsils, and vocal cords.

Pharmacological implications: Effects of chemotherapy on cardiac and respiratory function.

Other conditions to be considered:

BACILLARY ANGIOMATOSIS: This is an infectious capillary proliferation and neutrophilic inflammation caused by the slow-growing gram-negative bacillus *Rochalimaea*, and difficult to distinguish from KS (skin biopsy is required).

HEMANGIOMAS AND DERMATOFIBROMA: Might occasionally and temporarily look like KS, especially in patients with Kast (also called Maffucci) syndrome (enchondroma with multiple angioma that may undergo malignant degeneration, caused by mesodermal dysplasia occurring early in life but with no established genetic transmission).

REFERENCES:

Antman K, Chang Y: Kaposi's sarcoma. *N Engl J Med* 342:1027, 2000.

Cottoni E, Masia IM, Masala MV, et al: Familial Kaposi's sarcoma: Case reports and review of the literature. *Acta Derm Venereol* 76:59, 1996.

Iscovich J, Boffetta P, Franceschi S: Classic Kaposi sarcoma: Epidemiology and risk factors. *Cancer* 88:500, 2000.

Kapur-Toriello Syndrome

At a glance: Long columella with cleft lip/palate; eye, heart, and intestinal anomalies, and mental retardation.

Genetic inheritance: Autosomal recessive.

History: First reported in 1991 (two cases).

Pathophysiology: Unknown.

Diagnosis: The presence of multiple congenital anomalies with coloboma of the iris, cardiac defects (atrial and/or and ventricular septal defects, tetralogy of Fallot), mental retardation, urogenital and ear abnormalities, and facial cleft will point to the diagnosis. Recurrent episodes of bowel obstruction. Abnormal EEG.

Clinical aspects: Severe mental retardation, congenital heart defect, cleft lip/palate, malrotation of intestines, displaced kidneys, flat-tipped, bulbous nose, long columella, microphthalmia, iris coloboma.

Precautions before anesthesia: Echocardiography to assess cardiac function. Esophageal dysfunction may lead to recurrent aspiration pneumonia.

Anesthetic considerations: As determined by cardiac function. The potential for pulmonary aspiration should be considered (rapid-sequence induction).

Patient cooperation may be limited secondary to mental retardation. Sedative and/or anxiolytic premedication and presence of the primary caregiver for induction of anesthesia may be helpful.

Pharmacological implications: Subacute bacterial endocarditis prophylaxis may be indicated.

REFERENCE:

Kapur S, Toriello HV: Apparently new MCA/MR syndrome in sibs with cleft lip and palate and other facial, eye, heart and intestine anomalies. *Am J Med Genet* 41:423, 1991.

Karandikar-Maria-Kamble Syndrome

At a glance: Genetically transmitted polymalformative syndrome characterized by cataract, mental retardation, anal atresia, and urinary defects.

Incidence and genetic inheritance: Exact incidence unknown. Autosomal recessive inheritance.

Clinical aspects: Some degree of mental retardation is usually present. Ocular abnormalities include nystagmus, ocular muscle paresis, and cataracts. Imperforate anus is common. Tetralogy of Fallot may be present. No information is available regarding other forms of congenital heart disease. The palate may be high and narrow. Genitourinary abnormalities include ectopic testes and hypospadias.

Anesthetic considerations: Considerations related to congenital heart disease and tetralogy of Fallot in particular: degree of palliation/correction, current myocardial function and medications. An abnormally shaped palate could affect ease of intubation. Patient cooperation may be limited secondary to mental retardation. Sedative and/or anxiolytic premedication and presence of the primary caregiver for induction of anesthesia may be helpful.

Pharmacological implications: Subacute bacterial endocarditis prophylaxis may be indicated.

Reference:

Karandikar S, Maria D, Kamble B: Congenital cataract with multiple congenital anomalies in a sibship. *Indian J Ophthalmol* 27:59, 1979.

Karsch-Neugebauer Syndrome

At a glance: Inherited polymalformative syndrome characterized by the presence of split-hand syndrome and nystagmus.

Incidence and genetic inheritance: A total of 15 cases have been reported in the literature. Autosomal dominant transmission, although some cases appear to occur as a consequence of gonadal mosaicism (unaffected parents giving rise to affected children).

Clinical aspects: Ocular signs include undulatory nystagmus, retinopathy, ocular muscle paresis, and, in some cases, cataracts. Classic split-hand/split-foot abnormality (ectrodactyly or lobster claw deformity), (occasionally with an articulating "cross bone") and monodactyly.

Anesthetic considerations: No significant anesthetic concerns directly associated with this medical condition. Peripheral vascular access may be challenging given the anatomical anomalies.

Other conditions to be considered: Split hand/foot deformity may also be present in the following conditions:

☞Acro-Renal-Mandibular Syndrome, ☞ADULT Syndrome, ☞Ectrodactyly Ectodermal Dysplasia and Cleft Lip-Palate (EEC) Syndrome, ☞Cleft Hand and Absent Tibia Syndrome, ☞Goltz Syndrome, and ☞Weyer Syndrome.

References:

Pilarski RT, Pauli RM, Bresnick GH, et al: Karsch-Neugebauer syndrome: Split-foot/split-hand and congenital nystagmus. *Clin Genet* 27:97, 1985.

Wong SC, Cobben JM, Hiemstra S, et al: Karsch-Neugebauer syndrome in two sibs with unaffected parents. *Am J Med Genet* 75:207, 1998.

Kartagener Syndrome

At a glance: Genetically transmitted polymalformative syndrome characterized by bronchiectasis, situs inversus, and chronic sinusitis.

Synonyms: Afzelius Syndrome; Dextrocardia-Bronchiectasis-Sinusitis; Immotile Cilia Syndrome, Kartagener type; Primary Ciliary Dyskinesia (PCD), Kartagener Type; Siewert Syndrome.

History: Genetic disorder first described by Siewert in 1904, but identified as a syndrome by the Swiss internist Manes Kartagener (1897–1975) in 1933.

Incidence: 1:32 000 live births. Primary ciliary dyskinesia (PCD), of which Kartagener's is a subtype, has an incidence of 1:16,000 live births. Only 20 to 25% of patients with situs inversus also have bronchiectasis and sinusitis.

Genetic inheritance: Autosomal recessive trait. The axoneme of cilia contains 200 different proteins, and defects in genes coding for any one of these products could conceivably be responsible for PCD and thus Kartagener syndrome. Classically, Kartagener syndrome is caused by mutations in the gene encoding axonemal dynein intermediate chain (DNAI1), which maps to 9p21-p13. Other linkage studies have mapped the phenotype to 19q and 5p in Arabic families. Another mutation causing Kartagener syndrome has been mapped to the DNAH5 gene (5p15-p14).

Pathophysiology: Kartagener syndrome is essentially a subtype of an inherited disorder called *primary ciliary dyskinesia (PCD)*, a heterogeneous disease characterized by functionally abnormal cilia that are "dysmotile" or, rarely, absent. Defects of all of the axonemal structures, alone or in combination, have been identified in association with PCD. Overly long, overly short, and normally appearing but randomly oriented cilia have been associated with PCD and Kartagener syndrome. Finally, normal ciliary ultrastructure has been described in patients with the clinical picture of Kartagener syndrome. Lack of dynein arms, which are structures that form temporary cross-bridges between adjacent ciliary filaments and are believed to be responsible for generating movement in cilia and sperm tails, remains the most common defect identified (type 1) and the one classically associated with Kartagener syndrome. Cilia of the respiratory tract and sperms are dysmotile or nonfunctional. It has also been postulated that normal visceral asymmetry is determined by movement of cilia in certain embryonic epithelial tissues; failure of embryonic cilia to function normally results in situs inversus.

Diagnosis: The most important historical fact is the onset of upper and lower respiratory tract symptoms shortly after birth in the presence of situs inversus. Family history of PCD or Kartagener syndrome is very helpful, but the diagnosis may require examination of ciliary ultrastructure. To confirm the diagnosis, biopsy of respiratory mucosa or microscopic examination of sperms is required. Measurements of airway mucociliary clearance may be a valuable screening tool for excluding PCD because absent mucociliary clearance is a hallmark of the syndrome.

Clinical aspects: Kartagener syndrome is a clinical triad of chronic bronchorrhea with bronchiectasis, chronic sinusitis, and situs inversus. It can be regarded as a subgroup of primary ciliary dyskinesia (male sterility, bronchiectasis, sinusitis) because the clinical consequences are the same. Clinical signs appear soon after birth or early in childhood. Chronic rhinitis with nasal polyposis (approximately 30% of patients), agenesis of the frontal sinuses, and repeated otitis media are common. Conductive hearing loss may result. Anosmia is a frequent finding. Repeated episodes of atelectasis and pneumonia occur. Bronchiectasis subsequently develops during childhood and adolescence and affects primarily the dependent parts of the lung. In contrast, bronchiectasis from cystic fibrosis tends to affect primarily the upper lobes of the lungs. Reactive airways disease is a common feature. The situs inversus is often complete, but may only be partial (isolated dextrocardia or isolated transposition of abdominal viscera). Presumably, in an embryo that is homozygous for the mutation causing primary ciliary dyskinesia, there is no ciliary control of organ position. Therefore, approximately 50% of patients have situs solitus of the heart (levocardia), lungs, and abdominal organs, and the other 50% have partial or complete situs inversus, that is, Kartagener syndrome. A large number of patients with situs inversus are undiagnosed and asymptomatic. Additional cardiac malformations, such as atrial septal defect, right pulmonary artery hypoplasia, and transposition of the great vessels, usually occur in patients with isolated dextrocardia, levocardia with partial situs inversus (abdominal contents transposed), and dextrocardia with situs ambiguous (abdominal contents neither left nor right sided). Up to 90% of such patients have associated congenital heart disease, whereas only approximately 3% of patients with Kartagener syndrome have additional cardiac anomalies. Headaches, often of unclear etiology, are common. Communicating hydrocephalus, possibly as a result of impaired ependymal cilia function preventing CSF resorption, can occur. Asplenia is an infrequent finding, usually only seen in patients with situs ambiguus. Males are almost universally sterile because of absent sperm motility. Most women with Kartagener syndrome are fertile, despite the belief that ciliary action moves the ovum down the Fallopian tubes. Heterozygotes have normal ciliary function and no clinical features of PCD. Defective leukocyte migration has been reported in PCD, apparently secondary to cytoplasmic microtubule defects. This leukocyte problem has not been shown to have significant implications for the clinical course. With respect to respiratory manifestations, management is directed at early and aggressive treatment of sinusitis and pulmonary infections to prevent the impairment of respiratory function. Major congenital cardiac malformations may require corrective surgery.

Precautions before anesthesia: Determine cardiac, thoracic, and abdominal anatomy prior to operation. Lung function by spirometry (forced expiratory volume at 1 second [FEV_1], forced vital capacity [FVC], FEV_1/FVC, total lung capacity, diffusing capacity of lung for carbon monoxide [DLCO]) may be normal or may show an obstructive pattern. A chest radiograph should be obtained to check for pneumonia and atelectasis. Arterial blood gases are useful if respiratory impairment is significant. Optimization of the respiratory function prior to surgery includes aggressive use of antibiotics to treat or prevent upper/lower respiratory tract infections, bronchodilators to reduce airway reactivity, and physiotherapy plus postural drainage to minimize secretions. Situs inversus, if present, is readily diagnosed by radiography. No treatment is required. If associated congenital heart disease is present, the usual considerations, such as current anatomy and functional state, current medications, endocarditis prophylaxis, and prevention of air embolism, apply. CT scan should be performed to rule out hydrocephalus and raised intracranial pressure, especially if the patient complains of headaches. Severe respiratory or cardiovascular compromise may dictate admission to an intensive care setting postoperatively or even preclude elective general anesthesia and surgery altogether.

Anesthetic considerations: Typical operations for patients with Kartagener syndrome include sinus surgery, pulmonary surgery, infertility investigations, or cardiac surgery. Local or regional anesthesia may be preferable to general anesthesia to minimize respiratory compromise. Nasal intubation may be relatively contraindicated if polyps with chronic sinusitis are present. Poor respiratory function and copious secretions secondary to bronchiectasis may make controlled ventilation and postoperative extubation difficult. Avoid increasing intracranial pressure or lowering cerebral perfusion pressure if raised intracranial pressure is a possibility. Transposed cardiac and respiratory anatomy must be kept in mind, for example, use of a right double-lumen tube instead of a left double-lumen tube and placement of an internal jugular line preferentially on the left instead of the right side.

Pharmacological implications: No specific implications are directly associated with this medical entity.

Other conditions to be considered:

☞**YOUNG SYNDROME:** Characterized by bronchiectasis, sinusitis, and obstructive azoospermia. Ciliary ultrastructure and function are normal in Young syndrome, as well as in cystic fibrosis, hypogammaglobulinemia, and allergic diathesis.

☞**PRIMARY CILIARY DYSKINESIA:** Characterized by immotility of the ciliary function in the respiratory system. Clinically, it is associated with chronic rhinitis, sinusitis, bronchitis, severely decreased mucociliary clearance of the lungs, and nasal polyps. However, there is no situs inversus in this condition.

☞**ALPHA₁-ANTITRYPSIN DEFICIENCY:** Relatively common inherited disorder and primarily presents with early-onset panacinar lung emphysema and in a minority of the patients also with liver cirrhosis.

☞**MUCOVISCIDOSIS:** Congenital multiorgan disease affecting mainly the lungs, liver, and pancreas. Frequent lung infections, hemoptysis, intolerance to exercise, presence of finger clubbing suggesting pulmonary hypertension.

REFERENCES:

Cowan MJ, Gladwin MT, Shelhamer JH: Disorders of ciliary motility. *Am J Med Sci* 321:3, 2001.

Ho AM, Friedland MJ: Kartagener's syndrome: Anesthetic considerations. *Anesthesiology* 77:386-8, 1992.

Reidy J, Sischy S, Barrow V: Anaesthesia for Kartagener's syndrome. *Br J Anaesth* 85:919, 2000.

Kasabach-Merritt Syndrome

At a glance: Characterized by the association of a vascular tumor with thrombocytopenia and coagulopathy. Histologically, it is either a kaposiform hemangioendothelioma or a tuft angioma, not a hemangioma.

Synonym: Hemangioma-Thrombocytopenia Syndrome.

Incidence: Approximately 300 cases have been reported in the literature since 1940. Slightly more frequent in females. No racial predilection.

Genetic inheritance: Unknown; seems to be more frequent in Asia.

Pathophysiology: Ecchymotic tumor develops on a vascular lesion; it usually starts in the neonatal period and grows very quickly; tumoral growth is accompanied by thrombocytopenia and hypofibrinogenemia. This disseminated intravascular coagulation (DIC) picture is secondary to entrapment of platelets within the vascular tumor.

Diagnosis: The triad of thrombocytopenia, coagulopathy, and a vascular tumor should be highly suggestive.

Clinical aspects: Enlarging hemangioma-like lesion, mainly cutaneous (especially on the extremities) but also visceral. DIC (decreased platelets and fibrinogen, presence of increased D–dimers). Often inoperable. Treatment options: vincristine, interferon-α, steroids, ticlopidine with aspirin, or radiotherapy. Untreated Kasabach-Merritt syndrome has a 10 to 37% mortality rate.

Precautions before anesthesia: Examine for airway involvement. Check complete blood count (platelet count), coagulation profile, bleeding time, and cross-match for blood even for minor surgical procedures.

Anesthetic considerations: Potential difficult airway if oropharyngeal or neck involvement is present. Anticipate the need for blood products to treat anemia and/or coagulopathy. Do not transfuse platelets because they will immediately be trapped within the tumor with an ensuing increase in size. Effect of chemotherapy on the cardiac and respiratory system must be considered.

Pharmacological implications No specific pharmacological implications with this condition; however, patients treated with chemotherapy and corticosteroids (perioperative stress dose) must be prepared for anesthesia accordingly. Avoid nonsteroidal anti-inflammatory drugs secondary to their effects on platelets.

Other conditions to be considered:

CONGENITAL HEMANGIOMAS: Share many similarities with Kasabach-Merritt syndrome, but without the coagulation disorders; they usually regress between 5 and 9 years of age.

☞KLIPPEL-TRENAUNAY SYNDROME: Congenital arteriovenous malformation usually located on a single extremity resulting in skeletal and soft tissue hypertrophy.

REFERENCES:

David TJ: Hemangioma with thrombocytopenia (Kasabach-Merritt syndrome). *Arch Dis Child* 58:1022, 1953.

Enjolras O, Wassef M, Mazoyer E, et al: Infants with Kasabach-Merritt syndrome do not have "true" hemangiomas. *J Pediatr* 130:631, 1997.

Maguiness S, Guenther L: Kasabach-Merritt syndrome. *J Cutan Med Surg* 6:335, 2002.

Kashani-Strom-Utley Syndrome

At a glance: Polymalformative syndrome characterized by hypoplastic pulmonary arteries and aorta and urinary tract malformations.

Synonyms: Hypoplastic Pulmonary Arteries and Aorta with Obstructive Uropathy; Pulmonary and Aortic Stenosis with Obstructive Uropathy.

Incidence and genetic inheritance: Two cases in siblings have been described. Autosomal recessive inheritance.

Clinical aspects: Diffuse hypoplasia of the pulmonary arteries and the ascending aorta resulted in progressive right heart failure, systemic hypertension, chronic malabsorption, and failure to thrive. Urinary tract abnormalities included obstructive uropathy with reflux and hydronephrosis. The authors characterized the disease as possibly representing hypoplasia of the arterial vascular system.

Anesthetic considerations: Evaluate current cardiac status by history, physical examination, and investigations (electrocardiogram,

echocardiogram). Consultation with cardiologist to evaluate and optimize management, especially if cor pulmonale is present. Endocarditis prophylaxis may be required. Evaluate renal function (creatinine, blood urea nitrogen levels). Anesthetic techniques that minimize myocardial depression and pulmonary vascular resistance may be tolerated best. Inotropic support may be required if cor pulmonale is present.

Pharmacological implications: Avoid drugs with predominantly renal elimination in the presence of renal insufficiency.

REFERENCE:

Kashani IA, Strom CM, Utley JE, et al: Hypoplastic pulmonary arteries and aorta with obstructive uropathy in 2 siblings. *Angiology* 35:252, 1984.

Kasznica-Carlson-Coppedge Syndrome

At a glance: Polymalformative syndrome characterized by multiple skeletal malformation reported in a single female stillbirth.

Synonyms: Ectrodactyly with Spina Bifida and Cardiomyopathy.

Incidence and genetic inheritance: Single case report of female fetus aborted at approximately 34 weeks' gestational age for intrauterine death.

Clinical aspects: Craniofacial abnormalities were mild retrognathia and high-arched palate. Ear structure was simplified. There was a membranous-type ventricular septal defect and single umbilical artery. Spina bifida with myelomeningocele was present, as was ectrodactyly (absent right second and third digits and absent left second, third, and fourth digits) of the feet.

Anesthetic considerations: The only case reported was stillborn; however, the anesthetic considerations would be as follows in case of surgery for a surviving person: retrognathia could make intubation difficult. Considerations for patients with congenital heart disease include cardiovascular anatomy and function, current medications, endocarditis prophylaxis, and prevention of air embolus. Patients with uncorrected myelomeningocele must be handled carefully to prevent damage to or rupture of the sac. Latex precautions or allergy are a concern in these patients. ☞Arnold-Chiari malformation (cerebellar tonsillar compression of brainstem) is commonly associated with spina bifida and may cause obstructive hydrocephalus.

REFERENCE:

Kasznica J, Carlson JA, Coppedge D: Ectrodactyly, retrognathism, abnormal ears, highly arched palate, spina bifida, congenital heart defect, single umbilical artery. *Am J Med Genet* 40:414, 1991.

Katsantoni-Papadakou-Lagoyanni Syndrome

At a glance: Polymalformative syndrome associated with ptosis, mental retardation, and hair anomalies.

Synonym: Trichodermal Syndrome with Mental Retardation.

Incidence and genetic inheritance: Exact incidence and pattern of inheritance unknown. There is only one report of two siblings who died of liver problems in infancy.

Clinical aspects: Ocular manifestations include blepharoptosis and nystagmus. Neurologic signs are torticollis and mental retardation. The tongue has hyperplastic papillae. Abnormally fine, sparse, brittle hair is present on the body, proximal phalanges of the fingers and toes, and the head. Hair on the body and digits disappeared by the third month of life, leaving behind large dermal pores.

Anesthetic considerations: Enlarged tongue caused by hyperplastic papillae may cause difficulty with face-mask ventilation and possibly endotracheal intubation. Torticollis, or contraction of the cervical muscles, may make airway management awkward, but the spasticity should resolve with administration of neuromuscular blockade. Liver function should be carefully assessed, since both patients died from liver problems. Developmentally delayed patients may be uncooperative.

Pharmacological implications: Careful dosage of drugs with predominantly hepatic metabolism/elimination.

REFERENCE:

Katsantoni A, Papadakou-Lagoyanni S, Micheloyannis J, et al: New syndrome of trichodermal defect and mental retardation. *Am J Med Genet* 18:329, 1984.

Katz Syndrome

At a glance: Inherited polymalformative syndrome characterized by typical facial features, enlarged viscera, and skeletal anomalies. Short stature, cranial hyperostosis, hepatomegaly, diabetes. Probably a variant of autosomal recessive type of craniometaphyseal dysplasia.

Incidence and genetic inheritance: Approximately 30 cases have been reported. Autosomal recessive inheritance with consanguinity being a risk factor. The genetic defect has been mapped to 6q21-q22.

Clinical aspects: Craniofacial abnormalities include thickening of the cranial bone with scaphocephaly (long, narrow cranium as a result of premature closure of the sagittal suture) and frontal bossing, micrognathia with an arched palate, and a beaked nose. This autosomal recessive form is clinically more severe than the autosomal dominant form (☞Craniodiaphyseal Dysplasia). Cranial hyperostosis frequently results in cranial nerve compressions (blindness, deafness, facial palsy) and nasal obstruction. Mild mental retardation is possible. Hepatosplenomegaly is common, as is diabetes mellitus. Abnormalities of the digits include brachydactyly and clinodactyly, and the metacarpal bones may be abnormal. Patients are usually small as a consequence of advanced bone age and early growth plate closure. Fine hair and diffuse skin pigmentation often complete the clinical picture.

Anesthetic considerations: Potential for difficult airway if micrognathia is present. Early closure of cranial suture lines may lead to intracranial hypertension. Liver function studies (aspartate aminotransferase, alanine aminotransferase, alkaline phosphatase, bilirubin, international normalized ratio [INR], partial thromboplastin time) and a complete blood count should be done; splenic sequestration of platelets may be present. Perioperative management of diabetes mellitus depends on the timing and duration of surgery; involvement of an endocrinologist may be helpful. Nasal breathing as well as nasal passage of tubes (nasogastric or endotracheal) may be impossible. Avoid medications and anesthesia techniques known to potentially increase intracranial pressure in patients with craniosynostosis.

Other condition to be considered:

☞**CRANIODIAPHYSEAL DYSPLASIA:** Progressive hyperostosis leading to lifelong thickening of craniofacial bones and widening of the metaphyses of long bones. Autosomal dominant.

REFERENCES:

Elcioglu N, Hall CM: Temporal aspects in craniometaphyseal dysplasia: Autosomal recessive type. *Am J Med Genet* 76:245, 1998.

Iughetti P, Alanso LG, Wilcox W, et al: Mapping of the autosomal recessive (AR) craniometaphyseal dysplasia locus to chromosome region 6q21-22 and confirmation of genetic heterogeneity for mild AR spondylocostal dysplasia. *Am J Med Genet* 95:482, 2000.

Kaufman Oculo-Cerebro-Facial Syndrome

At a glance: Polymalformative syndrome of unknown origin characterized by particular facial features and mental retardation.

Synonym: Mental Retardation-Microcornea-Microcephaly Syndrome.

Incidence and genetic inheritance: No more than 10 cases have been described to date. Autosomal recessive.

Pathophysiology: Unknown.

Diagnosis: Based on clinical features. Radiologic examination reveals a turricephalic skull, marked craniofacial disproportion, mild kyphoscoliosis, coxa valga, bilateral hypoplasia of the first ray of both hands, and mild bilateral hypoplasia of the terminal and intermediate phalanges of the hands and feet.

Clinical aspects: Intrauterine and postnatal growth retardation. Neonatal respiratory distress. Lack of specific manifestations in early infancy, together with a changing phenotype. Congenital hypotonia, mental retardation, and microcephaly. Ophthalmologic features include hypertelorism, telecanthus, epicanthus, eyelid ptosis, blepharophimosis, up-slanting palpebral fissures, nystagmus, exotropia, strabismus, amblyopia, myopia, microcornea, optic atrophy, and sparse and laterally broad eyebrows. Other facial features may include a flat philtrum, micrognathia, poorly formed teeth, high and narrow palate, preauricular tags, and small and low-set ears. Lordosis, flat feet, joint contractures, constipation, large clitoris, edema, and cutis laxa may occasionally be present.

Precautions before anesthesia: Careful assessment of respiratory function and neuromuscular development.

Anesthetic considerations: Expect difficult laryngoscopy because of micrognathia and high, narrow palate. Peripheral vascular access may be difficult secondary to joint contractures and cutis laxa. The presence and severity of the congenital hypotonia dictates the management of intraoperative and postoperative ventilation support and intensive care plan.

Pharmacological implications: Use of succinylcholine in presence of generalized hypotonia is better avoided. No reports associated with malignant hyperthermia exist.

Other conditions to be considered:

CONGENITAL RUBELLA SYNDROME: Microcephaly, cataracts/congenital glaucoma, congenital heart disease, deafness, purpura, splenomegaly, jaundice, and mental retardation; a result of maternal infection in early pregnancy (☞TORCH-syndrome).

☞LOWE SYNDROME: Congenital disorder characterized by cataracts, infantile glaucoma, renal dysfunction and intellectual impairment.

☞**DE TONI DEBRÉ FANCONI SYNDROME:** An inherited condition involving a generalized transport defect in the proximal tubules resulting in renal losses of glucose, calcium, phosphate, uric acid, amino acids, and bicarbonate leading to renal failure, osteomalacia, and short stature.

REFERENCES:

Briscioli V, Manoukian S, Selicorni A, et al: Kaufman oculocerebrofacial syndrome in a girl of 15 years. *Am J Med Genet* 58:213, 1995.

Kaufman R, Rimoin DL, Prensky AL, et al: An oculocerebrofacial syndrome. *Birth Defects Orig Artic Ser* 7:135, 1971.

Kaveggia Syndrome

At a glance: Microcephaly with severe mental retardation and spastic disturbances of movements with athetoid cerebral palsy, dwarfism, and facial dysmorphism.

Synonyms: Kaveggia-Neuhäuser Syndrome; Mental Retardation-Athetosis-Megalocornea Syndrome; BD Syndrome. The name BD syndrome derives from the initials of the last name of the two described individuals (J.B. and D.D.).

Incidence and genetic inheritance: Approximately 20 cases have been reported. Only two of them were sporadic cases. Possibly autosomal recessive inheritance. However, the suspicion of a new autosomal dominant mutation has been considered.

Clinical aspects: Mental retardation may be mild to severe. Congenital hypotonia is one of the key features of this disorder. Other neurological findings include seizures, athetoid cerebral palsy with poor coordination, swallowing difficulties, and delayed myelination. Facial anomalies include macro- or microcephaly, frontal bossing, antimongoloid slanting of the eyes, epicanthal folds, widened nasal root, small mandible, and elongated upper lip. Megalocornea (corneal diameter ≥ 13 mm) is another key finding. (Mental retardation and megalocornea are the two minimal diagnostic criteria.) Iris hypoplasia may be present. Short stature, scoliosis, asteopenia, obesity, primary hypothyreoidism, and fleshy ears have been described in some patients.

Anesthetic considerations: Airway management might be difficult, depending on the severity of facial malformations. Given the possibility of swallowing difficulties, it seems appropriate to do a rapid-sequence induction technique. Protect the eyes with lubricants and keep them shut with tape. Muscle relaxants should only be used once the airway has been secured. Hypotonia makes the use of a peripheral nerve stimulator almost mandatory. Avoid drugs that may potentially trigger seizures. Careful positioning and padding is required (spasticity, osteopenia). Cooperation in mental retardation patients may be limited and sedative/anxiolytic premedication as well as the presence of the primary caregiver for induction of anesthesia may be helpful. Postoperative mechanical ventilation should be considered.

REFERENCES:

Antinolo G, Rufo M, Borrego S, et al: Megalocornea-mental retardation syndrome: An additional case. *Am J Med Genet* 52:196, 1994.

Neuhäuser G, Kaveggia EG, Opitz JM: The BD syndrome. A "new" multiple congenital anomalies/mental retardation syndrome with athetoid cerebral palsy. *Z Kinderheilkd* 120:191, 1975.

Neuhäuser G, Kaveggia EG, France TD, et al: Syndrome of mental retardation, seizures, hypotonic cerebral palsy and megalocorneae, recessively inherited. *Z Kinderheilkd* 120:1, 1975.

Kawasaki Disease

At a glance: Self-limited vasculitic syndrome of unknown etiology characterized by fever, cervical adenopathies, and cardiac involvement.

Synonym: Mucocutaneous Lymph Node Syndrome.

Incidence: Asian people are at greater risk: 5000–6000 new cases per year occur in Japan versus 3000 in the United States. Males are affected 1.5 times more often than females. Kawasaki disease (KD) is currently the leading cause of acquired heart disease in the United States among children younger than 5 years. Mortality from coronary artery abnormalities, including coronary aneurysms, is reported in 20 to 25% of untreated individuals.

Genetic inheritance: Etiology of KD is unknown. Several possibilities are considered, including an infectious etiology (retrovirus?), an immunologic abnormality, and even a toxic cause (carpet shampoo). Clinical and epidemiologic data support an infectious etiology, but many authors think that an autoimmune component or genetic predisposition also exists.

Pathophysiology: Necrotizing vasculitis of medium-size muscular arteries, including coronary and cerebral vessels. Arteries show focal segmental destruction, with subsequent ectasia and formation of aneurysms in 15 to 25% of children. Several infectious causes of KD have been theorized and include Ebstein-Barr virus, retroviruses, *Streptococcus pyogenes* and *viridans*, *Staphylococcus*, *Chlamydia*, *Propionibacterium,* and *Pseudomonas* species. However, conventional bacterial and viral cultures and serologic studies have not confirmed an infectious cause. Other postulated etiologic agents are immunizations, medications, and environmental agents, such as exposure to rug shampooing agents or house dust mites. The finding of a skewed T-cell receptor response in the myocardium and the coronary arteries led to a search for superantigens, such as toxic shock syndrome toxin-1 produced by *Staphylococcus aureus*. Immunohistochemical findings lend support to the hypothesis of a proinflammatory cell-mediated immune reaction possibly triggered by a superantigen or a conventional antigen.

Diagnosis: Clinical diagnosis. No diagnostic laboratory tests are available. The Centers for Disease Control and Prevention in Atlanta (USA) defines a case of KD as illness in a patient with fever of

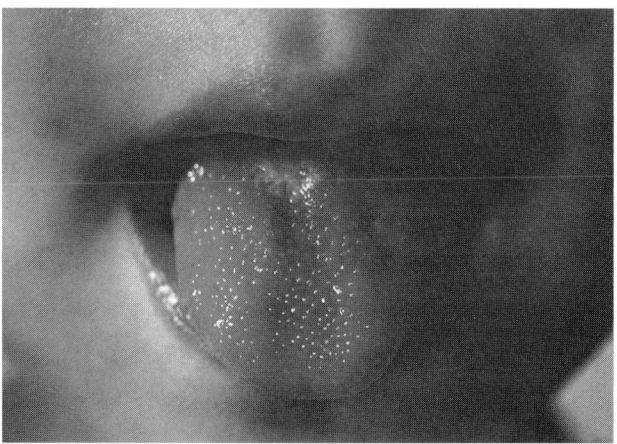

Kawasaki disease   Strawberry tongue in a child with Kawasaki disease. See color plates.

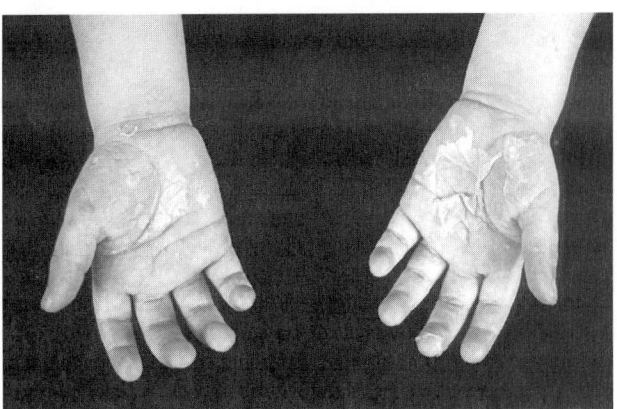

Kawasaki disease Palmar erytherma and desquamation of the skin in a child with Kawasaki disease.

5 or more days' duration (or fever until the of administration of intravenous immunoglobulin, if this is given before the fifth day of fever), and the presence of at least 4 of the following 5 clinical signs:

- Rash
- Cervical lymphadenopathy (at least one lymph node ≥ 1.5 cm in diameter)
- Bilateral conjunctival injection
- Oral mucosal changes (injected or fissured lips, injected pharynx, "strawberry" tongue)
- Peripheral extremity changes (erythema of palms or soles, edema of the hands or feet, or generalized or periungual desquamation).

Patients whose illness does not meet the above KD case definition but who have fever and coronary artery abnormalities are classified as having atypical or incomplete KD.

Clinical aspects: Occurs primarily in children within the first years of life. Main clinical signs are fever, conjunctivitis, inflammation of the mucous membranes and tongue (strawberry tongue), swollen erythematous hands and feet, truncal rashes, and diffuse lymphadenopathy. Cardiac complications include pericarditis, myocarditis, myocardial infarction, or ischemia as a result of coronary artery thrombosis or stenosis, and valvular dysfunction. Pneumonitis and pleural effusions can occur. Cerebral hemorrhage caused by aneurysm rupture has been reported. Other CNS complications are cranial nerve palsies, aseptic meningitis, and subdural effusions. Aneurysmal rupture of any affected vessel present with hemorrhage. Stenosis of vessels can cause hypoperfusion of distal extremities or other organs. Hepatic involvement occurs in less than 10% of cases, and renal involvement occurs in less than 1%. Anemia may be present. Management consists of γ-globulin and aspirin. Corticosteroids, pentoxifylline (a methyl-xanthine compound that inhibits TNF-α messenger RNA-transcription), ulinastatin (a human trypsin inhibitor that inhibits neutrophil elastase), abciximab (a platelet glycoprotein IIb/IIIa receptor antagonist), monoclonal antibodies, and cytotoxic agents (cyclophosphamide) have all been used with variable success in these patients.

Precautions before anesthesia: No elective procedures during the course of the disease. Rule out cardiac involvement prior to anesthesia: history and physical examination, electrocardiogram (dysrhythmias), echocardiogram to detect myocardial or valvular

dysfunction (usually mitral or tricuspid regurgitation), and even coronary angiogram to confirm myocardial ischemia caused by coronary artery aneurysms or stenosis. Cardiac medications should be continued throughout the perioperative period. Radiography or CT scan of the chest to rule out pulmonary involvement. Any neurologic deficits should be documented prior to anesthesia. If cerebral hemorrhage has occurred, check for signs of raised intracranial pressure. Complete blood count to check for anemia; electrolyte levels to rule out abnormalities that may occur with some cardiac medications (diuretics, angiotensin-converting enzyme inhibitors) and renal dysfunction.

Anesthetic considerations: Maintain optimum balance of myocardial oxygen supply to demand ratio if myocardial perfusion is compromised. Five-lead ECG monitoring (leads II and V_5) for signs of myocardial ischemia is mandatory. Avoid myocardial depressants if cardiac function is depressed. Have vasoactive and antidysrhythmic medications readily available to manage complications. Avoid hemodynamic instability at any stage of anesthesia to minimize the risk of aneurysm rupture. Maintenance of normal cerebral perfusion pressure in the presence of cerebral hemorrhage with raised intracranial pressure. Use of invasive arterial and central venous monitoring may be useful. Platelet dysfunction as a consequence of treatment with aspirin may predispose to increased blood loss. Careful laryngoscopy should be performed to avoid injury to inflamed lips, tongue, and oropharynx. Patients should be monitored for myocardial ischemia postoperatively.

Pharmacological implications: Avoid cardiodepressive drugs. Steroid supplementation if necessary. Some patients may be on antiplatelet drugs, heparin, or oral anticoagulation therapy. Check before (regional) anesthesia.

Other conditions to be considered: Other vasculitic diseases of children, particularly the following:

☞**SYSTEMIC LUPUS ERYTHEMATOSUS:** Characterized by unpredictable exacerbations and remissions of inflammatory multisystemic disorder of connective tissue. The circulation of immune complexes and activation of complement leads to involvement mainly of the skin, joints, kidneys, serosal membranes, lungs, gastrointestinal tract, and heart.

☞**CHAUFFARD SYNDROME:** Chronic inflammatory disease of variable severity that involves the joints and potentially also the connective tissues and viscera.

☞**POLYARTERITIS NODOSA:** Severe condition very similar to Kawasaki disease with unexplained fever, major alteration of physical status, and histologic lesions of arteritis nodosa (often discovered on postmortem examinations only).

REFERENCES:

Gedalia A: Kawasaki disease: An update. *Curr Rheumatol Rep* 4:25, 2002.

Newburger JW, Takahashi M, Gerber MA, et al: Committee on Rheumatic Fever, Endocarditis, and Kawasaki Disease, Council on Cardiovascular Disease in the Young, American Heart Association. Diagnosis, treatment, and long-term management of Kawasaki disease: A statement for health professionals from the Committee on Rheumatic Fever, Endocarditis, and Kawasaki Disease, Council on Cardiovascular Disease in the Young, American Heart Association. *Pediatrics* 114:1708, 2004.

National Center for Infectious Diseases. Kawasaki Syndrome. http://www.cdc.gov./ncidod/diseases/kawasaki/index.htm

Waldron RJ: Kawasaki disease and anaesthesia. *Anaesth Intensive Care* 21:213, 1993.

Kawashima-Tsuji Syndrome

At a glance: Polymalformative syndrome characterized by microcephaly, typical facial features, deafness, and mental retardation.

Synonym: Microcephaly-Deafness Syndrome.

Incidence and genetic inheritance: Exact incidence unknown; one case report of an affected mother and son. Suggested autosomal dominant inheritance.

Clinical aspects: Microcephaly, which apparently resolved in the mother by age 26 years. Facial asymmetry with prominent glabella, protruding lower lip, micrognathia, and low-set, cup-shaped ears were described. Both subjects suffered from mental retardation and deafness.

Anesthetic considerations: Primary concern is possible difficult airway management because of micrognathia. Patients with developmental delay may be uncooperative and be better off with sedative premedication.

REFERENCE:

Kawashima H, Tsuji N: Syndrome of microcephaly, deafness/malformed ears, mental retardation and peculiar facies in a mother and son. *Clin Genet* 31:303, 1987.

KBG Syndrome

At a glance: Polymalformative syndrome characterized by short stature (dwarfism), mental retardation, and skeletal anomalies.

Synonyms: Herrmann-Pallister Syndrome; Herrmann-Pallister-Opitz Syndrome.

History: First described in 1975 by J. Herrmann, P.D. Pallister, W. Tiddy, and J.M. Opitz in two families with multiple affected members. The designation "KBG-Syndrome" reflects Opitz's preference of using the initials of patients' last names.

Incidence and genetic inheritance: To date, about 41 cases have been reported. Autosomal dominant, but also autosomal recessive transmission has been suspected in some cases.

Clinical aspects: These patients have short stature (often below the third percentile; particularly short trunk, which may in part be due to anterior wedging and abnormal upper and lower plates of the vertebrae) and typical facial features that may include brachycephaly, hypertelorism, wide and bushy eyebrows, large prominent ears, anteverted nostrils with small alae nasi, long philtrum, and oligo- and/or macrodontia. Cryptorchidism seems to be quite common in male patients. Other features that have been described in some of the patients include low anterior and posterior hairline, fused or wide upper central incisors, short metacarpalia and clinodactyly, accessory cervical ribs, thoracic kyphosis, and cardiac defects (e.g., ventricular septal defect).

Mental retardation, however, is a constant finding and may be severe and accompanied by seizures. Hypoplasia of the cerebellar vermis or the posterior fossa could be demonstrated in some patients.

Anesthetic considerations: If kyphosis is severe, a chest radiograph should be obtained. Lung function tests are most likely difficult to perform on these mentally delayed patients. Echocardiography may not only be required to exclude structural cardiac lesions, but also to determine the presence of signs of cor pulmonale. Central neuraxial anesthesia techniques may be difficult to perform due to the vertebral anomalies. Patient cooperation could be limited secondary to mental retardation. Sedative and/or anxiolytic premedication and the presence of the primary caregiver for induction of anesthesia may be helpful.

Pharmacological implications: Subacute bacterial endocarditis prophylaxis may be required. Consider interactions of anesthetics with chronic anti-seizure therapy.

REFERENCES:

Bracanti F, D'Avanzo MG, Digilio MC, et al: KBG syndrome in a cohort of Italian patients. *Am J Med Genet* 131A:144, 2004.

Smithson SF, Thompson EM, McKinnon AG, et al: The KGB syndrome. *Clin Dysmorphol* 9:87, 2000.

Zollino M, Battaglia A, D'Avanzo MG, et al: Six additional cases of the KBG syndrome: Clinical reports and outline of the diagnostic criteria. *Am J Med Genet* 52:302, 1994.

Kearns-Sayre Syndrome

At a glance: Kearns-Sayre Syndrome (KSS) is a mitochondrial encephalomyopathy characterized by progressive external ophthalmoplegia, atypical retinitis pigmentosa, and cardiomyopathy.

Synonyms: Chronic Progressive External Ophthalmoplegia (CPEO) with Myopathy; CPEO with Ragged-Red Fibers; Progressive External Ophthalmoplegia with Ragged-Red Fibers; Kearns Syndrome; Kearns-Sayre Mitochondrial Cytopathy; Kearns-Sayre-Shy-Daroff Syndrome; Ophthalmoplegia Pigmentary Degeneration of Retina and Cardiomyopathy Syndrome; Oculo-Cranio-Somatic Syndrome; Ophthalmoplegia Plus Syndrome; Barnard-Scholz Syndrome.

History: The combination of ophthalmoplegia and retinal degeneration was first described by the two American ophthalmologists R.I. Barnard and R.O. Scholz in 1944; however, the syndrome now bears the names of the two Americans Thomas P. Kearns, a neuro-ophthalmologist, and George P. Sayre, an ophthalmologist, who published their findings in two patients in 1958.

Incidence: Approximately 300 cases have been reported. No sex or race predilection.

Genetic inheritance: Mitochondrial (deletions in mitochondrial DNA). Incidence of affected children is dependent upon maternal mutant load. Mitochondrial DNA encodes proteins that are part of the respiratory chain complexes.

Pathophysiology: In vitro studies of mitochondrial metabolism have identified defects in the respiratory chain and in the oxidative phosphorylation system. These defects are responsible for the elevated levels of serum lactate found during and after exercise.

Diagnosis: Clinical and laboratory confirmation of elevated pyruvate and lactate. Light microscopy reveals "ragged-red muscle fibers," which are caused by the presence of abnormal mitochondria. Electron microscopy demonstrates clusters of cells filled with abnormally enlarged mitochondria (paracrystalline inclusions). The biochemical defect often appears segmental on histochemistry.

Clinical aspects: KSS is a multiorgan disease characterized by the clinical triad of a chronic, progressive, external ophthalmoplegia, retinal pigment degeneration (with progressive loss of vision), and onset before the age of 20 years. Significant other clinical findings may include increased levels of protein in the cerebrospinal fluid, dementia, encephalopathy, cerebellar ataxia, bulbar weakness (dysphagia, which may also be related to cricopharyngeal achalasia), electroencephalographic anomalies (including seizures), sensorineural hearing loss, corneal anomalies (with increased risk of spontaneous perforation), but also cardiac anomalies (e.g., high-degree atrioventricular heart blocks, QT prolongation with the risk of sudden death, dilated cardiomyopathy, mitral valve prolapse, congestive heart failure), endocrine anomalies (hypogonadism, short stature due to growth hormone deficiency, hyperaldosteronism, diabetes mellitus, hypoparathyroidism, hypothyroidism), renal tubular acidosis, and myopathy with weakness. The clinical spectrum is related to the proportion of normal and mutant DNA.

Precautions before anesthesia: Due to the fact that KSS may affect many organ systems, a thorough review of the patient history and the actual clinical findings is necessary. Special attention has to focus on the cardiac, endocrine, and renal issues (check electrolytes and acid–base balance). Also assess the degree of muscle weakness to decide if postoperative mechanical ventilation may be required.

Mental retardation, loss of vision and hearing may affect patient cooperation. Sedative premedication and/or the presence of the primary caregiver for induction of anesthesia may be helpful.

Anesthetic considerations: The major anesthetic complication is sudden third-degree atrioventricular block. The patient should therefore be closely monitored at all times and a transcutaneous cardiac pacemaker should be easily available throughout the perioperative period. Avoid profound sedation with spontaneous ventilation. Meticulous care should be paid to temperature control (shivering may significantly increase lactate production and result in metabolic acidosis), glucose homeostasis, and ventilation with proper airway management and oxygenation. Avoid hypocarbia since it inhibits the pyruvate decarboxylase, which may further increase the serum lactate levels. Regular blood gas analyses (including lactate and glucose measurements) are recommended. A rapid-sequence induction may be necessary in the presence of dysphagia. Postoperative respiratory failure is a known risk in these patients and, depending on the surgical procedure, an intensive care unit bed with the possibility of mechanical ventilation should be available. A stress-free anesthesia technique reduces not only the metabolic response to surgery, but also lactate production.

Pharmacological implications: Patients are extremely sensitive to induction agents. Caution with benzodiazepines in view of myopathy. Extreme caution with opioids in spontaneously breathing patients. Careful inhalation anesthesia with isoflurane has been found to be safe. Local anesthetic techniques may be used. In order of preference, these agents are chloroprocaine, procaine, prilocaine, lignocaine, mepivacaine, etidocaine, bupivacaine, tetracaine, dibucaine, and cocaine. However, articaine administration for a tooth extraction resulted in transient exacerbation of neuromuscular symptoms in one patient. Because of muscle wasting, neuromuscular blockers should be used with a nerve stimulator only. Although the pathways of malignant hyperthermia and mitochondrial myopathy are different, the potential for malignant hyperthermia has been suggested after succinylcholine; consequently, it might be wise to avoid this agent. No reports of malignant hyperthermia with use of volatile anesthetic in these patients, but caution should be used. Avoid proepileptic drugs. Large doses of propofol should be avoided because of its blocking effects on mitochondrial complex 1.

Other conditions to be considered: Other mitochondrial myopathies, especially the following:

☞**MELAS Syndrome:** Progressive neurodegenerative disorder with lactic acidosis, stroke-like episodes. Deafness and diabetes mellitus are frequent.

☞**MERFF Syndrome:** Mitochondrial encephalopathy characterized by myoclonic epilepsy, muscle weakness, and progressive external ophthalmoplegia.

☞**Pearson Syndrome:** A mitochondrial disease presenting in infancy with sideroblastic anemia or pancytopenia, defective oxidative phosphorylation, exocrine pancreatic insufficiency and variable degrees of hepatic, renal, and endocrine failure.

REFERENCES:

Lauwers MH, Van Lersberghe C, Camu F: Inhalation anesthesia and the Kearns-Sayre syndrome. *Anaesthesia* 49:876, 1994.

Maslow A, Lisbon A: Anesthetic consideration in patients with mitochondrial dysfunction. *Anesth Analg* 76:884, 1993.

Wallace JJ, Perndt H, Skinner M: Anesthesia and mitochondrial disease. *Paediatr Anaesth* 8:249, 1998.

Kennedy Disease

At a glance: X-linked disorder characterized by degeneration of both sensory and lower motor neurons supplying the limb and bulbar musculature caused by a defect in the androgen receptor. Extraocular muscles are spared, possibly because of reduced numbers of androgen receptors in these muscles.

Synonyms: Bulbospinal Neuronopathy; Kennedy Spinal and Bulbar Muscular Atrophy; X-Linked Bulbospinal Muscular Atrophy.

Incidence: Approximately 1:40–50,000 males are affected worldwide (seems consistently more frequent in western Finland).

Genetic inheritance: X-linked recessive (only males can express the full phenotype). Affects mainly Caucasians and Asians, but not Africans. The genetic defect is located at the *DXYS1* marker on the proximal long arm of the X chromosome (Xq11-12). Females are carriers.

Pathophysiology: Degeneration of sensory and motor neurons supplying the limb and bulbar musculature, sparing extraocular muscles (possibly because of reduced numbers of androgen receptors in these muscles). Caused by an expanded trinucleotide (cytosine-adenine-guanine [CAG]) repeat in the androgen receptor within the first exon of the gene. The disease mechanism likely involves toxicity of an expanded polyglutamine tract in the androgen receptor protein. Electromyography and muscle histology demonstrate neurogenic atrophy. Necropsy shows diffuse loss and atrophy of anterior horn cells in the spinal cord.

Diagnosis: Laboratory findings include elevated serum creatine kinase, pronounced involutional changes in Leydig cells, hypobetalipoproteinemia, and abnormalities in the androgen receptor gene.

Clinical aspects: This is a slowly progressing muscle atrophy associated with mild androgen insensitivity that affects only males. Muscle atrophy is initially not obvious and usually starts between 20 and 50 years of age. Its onset is insidious and early signs may include difficulties with walking and a tendency to fall. Deep tendon reflexes are decreased and some patients complain about muscle cramps and/or intention tremor. The muscle weakness not only involves the extremities, but also the facial muscles (including facial fasciculations). Calf hypertrophy may occur. Over the following 10–20 years, most patients will start to experience difficulties with climbing stairs or other strenuous efforts, while about one third will even be wheelchair-bound. Most patients will also suffer from involvement of bulbar muscles with dysphagia, dysarthria (with a change in the voice character, e.g., a more nasal sound) and drooling. Bulbar palsy results in increased risk for aspiration and consecutive pneumonias, which can rarely be life-threatening. Lower motor and primary sensory neuropathy have been described and are due to degeneration of anterior horn cells and dorsal root ganglia, respectively. The disease may be symmetrical or asymmetrical.

Gynecomastia is an almost constant finding and usually the first sign of androgen insensitivity, manifesting already in adolescence. Testicular atrophy, erectile dysfunction, oligospermia/azoospermia with decreased fertility or sterility, as well as diminished secondary sex characteristics are frequently found. Diabetes mellitus has been described in some patients. Life expectancy is usually not affected, except when complications from aspiration/pneumonia arise.

Precautions before anesthesia: Preoperative assessment should evaluate the degree of muscle weakness and assess the neurologic function. Lung function tests may be indicated. Check fasting blood glucose concentration.

Anesthetic considerations: A rapid-sequence induction technique is recommended if bulbar symptoms are present. Depending on the degree of muscle weakness and the extent of surgery, postoperative mechanical ventilation may be required.

Pharmacological implications: To date, there have been no indications that this disease is associated with malignant hyperthermia. Nevertheless, succinylcholine should not be used, since it could result in an acute hyperkalemic response with cardiovascular collapse. Although this risk most likely decreases with progression of muscle atrophy (less muscle mass), this should not encourage the use of succinylcholine. The sensitivity to neuromuscular blockers may be altered and the use of a peripheral nerve stimulator is recommended. Opioids should be titrated carefully. Central neuraxial anesthesia techniques are controversial in this kind of disease, however, they have been used successfully.

Other conditions to be considered: Several syndromes resemble Kennedy syndrome, including the following:

☞**Amyotrophic Lateral Sclerosis:** Upper motor involvement and weakness more distal than proximal.

☞**Landouzy-Dejerine Syndrome:** Hereditary motor neuropathy, typical muscle biopsy and EMG patterns. Weakness of facial, shoulder, and arm muscles.

☞**Myasthenia Gravis:** A neuromuscular disorder characterized by muscle weakness and rapid muscle fatigue. Suggestive EMG tracings, involvement of extraocular muscles and presence of antibodies.

Oculopharyngeal Muscular Dystrophy (OPMD): Autosomal dominant, slow progression with dysphagia to solids and water. Other features include ptosis and ophthalmoparesis, suggestive muscle biopsy, and genetic marker. Characterized by late-onset (usually after age 45 years).

☞**Progressive Bulbar Palsy of Childhood:** Inherited motor neuropathy affecting the lower six cranial nerves but sparing the limbs; deafness; X-linked or autosomal recessive. Age of onset in late childhood. Other features include excessive drooling, dysarthria, recurrent pulmonary aspiration, and pneumonia eventually evolving to pulmonary failure. Limb involvement and pyramidal tract signs may develop. Most often fatal within the first two decades of life.

References:

Dejager S, Bry-Gauillard H, Bruckert E, et al: A comprehensive endocrine description of Kennedy's disease revealing androgen insensitivity linked to CAG repeat length. *J Clin Endocrinol Metab* 87:3893, 2002.

Okamoto E, Nitahara K, Yasumoto M, et al: Use of epidural anaesthesia for surgery in a patient with Kennedy's disease. *Br J Anaesth* 92:432, 2004.

Schmidt BJ, Greenberg CR, Allingham-Hawkins DJ, et al: Expression of X-linked bulbospinal muscular atrophy (Kennedy disease) in two homozygous women. *Neurology* 59:770, 2002.

Kennerknecht-Vogel Syndrome

At a glance: Polymalformative syndrome with numerous musculoskeletal anomalies and absent gonads.

Synonyms: Agonadism with Short Stature Mental Retardation and Delayed Bone Age and multiple extragenital malformations.

Incidence and genetic inheritance: Exact incidence unknown. One case report of two sisters with 46,XY genotype but phenotypically female with no gonadal tissue. Presumed autosomal recessive inheritance. The parents were consanguineous.

Clinical aspects: The children were 14 and 16 years old with short stature secondary to markedly reduced bone age. Other musculoskeletal abnormalities included thoracolumbar scoliosis, hip dysplasia, and partial clinosyndactyly of the toes. The face has been described as "peculiar" with a short neck and hypodontia. The older sibling had an omphalocele, right renal agenesis, and intestinal malrotation, but otherwise the internal organs were normal. External genitalia were normal female, but gonadal tissue was absent in both children. Both had significant developmental delay.

Anesthetic considerations: Abnormal facies and short neck may cause difficulties with face-mask ventilation and/or laryngoscopy for tracheal intubation. Progressive scoliosis may lead to restrictive lung disease resulting in hypoxemia, pulmonary hypertension, and limited respiratory reserve. Such patients are at increased risk for perioperative respiratory complications and may require prolonged ventilatory support. Evaluation should include a history for exertional dyspnea, physical examination for signs of respiratory dysfunction and pulmonary hypertension or cor pulmonale, and appropriate investigations. These would include arterial blood gas analysis, chest radiography, pulmonary function testing (FEV_1, FVC, FEV_1/FVC, total lung capacity, diffusing capacity), and formal exercise testing. Positioning of the patient with scoliosis can be awkward because of the kyphosis. Affected internal organs may result in metabolic abnormalities. Developmental delay may limit cooperation and sedative/anxiolytic premedication and the presence of the primary caregiver for induction of anesthesia may be helpful.

Reference:

Kennerknecht I, von Saurma P, Brenner R, et al: Agonadism in two sisters with XY gonosomal constitution, mental retardation, short stature, severely retarded bone age, and multiple extragenital malformations: A new autosomal recessive syndrome. *Am J Med Genet* 59:62, 1995.

Kenny-Caffey Syndrome

At a glance: Hereditary skeletal dysplasia resulting in proportionate dwarfism characterized by thickening of the inner corticalis and stenosis of the medullary cavities of the tubular bones.

Synonyms: Dwarfism-Congenital Medullary Stenosis Syndrome; Dwarfism-Tubular Bone Stenosis; Hypoparathyroidism-Retardation-Dysmorphism Syndrome (HRD); Kenny Syndrome;

Kenny-Linarelli Syndrome; Tubular Stenosis-Hypocalcemia-Convulsions-Dwarfism Syndrome; Tubular Stenosis-Periodic Hypocalcemia Syndrome; Tubular Stenosis with Hypocalcemia.

Incidence: Approximately 55 cases have been described. Both sexes are affected with equal severity.

Genetic inheritance: A genetic disorder caused by truncation mutations of the TBCE (tubulin-specific chaperone E) gene. Autosomal recessive; reported almost exclusively in Middle Eastern populations. Autosomal dominant and X-linked transmission is also possible. Sporadic cases may be a result of new mutations. Genetic defect located on chromosome 1 (locus 1q42-q43).

Pathophysiology: The most striking biochemical finding is hypocalcemia, which is related to hypoparathyroidism in 46% of cases. The hypocalcemia is frequently associated with seizures or episodes of tetany. Thickening of long bone cortices and the calvaria of the skull are common findings. The cortical thickening is associated with medullary stenosis.

Diagnosis: Based on a constellation of clinical findings in addition to persistent hypocalcemia and low-to-normal parathyroid hormone assays. Growth hormone and thyroid hormone levels usually are normal. Anemia is present in 30% of patients.

Clinical aspects: Proportionate growth retardation (prenatal and postnatal) associated with delayed bone age is the most common feature. Medullary stenosis of the long bones is common, and delayed closure of the anterior fontanelle occurs in 90% (fontanelle may remain open into teenage years). Sixty percent of patients have convulsions and tetany. Fatal outcome of these convulsions has been reported. Ophthalmic abnormalities are common: most frequently microphthalmia and hyperopia, as well as strabismus, congenital glaucoma, and pseudopapilledema. Intelligence usually is normal, but psychomotor delay may be present.

Precautions before anesthesia: Obtain a complete blood count and check the electrolytes. Evaluation of the eyes, particularly for presence of glaucoma.

Anesthetic considerations: Calcium levels should be closely monitored during long procedures. Hypocalcemia should be considered in the differential diagnosis of postoperative seizures or tetany. In the presence of glaucoma, avoid eye compression and other measures that may potentially increase intraocular pressure.

Pharmacological implications: Succinylcholine should be avoided in the presence of glaucoma.

Other conditions to be considered:

☞**DiGeorge Syndrome:** An inherited disorder with recurrent infections, defective thymus functions, heart defects, and characteristic facial features.

☞**Velocardiofacial Syndrome:** A hereditary disease characterized by heart defects, cleft palate or velopharyngeal insufficiency, typical facies, learning disabilities, and multiple other physical anomalies.

☞**Camurati-Engelmann Syndrome:** A musculoskeletal syndrome leading to enhanced bone formation, hyperostosis and sclerosis of the diaphyses of the long bones.

☞**Craniodiaphyseal Dysplasia:** A bone disorder characterized by marked hyperostosis of the craniofacial bones and diaphyseal expansion of the tubular bones resulting in significant clinical complications.

REFERENCES:

Abdel-Al Y, Auger T, El-Gharbawy F: Kenny-Caffey syndrome: Case report and literature review. *Clin Pediatr* 28;4:175, 1989.

Parvari R, Hershkovitz E, Grossman N, et al: Mutation of TBCE causes hypoparathyroidism-retardation-dysmorphism and autosomal recessive Kenny-Caffey syndrome. *Nat Genet* 32:448, 2002.

Keratitis Ichthyosis Deafness (KID) Syndrome

At a glance: A form of ectodermal dysplasia characterized by inflammation of the corneae (keratitis), skin scales, and deafness.

Synonyms: *Autosomal Dominant Form:* Senter Syndrome; Ichthyosiform Erythroderma with Corneal Involvement and Deafness. *Autosomal Recessive Form:* Desmons Syndrome; Desmons-Britton Syndrome.

Incidence: Exact incidence of either type unknown. Approximately 70 cases of the autosomal dominant form have been reported. The autosomal-recessive form is less common (approximately 35 cases have been described.)

Genetic inheritance: The dominant form of KID is caused by heterozygous missense mutations in the connexin-26 gene GJB2 ("gap junction beta 2"). A deletion in the GJB6 gene, which is very close to GJB2, can also be responsible for the disorder (especially the recessive form). Sporadic cases are frequent.

Pathophysiology: Dominant GJB2 mutations can disturb the gap junction system of one or several ectodermal epithelia, resulting in erythrokeratoderma, sensorineural hearing loss, and

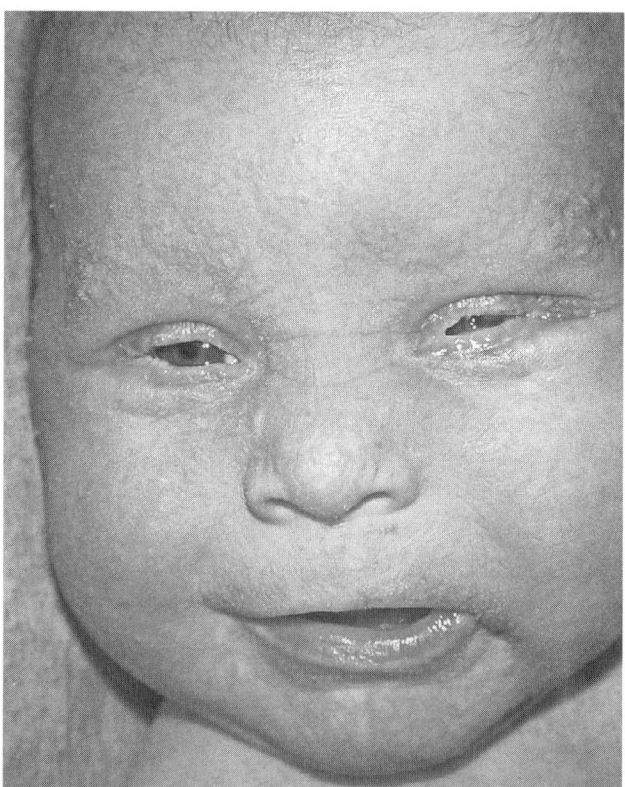

Keratitis ichthyosis deafness (KID) syndrome Erythermatous skin changes with scaly patches and lichenification in the face of a newborn with keratitis ichtyosis deafness (KID) syndrome. See color plates.

keratitis. The GJB2 protein allows the creation of gap junctions between cells. The absence of these channels prevents potassium flux between cells of the inner ear, a process necessary for normal hearing.

Diagnosis: Clinical picture and genetic testing (Cx26 test).

Clinical aspects: Common characteristics of both types of this syndrome include hyperkeratotic skin lesions, congenital sensorineural hearing deficits, and corneal opacity often requiring corneal transplant. The skin lesions start as erythematous, scaly patches on the face, ears, extensor surfaces of the limbs, palms, and soles, which later become brownish-yellow plaques. Ectodermal dysplasia is another major manifestation of KID syndrome. Most patients have partial alopecia, fragile and malformed nails, and small, malformed teeth. The recessive form also presents with hepatic cirrhosis, which may progress to the point of requiring liver transplantation by middle age, short stature, and mental retardation. Epidermal glycogen deposits were present in some patients with the recessive form.

Precautions before anesthesia: Check mouth opening in the presence of perioral skin lesions. Check liver function in patients affected by the autosomal recessive form and also obtain a complete blood count (thrombocytopenia secondary to hypersplenism). Mental retardation may limit patient cooperation, and sedative/anxiolytic premedication as well as the presence of the primary caregiver for induction of anesthesia may be helpful.

Anesthetic considerations: Perioral hyperkeratotic plaques may limit mouth opening, making glottic visualization difficult. Hyperkeratotic, erythematous skin may prevent ECG electrodes or tape from adhering to the skin, thus making the securing of endotracheal tubes and IV catheters difficult. Needle electrodes, sutures, and/or rolls of gauze dressing to secure devices are options. Intravenous access may be difficult as a consequence of skin plaques. Hepatic dysfunction or failure should be evaluated. Generalized edema, ascites, high-output cardiac failure, impaired coagulation, electrolyte and glucose abnormalities, and altered pharmacodynamics and kinetics are a few of the many considerations in patients with liver dysfunction. Careful insertion of nasogastric tubes in the presence of esophageal varices.

Pharmacological implications: Avoid drugs with predominantly hepatic metabolism and elimination if possible in patients with hepatic failure or use reduced doses (also applies for highly protein-bound drugs).

Other conditions to be considered:

ERYTHROKERATODERMIA VARIABILIS: Genetic syndrome associated with deafness and keratosis caused by a mutation in connexin 31 (GJB3) (gene map locus at 1p32-p36).

PROGRESSIVE SYMMETRIC ERYTHROKERATODERMIA: Autosomal dominant disorder of cornification characterized by hyperproliferation of erythematosquamous plaques, symmetrically distributed on the head, extremities, and buttocks; penetrance is variable, and sporadic new mutations may represent 40% of cases.

PALMOPLANTAR KERATODERMA DEAFNESS SYNDROME: Genetic disorder characterized by early deafness, progressive keratosis of the palms and soles in mid-childhood; both a mutation in the gene encoding connexin-26 (13q11-q12) and the 7445A-G mutation of the mitochondrial serine tRNA gene MTTS1 can cause this disorder.

☞ECTODERMAL DYSPLASIA: A group of inherited disorders affecting at least two derivatives of the ectoderm.

REFERENCES:

Miteva L: Keratitis, ichthyosis, and deafness (KID) syndrome. *Pediatr Dermatol* 19:513, 2002.

Richard G, Rouan F, Willoughby CE, et al: Missense mutations in GJB2 encoding connexin-26 cause the ectodermal dysplasia keratitis-ichthyosis-deafness syndrome. *Am J Hum Genet* 70:1341, 2002.

Keratitis, Hereditary

At a glance: Inherited inflammatory corneal disease. Corneal clouding of childhood, characterized by recurrent stromal keratitis and vascularization.

Synonym: Autosomal Dominant Keratitis.

Genetic inheritance: Autosomal dominant. Gene map locus is 11p13 (PAX6 gene). Variable penetrance and expressivity.

Pathophysiology: Characterized by the presence of a circumferential band of opacification and vascularization at the level of the Bowman membrane adjacent to the corneal limbus.

Diagnosis: Histopathologic studies confirm the inflammatory nature and anterior stromal localization of the keratitis.

Clinical aspects: Hereditary childhood corneal clouding. Recurrent episodes of "keratoendothelitis" associated with mild iritis and stromal edema. Propensity for early recurrence after keratoplasty.

Anesthetic considerations: No known specific consideration with this condition.

Other conditions to be considered:

☞KERATITIS ICHTHYOSIS DEAFNESS (KID) SYNDROME: A form of ectodermal dysplasia characterized by inflammation of the corneae (keratitis), skin scales, and deafness.

KERATOENDOTHELIITIS FUGAX HEREDITARIA: Condition distinct from hereditary keratitis in that it is characterized by

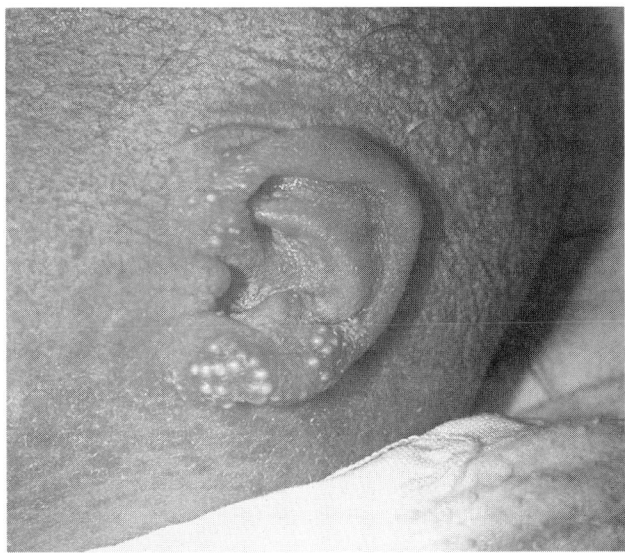

Keratitis ichthyosis deafness (KID) syndrome Skin lesions in keratitis ichthyosis deafness (KID) syndrome extend to the rest of the head and lead to alpecia and hyperkeratosis.

self-limiting intermittent attacks of keratoendotheliitis affecting one or the other eye.

OTHER PAX6 MUTATION SYNDROMES: Include ☞Aniridia, Peters anomaly, congenital cataracts, and isolated foveal hypoplasia.

REFERENCES:

Mirzayans F, Pearce WG, MacDonald IM, Walter MA: Mutation of the PAX6 gene in patients with autosomal dominant keratitis. *Am J Hum Genet* 57:539, 1995.

Singh S, Chao LY, Mishra R, et al: Missense mutation at the C-terminus of PAX6 negatively modulates homeodomain function. *Hum Mol Genet* 10:911, 2001.

Keratosis Palmaris et Plantaris: Overview

Diffuse hereditary palmoplantar keratoderma types without associated features are summarized in Table K-1.

Diffuse hereditary palmoplantar keratoderma types with associated features are summarized in Table K-2.

Focal (or nummular) hereditary palmoplantar keratoderma types with associated features are summarized in Table K-3.

Keratosis Palmoplantaris with Esophageal Cancer

At a glance: Most often autosomal dominant inherited disorder characterized by palmoplantar keratosis in combination with gastrointestinal cancer.

Synonyms: Tylosis with Esophageal Cancer; Keratosis Palmoplantaris with Adenocarcinoma of the Colon/Esophagus; Clarke Howel-Evans Syndrome; Clarke Howel-Evans-McConnell Syndrome; Howel-Evans Syndrome; Bennion Patterson Syndrome.

History: First reported by Clarke and McConnell in 1954 and further studied by William Howel-Evans et al. in 1958.

Incidence: Unknown. Originally described in two families from Liverpool, UK. The syndrome has now also been described in many other countries and ethnicities.

Genetic inheritance: A wide heterogeneity and variety of genes have been implicated. It is most often inherited as an autosomal dominant trait with full penetrance. The tylosis with esophageal cancer gene (TOC) is located in the 17q23-qter region, telomeric to the type I keratin gene cluster. Regions 17q24 and 17q25 may also be involved.

Pathophysiology: The cause of tylosis and esophageal carcinoma is unknown, but the association with cancer may represent a contiguous gene syndrome.

Diagnosis: Based on the findings of palmoplantar keratosis, oral leukoplakia, and squamous cell carcinoma of the esophagus. Hyperkeratosis limited to palms and soles, with the keratoderma stopping abruptly at the lateral margins and not extending onto the dorsum. The epidermis from biopsies of affected skin sites shows gross acanthosis, hyperkeratosis, and hypergranulosis.

Clinical aspects: The association of hyperkeratosis of soles and palms with various malignancies in several members of a family is characteristic for this syndrome. Tylosis usually appears between 5 and 15 years of age. The typical neoplastic manifestation is carcinoma of the esophagus and colon, but there is also an increased risk for other malignancies such as endometrial carcinoma or melanoma. Hyperkeratosis can also be found in other areas that are repeatedly exposed to mechanical trauma, and enoral leukoplakia is common. Typically, hyperkeratosis appears in

---

Table K-1   Diffuse Hereditary Palmoplantar Keratoderma Without Associated Features

Usual Name	Synonyms	Typical Features	Genetics
Diffuse non-epidermolytic palmoplantar keratoderma (NEPPK)	Diffuse NEPPK; Thost-Unna disease; PPK diffusa circumscripta	Onset: <2 years	Autosomal dominant
		Palmoplantar hyperkeratosis, hyperhidrosis, thick nails	Mutation in type II keratin locus (12q11-13)
Diffuse epidermolytic palmoplantar keratoderma (EPPK)	Diffuse EPPK; Vorner disease; PPK cum degeneratione granulosa	Onset: <1 year	Autosomal dominant
		Same phenotype as NEPPK but with epidermolytic hyperkeratosis	Mutation in 1A rod domain segment of the keratin 9 gene (chromosome 17)
Progressive palmoplantar keratoderma (PPPK)	Greither disease, PPK transgrediens et progrediens	Onset: 8–10 years	Autosomal dominant
		Extension onto dorsum of hands and feet, hyperhidrosis; improves after 50 years of age	
Palmoplantar keratosis Gamborg-Nielson	Gamborg-Nielson keratoderma	Mutilating constriction bands surrounding fingers	Autosomal recessive

Table K-2   *Diffuse Hereditary Palmoplantar Keratoderma with Associated Features*

Usual Name	Synonyms	Typical Features	Genetics
Meleda disease	Keratosis extremitatum hereditaria transgrediens et progrediens; Mal de Meleda; Mljet disease	Onset: early infancy Keratoderma with erythematous border, hyperhidrosis, periorbital erythema, lingua plicata, syndactyly, hairy palms and soles	Autosomal recessive Gene map locus: 8qter Greither variant: autosomal dominant
Palmoplantar keratoderma with periodontitis and onychogryposis	☞Haim-Munk syndrome; prepubertal periodontitis syndrome	Onset: 1–5 years Periodontosis, disorder of leukocyte function (increased infections), hyperhidrosis, malodor, lipid-like vacuoles in corneocytes and granulocytes	Autosomal recessive Gene map locus: 11q14-q21
Palmoplantar keratoderma with periondotopathia	☞Papillon-Lefèvre syndrome		
PPK mutilans Vohwinkel	Mutilating keratoderma; ☞Vohwinkel syndrome; palmoplantar keratoderma mutilans	Onset: infancy Fibrous digital bands with progressive autoamputation, alopecia, deafness, spastic paraplegia, myopathy, ichthyosis	Autosomal dominant Gene map locus: 1q21
Palmoplantar keratoderma with sclerodactyly	Huriez syndrome	Onset: infancy Sclerodactyly, nail dystrophy, hypohidrosis, squamous cell carcinomas Biopsy: acanthosis, orthohyperkeratosis	Autosomal dominant
Mutilating palmoplantar keratoderma with periorificial keratotic plaques	Olmsted syndrome	Onset: <1 year Onychodystrophy, periorificial keratosis, variable leukokeratosis	Autosomal dominant
Hidrotic ectodermal dysplasia	Clouston syndrome	Onset: infancy Papillomatous PPK, dystrophic nails, sparse hair, deafness, polydactyly, syndactyly, mental retardation, short stature, photophobia, strabismus Caused by depletion of hair matrix protein	Autosomal dominant Gene map locus: 13q11-q12.1
Palmoplantar keratoderma and cardiomyopathy	Naxos disease	Diffuse NEPPK, arrhythmogenic right ventricular cardiomyopathy, woolly hair	Gene map locus: 17q21
Diffuse NEPPK and sensorineural deafness		Progressive hearing loss preceding skin disorders	Autosomal dominant Connexin 26 mutation

Table K-3   Foċal (or Nummular) Hereditary Palmoplantar Keratoderma with Associated Features

Usual Name	Synonyms	Typical Features	Genetics
Pachyonychia congenita (four types described)	Type I: Jadassohn-Lewandowsky Type II: Jackson-Lawler Type III: Schafer-Brunauer Type IV	Nail discoloration and thickening	Autosomal dominant (occasionally autosomal recessive) Type 1: keratin 16 and 6a gene mutations Type II: keratin 17 and 6b gene mutations
Oculocutaneous tyrosinemia	Richner-Hanhart disease; tyrosinemia type II	Painful keratosis, pseudoherpetic corneal ulcerations, mental retardation, bullous lesions (inconstant), increased levels of serum tyrosine	Autosomal recessive Deletion of tyrosine aminotransferase gene (16q21.1-q22.3)
Keratosis palmoplantaris with esophageal cancer	Bennion Patterson syndrome; Clarke-Howell syndrome; Howel-Evans syndrome; tylosis with esophageal cancer	Onset: 2–4 years Hyperkeratosis of soles and palms with various malignancies	Autosomal dominant Gene map locus: 17q24
Focal palmoplantar and oral mucosa hyperkeratosis		Onset: early childhood Oral hyperkeratosis (sometimes subungual and circumungual) Paranuclear bodies in keratinocytes (condensations of tonofilaments)	Autosomal dominant Keratin 16 gene mutation

adolescence, and malignancies occur after the third decade of life. Development of esophageal carcinoma after the third decade is almost certain, estimated to be 95% by age 65 years. Recognition of tylosis allows better surveillance for the development of esophageal cancers.

Precautions before anesthesia: During childhood, the syndrome is unlikely to have any specific implications for anesthesia, as these are related to the presence of malignancies and their medical and surgical treatment. Determine the competency of the lower esophageal sphincter. A history of heartburn, reflux, or regurgitation may be elicited. Determine whether obstruction of the esophagus is present. Malnutrition is common in patients with esophageal carcinoma, and preoperative parenteral nutrition may have a role in improving the reserves and immunity status. Preoperative investigations in these patients should include chest radiographs, lung function tests including arterial blood gas analysis to evaluate if one-lung anesthesia would be tolerated, a complete blood count, coagulation status, urea and electrolyte levels, nutritional markers (e.g., serum protein, albumin), and an electrocardiogram.

Anesthetic considerations: During childhood, the syndrome is unlikely to have any specific implications for anesthesia, as these are related to the presence of malignancies and their medical and surgical treatment.

Other conditions to be considered: Palmoplantar keratoderma with esophageal cancer is only one form of a variety of autosomal dominant and recessively inherited palmoplantar keratoderma syndromes, some of which are associated with malignancy. The onset of hyperkeratosis might be as early as infancy in some variants. Some families with palmoplantar keratoderma without increased risk for malignancy were found to have mutations in the keratin gene on chromosome 12q.

☞**TYROSINEMIA (TYPE II):** An example of an autosomal recessive form of palmoplantar keratosis that is associated with photophobia, corneal ulcers, and callous keratosis developing between 2 and 4 years of age and with mental retardation.

REFERENCES:

Itin PH, Fistarol SK: Palmoplantar keratodermas. *Clin Dermatol* 23:15, 2005.

Kimyai-Asadi A, Kotcher LB, Jih MH: The molecular basis of hereditary palmoplantar keratodermas. *J Am Acad Dermatol* 47:327, 2002.

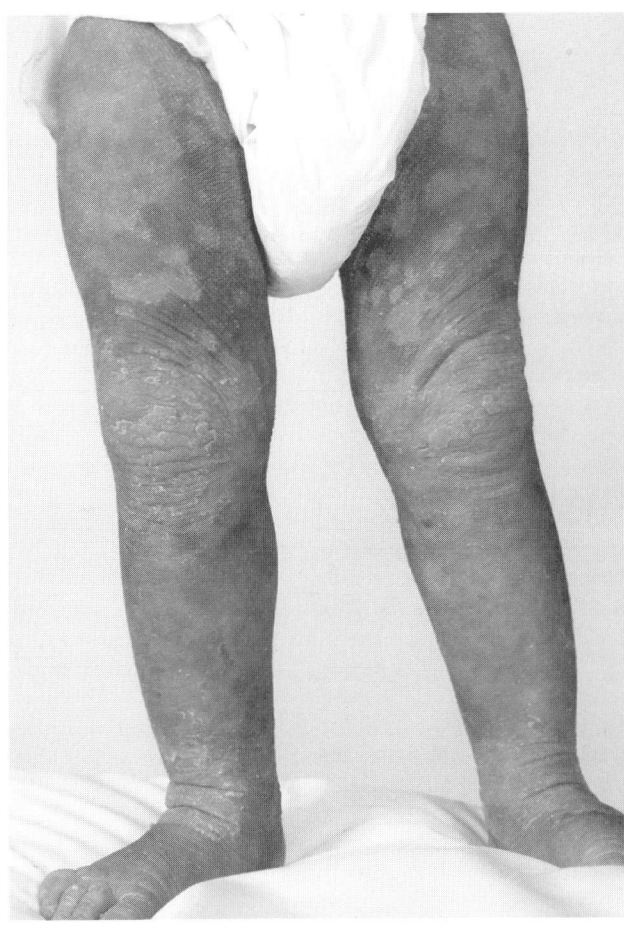

Keratosis palmaris et plantaris   Epidermolytic hyperkeratosis in an infant.

Stevens HP, Kelsell DP, Bryant SP, et al: Linkage of an American pedigree with palmoplantar keratoderma and malignancy (palmoplantar ectodermal dysplasia type III) to 17q24. *Arch Dermatol* 132:640, 1996.

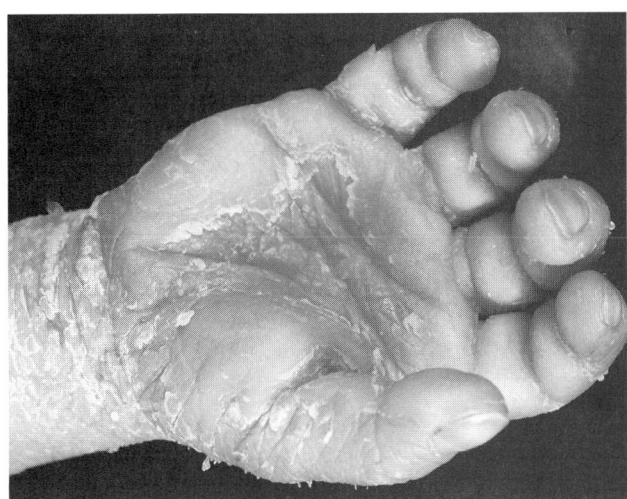

Keratosis palmaris et plantaris   Marked hyperkeratosis and scaling of the palm in a child with keratosis palmaris et plantaris.

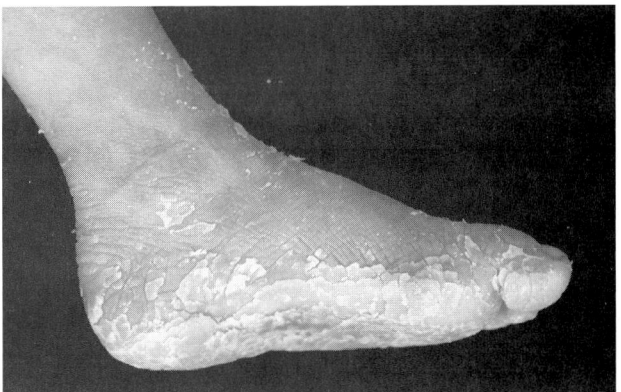

Keratosis palmaris et plantaris   The same lesions are found on the sole of this patient.

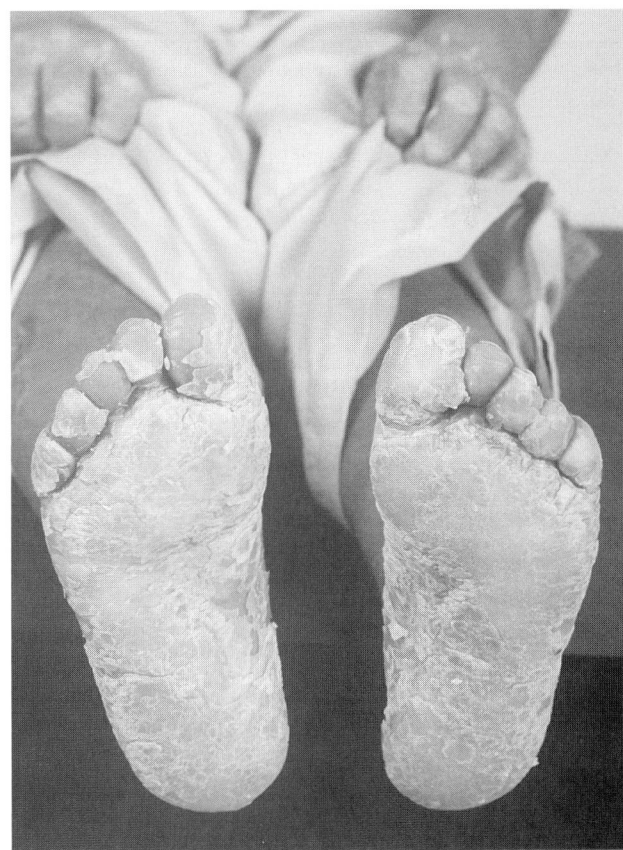

Keratosis palmaris et plantaris   Diffuse epidermolytic palmoplantar keratoderma with hyperkeratosis that was also involving the dorsum of the hands and other skin areas in a 5-year-old girl.

Kersey Syndrome

At a glance: Genetically transmitted syndrome characterized by disorders of hair (short anagen growth phase of hair follicles) and teeth growth.

Synonyms: Short (or Loose) Anagen Syndrome; Trichodental Syndrome; Trichodental Dysplasia-Microcephaly-Mental Retardation Syndrome.

Incidence and genetic inheritance: Unknown but probably not uncommon (often misdiagnosed as alopecia areata or trichotillomania). Only reported in whites; more common in females than in males. Autosomal dominant transmission.

Diagnosis: Suspected by "gentle hair pull" that yields much more hairs than the zero to two hairs per pull in normal patients; confirmed microscopic examination. Affected patients do not feel discomfort as hairs are extracted.

Clinical aspects: Onset between 2 and 5 years of age. The most common dental abnormalities are missing teeth, peg-shaped incisors, and shell teeth. The hair is sparse, brittle, and slow-growing because of a short anagen phase of the hair cycle (hair cannot grow long and affected patients almost never need to have their hair cut). Eyebrows and eyelashes are typically curly. Microcephaly with biparietal narrowing and a thin nose are usually seen. Mild mental retardation is common.

Anesthetic considerations: Careful manipulation of the airway must be provided to avoid damaging potentially brittle teeth. Craniofacial abnormalities must be evaluated for abnormal airway anatomy that could render face-mask ventilation and/or laryngoscopy difficult. Patients with mental retardation may be uncooperative and sedative premedication as well as the presence of the primary caregiver for induction of anesthesia may be helpful.

Other conditions to be considered:

ALOPECIA AREATA: Autoimmune disease resulting in varying amounts of patchy hair loss (can be a variant of vitiligo).

PSEUDOPELADE OF BROCQ: Scarring alopecia resembling alopecia areata resulting in dermal atrophy ("footprints in the snow"), mostly because of lichen planopilaris and chronic cutaneous lupus erythematosus.

TELOGEN EFFLUVIUM: Nonscarring alopecia with diffuse hair shedding caused by metabolic or hormonal stress or by drug absorption.

TINEA CAPITIS: Superficial fungal infection of the skin of the scalp, eyebrows, and eyelashes.

REFERENCES:

Barraud-Klenovsek MM, Trueb RM: Congenital hypotrichosis due to short anagen. *Br J Dermatol* 143:612, 2000.

Giannotti A, Digilio MC, Albertini G, et al: Sporadic trichodental dysplasia with microcephaly and mental retardation. *Clin Dysmorphol* 4:334, 1995.

Ketoacidosis of Infancy

At a glance: An inborn error of ketone body catabolism resulting in intermittent episodes of ketoacidosis.

Synonyms: SCOT Deficiency; Succinyl-CoA:3-Oxoacid-CoA Transferase Deficiency; Succinyl-CoA: Ketoacid-CoA Transferase Deficiency; Succinyl-CoA:Acetoacetate Transferase Deficiency.

Incidence: Less than 25 cases have been reported in the literature.

Genetic inheritance: Autosomal recessive. Gene map location is chromosome 5p12-p13. Prenatal diagnosis can be made because cultured amniocytes have measurable succinyl-CoA:3-ketoacid CoA transferase (SCOT) activity.

Pathophysiology: SCOT, the key enzyme of ketone body utilization, is an extrahepatic mitochondrial matrix enzyme necessary for synthesis of acetoacetyl-CoA by transfer of a CoA moiety from succinyl-CoA to acetoacetate. Ketoacidosis is caused by SCOT deficiency resulting in reduced ketone body utilization.

Diagnosis: Laboratory findings include succinyl-CoA:3-ketoacid-CoA transferase deficiency, together with ketonuria. Normal levels of plasma amino acids, lactic acid, ammonia, glucose, and organic acids other than beta-hydroxybutyrate and acetoacetate.

Clinical aspects: Severe intermittent ketoacidosis in ketogenic situations (fasting, febrile illness, any cause of stress) with no symptoms between episodes. There is persistent ketonuria, even in postprandial times. Age of onset is variable; however, a neonatal onset is common. The main clinical symptoms are vomiting and tachypnea.

Precautions before anesthesia: Need to exclude diabetes mellitus and type I glycogen storage disease. Ensure adequate fluid resuscitation and treatment. Treatment consists of limiting protein intake, providing adequate calorie intake, and preventing aggravation of ketosis by providing alkaline therapy at the onset of any intercurrent infection. Check blood glucose, electrolyte levels, and blood gases with acid–base status.

Anesthetic considerations: Risk of pulmonary aspiration during induction of anesthesia is increased. Maintain adequate hydration. Close monitoring of blood gases in the perioperative period is required.

Pharmacological implications: No known specific pharmacological implications with this condition. Infections may exacerbate ketoacidosis further. The threshold to use antibiotics should therefore be low.

Other conditions to be considered: Other constitutional causes of ketosis in children (differential diagnosis is made by enzyme assay), namely the following:

KETOTIC HYPOGLYCEMIA: Unclear disorder associating ketosis and hypoglycemia; there is a carbohydrate deprivation with dependence on adipose tissue as sources of energy.

☞MITOCHONDRIAL ACETOACETYL-CoA THIOLASE DEFICIENCY: Autosomal recessive disorder of isoleucine and ketone body metabolism characterized by recurrent episodes of metabolic acidosis, hypoglycemia, lethargy, and coma as a consequence of the defective mitochondrial enzyme acetoacetyl-CoA thiolase that allows conversion of fat to energy (especially in fasted patients).

REFERENCE:

Snyderman SE, Sansaricq C, Middleton B: Succinyl CoA:3-ketoacid CoA transferase deficiency. *Pediatrics* 101:709, 1998.

Keutel Syndrome

At a glance: Polymalformative syndrome characterized by characteristic facies, brachytelephalangism, calcification of the cartilage, deafness, and pulmonary stenosis.

Synonyms: Keutel Syndrome I; Pulmonic Stenosis, Brachytelephalangism, and Calcification of Cartilages.

(*NB:* Another Keutel syndrome (termed *Keutel syndrome II*) is characterized by humeroradial synostosis transmitted as an autosomal recessive trait.)

Incidence: Approximately 21 cases have been reported to date.

Genetic inheritance: Autosomal recessive inheritance. Gene map locus is short arm of chromosome 12 (12p13.1-p12.3). Consanguineous parents are common.

Pathophysiology: Phenotype related to faulty encoding of the human matrix Gla protein (MGP), which plays an important role in regulation of extracellular matrix calcification.

Diagnosis: Clinical diagnosis.

Clinical aspects: Macro-, normo-, and microcephaly have been described in these patients. A depressed nasal bridge, often combined with midface and maxillary hypoplasia are typical. Sensorineural hearing loss, optic nerve atrophy, and mental delay may be present. Electroencephalography may document a diffuse cerebral disturbance with epileptiform discharges, and scattered punctate foci of calcification in the subcortical white matter and cortex have been demonstrated. Calcification of cartilage may affect the ears, nose, epiglottis, larynx, trachea (see below), and ribs. Stippled epiphyses, which represent calcifications of the knees and elbows, may occur as early signs of the disease. Brachytelephalangism (short terminal phalanges) with short nails results in a drumstick-like shape of the fingers, which is often combined with mild-to-moderate distal interphalangeal stiffness. Most of these patients have cardiac issues, typically increased right ventricular pressures and pulmonary artery hypertension either due to pulmonary (valvular or supravalvular) stenosis or cor pulmonale as a consequence of calcification of tracheal, paratracheal, bronchial, and rib cartilages. These calcifications may lead to significant obstruction of the tracheobronchial tree down to the level of the lobular bronchi. Renal calcifications and bilateral hydronephrosis as a result of narrowing of the urethrovesicular junction or bladder outlet obstruction with vesicoureteral reflux have also been reported.

Precautions before anesthesia: Identify which sites or organs are affected by abnormal calcifications. Evaluate for pulmonary hypertension and/or cor pulmonale caused by chronic airway obstruction and/or pulmonary artery stenosis. Electrocardiogram and echocardiogram should be considered prior to anesthesia. Right heart and pulmonary angiograms may be required to diagnose peripheral pulmonary artery stenosis. Voice changes or stridor may indicate calcification of laryngeal cartilage and/or epiglottis. Theoretically, calcification of the costochondral joints could lead to a restrictive-type pulmonary disease if chest expansion is limited. Arterial blood gases, chest radiography, and pulmonary function tests are indicated if sufficient suspicion exists. Check renal function because of possible calcifications and hydronephrosis. Type of seizure activity, current management, and degree of control should be evaluated. Deaf patients may be more anxious and difficult to communicate with. Sedative premedication and/or the presence of the primary caregiver (sign language) for induction of anesthesia may be helpful.

Anesthetic considerations: Midfacial hypoplasia may render airway management, especially placement of a nasal endotracheal tube, difficult. These patients may require airway support postoperatively if prone to obstruction. A smaller endotracheal tube than expected may be required if the glottis or trachea is stenotic. May be more prone to postoperative laryngeal edema. If laryngeal function is compromised, patients should be extubated awake so that protective airway reflexes are intact. If pulmonary hypertension is present, avoid increased pulmonary vascular resistance (aim for mild alkalosis and hypocapnia and avoid hypoxia and high airway pressures) or depressed right ventricular function. If respiratory function is compromised because of restricted chest wall expansion, postoperative respiratory support in an intensive care unit may be required.

Pharmacological implications: Some antiseizure medications, such as phenytoin, can inhibit nondepolarizing muscle relaxant function. Phenobarbital up-regulates liver enzymes and may cause increased hepatic clearance of anesthetic agents. Doses should be titrated to desired effect.

Other condition to be considered:

Binder Syndrome (Maxillonasal Dysplasia Syndrome): Mild form of chondrodysplasia punctata with maxillonasal dysplasia and teeth malocclusion that may be an allelic variant of Keutel syndrome.

REFERENCES:

Hur DJ, Raymond GV, Kahler SG, et al: A novel MGP mutation in a consanguineous family: Review of the clinical and molecular characteristics of Keutel syndrome. *Am J Med Genet A* 135:36, 2005.

Keutel J, Jorgensen G, Gabriel P: A new autosomal recessive syndrome: Peripheral pulmonary stenoses, brachytelephalangism, neural hearing loss and abnormal cartilage calcifications-ossification. *Birth Defects Orig Artic Ser* VIII:60, 1972.

Teebi AS, Lambert DM, Kaye GM, et al: Keutel syndrome: Further characterization and review. *Am J Med Genet* 78:182, 1998.

Khalifa-Graham Syndrome

At a glance: An inherited polymalformative syndrome characterized by pterygium colli, anomalies of fingers and toes, and mental retardation.

Synonym: Pterygium Colli, Mental Retardation, and Digital Anomalies.

Incidence and genetic inheritance: Exact incidence unknown. One reported case. Presumed autosomal dominant or X-linked inheritance.

Clinical aspects: In the one reported case, craniofacial abnormalities included brachycephaly, inverted epicanthal folds, angulated eyebrows, severe webbing of the neck (pterygium colli), up-slanting of the palpebral fissures, ptosis, hypertelorism, and prominent, low-set ears rotated posteriorly. The hands and feet were edematous at birth, but this resolved soon after. Hypotonia was present at birth. At the age of 18 years the patient had proximally displaced small thumbs, widened interphalangeal joints, and broad terminal phalanges. The patient suffered from mental retardation.

Anesthetic considerations: Potential for difficult airway management should always be considered in patients with craniofacial abnormalities. In this patient, a short webbed neck may make visualization of the larynx difficult. Difficult placement of a peripheral venous cannula should be expected in the presence of edemas. Developmentally delayed patients may lack the ability to cooperate.

REFERENCE:

Khalifa MM, Graham G: New dominant syndrome of pterygium colli, mental retardation, and digital anomalies. *Am J Med Genet* 52:55, 1994.

Kikuchi-Fujimoto Disease

At a glance: Benign, histiocytic necrotizing lymphadenitis usually affecting young women. Unknown cause. Often mistaken for lymphoma or Hodgkin disease. The disease resolves spontaneously within 2 to 3 months, and relapse is uncommon.

Synonym: Histiocytic necrotizing lymphadenitis.

Incidence: It may account for 5 to 7% of all diagnoses among pathologic specimens of abnormal lymph nodes. The majority of patients are younger than 30 years but only 5 to 10% are younger than 21 years, although patients from 19 months to 75 years of age have been reported. Male-to-female ratio is 1:4. Most frequent in Japan where it was first described.

Pathophysiology: Unknown. Cytotoxic T cells expressing the cytolytic protein perforin infiltrate the affected lymph node(s); apoptosis induced by those T cells probably is the cause of the necrosis. The cause of this hyperimmune or autoimmune reaction has not been identified, yet.

Diagnosis: By histologic examination of the lymph node: paracortical patchy zones of eosinophilic fibrinoid necrosis and abundant karyorrhexis. Necrotic areas are surrounded by a mixed lymphohistiocytic infiltrate.

Clinical aspects: The most frequent presentation is cervical lymphadenopathy, which often is tender or painful on palpation. It may fluctuate in size. Hepatosplenomegaly may be present. Fever is predominant in 30 to 50% of cases. Weight loss, night sweats, and a rash may occur. Hematologic investigations show leukopenia, often with lymphocytosis, and atypical lymphocytes in the peripheral blood; levels of C-reactive protein, lactate dehydrogenase, and transaminases are raised. Spontaneous resolution of signs and symptoms occurs within a few months; no specific therapy is needed. Relapsing bouts of lymphadenopathy occur in 3 to 4% of cases. A beneficial effect of systemic steroids has been reported. Rare cases of associated myocarditis, aseptic meningitis, or ataxia have been described.

Precautions before anesthesia: Because the patient usually is anesthetized for biopsy of a lymphadenopathy with a possible diagnosis of lymphoma, a complete blood count (anemia, platelets) and chest radiography (mediastinal mass or adenopathies) are mandatory. Exclude the presence of associated myocarditis (echocardiography).

Anesthetic considerations: Large cervical lymph nodes can make face-mask ventilation, direct laryngoscopy, and tracheal intubation difficult. The risk of myocarditis is increased, so special anesthetic consideration must be considered in case of cardiomyopathy-like symptoms.

Pharmacological implications: No known specific pharmacological implication with this condition. However, patients receiving chronic steroid therapy may require perioperative supplementation.

REFERENCES:

Jang YJ, Park KH, Seok HJ: Management of Kikuchi's disease using glucocorticoid. *J Laryngol Otol* 114:709, 2000.

Payne JH, Evans M, Gerrard MP: Kikuchi-Fujimoto disease: Rare but important cause of lymphadenopathy. *Acta Paediatr* 92:261, 2003.

Kindler Syndrome

At a glance: Inherited syndrome of unknown inheritance pattern characterized by neonatal skin blistering on the extremities, appearing spontaneously and after minor trauma. Other features include limb hyperkeratosis, mucous membrane fragility with esophageal and urethral strictures, and webbing of the fingers and the toes.

Synonyms: Bullous Acrokeratotic Poikiloderma of Kindler and Weary; Congenital Bullous Poikiloderma; Congenital Poikiloderma with Bullae, Weary Type; Hereditary Acrokeratotic Poikiloderma.

Incidence and genetic inheritance: The exact number of affected individuals unknown. Approximately 15 cases have been reported in the literature. Presumed autosomal recessive inheritance.

Pathophysiology: Ultrastructural examination of the skin of affected patients shows marked basement membrane reduplication and variable levels of cleavage at the dermal–epidermal junction. It has been shown that the underlying molecular pathology involves loss-of-function mutations in a novel gene, KIND1, encoding kindlin-1, which is mainly expressed in basal keratinocytes and plays a role in the attachment of the actin cytoskeleton to the extracellular matrix via focal contacts. This makes Kindler syndrome the first genodermatosis that is caused by a defect in actin–extracellular matrix linkage rather than the classic keratin–extracellular matrix linkage underlying the pathology of other inherited skin fragility disorders such as epidermolysis bullosa.

Clinical aspects: Characteristic skin lesions that vary considerably in their expression: vesiculopustular lesions on the hands and feet that resolve by late childhood; widespread eczematoid dermatitis that resolves by age 5 years; diffuse poikiloderma with striate and reticulate atrophy that develops gradually, but spares the face, scalp, and ears, and persists into adulthood; keratotic papules on the hands, feet, elbows, and knees that appear before the age of 5 years and persist indefinitely; traumatic bullae at pressure sites that heal with atrophic scars. Patients are extremely photosensitive.

Anesthetic considerations: Intravenous access may be difficult. Adhesive tape used to secure intravascular catheters, endotracheal tubes, and other monitoring devices may cause skin damage. Repeated scarring from healed bullae on the skin and mucosal surfaces can result in reduced mobility of joints and narrowed mouth opening. Individuals affected with this condition have limited mouth opening, ankyloglossia, dental overbite, and atrophy of the buccal mucosa. Difficult airway management is expected in such a case. Bullae in the oropharynx and hypopharynx may be ruptured with spillage of serosanguineous fluid into the airway. Contracture of other joints makes proper positioning difficult. Application of a face mask or noninvasive blood pressure cuff may cause trauma and bullae formation. Needle electrodes, sutures, and/or rolls of gauze dressing to secure devices are options. Careful lubrication and padding of contact surfaces to reduce shearing forces and epithelial injury.

Other conditions to be considered:

☞**EPIDERMOLYSIS BULLOSA:** A genetic disorder characterized by cutaneous blistering and scarring following already minor trauma. There are more than 20 different subtypes of the disease.

☞**PEMPHIGOID:** A chronic, nonhereditary blistering disease of skin and mucosae.

☞**PEMPHIGUS:** An autoimmune blistering disease of the skin and mucous membranes.

☞**ROTHMUND-THOMSON SYNDROME:** Autosomal recessive disorder characterized by early photosensitivity as a consequence of a gene defect on chromosome 8.

REFERENCES:

Al Aboud K, Al Githami A: Kindler syndrome in a Saudi kindred. *Clin Exp Dermatol* 27:673, 2002.

Ashton GH: Kindler syndrome. *Clin Exp Dermatol* 29:116, 2004.

Haber RM, Hanna WM: Kindler syndrome. Clinical and ultrastructural findings. *Arch Dermatol* 132:1487, 1996.

King-Denborough Syndrome

At a glance: Noonan-like features identified in infancy and associated with a significant risk of malignant hyperthermia. Males are affected five times more often than females. However, in contrast to Noonan Syndrome, there is no congenital heart disease, mental retardation, or webbed neck. Serum creatinine kinase (CK) might be elevated.

Synonyms: King Syndrome; Malignant Hyperthermia Susceptibility, Noonan-like Syndrome.

Genetic inheritance: Autosomal dominant, but recessive modes have also been suggested. Genetically heterogeneous. Phenotypic manifestations of King-Denborough syndrome can result from different congenital myopathies. In all cases, there is probably an increased risk of malignant hyperthermia susceptibility. Most common gene locus for malignant hyperthermia is a mutation on the long arm of chromosome 19 at position 13.1 (19q13.1) (malignant hyperthermia susceptibility type 1 or MHS1). This corresponds with an abnormal type 1 ryanodine receptor (RyR1).

Pathophysiology: The etiology of King-Denborough syndrome is unknown. Multiple different pathophysiologies are possible, depending on the particular myopathy. The physical signs may reflect fetal hypokinesia. Malignant hyperthermia susceptibility is a result of abnormal sarcoplasmic reticulum calcium channel (RyR1). Hyperthermia results from sustained increase in myoplasmic Ca^{2+}, resulting in sustained muscle contraction and a hypermetabolism. Exposure to a triggering agent results in massive and sustained release of calcium, which results in excessive muscle contraction. Twenty percent of all malignant hyperthermic reactions result from mutation in the ryanodine receptor (chromosome 19); in other cohorts, malignant hyperthermia has been linked to mutations in chromosomes 17, 7, 5, 3, and 1.

Diagnosis: King-Denborough syndrome phenotype is a clinical diagnosis. Definitive diagnosis of associated MH susceptibility requires a muscle biopsy for halothane-caffeine contracture testing. However, a positive family history of malignant hyperthermia, the presence of muscle wasting, and/or an elevated CK level should make the clinician highly suspicious of malignant hyperthermia susceptibility. If the diagnosis is not determined prior to exposure to triggering agents, onset of malignant hyperthermia may be the event that initiates a diagnosis.

Clinical aspects: Typical features include an unusual facies often described as "Noonan-oid" with low-set ears, hypertelorism, downslanting palpebral fissures, ptosis, strabismus, a high-arched palate or cleft palate, micrognathia, crowded teeth, and short, webbed neck. Orthopedic findings include short stature, thoracic kyphosis, lumbar hyperlordosis, pectus carinatum, frequent dislocations of shoulders and patellae, and pes cavus. Cryptorchidism and mental delay are other frequent findings. There is one case report about a patient with dilatation of the aorta, pulmonary artery, and the cardiac ventricles. Malignant hyperthermia presents as a hypermetabolic response of the skeletal muscles to triggering agents, namely, inhalational anesthetic agents and succinylcholine. Combined metabolic and respiratory acidosis, tachycardia, hypertension, hypoxia, muscle rigidity, and myoglobinuria occur as a result of sustained muscle contraction. Hyperthermia is often a late sign in the course of malignant hyperthermia. Not all exposures will trigger a malignant hyperthermia response: approximately half of the patients who are susceptible to malignant hyperthermia had uneventful general anesthetics with trig-

gering agents prior to the triggering event (in some patients more than 10 uneventful non–trigger-free anesthetics have been administered).

Precautions before anesthesia: Careful airway assessment is recommended. Significant kyphoscoliosis may result in restrictive lung disease. Pulmonary function tests such as forced expiratory volume in 1 second (FEV_1), forced vital capacity (FVC), FEV_1/FVC, and diffusing capacity of the lungs for carbon monoxide (DLCO), arterial blood gases, and chest radiography, in addition to history and physical examination, may be done to evaluate pulmonary reserve. Although cardiovascular disease is unusual in this syndrome, a thorough history and physical examination with appropriate investigations (ECG, echocardiogram) should be done. Malignant hyperthermia susceptibility can be evaluated with a family or patient history of malignant hyperthermia reactions, creatine phosphokinase (CPK) levels (for screening), and, if deemed appropriate, muscle biopsy for halothane-caffeine contracture testing. Consultation to an anesthesia or malignant hyperthermia clinic is highly recommended. Dantrolene premedication is no longer indicated prior to anesthesia, but should definitely be available in the room.

Anesthetic considerations: Potential for difficult airway because of dysmorphic facies and short neck. Limited pulmonary reserve may indicate the need for postoperative ventilatory support. Use of regional anesthesia may be helpful by limiting use of respiratory depressant analgesics. Considerations for congenital heart disease include knowledge of the anatomy and pathophysiology of the lesion, endocarditis prophylaxis when appropriate, and avoidance of paradoxical air embolus. A malignant hyperthermia "trigger-free" anesthetic should be given unless the patient had a negative halothane-caffeine contracture test. Patients should be monitored at least 6 to 8 hours prior to discharge after an uneventful, trigger-free, day surgery operation.

Pharmacological implications: Inhalational anesthetic agents and succinylcholine are absolutely contraindicated. Judicious use of nondepolarizing muscle relaxants and opioids if significant muscle weakness or respiratory impairment is present. Avoid verapamil and diltiazem because of potential hyperkalemia and ventricular fibrillation if dantrolene has been given.

REFERENCES:

Chitayat D, Hodgkinson KA, Ginsburg O, et al: King syndrome: A genetically heterogenous phenotype due to congenital myopathies. *Am J Med Genet* 43:954, 1992.

Graham GE, Silver K, Arlet V, et al: King syndrome: Further clinical variability and review of the literature. *Am J Med Genet* 78:254, 1998.

Habib AS, Millar S, Deballi P 3rd, et al: Anesthetic management of a ventilator-dependent parturient with the King-Denborough syndrome. *Can J Anaesth* 50:589, 2003.

Kinky Hair Syndrome

At a glance: Inherited metabolic disorder with clinical expression in males only. Caused by defective intestinal copper absorption that results in severe mental retardation, failure to thrive, sparse hair, and osteoporosis.

Synonyms: Menkes Disease; Menkes Syndrome; Steely Hair Syndrome.

Incidence: Worldwide the incidence is estimated at 1:300,000 in the general population, however, in Australia the condition occurs in 1:35,000 in the general population.

Genetic inheritance: X-linked recessive; caused by a mutation in the gene encoding Cu^{2+}-transporting ATPase, alpha polypeptide (gene map locus is Xq12-q13).

Pathophysiology: Defective coding for an intracellular copper-transporting protein called MNK, which travels between the Golgi apparatus and the cell membrane, transporting copper to the exterior of the cell. Defective MNK prevents proper intestinal absorption of copper. The resultant free-copper deficiency affects the function of copper-dependent enzymes such as cytochrome oxidase, tyrosinase, and lysyl oxidase, which results in symptoms and signs of disease.

Diagnosis: Should be considered in any male infant with unexplained seizures, hypothermia, and mental retardation. Serum copper and ceruloplasmin concentrations are low. The copper levels are elevated in fibroblasts and the placenta. Carrier status for the abnormal gene usually can be determined by microscopic examination of multiple hairs from scattered scalp sites for pili torti (twisted hair). Prenatal diagnosis is available (DNA probe).

Clinical aspects: Intrauterine growth retardation, which persists after birth. Neurologic deterioration begins approximately 2 months after birth. Focal cerebral and cerebellar degeneration progress rapidly to decerebration, with characteristic hypotonia, spasticity, and partial and generalized seizures. Strabismus, myopia and poor visual acuity are common findings. Abnormal thermoregulation with resultant hypothermia is common. Microcephaly occurs as a result of gliosis. The hair is sparse, dull, hypopigmented, brittle, and twisted (pili torti). Hypotonus of the facial musculature gives a chubby-cheek appearance. Micrognathia may be present. Typically, the long bones are osteoporotic. Blood vessels (systemic arteries) become long and tortuous with irregular lumens because of abnormal development of the elastic lamina and thickening of the intima. Aneurysms subsequently develop that may lead to subdural, cerebral, and intestinal hemorrhages. Orthostatic hypotension may develop. The skin is thick and dry and has irregular pigmentation. These patients may also suffer from gastroesophageal reflux with recurrent aspiration pneumonias. Chronic diarrhea is common. Death usually occurs in early childhood (at around two years of age). Parenteral injections of copper-histidine may slow the disease progression and prevent neurologic signs.

Precautions before anesthesia: Anticonvulsant therapy should be assessed and optimized preoperatively and continued throughout the perioperative period. Consider raised intracranial pressure if previous intracranial hemorrhage. Repeated aspiration pneumonias plus hypotonia may compromise respiratory function. A chest radiograph, arterial blood gases, and other tests may be required. Rule out ongoing pneumonia. Check for anemia secondary to aneurysmal bleeding. Hypovolemia and/or electrolyte disturbances may be present if diarrhea is severe. Postural vital signs to check for orthostatic hypotension.

Anesthetic considerations: Pretreatment with H_2-antagonists and/or metoclopramide to reduce the risk of reflux and aspiration. Consider rapid-sequence induction, although keep in mind that intubation may be difficult if the patient is micrognathic. Avoid significant increases in blood pressure if cerebral aneurysms are present or suspected. Respiratory compromise because of repeated pneumonias, in combination with low muscle tone, may make the patient susceptible to perioperative respiratory failure. Postoperative respiratory support may therefore be necessary. Minimizing the use of opioid analgesics while providing good analgesia with regional anal-

gesia may be beneficial in this regard. Active warming is necessary to prevent hypothermia. The patient may be unable to compensate for hypovolemia by increasing systemic vascular resistance, hence maintaining normovolemia is important. Thick skin makes insertion of intravenous catheters and other lines more difficult. Osteoporotic bones may be brittle and prone to fracture during positioning.

Pharmacological implications: Avoid triggers that potentiate occurrence of seizures (enflurane with hypocapnia, methohexital, ketamine). Anticonvulsant therapy results in induction of hepatic enzymes, and some anticonvulsants, such as phenytoin, can reduce the efficacy of nondepolarizing muscle relaxants.

Other conditions to be considered:

☞**AMISH HAIR BRAIN SYNDROME:** Sulfur-deficient brittle hair, short stature, mental deficiency, sexual infantilism, and infertility originally observed in the Amish kindred.

HEREDITARY WOOLY HAIR SYNDROME (Salamon Syndrome): Autosomal dominant, characterized by the presence of presence of woolly, kinky hair often associated with ocular disorders or atrophic keratosis of the hair (with partial or complete axillary or pubic alopecia).

☞**BRITTLE HAIR AND MENTAL DEFICIT SYNDROME:** Autosomal recessive disorder with fragile hair, onychodystrophy, mental retardation, and scalp hypotrichosis.

TAY SYNDROME (Ichthyosis-Brittle Hair-Impaired Intelligence-Decreased Fertility-Short Stature [IBIDS] Syndrome): Photosensitivity, ichthyosiform erythrodrema, progeria-like facies, failure to thrive, mental retardation, occasional infertility, and trichothiodystrophy (sulfur-deficient brittle hair) characterize this disorder.

REFERENCES:

Kazim R, Weisberg R, Sun LS: Upper airway obstruction and Menkes syndrome. *Anesth Analg* 77:856, 1993.

Llanos RM, Mercer JF: The molecular basis of copper homeostasis copper-related disorders. *DNA Cell Biol* 21:259, 2002.

Tobias JD: Anaesthetic considerations in the child with Menkes' syndrome. *Can J Anaesth* 39:712, 1992.

Kinsbourne Syndrome

At a glance: Rare neurologic disorder usually affecting infants and young children. Characterized by sudden onset of brief, repeated, shock-like spasms of several muscles within the arms, legs, or the entire body. Impaired ability to control voluntary movements. Jerking movements of the eyes are most often present. In 50% of patients, a malignant tumor (neuroblastoma) is responsible for the symptoms associated with this syndrome. A viral infection may also be responsible.

Synonyms: Ataxia-Opsoclonus-Myoclonus Syndrome; Dancing Eyes Syndrome; Dancing Eyes-Dancing Feet Syndrome; MEI Syndrome (Myoclonic Encephalopathy of Infants or Infancy Syndrome); Neuroblastoma Paraneoplastic Syndrome; Opsoclonic Encephalopathy; Opsoclonus-Myoclonus Syndrome.

Genetic inheritance: None. Sometimes chromosome 1 deletions are found in the associated neuroblastoma tissue.

Pathophysiology: Autoimmune disease initiated by a viral infection or a neuroblastoma and attacking the cerebellum (similarity of antigens).

Diagnosis: Mainly clinical. Brain histology reveals widely distributed perivascular lymphocyte infiltration in the brain.

Clinical aspects: Kinsbourne syndrome occurs either spontaneously, in association with a neuroblastoma, or following an infectious process. Approximately 50% of cases are linked to an occult neuroblastoma, but the clinical features and the response to therapy are comparable with or without neuroblastoma. However, neuroblastoma associated with Kinsbourne syndrome has a better prognosis than without it. Several investigations point towards an immunologic process. Children usually present with an encephalopathy with progressive ataxia, uncontrolled movements of the head, myoclonic jerks, and chaotic jerking movements of the eyes. Sometimes it is associated with mental retardation. In 60% of cases, Kinsbourne syndrome improves with steroid or adrenocorticotropic hormone (ACTH) administration. Recurrences and sequelae such as speech problems and mental deficiency are found in approximately 90% of the cases and are severe in 60%. Usually, Kinsbourne syndrome features improve with treatment of the underlying neuroblastoma.

Precautions before anesthesia: Usually these children present for surgery of neuroblastoma or for radiotherapy. Hyperfractionated radiotherapy (twice daily) is used in some of these patients. Check for neuroblastoma location and catecholamine levels. Check for deviation or compression of the airways and great vessels, pneumonia, or pleural effusion with mediastinal or cervical neuroblastomas.

Anesthetic considerations: No optimal anesthetic regimen can be recommended. Even if no catecholamine secretion is detected, hypotension may immediately follow tumor excision. Central neuraxial anesthesia should be avoided in case of paravertebral tumor invading the intravertebral space.

Pharmacological implications: No known specific pharmacological implications. Often individuals affected with this condition receive chronic corticosteroid therapy and may require perioperative supplements.

Other condition to be considered:

Sᴘᴅᴇɴʜᴀᴍ Cʜᴏʀᴇᴀ: Emotional instability, purposeless movements, muscular weakness; autoimmune response to acute rheumatic fever.

REFERENCES:

Kain ZN, Shamberger RS, Holzman RS: Anesthetic management of children with neuroblastoma. *J Clin Anesth* 5:486, 1993.

Plantaz D, Michon J, Volteau-Couanet D, et al: [Opsoclonus-myoclonus syndrome associated with non-metastatic neuroblastoma. Long-term survival. Study of the French Society of Pediatric Oncologists]. *Arch Pediatr* 7:621, 2000.

Pranzatelli MR, Tate ED, Kinsbourne M, et al: Forty-one year follow-up of childhood-onset opsoclonus-myoclonus-ataxia: Cerebellar atrophy, multiphasic relapses, and response to IVIG. *Mov Disord* 17:1387, 2002.

Kleine-Levin Hibernation Syndrome

At a glance: Intermittent disorder affecting the behavior during adolescence characterized by hypersomnolence (up to 20 hours/day), excessive food intake, and abnormally uninhibited sexual drive.

Synonyms: Critchley Syndrome; Familial Hibernation Syndrome; Hypersomnia-Bulimia Syndrome; Kleine-Levin-Critchley Syndrome; Periodic Somnolence and Morbid Hunger Syndrome.

Incidence and genetic inheritance: Approximately 200 cases have been reported. About 2/3 of patients are males. Autosomal dominant inheritance. Human leukocyte antigen (HLA)-DQB1*0201 allele frequency was significantly increased in patients with Kleine-Levin syndrome.

Pathophysiology: Unknown. Hypotheses include a hypothalamic dysfunction and abnormalities in the central serotonin and dopamine metabolism. Several clinical symptoms also suggest an underlying autoimmune process.

Clinical aspects: Episodic attacks of aberrant behavior with normal behavior between episodes. Attacks may last for several weeks and are characterized by hypersomnia, hyperphagia with subsequent vomiting, hallucinations with disorientation, increased sexual drive, and mood depression. Attacks may be precipitated by infections, head trauma, or alcohol consumption.

Anesthetic considerations: Repeated episodes of bulimia may lead to electrolyte disorders. Mallory-Weiss tears can result from repetitive vomiting, which may lead to anemia from chronic upper gastrointestinal blood loss.

Pharmacological implications: These patients may be treated with amphetamines or lithium. Their interference with anesthetic drugs should be kept in mind.

REFERENCES:

Arnulf I, Zeitzer JM, File J, et al: Kleine-Levin syndrome: A systematic review of 186 cases in the literature. *Brain* 128:2763, 2005.

Dauvilliers Y, Mayer G, Lecendreux M, et al: Kleine-Levin syndrome: An autoimmune hypothesis based on clinical and genetic analyses. *Neurology* 59:1739, 2002.

Gadoth N, Kesler A, Vainstein G, et al: Clinical and polysomnographic characteristics of 34 patients with Kleine-Levin syndrome. *J Sleep Res* 10:337, 2001.

Kleiner-Holmes Syndrome

At a glance: Malformative syndrome characterized by the association of polysyndactyly and hallux valgus.

Synonym: Hallux varus and Preaxial Polysyndactyly.

Incidence and genetic inheritance: One case report of two siblings. Exact incidence unknown. Autosomal recessive inheritance.

Clinical aspects: In 1980, Kleiner and Holmes described two brothers with bilateral hallux varus. One brother had duplication-triplication of the great toes and the other had unusually broad great toes with incomplete duplication of the phalanges. The parents were not related and showed no skeletal abnormality.

Anesthetic considerations: No specific anesthetic considerations.

REFERENCE:

Kleiner BC, Holmes LB. Hallux varus and preaxial polysyndactyly in brothers. *Am J Med Genet* 6:113-7, 1980.

Klinefelter Syndrome XXY/XYY

At a glance: Chromosomal disorder characterized by supernumerary X chromosome(s) in male subjects associated with infertility and hypogonadism.

Synonyms: 47-XXY Syndrome; Hypogonadotropic Hypogonadism; Klinefelter-Reifenstein Syndrome; Klinefelter-Reifenstein-Albright Syndrome; Seminiferous Tubule Dysgenesis; Xq Klinefelter Syndrome.

History: First described in 1942 by the American physicians H.F. Klinefelter, Jr., E.C. Reifenstein, Jr., and F. Albright.

Incidence: Chromosomal disorder affecting only males. Estimated prevalence of 1:600–700 in the male population. No racial predilection. This disorder is the most common chromosomal cause of male hypogonadism and infertility.

Genetic inheritance: Nondisjunction of sex chromosomes during maternal meiosis (53%) or paternal meiosis (47%) results in 47,XXY genotype classically, although variants such as XXYY, XXXY, and XXXXY, and mosaic patterns, such as XXX/XY, also exist.

Pathophysiology: Additional X chromosome(s) result in cognitive abnormalities and affect the development of secondary sexual characteristics (proportionally to the extra number of X chromosomes). Extra sex chromosomes usually result from an error of nondisjunction during parental gametogenesis. The primary testicular failure causes elevation of gonadotropin levels because of a lack of feedback inhibition on the pituitary gland. In addition to androgen deficiency, which causes eunuchoid body proportions with gynecomastia, there is an increased incidence of autoimmune disorders (e.g., systemic lupus erythematosus, rheumatoid arthritis).

Diagnosis: Clinical characteristics and genotyping.

Clinical aspects: Phenotypically male. Physical manifestations of this syndrome develop at puberty. Typically small, soft testes with underdeveloped secondary sex characteristics, such as sparse facial and body hair. Affected men are infertile as a consequence of azoospermia caused by sclerosed seminiferous tubules. Patients may be tall with long limbs. Osteoporosis may lead to vertebral collapse and even scoliosis. Unless treated with exogenous testosterone starting at puberty, patients can become obese and develop diabetes mellitus. A recent study from Britain showed that these patients have a reduced life expectancy. The main reasons were peripheral vascular disease, pulmonary embolism, diabetes mellitus (secondary to insulin resistance), respiratory disease (restrictive pneumopathy), and nervous system disease (e.g., subarachnoid hemorrhage, epilepsy). Mortality from ischemic heart disease, however, was reduced.

Precautions before anesthesia: Evaluate and optimize control of diabetes mellitus if necessary. Assess for long-term complications of diabetes (atherosclerosis, renal disease). Vertebral body fractures can result in decreased mobility of spine and/or compression of nerves or spinal cord. Any neurologic abnormalities should be documented preoperatively. Cervical spine mobility should be evaluated. Patient cooperation may be limited if mental retardation is present and sedative/anxiolytic premedication and/or the presence of the primary caregiver for induction of anesthesia may be helpful.

Anesthetic considerations: Perioperative control of blood glucose levels to prevent hypoglycemia or severe hyperglycemia. Difficult intubation if cervical spine mobility is limited. Consider awake intubation or avoid airway manipulation altogether if there is risk of neurologic injury with movement of the cervical spine. Central neuraxial anesthesia techniques are controversial if spinal problems are present and if in doubt should best be avoided. Scoliosis makes proper positioning more difficult.

Pharmacological implications: No specific implications.

Other conditions to be considered:

☞**FRAGILE X SYNDROME:** Mental retardation, joint hyperlaxity, attention deficit, unstable mood, autistic-like behavior, epilepsy in 25% of patients. Boys are more severely affected than girls. Caused by a mutation on the FMR1 gene, which is located on the long arm of the X chromosome.

HYPOGONADISM IN MALES: Features of eunuchoidism (sparse body hair, underdevelopment of skeletal muscles, delayed epiphyseal closure resulting in long arms and legs) caused by interruption of the hypothalamic–pituitary–gonadal axis, which can be genetic (☞Kallmann syndrome, congenital adrenal hypoplasia, several gene mutations) or secondary to other disorders (particularly brain tumors).

REFERENCES:

Manning MA, Hoyme HE: Diagnosis and management of the adolescent boy with Klinefelter syndrome. *Adolesc Med* 13:367, 2002.

Swerdlow AJ, Higgins CD, Schoemaker NJ, et al: Mortality in patients with Klinefelter syndrome in Britain. A cohort study. *J Clin Endocrinol Metab* 90:6516, 2005.

Visootsak J, Aylstock M, Graham JM Jr: Klinefelter syndrome and its variants: An update and review for the primary pediatrician. *Clin Pediatr (Phila)* 40:639, 2001.

Klippel-Feil Syndrome

At a glance: Syndrome characterized by the congenital fusion of any two of the seven cervical vertebrae resulting in shortness of the neck, restricted neck movements, and low posterior hair line. Other features include congenital heart defect (e.g., ventricular septal defect) and hearing loss.

History: Although this syndrome was first described in 1743 by the Swiss physician Albrecht von Haller (1708–1777), it now bears the name of the two French neurologists, Maurice Klippel (1858–1942) and André Feil (born 1884), who described the disorder in 1912.

Incidence: Estimated at approximately 1:42,000 live births. Females account for approximately 65%.

Genetic inheritance: Autosomal dominant and autosomal recessive inheritance do occur, but most cases are sporadic. Gene map locus is 8q22.2.

Pathophysiology: Vertebral malformation caused by failure of normal segmentation of cervical somites during the third and eighth week of gestation with resulting associated primary or secondary neurologic defects. Four types are described:

- *Type I:* Extensive cervical and upper thoracic spinal fusion
- *Type II:* One to two interspace fusions often associated with occipitoatlantal fusion and hemivertebrae
- *Type III:* Coexisting fusion in the lower thoracic or lumbar spine
- *Type IV:* Klippel-Feil anomaly associated with sacral agenesis

Type I is 50 times less common than type II, but tends to present with the classic triad (see *Clinical Aspects*) and is frequently associated with birth injuries and other major organ abnormalities. Practically, the presence of spine anomalies in the form of hypermobility or spondylosis places these patients at higher risk for spinal cord injury with minor trauma.

Diagnosis: Clinical suspicion is confirmed by radiography. Lateral flexion-extension radiographs of the cervical spine should be

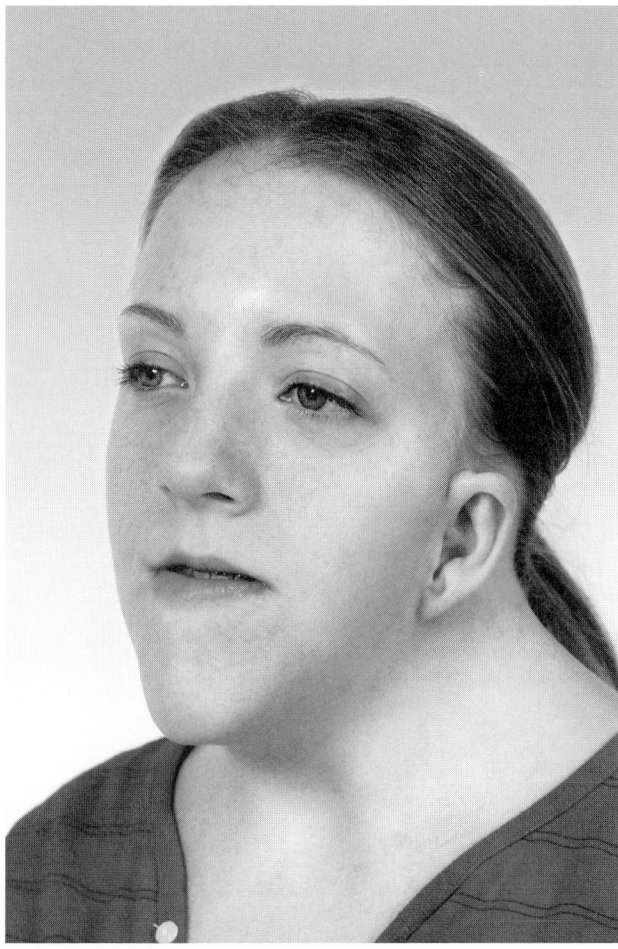

Klippel-Feil syndrome   Facial asymmetry and short, webbed neck in a 17-year-old girl with Klippel-Feil syndrome.

performed to determine the motion range at each interspace. Once diagnosed, patients should be followed with radiographic assessment at least annually.

Clinical aspects: The classic triad consists of short neck, restriction of neck movement, and low posterior hair line. Of these, restriction of movement is most common and occurs in up to 50% of cases. The syndrome often remains unrecognized because the neck may appear normal and the patient is asymptomatic until later in life. Presentation may be with neurologic deficit that occurs either spontaneously or after minor trauma. Syncopal attacks may be precipitated by sudden rotary movements of the neck. Other skeletal anomalies include cervical vertebral fusion, hemivertebrae, sacral agenesis, scoliosis (either primary or secondary) in up to 60% of cases, spinal canal stenosis, and torticollis. Other findings include webbed neck, Sprengel deformity (both, small and elevated scapula) in 30%, genitourinary abnormalities in 35 to 65% (hydronephrosis, renal ectopia, renal agenesis, horseshoe kidney, anomalies of the collecting system), congenital heart disease in 15% (particularly ventricular septal defect), deafness in 30% (conductive and/or sensorineural), synkinesia (mirror movements) in 20%, and, rarely, paraplegia or hemiplegia. Cleft palate is common, as is the association with malformation of laryngeal cartilage and mild-to-severe vocal cord paresis.

Precautions before anesthesia: Clinical suspicion based on history and examination to assess the degree of instability. Lateral cervical radiographs in flexion-extension are essential preoperatively. Assessment of associated abnormalities at the atlantooccipital junction and presence of spinal canal stenosis or scoliosis also increase the risk of neurologic damage. Assessment of neurologic function with documentation of preexisting abnormalities. Assessment of related abnormalities, particularly of the airway in terms of difficulties with intubation, and cardiac system for evidence of congenital heart defects, cardiac failure, and possible optimization of cardiac state preoperatively. An echocardiogram may be required and cardiac surgery may be necessary as the primary procedure. Check renal function, electrolytes, and a complete blood count. Depending on the degree of scoliosis, lung function tests are recommended. A preoperative anesthesia consultation is recommended.

Anesthetic considerations: Patients have cervical instability and are at high risk for spinal cord injury during direct laryngoscopy, tracheal intubation, and positioning for surgery. Alternative anesthetic techniques, if possible, should be considered preferable to induction of general anesthesia with intubation. Patients should be managed as an unstable cervical spine and should have inline stabilization for laryngoscopy and intubation. Awake, nasal fiberoptic-guided intubation is the technique of choice, but is often difficult in children, especially if a pediatric-size fiberoptic bronchoscope is not available. Use of inhalational induction in a spontaneously breathing child with use of fiberoptic bronchoscope is the technique of choice in this case. Otherwise, intubation via direct laryngoscopy should be performed to ensure intubation is possible before neuromuscular blockade is given. Meticulous attention must be paid to positioning, particularly if the patient will be turned prone. Use of spinal cord monitoring showing ongoing neurologic response prevents the need for wake-up tests, which are difficult and dangerous in the presence of an unstable spine. Postoperative extubation should occur in the fully awake patient with stabilization of the neck during emergence. Associated abnormalities may have other considerations.

Pharmacological implications: Preinduction use of atropine should be considered for antisialagogue activity and prior to inhalational induction. Neuromuscular blockade is relatively contraindicated because of anticipated difficult intubation until the airway is secured. Prophylactic antibiotics should be used if indicated for cardiac or renal abnormalities. With significant cardiac failure, halothane should be avoided postinduction and fluid balance should be carefully controlled.

Other conditions to be considered:

☞ **ULLRICH-TURNER SYNDROME:** X-linked or autosomal dominant pterygium colli with limb lymphedema, short stature, skin laxity, dystrophic nails, and motor dysfunction of cranial nerves.

☞ **CERVICO-OCULO-ACOUSTIC SYNDROME:** Fused cervical vertebrae with torticollis, congenital deafness, and abducens palsy.

REFERENCES:

Clarke RA, Catalan G, Diwan AD, et al: Heterogeneity in Klippel-Feil syndrome: A new classification. *Pediatr Radiol* 28:967, 1998.

Farid IS, Omar OA, Insler SR: Multiple anesthetic challenges in a patient with Klippel-Feil Syndrome undergoing cardiac surgery. *J Cardiothorac Vasc Anesth* 17:502, 2003.

Rouvreau P, Glorion C, Langlais J, et al: Assessment and neurologic involvement of patients with cervical spine congenital synostosis as in Klippel-Feil syndrome: Study of 19 cases. *J Pediatr Orthop B* 7:179, 1998.

Klippel-Trenaunay Syndrome

At a glance: Congenital malformation characterized by the association of soft tissue and bony hypertrophy, venous malformations, lymphatic abnormalities, and cutaneous capillary malformations.

Synonyms: Angio-Osteohypertrophy; Klippel-Trenaunay-Weber Syndrome.

History: First described in 1900 by two French physicians, Maurice Klippel and Paul Trénaunay, under the name of "naevus varicosus osteohypertrophicus" ("Du naevus variqueux osteohypertrophique").

Incidence: Unknown, but very rare. No racial predilection. Males and females equally affected.

Genetic inheritance: Causes unknown, may be multifactorial, but usually assumed to be a sporadic disorder.

Pathophysiology: The cause of the soft tissue and bony hypertrophy has not been elucidated, but is postulated to result from the increased blood supply and local growth factors. The disorder may be caused by a genetic mutation or by mesodermal abnormalities during fetal development, intrauterine damage to the sympathetic ganglia (or intermediolateral tract) leading to dilated microscopic arteriovenous anastomoses.

Diagnosis: A port-wine stain and venous varicosities in association with bony and soft tissue hypertrophy, radiology (elongation and cortical thickening of affected bones), and arterial and venous evaluation (angiography, venography) are characteristic. Histology shows capillary spread of the papilla dermis adjacent to the lesion, but also in deeper layers of dermis and subcutis.

Clinical aspects: The cutaneous stains are the earliest signs, with lateral plain hemangiomas (85% of cases), often affecting the lower limbs (95% of cases). Osteohypertrophy, usually affecting the involved bone, is often not present at birth, but appears within the first few months of life. Associated anomalies include ocular anomalies, glaucoma, cerebral aneurysm, spinal cord arteriovenous malformations, gastrointestinal hemorrhage, and severe menorrhagia. Eighty percent of the cord lesions may bleed spontaneously or after straining or coughing at some time during the patient's life. Often the bleeding is contained within the lesion, and no neurologic deficit occurs. Treatment usually is symptomatic and, in general, conservative. Specific embolization of extensive varicoses improves the clinical picture. Intracutaneous laser surgery for angiokeratomas is also used.

Precautions before anesthesia: Exclude anemia caused by recent or ongoing hemorrhage from the abnormal vessels; obtain full neurologic assessment; may require CT scan, MRI, or, angiography to locate presence of cerebral or spinal vascular malformations. Assess presence of ocular vascular masses and glaucoma.

Anesthetic considerations: Loss of autoregulation in the abnormal vessels predisposes to hemorrhage, especially in the presence of hypertension that may occur intraoperatively. Measures to obtund the hemodynamic responses to direct laryngoscopy and tracheal intubation, noxious surgical stimuli, and extubation should be performed. Avoidance of coughing, straining, retching, and vomiting is important to prevent rupture of the abnormal vessels. Extubation should be accomplished before the tendency to cough arises. Central neuraxial anesthesia techniques are contraindicated in the presence of spinal lesions.

Pharmacological implications: Succinylcholine, when used, should be administered after careful pretreatment with a nondepolarizer to minimize fasciculations and the increase in intraocular

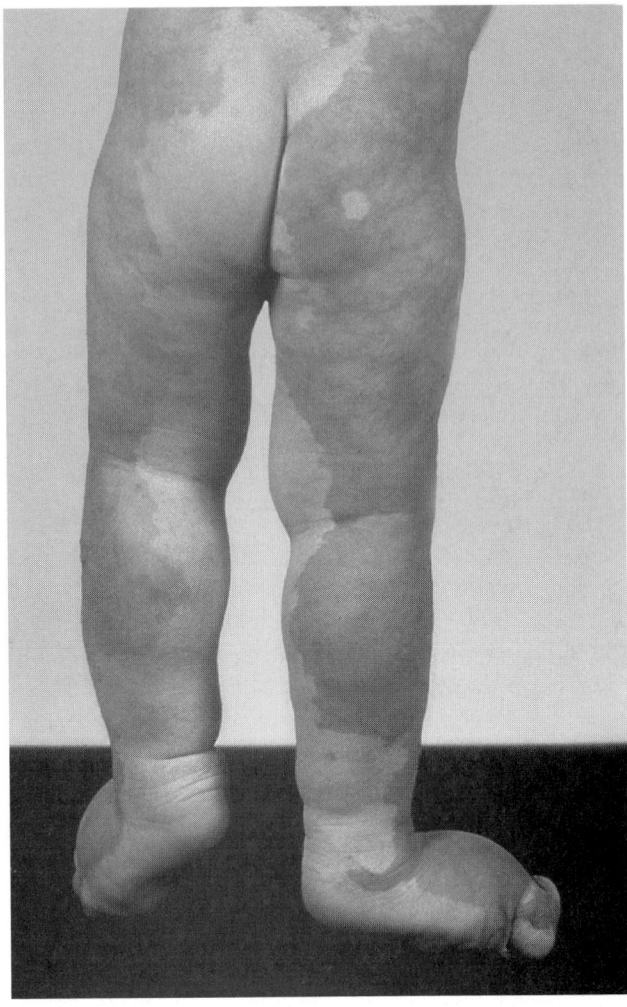

Klippel-Trenaunay syndrome Extensive and bilateral form of Klippel-Trenaunay syndrome in a 2-year-old boy. Note hypertrophy of the feet and leg length difference.

pressure. Intravenous lidocaine prior to tracheal extubation may be helpful to attenuate coughing. In small infants, intravenous lidocaine must be administered cautiously to avoid sudden cardiac arrest (dose <0.5 mg/kg). Use of antiemetics is valuable in reducing the incidence and severity of nausea and vomiting postoperatively.

Other conditions to be considered:

☞**MAFFUCCI SYNDROME:** A genetic disorder characterized by enchondromas, multiple cavernous hemangiomas often involving head and neck. Bone and cartilage deformities appear during childhood. Pathological fractures and progression to chondrosarcoma are common.

☞**PROTEUS SYNDROME:** Hamartomatous disorder with multisystem involvement, such as partial bilateral gigantism of hands and feet, naevi, subcutaneous tumors, hemihypertrophy, and macrocephaly.

REFERENCES:

Capraro PA, Fisher J, Hammond DC, et al: Klippel-Trenaunay syndrome. *Plast Reconstr Surg* 109:2052, 2002.

Ezri T, Szmuk P, Panksy A, et al: Anaesthetic management for Klippel-Trenaunay-Weber syndrome. *Paediatr Anaesth* 6:81, 1996.

Jacob AG, Driscoll DJ, Shaughnessy WJ: Klippel-Trenaunay syndrome: Spectrum and management. *Mayo Clin Proc* 73:28, 1998.

Kniest Syndrome

At a glance: Severe chondrodysplasia caused by the defective formation of type II collagen characterized by dwarfism, skeletal anomalies, and often cleft palate and deafness.

Synonyms: Kniest Dysplasia; Metatropic Dysplasia II (name given by "accident," because Metatropic Dwarfism is a completely different entity); Swiss Cheese Cartilage Syndrome; Pseudometatropic Dysplasia.

Incidence: Unknown, but very rare. Males and females equally affected.

Genetic inheritance: Autosomal dominant inheritance. The genetic defect has been mapped to 12q13.11-q13.2. Many cases, however, seem to be sporadic.

Pathophysiology: Mutations of this genetic segment lead to abnormal type II collagen with specifically shorter monomers. Grossly, the cartilage feels soft. Histologically, the cartilage has lacunae throughout, giving it the appearance of "Swiss cheese." As a result, all tissues containing cartilage are affected with respect to growth, structure, and function.

Diagnosis: Characteristic phenotype. Some patients excrete keratan sulfate (a mucopolysaccharide) in the urine. Cartilage histology and electron microscopy are characteristic.

Clinical aspects: Phenotype is apparent at birth. Craniofacial abnormalities include macrocephaly, flat midface, flat nose root, and cleft palate. Occasional association with Pierre-Robin syndrome has been reported. Tracheal cartilage is abnormal, and tracheomalacia may occur as a result. The chest may be short and narrow, but ventilation and perfusion of the lungs usually remain unaffected. The vertebral column often has platyspondylia with anterior wedging of the vertebral bodies, coronal clefting of the thoracolumbar vertebral bodies, and occipitoatlantal instability. Kyphoscoliosis and/or lumbar hyperlordosis may develop. In an extensively studied patient, there was bony fusion between the anterior arch of the atlas and the odontoid and between the posterior arch of the atlas and the cranial base. Growth usually is retarded. The limbs are characteristically very short secondary to short tubular bones. The epiphyses are large and deformed and the metaphyses broad resulting in so-called "dumbbell" shape, as a consequence of delayed epiphyseal ossification resulting in mega-epiphyses. The joint space is narrow with limited joint mobility. Early-onset myopia, retinal detachment, and sensorineural hearing loss are common findings. Patients often present for repair of umbilical and inguinal hernias.

Precautions before anesthesia: Assessment for potential difficult intubation. Presence of respiratory distress, especially stridor, may signify tracheomalacia. Preoperative arrangement for close postoperative supervision and the possibility for postoperative mechanical ventilation is advisable if one or both of the above conditions are present. Documentation of cervical spine instability with lateral flexion and extension cervical spine radiographs, if possible.

Anesthetic considerations: Potentially difficult airway management. Passage of nasotracheal tubes may be difficult if midface hypoplasia is present. If there is atlantooccipital instability, utmost care must be taken to avoid excessive, if any, movement of the cervical spine in an anesthetized patient. Manual inline stabilization of the cervical spine during direct laryngoscopy and tracheal intuba-

tion attempts is crucial. Techniques that minimize movement, such as fiberoptic intubation, are the best approach. Awake intubation in a cooperative patient, with documentation of intact neurologic status after intubation and positioning, is ideal. The combination of difficult airway with an unstable cervical spine is potentially disastrous, so anesthetic techniques that require manipulation of the airway should be avoided if possible. However, central neuraxial anesthesia techniques could be difficult given the anatomical anomalies of the spine. Airway obstruction can occur intra- and postoperatively because of tracheomalacia. Judicious use of opioids and other sedating drugs and close supervision with oxygen saturation and apnea monitoring in the postoperative period are highly recommended. Careful positioning of stiff and painful joints is important for preventing pressure sores and nerve palsies. Patients with visual or hearing impairment may suffer from a greater degree of anxiety and may not be as cooperative.

Pharmacological implications: Use of agents that may affect respiration and airway patency should be used cautiously in patients with abnormal airway anatomy. Avoid neuromuscular blockers and maintain spontaneous ventilation until the airway has been secured.

Other conditions to be considered:

☞**ACHONDROGENESIS:** Short trunk and limbs, large head, and usually a cleft palate and small chin; also a result of defective type II collagen.

METATROPIC DYSPLASIA TYPE I: Severe dwarfism with short arms and legs, narrow thorax, short ribs, kyphoscoliosis, joint anomalies, and tail-like skin fold over sacrum; both autosomal dominant and autosomal recessive forms exist.

☞**MORQUIO DISEASE:** Autosomal recessive mucopolysaccharidosis with dwarfism, kyphosis, platyspondyly, and severe disability but normal intelligence.

REFERENCES:

Cole WG: Abnormal skeletal growth in Kniest dysplasia caused by type II collagen mutations. *Clin Orthop* 341:162, 1997.

Hicks J, De Jong A, Barrish J, et al: Tracheomalacia in a neonate with Kniest dysplasia: Histopathologic and ultrastructural features. *Ultrastruct Pathol* 25:79, 2001.

Wilkin DJ, Artz AS, South S, et al: Small deletions in the type II collagen triple helix produce Kniest dysplasia. *Am J Med Genet* 85:105, 1999.

Knobloch Syndrome

At a glance: An inherited disorder characterized by encephalocele, vitroretinal degeneration with retinal detachment, high myopia, and normal intelligence. Because all patients have normal intelligence, it is suggested that the cephalocele is a meningocele rather than an encephalocele.

Synonyms: Vitreoretinal Degeneration with Retinal Detachment, and Occipital Cephalocele; Knobloch-Layer Syndrome; Retinal Detachment and Occipital Encephalocele Syndrome.

Incidence: Approximately 35 patients have been reported in the literature.

Genetic inheritance: Autosomal recessive, caused by defective collagen XVIII. Gene map locus is 21q22.3. Penetrance seems to be 100%; however, variability (intra- and interfamilial) is considerable.

Pathophysiology: Condition controlled by a mutation in the COL18A1 collagen gene that is of variable expressivity. The cranial and eye alterations in this syndrome may occur early in embryogenesis, suggesting that developmental genes may be involved in the pathogenesis of this syndrome.

Diagnosis: Made based on the clinical findings. Histology may reveal heterotopic neuronal tissue in the skull lesions (thereby distinguishing between scalp defect and encephalocele).

Clinical aspects: The most common findings are high myopia, vitreoretinal degeneration with retinal detachment, and occipital encephalocele. Intellegence is usually normal. This led to the assumption, that in many cases the encephalocele may in fact be either a meningocele or a scalp defect. Heterotopic neuronal tissue could be found in the scalp lesions of some patients. Other reported, but inconstant findings include ☞Scimitar Syndrome, patent ductus arteriosus, single umbilical artery, mild congenital pulmonary lymphangiectasia (visible on chest radiographs as interstitial changes), and abnormal palmar creases.

Precautions before anesthesia: A complete history and thorough examination is required. Ask about pulmonary problems (respiratory distress, cyanosis, cough) and rule out encephalocele (important for positioning of the patient).

Anesthetic considerations: If an occipital encephalocele/meningocele is present, induction of anesthesia is best performed in the left lateral position or alternatively on bolsters avoiding any pressure on the lesion. Congenital pulmonary lymphangiectasia is often fatal in the neonatal period; respiratory distress has not been described in these patients, which probably indicates a mild form of congenital pulmonary lymphangiectasia. However, the threshold for a chest radiograph and/or an arterial blood gas analysis should be kept low. Increases in intraocular pressure should be avoided in patients at risk for retinal detachment.

Pharmacological implications: Since succinylcholine is known to potentially increase intraocular pressure, it should best be avoided in these patients with a high risk of retinal detachment.

Other condition to be considered:

☞**MECKEL GRUBER SYNDROME:** Autosomal recessive disorder characterized by the presence of renal cysts, developmental anomalies of the central nervous system (e.g., posterior encephalocele most often defined as an occipital scalp defect), hepatic ductal dysplasia and cysts, and polydactyly.

REFERENCES:

Myllyharju J, Kivirikko KI: Collagens and collagen-related diseases. *Ann Med* 33:7, 2001.

Sniderman LC, Koenekoop RK, O'Gorman AM, et al: Knobloch syndrome involving midline scalp defect of the frontal region. *Am J Med Genet* 90:146, 2000.

Suzuki OT, Sertie AL, Der Kaloustian VM, et al: Molecular analysis of collagen XVIII reveals novel mutations, presence of a third isoform, and possible genetic heterogeneity in Knobloch syndrome. *Am J Hum Genet* 71:1320, 2002.

Köbberling-Dunnigan Syndrome

At a glance: An inherited metabolic disorder mainly affecting young female adults characterized by insulin resistance with glucose intolerance, hypertriglyceridemia, and partial lipodystrophy. Slow onset initially presenting with progressive loss of subcutaneous adipose tissue. Other features include hypocomplementemia, glomerulonephritis, and autoimmune disorders.

Synonyms and classification: Familial Partial Lipodystrophy (FPLD).

Familial Partial Lipodystrophy Type I (Köbberling Type): Characterized by loss of adipose tissue confined to the extremities, with normal or increased amounts of fat on the face, neck, and trunk. So far, this type has been reported only in females.

Familial Partial Lipodystrophy Type II (Dunnigan Type; Familial Lipodystrophy of Limbs and Lower Trunk; Reverse Partial Lipodystrophy; Lipoatrophic Diabetes): Characterized by partial lipodystrophy with onset around puberty after a normal fat distribution in early childhood. The subcutaneous adipose tissue gradually disappears from the upper and lower extremities and the gluteal and truncal regions. Clinical features include a muscular appearance with prominent superficial veins, a double chin, fat neck, or cushingoid appearance. Adipose tissue may accumulate in the axillae, back, labia majora, and intraabdominal region. Acanthosis nigricans, hirsutism, and menstrual abnormalities (polycystic ovary syndrome) occur occasionally. Affected patients are insulin resistant and may develop glucose intolerance and diabetes mellitus after age 20 years.

Familial Partial Lipodystrophy Type III (Familial Partial Lipodystrophy Associated with PPARG Mutations): Characterized by frank type II diabetes requiring insulin treatment and severe sustained hypertension.

Incidence: Approximately 20 patients with FPLD I have been reported in the literature. More than 200 cases of FPLD II have been described. Females are approximately 5 times more often affected than men. Both types, but particularly FPLD I, are most likely far more common than previously thought.

Genetic inheritance: All forms of FPLD (type I–III) are autosomal dominant inherited, although for some cases of FPLD II X-linked dominant transmission has been discussed. The genetic defects map to 1q21.2 and 3p25 for FPLD II, to 7q11.23-q21 and 3p25 for FPLD III, while for type I the locus has not been determined, yet.

Pathophysiology: A missense mutation in the gene encoding lamins A and C (LMNA). Lamins provide structural integrity of the nuclear envelope and are associated with chromatins and other nuclear proteins. The exact mechanism by which lamins affect the fat distribution remains to be elucidated.

Diagnosis: Phenotype is characteristic, although it has been confused with Cushing syndrome. MRI studies verify virtual absence of subcutaneous fat in extremities with or without trunk involvement with excessive collection of adipose tissue in the head and neck region. Hypertriglyceridemia and hyperinsulinemia.

Clinical aspects: Type I is characterized by the gradual disappearance of most subcutaneous adipose tissue from the lower extremities and gluteal areas at puberty. Muscles and superficial veins become prominent in these areas. In type II, there is also disappearance of adipose tissue from the upper extremities and trunk, with simultaneous accumulation of adipose tissue on the face and neck, giving a cushingoid appearance. Adipose tissue may accumulate in the axillae, back, labia majora, and intraabdominal region. Acanthosis nigricans and hirsutism occur infrequently in both types. Females may have menstrual abnormalities as a result of polycystic ovaries. After the age of 20 years, affected patients become insulin resistant and may develop glucose intolerance or type II diabetes mellitus. Lipid abnormalities include hypertriglyciceridemia and low levels of high-density lipoprotein (HDL) cholesterol. Hypertriglyceridemia may result in acute pancreatitis. Affected patients have a higher incidence of atherosclerosis leading to hypertension and coronary artery disease. Women have a higher incidence of atherosclerosis and diabetes mellitus than men. Females are more

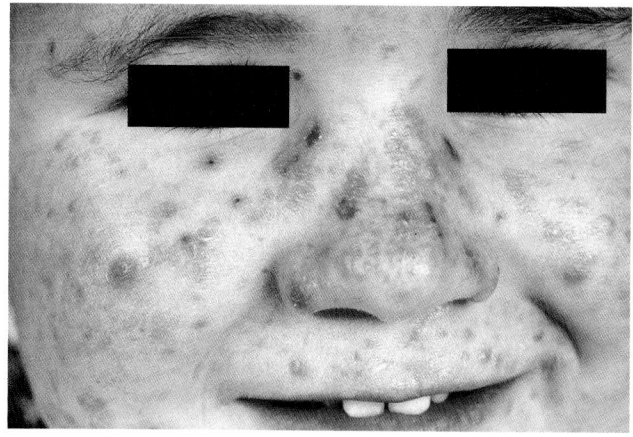

AEC syndrome Skin features in the face of a young boy suffering from AEC syndrome.

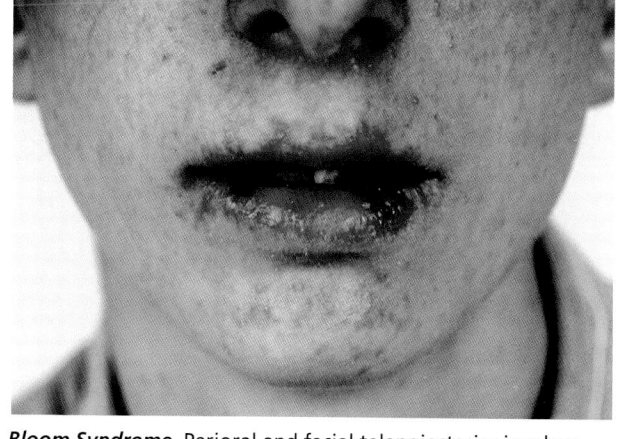

Bloom Syndrome Perioral and facial telangiectasias in a boy with Bloom syndrome.

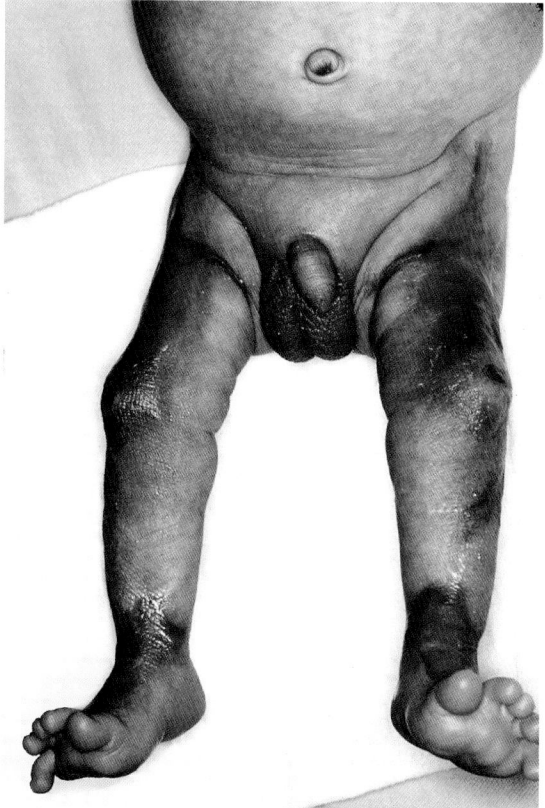

Aplasia cutis congenita Skin defects in a boy with aplasia cutis congenita.

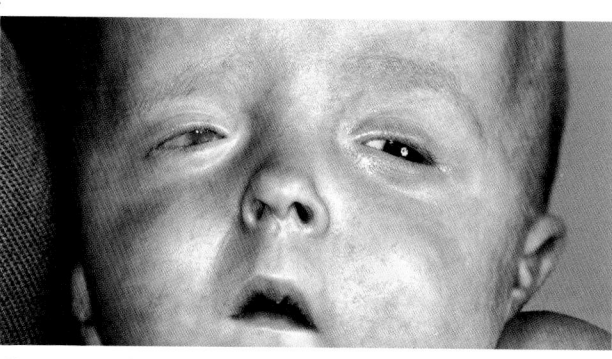

CHARGE Syndrome Eye anomalies in a 3-month-old boy with CHARGE syndrome.

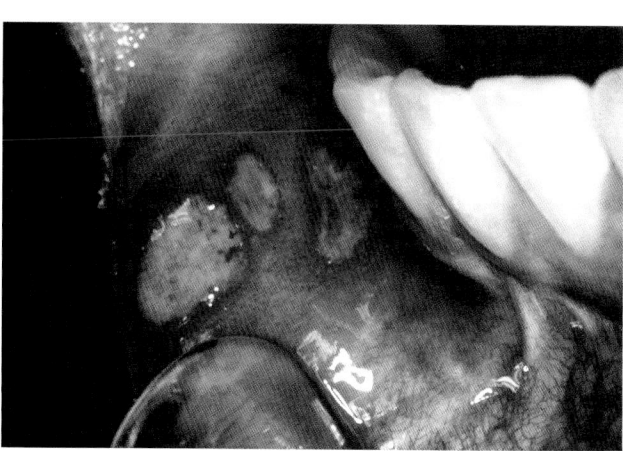

Behçet Disease Ulcerations on the mucosa of the lower lip of a patient with Behçet disease.

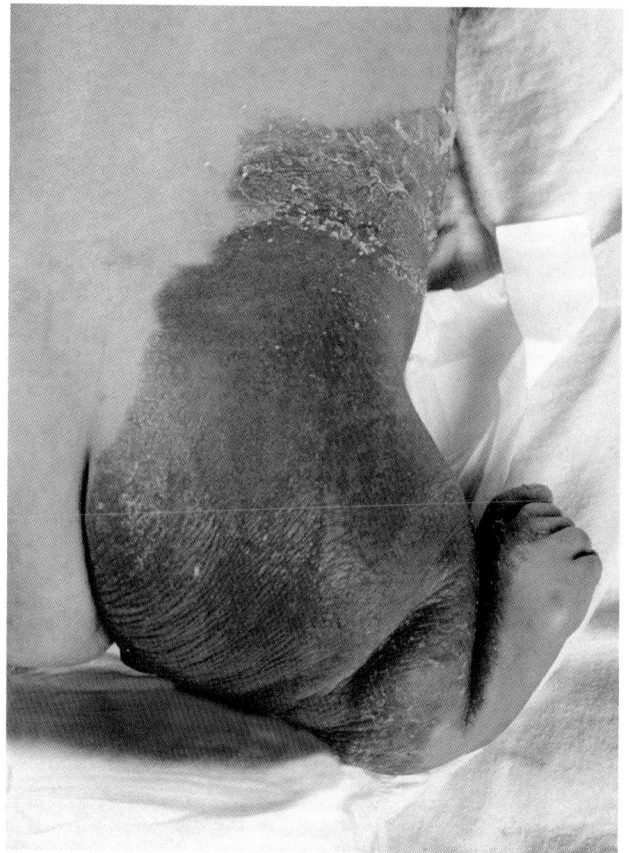

CHILD Syndrome Unilateral inflammatory nevus with hemidysplasia of the leg in a newborn with CHILD Syndrome.

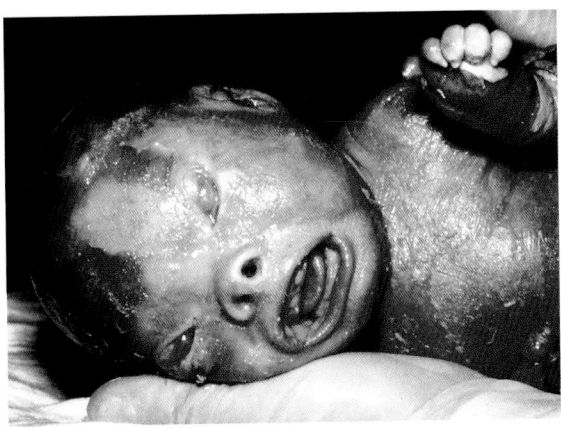

Collodion Baby Newborn with the most severe form of collodion baby.

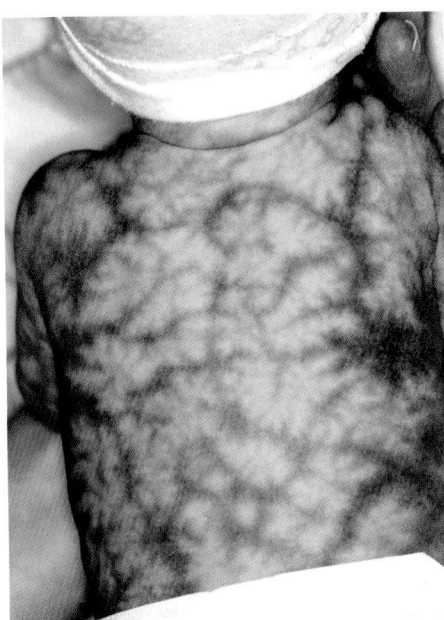

Cutis Marmorata Cutis marmorata telangiectatica congenita in a newborn.

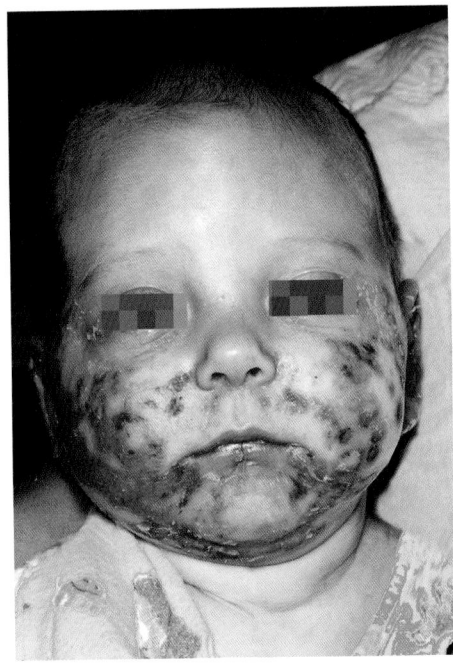

Danbolt-Closs Syndrome Periorificial skin lesions in the face of a toddler.

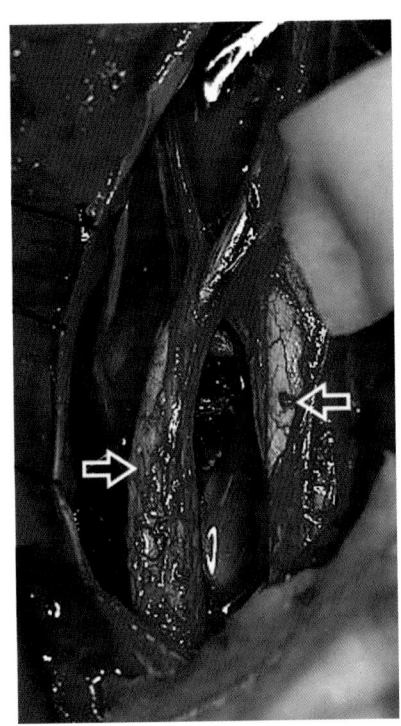

Diastematomyelia Asymmetrical splitting of the spinal cord into two hemicords (*arrows*) in a patient with diastematomyelia.

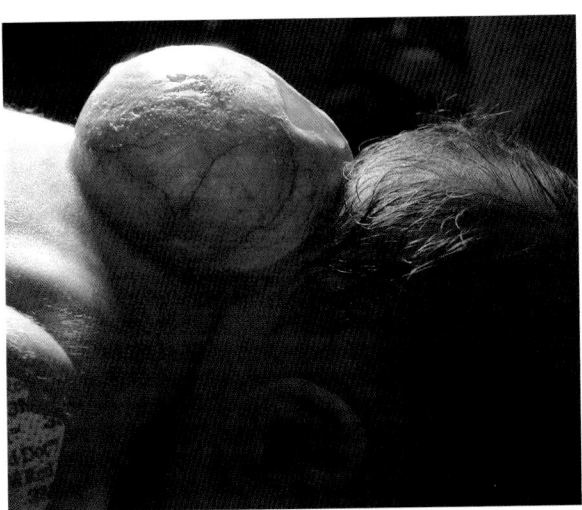

Encephalocele Transilluminated nuchal encephalocele in a newborn baby positioned in the prone position for operation.

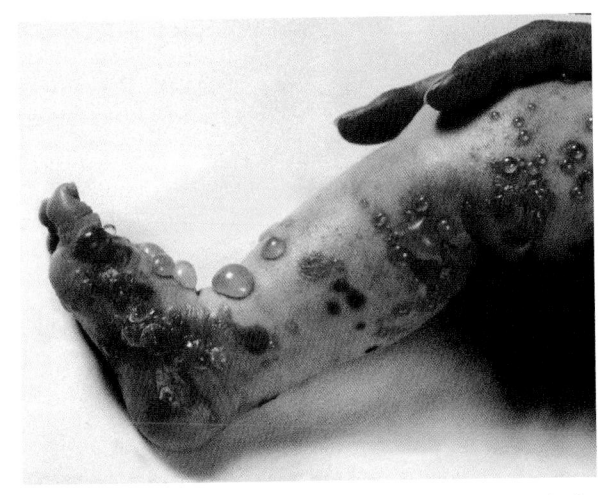

Epidermolysis Bullosa Different stages of epidermolysis bullosa on the leg of an infant.

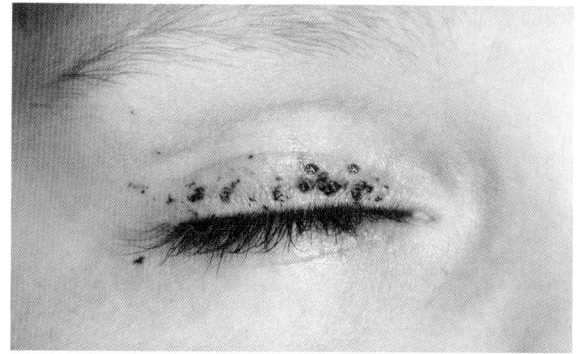

Fabry Disease Angiokeratomata on the eyelids in a patient with Fabry disease.

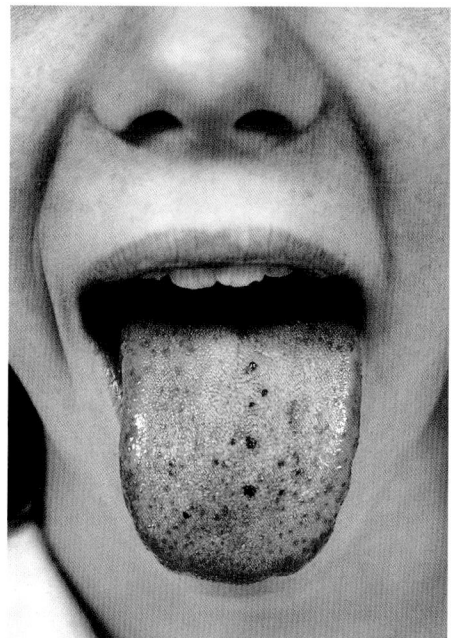

Hereditary telangiectasia Pinpoint and nodular telangiectasias on the tongue of a patient with hereditary telangiectasia.

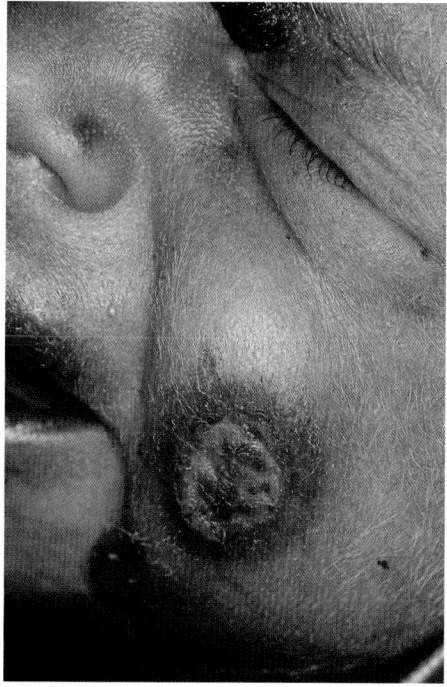

Histiocytosis Ulceration, infiltrates, and bronzing of the skin in a 3-month-old girl with congenital, self-healing histiocytosis.

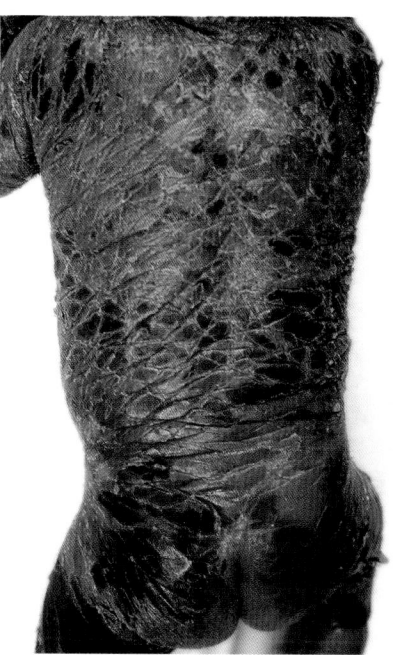

Ichthyosis lamellaris 2 Severe form of ichthyosis lamellaris in an infant.

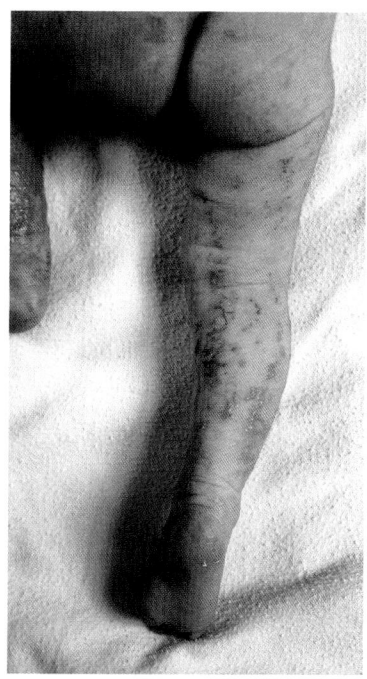

Incontinentia pigmenti First stage of incontinentia pigmenti with spiral lines and blisters on the skin of the legs in a 5-month-old infant.

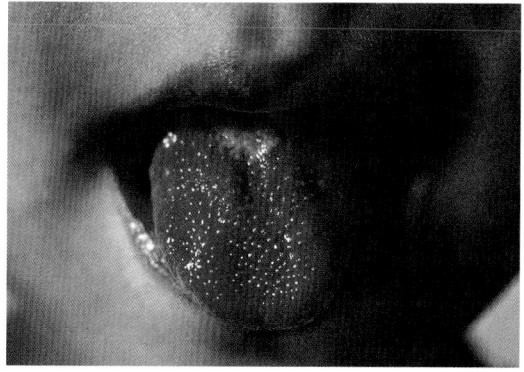

Kawasaki disease Strawberry tongue in a child with Kawasaki disease.

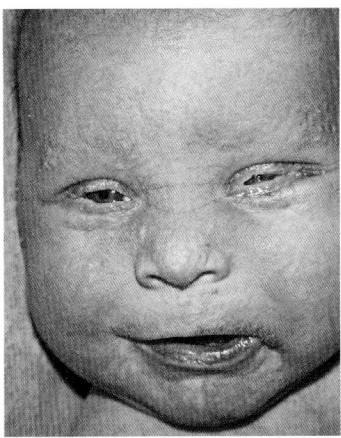

Keratitis ichthyosis deafness (KID) syndrome Erythermatous skin changes with scaly patches and lichenification in the face of a newborn with keratitis ichtyosis deafness (KID) syndrome.

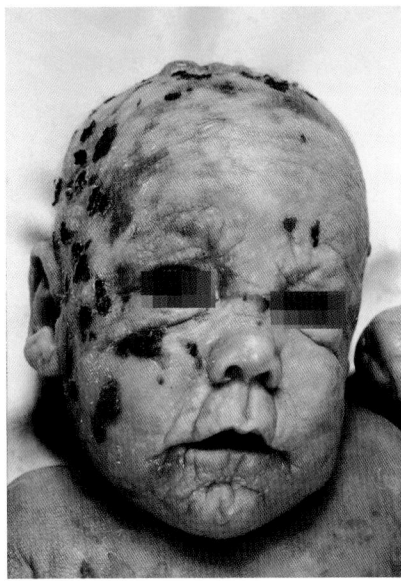

Mastocytosis Severe form of diffuse cutaneous mastocytosis in an infant.

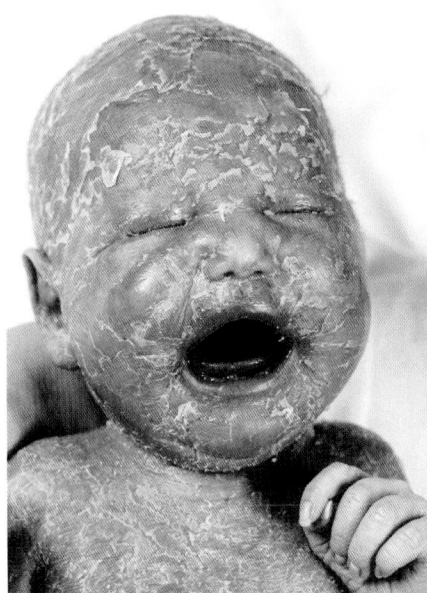

Netherton syndrome Generalized scaling of the skin of a newborn girl with Netherton syndrome.

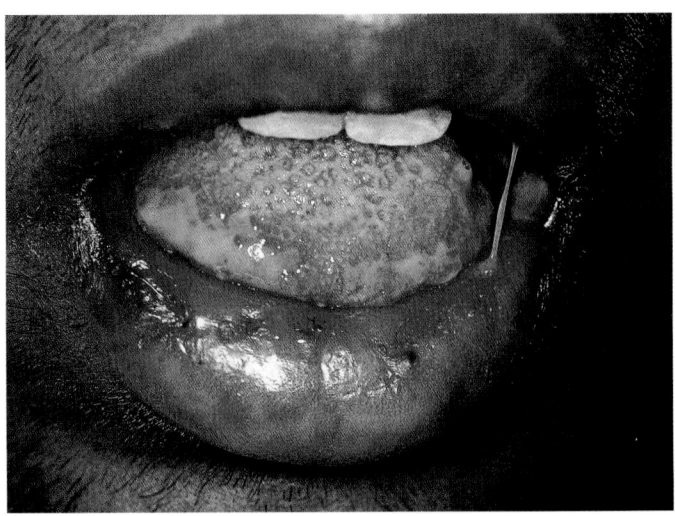

Parry-Romberg syndrome This adolescent girl with Parry-Romberg syndrome presents with a severe form of left-sided hemifacial atrophy involving the skin, subcutaneous tissue, and the osseous structures. This results in left-sided enophthalmos (not shown) and profound atrophy of the skin and the left side of the tongue.

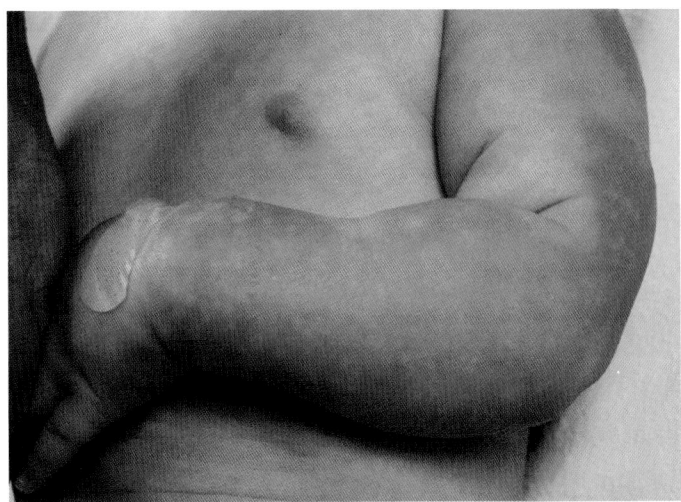

Rothmund-Thomson syndrome These erythematous skin changes are caused by photosensitivity in an infant with Rothmund-Thomson syndrome.

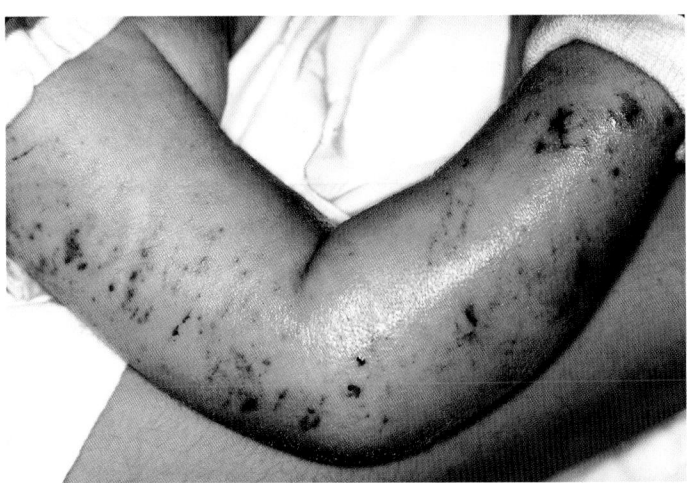

Wiskott-Aldrich syndrome I Eczematous and hemorrhagic skin changes in an infant boy with Wiskott-Aldrich syndrome.

likely to be diagnosed because of the relative muscularity and reduced body fat in normal males. Characterization of affected or unaffected status is not possible in prepubertal children. In type III, insulin-dependent diabetes mellitus and severe hypertension have been reported.

Precautions before anesthesia: Assess for potential difficult airway caused by excessive subcutaneous adipose tissue and for symptoms and signs of obstructive sleep apnea, coronary artery disease, peripheral arterial disease, and cerebrovascular disease. Obtain an electrocardiogram to look for signs of right and left ventricular hypertrophy and ischemic changes suggestive of coronary artery disease. An echocardiogram may help to evaluate cardiac function and estimate pulmonary artery pressure. A cardiology consult may be indicated to optimize management of myocardial ischemia and hypertension prior to anesthesia. Assess management and stability of diabetes mellitus. Consult with endocrinology about perioperative management of blood glucose levels.

Anesthetic considerations: Potentially difficult airway management. Patients with obstructive sleep apnea may be very sensitive to sedatives, especially opioids. They may require supplemental oxygen therapy or noninvasive airway support postoperatively (continuous positive airway pressure or bilevel positive airway pressure) to prevent desaturation. Patients with coronary artery disease benefit from slower heart rates, reduced contractility, and reduced afterload. Monitor for myocardial ischemia with five-lead electrocardiogram. Continue cardiac medications perioperatively. Intraoperative management of diabetes mellitus requires serial blood glucose measurements to avoid hyper- or hypoglycemia, especially if an insulin infusion is used. The lack of subcutaneous tissue in the extremities may increase the risk of hypothermia, nerve compression, and pressure sores, necessitating careful positioning and padding of all pressure points. Difficult placement of neck and subclavian central venous catheters should be expected.

Pharmacological implications: No specific contraindications.

Other conditions to be considered: Other lipodystrophies, especially the following:

BARRAQUER-SIMONS SYNDROME (Acquired Partial Lipodystrophy; Cephalothoracic Lipodystrophy): Begins in childhood, affects females predominantly, and is not genetically transmitted.

PROGRESSIVE LIPODYSTROPHY: Progressive disappearance of subcutaneous fat in the upper part of the body with low C3 serum complement levels, presence of C3 nephritic factor, glomerulonephritis, and other autoimmune disorders.

☞**APOLIPOPROTEIN C-II DEFICIENCY:** Inborn error of metabolism characterized by the deficiency in a cofactor necessary for activation of lipoprotein lipase. Diabetes mellitus, pancreatitis, and epigastric pain do not exclude the possibility of angina in early age and congestive heart failure.

☞**BERARDINELLI-SEIP SYNDROME:** Inherited disorder with hyperinsulinemia resulting from insulin resistance combined with lipodystrophy and acromegaloid features.

☞**FAMILIAL HYPERLIPOPROTEINEMIA TYPE I:** Inherited inborn error of metabolism characterized by massive accumulation of chylomicrons and triglycerides in plasma resulting in recurrent abdominal pain and hepatosplenomegaly.

☞**FAMILIAL HYPERLIPIDEMIA TYPE IIA:** Genetic disorder of lipid metabolism causing accumulation of cholesterol and thus increasing the risk of cardiovascular diseases. Hypercholesterolemia, Low Density Lipoprotein–LDL–Receptor Disorder.

☞**PHYTOSTEROLEMIA:** Rare inherited disorder characterized by congenital hypercholesterolemia, presenting clinically with tendon xanthomas, premature coronary artery disease, and atherosclerosis.

REFERENCES:

Garg A: Acquired and inherited lipodystrophies. *N Engl J Med* 350:1220, 2004.

Garg A: Gender differences in the prevalence of metabolic complications in familial partial lipodystrophy (Dunnigan variety). *J Clin Endocrinol Metab* 85:1776, 2000.

Herbst KL, Tannock LR, Deeb SS, et al: Köbberling type of familial partial lipodystrophy: An underrecognized syndrome. *Diabetes Care* 26:1819, 2003.

Kocher-Debré-Sémélaigne Syndrome

At a glance: Congenital infantile disorder characterized by hypothyroidism with myxedema, muscular hypertrophy, short stature, macroglossia, cretinism, and mental retardation.

Synonyms: Brissaud Syndrome I; Cretinism Muscular Hypertrophy Syndrome; Hypothyroid Myopathy; Hypothyroidism-Large Muscle Syndrome; Hypothyreotic Muscular Hypertrophy of Childhood; Infantile Myxedema-Muscular Hypertrophy; Myopathy-Myxedema Syndrome; Myxedema-Muscular Hypertrophy Syndrome; Myxedema-Myotonic Dystrophy Syndrome.

History: This syndrome is named after the famous Swiss surgeon and Nobel Prize winner Emil Theodor Kocher (1841–1917) and the two French pediatricians, Robert Debré (1882–1978) and Georges Sémélaigne (born 1892).

Incidence and genetic inheritance: Usually sporadic. Has also been associated with autosomal recessive inheritance.

Pathophysiology: Caused by a deficiency of iodotyrosine deaminase with subsequent leakage of iodotyrosine into the circulation and failure of iodine recirculation into the thyroid gland resulting in loss of iodine, initiating a vicious circle of thyroid stimulation, hyperplasia, goiter, and increased synthesis and leakage of hormone precursors.

Clinical aspects: Muscular pseudohypertrophy particularly involves the muscles of the extremities, leading to a "Herculean" appearance of these patients. The term pseudohypertrophy is preferred since histological examination of the affected muscles shows patchy atrophy, necrosis, and increased interstitial connective tissue without signs of muscle fiber hypertrophy. This myopathy associated with hypothyroidism typically presents with proximal weakness and fatigue, exertional pain, muscle cramps and myalgia, slowed movements, diminished deep tendon reflexes (prolongation of the muscle contraction produces a slow relaxation phase of the tendon relaxation phase), stiffness, and myxedema. Mental and growth retardation and macroglossia are further findings reported.

Anesthetic considerations: Evaluate the airway with respect to macroglossia. The relevance of the muscular "hypertrophy" (which mainly affects the limbs) to the use of muscle relaxants is not known. Faced with this myopathy, it is recommended to avoid succinylcholine due to the risk of hyperkalemia. Achieving pharmacological and clinical euthyroidism is desirable from an anesthetic point of view and seems to improve the long-term prognosis.

Other condition to be considered:

HOFFMAN SYNDROME: Same clinical presentation with the addition of painful spasms and pseudomyotonia.

REFERENCES:

Mehrotra P, Chandra M, Mitra MK: Kocher Debre Semelaigne syndrome: Regression of pseudohypertrophy of muscles on thyroxine. *Arch Dis Child* 86:224, 2002.

Tashko V, Davachi F, Baboci R, et al: Kocher-Debre Semelaigne syndrome. *Clin Pediatr (Phila)* 38:113, 1999.

Konigsmark Syndrome

At a glance: Inherited progressive sensorineural hearing loss and the presence of malformed middle ears. Other features include mental retardation, narrow palate, and hypogonadism.

Synonyms: Autosomal Dominant, Nonsyndromic Sensorineural Deafness; Hereditary Low-Frequency Hearing Loss; Konigsmark-Hollander-Berlin Syndrome; Konigsmark-Knox-Hussels Syndrome.

Genetic inheritance: Autosomal dominant. Gene map locus is 5q31.

Pathophysiology: Short increment sensitivity index (SISI) examination suggests a cochlear lesion as the source of the hearing loss.

Diagnosis: Familial occurrence of low-frequency sensorineural hearing loss.

Clinical aspects: Sensorineural hearing loss that shows moderate variation in affected persons. In general, the hearing loss begins in childhood, but postlingual (after language and speaking have been acquired), affecting first the low frequencies and progressing slowly to involve all frequencies in the latter decades of life.

Precautions before anesthesia: No specific precautions associated with this syndrome other than the usual preoperative preparation for an anesthesia.

Anesthetic considerations: Anesthetic considerations for any individual affected with this syndrome are those associated with the surgical procedures rather than the syndrome itself.

Pharmacological implications: No known specific pharmacological implications.

REFERENCES:

Konigsmark BW, Mengel MC, Berlin CI: Dominant low-frequency hearing loss: Report of three families. *Laryngoscope* 81:759, 1971.

Willems PJ: Genetic causes of hearing loss. *N Engl J Med* 342:1101, 2000.

Korula-Wilson-Salomon Syndrome

At a glance: An inherited syndrome involving mainly the face (incomplete closure of eyelids, cleft lip/palate, hypodontia), the existence of which, as a separate entity, is questionable.

Synonyms: Lagophthalmia with Cleft Lip and/or Palate.

Incidence and genetic inheritance: Less than 10 cases have been reported. Autosomal dominant inheritance. Gorlin et al. suggested in 1996 that the family reported by Korula et al. in 1995 actually had blepharo-cheilo-dontic syndrome. Both genders are affected.

Clinical aspects: Lagophthalmia or pathologic incomplete closure of the eyelids is the common finding. Other ocular findings include megaloblepharon (large eyelids), distichiasis (double row of eye-lashes), and ectropion of the lower eyelids. Bilateral cleft lip and palate is usually present. Hypodontia or delayed dentition occur less commonly. Clinodactyly and hypoplastic fingernails have occurred only in the three cases reported from one family.

Anesthetic considerations: The main considerations relate to cleft lip and palate. Affected children may suffer from repeated episodes of upper respiratory tract infections. Anemia and malnourishment may be present because of feeding difficulties. A large or bilateral cleft palate may cause difficulties with intubation. Cleft palate repair is rarely complicated by excessive blood loss or swelling of the tongue causing obstruction after extubation. Although not a specific feature of this syndrome, congenital heart disease has been associated with cleft lip and/or palate. Protect the eyes during anesthesia with lubricants and tape to keep them shut.

Other condition to be considered:

BLEPHARO-CHEILO-DONTIC SYNDROME: Very similar syndrome with cleft lip and/or palate, ectropion of lower eye-lids, hypertelorism, abnormal teeth, and autosomal dominant transmission.

REFERENCES:

Gorlin RJ, Zellweger H, Curtis MW, et al: Blepharo-cheilo-dontic (BCD) syndrome. *Am J Med Genet* 65:109, 1996.

Korula S, Wilson L, Salomonson J: Distinct craniofacial syndrome of lagophthalmia and bilateral cleft lip and palate. *Am J Med Genet* 59:229, 1995.

Kostmann Syndrome

At a glance: This rare blood disorder is characterized by severe chronic neutropenia. Symptoms associated with severe chronic neutropenia include recurring fevers, mouth ulcers, and periodontitis. Life-threatening recurrent infections are common complications that may last for months or years and can affect both children and adults.

Synonyms: Kostmann Disease; Severe Neutropenia Syndrome; Infantile Agranulocytosis; Congenital autosomal dominant (or sporadic) neutropenia.

Incidence and genetic inheritance: It is estimated to affect approximately 2000 to 5000 individuals in the United States. Severe chronic neutropenia may be inherited as an autosomal dominant or an autosomal recessive genetic trait. It can be acquired or may be idiopathic for unknown reasons. It affects males and females equally. Both children and adults can be affected.

Classification: The three main forms are congenital, idiopathic, and cyclic neutropenia. *Congenital forms* are typically apparent at birth or during early childhood and are considered the most severe form. *Chronic idiopathic neutropenia* usually affects adults. However, in some cases, the disorder has been demonstrated during childhood, but remains clinically undetected until adulthood. *Cyclic neutropenia* in most cases is thought to be present at birth. However, in some cases, symptoms may not become apparent until childhood, adolescence, or even early adulthood. The disorder may also be acquired.

Clinical aspects: *Congenital forms of severe chronic neutropenia:* Characterized by fevers, recurrent pneumonia, ear infections, gingivitis, and stomatitis. Periodontitis is often present. Recurrent oral ulcerations are common. Bacterial infections often affect the skin, gastrointestinal tract, and respiratory system and can be life-threatening. The most severe form of congenital neutropenia is known as Kostmann Syndrome. Treatment of Kostmann Syndrome consists of G-CSF for life. Some patients unfortunately may progress to myclodysplastic syndrome or acute myelogenous leukemia under this G-CSF therapy.

Chronic idiopathic neutropenia: Symptoms are less severe than those observed with congenital neutropenia; however, infections may also be life-threatening.

Cyclic neutropenia: Severe chronic decrease of neutrophils, presenting as episodes recurring on an average every 21 days and lasting for approximately 3 to 6 days. The cycling period usually remains constant and is consistent among affected individuals.

Anesthetic considerations: A complete blood count should be obtained for all these patients prior to anesthesia. Meticulous attention to sterility and asepsis is mandatory. Appropriate antibiotics must be used for all surgical procedures, including laryngoscopy and tracheal intubation.

Pharmacological implications: Several drugs (and other chemicals) may induce neutropenia/agranulocytosis in even healthy people. It seems therefore reasonable, to avoid these drugs in these patients. Some of these drugs include chemotherapeutics, antimicrobials (macrolides), non-steroidal anti-inflammatory drugs, antipsychotics, antithyroid drugs, anticonvulsants, antihistamines and many more.

REFERENCES:
Fujiu T, Maruyama K, Koizumi TL Early-onset group B streptococcal sepsis in a preterm infant with Kostmann syndrome. *Acta Paediatr* 91:1397, 2002.

Zetterstrom R: Kostmann disease–infantile genetic agranulocytosis: Historical views and new aspects. *Acta Paediatr* 91:1279, 2002.

Kosztolanyi Syndrome

At a glance: Polymalformative syndrome characterized by Marfan-like appearance (arachnodactyly), ossification disorders, and mental retardation.

Synonym: Arachnodactyly with Abnormal Ossification and Mental Retardation.

Incidence and genetic inheritance: Five reported cases in the literature. Possible association with chromosome 10 abnormality.

Pathophysiology: Unknown.

Clinical aspects: Numerous craniofacial abnormalities, including protruding eyes with downward-slanting palpebral fissures, midface hypoplasia, short, upturned nose, micrognathia, and abnormal, severely underdeveloped epiglottis. Arachnodactyly was present in all cases. Severe developmental delay. Recurrent apneic episodes and feeding difficulties are common.

Anesthetic considerations: The main concerns are related to craniofacial abnormalities. Potential difficult airway in terms of mask ventilation and laryngoscopy. Since these patients are prone to airway obstruction and apneas, minimizing or avoiding exposure to opioids or other sedatives is desirable. Close monitoring postoperatively is a requirement. Respiratory function may be compromised as a result of repeated aspiration pneumonias. The ability to protect the airway from aspiration is probably impaired as a result of the abnormal epiglottis. Malnutrition because of feeding difficulties may alter drug binding and clearance and impair the immune system function. Malnourished patients may also suffer from electrolyte disturbances and dehydration.

Other conditions to be considered:

Congenital Contractural Arachnodactyly: Marfanoid presentation. Other features include flexion contractures of multiple and major joints (including elbows, knees, hips, and fingers), often severe kyphoscoliosis accompanied by ventilation impairment, muscular hypoplasia, cardiovascular abnormalities (atrial septal defect, ventricular septal defect, interrupted aortic arch, single umbilical artery, and, rarely, aortic root dilatation); duodenal and esophageal atresia, intestinal malrotation; and camptodactyly. Thought to be associated with mutations in the fibrillin 2 gene.

☞**Marfan Syndrome:** Generalized connective tissue disorder with impaired structural integrity of the skeletal (hyperextensible joints), ocular, pulmonary (spontaneous pneumothorax), and cardiovascular systems (risk of valvular/aortic disease) caused by mutations in the fibrillin 1 gene.

REFERENCE:
Kosztolanyi G, Weisenbach J, Mehes K: Syndrome of arachnodactyly, disturbance of cranial ossification, protruding eyes, feeding difficulties, and mental retardation. *Am J Med Genet* 58:213, 1995.

Kousseff-Nichols Syndrome

At a glance: Often neonatal lethal syndrome with facial malformations and myopathy with high risk of malignant hyperthermia.

Synonym: Noonan-Like Contracture Myopathy Hyperpyrexia.

Incidence and genetic inheritance: Extremly rare syndrome with most likely autosomal recessive inheritance.

Clinical aspects: Patients present with short stature and myopathy. Clinical features may involve head and neck (webbed short neck with excess nuchal skin, expressionless face, epicanthic folds, down-slanted fissures, micrognathia, high-vaulted, narrow palate, low-set, posterior ears), and the musculoskeletal system (restricted joint mobility, scoliosis, webbing of joints, symphalangy, abnormal rib structure, abnormal scapula position, terminal hypoplasia of fingers, and camptodactyly). Absent nipples, abnormal scarring, and abnormal dental position can be associated. Death is frequent in neonatal period secondary to respiratory distress.

Anesthetic considerations: No literature is available. Evaluate intubation because of facial malformations and preserve spontaneous ventilation until the airway has been secured. Careful intraoperative positioning because of orthopedic features. Evaluate respiratory function because of skeletal deformations and myopathy. Postoperative ventilatory support may be necessary. Malignant hyperthermia can occur and requires avoidance of all triggering drugs. Volatile agents and succinylcholine therefore are contraindicated. Dantrolene should be easily available.

REFERENCE:
Kousseff BG, Nichols P: A new autosomal recessive syndrome with Noonan-like phenotype, myopathy with congenital contractures and maligant hyperthermia. *Birth Defects Orig Artic Ser* 21:111, 1985.

Kousseff Syndrome

At a glance: Severe polymalformative syndrome involving the nervous system (sacral meningocele), heart (conotruncal heart defect), unilateral renal agenesis, significant craniofacial deformities, low-set and posteriorly angulated ears, retrognathia, and short neck with low posterior hairline.

Synonym: Sacral Meningocele and Conotruncal Heart defects Syndrome.

Incidence: Only four reported cases in the literature. However, Toriello et al. suggested in 1985 that the incidence may be under-diagnosed and may represent as many as one in 100 cases of spina bifida cystica.

Genetic inheritance: Autosomal recessive. No single gene defect has been identified. Chromosomal studies in affected patients were normal.

Pathophysiology: Unknown.

Diagnosis: Significant cardiac and neural tube defects may be diagnosed in utero by ultrasonography. Elevated amniotic α-feto-protein levels are suggestive of open neural tube defects. Postpartum diagnosis is made based on phenotypical findings, including cardiac imaging with echocardiogram and/or cardiac catheterization.

Clinical aspects: Craniofacial features common to all cases included low-set, posteriorly rotated ears, retrognathia, depressed nasal tip, and short neck with low posterior hairline. Myelomeningocele with hydrocephalus was present in at least three of the four cases. Cardiac abnormalities have been described as truncus arteriosus in two cases and transposition of the great arteries in one case. The fourth patient had no cardiac abnormalities. Left renal and ureter agenesis was present in one case. The fingers may be long, and the space between the first and second toes may be large.

Precautions before anesthesia: Evaluation for congenital heart disease is mandatory. Presence of a harsh systolic and/or diastolic murmur, respiratory distress with cyanosis, and low oxygen saturation are signs of underlying cardiac disease. Electrocardiogram, echocardiogram, and consultation with a cardiologist to optimize cardiovascular therapy preoperatively are recommended. Patients with myelomeningocele may have neurologic deficits prior to or, especially, after repair. Any deficits should be documented prior to anesthesia and surgery. If renal anomalies are suspected, renal function and electrolyte status should be checked preoperatively.

Anesthetic considerations: Potentially difficult direct laryngoscopy and tracheal intubation because of retrognathia and short neck should be expected. Considerations for myelomeningocele (MMC) include protection of the defect while the patient is lying supine. Some MMC patients have a short trachea. There is a potential for considerable blood loss, especially if skin undermining is required to release subcutaneous fat and facilitate closure of the defect. Hydrocephalus and raised intracranial pressure secondary to Arnold-Chiari malformation may be present. Anatomy, pathophysiology, and particular hemodynamic goals for the specific form of congenital cardiac defect should be determined prior to anesthesia.

Pharmacological implications: Succinylcholine is not contraindicated because denervation is congenital. Endocarditis prophylaxis and prevention of paradoxical air embolus are additional considerations in such patients. Impaired renal function affects the pharmacokinetics and pharmacodynamics of drugs, particularly those that are water soluble and predominantly excreted via the kidney.

Other conditions to be considered:

☞**DiGeorge Syndrome:** Disorder characterized by hypocalcemia arising from parathyroid hypoplasia, thymic hypoplasia, and complex congenital heart defects. These include tetralogy of Fallot, type B interrupted aortic arch, truncus arteriosus, right aortic

arch, and aberrant right subclavian artery. Micrognathia may be present in infancy.

Conotruncal Anomaly Face Syndrome (Takao Velocardiofacial Syndrome): Japanese syndrome defined as "conotruncal anomaly face syndrome" with similar congenital heart defect as observed in the DiGeorge syndrome, but without the low T-cell count and hypocalcemic presentation in infancy and the craniofacial and palatal abnormalities typical of velocardiofacial syndrome.

☞**Velocardiofacial Syndrome:** Characterized by conotruncal anomaly and isolated outflow tract defects of the heart, including tetralogy of Fallot, truncus arteriosus, and interrupted aortic arch. Other clinical features include microcephaly, mental retardation, learning disabilities, minor auricular anomalies, bulbous nose, cleft palate, short stature, slender hands and digits, and inguinal hernia.

Gardner-Silengo-Wachtel Syndrome (Genitopalatocardiac Syndrome; Male Pseudohermaphroditism with Micrognathia, Cleft Palate and Conotruncal Cardiac Defect Syndrome): Autosomal-recessive transmitted disorder characterized by micrognathia, low-set ears, double-outlet right ventricle, transposition of the great vessels, ventricular septal defect, right-sided aortic arch, and 46,XY gonadal dysgenesis. Other clinical features may include cleft lip and palate, polycystic kidneys, and hypospadias.

REFERENCES:

Kousseff BG: Sacral meningocele with conotruncal heart defects: A possible autosomal recessive trait. *Pediatrics* 74:395, 1984.

Maclean K, Field MJ, Colley AS, et al: Kousseff syndrome: A causally heterogenous disorder. *Am J Med Genet A* 124:307, 2004.

Toriello HV, Sharda JK, Beaumont EJ: Autosomal recessive syndrome of sacral and conotruncal developmental field defects (Kousseff syndrome). *Am J Med Genet* 22:357, 1985.

Kowarski Syndrome

At a glance: Nanism caused by functional growth hormone deficiency.

Synonym: Pituitary Dwarfism Type IV.

Incidence: Exact incidence unknown. Less than 10 cases have been reported in the literature.

Genetic inheritance: Autosomal recessive inheritance. Presumed mutation is in the growth hormone gene on chromosome 17.

Pathophysiology: A structural abnormality of growth hormone causes low levels of somatomedin, which results in delayed bone age and growth retardation. Administration of exogenous growth hormone results in normal somatomedin levels and a significant increase in growth rate.

Diagnosis: Phenotypical findings. Low levels of somatomedin.

Clinical aspects: Typical clinical findings in patients with achondroplastic dwarfism may be absent in patients with Kowarski syndrome who have been treated with exogenous growth hormone. Neurological findings in achondroplastic dwarfs include foramen magnum stenosis and odontoid hypoplasia causing spinal cord compression, central sleep apnea, and obstructive hydrocephalus. Facial features are short maxilla, large tongue, and flat nose, which may predispose to obstructive sleep apnea. Pulmonary hypertension and cor pulmonale secondary to kyphoscoliosis and sleep apnea have been reported.

Precautions before anesthesia: Although none of the typical findings of achondroplasia are described in the referenced cases, any patient with abnormal growth should be carefully evaluated for potential difficult airway management, unstable cervical spine and/or spinal cord compression, and potential adverse effects of delayed growth on the respiratory and cardiovascular systems.

Anesthetic considerations: No specific considerations for isolated short stature are required, especially if treated. If untreated, considerations may include difficult laryngoscopy and avoidance of excessive airway manipulation, which may further compress the spinal cord. If the patient is at risk for apnea, judicious use of sedating medications and close postoperative monitoring may be necessary. Respiratory and cardiovascular compromise may increase complication rates and necessitate admission to an intensive care unit postoperatively. Thick, lax skin can make vascular access challenging.

Other conditions to be considered: Other types of dwarfism, especially the following:

☞**LARON SYNDROME:** Features of this autosomal-recessive transmitted disorder include severe dwarfism with sparse hair caused by primary (not acquired) abnormally high concentrations of immunoreactive serum growth hormone and insensitivity to exogenous growth hormone. Other features include craniofacial abnormalities, relative obesity (mostly reflected by excess of adipose tissue in the context of thin bones and diminished muscle mass), and hypotonia. More than 250 cases reported worldwide, but 65% of patients are of Semitic descent.

REFERENCES:

Kowarski AA, Schneider JJ, Ben-Galim E, et al: Growth failure with normal serum RIA-GH and low somatomedin activity: Somatomedin restoration and growth acceleration after exogenous GH. *J Clin Endocrinol* 47:461, 1978.

Takahashi Y, Chihara K: Clinical significance and molecular mechanisms of bioinactive growth hormone (review). *Int J Mol Med* 2:287, 1998.

Valenta LJ, Sigel MB, Lesniak MA, et al: Pituitary dwarfism in a patient with circulating abnormal growth hormone polymers. *N Engl J Med* 312:214, 1985.

Kozlowski-Brown-Hardwick Syndrome

At a glance: Polymalformative syndrome characterized by multiple skeletal anomalies, hydrocephalus, ptosis, myopia, micrognathia, and retrognathia.

Incidence and genetic inheritance: Only two reported cases involving dizygotic female twins have been described. Presumed autosomal recessive inheritance.

Clinical aspects: Craniofacial abnormalities included a long narrow head with communicating hydrocephalus, prominent forehead, large anterior fontanelle, midface hypoplasia, proptosis and hypertelorism, grooved chin and small upturned nose, and mandibular hypoplasia (micrognathia). Musculoskeletal abnormalities included hooked clavicles, 13 pairs of ribs, large hands and feet with long, slender fingers, widened metaphyses, and square-shaped vertebral bodies, which developed over time as a sign of muscular hypotonia. Both patients were developmentally delayed and suffered from gastroesophageal reflux and recurrent respiratory infections. The only cardiac finding was a functional systolic murmur.

Anesthetic considerations: Possibly difficult face-mask ventilation and direct laryngoscopy. These patients may be prone to upper airway obstruction. Raised intracranial pressure secondary to hydrocephalus should be considered. Hypotonia may predispose to respiratory fatigue and failure with increased work of breathing for same reason. Sensitivity to muscle relaxants may be increased. Additional respiratory compromise should be expected from repeated aspiration pneumonias due to gastroesophageal reflux. Reduced cooperation because of developmental delay is likely. Sedative premedication and/or the presence of the primary caregiver for induction of anesthesia may be helpful.

REFERENCE:

Kozlowski K, Brown J, Hardwick R, et al: A new syndrome? Unusual facies, hooked clavicles, 13 pairs of ribs, widened metaphyses, square shaped vertebral bodies and communicating hydrocephalus. *Pediatr Radiol* 22:328, 1992.

Kozlowski-Celermajer Syndrome

At a glance: Malformative syndrome characterized by musculoskeletal anomalies (humerospinal dysostosis) associated with cardiac malformation (cardiomegaly, tricuspid regurgitation, and pulmonary hypertension).

Synonyms: Humerospinal Dysostosis; Humerospinal Dysostosis with Congenital Heart Disease.

Incidence and genetic inheritance: Four cases are reported in the literature, two of which were half-siblings. Presumed autosomal dominant inheritance with variable penetrance.

Clinical aspects: Musculoskeletal anomalies were the primary findings and included dysplastic vertebrae with midcoronal clefts, shortened humeri with distal bifurcation, subluxated elbow and knee joints, shortened and hypotubular long bones of the lower extremities that were often bowed, widened iliac bones, and talipes equinovarus. Range of motion of affected joints was limited. Scoliosis developed in one patient. All three patients had murmurs and two had cardiomegaly on the chest radiograph. Tricuspid regurgitation and pulmonary hypertension were diagnosed by cardiac catheterization in the second half-sibling at age 2 years. Both half-siblings, who died at ages of 7 months and 8 years, respectively, were found to have thickened and stenotic mitral and tricuspid valves, right atrial and ventricular hypertrophy with dilatation and endocardial fibrosis on autopsy. The pulmonic and aortic valves were only mildly affected.

Anesthetic considerations: Cardiac evaluation, particularly echocardiography, prior to anesthesia to identify valvular anomalies and pulmonary hypertension is required. Patients with pulmonary hypertension are at greater risk for perioperative cardiac morbidity. Anesthetic management should be directed toward lowering, or at least preventing a rise in, pulmonary artery pressure. Endocarditis prophylaxis may be required, depending on the proposed procedure. Extremities with contracted joints require careful positioning and padding to maintain the limb in the usual position and prevent injury to pressure points.

REFERENCES:

Cortina H, Vidal J, Vallcanera A, et al: Humero-spinal dysostosis. *Pediatr Radiol* 8:188, 1979.

Hall BD: Humero-spinal dysostosis: Report of the fourth case with emphasis on generalized skeletal involvement, abnormal craniofacial features, and mitral valve thickening. *J Pediatr Orthop B* 6:11, 1997.

Kozlowski KS, Celermajer JM, Tink AR: Humero-spinal dysostosis with congenital heart disease. *Am J Dis Child* 127:407, 1974.

Kozlowski-Ouvrier Syndrome

At a glance: Malformative syndrome characterized by corpus callosum agenesis associated with multiple skeletal anomalies.

Synonym: Bone Dysplasia with Corpus Callosum Agenesis.

Incidence and genetic inheritance: One case reported in the literature. No mention of possible chromosomal abnormalities or method of genetic transmission.

Clinical aspects: Agenesis of the corpus callosum with significant gross motor and developmental delay. Circular-shaped head with lambdoid synostosis (no surgical correction was required), broad forehead, and triangular-shaped face. Diffuse bony abnormalities, including multiple "Wormian" bones (named after the Danish anatomist Ole Worm [1588–1654], describing small intrasutural bones [most commonly lambdoid suture], that can appear in significant numbers), osteopenic vertebrae, thin ribs, short, straight and laterally tapering clavicles, abnormal phalanges, and retarded bone age.

Anesthetic considerations: Developmentally delayed patients may be uncooperative. Cranial synostosis can lead to raised intracranial pressure, although this was not the case in this patient. Osteopenic bones may be fragile and prone to fracture during handling and positioning of anesthetized patients.

REFERENCE:

Kozlowski K, Ouvrier RA: Agenesis of the corpus callosum with mental retardation and osseous lesions. *Am J Med Genet* 48:6, 1993.

Kozlowski-Rafinski-Kucharska Syndrome

At a glance: Congenital cataract with epimetaphyseal dysplasia and facial anomalies.

Synonym: Epimetaphyseal Dysplasia with Cataract.

Incidence and genetic inheritance: One reported case. Mode of inheritance unknown.

Clinical aspects: Peculiar, "old-looking," face with small mouth opening, small jaw with hypoplastic mandibular rami, small and irregular teeth, narrow, sharp nose, and cataracts in both eyes. The chest was small with protruding sternum and scapulae. Lumbar lordosis was present, but no kyphoscoliosis. The extremities were relatively long and thin, with large hands and feet and muscle tone was decreased. Skeletal radiographs showed marked, generalized epiphyseal and metaphyseal ossification disturbances. Mental and developmental delay were present. The electrocardiogram showed signs of right ventricular hypertrophy. All laboratory investigations were normal except for elevated gonadotropins and sustained elevation of blood glucose levels after glucose tolerance tests.

Anesthetic considerations: The facial abnormalities could make airway management difficult. Micrognathia and a small mouth opening may interfere with laryngoscopy. The cause of the right ventricular hypertrophy is unknown. Congenital heart defects and pulmonary hypertension resulting from an abnormally shaped chest are two possibilities. The exact cause needs to be determined prior to anesthesia and surgery. Significant lumbar lordosis and skeletal abnormalities make proper positioning more difficult, and special attention must be paid to careful padding of susceptible pressure points. Patients with glucose intolerance may develop overt diabetes mellitus perioperatively and require insulin therapy to maintain normal blood glucose levels.

REFERENCE:

Kozlowski K, Rafinski T, Kucharska K: Metaphyseal and epiphyseal dysplasia with unusual facies and cataract. *Am J Dis Child* 125:553, 1973.

Kozlowski-Tsuruta-Taki Syndrome

At a glance: Lethal neonatal dwarfism characterized by microcephaly, cortical hyperostosis, and multiple vital organ malformations.

Synonym: Dysplastic Cortical Hyperostosis.

Incidence and genetic inheritance: One reported case of a stillborn infant of 28 weeks' gestational age. The mode of inheritance, if any, is unknown.

Clinical aspects: Microcephaly with poor cerebral sulci development, normal-size mandible, but small mouth opening, severe facial edema, hypoplastic lungs, left renal duplication, high position of the right coronary artery orifice, hepatosplenomegaly, generalized, symmetrical cortical bone thickening with shortened tubular bones, and poorly developed vertebral bodies.

Anesthetic considerations: Lethal disease with intrauterine death.

REFERENCE:

Kozlowski K, Tsuruta T: Dysplastic cortical hyperostosis: A new form of lethal neonatal dwarfism. *Br J Radiol* 62:376, 1989.

Kozlowski-Warren-Fisher Syndrome

At a glance: Lethal malformative syndrome characterized by cloverleaf skull and bone dysplasia in stillborns.

Synonym: Cloverleaf Skull with Generalized Bone Dysplasia.

Incidence and genetic inheritance: One reported case. Male infant stillborn at 35 weeks' gestation. Mode of genetic inheritance unknown.

Clinical aspects: Cloverleaf deformity of the skull, with extremely broad anterior fontanel, frontal, and coronal sutures, small posterior fossa and foramen magnum, and gross hydrocephaly. Midfacial hypoplasia with shallow orbits, a narrow chest with long, narrow lungs, normal heart except for a large foramen ovale with a fenestrated, diaphanous flap were further findings. The limbs were short with the proximal segment being most severely affected. The abdominal contents were morphologically normal, but there were widespread petechial hemorrhages of the organs.

Anesthetic considerations: Lethal in utero.

REFERENCE:

Kozlowski K, Warren PS, Fisher CC: Cloverleaf skull with generalised bone dysplasia. Report of a case with short review of the literature. *Pediatr Radiol* 15:412, 1985.

Krasnow-Qazi Syndrome

At a glance: Disorder characterized by the association of cataracts, cardiomyopathy and multiple joint disorders.

Synonym: Cardiomyopathy with Cataract and Hip Spine Disease.

Incidence and genetic inheritance: Three of seven children from consanguineous parents had a triad of cardiomyopathy, joint disease, and cataracts. Several relatives in the previous and following generations had one or two conditions of the triad. Autosomal recessive inheritance, with variable penetrance and expressivity has been suggested.

Clinical aspects: Dilated cardiomyopathy secondary to myocardial infiltration with basophilic periodic acid–Schiff (PAS)-positive granulofilamentous deposits resulting in hypokinetic left ventricular function. Electrocardiographic changes, including Q-waves in inferior leads, right bundle branch block, and long-QT interval, were common, but dysrhythmias were not a frequent feature of the clinical course. Bilateral degenerative disease of the hips and intervertebral disks of the thoracolumbar spine, which caused mild scoliosis was noted. Platyspondyly and anterior wedging of the vertebrae were seen on spine radiographs. Cataracts appeared in the young adults prior to other manifestations of the syndrome.

Anesthetic considerations: Evaluate and optimize cardiac status preoperatively. Obtain an echocardiogram to check for dysrhythmias. Echocardiogram to assess myocardial function (ejection fraction) and valvular function. Some cardiac medications may cause electrolyte abnormalities (angiotensin-converting enzyme inhibitors, diuretics). Tolerance of myocardial depressants, hyper- or hypovolemia may be limited. Invasive monitoring with arterial line, central line with or without pulmonary artery catheter may be useful to optimize myocardial function. Postoperative intensive care unit care for monitoring and inotropic support may be required. Patients with degenerative joint disease may have contractures that are painful and require careful positioning and padding. Although not a significant feature of this syndrome, severe thoracolumbar disk disease could lead to kyphoscoliosis, which may affect respiratory and later on also cardiac function.

REFERENCE:

Krasnow N, Qazi QH, Yermakov V: A familial dilated cardiomyopathy associated with cataracts and hip-spine disease. *Chest* 87:56, 1985.

Krause-Kivlin Syndrome

At a glance: This congenital syndrome is characterized by the combination of short limb dwarfism, facial anomalies, and mental retardation with ophthalmologic anomalies. Corneal opacification and shallow anterior chamber with synechiae are summarized as Peters anomaly. Other features may include cardiac anomalies, hydrocephalus, seizures, and urogenital anomalies.

Synonyms: Krause-Van Schooneveld-Kivlin Syndrome; Peters Anomaly with Short-Limb Dwarfism; Peters-Plus Syndrome.

Incidence and Genetic Inheritance: Approximately 50 cases have been described so far. Autosomal recessive inheritance. Consanguinity is a common feature.

Clinical aspects: Intrauterine and postnatal growth retardation with birth weight and length below the third percentile and postnatal length also below the third percentile. Mental retardation of variable degree affects the majority of these patients and seizures have been reported in a minority. Peters anomaly of the eye refers to abnormal embryonic development of the eye, resulting in corneal opacification (central corneal leukoma, central defect of Descemet's membrane) and adhesions involving the iris, lens, and cornea. Glaucoma is the main cause of loss of vision in many of these patients. Abnormal facial features include round face, microcephaly (less commonly macrocephaly), hydrocephalus with cerebral atrophy, hypertelorism, abnormal ears, depressed nasal bridge, mild micrognathia, cleft lip and/or palate, thin upper lip, and hypoplastic columella. Brachymorphism, especially of the hands, tapering brachydactyly, and fifth finger clinodactyly are prominent findings. Cardiac defects such as ventricular and/or atrial septal defects occur in about one third of patients. Urogenital abnormalities frequently occur and may include pyelonephritis, hydronephrosis, and duplication of the ureters and hypospadias. Spina bifida and anal atresia have been reported in some patients. A recent case report showed that these patients may be growth hormone deficient and respond well to its exogenous substitution.

Anesthetic considerations: Assess the patient for cardiac defects (clinically, echocardiogram) and for renal anomalies (creatinine, urea, ultrasound). Dysmorphic facial features, especially micrognathia, may make airway management difficult. Raised intracranial pressure may be present. Mental retardation may limit patient cooperation. Sedative and/or anxiolytic premedication and the presence of the primary caregiver for induction of anesthesia may be helpful. Avoid succinylcholine in the presence of glaucoma. Glaucoma therapy may include topical β-blockers that can exert systemic effects.

Other condition to be considered:

PETERS ANOMALY: Most often characterized by central corneal leukoma, absence of the posterior corneal-stroma and Descemet membrane (the membrane limiting the posterior aspect of the cornea), amblyopia, visual impairment, and a variable degree of iris and lenticular synechiae with the central aspect of the posterior cornea. Severe glaucoma is common.

REFERENCES:

Frydman M, Weinstock AL, Cohen HA, et al: Autosomal recessive Peters anomaly, typical facial appearance, failure to thrive, hydrocephalus, and other anomalies: Further delineation of the Krause-Kivlin syndrome. *Am J Med Genet* 40:34, 1991.

Lee KW, Lee PD: Growth hormone deficiency (GHD): A new association in Peters' Plus Syndrome (PPS). *Am J Med Genet A* 124:388, 2004.

Maillette de Buy Wenninger-Prick LJ, Hennekam RC: The Peters' plus syndrome: A review. *Ann Genet* 45:97, 2002.

Krause-Reese Syndrome

At a glance: Inherited syndrome characterized by multiple ocular malformations and microcephaly, more commonly found in premature infants.

Synonyms: Encephalo-Ophthalmic Dysplasia; Congenital Encephalo-Ophthalmic Dysplasia; Encephalo-Ophthalmic Syndrome; Ophthalmo-Encephalic Dysplasia; Reese-Blodi Retinal Dysplasia; Reese-Blodi-Krause Syndrome.

Incidence and genetic inheritance: Extremely rare. Autosomal recessive inheritance has been suggested, although in one family inheritance was described as autosomal dominant with variable expressivity.

Clinical aspects: Microcephaly and retinal and cerebral dysplasia, more commonly found in premature infants and single infants of multiple birth. Ocular findings include microphthalmos, enophthalmos, persistence of the primary vitreous, intraocular hemorrhages, retinal choroid and optic nerve malformations, glaucoma, cataracts, strabismus, retinal atrophy, and blindness. Hyperplasia or aplasia of the cerebrum and cerebellum can occur, resulting in hydrocephalus and mental retardation.

Anesthetic considerations: Increased intracranial pressure may be present. Developmental delay may make cooperation more difficult. Avoid succinylcholine in the presence of glaucoma.

Other condition to be considered:

☞**HARD (±) E SYNDROME:** An acronymic syndrome (*H*ydrocephalus, *A*gyria, *R*etinal *D*ysplasia) that is occasionally associated with an occipital *E*ncephalocele (± E). Other features include micropenis, cryptorchism, hydronephrosis, pelviureteral junction obstruction, anoperineal fistula. Usually lethal within the first months of life. Inheritance is autosomal recessive.

REFERENCES:

Krause AC: Congenital encephalo-ophthalmic dysplasia. *Arch Ophthalmol* 36:387, 1946.

Reese AB, Blodi FC: Retinal dysplasia. *Am J Ophthalmol* 33:23, 1950.

Reese AB, Straatsma BR: Retinal dysplasia. *Am J Ophthalmol* 45:199, 1958.

Krauss-Herman-Holmes Syndrome

At a glance: Malformative syndrome of the skeleton characterized by hypoplasia of carpal bones, microstomia, and micrognathia.

Synonyms: Carpal Deformity with Micrognathia and Microstomia.

Incidence and genetic inheritance: Two reported cases, a mother and her son, have been described. Presumed autosomal dominant inheritance.

Clinical aspects: Main feature is a unilateral congenital hypoplasia of the proximal row of carpal bones in the right hand. Dysplasia of the distal carpal bones, radius, and ulna on the right side were also present. Both patients had marked micrognathia, high-arched palate, and small mouth opening (microstomia). However, several otherwise healthy family members (i.e., no limb abnormalities) were retrognathic, thus, it is difficult to unequivocally link this feature to the congenital carpal bone hypoplasia.

Anesthetic considerations: Primary concern is potential difficult direct laryngoscopy and tracheal intubation because of retrognathia and microstomia. Awake fiberoptic intubation, or other similar techniques, may be necessary to secure the airway.

REFERENCE:

Krauss CM, Herman TE, Holmes LB: Unilateral carpal bone deformity in mother and son. *Am J Med Genet* 26:557, 1987.

Krieble-Bixler Syndrome

At a glance: Inherited syndrome characterized by ocular hypotelorism, submucosal cleft palate, clinodactyly of the fifth finger,

and hypospadias. May present with tetralogy of Fallot and short stature (dwarfism).

Synonyms: Hypotelorism with Cleft Palate and Hypospadias; Ocular Hypotelorism, Submucosal Cleft Palate, and Hypospadias Syndrome.

Incidence and genetic inheritance: One case report of a father and his son. Autosomal dominant inheritance.

Clinical aspects: Ocular manifestations include hypotelorism, blepharophimosis, epicanthus and upslanting of the palpebral fissures. Submucosal cleft palate, inguinal hernia and hypospadias, syndactyly of the third and fourth fingers and second and third toes and clinodactyly of the fifth finger were other characteristic features. Tetralogy of Fallot was present in the boy only.

Anesthetic considerations: Infants with cleft palate may suffer from feeding difficulties resulting in failure to thrive, anemia, and repeated respiratory infections. Preoperative screening for hemoglobin level and signs of ongoing infection may be warranted. Cleft palate may make laryngoscopy awkward, although not usually difficult. Cardiac assessment is recommended and echocardiography may be indicated to rule out structural lesions.

Other conditions to be considered:

SCHILBACH-ROTT SYNDROME (Ocular Hypotelorism-Cleft Palate-Hypospadias Syndrome; Cleft Palate-Hypotelorism-Hypospadias Syndrome): Ten patients in one family (over 5 generations) have been reported. Characterized by ocular hypotelorism, submucosal cleft palate, and hypospadias. Other clinical features include blepharophimosis, upslanted palpebral fissures, cutaneous syndactyly of fingers 3 and 4 and toes 2 and 3. No known congenital heart defects associated.

HARROD SYNDROME: Characterized by mental retardation, large protruding ears, arachnodactyly, hypogenitalism, failure to thrive, unusual facial appearance (hypotelorism, long nose, highly arched palate, pointed chin, microstomia), and hypospadias.

REFERENCES:

Krieble BF, Bixler D: Autosomal dominant blepharophimosis with multiple congenital anomalies. *J Clin Dysmorphol* 2:24, 1984.

Schilbach U, Rott H-D: Ocular hypotelorism, submucosal cleft palate, and hypospadias: A new autosomal dominant syndrome. *Am J Med Genet* 31:863, 1988.

Kudo-Tamura-Fuse Syndrome

At a glance: Severe polymalformative syndrome leading to death within the newborn period and characterized by malformations of kidneys, facial features, and multiple visceral and cerebral anomalies.

Synonym: Renal Dysplasia with Hepatic Fibrosis and Dandy-Walker.

Incidence and genetic inheritance: Two reported cases of premature babies who died in the early neonatal period. Unknown mode of inheritance.

Clinical aspects: Characteristic cystic dysplastic kidneys. Congenital hepatic fibrosis, Dandy-Walker malformation, and hydrocephalus complete the syndrome. The fourth ventricle in both patients was cystic, with dilated third and lateral ventricles. The vermis cerebelli was absent in both patients. Dysmorphic facies, including low-set ears, flattened nose, hypertelorism, and microphthalmos were present.

Anesthetic considerations: Both, dysplastic kidneys and fibrotic liver most likely have impaired function. Kidney dysfunction may cause electrolyte abnormalities, hyper- or hypovolemia, and abnormal platelet function. Liver dysfunction may cause abnormal glucose regulation, coagulation status, ascites, and many other problems. Pharmacodynamics and pharmacokinetics of anesthetic and other drugs will be affected. Hydrocephalus and raised intracranial pressure may be present.

Other conditions to be considered:

☞**GOLDSTON SYNDROME:** Characterized by a combination of central nervous malformations (including Dandy-Walker malformation), renal dysplasia, and hepatic and pancreatic malformation.

☞**MECKEL-GRUBER SYNDROME:** Characterized by a combination of sloping forehead, occipital encephalocele, Dandy-Walker malformation, renal cysts, hepatic ductal dysplasia and cysts, polydactyly and polycystic kidneys. Genetically transmitted as an autosomal recessive trait.

REFERENCE:

Kudo M, Tamura K, Fuse Y: Cystic dysplastic kidneys associated with Dandy-Walker malformation and congenital hepatic fibrosis. Report of two cases. *Am J Clin Pathol* 84:459, 1985.

Kumar-Levick Syndrome

At a glance: Inherited syndrome associated with mild mental retardation, malformations of the extremities and occasionally deafness.

Synonym: Anonychia Onychodystrophy Brachydactyly, Type B.

Incidence and genetic inheritance: Reported in only one kindred across five generations. Autosomal dominant inheritance with variable penetrance.

Clinical aspects: The malformations are confined to the limbs: absent or dystrophic finger- and toenails, hypoplastic metacarpals, metatarsals, and distal phalanges, clinodactyly, and long, broad finger-like thumbs. Two individuals had absent metacarpals and phalanges. Mild mental retardation occurred in some individuals.

Anesthetic considerations: Mental retardation may limit cooperation. Sedative/anxiolytic premedication and/or the presence of the primary caregiver for induction of anesthesia may be helpful.

REFERENCE:

Kumar D, Levick RK: Autosomal dominant onychodystrophy and anonychia with type B brachydactyly and ectrodactyly. *Clin Genet* 30:219, 1986.

Kunze-Riehm Syndrome

At a glance: A disorder characterized by dystrophic skin (deep circumferential creases), mental retardation, hypertrichosis, and, occasionally, congenital heart defects. Other features include cleft palate and neuroblastoma.

Synonyms: Michelin Tire Baby Syndrome; Multiple Benign Ring-Shaped Skin Creases of Limbs.

Incidence: Approximately 25 cases have been reported in the literature.

Genetic inheritance: Presumed autosomal dominant inheritance with variable penetrance and expression.

Pathophysiology: Unknown. Explanations for deep circumferential skin creases include diffuse underlying lipomatous nevus, underlying smooth muscle hamartoma, and a disorder of "elastic fiber" formation.

Diagnosis: Primarily clinical. Biopsy to show the presence of a smooth muscle hamartoma has been suggested. Histologic examination to determine the presence of elastic fiber abnormalities has been proposed, whereas electronic microscopy may show decreased elastin deposition.

Clinical aspects: Primary features include deep circumferential skin creases on the forearms and sometimes neck and lower limbs. Gyrus-like creases may be seen on the back. The skin is loose and may seem thick. The creases resolve spontaneously during childhood, although remnants may be visible in adults. Numerous other congenital abnormalities have occurred in association with this disorder: cleft palate, congenital heart disease, localized neuroblastoma, craniofacial anomalies (micrognathia), inguinal and umbilical hernias, and psychomotor retardation.

Precautions before anesthesia: The infant or young child presenting with deep skin creases should be investigated for associated anomalies. A full history and physical examination must be done to assess for cleft palate, congenital heart disease, and craniofacial abnormalities. Developmental delay may be present. Investigations should include hemoglobin level, electrocardiogram, chest radiograph, and echocardiogram if necessary. Workup for neuroblastoma would include urine and plasma catecholamine levels and imaging studies. Uncommonly, hypertension is present, which should be well controlled prior to anesthesia.

Anesthetic considerations: Potential for difficult airway management must be anticipated because of micrognathia and/or cleft palate. Difficult placement of intravenous, intraarterial, and central venous catheters is most probable because of deep folds of loose, thick skin. Considerations for congenital heart disease include knowledge of the anatomy and pathophysiology of the lesion and strict avoidance of air embolism. Fluctuations in blood pressure caused by release of catecholamines and/or blood loss can occur during manipulation of a neuroblastoma tumor. Careful padding for intraoperative positioning is required.

Pharmacological implications: No specific pharmacological implications. In the presence of congenital heart defect, anesthetic drug implications are dictated by the cardiovascular pathophysiology. Subacute bacterial endocarditis prophylaxis must be considered in presence of a congenital heart defect.

REFERENCES:

Kunze J, Riehm H: A new genetic disorder: Autosomal-dominant multiple benign ring-shaped skin creases. *Eur J Pediatr* 138:301, 1982.

Sardana K, Mendiratta V, Kakar N, et al: Spontaneously improving Michelin tire baby syndrome. *Pediatr Dermatol* 20:150, 2003.

Sato M, Ishikawa O, Miyachi Y, et al: Michelin tyre syndrome: A congenital disorder of elastic fibre formation? *Br J Dermatol* 136:583, 1997.

Kurczynski-Casperson Syndrome

At a glance: Congenital polymalformative syndrome characterized by craniosynostosis, mild mental retardation, hearing loss, symmetric syndactyly of the toes, and possible congenital heart defect.

Synonym: Auralcephalosyndactyly.

Incidence and genetic inheritance: Five cases have been documented in the literature. Presumed autosomal dominant inheritance. Normal karyotype.

Clinical aspects: Facial anomalies include bilateral coronal craniosynostosis without neurologic sequelae, relatively narrow pinnae inferiorly and short columella, and symmetrical syndactyly of the fourth and fifth toes. Two of the five cases developed mild mental retardation and hearing loss. One case died in infancy as a consequence of congenital heart disease (unknown type).

Anesthetic considerations: Isolated craniosynostosis usually does not interfere with airway management, but it may be associated with other craniofacial abnormalities. Raised intracranial pressure can occur secondary to fused cranial sutures. If more than two sutures are affected, up to 38% of patients will have increased intracranial pressure. Cranial vault reconstruction involves large volume blood product transfusion and risk of air embolus. Large-bore venous access and invasive pressure monitoring is therefore recommended. Congenital heart disease may be associated with this syndrome, and the patient should be evaluated appropriately (history and physical examination, electrocardiogram, echocardiogram). Considerations for the patient with a congenital cardiac lesion include knowledge of the anatomy and pathophysiology, subacute bacterial endocarditis prophylaxis, and strict avoidance of air embolus. Mental retardation and hearing loss may compromise cooperation.

REFERENCE:

Kurczynski TW, Casperson SM: Auralcephalosyndactyly: A new hereditary craniosynostosis syndrome. *J Med Genet* 25:491, 1988.

Legius E, Fryns JP, Van den Berghe H: Auralcephalosyndactyly: A new craniosynostosis syndrome or a variant of the Saethre-Chotzen syndrome? *J Med Genet* 26:522, 1989.

Kuster-Majewski-Hammerstein Syndrome

At a glance: Characterized by alopecia, macular degeneration, growth retardation, cleft hand, ectrodactyly syndactyly, and ectodermal dysplasia.

Synonym: Alopecia with Macular Degeneration and Growth Retardation.

Incidence and genetic inheritance: One case report exists. Autosomal recessive inheritance most probable.

Clinical aspects: Repeated loss of scalp and body hair with some regrowth (hypotrichosis) started at the age of 20 years. Ring-shaped ("bull's-eye") degeneration of the retinal pigmentary epithelium of both eyes with poor visual acuity was noted. Short stature (proportional dwarfism) but otherwise normal musculoskeletal examination. Intelligence was normal.

Anesthetic considerations: No significant anesthetic considerations specific to this condition.

Other condition to be considered:

☞**EEM SYNDROME:** Main features are syndactyly and other abnormalities of the fingers and toes, sparse head hair from birth, bilateral macular degeneration, and small widely spaced teeth.

REFERENCE:

Kuster W, Majewski F, Hammerstein W: Alopecia, macular degeneration, and growth retardation: A new syndrome? *Am J Med Genet* 28:477, 1987.

Ohdo S, Hirayama K, Terawaki T: Association of ectodermal dysplasia, ectrodactyly, and macular dystrophy: The EEM syndrome. *J Med Genet* 20:52, 1983.

Senecky Y, Halpern GJ, Inbar D, et al: Ectodermal dysplasia, ectrodactyly and macular dystrophy (EEM syndrome) in siblings. *Am J Med Genet* 101:195, 2001.

Kuzniecky Syndrome

At a glance: Neurologic syndrome with mental retardation, epilepsy, and enlarged gyri (pachygyria).

Synonym: Pachygyria Mental Retardation Epilepsy.

Incidence and genetic inheritance: Two brothers have been described with this disease. Presumed autosomal recessive inheritance. Normal chromosomal studies.

Clinical aspects: Severe nonprogressive encephalopathy characterized by impairment of motor and intellectual development with atypical, absence, and generalized tonic-clonic seizures. The parietal cortex was enlarged to 10 to 12 mm on MRI, which suggested pachygyria (enlarged gyri).

Anesthetic considerations: Type, severity, and control of seizure disorder should be evaluated. Antiepileptics should be continued throughout the perioperative period. Some antiseizure medications affect the pharmacodynamic properties of some commonly used anesthetic drugs (e.g., phenytoin increases the requirements for nondepolarizing muscle relaxants).

Other conditions to be considered:

CONGENITAL BILATERAL PERISYLVIAN SYNDROME: This disorder is characterized by diplegia of the face, tongue, jaws, and pseudobulbar palsy, dysarthria, inability to chew, dysphagia, and epilepsy. In most cases, mild-to-severe mental retardation is present. The clinical picture is influenced by the age of onset. It is thought to result from neuronal dysmigration in the cortex. Three types have been suggested: congenital, infantile, and childhood form. The disorder appears to occur sporadically. Histopathologically, polymicrogyria with cortical thickness of 5 to 7 mm can be demonstrated.

DOUBLE CORTEX SYNDROME: Clinically similar, but differentiated by the presence of a band of subcortical heterotopic gray matter underlying the cortical mantle. This disorder must be considered to be transmitted in an X-linked dominant way causing classic lissencephaly with severe mental retardation and epilepsy in hemizygous males and subcortical laminar heterotopia associated with milder mental retardation and epilepsy in heterozygous females.

REFERENCE:

Kuzniecky R: Familial diffuse cortical dysplasia. *Arch Neurol* 51:307, 1994.

Kwashiorkor

At a glance: Acquired disorder caused by malnutrition secondary to insufficient protein intake resulting in multisystemic chronic failure with generalized edemas.

Genetic inheritance: No genetic component. Acquired malnutrition disease.

Pathophysiology: A condition in which almost all systems may be involved. A multifactorial process related primarily to dietary and environmental factors. The presence of edema is an important criteria in making the diagnosis.

Diagnosis: Decreased protein intake, and thus production, results in a decrease in albumin. Increase in total body water (particularly extracellular) relative to body weight. Decreased total body potassium and magnesium. Low plasma sodium, but increased total body sodium. Bone demineralization. Anemia is common and is related to iron, protein, and vitamin deficiencies. Impaired immune status as a result of thymic atrophy and impaired polymorphonuclear cell chemotaxis. Hepatocellular damage is a poor prognostic sign.

Clinical aspects: Presence of edema is necessary to make the diagnosis. Patients usually have stunted growth and wasting. There is relative sparing of subcutaneous adipose tissue. Anorexia, diarrhea, and skin excoriation are common. Wasting of cardiac muscle with decrease in stroke volume and prolongation of circulation time. Concentrating and diluting ability of the kidneys may be impaired.

Precautions before anesthesia: Evaluate cardiac function. Obtain echocardiography if necessary. Blood examination: should include a complete blood count, electrolytes, acid–base status, and liver function tests, including albumin. Coagulation profile and bleeding time should be obtained.

Anesthetic considerations: Low albumin concentration may increase the free fraction of protein-bound drugs, but this may be offset by an increase in total body water. Low cardiac output may slow induction with intravenous induction agents. Children with Kwashiorkor are unable to control their body temperature within a narrow range and may develop hypothermia or hyperthermia depending on the circumstances. Pressure points must be well protected in view of the friable skin.

Pharmacological implications: Consider altered hepatic and renal function and albumin concentration when selecting anesthetic agents and other drugs.

Other conditions to be considered:

☞**DANBOLT-CLOSS SYNDROME:** An inherited vesiculobullous disorder characterized by intermittent simultaneous occurrence of diarrhea and bullous dermatitis (dry lesions surrounding the mouth, ears, nose and eyes, but also affecting the fingers, feet, and knees) and failure to thrive in premature babies. In children, periorificial lesions of the face and anogenital region occur. Alopecia and absence of eyebrows, eyelashes, and thymus are common.

KESHAN DISEASE: A condition caused by a deficiency of the essential trace mineral selenium as well as an infection with an enterovirus (coxsackie). It is named after the Chinese province Keshan, where this disease is endemic and was first described. It has since been reported from other parts of the world (e.g., New Zealand, Finland). The clinical picture consists of a potentially fatal cardiomyopathy of childhood characterized by multiple patchy areas of myocardial necrosis (later fibrosis) mainly affecting the left ventricle, but also the atria and the right ventricle. The necrotic lesions are isolated and lack a vascular or inflammatory reaction.

REFERENCES:

Collins S, Sadler K: Outpatient care for severely malnourished children in emergency relief programmes: A retrospective cohort study. *Lancet* 360:1824, 2002.

Jackson A, Golden M: Protein energy malnutrition: Kwashiorkor and marasmic Kwashiorkor: Physiopathology, in Brunser O, Carrazza FR, Gracey M, et al. (eds): *Clinical Nutrition of the Young Child.* New York, Raven Press, 1991, p 133.

Liu T, Howard RM, Mancini AJ, et al: Kwashiorkor in the United States: Fad diets, perceived and true milk allergy, and nutritional ignorance. *Arch Dermatol* 137:630, 2001.

Nezelot C, Bouvier R, Dijoud F: Multifocal myocardial necrosis: A distinctive cardiac lesion in cystic fibrosis, lipomatous pancreatic atrophy, and Keshan disease. *Pediatr Pathol Mol Med* 21:343, 2002.

Kyrle Disease

At a glance: Skin disease usually associated with systemic disorders such as chronic renal failure, diabetes mellitus, hepatic abnormalities, and congestive heart failure. Characterized by widespread development of large papules with central keratin plugs. Intense itching is often present. Skin lesions are present for 4 months to 4 years, but most often respond to the treatment of the underlying cause. Other features include coagulation disorders, albuminemia, elevated serum creatinine, and polyuria. Onset age is approximately 30 years.

Incidence: Rare, except in the setting of diabetes mellitus, chronic renal failure, or hepatic anomalies of metabolism. The most commonly affected patients are diabetics undergoing hemodiolysis for chronic renal failure.

Genetic inheritance: Most likely not a genetic disorder in most instances, but some reports suggest an autosomal dominant transmission. Most often associated with systemic disorders such as diabetes mellitus, hepatic abnormalities (alcoholic cirrhosis), congestive heart failure, and renal disease.

Pathophysiology: Not clearly established. Characterized by multiple hyperkeratotic papules with penetration of a keratotic plug into the dermis, resulting in transepidermal elimination of keratin, cellular material, and connective tissue elements triggered by an inflammatory reaction. The initiating step may be an alteration of dermal connective tissue, which then is recognized and eliminated by proliferative epidermis.

Diagnosis: Histopathologic examination shows a central, thick hyperkeratotic and parakeratotic plug embedded in an epidermal invagination. The plug consists of basophilic material. Abnormal (parakeratotic) keratinization of all the epithelial cells, including the basal cells, is present in at least one deep region of the plug.

Clinical aspects: The average age at presentation is 30 years, however, childhood cases have also been described. Flesh-colored, hard, horny papules may develop anywhere on the body except for palms and soles. Most commonly the extensor surfaces of the extremities are affected. Rarely, it may also involve the mucous membranes (conjunctivae, buccal mucosa). The papules eventually acquire a central keratotic plug that, upon removal, leaves a crater that matches the shape of the plug (Kyrle sign). The lesions come in crops, last for several weeks, and eventually disappear with minimal or no scarring. The lesions are asymptomatic. Posterior subcapsular cataracts may occur, as may multiple, tiny, yellow-brown stromal corneal opacities.

Precautions before anesthesia: Hepatic functions must be evaluated for coagulation disorders and hypoalbuminemia. Glucose homeostasis should be established prior to anesthesia. Creatinine level and clearance must be assessed. A complete blood count is recommended (renal anemia). In presence of severe itching, skin infections should be ruled out.

Anesthetic considerations: Difficult venous access should be expected because of the skin condition. In presence of congestive heart failure, chronic renal failure, and/or hepatic dysfunction, all considerations specific to these underlying conditions apply (rather than to Kyrle disease itself).

Pharmacological implications: Renal and/or hepatic insufficiency should be kept in mind when selecting drugs. Hypoalbuminemia may alter protein-binding characteristics of drugs and reduced drug doses may be required.

REFERENCES:

Alyahya GA, Heegaard S, Prause JU: Ocular changes in a case of Kyrle's disease: 20-year follow-up. *Acta Ophthalmol Scand* 78:585, 2000.

Chang P, Fernandez V: Acquired perforating disease associated with chronic renal failure. *Int J Dermatol* 31:117, 1992.

Sehgal VN, Jain S, Thappa DM, et al: Perforating dermatoses: A review and report of four cases. *J Dermatol* 20:329, 1993.

L

L-2-Hydroxyglutaric Aciduria

At a glance: Inborn error of metabolism manifesting as progressive neurodegenerative disorder with psychomotor retardation.

Incidence and genetic inheritance: The incidence is unknown, but approximately 20 cases have been reported. Transmission is autosomal recessive.

Clinical aspects: The enzymatic defect causing this progressive neurometabolic disorders is yet to be found. L-2-Hydroxyglutaric acid is a stereoisomer of D-2-hydroxyglutaric acid. Elevated levels of L-2-hydroxyglutaric acid are found in the urine, cerebrospinal fluid (CSF), and, to a lesser degree, in the serum. Plasma and CSF levels of lysine are elevated in some of these patients. In most patients, the initial symptoms are a delay of speech, unsupported walk and febrile seizures within the first 2 years of life. Over the following years, mental retardation associated to cerebellar ataxia with or without dystonia, pyramidal signs, and seizures develop. However, onset can be as early as neonatal age or as late as adolescent age. The oldest patient reported with this disorder was 57 years old. MRI scans reveal a consistent pattern with symmetrical subcortical leukoencephalopathy and cerebellar atrophy (vermis more than hemispheres). Furthermore, pathologic changes can—although inconsistently—be detected in the dentate nuclei, putamina, and globus pallidus.

Anesthetic considerations: Macrocephaly is a common feature, but no other facial anomalies have been reported, so airway management should not be affected. Keep in mind that these patients may be taking antiseizure medication, and potential interaction with other drugs and altered hepatic metabolism can occur.

Other conditions to be considered:

☞**CANAVAN SYNDROME:** Progressive leukodystrophy caused by spongy degeneration of the central nervous system. It is uniformly fatal.

☞**D-2-HYDROXYGLUTARIC ACIDURIA:** Metabolic disease resulting in abnormal MRI findings and psychomotor retardation, hypotonia, and non neurologic signs.

REFERENCES:

Barth PG, Hoffmann GF, Jaeken J, et al: L-2-Hydroxyglutaric acidemia: A novel inherited neurometabolic disease. *Ann Neurol* 32:66, 1992.

Fujitake J, Ishikawa Y, Fujii H, et al: L-2-Hydroxyglutaric aciduria: Two Japanese adult cases in one family. *J Neurol* 246:378, 1999.

Topcu M, Erdem G, Saatci I, et al: Clinical and magnetic resonance imaging features of L-2-hydroxyglutaric acidemia: Report of three cases in comparison with Canavan disease. *J Child Neurol* 11:373, 1996.

Laband Syndrome

At a glance: Inherited polymalformative syndrome characterized by craniofacial anomalies with gingival fibromatosis, dystrophic fingers and fingernails.

Synonym: Zimmermann-Laband Syndrome.

Incidence: Unknown; 29 cases reported in the literature up until 2004.

Genetic inheritance: Autosomal dominant.

Pathophysiology: Findings are suggestive of a storage disorder, but no biochemical defect has been identified.

Diagnosis: Clinical features first observed in infancy, with evolution during childhood. Radiologic evidence of hypoplastic terminal phalanges of the toes, with the most postaxial digits most markedly affected. The terminal phalanges of the hands may have narrow shafts and are hypoplastic. There may also be narrowing of the distal interphalangeal joint spaces in both hands and feet, with the narrowing being more pronounced in the feet.

Clinical aspects: Coarse facial appearance, gingival fibromatosis. Variable intellectual deficit, hepatosplenomegaly, hirsutism, small joint hyperextensibility, and "dystrophic" fingernails and toenails. Association with proximal aortic dilatation and cardiomyopathy.

Precautions before anesthesia: Echocardiography may be required to assess cardiac function. Laboratory investigation should include coagulation profile, liver function, and renal excretion.

Anesthetic considerations: As determined by cardiac function. Gingival fibromatosis may make tracheal intubation or insertion of a laryngeal mask difficult.

Pharmacological implications: No known pharmacological implications.

Other condition to be considered:

☞**RAMON SYNDROME:** Gingival fibromatosis associated with maxillary fibrous dysplasia, seizures, mental retardation, rheumatoid arthritis, and hypertrichosis. An autosomal recessive transmission has been suggested.

REFERENCES:

Katz J, Guelmann M, Barak S: Hereditary gingival fibromatosis with distinct dental, skeletal and developmental abnormalities. *Pediatr Dent* 24:253, 2002.

Robertson SP, Lipp H, Bankier A: Zimmermann-Laband syndrome in an adult. Long-term follow-up of a patient with vascular and cardiac complications. *Am J Med Genet* 78:160, 1988.

Lacrimo-Auriculo-Dento-Digital Syndrome (LADD Syndrome)

At a glance: Genetically transmitted syndrome characterized by the association of eye, ear, teeth, and hand abnormalities. The potential association of cardiac defects cannot be excluded.

Synonyms: Levy Hollister Syndrome; Limb Malformations-Dento-Digital Syndrome.

Incidence: Exact incidence unknown. Only 12 cases reported in the literature.

Genetic inheritance: Autosomal dominant inheritance with variable expression.

Pathophysiology: Suspected disorder of mesomelic development.

Clinical aspects: Wide variability in clinical expression. Persistent dry mouth because of decreased salivation caused by aplasia or hypoplasia of the salivary glands. Other features include severe dental caries; nasolacrimal duct obstruction with chronic epiphora and dacryocystitis; absent lacrimal gland; peg-shaped teeth with enamel hypoplasia; cup-shaped ear(s) and sometimes hearing loss; preaxial digital anomalies (triphalangeal thumb, digitalization of thumb, syndactyly, radial hypoplasia) and clinodactyly of the fifth digit. Other features less commonly associated include congenital renal disease (bilateral renal agenesis, cystic dysplastic kidneys) and dysmorphic facies with retrognathia, high forehead, and deep metopic fissure. One patient was reported to have a complex cardiopulmonary malformation: right diaphragmatic palsy (which was present in asymptomatic form in the mother also), hypoplasia of the left lung vasculature without bronchial anomalies, mild hypoplasia of the left pulmonary artery, and, on echocardiography, aneurysm of the interventricular septum.

Precautions before anesthesia: The potential for difficult direct laryngoscopy and tracheal intubation must be evaluated carefully clinically and radiologically if needed. A thorough examination of the renal, pulmonary, and cardiac systems must be performed, although the association of anomalies is not frequent but significant when part of the clinical picture. Pulmonary hypertension may be present because of pulmonary vascular hypoplasia and should be specifically investigated (e.g., arterial blood gases, chest radiographs, ultrasound, CT scan, and echocardiography). The laboratory investigation should include electrolytes, creatinine, blood urea nitrogen (BUN), and coagulation profile.

Anesthetic considerations: The possibility of difficult laryngoscopy and tracheal intubation is present. Brittle teeth may damage easily; therefore dentition must be checked prior to oral instrumentation. The presence of feet and hands abnormalities may make placement of intravenous and arterial catheters difficult. Diaphragmatic palsy may increase postoperative respiratory complications. Pulmonary hypertension may be present because of pulmonary vascular hypoplasia, and the anesthetic management should be adapted according to this clinical presentation. The fluid regimen should be adapted to the renal function.

Pharmacological implications: Preservation of spontaneous ventilation until confirmation that either face-mask ventilation or tracheal intubation can be achieved easily must be ensured before neuromuscular blocking agents are used. Avoid atropine if possible because of the presence of hypoplasia of the salivary glands and potential consequences of severely drying lung secretions.

REFERENCES:

Azar T, Scott JA, Arnold JE, Robin NH: Epiglottic hypoplasia associated with lacrimo-auriculo-dental-digital syndrome. *Ann Otol Rhinol Laryngol* 109:779, 2000.

Francannet C, Vanlieferinghen P, Dechelotte P, et al: LADD syndrome in five members of a three-generation family and prenatal diagnosis. *Genet Counsel* 5:85, 1994.

Heinz GW, Bateman JB, Barrett DJ, et al: Ocular manifestations of the lacrimo-auriculo-dento-digital syndrome. *Am J Ophthalmol* 115:243, 1993.

Lafora Syndrome or Disease

At a glance: Very rare congenital progressive myoclonic syndrome associated with seizures and severe mental deterioration. Fatal outcome in few years.

Synonyms: Myoclonus Epilepsy of Lafora (MELF); Progressive Myoclonus Epilepsy (EPM II).

Incidence: Very rare; more common in Turkey, India, and Iran.

Genetic inheritance: Autosomal recessive; belongs to the myoclonic progressive familial epilepsy disorder. Gene located on 6q24.

Pathophysiology: Enzyme defect leads to deposition of polyglucosans near their site of synthesis in the agranular endoplasmic reticulum. Lafora bodies are found within the eccrine sweat gland ducts on skin biopsy. They are periodic acid–Schiff (PAS)-positive inclusions. In biopsy performed in the central nervous system, Lafora bodies are typically found in the substantia nigra, superior olive, dentate nucleus, globus pallidus, and sensorimotor cortex. Intracellular Lafora bodies suggest amyloid in brain, heart, and liver.

Diagnosis: Clinical and from evidence of Lafora bodies on biopsy obtained from the axilla skin. The onset is reported during the second decade of life when grand mal seizures with rapidly progressive severe mental retardation occurs.

Clinical aspects: Principal features involve the neurologic function. Myoclonic seizures (worse with stress or preceding a generalized seizure) and tonic-clonic seizures (associated with photosensitivity and complex visual aura) tend to be progressive. Mental deterioration, psychosis, and dementia appear within months of onset. Other neurologic signs can include dysarthria, increased deep tendon reflexes, rigidity, hypotonia, and quadriplegia. Fatal outcome is usual 2 to 10 years after onset. There is no specific treatment.

Precautions before anesthesia: Evaluate neurologic status (age of onset, full history, clinical, CT/MRI will show cerebral atrophia). Make sure that the therapy for seizure control is continued until the day of surgery and anesthesia.

Anesthetic considerations: Careful intraoperative positioning is needed because of rigidity. Avoid central regional anesthesia (medullar blockade) because of the quadriparesis that is often observed.

Pharmacological implications: Consider drug interactions between antiepileptic treatment and anesthetics drugs. For long surgical procedure, intravenous administration of anticonvulsant must be considered.

Other conditions to be considered:

☞**Juvenile Myoclonic Epilepsy:** Characterized by early onset of age and isolated myoclonic jerks that occur mostly in the morning and do not become major seizures. Familial history of epilepsy is frequent. It is often diagnosed during an electroencephalogram (EEG). This disorder is chronic but not progressive. It is inherited as an autosomal dominant trait manifested on gene 5q34-q35 and 2q22-q23. All individuals affected with this medical condition have normal intelligence.

Myoclonus Epilepsy of Unverricht and Lundborg (Progressive Myoclonus Epilepsy; Baltic Myoclonic Epilepsy): Syndrome characterized by myoclonic seizures in which the patient may experience more than one type of seizure activity, such as petit mal or grand mal. It is progressive, and the rate of progression may be slow or rapid depending on the underlying disease. Phenytoin and carbamazepine tend to worsen the myoclonic activities. It is inherited as an autosomal recessive trait manifested on gene 21q22.3. The incidence of this disease is particularly frequent in Finland, where is it estimated at 1:20,000 general population.

REFERENCES:

Ganesh S, Delgado-Escueta AV, Suzuki T, et al: Genotype-phenotype correlations for EPM2A mutations in Lafora's progressive myoclonus epilepsy: Exon 1 mutations associate with an early-onset cognitive deficit subphenotype. *Hum Mol Genet* 11:1263, 2002.

Sainz J, Minassian BA, Serratosa JM, et al: Lafora progressive myoclonus epilepsy: Narrowing the chromosome 6q24 locus by recombinations and homozygosities [letter]. *Am J Hum Genet* 61:1205, 1997.

Lambert Syndrome

At a glance: Inherited polymalformative syndrome characterized by the association of branchial arch dysplasia, clubfoot, inguinal hernia, and intrahepatic biliary atresia.

Synonym: Branchial Dysplasia Club Foot Inguinal Hernia Biliary Atresia Syndrome.

Incidence: Unknown; ten cases reported in the literature.

Genetic inheritance: Autosomal recessive.

Pathophysiology: Abnormal development of the first and second branchial arches. Liver biopsy shows paucity of interlobular bile ducts.

Diagnosis: Familial occurrence of branchial dysplasia in association with cholestasis.

Clinical aspects: Patients with Lambert syndrome present with facial dysmorphism related principally to abnormal development of the first branchial arch (malar hypoplasia, macrostomia, preauricular tags, and/or auricular atresia). Other malformation may include clubfeet, inguinal hernia, and hypospadias. Congenital heart defects (e.g., ventricular septal defect) have been reported. Patients develop cholestatic jaundice related to a paucity of intrahepatic biliary ducts and moderate-to-severe mental retardation.

Precautions before anesthesia: Assess airway and cardiac and liver function. Check coagulation profile.

Anesthetic considerations: Because of facial dysmorphism, direct laryngoscopy and tracheal intubation might be difficult.

Pharmacological implications: Determined by liver function tests.

Other condition to be considered:

☞**ALAGILLE SYNDROME:** Characterized by neonatal jaundice, ophthalmologic anomalies (e.g., posterior embryotoxon and retinal pigmentary changes), pulmonary valvular stenosis, peripheral arterial stenosis, "butterfly" vertebrae on x-ray film, absent deep tendon reflexes, broad forehead, and pointed mandible and bulbous nose.

REFERENCE:

Lambert JC, Saint-Paul MC, Bastiani F, et al: Branchial dysplasia, mental deficiency, club feet and inguinal herniae: A report of two further cases associated with paucity of interlobular bile ducts. *J Med Genet* 27:330, 1990.

Landau-Kleffner Syndrome (LKS)

At a glance: Rare syndrome of childhood period characterized by aphasic epilepsy of unknown origin resulting in severe language dysfunction (e.g., loss of previously acquired speech and language skills [aphasia]) and auditory agnosia.

Synonyms: Acquired Epileptiform Aphasia; Epileptic Aphasia; Infantile Acquired Aphasia.

History: Neurologic disorder first described in 1957 under the name of *Acquired Epileptic Aphasia.*

Incidence: No data available, but a rare form of epilepsy. Male predominance (2:1).

Genetic inheritance: None.

Pathophysiology: The cause of LKS is not known. Possible suggested mechanisms include a dysfunctional immune system, exposure to a virus, and brain trauma.

Diagnosis: Electroencephalography (EEG) tracings are typical (present even in children with no clinical seizures); there is an epileptiform electrical activity in one but sometimes both temporal lobes, particularly when the child is asleep ("continuous spike waves of sleep" or "electrical status epilepticus of sleep").

Clinical aspects: LKS usually starts between the ages of 3 and 8 years and may develop either slowly over months or rapidly overnight. Most children have seizures that are readily controlled by antiepileptic drugs, but some children never have obvious seizures. Children with LKS have a language disorder that affects comprehension and/or understanding. They become unable to understand their own name, to identify environmental sounds such as telephone ringing, and to recognize family and friends or common objects, such as food and clothes. They may appear to be deaf. Some patients lose their speech completely and have behavioral problems (hyperactivity, poor attention, depression, and irritability). Occasionally, they have other neurologic problems, such as loss of bladder and bowel control, and visual disturbances (they can see but are unable to understand what they see). In some children who do not respond to steroids, a new brain surgery procedure called *multiple subpial transection* may be successful. Some affected children may regain some of their language abilities (over months or years), sometimes with remissions and relapse. Seizures generally disappear by adulthood.

Precautions before anesthesia: An anesthesiology consultation before elective surgical procedures is highly recommended. Complete evaluation of the epileptic disorder and the pharmacological therapy used to control the disease must be obtained before anesthesia.

Anesthetic considerations: The induction of anesthesia must take into consideration the possibility of behavioral problems, communication, and sudden burst of epileptic activities under stress. Use of sedation as premedication must be considered to reduce the risk of epilepsy.

Pharmacological implications: It is important to review the list of anticonvulsant medications used to control the disease and assess their potential interactions with the anesthetic agents. Special consideration must be given to the patient receiving chronic corticosteroid administration when intraoperative steroid supplementation must be given.

Other conditions to be considered:

ASPERGER SYNDROME: Nonverbal learning disability, marked deficiencies in social skills, normal intelligence and language.

PERVASIVE DEVELOPMENTAL DELAY: Mild form of autism with a central auditory processing defect and quite specific areas of difficulty.

☞**WEST SYNDROME:** Sudden generalized muscle contractions in addition to autistic manifestation, usually beginning between ages 3 and 8 months.

REFERENCES:

Chung PW, Seo DW, Kwon JC, et al: Nonconvulsive status epilepticus presenting as a subacute progressive aphasia. *Seizure* 11:449, 2002.

Kolski H, Otsubo H: The Landau-Kleffner syndrome. *Adv Exp Med Biol* 497:195, 2002.

Landouzy-Dejerine Dystrophy

At a glance: Genetically transmitted neuromuscular disease characterized by weakness of facial, shoulder, and/or upper arm muscles.

Synonyms: Duchenne Landouzy Disease; Facio-Scapulo-Humeral Muscular Atrophy (or Dystrophy).

Incidence: 5:1,000,000 live births, $\frac{1}{10}$ and $\frac{1}{50}$ the incidence of limb-girdle and Duchenne types, respectively.

Genetic inheritance: Autosomal dominant; gene located on 4q35. Up to 30% of cases have no apparent family history of the disease and probably are related to new mutations.

Pathophysiology: Progressive muscle degeneration occurs. Histologic features are variations in fiber size, areas of necrosis, and deposition of fat and connective tissue.

Diagnosis: Diagnosis is made based on the clinical picture, elevated creatine kinase, abnormalities on muscle biopsy, and electromyography. Electrophoretic measurement of restriction enzyme can be useful. DNA fragments associated with the responsible gene can confirm the diagnosis in presymptomatic and prenatal patients. Fragments shorter than 35 kb are associated with the disease, and the shorter the fragments, the earlier the onset and more severe the disease.

Clinical aspects: The onset is in adolescence. The course is slower and more benign than the other dystrophies. Features involve the _eyes and ears_ (sensorineural hearing loss, eyelid drooping, retinal detachments, and telangiectasia), _cardiac system_ (atrial tachycardia, cor pulmonale), _thoracic system_ (restrictive lung disease, winged scapula), and _neuromuscular system_ (facial, scapular, and humeral muscular dystrophy, abdominal wall weakness; inability to raise the arms is an early feature and facial weakness is characteristic). The lower limbs are affected later.

Precautions before anesthesia: Although respiratory and cardiac complications are lesser issues than observed with Duchenne muscular dystrophy, a detailed evaluation of these systems, including ECG and lung function tests, is indicated. Assess baseline serum potassium and creatinine kinase and consider arterial blood gases.

Anesthetic considerations: Little has been published regarding anesthesia in this group, although the general principles pertaining to the other muscular dystrophies apply (see _Duchenne Muscular Dystrophy_).

Pharmacological implications: Depolarizing muscle relaxants are contraindicated for all patients with muscular dystrophy because of the risk of acute hyperkalemia and rhabdomyolysis and its sequelae. In a case report, a patient had normal sensitivity to, but faster recovery from, atracurium than that observed in the general population. Despite this unexpected finding, it is prudent to use nondepolarizing agents sparingly in these patients and monitor closely the response with a neuromuscular blockade monitor. There is controversy about the overlap between malignant hyperthermia and some of the muscular dystrophies. Consequently, many anesthetists avoid volatile anesthetic drugs in all these patients.

Other conditions to be considered: This disease is clinically and histologically related to the other muscular dystrophies (which, in comparison, are all predominant in the lower extremities). The reader will find them all described in this book.

REFERENCES:

Dresner DL, Ali HH: Anaesthetic management of a patient with facioscapulohumeral muscular dystrophy. _Br J Anaesth_ 62:331, 1989.

Fitzsimons RB: Facioscapulohumeral muscular dystrophy. _Curr Opin Neurol_ 12:501, 1999.

Kissel JT: Facioscapulohumeral dystrophy. _Semin Neurol_ 19:35, 1999.

Upadhyaya M, Cooper DN: Molecular diagnosis of facioscapulohumeral muscular dystrophy. _Expert Rev Mol Diagn_ 2:160, 2002.

Laron Syndrome

At a glance: Genetically transmitted endocrine disorder characterized by congenital insensitivity to growth hormone (GH). It is characterized by short stature, blue sclerae, hip degeneration, and delayed bone age.

Synonyms: Growth Hormone Insensitivity Syndrome; Laron Dwarfism (or Laron-type Dwarfism); Primary GH Insensitivity (Primary GH Resistance); Pituitary Dwarfism II.

Nature: Genetic disorder first reported by Laron et al. in 1966. Most patients are of Jewish descent (including many individuals who converted to Christianity during the Spanish Inquisition and emigrated to the New World).

Incidence: More than 250 cases have been reported worldwide. Male-to-female ratio varies based on geographic area.

Genetic inheritance: Autosomal recessive; gene locus at 5p13.1-p12 (33 mutations have been reported).

Pathophysiology: Mutation of the gene encoding the GH receptor (type I dwarfism) or a defect in the postreceptor signaling mechanism (type II dwarfism), resulting in complete resistance to the action of GH and failure to generate somatomedin or insulin-like growth factor-1 (IGF-1). Lack of feedback causes pituitary oversecretion of GH.

Diagnosis: Clinical signs of GH deficiency including biochemical (normal or increased plasma GH levels, low IGF-1 levels unresponsive to exogenous GH, and low GH-binding protein levels) and radiologic (delayed bone age, markedly advanced osseous maturation for height and age).

Clinical aspects: Clinical hyposomatotropism manifested by proportionate short stature, delayed bone age, limited elbow extension, and hip degeneration. An important characteristic is the more pronounced decrement in body size than in head size, resulting in child-like body proportions in adults, small face, prominent forehead, occasionally blue sclerae, flat nasal bridge, and delayed tooth development. Patient may have micrognathia, sparse hair, high-pitched voice (caused by a narrow larynx), delayed menarche in girls, a small-size penis (which reaches normal adult size) in boys, and normal intelligence. Adult stature is severely affected (ranging from −4 to −12 standard deviation). Approximately 50% of infants and children with Laron syndrome present with overt symptoms of hypoglycemia (especially fasting hypoglycemia), including seizures. Hip dysplasia, especially avascular necrosis of the femoral head (Legg-Calvé-Perthes disease) is common.

Precautions before anesthesia: Because of increased risk for spinal cord compression and atlantoaxial odontoid subluxation, all patients must be assessed very carefully prior to anesthesia (e.g., clinically and radiologically). The investigation should include a complete endocrinologic evaluation, including and lung ventilation glucose level and tolerance to fasting. Avoid long periods of fasting.

Anesthetic considerations: Intelligence usually is normal for chronologic age. Limited elbow movement and hip degeneration calls for extra care during positioning of the patient. A difficult airway may be encountered in the presence of micrognathia. Manipulate patient's head very cautiously, especially during tracheal intubation (possible cervical spine instability) and positioning for surgery. Check blood glucose intraoperatively and postoperatively.

Pharmacological implications: No known specific pharmacological implications; however, the basic principles of safe airway management in these patients dictate that spontaneous ventilation should be maintained until an easy tracheal intubation and lung ventilation can be confirmed. Therefore, neuromuscular blockade agents must be used judiciously.

Other conditions to be considered:

☞**COFFIN SIRIS SYNDROME:** Present at birth and affects both sexes equally. Characterized by severe failure to thrive, frequent respiratory infections, and growth deficiencies.

☞**COCKAYNE SYNDROME:** Progressive disorder presenting with onset during the second year of life and characterized by photosensitivity and growth retardation.

☞**PITUITARY DWARFISM III:** Panhypopituitary dwarfism is not considered a rare condition, considering that approximately 7000 to 10,000 cases have been diagnosed in the United States. Most cases are the result of craniopharyngioma and other nongenetic causes. If inherited, it is believed to be autosomal recessive, but rare.

REFERENCES:

Hull KL, Harvey S: Growth hormone resistance: Clinical states and animal models. *J Endocrinol* 163:165, 1999.

Kornreich L, Horev G, Schwarz M, et al: Laron syndrome abnormalities: Spinal stenosis, os odontoideum, degenerative changes of the atlanto-odontoid joint, and small oropharynx. *Am J Neuroradiol* 23:625, 2002.

Laron Z: Growth hormone insensitivity (Laron syndrome). *Rev Endocr Metab Disord* 3:347, 2002.

Larsen Syndrome

At a glance: Congenital dysmorphic syndrome associated with characteristic anomalies of face, hands, and feet, and multiple congenital dislocations. Spine, airway, and cardiac abnormalities are also present.

Synonym: Multiple Congenital Dislocation Syndrome.

Classification:

Larsen Syndrome, Autosomal Dominant: Characterized by short stature, flat facies, prominent forehead, hypertelorism, cataracts, cleft lip/palate, congenital heart defects (e.g., aortic dilatation, atrial septal defect and ventricular septal defect), respiratory abnormalities (e.g., tracheal stenosis and malacia, bronchomalacia), and potentially severe cervical spine anomalies leading to spinal cord compression.

Larsen Syndrome, Autosomal Recessive: Characterized by multiple congenital dislocations, craniofacial abnormalities (e.g., prominent forehead, depressed nasal bridge, hypertelorism) and clubfeet. Other clinical features include cleft palate, hydrocephalus, and atlantoaxial joint and cervical spine abnormalities.

Larsen-like Syndrome (LRSL): Very rare disorder characterized by facial dysmorphism, multiple joint dislocations suggesting the presence of a Larsen syndrome but presenting as a partial trisomy 1q and partial monosomy 6p.

Larsen-like Lethal Syndrome: Characterized by multiple joint dislocations and neonatal death as a result of pulmonary insufficiency, laryngomalacia, tracheomalacia, and pulmonary hypoplasia.

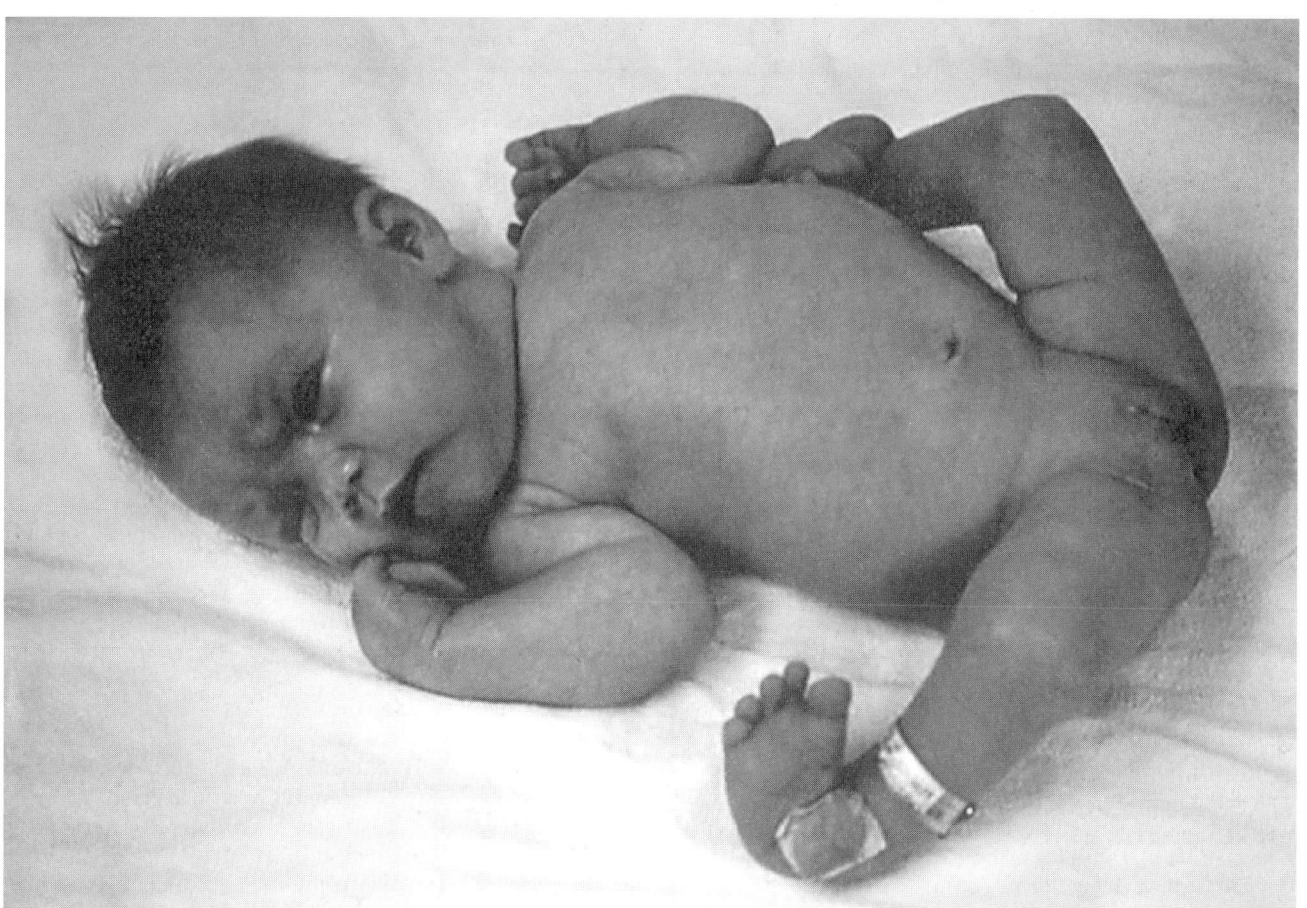

Larsen syndrome   Joint hyperlaxity with multiple congenital dislocations in an infant with Larsen syndrome.

Incidence: Approximately 1:100,000 live births; both sexes affected equally. However, in La Réunion Island in the Indian Ocean, the incidence is 1:1500 all births.

Genetic inheritance: The syndrome occurs sporadically. Most often it is inherited an autosomal dominant trait, although an autosomal recessive transmission has also been described. The responsible gene maps to 3p21.1-p14.1.

Pathophysiology: The exact mechanism is unknown, but it most likely is the result of an error in collagen synthesis.

Diagnosis: Usually made by the typical clinical features of association of musculoskeletal abnormalities with a typical flat facies and the presence of a double ossification center in the calcaneum (see *Clinical Aspects*).

Clinical aspects: Differentiation between the recessive and the dominant form can be difficult because both show a wide clinical variability; however, the recessive form is generally more severe. The typical features include anomalies of the *face* (flat-profiled face with frontal bossing and depressed nasal bridge, hypertelorism, cleft palate), *the spine* (abnormal segmentation of vertebrae, cervical spina bifida occulta, hypoplastic cervical vertebrae with cervical instability, and progressive cervical kyphosis), the *skeletal system* (short stature, joint hyperlaxity with multiple congenital dislocations—most often knee, hip, elbow [radiohumeral and ulnohumeral]—an accessory ossification center in the calcaneus, syndactyly, and cylindrically shaped fingers with short end phalanges giving a pseudoclubbing aspect), *the airway* (hypoplastic lungs, cartilage anomalies resulting in decreased chest wall stability, floppy epiglottis, laryngotracheomalacia, and respiratory failure), and *the heart* (congenital [atrial septal defect, ventricular septal defect, patent ductus arteriosus] and—depending on the age of the patient—acquired [marfanoid] cardiac lesions such as aortic dilatation and regurgitation, subaortic stenosis, mitral valve prolapse, mitral regurgitation, and cardiomyopathy). Most of these patients are mentally normal, although some suffer from hydrocephalus and their motor skills are delayed because of the orthopedic problems.

Precautions before anesthesia: Patients often present for management of congenital dislocations, posterior cervical arthrodesis, clubfoot, serpentine, or pes equinovalgus repair. Cervical spine anomalies are frequent and require thorough clinical and radiologic evaluation. It may be necessary to obtain lateral flexion and extension radiographs or MRI scans of the neck. Cervical kyphosis is progressive and may result in impingement of the spinal cord at the apex of the kyphosis, which is a serious and potentially life-threatening condition. Postoperatively, these patients are prone to airway complications with a high incidence of croup-like symptoms secondary to subglottic stenosis, laryngotracheomalacia, and airway edema. Thoracolumbar kyphoscoliosis may result in chronic chest disease. It is therefore recommended that arrangements for postoperative mechanical ventilation be made in advance. Evaluate respiratory function because of chest and rachis anomalies (clinical, radiographic, CT, arterial blood gas examination, respiratory function tests). Evaluate cardiac function (clinical, echography, radionuclide examination). Evaluate neurologic and spinal function (clinical, CT/MRI, somatosensory-evoked potentials).

Anesthetic considerations: Death as a consequence of anesthetic complications has been described. If endotracheal intubation is required, either inline cervical stabilization or fiberoptic intubation is recommended. Difficult airway management must be expected. Careful handling and positioning of these patients are mandatory in the presence of cervical instability, contractures, and skeletal deformities. Depending on the type of surgery, short-latency somatosensory-evoked potentials during induction, but especially

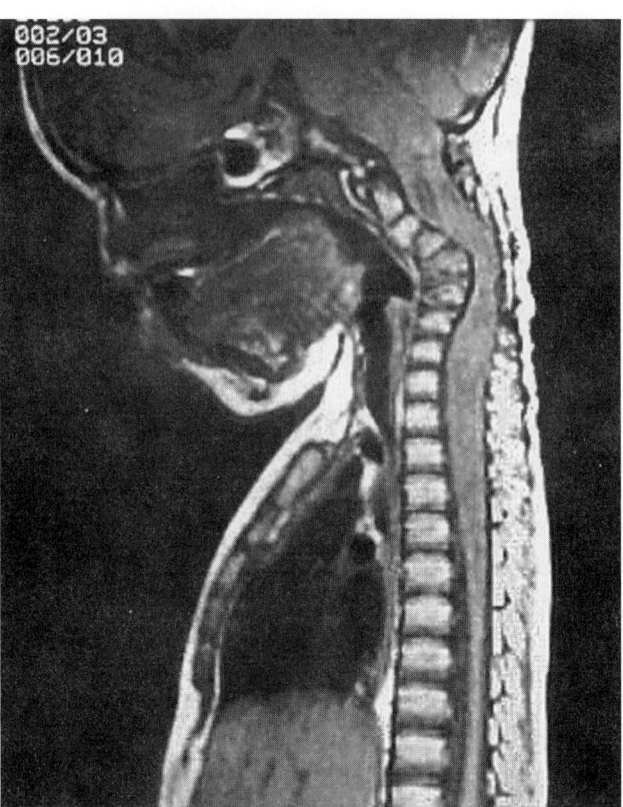

Larsen syndrome   Magnetic resonance imaging scan shows severe cervical kyphosis and compression of the cervical spinal cord in a patient with Larsen syndrome.

for positioning, have been recommended in patients with cervical instability to monitor for signs of cord compression. Because of subglottic stenosis and the high incidence of postoperative croup-like symptoms, it is recommended that an endotracheal tube size be chosen that allows for an audible leak at airway pressures approximately 20 cm H_2O. If tracheal intubation is not mandatory, a face mask or, alternatively, a laryngeal mask, is considered a good alternative, avoiding not only tracheal but also cervical spine manipulations. However, care should be taken with laryngeal masks (#1.0 and #1.5), which often lead to loss of airway patency. Instrumenting the trachea in this situation could lead to a catastrophy in these infants. Continuous positive airway pressure may be required secondary to laryngotracheobronchomalacia.

Pharmacological implications: Cervical instability may result in spinal cord compression and consecutive weakness of distal muscles. Succinylcholine could lead to a hyperkalemic response. Prophylactic antibiotics in case of cardiopathy as indicated. For scoliosis surgery, anesthetic management must consider interaction with somatosensory-evoked potential monitoring. Level of intracranial pressure should be considered each time.

Other conditions to be considered:

☞ **DESBUQUOIS SYNDROME:** Osteochondrodysplastic disease characterized clinically by micromelic dwarfism, narrow chest, vertebral and metaphyseal abnormalities, and advanced carpotarsal ossification. There is a high mortality during the first year of life. It is believed to be inherited as an autosomal recessive trait.

☞ **DIASTROPHIC DYSPLASIA:** Autosomal recessive inherited form of short-limb dwarfism associated with spine anomalies and cervical spine compression.

Rotter-Erb Syndrome: Some authors consider Rotter-Erb syndrome to be the same as Larsen syndrome.

REFERENCES:

Lauder GR, Sumner E: Larsen's syndrome: Anaesthetic implications. Six case reports. *Paediatr Anaesth* 5:133, 1995.

Malik P, Choudry DK: Larsen syndrome and its anaesthetic considerations. *Paediatr Anaesth* 12:632, 2002.

Morishima T, Sobue K, Tanaka S, et al: Sevoflurane for general anaesthetic management in a patient with Larsen syndrome. *Paediatr Anaesth* 14:194, 2004.

Saricaoglu F, Dal D: Cardiac arrest in a patient with Larsen syndrome under sevoflurane anesthesia. *Paediatr Anaesth* 14:889, 2004.

Tobias JD: Anesthetic implications of Larsen syndrome. *J Clin Anesth* 8:255, 1996.

Laryngo-Onycho-Cutaneous (LOC) Syndrome

At a glance: Severe progressive multisystem disorder involving the skin (dermal granula and ulcerations) and larynx (vocal cord granuloma). It is often lethal during childhood.

Synonyms: Laryngeal and Ocular Granulation in Indian Children; LOGIC Syndrome.

Incidence: Unknown; fewer than 50 cases reported in the literature.

Genetic inheritance: Autosomal recessive.

Pathophysiology: Caused by an inherited defect affecting the lamina lucida of the skin basal membrane layer.

Diagnosis: Demonstration of dermal and submucosal granulation with vocal cord involvement.

Clinical aspects: Onset within 2 weeks of birth; death common in childhood. Hoarse, weak cry, vocal cord granulation, dystrophic changes in the nails, with recurrent loss of toenails and fingernails, dermal granuloma, skin ulceration, conjunctival scarring, amelogenesis imperfecta.

Precautions before anesthesia: Significant risk of airway obstruction because of the presence of a laryngeal web and large supraglottic and glottic nodules; epiglottic and supraglottic edema may be present with ulceration and contact bleeding, together with swollen and poorly defined cords.

Anesthetic considerations: Permanent tracheotomies may be required, which may lead to granulation formation and obstruction distally in the trachea.

Pharmacological implications: Determined by degree of airway obstruction.

REFERENCES:

Hodges UM, Lloyd-Thomas A: Anaesthesia for airway obstruction in laryngo-onycho-cutaneous syndrome. *Anaesthesia* 48:503, 1993.

Phillips RJ, Atherton DJ, Gibbs ML, et al: Laryngo-onycho-cutaneous syndrome: An inherited epithelial defect. *Arch Dis Child* 70:319, 1994.

Launois Syndrome

At a glance: Gigantism caused by excessive GH secretion usually because of a pituitary adenoma that normally occurs before the epiphyses are fused in comparison with acromegaly that occurs after fusion of the epiphyses.

Synonyms: Acromegaloid Gigantism; Fractional Hypopituitarism-Gigantism Syndrome; Neurath-Cushing Syndrome; Pituitary Gigantism; Launois-Bensaude Syndrome.

Incidence: Very rare cause of tall stature in children. Reports are limited to sporadic cases. Peak incidence in teenagers, although it has been reported in a child as young as 21 months.

Genetic inheritance: Not a genetic syndrome.

Pathophysiology: Almost always caused by pituitary adenoma, producing excessive GH. Some tumors are mixed and produce both prolactin and GH. Very rarely it is caused by excessive secretion of GH-releasing factor from an ectopic source.

Clinical aspects: Rapid linear growth, tall stature, large hands and feet, coarsening of facial features, prognathism, macroglossia, widely spaced teeth, and husky voice. Other features include greasy thick skin, slipped epiphyses with joint pain, kyphoscoliosis, myopathy, nerve entrapment syndromes; headaches and visual field defects, usually hemianopsia, pale optic discs and optic atrophy. Patients may have behavioral problems and mental retardation, early pubertal signs, galactorrhea, glucose intolerance, obesity, or diabetes mellitus.

Diagnosis: Clinical features; *biochemical* (elevated serum levels of GHs not suppressed by oral glucose loading, elevated levels of IGF-1, high prolactin and gonadotropin levels); *radiology* (advanced bone age, enlarged sella turcica on skull radiograph, CT scan demonstrates pituitary tumor).

Anesthetic considerations: May be anxious and uncooperative in the presence of visual defects, mental retardation, or behavioral problems. Airway problems should be anticipated, but, unlike acromegaly, glottic stenosis and vocal cord paresis have not been reported in gigantism. Presence of myopathy may predispose to postoperative respiratory insufficiency. Close monitoring of preoperative glucose level necessary in the presence of diabetes mellitus. If the patient is already being treated, complications of medical and/or irradiation therapy, such as pituitary insufficiency, should be evaluated preoperatively.

Other condition to be considered:

Acromegaly: Hormonal disorder caused by overproduction of GH in adults, not resulting in gigantism but enlargement of extremities, usually a result of a benign tumor of the pituitary gland.

REFERENCES:

Alvi NS, Kirk JM: Pituitary gigantism causing diabetic ketoacidosis. *J Pediatr Endocrinol Metab* 12:907, 1999.

Daughaday WH: Pituitary gigantism. *Endocrinol Metab Clin North Am* 21:633, 1992.

Lu PW, Silink M, Johnston I, et al: Pituitary gigantism. *Arch Dis Child* 67:1039, 1992.

Laurence Moon Syndrome (LMS)

At a glance: Association of ophthalmoplegia, pigmentary degeneration of retina (rod cone dystrophy), mental retardation, and cardiomyopathy.

Synonyms: Adipogenital-Retinitis Pigmentosa Syndrome; Laurence Syndrome

NB: Although Laurence-Moon-Bardet-Biedl syndrome has been split into two syndromes—LMS and Bardet-Biedl syndrome (rod cone dystrophy, obesity, postaxial polydactyly, learning disabilities and hypogenitalism)—many cases overlap.

History: First reported by ophthalmologist Laurence and surgeon Moon in 1866. Often confused with Bardet-Biedl Syndrome and called LMBB (Laurence-Moon-Bardet-Biedl syndrome).

Incidence: Rare; more frequent in some places (Arabic population of Kuwait, among the Bedouins, often as Bardet-Biedl syndrome).

Genetic inheritance: Autosomal recessive.

Pathophysiology: Not known. Pituitary gland is morphologically and immunohistologically normal.

Diagnosis: Based on the clinical features: mental retardation, pigmentary retinopathy, hypogonadism, hypogenitalism, and spastic paraplegia. No obesity or polydactyly observed (as observed in Bardet-Biedl syndrome, with which the syndrome should not be confused even though it has strong similarities and overlap).

Clinical aspects: Symptoms usually occur in early or late childhood. Strabismus is often present and the cause of visual difficulties. Other clinical manifestations include night blindness, cataracts, and retinitis pigmentosa occurring during childhood. There is a decreased level of gonadotrophic hormone production because of hypogonadism, which contributes to delay of onset of puberty and development of secondary sex characteristics. Males usually are infertile and may develop pseudogynecomastia. Females have amenorrhea and fail to develop breasts. Other signs include mental retardation, ataxia, muscle rigidity, and spastic paraplegia. Renal disease is common because of abnormalities in the structure or function of the kidneys. In some rare cases, diabetes, congenital heart defects, and breathing problems may occur.

Precautions before anesthesia: It is recommended to obtain a consultation in anesthesiology before elective surgery. Patients affected with morbid obesity will require complete evaluation of cardiovascular and respiratory functions prior to anesthesia and surgery. Pulmonary function tests (when possible) will be needed to determine the presence of obstructive respiratory function and to evaluate the possible need for postoperative mechanical ventilation. The investigation should include a complete cell blood count, glucose level, coagulation profile, and renal functions. The fasting period might require a longer time to allow complete gastric transit because these patients are more susceptible to maintain higher gastric volumes than others.

Anesthetic considerations: Anesthetic considerations are mostly influenced by the obesity status and the surgical procedure plan for the patient. In presence of severe obesity, use of invasive monitoring to ensure proper management of cardiovascular and respiratory functions might be appropriate. The potential for difficult direct laryngoscopy and tracheal intubation because of severe obesity and the risk of pulmonary aspiration complicate the management. The anesthetic management per se is not specific to the disease but rather to the anomalies associated with it. The presence of diabetes necessitates proper preoperative management and frequent measurement of glucose levels. Postoperative ventilatory support might be necessary to facilitate pain management and reduce risk of hypoventilation in these patients. The necessity for intermittent positive-pressure ventilation in the postoperative period should be organized ahead of the procedure.

Pharmacological implications: No specific implications with this condition. Use of medication preventing increase of the plasma glucose level and administration of antibiotics in presence of cardiac defects are recommended.

Other conditions to be considered:

☞**ALSTRÖM SYNDROME:** Photophobia, nystagmus, cone-rod dystrophy, dilated cardiomyopathy leading to congestive heart failure, acanthosis nigricans, short stature, hearing loss, hyperinsulinemia with insulin resistance, and renal tubular dysfunction.

☞**BIEMOND SYNDROME TYPE II:** Mental retardation, coloboma, obesity, polydactyly, hypogonadism, hydrocephalus, and facial dysostosis; closely related to Laurence Moon syndrome (might be a variant).

☞**BARDET-BIEDL SYNDROME:** Rod-cone dystrophy, obesity, post-axial polydactyly, learning disabilities, and hypogenitalism; also closely related to Laurence Moon syndrome.

☞**PRADER WILLI SYNDROME:** Diagnosed more often in males born after a prolonged, delayed birth in the breech position. Characterized by muscular weakness, failure to thrive during infancy, hypogonadism, dwarfism, and psychomotor retardation. Onset of age is between 1 and 3 years, when hyperphagia usually develops. Left uncontrolled, morbid obesity develops and leads to life-threatening heart and lung complications.

☞**BORJESON-FORSSMAN-LEHMAN SYNDROME:** Inherited as an X-linked dominant trait and characterized by unusual facial appearance, mental retardation, seizures, short stature, slowed sexual development, muscle weakness, and obesity.

HYPOGONADOTROPHIC HYPOGONADISM SYNDROME (Secondary Hypogonadism): Disorder that affects the hypothalamus and production of gonadotropins. Characterized by the absence of secondary sexual characteristics.

WEISS SYNDROME: Extremely rare disorder characterized by hypogonadism, mental retardation, obesity, and deafness.

REFERENCES:

Farag TI, Teebi AS: Bardet-Biedl and Laurence-Moon syndromes in a mixed Arab population. *Clin Genet* 33:78, 1988.

Whitaker MD, Scheithauer BW, Kovacs KT, et al: The pituitary gland in the Laurence-Moon syndrome. *Mayo Clin Proc* 62:216, 1987.

Leber Congenital Amaurosis (LCA)

At a glance: Inherited degenerative disease of the retina characterized by severely decreased vision manifesting at birth or shortly thereafter. Other ocular anomalies may include sensory (wandering) nystagmus, amaurotic pupils, deep-set eyes, and photophobia. Central nervous system anomalies have been described in some patients. Do not confuse with Leber hereditary optic neuropathy (see ☞Leber Hereditary Optic Neuropathy).

History: First described by the German ophthalmologist Theodor von Leber in 1869.

Incidence and genetic inheritance: Approximately 3:100,000 neonates are born with this autosomal recessive transmitted disorder. Nine genetic loci for LCA have been discovered, of which six genes have identified. LCA is now no longer considered one disorder but rather multiple disorders, which can be classified into three different categories: (1) aplasia, resulting in abnormal embryologic formation of photoreceptors; (2) early degeneration of photoreceptors with progressive cell death; and (3) dysfunction of the photoreceptors with normal retinal anatomy.

Clinical aspects: Vision is already significantly reduced at birth or shortly thereafter. Sensory (wandering) nystagmus and lack of visual responsiveness alert the parents, usually within the first months of life. Initial examination may reveal a normal retina and a fundus appearance that either is essentially normal or reveals a progressive pigmentary retinopathy. The pupils are amaurotic and the eyes deep sunken. However, the final diagnosis is made by elec-troretinography, which shows only small (at high intensities) or no photopic responses. Both cone and rod responses are affected. Patients are described as frequently poking and rubbing their eyes (the so-called "Oculodigital Reflex" of Leber and Franceschetti), which is not specific to LCA because it is observed in other forms of amaurosis (Leber was the first to describe this phenomenon). Other associated ocular features may include ptosis, strabismus, kerato-conus/keratoglobus, cataracts, microphthalmos, macular coloboma, pigmentary retinopathy and maculopathy, optic disc edema, retinal vascular changes, and high-grade hyperopia or myopia (less common). By early adolescence, the retina of LCA patients may undergo significant changes. Retinal blood vessels often become narrow and constricted, and pigmentary changes similar to those found in retinitis pigmentosa may affect the retinal pigment epithelium. Despite these changes, vision does not usually deteriorate further. Visual acuity in LCA patients is most often limited to the level of finger counting or detection of bright light. Some patients are extremely photophobic. At this time, no treatment is available; however, current research is focusing on gene therapy. On rare occasion, LCA is associated with central nervous system symptoms such as delayed psychomotor development and seizures.

Anesthetic considerations: In patients with isolated LCA (i.e., not associated with a syndrome or central nervous system findings), no specific anesthetic concerns should arise from this disorder. In the presence of seizures, keep in mind that antiseizure medications can alter the metabolism and elimination of anesthetic drugs. Cooperation of mentally delayed patients may be limited. Sedative and/or hypnotic premedication and the presence of the primary caregiver may be helpful during induction of anesthesia. Dealing with a blind patient who cannot see what is happening requires more explicit explanations in general and particularly warnings before painful procedures. Severely photophobic patients will appreciate having the operating theater lights dimmed during induction and emergence of anesthesia and afterward in the postanesthesia care unit. In cases where LCA is part of a syndrome, the specific anesthetic considerations for that syndrome apply.

Other conditions to be considered:

☞**Cone-Rod Retinal Dystrophies:** Inherited dystrophy of retinal photoreceptors and pigment epithelium; simultaneous abiotrophic degeneration of rods and cones.

LCA can be associated with the following syndromes:

☞**Alström Syndrome:** Inherited syndrome with diabetes mellitus, cardiac, hepatic, and renal involvement and progressive visual and hearing loss.

☞**Bardet-Biedl Syndrome:** Mental retardation, pigmentary retinopathy, polydactyly, obesity, renal anomalies, and hypogenitalism.

☞**Joubert Syndrome:** Genetic disorder characterized by cerebral malformations (vermis and brainstem) resulting in severe coordination (ataxia) and breathing (sleep apnea, hyperpnea) disorders.

☞**Neuronal Ceroid Lipofuscinoses (NCLs):** Hereditary progressive neurodegenerative disorders with mental retardation, visual loss, and seizures. The NCLs are probably the most common class of neurodegenerative disease in children.

☞**Loken Senior Syndrome:** Inherited disorder characterized by rapidly progressive renal insufficiency (nephronophthisis) and eye disease (retinitis pigmentosa).

☞**Zellweger Syndrome:** Disorder characterized by the congenital absence of functioning peroxisomes (cellular structures

responsible for elimination of toxic substances) resulting in a cerebrohepatorenal syndrome. The disease affects brain development, particularly myelination. Most important features include hepatomegaly, polycystic kidney disease, visual disturbances, and high plasma levels of iron and copper. Other features include muscular hypotonia already noticeable at birth, mental retardation, seizures, coagulopathy, and dysphagia with recurrent aspiration. Congenital heart defects have been described. Life expectancy is approximately 6 months.

Reference:

Koenekoop RK: An overview of Leber congenital amaurosis: A model to understand human retinal development. *Surv Ophthalmol* 49:379, 2004.

Leber Hereditary Optic Neuropathy (LHON)

At a glance: Rare hereditary form of optic atrophy that usually affects young males. Characterized by sudden bilateral cloudiness of vision, followed by scotoma, rapid deterioration of central vision, and occasional color vision disorders. Associated with atrophy of the optic nerve fibers and retinae. Considered a mitochondrial disease. Cardiac conduction defects have been reported with this condition.

Synonyms: Leber Disease; Leber Optic Atrophy.

> *NB:* Do not confuse with Leber congenital amaurosis, another inherited condition (without mitochondrial DNA involvement), resulting from a mutation in the CRX gene.

History: Originally described by Theodore von Leber, a German Ophthalmologist, in the 19th century.

Incidence: Incidence is not established, however, the disease is present worldwide. Male predominance (2:1).

Genetic inheritance: Genetic disorder related to mitochondrial DNA transmission (i.e., exclusively from mother to child, either male or female). At least four mutations in mitochondrial DNA (including G11778A, T14484C, and G3460A) are associated with this clinical abnormality. Different family pedigrees show different mutations but with clinically similar pictures. The pattern of transmission within a kindred are not in accordance with mendelian principles, and it is apparent that a complex mechanism of inheritance is in operation. The disease is never transmitted by affected men; it is transmitted by affected women or, most frequently, by female carriers of the gene.

Pathophysiology: The mutation in mitochondrial DNA results in lowering of the amount of energy available to the cells of the optic nerve and retina, thus leading to severe cell damage. Fundal changes are described as opacification of the disc margin, hyperemia of the disc vessels, circumpapillary telangiectatic microangiopathy, and swelling of the peripapillary nerve fiber layer.

Diagnosis: Visual field testing reveals enlarging centrocecal scotoma. Fluorescein angiography shows pseudoedema of the nerve fiber layer, peripapillary telangiectasia, and increased tortuosity of the retinal vessels. Pattern electroretinogram and visual-evoked potentials show optic nerve dysfunction not associated with retinal disease. Magnetic resonance imaging may reveal a high signal within the optic nerves. Molecular genetic testing for the mutations can be decisive.

Clinical aspects: There is a wide spectrum of ages at onset of the disorder. However, the most frequent age at onset is in the late teens. Typically, vision fails from normal to severely impaired over a period of weeks, beginning with one eye and then the other eye a few weeks later. Some improvement may occur over months or years, however, vision is permanently impaired. There is probably no association between this disorder and other organ systems. A link between this and multiple sclerosis has been suggested but remains unproved. Similarly, some patients have demonstrated both optic neuropathy and cardiac preexcitation, but any link may be purely chance.

Precautions before anesthesia: Thorough history and examination should exclude any coexisting pathology. A 12-lead electroencephalogram should be performed to exclude cardiac preexcitation or conduction defects.

Anesthetic considerations: No specific anesthetic techniques are recommended or contraindicated. As with all neurologic conditions, it is prudent to demonstrate the extent of disability before anesthesia in order to be confident in making postoperative assessments.

Pharmacological implications: Use of sodium nitroprussiate should be avoided because of the increase in cyanide anions in this specific condition. The mechanism is unknown.

Other conditions to be considered: Other forms of optic atrophy: coloboma and other congenital defects of optic nerve, congenital optic atrophy, juvenile optic atrophy, Behr optic atrophy (with ataxia), demyelinating neuropathies.

REFERENCES:

Man PY, Turnbull DM, Chinnery PF: Leber hereditary optic neuropathy. *J Med Genet* 39:162, 2002.

Riordan-Eva P, Sanders MD, Govan GG, et al: The clinical features of Leber's hereditary optic neuropathy defined by the presence of a pathogenic mitochondrial DNA mutation. *Brain* 118:319, 1995.

Legg-Calvé-Perthes Disease

At a glance: Self-limited idiopathic osteonecrosis of the capital femoral epiphysis of the femoral head. Can be bilateral in 10% of patients.

Synonyms: Aseptic or Avascular Necrosis of the Femoral Head; Calvé Disease; Calvé-Perthes Disease; Legg Disease; Maydl Disease; Perthes-Calvé-Legg Disease; Perthes Disease; Perthes-Calvé-Legg-Waldenström Syndrome; Waldenström Syndrome.

History: First described by Karel Maydl in 1897.

Incidence: 1:1200 children younger than 15 years. Racial predominance in white children. Male predominance (4–5:1).

Genetic inheritance: Not a genetic syndrome.

Pathophysiology: Unknown. The disease goes through four phases. (1) Interruption of the blood supply to the capital femoral epiphysis; the hip joint becomes inflamed, stiff, and painful as a result of bone infarctions, especially in the subchondral cortical bone, while articular cartilage continues to grow (several months up to 1 year). (2) Remodeling of the femoral head with occurrence of subchondral fracture (usually the result of normal physical activity, not direct trauma); the joint remains irritated and painful (1 to 3 years). (3) Rebuilding of the femoral head by new bone cells as a result of changes of the epiphyseal growth secondary to the subchondral fracture (1 to 3 years). (4) Normalization process in which normal bone cells replace the new bone cells (several years).

Diagnosis: Established by radiographic findings (plain and frog-leg views). Five radiographic stages, from better (early stages) to worse (late stages): (1) smaller femoral head epiphysis and widening of articular space on affected side; (2) subchondral fracture; (3) bone resorption; (4) reossification of new bone; (5) healed stage. Technetium-99 bone scan helps delineate the extent of avascular changes, and dynamic arthrography allows assessment of the sphericity of the head of the femur.

Clinical aspects: Usually affects children between the ages of 3 and 12 years. Progressive hip and groin pain that may be referred to the thigh or the knee. Physical examination shows decreased range of motion (limited hip rotation and abduction), atrophy of thigh muscles (secondary to disuse), muscle spasm, and occasionally limb length inequality (because of collapse). Radiographs often show delayed bone age. Children older than 10 years are at high risk for developing osteoarthritis (coxa plana).

Precautions before anesthesia: Careful mobilization of the patient to avoid favoring acute slipping of the femoral head.

Anesthetic considerations: No specific anesthetic considerations with this disorder.

Pharmacological implications: Although there are no known pharmacological implications with this condition, special attention needed in that chronic use of corticosteroid in the initial phase of the disease requires supplementation intraoperatively.

Other conditions to be considered:

☞**OSGOOD-SCHLATTER DISEASE:** Benign, self-limited knee condition associated with traction apophysitis in adolescents.

☞**PSEUDOACHONDROPLASTIC DYSPLASIA:** Rare inherited disorder characterized by skeletal malformations resulting in short-limbed dwarfism. Affected individuals present brachydactyly, genu varum, and genu valgum. In addition, they may have lumbar lordosis and kyphosis. Cases of pseudoachondroplastic dysplasia are the result of mutations of the COMP gene, indicating this disorder is allelic to some cases of multiple epiphyseal dysplasia. Pseudoachondroplastic dysplasia is inherited as an autosomal dominant trait.

☞**MULTIPLE EPIPHYSEAL DYSPLASIA (MES):** Very rare genetic disorder characterized by irregular epiphyseal growth, skeletal deformities, short-limbed dwarfism, and pain and stiffness of affected joints. There are two types of MES: a mild and a severe form. In the mild form, the hands and wrists are usually normal, whereas in the severe form the hands and feet are short and stubby.

REFERENCES:

Roy DR: Current concepts in Legg-Calvé-Perthes disease. *Pediatr Ann* 28:748, 1999.

Thompson GH, Price CT, Roy D, et al: Legg-Calvé-Perthes disease: Current concepts. *Instr Course Lect* 51:367, 2002.

Wiig O, Terjesen T, Svenningsen S: Inter-observer reliability of radiographic classifications and measurements in the assessment of Perthes' disease. *Acta Orthop Scand* 73:523, 2002.

Leigh Syndrome

At a glance: Severe progressive necrotizing encephalopathy occurring between the age of 3 months and 2 years. Caused by a mitochondrial disorder impeding oxidative phosphorylation. Symptoms include loss of previously acquired motor skills, muscle weakness, hypotonia, lactic acidosis associated with respiratory and kidney dysfunction.

Synonyms: Cytochrome Oxidase Deficiency Disease; Infantile Subacute Necrotizing Encephalopathy; Necrotizing Encephalopathy; Pyruvate Decarboxylase Deficiency; Subacute Necrotizing Encephalomyelitis, X-Linked Infantile Necrotizing Encephalopathy.

Nature: Mutation in the oxidative phosphorylation system resulting in necrotizing encephalopathy transmitted either as an autosomal trait or via mitochondrial DNA (maternal transmission only).

Incidence: Unknown. Male-to-female ratio is 3:2.

Genetic inheritance: Genetic inheritance is variable: about half of cases are autosomal recessive with multiple loci, a few are dominant or X-linked, and the remainder are a result of mitochondrial DNA defects (and thus maternally inherited only).

Pathophysiology: When related to a mutation in the mitochondrial DNA, a single base pair is changed from thymine to either cytosine or guanidine in the gene coding for ATPase, an enzyme involved in the electron transfer chain allowing oxidative phosphorylation (resulting in deficiency of cytochrome C oxidase, which is the terminal enzyme of the mitochondrial respiratory chain). Because of the vital nature of this process, ATPase is only partially defective in Leigh syndrome, or several types of mitochondria coexist, some with normal ATPase and some with the defective version. Brain neurons are mainly affected, but liver and heart cells also may deteriorate.

Diagnosis: Diagnosis is usually made during the first or second year of life with delayed psychomotor development or regression of already acquired skills. Ophthalmoplegia and hypotonia are often associated. Further neurologic signs include poor vision, nystagmus, tremor, ataxia, seizures, positive Babinski sign, and absent tendon reflexes. Respiratory signs include alternation of polypnea "sine materia" and bradypnea, poor response to hypoxia or hypercarbia, and eventually respiratory failure.

Clinical aspects: Leigh syndrome is a progressive necrotizing encephalopathy, usually presenting with feeding and swallowing problems, dysautonomia, weakness, ataxia, and convulsions. There are several foci of necrosis in the brainstem, putamen, and globus pallidus. Respiratory involvement is late in the evolution and is associated with poor prognosis. Laboratory investigations include elevated lactate and pyruvate levels and low glucose levels in blood and cerebrospinal fluid (CSF). Several enzymes have been involved in Leigh syndrome: a decrease of pyruvate decarboxylase, inhibition of thiamine pyrophosphate–ATP phosphoryl transferase, or blockade of pyruvate dehydrogenase. Pyruvate dehydrogenase is itself a complex of six enzymes. Other mitochondrial genetic defects can lead to the clinical picture of Leigh syndrome. These enzymatic defects prevent entry of pyruvate in the Krebs cycle.

Precautions before anesthesia: Assess blood lactate and glucose levels. Evaluate breathing pattern. Define a strategy in case of respiratory failure, especially with postoperative management. Check preoperative diet and carbohydrate intake.

Anesthetic considerations: Because the brainstem is often involved, meticulous care should be devoted to temperature, airway, and control of ventilation. Prevent hypocarbia because hypocarbia inhibits pyruvate decarboxylase and further increases lactate levels. Prevent hypothermia because hypermetabolism caused during rewarming can lead to severe metabolic acidosis and hypoglycemia. Maintain normal blood glucose levels at all times, with frequent measurement of glucose concentration. A stress-free anesthesia decreases metabolic response to surgery and lactate production. Maintain adequate preload and prevent tachycardia, which may lead to obstructive cardiomyopathy because of septal hypertrophy. Patients with Leigh syndrome have elevated endorphin levels in CSF and are highly sensitive to intravenous narcotics. These patients should be carefully observed postoperatively. Postoperative respiratory failure is common following general anesthesia or even sedation, especially in the presence of preoperative respiratory impairment; general anesthesia carries a significant risk of postoperative apnea or respiratory failure, and postoperative mechanical ventilation must be considered. Regional anesthetic techniques such as spinal anesthesia may minimize postoperative respiratory complications.

Pharmacological implications: Avoid lactate-containing solutions (Ringer lactate). Thiopental, halothane, and possibly other volatile anesthetic agents may inhibit neoglucogenesis and worsen hypoglycemia. Isoflurane should be preferred to sevoflurane because of the central nervous system (CNS) excitatory effect of sevoflurane in patients susceptible to convulsions. Nitrous oxide and benzodiazepines seem safe. Because of the increased opiate sensitivity, these drugs should be used with caution; short-acting opiates are preferred. Because of the muscular involvement observed with Leigh syndrome patients, succinylcholine may be contraindicated. Short-acting agents such as mivacurium are better indicated. Short-acting agents, remifentanil and desflurane, offer the advantages of quick recovery with limited postoperative CNS and respiratory depression. The potential inhibition of mitochondrial function caused by propofol may preclude its use.

Other conditions to be considered:

☞**Creutzfeldt-Jakob Disease:** Degenerative, invariably fatal brain disorder typically developing in patients older than 60 years; the variant transmitted from cattle contamination ("mad cow disease") can affect young adults and even children.

☞**Wilson Disease:** Progressive multivisceral failure as a result of copper accumulation resulting from an inability to produce sufficient levels of ceruloplasmin. Gene map locus is 13q14.3.

☞**Neuronal Ceroid Lipofuscinoses:** *Kufs Disease*, also known as *Juvenile Neuronal Ceroid Lipofuscinosis type IV*, is characterized by an onset in late adolescence or early adulthood. The clinical symptoms include muscle weakness, ataxia, lack of muscle coordination, chorea, confusion, behavioral changes, and seizures. *Batten Disease*, also known as type III juvenile form of Neuronal Ceroid Lipofuscinosis, is characterized by an onset during childhood or early adolescence and most often presenting clinical features of rapid visual loss, deterioration of earlier psychomotor development, behavior changes, and severe seizure activities. Individuals affected with this condition often develop kyphoscoliosis. It is inherited as an autosomal recessive trait.

Tay-Sachs Disease (☞Gangliosidosis G$_{M2}$ Type II): Caused by accumulation of G$_{M2}$ gangliosides in the brain because of absence of the enzyme hexosaminidase A. The consequence of this metabolic disorder is progressive destruction of the central nervous system. Clinically, the symptoms begin at approximately age 4 months and may include mild muscle weakness, abnormal startle response, and muscle spasms. Between 6 and 10 months of age, feeding difficulties, severe muscle weakness, restlessness, and visual abnormalities (e.g., staring episodes, unusual eye movements, cherry red macular spots) are present. It is generally observed among children of Eastern European Jewish descent.

Sandhoff Disease (☞Gangliosidosis G$_{M2}$ Type II): Rare lipid storage disorder resulting in progressive deterioration of the central nervous system because of deficiency in the enzyme hexosaminidase (β subunit). Sandhoff disease is known as a severe form of Tay-Sachs Disease and is not limited to any particular ethnic group. The clinical features include feeding problems, general muscle weakness and hypotonia, and an exaggerated startle reflex in response to sudden loud noises. Other symptoms may include red spots in the eyes, motor delays, mental deterioration, spasticity, heart murmurs, seizures, blindness, and splenomegaly.

☞**NIEMANN-PICK DISEASE:** Affects most frequently infants and children. Symptoms may include poor feeding habits, physical and mental impairment, hepatosplenomegaly, severe abdominal distension, and vomiting. Some children experience neurologic impairment, including loss of speech, inability to coordinate voluntary muscle movements, convulsions, and dementia.

☞**ALPERS DISEASE:** Affects infants and children. It is a rare progressive neurologic disorder characterized by degeneration of the gray matter of the brain. The clinical features include psychomotor retardation, partial paralysis, growth delays, severe seizures, and myoclonus. Liver damage and blindness may develop. The symptoms may be intensified by stress (e.g., anesthesia and surgical stress) or other illnesses.

REFERENCES:

Grattan-Smith PJ, Sjield LK, Hopkins IJ, et al: Acute respiratory failure precipitated by general anesthesia in Leigh's syndrome. *J Child Neurol* 5:137, 1990.

Shear T, Tobias JD: Anesthetic implications of Leigh's syndrome. *Paediatr Anaesth* 14:792, 2004.

Shenkman Z, Krichevski I, Elpeleg ON, et al: Anaesthetic management of a patient with Leigh's syndrome. *Can J Anaesth* 44;1091, 1997.

Yasaki E, Saito Y, Nakano K, et al: Characteristics of breathing abnormality in Leigh and its overlap syndromes. *Neuropediatrics* 32:299, 2001.

Leiner Syndrome

At a glance: Severe seborrheic dermatitis with systemic infection, diarrhea, and central nervous system deficiency as a consequence of complement C5 deficiency (acquired deficiency in most patients).

Synonyms: Complement C5 Deficiency; Dermatitis Exfoliativa Generalisata; Desquamative Erythroderma in Infants; Eczema Universale Seborrhoeicum; Erythrodermia Desquamativa of Leiner; Erythrodermia Desquamativa in Infants; Erythroderma Desquamativum; Erythrodermic Seborrheic Dermatitis in the Trianon of Life; Exfoliative Dermatitis; Seborrhoic Diathesis in Infants; Leiner-Moussous Disease.

History: First described in 1908 by Karl Leiner, an Austrian pediatrician.

Incidence: Prevalent in infant females. Breast-fed infants are most frequently affected.

Genetic inheritance: Not a genetic disorder in most patients. Gene map locus of hereditary complement C5 deficiency is 9q34.1.

Pathophysiology: Leiner disease includes a heterogeneous group of disorders. A common feature of these disorders is temporary or permanent (hereditary forms) plasma deficiency in complement C5 activity resulting in decrease of opsonic properties of plasma (deficiency in phagocytosis).

Diagnosis: Clinical picture. Deficiency in complement C5 activity in plasma.

Clinical aspects: Syndrome characterized by desquamation (severe generalized seborrheic dermatitis), recurrent local and systemic infection, severe diarrhea, marked wasting, central nervous system deficiency, and failure to thrive. It begins as seborrheic eczematoid lesions of the scalp and face or the gluteal region, eventually spreading to other areas. Keratitis and corneal ulcers may occur. Caused by complement C5 deficiency in infancy; rapid onset in second to fourth month of life.

Precautions before anesthesia: Elective anesthesia and surgery should be postponed until skin covering is restored in relevant areas.

Anesthetic considerations: Patients with Leiner disease are prone to severe bacterial contamination as a consequence of their extensive skin lesions and deficiency in phagocytosis. Large spectrum antibioprophylaxis should be considered. Because of extended skin lesions, there is a danger of systemic toxicity with topical agents (especially disinfectants and skin preparation solutions).

Pharmacological implications: Use topical agents with extreme care because of increase systemic absorption and toxicity. Avoid any solution containing potentially toxic components, either topical or systemic. Some patients receive high-dose corticosteroid in the acute phase, so intraoperative supplementation will be needed.

Other conditions to be considered: Other disorders with erythroderma (some of which are included in the general term of Leiner disease), including the following:

ATOPIC ECZEMA: Later onset, familial context of atopy.

INFANTILE SEBORRHEIC DERMATITIS: "Cradle cap," usually self-limiting, subsiding by age 6 months; no complement C5 deficiency; cured by topical cortisone.

ICHTHYOSIFORM ERYTHRODERMA: Autosomal dominant; bullous ichthyosis.

☞**NETHERTON SYNDROME:** Recessive skin atopy disorder, bamboo hair, mostly in females.

IMMUNODEFICIENCY SYNDROMES: Group of syndromes that have in common a dysfunction of the immune system. They are divided into T-cell system deficiency or B-cell deficiency. For instance, Idiopathic Thrombocytopenic Purpura (ITP), X-linked Agammaglobulinemia, Severe Combined Immunodeficiency, Nezelof Syndrome, and Wiskott-Aldrich Syndrome are all considered immunodeficiency syndromes.

REFERENCES:

Bykowsky MJ: Generalized seborrheic dermatitis in an immunodeficient newborn. *Cutis* 70:324, 2002.

Moises-Alfaro CB, Caceres-Rios HW, Rueda M, et al: Are infantile seborrheic and atopic dermatitis clinical variants of the same disease? *Int J Dermatol* 41:349, 2002.

Whaley K, Schwaeble W: Complement and complement deficiencies. *Semin Liver Dis* 17:297, 1997.

Lemierre Syndrome

At a glance: Anaerobic sepsis after oropharyngeal infection leading to septic thrombophlebitis of the internal jugular vein.

History: Bacterial infection by gram-negative bacillus *Fusobacterium necrophorum* (*Bacteroides melaninogenicus, Eikenella corrodens,* and nongroup A streptococcus have also been isolated from patients with this syndrome) reported in 1936 by Lemierre, who called the syndrome "postanginal septicemia."

Incidence: Rare but probably frequently overlooked. Occurs more frequently in teenagers and young adults but has also been described in children.

Genetic inheritance: Not a genetic disorder.

Pathophysiology: Untreated *F. necrophorum* tonsillitis or peritonsillar abscess may cause septic thrombophlebitis of the ipsilateral internal jugular vein that rapidly progresses to septicemia because of septic emboli in the lungs or other organs. The proliferation of these bacteria is favored by disruption of normal host mucosal defenses through trauma or hypoxia. Release of proteolytic enzymes, lipopolysaccharide endotoxin, leukocidin, and hemagglutinin accounts for the pathogenicity of *F. necrophorum,* which usually invades the regional veins. The hemagglutinin moiety can aggregate bovine platelets, and this phenomenon may play a role in the development of internal jugular vein thrombosis.

Diagnosis: Cervical Doppler ultrasound shows thrombophlebitis of the internal jugular vein, and high-resolution CT scanning shows nodules abutting the pleura with or without cavitation. Positive blood cultures for *F. necrophorum* confirm the diagnosis.

Clinical aspects: Fever and neck pain; moderate dyspnea; pharyngotonsillar inflammation and ipsilateral tender swelling of the cervical region; often complicated by distant metastatic infections; chest radiograph usually shows ill-defined infiltrates or round opacities but also signs of septic lung emboli (wedge-shaped peripheral densities, nodular or cavitary lesions). Overall mortality rate approximately 15% (but > 80% if no antibiotics are given).

Precautions before anesthesia: Check room air pulse oximetry and chest radiograph. Appropriate antibiotic treatment should have been started. If central venous catheterization is foreseen, ultrasound examination of the jugular and subclavian vessels must be obtained to check the potency of these vessels.

Anesthetic considerations: All anesthetic considerations for management of anesthesia of a septic patient with pulmonary ventilation/perfusion mismatch and potential cardiovascular instability must be clearly established and considered in designing the anesthetic plan.

Pharmacological implications: No known specific pharmacological implications; however, patients treated by antibiotics and, occasionally, by anticoagulants, which occasionally interfere with other treatments, may affect anesthetic agents and techniques. For instance, the use of antibiotics may significantly affect the pharmacokinetics of neuromuscular blockade agents.

Other condition to be considered:

☞**GRISEL SYNDROME:** Infectious complication of upper neck inflammatory processes (pharyngitis and pharyngeal abscess) and head and neck surgery resulting in subluxation of the atlantoaxial joint.

REFERENCES:

Armstrong AW, Spooner K, Sanders JW: Lemierre's syndrome. *Curr Infect Dis Rep* 2:168, 2000.

Hoehn S, Dominguez TE: Lemierre's syndrome: An unusual cause of sepsis and abdominal pain. *Crit Care Med* 30:1644, 2002.

Klinge L, Vester U, Schaper J, Hoyer PF: Severe Fusobacteria infections (Lemierre syndrome) in two boys. *Eur J Pediatr* 161:616, 2002.

Lennox-Gastaut Syndrome

At a glance: Severe form of intractable epilepsy resulting in severe learning disabilities and impaired organization of movements. Poor prognosis: 5% of patients die within 10 years; 50% of affected adults are completely dependent and less than 20% are independent.

Synonym: Childhood Epileptic Encephalopathy.

History: First described in 1770 by Tissot, who reported an 11-year-old boy with frequent drop attacks, myoclonus, and progressive functional impairment.

Incidence: From 3 to 10% of children with epilepsy. Male predominance. No racial predominance.

Genetic inheritance: Commonly, there is a history of epilepsy in the family of children with Lennox-Gastaut syndrome, but no familial case of this syndrome has been reported.

Pathophysiology: Unknown even though many favoring factors have been suggested, such as brain injury at birth, brain infections, genetic brain diseases (e.g., tuberous sclerosis and inherited metabolic brain diseases), brain malformations, and West syndrome. Excessive permeability in the excitatory interhemispheric pathways in the frontal areas might play a role. Immunogenetic mechanisms may be involved in triggering or maintaining some cases of Lennox-Gastaut syndrome. One study found a strong association between Lennox-Gastaut syndrome and the human lymphocyte antigen class I antigen B7, but a second study did not.

Diagnosis: Clinical presentation and characteristic electroencephalographic (EEG) pattern. The EEG shows spikes and slow frequency waves of 1.5 to 2.5 Hz. The background rhythm is slow with multifocal spikes. The maximal voltage area is usually anterior.

Clinical aspects: Peak age for onset is between 3 and 5 years (extremes: 1–10 years). The syndrome consists of the triad of intractable seizures (tonic seizures, drop attacks, atypical absences), mental retardation, and characteristic EEG. Affected patients have a large variety of seizures that occur at any time (day and night). Consciousness may be only partially affected, and patients may remain rather active but "distant," with loss of tone of muscles of the face and neck resulting in impaired balance or abnormal posture. Severe cases of status epilepticus may develop. Lennox-Gastaut syndrome may be preceded by infantile spasms (West syndrome), which worsens the prognosis. Antiepileptic agents are not effective against this baffling disorder. Felbamate currently seems to be the only agent with some efficacy.

Precautions before anesthesia: Proper evaluation of the degree of epilepsy and the medications used in this situation. No known specific precautions other than the evaluation of the potential complications associated with this form of intractable seizure disease. Most patients are resistant to medications. In patients with frequent seizures, a ketogenic diet may be considered, and less conventional therapies such as intravenous immunoglobulin therapy may be worth considering.

Anesthetic considerations: No specific anesthetic considerations except for the importance and the frequency of seizure activities, which may affect the anesthetic management. Patients may be anxious and uncooperative. Induction of anesthesia should be performed in conditions adapted to the behavior of the patient. Use of preoperative sedative medication should be considered if there are no contraindications from the cardiopulmonary and intracranial clinical condition.

Pharmacological implications: It is essential to avoid anesthetic medications that could trigger seizure activities (e.g., methohexital, enflurane, high and sustained concentration of sevoflurane during induction of anesthesia). The only treatment for this medical condition is felbamate, which is associated with a significant risk of hepatotoxicity. Therefore, anesthesia drugs with considerable hepatic metabolism probably should be avoided or used with great caution (e.g., halothane).

Other conditions to be considered: Other forms of infantile epilepsy include the following:

☞**WEST SYNDROME:** Rare form of infantile spasm that manifests during the first months of life and is characterized by hypsarrhythmia (abnormal brain waves) and mental retardation. There are two forms: *cryptogenic*, which has no known cause, and *symptomatic*, which results from an underlying condition or factor. The cryptogenic form usually follows a normal pregnancy, birth, and development and is associated with a more favorable outcome. Patients affected with the symptomatic form often develop mental retardation. Clinical features include involuntary muscle spasms occurring during seizures, typically beginning suddenly and lasting a few seconds. They may occur during sleep or upon awakening, are characterized by sudden, involuntary contractions of the head, neck, and trunk, with uncontrolled extension of the legs and arms. The syndrome often develops into the Lennox-Gastaut form of epilepsy with seizures that are difficult to control, making early diagnosis very important.

DOOSE SYNDROME (Photogenic Seizures): Characterized by myoclonic-astatic epilepsy occurring during childhood that is triggered by light and often called "cerebral light sensitivity" syndrome. It is inherited as an autosomal dominant pattern.

☞**AICARDI SYNDROME:** Rare disorder characterized by partial or complete agenesis of the corpus callosum, infantile spasms (spasm-like epilepsy), mental retardation, and an ocular abnormality called *lacunae of the retina*. Often associated with other features such as microcephaly and porencephalic cysts. Onset is generally between the age of 3 and 5 months. The disorder affects only females.

REFERENCES:

Camfield P, Camfield C: Epileptic syndromes in childhood: Clinical features, outcomes, and treatment. *Epilepsia* 43(suppl 3):27, 2002.

Gates JR: Surgery in Lennox-Gastaut syndrome. Corpus callosum division for children. *Adv Exp Med Biol* 497:87, 2002.

Niedermeyer E: Lennox-Gastaut syndrome. Clinical description and diagnosis. *Adv Exp Med Biol* 497:61, 2002.

Lenz Syndrome

At a glance: Syndrome characterized by unilateral or bilateral microphthalmos and blepharoptosis. In rare cases, affected infants present anophthalmia, severe mental retardation, microcephaly, and malformations of the teeth, ears, and digits.

Synonyms: Lenz Dysplasia; Lenz Syndrome II; Lenz Dysmorphogenic Syndrome; Lenz Microphthalmia Syndrome; Microphthalmia with Associated Anomalies (MAA).

Incidence: Twenty case reports in the literature.

Genetic inheritance: Genetic inheritance is controversial. Most cases are X-linked (gene map locus is Xq27-Xq28), but an autosomal inheritance cannot be excluded in some cases.

Pathophysiology: Pathophysiologic background has not been determined.

Diagnosis: Based on clinical features.

Clinical aspects: Microcephaly with mental retardation, and various anomalies of external ear, digits (double thumbs), heart, skeleton, and urogenital system. Features of the syndrome include severe ophthalmic abnormalities possibly including microphthalmia (even anophthalmos), absent pupil, microcornea, and a variety of craniofacial anomalies such as microcephaly, auricular malformations, and dental abnormalities. Other features include skeletal anomalies with underdeveloped shoulders, webbed neck, cardiac malformations (bicuspid aortic valve), hypospadias, and other severe urogenital anomalies. Most patients are mentally retarded with dilatation of

the lateral ventricles (hydrocephalus) and dysgenesis of the corpus callosum.

Precautions before anesthesia: Thorough history and examination are necessary to determine the extent of the syndrome. Particular note should be made of the following:

- Central nervous system involvement including epilepsy, mental retardation, and possible blindness
- Respiratory system involvement as a result of restrictive skeletal abnormalities
- Urogenital involvement, possibly to the point of renal impairment
- Craniofacial abnormalities that may cause airway difficulties
- Cardiac evaluation (echocardiography, electroencephalography) to eliminate associated defects

Anesthetic considerations: Because of the versatility in the expression of the syndrome, each patient must be evaluated individually. The potential association with multiple organ system involvement and anesthesia raises numerous considerations and challenges. Based on proper preoperative evaluation of the cardiovascular and respiratory systems, including the airway, anesthesia considerations are directed by the associated anomalies rather than the syndrome itself. The association of microcephaly, cleft lip and palate, and respiratory problems may lead to difficult induction of anesthesia.

Pharmacological implications: No specific implications reported for this medical condition. However, in the presence of difficult airway management, use of muscle relaxants should be postponed until the trachea has been secured and lung ventilation confirmed. The presence of microcephaly should indicate a need to reduce the amount of anesthetic used to maintain hemodynamic stability and a proper depth of surgical anesthesia.

Other conditions to be considered:

☞**AICARDI SYNDROME:** X-linked syndrome affecting females only, characterized by the absence of corpus callosum, infantile spasms by age 3 months because of closure of the final neural synapses in the brain, mental retardation, and lacunae of the retina.

☞**GOLTZ SYNDROME:** X-linked dominant disease with in utero lethality in males characterized by focal dermal hypoplasia, asymmetrical limb defects, and a variety of additional anomalies; very similar to Aicardi syndrome.

☞**MIDAS SYNDROME:** X-linked phenotype distinct from Goltz syndrome; characterized by microphthalmia, dermal aplasia, and sclerocornea.

REFERENCES:

Ng D, Hadley DW, Tifft CJ, et al: Genetic heterogeneity of syndromic X-linked recessive microphthalmia-anophthalmia: Is Lenz microphthalmia a single disorder? *Am J Med Genet* 110:308, 2002.

Ozkinay FF, Ozkinay C, Yuksel H, et al: A case of Lenz microphthalmia syndrome. *J Med Genet* 34:604, 1997.

Lenz-Majewski Syndrome

At a glance: Characterized by multiple congenital anomalies (delayed closure of fontanel, proximal symphalangism, prominent scalp cutaneous veins), mental retardation, and progressive skeletal sclerosis with severe growth retardation and a progeroid appearance. Other clinical features include dysplastic teeth, skin hypoplasia, joint laxity, choanal atresia, short digits, and partial syndactyly.

Synonyms: Braham-Lenz Syndrome; Lenz Syndrome I; Lenz-Majewski Hyperostotic Dwarfism.

History: First described by Braham in 1969 as Camurati-Engelmann syndrome.

Genetic inheritance: Autosomal dominant.

Pathophysiology: Nature of the disorder is obscure. Possibly caused by a dominant mutation leading to disturbance of connective tissue.

Diagnosis: Radiologic evidence of progressive skeletal sclerosis (skull, facial bones, and vertebrae), broad clavicles and ribs, short or absent middle phalanges. Diaphyseal undermodeling and midshaft cortical thickening. Retarded skeletal maturation, humeroradial synostosis.

Clinical aspects: Delayed closure of fontanelle, proximal symphalangism, short digits, partial syndactyly, prominent cutaneous veins, loose and wrinkled atrophic skin of hands, skin hypoplasia, mental retardation, progeroid appearance, dysplastic dental enamel, joint laxity, choanal atresia, nasolacrimal duct obstruction, sporadic occurrence, advanced paternal age.

Precautions before anesthesia: No specific precautions before anesthesia have been reported for this medical condition. Because of the progeroid appearance, it is recommended to review carefully the history and physical characteristics for possible association of anomalies with the cardiovascular system and the airway. However, these possible complications are not directly related to the description of this syndrome but are considered circumstantial.

Anesthetic considerations: No specific anesthetic considerations for this medical condition rather than the usual patient management. However, positioning might require special attention because of the leg problems and the exquisite pain manifested by the patient.

Pharmacological implications: No known pharmacological implications for this syndrome.

Other conditions to be considered:

☞**CAMURATI-ENGELMANN DISEASE:** Characterized by diaphyseal dysplasia, bone pain most often in the legs, skeletal abnormalities, and a "waddling" gait caused by severe hypoplasia of various muscles in the legs. It may become apparent as early as age 3 months or as late as the sixth decade of life. In some cases, fatigue, headaches, poor appetite, exophthalmos, reduced subcutaneous fat, and hepatosplenomegaly have been reported. It is inherited as an autosomal dominant trait and is the result of a mutation in the beta 1-LAP gene.

LENZ-MAJEWSKI–LIKE SYNDROME: Mesoectodermal dysplasia with macrocephaly, specific facial features (exophthalmos, broad nasal root, anteverted nostrils, large auricles, thick lips, micrognathia), failure to thrive, mental retardation, sparse hair, enamel hypoplasia, loose skin, and skeletal abnormalities.

REFERENCES:

Majewski F: Lenz-Majewski hyperostotic dwarfism: Reexamination of the original patient. *Am J Med Genet* 93:335, 2000.

Robinow M, Johanson AJ, Smith TH: The Lenz-Majewski hyperostotic dwarfism: A syndrome of multiple congenital anomalies, mental retardation, and progressive skeletal sclerosis. *J Pediatr* 91:417, 1977.

LEOPARD Syndrome

At a glance: Acronym for *l*entigines (multiple), *e*lectrocardiographic conduction abnormalities, *o*cular hypertelorism, *p*ulmonary stenosis, *a*bnormal genitalia, *r*etardation of growth, and *d*eafness (sensorineural). Complex congenital dysmorphogenetic disorder associating mainly skin lesions (lentigines), severe cardiac anomalies (dysrhythmias, pulmonary valve stenosis), ocular hypertelorism, abnormalities of genitalia, sensorineural deafness, and severe retardation of growth.

Synonyms: Cardiocutaneous Syndrome; Cardiocutaneous Lentiginosis Syndrome; Cardiomyopathic Lentiginosis; Centrofacial Lentiginosis; Generalized Lentiginosis; Lentiginosis-Deafness-Cardiopathy Syndrome; Lentiginosis Profusa Syndrome; Moynahan Syndrome; Multiple Lentigines Syndrome; Progressive Cardiomyopathic Lentiginosis.

History: First described by Zeisler and Becker in 1936. It has many similarities to Noonan syndrome, except in the most striking features, from which its name is derived. The mnemonic was first used by Gorlin et al. in 1969.

Incidence: Rare; slightly more than 80 cases reported. Life expectancy is normal.

Genetic inheritance: Sporadic or autosomal dominant. Single mutant gene with high penetrance and variable expression produces the defects in this syndrome. Slight male predominance.

Pathophysiology: Mutation in the stem cell pool of the neural crest in embryonic life is regarded as a common cause of cutaneous (producing lentigines), neurologic, cardiac (resulting in cardiomyopathy), and possibly urogenital defects. Metabolism of dihydroxyphenylalanine (DOPA), epinephrine, and norepinephrine is altered, which may result in abnormal skin pigmentation.

Diagnosis: Diagnostic criteria included skin lentigines plus two other recognized features or a first-degree relative with lentigines plus three other features in the patient. Histologic examination of the lentigines shows pigment accumulation in the dermis and in the deeper layers of epidermis. There is an increase in melanocytic density owing to corrugation of the dermoepidermal junction.

Clinical aspects: Lentigines (1–2 mm; flat, dark brown-to-black cutaneous lesions) can be present at birth and increase in number until puberty. They are most numerous on the face, neck, and upper trunk but spare the mucous membranes. Valvular pulmonary stenosis is the most common (40% of cases) cardiovascular abnormality. Hypertrophic obstructive cardiomyopathy is a major concern with onset usually in childhood. Subsequent progression may be mild and slow or severe and florid with rapid decompensation. Conduction abnormalities are common and result from combinations of blocks in the bundle branch system. These abnormalities may be asymptomatic or sufficiently severe to provoke sudden death. The conduction impairment develops gradually and is progressive. Ocular hypertelorism, mandibular prognathism, and short stature are the most common skeletal abnormalities. Pectus excavatum and carinatum are common, as is scoliosis (10% of cases). Sensorineural hearing loss may be severe and may appear late in life.

Precautions before anesthesia: Echocardiographic examination to look for the presence of cardiomyopathy, pulmonary valve stenosis, and subaortic stenosis (with outflow tract obstruction) is mandatory. Evaluate pulmonary function (when feasible as a function of patient's age) in the presence of thoracic abnormalities (forced vital capacity [FVC], peak expiratory flow rate [PEFR], forced expiratory volume in 1 second [FEV_1], FEV_1/FVC ratio, arterial blood gas analysis, and chest radiographs).

Anesthetic considerations: Of primary importance is the high incidence of associated disorders affecting the cardiovascular system, such as congenital heart diseases, conduction disturbances, and hypertrophic obstructive cardiomyopathy. All children presenting with

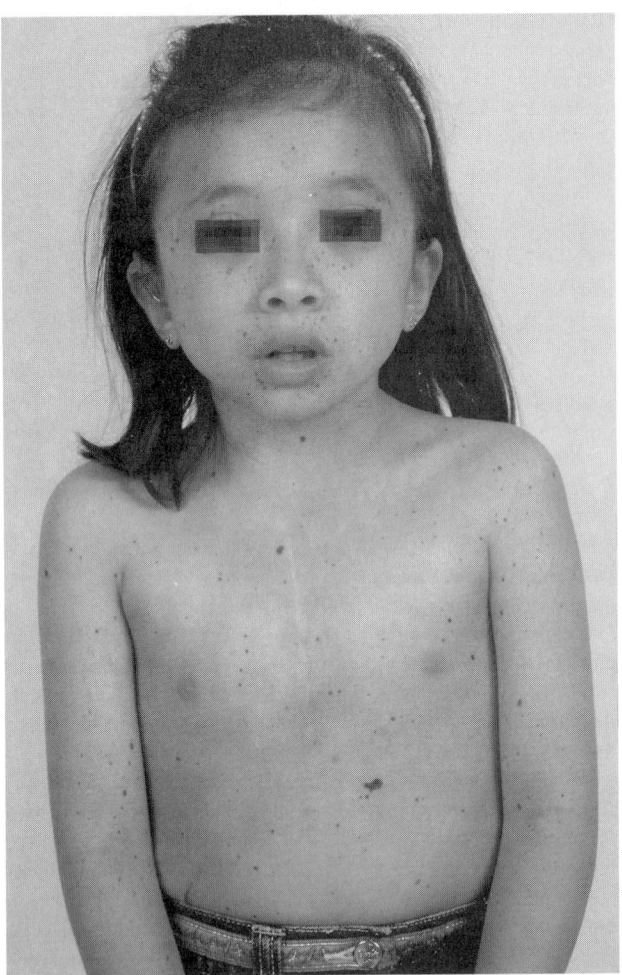

LEOPARD syndrome Young girl with hypertelorism and multiple lentigines has LEOPARD syndrome. Note the scar from sternotomy for repair of severe right ventricular outflow tract obstruction.

multiple cutaneous lentigines should be considered to have Leopard syndrome until proven otherwise. Special consideration given to factors that may produce changes in intravascular volume, ventricular contractility, and transmural distending pressure of the outflow tract. Avoid prolonged preoperative fasting that produces volume depletion. Tachycardia and positive inotropic agents may be deleterious because they decrease diastolic filling time and stroke volume and increase turbulent flow across the outflow tract. Elective surgery under general anesthesia is contraindicated when respiratory and/or cardiac functions are severely impaired (ventricular ejection fraction <0.5, FVC <25%, PEFR <30%). Regional anesthesia (central neuraxial) should be used with great caution in children older than 5 years of age.

Pharmacological implications: Avoid anticholinergic premedication but provide adequate anxiolysis. Halothane is preferred by some because it decreases more ventricular contractility and heart rate compared to isoflurane or sevoflurane. The use of total intravenous anesthesia maintaining the patient's preoperative hemodynamic condition is also an alternative.

Other conditions to be considered:

☞**Neurofibromatosis Generalisata Type I:** Café-au-lait spots, freckles, development of benign neurofibromas. Autosomal dominant. Caused by a mutation on chromosome 17.

Central Neurofibromatoses: Development of schwannomas on the eighth cranial nerve and many other nerves, early cataract, and few (inconstant) café-au-lait spots. Autosomal dominant. Caused by a mutation on chromosome 22.

☞**Noonan Syndrome:** Unusual facies mimicking Turner syndrome, short stature, chest deformity, and inconstantly mental retardation. Autosomal dominant (gene defect probably located on chromosome 12q). Multiple lentigines are found in 3% of cases (thus mimicking LEOPARD syndrome and neurofibromatosis).

Forney Syndrome: Rare syndrome characterized by familial mitral insufficiency, congenital conductive hearing loss because of stapes footplate fixation, short stature, and bony fusion of carpal and tarsal bones and cervical vertebrae. The latter could lead to difficult airway management.

References:

Coppin BD, Teple IK: Multiple lentigines syndrome. *J Med Genet* 34:582, 1997.

Digilio MC, Conti E, Sarkozy A, et al: Grouping of multiple-lentigines/LEOPARD and Noonan syndromes on the PTPN11 gene. *Am J Hum Genet* 71:389, 2002.

Rodrigo MRC, Cheng CH, Tai YT, et al: "LEOPARD" syndrome. *Anaesthesia* 45:30, 1990.

Torres J, Russo P, Tobias JD: Anesthetic implications of LEOPARD syndrome. *Paediatr Anesth* 14:352, 2004.

Leri Pleonosteosis

At a glance: Congenital disorder of the bone and joints with characteristic facial features. The presence of laryngeal stenosis may be a significant anesthetic consideration.

Incidence: Only a few cases reported in the literature.

Genetic inheritance: Autosomal dominant.

Pathophysiology: Etiology unknown. Primary pathology may be in the joint capsules rather than the bone itself. A characteristic feature is bony overgrowth of the cartilaginous skeleton, which produces increased width rather than length of the bones, together with enlargement of the bone ends.

Diagnosis: Based on clinical features. Radiologic features include evidence of delayed bone age, marked broadening of the phalanges with evidence of flexion deformity, increase in width of the vertebrae, and bizarre enlargement of the posterior neural arches of the cervical vertebrae.

Clinical aspects: Short stature; mongoloid facies; brachydactyly; genu recurvatum; short, spade-like hands; broad thumbs in valgus position; thick palmar and forearm fasciae; shuffling, short-stepped gait; decreased joint mobility; and laryngeal stenosis.

Precautions before anesthesia: Assess airway and neck mobility.

Anesthetic considerations: Difficult tracheal intubation because of limited neck movement and laryngeal stenosis.

Pharmacological implications: No known specific pharmacological implications; however, several patients will be on chronic corticosteroid therapy and will require intraoperative supplementation.

Other conditions to be considered:

☞**Acromicric Dysplasia:** Mild facial abnormalities, short hands and feet, short stature with delayed bone maturation (may be the same disease as Moore-Federman syndrome).

☞**LÉRI-WEILL SYNDROME:** Dominant pseudoautosomal skeletal dysplasia with mesomelic short stature as a result of the loss of one copy of the short stature homeobox gene (SHOX) located on the short arm of the X or Y chromosome.

☞**MOORE-FEDERMAN SYNDROME:** Short stature with disproportionately short legs, joint limitations, ocular anomalies, laryngeal stenosis. Autosomal dominant transmission.

REFERENCES:

Greenspan A, Azouz EM: Bone dysplasia series. Melorheostosis: Review and update. *Can Assoc Radiol J* 50:324, 1999.

Hoshi K, Amizuka N, Kurokawa T, et al: Histopathological characterization of melorheostosis. *Orthopedics* 24:273, 2001.

Léri-Weill Syndrome

At a glance: Disproportionate moderate dwarfism with Madelung wrist deformity and multiple skeletal deformities.

Synonyms: Lamy Bienenfeld Syndrome; Lery-Weill Dyschondrosteosis Syndrome.

History: First described by A. Léri and J.A. Weill in 1929.

Incidence: Very rare.

Genetic inheritance: Pseudoautosomal dominant (mutation in the pseudoautosomal genes SHOX or SHOXY, located on Ypter-p11.2, Xpter-p22.32).

Diagnosis: Disease characterized by bowed radius and ulna, with small stature mainly from mesomelic origin. Can be evocated at the end of fetal growth. Predominant and more severe in female (female-to-male ratio = 4:1).

Clinical aspects: Stature is short and disproportionate (adult height 135 cm [53.1 inches]). Multiple skeletal deformities are observed. Radiologically the bones present cone epiphyses, enlarged diaphysis, metaphyseal anomaly, and multiple exostoses. Fingers and toes are abnormal. Superior limb anomalies include mesomelia, increased carrying angle, limited elbow mobility, dorsal-limited wrist mobility, subluxation of ulna, Madelung wrist deformity (occurring after 10 years and described as a displacement of the hand to the radial side as the result of dorsolateral distortion of the lower end of the radius because of relative overgrowth of the ulna). Inferior limb can present coxa vara, hip and pelvis anomalies, abnormal femur and patella, genu varum, flat foot that restricts joint mobility. Scoliosis is frequent. The face presents with a broad nose, depressed nasal bridge, and flat occiput brachycephaly.

Precautions before anesthesia: Although there are multiple skeletal deformities, there are no indications that a difficult airway must be expected. However, it is recommended to assess carefully this aspect.

Anesthetic considerations: Consider chronologic age and not physical stature to determine the airway size. Careful intraoperative positioning is difficult but necessary because of deformations. Regional anesthesia is not contraindicated but can be difficult because of skeletal anomalies.

Pharmacological implications: No known pharmacological implications.

Other conditions to be considered:

☞**ARKLESS-GRAHAM SYNDROME:** Characterized by short hands and feet, stubby fingers and toes, broad short nails, flat nasal bridge, underdeveloped jaw, improper alignment of the teeth, widely spaced eyes, mental retardation, and deformity of the bones in the arms, legs, and elbows. It is inherited as an autosomal dominant trait. Females are affected twice as often as males.

☞**ELLIS-VAN CREVELD SYNDROME:** Characterized by short limb dwarfism, polydactyly, abnormal fingernails, and congenital heart defects. It is a form of ectodermal dysplasia that involves the skin, hair, teeth, and nails. It is inherited as an autosomal recessive trait.

MADELUNG DEFORMITY: Results from partial dislocation of the bones of the forearm because of trauma or infection. Short stature is not involved.

LANGER MESOMELIC DYSPLASIA TYPE: Affects males and females equally and is inherited as an autosomal recessive trait. Clinical features include typically short, thick, curved bones of the radius and tibia. Other features include restricted elbow and forearm movement, underdeveloped jaw, and abnormal degree of forward curvature of the lower back.

NIEVERGELT MESOMELIC DYSPLASIA TYPE: Rare form of dwarfism characterized by shortening of the limbs and restricted movement of the elbows and forearms, unusual clubfeet, and metatarsal synostosis. Affects males and females equally.

REINHARDT-PFEIFFER MESOMELIC DYSPLASIA TYPE: Inherited as an autosomal dominant trait and affects females more often than males. Ulna and fibula are underdeveloped.

WERNER MESOMELIC DYSPLASIA TYPE: Affects males and females equally and is inherited as an autosomal dominant trait. The tibia is typically underdeveloped or absent, and polydactyly is present. Other features include absent thumbs, limited movement of the wrist, and deformed ankle.

☞**ROBINOW SYNDROME:** Characterized by shortened fingers, toes, and forearms and moderately short stature. There may be an enlarged head and forehead associated with hypertelorism, a broad, short, upturned nose, triangular-shaped mouth with a cleft lower lip, a small jaw, and crowded teeth.

REFERENCES:

Huber C, Cusin V, Le Merrer M, et al: SHOX point mutations in dyschondrosteosis. *J Med Genet* 38:323, 2001.

Léri A, Weill JA: Une affection congénitale et symétrique du développement osseux. La dyschondrostéose. *Bulletins et mémoires de la Société médicale des hôpitaux de Paris* 53:1491, 1929.

Ross JL, Bellus G, Scott CI Jr, et al: Mesomelic and rhizomelic short stature: The phenotype of combined Leri-Weill dyschondrosteosis and achondroplasia or hypochondroplasia. *Am J Med Genet* 116A:61, 2003.

Lesch-Nyhan Syndrome

At a glance: Rare inborn error of purine metabolism that becomes apparent between the ages of 3 and 6 months. Characterized by the presence of orange crystal-like deposits ("orange sand") in the diapers of infants with the disorder. This is frequently the first symptom of Lesch-Nyhan syndrome. Other clinical features include hematuria, urinary tract infections, arthritis, choreoathetosis manifested by raising and lowering of the shoulders, and facial grimacing. Hypotonia, hypertonia, hyperreflexia, and spasticity have been reported. Megaloblastic anemia, self-mutilating behavior, irritability, screaming, uncontrolled aggressiveness, and compulsive actions complete the clinical presentation.

Synonyms: Hyperuricemia Syndrome; Hypoxanthine-Phosphoribosyl-Transferase Deficiency Disease; Complete HGPRT Deficiency Disease; Kelley-Seegmiller Syndrome; Hyperuricemia-Oligophrenia Syndrome.

Nature: Genetically transmitted error of metabolism of purine bases.

Incidence: Estimated at 1:380,000 live births in the United States; almost exclusively males, although a few females are reported (heterozygotes, mild form of the disease).

Genetic inheritance: X-linked (Xq26-Xq27) recessive disorder caused by a mutation in the gene coding for the enzyme hypoxanthine phosphoribosyltransferase (HPRT). Different mutations have been described.

Pathophysiology: The mutation leads to total or partial loss of function of HPRT, which normally catalyzes the conversion of hypoxanthine and guanine to inosinic and guanylic acid, a reaction that allows reuse of preformed purine bases resulting from cell turnover and catabolism. The absence of this reaction results in overproduction of uric acid and leads to hyperuricemia and uricosuria and thus urate nephropathy, urinary tract calculi, and gout. The neurologic features of the syndrome (choreoathetosis, self-mutilation, spasticity) are caused by abnormalities in brain neurotransmitters, mainly decreased dopaminergic activity in the basal ganglia. Treatment with inhibitors of xanthine oxidase (allopurinol 10 mg/kg/day, maximum 800 mg/day) can control hyperuricemia but does not prevent the effect on neurologic system. Poor prognosis (few patients live beyond age 40 years).

Diagnosis: Patients are normal at birth; onset after a few months. Diagnosis can be clinically evocated by the observation of orange crystals in the diapers or crystalluria with obstruction of the urinary tract. Psychomotor retardation appears quickly (delay in acquisition of sitting and head support), followed by spasticity and athetoid movements. Self-mutilation is characteristic and can start as soon as teeth are present. Enzyme and molecular studies confirm diagnosis.

Clinical aspects: Boys only are affected; the first symptom is often the presence of orange-colored crystal-like deposits ("orange sand") of urates in the diapers of affected infants.

Total Deficit in HPRT: Manifests during the first year of life with motor development delays. Thereafter, choreoathetotic movements with dysphagia and dysarthria; later, axial hypotonia and limb spasticity. Compulsive self-mutilation (biting of lips, fingers, and hands) and aggressive behavior usually appear between ages 2 and 4 years, Nephrolithiasis and gouty arthritis occur if no allopurinol treatment is given. Mental retardation is present, but the severity is difficult to determine because IQ testing is problematic.

Partial Deficit in HPRT: The child presents with juvenile gout with nephrolithiasis; there is no self-mutilation and the neurologic signs are mild (some choreic or athetotic involuntary movements). Partial Lesch-Nyhan syndrome should be excluded in children with uric nephrolithiasis.

Precautions before anesthesia: Evaluate neurologic status (obtain full history, clinical, electroencephalogram, CT/MRI), particularly concerning dysphagia and extrapyramidal signs. Evaluate hyperuricemia consequences (clinical, laboratory investigations including blood and urinary uric acid, echography, CT, radiography). Coagulation disorder is possible in severe cases.

Anesthetic considerations: Careful intraoperative positioning is necessary. Strict asepsis is needed considering infectious risk. The risk of pulmonary aspiration is high because of oropharyngeal abnormal motility. Perioperative observation of the patient is needed

considering the degree of aggressivity, explosive compulsive action, and severe behavioral problems. Cooperation is not possible, and sedation should be considered.

Pharmacological implications: Although propofol may increase urinary acid excretion in normal subjects, it has been used without problems in patients with Lesch-Nyhan syndrome. Nevertheless, prolonged propofol infusion probably should be avoided. There is some evidence of abnormal adrenergic function and diminished sympathetic response to stress; consequently, exogenous catecholamines should be administered with care (titration to effect).

Other conditions to be considered: Inherited chorea syndromes may rarely be confused with Lesch-Nyhan syndrome, the diagnosis of which is easy (orange crystal in the diaper).

REFERENCES:

Larson LO, Wilkins RG: Anesthesia and the Lesch-Nyhan syndrome. *Anesthesiology* 63:197, 1985.

Mak BS, Chi CS, Tsai CR, et al: New mutations of the HPRT gene in Lesch-Nyhan syndrome. *Pediatr Neurol* 23:332, 2000.

Williams KS, Hankerson JG, Ernst M, et al: Use of propofol anesthesia during outpatient radiographic imaging studies in patients with Lesch-Nyhan syndrome. *J Clin Anesth* 9:61, 1997.

Letterer-Siwe Disease (LSD)

At a glance: Childhood immunologic disorder characterized by pathologic proliferation of histiocytes caused by the Langerhans cells. Involves mainly the skin, bones, brain, lungs, spleen, and liver. The presence of diabetes insipidus must be considered. Presents nonmalignant growths that represent accumulation of histiocytes. Poor prognosis (70% mortality).

Synonyms: Letterer-Siwe Syndrome; Abt-Letterer-Siwe Syndrome; Siwe Disease.

Incidence: Reported between 1:200,000 and 1:3,300,000 live births. Most cases are sporadic.

Genetic inheritance: Evidence supporting both autosomal dominant and recessive inheritance in different families.

Pathophysiology: Letterer-Siwe disease (LSD) is one of the Langerhans cell histiocytoses (LCH). Physiologically, Langerhans cells detect non–self-antigens and present them to the cells of the immune system (T cells), thus allowing an appropriate immune response from the body. They are normally found in the epidermis of the skin, but in LSD they spread to bone and other tissues and become associated with eosinophils. Lesions arise in many organs, including bone, skin, spleen, liver, lungs, lymph nodes, and brain. Granulomatous inflammatory lesions develop and may proliferate and become destructive. These lesions later become less cellular, necrotic, and fibrotic.

Diagnosis: The hallmark of LSD is the presence of pathologic Langerhans cells in involved tissues. Specific histochemical, immunologic, and protein markers have been identified (Birbeck granules or positive S-100 beta protein and CD Ia antigen). These biochemical findings in addition to multiorgan involvement help make the diagnosis.

Clinical aspects: Although LSD has been described in adult patients, it is predominantly a condition affecting children age 2 months to 3 years. Clinical features include fever, anemia, thrombocytopenia, and the manifestations of histiocyte proliferation, including skin disorders (seborrheic, eczematous, pustular or nodular lesions particularly on the scalp), lytic lesions of the bones, and splenogenic thrombocytopenia. The lungs can be involved (nonproductive cough, dyspnea, pleural effusion, interstitial pneumonitis, and spontaneous pneumothorax). Hypothalamic involvement resulting in diabetes insipidus (DI). Eye protrusion may be present. The clinical course is very variable, and spontaneous remissions have occurred. Prognosis is generally poor. Treatment may include use of glucocorticoids, chemotherapeutic agents, bone marrow transplantation, and desmopressin for DI.

Precautions before anesthesia: Blood examination: cell blood count, platelet count must be obtained. Determine whether DI is present; evaluate electrolytes. Evidence of long bone involvement should be sought. Consider perioperative glucocorticoid coverage. A chest x-ray film should be obtained. Coagulation profile and bleeding time must be available.

Anesthetic considerations: Correction of anemia and thrombocytopenia may be necessary. Be vigilant for presence of DI. Care should be taken when moving patients to prevent pathologic fractures where bony lesions are present. In the presence of lung involvement, the potential for pneumothorax, and/or pleural fusion, mechanical ventilation must be used judiciously.

Pharmacological implications: Perioperative glucocorticoid coverage may be necessary. Consider side effects of chemotherapeutic agents.

Other conditions to be considered:

☞**HISTIOCYTOSIS:** Rare spectrum of disorders characterized by proliferation and accumulation of histiocyte in various lesions within the body. Lesions may include Langerhans cells, monocytes, and eosinophils. Most affected individuals have single or multiple bone lesions characterized by degenerative changes and osteolysis. Although the skull is most commonly affected, there may be involvement of the vertebrae and the long bones of the arms and legs. Some individuals present with DI. The exact cause of LCH cell histiocytosis is unknown. Langerhans cell histiocytosis has replaced the older, less specific term *histiocytosis X. Histiocytosis X* encompassed three entities known as eosinophilic granuloma, Hand-Schüller-Christian disease, and LSD, which are all characterized by the accumulation of histiocytes. The *X* denoted that the cause and development of the disorder were not understood.

HASHIMOTO-PRITZKER DISEASE: Specific form of LCH occurring in newborns or young infants and characterized by the formation of papules, nodules, or vesicles eventually leading to ulcerations. The face, limbs, palms, and soles are most often affected. These skin lesions usually heal without treatment within a few weeks or months. These cases may also be referred to as *congenital self-healing histiocytosis* or *pure cutaneous histiocytosis.*

HAND-SCHÜLLER-CHRISTIAN DISEASE: Old term used to describe multifocal LCH occurring in association with DI and exophthalmos. Multiple bony lesions most often affect the skull. In affected individuals with this form of LCH, bony lesions may affect the liver, spleen, and lymph nodes.

ROSAI-DORFMAN DISEASE: Characterized by histiocytosis affecting the sinuses and the lymph nodes, resulting in lymphadenopathy. Organs affected include the central nervous system, skin, and kidneys. The exact cause is unknown. The disorder may also be known as *sinus histiocytosis with massive lymphadenopathy.*

☞**MASTOCYTOSIS:** Characterized by the accumulation of mast cells in skin, bone marrow, and internal organs such as the liver, spleen, and lymph nodes. Also known as *urticaria pigmentosa* and characterized by small, brownish, flat or elevated lesions that may

be surrounded by reddened, itchy skin. Hepatosplenomegaly, abdominal pain and diarrhea, and hypertension are present. The exact cause of mastocytosis is unknown.

☞**ERDHEIM-CHESTER DISEASE:** Multisystem disorder of adulthood characterized by the accumulation of histiocytes. It affects the long bones, skin, ophthalmic regions, lungs, brain, pituitary gland, and additional tissues and organs.

REFERENCES:

Lebeau A, Zeindl-Eberhart E, Muller EC, et al: Generalized crystal-storing histiocytosis associated with monoclonal gammopathy: Molecular analysis of a disorder with rapid clinical course and review of the literature. *Blood* 100:1817, 2002.

Lichtman M, Komp D: Inflammatory and malignant histiocytosis, in Beutler E, Lichtman M, Coller B, Kipps T (eds): *Williams Hematology.* 5th ed. New York, McGraw-Hill, 1995, p 885.

Leukocyte Adhesion Deficiency (LAD) Syndrome

At a glance: Inherited disorder affecting leukocytes resulting in localized bacterial infections rapidly progressing to an extensive life-threatening level.

Synonyms: Lymphocyte Function-Associated Antigen-1 Immunodeficiency; LFA-1 Deficiency.

Nature: Immunologic disorder affects phagocytic properties of leukocytes as a consequence of lack of expression of β_2 integrin CD18 (LAD I) or of its selective ligand (LAD II).

Incidence: Fewer than 200 cases of LAD I and 10 cases of LAD II have been reported in the literature. No racial predominance for LAD I; LAD II has been reported only in people of Middle Eastern descent.

Genetic inheritance: Both forms are autosomal recessive (equal number of males and females). LAD I is caused by mutations in the gene for CD18 (β chain of β_2 integrins). Gene map locus is 21q22.3. LAD II is caused by mutations in a gene that fucosylates sialyl Lewis X (ligand for E selectin), resulting in a defect in fucose metabolism.

Pathophysiology: β Integrins are transmembrane glycoproteins that transmit signals from the extracellular surface to cytoskeletal proteins, thus playing a critical role in phagocytic functions. The β_2 integrin CD18 is expressed on leukocytes, and its ligands are expressed on endothelial cells. Binding of CD18 to ligands also mediates cytokine production, cytotoxicity, apoptosis, and proliferation. LAD I is a result of a mutation in CD18 gene, the expression of which is severely diminished (<1% in 75% of affected patients).

Sialylated Lewis X (SleX or CD15) is the major selectin ligand; both the sialic acid and the fucose moieties of SleX are needed for binding to selectins. This ligand is missing in LAD II; affected patients also have a defect in fucose metabolism.

Diagnosis: Neutrophilia (>20 × 10^9 WBC/l) in the absence of infection; impaired microbicidal activity and oxidative responses against bacteria and *Candida* (in LAD I); flow cytometry shows a considerable decrease in β_2 integrin CD18 on leukocytes (LAD I). In LAD II, Bombay blood group phenotype is detected and biochemical activity of GMD is decreased.

Clinical aspects: Patients with LAD I present with delayed umbilical cord separation followed by various types of localized infection caused by *Staphylococcus* bacteria (plus fungal organisms, usually

Candida albicans) without pus (omphalitis, perirectal and labial cellulitis, classic infections in neutropenic patients, otitis media with minimal inflammation, and other indolent necrotic skin infections) prone to generalization. In less severely affected patients, periodontitis accompanying tooth eruption and oral ulcerations may be the presenting symptoms. Patients with severe LAD I die before age 1 year as a consequence of severe bacterial or, less frequently, life-threatening viral infections. Patients with LAD II do not have delayed umbilical cord separation and usually do not die of infection. They have severe mental retardation, neurologic impairment, and short stature.

Precautions before anesthesia: Blood examination: white blood cells and platelet count must be obtained. Consider fucose supplementation in patients with LAD II.

Anesthetic considerations: None specific. Administer broad-spectrum IV antibiotic therapy.

Pharmacological implications: Epinephrine and corticosteroids are responsible for adhesion defects by demarginating neutrophils from the peripheral vasculature. These agents must be avoided in LAD patients.

Other condition to be considered:

☞**GLANZMANN THROMBOASTHENIA:** An autosomal recessive bleeding disorder characterized by failure of platelet aggregation and absent or diminished clot retraction. It has been classified clinically into types I and II. In type I, platelets show absence of the glycoprotein IIb/IIIa (GPIIb-IIIa) complexes at their surface and lack fibrinogen and clot retraction capability. In type II, the platelets express the GPIIb-IIIa complex at reduced levels (5–20% controls), have detectable amounts of fibrinogen, and have low or moderate clot retraction capability. The disorder is manifest soon after birth with episodic mucocutaneous bleeding and unprovoked bruising. Epistaxis frequently occurs. Women experience copious menstrual hemorrhage. Intracranial bleeding may occur. Bleeding time is prolonged, with normal platelet count, platelet morphology, and coagulation times. Platelets fail to aggregate, either spontaneously or in response to agonists, such as ADP, thrombin, or epinephrine, although there may be a transient response to ristocetin.

REFERENCES:

Lakshman R, Finn A: Neutrophil disorders and their management. *J Clin Pathol* 54:7, 2001.

Marquardt T, Brune T, Luhn K, et al: Leukocyte adhesion deficiency II syndrome, a generalized defect in fucose metabolism. *J Pediatr* 134:681, 1999.

Wild MK, Luhn K, Marquardt T, et al: Leukocyte adhesion deficiency II: Therapy and genetic defect. *Cells Tissues Organs* 172:161, 2002.

Leukodystrophies: Overview

See Table L-1.

Leukonychia and Other Nail Discoloration: Overview

See Table L-2.

Leukonychia Totalis

At a glance: Genetically transmitted anomaly of nails (presence of white nails).

Synonyms: Gorlin Bushkell Jensen Syndrome; Porcelain Nails Disease.

Incidence and genetic inheritance: Incidence is unknown. Inherited as an autosomal dominant; however, an autosomal recessive inheritance as been suggested.

Pathophysiology: Incomplete keratinization in the intermediate part of the nail plate.

Clinical aspects: Clinical presence of completely white nails, together with histologic evidence of a defect in the nail plate. Leukonychia totalis, koilonychia, multiple sebaceous cysts, renal calculi.

Anesthetic considerations: No specific precautions before anesthesia and perioperative considerations except for patients receiving chronic corticosteroid therapy, in whom intraoperative supplementation might be required.

Other conditions to be considered: See Table L-2 comparing leukonychia and other nail discoloration syndromes.

REFERENCES:

Claudel CD, Zic JA, Boyd AS: Idiopathic leukonychia totalis and partialis in a 12-year-old patient. *J Am Acad Dermatol* 44(suppl):379, 2001.

Frydman M, Cohen HA: Leukonychia totalis in two sibs. *Am J Med Genet* 47:540, 1993.

Liddle Syndrome

At a glance: Renal tubular defect causing severe heritable hypertension with hypokalemia and metabolic alkalosis.

Synonym: Pseudohyperaldosteronism.

Genetic inheritance: Autosomal dominant trait with variable penetrance. The variability is particularly evident with regard to serum potassium concentration. Complete linkage of the disorder localized to gene 16p13-p12.

Pathophysiology: Liddle syndrome is the result of specific mutations that prevent the binding of a regulatory protein to a specific proline-rich region in the carboxyl terminal of the three subunits that compose the epithelial sodium channel SCNN1. This prevents normal degradation of the sodium channel so that the total number of channels is increased, giving rise to constitutive activation of the channel, which increases renal sodium absorption and excretes potassium despite the virtual absence of mineralocorticoids, accounting for the clinical and biochemical abnormalities.

Diagnosis: Liddle syndrome is characterized by hypertension, hypokalemia, severe metabolic acidosis, decreased renin, and angiotensin. The hallmark is the finding of markedly suppressed serum aldosterone levels and the lack of response to administration of the mineralocorticoid receptor blocker spironolactone.

Clinical aspects: Clinically, patients resemble those with primary hyperaldosteronism. They may present with severe hypertension in their teenage years, and this is usually the presenting symptom. Amiloride and triamterene, but not spironolactone, are effective treatments for hypertension and hypokalemia in patients with this syndrome as long as dietary sodium intake is restricted. Hypokalemic metabolic alkalosis is present. Renal function is normal apart from the inability to conserve potassium. However, renal

Table L-1   *Leukodystrophies*

Name	Synonyms	Inheritance	Defective Protein/Gene
Adrenoleukodystrophy	☞Schilder disease; Bronze-Schilder syndrome; sudanophilic leukodystrophy	X-linked	ALD protein
Adrenomyeloneuropathy (minor form of adrenoleukodystrophy)		X-linked	ALD protein
☞**Aicardi-Goutieres syndrome**		Autosomal recessive	Unknown
☞**Alexander syndrome**		Autosomal recessive	Unknown
CACH	Childhood ataxia with central nervous system hypomyelination; vanishing white matter disease	Autosomal recessive	Unknown
☞**CADASIL**	Cerebral autosomal dominant arteriopathy with subcortical infarcts and leukoencephalopathy	Autosomal dominant	Chromosome 19p13.1 (Notch3 gene)
☞**Canavan syndrome** (several clinical forms reported)	Spongy degeneration of the brain	Autosomal recessive	Deficiency of aspartoacylase (accumulation of N-acetylaspartic acid)
Cerebrotendinous xanthomatosis		Autosomal recessive	Unknown (accumulation of cholestanol)
Krabbe disease (several clinical forms reported)	Globoid cell leukodystrophy	Autosomal recessive	Chromosome 14; deficiency of galactocerebrosidase (GALC)
☞**Metachromatic leukodystrophies** (many subtypes)		Autosomal recessive	Chromosome 22; deficiency in arylsulfatase A (also called sulfatase A or cerebroside sulfate sulfohydrolase) Occasionally chromosome 10; deficiency in cerebroside sulfatase activator (or saponin B)
Ovarioleukodystrophy syndrome		Possibly autosomal recessive	Unknown
☞**Pelizaeus-Merzbacher disease** (several subtypes)	X-linked spastic paraplegia; PMD/SPG2	X-linked	Duplication of or other mutation in the proteolipid protein gene
☞**Refsum disease**	Refsum syndrome	Autosomal recessive	Deficiency in phytanoyl-CoA hydroxylase (accumulation of phytanic acid)
Van der Knaap syndrome	Vacuolating leukoencephalopathy with subcortical cysts	Autosomal recessive	Unknown
☞**Zellweger syndrome**		Autosomal recessive	At least 10 different gene abnormalities (resulting in decreased or missing peroxisomes in liver, kidney, and brain cells)

Table L-2   Leukonychia and Other Nail Discoloration

Nail Discoloration (Name)	Clinical Aspect and Causes
☞**Leukonychia** (partial or totalis white nails)	Congenital (leukonychia totalis): autosomal dominant syndrome
	Terry nails (either all or only proximal 80% of nail bed is white): liver disease (cirrhosis)
	Half-and-half nails (pink proximally, white distally): renal failure, uremia
Leukonychia punctata (white spots)	Minor trauma to nail cuticle or matrix
Transverse striate leukonychia (white lines)	Muehrcke lines (transverse white lines): hypoalbuminemia
	Mees lines (transverse white lines): heavy metal poisoning (arsenic), renal failure
Green nails	*Pseudomonas pyocyanea* infection (candidiasis)
Blue and brown nails	Medication side effect (quinacrine, chloroquine, minocycline [blue nails], doxorubicin, melphalan, bleomycin, daunorubicin)
	Wilson disease
	Ochronosis
	Psoriasis
	Alopecia areata
	Consider staining (nicotine, potassium permanganate, varnish)
Black nails (melanonychia)	Medication side effects (cyclophosphamide)
	Melanonychia striata: common in dark-skinned persons; idiopathic or secondary to trauma or chemotherapy
	Nevus (uniform brown longitudinal streak localized to nail)
	Melanoma (longitudinal brown-black streak that may encompass entire nail
	Hematoma
☞**Yellow nails**	Lymphedema
	AIDS
	Bacterial infection
	Fungal infection (onychomycosis)
	Psoriasis
	Alopecia aerata
	Cardiopulmonary diseases
Red nails (including red and white streaks)	Darier disease
	Glomus tumor

failure may occur secondary to hypertension. The metabolic defects are completely corrected with renal transplantation.

Precautions before anesthesia: Evaluate the extent and severity of end-organ damage secondary to long-standing hypertension, in particular the cardiorespiratory and neurologic systems. Optimize antihypertensive therapy; addition of triamterene may help reverse the biochemical abnormalities. Treatment of any volume deficit helps in the correction of a persistent metabolic alkalosis and hypokalemia. Investigations: urea, creatinine, electrolytes, ECG, chest radiography, echocardiography. A sedative premedicant to reduce anxiety and its hypertensive response should be prescribed.

Anesthetic considerations: The anesthetic technique should avoid hypotensive and hypertensive events. Invasive arterial and central venous pressure monitoring should be determined by the severity of cardiovascular, neurologic, and renal impairment secondary to hypertension. Esmolol and labetalol are useful antihypertensive agents. Regional techniques, by itself or in conjunction with general anesthesia, offer excellent intraoperative and postoperative analgesia and reduce considerably the stress response to surgery. Capnography monitoring is essential as hyperventilation exacerbates a preexisting metabolic alkalosis.

Pharmacological implications: Hypokalemia and metabolic acidosis may not only increase sensitivity to but may also prolong the duration of action with nondepolarizing muscle relaxants. These problems should be corrected before anesthesia.

Other condition to be considered:

☞**CONN SYNDROME:** Potentially curable endocrine disorder resulting from hyperaldosteronism; presents with symptoms associated with hypertension and hypokalemia.

REFERENCES:

Botero-Velez M, Curtis JJ, Warnock DG: Liddle's syndrome revisited—A disorder of sodium reabsorption in the distal tubule. *N Engl J Med* 330:178, 1994.

Palmer BF, Alpern RJ: Liddle's syndrome. *Am J Med* 104:301, 1998.

Li-Fraumeni Syndrome (LFS)

At a glance: Genetically transmitted cancer predisposition syndrome associated with soft tissue sarcoma, breast cancer, leukemia, osteosarcoma, melanoma, and cancer of the colon, pancreas, adrenal cortex, and brain.

Synonyms: Sarcoma, Breast Syndrome, Leukemia, and Adrenal Gland (SBLA) Syndrome; Sarcoma Family Syndrome.

History: Li-Fraumeni syndrome is defined by the association of a proband with a sarcoma who is diagnosed before the proband, i.e., the affected person who ascertains independently of his relatives in a genetic study, is age 45 years, a first-degree relative with any cancer who is younger than 45 years, and a first- or second-degree relative with any cancer who is younger than 45 years or who has a sarcoma at any age.

Incidence: Fewer than 400 families reported worldwide.

Genetic inheritance: Autosomal dominant. More than 50% of LFS patients have an identifiable disease-causing mutation in the *TP53* gene (gene map locus is 17p13.1), 95% of which can be detected by direct sequence-based DNA testing (clinically available). The *CHEK2* gene is also known to be associated in a few families with LFS, but *CHEK2* testing is only available on a research basis.

Pathophysiology: The *TP53* gene encodes a cellular tumor antigen protein (the "guardian of the genome") that complexes to the large T antigen of SV40. This protein determines whether cells undergo arrest for purposes of DNA repair or programmed cell death (apoptosis). In case of damaged DNA, the normal cellular tumor antigen p53 protein either (1) transcriptionally activates downstream genes to repair the DNA or (2) directly signals a "sensor" molecule that proceeds with apoptosis. Mutant cellular tumor antigen p53 is able to cooperate with *RAS* oncogene products and blocks normal cellular tumor antigen p53 protein from appropriately binding, thus favoring the development or maturation of many tumor types.

Diagnosis: Molecular genetics (direct sequence-based DNA testing).

Clinical aspects: Li-Fraumeni syndrome is a highly penetrant cancer syndrome. Original descriptions of LFS consisted of autosomal dominant patterns of osteosarcomas, soft tissue sarcomas, premenopausal breast cancer, brain tumors, adrenal cortical tumors, and acute leukemias. Since then, reports of LFS families suggest excess rates of melanoma; cancer of the stomach, colon, pancreas, and esophagus; and gonadal germ cell tumors diagnosed at early ages. At-risk children should undergo examination on an annual basis: complete physical examination, blood cell count, urinalysis, abdominal ultrasonography examination, and organ-targeted surveillance based on family history.

Precautions before anesthesia: No specific precautions to be taken before anesthesia. However, a thorough evaluation of possible complications associated with the type of malignancy diagnosed must be done. Proper laboratory investigations for coagulation disorders, anemia, and electrolyte imbalances must be performed prior to surgery and anesthesia.

Anesthetic considerations: Anesthetic considerations are those indicated by the pathology involved.

Pharmacological implications: No specific pharmacological implications other than those associated with the pathology involved and the treatment performed preoperatively.

REFERENCES:

Birch JM, Alston RD, McNally RJ, et al: Relative frequency and morphology of cancers in carriers of germline TP53 mutations. *Oncogene* 20:4621, 2001.

Chompret A: The Li-Fraumeni syndrome. *Biochimie* 84:75, 2002.

Chompret A, Brugieres L, Ronsin M, et al: p53 Germline mutations in childhood cancers and cancer risk for carrier individuals. *Br J Cancer* 82:1932, 2000.

Ganjavi H, Malkin D: Genetics of childhood cancer. *Clin Orthop* 401:75, 2002.

Lightwood Syndrome

At a glance: Transient renal tubular acidosis in infants.

Synonyms: Distal Renal Tubular Acidosis; Transient Renal Tubular Acidosis (Infantile form).

Pathophysiology: Defect in urinary acidification with a reduction in urinary secretion of titratable acid and ammonium associated with bicarbonate wasting. By definition, this condition is transient and may be characterized by distal renal tubular acidosis (with or without bicarbonate wasting) and proximal renal tubular acidosis. Typical biochemical findings include acidemia, which may be severe, hyperchloremia, and marked base deficit. The severe acidosis may induce hyperparathyroidism, which in turn results in hypercalcemia.

Diagnosis: The typical clinical picture, in association with the following biochemical changes, is used to make the diagnosis: metabolic acidosis, hyperchloremia, hyperparathyroidism and hypercalcemia, large base deficit, high urinary pH, and reduced renal excretion of titratable acid. Treatment with alkali replacement results in an improvement in the hyperchloremia and hypercalcemia. The transient need for alkali replacement therapy distinguishes this condition from other forms of renal tubular acidosis in which lifelong treatment may be required.

Clinical aspects: Lightwood syndrome occurs in neonates and is a self-limiting condition that rarely requires treatment beyond 18 months. Males are most commonly affected. Clinical findings include lethargy and reduced muscle tone, vomiting, constipation, anorexia, failure to thrive, polyuria, polydipsia, wasting. The clinical and biochemical findings are reversed by the administration of alkali (up to 25 mEq/kg/day). Nephrocalcinosis may be a feature, particularly in untreated patients. Gastroenteritis associated with prolonged dehydration may mimic the biochemical findings.

Precautions before anesthesia: Clinical evaluation should confirm the absence of any clinical findings in adequately treated patients. Evaluate serum acid–base and electrolyte status. Serum calcium and parathyroid hormone activity should be normal. Evaluate renal function, particularly if there is a history of renal calculi.

Anesthetic considerations: Electrolyte and intravascular fluid status must be corrected prior to administration of anesthesia.

Pharmacological implications: No known specific considerations.

Other conditions to be considered: Others diseases associated with renal tubular acidosis are as follows:

☞**DE TONI DEBRÉ FANCONI SYNDROME:** Rare acquired or inherited condition involving a generalized transport defect in the proximal tubules with renal losses of glucose, phosphate, calcium, uric acid, amino acids, and bicarbonates leading to short stature, osteomalacia, and renal failure.

☞**PERIODIC PARALYSIS:** Congenital abnormality in membrane electrolyte conductance leading to episodic muscle weakness.

☞**ALBRIGHT BUTLER SYNDROME:** Patients present with renal tubular acidosis, nephrocalcinosis, and renal failure. Hypokalemia with muscle weakness and periodic paralysis is frequent. Polyuria, vomiting, and dehydration lead to fluid and electrolyte imbalances.

☞**ADENOSINE DEAMINASE DEFICIENCY:** Heterogeneous systemic disorder caused by the deficiency of adenosine deaminase resulting primarily in severe combined (cellular and humoral) immunodeficiency but also systemic abnormalities.

☞**GITELMAN SYNDROME:** Inherited renal tubular defect resulting in urinary loss of magnesium, sodium, potassium, and chloride with otherwise normal kidneys.

☞**LOWE SYNDROME:** Genetically transmitted polymalformative syndrome characterized by the association of ocular problems with renal dysfunction and mental retardation.

☞**PHOSPHOENOLPYRUVATE CARBOXYKINASE DEFICIENCY:** Congenital metabolic disease leading to a defect in gluconeogenesis.

☞**PROPIONIC ACIDEMIA:** Inborn error of metabolism affecting the mitochondrial catabolism of valine and isoleucine that, left untreated, results in ketoacidosis, lethargy, coma, and finally death.

☞**PYRUVATE CARBOXYLASE DEFICIENCY:** Mitochondrial disease impairing synthetic pathways and leading to hypoglycemia and severe lactic acidosis.

☞**TYROSINEMIA:** Elevated blood tyrosine levels are present in several clinical entities. The term *tyrosinemia* is used to describe several syndromes. In general, the association of liver and renal failure, marked edema, epistaxis, and distinctive cabbage-like odor are characteristic of the disease.

REFERENCES:

Igarashi T, Sekine Y, Kawato H, et al: Transient neonatal distal renal tubular acidosis with secondary hyperparathyroidism. *Pediatr Nephrol* 6:267, 1992.

Rodriguez-Soriano J: Renal tubular acidosis, in Edelman C (ed): *Pediatric Kidney Disease*. 2nd ed. Boston, Little, Brown and Company, 1992, p 1756.

Zelikovich I: Renal tubular acidosis. *Pediatr Ann* 24:48, 1995.

Limb Deficiency–Heart Malformation Syndrome

At a glance: Genetically transmitted limb malformation leading to terminal transverse limb defect in association with congenital heart disease.

Synonym: Hecht-Scott Syndrome.

Incidence and genetic inheritance: Incidence is estimated at 1:30,000–75,000 live births. It is inherited as an autosomal recessive trait. Also believed that it may be a gonadal mosaicism for a dominant mutation.

Pathophysiology: The defect may be isolated or part of a malformation syndrome. The severity may vary for a particular segment or as a result of the number of extremities involved. The etiology of limb malformations is diverse: they may be sporadic, single gene in origin, or occasionally the result of chromosome aneuploidy.

Clinical aspects: Severe terminal transverse defects involving all extremities, with radiologic evidence that the malformations are not the intercalary defects associated with the genetic and drug-induced phocomelia syndromes nor the quadruple amputations seen in Brazilian acheiropody-type syndrome. The presence of congenital heart malformation confirms the diagnosis.

Anesthetic considerations: Echocardiography should be required to identify any congenital heart defect. The anesthetic and pharmacological considerations are determined by the cardiac anomaly and function.

Other condition to be considered:

☞**HOLT-ORAM SYNDROME:** Characterized by an atrial septal defect with upper limb abnormalities. It is transmitted as an autosomal dominant trait.

REFERENCE:

Hecht JT, Scott CI Jr: Limb deficiency syndrome in half-sibs. *Clin Genet* 20:432, 1981.

Limb-Girdle Muscular Dystrophy (LGMD)

At a glance: Genetically transmitted neuromuscular disorder characterized by progressive proximal muscle weakness.

Synonyms and classification: There are two types and numerous variants of LGMD.

Type I

- *Limb-Girdle Muscular Dystrophy Type IA (Proximal Muscular Dystrophy):* Autosomal dominant disorder characterized by adult onset of proximal muscle weakness, beginning in the hip girdle region and later progressing to the shoulder girdle region. Distal muscle weakness may occur later. Some affected individuals exhibit a distinctive nasal, dysarthric pattern of speech.

- *Limb-Girdle Muscular Dystrophy Type IB:* Characterized by cardiac involvement and symmetrical weakness in the proximal lower-limb muscles before age 20 years. In the third or fourth decade, upper-limb muscles gradually become affected. Early contractures of the spine and contractures of elbows and Achilles tendons are minimal or late, distinguishing this disorder from Emery-Dreifuss muscular dystrophy.

- *Limb-Girdle Muscular Dystrophy Type IC:* Characterized with onset of disease around age 5 years. Calf hypertrophy, mild-to-moderate proximal muscle weakness, multiple episodes of muscle cramps after physical effort, and serum creatinine kinase levels more than 4- to 25-fold normal values are present.

- *Limb-Girdle Muscular Dystrophy Type ID:* Characterized with a slowly progressive LGMD. Onset is believed to occur between the second and sixth decade, with hip girdle involvement preceding shoulder girdle involvement. It is inherited as an autosomal dominant pattern.

- *Limb-Girdle Muscular Dystrophy Type IE:* Characterized by severe dilated cardiomyopathy with conduction defect. The age of onset is during the adulthood period and most often presents as progressive and severe muscle weakness of the lower extremities. Other clinical features include progressive dyspnea over years, becoming very severe even at rest, syncopal episodes due to complete heart block, and sudden death. An echocardiography always demonstrates dilatation of all four chambers of the heart.

- *Limb-Girdle Muscular Dystrophy Type IF:* Characterized by pelvic and shoulder girdle proximal weakness. Pelvic girdle impairment is more severe and occurs earlier than shoulder girdle weakness. Distal weakness often occurs later. Respiratory muscles are clinically affected, especially in the juvenile onset group.

Type II

- *Limb-Girdle Muscular Dystrophy Type IIA (Pelvofemoral Muscular Dystrophy; Leyden-Moebius Muscular Dystrophy; Calpainopathy):* Occurs usually in childhood but sometimes in young adult or middle age period. Muscular involvement is first evident in either the pelvic or, less frequently, the shoulder girdle. It manifests often with asymmetry of muscle wasting when the upper limbs are first involved.

- *Limb-Girdle Muscular Dystrophy Type IIB:* Characterized by slowly progressive muscular weakness of the lower limbs (distal and proximal) beginning in the late part of the second decade of life. Patients had markedly elevated serum creatine kinase levels, and two of the four patients from whom muscle biopsies were available demonstrated an inflammatory process, a finding not previously described in LGMD.

- *Limb-Girdle Muscular Dystrophy Type IIC (Duchenne-like Muscular Dystrophy; Secondary Adhalin Deficiency; North African Severe Childhood Autosomal Recessive Muscular Dystrophy type; Sarcoglycan Deficiency):* Autosomal recessive inheritance of muscular dystrophy resembling the X-linked Duchenne type with onset before 5 years, confinement to wheelchair by 12 years, and death usually before 20 years. Pseudohypertrophy is present. Chronic congestive heart failure and severe arrhythmias have been described.

- *Limb-Girdle Muscular Dystrophy Type IID (Duchenne-like Autosomal Recessive Muscular Dystrophy; Primary Adhalinopathy):* Characterized by a progressive form of muscular dystrophy including proximal muscle weakness beginning at approximately age 10 years, associated with calf hypertrophy and elevated serum creatine kinase.

- *Limb-Girdle Muscular Dystrophy Type IIE:* Characterized by severe cardiomyopathy resulting from mutations in β-sarcoglycan. Cardiac function should be monitored in patients with LGMD and defective sarcoglycan expression.

- *Limb-Girdle Muscular Dystrophy Type IIF:* Characterized by a severe clinical phenotype and muscle biopsy revealing the absence of α-sarcoglycan.

- *Limb-Girdle Muscular Dystrophy Type IIG:* Characterized by early involvement of the distal muscles, mildly elevated serum creatine kinase levels, and rimmed vacuoles in muscle biopsies. It has been suggested that this form resembled autosomal recessive Kugelberg-Welander disease. The mean age at onset has been 12.5 years in most patients. All had difficulty with

walking, running, and climbing stairs. Extraocular and facial muscles are spared.

- *Limb-Girdle Muscular Dystrophy Type IIH (Hutterite Muscular Dystrophy):* Characterized by the combination of a slowly progressive muscular dystrophy with facial features of the facioscapulohumeral type and the proximal distribution of the limb-girdle type. Onset is between 1 and 9 years of age, and the quadriceps and pelvic girdle musculature are most involved. Waddling gait and difficulty rising from the squatting position result.

- *Limb-Girdle Muscular Dystrophy Type II I:* Characterized by late clinical onset with absence of merosin on immunoblotting but normal merosin on immunocytochemistry. It involves muscle weakness, initially the proximal muscles of the lower limbs between the ages of 17 and 40 years. Hypertrophy of the calf muscles, absence of scapular winging, and predominant involvement of hip flexors and hamstrings more than quadriceps. Serum creatine kinase is at least 10 times normal, and muscle biopsies show nonspecific dystrophic features.

- *Limb-Girdle Muscular Dystrophy Type IIJ:* Characterized by late-onset distal tibial myopathy. It is confirmed by nonspecific myopathic changes on muscle biopsy and progressive fatty infiltration of involved muscles. Onset of the severe LGMD phenotype form usually presents between the first and third decades and involves weakness of all proximal muscles. Within 20 years, patients present with severe disability and complete loss of ambulation. There is no facial muscle involvement or cardiomyopathy in this type of muscular dystrophy. It has been suggested that the mild form of the disease is inherited as an autosomal dominant pattern, whereas the severe limb-girdle muscular dystrophy is inherited as an autosomal recessive pattern.

- *Limb-Girdle Muscular Dystrophy Type IIK:* Characterized by an autosomal recessive muscular dystrophy and severe mental retardation. All patients acquire early motor milestones; however, there is no congenital muscular dystrophy. The age at onset ranges from 1 to 6 years, and the clinical presentation is confirmed by difficulty in walking and climbing stairs. Other clinical features include slow progression, proximal muscle weakness, mild muscle hypertrophy, increased serum creatine kinase, microcephaly, and mental retardation (IQ range 50–76). Magnetic resonance imaging of the brain shows normal structures in all cases. Skeletal muscle biopsy shows dystrophic changes, including mild fibrosis with many regenerating and few necrotic fibers, increased fiber size variability, and multiple central nuclei.

Incidence: Overall frequency ranges between 5 and 70 per one million population. No sex or racial predominance in either autosomal dominant or recessive forms.

Genetic inheritance: LGMDs are classified as autosomal dominant (LGMD I, A–F) and recessive (LGMD II, A–H) syndromes. Additionally, there are rare X-linked forms (Barth syndrome, McLeod syndrome). Autosomal dominant, recessive, and familial variants. *Type I* is familial and is transmitted as an autosomal dominant trait: type IA is linked to the chromosome 5 (gene unidentified); type IB to chromosome 1 (gene unidentified); type IC to chromosome 3 (caveolin-3 gene); and type ID to chromosome 7 (gene unidentified). *Type II* is transmitted as an autosomal recessive trait: type IIA is caused by a mutation in the calpain-3 gene of chromosome 15 (15q15.1-q21.1); type IIB is caused by a mutation in the dysferlin gene on chromosome 2; type IIC is caused by a mutation in the γ-sarcoglycan gene on chromosome 13; type IID is caused by a mutation in the α-sarcoglycan (adhalin) gene on chromosome 17; type IIE is caused by a mutation in the β-sarcoglycan gene on chromosome 4; type IIF is caused by a mutation in the δ-sarcoglycan gene on chromosome 5; type IIG is caused by an unidentified gene mutation on chromosome 17; and type IIH is caused by an unidentified gene mutation on chromosome 9 in Manitoba Hutterites.

Bethlem myopathy is caused by mutations on either chromosome 21 or 2 in one of the three subunits of type VI collagen; dilated cardiomyopathy with conduction defect and muscular dystrophy has been linked to chromosome 6 (gene unidentified).

Pathophysiology: LGMD result in abnormal dystrophin-glycoprotein complex that bridges the inner cytoskeleton (F-actin) and the basal lamina. Mutations in all the sarcoglycans and several other members of the complex result in a muscular dystrophy. Limb-girdle muscular dystrophy is a generic term for muscular dystrophies that are distinct from the much more common X-linked dystrophinopathies (Duchenne muscular dystrophy). Patients with LGMD generally show weakness and wasting restricted to the limb musculature, proximal greater than distal. Most patients with LGMD show relative sparing of the heart and bulbar muscles, although exceptions occur, depending on the genetic subtype. Onset, progression, and distribution of the weakness and wasting vary considerably among patients and genetic subtype. This produces a progressive disorder involving pelvic and scapular girdle muscles marked by weakness of proximal muscles of hip and shoulder areas with variable psychiatric disorders and occasional mild mental retardation. The disorder is bilateral, symmetrical, and very selective; the face muscles are not affected. The muscle selectivity persists throughout the course of the disease. Muscle wasting tends to be asymmetrical when the upper limbs are first involved. The progression of the disease varies with inability to walk, usually occurring approximately 20 to 30 years after onset. Facial weakness and contractures may occur later. Limb-girdle muscular dystrophy Type II I is a slowly progressive form of muscular dystrophy that involves the pelvic girdle, with onset in the late teens.

Diagnosis: Elevated creatine phosphokinase (CPK) in plasma. Limb-girdle muscular dystrophy typically shows degeneration/regeneration of muscle (dystrophic biopsy) without dystrophin disorders. Biochemical testing (i.e., protein testing by immunostaining) performed on a muscle biopsy can establish the diagnosis of sarcoglycanopathy, calpainopathy, dysferlinopathy, and telethoninopathy. Demonstration of complete or partial deficiencies of any particular protein can be followed by mutation studies of the corresponding gene on a research basis only.

Clinical aspects: Progressive dystrophy of muscles forming the pelvic and shoulder girdles, pseudohypertrophy of calves, facial weakness, and weakness of proximal leg, shoulder, biceps, and brachioradialis muscles. Mental retardation, with depression, substance abuse, depersonalization, psychotic disorders, dysthymia, and obsessive behavior are frequent. Difficulty in climbing stairs and holding hands above head are typical.

Precautions before anesthesia: There does not appear to be any literature specifically about this condition and anesthesia, but certain considerations are very important to mention. Weakness of muscles can be extensive and generalized. Complete workup is required, including neurologic and motor milestones, family history, and previous problems. Cardiac function should be assessed in light of the potential for cardiomyopathy (although rare with limb-girdle variants). Respiratory function should be checked by chest radiographs and arterial blood gas analysis the need for physiotherapy preoperatively likely will be of benefit to those with affected respiratory muscles (rare).

Anesthetic considerations: Postoperative mechanical ventilation may be necessary in severe patients. Delayed respiratory failure may occur. Favor regional techniques whenever possible for postoperative pain relief instead of opiates. Remember the possibility of severe cardiac disease. There may be a need for pacing and pharmacological therapies, so equipment for pacing should be ready. However, these interventions may not be necessary because there is a low incidence of cardiac and respiratory muscle disease. Realize that cardiac, respiratory, and other system involvement is common with closely related syndromes and should be planned for if not ruled out.

Pharmacological implications: Succinylcholine use may cause rhabdomyolysis, cardiac arrest as a result of hyperkalemia, and possibly malignant hyperpyrexia, so it is not recommended. Use minimal drug dosages. Avoid respiratory depressants or muscle relaxants as much as possible.

Other conditions to be considered:

☞**DUCHENNE AND BECKER MUSCULAR DYSTROPHIES:** X-linked recessive inherited dystrophinopathies (dystrophin is normal in LGMD patients).

FASCIOSCAPULOHUMERAL MUSCULAR DYSTROPHY (FSH): Autosomal dominant disorder, often included in LGMD, that is characterized by marked weakness of the facial muscles and the stabilizers of the scapula or the dorsiflexors of the foot. The diagnosis is established by molecular genetic testing. Approximately 95% of patients have detection of integral copies of a 3.3-kb DNA repeat motif termed D4Z4.

☞**EMERY-DREIFUSS MUSCULAR DYSTROPHY:** Often included in LGMD. It can be inherited as an autosomal recessive, autosomal dominant, or X-linked recessive manner. It is a degenerative myopathy characterized by weakness and atrophy of muscle without involvement of the nervous system. It is caused by an autosomal dominant mutation in the laminin A/C gene (LMNA). There is an autosomal recessive form without cardiac involvement that is caused by a mutation in the emerin gene.

☞**CONGENITAL MUSCULAR DYSTROPHY:** Dystrophy caused by a complete loss of function of the laminin alpha 2 gene in 50% of cases. Patients typically have white matter changes in the brain that are visible on MRI as a result of altered water distribution in the white matter secondary to blood-brain barrier dysfunction, which is a result of merosin deficiency in the vasculature.

REFERENCES:

Bonnemann CG: Limb-girdle muscular dystrophy in childhood. *Pediatr Ann* 34:569, 2005.

Bonnemann CG, Finkel RS: Sarcolemmal proteins and the spectrum of limb-girdle muscular dystrophies. *Semin Pediatr Neurol* 9:81, 2002.

Mathews KD, Moore SA: Limb-girdle muscular dystrophy. *Curr Neurol Neurosci Rep* 3:78, 2003.

Wagner KR: Genetic diseases of muscle. *Neurol Clin* 20:645, 2002.

Lipofuscinoses, Neuronal Ceroid: Overview

At a glance: Group of inherited, neurodegenerative, lysosomal storage disorders characterized by progressive mental and motor deterioration, seizures, and early death. Visual loss is a feature

Table L-3   Lipofuscinoses, Neuronal Ceroid

Type	Age of Onset	Clinical Features	Gene Locus and Chromosomal Location	Defective Enzyme
Infantile	6–18 months	Early psychomotor and visual deterioration, late-onset seizures	CLN1 on 1p32	Lysosomal palmitoyl-protein thioesterase
Late infantile (classic)	2–4 years	Early psychomotor and late visual deterioration, early-onset seizures	CLN2 on 11p15	Lysosomal pepstatin-insensitive protease
Variant late infantile	2–6 years	Early psychomotor and visual deterioration, early-onset seizures	CLN6 on 15q21-23	Unknown
Turkish variant late infantile	2–4 years	Early psychomotor deterioration, variable-onset visual deterioration and seizures	CLN7 on unknown chromosome	Unknown
Finnish late infantile	5–7 years	Early psychomotor and visual deterioration, late-onset seizures	CLN5 on 13q21-q32	Novel membrane protein (not an enzyme)
Juvenile	4–8 years	Late-onset psychomotor deterioration and seizures, variable-onset visual deterioration	CLN3 on 16p12	Novel membrane protein (not an enzyme)
Progressive epilepsy with mental retardation	5–10 years	Early-onset seizures, late psychomotor deterioration, no visual deterioration	CLN8 on 8p23	Unknown
Kufs disease	>20 years	Early-onset psychomotor deterioration and seizures (or no seizures), no visual involvement	CLN4 on unknown chromosome	Unknown

of most forms. The phenotypes have been classified clinically by age of onset and order of appearance of the clinical features. See Table L-3.

Lissencephaly

At a glance: Group of disorders involving the neuronal migration during the period at 9 to 13 weeks' gestation. It is characterized by the absence of sulcation of the cerebral hemispheres resulting in smooth brain surface (absence of gyri). Neurologic disorder caused by incomplete development of the brain, which is caused by abnormalities in the neural migration process. The name comes from the Greek *lissos* (smooth) and *enkephale* (brain).

Synonyms and classification: There are many types of lissencephaly:

Type I

- *Miller-Dieker Syndrome:* with facial abnormality
- X-linked lissencephaly (gene located on Xp22.13)
- X-Linked lissencephaly with ambiguous genitalia
- Isolated lissencephaly sequence
- Lissencephaly Norman-Roberts type syndrome

Type II

- Walker-Warburg or *HARD syndrome*

Type III

- Lissencephaly and bone dysplasia
- Familial lissencephaly with cleft palate and cerebellar hypoplasia (three cases described)

Incidence: Unknown. A global incidence of 1.2:100,000 live births has been proposed.

Genetic inheritance: Lissencephaly can be acquired (cytomegalovirus infection) as in the isolated lissencephaly sequence or genetically transmitted as in the other lissencephalies.

Pathophysiology: Lissencephaly results from a neuronal development insult before 12 weeks of gestational age. This interrupts further migration of neurons, preventing them from reaching the cerebral cortex and leading to agyria and a thickened smooth cortical surface. The causal factor can be infectious (congenital cytomegalovirus infection), genetic, or chromosomic.

Diagnosis: CT/MRI: smooth cerebral cortex with few primary fissures but no secondary sulci; symmetrical enlargement of ventricles; structure of hemispheres and ventricles similar to the 3- to 4-month-old fetal brain. Even though most of the syndromes resulting in lissencephaly are inherited, genetic examinations are inconclusive because most of the genes involved are still unknown.

Clinical aspects: Presenting symptoms are mainly neurologic: infantile hypotonia; various types of seizure disorders (West syndrome, Lennox-Gastaut syndrome, massive myoclonus, tonic-clonic seizures), severe mental retardation with microcephaly; motor dysfunction with hypotonia, but also rigidity and opisthotonos. Patients also have various nonneurologic anomalies, including congenital heart disease; cataracts and various ocular anomalies; duodenal atresia; renal agenesis; polydactyly or syndactyly; cryptorchidism. Other migration disorders, such as macrogyria, micropolygyria, or gray matter heterotopias, are not uncommon.

Precautions before anesthesia: It is recommended to obtain an anesthesiology consult for patients affected with this condition and undergoing elective surgery. Complete evaluation of the anticonvulsant therapy must be obtained. Cardiac function must be assessed to eliminate the association of congenital heart defect, chronic congestive heart failure, and other anomalies (ECG, echocardiography, chest radiograph). Consultation with an ophthalmologist is important.

Anesthetic considerations: No specific anesthetic considerations except for those necessary for patients with heart problems. Patients presenting with behavioral problems might benefit from a sedative premedication that will facilitate induction of anesthesia.

Pharmacological implications: Anticonvulsant therapy should be continued until the day of surgery and an intravenous anticonvulsant should be administered for long surgical procedures. Prophylactic antibiotics might be needed in presence of a cardiac anomaly.

REFERENCES:

Cardoso C, Leventer RJ, Dowling JJ, et al: Clinical and molecular basis of classical lissencephaly: Mutations in the LIS1 gene (PAFAH1B1). *Hum Mutat* 19:4, 2002.

Kato M, Dobyns WB: Lissencephaly and the molecular basis of neuronal migration. *Hum Mol Genet* 12(suppl 1):R89, 2003.

Pilz D, Stoodley N, Golden JA: Neuronal migration, cerebral cortical development, and cerebral cortical anomalies. *J Neuropathol Exp Neurol* 61:1, 2002.

Loken Senior Syndrome

At a glance: Inherited disorder characterized by rapidly progressive renal insufficiency (nephronophthisis) and eye disease (retinitis pigmentosa).

Synonyms: Familial Juvenile Nephronophthisis with Associated Ocular Anomaly; Hereditary Renal Dysplasia-Blindness; Renal Dysplasia-Retinal Aplasia, Loken-Senior type; Familial Renal-Retinal Dystrophy; Renal-Retinal Syndrome; Senior-Biochi Syndrome; Senior-Loken Syndrome.

Incidence: Incidence of all nephrophthisis disorders is approximately 1:1,000,000 population in the United States and still more in Europe. No racial predilection; both sexes are equally affected.

Genetic inheritance: Autosomal recessive. Gene map locus mostly unknown. Candidate loci are 1p36, 2q12-q13, and 15q.

Pathophysiology: The function of α_6 integrin is defective. Probably as a compensatory mechanism, there is also an abnormal expression of the α_5 integrin fibronectin receptor in the tubular basement membrane. This process may lead to destruction of the tubular basement membrane, resulting in gradual loss of kidney function and development of cysts in the renal medulla.

Diagnosis: Renal insufficiency and severe normocytic and normochromic anemia. Serum erythropoietin concentration is lower than in patients with other progressive renal diseases. Laboratory findings indicative of renal failure: metabolic acidosis, hypocalcemia, hyperphosphatemia, elevated serum BUN and creatinine concentrations. Imaging studies showing multiple cysts, typically in the medulla and corticomedullary region. Ophthalmoscopy and electroretinography are consistent with tapetoretinal degeneration. Renal biopsy shows typical lesions. The prognosis is poor (death before age 10 years in most patients).

Clinical aspects: Symptoms include high urine output (patient cannot concentrate the urine), nocturia, headache, anorexia, progressive weakness, and weight loss. The disease progresses from chronic renal failure to end-stage renal disease. No curative treatment is available except for renal transplant.

Precautions before anesthesia: Check severity of renal failure (blood and urine tests). Request preoperative dialysis in patient with severe renal insufficiency. Check red blood cell count. Consider preoperative treatment with erythropoietin to improve anemia. Preoperative eye examination is recommended.

Anesthetic considerations: Presence of chronic renal failure leads to increased sensitivity to opioid analgesic agents. Danger of fluid overload (or hypovolemia after dialysis therapy). Severe anemia may require intraoperative transfusion.

Pharmacological implications: Unable to metabolize nitroprusside.

Other conditions to be considered:

    S<small>ALDINO</small>-M<small>AINZER</small> S<small>YNDROME</small> (Conorenal Syndrome; Retinal Pigmentary Dystrophy-Cerebral Ataxia-Skeletal Dysplasia Syndrome): Characterized by chronic renal faliure and the presence of prominent cone-shaped epiphyses in the distal phalanges and cone-shaped epiphyses in the middle phalanges of the hands. The clinical association has led to name this medical condition as "conorenal syndrome." Other clinical features include retinitis pigmentosa, cerebellar ataxia, nephronophthisis (medullary cystic kidney disease), often evolving to end-stage renal disease. Percutaneous renal biopsy showed global scarring and acellularity of many glomeruli in both sibs.

    ☞P<small>OLYCYSTIC</small> K<small>IDNEY</small> D<small>ISEASE</small>: Usually with congenital hepatic fibrosis and prone to result in severe renal failure.

REFERENCES:

Fleischhauer J, Njoh WA, Niemeyer G: Syndromic retinitis pigmentosa: ERG and phenotypic changes. *Klin Monatsbl Augenheilkd* 222:186, 2005.

Schuermann MJ, Otto E, Becker A, et al: Mapping of gene loci for nephronophthisis type 4 and Senior-Loken syndrome, to chromosome 1p36. *Am J Hum Genet* 70:1240, 2002.

Tanaka H, Waga S, Tateyama T, et al: Senior-Loken syndrome associated with mental retardation and microcephaly. *Pediatr Int* 43:310, 2001.

Warady BA, Cibis G, Alon V, et al: Senior-Loken syndrome: Revisited. *Pediatrics* 94:111, 1994.

Long QT Syndrome (LQTS)

At a glance: Congenital or acquired adrenergic-induced ventricular arrhythmias.

Synonyms: Romano-Ward Syndrome; Long QT Syndrome (1-2-3-4-5); Prolonged QT Interval Syndrome; Protracted QT; QT Interval Prolongation; QT Prolongation Syndrome; Ventricular Fibrillation Prolonged QT Interval Syndrome.

Classification: Seven different genetic defects have been identified, all involving potassium and sodium transmission.

LQT1 is the most common type. It corresponds to a defect of chromosome 11, encoding for the potassium channel.

LQT2 is the second most common form of LQTS. It is reported to be a defect on chromosome 7, again encoding for the potassium channel. LQT1 and LQT2 are thought to represent 95% of all cases of LQTS. The standard treatment for LQT1 and LQT2 is β-adrenergic blockade, which has been confirmed to reduce mortality.

LQT3 represents 3 to 4% of cases and corresponds to a defect on chromosome 3. It is encoding the sodium channel. β-Blockade is contraindicated in this type of LQTS because bradycardia can further prolong the QT interval and lead to ventricular arrhythmias. Therefore, it has been suggested that increasing the heart rate probably would be beneficial in LQT3.

LQT4, LQT5, and *LQT6* all involve defects on the potassium transmission and are located on chromosomes 4, 21, and 21, respectively. They are very rare.

LQT7 (Andersen Cardiodysrhythmic Periodic Paralysis Syndrome) is discussed in Section A under this name.

All types are characterized by a corrected QT interval of at least 440 ms on the electrocardiogram. The manifestation is recurrent syncope associated with documented ventricular arrhythmia and sudden death.

Incidence: 1:10,000 in the general population (= 90% of congenital LQTS).

Genetic inheritance: Romano-Ward by autosomal dominant inheritance. LQT1 has been mapped to chromosome 11. Other mutated genes located on chromosomes 3, 6, and 11 may contribute to or cause LQTS.

Pathophysiology: Long QT syndrome results from structural of acquired/transient (therapeutic) abnormalities in the potassium channels of the heart.

Acquired LQTS may be caused by the following:

- *Drugs:* A list of drugs known or suspected to prolong the QT interval is given in Table L-4. A more extensive list of drugs that prolong the QT interval can be found on the web site of either The University of Arizona Center for Education and Research on Therapeutics at *http://qtdrugs.org* or *http://www.torsades.org*
- *Electrolyte Disturbances:* Acute or chronic hypokalemia, chronic hypocalcemia, and chronic hypomagnesemia.

Table L-4 *Drugs Known or Suspected to Prolong the QT Interval*

Albuterol	Granisetron
Alfuzosin	Haloperidol
Amantadine	Imipramine
Amiodarone	Isoproterenol
Amitripyiline	Ketoconazole
Ampicillin	Levalbuterol
Astemizole	Lithium
Azithromycin	Methadone
Bretylium	Methylphenidate
Chloral hydrate	Mexiletine
Chloroquine	Midodrine
Chlorpromazine	Nicardipine
Ciprofloxacin	Norepinephrine
Cisapride	Octreotide
Clarithromycin	Ondansetron
Clomipramine	Quinidine (5%)
Cocaine	Pentamidine
Desipramine	Phenylephrine
Disopyramide	Procainamide
Dobutamine	Risperidone
Dofetilide	Ritodrine
Dolasetron	Salmeterol
Domperidone	Sertraline
Dopamine	Sotalol
Doxepin	Tacrolimus
Droperidol	Tamoxifen
Ephedrine	Terbutaline
Epinephrine	Terfenadine
Erythromycin	Thioridazine
Flecainide	Tizanidine
Fluconazole	Trimethoprim-sulfamethoxazole
Fluoxetine	Vardenafil
Foscarnet	Venlafaxine
Fosphenytoin	Voriconazole
Gatifloxacin	Ziprasidone
Glibenclamide	

Note: Female patients usually are more sensitive to the effect of these medications than are their male counterparts.

- *Associated Medical Conditions:* Atrioventricular block, sick sinus syndrome, myocarditis, hyperparathyroidism, hypothyroidism, subarachnoid hemorrhage, encephalitis, head trauma, starvation, and anorexia nervosa.

Congenital LQTS presents a large genetic heterogeneity: at least six genes have been identified that code for subunits of K or Na ionic channels. Six genotypes have been identified for the Romano-Ward syndrome (LQTS 1–6). Mutations have been identified in the KVLQT1, HERG, and KCNE1 genes (coding for a K$^+$ channel controlling cardiomyocyte repolarization during phases 3 and 4 of the cardiac muscle action potential). A mutation of the SCN5A gene has been identified and affects Na^+ influx during phase 1 of depolarization.

Diagnosis: Patient history, family history. Corrected QT (QTc) greater than 0.46 seconds has a positive predictive value greater than 90%. A QTc greater than 0.42 seconds needs to be taken in context of history. Some patterns of repolarization abnormalities reflected by T-wave morphology on surface ECG (wide base, double hump) could indicate which mutation is involved.

Clinical aspects: Forty percent of patients remain asymptomatic. Ten percent of patients will have as first clinical sign, a cardiac arrest. Symptoms include syncope, "epilepsy," and palpitations precipitated by stressful events (intense emotion or physical activity). Swimming appears to be a potent trigger. Sudden death or cardiac arrest secondary to ventricular dysrhythmia can be the presentation. ECG findings include long QTc interval (QTc = QT interval/square root of R-R interval) calculated in lead II or V_5 and abnormal T-wave morphology. Ventricular dysrhythmias, torsades de pointes, and ventricular tachycardia are common causes of collapse. Medical management includes beta blockade, pacemaker insertion, implantable cardioverter-defibrillator placement, and rarely left stellate ganglion excision/ablation. Genotyping may allow targeting drugs at specific ion channels in the future.

Precautions before anesthesia: Full history regarding episodes of collapse and current medical management. Check pacemaker specifications if present. Exclude obvious signs of endocrine disease. Review drug history for medications associated with the syndrome. Check Na, K, Ca, and Mg electrolytes. Correct abnormalities preoperatively. Review ECG. Continue beta blockade preoperatively (IV if necessary). Check QT duration on ECG in infants presenting with deafness or syndactyly. Defibrillator cardiac and resuscitation drugs should be present in the same room as the patient. Preoperative laboratory investigations must include kalemia, magnesemia, and calcemia, which can increase arrhythmia.

Anesthetic considerations: Death can occur at any age and at any stage of anesthesia. Increased rhythm troubles are observed with light anesthesia, hypoxemia, hypercarbia, and hypocarbia. Tracheal intubation and extubation should be performed with deep anesthesia. The number of episodes of induced arrhythmias during induction and intubation is given in Table L-5. Prevent any electrolytic disorders. Premedication is desirable to prevent any stress to the patient. Hypoglycemia has been reported after preoperative fasting associated with beta blockade. Monitor blood glucose and consider administration of dextrose-containing fluids. Full monitoring preinduction! Aim to minimize surges in endogenous catecholamines. Cover stress response to laryngoscopy. Prevent hypocalcemia and hypokalemia. Ensure optimal postoperative analgesia.

Pharmacological implications: Although thiopental, succinylcholine, and propofol all increase QT interval in normal patients, the effect is least with propofol. Because sevoflurane prolongs QT interval in both normal and congenital LQTS patients, it should be used very cautiously. Esmolol should be available at induction. Magnesium sulfate should be used to treat torsades de pointes. Ketamine and pancuronium are contraindicated because of their sympathomimetic effects. Vasopressors are relatively contraindicated. Halothane is contraindicated because of sensitization of myocardium.

Avoid drugs known to prolong QT duration (see Table L-4). Stellate ganglion block should be considered in patients who are at particularly high risk for arrhythmia. Treatment of cardiac ventricular arrhythmia can include β-adrenergic blockade, internal atrial

pacing, isoproterenol (increases heart rate to reduce QT interval), and cardioversion.

Other conditions to be considered:

Jervell and Lange-Nielsen Syndrome (JLN 1-2): Two genotypes have been described; one results in mutation of the cardiac potassium channel KCNQ1 (K channel involved in phase 3 of cardiac action potential). This gene is involved in endolymph homeostasis explaining the association of the syndrome with deafness. Although congenital LQTS typically occurs in patients with normal cardiac morphology, a new variant with congenital heart disease and bilateral syndactyly has been described. Epidural anesthesia has been used successfully for cesarean section in Jervell and Lange-Nielsen syndrome: lidocaine might be a better choice than bupivacaine. No experience with ropivacaine or levobupivacaine have been reported.

☞**Andersen Cardiodysrhythmic Periodic Paralysis Syndrome:** Characterized by the clinical triad of potassium-sensitive periodic paralysis (low, normal, or high potassium levels), ventricular arrhythmias (bigeminy, long QT interval, ectopy, and bidirectional ventricular tachycardia), and dysmorphic facial features. Sudden death has been reported. Andersen syndrome must not be confused with Andersen disease (glycogen storage disease type IV).

☞**Periodic Paralysis:** Congenital abnormality in membrane electrolyte conductance leading to episodic muscle weakness.

☞**Thyrotoxic Periodic Paralysis:** Acquired disorder characterized by intermittent episodes of muscle weakness alternating with periods of normal muscular function. Occurs during hyperthyroidism and thyrotoxicosis. During attacks, hypokalemia is present. May be precipitated by low plasma concentration of insulin. Occurs predominantly in Asian males but has been found in Latin American males.

REFERENCES:

Gallagher JD, Weindling SN, Anderson G, et al: Effects of sevoflurane on QT interval in a patient with congenital long QT syndrome. *Anesthesiology* 89:1569, 1998.

Johnston AJ, Hall JM, Levy DM: Anaesthesia with remifentanil and rocuronium for caesarean section in a patient with long-QT syndrome and an automatic implantable cardioverter-defibrillator. *Int J Obstet Anesth* 9:133, 2000.

Joseph-Reynolds AM, Auden SM, Sobczyzk WL: Perioperative considerations in a newly described subtype of congenital long QT syndrome. *Paediatr Anaesth* 7:237, 1997.

Kies SJ, Pabelick CM, Hurley HA, et al: Anesthesia for patients with congenital long QT syndrome. *Anesthesiology* 102:204, 2005.

Louis-Bar Syndrome

At a glance: Heredofamilial neurocutaneous progressive syndrome characterized by cerebellar ataxia (early childhood), oculocutaneous telangiectasia (adolescence), and impairment of the immune system. Recurrent infections of the lung (pulmonary restrictive disease) and sinuses.

Synonym: Ataxia Telangiectasia Syndrome.

History: Described by Denise Louis-Bar, a Belgian neuropathologist, in 1941.

Genetic inheritance: Autosomal recessive. The ataxia telangiectasia (AT) gene has been localized to chromosome 11q23.

Table L-5   Number of Episodes of Induced Arrhythmias During Induction or Maintenance of Anesthesia in Patient with Long QT Syndrome Presenting Preoperatively with Symptoms Controlled or Not Controlled

Anesthetic Agents	Symptoms Controlled (n)		Symptoms Not Controlled (n)	
	Arrhythmia	No Arrhythmia	Arrhythmia	No Arrhythmia
Halothane	0	4	6	0
Isoflurane	0	5	2	1
Sevoflurane	0	0	2	0
Enflurane	0	1	1	0
N₂O/narcotic	1	3	0	0
Ketamine	1	0	1	0
On induction	0	1	3	2

Modified from Katz RI, Quijano I, Barcelon N, et al: Ventricular tachycardia during general anesthesia in a patient with congenital long QT syndrome. *Can J Anaesth* 50:398, 2003.

Pathophysiology: Ataxia telangiectasia is a syndrome with multiorgan involvement. Pathophysiology cannot be explained by a single cellular mechanism. *Neurologic:* Cerebellar dysfunction, progressive neurologic deterioration, developmental delay; *mucocutaneous:* telangiectasia on conjunctiva and exposed areas; *endocrine:* glucose intolerance, hypogonadism.

Diagnosis: Based on clinical features. Immunodeficiency as evidenced by low or absent IgA and IgE and atypical IgM. Slight elevation of liver enzymes in 50% of patients. May have raised α-fetoprotein. Glucose intolerance and hypogonadism particularly seen in females. Marked progressive cerebellar atrophy usually is demonstrated early by CT scan or MRI and characteristically defined as enlarged cerebellar sulci and cisterns and fourth ventricle.

Clinical aspects: Initial presentation usually is neurologic as evidenced by problems with development of walking, oculomotor abnormalities, and progressive neurologic disability. Risk of recurrent aspiration of oral secretions. In addition to telangiectasia, vitiligo, café-au-lait spots, and premature graying may be present. Absence of secondary sexual characteristics in females. Elevated liver enzymes associated with fatty infiltration of the liver. Ataxia telangiectasia patients are at increased risk for developing malignancies, particularly lymphoma and leukemia in children and gastric carcinoma in adults. Chronic respiratory infections and bronchiecta-

sis, unresponsive to antibiotics, are frequently the ultimate cause of death. Unusual to survive beyond the third decade.

Precautions before anesthesia: Neurologic evaluation, particularly cerebellar and bulbar function. Evaluate pulmonary and cardiac function in light of chronic lung disease. Objective evaluation

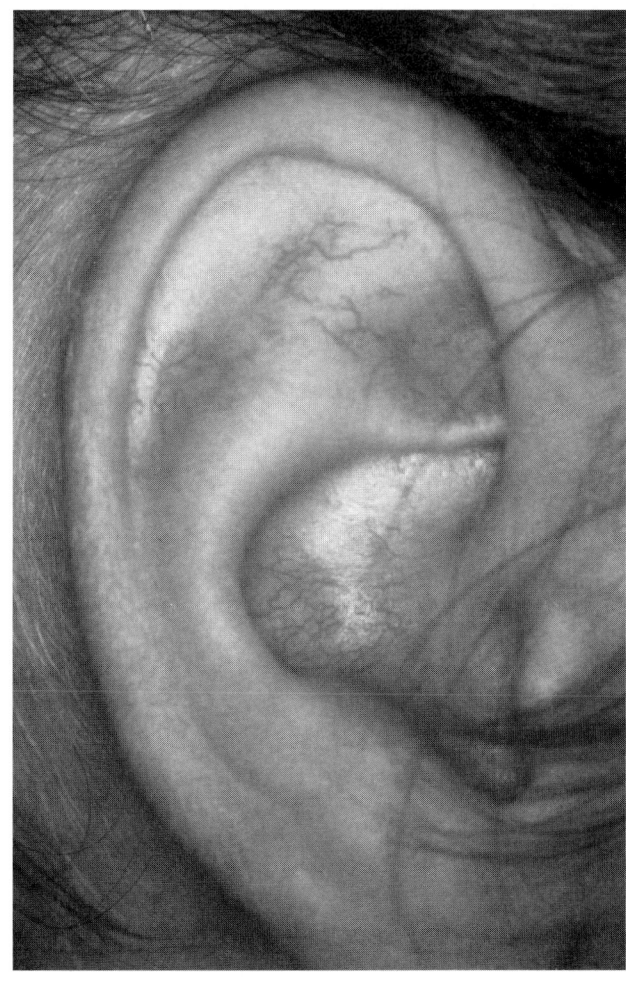

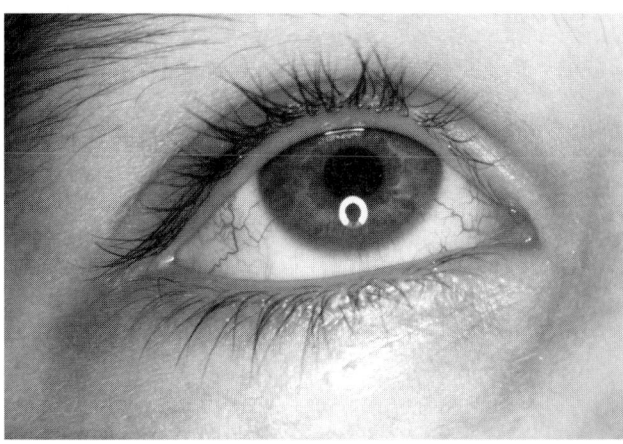

Louis-Bar syndrome Ocular telangiectasias in a patient with ataxia telangiectasia.

Louis-Bar syndrome Similar telangiectases in Louis-Bar syndrome can also be found on the ear.

of respiratory system may be difficult because of neurologic disease. Hematologic evaluation should look for malignancies that may result in pancytopenia, requiring blood or platelet transfusions preoperatively. Evaluation of hepatic function, glucose homeostasis, and coagulation profile.

Anesthetic considerations: Patient cooperation may be limited because of mental deficiency. Ventilation/oxygenation may be challenging because of chronic lung disease. May need postoperative ventilation. Increased risk of aspiration because of neurologic disease. Although there are no known direct cardiac anomalies, the presence of chronic lung disease and the potential effect of increased pulmonary vascular resistance on cardiac function must be evaluated.

Pharmacological implications: Drugs that depend on hepatic metabolism should be used with care in the presence of hepatic dysfunction. Use muscle relaxants judiciously in presence of progressive neurologic disease.

REFERENCES:
Jones KL: Ataxia telangiectasia syndrome, in Lyons K (ed): *Smith's Recognisable Patterns of Human Malformation.* 5th ed. WB Saunders, Philadelphia, 1997, p 196.

Gatti RA: Ataxia telangiectasia. in Scriver CR, Beaudet AL, Sly WS, et al. (eds): *The Metabolic and Molecular Bases of Inherited Disease.* 6th ed. New York, McGraw-Hill, 1989, p 2702.

Lowe Syndrome

At a glance: Genetically transmitted polymalformative syndrome characterized by the association of ocular problems with renal dysfunction and mental retardation.

Synonyms: Lowe Oculocerebrorenal Syndrome; Oculocerebrorenal Syndrome; Lowe-Terrey-MacLachlan Syndrome; OCRL I.

Genetic inheritance: X-linked disorder (Xq26.1). However, a few cases have been reported in females.

Pathophysiology: Lack of the enzyme phosphatidylinositol 4,5-biphosphate 5-phosphatase, which is located in the Golgi apparatus and controls the intracellular level of phosphatidylinositol 4,5-biphosphate. This enzyme deficiency may impair normal intracellular protein sorting (including second messengers), especially within polarized cells, and could be responsible for the observed ocular, renal, and cerebral abnormalities.

Diagnosis: Cataracts associated with renal tubular acidosis. In the blood, hypophosphatemia and elevated α_2-globulin help confirm the diagnosis. Creatine kinase is sometimes increased. Deficiency of Phosphatidylinositol 4,5-Bisphosphate 5-Phosphatase.

Clinical aspects:

Infancy: Neonatal cataracts (100%), glaucoma, megacornea, enophthalmos and nystagmus caused by poor vision. The problems caused by renal tubular acidosis appear during the first year. Approximately 50% of patients experience seizures.

Childhood: Renal tubular acidosis, aminoaciduria, proteinuria (Fanconi syndrome); failure to thrive; vitamin D-resistant rickets; corneal scarring.

Late Childhood: Progressive renal failure.

Patients have typical facies characterized by large forehead, sunken eyes, large, poorly shaped ears, and sometimes retrognathism. They have mild-to-moderate mental retardation with ma-

jor hypotonia and behavioral problems (stereotypical behavior); cryptorchidism is common.

Precautions before anesthesia: Check serum electrolytes, acid–base status, calcium and phosphate levels, and renal function. Some patients receive chronic oral bicarbonate therapy; treatment for glaucoma usually involves eye drops of a beta-blocking agent. Check intraocular pressure and presence of retrognathism.

Anesthetic considerations: Retrognathism may make direct laryngoscopy and tracheal intubation difficult. Careful titration of perioperative IV fluids to prevent hyperhydratation or dehydration. Ophthalmic beta blockade may lead to some systemic effects following local resorption.

Pharmacological implications: Related to the medical treatment of glaucoma (topical beta blockers) and to the extent of renal insufficiency or failure. Avoid succinylcholine in the presence of glaucoma.

Other condition to be considered:

CONGENITAL CATARACTS AND FANCONI SYNDROME: Characterized by alteration of renal tubular function resulting in severe rickets, hypokalemia, acidosis, and severe growth failure; several diseases (usually autosomal recessive) are associated with Fanconi syndrome, including cystinosis, glycogenosis, galactosemia, and tyrosinemia.

REFERENCES:
Charnas LR, Bernardini I, Rader D, et al: Clinical and laboratory findings in the oculocerebrorenal syndrome of Lowe, with special reference to growth and renal failure. *N Engl J Med* 324:1318, 1991.

Saricaoglu F, Demirtas F, Aypar U: Preoperative and perioperative management of a patient with Lowe syndrome diagnosed to have Fanconi's syndrome. *Paediatr Anaesth* 14:530, 2004.

Suchy SF, Olivos-Glander IM, Nussabaum RL: Lowe syndrome, a deficiency of phosphatidylinositol 4,5-bisphosphate 5-phosphatase in the Golgi apparatus. *Hum Mol Genet* 4:2245, 1995.

Lown-Ganong-Levine Syndrome

At a glance: Ventricular preexcitation syndrome.

Synonyms: Accelerated Atrioventricular Nodal Conduction; Enhanced Atrioventricular Nodal Conduction Syndrome; Short PR/Normal QRS Syndrome; Short PR/Narrow QRS Syndrome.

History: Occurrence of frequent paroxysms of tachycardia in patients with short PR interval was described by A. Clerc in 1938, but B. Lown, W.F. Ganong, and S.A. Levine gave it their eponym in 1952.

Nature: Ventricular preexcitation syndrome (other types include Wolff-Parkinson-White syndrome via Kent fibers and preexcitation via Mahaim fibers).

Incidence: 0.5% of the overall adult population. Retrospective analysis has suggested that paroxysmal supraventricular tachycardia occurs in approximately 9.5% of patients with short PR and normal QRS duration.

Genetic inheritance: Unknown. A familial occurrence has been suggested.

Pathophysiology: Atriofascicular tracts (called *James fibers*) completely or partially bypass the atrioventricular node, resulting in a short PR interval (<0.12 seconds). These tracts insert into the bundle of His or its branches; thus, the ventricles are depolarized in a normal sequence and the QRS complex appears normal on ECG (no delta wave as in Wolff-Parkinson-White syndrome). Paroxysmal tachycardias classically arise from reentry through the bypass tract. Direct atrioventricular connections have been suggested to be part of the syndrome; such connections could allow tachycardias to develop as a result of antegrade, rather than retrograde, conduction.

Diagnosis: History; ECG; short PR interval with normal QRS complex; electrophysiologic studies.

Clinical aspects: Patients may remain asymptomatic. Episodes of paroxysmal palpitation (atrial flutter, supraventricular tachycardia) may be associated with shortness of breath, signs of ventricular failure, and syncope. Investigations include ECG and electrophysiologic studies to define the site of accessory conducting tissue and the individual mechanism for tachycardia generation. The tachycardia is usually a narrow complex, but functional right bundle or left bundle branch block may cause a wide complex tachycardia. Several drugs may be used in the management of the condition, including adenosine (acutely), verapamil, beta blocker, procainamide, amiodarone, or digitalis. However, verapamil and digoxin are contraindicated for treatment of atrial fibrillation or flutter in these patients because they might accelerate conduction through the bypass tract and induce ventricular fibrillation. Surgical or catheter pathway ablation or pacemakers (overdrive pacing) may be used.

Precautions before anesthesia: Obtain a history of the frequency of dysrhythmias and the current treatment regimen. Continue antidysrhythmic drugs perioperatively. In case of chronic amiodarone therapy, check thyroid function and exclude pulmonary fibrosis. Review the results of electrophysiologic studies if available. Preoperative ECG mandatory. Data regarding pacemaker if overdrive pacing is being used to control supraventricular tachycardias. Correct any electrolyte disturbance (sodium, potassium, and magnesium).

Anesthetic considerations: Minimize perioperative catecholamine surges. Premedication may be beneficial. Atropine is relatively contraindicated. Hypoxia, hypercarbia, or acidosis must be prevented because all these complications render cardiac muscle membranes unstable and ectopic depolarization more likely.

Pharmacological implications: Same as for Wolff-Parkinson-White syndrome. Enflurane is the volatile agent that probably is least likely to induce arrhythmia. Halothane is contraindicated (proarrhythmogenic, myocardial depressant). Isoflurane and sevoflurane have been used without problem in patients with Wolff-Parkinson-White syndrome. Desflurane has a sympathomimetic effect that is undesirable. Because propofol has no effect on the refractory period of normal and accessory tissue, it is useful for electrophysiologic studies and ablation procedures. Pancuronium is relatively contraindicated. Extreme care if administering a beta blocker to a patient already taking verapamil (may precipitate extreme bradycardia or heart block); in case of need, esmolol probably is the perioperative beta blocker of choice. Amiodarone therapy may induce intense vasoplegia after induction of anesthesia.

Other conditions to be considered:

☞ **WOLFF-PARKINSON-WHITE SYNDROME:** Preexcitation syndrome caused by the presence of a track bypassing the atrioventricular node, thus shortening the PR interval and leading to paroxystic access of tachycardia.

PAROXYSMAL ATRIAL TACHYCARDIA: Often a complication of Wolff-Parkinson-White syndrome.

REFERENCES:

Durakovic Z, Durakovic A, Kastelan A: The preexcitation syndrome: Epidemiological and genetic study. *Int J Cardiol* 35:181, 1992.

Jones R, Broadbent M, Adams A: Anaesthetic considerations in patients with paroxysmal supraventricular tachycardia. *Anaesthesia* 39:307, 1984.

Sharpe M, Dobkowski W, Murkin J, et al: Propofol has no direct effect on sinoatrial node function or on normal atrioventricular and accessory pathway conduction in Wolff-Parkinson-White syndrome during alfentanil/midazolam anesthesia. *Anesthesiology* 82:888, 1995.

Lowry-Wood Syndrome

At a glance: Genetic syndrome with multiple epiphyseal dysplasia, microcephaly, nystagmus, retinitis pigmentosa, and growth retardation.

Synonyms: Epiphyseal Dysplasia, Microcephaly, and Nystagmus; Epiphyseal Dysplasia-Short Stature-Microcephaly-Nystagmus Syndrome; Short Stature-Microcephaly-Mental Retardation-Multiple Epiphyseal Dysplasia Syndrome.

Incidence: Incidence remains uncommon; only a few cases have been reported in the literature.

Genetic inheritance: Autosomal recessive.

Pathophysiology: Radiographic changes are consistent with multiple epiphyseal dysplasia. The changes are mainly irregular and fragmented epiphyses in the long bones, especially the femoral heads.

Diagnosis: Radiologic evidence of microcephaly without thickening of the skull vault. Delayed ossification of all long bone epiphyses.

Clinical aspects: Neonates and infants are small for gestational age, short stature, epiphyses small and irregular, square iliac bones, flattened acetabula, microcephaly, nystagmus, mild mental retardation.

Precautions before anesthesia: In the presence of microcephaly, the facial features must be reviewed in case of anomalies that may lead to difficult airway management. The extent of mental retardation must be assessed to determine the impact on the patient's behavior during induction of anesthesia.

Anesthetic considerations: In the presence of mental retardation and lack of communication, use of a sedative premedication might be appropriate to reduce patient's stress during induction of anesthesia. No anesthetic considerations specific to this medical condition.

Pharmacological implications: No known pharmacological implications to this syndrome.

REFERENCES:

Nevin NC, Thomas PS, Hutchinson J: Syndrome of short stature, microcephaly, mental retardation and multiple epiphyseal dysplasia—Lowry-Wood syndrome. *Am J Med Genet* 24:33, 1986.

Yamamoto T, Tohyama J, Koeda T, et al: Multiple epiphyseal dysplasia with small head, congenital nystagmus, hypoplasia of corpus callosum, and leukonychia totalis: A variant of Lowry-Wood syndrome? *Am J Med Genet* 56:6, 1995.

Lucey-Driscoll Syndrome

At a glance: Benign disorder of metabolism of bilirubin resulting in transient neonatal hyperbilirubinemia (unconjugated bilirubin).

Synonym: Transient Familial Neonatal Hyperbilirubinemia.

NB: Lucey-Driscoll syndrome is occasionally misspelled "Lucy-Driscoll syndrome."

Incidence: Rare; 24 cases reported.

Genetic inheritance: Familial or sporadic. Usually all siblings are affected. Cases transmitted as an autosomal recessive trait (gene map locus is 2q37) have been reported.

Pathophysiology: A substance, probably a metabolite of gestational hormones (inhibitor of uridine diphosphate [UDP]-glucuronosyltransferase activity), that inhibits bilirubin conjugation is responsible for the disease. This inhibitor is present in the sera of both mother and infant. Unconjugated hyperbilirubinemia, which is more severe than the form observed in breast milk jaundice, is present. Serum bilirubin may reach 40 mg/dl (680 μmol/l).

Diagnosis: The presence of significant neonatal jaundice frequently associated with a familial pattern. All siblings are usually affected, and there is frequently a history of the phenomenon occurring in previous generations. Other causes of hyperbilirubinemia should be excluded.

Clinical aspects: Unconjugated hyperbilirubinemia resulting in jaundice usually presenting on the third to fifth day of life and persisting for 3 weeks. Left untreated, kernicterus may develop. Phototherapy is used to treat the hyperbilirubinemia.

Precautions before anesthesia: Exclude other causes of hyperbilirubinemia, such as sepsis, hemolytic disease of the newborn, and biliary atresia. Ensure adequate hydration. Obtain coagulation profile and bleeding time.

Anesthetic considerations: This syndrome occurs only in neonates; therefore, basic principles of safe neonatal anesthesia must be applied.

Pharmacological implications: Drugs that interfere with metabolism of bilirubin or that may displace bilirubin from albumin could increase the risk of hyperbilirubinemia or kernicterus. Sulfonamides, ceftriaxone, pancuronium, and chloral hydrate are associated with hyperbilirubinemia.

Other conditions to be considered: The hereditary hyperbilirubinemias include (1) those resulting in predominantly unconjugated hyperbilirubinemia, such as Gilbert or Arias syndrome, Crigler-Najjar syndrome type I, and Crigler-Najjar syndrome type II; and (2) those resulting in predominantly conjugated hyperbilirubinemia, such as Dubin-Johnson syndrome, Rotor syndrome, and other forms of intrahepatic cholestasis.

BREAST MILK JAUNDICE: Jaundice occurring in breast-fed neonate around the fourth to seventh day of life, persisting beyond physiologic jaundice, and with no other identifiable cause, probably resulting from a milk component that inhibits uridine diphosphoglucuronic acid (UDPGA) glucuronyl transferase, thus resulting in a prolonged unconjugated hyperbilirubinemia.

☞**CRIGLER-NAJJAR SYNDROME:** Inherited error of bilirubin metabolism in which bilirubin cannot be converted into water-soluble bilirubin glucuronide because of a defect of hepatic glucuronyl transferase. Crigler-Najjar syndrome type II is less severe than type I.

☞**GILBERT SYNDROME:** Characterized by normal liver function tests, normal liver histology, delayed clearance of bilirubin from the blood, and mild jaundice that tends to fluctuate in severity, particularly after fasting. It is defined as a mild unconjugated hyperbilirubinemia resulting from a mutation in the promoter of the UDP-glucuronosyltransferase gene (allelic to the mutation for Crigler-Najjar syndrome type I).

☞**DUBIN-JOHNSON SYNDROME:** Occurs with a minimal frequency of 1:1300 among Iranian Jews. It is characterized by hyperbilirubinemia, deposition of melanin-like pigment in otherwise normal liver cells, hepatomegaly and abdominal pain, and otherwise normal liver function.

☞**ROTOR SYNDROME:** Considered similar to the Dubin-Johnson syndrome; however, it shows no abnormal hepatic pigmentation and oral cholecystography is often normal. Total coproporphyrin excretion in the urine is markedly increased.

REFERENCES:

Colón AR: Hyperbilirubinaemia syndromes, in Colón AR (ed): *Textbook of Pediatric Hepatology.* 2nd ed. Chicago, Year Book Medical Publishers, 1990, p 173.

Maruo Y, Nishizawa K, Sato H, et al: Prolonged unconjugated hyperbilirubinemia associated with breast milk and mutations of the bilirubin uridine diphosphate-glucuronosyltransferase gene. *Pediatrics* 106:E59, 2000.

Oski F: Unconjugated hyperbilirubinemia, in Tadeusch HW, Ballard R, Avery M (eds): *Schaffer and Avery's Diseases of the Newborn.* 6th ed. Philadelphia, WB Saunders, 1991, p 173.

Lujan Fryns Syndrome

At a glance: Inherited syndrome with marfanoid features and X-linked mental retardation.

Synonym: X-Linked Mental Retardation with Marfanoid Habitus Syndrome.

Incidence: Approximately 59 cases reported up to 2005, almost exclusively in males.

Genetic inheritance: X-linked dominant transmission with a greater expressivity and penetrance in males has been suggested.

Diagnosis: Major criteria include mild-to-moderate mental retardation; marfanoid habitus; generalized hypotonia; hypernasal voice; normal secondary sexual development and normal or enlarged testicular size; characteristic craniofacial appearance with large forehead; contrasting long and narrow face; maxillary hypoplasia; long nose with high and narrow nasal bridge; short and deep philtrum; thin upper lip; and high-arched palate.

Clinical aspects: Patients appear tall and slender with long limbs and fingers (arachnodactyly). General muscular hypotonia and hyperlaxity of the joints are further features. Seizures are possible, and mental retardation is described as mild to severe. Partial or complete agenesis of the corpus callosum has been reported in some cases. A high forehead and a long, narrow face with hypoplastic mandible and micrognathia with a narrow and high-arched palate are typical. The nasal bridge is high, and the ears are low set and posteriorly rotated. Kyphoscoliosis and pectus excavatum are present in some cases. Cardiac defects (atrial septal defect) have been described, and two (related) patients were reported to have dilatation of the aortic root and a ventricular septa defect.

Precautions before anesthesia: Depending on the severity of kyphoscoliosis, restrictive lung disease and cor pulmonale may be present. If kyphoscoliosis is significant, pulmonary investigations should include a chest radiograph, arterial blood gas analysis, and lung function tests (although they may be difficult to obtain in a mentally delayed patient). Preoperative assessment should include echocardiography to rule out congenital heart defects and to determine the size of the aortic root. Finally, the association of a hypoplastic mandible and micrognathia should prompt complete evaluation of the airway.

Anesthetic considerations: No reports referring to anesthesia were found. However, airway management could be challenging in the presence of the aforementioned facial anomalies. Therefore, proper preparation for difficult direct laryngoscopy and tracheal intubation should be planned. Patient compliance is likely to increase with sedative and anxiolytic premedication given that psychotic, autistic-like, and aggressive behavior have been reported.

Pharmacological implications: Some patients are taking antiseizure medication. These drugs can induce hepatic enzymes, thereby altering the metabolism of other drugs with predominant hepatic clearance. Because of aortic root dilatation, these patients may also be on beta-blocker therapy.

Other conditions to be considered:

☞DE DIE-SMULDERS VLES FRYNS SYNDROME: Genetic disorder characterized by a characteristic facies, marfanoid habitus, and mental delay.

☞MARFAN SYNDROME: Autosomal dominant connective-tissue disorder linked to the FBN1 gene on chromosome 15 that encodes fibrillin 1. Without fibrillin, many tissues are weakened, especially the joints, tendons, lens, and walls of major arteries. Aortic regurgitation and dissection are responsible for premature death in the third to fifth decade.

CONGENITAL CONTRACTURAL ARACHNODACTYLY: Marfan-like appearance, "crumpled" ears, contractures of major joints, kyphoscoliosis, and camptodactyly. It is caused by a defective FNB2 gene (chromosome 5q23-q31) that encodes the extracellular matrix microfibril, fibrillin 2.

SHPRINTZEN-GOLDBERG (OR MONTEFIORE) SYNDROME: Craniosynostosis associated with marfanoid habitus (tall stature, arachnodactyly, joint hyperextensibility, narrow face, hypotonia), abdominal hernia, developmental delay, and other anomalies. It is caused by mutations in the same gene as that involved in the Marfan syndrome, fibrillin-1.

REFERENCES:

Lacombe D, Bonneau D, Verloes A, et al: Lujan-Fryns syndrome (X-linked mental retardation with marfanoid habitus): Report of three cases and review. *Genet Counsel* 4:193, 1993.

Lujan JE, Carlis ME, Lubs HA: A form of X-linked mental retardation with marfanoid habitus. *Am J Med Genet* 17:311, 1984.

Wittine LM, Josephson KD, Williams MS: Aortic root dilation in apparent Lujan-Fryns syndrome. *Am J Med Genet* 86:405, 1999.

Lutembacher Syndrome

At a glance: Congenital heart disease characterized by the association of an atrial septal defect with a mitral stenosis (left-to-right shunt at the atrial level).

Synonym: Lutembacher Disease.

History: First reported by anatomist Johann Friedrich Meckel in a letter to Albrecht von Haller in 1750.

Incidence: Uncommon. Prevalence among cases of atrial septal defect is estimated to be 4%. Prevalence among cases of mitral stenosis is estimated to be 0.6 to 0.7%. Occurs more frequently in females than in males.

Genetic inheritance: Unknown. A reported kindred suggested autosomal dominant inheritance with almost complete penetrance. The condition is thought to represent a disorder of midline development.

Pathophysiology: Lutembacher syndrome is classically described as a secundum atrial septal defect associated with mitral stenosis. The mitral stenosis is often rheumatic rather than congenital in ori-

gin. An atrial septal defect may be protective in mitral stenosis by providing a conduit for decompression of the left atrium and pulmonary venous system. However, mitral stenosis worsens the prognosis of an uncomplicated atrial septal defect by increasing right ventricular work and pulmonary blood flow, resulting in pulmonary hypertension. Central venous pressure is elevated in this syndrome.

Diagnosis: Clinical examination suggests the diagnosis and echocardiography confirms the diagnosis.

Clinical aspects: Patients may not become symptomatic until adult life. Symptoms include dyspnea, orthopnea, paroxysmal nocturnal dyspnea, decreased exercise tolerance, and palpitations. There may be signs of right ventricular failure. A loud S_1 (mitral stenosis) with fixed splitting of S_2 (atrial septal defect) is usually heard. A diastolic parasternal murmur may be heard and represents increased flow across the tricuspid valve. Electrocardiographic findings include atrial flutter, atrial fibrillation, incomplete or complete right bundle branch block, right ventricular hypertrophy, and right-axis deviation. The chest radiograph demonstrates right atrial enlargement and prominent pulmonary vasculature and may show signs of pulmonary venous congestion.

Precautions before anesthesia: Full history and examination to establish cardiac and pulmonary reserve. Chest radiograph to exclude pulmonary edema. Preoperative ECG and review of recent echocardiographic examinations. Laboratory investigations as indicated by surgical procedure and patient medications.

Anesthetic considerations: Maintain left ventricular preload. Avoid increases in systemic vascular resistance. Avoid tachycardia, which will decrease time for left ventricular filling through the stenotic valve. Maintain ventricular contractility. Use a technique to prevent an increase in pulmonary vascular resistance and potential reversal of the left-to-right shunt. Strict precautions regarding air in intravenous lines because of increased risk of paradoxical embolism.

Pharmacological implications: Anesthetic agents favoring a sympathomimetic discharge (e.g., pancuronium, desflurane) and anticholinergic actions (e.g., atropine) are relatively contraindicated. Consider need for antibiotic prophylaxis against bacterial endocarditis.

REFERENCES:

Megarbane A, Stephan E, Kassab R, et al: Autosomal dominant secundum atrial septal defect with various cardiac and noncardiac defects: A new midline disorder. *Am J Med Genet* 83:193, 1999.

Steinbrunn W, Cohn K, Selzer A: Atrial septal defect associated with mitral stenosis. The Lutembacher syndrome revisited. *Am J Med* 48:295, 1970.

Lyell Syndrome

At a glance: Severe allergic syndrome caused by an allergic reaction (hypersensitivity) to pharmacological agents, infections, or illnesses such as lymphoma and graft-versus-host disease. It is characterized by extensive bullous eruption of the skin and mucous membranes, fever, malaise, conjunctivitis, and diffuse erythema; often lethal in children.

Synonyms: Acute Toxic Epidermolysis Syndrome; Brocq-Debré-Lyell Syndrome; Bullous Erythroderma Epidermolysis; Debré-Lamy-Lyell Syndrome; Dermatitis Medicamentosa Syndrome; Epidermolysis Acuta Combustiformis; Epidermolysis Combustiformis; Epidermolysis Acuta Toxica; Epidermolysis Necroticans

Combustiformis; Erythrodermia Bullosa with Epidermolysis; Fuchs-Salzmann-Terrier Syndrome; Scalded Skin Syndrome; Toxic Epidermal Necrolysis, Toxic-Allergic Epidermal Necrolysis.

Genetic inheritance: Not a genetic syndrome.

Pathophysiology: Hypersensitivity reaction in response to medications (sulfonamides, penicillins, barbiturates, and phenytoin), infections (herpes simplex, mycoplasma, staphylococcal, viral and fungal infections), malignant diseases, radiation, or vaccination.

Diagnosis: Primarily based on skin lesion appearance and symmetrical distribution in the context of history of risk factors or associated diseases. Positive Nikolsky sign (i.e., separation of the center layer of the epidermis from the basal layer with sloughing of the skin produced by minor trauma). Skin biopsy occasionally is useful to exclude other skin disorders and may show significant deposits of immune complexes.

Clinical aspects: Development of multiple and large blisters (bullae) that coalesce and result in sloughing of most of the skin and mucous membranes. Associated symptoms may consist of fever, itching, painful joints, visual disorders and pain, and general ill feeling. Lesions of internal organs may occur (pneumonitis, myocarditis, hepatitis, nephritis). Secondary skin infection (cellulitis), septicemia, loss of body fluid (as in extended burns), and shock are common complications. The death rate is high in children and in elderly patients.

Precautions before anesthesia: Assess airway patency with regard to the presence of mucosal lesions and bullae. Protect skin lesions with moist compresses. Consider symptomatic treatment to prevent further aggravation: antihistamines to control itching, acetaminophen to reduce fever, pain killer including opiates to treat pain, topical anesthetics (especially for oral lesions) to ease discomfort. Severe cases should be managed in an intensive care or burn care unit. Intravenous corticosteroids (to control inflammation), immunoglobulins (to stop the allergic process), and antibiotics (to control secondary skin infections) must be used. Considerable precaution should be taken to prevent bacterial contamination. Extended skin lesions may cause loss of large quantities of body fluids with shock and require intensive care with support of body systems.

Anesthetic considerations: Prevent any trauma to skin and mucosal surfaces by appropriate positioning and padding. Monitoring should be applied without use of adhesive gels or tapes; the sticky surround of ECG electrodes must be removed. The use of ECG needles might be considered as alternatives. Wrap limb in soft padding prior to use of automated blood pressure recording devices. Venous access may be difficult, and intravenous (IV) cannulas may need to be sutured in place. The pressure from an anesthetic face mask may be damaging, so it should be held lightly just above the face and spontaneous ventilation maintained. The application of vaseline ointment to reduce shearing forces between the face mask and the skin is another option. Oral airways should be avoided if possible. Intratracheal lesions do not occur often if intubation proceeds cautiously with a well-lubricated undersized tube. Because endotracheal tube securing may be complicated, suturing the tube in place may be the best choice. Whenever possible, spontaneous ventilation without tracheal intubation or placement of an airway (including a laryngeal mask) is mandatory; use of IV ketamine or volatile agents delivered through a head box (or a gently applied face mask) is recommended when applicable. Because hypothermia may develop rapidly, temperature should be carefully monitored and every measure taken to ensure normothermia. It is mandatory to avoid oropharyngeal suctioning because it can lead to bullae formation and post-

operative airway obstruction. Regional anesthesia is not contraindicated if the skin over the region is unaffected, but it is imperative to use a sterile technique because these patients are more prone to infection. Because of the esophageal scarring, there is a danger of regurgitation and aspiration; consequently, antacid prophylaxis is recommended prior to surgery. Infection is more common because of the broken epidermal barrier, which should be treated prior to the patient going to the operating room. Because there is a greater risk of corneal abrasion, lubricant and petroleum jelly gauzes should be applied.

Pharmacological implications: It might be prudent to avoid succinylcholine in case of hyperkalemia caused by acute renal failure and shock.

Other conditions to be considered:

☞**Epidermolysis Bullosa:** Group of skin diseases characterized by recurring painful blisters and open sores, often in response to minor trauma, as a result of the unusually fragile nature of the skin. There are three major forms: epidermolysis bullosa simplex, the most common; junctional epidermolysis bullosa; and dystrophic epidermolysis bullosa. In *epidermolysis bullosa simplex (nonscarring),* the blisters occur within the epidermis. In the Weber-Cockayne variant, blisters are usually confined to the hands and the feet. The Dowling-Meara variant is characterized by the presence of blisters on the entire body. About one third of all epidermolysis bullosa simplex patients experience blisters and sores within the oral cavity that impair feeding and swallowing. Growth retardation and anemia can be present. Children usually have normal mental and physical development. In *junctional epidermolysis bullosa (JEB),* the blisters occur deeper within the lamina lucida of the basement membrane zone. Herlitz JEB and non-Herlitz JEB are the two subtypes. Patients present with widespread painful blisters and skin erosions. The skin is very fragile and may peel off easily. *Dystrophic epidermolysis bullosa (DEB)* is characterized by blisters that develop beneath the basement membrane zone and are present at, or shortly after, birth. Patients have widespread painful blisters and sores. The two major subtypes are dominant DEB and recessive DEB. The Hallopeau-Siemens variant, a recessive form, is the most severe. Blisters appear on the arms and legs and are widespread, affecting mucous membranes and skin. Blisters leave scars and small "seed-like" cysts after healing.

☞**Erythema Multiforme:** Characterized by inflammation of the oropharynx and hypopharynx membranes, anogenital region, intestinal tract, and conjunctiva. Macules or papules are present. Bullae or blisters may develop. Abnormalities of the eyes may lead to ocular damage as a result of purulent conjunctivitis.

References:

Rabito SF, Sultana S, Konefal TS, et al: Anesthetic management of toxic epidermal necrolysis: Report of three adult cases. *J Clin Anesth* 13:133, 2001.

Ringheanu M, Laude TA: Toxic epidermal necrolysis in children—An update. *Clin Pediatr (Phila)* 39:687, 2000.

Tristani-Firouzi P, Petersen MJ, Saffle JR, et al: Treatment of toxic epidermal necrolysis with intravenous immunoglobulin in children. *J Am Acad Dermatol* 47:548, 2002.

Lyme Disease

At a glance: Infectious disease caused by a spirochete with significant immune response possibly leading to neurologic problems.

Synonyms: Erythema Migrans Disease; Tick-Borne Disease.

History: Named after the town of Lyme, Connecticut, USA, where a mysterious clustering of arthritis cases was reported in 1970.

Incidence: 0.15–4.4:1000 population. Lyme disease is the most common disease transmitted by an insect in the United States. It is also prevalent in Europe and Asia.

Genetic inheritance: None (infectious disorder).

Pathophysiology: Results from both direct infection and the host's immune response to the spirochete *Borrelia burgdorferi*, which is carried by the tick *Ixodes dammini*. The spirochete is injected into the bloodstream through the saliva of the tick or deposited on the skin with fecal material. After incubation period of 3 to 32 days, which the spirochete may migrate to the skin, causing erythema chronicum migrans, or it may enter the bloodstream, thereby migrating to other organs. The first clinical sign of the disease can be a facial nerve palsy, followed by arthritis and a meningitis-like symptom. The late complications are probably caused by a direct effect of infection with viable organisms and the immunologic response to them. The arthritis is thought to be a result of localization of immune complexes to the synovium, resulting in joint inflammation. The B-cell alloantigen HLA-DR4 is common in patients with severe and prolonged illness, particularly arthritis or neurologic disease.

Diagnosis: Clinical evidence of erythema chronicum migrans together with symptoms of influenza or meningitis.

Clinical aspects: Skin lesions are prominent in the first stage of the disease, with cardiac and neurologic abnormalities occurring in the second stage. Arthritis is most common in the third stage. Hepatitis, myositis, eosinophilic lymphadenitis, respiratory distress syndrome, and facial nerve palsies may occur.

Precautions before anesthesia: Full history of disease progression and any antibiotic therapy. Assessment of cardiac, hepatic, and respiratory function must be obtained. Coagulation profile should be obtained.

Anesthetic considerations: Cardiac abnormalities are present in approximately 10% of patients and include atrioventricular block, myopericarditis, and left ventricular dysfunction. Temporary cardiac pacing may be required.

Pharmacological implications: No known specific pharmacological implications.

REFERENCES:

Doughty RA: Lyme disease. *Pediatr Rev* 6:20, 1984.

Hayes E: Lyme disease. *Clin Evid* 7:652, 2002.

Montiel NJ, Baumgarten JM, Sinha AA: Lyme disease—Part II: Clinical features and treatment. *Cutis* 69:443, 2002.

Lymphedema

At a glance: Primary or secondary disorder of lymphatic drainage.

Synonyms and classifications: Hereditary Lymphedema.

Hereditary Lymphedema Type I (Nonne-Milroy Syndrome; Milroy Syndrome; Congenital Hereditary Lymphedema type): Present at birth with areas of swelling. The importance of the swelling tends to increase with age, especially during infancy.

Hereditary Lymphedema Type II (Meige Lymphedema; Familial Lymphedema Praecox; Hereditary Lymphedema Tarda): Usually develops during childhood, adolescence, or early adulthood. It produces severe swelling in areas below the waist. It usually includes red skin over areas of swelling and associated discomfort and/or inflammation.

Secondary Lymphedema: Results from inadequate lymphatic drainage as a result of various causes, such as surgery, recurrent lymphangitis, cellulitis, neoplastic invasion of lymphatics, fibrosis following radiotherapy, or scar formation.

Incidence: Incidence for hereditary lymphedema is estimated at 1:10,000 individuals. However, the incidence for secondary lymphedema is significantly higher. Meige lymphedema represents 80% of all hereditary lymphedema.

Genetic inheritance: Hereditary lymphedemas that are not associated with other malformations usually affect the lower limbs and are inherited as an autosomal dominant trait with variable penetrance (autosomal or sex-linked recessive forms are less common). These nonsyndromic hereditary lymphedemas are categorized by their age of onset, being either congenital (Milroy disease) or having an onset in childhood or around puberty (Meige disease). Lymphedema can been associated with various other anomalies, many of which are genetic (autosomal recessive, autosomal dominant or X-linked recessive inheritance), and with Turner and Noonan syndromes.

Several genes may be involved in the development of hereditary lymphedema, including the following:

- Vascular endothelial growth factor receptor 3 (VEGFR3), formerly known as FLT4, is located on chromosome 5.
- FOXC2, which is responsible for causing the lymphedema-distichiasis syndrome (16q24.3).
- At least one (more likely, several) other gene can be responsible for other forms of hereditary lymphedema.

Pathophysiology: In the primary forms, aplasia or hypoplasia of the lymphatic vessels results in dilatation of extralymphatic spaces. In both primary and secondary forms, lymphatic obstruction from any cause results in increased protein content of the extravascular tissue and, because of its osmotic effect, retention of additional water. This excess extravascular protein often leads to proliferation of fibroblasts and organization of the edema fluid, giving rise to a characteristic firm, nonpitting swelling.

Diagnosis: Clinical findings, results of the patent blue test and fluorescence microlymphography, indirect lymphography, or isotope studies suffice for correct diagnosis. In hereditary lymphedema present at birth (Milroy disease), the lymphatic capillaries and precollectors are aplastic, whereas in sporadic lymphedema with postpubertal onset, the large collectors are hypoplastic or aplastic, and a well-developed superficial capillary network is detected.

Clinical aspects: The edema in Milroy disease is present from birth in contrast to the edema, particularly severe below the waist, that develops around puberty in Meige syndrome. Involvement of the upper limbs, face, and larynx are notable features in Meige syndrome. There is also an association with deafness, cleft palate, primary pulmonary hypertension, and cerebrovascular malformations. In the autosomal recessive form, there is intestinal lymphedema, facial anomalies (antimongoloid slant of palpebral fissures, euryblepharon, retrognathia, chemosis), coarctation of aorta, patent ductus arteriosus, and hypoalbuminemia. At the beginning, the edema is pitting and disappears with elevation of the affected part. Subsequently, with development of fibrosis, the edema becomes nonpitting. The overlying skin becomes hyperkeratotic and waters. Fissures and secondary infections often occur. Treatment is often symptomatic with elastic stocking, active muscle exercises, and centripetal massage. Diuretics may be used. Antibiotics are often required for recurrent infection. Surgical management of lymphedema does not amount to more than 10% of cases. Excisional procedures, such as the Thompson operation, are done. Liposuction is an attractive alternative. The most effective types of surgical treatment are microsurgical lymphovenous or lymphovenous-lymphatic bypass. Secondary lymphedema of the lower extremities (more rarely of the upper limbs) is the primary indication for surgical treatment.

Precautions before anesthesia: Depending on the form of lymphedema, a detailed systematic review of the known involvement is necessary. In Milroy disease, particular attention should be paid to the presence of respiratory impairment potentially caused by pleural effusions and the hypoproteinemia secondary to chronic gastrointestinal protein loss. In Meige syndrome, the airway should be assessed with regard to the presence of cleft palate, laryngeal edema, and facial edema. Pulmonary hypertension should be excluded and any neurologic history or deficits noted. Investigations include complete cell blood count, coagulation status, serum protein and albumin levels, chest radiography, arterial blood gas analysis, serum electrolytes, ECG, echocardiography, and radionuclide imaging, if necessary, in the presence of pulmonary hypertension.

Anesthetic considerations: Monitoring and the anesthetic technique depend on the involvement of the various systems with regard to the type of lymphedema. In general, adequate venous access should be obtained if excision of the lymphatic system is to be performed. Adequate analgesia should be provided in such instances, as the amount of postoperative pain is significant. In all cases, proper positioning of the edematous parts is necessary to prevent trauma and sores. Stockings and pneumatic devices to reduce further dependency-related edema are useful for long operations. Thromboembolic prophylaxis should be considered.

Pharmacological implications: Low serum protein levels result in a higher free drug concentration; consequently, the dose of drugs that are highly protein bound (e.g., thiopentone) needs to be carefully titrated. Potassium supplementation perioperatively may be required in those on long-term diuretic therapy.

Other conditions to be considered:

HEREDITARY ANGIOEDEMA: Vascular disorder characterized by edema on the back of the hands or feet, eyelids, lips, and genitals. Pruritus and urticaria are rarely present. It is inherited as an autosomal dominant trait.

TRAUMATIC LYMPHEDEMA: Caused by injury to the lymph system. It is a localized lymphedema and is secondary to postinfectious syndromes, postradiation fibrosis, tumor growth, and surgery (e.g., mastectomy). Symptoms may include swelling, pitting, redness, discomfort, and/or tingling sensations.

ELEPHANTIASIS: An infectious tropical disease of the lymphatic system that is characterized by gross enlargement of an arm or leg or other areas of the trunk or head.

REFERENCES:

Fang J, Dagenais SL, Erickson RP, et al: Mutations in FOXC2 (MFH-1), a forkhead family transcription factor, are responsible for the hereditary lymphedema-distichiasis syndrome. *Am J Hum Genet* 67:1382, 2000.

Ferrell RE, Levinson KL, Esman JH, et al: Hereditary lymphedema: Evidence for linkage and genetic heterogeneity. *Hum Mol Genet* 7:2073, 1998.

Goodman RM: Familial lymphedema of the Meige's type. *Am J Med* 32:651, 1962.

Witte MH, Erickson R, Bernas M, et al: Phenotypic and genotypic heterogeneity in familial Milroy lymphedema. *Lymphology* 31:145, 1998.

Lymphedema Hypoparathyroidism Syndrome

At a glance: Rare polymalformative syndrome with lymphedema, endocrine disorders, and progressive renal failure.

Synonym: Dahlberg Borer Newcomer Syndrome.

Genetic inheritance: Either autosomal recessive or X-linked recessive.

Pathophysiology: Not known. Some similarities to Noonan syndrome.

Diagnosis: Evidence of lymphedema occurring shortly after birth, together with clinical and laboratory evidence of hypoparathyroidism. Clinical, radiologic, and/or histologic evidence of nephropathy and pulmonary lymphangiectasia.

Clinical aspects: Congenital lymphedema, hypoparathyroidism, nephropathy, progressive renal failure, mitral valve prolapse, brachytelephalangy, cataracts, broad nasal bridge, telecanthus.

Precautions before anesthesia: Echocardiography to assess cardiac function. Check electrolytes and renal function. It is very important to measure calcium level.

Anesthetic considerations: As determined by cardiac and parathyroid functions.

Pharmacological implications: No specific pharmacological implications except for patients with renal impairment.

Other conditions to be considered:

NONNE-MILROY SYNDROME: Hereditary onset type I (onset before age 35 years), congenital lymphedema, noninfectious hereditary elephantiasis. Severe swelling of the soft tissue secondary to obstruction of lymphatic drainage. Extravasation of significant amount of protein to the interstitial space, leading to stimulation of fibroblasts and development of "woody feeling"; nonpitting edema of the affected extremities.

MEIGE SYNDROME: Same as Nonne-Milroy syndrome but considered the hereditary onset type II with onset after age 35 years.

PULMONARY CYSTIC LYMPHANGIECTASIS (Pulmonary Lymphangiomatosis): Characterized by a congenital pulmonary lymphangiectasis with bilateral pneumothorax. It is often complicated by chylous pleural effusions, which is associated pulmonary hypoplasia. The basic defect is not an intrinsic lung abnormality but a developmental error of the lymphatic system resulting in a pulmonary lymphatic obstruction sequence.

REFERENCE:

Dahlberg PJ, Borer WZ, Newcomer KL, et al: Autosomal or X-linked recessive syndrome of congenital lymphedema, hypoparathyroidism, nephropathy, prolapsing mitral valve and brachytelephalangy. *Am J Med Genet* 16:99, 1983.

Lymphedema with Distichiasis

At a glance: Very rare congenital disorder presenting with double row of eyelashes, lymphatic drainage dysfunction and sometimes cardiac and spinal anomalies.

Synonym: Lymphedema-Distichiasis Syndrome.

History: In 1964, H.F. Falls and E.D. Kertesz described this hereditary disorder of lymphatic drainage combined with ocular and systemic complications, including spinal arachnoid cysts and congenital heart defects.

Genetic inheritance: Autosomal dominant with incomplete penetrance and variable expression caused by mutations in the FOXC2 gene on chromosome 16.

Diagnosis: Features are late-onset lymphedema (end of first decade of life) mainly involving the lower limbs and distichiasis (a double row of eyelashes). Lymphography shows abundant and dilated lymphatics in both legs and an absent or deformed thoracic duct.

Clinical aspects: Lymphedema is present from the knees downward and scrotal swelling may be considerable in males. Lymphedema usually presents during the second half of the first decade of life. One side may be affected many years before the other. Irritation of the cornea caused by the eyelashes, with corneal ulceration and scarring in some cases, brings the patient to the attention of an ophthalmologist. This form of lymphedema is associated with other congenital malformations, including (a) congenital heart disease (tetralogy of Fallot, patent ductus arteriosus, ventricular septal defect, atrial septal defect, coarctation of aorta, and pulmonary stenosis) and development of dilated cardiomyopathy; (b) spinal arachnoid cysts (in some patients, neurologic signs may be present); and (c) diverse anomalies of the vertebral column. The course and prognosis depend upon the extent and severity of the edema and the development of spinal column complications. Symptomatic management (compression, elevation, diuretics) of the edema is common. Removal of the lid hair to prevent ocular complications is done.

Precautions before anesthesia: Complete history and physical examination with special attention to the cardiac and spinal systems must be obtained. Investigations should be directed by history and clinical examination and may include hematocrit, ECG, chest radiography, echocardiography, and radionuclide imaging when necessary. Assess and document any neurologic deficits. Investigations include serum potassium (to exclude diuretic-induced hypokalemia), serum protein and albumin levels, and arterial blood gas analysis. Antibiotics for active infection of the edematous areas are to be continued, but suitable antibiotic prophylaxis for cardiac lesions should also be used. Use of sedative premedication should be assessed on an individual basis. Dehydration should be prevented at all times in patients who are polycythemic (hematocrit >45%).

Anesthetic considerations: Venous cannulation is difficult in the affected areas. Careful positioning of the affected limbs is required to prevent pressure sores and trauma. Stockings and pneumatic devices can be useful to reduce further dependency-related edema during long operations. Antithromboembolic prophylaxis should be considered. Induction and maintenance of anesthesia in patients with cardiac lesions is dictated by the underlying pathophysiology. Elective admission to the intensive care unit should be provided for all patients undergoing major surgical procedures and for those with advanced cardiac disease. Eye ointment and padding should be provided in patients with ophthalmic lesions.

Pharmacological implications: Low serum protein levels result in a higher free drug concentration; consequently, the dose of drugs that are highly protein bound (e.g., thiopentone) needs to be carefully titrated. Perioperative potassium supplementation may be required in patients on long-term diuretic therapy. In patients with cardiac lesions and dilated cardiomyopathy, avoid drugs known to induce myocardial depression and decrease preload. In presence of polycythemia, the use of dextran 40 or 70 should be considered as part of fluid management to reduce blood rheology.

REFERENCES:

Brice G: Diagnostic difficulties in lymphedema distichiasis. *Pediatr Dermatol* 20:89, 2003.

Fang J, Dagenais SL, Erickson RP, et al: Mutations in FOXC2 (MFH-1), a forkhead family transcription factor, are responsible for the hereditary lymphedema-distichiasis syndrome. *Am J Hum Genet* 67:1382, 2000.

Kolin T, Johns KJ, Wadlington WB, et al: Hereditary lymphedema and distichiasis. *Arch Ophthalmol* 109:980, 1991.

Lymphoreticular Syndrome

At a glance: Idiopathic enlargement of mesenteric lymph nodes associated with debilitating sprue.

Incidence: Extremely rare; only occurs in association with celiac sprue (or disease).

Genetic inheritance: Unknown.

Pathophysiology: Uncertain. Debilitated patients with celiac sprue develop mesenteric lymph node enlargement and cavitation, anemia, and duodenal ulcerations. This leads to worsening of the failure to thrive most often associated with celiac sprue.

Diagnosis: Based on the clinical picture. Patients may have repeated negative biopsies for lymphoma, despite a highly suspicious presentation. Lymphoreticular syndrome is diagnosed in the presence of celiac sprue.

Clinical aspects: Anemia, diarrhea, electrolyte derangement, hyposplenism, duodenal ulceration, total parenteral nutrition are the most frequent features.

Precautions before anesthesia: Check volemia, baseline cell blood count, and electrolytes.

Anesthetic considerations: The anesthetic considerations must be adapted according to the procedure. For instance, discontinue total parenteral nutrition perioperatively and adapt intravenous glucose administration (10% solution might be necessary) to prevent hypoglycemia.

Pharmacological implications: No reported pharmacological implications.

REFERENCES:

Cardenas A, Kelly CP: Celiac sprue. *Semin Gastrointest Dis* 13:232, 2002.

Freeman HJ: Small bowel malignant lymphoma complicating celiac sprue and the mesenteric lymph node cavitation syndrome. *Gastroenterology* 90:2008, 1986.

Lynch Syndrome

At a glance: Genetically transmitted predisposition to develop colorectal cancers.

Synonyms: Cancer Family Syndrome; Familial Cancer Syndrome; Hereditary Nonpolyposis Colorectal Cancer (HNPCC); Hereditary Nonpolyposis Colorectal Carcinoma.

History: First described by Alder Scott Warthin, an American pathologist, in 1913.

Incidence: Five percent of the colorectal cancer population.

Genetic inheritance: Both clinical forms of HNPCC are autosomal dominant with a penetrance of 85 to 90%. Two DNA mismatch repair genes are closely linked to the disease: hMSH2 gene in chromosome 2p and hMLS1 gene in chromosome 3p. Mutations in these genes account for 90% of all known HNPCC families.

Pathophysiology: Defective DNA mismatch repair leads to accumulation of mutations. The mutation load can be identified as errors in long tandem repeat sequences, which produce microsatellite instability.

Diagnosis: Familial history, colonic screening examinations, DNA genetic testing.

Clinical aspects: Two clinical forms described:

- *Lynch Syndrome I:* Familial predisposition to early-onset colorectal cancer (mainly right colon).
- *Lynch Syndrome II:* Same features and familial predisposition with an associated predisposition for other primary cancers (often female reproductive organs, particularly endometrial carcinoma). This variant is not easily recognized because of the lack of phenotypical expression as familiar adenomatous polyposis.

Precautions before anesthesia: All precautions before anesthesia will be dictated by those associated with the patient's underlying medical condition.

Anesthetic considerations: Anesthetic considerations are those associated with the surgical procedure only or any associated medical conditions.

Pharmacological implications: No specific pharmacological implications except for patients receiving chemotherapy.

REFERENCES:

de Vos tot Nederveen Cappel WH, Nagengast FM, Griffioen G, et al: Surveillance for hereditary nonpolyposis colorectal cancer: A long-term study on 114 families. *Dis Colon Rectum* 45:1588, 2002.

Mitchell RJ, Farrington SM, Dunlop MG, et al: Mismatch repair genes hMLH1 and hMSH2 and colorectal cancer: A HuGE review. *Am J Epidemiol* 156:885, 2002.

Wagner A, Tops C, Wijnen JT, et al: Genetic testing in hereditary non-polyposis colorectal cancer families with a MSH2, MLH1, or MSH6 mutation. *J Med Genet* 39:833, 2002.

Lysinuric Protein Intolerance

At a glance: Autosomal recessive disease characterized by defective transport of the dibasic amino acids. Failure to thrive, poor growth during childhood, hepatomegaly, splenomegaly, sparse hair, and muscle hypotonia. Normal development to moderate mental retardation.

Synonym: Hyperdibasic Aminoaciduria type II.

Incidence: The highest known incidence is observed in Finland with 1:60,000 live births. Other areas with a high incidence are Japan, Italy, and Turkey; however, only approximately 100 patients have been described in the literature.

Genetic inheritance: Transmission is autosomal recessive, with the defect linked to chromosome 14q11.2.

Diagnosis: Caused by a defect in the renal and intestinal transport system for lysine and for ornithine and arginine (dibasic amino acid transport). In contrast to patients with cystinuria, these patients do not have increased urinary cystine excretion.

Clinical aspects: Symptoms can become apparent any time after birth, although breast-feeding seems to delay the onset (probably because of its low-protein content). However, as soon as these patients receive nutrition with a higher protein content, hyperammonemia, diarrhea, nausea, vomiting, and even coma may occur. If undiagnosed, additional clinical symptoms, including failure to thrive as a consequence of the episodes of diarrhea and vomiting, mild-to-moderate hepatosplenomegaly, osteoporosis, and sparse scalp hair,

may develop. Hyperammonemia is usually present only after protein feeding, which is thought to be the result of a disturbance in the urea cycle secondary to decreased levels of arginine and ornithine. Mild-to-severe anemia has been reported in some of these patients who are on a low-protein diet with citrulline replacement. Osteoporosis is often severe and in childhood results in fractures after only minor trauma. Glomerulosclerosis and chronic interstitial lung disease are not uncommon. A potential fatal complication in these patients is an interstitial pneumonia with alveolar proteinosis. The cause for complication is unknown. Intermittent hemophagocytotic lymphohistiocytosis with increased levels of ferritin and lactate dehydrogenase and an association with systemic lupus erythematosus have been reported to be a regular feature of this syndrome. L-Arginine deficiency was also responsible for vascular endothelial dysfunction via a decrease in nitric oxide production, which became normal after an L-arginine infusion. In another report, the L-arginine deficiency was found to be responsible for thrombocytopenia and increased antithrombin III levels, which normalized after an L-arginine infusion or transdermal nitroglycerin application. Mental development is usually normal, although frequent and long-lasting episodes of hyperammonemia are considered deleterious for the brain, and amazing recoveries have been reported under strict diet.

Precautions before anesthesia: An anesthesiology consultation is highly recommended before elective surgical procedures. Proper evaluation of intravascular volemia, electrolyte imbalance, and feeding habits. The patient should be admitted the day before surgery to allow proper fluid resuscitation and electrolyte correction. Obtain a coagulation profile and bleeding time; if abnormal, correct immediately. Anemia is often present and requires correction. In the presence of moderate-to-severe hyperammonemia, elective surgery should be delayed until proper correction, to avoid neurologic deficit.

Anesthetic considerations: No reports about anesthesia in these patients were found. Obtain a complete cell blood count, clotting screen, electrolytes, BUN, and creatinine, as well as pulmonary, liver, and kidney function tests. Depending on the severity of the interstitial lung disease and the planned procedure, the need for postoperative mechanical ventilation support should be anticipated. Be cautious if the patient is on total parental nutrition; it must be maintained or replaced by properly adjusted glucose fluid administrations. Careful positioning is required to prevent fractures in the presence of severe osteoporosis. Immunologic problems have been reported in some of these patients; consequently, a strict aseptic technique is recommended.

Pharmacological implications: No known specific pharmacological implication to anesthetic agents.

Other conditions to be considered:

☞**BLUE DIAPER SYNDROME:** Genetic disorder with defective transport for L-tryptophan resulting in blue urine. It is characterized by the presence of hypercalcemia and nephrocalcinosis. Bacterial degradation of the tryptophan leads to excessive indole production and to indicanuria that, on oxidation to indigo blue, causes a peculiar bluish discoloration of the diaper. Although almost certainly recessive, the disorder could be X-linked. It has also been suggested that it results from blue-green discoloration of the stools by a pigment elaborated by *Pseudomonas aeruginosa*.

☞**HARTNUP SYNDROME/DISEASE:** Autosomal recessive disorder caused by a defective transport of tryptophan and other neutral (i.e., monoamino-monocarboxylic) amino acids in the small intestine and kidney. Patients may present with a pellagra-like skin condition, cerebellar ataxia, and gross aminoaciduria.

☞**DIAMINOPENTANURIA:** Increased renal clearance of cystine, lysine, arginine, and ornithine as a result of dysfunction of the reabsorptive capacity of the renal tubules. In addition, defective intestinal absorption results in increased degradation of these amino acids by bacteria in the intestine.

☞**HYPERPROLINEMIA:** Autosomal recessive inherited disorder with decreased renal tubular reabsorption of glycine and the amino acids proline and hydroxyproline. Patients with type II of the disease may be taking antiseizure medication, so epileptogenic drugs should be avoided.

REFERENCES:

Duval M, Fenneteau O, Doireau V, et al: Intermittent hemophagocytic lymphohistiocytosis is a regular feature of lysinuric protein intolerance. *J Pediatr* 134:236, 1999.

Kamada Y, Nagaretani H, Tamura S, et al: Vascular endothelial dysfunction resulting from L-arginine deficiency in a patient with lysinuric protein intolerance. *J Clin Invest* 108:717, 2001.

Kayanoki Y, Kawata S, Yamasaki E: Reduced nitric oxide production by L-arginine deficiency in lysinuric protein intolerance exacerbates intravascular coagulation. *Metabolism* 48:1136, 1999.

Machado-Joseph Disease

At a glance: Rare hereditary neurodegenerative disorder, also called *spinocerebellar ataxia type III,* which is characterized by weakness of arms and legs, spasticity, and a staggering lurching gait easily mistaken from drunkenness. Other clinical features include dysphagia, severe nystagmus, dystonia, and twitching of the tongue. Some patients have peculiar exophthalmos.

Synonyms: Spinocerebellar Ataxia Type III; Machado Disease; Joseph Disease; Portuguese-Azorean Disease; Azorean Neurologic Disease; Spinocerebellar Atrophy Type III; Spinopontine Atrophy; Nigro-Spino-Dental Degeneration.

Classification: The differences in the types of Machado-Joseph disease (MJD) relate to the age of onset and severity.

Machado-Joseph Disease Type I (MJD-I): Characterized by age of onset between 10 and 30 years and presents a rapid evolution. Clinical features include a combination of dystonic and spastic muscle in the arms and legs, ataxia often associated with athetosis and dysarthria (as observed with drunkenness, slurred speech), ophthalmoplegia, and exophthalmia. Mental alertness and intellectual capacities are unaffected.

Machado-Joseph Disease Type II (MJD-II): Characterized by a symptomatology similar to that observed in type I; however, the progression of the disease is slower. The age of onset is usually between 20 and 50 years. The distinctive characteristic of MJD-II is the presence of ataxia associated with increasing hypertonicity in the arms and legs, leading to significant difficulties in controlling movements.

Machado-Joseph Disease Type III (MJD-III): Characterized by a late onset between ages 40 and 70 years, severe ataxia, and slow degeneration of the central nervous system, particularly the hindbrain, motor polyneuropathy, and lateral amyotrophy. Individuals affected with this condition may become paralyzed early in their teens or during early adulthood. Individuals affected with this condition present with loss of feeling, lack of sensitivity to pain, impaired ability to coordinate movement of the arms and legs, and diabetes. The progression of type III disease is slowest of the three types.

Incidence: Machado-Joseph disease is one type of autosomal dominant spinocerebellar ataxia. More than 100 families worldwide have been described. Many of them live in the eastern United States and in Japan and have ancestors from Portugal or the Azorean Islands. Estimated to be 0.1:100,000 persons in Japan.

Genetic inheritance: Machado-Joseph disease reflects a CAG triplet expansion on chromosome 14q32.1. Studies of numerous kindreds suggest the heterogeneous phenotypic expression of MJD may be related to the number of CAG repeats. A phenomenon of anticipation is associated a higher number of repeats with earlier onset.

Pathophysiology: Histologically, degenerative changes with neuronal loss and astrocytosis are seen in various loci of the cerebellum, midbrain, brainstem, and medulla.

Diagnosis: Based on the clinical manifestations, family history, and genetic analysis.

Clinical aspects: Except for type I in which teens can begin to show symptoms, the onset age of symptoms in MJD is most often during adulthood. Manifestations of MJD are variable and include progressive ataxia, dystonia, spasticity, facial and lingual fasciculations, bulbar signs with impaired speech and dysphagia, and ocular findings, such as bulging and injected eyes, nystagmus, or external ophthalmoplegia. Intellectual function remains intact. The disease is progressive and generally leads to death within 15 years on average, usually from respiratory failure and pneumonia. Diabetes mellitus can be present.

Precautions before anesthesia: The presence of pharyngeal dysfunction and muscular weakness should be assessed. Chest radiography should be performed, looking for signs of aspiration and pneumonia. Pulmonary function testing with measurement of maximum inspiratory and expiratory flows allows a more objective assessment of respiratory muscle function. Current medication with a potential for drug interactions with anesthetic agents must be expected. Check if the patient is receiving dopaminergic or monoamine oxidase inhibitor medication. Inquire if the patient has diabetes mellitus.

Anesthetic considerations: No reports about anesthesia in these patients have been published. In case of bulging eyes, perioperative eye care should be provided to prevent corneal injury. Impaired airway protection from pharyngeal dysfunction and alveolar hypoventilation from respiratory muscle weakness should be expected in advanced disease. Weaning from mechanical ventilation might be difficult. Patient's perception of impaired control over airways and breathing might increase anxiety. Continue dopaminergic medication up to the morning of the operation. Treat diabetes mellitus in a standard manner. There may be cardiovascular instability because of autonomic defects.

Pharmacological implications: Avoid drugs with antidopaminergic effects such as phenothiazines, butyrophenones (droperidol), or ketamine. Because of diffuse axonal changes and muscular denervation, hyperkalemic cardiac arrest following succinylcholine is a possibility. If muscle relaxation is necessary, small doses of short-acting agents should be titrated. Succinylcholine should be regarded as contraindicated.

Other conditions to be considered: Machado-Joseph disease is part of many different inherited types of spinocerebellar ataxia with variable phenotypic expression.

SANCHEZ-CORONA SYNDROME (**Spinocerebellar Ataxia-Dysmorphism Syndrome**): Presents with characteristic craniofacial features (dolichocephaly, exophthalmos, blepharoptosis, downslanting corners of the mouth), delayed psychomotor development, dysarthria, delayed psychomotor development, scoliosis, foot deformities, and peculiar gait.

☞HALLERVORDEN-SPATZ DISEASE: Rare inherited disorder characterized by a slow and steady hypertonia of the muscles of the arms, legs, neck, face, mouth, or trunk. Other clinical features include muscle spasms, dysarthria, mental retardation, dysphasia, and amyotrophy.

OLIVOPONTOCEREBELLAR ATROPHY TYPES I AND II (**Spinocerebellar Atrophy Type II; Holguin Olivopontocerebellar Atrophy Syndrome; Cuban Spinocerebellar Ataxia Syndrome**): Group of rare inherited neurologic disorders characterized by progressive neurologic degeneration. The clinical symptomatology includes ataxia, muscle spasms, athetosic movements, abnormal posture, dysarthria, and extrapyramidal behavioral signs. Age of onset varies according to the type.

PROGRESSIVE SUPRANUCLEAR PALSY (Steele-Richardson-Olszewski Syndrome): An autosomal dominant inherited disorder characterized by muscular spasticity of the face, throat and tongue, axial rigidity, slowness of movement, and gait difficulty. The age of onset begins during middle age. Presents as severe ataxia and most often unexplained falls.

MARIE ATAXIA: Rare inherited neurologic disorder characterized by progressive loss of muscle coordination, severe ataxia, and progressive spinal nerve degeneration leading to amyotrophy in the arms, legs, head, and neck.

PARENCHYMATOUS CORTICAL DEGENERATION OF THE CEREBELLUM (Cerebelloparenchymal Disorder Syndrome Types I and II): Characterized by ataxia and dysarthria developing in the fourth or fifth decades of life. Estimated prevalence in the Japanese population has been established at 4.53:100,000 population. Fifteen percent of patients affected with this disorder are believed to have a late-onset pure cerebellar condition that is most often referred to as late cortical cerebellar atrophy. It may be inherited or acquired.

REFERENCES:

Evidente VG, Gueinn-Hardy KA, Caviness JN, et al: Hereditary ataxia. *Mayo Clin Proc* 75:475, 2001.

Kawaguchi Y, Okamoto T, Taniwaki M, et al: CAG expansions in a novel gene for Machado-Joseph disease at chromosome 14q32.1. *Nat Genet* 8:221, 1994.

Sanchez-Corona J, Garcia-Cruz D, Gonzalez-Angulo A, et al: A distinct dysmorphic syndrome with spinocerebellar ataxia and probable autosomal recessive inheritance. *Hum Genet* 69:243, 1985.

Sudarsky L, Coutinho P: Machado-Joseph disease. *Clin Neurosci* 3:17, 1995.

Macrocephaly, Hypertelorism, Short Limbs, and Hearing Loss Syndrome

At a glance: Rare association of macrocephaly, hypertelorism, short stature, and hearing loss. Other clinical features include sparse hair, hypertelorism, dowslanting palpebral fissures, and delayed psychomotor development.

Synonym: Bagatelle Cassidy Syndrome.

History: First described by R. Bagatelle and S.B. Cassidy in 1995.

Incidence and genetic inheritance: One case report has been published. The parents were of European and Native American descent. Chromosomal and metabolic workup was normal.

Clinical aspects: Features of the described child included macrocephaly, widely open fontanelles, hypertelorism, broad and flat nasal bridge, mild macroglossia, and mild micrognathia. Other features included mild to moderate and static neurosensory hearing loss, hoarse and low-pitched voice, short stature with short metacarpals, and mild developmental delay. The child had a few apneic spells with feeding during early infancy.

Anesthetic considerations: Features of midface dysplasia, mild macroglossia, and mild micrognathia might lead to difficult direct laryngoscopy and tracheal intubation. However, the described boy had surgery for chronic nasal and sinus congestion and no anesthetic difficulties were reported.

REFERENCE:

Bagatelle R, Cassidy SB: New syndrome of macrocephaly, hypertelorism, short limbs, hearing loss, and developmental delay. *Am J Med Genet* 55:367, 1995.

Maffucci Syndrome

At a glance: Genetic disorder characterized by enchondromas (benign tumors of cartilage), and multiple cavernous hemangiomas, often involving the head and neck. Bone and cartilage deformities appear during childhood in the years before puberty. Pathologic fractures and sarcomas. Normal intelligence.

Synonyms: Maffucci-Kast Syndrome; Kast Syndrome; Chondrodysplasia-Hemangioma Syndrome.

History: First reported in 1881 by Angelo Maffucci, an Italian pathologist. This congenital disorder is characterized by dyschondroplasia of one or more limbs, multiple enchondromas, and soft tissue hemangiomas.

Incidence: Rare; fewer than 100 cases have been reported in the United States, whereas approximately 160 case reports have been discussed in the English literature. There is no increased frequency because of race, no sexual bias, and the lesions are first noted by age 4 or 5 years.

Genetic inheritance: Genetic disorder that is expressed in both sexes, but males are more frequently affected. Sporadic occurrence (noninherited), although familial cases have been reported. Gene locus is short arm of chromosome 3 (3p22-p21.1).

Pathophysiology: Medical condition that affects the skin and the skeletal systems. Asymmetrical hemangiomas (blue subcutaneous nodules) often protrude as soft nodules or tumors usually on the distal extremities. Thrombi often form within vessels and develop into phleboliths. These phleboliths appear as calcified vessels under microscopic examination. Venous-lymphatic malformations can occur but are much less common. Enchondromas are benign cartilaginous tumors that can appear anywhere but are usually found on the phalanges and the long bones. Neoplastic changes occur in enchondromas. Approximately 30 to 37% of enchondromas can develop into a chondrosarcoma, which is the most common neoplasm. The average age for neoplastic change is 40 years.

Diagnosis: Based on clinical findings. Biopsy of soft tissue and bony lesions that are rapidly growing is mandatory to exclude malignant changes. Characteristic radiographic findings of ovoid, pyramidal-shaped, and linear translucent defects in the metaphyses of affected long bones and in flat bones.

Clinical aspects: Manifestations usually after second year of life. Vascular lesions (usually cavernous sometimes capillary and mixed capillary-venous anomalies) often appear in infancy and commonly involve hands and feet. They are soft, compressible blue or purple vascular malformations that enlarge in proportion to the child's growth. Twenty-five percent of patients have hemangiomas in the head and neck region, including pharynx, tongue, and trachea. Hemangiomas in the cervical spine may result in paraplegia, whereas those involving the gastrointestinal tract may cause severe bleeding. Skeletal changes consist of multiple enchondromas, exostoses, and recurrent fractures (phalangeal and metacarpal bones). Long bone involvement is common and leads to progressive skeletal deformity and pathologic fractures. Scoliosis occurs in one third of patients. Encroachment of cranial enchondromas on the cerebral cortex may result in neurologic deficits or intracranial hypertension. Endocrine

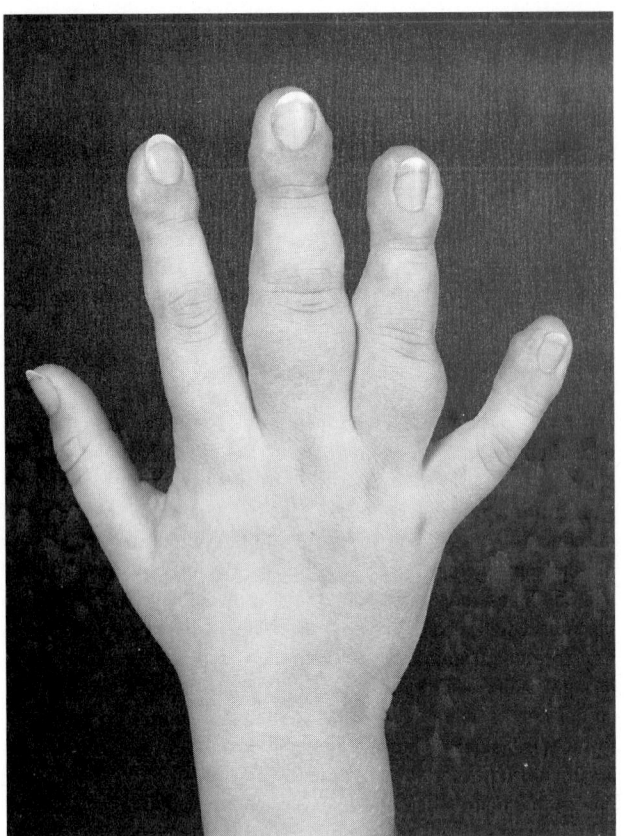

Mafucci syndrome   Gross deformity of the hand as a result of multiple enchondromas in a woman with Mafucci syndrome.

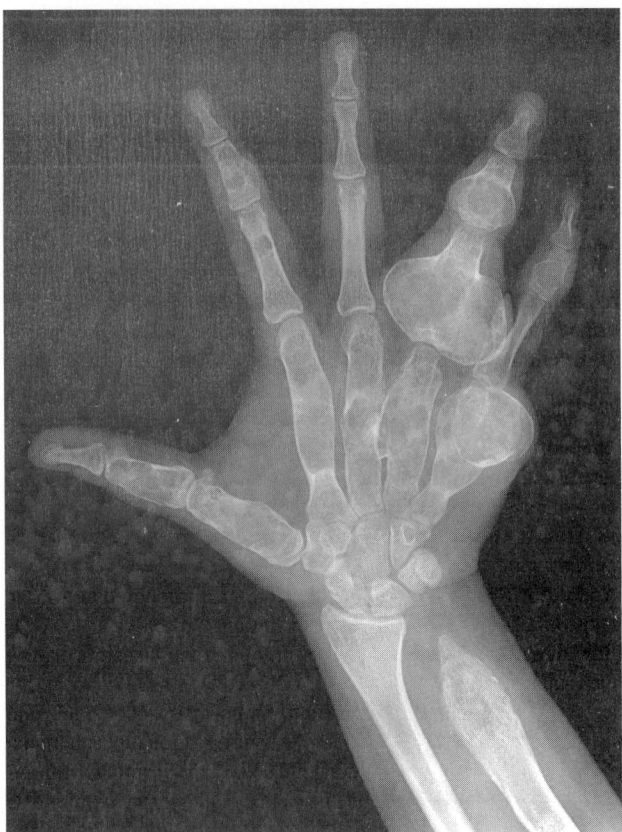

Mafucci syndrome   Radiograph of the hand showing multiple enchondromas in the fingers, metacarpalia, and the ulna (with bone destruction).

abnormalities have been described, such as pituitary adenoma and Cushing syndrome. Malignant changes of the lesions have been reported in 5 to 15% of patients. Chondrosarcomas are especially common and occur in 30% of patients. Careful clinical and radiologic follow-up in patients with this syndrome is necessary to allow early detection of malignant changes. Surgical resection of enchondromas for patients with marked impairment of function, disfigurement, or suspected malignant changes.

Precautions before anesthesia: Examine the oral cavity and upper airway for the presence of hemangiomas. If significant scoliosis is present, a detailed respiratory evaluation is necessary (chest radiography, arterial blood gas analysis, pulmonary function test). Examine for CNS deficits indicative of intracranial or spinal canal lesions. Investigations: complete blood count, coagulation status.

Anesthetic considerations: Long bones are prone to pathologic fractures, requiring careful handling of the patient. In case of severe scoliosis, consider restrictive lung disease and difficult positioning. Adequate padding needed for vascular lesions. Use of a central neuraxial block may be complicated by bony abnormalities or increased risk of perimedullar hematoma (asymptomatic spinal hemangioma). Acute bleeding from surgically disrupted hemangiomas could be significant. Hemangiomas may be present in the airway and could make tracheal intubation difficult. High-output cardiac failure if hemangiomas are large. Intracranial chondrosarcomas may cause raised intracranial pressure. Limited joint mobility may make airway management difficult and positioning awkward. May be more prone to pathologic fractures and must be handled carefully. Hemangiomas

on extremities could interfere with placement of intravenous and arterial catheters.

Pharmacological implication: Patients may be sensitive to cardiovascular-depressant medications, and inotropic support may be required.

Other conditions to be considered:

OLLIER DISEASE (Multiple Spondyloenchondromatosis Syndrome; Spondyloenchondrodysplasia Syndrome): Characterized by multiple enchondromas. Clinical problems caused by enchondromas include skeletal deformity and the potential for malignant change to osteosarcoma. It appears to be inherited as autosomal recessive. In comparison to the Mafucci syndrome, Ollier disease does not have hemangiomata.

☞**KLIPPEL-TRENAUNAY SYNDROME:** Characterized by large cutaneous hemangiomata with hypertrophy of the related bones and soft tissues. It is often considered a blood vessel disorder combining nevus flammeus (port-wine stain), excessive growth of soft tissue and bone, and varicose veins. Onset usually occurs before birth or during infancy or early childhood.

☞**BLUE RUBBER BLEB NEVUS SYNDROME:** Blood vessel disorder characterized by benign growths in the skin and gastrointestinal tract present at birth. The skin lesions are usually elevated and blue or purplish-red in color. Other clinical features include nocturnal pain and regional hyperhidrosis. Bleeding hemangiomas of the gastrointestinal tract are an important complication. Angiomatous gigantism of a limb and the presence of multiple enchondromata have been reported. Blue rubber bleb nevi can be seen over the entire surface of the body and in the mucosa of the oropharynx, esophagus, distal ileum, and anus.

☞**PROTEUS SYNDROME:** Characterized by multiple, diverse, somatic manifestations, partial bilateral gigantism of hands and feet, nevi, hemihypertrophy, subcutaneous tumors, macrocephaly, and cranial hyperostoses.

REFERENCES:

Akagi S, Saito T, Ogawa R: Maffucci's syndrome involving hemangioma in the cervical spine. *Spine* 20:1510, 1995.

Chan SK, Ng SK, Cho AM, Oh TE: Anaesthetic implications of Maffucci's syndrome. *Anaesth Intensive Care* 26:586, 1998.

Kaplan RP, Wang JT, Amron DM, et al: Maffucci's syndrome: Two case reports with a literature review. *J Am Acad Dermatol* 29:894, 1993.

Majocchi Disease

At a glance: Rare idiopathic disorder characterized by pigmented purpuric dermatitis caused by chronic inflammation of capillaries. A chronic disease of mostly unknown etiology showing very distinctive clinical appearance (extravasation of erythrocytes in the skin with marked hemosiderin deposition).

Synonym: Purpura Annularis Telangiectodes; Pigmented Purpuric Eruption.

Incidence: Uncommon disease that occurs predominantly in children and young adults; seems to affect males more frequently. During a 10-month period, ten cases were reported in the United kingdom from a dermatology practice that serves a population of 300,000 persons. Five patients were diagnosed with lichen aureus and the remainder had more extensive capillaritis.

Genetic inheritance: None.

Pathophysiology: Chronic inflammation of capillaries in the upper dermis. Venous hypertension, exercise, and gravitational dependency are important cofactors that appear to influence disease presentation. There is perivascular T-cell lymphocytic infiltrate centered on the superficial small blood vessels of the skin, which show signs of endothelial cell swelling and narrowing of the lumen.

Diagnosis: Characteristic small, reddish macules that vary in shape and distribution, ranging from 2 mm to more than 2 cm, and found predominantly on the buttock and lower extremities. Biopsy demonstrates capillary telangiectasis, pericapillary infiltration of mononuclear cells, erythrocyte extravasation into superficial dermal connective tissue, and (rare) hemosiderin deposition into macrophages.

Clinical aspects: Although this disease has a benign nature, it must be distinguished from other systemic purpuric diseases.

Precautions before anesthesia: Check cell blood count to rule out thrombocytopenia and anemia.

Anesthetic considerations: Per procedure. There are no case reports of anesthetics in patients with this disease.

Pharmacological implications: No known pharmacological implications. However, pigmented purpuric dermatoses may show hypersensitivity to drugs such as carbamazepine, furosemide, and nitroglycerin.

Other conditions to be considered:

SCHAMBERG DISEASE: Pigmented purpuric dermatitis that may occur at any age. It is a chronic discoloration of the skin that usually affects the legs and spreads slowly. Leaky blood vessels al-

low red cells to extravasate into the skin. It gives an appearance of "cayenne pepper" spots because of the hemosiderin deposits. Some itching may be present. It was described by J. Schlamberg in 1901.

GOUGEROT BLUM DISEASE: Mainly affects men between 40 and 50 years old. It is characterized by a peculiar form of hemorrhagic pigmentary dermatosis and lichenoid plaques on the legs. Rust-colored papules, purpuric and telangiectatic. Both sexes affected; prevalent in females, onset in middle life. First described by H. Gougerot, French dermatologist, in 1925.

LICHEN AUREUS DISEASE: Similar to Majocchi disease because of its increased incidence in children and young adults. Characterized by yellowish/red papules or patches appearing bilaterally on the lower limbs; can also be seen on the trunk and upper limbs. Usually responds to high-dose steroids.

REFERENCE:

Nichamin SJ: Chronic progressive pigmentary purpura: Purpura annulares telangiectodes of Majocchi-Schamberg. *Am J Dis Child* 116:429, 1968.

Mallory-Weiss Syndrome

At a glance: Sporadic condition characterized by esophageal bleeding caused by a mucosal tear in the esophagus as a result of forceful or prolonged vomiting.

History: First described in 1929 by George Kenneth Mallory and Soma Weiss, American physicians.

Incidence: Uncommon in children. Responsible for 11 to 13% of significant upper gastrointestinal bleedings in adults.

Genetic inheritance: No genetic component.

Pathophysiology: Prolonged or forceful vomiting can increase intraesophageal pressure significantly. This may result in lacerations, usually at the gastroesophageal junction. In adults the tears are usually confined to the gastroesophageal junction (49%) but may extend into the esophagus (15%) and stomach (33%). Significant bleeding is unusual and is most likely to occur if the tear extends into the vascular cardia.

Diagnosis: Endoscopy of the upper gastrointestinal tracts reveals superficial, longitudinal tears in the esophageal mucosa in the acute phase. Granulation tissue forms later, and the lesion may appear as a white raised streak.

Clinical aspects: Patients usually present with hematemesis after an episode of acute, severe and prolonged vomiting. Bleeding is usually painless and is rarely significant enough to require blood transfusion. In children, specific treatment is rarely required. If bleeding persists, then treatment modalities include vasopressin, angiographic-guided embolization, and, rarely, surgical control of the bleeding. Pediatric patients usually require anesthesia for endoscopy.

Precautions before anesthesia: Careful history to determine cause of vomiting and the extent of bleeding. Blood examination: hemoglobin to determine blood loss; blood transfusion if necessary. Consider patient to have full stomach, particularly if bleeding has been extensive.

Anesthetic considerations: Correction of anemia and hypovolemia if necessary. Rapid-sequence induction.

Pharmacological implications: May require perioperative antiemetic therapy.

REFERENCES:

Gryboski J: Traumatic injury of the esophagus, in Walker W, Durie P, Hamilton J, Walker-Smith J, Watkins J (eds): *Pediatric Gastrointestinal Disease.* 2nd ed. Mosby, St. Louis, 1996, p 444.

Michel L, Serrano A, Malt R: Mallory-Weiss syndrome: Evolution of diagnostic and therapeutic patterns over two decades. *Ann Surg* 192:716, 1980.

Crisponi G, Marras AR, Corrias A: Two sibs with Malpuech syndrome. *Am J Med Genet* 86:294, 1999.

Guion-Almeida ML: Apparent Malpuech syndrome: Report of three Brazilian patients with additional signs. *Am J Med Genet* 58:13, 1995.

Malpuech Syndrome

At a glance: Genetic disorder characterized by an association of mental retardation, dwarfism, hypertelorism, facial clefting, and urogenital abnormalities. Other features include malar hypoplasia, large fontanelle, cleft lip and palate, omphalocele, seizures, polycystic kidneys, and deafness.

Synonym: Facial Cleft Syndrome, Gypsy type.

Incidence: Rare.

History: First was described in 1983 by G. Malpuech, a French pediatrician, in four sibs of a Gypsy family. Ten patients, seven males and three females, have been reported.

Genetic inheritance: Inherited in an autosomal recessive mode.

Pathophysiology: Unknown.

Diagnosis: Based on clinical stigmata and family history.

Clinical aspects: All individuals had facial malformations, including cleft lip and palate, hypertelorism, and a wide forehead. All had growth retardation, and 8 of 10 were mentally retarded. Other common findings were arched eyebrows, proptosis, malar hypoplasia, and urogenital malformations. Tear duct atresia, omphalocele or umbilical hernia, caudal spine anomalies, and hearing loss are less common.

Precautions before anesthesia: Facial malformations and associated anomalies must be assessed prior to anesthesia.

Anesthetic considerations: Expect a difficult tracheal intubation from malar hypoplasia and midline cleft. Whether Malpuech syndrome patients with spinal malformations have an increased risk of latex allergy, as do spina bifida patients, is not known.

Pharmacological implications: No known implication with this condition.

Other conditions to be considered:

☞**KRIEBLE-BIXLER SYNDROME:** Rare autosomal recessive disorder; nine cases in seven families have been reported. Hypertelorism, microtia, and clefting of lip or palate are the hallmarks of this syndrome. Other associated features may include cardiac and urogenital defects, cleft nose, limb anomalies, and possible (mild) mental retardation.

CRANIOSYNOSTOSIS-MENTAL RETARDATION-CLEFTING SYNDROME (Baraitser Rodeck Garner Syndrome): In 1982, Baraitser et al. described a 5-year-old girl with cleft lip and palate, bat ears, an oddly shaped skull, hypertelorism, a prominent nasal bridge, bilateral coloboma, short forearms and legs with stubby fingers, cystic dysplasia of the kidneys, and a seizure disorder with developmental delay. In addition, her mother had another pregnancy terminated because fetoscopy revealed similar malformations in a male fetus.

REFERENCES:

Amiel J, Faivre L, Marianowskl R, et al: Hypertelorism-microtia-clefting syndrome (Bixler syndrome): A report of two unrelated cases. *Clin Dysmorphol* 10:15, 2001.

Mannosidosis

At a glance: Lysosomal glycoprotein storage disease with mental retardation, hearing loss, and recurrent infections (upper or lower respiratory tract, and gastrointestinal tract). Other clinical features include coarse face, prominent forehead, prominent jaw, diffuse dysfunction of the brain, severe ataxia, deafness, scoliosis, rheumatoid arthritis, hypotonia, and muscle pain. Two types are described: α and β. α-Mannosidosis displays clinical heterogeneity, ranging from very serious to very mild forms. β-Mannosidosis causes a severe disorder that affects the peripheral and central nervous systems.

Synonym: Lysosomal Mannosidosis Deficiency Syndrome.

History: First reported in 1967 by Oeckerman in Lund, Sweden, who described a boy affected with mental retardation, increased tissue total mannose concentration, and susceptibility to infection.

Incidence: Rare; approximately 100 cases of α-mannosidosis and 10 to 15 cases of β-mannosidosis have been described. Found in all ethic groups in Europe, America, Africa, and Asia.

Genetic inheritance: Autosomal recessive genetic disorder, 2.5:1 male preponderance. The α-mannosidase gene maps to chromosome 19p13.2-q12. The β-mannosidase gene is located at chromosome 4q22-25. Prenatal diagnosis is possible.

Pathophysiology: α-Mannosidosis is a disorder of glycoprotein catabolism associated with abnormal levels and excretion of mannose-rich oligosaccharides, caused by a deficiency of its catabolic enzyme α-mannosidase. β-Mannosidosis results from β-mannosidase deficiency with an increase in the corresponding oligosaccharide. Both enzymes are located in the lysosomes.

Diagnosis: Usually made by measuring enzyme activity in white blood cells and eventually by measuring certain substances in urine. Increased urinary oligosaccharides as measured by thin-layer chromatography confirms the type. Measuring activity in lymphoblasts correlates with severity. Pathology shows multiple vacuoles in lymphocytes and hepatocytes. Clinical history and physical findings are considered important in the diagnosis.

Clinical aspects: *Facies:* The very typical facial characteristics of mannosidosis are a coarse face, a prominent forehead, a flattened nasal bridge, a small nose, and prominent jaw. *Cerebral symptoms:* The disease causes a diffuse dysfunction of the brain characterized by delayed early landmarks of neural development and severe ataxia. *Hearing problems:* Central and peripheral deafness. *Immunodeficiency:* Recurrent infections are a main feature of the disease. These infections are in the upper or lower respiratory tract, middle ear, or gastrointestinal tract. *Skeletal:* Scoliosis, rheumatoid arthritis, ataxia. *Muscular:* Muscular pain and weakness, which is caused by accumulation of storage material in the muscle and usually contributes to the immobilization of the patient.

α-*Mannosidosis:* Type I or severe infantile phenotype (onset between 3 and 12 months) includes rapid, progressive mental retardation, coarse facies resembling mucopolysaccharidosis, hepatosplenomegaly, dysostosis multiplex, recurrent bacterial infections with death between 3 and 12 years. Type II or juvenile-adult phenotype (onset between 1 and 4 years) is milder and slowly progressive with survival into adulthood. Other clinical features include spastic paraplegia (vertebral bodies abnormalities) and pancytopenia. In both types, deafness, cataracts, corneal opacifications, and vacuolated lymphocytes are present. Recurrent infections could be caused by a defect in leukocyte chemotaxis. Dysostosis multiplex causes skeletal dysplasia, ovoid configuration or flattening of the vertebral bodies, and kyphosis.

β-Mannosidosis: Rarer, and ranges from mild features (mental retardation, behavioral problems, angiokeratomas, mild facial dysmorphism) to severe (status epilepticus, quadriplegia, and early death). Respiratory infections are common, caused by swallowing difficulties or abnormal esophageal motility.

Successful bone marrow transplantation has been reported in both cases.

Precautions before anesthesia: Chest radiography and SpO$_2$ (arterial oxyhemoglobin saturation) because frequent respiratory infections. Check neurologic and stability of the vertebral spine. ECG may be indicated (short PR interval reported). Liver function tests, CBC, coagulation screen if hepatosplenomegaly.

Anesthetic considerations: Airway manipulation may be problematic if the cervical spine is unstable. Gingival hyperplasia is sometimes present. Neuraxial regional blockade might be difficult because of skeletal dysplasia. Avoid tachycardia if short PR interval. Postoperative ventilation and reverse isolation (pancytopenia) might be necessary.

Pharmacological implications: Avoid succinylcholine if there is paraparesis. Interactions with antiepileptic drugs.

Other conditions to be considered:

☞**Hurler Syndrome:** Most severe form of mucopolysaccharidosis. It is characterized by a deficiency of the enzyme α-L-iduronidase, which results in accumulation of dermatan and heparan sulfates. Symptoms of the disorder first become evident at age 6 months to 2 years. Affected infants may experience developmental delays, recurrent urinary and upper respiratory tract infections, noisy breathing, and persistent nasal discharge. Additional physical problems may include clouding of the cornea of the eye, an unusually large tongue, severe deformity of the spine, and joint stiffness. Mental development begins to regress at approximately age 2 years. The clinical features observed with α-mannosidosis resemble closely the Hurler syndrome.

☞**Sialidosis:** Characterized by progressive lysosomal storage of sialidated glycopeptides and oligosaccharides caused by deficiency of the enzyme neuraminidase. There are two types of mucoliposis: type I and type II. Type I is the milder form, also known as the *normosomatic type* or the *cherry-red spot myoclonus syndrome.* Some patients classified as mucolipidosis I proved to have mannosidosis. Sialidosis type II is the more severe form with an earlier onset; it is also known as the *dysmorphic type.* Type II has been subdivided into juvenile and infantile forms. The clinical characteristics of mucoliposis type I include neurologic abnormalities, muscular hypotonia and hypotrophy, ataxia, myoclonus, seizures, coarse facies (Hurler-like facies), short trunk, barrel chest, spinal deformity, deafness, cherry-red spot, and severe mental retardation.

Mucolipidosis III (Pseudo-Hurler Polydystrophy): Characterized by painless joint stiffness, decreased mobility, dwarfism, coarse Hurler-like facial features, mild mental retardation, multiple defective bone formations, and aortic valve heart disease. Mobility may gradually diminish until puberty and then stabilize. It is considered a milder form of I-cell disease (mucolipidosis II).

☞**Mucopolysaccharidosis Type III:** Characterized by hyperactivity, sleep disorders, mental retardation, dysarthria (progressive loss of previously acquired skills), sensory hearing loss, and delays in attaining developmental milestones (e.g., crawling and walking). Affected individuals may experience seizures, ataxia, and aggressive behavior. Affected individuals may eventually lose the ability to walk. Four types have been described (A, B, C, and D), which are identified according to the enzyme deficiency. Many of the clinical findings observed in patients affected with mannosidosis resembled those in patients with mucopolysaccharidosis III.

References:

Gerards AM, Winia WP, Mesterga J, et al: Destructive joint disease in alpha-mannosidosis. A case-report and review of the literature. *Clin Rheumatol* 23:40, 2004.

Thomas G, Beaudet A: Disorders of glycoprotein degradation and structure, in Scriver CR, Baudet AL, Sly WS (eds): *The Metabolic and Molecular Basis of Inherited Disease.* 7th ed. New York, McGraw-Hill, 1995, p 2529.

Maple Syrup Urine Disease (MSUD)

At a glance: Inherited inborn error of metabolism caused by a complex enzymatic deficiency of branched-chain α-ketoacid dehydrogenase leading to the production of urine and sweat that smell like maple syrup. Clinical features include lethargy, hypotonia, seizures, bulging fontanelles, and progressive neurologic deterioration. Severe metabolic acidosis is the cause of death in the newborn.

Synonym: Branched-Chain Ketonuria.

History: First described in 1954 by Menkes et al., who lost 4 infants because of neurodegenerative disorder. The urine of these infants had a burned sugar smell. In 1955, Dancis et al., identified the pathogenic compounds as branched chain amino acids and in 1960 confirmed that decarboxylation was responsible.

Classification: Several conditions are described based on the clinical presentation and enzymatic defects for the MSUD.

Classic Severe Maple Syrup Urine Disease (Classic Severe MSUD; MSUD Type IA): Characterized by a progressive infantile cerebral dysfunction defined as lethargy, failure to thrive and weight loss, severe metabolic derangement, hypotonia and/or hypertonia, progressive encephalopathy, seizures, and rapidly coma. Affected newborns appear normal at birth, with symptoms developing between 4 and 7 days of age. Left untreated, death occurs by age 3 months. This is the most common form of the disorder, 50% or more of the ketoacids are derived from leucine.

Intermediate Maple Syrup Urine Disease (Intermediate MSUD; MSUD Type IB): Characterized by mental retardation, severe psychomotor delay, mild systemic acidosis, and markedly increased plasmatic levels of branched-chain amino acids and urinary branched-chain ketoacids. Other clinical features may include ophthalmoplegia, history of irritability, poor feeding, and failure to thrive.

Intermittent Maple Syrup Urine Disease (Intermittent MSUD; MSUD Type II): Characterized by episodic ataxia, lethargy, semicoma, and elevated urinary branched-chain ketoacids. Transient neurologic disorder can be a mode of presentation. Late onset of symptoms and clinical normality between attacks differentiate the condition from classic MSUD.

E3-Deficient Maple Syrup Urine Disease (MSUD Type III): Combined deficiency of the branched-chain α-ketoacid dehydrogenase pyruvate dehydrogenase and the α-ketoglutarate dehydrogenase complexes. Clinical features include progressive neurologic deterioration, irregular and difficult respiration, hypertonia, bilateral optic nerve atrophy, and persistent metabolic acidosis.

Thiamine-Responsive Maple Syrup Urine Disease (Thiamine-Responsive MSUD): Thiamine-responsive MSUD is approximately 30 to 40% the normal rate.

Incidence: 1:120,000 live births. Affects both males and females. All ethnic backgrounds. Increased incidence in the Mennonite (Amish) community in Pennsylvania, USA.

Genetic inheritance: Autosomal recessive.

Pathophysiology: Deficiency of the mitochondrial branched-chain α-ketoacid dehydrogenase enzyme system, which is responsible for decarboxylation of the three neutral branched-chain amino acids: leucine, isoleucine, and valine.

Diagnosis: Maple syrup odor of urine. Metabolic acidosis with elevated ketone bodies and sometimes hypoglycemia. Elevated plasma and urine levels of leucine, isoleucine, and valine. CT scan shows hypodensity and swelling of the cerebellar hemispheres, dorsal part of the pons and mesencephalon, posterior limb of the internal capsule, globus pallidus, and often the thalami.

Clinical aspects: Severity of clinical presentation varies according to the proportion of residual activity of the enzyme system. In the classic form, there is no enzymatic activity. Affected infants are normal at birth, but they develop poor feeding during the first week and progress to lethargy and coma. Convulsions occur frequently. Severe metabolic acidosis develops. Untreated patients die in infancy. In the other forms, which are called "mild" or "intermittent," acute crisis of metabolic acidosis occur in case of metabolic stress. These late forms are often responsive to chronic oral thiamine therapy (5–20 mg/kg/day). Treatment of the acute state involves removing amino acids, if necessary by peritoneal dialysis or hemodialysis, and providing sufficient calories to prevent catabolism (glucose, lipids, mixture free of branched-chain amino acids) and hypoglycemia. Long-term management involves administration of a low branched-chain amino acid and low protein (2 g/kg/day) diet and thiamine therapy. Dietary indiscretion and any situation resulting in a catabolic state, such as poor oral intake, vomiting, diarrhea, infection, or surgery, may precipitate acute deterioration with ketoacidosis and cerebral edema.

Precautions before anesthesia: Avoid prolonged fasting. Establish infusion of dextrose with or without lipid preoperatively. Assess blood glucose and acid–base status on a regular basis.

Anesthetic considerations: Acute deterioration may occur with stress of surgery, particularly in emergency situations. Adequate calorific intake should be maintained perioperatively to prevent hypoglycemia and catabolism. Acid–base status and blood glucose should be monitored perioperatively. Patients may develop cerebral edema, so excessive administration of intravenous fluid should be avoided. Gastric content should be aspirated in surgery with the potential for oral, nasal, or gastric bleeding because ingested blood presents a protein load and might trigger acute metabolic decompensation. Postoperatively, the patient should return to a normal dietary regimen as soon as possible.

Pharmacological implications: No pharmacological agents are specifically contraindicated.

REFERENCES:
Delaney A, Gal TJ: Hazards of anesthesia and operation in maple-syrup-urine disease. *Anesthesiology* 44:83, 1976.

Kahraman S, Ercan M, Akkus Ö, et al: Anaesthetic management in maple syrup urine disease. *Anaesthesia* 51:575, 1996.

Marden-Walker Syndrome

At a glance: Very rare inherited disorder characterized by blepharophimosis, immobile facies, abnormal jaw, microcytic disease of the kidney, and severe joint contractures. Other clinical features include curvature of the spine causing a hunchback, cleft lip and palate or high-arched palate, growth delay, and slow muscle movement.

Genetic inheritance: Autosomal recessive.

Clinical aspects: Prenatal and severe postnatal growth deficiency; moderate-to-severe mental retardation with hypotonia; microcephaly with fixed facial expression and blepharophimosis; micrognathia and small mouth; seizures, ventricular dilation, cerebellar hypoplasia, agenesis of corpus callosum; multiple joint contractures present at birth; scoliosis, arachnodactyly; clubfeet; pectus excavatum or carinatum, absent clavicles (rare); pulmonary hypoplasia (rare). Most children die in early infancy as a consequence of aspiration, infection, or cardiac failure.

Precautions before anesthesia: Check antiepileptic treatment, chest radiograph (chronic aspiration, lung hypoplasia). Proper cardiac investigation must be obtained. Kidney function should be evaluated.

Anesthetic considerations: Be prepared for difficult direct laryngoscopy and tracheal intubation; patients are at risk for perioperative aspiration; difficult venous access and positioning caused by joint contractures.

Pharmacological implications: No specific implications, except in patients with kidney dysfunction and those receiving medications for seizures and cardiovascular problems.

Other conditions to be considered:

☞**ARTHROGRYPOSIS MULTIPLEX CONGENITA:** Congenital disease characterized by reduced mobility of multiple joints at birth as a consequence of proliferation of fibrous tissue. Severe joint contractures.

☞**SCHWARTZ-JAMPEL SYNDROME:** Characterized by the inability of muscles to relax after contractures (myotonia). Typical are abnormal bone formation and abnormalities of the face and eyes, short stature, low birth weight, short neck, pectus carinatum, and hunchback curvature.

REFERENCE:
Williams MS, Josephson KD, Wargowski DS: Marden-Walker syndrome: A case report and a critical review of the literature. *Clin Dysmorphol* 2:211, 1993.

Marfan Syndrome

At a glance: Familial disorder of generalized connective tissue abnormalities leading to connective tissue weakness with hyperextensible joints, eyes (dislocation of the lens), increased risk of valvular/aortic dissection disease, and spontaneous pneumothorax. The leading cause of mortality in the infancy period is progression from mitral valve prolapse to regurgitation often in conjunction with tricuspid regurgitation.

History: First described in 1896 in a 5-year-old girl, Gabrielle P, by Antoine B. J. Marfan, a French pediatrician. The girl had disproportionately long limbs, hands, and feet. Marfan used the term "pattes d'araignée" (spider's legs) and originally called the condition "dolichostenomely" (Greek: stenos = narrow; slender; melos = limb). In 1902, H. Méry and L. Baboneix confirmed radiologically the skeletal anomalies. The first person to use the term "Marfan's syndrome" was Henriculus J. M. Weve of Utrecht in 1931.

Incidence: In the United States, this medical condition affects about 1:10,000 individuals and possibly as many as 1:3000–5000 individuals. It is estimated that in 2004 at least 200,000 people had Marfan syndrome. Internationally, there are no geographic predilections.

Genetic inheritance: Autosomal dominant trait with variable expression. Approximately 15% of cases occur sporadically. In fewer than 1% of cases, it is autosomal recessive.

Pathophysiology: Mutations in the gene for fibrillin-1 on chromosome 15 (15q21.1). Fibrillin is a major component of microfibrils, which are structural components of the zonular fibers of the lens and associated with elastic fibers in the aorta and skin. Tensile strength of collagen is reduced, while its elasticity is increased. Degeneration of media of the pulmonary artery, aorta, and distal arteries lead to "cystic medial necrosis" and weakness. Aneurysm formation results. Disproportionate growth of long bones is present, leading to arachnodactyly with hyperextensible joints. Emphysema and spontaneous pneumothorax may occur.

Diagnosis: The thumb and wrist signs are screening tests for the joint hypermobility of Marfan syndrome. The former is positive when the thumb extends well beyond the ulnar border of the hand when overlapped by fingers and the latter positive when the thumb overlaps the fifth finger as they grasp the opposite wrist. The definitive diagnosis is made on clinical grounds; at least two of the four criteria should be present: a positive family history of the condition, the skeletal, cardiovascular, or ocular features. There is no diagnostic laboratory test.

Clinical aspects: In persons younger than 20 years, the prevalence of serious cardiac complications is low, but aortic root diameter increases with age and aortic regurgitation and type II dissection are responsible for premature death in the third to fifth decade. Regular cardiovascular assessment (mitral and aortic valves) and aggressive surgery have improved prognosis. Significant pulmonary problems include restriction of lung function because of pectus excavatum or kyphoscoliosis and intrinsic pulmonary involvement with emphysema, bronchogenic cysts, and "honeycomb lung." This leads to a significant incidence of spontaneous pneumothorax and the danger of tension pneumothorax with positive-pressure ventilation. Optic lens dislocation is common and can result in cataracts; there is an increased risk of retinal detachment.

The neonatal or infantile form of Marfan syndrome has similar body disposition and, in addition, lax skin, scoliosis, adducted thumbs, large floppy ears, flexion contractures, micrognathia, dolichocephaly, muscle hypoplasia, ectopia lentis, megalocornea, and deficient subcutaneous fat over joints. Severe cardiac valve insufficiency and aortic dilatation result in death during the first 2 years of life.

Precautions before anesthesia: Detailed cardiovascular assessment for the presence of mitral valvular disease (mitral valve prolapse is present in 80% of cases) and aortic valvular disease; presence of angina and heart failure. Preoperative assessment should include echocardiography to determine aortic root size. Pulmonary investigation should include chest radiograph; perform arterial blood gas analysis and lung function test only in the presence of significant kyphoscoliosis.

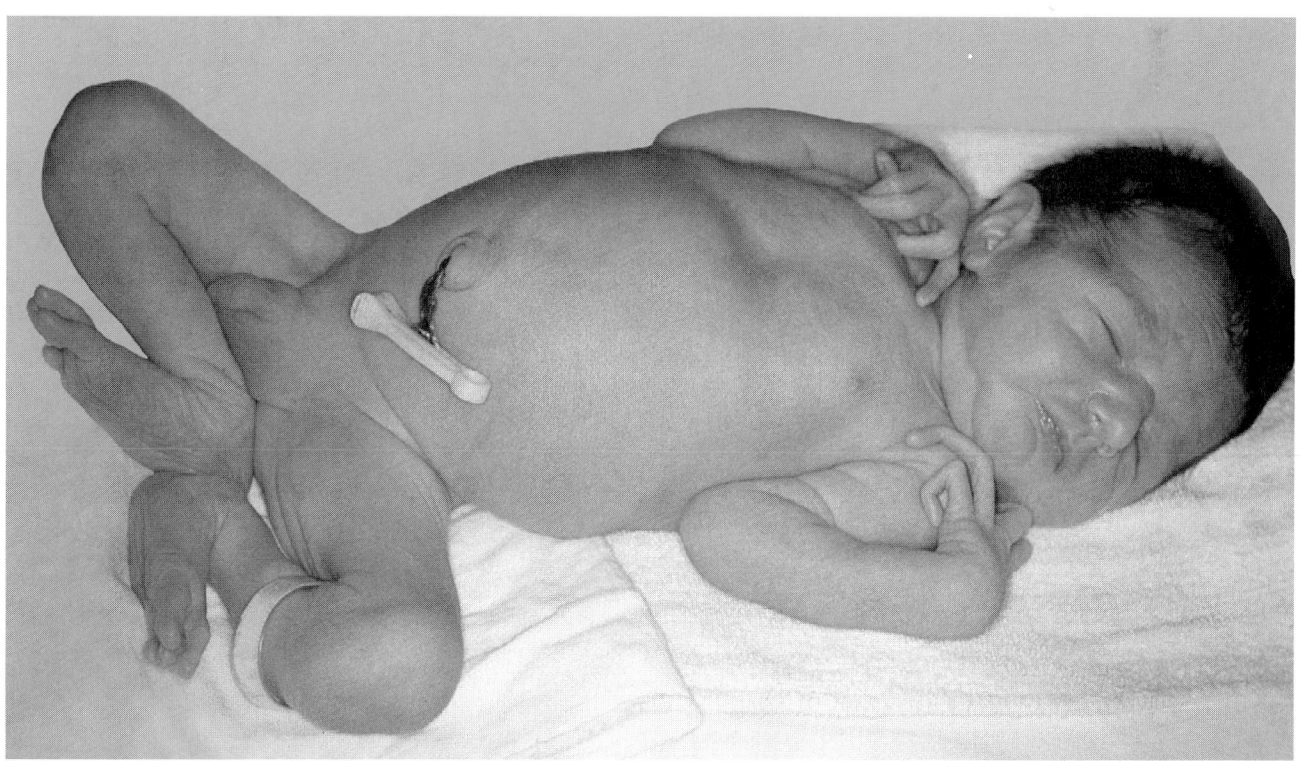

Marfan syndrome   Hyperlaxity of the joints (wrist, ankles) and arachnodactyly (finger and toes) in a newborn with Marfan syndrome.

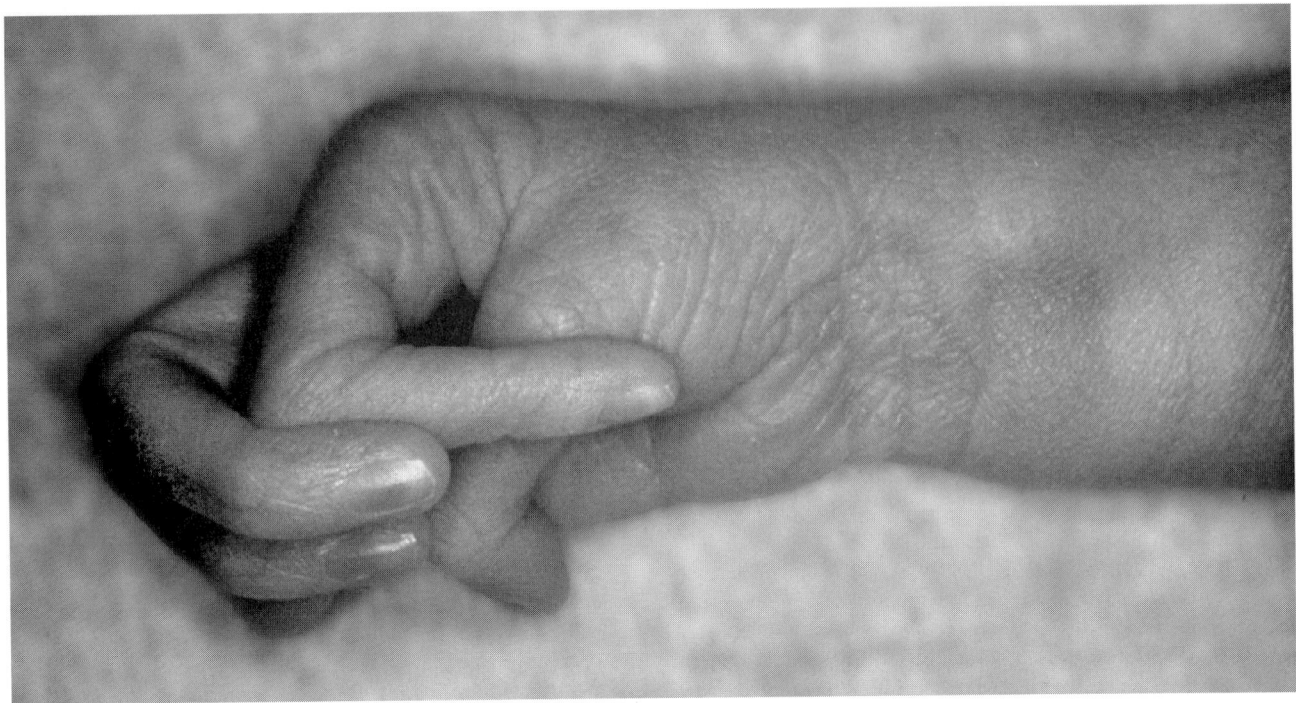

Marfan syndrome   Characteristic adduction of the thumb and arachnodactyly in the same child with Marfan syndrome.

Anesthetic considerations: Prophylactic antibiotics must be given because of the high risk of bacterial endocarditis. Careful handling and positioning are essential to prevent joint trauma and dislocation and eye trauma. Tracheal intubation may be difficult, and the temporomandibular joint may sublux or dislocate. To minimize the risk of aortic dissection or rupture, the anesthetic technique chosen should be designed to minimize sudden changes in blood pressure. Ventilatory pressures should be kept low to prevent barotrauma and creation of pneumothoraces. Tracheomalacia has been reported as a potential complication during and after anesthesia in patients with Marfan syndrome. Regional anesthesia is not contraindicated; however, reports of dural ectasia may be responsible for inadequate spinal anesthesia.

Pharmacological implications: No specific choice of anesthetic agents is indicated, except cardiodepressive drugs should be avoided in patients with significant cardiac disease.

Other conditions to be considered:

☞**EHLERS-DANLOS SYNDROME:** Presents in 10 different connective tissue disorders. Clinically, it is characterized by hyperextensibility, fragile skin, bruising, and bleeding. Individuals affected with this syndrome can present (depending on the type) with serious cardiovascular manifestations such as acute mitral valve regurgitation, aortic root dissection, carotid-cavernous fistula, rupture of large vessels, hiatus hernia, spontaneous rupture and diverticula of the bowel, and retinal detachment.

☞**HOMOCYSTINURIA:** Rare metabolic disorder characterized by ectopia lentis, cataracts, osteoporosis, mental retardation, coagulation disorder (i.e., systemic spontaneous thrombotic responses), and mitral valve prolapse. Patients present with signs and symptoms of Marfan syndrome, such as an elongated body and extremities, pectus excavatum, and cardiovascular anomalies.

☞**BEALS SYNDROME:** Characterized by long, thin, "spider-like" fingers and toes, kyphoscoliosis, pectus excavatum, and mitral valve prolapse.

FAMILIAL THORACIC AORTIC ANEURYSM: Characterized by sudden aortic aneurysm or any major thoracic vessels. Aortic dilatation accounts for approximately 50% of all aneurysms. In the presence of aortic root dilatation, acute aortic valve regurgitation and cardiac failure could cause death. More than half of people with this medical entity have Marfan syndrome or a variation of it.

REFERENCES:

Beighton P, de Paepe A, Danks D, et al: International nosology of heritable disorders of connective tissue. *Am J Med Genet* 29:581, 1988.

Ben Letaifa D, Slama A, Methamem M, et al: Anesthesia for cesarean section in a Marfan patient with complicated aortic dissection. *Ann Fr Anesth Reanim* 21:672, 2002.

Lacassie HJ, Miller S, Leithe LG, et al: Dural ectasia: A likely cause of inadequate spinal anesthesia in two parturients with Marfan's syndrome. *Br J Anaesth* 94:300, 2005.

Oh AY, Kim YH, Kim BK, et al: Unexpected tracheomalacia in Marfan syndrome during general anesthesia for correction of scoliosis. *Anesth Analg* 95:331, 2002.

Marinesco-Sjögren Syndrome

At a glance: Very rare genetic disorder characterized by the association of cerebellar ataxia with postnatal congenital cataracts, delayed mental and physical development (spasticity), very small stature, and hypotonia. The designation "hereditary oligophrenic cerebellolental degeneration" has been suggested.

Synonyms: Marinesco-Garland Syndrome; Marinesco-Sjögren-Garland Syndrome; Marinesco-Sjögren-Garland Myopathy; Marinesco-Sjögren-Garland Neuropathy; Moravcsik-Marinesco-Sjögren Syndrome; Hereditary Oligophrenic Cerebellolental Degeneration.

Incidence: Approximately 100 cases have been described worldwide. It occurs more often in Italy, Scandinavia, and part of Alabama in the United States.

Genetic inheritance: Autosomal recessive.

Pathophysiology: It could be a lysosomal disease. Electronic microscopy demonstrates vacuolization with myeloid bodies derived from the dense sarcoplasmic reticulum.

Diagnosis: Clinical examination and MRI picture of cerebellar cortical atrophy; conjunctival biopsy shows marked increase in the number of lysosomes in the fibroblasts.

Clinical aspects: Microcephaly with congenital cataracts; often strabismus or nystagmus. Cerebellar ataxia with dysarthria. Hypotonia with progressive muscle weakness of neurogenic origin. Short stature with kyphoscoliosis and contractures.

Precautions before anesthesia: Assessment of residual muscular power; chest radiograph: scoliosis, infection.

Anesthetic considerations: Kyphoscoliosis and contractures make positioning difficult. Increased risk of postoperative pulmonary complications.

Pharmacological implication: Succinylcholine should be used with extreme caution or not at all in presence of severe myopathy.

Other conditions to be considered:

☞**FRIEDREICH ATAXIA:** Characterized by slow degenerative changes of the central nervous system that affect coordination of the muscles in the limbs. Dysarthria, hypotonia, and/or hypertonia (spasticity) in the arms and legs are pathognomonic features. It is inherited as an autosomal recessive trait, although it does not manifest clinically during infancy.

☞**LOWE SYNDROME:** Characterized by hydrophthalmia, congenital cataract, glaucoma, mental retardation, vitamin D-resistant rickets, and aminoaciduria. It affects only males with fair complexion. Hyperextensibility of the joints, hypotonic (floppy) muscles, and absence of muscle reflex are classic features. Other clinical features include bowed legs, hypogonadism, excess fatty tissue, and wide-ranging weight fluctuation.

☞**LOUIS-BAR SYNDROME:** Inherited progressive form of cerebellar ataxia that usually begins during infancy. The clinical features include progressive loss of coordination in the limbs, head, and eyes and recurrent systemic infection because of immunologic dysfunction. It is inherited as an autosomal recessive trait.

REFERENCES:

Merlini L, Gooding R, Lochmüller H, et al: Genetic identity of Marinesco-Sjögren/myoglobinuria and CCFDN syndromes. *Neurology* 58:231, 2002.

Tachi N, Nagata N, Wakai S, et al: Congenital muscular dystrophy in Marinesco-Sjögren syndrome. *Pediatr Neurol* 7:296, 1991.

Maroteaux Cohen-Solal Bonaventure Syndrome

At a glance: Severe congenital genetic disease characterized by undermineralization of skull and bones, thin ribs, thoracic collapse, multiple fractures, short stature, and prenatal onset. It is not believed to be linked to collagen metabolism defects. Facies is peculiar.

Synonym: Lethal Type of Brittle Bone Syndrome.

Genetic inheritance: Autosomal recessive inheritance.

Pathophysiology: Unknown but probably not linked to collagen metabolism.

Diagnosis: Clinically evocated at birth, or before birth in case of intrauterine growth retardation with fracture.

Clinical aspects: Bone anomalies include multiple fractures, asymmetry of the body, abnormal ossification. Skeletal deformations concern head and face with unusual Larsen-like facies, including high forehead, microstoma, hypertelorism, flat supraorbital ridges, anteverted nares, broad nasal root, and small nose. Limbs are involved with pes talus, metaphyseal enlargement, overlapping fingers. Other features concern spleen and metabolism anomalies. Respiratory distress is often observed because of thin chest and frequent and multiple ribs fractures.

Precautions before anesthesia: Evaluate phosphocalcic metabolism. Evaluate tracheal intubation (clinical, radiographic) and respiratory function (clinical, chest radiographs, CT scan, pulmonary function tests, arterial blood gas).

Anesthetic considerations: Direct laryngoscopy and tracheal intubation can be difficult because of microstoma and is always dangerous to perform because of the risk of fracture. Perioperative respiratory monitoring should be useful because of frequency of respiratory distress. Cautious intraoperative positioning is needed because of skeletal deformation.

Pharmacological implications: Avoid succinylcholine because the risk of fractures during fasciculation.

REFERENCES:

Bonaventure J, Zylberberg L, Cohen-Solal L, et al: A new lethal brittle bone syndrome with increased amount of type V collagen in a patient. *Am J Med Genet* 33:299, 1989.

Maroteaux P, Cohen-Solal L, Bonaventure J, et al: Lethal syndromes with thin bones. *Arch Fr Pediatr* 45:477, 1988.

Maroteaux-Lamy Syndrome

At a glance: The three variants of Maroteaux-Lamy syndrome (mucopolysaccharidosis type VI) are severe, intermediate, and mild. The severe form of this condition is similar to the severe form of Hurler syndrome, except for the preservation of intelligence in these patients. Other clinical features include macrocephaly, coarse facial features, and short stature. Corneal opacities are often present. Stubby fingers, joint restrictions, clawhands, lumbar lordosis, and hip pain occur after age 3 or 4 years.

Synonyms: Mucopolysaccharidosis Type VI; Arylsulfatase B Deficiency; N-Acetylgalactosamine-4-Sulfatase Deficiency; Polydystrophic Dwarfism; Pyknodysostosis of Maroteaux-Lamy.

Incidence: Unknown. Seems to affect males and females equally. Patients affected with the severe form of this disease usually die by early adulthood. One survey in British Columbia, Canada, reported a frequency estimated at 1:216,000 live births.

Genetic inheritance: Autosomal recessive trait.

Pathophysiology: Deficiency of N-acetylglucosamine-4-sulfate sulfatase B leads to excessive accumulation of dermatan sulfate in the urine. Continuous storage of dermatan sulfate in the skeleton, heart valves, spleen, liver, and cornea. The enzyme deficiency results in an inability to metabolize mucopolysaccharides.

Diagnosis: Phenotype. Dermatan sulfituria. Specific enzyme assay.

Clinical aspects: Resembles Hurler syndrome but is not usually associated with mental retardation. Patients have coarse facial features, short neck and trunk, skeletal abnormalities (hypoplasia of hip acetabula, flared iliac wings, hypoplasia of L1 to L2 vertebral bodies, and lumbar kyphosis), hernias, and corneal clouding. Sleep apnea syndrome is common. Mitral or aortic insufficiency may occur; heart failure is the most common cause of death (second or third decade). Hepatosplenomegaly.

Precautions before anesthesia: Assess cardiorespiratory status carefully and obtain chest radiography, echocardiography. Assess airway and cervical spine.

Anesthetic considerations: As in other forms of mucopolysaccharidosis, the main considerations are related to difficulty with airway maintenance and tracheal intubation. If difficulties are predicted, spontaneous ventilation should be preserved until the airway is secured and lung ventilation is confirmed. A laryngeal mask airway suitable for the patient's size should be readily available in case of failure to ventilate or intubate. Fiberoptic airway equipment can also be useful. Appropriate equipment should be available. See *Mucopolysaccharidoses* for further discussion.

Pharmacological implications: Avoid sedation in the postoperative period.

Other conditions to be considered: See other forms of mucopolysaccharidoses.

REFERENCE:

Walker RWM, Darowski M, Morris P, et al: Anesthesia and mucopolysaccharidoses. A review of airway problems in children. *Anesthesia* 49:1078, 1994.

Marshall Syndrome

At a glance: Association of ocular disorders, distinctive facies characterized by a flattened nasal bridge, anteverted nares, hypertelorism, myopia, cataracts, and sensorineural deafness. Other clinical features include protruding upper incisors, retinal detachment, glaucoma, and esotropia.

Synonym: Deafness-Myopia-Cataract-Saddle Nose Syndrome.

Genetic inheritance: Autosomal dominant.

Clinical aspects: Diagnosis based on clinical examination, familial history, and typical radiograph: absent frontal sinuses; tentorial, falx and meningeal calcifications; flat midface with shallow orbits. Eyes appear prominent with some hypertelorism. Cataracts, congenital glaucoma, myopia, lens dislocation, and retinal detachment have been observed. Sensorineural deafness. Short nose with upturned tip and anteverted nares. May have cleft palate, mental deficiency, and short stature (anomalies of vertebral epiphyses). Associated ectodermal dysplasia has been described.

Anesthetic considerations: Check medical treatment of glaucoma: inhibitor of carbonic anhydrase (serum electrolytes), topical beta blockers (consider systemic effects). Careful protection of eyes. Skin padding in case of ectodermal dysplasia.

Other conditions to be considered:

☞**STICKLER SYNDROME:** Autosomal dominant hereditary progressive arthro-ophthalmology condition characterized by congenital abnormalities of the eye, micrognathia, and cleft palate. Other clinical features include flat midface, intracranial calcifications, and deafness. More than 50% patients affected with this condition have a mitral valve prolapse, and authors have suggested that in the presence of an autosomal dominant inherited mitral valve prolapse, a Stickler syndrome should be suspected until proven otherwise.

☞**WAGNER SYNDROME:** Inherited as an autosomal dominant pattern and characterized by facial abnormalities, an underdeveloped jaw, saddle nose, cleft palate, and vision abnormalities. Joint hyperextensibility and hip deformities may occur. Patients with Wagner syndrome do not have retinal detachment as reported with Marshall and Stickler syndromes. Three types of Wagner syndrome are defined as mild, moderate, or severe.

WEISSENBACHER-ZWEYMULLER SYNDROME (PIERRE ROBIN WITH FETAL CHONDRODYSPLASIA SYNDROME): Characterized by neonatal micrognathia and rhizomelic chondrodysplasia with dumbbell-shaped femora and humeri. Other clinical features may include proximal limb shortness, midface hypoplasia, myopia, high incidence of parietal-occipital encephalocele or meningocele, and cleft palate.

☞**OTOSPONDYLOMEGAEPIPHYSEAL DYSPLASIA:** Characterized by midfacial hypoplasia, saddle-like nose, deafness, and severe degenerative joint disease of the osteoarthritis type affecting predominantly the hips, knees, elbows, and shoulders.

REFERENCE:

Stratton RF, Lee B, Ramirez F: Marshall syndrome. *Am J Med Genet* 41:35, 1991.

Marshall-Smith Syndrome

At a glance: Genetic disorder characterized by the association of facial dysmorphism, failure to thrive, and accelerated osseous maturation and linear growth. Accompanied by severe respiratory problems that are often fatal during the first year of life, mental retardation, hypotonia, muscle weakness, and psychomotor retardation. Craniofacial abnormalities include prominent forehead and eyes, maldevelopment of the epiglottis, and laryngomalacia.

History: First described in 1971 by Richard E. Marshall, an American pediatrician, and David W. Smith, an American pediatrician and dysmorphologist.

Incidence: Rare; 25 cases described in the literature through 2000.

Genetic inheritance: None; all cases reported were sporadic.

Pathophysiology: Unknown.

Diagnosis: Based on clinical aspect and typical radiograph of bones: markedly advanced osseous maturation, widening of the middle and proximal phalanx, and multileveled platyspondylia (thin anterior part of vertebral bodies).

Clinical aspects: Orofacial dysmorphism: prominent forehead, shallow orbits with prominent eyes, megalocornea, micrognathia caused by hypoplastic mandibular ramus, upturned nose with anteverted nostrils, large overflexed ears. Stridor caused by laryngeal anomalies or hypoplasia with rudimentary epiglottis. Scoliosis. Atlantoaxial instability. Hypoplastic thorax. Choanal atresia and/or functional obstruction of the upper airway leading to sleep apnea. Mental retardation. Most patients die before age 2 years as a consequence of recurrent pulmonary infections (chronic aspiration).

Precautions before anesthesia: Check for presence or history of stridor and/or laryngomalacia; probable sleep apnea syndrome: consider insertion of a nasopharyngeal airway before sleep during a few days before anesthesia; echocardiography to rule out associated cardiac malformation and pulmonary hypertension caused by chronic upper airway obstruction. Check patency of both nostrils. Cervical spine radiograph to check atlantoaxial stability. Chest radiograph to check for infection and hypoplasia.

Anesthetic considerations: Difficult face-mask ventilation. Direct laryngoscopy may be complicated by the presence of macroglossia, malformed epiglottis, and laryngomalacia. Difficult tracheal intubation should be anticipated. An induction technique maintaining spontaneous breathing is indicated; upper airway collapse at the beginning of induction and at awakening can be prevented by use of a nasopharyngeal airway; have laryngeal mask airway and fiberoptic bronchoscope ready for use.

Other conditions to be considered:

☞McCUNE-ALBRIGHT SYNDROME: Fibrous dysplasia of bones associated with endocrine disorders, mainly precocious puberty.

☞SOTOS SYNDROME: Characterized by excessively rapid growth during the first year of life, acromegalic craniocerebral features (macrocephaly, prominent forehead), and a nonprogressive cerebral disorder with mental retardation. Other features include high-arched palate and prognathism with premature eruption of teeth, hypotonia, hyperthyroidism or hypothyroidism, delayed motor and cognitive development.

☞WEAVER SYNDROME: Syndrome characterized by accelerated maturation of bone and physical growth accompanied by developmental delay and specific facial abnormalities (micrognathia, hypertelorism, down-slanting of palpebral fissures), hypertonia, progressive spasticity, and a typical low-pitched and hoarse cry in infants.

REFERENCES:

Antilla H, Laitio T, Aantaa R, et al: Difficult airway in a patient with Marshall-Smith syndrome. *Paediatr Anaesth* 8:429, 1998.

Charon A, Gillerot Y, Van Maldergem L, et al: The Marshall-Smith syndrome. *Eur J Pediatr* 150:54, 1990.

Dernedde G, Pendeville P, Veyckemans F, et al: Anaesthetic management of a child with Marshall-Smith syndrome. *Can J Anaesth* 45:660, 1998.

MASA Syndrome

At a glance: MASA is an acronym for *m*ental retardation, *a*phasia, *s*huffling gait, and *a*dducted thumbs. Hydrocephalus associated with aqueductal stenosis. Extremely rare inherited disorder that is one of several disorders known as X-linked mental retardation (XLMR) syndromes.

Synonyms: Clasped Thumb and Mental Retardation Syndrome; Gareis-Mason Syndrome; Spastic Paraplegia Type I Syndrome; Crash Syndrome.

Incidence: Rare; it is responsible for approximately 10% of cases of hydrocephalus in males.

Genetic inheritance: X-linked recessive; locus at Xq28. Caused by a mutation in the gene for the neural L1 cell adhesion molecule (L1-CAM).

Pathophysiology: Seems to be associated with a mutation in L1-CAM, which is an axonal glycoprotein that is essential for normal development of the central and peripheral nervous systems during the fetal period and postnatally. However, the exact function of the L1-CAM protein is not fully understood.

Diagnosis: Clinical picture; prenatal-onset hydrocephalus in males. Female carriers may have mild mental retardation or slightly adducted thumbs.

Clinical aspects: Varies from extreme macrocephaly following hydrocephalus caused by in utero stenosis of the sylvian aqueduct to absence of hydrocephalus with mental retardation and aphasia. Shuffling gait secondary to spastic paraplegia. Adducted thumbs (i.e., flexed over the palms or "cortical thumb"). Small stature. Lumbar lordosis.

Precautions before anesthesia: Risk of raised intracranial pressure should be well assessed. Neurologic and cardiovascular status should be evaluated.

Anesthetic considerations: Prevent elevation of intracranial pressure.

Pharmacological implications: Avoid anesthetic agents with known potential to increase intracranial pressure.

Other conditions to be considered:

X-LINKED HYDROCEPHALUS (Bickers Adams Syndrome): Characterized by severe hydrocephalus and caused by congenital stenosis of the aqueduct of Sylvius (HSAS). Other clinical features include macrocephaly, mental retardation, hypoplastic clasped or adducted thumbs, and/or spastic paraplegia. It is inherited as an X-linked recessive pattern. X-linked hydrocephalus and MASA syndrome result from different mutations of the same L1-CAM gene and are considered allelic disorders.

COMPLICATED X-LINKED SPASTIC PARAPLEGIA (SPG1): Characterized by early onset and slow progression of symptoms such as muscle weakness, legs spasticity, mental retardation, optic nerves atrophy, and/or neurodegeneration of certain parts of the brain (e.g., cerebellum, cerebral cortex). It affects primarily males. Other clinical features include ataxia, spastic paraplegia, and hydrocephalus. Complicated X-linked spastic paraplegia (SPG1) and MASA syndrome are thought to result from different mutations of the same gene (allelic disorders) on the X chromosome (L1-CAM).

UNCOMPLICATED X-LINKED SPASTIC PARAPLEGIA (SPG2): Milder form characterized by late onset, severe hyperreflexia, and spastic gait. Nystagmus, optic nerve atrophy, mild intellectual disability, and/or coordination problems are significant features. The genetic mutations that cause this disorder do not occur in the same region of the X chromosome as those occurring in MASA syndrome, X-linked hydrocephalus, and complicated X-linked spastic paraplegia.

RENPENNING SYNDROME: Affects only males; characterized by moderate-to-severe mental retardation, microcephaly, short stature, and/or microgenitalia. Renpenning type is thought to be inherited as an X-linked recessive genetic trait.

ESCALANTE SYNDROME: Similar to Renpenning syndrome; associated with macroorchidism.

☞ALLAN-HERNDON SYNDROME: Although most neonates and infants with this disorder appear to develop normally in the first few months of life, the presence of poor muscle tone is most often already present at birth. By age 6 months, hypotonia, inability to hold the head, and severe muscle atrophy are detectable. Severe mental retardation is associated with multiple congenital anomalies.

☞FRAGILE X SYNDROME: Most common form of X-linked mental retardation; affects males more often and more severely than females. Only subtle dysmorphic features; behavioral issues may be more pronounced.

☞JUBERG-MARSIDI SYNDROME: X-linked recessive inherited syndrome characterized by severe mental retardation, deafness, failure to thrive, microgenitalism, and early death.

☞HAPPY PUPPET SYNDROME: Rare disorder characterized by developmental delay, ataxia, dysmorphic facial features, and seizures associated with a happy, sociable disposition.

SUTHERLAND-HAAN SYNDROME (Sutherland-Haan X-Linked Mental Retardation Syndrome; X-Linked Mental Retardation with Spastic Diplegia): Extremely rare form of X-linked severe mental retardation. Features include short stature, spastic diplegia, significant congenital heart defects, and craniofacial abnormalities (microcephaly, cleft palate or high-arched palate, abnormal ears, bulbous nose, broad nasal bridge, malar hypoplasia, micrognathia, and a small mouth). No reports exist about anesthesia in these patients; however, difficult airway management seems likely.

REFERENCE:

Fryns JP, Spaepen A, Cassiman JJ: X-linked complicated spastic paraplegia, MASA syndrome and X-linked hydrocephalus owing to congenital stenosis of the aqueduct of Sylvius: Variable expression of the same mutation at Xq28. *J Med Genet* 28:429, 1991.

Mastocytosis

At a glance: Accumulation and degranulation of mast cells (mastocytosis) in the skin or other organs. A group of disorders characterized by accumulation of mast cells in the skin with or without other organ system involvement. Systemic mastocytosis occurs in approximately 10% of all cases, with proliferation of mast cells in other tissues such as bone, liver, and spleen.

Synonym: Mast Cell Disease; Systemic Mast Cell Disease (SMCD).

Classification: A classification of mastocytosis has been proposed based on clinical presentation and prognosis (see the WHO Classification of Mastocytosis in Table M-1).

History: The cutaneous manifestation, urticaria pigmentosa, is the most common form and was first described in 1869.

Incidence: Rare; approximately 1–4:10,000 live births.

Genetic inheritance: Usually not considered an inherited disease, although there is some evidence of an autosomal dominant pattern in the diffuse cutaneous form. Males and females are affected equally.

Pathophysiology: There is an excess of mast cells in body tissues, and the clinical expression of the disorder depends upon the pattern of localization of the mast cells to specific organs. Dysregulation of production and function of mast cells is caused by distinct mutations in c-Kit, a type III transmembrane tyrosine kinase. Mediator release by mast cells may occur spontaneously or be triggered by a variety of stimuli. These biochemical substances include histamine and heparin, thought to be the most important, and other enzymes such as chymases, tryptases, and hydrolases. Prostaglandin D_2, cytokines (tumor necrosis factor [TNF]-α and TNF-β, interleukin [IL]-3, IL-5, and IL-16), serotonin, leukotrienes, and platelet-activating factor are also released. Among the precipitating factors are trauma, surgery, extremes of temperature, toxins, alcohol, and a variety of drugs (including acetylsalicylic acid, morphine, codeine, thiopentone, lignocaine, gallamine, and D-tubocurarine).

Diagnosis: History of recurrent flushes, urticarial wheals, pruritus, dizziness, and headaches. Darier sign is pathognomonic and is defined as development of an urticarial wheal on a lesion after it is stroked. Skin or gastric mucosa biopsies show an increased number of mast cells (>5 per high-power field). Increased blood and urinary levels of histamine. Bone marrow biopsy is not recommended unless there is evidence of systemic disease.

Clinical aspects: Approximately 65% of patients with mastocytosis present with the disease in childhood (more than half before age

Table M-1   WHO Classification of Mastocytosis

Cutaneous Mastocytosis
 1. ☞Urticaria pigmentosa
 2. Diffuse cutaneous mastocytosis
 3. Mastocytoma of the skin

Systemic Mastocytosis without Associated Hematologic Non-Mast Cell Disorder
 1. Systemic indolent mastocytosis
 2. Systemic smoldering mastocytosis

Systemic Mastocytosis with Associated Hematologic Non-Mast Cell Disorder
 1. Myeloproliferative syndrome
 2. Myelodysplastic syndrome
 3. Acute myeloid leukemia
 4. Non-Hodgkin lymphoma

Systemic Aggressive Mastocytosis
 1. Mast cell leukemia
 2. Mast cell sarcoma
 3. Extracutaneous mastocytoma

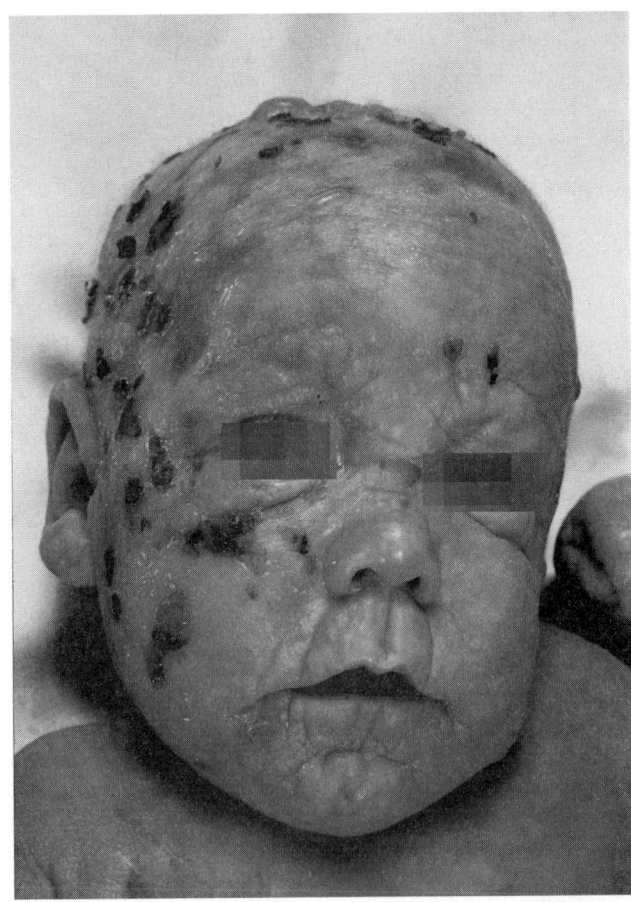

Mastocytosis   Severe form of diffuse cutaneous mastocytosis in an infant.

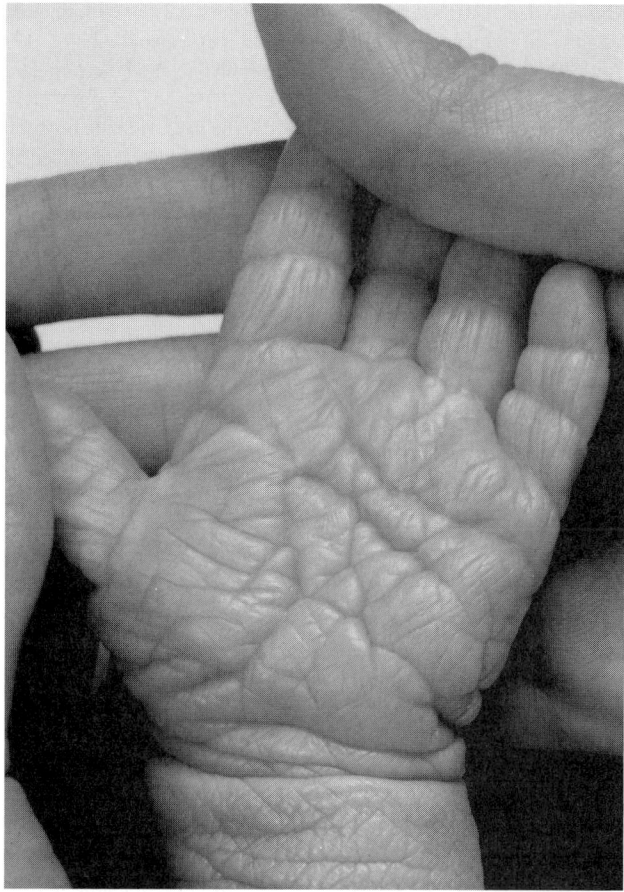

Mastocytosis Thickening of the palms in an infant with diffuse cutaneous mastocytosis.

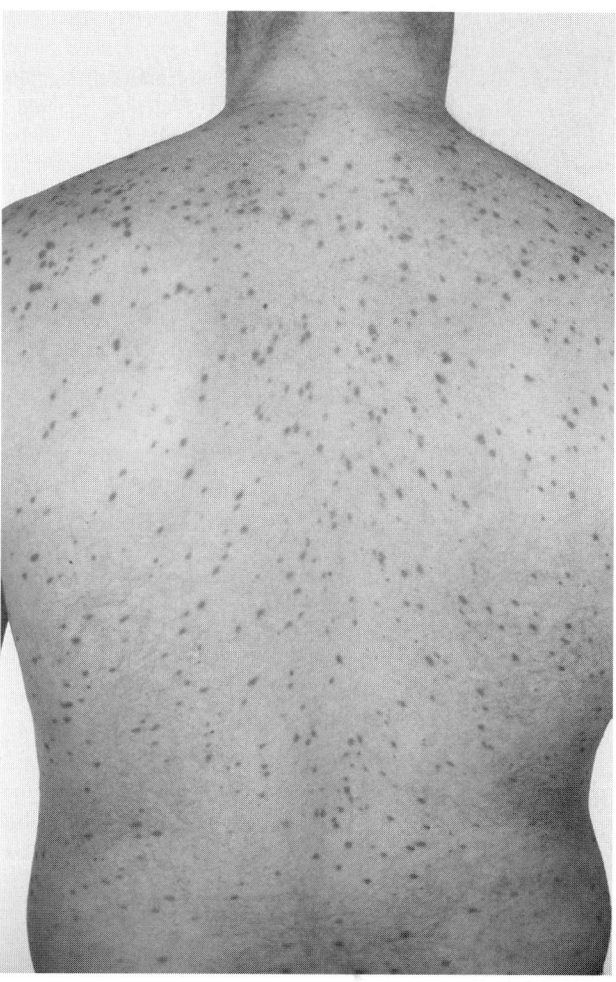

Mastocytosis Multiple mastocytomas on the back of an adult man.

2 years). The remaining 35% develop the disease after puberty and are classified as adult-onset cases. Mastocytosis limited to the skin is primarily a benign disease of children. Systemic internal mastocytosis is more common in adults with infiltration of mast cells in the gastrointestinal tract, skeletal system, lung, kidney, myocardium, and other tissues.

Urticaria pigmentosa is the most frequent form: lesions are red-brown macules, papules, or plaques showing Darier sign. Darier's sign is defined by skin lesions caused by mast cell urtication on rubbing. Described by Ferdinand-Jean Darier, a French dermatologist. Symptoms are pruritus, flushing associated with bathing in cold or hot water, or exercise. Bullae and blistering may appear. It has a favorable outcome.

Mastocytomas are brownish solitary or multiple nodules that can cause flushing and hypotension when traumatized. The course of an isolated mastocytoma is usually spontaneous regression in several years.

Diffuse cutaneous mastocytosis is seen almost only in infants: skin has a thickened appearance and/or a reddish-brown discoloration. Increased risk of flushing, hypotension, and shock; diarrhea and other gastrointestinal manifestations are common.

Bronchospasm may occur. Anemia, leukocytosis, and thrombocytopenia are common problems. Hematologic abnormalities are rare in children with mastocytosis; however, cases of acute lymphocytic leukemia have been observed in children with rapidly progressive and late-onset mastocytosis. Children and adults who

have serious systemic involvement have a guarded prognosis, as do neonates with diffuse cutaneous involvement.

Precautions before anesthesia: Because the main preoperative aim is to reduce the risk of mast cell degranulation, H_1 and H_2 antagonists can be given. Some patients are on steroid therapy; check for perioperative coverage. High-dose acetylsalicylic acid inhibits prostaglandin synthetase and is effective in controlling episodes of severe vasodilatation normally associated with prostaglandin D_2 release. In approximately 5% of patients, however, severe hypotension may be precipitated by acetylsalicylic acid itself. In addition, aspirin has a detrimental effect on bleeding time and must be carefully assessed. Preoperative intradermal skin testing with drugs likely to be used during anesthesia has been recommended but is not useful if known histamine-releasing drugs are avoided. Blood investigations: hemoglobin, platelet count, coagulation studies, and serum electrolytes. Stress can precipitate a reaction, so an appropriate sedative/hypnotic premedicant should be prescribed.

Anesthetic considerations: Both regional anesthesia and general anesthesia have been reported. Care should be taken when handling and positioning the patient to prevent skin irritation and trauma. Core temperature should be measured and actions to maintain normothermia should be continued into the postoperative period. Large-bore intravenous cannula to allow rapid volume replacement.

Pharmacological implications: Avoid use of medications known to trigger histamine release (e.g., morphine, codeine, ketorolac tromethamine, D-tubocurarine, atracurium, thiopentone). Use of propofol as an intravenous anesthetic induction agent has been found to be safe. Inhalational anesthetics tend to inhibit mast cell degranulation, so general anesthesia may be preferred. Adrenaline, antihistamines, bronchodilators, and intravenous fluids should be available for immediate use to treat severe hypotension and bronchospasm or cardiovascular shock.

Other conditions to be considered:

CARCINOID SYNDROME (Thorson-Biörck Syndrome; Flush Syndrome; Cassidy-Scholte Syndrome): Characterized by hot, red flushing of the face, severe and debilitating diarrhea, and asthma attacks. Malignant carcinoid syndrome occurs in fewer than 10% of patients with a carcinoid tumor. Typically, 90% of cases originate from the distal ileum or appendix (the embryologic midgut) and represent 90% of appendiceal tumors.

ZOLLINGER ELLISON SYNDROME: Caused by a non-beta islet cell, gastrin-secreting tumor of the pancreas; occurs sporadically or as part of an autosomal dominant familial syndrome called multiple endocrine neoplasia type I (MEN I: hyperparathyroidism, pancreatic endocrine tumors, and pituitary tumors). The primary tumor usually is located in the duodenum, pancreas, and abdominal lymph nodes, but ectopic locations have also been described (e.g., heart, ovary, gallbladder, liver, kidney). Abdominal pain is the most common symptom, present in 75% of patients. Diarrhea, abdominal pain, nausea, vomiting, gastrointestinal bleeding, and weight loss.

REFERENCES:

Anurag L, Letourneau B. Mastocytosis: General anesthesia with remifentanil and sevoflurane. *Ann Fr Anesth Reanim* 20:635, 2001.

Borgeat A, Ruetsch YA: Anesthesia in a patient with malignant systemic mastocytosis using total intravenous anesthetic technique. *Anesth Analg* 86:442, 1998.

Carter MC, Metcalfe DD: Pediatric mastocytosis. *Arch Dis Child* 86:315, 2002.

James PD, Krafchick BR, Johnston AE: Cutaneous mastocytosis in children: Anaesthetic considerations. *Can J Anaesth* 34:522, 1987.

Mauriac Syndrome

At a glance: Rare metabolic disorder characterized by early onset of diabetes mellitus in the infancy period, multiple epiphyseal dysplasia, multiple fractures, microcephaly, short stature, hypertonia, barrel-shaped chest, hepatomegaly, tooth discoloration, gray-blue sclerae, high-arched palate, and skin abnormalities. Epiphyseal dysplasia and growth retardation have onset within the first 2 years of life.

Synonyms: MED-IDDM Syndrome; IDDM-MED Syndrome; Wolcott-Rallison Syndrome.

Genetic inheritance: Acquired condition only in diabetics.

Pathophysiology: Mauriac syndrome is primarily of historic interest. It occurred in poorly controlled diabetics when only short-acting insulin was used. Insufficient tissue glucose results in gluconeogenesis and fat metabolism and therefore a catabolic state. In addition, somatomedin production is reduced, resulting in relatively short stature. Although the pituitary–adrenal axis remains intact, high cortisol levels are typical.

Diagnosis: This syndrome should be suspected in poorly controlled diabetics with cushingoid appearance.

Clinical aspects: Mauriac syndrome occurs only in children and adolescents with poorly controlled insulin-dependent diabetes mellitus. They present with dwarfism, hepatomegaly, and a cushingoid appearance, including truncal obesity and "buffalo hump." Hepatomegaly is caused by fatty deposition in the liver. Hepatic function is usually normal. These findings are almost completely reversed by improved diabetic control. However, diabetic end-organ damage, including retinopathy and nephropathy, may be present.

Precautions before anesthesia: Preoperative evaluation of diabetic control is essential. Careful evaluation of end-organ damage. Kidney function must be assessed because these patients are susceptible to renal failure.

Anesthetic considerations: Perioperative control of blood sugar must be accomplished in cooperation with endocrinologists.

Pharmacological implications: Doses of anesthetic agent may require adjustment in the presence of renal dysfunction. Medication with renal excretion only should better be avoided.

REFERENCES:

Najjar S, Ayash MA: The Mauriac syndrome. *Clin Pediatr* 13:723, 1974.

Traisman HS, Traisman ES: Mauriac's syndrome revisited. *Eur J Pediatr* 142:296, 1984.

Mayer-von Rokitansky-Kuster-Hauser Syndrome

At a glance: Syndrome characterized by congenital absence of vagina, rudimentary cornua uteri, and morphologically normal ovaries and Fallopian tubes situated on the pelvic sidewall. Primary amenorrhea, normal ovulation, breast development, body, and hair. Women are infertile. Frequently associated with urinary tract anomalies, skeletal abnormalities, congenital heart conditions, and inguinal hernia.

Synonyms: von Rokitansky Syndrome; Uterus Bipartitus Solidus Rudimentarius cum Vagina Solida.

History: The first description of this disorder dates back to 1820, when the German anatomist Auguste Franz Joseph Karl Mayer described this kind of anomaly, followed by a report by the Austrian pathologist Karl Freiherr von Rokitansky in 1838. The detailed description by the German gynecologist Hermann Küster was published no earlier than 1910. Another German gynecologist, G.A. Hauser, published one article each about the Küster-von Rokitansky syndrome and the Mayer-von Rokitansky-Küster syndrome in 1961. Thus, it seems the correct order of names is "Mayer–von Rokitansky–Küster–(Hauser) syndrome."

Incidence: 1:4000–5000 female newborns.

Genetic inheritance: Congenital disorder that usually occurs sporadically. Few familial cases have been described with an autosomal recessive inheritance trait.

Pathophysiology: There is an arrest, for unknown reasons, of the müllerian duct development at the fifth gestational week. Structures deriving from the mesoderm can be involved (uterus, cervix, and upper 75% of the vagina). Ovarian function is preserved because the ovaries originate in the primitive ectoderm. Skeleton development from mesoderm is highly sensible at this period.

Diagnosis: Clinically evocated on functional complaints of primary amenorrhea and unsatisfactory or impossible sexual intercourse. Sonography can confirm diagnosis.

Clinical aspects: Female phenotype with normal secondary sexual characteristics (breast and pubic hair growth). Pituitary and ovarian function is normal, and ovulatory progesterone levels can be detected. Features can involve the *genitourinary system* (congenital absence of the vagina, rudimentary uterus, bipartite uterus, hypoplasia of kidneys, ectopic malformed kidneys). Other frequent signs are short neck, low hair line, short stature, abnormal rib scapula, abnormal position, and vertebral segmentation anomaly. Hearing loss can occur. Two sisters with the syndrome have been described, both also suffering from pulmonary valvular stenosis. Use echocardiography if cardiac lesions are suspected.

Precautions before anesthesia: Evaluate renal function (clinical, echography, biology); assess the airway in view of tracheal intubation because of associated skeletal anomalies (clinical, radiographs).

Anesthetic considerations: Careful intraoperative positioning is needed because of skeletal deformities. Direct laryngoscopy and tracheal intubation could be difficult because of short neck. It is recommended to maintain spontaneous respiration until the trachea has been secured and lung ventilation is confirmed. Care with urinary catheter insertion, which can be difficult.

Pharmacological implications: Avoid muscle relaxants until airway is secured. Nonnephrotoxic drugs are preferred. Aminoglycosides should be used with care, considering renal function and hearing loss. Subacute bacterial endocarditis prophylaxis may be required.

Other condition to be considered:

☞**COMPLETE ANDROGEN INSENSITIVITY SYNDROME:** Inherited disorder caused by androgen insensitivity. Affected males have a female phenotype with normal female external genitalia but abnormal or absent internal female organs. Testes are often intraabdominal, in the inguina, or in the labia. Newborns are identified by the presence of inguinal masses corresponding to enlarged testes. Some patients are first seen in the teenage years for evaluation of amenorrhea. Normal male (46,XY) karyotype.

REFERENCE:

Chervenak FA, Stangel JJ, Nemec M: Mayer-Rokitansky-Kuster-Hauser syndrome. Congenital absence of vagina. *N Y State J Med* 82:23, 1982.

McCune-Albright Syndrome

At a glance: Characterized by the triad of polyostotic fibrous dysplasia, café-au-lait skin pigmentation, and autonomous endocrine hyperfunction. The most common form of autonomous endocrine hyperfunction is gonadotropin-independent precocious puberty, but affected individuals also may have hyperthyroidism, hypercorticism, pituitary gigantism, or acromegaly. Nonendocrine abnormalities in this disorder include hypophosphatemia, chronic liver disease, tachycardia, and rarely sudden death, possibly from cardiac arrhythmias.

Synonym: Polyostotic Fibrous Dysplasia; Osteitis Fibrosa Cystica; McCune Syndrome; Albright Syndrome; Osteitis Fibrosa Disseminata.

History: Genetic disorder first described in 1936 by Donovan James McCune, an American pediatrician, and then in 1937 by Fuller Albright, an American physician.

Incidence: Occurs sporadically; more common in females.

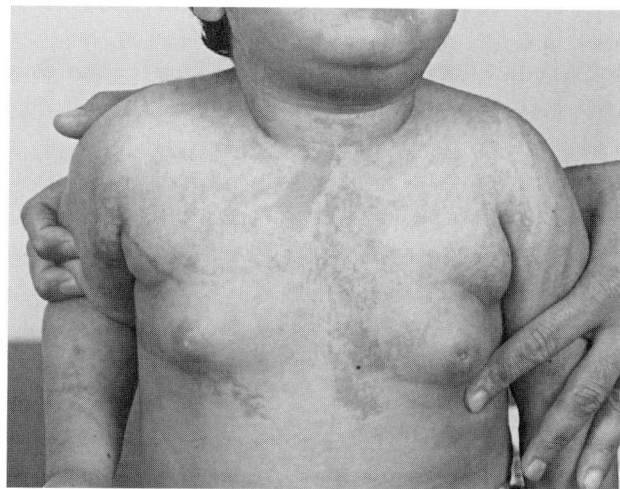

McCune–Albright syndrome Cushing-like habitus and café-au-lait skin pigmentation in a small girl with McCune-Albright syndrome. Note precocious breast development.

Genetic inheritance: Autosomal dominant lethal mosaic postzygotic somatic mutation in the GNAS 1 gene located on chromosome 20q13.2.

Pathophysiology: Described as a mosaicism for a mutation in the gene encoding the subunit of the G protein stimulating cyclic adenosine monophosphate (cAMP) formation. This results in activation of various cAMP-dependent receptors including adrenocorticotropic hormone (ACTH), thyroid-stimulating hormone (TSH), follicle-stimulating hormone (FSH), and luteinizing hormone (LH) receptors leading to autonomous and aberrant behavior toward otherwise normal stimuli.

Clinical aspects: Classic triad of endocrine dysfunction, bone lesions, and pigmented skin lesions. Average age of onset is 3 years. Precocious pseudopuberty (F > M); vaginal bleeding may begin as early as age 4 months and secondary sexual characteristics as early as 6 months. Acromegaly (F = M). Cushing syndrome may occur in early infancy before onset of precocious pseudopuberty and is associated with adrenocortical hyperplasia. Multinodular goiter (M = F) and hyperthyroidism in 20 to 40% of patients. Pathologic fractures and deformities of long bones resulting from hypophosphatemic osteomalacia. Shepherd crook deformity of the proximal femur is particularly characteristic, and bony lesions in the base of skull may result in cranial nerve compression, blindness, and deafness. Large, patchy cutaneous pigmentation with irregular margins on neck, face, back, and shoulders are found in approximately 90% of children with this syndrome. Both the bony and skin lesions are limited predominantly to one side.

Diagnosis: Clinical features of endocrine abnormalities, café-au-lait spots, and polyostotic fibrous dysplasia. Biochemical: Thyroid (mildly elevated T_3, low TSH); adrenal (raised cortisol and low ACTH levels, adrenal function not suppressed by dexamethasone); pituitary (elevated growth hormone and prolactin levels); hypophosphatemia as a result of decreased resorption of phosphate in the renal tubule; ovaries (estradiol varies from normal to markedly elevated levels, suppressed levels of LH and FSH, no response to luteinizing hormone-releasing hormone stimulation). Imaging studies: Ultrasonography (ovarian cysts, nodular adrenal hyperplasia); skeletal radiography (widespread cystic bony lesions, advanced bone age, fractures and deformities of long bones, bony lesions in base of skull).

Anesthetic considerations: Direct laryngoscopy and tracheal intubation may be difficult in the presence of acromegaly. Possibility of airway compression and tracheomalacia must be considered with long-standing multinodular goiter. Hyperthyroidism, if present, should be controlled before anesthesia to avoid thyroid storm crisis. Cushing syndrome requires preoperative correction of hypokalemia. Intraoperative monitoring and control of blood sugar levels, hypertension, and/or heart failure must be managed accordingly. Venous access may be difficult because of fragility of veins.

Pharmacological implications: Supplementation corticosteroids must be considered preoperatively. All supplemental endocrinologic medication must be administered.

Other conditions to be considered:

ACROMEGALY AND GIGANTISM: Gigantism is extremely rare in the United States, with approximately 100 reported cases. Acromegaly is found more frequently, with an incidence of 3–4:1,000,000 people per year and a prevalence of 40–70:1,000,000 population. It is associated with chronic exposure to excessive growth hormone production and clinically characterized with overgrowth of the extremities in adulthood.

☞CHERUBISM: Characterized by bilateral displacement of normal bone tissue with areas of fibrous dysplasia within the maxilla and mandible. Clinical presentation includes swelling of the face, "upturning" of the eyes, café-au-lait spots, and/or significant nevi. Age of onset is usually between the third and fourth year of life. It is inherited as an autosomal dominant trait with variable expressivity and penetrance. One hundred percent of males are fully affected (high penetrance), whereas 50 to 75% of females have signs of the disease (reduced penetrance).

☞ALBRIGHT HEREDITARY OSTEODYSTROPHY: Syndrome presenting with round face, short stature and neck, and obesity. Subcutaneous and intracranial calcifications, seizures, and neuromuscular problems such as fatigue and muscle cramps. Pseudohypoparathyroidism and hypocalcemia.

REFERENCES:

DiMeglio LA, Pescovitz OH: Disorders of puberty: Inactivating and activating molecular mutations. *J Pediatr* 131:S8, 1997.

Happle R: The McCune-Albright syndrome: A lethal gene surviving by mosaicism. *Clin Genet* 29:321, 1986.

Langer RA, Yook I, Capan LM: Anesthetic considerations in McCune-Albright syndrome: Case report with literature review. *Anesth Analg* 80:1236, 1995.

McKusick-Kaufman Syndrome

At a glance: Hydrometrocolpos develops in females and is associated with anomalies of the limbs (postaxial polydactyly) and congenital heart malformation. However, the same presentation associated with urogenital anomalies (e.g., hypospadias, prominent scrotal raphe) has been reported in males.

Synonyms: MKKS; Hydrometrocolpos Syndrome; Hydrometrocolpos, Postaxial Polydactyly, and Congenital Heart Malformation; HMCS; Kaufman-McKusick Syndrome.

Incidence: Approximately 100 cases described.

Genetic inheritance: Autosomal recessive; probably caused by a mutation. It has the same map locus (chromosome 20p12) and is similar to the Bardet-Biedl syndrome.

Pathophysiology: Hydrometrocolpos develops in the female fetus. It is a result of transverse vaginal membranes and excessive cervical secretions in response to maternal hormone. Intrauterine maternal hormone stimulation causes cervical gland secretion, which, in association with high vaginal obstruction, results in hydrometrocolpos. External compression of ureters by hydrometrocolpos may cause hydroureter and hydronephrosis. McKusick-Kaufman syndrome-predicted protein showed amino acid similarity to the chaperonin family of proteins, suggesting a role for protein processing in limb, cardiac, and reproductive system development.

Diagnosis: Clinically and by gene mapping.

Clinical aspects: Female infants usually present with intraabdominal swelling (hydrometrocolpos) arising from the pelvis. This is associated with other abnormalities, including imperforate anus, malrotation of the gut, polydactyly, syndactyly, obesity, and congenital heart disease (septal defects). Less common features are abnormalities of the upper airway (larynx), pituitary dysplasia, and developmental delay. Males usually present with isolated polydactyly, but cryptorchidism and hypospadias have been described. Ellis van Creveld syndrome may be a phenotype for the male.

Precautions before anesthesia: Some patients with Bardet-Biedl syndrome are described but never with the McKusick-Kaufman syndrome. Consequently, each system involved should be assessed, and good preoperative evaluation of the kidneys, larynx, and heart is advisable. Evaluation of cardiovascular system must include echocardiogram. Preoperative abdominal and renal ultrasonography. Evaluation of renal function with electrolytes, urea, and creatinine.

Anesthetic considerations: Direct laryngoscopy and tracheal intubation can be difficult if laryngeal anomalies are present. Neonates with severe hydrometrocolpos may present with diaphragm compression necessitating gastric decompression. Most patients will be tachypneic, tachycardiac, and cyanotic because of the large cystic mass. Anesthetic management must take into consideration the presence of congenital heart defects and be adapted accordingly. Surgical resection of an hydrometrocolpos may be associated with significant fluid shift and electrolyte imbalance.

Pharmacological implications: Drugs requiring renal excretion should be avoided in the presence of kidney dysfunction. Endocarditis prophylaxis may be required for congenital heart disease.

Other conditions to be considered:

☞PALLISTER-HALL SYNDROME: Hypothalamic hamartoblastoma, hypopituitarism, imperforate anus, and postaxial polydactyly.

☞BARDET-BIEDL SYNDROME: Diagnostic pitfall: all McKusick-Kaufman syndrome patients should be reevaluated for retinitis pigmentosa and other signs of this syndrome in later childhood.

☞ELLIS-VAN CREVELD SYNDROME: Achondroplastic disorder associated with polydactyly, abnormal development of fingernails, and cardiac defects (atrial septal defect [ASD] is the most common). Dandy-Walker malformation, epispadias, mental retardation, and renal agenesis are also considered features of this syndrome.

REFERENCES:

Kumar D, Primhak RA, Kumar A: Variable phenotype in Kaufman-McKusick syndrome: Report of an inbred Muslim family and review of the literature. *Clin Dysmorphol* 7:163, 1998.

Tekin I, Ok G, Genc A, et al: Anaesthetic management in McKusick-Kaufman syndrome. *Paediatr Anaesth* 13:167, 2003.

McPherson-Clemens Syndrome

At a glance: Very rare, autosomal recessive disorder characterized by bilateral cleft lip and palate, hypertelorism, flat facial profile, bifid thumbs, flat occiput, complex congenital heart defect, and malrotation of the intestine.

Synonym: Cleft lip/palate-intestinal malrotation-lethal congenital heart disease association.

Genetic inheritance: Autosomal recessive.

Clinical aspects: The clinical features of the syndrome include the association of bilateral cleft lip and palate with severe and atypical congenital heart defect. Other clinical features are hypertelorism, flat facial profile (flat face, flat occiput), and malrotation of the intestine. All patients are affected with complex congenital heart defects. Three patients had bilobed tongues, bifid thumbs, and bilateral cleft lip and palate.

Precautions before anesthesia: Complete evaluation of the cardiovascular system must be done, and a cardiology consultation (if possible) should be obtained.

Anesthetic considerations: Direct laryngoscopy and tracheal intubation may be difficult in the presence of dysmorphic facial features. The most challenging considerations are those associated with congenital heart defect.

Other conditions to be considered:

☞**FRYNS SYNDROME:** Presents similar features and the presence of diaphragmatic hernia found in more than 90% of patients.

☞**ROBINOW SYNDROME:** Similar presentation except for the severity of heart defects. Other clinical features include hemivertebrae or short arms.

REFERENCES:

McPherson E, Clemens M: Cleft lip and palate, characteristic facial appearance, malrotation of the intestine, and lethal congenital heart disease in two sibs: A new autosomal recessive condition? *Am J Med Genet* 62:58, 1996.

Nevin NC, Craig BG, Mullholland HC, et al: Cleft lip and palate, hypertelorism, brachycephaly, flat facial profile, and congenital heart disease in three brothers. *Am J Med Genet* 73:412, 1997.

Meckel-Gruber Syndrome (MKS)

At a glance: Characterized by postaxial polydactyly and central nervous system malformation (encephalocele, severe hydrocephalus), large polycystic kidneys, and liver failure (fibrosis). Other clinical features include microcephaly, abnormality of the larynx and tongue, severe mandibular micrognatism, obesity, and cleft lip/palate. Associated abnormalities include oral clefting and genital anomalies. Pulmonary hypoplasia is the leading cause of death.

Synonyms: Meckel Syndrome; Gruber Syndrome; Dysencephalia Splanchnocystica; MKS.

Nature: Genetic disorder characterized mainly by encephalocele, polydactyly, and polycystic kidneys, but with a wide phenotypic variation.

Incidence: Worldwide incidence of Meckel-Gruber syndrome varies from 1:13,250–140,000 live births. There is a predilection for the Finnish population, in whom the birth incidence is 1:9000. More than 200 cases have been described in the literature.

Genetic inheritance: Autosomal recessive; a gene has been identified on chromosome 17q21-q24.

Pathophysiology: It has been suggested that a failure of mesodermal induction causes MKS. The induction cascades of early morphogenesis involve numerous growth factors, homeobox genes, and paired domain genes.

Diagnosis: Some authors consider that the minimal diagnostic criteria for the syndrome consist of cystic dysplasia of the kidney, fibrotic changes of the liver, and occipital encephalocele. Thus histologic studies are needed to confirm the diagnosis. Clinical features are highly variable among patients.

Clinical aspects: The main features are *central nervous system* malformations consisting usually of occipital encephalocele (with holoprosencephaly, agenesis of corpus callosum and/or hydrocephalus); seizures; *postaxial polydactyly* always involving the hand and occasionally the feet and *polycystic kidneys; other urologic anomalies* include absent or hypoplastic ureters or bladder. Often the liver shows cystic changes with duct proliferation and fibrosis. Other anomalies include microcephaly, microphthalmia or anophthalmia, cleft lip and/or palate, genital anomalies, lung hypoplasia, and congenital heart disease such as atrial septal defect (ASD), ventricular septal defect (VSD), coarctation of the aorta, and patent ductus arteriosus (PDA). Patients also present a typical "Meckel appearance" with micrognathia, flat nose, hypertelorism, a sloping forehead, wide mouth with full lips, low-set ears, and short neck.

Precautions before anesthesia: A complete medical history must be obtained. Assess the neurological system, especially for seizures and the presence of encephalocele and raised intracranial pressure. The renal function must be evaluated. Because of the facial anomalies, the airway must be carefully examined. Finally, the cardiac system needs a thorough examination because of the high incidence of congenital heart defects. An ECG and echocardiogram must be obtained. Medications should be continued until the morning of surgery.

Anesthetic considerations: It is highly improbable that children with Meckel syndrome will come to the operating room. If they do, remember that all the main systems, such as the heart, liver, kidneys, and lungs, may be involved, so these children can be very unstable. Also, they present many features, such as micrognathia, short neck, and occipital encephalocele that can render intubation difficult.

Pharmacological implications: Implications are related to decreased renal and liver function in the setting of neonatal anesthesia.

REFERENCES:

Farag TI, Usha R, Uma R, et al: Phenotypic variability in Meckel-Gruber syndrome. *Clin Genet* 38:176, 1990.

Fraser FC, Lytwyn A: Spectrum of anomalies in the Meckel syndrome, or: "maybe there is a malformation syndrome with at least one constant anomaly." *Am J Med Genet* 9:67, 1981.

Miyasu M, Sobue H, Azami T, et al: Anesthetic and airway management of general anesthesia in a patient with Meckel-Gruber syndrome. *J Anesth* 19:309, 2005.

Salonen R: The Meckel syndrome: Clinicopathological findings in 67 patients. *Am J Med Genet* 18:671, 1984.

Median Cleft Facial Syndrome

At a glance: Syndrome manifested by cleft lip and anterior cleft palate, microcephaly, mental retardation, hypertelorism, bifid uvula, and absence of the nasal septal cartilage.

N.B: This is also known as *holoprosencephaly type I*. This medical condition should not be confused with *holoprosencephaly type II* in which hypotelorism and the possibility of cebocephaly (cyclopia) may be encountered.

Synonyms: Frontonasal Dysplasia Sequence; Median Cleft Face Syndrome; DeMyer Syndrome; Holoprosencephaly Type I.

Incidence: Rare; male-to-female ratio is 2:1; increased paternal and maternal ages at the time of conception.

Genetic inheritance: Most often a sporadic condition limited to the face and head. A dominant form with associated spinal anomalies has been reported; other reports suggest a multifactorial transmission. Translocation involving chromosomes 3, 7, and 11 and four breakpoints have been reported in one 4-year-old boy. For some unknown reason, instances of twinning are greater in families with frontonasal dysplasia than in the general population.

Pathophysiology: Facial dysplasia with dysostosis (craniofacial helix) and clefting. True or primary clefts are caused by the persistence of epithelium between the borders of the facial processes (deficient epithelial cell degeneration).

Diagnosis: Clinical features (wide midline cleft of the facial skeleton, hypertelorism of eyes, and possible coexisting severe deformity of lower extremities) in conjunction with certain roentgenographic findings (anterior cranium bifidum, hypoplastic frontal sinuses, dense calcification of the falx, interhemispheric lipoma) and ophthalmologic examinations (refractive errors, strabismus, nystagmus, and eyelid ptosis).

Clinical aspects: *Facies:* Frontonasal dysplasia; narrowing of palpebral fissures; hypertelorism; broad nasal root; median nasal groove; absent nasal tip; separated slit-like nares, bifid nose; widow's peak; strabismus; nystagmus; eyelid ptosis. *Skeleton:* Tibial aplasia; hallucal polydactyly; varus deformity; anterior cranium bifidum occultum. *Other Anomalies:* Median cleft palate; encephalocele; duplication of labial frenulum; tetralogy of Fallot; mental retardation (10–15% of patients). In severe cases, the central nervous system may be affected, and there is a mental deficiency. The severity of reported examples can be graded in a logical sequence. The patients may have bifidity of the tip or dorsum of the nose, sometimes in association with a median cleft lip or median notch of the cupid's bow and with a duplication of the labial frenulum. Frontonasoethmoidal dysplasia and even transsphenoidal encephalocele with pituitary herniation and orbital hypertelorism are common. The maxilla may show a keel-shaped deformity with rotation of the incisors. A median cleft of the palate may be observed, with other anomalies including mental retardation.

Precautions before anesthesia: Evaluate carefully for difficult laryngoscopy and tracheal intubation. Physical examination directed primarily toward the central nervous system, cardiovascular system (tetralogy of Fallot), lungs, and upper airway. Standard preoperative laboratory examinations are appropriate in most patients (blood chemistries, blood group, hemoglobin, coagulation profile).

Anesthetic considerations: The potential for difficult direct laryngoscopy and tracheal intubation is very high. It is important to maintain spontaneous ventilation at all times, and other technical means of airway management, such as laryngeal mask airway and fiberoptic airway equipment, must be available. No other specific anesthetic considerations other than those associated with the surgical procedure itself.

Pharmacological implications: No known pharmacological contraindications.

Other conditions to be considered:

TEEBI HYPERTELORISM (Brachycephalofrontonasal Dysplasia): Characterized by hypertelorism, craniofrontonasal dysplasia, short stature, joint laxity, prominent forehead, mild antimongoloid slant, long palpebral fissures, heavy and broad eyebrows, widow's peak, broad and depressed nasal bridge, short nose, and slightly small, broad hands, mild syndactyly, and genital anomalies. Other clinical features may include congenital heart defects (e.g., ventricular septal defect), lipoma of the occipital area, and hypoplastic left cerebellar hemisphere. It has been suggested to be inherited as an autosomal dominant pattern.

☞**TORIELLO-CAREY SYNDROME:** Characterized by multiple congenital anomalies. The association of agenesis of the corpus callosum, telecanthus, short palpebral fissures, small nose with anteverted nares, Pierre Robin sequence, abnormally shaped ears, redundant neck skin, laryngeal anomalies, congenital heart defects, short hands, and hypotonia form this medical entity.

PAI SYNDROME: Characterized by median cleft of the upper lip, pedunculated skin masses on the face, and midline lipomas of the central nervous system. The cause of this syndrome is unknown, although autosomal dominant inheritance has been proposed. First described in 1987.

REFERENCE:

Guion Almeida ML, Richieri Costa A, Saavedra D, et al: Frontonasal dysplasia: Analysis of 21 cases and literature review. *Int J Oral Maxillofac Surg* 25:91, 1996.

Meier-Gorlin Syndrome

At a glance: Inherited disorder characterized by short stature, craniofacial anomalies, bilateral microtia, and absence of patellae. Other clinical features include complete dislocation of the elbow, hooked clavicle, and clinodactyly.

Synonyms: Ear, Patella, Short Stature (EPS) Syndrome; Microtia, Absent Patellae Syndrome; Micrognathia Syndrome; Meier Rothschild Syndrome.

Incidence: Unknown.

Genetic inheritance: Autosomal recessive genetic disorder.

Pathophysiology: Unknown.

Diagnosis: Clinically; neuroradiographic imaging and functional inner ear investigations are recommended.

Clinical aspects: Short stature, very slender, poor weight gain, delayed bone age, and absent patellae may be signs, but they are more part of the delayed bone age. Habitual elbow dislocation, slender ribs, slender long bones, abnormal glenoid fossas, hooked clavicles, clinodactyly, epiphyseal flattening, camptodactyly, blunt osteochondritis dissecans, aseptal necrosis of the lateral femoral condyles, bilateral microtia with dysplasia of the labyrinthus, micrognathia.

Precautions before anesthesia: Evaluation of the airway for potential difficult laryngoscopy and tracheal intubation. Preoperative assessment should include radiography of the cervical spine and mobility of the neck. In the presence of craniofacial anomalies, an anesthesia consultation should be obtained before any elective surgical procedures.

Anesthetic considerations: Careful assessment of the upper airway abnormalities combined with cervical spine mobility that may affect direct laryngoscopy and tracheal intubation. Positioning and intravenous access may be difficult. If the craniofacial anomalies are significant, consider the presence of raised intracranial pressure (e.g., craniosynostosis).

Pharmacological implications: If raised *intracranial pressure* is suspected, then a rapid-acting nondepolarizing muscle relaxant is preferable. In the case of major craniofacial surgery, *hypotensive anesthesia* technique may be considered. If venous gas embolism is a possibility, nitrous oxide should not be used.

REFERENCES:

Cohen A, Mulas R, Seri M, et al: Meier-Gorlin syndrome (ear-patella-short stature syndrome) in an Italian patient: Clinical evaluation and analysis of possible candidate genes. *Am J Med Genet* 197:48, 2002.

Feingold M: Meier-Gorlin syndrome. *Am J Hum Genet* 109:338, 2002.

Loeys BL, Lemmerling MM, Van Mol CE, et al: The Meier-Gorlin syndrome, or ear-patella-short stature syndrome, in sibs. *Am J Med Genet* 84:61, 1999.

Meigs Syndrome (Including Pseudo-Meigs Syndrome)

At a glance: Acquired disorder associated with a triad presentation of benign tumors of the ovary or other female pelvic organs, leading to ascites and pleural effusion. Histologically, the benign ovarian tumor might be a fibroma, thecoma, cystadenoma, or granulosa cell tumor.

Synonym: Meigs Salmon Syndrome.

History: In 1934, Salmon described the association of pleural effusion with benign pelvic tumors. In 1936, Joe Vincent Meigs, an American obstetrician, and John W. Cass, an American physician, described seven cases of ovarian fibromas associated with ascites and pleural effusion.

Incidence: In the United States, ovarian tumors are more prevalent in upper socioeconomic groups. Ovarian fibroma is found in 2 to 5% of surgically removed tumors and Meigs syndrome represents 1%. The prevalence is unknown. It is seen from the third decade, with a peak in the seventh decade.

Genetic inheritance: Acquired disorder.

Pathophysiology: Meigs syndrome is characterized by the presence of ascites and pleural effusion in the presence of a benign ovarian tumor. Pseudo-Meigs syndrome presents in a similar fashion and is associated with benign tumors of other pelvic organs. The cause of the ascites is uncertain but may be a result of mechanical irritation of the peritoneum, venous or lymphatic obstruction, or production of vasoactive substances by the tumor. The development of pleural effusions, which are usually right sided and may be massive, probably is caused by passage of ascitic fluid via transdiaphragmatic lymphatics or directly via diaphragmatic defects. Classically, the ascites and pleural effusions disappear following tumor removal. Development of ascites may be caused by release of mediators (e.g., activated complements, histamines, fibrin degradation products) from the tumor, leading to increased capillary permeability.

Diagnosis: The presence of a pleural effusion and ascites in the presence of a benign pelvic tumor and the disappearance of effusions following excision of the tumor are a sine qua non in making the diagnosis. Other causes of ascites and/or pleural effusions must be excluded. The presence of elevated CA125 levels usually is suggestive of ovarian malignancy. Elevated levels of CA125 have been reported in Meigs syndrome in the absence of malignancy.

Clinical aspects: *Meigs Syndrome:* Usually presents as abdominal pain and/or distension. If the ascites is significant or in the presence of a pleural effusion, dyspnea may be a presenting feature. Nonpro-ductive cough, malaise, and weight loss may accompany the other clinical features.

Pseudo-Meigs Syndrome: Consists of pleural effusion, ascites, and benign tumors of the ovary other than fibromas. These benign tumors include those of the fallopian tube or uterus and mature teratomas, struma ovarii, and ovarian leiomyomas.

Atypical Meigs Syndrome: Characterized by a benign pelvic mass with right-sided pleural effusion but without ascites. As in Meigs syndrome, pleural effusion resolves after removal of the pelvic mass.

Precautions before anesthesia: Respiratory status must be evaluated. A recent chest radiograph is mandatory; if the pleural or peritoneal fluid is interfering with respiratory mechanics, preoperative drainage of the collections must be considered. Other causes of pleural effusions must be excluded, including other malignancies and infections.

Anesthetic considerations: Respiratory function must be optimized. Laparotomy will be required for removal of the ovarian or pelvic tumor.

Pharmacological implications: No known specific implications with this condition.

REFERENCES:

Abad A, Cazorla E, Ruiz F, et al: Meigs' syndrome with elevated CA125: Case report and review of the literature. *Eur J Obstet Gynecol* 82:97, 1999.

Agranoff D, May D, Jameson C, et al: Pleural effusion and a pelvic mass. *Postgrad Med J* 74:265, 1998.

Hirota M, Noda J, Katoh S, et al: Perioperative management of patients with Meigs syndrome. *Masui* 44:874, 1995.

O'Flanagan SJ, Tighe BF, Egan TJ, et al: Meigs' syndrome and pseudo-Meigs' syndrome. *J R Soc Med* 80:252, 1987.

Melanoma-Astrocytoma Syndrome

At a glance: Inherited disorder characterized by numerous cutaneous malignant melanomas associated with tumors of the nervous system, including astrocytoma, medulloblastoma, glioblastoma multiforme, ependymoma, glioma, meningioma, and acoustic neurilemmoma.

Synonyms: Melanoma and Neural System Tumor Syndrome.

Incidence: Unknown.

Genetic inheritance: Autosomal dominant. The gene has been mapped to 9p21 with germ-like mutation in the cyclin-dependent kinase inhibitor 2A (CDKN2A)

Pathophysiology: Chromosome region 9p21 is involved in chromosomal inversions, translocations, heterozygous deletions, and homozygous deletions in a variety of malignant cell lines. These findings suggest that 9p21 contains a tumor suppressor locus that may be involved in the genesis of several tumor types.

Diagnosis: Clinical predictive genetic testing for mutation in the CDKN2A gene is available commercially.

Clinical aspects: Generally, most individuals affected with this syndrome present with more nevi than normal, and the tendency to dysplastic transformation is significantly higher. The association with neural tumor may be higher, and more pancreatic cancers are associated.

Anesthetic considerations: Anesthetic considerations will be determined by the presence of brain tumor and its type. Raised intracranial pressure, vascularization (e.g., medulloblastoma), and seizures. Anesthesia may be challenging when isolated limb perfusion is indicated to prevent cardiovascular instability, called "distributive shock", which is caused by the injection of tumor necrosis factor.

Pharmacological implications: No known specific implications with this condition.

Other conditions to be considered: All of the following conditions are allelic variants of CDKN2A mutation.

MELANOMA-PANCREATIC CANCER SYNDROME: Atypical familial multiple mole that can be caused by mutations in the gene encoding cyclin-dependent kinase inhibitor-2A (CDKN2A). Standard anesthetic considerations.

CUTANEOUS MALIGNANT MELANOMA: Mostly associated with fair complexion, blue eyes, multiple ephelides, and familial history of melanoma.

☞**LI-FRAUMENI SYNDROME:** Childhood sarcoma that usually is family related. This association often involves brain tumors, osteosarcoma, leukemia, and adrenocortical carcinoma. Precautions before anesthesia should include proper evaluation of intracranial pathology, intracranial pressure, and cortisol functions.

REFERENCES:

Fraser M, Marentay P, Bertha R: A collaborative approach to isolated limb perfusion. *AORN J* 70:642, 649, 651, 1999.

Greene MH: The genetics of hereditary melanoma and nevi. 1998 Update. *Cancer* 86(11 suppl):2464, 1999.

MELAS Syndrome

At a glance: MELAS is an acronym for *m*itochondrial myopathy, *e*ncephalopathy, *l*actic *a*cidosis, and *s*troke. It is a progressive neurodegenerative disorder. Other clinical features include diabetes mellitus, deafness, episodic vomiting, seizures, and cortical blindness.

Incidence: In the US adult population, the frequency is approximately 16.3:100,000. Internationally, the prevalence is approximately 10.2:100,000 in the Finnish population. Affects males and females between the ages of 4 and 15 years.

Genetic inheritance: Mitochondrial; the incidence of affected children is dependent upon maternal mutant load. It is a large heterogeneic syndrome with possible mutation of many genes such as MTTL1, MTND6, and MTTQs.

Pathophysiology: Multiple organ systems involved are the central nervous system, skeletal muscle, eye, cardiac muscle, and, more rarely, the gastrointestinal system. Approximately 80% of patients with the clinical characteristics of MELAS have a heteroplasmic A-to-G point mutation in the dihydrouridine loop of the tRNALeu (UUR) gene at base pair 3243 (i.e., A3243G mutation). Mitochondrial angiopathy of a small vessel is responsible for contrast enhancement of affected regions and mitochondrial abnormalities of endothelial cells and smooth muscle cells of blood vessels. The multisystem dysfunction may be a result of both parenchymal and vascular oxidative phosphorylation defects. The effect of potent vasodilators (e.g., nitric oxide) may be offset by increased production of free radicals in association with an oxidative phosphorylation defect leading to vasoconstriction. Defect of the respiratory chain enzymes, mainly the reduced form of nicotinamide adenine dinucleotide (NADH)-cytochrome *c* reductase (complex I).

Diagnosis: Usually based on clinical criteria; lactate levels are elevated at rest and increase further with minimal exercise. Demonstration of ragged-red fibers on muscle biopsy. Electronic microscopy may show abnormal mitochondria and mitochondrial DNA (mtDNA) testing (80% have a mutation at base 3243 and 10% at base 3271). The stroke-like episodes usually are associated with infarcts exhibited on head CT scan or MRI. These infarcts have been hypothesized to be nonvascular and caused by transient oxidative phosphorylation dysfunction within the brain parenchyma.

Clinical aspects: These children have normal early development. Onset is most often during the second decade but can be seen as early as age 4 years. The severity and form of presentation vary considerably and depend on maternal mutant mitochondrial load. The main features include subsequently poor growth and fatigability with muscle weakness. There is progressive episodic vomiting, seizures, and recurrent cerebral insults mimicking strokes and causing hemiparesis, hemianopsia, or cortical blindness. The most frequent symptom is episodic sudden headaches with vomiting and convulsions. Myopathy is associated with lactic acidosis in blood and cerebrospinal fluid. Most of the allelic variants are described with atrioventricular block, Wolff-Parkinson-White syndrome, or cardiomyopathy. Multihormonal hypopituitarism may be present. Alterations of the skin (purpura and hirsutism) occur in 45% of cases. The clinical diagnosis is based on five cardinal manifestations: clinical stroke, seizures, lactic acidosis, ragged-red fibers, and exercise intolerance.

Precautions before anesthesia: The diagnosis of mitochondrial disease should be considered in any child with a multisystem neurologic disorder or who is being investigated for hypotonia. Anesthesia-related morbidity and mortality risk is essentially linked to the preoperative status of the child, that is, the number and extent of organ dysfunction. A preoperative electrocardiogram should be considered at any age. The elevated serum lactate resulting from defects in the respiratory chain necessitate maintenance of a normal glucose level, normothermia, normocapnia, and more stable possible cardiovascular function. Allelic variants are diabetic, so serum glucose must be closely measured. Avoid any elective anesthesia/ surgery in the presence of infection or raised temperature because cytokines (mainly tumor-necrosis factor) inhibit some complex of the respiratory chain. The following should be checked: *central nervous system* (seizures, myoclonus, strokes, swallowing problems); *metabolic* (usual venous or arterial concentration of lactates and glucose); *muscles* (hypotonia, contractures, scoliosis); *cardiac* (even if the child is asymptomatic, ECG and echocardiography to exclude conduction disorders and cardiomyopathy, respectively; check functioning of pacemaker, if present; *pulmonary* (frequent infections, chronic aspiration, pulse oximetry breathing room air, obstructive and/or central apnea; reduced ventilatory drive is common and many patients have an abnormal response to both hypoxia and hypercarbia, and deaths have been reported following sedation with chloral hydrate or diazepam); *hepatic* and *renal* function; and *nutritional status* and *diet* (glucose and/or lipid-rich, tolerance to fasting and treatment [carnitine, vitamin Q, antiepileptic drugs]).

Anesthetic considerations: Usual treatment up to the day of surgery. Preoperative fasting as short as possible; if fasting is usually poorly tolerated, a glucose-containing solution should be started when the fasting period starts. A sedative premedication is best avoided because of the possible abnormal response to hypoxia/ hypercarbia. *Induction:* No contraindication to choice of anesthetic; however, the dosage of sedative agents might require reduction; sevoflurane is the best choice for inhalation induction; propofol seems the best choice for IV induction, but a 2% solution should be used to lessen the lipid load. *Opiates:* Dose should be carefully titrated according to the patient's needs. *Muscle Relaxant:* Published data are contradictory. Even in the absence of clinical myopathy, the patient's muscular response to nerve stimulation should be measured before administering a muscle relaxant. Atracurium and *cis*-atracurium are the best choices because of their spontaneous degradation. In case of myopathy, succinylcholine should not be used to avoid producing rhabdomyolysis. *Intraoperative Fluids:* Avoid infusion containing lactates, such as lactated Ringer or Hartmann solution, but the patient should receive a glucose solution (5 or 10% according to blood sugar level). Aim for normoglycemia because hyperglycemia can increase lactate production. Monitor (arterial or venous) blood gases and lactates level. In case of severe lactic acidosis, use dichloroacetate 50 mg/kg IV over 30 minutes to stimulate pyruvate dehydrogenase to metabolize lactate in pyruvate. Perimedullar locoregional anesthesia can be used, but its cost-to-benefit ratio should be evaluated, taking into account the presence of severe scoliosis or degenerative lesions in the spinal cord. Some patients with mitochondrial disease also present with axonal neuropathy of peripheral nerves; the possible effects of local anesthetics on these nerves are unknown. Prevention of hypothermia is important to avoid shivering and increased oxygen consumption upon awakening.

Pharmacological implications: Patients with mitochondrial disease are very sensitive to the respiratory effects of sedatives. It also seems, according to the Bispectral index (BIS) measurement, that children with an anomaly of complex I of the respiratory chain are much more sensitive to the hypnotic effects of sevoflurane. Most studies performed on isolated mitochondria use doses of anesthetic agents far in excess of those used in daily practice; thus their clinical relevance is often dubious. The sensitivity to neuromuscular blocking agents is controversial. It would be advisable to avoid succinylcholine and to carefully monitor short-duration drugs.

Other conditions to be considered:

☞**Kearns-Sayre Syndrome:** Mitochondrial encephalomyopathy characterized by progressive external ophthalmoplegia, atypical retinitis pigmentosa, and cardiomyopathy.

☞**MERRF Syndrome:** Mitochondrial cytopathy that stands for myoclonus epilepsy associated with Ragged-Red fibers. It is characterized by severe myoclonic seizures that are usually brief, sudden, and defined as jerking spasms that affect the limbs and/or the entire body. Severe lactate acidosis is often present. Dysarthria, ataxia, short stature, hearing loss, and dementia are also features.

☞**Leber Hereditary Optic Neuropathy:** Rare hereditary form of optic atrophy that usually affects young males. Characterized by sudden bilateral cloudiness of vision, followed by scotoma, rapid deterioration of central vision, and occasional color vision disorders. Associated with atrophy of the optic nerve fibers and the retinae. Considered a mitochondrial disease.

☞**Alström Syndrome:** Inherited syndrome with diabetes mellitus, cardiac, hepatic and renal involvement, and progressive visual and hearing loss.

References:

Hirano M, Pavlakis SG: Mitochondrial myopathy, encephalopathy, lactic acidosis, and stroke-like episodes (MELAS): Current concepts. *J Child Neurol* 9:4, 1994.

Thompson VA, Wahr JA: Anesthetic consideration in patients presenting with mitochondrial myopathy, encephalopathy, lactic acidosis and

stroke-like episodes (MELAS) syndrome. *Anesth Analg* 85:1404, 1997.

Vilela H, Garàa-Fernandez J, Parodi E, et al: Anesthetic management of a patient with MERRF syndrome. *Paediatr Anaesth* 15(1):77, 2005.

Wallace JJ, Perndt H, Skinner M: Anesthesia and mitochondrial disease. *Paediatr Anaesth* 8:249, 1998.

Melkersson-Rosenthal Syndrome

At a glance: *Melkersson-Rosenthal syndrome* is the term used when there is cheilitis (chronic swelling of the face), peripheral facial palsy, and lingua plicata ("scrotal" tongue). Granulomatous cheilitis is a chronic swelling of the lip caused by granulomatous inflammation. *Miescher cheilitis* is the term used when the granulomatous changes are confined to the lip. Miescher cheilitis generally is regarded as a monosymptomatic form of the Melkersson-Rosenthal syndrome, although the possibility remains that they are separate diseases.

Synonym: Melkersson Syndrome; Cheilitis Granulomatosis; Orofacial Granulomatosis Syndrome; Wiescher-Melkersson-Rosenthal Syndrome.

Incidence: Unknown. Condition is rare. No racial or gender predilection. Onset usually is in young adult life.

Genetic inheritance: Autosomal dominant; gene on chromosome 9.

Pathophysiology: Probably of autoimmune origin related to HLA-DR histocompatibility complex. Normal lip architecture eventually is altered by the presence of lymphedema and noncaseating granulomas in the lamina propria.

Diagnosis: Episodic swelling of the face with relapsing peripheral nerve palsy; uveitis is accompanied by granulomas elsewhere. The main differential diagnosis is with sarcoidosis. However, the Kveim test is negative.

Clinical aspects: Characterized by episodic swelling of the face and orofacial granulomatosis. The eyelids, pharynx, oral mucosa, and larynx may be affected by granuloma formation. The tongue is said to be "scrotal" in appearance. Recurrent peripheral facial paralysis as a result of involvement of the facial nerve.

Precautions before anesthesia: History and examination should assess the extent of airway involvement by granulomas.

Anesthetic considerations: Even in the presence of a normal upper airway, the possibility of laryngeal and upper tracheal granulomas must be considered. Upper airway and facial swelling may cause considerable problems with face-mask fit and tracheal intubation. Postoperative airway obstruction has been reported.

Pharmacological implications: No specific considerations have been demonstrated.

Other condition to be considered:

Iceland Amyloidosis (Amyloiosis Type VI; Cerebral Amyloid Angiopathy Syndrome; Icelandic Cerebroarterial Amyloidosis Syndrome): Autosomal dominant disorder characterized by facial paralysis or swelling around the mouth, which is similar to Melkersson-Rosenthal syndrome. Other clinical features include premature stroke, intracranial hemorrhage, and dementia with an onset during the third or fourth decade of life. Death occurs before age 40 years and most often related to intracerebral hemorrhage. There is evidence that the disorder is caused by mutation in the gene encoding cystatin C in some patients. Cerebral amyloid angiopathy has also been observed with high-density lipoprotein deficiency. The British type of cerebral amyloid angiopathy is caused by mutations in the ITM2B gene.

REFERENCES:

James DG: All that palsies is not Bell's. *J R Soc Med* 89:184, 1996.

Jayamaha JEL: Respiratory obstruction in a patient with Melkersson-Rosenthal syndrome. *Anesth Analg* 77:395, 1993.

Melnick-Fraser Syndrome

At a glance: Very rare genetic disorder characterized by distinctive malformations of the head and facial area, with skin lesions and abnormalities of the eyes. Other clinical features may include renal anomalies (bilateral renal dysplasia), Mendini-type cochlear malformation (hypoplasia of cochlear apex on CT scan), bilateral prehelical pits, and bilateral branchial cleft fistulas.

Synonym: Branchio-Oto-Renal (BOR) syndrome.

Incidence: Rare; 1:40,000 live births; approximately 2% of profoundly deaf children.

Genetic inheritance: Autosomal dominant; gene located on 8q13.3.

Pathophysiology: Not clearly defined, probably caused in great part by mutation of human EYA 1 gene homologue of the *Drosophila* "eyes absent" gene (EYA). This gene is expressed in all areas of the developing inner ear and in the metanephric cells of the developing kidney, early in fetal development.

Diagnosis: Clinically evocated by pits or ear tags in front of the outer ear, branchial fistulas, branchial cysts, hearing loss, and abnormal development of the kidneys (polycystic or dysplasia). Prenatal diagnosis is possible.

Clinical aspects: This bipolar disease involves head and neck with auricular pits (77%); deafness that is perceptive, conductive, or mixed (89%); narrow auditory canal; and branchial cleft or cysts (63%). Cleft palate or uvula, facial paresis, microphthalmia, and absent nasolacrimal duct can be observed. Occasional deep prognathism. Genitourinary tract is the second pole of the disease (66%), ranging from minor dysplasia (double ureters, hydronephrosis, polycystic kidneys, supernumerary, ectopic or small kidneys) to bilateral renal agenesis.

Precautions before anesthesia: Evaluate deafness (clinical, auditory evoked potentials, ear, nose, throat investigations). Evaluate renal function (clinical; echography/CT scan; scintigraphy; laboratory blood and urinary investigations, including urea and electrolytes).

Anesthetic considerations: Comprehension and cooperation of the patient is not always evident in case of deafness. Prognathism may make direct laryngoscopy and tracheal intubation difficult.

Pharmacological implications: Perioperative fluid regimen should be adapted to renal status. Avoid drugs with renal metabolism in case of renal insufficiency. Use of aminosides should be carefully evaluated considering deafness and renal status.

Other conditions to be considered:

☞**BRANCHIO-OCULO-FACIAL SYNDROME:** Very rare genetic disorder apparent at birth. May be characterized by low birth weight; presence of an abnormal pit, cleft, or hemangiomatous or atrophic postauricular skin lesion. Distinctive craniofacial malformations; abnormalities of the eyes; and premature graying of the scalp hair during adolescence. Other features might include cleft palate and lip and prominent philtrum that resembles a surgically repaired cleft lip (pseudocleft). Characteristic eye includes microphthalmia, cataracts, congenital strabismus, ocular hypertelorism, and coloboma of the iris, giving the iris a "keyhole" appearance. Inherited as an autosomal dominant genetic trait.

BRANCHIO-OTO-URETERAL SYNDROME: Rare disorder inherited as an autosomal dominant trait with variable expression. The main characteristics are ear and kidney abnormalities. The outer ear may have pits or tags, be cone shaped, or be smaller than normal. Ureteral duplication or misposition is always present, and the kidney collecting system may be split in two.

REFERENCE:

Chitayat D, Hodgkinson KA, Chen MF, et al: Branchio-oto-renal syndrome: Further delineation of an underdiagnosed syndrome. *Am J Med Genet* 43:970, 1992.

Melnick-Needles Syndrome (MNS)

At a glance: Genetic disorder characterized by abnormal bone development. Bowing of the bones in the arms and legs is characteristic. Particular facial appearance includes hypertelorism, full cheeks, small facial bones, and severe micrognathia. Other clinical features include a relatively small chest cavity with irregular ribbon-like ribs, short clavicle, short stature, and narrow shoulders. Pectus excavatum is often present. Occasionally, dislocation of the hip occurs. May present hydronephrosis caused by urinary retention caused by small ureters. There is some suggestion that the entity is a form of the fronto-otopalatodigital osteodysplasia syndrome.

Synonyms: Osteodysplasty of Melnick and Needles; Melnick-Needles Osteodysplasty.

History: First described in 1966 by John Welnick, an American radiologist, and Carl F. Needles, an American physican.

Incidence: Fewer than 50 persons described; seems to affect more females than males.

Genetic inheritance: Either an X-linked dominant or autosomal sex-limited dominant trait. Otopalatodigital syndrome type II and MNS likely result from mutations in the same gene. The difference in expression would be explained by allelic heterogeneity in expression. Most patients are female, but disease severity is greater in males.

Pathophysiology: Some cases suggest that this condition is a generalized connective tissue disorder in which an increased content of collagen is found.

Diagnosis: Clinically and radiologically.

Clinical aspects: Considerable heterogeneity, short stature, generalized bone dysplasia. Facial anomalies include a small face with prominent eyes appearing hyperteloric; broad nasal bridge with anteverted nares; micrognathia; sometimes cleft palate; full cheeks; and gingival hypertrophy. Small chest with ribbon-like ribs, sometimes pectus excavatum; bowing of long bones, mainly tibia and radius (metaphyseal flaring on radiograph), and short upper limbs; vertebral anomalies leading to scoliosis. In case of severe lung disease, secondary pulmonary hypertension. Mitral and/or tricuspid valve prolapse, hydronephrosis, omphalocele, hypoplastic kidneys, and urethral obstruction can be associated in some described cases.

Precautions before anesthesia: Check airway for possible difficult laryngoscopy and tracheal intubation. It is important to obtain an echocardiography to exclude associated cardiac problem (mitral and/or tricuspid valve prolapse) or pulmonary hypertension. Preoperative chest physiotherapy to prevent postoperative complications.

Anesthetic considerations: The anesthetic management of a patient with mitral or tricuspid valve prolapse must be applied. In the presence of a child with recurrent pulmonary infection, special care must be taken because of increased risk for postoperative pulmonary complications. Be prepared for difficult tracheal intubation.

Pharmacological implications: No known pharmacological implications.

Other conditions to be considered:

☞**OTOPALATODIGITAL SYNDROME TYPE I:** Congenital association of coarse facies, posterior cleft palate, conduction deafness, clinodactyly on the fifth fingers, and broad big toes. The skull and limb are most often abnormal.

☞**OTOPALATODIGITAL SYNDROME TYPE II:** Congenital association of craniofacial and limb anomalies.

☞**FRONTOMETAPHYSEAL DYSPLASIA:** Congenital syndrome involving multiple abnormalities of the face and airway, poorly developed musculature, and limited joint mobility.

☞**SERPENTINE FIBULA-POLYCYSTIC KIDNEY SYNDROME:** Probably X-linked dominant inherited disorder with normal intelligence characterized by S-shaped (serpentine-shaped) elongation of the fibulas, bowed long bones of forearms and lower legs, proportionate short stature, short neck, shield thorax with pectus excavatum and increased intermamillary distance (some features similar to ☞Ullrich-Turner Syndrome), polycystic kidneys, large head with low-set ears, full cheeks, prominent eyes with megalocornea and ptosis, and micrognathia. Sensorineural deafness is not uncommon. Other features may include congenital cardiac defects (e.g., ASD and/or VSD, PDA), intestinal malrotation, joint laxity, and hirsutism. It has been suggested that SFPKS and ☞Melnick-Needles Syndrome are allelic disorders.

☞**HAJDU CHENEY SYNDROME:** Very rare diffuse connective tissue disorder with osteolysis involving mainly head and musculoskeletal system.

REFERENCE:

Verloes A, Lesenfants S, Barr M, et al: Fronto-otopalatodigital osteodysplasia: Clinical evidence for a single entity encompassing Melnick-Needles syndrome, otopalatodigital syndrome types 1 and 2, and frontometaphyseal dysplasia. *Am J Med Genet* 90:407, 2000.

Meltzer Syndrome

At a glance: Cryoglobulinemia leading to hematuria, anasarca, and progressive deterioration of the renal function. As the patient ages, hypertension, proteinuria, and elevated serum creatinine are present. Special attention to hypothermia and the possibility of hepatitis C.

Synonym: Mixed Familial Cryoglobulinemia.

Incidence and genetic inheritance: Autosomal dominant.

Clinical aspects: Cryoglobulinemia with systemic manifestations has acquired the name *Meltzer syndrome*. Cryoglobulins are immunoglobulins that persist in the serum, precipitate at cold temperature, and resolubilize when rewarmed. Type I is often associated with hematologic disorders. Types II and III are mixed, composed of different immunoglobulins with a monoclonal component in type II and only polyclonal immunoglobulins in type III. Hepatitis C virus is involved in most previously called *essential mixed cryoglobulinemia*. Dermatologic, rheumatologic, and nephrologic manifestations are the most frequent; neurologic complications are found

in 20% of cases. End-stage cases may lead to renal insufficiency, hypertension, and anasarca.

Anesthetic considerations: Assessment of renal function is mandatory; check for hepatitis C. Keep all the perfused fluids (blood and electrolytes solutions) warm and pay attention to normothermia. In procedures that require hypothermia, plasma exchanges may help.

REFERENCE:

Maisonobe T, Leger JM, Musset L, et al: Neurological manifestations in cryoglobulinemia. *Rev Neurol (Paris)* 158:920, 2002.

Menkes Syndrome

At a glance: Genetic disorder of copper metabolism beginning before birth. Copper accumulates in excessive amounts in the liver and is deficient in most other tissues of the body. Structural changes occur in the hair, brain, bones, liver, and arteries. Other clinical features include spontaneous hypothermia, severe developmental delay, loss of early development skills, and seizures. Spontaneous subdural hematoma and/or rupture or thrombosis of arteries in the brain may occur. Spastic dementia may eventually arise. Osteoporosis as a result of abnormal copper metabolism can result in pathologic fractures. The combination of subdural hematoma and bone fractures may lead to an incorrect diagnosis of child abuse. Emphysema, bladder abnormalities, degeneration of the retina, and cysts of the iris have been described.

Synonyms: Kinky Hair Disease; Steely Hair Disease; X-Linked Copper Malabsorption; Trichopoliodystrophy.

History: Neurodegenerative and connective tissue disorder first described by John H. Menkes, an American neuropediatrician, in 1962.

Incidence: In the early 1970s, an incidence of 1:35,000 male births was suggested. However, in the 1980s, this frequency was reviewed at 1:90,000 live births. Finally, most agree that the incidence is estimated at 1:50,000–100,000 live births.

Genetic inheritance: X-linked recessive. Caused by mutation in the gene encoding the Cu^{2+}-transporting ATPase α-polypeptide. Gene map locus is X-q12-q13.

Pathophysiology: Defective coding for an intracellular copper-transporting protein called the human Menkes protein (MNK or ATP7A), which travels between the Golgi apparatus and the cell membrane, transporting copper to the exterior of the cell. Defective MNK prevents proper intestinal absorption of copper. Resultant free-copper deficiency affects function of copper-dependent enzymes such as cytochrome oxidase, tyrosinase, and lysyl oxidase, which results in symptoms and signs of disease.

Diagnosis: Menkes syndrome should be considered in any male infant with unexplained seizures, hypothermia, and mental retardation. Hair changes (stubby, tangled, sparse, steely, or kinky hair that is easily broken), low serum copper and ceruloplasmin concentrations, and radiologic findings are characteristic. Copper levels are elevated in fibroblasts and the placenta. Carrier status for the abnormal gene can usually be determined by microscopic examination of multiple hairs from scattered scalp sites for pili torti (twisted hair). Prenatal diagnosis is available (DNA probe).

Clinical aspects: In the classic form, the disease starts before age 3 months by loss of neurologic development (hypotonia progressively evolving to spasticity), severe seizures, and subdural hematoma. Patients manifest hypopigmentation, growth failure, skeletal defects, arterial aneurysms, and progressive cerebral and cerebellar degeneration. Myoclonic seizures and hypothermia are frequent. Fragile steely depigmented (grayish or ivory colored) hair is present in the newborn period; they appear as pili torti at microscopic examination. Typical facies consist of frontal or occipital bossing, abnormal or absent eyebrows, pudgy cheeks with sagging jowls, micrognathia, and pallor. Characteristic radiographic changes include wormian bones in lamboid and sagittal sutures, anterior rib flaring, spur formation on the femoral and humeral metaphysis, and osteoporosis. Arteriography shows elongation, tortuosity, narrowing, and dilatation of cerebral, visceral, and limbs arteries. Gastroesophageal reflux and recurrent aspiration frequently accompany progressive central nervous system deterioration. Joint hyperlaxity and capillary fragility caused by defective lysyl oxidase, a copper-containing enzyme involved in the cross-linking of collagen similar to Ehlers-Danlos syndrome. Diverticular malformations of the bladder and ureters. Treatments have been generally unsuccessful; oral copper helps control the seizures but has no effect on progression of neurologic damage. Death within 3 years as a consequence of intractable seizures or pneumonia.

Precautions before anesthesia: Anticonvulsant therapy should be assessed and optimized preoperatively and continued through the perioperative period. Consider raised intracranial pressure if previous intracranial hemorrhage. Repeated aspiration pneumonias plus hypotonia may compromise respiratory function. May need evaluation with chest radiograph, arterial blood gases, and other tests. Rule out ongoing pneumonia. Check for anemia secondary to aneurysmal bleeding. Hypovolemia and/or electrolyte disturbances may be present if diarrhea is severe. Postural vital signs to check for orthostatic hypotension.

Anesthetic considerations: Risk of pulmonary aspiration because of gastroesophageal reflux. Postoperative upper airway obstruction secondary to hypotonia: the two infants reported in the anesthetic literature eventually needed a tracheostomy. Therefore, overnight admission in the pediatric intensive care unit should be planned, as well as prolonged tracheal intubation or the use of a nasopharyngeal airway. Difficult tracheal intubation caused by redundancy of pharyngeal soft tissue has been described. As a consequence of capillary fragility, patients are at increased risk for hemorrhage during surgery and regional anesthetic techniques, especially the central neuraxial blocks, which are relatively contraindicated. Measures to prevent hypothermia should be instituted vigorously. Thick skin makes insertion of intravenous catheters and other lines more difficult. Osteoporotic bones may be brittle and prone to fracture during positioning.

Pharmacological implications: Anesthetic agents known to trigger the occurrence of seizures must be avoided (enflurane with hypocapnia, methohexital, ketamine, and sustained high concentration of sevoflurane). Anticonvulsant therapy results in induction of hepatic enzymes, so the metabolism of anesthetic agents (e.g., local anesthetics) might be affected.

Other conditions to be considered: A forme fruste of Menkes syndrome presents with cerebellar ataxia and mild mental retardation.

OCCIPITAL HORNS SYNDROME: A phenotypic overlap between Menkes syndrome and occipital horns syndrome that is caused by a mutation of the same ATP7A gene. Clinical findings include mild mental retardation, joint hyperlaxity, dysfunction of the autonomous nervous system (chronic diarrhea, orthostatic hypotension), bladder anomalies, and ossified occipital horns on skull radiographs.

☞**WILSON DISEASE:** Copper and ceruloplasmin metabolic disorder characterized by liver disease, brain dysfunction, and a char-

acteristic rusty-brown colored ring around the cornea of the eye (Kayser-Fleischer ring). Individual affected with this disease do not have the characteristic kinky hair of Menkes syndrome.

☞**AMISH HAIR BRAIN SYNDROME:** Sulfur-deficient brittle hair, short stature, mental deficiency, sexual infantilism, and infertility originally observed in the Amish kindred.

HEREDITARY WOOLY HAIR SYNDROME (Salamon Syndrome): Autosomal dominant; characterized by the presence of woolly, kinky hair often associated with ocular disorders or atrophic keratosis of the hair (with partial or complete axillary or pubic alopecia).

☞**BRITTLE HAIR AND MENTAL DEFICIT SYNDROME:** Autosomal recessive disorder with fragile hair, onychodystrophy, mental retardation, and scalp hypotrichosis.

TAY SYNDROME (Ichthyosis-Brittle Hair-Impaired Intelligence-Decreased Fertility-Short Stature [IBIDS] Syndrome): Photosensitivity, ichthyosiform erythroderma, progeria-like facies, failure to thrive, mental retardation, occasional infertility, and trichothiodystrophy (sulfur-deficient brittle hair). First described by Chong H. Tay, a Singapore physician, in 1971.

REFERENCES:

Kazim R, Weisberg R, Sun LS: Upper airway obstruction and Menkes syndrome. *Anesth Analg* 77:856, 1993.

Llanos RM, Mercer JF: The molecular basis of copper homeostasis copper-related disorders. *DNA Cell Biol* 21:259, 2002.

Tobias JD: Anaesthetic considerations in the child with Menkes' syndrome. *Can J Anaesth* 39:712, 1992.

Meretoja Syndrome

At a glance: Primary hereditary systemic amyloidosis (type V) characterized by cardiac and airway implications. Clinical features include corneal lattice dystrophy and cranial neuropathy (e.g., facial paresis), nephrotic syndrome and renal failure, and cutis laxa. Peripheral polyneuropathy mainly affecting vibration and touch senses may be present in these individuals.

Synonyms: Amyloidosis Type V; Finnish Type Amyloidosis; Meretoja Type Amyloidosis; Amyloid Cranial Neuropathy with Lattice Corneal Dystrophy; Amyloidosis due to Mutant Gelsolin; Generalized Amyloid Disease.

Genetic inheritance: Autosomal dominant.

Pathophysiology: Amyloidosis type V results from the extracellular deposition of gelsolin, a proteinaceous material. These deposits impair organ function.

Diagnosis: Amyloid deposits in the skin, kidneys, and heart. Genetic mutation in gelsolin (asp187-to-asn) found in all Finnish families and in several Scottish American cases studied and can therefore be diagnostic. The Melkersson-Rosenthal syndrome may be considered in the differential diagnosis.

Clinical aspects: Arises from infiltration of all tissues by amyloid deposits. Functional impairment may lead to death, particularly when the liver, kidney, brain, or heart is affected. Cardiac conduction system dysfunction with bradyarrhythmia and hypotension. This amyloidosis is often associated with macroglossia and benign tumors of the tracheobronchial tree.

Precautions before anesthesia: Assess the airways because of the extensive amyloidosis deposits. In adults, if possible obtain an endoscopic status down to the carina. Obtain a detailed cardiac history; look for dysrhythmias, syncopes, pacemaker. Ask for signs of diastolic dysfunction, sudden dyspnea attacks, orthopnea. Obtain ECG and echocardiogram.

Anesthetic considerations: Be prepared for difficult laryngoscopy and tracheal intubation (fiberoptic intubation). Be prepared for (complete) heart block: atropine, isoprenaline, dopamine, and/or external pacemaker should be available and ready for use. Arterial line. Be prepared for diastolic dysfunction; titrate fluids carefully. Pulmonary artery catheter and/or echocardiography can be useful.

Pharmacological implications: Avoid drugs that may exacerbate bradycardia. Avoid cardiac ischemia and cardiodepressant drugs.

REFERENCES:

Meretoja J: Genetic aspects of familial amyloidosis with corneal lattice dystrophy and cranial neuropathy. *Clin Genet* 4:173, 1973.

Rothstein A, Auran J, Wittpen JR, et al: Confocal microscopy in meretoja syndrome. *Cornea* 21:364, 2002.

Seguin P, Freidel M, Perpoint B: Amyloid disease and extreme macroglossia. Apropos of a case. *Rev Stomatol Chir Maxillofac* 95:339, 1994.

Shah H, Garbe L, Nussbaum E, et al: Benign tumors of the tracheobronchial tree. Endoscopic characteristic and role of laser resection. *Chest* 107:1744, 1995.

Merlob Syndrome

At a glance: Inherited disorder characterized by coloboma, microcephaly, porencephaly, and hydronephrosis, in which an affected individual has a head circumference less than 3 standard deviations below the age- and sex-related mean. All affected individuals are mentally retarded.

Synonyms: Primary Autosomal Recessive Microcephaly; MCPH Syndrome.

Incidence and genetic inheritance: Approximately 1:250,000 live births. True microcephaly is inherited as an autosomal recessive trait. It is genetically heterogenous, with at least five loci mapped: MCPH1 to chromosome 8p23; MCPH2 to locus 19q13.1-q13.2; MCPH3 at 9q34; MCPH4 at 15q15-q21; and MCPH5 to 1q31, which is a mutant of the ASPM (abnormal spindle-like, microcephaly associated) gene.

Clinical aspects: Microcephaly with sloping forehead, narrow forehead, and flat occiput. It is associated with mental deficiency and seizures. A small but apparently normally formed brain is the reason for the reduced head circumference.

Anesthetic considerations: There are no specific considerations reported. Assessment of severity of seizures and knowledge of treatment.

REFERENCE:

Pattison L, Crow YJ, Deeble VJ, et al: A fifth locus for primary autosomal recessive microcephaly maps to chromosome 1q31. *Am J Hum Genet* 67:1578, 2000.

MERRF Syndrome

At a glance: Acronym for *m*yoclonus *e*pilepsy with *r*agged-*r*ed *f*ibers. Belongs to a group of rare muscular disorders called *mitochondrial encephalomyopathies*. The most characteristic symptom is myoclonic seizures that are usually sudden, brief, jerking spasms that can affect the limbs or the entire body. Ataxia, lactic acidosis, dysarthria, optic atrophy, short stature, hearing loss, dementia, and nystagmus may occur.

Synonym: Fukuhara Syndrome.

Genetic inheritance: Mitochondrial; incidence of affected children is dependent upon maternal mutant load.

Pathophysiology: Defect of the respiratory chain enzymes, mainly complexes I and IV.

Diagnosis: Clinical and laboratory confirmation of elevated pyruvate and lactate. Muscular biopsy shows ragged-red muscle fibers, and the biochemical defect is often segmental on histochemistry.

Clinical aspects: Clinical spectrum is proportional to the amount of normal and mutant DNA. Onset is in the neonatal period, with mental deterioration, intention tremor, myoclonic epilepsy, spasticity, ataxia, muscle weakness and atrophy, myopathy, and sensory neural hearing loss. The neuropathologic findings are (a) degeneration of dentate nucleus, red nucleus, globus pallidus, subthalamic nucleus, and pontine tegmentum; (b) degeneration of the Clarke column (the dorsal nucleus of the spinal cord), spinocerebellar tract, posterior column and corticospinal tract, and posterior spinal nerve root and sural nerve; and (c) degeneration of substantia nigra, locus caeruleus, cerebellar cortex, and inferior olivary nucleus.

Precautions before anesthesia: Diagnosis of mitochondrial disease should be considered in any child with a multisystem neurologic disorder or who is being investigated for hypotonia. Anesthesia-related morbidity and mortality risk is essentially linked to the preoperative status of the child, that is, the number and extent of organ dysfunction. The presence of a mitochondrial disease is not considered a risk for malignant hyperthermia. Avoid any elective anesthesia/surgery in the presence of infection or temperature because cytokines (mainly tumor necrosis factor (TNF)), inhibit some complex of the respiratory chain. The following should be checked: central nervous system (seizures, myoclonus, strokes, swallowing problems); *metabolic* (usual venous or arterial concentration of lactates and glucose); *muscles* (hypotonia, contractures, scoliosis); *cardiac* (even if the child is asymptomatic, ECG and echocardiography to exclude conduction disorders and cardiomyopathy, respectively; check functioning of pacemaker, if present); *pulmonary* (frequent infections, chronic aspiration, pulse oximetry breathing room air, obstructive and/or central apnea; reduced ventilatory drive is common, and many patients have an abnormal response to both hypoxia and hypercarbia, and deaths have been reported following sedation with chloral hydrate or diazepam); *hepatic* and *renal* dysfunctions; *nutritional status* and *diet* (glucose and/or lipid rich; tolerance to fasting and treatment [carnitine, vitamin Q, antiepileptic drugs]).

Anesthetic considerations: Usual treatment until the morning of surgery. Preoperative fasting as short as possible; if fasting is usually poorly tolerated, a glucose-containing solution should be started when fasting period starts. A sedative premedication is best avoided because of the possible abnormal response to hypoxia/hypercarbia. *Induction:* No contraindication to choice of anesthetic; however, the dosage of sedative agents might require reduction; sevoflurane is the best choice for inhalation induction; propofol seems the best choice for IV induction, but a 2% solution should be used to lessen the lipid load. *Opiates:* Dose should be carefully titrated according to the patient's needs. *Muscle Relaxant:* Published data are often contradictory. Even in the absence of clinical myopathy, the patient's muscular response to nerve stimulation should be measured before administering a muscle relaxant. Atracurium and *cis*-atracurium are the best choice because of their spontaneous degradation. In case of myopathy, succinylcholine should not be used to avoid producing rhabdomyolysis. *Intraoperative Fluids:* Avoid infusion containing lactates, such as Ringer lactate or Hartmann solution, but the patient should receive a glucose solution (5 or 10% according to blood sugar level). Aim for normoglycemia because hyperglycemia can increase lactate production. Monitor (arterial or venous) blood gases and lactate levels; in case of severe lactic acidosis, use dichloroacetate 50 mg/kg IV over 30 minutes to stimulate pyruvate dehydrogenase to metabolize lactate in pyruvate. Perimedullar locoregional anesthesia can be used, but its cost-to-benefit ratio should be evaluated, taking into account the presence of severe scoliosis or degenerative lesions in the spinal cord. Some patients with mitochondrial disease also present with axonal neuropathy of peripheral nerves: the possible effects of local anesthetics on these nerves are unknown. Prevention of hypothermia is important to avoid shivering and increased oxygen consumption at awakening.

Pharmacological implications: Patients with mitochondrial disease are very sensitive to the respiratory effects of sedatives. It also seems, according to BIS measurement, that children with an anomaly of complex I of the respiratory chain are much more sensitive to the hypnotic effects of sevoflurane. Most studies performed on isolated mitochondria use doses of anesthetic agents far in excess of those used in daily practice; thus their clinical relevance is often dubious.

Other conditions to be considered:

☞**KEARNS-SAYRE SYNDROME:** Neuromuscular disorder characterized by chronic progressive external ophthalmoplegia, atypical retinitis pigmentosa, cardiomyopathy, and conduction defects (e.g., heart block). Other findings may include muscle weakness, short stature, hearing loss, and ataxia.

☞**MELAS SYNDROME:** Mitochondrial encephalomyopathy. The most characteristic presentation is recurring, stroke-like episodes associated with sudden headaches, vomiting, and seizures. Short stature, lactic acidosis, and seizures are typically present. Hemianopsia and cortical blindness may affect individuals with this medical entity.

☞**LEIGH SYNDROME:** Neurometabolic disorder characterized by progressive neurologic degeneration (i.e., brain, spinal cord, and optic nerve), generalized weakness, hypotonia, lactic acidosis, and impairment of respiratory and kidney function. It is inherited as an autosomal recessive pattern and usually begins between the ages of 3 months and 2 years. However, X-linked recessive and mitochondrial inheritance have also been suggested.

REFERENCES:

Bindoff LA, Desnuelle C, Birch-Machin MA, et al: Multiple defects of the mitochondrial respiratory chain in a mitochondrial encephalopathy (MERRF): A clinical, biochemical and molecular study. *J Neurol Sci* 102:17, 1991.

Vilela H, Garcia-Fernandez J, Parodi E, et al: Anesthetic management of a patient with MERRF syndrome. *Paediatr Anaesth* 15:77, 2005.

Wallace JJ, Perndt H, Skinner M: Anesthesia and mitochondrial disease. *Paediatr Anaesth* 8:249, 1998.

Mesomelia-Synostoses Syndrome

At a glance: Mesomelic shortness of stature with severe skeletal changes in the vertebrae, ankles, knees, and elbows. Present agenesis of the palate, broad nose, and small mouth.

Synonym: Facio-Renal-Acromesomelic Syndrome.

History: First described in 1995 as a newly autosomal dominant inherited form of mesomelic shortness of stature by A Verloes and A David.

Incidence and genetic inheritance: Autosomal dominant; two families described.

Clinical aspects: Mesomelic short stature, shorts limbs with severe skeletal changes in the ankles, knees, and elbows, progressive curvature of the forearm, microretrognathia, beaked nose, transverse agenesis of soft palate, nasal speech, down-slanting of palpebral fissures with hypertelorism and ptosis. Hydronephrosis and mild vertebral anomalies. At birth, is associated with short umbilical cord having unusually long skin coverage.

Anesthetic considerations: Vertebral anomalies can lead to difficulties in locoregional anesthesia. Renal function should be assessed with the association of hydronephrosis. Difficulty with the upper airways is anticipated given the retromicrognathia and agenesis of the soft palate.

Other condition to be considered:

☞**KANTAPUTRA GORLIN SYNDROME:** Characterized by bilateral, symmetrical marked shortening of the ulna and shortening and bowing of the radius. Synostoses between the tibia and fibula are present because of an unusually short proximal fibula. The most characteristic feature is the presence of a prominent calcaneus on the ventral surface of the distal fibula. Carpal and tarsal synostoses are present. The average height of affected male adults was 152 cm. This medical entity is very similar to the mesomelia-synostosis syndrome.

REFERENCE:

Verloes A, David A: Dominant mesomelic shortness of stature with acral synostoses, umbilical anomalies, and soft palate agenesis. *Am J Med Genet* 55:205, 1995.

Metachromatic Leukodystrophy

At a glance: Inherited disorder of the myelin metabolism with progressive loss of white matter in the central and peripheral nervous system. It is the most common form of leukoencephalopathy and is characterized by sulfatide accumulation in the brain and other areas of the body (liver, gall bladder, kidneys, and/or spleen). Clinical manifestations may include seizures, behavioral changes, spasticity, progressive dementia, psychomotor dysfunction leading to paralysis, and visual impairment leading to blindness.

Synonyms: Arylsulfatase A Deficiency; Cerebroside Sulfatase Deficiency; Diffuse Cerebral Sclerosis; Greenfield Disease; Sulfatide Lipidosis; Sulfatidosis.

Classification: *Late Infantile Metachromatic Leukodystrophy:* Characterized by onset usually in the second year of life, most commonly before age 30 months. It is associated with rapid progression leading to death before age 5 years in most cases. The clinical features include psychomotor disturbances, spasticity, mental deterioration, progressive blindness, hypotonia, ataxia, and seizures. The cerebrospinal fluid contains elevated protein.

Juvenile Metachromatic Leukodystrophy: Typically begins between the ages of 4 and 10 years, presenting symptomatology similar to the late infantile form.

Adult Metachromatic Leukodystrophy: Begins after age 16 years with severe psychiatric behavioral disorders by age 30 years.

Abdominal distension, dysarthria, loss of previously acquired intellectual skills, behavioral abnormalities, and dementia are particularly pronounced in this form of the disease.

Incidence: Estimated at 1:100,000 live births.

Genetic inheritance: Autosomal recessive. Gene locus: long arm (q13) of chromosome 22 codes for the arylsulfatase A gene (3.2 kb). Gene mutations can lead to low (group A) or absent (group I) enzyme activity with the following phenotypes: late infantile (alleles II), juvenile (IA), and adult (AA). The saposin B gene is located on chromosome 10.

Pathophysiology: Galactosyl-3-sulfatide (cerebroside sulfate) is normally located on the surface of the myelin sheath, maintaining electrical neutrality, sodium transport, and opioid receptor function. It is hydrolyzed by the lysosomal arylsulfatase A with saposin B (a glycoprotein) as coenzyme. Enzyme deficiency leads to galactosyl sulfatide accumulation in myelin (demyelination), kidney (excess excretion), and gallbladder (cholecystitis). Rarely, saposin B deficiency causes metachromatic leukodystrophy.

Diagnosis: Clinical course. *Biochemical:* (a) Decreased arylsulfatase A activity in peripheral leukocytes and cultured skin fibroblasts; (b) increased sulfatide in cerebrospinal fluid and urine. Delayed nerve conduction and evoked potentials. Characteristic CT scan and MRI images show white matter lesions and cortical atrophy. *Histology:* Spherical metachromatic granules in the central and peripheral nervous systems (sural nerve). Prenatal and heterozygote diagnosis is possible.

Clinical aspects: Progressive white matter disease, starting with gait disturbance, mental regression, and urinary incontinence. Congenital form results in early death. Late infantile form is usually recognized during the second year of life: common manifestations are progressive blindness, loss of speech, quadriparesis, posturing, peripheral neuropathy, and seizures. The disease process lasts 2 to 6 years. The juvenile form starts between 4 and 12 years. The adult form is slowly progressive with mental dysfunction, dementia, and behavioral problems. Multiple sulfatase deficiency is a rare form of metachromatic leukodystrophy, with features resembling mucopolysaccharidosis and deficiency of at least seven sulfatases. Other categories include (a) metachromatic leukodystrophy without arylsulfatase A deficiency and (b) arylsulfatase A pseudodeficiency. In all cases, there is no dysfunction of the heart, lungs, adrenal cortex, liver, and kidneys. *Treatment:* (a) symptomatic with vigabatrin (reduce spasticity); (b) bone marrow transplantation before clinical symptoms may be useful; (c) gene or enzyme replacement and protease inhibitor treatments are experimental.

Precautions before anesthesia: Evaluate the extent of demyelination, evidence of cord compression (vertebral body hypoplasia), and bulbar palsy. Evidence of aspiration pneumonitis: SpO_2 (arterial oxyhemoglobin saturation), gases, chest radiography. Electrolytes if dehydration is a factor, but adrenal function is normal. Assess carefully the medical management of seizures and dysphagia and the potential for recurrent pulmonary aspiration.

Anesthetic considerations: Rapid-sequence induction if airway reflexes are impaired. Antisialagogue indicated if copious secretions. Prevention of hypothermia. Postoperative respiratory failure possible if patient is hypotonic. Preexisting mental dysfunction may prolong recovery, especially after opioid use. Prevention of gastrointestinal regurgitation during induction must be a prime concern.

Pharmacological implications: Succinylcholine should be avoided in the presence of spinal cord compression. Although vigabatrin is an anticonvulsant, causing an irreversible inhibition of gamma-aminobutyric acid (GABA) transaminase (increasing GABA level as a result), it does not induce liver cytochrome enzymes. Meperidine, ketamine, and enflurane are relative contraindications if seizures present. Ensure administration of intravenous anticonvulsant medications.

Other conditions to be considered:

☞**TAY-SACHS DISEASE:** Autosomal recessive progressive neurodegenerative disorder that, in the classic infantile form, is usually fatal by age 2 or 3 years. In the absence of hexosaminidase A, the brain accumulates significant amounts of G_{M2} gangliosidosis. Clinical features include myoclonic jerks (seizure-like activities) at birth and between the age of 6 and 10 months, feeding difficulties that have become apparent, hypotonia, restlessness, unusual eye movements, and presence of cherry-red macular spots. After age 12 months, there is noticeable loss of previously acquired skills and coordination. It is generally found among children of Eastern European Jewish heritage.

SANDHOFF DISEASE (☞Gangliosidosis Type II): Manifested by progressive deterioration of the central nervous system because of a deficiency in the β-subunit of hexosaminidase. Sandhoff disease is considered the severe form of Tay-Sachs disease and is not limited to any particular ethnic group. It typically begins between the ages of 3 and 6 months and is clinically manifested by dysphagia, general weakness, motor weakness, progressive mental deterioration, spasticity, heart murmurs, seizures (myoclonic and generalized), blindness, and splenomegaly and cherry macules in the eyes.

☞**ALEXANDER SYNDROME:** Progressive metabolic disorder classified as a leukodystrophy. It is characterized by rapid loss of myelin. The clinical manifestations usually begin during infancy and may include muscle spasms, developmental delays, seizures, and mental retardation. When it begins during childhood, the symptoms may include dysphagia, arthritis, severe vomiting, respiratory problems because of the inability to cough, and muscle spasms.

☞**PELIZAEUS-MERZBACHER SYNDROME:** Associated with progressive deterioration of the white matter of the brain. The classic form of the disease usually detected during infancy is characterized by the absence of normal psychomotor development, failure to control the head and eyes, severe growth retardation, muscle tremors, weakness, involuntary jerky muscle movements, facial grimacing, unsteadiness, and joints contractures.

☞**ADRENOLEUKODYSTROPHY:** Association of cerebral demyelination and progressive adrenal atrophy. The most common form of the disease occurs during childhood. Clinical manifestations include seizures, ataxia, hyperreflexia, hemiparesis, dysarthria, deafness, behavioral problems, and visual difficulties. This medical condition was the basis of the story in the 1993 film "Lorenzo's oil" depicting the life of Lorenzo Odone, afflicted with the disease.

☞**CANAVAN SYNDROME:** Characterized by spongy degeneration of the central nervous system associated with hypotonia, poor head control (atonicity), megalocephaly, involuntary muscle contractions of limbs, exaggerated reflex responses, paralysis, and blindness.

KRABBE DISEASE: Characterized by abnormal accumulation of ceramide galactoside in the brain; associated with irritability, vomiting, episodes of partial unconsciousness, leg spasticity, dysphagia, mental deterioration, and seizures.

☞**ZELLWEGER SYNDROME:** Characterized by the congenital absence of functioning peroxisomes (cellular structures responsible for elimination of toxic substances) resulting in a cerebrohepatorenal syndrome. The disease affects brain development, particularly myelination. Most important features include hepatomegaly, polycystic kidney disease, visual disturbances, and high plasma levels of iron and copper. Other clinical features include muscular hypotonia already noticeable at birth, mental retardation, seizures, coagulopathy, and dysphagia with recurrent aspiration. Congenital heart defects have been described. Life expectancy is approximately 6 months.

REFERENCES:

Hernandez-Palazon J: Anaesthetic management in children with metachromatic leukodystrophy. *Paediatr Anaesth* 13:733, 2003.

Kolodny EH, Fluharty AL: Metachromic leukodystrophy and multiple sulfatase deficiency: sulfatide lipidosis, in Scriver CR, Beaudet AL, Sly WS (eds): *The Metabolic and Molecular Bases of Inherited Disease.* 7th ed. New York, McGraw-Hill, 1995, p 2693.

Malde AD, Naik LD, Pantvaidya SH, et al: An unusual presentation in a patient with metachromatic leukodystrophy. *Anesthesia* 52:690, 1997.

Tobias JD: Anaesthetic considerations for the child with leukodystrophy. *Can J Anaesth* 39:394, 1992.

Metaphyseal Chondrodysplasia, Jansen Type

At a glance: Extremely rare progressive disorder in which portions of the bones of the arms and legs develop abnormally with unusual cartilage formations and subsequent abnormal bulbous metaphyses (metaphyseal chondrodysplasia). Affected individuals exhibit unusually short arms and legs and short stature (short-limbed dwarfism), findings that typically become apparent during early childhood. Infants with Jansen-type metaphyseal chondrodysplasia may have characteristic facial abnormalities and additional skeletal malformations. Hypercalcemia is present.

Synonyms: Jansen Metaphyseal Dysplasia; Murk Jansen Metaphyseal Chondrodysplasia; Chondrodysplasia Jansen type

Incidence: Fewer than 25 cases have been reported in the literature.

Genetic inheritance: Autosomal dominant. Majority of cases are sporadic.

Pathophysiology: Caused by mutation in parathyroid hormone receptor 1 gene (PTHR1), which has been mapped to 3p22-p21.1.

Diagnosis: Clinically evocated by the postnatal onset of severe short stature with joint dysfunction. Radiologic signs vary with age, showing diffuse radiolucency at birth, irregular calcification in childhood, and bulbous deformations of long bone extremities.

Clinical aspects: Severe short stature (adult height: 125 cm [49.2 inches]) and enlarged joints with flexion contractures (knees, hips). Small thorax, kyphoscoliosis. Irregular and disorganized metaphyses but normal epiphyses. Small face with prominent supraorbital ridges; micrognathia; sometimes choanal atresia, high-arched palate, mandibular cyst. Wide cranial sutures with hyperostosis of calvaria and cranial bone sclerosis. Variable deafness. Waddling gait. *Biochemistry:* Hypercalcemia, hypercalciuria, hypophosphatemia. Increased urinary cAMP; elevated $1,25(OH_2D_3$, alkaline phosphatase; low/absent parathyroid hormone.

Precautions before anesthesia: Assess renal function and serum calcium and phosphate levels. Hypercalcemia may be asymptomatic or may be associated with polyuria, dehydration, thrombosis, muscle weakness, and hyporeflexia. ECG is recommended. In the presence of symptomatic or clinically significant hypercalcemia, active steps should be taken to lower the serum levels (i.e., with saline rehydration/diuresis). Phosphate supplementation may be required.

Evaluate carefully the airway for potential difficult tracheal intubation (clinical, radiograph). Evaluate severity of the disease (clinical, full history, radiographs).

Anesthetic considerations: Anesthesia in this condition has not been described. The features of the disease suggest that face-mask ventilation, direct laryngoscopy, and tracheal intubation may be difficult. If it is the case, spontaneous respiration should be maintained until confirmation that face-mask ventilation can support gas-exchange or until the trachea has been secured and lung ventilation confirmed. Renal dysfunction may be present. Patient positioning may be difficult because of contractures. Patients may be prone to fractures. Hypercalcemia may lead to arrhythmias and hypertension. Hyperventilation may be useful in life-threatening hypercalcemia. Neuromuscular monitoring is recommended to facilitate titration of muscle relaxants.

Pharmacological implications: Metabolism/excretion of some drugs may be altered in the presence of renal dysfunction. Digitalis toxicity is exacerbated by hypercalcemia. The response to neuromuscular blockers may be potentialized by hypercalcemia. Consider renal function before using aminoside antibiotics.

REFERENCES:

Aguilera IM, Vaughan RS: Calcium and the anaesthetist. *Anaesthesia* 55:779, 2000.

Schipani E, Langman C, Hunzelman J, et al: A novel parathyroid hormone (PTH)/PTH-related peptide receptor mutation in Jansen's metaphyseal chondrodysplasia. *J Clin Endocrinol Metab* 84:3052, 1999.

Kruse K, Schutz C: Calcium metabolism in the Jansen type of metaphyseal dysplasia. *Eur J Pediatr* 152:912, 1993.

Metaphyseal Chondrodysplasia, McKusick Type

See *Cartilage-Hair Hypoplasia Syndrome.*

Metaphyseal Chondrodysplasia, Schmid Type

At a glance: Very rare inherited disorder characterized by short stature with abnormally short arms and legs (short-limbed dwarfism). Other physical characteristics may include outward "flaring" of the lower rib cage, genu varum, pain in the legs, and/or hip deformities (coxa vara). Such abnormalities of the legs and hips typically result in an unusual "waddling" gait.

Synonyms: Metaphyseal Dysplasia, Schmid Type; Schmid Metaphyseal Dysplasia.

Nature: Congenital anomaly of collagen located in the metaphyses.

Genetic inheritance: Autosomal dominant with variable expression; de novo mutations not rare.

Pathophysiology: Mutation in COL10A1 gene for collagen type X, the expression of which is restricted to the hypertrophic zone of the growth plate. This explains the metaphyseal location of the disease and the mechanical weakness of the growth plates in these patients.

Diagnosis: Clinical picture, but rickets and causes of hypophosphatasemia should be excluded.

Clinical aspects: Moderate short stature, bowed legs, coxa vara, waddling gait. Irregular metaphyses, but the radiological picture can temporarily disappear after prolonged bed rest. Enlarged femoral capital epiphyses. No vertebral anomalies. Adult height: approximately 130 to 160 cm (51.2–63 inches).

Anesthetic considerations: Because of the numerous skeletal anomalies, positioning of the patient must require special attention.

REFERENCE:

Lachman RS, Rimoin DL, Spranger J: Metaphyseal chondrodysplasia, Schmid type. Clinical and radiographic delineation with a review of the literature. *Pediatr Radiol* 18:93, 1988.

Methemoglobinemia (Congenital)

At a glance: Congenital presence of high levels of methemoglobin in blood. Presence of abnormally high levels of methemoglobin in the blood because of a congenital anomaly of one chain of hemoglobin (hemoglobins M) or congenital deficit in NADH-cytochrome b_5 reductase.

Classification:

- Hemoglobins M
- Congenital Deficit in NADH-Cytochrome b_5 Reductase

History: Mutations in cytochrome $b5$ reductase activity were identified in 1943 by Quentin Gibson, which was considered a "Tour de Force" of clinical investigation. Gibson subsequently went on to become one of the world's leading biochemists.

Incidence: Rare. There are no epidemilogical studies on congenital methemoglobinemia.

Genetic inheritance: Autosomal dominant (hemoglobins M) but a high rate of new mutations or recessive (congenital deficit in cytochrome $b5$ reductase) with a gene located on chromosome 22 q 13.31-qter.

Pathophysiology: *Hemoglobins M:* Five different mutations of hemoglobin (Hb) are known to produce congenital methemoglobinemia: Hb M_{Boston}, Hb M_{Iwate}, Hb $M_{Saskatoon}$, Hb $M_{Hyde Park}$, and Hb $M_{Milwaukee}$. *Congenital Deficit in NADH-Cytochrome $b5$ Reductase:* Two types: type I in which the deficit is limited to the red blood cells, and type II in which the deficit is generalized (brain, liver, muscle, etc.). In red blood cells, the enzyme is present in its soluble form and is responsible for reversing the spontaneous oxidation of hemoglobin to methemoglobin. In other cells, it is located in the membrane of many organelles (Golgi system, microsomes, mitochondria) and is involved in the recycling of vitamin E and in the synthesis of cholesterol and cerebral lipids.

Diagnosis: Measurement of dyshemoglobins with a co-oximeter. *Hemoglobins M:* Methemoglobinemia above 25% leads to cyanosis unaffected with oxygen administration, blood that is chocolate color, headache, confusion, chest pain, and weakness. *Congenital Deficit in NADH-Cytochrome $b5$ Reductase:* Measurement of enzymatic activity in red cells and fibroblasts

Clinical aspects: The patient's coloring is more grayish than truly cyanotic and the blood appears brown on inspection.

Hemoglobins M: Cyanosis is present from birth if mutation is on the α chain, later if mutation is on the β chain of hemoglobin (when hemoglobin F is replaced by hemoglobin A). It is well tolerated and requires no treatment.

Congenital Deficit in Cytochrome $b5$ Reductase: Type I: Cyanosis from birth; it is very well tolerated and varies with temperature and exercise. Headache and palpitations when methemoglobinemia is greater than 50%. Patients are very sensitive to exogenous methemoglobin-producing agents.

Congenital reductase Type II: Cyanosis from birth but accompanied by irritability, vomiting, and feeding problems. By age 6 to 9 months, profound mental retardation is present, with microcephaly, nystagmus, athetosis, and attacks of hypertonia. Seizures are frequent, and death usually occurs before age 10 years as a consequence of pulmonary infections (chronic aspiration).

Precautions before anesthesia: Determine the precise cause of methemoglobinemia.

Anesthetic considerations: Monitoring of hemoglobin oxygen saturation with pulse oximetry is unreliable. In case of worsening hemoglobinemia in a patient with type I congenital deficit of NADH-cytochrome $b5$ reductase, methylene blue 1 to 3 mg/kg should be administered intravenously (more than 5 mg/kg could induce hemolysis or methemoglobinemia by itself).

Pharmacological implications: Methemoglobinizing agents such as benzocaine, prilocaine, quinine, metoclopramide, sulfamides, dapsone, and chloral hydrate should be avoided.

Other condition to be considered: Rare cases of abnormal fetal hemoglobin M have been described. Cyanosis disappears in infancy when hemoglobin F is replaced by hemoglobin A.

REFERENCES:

Baraka AS, Chakib A, Kaddoum R, et al: Severe oxyhemoglobin desaturation during induction of anesthesia in a patient with congenital methemoglobinemia. *Anesthesiology* 95:1296, 2001.

Beauvais P: Les méthémoglobinémies héréditaires. *Arch Pediatr* 7:513, 2000.

Vadgama S, Wallace J: Methemoglobinemia as a complication of topical anesthesia during bronchoscopy. *J Bronchology* 12:111, 2005.

Methionine Malabsorption Syndrome

At a glance: An inherited disease caused by malabsorption of methionine and secondary malabsorption of other amino acids. The unabsorbed methionine is converted to α-hydroxybutyric acid by intestinal bacteria. Urine has characteristic smell of dried malt. Clinical characteristics include mental retardation, seizures, white hair, diarrhea, and episodes of generalized edema.

Incidence and genetic inheritance: Only a single case described. Autosomal recessive.

Clinical aspects: Patient had white hair, rapid breathing, convulsions, and mental retardation. Urine had characteristic oasthouse smell. Another patient who may have had this condition had mental retardation, diarrhea, convulsions, and white hair.

Anesthetic considerations: Anesthetic management in this condition has not been described. No particular problems are anticipated based on the clinical description. Agents that may precipitate seizures, such as enflurane, should be avoided.

REFERENCE:

Ulshen M: Malabsorptive disorders, in Behrman RE, Kliegman RM, Arvin AM (eds): *Nelson Textbook of Pediatrics.* 15th ed. Philadelphia, WB Saunders, 1995.

Methylmalonic Acidemia (MMA)

At a glance: Heterogeneous inborn error of metabolism affecting amino acid metabolism, leading to metabolic acidosis and accumulation of methylmalonic acid (MMA) and its by-products.

Synonyms: Methylmalonic Aciduria, Methylmalonic-Coenzyme A Mutase Deficiency; MMA.

History: First reported in 1967 by Oberholzer and Stokke.

Incidence: Approximately 1:25,000–50,000 (all types of MMA included). Consanguinity is a risk factor. No gender predilection has been reported.

Genetic inheritance: Autosomal recessive (for all types). The gene encoding the enzyme methylmalonyl-CoA mutase has been mapped to 6p12-21.1. Two forms of this mutase deficiency exist: the mut^0 form with complete absence of mutase activity, and the mut^- form with reduced mutase activity. The mutase defect accounts for approximately 50% of patients with MMA. The defect in adenosylcobalamin synthesis has been mapped to chromosome 4q31.1-2.

Pathophysiology: Methylmalonic-coenzyme A mutase is a vitamin B_{12}-dependent enzyme involved in the catabolism of leucine, isoleucine, and valine; its deficiency leads to increased amounts of MMA in plasma and urine. Because of secondary inhibition of propionyl-CoA carboxylase, propionic acid also accumulates, as do other organic acids. Accumulation of propionyl-CoA results in inhibitory effects on various pathways of intermediary mitochondrial metabolism and secondary carnitine deficiency, thus explaining hypoglycemia, hyperammonemia, and hyperlactacidemia and the synthesis of odd-numbered abnormal fatty acids. Moreover, gut bacteria produce approximately 25% of the propionate to be metabolized.

Diagnosis: Neonatal screening for inborn errors of metabolism should detect all genetic variants of MMA. Large amounts of MMA, methylcitrate, propionic acid, and 3-hydroxy propionic acid can be detected in the urine by gas chromatography–mass spectrometry. However, once other causes for neonatal or infantile ketoacidosis have been ruled out, simple colorimetric assays for urinary MMA for suspected MMA are also available. Enzyme analysis in fibroblasts is used to detect the specific enzyme abnormality and finalize the diagnosis. Cultured amniotic cells are used for prenatal diagnosis.

Clinical aspects: The clinical picture has a high variability, and asymptomatic children with mutase apoenzyme deficiency have been identified through newborn screening. Although the signs in symptomatic children are basically similar to those of ☞Propionic Acidemia, complications and prognosis are worse in MAA. In 80%, manifestation of mut^0 patients occurs in the first week of life and the remainder by 6 months of life. In contrast, mut^- and cobalamin disorder patients most often present after the first month of life. The most common signs and symptoms at onset after a period of normal feeding are lethargy or coma, poor feeding with failure to thrive, recurrent vomiting with dehydration, hepatosplenomegaly, respiratory distress, and muscular hypotonia. MMA caused by a cobalamin-related defect usually has onset later in childhood or adolescence, starting with decreased lower leg sensitivity, thrombosis secondary to persistent homocystinuria, and progressive myopathy leading to chronic gait disturbances, which may not be irreversible. The majority of patients present with metabolic acidosis with a blood pH less than 6.9 and bicarbonate concentrations as low as 5 mmol/l. Ketonemia and ketonuria, hyperammonemia, anemia, leukopenia, and thrombocytopenia are found in more than 50% and hypoglycemia in 40% of the patients at presentation. Hyperglycinemia has been

reported in some patients. All patients with isolated MMA have in common the high plasma and urine concentrations of MMA, with urine concentrations up to 1000 times higher than normal. Infections and high-protein diet are known triggers for acute exacerbation, and many children with MMA may die in the first weeks of life, often before a diagnosis has been established secondary to ketoacidosis and/or hyperammonemia. The risk is significantly lower in MMA resulting from cobalamin deficiency. The median life expectancy for mut^0 patients is approximately 6 years. Mental retardation, seizures, and stroke are common features in MMA. The reasons for increased risk for stroke remain to be determined, but several hypotheses exist: severe acidosis may result in reduced cerebral blood flow secondary to hypocapnia or direct toxicity to the brain (glial and neuronal cells) from MMA and odd-chain fatty acids, or iatrogenic by treatment with high doses of cyanocobalamin, which is metabolized to the highly toxic cyanide. A stroke should always be excluded in MMA patients with acute onset of dystonia, dysarthria, dysphagia, or choreoathetosis. Acute exacerbation requires symptomatic treatment (rehydration, acid-base correction) and parenteral hyperalimentation with minimal amounts of proteins and high doses of vitamin B_{12} and L-carnitine. Hemo- or peritoneal dialysis may be required to correct hyperammonemia effectively. Long-term treatment consists of a low-protein diet and supplements of vitamin B_{12} and L-carnitine. Often chronic bicarbonate supplements are required to correct the metabolic acidosis. High forehead, epicanthal folds, broad nasal bridge, long philtrum, and a triangular mouth are the features responsible for facial dysmorphism. Skin lesions similar to acrodermatitis enteropathica have been described repeatedly. Chronic tubulointerstitial nephritis with progressive decline of renal function is a frequent long-term complication (20–60% of adolescents with MMA) and may require either hemodialysis or kidney transplantation.

Precautions before anesthesia: Obtain a full neurologic status and ask particularly about strokes, seizures pattern and frequency (and efficacy of treatment), and degree of mental retardation. Laboratory investigations should include a complete blood count (anemia, thrombocytopenia, leukopenia), blood glucose, electrolytes, acid–base status (blood gas analysis), and urine analysis for ketones. Renal function should be checked. For elective surgery, patients must be optimized as much as possible. Muscular hypotonia may require prolonged postoperative mechanical ventilation, and appropriate arrangements should be made in advance. During periods of increased catabolism, patients with MMA are at increased risk for metabolic decompensation (e.g., stress, intercurrent infections, trauma, surgery). The appropriate treatment is directed toward stopping catabolism and promoting anabolism. This can be achieved by intravenous administration of dextrose-containing solutions and maintenance of normovolemia. Provision of a stress-free anesthetic helps prevent acute exacerbations. Careful sedative and/or anxiolytic premedication may be helpful in the absence of lethargy and/or muscular hypotonia.

Anesthetic considerations: Dehydration, arterial hypotension, hypoxia, inappropriate caloric intake (catabolism, high-protein diet), and inadequate anesthesia technique can result in severe metabolic acidosis. Lactate-containing solutions (e.g., Ringer lactate, Hartmann or Stocker [swiss modification of Hartman solution]) should be avoided because they may not be metabolized appropriately in the presence of dysfunctional mitochondria and therefore contribute to the acid load. The regular bicarbonate requirements of the patients should be replaced intravenously in the perioperative period. Depending on the length of the procedure, an arterial line may be inserted to facilitate mandatory perioperative monitoring of acid–base status, blood glucose, ammonia, and lactate levels. Often, patients show lethargy and muscle hypotonia preoperatively. If there is risk of nasal, pharyngeal, or gastric bleeding, a gastric tube should be inserted to remove swallowed blood, which may otherwise provide a significant protein load and trigger an acute metabolic decompensation. Perioperative gastroduodenal ulcer prophylaxis with an H_2 antagonist or proton pump inhibitor may be indicated. Osteoporosis (secondary to malnutrition resulting from low-protein diet) requires careful positioning. Prolonged postoperative metabolic monitoring for early diagnosis of acute decompensation is recommended.

Pharmacological implications: Nitrous oxide inhibits vitamin B_{12}-dependent enzymes and so should be avoided in these patients. Drugs containing or metabolized to MMA, odd-chain organic acids, odd-chain fatty acids, odd-chain alcohols, or acrylic acids must be avoided because they can be metabolized to MMA, inhibit citric acid cycle enzymes, and result in ketoacidosis. These drugs include muscle relaxants metabolized by ester hydrolysis (succinylcholine, atracurium, *cis*-atracurium, mivacurium). Furthermore, propionic acid–derived nonsteroidal antiinflammatory drugs (e.g., naproxen, ketoprofen, ibuprofen) should be avoided. Propofol contains polyunsaturated fat (soybean oil) and should not be used. Avoid potentially epileptogenic drugs such as methohexital, ketamine, enflurane, atracurium, and meperidine (the last two in large quantity because of their respective metabolites of laudanosine and normeperidine) in patients with known seizures.

Other conditions to be considered:

☞**PROPIONIC ACIDEMIA:** Inborn error of metabolism affecting mitochondrial catabolism of valine and isoleucine that left untreated results in ketoacidosis, lethargy, coma, and finally death.

☞**HOMOCYSTINURIA:** Genetically transmitted error of metabolism of the amino acid methionine characterized by severe myopia, Marfan-like stature with pectus excavatus, slight mental retardation, and tendency to develop spontaneous generalized arterial and venous thromboses under stress.

☞**MAPLE SYRUP DISEASE:** Autosomal recessive transmitted inborn error of metabolism caused by a defect in the branched-chain α-ketoacid dehydrogenase resulting in the characteristic smell of the urine. Untreated, this disorder leads to mental retardation, seizures, and most often death.

☞**MULTIPLE CARBOXYLASE DEFICIENCY:** Inborn error of metabolism characterized by defective activity of all biotin-dependent carboxylases. Characterized by seizures, developmental delay, eczema, and hearing loss when left untreated.

☞**ARGININEMIA:** Urea cycle disorder that leads to hyperammonemia and neurologic symptoms, which are less severe than in other forms of urea cycle abnormalities. Clinical features include spastic paraplegia, seizures, and severe mental retardation. The triad of hyperammonemia, encephalopathy and respiratory alkalosis may be present.

☞**CITRULLINEMIA:** Syndrome arising from argininosuccinate synthetase deficiency leading to hyperammonemia and neurologic consequences. Severe vomiting spells beginning in infancy and the presence of mental retardation are characteristic features.

☞**HHH SYNDROME:** Genetically transmitted inborn error of metabolism resulting from a defect in the transport of ornithine into the mitochondrial matrix, clinically characterized by early growth retardation, learning disabilities, periodic confusion, and ataxia.

☞**N-ACETYLGLUTAMATE SYNTHETASE DEFICIENCY:** Congenital mitochondrial disorder affecting the metabolism of ammonium and resulting in hyperammonemia. Clinical features include cerebral edema, raised intracranial pressure, lethargy, heavy and rapid breathing, irritability, and coma leading to death if untreated.

☞**ORNITHINE CARBAMOYLTRANSFERASE DEFICIENCY:** Rare genetic disorder characterized by complete or partial lack of the enzyme ornithine transcarbamylase. The lack of this enzyme results in excessive hyperammonemia, which is a known neurotoxin. Clinically, patients present with vomiting, refusal to eat, progressive lethargy, and coma.

☞**CARNITINE DEFICIENCY:** Disorder resulting from decreased carnitine concentrations in plasma and tissues preventing mitochondria from adequate beta oxidation. Primary and secondary defects have been described. The manifestations are cardiomyopathy, encephalopathy, and myopathy.

☞**ISOVALERIC ACIDEMIA:** Genetic disorder affecting the branched-chain organic acids, the most frequent form of leucine metabolism disorders. It results in accumulation of isovaleric acid (and its metabolites), leading to vomiting, dehydration, severe metabolic acidosis, and neurologic manifestations.

REFERENCES:

Fenton WA, Gravel RA, Rosenblatt DS: Disorders of propionate and methylmalonate metabolism, in Scriver CR, Beaudet AL, Sly WS, et al (eds.): *The Metabolic and Molecular Bases of Inherited Disease.* 8th ed. New York, McGraw Hill, 2001, p 2165.

Harker HE, Emhardt JD, Hainline BE: Propionic acidemia in a four-month-old male: A case report and anesthetic implications. *Anesth Analg* 91:309, 2000.

Matsui SM, Mahoney MJ, Rosenberg LE: The natural history of the inherited methylmalonic acidemias. *N Engl J Med* 308:857, 1983.

Van't Hoff WG, Dixon M, Taylor J, et al: Combined liver-kidney transplantation in methylmalonic acidemia. *J Pediatr* 132:1043, 1998.

Meyer-Betz Disease

At a glance: Rare metabolic disorder characterized by an idiopathic myoglobinuria. The two clinical entities of this disease are *type I*, which is associated with onset after exertion, and *type II*, which occurs after infection.

Synonym: Idiopathic Paroxysmal Myoglobinuria.

Pathophysiology: Focal necrosis of skeletal muscle leads to rhabdomyolysis and myoglobinuria. Death may occur secondary to immediate hyperkalemia or subsequent renal tubular necrosis.

Diagnosis: No specific test for this disorder. Diagnosis is based on clinical and laboratory findings, specifically hyperkalemia, myoglobinuria, renal failure, and muscle weakness associated with either exertion or febrile illness.

Clinical aspects: Hyperkalemia, myoglobinuria, renal failure, muscle weakness that may lead to respiratory failure, association with exertion or febrile illness.

> *NB:* This disease mimics disorders of lipid metabolism, in which similar signs and symptoms occur with hypoglycemia.

Precautions before anesthesia: Obtain baseline serum electrolytes, glucose, blood urea nitrogen, and creatinine. Check temperature. Avoid prolonged fasting; start dextrose infusion while administering nothing by mouth.

Anesthetic considerations: Anticipate need to treat intraoperative hyperkalemia and renal failure. Frequently check glucose and supplement if needed. Prevent hyperthermia and cool aggressively if it occurs. Although few data on the use of succinylcholine in Meyer-Betz disease are available, prudence suggests substitution with nondepolarizing neuromuscular blocking agents in reduced doses in the presence of muscle weakness.

Pharmacological implications: Avoid succinylcholine. Titrate nondepolarizing neuromuscular blocking agents with a nerve stimulator.

REFERENCE:
Savage DCL: Idiopathic rhabdomyolysis. *Arch Dis Child* 46:594, 1971.

Michels Syndrome

At a glance: Triad of blepharophimosis, blepharoptosis, and epicanthus inversus. Occasional presence of spinal bifida occulta, cranial asymmetry, occipital bone flattening, and cleft lip/palate.

Synonyms: Oculopalatoskeletal Syndrome; Clefting-Ocular Anterior Chamber Defect-Lid Anomalies Syndrome.

Genetic inheritance: Autosomal recessive.

Clinical aspects: Eyelid traits are usually blepharophimosis, blepharoptosis, and telecanthus inversus, plus a developmental defect of the anterior segment of the eye. Craniosynostosis with cranial asymmetry, skeletal defects, hearing deficit, cleft lip and palate, and mild mental retardation; hydronephrosis is described.

Anesthetic considerations: Creatinine and blood urea nitrogen should be obtained. The presence of raised intracranial pressure cannot be excluded in presence of craniosynostosis. It is reported that in presence of a one-suture fusion, the intracranial pressure is elevated in 18% of patients and when two or more are involved, 40% of patients have an increase in intracranial pressure.

REFERENCE:
Sculerati N, Gottlieb MD, Zimbler MS, et al: Airway management in children with major craniofacial anomalies. *Laryngoscope* 108:1806, 1998.

Microgastria-Limb Reduction Defects Association

At a glance: Very rare syndrome characterized by splenic and intestinal anomalies associated with hypoplastic or absent upper limb. Severe congenital heart defect (e.g., truncus arteriosus) and pulmonary anomalies can be present.

Synonyms: MLRD; Congenital Microgastria Limb Reduction Complex.

History: First described by Robert in 1842.

Incidence and genetic inheritance: Fewer than 20 cases have been described. Genuine association, but no evidence of mendelian inheritance.

Clinical aspects: Features involve *gastrointestinal* (microgastria, asplenia, splenic hypoplasia, splenogonadal fusion, failure to thrive, gastric ulcer, malrotation of the gut, congenital megacolon), *limbs* (absent thumbs, radius, ulna, arm with single digit at the shoulder), and *genitourinary* (dysplastic or ectopic kidney). Torticollis, plagiocephaly, frontal bossing, paresis of ocular muscles, microphthalmos or anophthalmia, mental retardation, arrhinencephaly, fused thalami, agenesis of corpus callosum, cranial nerve anomalies, lissencephaly, absent clavicle, complex heart disease (Atrial septal defect, truncus arteriosus), imperforate anus, absent lobe lung, and segmentation defect can occur.

Anesthetic considerations: High rate of anesthetic implications. Major considerations are dictated by the preoperative evaluation of cardiac and respiratory anomalies. Aspiration risk may require rapid-sequence induction. Both central/peripheral venous and arterial access can be difficult. Careful intraoperative positioning is needed. Preoperative assessment, anesthetic management, and prophylactic antibiotics should be considered in presence of cardiopathy.

REFERENCES:
Cunniff C, Williamson-Kruse L, Olney AH: Congenital microgastria and limb reduction defects. *Pediatrics* 91:1192, 1993.

Stewart C, Stewart M, Stewart F: Microgastria-limb reduction anomaly with total amelia. *Clin Dysmorphol* 11:187, 2002.

Microvillous Inclusion Syndrome

At a glance: Extremely rare inherited enteropathy that is typically apparent within hours or days after birth. The disorder is characterized by chronic, severe, watery diarrhea and malabsorption caused by hypoplasia and/or atrophy of the wall of the small intestine (e.g., hypoplastic villus atrophy, defective brush-border assembly and differentiation). In infants, chronic diarrhea and malabsorption may result in severe dehydration, electrolyte imbalance, malnutrition, failure to thrive, and acidosis.

Synonyms: Congenital Microvillous Atrophy; Davidson Disease.

Incidence: Very rare but seems to be the most common cause of severe protracted diarrhea of neonatal onset in developed countries. In 1987, 30 cases were reported worldwide in a survey among centers specializing in pediatric gastroenterology. More recent reports indicate that typical congenital microvillous atrophy accounts for 80% of cases. In the Navajo reservation in Northern Arizona, the incidence is reported at 1:12,000 live births.

Genetic inheritance: Probably an autosomal recessive trait.

Pathophysiology: It seems that the brush-border lesion is associated with a disorder of the enterocyte cytoskeleton; it results in failure of reabsorption of the large volumes of endogenous gastric, pancreatic, and biliary secretions.

Diagnosis: History; absence of serosal (e.g., vasoactive intestinal peptide-secreting tumor, Zollinger-Ellison syndrome) or infectious (bacterial toxins) causes; fecal electrolyte concentrations similar to those seen in small intestinal fluid. Jejunal biopsies complete the diagnosis: on light microscopy, hypoplastic villus atrophy with abnormal brush-border pattern and positive staining material within the apical cytoplasm of enterocytes. On electronic microscopy, surface cells show absent or grossly abnormal microvilli with numerous vesicular bodies and characteristic microvillus inclusions; crypt cells appear normal but contain increased numbers of apical vesicles and vesicular bodies.

Clinical aspects: Infants develop severe secretory diarrhea within days of birth; more than 140 ml/kg body weight of feces can be produced every day. The disease is fatal without parenteral nutrition and even with such supplementation, most children die in infancy or early childhood. The only treatment is small bowel transplantation.

Precautions before anesthesia: In infant or child on total parenteral nutrition (TPN), check hydration, levels of blood glucose and electrolytes, liver enzymes (TPN-associated cholestasis), and coagulation (vitamin K deficit). In patients at risk for thromboembolic complications (catheter-related sepsis, serum protein imbalance), ascertain patency of the great veins if a new central venous access has to be inserted. Patient may be on intravenous octreotide therapy. The presence of an altered gastrointestinal barrier increases the risk of systemic sepsis.

Anesthetic considerations: Blood glucose and electrolytes should be monitored intraoperatively on a regular basis. Patients on TPN must be maintained intraoperatively and serial measurements of electrolytes and glucose are needed.

Pharmacological implications: No known implications.

Other conditions to be considered:

CONGENITAL CHLORIDE DIARRHEA: Caused by a defect in the Cl^-/HCO_3^- exchangers in the brush-border membrane in the ileum and colon. Autosomal recessive inheritance. Higher incidence in Finland and the Middle East. Parenteral replacement of fluids and electrolytes during the neonatal period, but oral compensation can be achieved with careful balancing of the intake of Na, K, and Cl. Normal life.

CONGENITAL SODIUM DIARRHEA: Caused by a defect in the Na^+/H^+ exchangers in the brush-border membrane in the small intestine. After initial parenteral treatment to restore normal hydration and blood electrolytes, oral Na citrate usually is effective in maintaining a normal electrolytic status.

REFERENCE:

Booth IW: Secretory diarrhoea, in Buts JP, Sokal EM (eds): *Management of Digestive and Liver Disorders in Infants and Children.* Amsterdam, Elsevier, 1993, p 351.

MIDAS Syndrome

At a glance: MIDAS is an acronym for *mi*crophthalmia, *d*ermal *a*plasia, and *s*clerocornea. This genetic disorder is characterized by irregular linear skin erythema of head and neck, microphthalmia, corneal opacities, diaphragmatic hernia, respiratory distress, and absent cerebral septum pellucidum leading to seizures.

Synonyms: Microphthalmia-Linear Skin Defects Syndrome; MLS.

Incidence and genetic inheritance: Approximately 20 cases described. Transmitted as an X-linked dominant trait; lethal in males. Mapped to the short arm of chromosome X (Xp22.31). It is considered as an X-linked phenotype distinct from ☞Goltz syndrome.

Clinical aspects: Midfacial hypoplasia and linear erythematous skin lesions, narrow and deformed ears, unilateral or bilateral microphthalmia, anterior chamber anomalies (corneal opacity, sclerocornea, orbital cysts, unplanted palpebral fissures and chorioretinal abnormalities). Focal dermal hypoplasia or aplasia affecting usually the face, scalp, and neck. Looks like linear burns or cuts at birth but heals without scar, or the skin can remain pigmented and depressed at those places. Mild short stature. Diaphragmatic hernia and rare occurrence of cardiac defects (atrial septal defect, ventricular septal defect, one case of cardiomyopathy, conduction defect, supraventricular tachycardia, and ventricular fibrillation). In one case, the autopsy showed persistent gross trabeculation of the left ventricle and an arteria lusoria. Hydrocephalus, agenesis of corpus callosum,

seizures, absence of septum pellucidum, and ectopic gray and white matter.

Precautions before anesthesia: Check for the presence of diaphragmatic hernia and cardiomyopathy. Ventricular fibrillation seems to result from polymorphic ventricular tachycardia and is refractory to medical treatment. Perform echocardiography to eliminate cardiac malformations and ECG to determine conduction defect. Elective surgery should be postponed until complete electrophysiologic study of the heart has been performed.

Anesthetic considerations: Anesthetic considerations are those associated with cardiac problems, potential peroperative threatening arrhythmias, and raised intracranial pressure.

Pharmacological implications: Use of anesthetic agents that increase risk of arrhythmia should be avoided. Patients presenting with seizures activities should receive their routine preoperative anticonvulsant medications and intraoperative supplementation of an intravenous antiepileptic agent may be needed for prolonged procedures.

Other conditions to be considered:

☞GOLTZ SYNDROME: Complex mesoectodermal hereditary disorder characterized by focal dermal atrophy with herniation of fat-producing multiple papillomas, in association with a skeletal, dental, ocular, and other anomalies.

☞AICARDI SYNDROME: Rare disorder characterized by partial or complete agenesis of the corpus callosum, infantile spasms (spasm-like epilepsy), mental retardation, and an ocular abnormality called *lacunae of the retina.* Often associated with other features such as microcephaly and porencephalic cysts. Onset generally begins between the ages of 3 and 5 months. The disorder affects only females.

REFERENCES:

Happle R, Daniels O, koopman RJ: MIDAS syndrome (microphthalmia, dermal aplasia, and sclerocornea). An X-linked phenotype distinct of Goltz syndrome. *Am J med Genet* 47:710, 1993.

Paul T, Laohakunakorn P, Long B, et al: Complete elimination of incessant polymorphic ventricular tachycardia in an infant with MIDAS syndrome. *J Cardiovasc Electrophysiol* 13:612, 2002.

Temple IK, Al-Gazali LI: Microphthalmia with linear skin defects and Xp22 deletions (MLS) syndrome, in Donnai D, Winter RM (eds): *Congenital Malformation Syndromes.* London, Chapman & Hall, 1995, p 386.

Miller-Dieker Lissencephaly Syndrome

At a glance: Malformation of the cerebral cortex with abnormal facies. Classic lissencephaly, also known as *lissencephaly type I,* is a brain malformation that may occur as an isolated abnormality (isolated lissencephaly sequence) or in association with certain underlying syndromes (e.g., Miller-Dieker syndrome, Norman-Roberts syndrome). The condition is characterized by agyria or pachygyria of the gyri of the cerebral cortex, causing the brain's surface to appear unusually smooth. In infants with classic lissencephaly, microcephaly is usually present. Other clinical features include seizures, severe or profound mental retardation, feeding difficulties, growth retardation, and impaired motor functions.

Synonym: Lissencephaly Syndrome, Type I; MDLS.

Incidence: It is undoubtedly a rare condition. In 1991, it was reported in the only published epidemiological study performed in the Dutch population that the prevalence was 11.7 per million live births. Since then, the larger use of MRI diagnosis has most certainly contributed to make the incidence and prevalence higher. It is suggested that 25–30% of patients with classical lissencephaly have Miller-Dieker syndrome.

Genetic inheritance: Usually sporadic cases with no familial inheritance; in most cases, changes (mutations) of at least two different genes have been implicated in isolated lissencephaly: a gene located on chromosome 17 (known as LIS1) and a gene located on the X-chromosome (deletions or mutations of gene LIS1 on chromosome 17 p13.3).

Pathophysiology: Various possible causes of isolated lissencephaly include viral infections, insufficient blood flow to the brain during fetal development, and certain genetic factors.

Diagnosis: Clinical picture and central nervous system imaging: smooth brain surface (with or without pachygyria), thickened cortex, absent or hypoplastic corpus callosum, small brainstem.

Clinical aspects: Postnatal failure to thrive with death before age 2 years. Microcephaly with bitemporal narrowing, vertical ridging, and furrowing of the skin on the forehead; up-slanted palpebral fissures; small nose with anteverted nostrils; protuberant upper lip and micrognathia. May have cardiac defect (atrial septal defect, ventricular septal defect, tetralogy of Fallot). Severe mental deficiency with hypotonia progressing to spasticity and seizures. Dysphagia and gastroesophageal reflux are common.

Precautions before anesthesia: Check for chronic aspiration pneumonia (radiography), presence of a cardiac defect and possible undernutrition; antiepileptic and antireflux treatment should be continued until the morning of anesthesia.

Anesthetic considerations: Classic considerations for infants at risk for difficult intubation and gastroesophageal reflux; adapt choice of drugs and technique to the cardiac defect.

Pharmacological implications: Antiepileptic treatment is usually complex: possible induction of cytochrome P-450 enzymes. In presence of cardiac anomalies, antibiotherapy must be considered.

Other conditions to be considered:

☞**HARD SYNDROME:** Characterized by type II lissencephaly in association with retinal dysplasia, obstructive hydrocephalus, and agenesis of the corpus callosum. Affected infants also typically have severe growth failure, severe microcephaly, seizures, microphthalmia, and cataracts. Some affected infants have an occipital encephalocele.

NEU-LAXOVA SYNDROME: Rare genetic disorder in which intrauterine growth retardation, polyhydramnios, and an unusually short umbilical cord occur. Typically characterized by severe microcephaly, joint contractures, generalized edema, and abnormalities of the brain and spinal cord. Affected infants may have a prominent nasal bridge, a sloped forehead, microstomia, micrognathia, malformed ears, exophthalmos, cataracts, and a short neck. Other clinical features include hypoplastic fingers and toes; polysyndactyly, camptodactyly, clinodactyly, and/or overlapping of fingers; and joint contractures. The central nervous system typically includes a form of lissencephaly with agenesis of the corpus callosum, hydrocephalus, and cerebellar hypoplasia. Infants may have abnormal yellowish ichthyotic skin and malformations of the genitals, kidneys, and/or heart.

☞**LISSENCEPHALY TYPE II:** Characterized by severe brain malformations and obstructive hydrocephalus leading to severe rise in intracranial pressure. Associated symptoms include rapid enlargement of the head and seizures. Often considered a major manifestation of Walker-Warburg syndrome.

REFERENCES:
Kholer A, Hain J, Muller U: Clinical and molecular genetic findings in five patients with Miller-Dieker syndrome. *Clin Genet* 47:161, 1995.

King A, Upadhyaya M, Penney C, et al: A case of Miller-Dieker syndrome in a family with neurofibromatosis type I. *Acta Neuropathol (Berl)* 99:425, 2000.

Miller Disease

At a glance: Pathologic fractures. Electrolyte disturbances, especially involving calcium and phosphate.

Synonyms: Calciferol Osteomalacia; Idiopathic Pseudofracture; Looser Syndrome; Looser Zones; Looser-Debray-Milkman Syndrome; Osteoporosis-Osteomalacia Syndrome.

Genetic inheritance: Not genetic.

Clinical aspects: Very old names for severe vitamin D deficiency. This can lead to decreased intestinal absorption of calcium and secondary hyperparathyroidism.

Anesthetic considerations: Electrolytes should be carefully screened, especially calcium and phosphate, and corrected before anesthesia. Careful positioning of the osteopenic patient is necessary to prevent pathologic bone fractures. There is no evidence that a specific anesthetic drug or technique has advantages over any other. The response to the neuromuscular blocking drugs may be unpredictable.

REFERENCE:
Barash PG, Cullen BF, Stoelting RK: *Clinical Anesthesia*. Philadelphia, Lippincott Williams & Wilkins, 2001.

Miller Fisher Syndrome

At a glance: Rare, acquired nerve disease considered to be a variant of Guillain-Barré syndrome. It is characterized by abnormal muscle coordination, ophthalmoplegia, and tendon areflexia. As with Guillain-Barré syndrome, the symptoms may be preceded by a viral illness. Other clinical features include generalized muscle weakness and respiratory failure. The prognosis is good, with recovery beginning within 2 to 4 weeks and almost completed within 6 months. Residual neurologic deficits may occur, and relapses occur in less than 3% of individuals affected. The majority of individuals with Miller Fisher syndrome have a unique antibody that characterizes the disorder.

Synonym: Fisher Syndrome.

History: First described in 1956 by Charles Miller Fisher, a Canadian neurologist.

Incidence: Rare; 223 cases reported in world literature; male-to-female ratio is 2:1.

Genetic inheritance: Not genetically inherited. Probably a viral etiology.

Pathophysiology: Precipitating factors of the Miller Fisher syndrome are an upper respiratory tract infection in the majority of cases but also include infection, surgery, vaccination, or insect bite. Diplopia and ataxia are the first signs of development of the syndrome. The exact nature of the clinical entity is unclear, but the following three interpretations have been suggested: (1) the Miller Fisher syndrome is a variant of the Guillain-Barré syndrome; (2) the Miller Fisher syndrome is a brainstem encephalitis without involvement of peripheral nerves; and (3) areflexia is caused by a lesion of the mesencephalon and the upper pontine reticular formation.

Diagnosis: Ophthalmoplegia, unilateral or bilateral ptosis, and cerebellar ataxia with lower limb areflexia are required for diagnosis.

Clinical aspects: Other cranial nerves may be involved in the process, causing facial palsy, dysarthria, or dysphagia. The course of the disease has a duration between 3 weeks and 18 months with spontaneous remission. Rarely is the cerebellar ataxia or areflexia severe enough to cause major problems; the major impediment to these patients is their vision. Steroids, plasmapheresis, and immunoglobulin therapy have all been attempted to reduce the course of this illness.

Precautions before anesthesia: History and physical examination should reveal the extent of problems caused by the syndrome. Autonomic neuropathy and its consequent problems have not been reported in these patients. Cranial nerve impairment must be carefully documented before anesthesia. Eye examination by the anesthetist is worthwhile in order to have a baseline against which to gauge recovery.

Anesthetic considerations: No specific measures must be undertaken in the anesthetic care of these individuals. Patients being treated with high-dose corticosteroids will require appropriate steroid therapy perioperatively.

Pharmacological implications: No specific indications or contraindications.

Other condition to be considered:

    GUILLAIN-BARRÉ SYNDROME: Acquired neurologic disorder preceded by a viral infection and leading to the destruction of posterior horn of the spinal cord neural tissue. It is clinically manifested with muscle weakness, areflexia, and numbness or tingling in the arms, legs, face, and other parts of the body. It may progress to complete paralysis. Difficulties in breathing and swallowing can occur, and intermittent positive-pressure ventilation can be required. It can be life-threatening; however, most people recover with few neurologic residual deficits. The clinical presentation is usually preceded by numbness or tingling in the fingers and toes, followed by weakness in the leg and arm muscles that develops over a period of hours to weeks. The muscle weakness gradually improves within months, and complete recovery may be expected within 1 year.

REFERENCE:
Berlit P, Rakicky J: The Miller Fisher syndrome. Review of the literature. *J Clin Neuroophthalmol* 12:57, 1992.

Miller Syndrome

At a glance: Congenital disorder characterized by postaxial acrofacial dysostosis in association with severe postaxial limb deficiencies. The craniofacial malformations may include malar hypoplasia, micrognathia, cleft palate, small, protruding, "cup-shaped" ears, eye colobomas and ptosis, and ectropion. The limb abnormalities include incomplete hypoplasia, syndactyly, clinodactyly (e.g., the fifth digits and, in some cases, the fourth and third digits) and hypoplasia of the ulna and occasionally the radius. It is believed to be transmitted in an autosomal recessive pattern.

Synonyms: Postaxial Acrofacial Dysostosis Syndrome (POADS); Genée-Wiedemann Syndrome (formerly).

Incidence: Very rare; fewer than 20 cases reported.

Genetic inheritance: Autosomal recessive.

Pathophysiology: Unknown.

Diagnosis: Clinical aspect similar to Treacher Collins syndrome but with postaxial upper and lower limb defects.

Clinical aspects: Craniofacial anomalies include malar hypoplasia with micrognathia, cleft lip or palate; down-slanting palpebral fissures with lower-lid ectropion; eyelid coloboma; absent superior orbital ridge; hypoplastic, low-set ears. Sometimes choanal atresia. Limbs demonstrate absence of fourth or fifth ray in hands and feet; forearm shortening caused by ulnar hypoplasia; syndactyly. Cardiac defects in 30% of patients (atrial septal defect, ventricular septal defect, patent ductus arteriosus). Sometimes pectus excavatum. Intelligence is normal but often questioned because of hearing deficit.

Precautions before anesthesia: Complete preoperative workup for associated cardiac anomaly must be conducted. Evaluation of the airway and anesthesia consultation are indicated.

Anesthetic considerations: Preparation for difficult tracheal intubation is the rule. Nasopharyngeal and laryngeal mask airway should be ready for use, as should special intubation devices such as fiberoptic laryngoscope, Bullard laryngoscope, and light wand, etc. Spontaneous ventilation should be maintained until airway is secured; venous access can be difficult because of limb defects. A laryngeal mask airway must be available in case of failure to ventilate or intubate. The presence of associated congenital heart defects also dictates the anesthetic plan. Hearing difficulties may complicate the induction period.

Pharmacological implications: Medicaments with ototoxicity must be avoided. In presence of cardiopathy, antibiotherapy must be considered.

Other conditions to be considered:

    ☞TREACHER COLLINS SYNDROME: Disorder of craniofacial development. The features include antimongoloid slant of the eyes, coloboma of the lid, micrognathia, microtia and other deformity of the ears, hypoplastic zygomatic arches, and macrostomia. Conductive hearing loss and cleft palate are often present.

    ☞ACROFACIAL DYSOSTOSIS NAGER TYPE: Characterized by limb deformities consisting of absence of radius, radioulnar synostosis, and hypoplasia or absence of the thumbs. The mandibulofacial dysostosis is characterized by severe micrognathia and malar hypoplasia. Most reported cases have been sporadic.

    ☞GOLDENHAR SYNDROME: Congenital disorder that involves partial absence or an unusual slant of the upper eyelid, skull asymmetry, hemifacial atrophy, microtia, and cleft palate.

    ☞JUBERG-HAYWARD SYNDROME: Disorder characterized by cleft lip and palate, microcephaly, hands deformities (e.g., thumbs and toes), and short stature.

    HEMIFACIAL MICROSOMIA: Incidence of 1:5000 live births and often considered a Treacher Collins–like syndrome. However, it is not genetic. It can cause abnormalities on both sides of the face, but they are always uneven, whereas in Treacher Collins syndrome both sides of the face appear equally affected. The facial nerve is frequently paralyzed in hemifacial microsomia. The clinical features include severe micrognathia, microtia, facial nerve paralysis, macrostomia, and hemifacial atrophy involving the ipsilateral eye. Other less common abnormalities include fatty tumors over the eye, abnormalities of the vertebrae and ribs, cleft lip/palate, congenital heart defects, and kidney abnormalities.

REFERENCES:

Donnai D, Hugues HE, Winter RM: Postaxial acrofacial dysostosis (Miller) syndrome, in Donnai D, Winter RM (eds): *Congenital Malformation Syndromes.* London, Chapman & Hall, 1995, p 333.

Stevenson GW, Hall SC, Bauer BS, et al: Anaesthetic management of Miller's syndrome. *Can J Anaesth* 8:1046, 1991.

Milroy Disease

At a glance: Familial primary congenital lymphedema involving mainly the lower limbs and present at birth. Other features include recurrent scrotal swelling, intestinal tract protein loss, persistent pulmonary pleural effusion, and hypoproteinemia.

Synonyms: Noone-Milroy-Meige Lymphedema; Primary Congenital Lymphedema; Hereditary Lymphedema, Type I.

Classification: Primary lymphedema is divided in three groups based on the age of onset:

* Milroy disease: Congenital lymphedema present at birth and autosomal dominant inheritance.
* Lymphedema praecox (Meige disease): Presents after birth but before the age of 35 years. The age of onset is usually during adolescence.
* Lymphedema tarda: After age of 35 years. Of patients with primary lymphedema, 10% have Milroy disease, 80% present with lymphedema praecox, and 10% lymphedema tarda.

History: First described in 1891 by Max Nonne, a German Neurologist, when he reported a case of hereditary lymphedemia of the legs. In 1892, William F. Milroy, an American physician, presented a 31-year-old man affected with a similar condition but which the mother also had. Following work by Milroy on 22 persons, Henri Meige, a French physician, described the condition in 1898.

Incidence: Twenty percent of all primary lymphedemas. In the United States, primary lymphedemas occur in 1:10,000 individuals. Approximately 200 cases have been described in the literature.

Genetic inheritance: Autosomal dominant inheritance with variable expression.

Pathophysiology: Results from inadequate lymphatic drainage because of congenital abnormalities of the lymphatic system. The protein content of the extravascular tissue rises and, because of its osmotic effect, additional water is retained. This excess of extravascular protein leads to proliferation of fibroblasts and organization of the edema fluid, giving rise to firm, nonpitting edema.

Diagnosis: Clinical findings, results of the patent blue test and possibly fluorescence microlymphography with fluorescent dextrans, indirect lymphography, or isotope studies are essential to establish the diagnosis. In Milroy disease, the lymphatic capillaries and precollectors are aplastic.

Clinical aspects: Milroy disease presents at birth; the edema is confined to legs and feet. Over time, with the development of fibrosis, the edema becomes nonpitting. The overlying skin becomes hyperkeratotic with fissures, and secondary infection occurs. Severe lymphedema is called *elephantiasis (filariasis).* Often associated with congenital chylous ascites, recurrent scrotal swelling, intestinal tract protein loss, persistent bilateral pleural effusion, and hypoproteinemia. Poor wound healing after trauma. In adulthood, development of lymphangiosarcomas and squamous epidermoid carcinomas, with 50% mortality within 24 months of diagnosis. Normal life expectancy in patients without tumors. Management is otherwise symptomatic; combined physical therapy with tight bandages and stockings, massage, and use of pneumatic devices for intermittent compression considerably reduces the edema and renders surgery unnecessary in most patients. Diuretics have a beneficial effect during early management and benzopyrones for long-term treatment. Surgical excision of subcutaneous tissue followed by skin graft is performed in selected patients.

Precautions before anesthesia: Evaluate the respiratory system for presence of ascites and pleural effusion; determine if the patient is able to lie supine comfortably. Antibiotics for active skin infection must be continued or started. Assess nutritional status in the presence of chronic intestinal protein loss. Investigations include serum potassium (exclude diuretic-induced hypokalemia), serum protein and albumin levels, arterial blood gas analysis, chest radiography. Obtain an oncotic pressure reducing to assist with fluid therapy.

Anesthetic considerations: Venous cannulation will be difficult in the affected areas. Careful positioning of the affected limbs is required to prevent pressure sores and trauma. Stockings and pneumatic devices to reduce further dependency-related edema would be useful for long operations. Respiratory impairment from gross ascites and pleural effusion may be exacerbated by supine position. A general anesthesia with controlled ventilation minimizes patient's discomfort and helps reduce ventilation/perfusion (V/Q) imbalance. Adequate preoxygenation should be allowed before tracheal intubation to minimize the rapid desaturation that may occur during induction. The presence of a large interstitial volume and third space influence the choice of anesthetic agents.

Pharmacological implications: Because low serum protein levels result in a higher free drug concentration, drugs that are highly protein bound (e.g., thiopentone) require dose reduction. Potassium supplementation may be required in those on long-term diuretic therapy. Thromboembolic prophylaxis should be considered.

REFERENCES:

Esterly JR: Congenital hereditary lymphedema. *J Med Genet* 2:93, 1965.

Lazareth I: Classification of lymphedema. *Rev Med Interne* 23:375, 2002.

Mallick A, Bodenham AR: Disorders of the lymph circulation: Their relevance to anaesthesia and intensive care. *Br J Anaesth* 91:265, 2003.

Milton Disease

At a glance: Disorder of complement regulation in which C1 esterase inhibitor (C1INH), an inhibitor of spontaneous activation of C1, is lacking. This produces circumscribed, nonpitting subepithelial edema involving the lips, eyelids, tongue, larynx, pharynx, respiratory tract, gastrointestinal tract, renal system, and occasionally the central nervous system.

Synonyms: Angioedema; Hereditary Angioneurotic Edema; HANE Syndrome; C1 Esterase Inhibitor Deficiency.

Incidence: Estimated incidence of the hereditary form is 1:50,000–150,000 live births in the United States.

Genetic inheritance: In the hereditary form, transmission is via an autosomal dominant pattern, with males affected twice as often as females. Human C1 inhibitor gene is localized to chromosome 11q11-q13.1. In more than 20% of patients with hereditary angioedema, the mutations are de novo; thus there is no family history of the disease.

Pathophysiology: Hereditary angioneurotic edema (HANE) is caused by either the absence of C1INH (type I) or the presence of inactive C1INH (type II). Acquired forms result from either consumption of C1INH in association with benign or malignant B-cell lymphoproliferative disorders, connective tissue diseases, and monoclonal gammopathies (type I), or the presence of antibodies to C1INH (type II).

Diagnosis: Positive family history and characteristic clinical presentation. Serum C1 esterase inhibitor deficiency in the hereditary form (5–30% of normal) and low C4.

Clinical aspects: Age at onset of HANE syndrome (Milton disease) is before 7 years in 50% of cases. Both inherited or acquired forms are characterized by recurrent attacks of nonpruritic and nonerythematous, often asymmetrical, edema affecting the extremities, abdomen, and face. Edema of the larynx and other portions of the airways is the most fearsome feature of this disorder and is the major cause of mortality, an outcome that could occur in up to 50% of these patients. Precipitating factors are minor trauma or emotional upset. Visceral involvement with crampy abdominal pain without peritoneal signs can lead to unnecessary laparotomy. Severe attacks of watery diarrhea are another manifestation of HANE. Edema of the airway is slowly progressive over hours, but local trauma, as in attempted tracheal intubation, can precipitate or aggravate the edema. During an attack, levels of C1 inhibitor and C4 and C2 are depressed. There are increased levels of thyroglobulin antibodies and thyroid microsomal antibodies in patients with hereditary angioedema. Androgen derivatives are useful for long-term prophylaxis because they increase hepatic synthesis of C1INH. Concentrates of C1 inhibitor are effective and without side effects in the treatment of severe acute attack.

Precautions before anesthesia: Skin testing for anesthetic drugs is useless. Suitable premedication to allay anxiety. Investigations include coagulation status, C1NH and C4 levels in HANE, and electrolytes when there is diarrhea associated with gastrointestinal attacks. Because androgen derivatives used for prophylaxis may affect hepatic function, liver function tests should be performed. In HANE, attempts should be made to increase C1NH levels preoperatively by using androgens, antifibrinolytics, fresh-frozen plasma (FFP), or purified C1NH concentrate. If the patient is not receiving long-term therapy with androgens (e.g., danazol 200 mg TID for 5 days can be used in adults but is contraindicated in children; stanazol 2 mg/kg/day to a maximum of 6 mg/kg/day), these agents should be administered for several days prior to surgery; they often require 1 to 2 weeks to reach maximum effect. Alternatively, in case of emergency, 2 units of FFP or purified C1INH concentrate (25 U/kg) will restore the C1NH to a safe level (>40% of normal) for a duration between 1 and 4 days.

Anesthetic considerations: There is no influence of anesthetic drug choice. Local and spinal/extradural anesthesia has always been preferred in these patients. Avoid airway manipulation and tracheal intubation to limit mucosal damage and severe edema, where possible. Use of a laryngeal mask airway probably is unsafe because of the large contact surface and the potential postoperative complications of airway obstruction. If tracheal intubation is necessary, prophylaxis is mandatory but may not be completely effective. Facilities and equipment to treat anaphylaxis or airway obstruction (e.g., drugs, intubation equipment, and tracheostomy) should be available. Treat attacks of angioedema caused by C1NH deficiency with FFP or purified C1NH concentrate (25 U/kg) because patients will not

respond to adrenaline, steroids, or antihistamines. Remember that C1NH levels will fall with hemodilution; this is especially important if the patient receives excessive fluids or undergoes cardiopulmonary bypass (level >50% of normal is necessary before bypass). Postoperative intensive care unit monitoring is recommended, depending on the type and extent of surgery.

Pharmacological implications: Avoid drugs that may aggravate disease, such as salicylates and nonsteroidal antiinflammatory drugs (NSAIDs). Use the most "immunologically benign" agents and avoid histamine-releasing drugs where possible.

REFERENCES:

Jensen NF, Weiler JM: C1 esterase inhibitor deficiency, airway compromise and anesthesia. *Anesth Analg* 87:480, 1998.

Wall RT, Frank M, Hahn M: A review of 25 patients with hereditary angioedema requiring surgery. *Anesthesiology* 71:309, 1989.

Minicore Disease with External Ophthalmoplegia

At a glance: Congenital myopathy associated with proximal extremity weaknesses, external ophthalmoplegia, and eventual respiratory failure. In the neonatal subgroup, severe hypotonia, delayed motor development, generalized muscle weakness and amyotrophy which may progress or remain stable. This presentation corresponds to a subgroup called "Central core disease" and susceptibility to malignant hyperthermia has been suggested.

Synonyms: MmD; Multicore Myopathy with External Ophthalmoplegia; Minicore Myopathy with External Ophthalmoplegia.

Incidence: Remains unknown. No more than 30 cases of this medical condition have been reported in the literature.

Genetic inheritance: Autosomal recessive; also a possible dominant form.

Pathophysiology: Myopathy characterized by the presence of multiple, short, core lesions (known as *minicores*) in most muscle fibers as a result of sarcomere disorganization and mitochondria depletion. Four subgroups have been identified. RYR1 mutations were recently identified in the moderate form—the central core disease. The genes responsible for the three other forms remain unknown, but a mutation of the selenoprotein N gene is implicated.

Clinical aspects: The most prevalent phenotype is characterized by the predominance of axial muscle weakness that leads, in two thirds of patients, to development of severe life-threatening respiratory insufficiency and scoliosis. The second group is the classic form with ophthalmoplegia, which occurs in only 10% of cases. The third group consists of the mild cases of central core disease. The fourth group is rare and probably consists of rigid spine dystrophy.

Precautions before anesthesia: Assessment of severity of respiratory failure and degree of cardiac involvement is necessary, with complete pulmonary function test, blood gas analysis, and echocardiography.

Anesthetic considerations: High complication rate because of muscle weakness, respiratory insufficiency, and cardiac myopathy (late onset). A risk for malignant hyperthermia has been suggested in the subgroup (e.g., central core disease) of the disease but remains unknown in the classic form. Positioning may be challenging because of often severe spinal deformity.

Pharmacological implications: Succinylcholine should be considered absolutely contraindicated. Muscle relaxants are usually not mandatory and must be carefully adjusted if used. Volatile halogenated agents are not advisable because of the possibility of malignant hyperthermia.

Other conditions to be considered: Central core disease of muscle, rigid spine muscular dystrophy. Association with short-chain acyl-CoA dehydrogenase deficiency has been described.

REFERENCES:

Docquer MA, Veyckemans F, Prudhomme S, et al: Anesthesia in a child presenting a anhydrotic ectodermic dysplasia associated with a multiminicore myopathy. *Can J Anaesth* 47:449, 2000.

Ferreiro A, Quijano-Roy S, Pichereau C, et al: Mutations of the selenoprotein N gene, which is implicated in rigid spine dystrophy, cause the classical phenotype of multiminicore disease: Reassessing the nosology of early-onset myopathies. *Am J Hum Genet* 71:739, 2002.

Jungbluth H, Sewry C, Brown SC, et al: Minicore myopathy in children: A clinical and histopathological study in 19 cases. *Neuromuscul Disord* 10:264, 2000.

Mitochondrial Acetoacetyl-CoA Thiolase (ACAT) Deficiency

At a glance: Inherited mitochondrial disease (inborn error of metabolism) affecting the isoleucine catabolism resulting in recurrent episodes of ketoacidosis.

Synonyms: Beta-Ketothiolase Deficiency *(note that beta-ketothiolase describes a group of enzymes, and patients with defects of different thiolases are known to have a different clinical picture);* T2 Deficiency; Alpha-Methyl-Acetoacetic Aciduria; Methionine S-Adenosyltransferase (MAT) Deficiency; 2-Alpha Methyl-3-Hydroxybutyricacidemia; 3-Alpha-Oxothiolase Deficiency; 3-Alpha Ketothiolase Deficiency; 3-Alpha KTD Deficiency.

Incidence: Approximately 60 cases have been described.

Genetic inheritance: Inherited in an autosomal recessive mode. The responsible acetoacetyl-CoA thiolase (ACAT) gene has been mapped to chromosome 11q22.3-23.1. The severity of the clinical features and the penetrance within families are variable.

Pathophysiology: Mitochondrial ACAT is responsible for cleavage of acetyl-CoA from acetoacetyl-CoA and 2-methylacetoacetyl-CoA, which is an intermediate in the isoleucine metabolism, but also for acetoacetyl-CoA formation in ketogenesis and acetoacetyl-CoA cleavage in ketolysis.

Diagnosis: Based on recurrent episodes of severe ketosis and acidosis without chronic ketosis. Urine analysis before and after an isoleucine challenge (showing 2-methyl-3-hydroxybutyric acid, 2-methylacetoacetic acid, butanone, and tiglylglycine) is helpful for diagnosis. Demonstration of the enzyme defect in fibroblasts or leukocytes confirms the definite diagnosis.

Clinical aspects: Children with this defect commonly present with failure to thrive, recurrent episodes of severe ketoacidosis with hyperventilation (caused by metabolic acidosis), vomiting, diarrhea (often bloody), and coma during the course of intercurrent infections or after excessive protein intake. Onset is rarely before age 4 months. Most patients (approximately 60%) can have normal mental development if severe metabolic decompensations can be prevented. However, ataxia and frequent headaches have been reported. One case with congestive cardiomyopathy has been described. Mainstay of therapy is moderate restriction of isoleucine intake, intravenous glucose, and sodium bicarbonate during decompensations and avoidance of fasting.

Precautions before anesthesia: Most importantly, hypoglycemia during preoperative fasting must be prevented. A dextrose-containing intravenous solution should be started before the preoperative fasting period and kept intraoperatively and postoperatively until regular oral feeds are tolerated again. Cardiomyopathy has been described, so cardiac assessment of the patient is recommended.

Anesthetic considerations: Regional anesthesia allows better monitoring of central nervous function. Lactated Ringer solution should be avoided in patients with mitochondrial diseases because these patients may already have increased lactate levels and acidosis. Glucose and lactate levels in the plasma, as well as ketone levels in the urine, should be monitored perioperatively. Prevent hypothermia, shivering, or other conditions that cause increased energy expenditure.

Pharmacological implications: No specific literature on anesthesia in patients with ACAT deficiency. Although not all of the various mitochondrial disorders can be summarized and unified, adverse anesthetic experiences in a particular mitochondrial disease should be considered for every patient with mitochondrial dysfunction until further information for specific metabolic defects is available. Most reports refer to anesthesia in patients with mitochondrial *myopathy*. Muscular sensitivity to muscle-relaxing agents might be enhanced in these patients, and malignant hyperthermia after succinylcholine has been reported on rare occasions. Therefore, although scientific evidence is lacking, it has been advocated that neuromuscular blockade should be instituted cautiously, and succinylcholine should best be avoided in patients with mitochondrial disease.

Other condition to be considered:

☞**SUCCINYL-COA:3-KETOACID COA-TRANSFERASE DEFICIENCY:** Inherited metabolic disorder resulting in ketoacidotic episodes. Clinical characteristics include lethargy, hypothermia, respiratory failure, metabolic acidosis, and infections. Upon treatment, complete recovery is expected.

REFERENCES:

Maslow A, Lisbon A: Anesthetic considerations in patients with mitochondrial dysfunction. *Anesth Analg* 76:884, 1993.

Mitchell GA, Fukao T: Inborn errors of ketone body catabolism, in Scriver CR, Beaudet AL, Sly WS, Valle D (eds): *The Metabolic and Molecular Bases of Inherited Disease.* 8th ed. New York, McGraw-Hill, 2001, p 2327.

Sharma AD, Erb T, Schulman SR, et al: Anaesthetic considerations for a child with combined Prader-Willi syndrome and mitochondrial myopathy. *Paediatr Anaesth* 11:488, 2001.

Mitochondrial Disease

At a glance: Progressive multiorgan disease. The mitochondrial myopathies are a rare group of conditions affecting the respiratory chain and oxidative phosphorylation. A total of five proteins complexes make up the mitochondrial electron transport chain (see Complex Diseases).

Mitochondria are the main source of adenosine tri-phosphate (ATP) in the cell. They depend on several metabolic pathways to supply ATP during varying cellular conditions: glycolysis is the main pathway during nutritional repletion state, and fatty acid oxidation is the main pathway during fasting. ATP is generated by five protein complexes, called the *respiratory chain,* contained in the inner mitochondrial membrane: NADH from the tricarboxylic cycle is a substrate for complex I, and the reduced form of flavin adenine dinucleotide ($FADH_2$) from fatty acid oxidation is a substrate for complex II. Strictly speaking, disorders of pyruvate metabolism, fatty acid oxidation, ketogenesis, or ketolysis, and defects of the urea cycle or of the respiratory chain, are mitochondrial pathologies; however, the term *mitochondrial diseases* is usually a synonym for respiratory chain or oxidative phosphorylation anomaly.

Synonyms: Mitochondrial Cytopathy; Mitochondrial Myopathy

Incidence: In the United States, it is estimated that one in 4,000 children will develop mitochondrial disease by the age of 10 years. The prevalence of the disease at birth is 1:4000 to have a type of mitochondrial disease.

Genetic inheritance: Any mode of inheritance may be observed: autosomal recessive, dominant, X-linked, maternal, or sporadic. This is a consequence of the high number of genes encoding respiratory chain proteins: most are located in the cell DNA but 26 are in the mtDNA. Consequently, mutations, depletion, deletions, or duplications can occur in both genetic materials. Transmission of mitochondrial diseases is complex because mtDNA is maternally inherited, has a different structure than complementary DNA, and is more subject to spontaneous mutations. Therefore, many mtDNA mutations accumulate with age and are probably the cause of some diseases (e.g., Parkinson, diabetes). Moreover, there are many mitochondria in each cell, and they are randomly partitioned between daughter cells during mitosis. Thus, if normal and mutant mtDNA are present in the initial cell (heteroplasmy), some lineages will have only abnormal mtDNA or normal mtDNA (homoplasmy). There are also cases of acquired reversible mitochondrial dysfunction caused by mtDNA depletion in *children with HIV treated with nucleoside analogues* (mainly zidovudine [AZT]); AZT inhibits DNA polymerase γ, a nuclear protein essential for mtDNA replication and maintenance.

Pathophysiology: Whether cells can generate enough ATP depends on the amount of dysfunctional mtDNA present in the mitochondria. Because cells of different organs have different metabolic needs, some organs can tolerate a greater burden of mutated mtDNA, and the first symptoms usually appear in the organs with the greatest metabolic needs (e.g., brain, heart, muscle, liver, kidney). This is called the *threshold effect.* The concepts of heteroplasmy and threshold effect explain how the same mutation can present with many different phenotypes and how some clinical phenotypes are caused by different mutations. If the segregation of abnormal cells occurs early during fetal development, a single organ may inherit cells containing only mutant mtDNA.

Clinical aspects: Mitochondrial diseases can affect almost every organ (see Table M-2 and the description of the disease under its

---

Table M-2 Most Usual Clinical Profiles in Defects of the Respiratory Chain

Neonates (<1 month)

- Ketoacidotic coma with seizures, hypotonia, hepatomegaly, and proximal tubulopathy
- Sideroblastic anemia with neutropenia and exocrine pancreatic dysfunction (*Pearson syndrome*)
- Hypertrophic cardiomyopathy (concentric) and muscle weakness
- Hypertrophic cardiomyopathy (concentric) with neutropenia and myopathic features in males (*Barth syndrome*)
- Hepatic failure with lethargy, hypotonia and, proximal tubulopathy
- Cholestasis
- Hypotonia, macroglossia, respiratory distress with spontaneous remission between 1 and 2 years (*"Benign infantile myopathy"*)

Infants (<2 years)

- Failure to thrive ± watery diarrhea and villous atrophy unresponsive to gluten-free and milk-free diet
- Episodes of acute myoglobinuria, hypertonia, and muscle stiffness
- Proximal renal tubulopathy (*De Toni-Fanconi-Debré syndrome*) with rickets, recurrent episodes of watery diarrhea, and photosensibility
- Tubulo-interstitial nephritis mimicking nephronoptosis with subsequent encephalomyopathy and leukodystrophy
- Insulin-dependent diabetes mellitus with diabetes mellitus, optic atrophy and deafness (*Wolfram or DIDMOAD syndrome*)
- Subacute necrotizing encephalomyopathy (*Leigh syndroshapeme*)
- Rapidly progressive encephalomyopathy with hypotonia, cerebral ataxia, muscle weakness

Children and Adults

- Muscle weakness with myalgia ± progressive external ophthalmoplegia
- Progressive sclerosing poliodystrophy (*Alpers disease*)
- Encephalomyopathy with myoclonus, ataxia, seizures and hearing loss (*MERRF syndrome*)
- Progressive external ophthalmoplegia (from pure ocular myopathy to *Kearns-Sayre syndrome*)
- Encephalomyopathy with stroke-like episodes (*MELAS syndrome*)
- Leber hereditary optic neuroretinopathy (*LHON*)
- Ataxia, retinitis pigmentosa, muscle weakness, sensory neuropathy with seizures or dementia (*NARP syndrome*)
- Myopathy with peripheral neuropathy, encephalopathy, and gastrointestinal disease (*MNGIE syndrome*)

precise denomination). Whatever the age of onset and the presenting symptoms, an increased number of organs are affected during the course of the disease. Initial symptoms usually persist and worsen but occasionally improve or disappear as other organs become involved (e.g., Pearson syndrome). Screening tests include *blood levels* of glucose, lactate, and pyruvate and their molar ratio (>20 is abnormal), β-hydroxybutyrate/acetoacetate molar ratio, carnitine; provocative tests if standard samples are inconclusive (e.g., glucose loading test to detect paradoxical postprandial hyperlactacidemia); *CSF:* lactate/pyruvate molar ratio; *urine:* organic acids and lactates; in vitro polarography or ^{31}P-NMR spectroscopy; *muscle biopsy:* light microscopy traditionally shows "ragged-red fibers" (subsarcolemmal accumulation of abnormal mitochondria) with Gomori trichrome staining, but the absence of these ragged-red fibers does not exclude the diagnosis. On electronic microscopy, mitochondria appear abnormal with increased size, abnormal cristae, or inclusions; *mitochondrial enzymology* in some tissues (muscle, liver) can be performed in some centers. The treatment, which usually is dietetic and supportive, does not markedly influence the usually unfavorable course of the disease.

Precautions before anesthesia: The diagnosis of mitochondrial disease should be considered in any child with a multisystem neurologic disorder or who is being investigated for hypotonia. Anesthesia-related morbidity and mortality risk is essentially linked to the preoperative status of the child, that is, the number and extent of organ dysfunction. The presence of a mitochondrial disease is not considered a risk for malignant hyperthermia. Avoid any elective anesthesia/surgery in the presence of infection or temperature because cytokines (mainly tumor necrosis factor [TNF]) inhibits some complex of the respiratory chain. The following should be checked: central nervous system (seizures, myoclonus, strokes, swallowing problems); *metabolic* (usual venous or arterial concentration of lactates and glucose); *muscles* (hypotonia, contractures, scoliosis); *cardiac* (even if the child is asymptomatic, ECG and echocardiography to exclude for conduction disorders and cardiomyopathy, respectively; check functioning of pacemaker, if present); *pulmonary* (frequent infections, chronic aspiration, pulse oximetry breathing room air, obstructive and/or central apnea; reduced ventilatory drive is common, and many patients have an abnormal response to both hypoxia and hypercarbia, and deaths have been reported following sedation with chloral hydrate or diazepam); *hepatic* and *renal* function must be evaluated; *nutritional status* and *diet* (glucose and/or lipid rich, tolerance to fasting and treatment [carnitine, vitamin Q, antiepileptic drugs]).

Anesthetic considerations: Maintain the usual treatment until the morning of surgery. Preoperative fasting as short as possible; if fasting is usually poorly tolerated, a glucose-containing solution should be started when the fasting period starts. A sedative premedication is best avoided because of the possible abnormal response to hypoxia/hypercarbia. *Induction:* No specific technique. Sevoflurane is the best choice for inhalation induction; propofol may be the best choice for intravenous induction, but a 2% solution should be used to lessen the lipid load. In a recent report, it was suggested that propofol for anesthetizing patients affected with severe mitochondrial diseases should not be used. The authors acknowledged using propofol for short-term administration (15–30 min) during muscle biopsy procedures or noninvasive diagnostic procedures and found in the more symptomatic patients that it prolonged anesthesia recovery and at times required intensive care unit admission. It seems that the duration of the infusion and the total dose of propofol may be the critical factors in these cases. Furthermore, it is reported that propofol in-

hibits mitochondrial metabolism and that the lipid component of the formulation may play a role in toxicity for those patients with fatty acid oxidation disorders. *Opiates:* Dose should be carefully titrated according to the patient's needs. *Muscle Relaxant:* Published data are often contradictory. Even in the absence of clinical myopathy, the patient's muscular response to nerve stimulation should be measured before administering a muscle relaxant. Atracurium and *cis*-atracurium are the best choices because of their spontaneous degradation. In case of myopathy, succinylcholine should not be used to avoid producing rhabdomyolysis. *Intraoperative Fluids:* Avoid infusion containing lactates such as lactated Ringer, Hartmann, and Stocker (Swiss) solution, but the patient should receive a glucose solution (5 or 10% according to blood sugar level). Aim for normoglycemia because hyperglycemia can increase lactate production. Monitor (arterial or venous) blood gases and lactate levels: in case of severe lactic acidosis, use dichloroacetate 50 mg/kg IV over 30 minutes to stimulate pyruvate dehydrogenase to metabolize lactate in pyruvate. Perimedullar locoregional anesthesia can be used, but its cost-to-benefit ratio should be evaluated taking into account the presence of severe scoliosis or degenerative lesions in the spinal cord. Some patients with mitochondrial disease present with axonal neuropathy of peripheral nerves; the possible effects of local anesthetics on these nerves are unknown. Prevention of hypothermia is important to avoid shivering and increased oxygen consumption at awakening.

Pharmacological implications: Patients with mitochondrial disease are very sensitive to the respiratory effects of sedatives. It also seems, according to BIS measurement, that children with an anomaly of complex I of the respiratory chain are much more sensitive to the hypnotic effects of sevoflurane. Most studies performed on isolated mitochondria use doses of anesthetic agents far in excess of those used in daily practice, so their clinical relevance is often dubious.

REFERENCES:

Church JA, Mitchell WG, Gonzalez-Gomze I, et al: Mitochondrial DNA depletion, near-fatal metabolic acidosis, and liver failure in an HIV-infected child treated with combination antiretroviral therapy. *J Pediatr* 138:748, 2001.

Farag E, Argalious M, Narouze S, et al: The anesthetic management of ventricular septal defect (VSD) repair in a child with mitochondrial cytopathy. *Can J Anesth* 49:958, 2002.

Farag E, Deboer G, Cohen B, et al: Metabolic acidosis due to propofol infusion. *Anesthesiology* 102:697, 2005.

Morgan PG, Hoppel C, Sedensky M: Mitochondrial defects and anesthetic sensitivity. *Anesthesiology* 96:1268, 2002.

Munnich A: Defects of the respiratory chain, in Fernandes J, Saudubray J-M, Van den Bergh G (eds): *Inborn Metabolic Diseases*. 3rd ed. Berlin, Springer, 2000, p 159.

Wallace JJ, Perndt H, Skinner M: Anesthesia and mitochondrial disease. *Paediatr Anaesth* 8:249, 1998.

Moebius Syndrome

At a glance: Rare developmental disorder characterized by facial paralysis (mask-like face) present at birth. Facial nerve development is absent, and the sixth (abducens) and seventh (facialis) cranial nerves are most often affected. Other features include numerous abnormalities of the orofacial region and malformations of limbs. Mental retardation occurs in approximately 10% of cases.

Synonyms: Congenital Oculofacial Paralysis; Congenital Facial Diplegia, Moebius Sequence.

History: First described by Henri M. Thomas, an American neurologist, in 1898.

Incidence: Rare. Affects males and females equally. Most cases of Moebius syndrome occur randomly for no apparent reason (sporadic cases).

Genetic inheritance: Usually sporadic. Cases of autosomal dominant inheritance described (1898). Gene map locus is 13q12.2-q13. Recurrence risk is low at less than 1 in 50. Clinically they can often be differentiated by lack of limb involvement. A Moebius syndrome type II has been described in a large Dutch family with strong autosomal dominant transmission. Gene map locus is 3q21-q22. It is associated with multiple vascular abnormalities and poor prognosis.

Pathophysiology: Etiology is unknown. Four possible pathologic causes have been suggested: (a) hypoplasia to absence of central brain nuclei; (b) destructive degeneration of the central brain nuclei (this is the most common form; it is likely caused by a transient brainstem hypoxic event occurring at a critical time in utero and affecting the structures supplied by the developing subclavian artery); (c) peripheral nerve involvement; and (d) a myopathy. Moebius syndrome is thus considered as a nonspecific sign.

Diagnosis: Based on clinical findings. Usually manifests soon after birth with sixth and seventh nerve palsies, which are either partial or complete and may be bilateral. Patients present with mask-like facies, incomplete closure of the eyelids during sleep, drooling of saliva, and difficulty sucking. Aspiration is common. On examination, multiple other abnormalities are usually detected. Important to differentiate from neuromuscular disorders occurring in early childhood.

Clinical aspects: Multiple cranial nerves may be involved (nerves V, VI, VII, IX, X, and XII can all be affected) and lead to orofacial malformations, abnormalities of tongue coordination, swallowing (bulbar muscle weakness), and drooling. Speech abnormalities are common. High risk for corneal abrasions. Usually the affected individuals are mentally normal. However, there is a 10% incidence of mild mental retardation. Occasionally peripheral neuropathy and pectoral muscle deficiency. Abnormalities of ventilation (central hypoventilation and idiopathic tachypnea) presumably result from brainstem abnormalities. Craniofacial features include micrognathia, microstomia, mandibular hypoplasia, tongue tethering, premaxillary overgrowth, and cleft lip and palate. Strabismus is common. Congenital cardiac anomalies include ventricular septal defect (VSD) and patent ductus arteriosus (PDA). Skeletal features are talipes equinovarus (in up to 50%), arthrogryposis, and terminal limb defects. Cervical spine anomalies have been described.

Precautions before anesthesia: Full assessment of the airway is particularly important in these children because of a high incidence of difficult direct laryngoscopy and failed tracheal intubation. The availability of a laryngeal mask airway is highly recommended in case of failure to ventilate or intubate. In this case, the use of a fiberoptic scope could be used through the laryngeal mask to facilitate tracheal intubation. Review of previous anesthetic records is important. Evaluation of respiratory function for acute and chronic pulmonary complications by clinical examination and chest radiographs. Involvement of bulbar muscles increases the risk of aspiration. Assessment and documentation of existing neurologic defects,

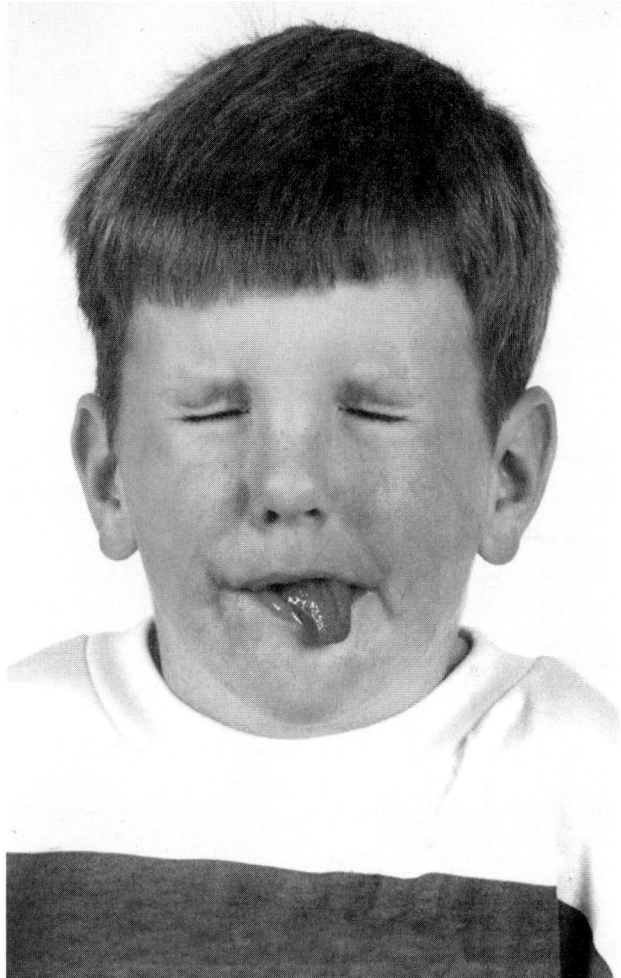

Moebius syndrome   A 5-year-old boy with Moebius syndrome and left-sided cranial nerve XII palsy manifesting with a deviation of the tongue to the affected side.

associated cardiac lesions (echocardiography may be required), or cervical spine abnormalities.

Anesthetic considerations: An anesthetic plan must be made considering whether or not tracheal intubation is necessary. Use of an antisialagogue is recommended for induction and recovery secondary to copious secretions. A number of cases with secretions causing airway obstruction and severe hypoxia and bradycardia postoperatively have been reported. Peripheral deformities may result in difficult intravenous access. Induction is most commonly accomplished by inhalational technique in a spontaneously breathing patient. Prepare for difficult or failed tracheal intubation by having additional equipment available. In a series of 41 attempted intubations by experienced anesthetists, 28 (68%) were unsuccessful. Face-mask anesthesia has been used successfully many times without complications and is the anesthetic technique of choice when appropriate. Attempts at intubation have been aided by use of intubating stylets, gum elastic bougies, a variety of laryngoscopes, and fiberoptic devices. Laryngeal mask airways have been used successfully (although correct placement was reported to be difficult in some cases) when intubation failed. Corneal protection with lubrication and tape is required. Careful positioning and padding. Close

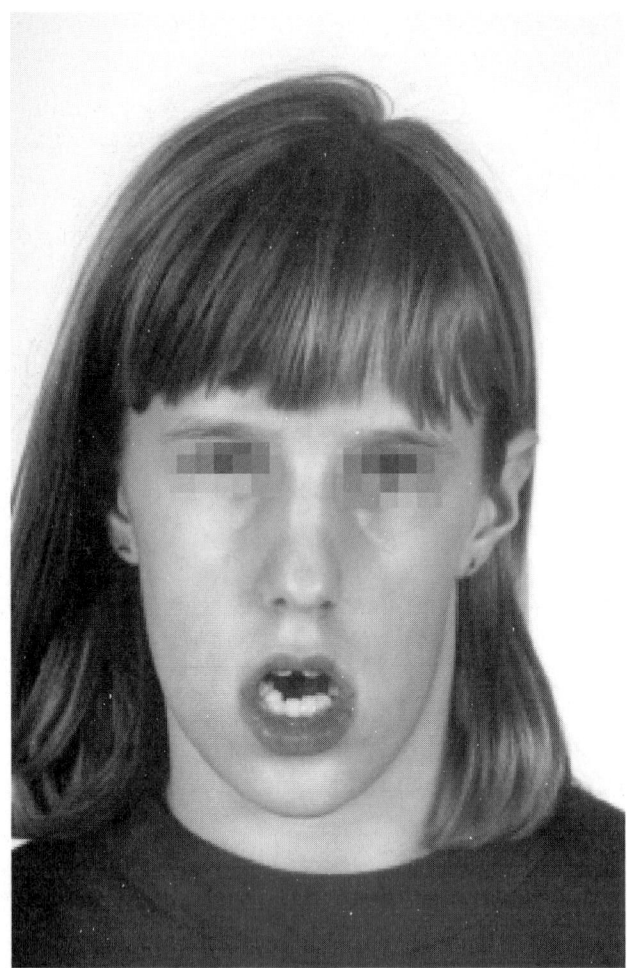

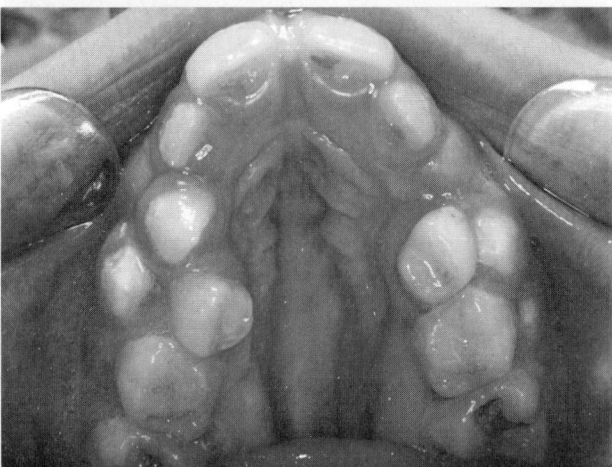

Moebius syndrome A 10-year-old girl with Moebius syndrome. Very narrow palate with a wide open cleft.

postoperative observation is mandatory for patients with a history of apneas and central hypoventilation.

Pharmacological implications: Avoid neuromuscular blockers until the airway has been secured. Caution with opioids may be appropriate if there is evidence of central hypoventilation and apneas. Depending on the planned procedure, subacute bacterial endocardi-

tis prophylaxis may be necessary in patients with congenital cardiac lesions.

Other condition to be considered:

☞**POLAND-MOEBIUS SYNDROME:** Characterized by the association of the abnormalities observed with the Moebius syndrome and the Poland syndrome. The clinical features of the Poland syndrome are agenesis or hypoplasia of the pectoralis major and pectoralis minor and symbrachydactyly. Additional findings may include underdevelopment or absence of one nipple and patchy axillary hair growth. In females, the presence of unilateral hypoplastic breast development or complete amastia.

REFERENCES:

Ames WA, Shichor TM, Speakman M, et al: Anesthetic management of children with Moebius sequence. *Can J Anesth* 52:837, 2005.

Ferguson S: Moebius syndrome: A review of anaesthetic implications. *Paediatr Anaesth* 6:51, 1996.

Krajcirik WJ, Azar I, Opperman S, et al: Anesthetic management of a patient with Moebius syndrome. *Anaesth Analg* 64:371, 1985.

Mohr Syndrome

At a glance: Very rare familial association of deafness with minor facial hypoplasia and minor midline cleft (tongue, lip, palate). Symptoms include frequent episodic neuromuscular disturbances, congenital malformations such as cleft palate, malformation of the hands and feet, shortened limbs, and differing degrees of mental retardation.

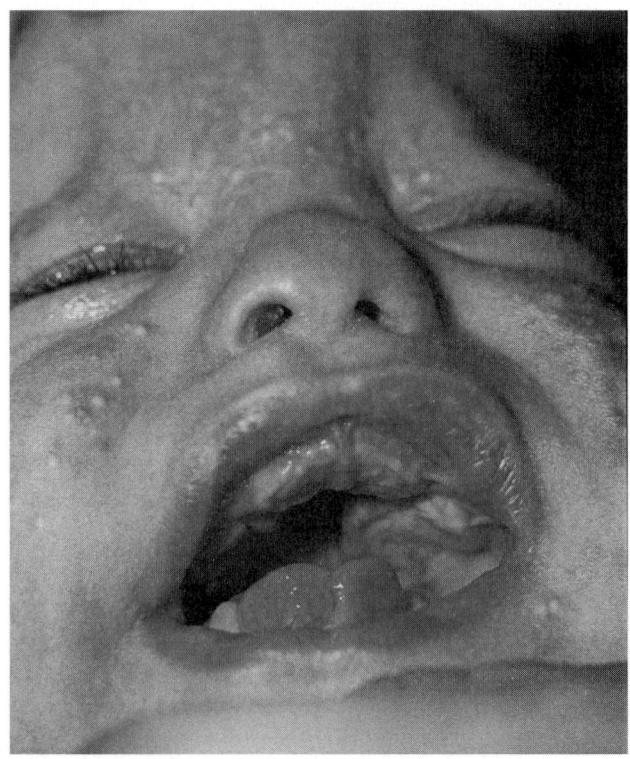

Mohr syndrome Neonate with partial cleft of the palate and the tongue and flat nasal bridge was diagnosed with Mohr syndrome (orofaciodigital syndrome type II).

Synonyms: Oral-Facial-Digital Syndrome Type II; ORF Syndrome II; Orofaciodigital Syndrome II.

Incidence: Remains unknown.

History: First described in 1941 by the Norwegian geneticist Otto L. Mohr, who was the uncle of Professor Jan Mohr of Copenhagen.

Incidence and genetic inheritance: Fewer than 50 cases reported. Affects male and female equally. Autosomal recessive.

Clinical aspects: Conductive hearing loss (anomaly of unci); mild hypoplasia of zygomatic arch, maxilla and body of mandible; flat nasal bridge; partial cleft of lip or palate, hyperplastic frenulum; midline cleft of tongue and/or nodules on the tongue; short stature, partial reduplication of big toe, polydactyly; flared epiphyses.

Anesthetic considerations: No report in the anesthetic literature, but the presence of maxillary and mandibular hypoplasia associated to a cleft palate may lead to difficult direct laryngoscopy and tracheal intubation. No other specific considerations with this condition.

REFERENCE:

Prpic I, Cekada S, Franulovic J: Mohr syndrome (oro-facial-digital syndrome type II): A familial case with different phenotypic findings. *Clin Genet* 48:304, 1995.

Mohr-Tranebjaerg Syndrome

At a glance: Novel rare genetic type of mitochondrial disease. Progressive deafness becomes evident at age 3 to 5 years. Severe dysarthria and occasional bizarre posturing of head and neck are possible. Dystonia, spasticity, dysphagia and optic atrophy appear in adult life. Patients are prone to seizures and lactate acidosis.

Synonyms: MTS; Dystonia-Deafness Syndrome; DDS; Deafness-Dystonia-Optic Atrophy Syndrome; DDP; Deafness Syndrome, Progressive, with Blindness, Dystonia, Fractures, and Mental Deficiency.

Incidence: There are few cases reported in the literature. Remains unknown.

Genetic inheritance: X-linked recessive inheritance; caused by a mutation on the TIMM8A (DDP) gene. A mutation in the same gene has been found as the cause of the Jensen syndrome.

Pathophysiology: Pathologic changes are represented mainly by neuronal loss and glioses in the basal ganglia. This illness is a novel type of mitochondrial disease consisting of a defect in mitochondrial oxidative phosphorylation (OXPHOS), specifically caused by deficiencies in carrier proteins.

Clinical aspects: Progressive deafness occurs at age 3 to 5 years. It is a progressive syndrome, which includes myopia, decreased visual acuity, and abnormal electroretinogram, leading to cortical blindness, dystonia, fractures, and mental deficiency. The female carrier showed signs of minor neuropathy and mild hearing impairment.

Precautions before anesthesia: No specific precautions; however, in comparison to the other mitochondrial illnesses, blood sugar level and electrocardiogram should be considered.

Anesthetic considerations: Patients may develop lactic acidosis and seizure peroperatively.

Pharmacological implications: As reported with other mitochondrial diseases, use of neuromuscular blocking drugs is associated with significant implications, so careful monitoring is advisable.

Other conditions to be considered:

JENSEN SYNDROME (Opticoacoustic Nerve Atrophy with Dementia Syndrome): Characterized by profound sensorineural hearing loss with onset in infancy, followed in adolescence by progressive optic nerve atrophy with loss of vision and in adulthood by progressive dementia. It is inherited as an X-linked recessive pattern. Extensive intracerebral calcification affecting meninges, vessels, and neurons has been reported. Moderate diffuse wasting of skeletal muscles is reported and should be carefully assessed before anesthesia.

☞**MITOCHONDRIAL DISEASE:** Progressive multiorgan disease. The mitochondrial myopathies are a rare group of conditions affecting the respiratory chain and oxidative phosphorylation. A total of five proteins complexes make up the mitochondrial electron transport chain (see ☞Diseases Complex).

REFERENCE:

Koehler CM, Leuenberger D, Merchant S, et al: Human deafness dystonia syndrome is a mitochondrial disease. *Proc Nat Acad Sci U S A* 96:2141, 1999.

Mollica Pavone Antener Syndrome

At a glance: Short stature/dwarfism, mental retardation, severe myopia, iris hypoplasia, cataracts, and increased body hair.

Synonyms: Dwarfism, Mental Retardation, and Eye Abnormality.

Incidence and genetic inheritance: Only three cases described. The mode of inheritance is uncertain but most probably autosomal recessive.

Clinical aspects: Short stature/dwarfism, mental retardation, microcephaly, and ocular abnormalities, including iris hypoplasia, nuclear cataracts, and severe myopia. The related syndromes are listed, but review showed overlapping manifestations. Increased body hair.

Anesthetic considerations: Usually the microcephaly does not lead to airway difficulties.

Other conditions to be considered:

RODRIGUES BLINDNESS: Severe mental retardation and ocular malformations including microphthalmos, short stature, dysmorphic facial features (narrow nasal bridge, prominent ears), and malaligned teeth.

☞**CAHMR SYNDROME:** Hypertrichosis, most often in the face and shoulders. Individuals affected have congenital lamellar cataracts.

MARTSOLF SYNDROME (Cataract, Mental Retardation, and Hypogonadism Syndrome): Short stature, minor digital and cephalic abnormalities. Microcephaly occasional. One patient reported with cardiomyopathy and another with cardiac failure.

REFERENCE:

Mollica F, Pavone L, Antener I: Short stature, mental retardation and ocular alterations in three siblings. *Helv Paediatr Acta* 27:463, 1972.

Moloney Syndrome

At a glance: Absent or decreased eyelashes and eyebrows; visual loss. Other clinical features include dysplastic and grooved nails and alopecia.

Synonym: Choroidal Atrophy; Alopecia Syndrome.

Incidence and genetic inheritance: Only two cases described. The mode of inheritance is uncertain, but mild macular disease in the father who may be a heterozygote representation of a recessive transmission.

Clinical aspects: Total regional choroidal atrophy and other signs of ectodermal dysplasia, dysplasia of the nails (grooved), and teeth. Fine hair, absent or decreased eyelashes, eyebrows. Visual loss must be suspected. Occasionally syndactyly of fingers.

Anesthetic considerations: Other than special attention to protection of the eye and its sensitivity to the light, no specific measures must be undertaken in the anesthetic care of this patient.

REFERENCE:

Moloney JB, Blake J, Denham B, et al: Regional choroidal atrophy and alopecia. A new syndrome. *Acta Ophthalmol* 66:272, 1988.

Molybdenum Cofactor Deficiency

At a glance: Extremely rare, congenital, severe neurologic anomalies including seizures, spastic tetraparesis, brain atrophy, mental retardation, abnormal muscle tone and myoclonic spasms, dislocated lenses, and xanthine urinary stones.

Synonym: MOCOD; Sulfite oxidase deficiency.

Incidence: Extremely rare; approximately 50 patients described.

Genetic inheritance: Autosomal recessive; heterozygotes show no symptoms.

Pathophysiology: This cofactor is essential for function of the enzymes sulfite oxidase, xanthine dehydrogenase, and aldehyde oxidase. Symptoms are the result of combined deficiencies of these enzymes. However, isolated deficiency in sulfite oxidase produces the same symptoms. Accumulation of toxic metabolites produces severe encephalopathy, demyelinization of white matter, gliosis, and diffuse spongiosis of the brain.

Diagnosis: Deficiency of sulfite oxidase in fibroblasts or of molybdenum cofactor in liver biopsy. High concentrations of sulfite, thiosulfate, taurine, xanthine, and hypoxanthine, but very low levels of uric acid in the urine. Antenatal diagnosis is possible.

Clinical aspects: Clinical manifestations are apparent within a few weeks of birth and were formerly called "infantile encephalopathy": mainly severe convulsions unresponsive to therapy and caused by sulfite production from oral protein intake. Poor feeding and vomiting, seizures, spastic quadriparesis, and severe developmental delay. Dilated ventricles, unresponsiveness to light. Bilateral dislocation of the ocular lens is a common finding. There is no effective treatment, and death usually occurs before age 2 years.

Precautions before anesthesia: Assess neurologic status until the day of surgery; optimize seizure therapeutic management.

Anesthetic considerations: Anesthetic management in this condition has not been described. The severity of neurologic defects determines anesthetic management. Patients may be at risk for pulmonary aspiration and recurrent infections. Poor feeding and vomiting may lead to electrolyte abnormalities, which should be corrected preoperatively.

Pharmacological implications: Succinylcholine should be avoided in presence of spastic tetraparesis. Seizure medications must be optimized intraoperatively and postoperatively.

REFERENCE:

Rezvani I: Defects in metabolism of amino acids, in Behrman RE, Kliegman RM, Arvin AM (eds): *Nelson Textbook of Pediatrics.* 16th ed. Philadelphia, WB Saunders, 1995, p 344.

MOMO Syndrome

At a glance: MOMO is an acronym for *m*acrosomia, *o*besity, *m*acrocephaly, and *o*cular abnormalities. Macrocephaly and tall stature, delayed bone development, generalized obesity, numerous ocular abnormalities (retinal coloboma and nystagmus), and mental retardation.

Incidence and genetic inheritance: Only three cases described; suggested to be a new mutation with autosomal dominant inheritance.

Clinical aspects: Two unrelated sibs were first described with significant obesity, mental retardation, macrocephaly, delayed bone maturation, retinal coloboma, nystagmus, and downward slant of palpebral fissures. Tall stature, macrostomia, and delayed eruption of teeth.

Anesthetic considerations: Based on the few cases described, special attention must be paid to the airways because of the generalized, often morbid obesity. The increased risk of gastric content regurgitation must be kept in mind in patients with severe obesity. The presence of macrocephaly may be associated with macroglossia and potential difficult tracheal intubation. Difficulty in mechanical ventilation preoperatively and postoperatively is possible in presence of severe obesity.

REFERENCES:

Moretti-Ferreira D, Koiffmann CP, Listik M, et al: Macrosomia, obesity, macrocephaly and ocular abnormalities (MOMO syndrome) in two unrelated patients: Delineation of a newly recognized overgrowth syndrome. *Am J Med Genet* 46:555, 1993.

Zannolli R, Mostardini R, Hadjistilianou T, et al: MOMO syndrome: A possible third case. *Clin Dysmorphol* 9:281, 2000.

Monilethrix

At a glance: Genetic disorder affecting the hair and occasionally the skin; does not belong to the group of ectodermal dysplasias.

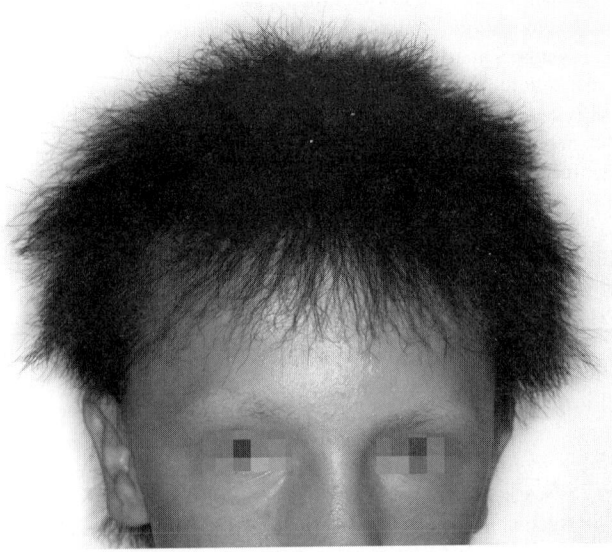

Monilethrix Brittle, dry hair in a teenager with monilethrix. The eyebrows and eyelashes are also affected.

Incidence and genetic inheritance: Unknown. It is an autosomal dominant disorder. The cause of this disease seems to be a mutation in the genes responsible for the hair keratin, which has been mapped to 12q13.

Clinical aspects: Although the symptoms of these syndromes may resemble ectodermal dysplasia, monilethrix does not belong to this group. It is characterized by a beaded appearance of the scalp hair caused by periodic narrowing of the hair shaft. Phenotypically, this results in breakage of the hair (brittle, dry, lusterless look) and patchy alopecia. The onset is usually in infancy, and symptoms may ameliorate to a certain degree after puberty and during pregnancy. Hair outside of the scalp area (pubis, axilla, eyelashes, eyebrows) is occasionally affected. Some patients show signs of koilonychia and follicular keratosis. Over the years, skin atrophy may develop in affected areas.

Anesthetic considerations: These patients are otherwise healthy and do not require any specific anesthetic precautions.

REFERENCES:

Despontin K, Krafchik B: What syndrome is this? Monilethrix syndrome. *Pediatr Dermatol* 10:192, 1993.

Ito M, Hashimoto K, Yorder FW: Monilethrix: An ultrastructural study. *J Cutan Pathol* 11:513, 1984.

Stevens HP, Kelsell DP, Bryant SP: Linkage of monilethrix to the trichocyte and epithelial keratin gene cluster on 12q11-q13. *J Invest Dermatol* 106:795, 1996.

Moore-Federman Syndrome

At a glance: Dwarfism with disproportionately short legs. Reduced joint mobility (or stiffness) and ocular anomalies (hyperopia, glaucoma, cataract, and retinal detachment).

Synonyms: Dwarfism with Stiff Joints and Ocular Abnormalities.

Incidence and genetic inheritance: Only a few families described. Autosomal dominant. Genetic disorder thought to be transmitted from male to male. Acromicric dysplasia, geleophysic dysplasia, and Moore-Federman syndrome may be allelic forms of the same disorder or different disturbances of the same metabolic pathway.

Clinical aspects: Disproportionate dwarfism, with short legs and fingers, delayed carpal bone age, stiff joints, and thickened forearm skin. Abnormalities of the eyes may include hyperopia, glaucoma, cataract, and retinal detachment. A comparison of these different related entities is difficult because of the small number of patients reported, and not all descriptions are of the same quality with regard to details of clinical features or radiography.

Anesthetic considerations: The true syndrome has no descriptions of association with any storage or metabolic disease, and no problems with tracheal stenosis have been reported. However, because of the small number of cases and the possible overlapping of several syndromes, pay special attention to the airway, and check cardiac and hepatic functions.

Other conditions to be considered:

☞**ACROMICRIC DYSPLASIA:** Mild facial anomalies, markedly shortened hands and feet, and severe growth retardation. Radiologic examination reveals short, stubby metacarpals and phalanges with notching of the second metacarpal.

☞**GELEOPHYSIC DYSPLASIA:** Characterized by the designation of the happy face of the affected child (*gelios* = happy, *physis* =

nature). This disorder is often considered a "focal" mucopolysaccharidosis. The clinical features include dysostosis multiplex-like changes, predominantly in the hands and feet, and the consequences of focal accumulation of acid mucopolysaccharides in the liver and possibly the cardiovascular system. Joint contractures, hepatomegaly, and cardiomegaly can be present. Aortic and mitral valves regurgitation have been reported.

☞**LERI PLEONOSTEOSIS:** Characterized by laryngotracheal-stenoses, short stature, mongoloid facies, short spadelike hands, broad thumbs in valgus position, genu recurvatum and generalized limitation of joint mobility, thickening of the palmar and forearm fasciae, enlargement of the posterior neural arches of the cervical vertebrae, and shuffling short-stepped gait. It is inherited as an autosomal dominant pattern.

☞**WEILL-MARCHESANI SYNDROME:** Rare, genetic disorder characterized by short stature, brachycephaly, hand defects, including brachydactyly, and unusually small, round lenses of the eyes (spherophakia) prone to ectopia lentis. Affected individuals may have varying degrees of visual impairment, ranging from myopia to blindness. Autosomal recessive or autosomal dominant inheritance.

REFERENCES:

Faivre L, Le Merrer M, Baumann C, et al: Acromicric dysplasia: Long-term outcome and evidence of autosomal dominant inheritance. *J Med Genet* 38:745, 2001.

Hennekam RCM, van Bever Y, Oorthuys JWE: Acromicric dysplasia and geleophysic dysplasia: Similarities and differences. *Eur J Pediatr* 155:311, 1996.

Winter RM, Patton MA, Challener J, et al: Moore-Federman syndrome and acromicric dysplasia: Are they the same entity? *J Med Genet* 26:320, 1989.

Moore-Smith-Weaver Syndrome

At a glance: Asymmetrical long bone bowing with a "beaten-metal" appearance of the skull, dolichomacrocephaly, and ocular hypertelorism.

Synonym: Bowing of Long Bones, Asymmetrical and Symmetrical.

Incidence: Very rare; only a few cases described.

Diagnosis and clinical aspects: Two sibs with congenital asymmetrical long bone bowing and one with congenital symmetrical long bone bowing were described. Other abnormalities included beaten-metal appearance of the skull, dolichomacrocephaly, ocular hypertelorism, and bone-within-bone appearance of vertebrae. Differential diagnosis must be made with camptomelic dysplasia, kyphomelic dysplasia, hypophosphatasia, Grant syndrome, and osteogenesis imperfecta.

Anesthetic considerations: This illness is a special mild form of the other bone dysplasia genetic syndromes and has no special repercussion on anesthesia technique, with the potential exception of positioning and access for locoregional anesthesia.

Other conditions to be considered:

☞**GRANT SYNDROME:** Persistent wormian bones, blue sclerae, mandibular hypoplasia, shallow glenoid fossae, camptomelia, and hypotonia. Apparently, it is an autosomal dominant trait.

☞**OSTEOGENESIS IMPERFECTA:** Inherited disease responsible for varying degrees of skeletal fragility. Minimal trauma is sufficient to cause fractures and bone deformities.

REFERENCE:
Moore LA, Moore CA, Smith JA, et al: Asymmetric and symmetric long bone bowing in two sibs: An apparently new bone dysplasia. *Am J Med Genet* 47:1072, 1993.

Morgagni-Stewart-Morel Syndrome

At a glance: Polyglandular endocrine syndrome characterized by the classic triad of (a) hyperostosis frontalis interna, (b) adipositas, and (c) virilism and hirsutism. A peculiar, noninflammatory, usually benign osteopathy with symmetrical thickening of the frontal, parietal, or occipital bones as a result of deposits on the internal aspects of the squama frontalis. Other clinical features include menstrual disorders, virilism, hirsutism, mental disorders, fatigue, somnolence, visual disorders, vertigo, tinnitus, obesity, polyphagia, polydipsia, polyuria, loss of sense of smell, decreased glucose tolerance, convulsions, and involvement of the second, fifth, and seventh cranial nerves with hemiplegia and hemiparesis.

Synonyms: Hyperostosis Frontalis Interna; Morel Syndrome.

History: The frontal bone lesions associated with obesity and virilism were first described in 1719 by Giovanni Battista Morgagni, an Italian anatomist. In 1928, Douglas Hunt Stewart emphasized the association with obesity. In 1930, Ferdinand Morel emphasized the accompanying menstrual disturbance, amenorrhea, and impotence. The term *Morgani triad* was introduced by Folke Henschen in 1937, but the term *Morgagni-Stewart-Morel syndrome* is now commonly used.

Incidence: Extremely uncommon. Occurs almost exclusively in females. Age of onset average about 45 years; incidence in females is approximately 90%.

Genetic inheritance: Probably autosomal dominant. No reported cases of male-to-male transmission.

Pathophysiology: Unknown. The underlying defect causing excess bone formation appears to be different from normal mechanisms. The biochemical response to calcitriol and bone biopsy findings (increased number of osteoblasts) has been shown to be different. Many of the endocrine features may be related to hyperprolactinemia, which is frequently found in these cases.

Diagnosis: Clinical supported by investigations and imaging. Hyperphosphatasemia is common. Radiologic, CT, and MRI scans confirm bony overgrowth. Audiology confirms changes in hearing.

Clinical aspects: May be almost symptomless and is found incidentally. *Skull:* Hyperostosis frontalis interna; as a result of progressive overgrowth, intracranial pressure may increase and lead to brain and nerve compression, cranial nerve palsies, and seizures; choanal stenosis; glaucoma. *Endocrine:* Obesity, hyperphosphatasemia, hyperprolactinemia, galactorrhea, diabetes mellitus, menstrual irregularity. *Neuropsychiatric:* "Treatable dementia." *Skin:* Hypertrichosis.

Precautions before anesthesia: Assessment of severity of condition; exclude raised intracranial pressure and neurologic abnormalities, including seizures and medications. Assessment of airway and evidence of choanal stenosis. Assessment of endocrine status and optimization of abnormalities with endocrine consultation and hormonal manipulation.

Anesthetic considerations: Usually minimal. Nasal intubation may be contraindicated. General considerations for obesity, including problems such as reflux, intravenous access, monitoring, positioning, and increased risk for sleep apnea syndrome. The possibility of raised intracranial pressure may modify the anesthetic technique.

Pharmacological implications: May require intraoperative endocrine manipulation, such as insulin and glucose monitoring.

REFERENCES:
Richards A, Brain C, Dillon MJ, et al: Craniometaphyseal and craniodiaphyseal dysplasia, head and neck manifestations and management. *J Laryngol Otol* 110:328, 1996.

Thurnau GR, Stein SA, Schaefer GB, et al: Management and outcome of two pregnancies in a woman with craniodiaphyseal dysplasia. *Am J Perinatol* 8:56, 1991.

Morning Glory Syndrome

At a glance: Very rare congenital disorder characterized by the association of strabismus, nonrhegmatogenous retinal detachment, or remnants of the hyaloid system of the eyes. Basal encephalocele has been encountered in a few cases. The CHARGE (*c*oloboma of iris, *h*eart deformities, choanal *a*tresia, *r*etarded growth, *g*enital and *e*ar deformities) association or isolated congenital defects have been demonstrated with this condition.

Synonym: Morning Glory Flower.

Incidence and genetic inheritance: Unknown; females affected twice as often as males.

Clinical aspects: Funnel-shaped, excavated optic disc surrounded by chorioretinal pigmentary anomalies; it is generally unilateral and isolated but has been observed in association with midline facial defects (cleft lip or palate, hypertelorism, basal meningomyelocele, agenesis of corpus callosum), renal anomalies, the CHARGE association, and isolated cardiac defects (i.e., atrial septal defect [ASD], ventricular septal defect [VSD], and patent ductus arteriosus [PDA]). In a few cases, basal encephalocele was also associated with the defect.

Anesthetic considerations: Check for associated anomalies, mainly airway and cardiac malformations. Anesthetic management is dictated by associated anomalies; one case of unexpected difficult tracheal intubation has been reported. The presence of a basal encephalocele might complicate airway management and positioning. Cardiac anomalies may be present and have their own considerations.

REFERENCES:
Eustis HS, Sanders MR, Zimmerman T: Morning glory syndrome in children. Association with endocrine and central nervous system anomalies. *Arch Ophthalmol* 2:204, 1992.

Shevchenko Y, Rehman M, Dorsey AT, et al: Unexpected difficult intubation in the patient with morning glory syndrome. *Paediatr Anaesth* 9:359, 1999.

Morquio Syndrome

At a glance: Inborn error of metabolism characterized by the deficiency of one of 10 specific lysosomal enzymes, resulting in an inability to metabolize complex carbohydrates (mucopolysaccharides) into simpler molecules. It exists in two forms: Morquio syndromes A and B are caused by a deficiency in the enzyme N-acetylgalactosamine-6-sulfatase and β-galactosidase, respectively. May be detected as early as 18 months to 2 years. The skeletal abnormalities may include macrocephaly, a broad mouth, prominent cheekbones, an unusually small nose, short necks, short barrel chests, disproportionately long arms, enlarged and possibly hyperextensible wrists, stubby hands, and "knock knees." The joint laxity and bony abnormalities of the spine can result in life-threatening spinal cord compression. The presence of a thoracic kyphoscoliosis may contribute to spinal cord ischemia risk during positioning. Aortic regurgitation and deafness have been reported.

Synonyms: Mucopolysaccharidosis Type IV; Morquio-Silfverskiöld Syndrome Morquio-Brailsford Syndrome; Morquio-Ullrich Syndrome; Atypical Chondrodystrophy; Dysotosis Enchondralis Metaepiphysaria; Eccentrochondrodysplasia; Eccentro-Osteochondrodysplasia; Familial Osseous Dystrophy; Hereditary Chondrodysplasia; Hereditary Osteochondrodystrophy; Hereditary Polytopic Enchondral Dysostosis; Keratansulfaturia; KS Mucopolysaccharidosis; Osteochondrodystrophia Deformans; Osteochondrodystrophy; Spondyloepiphyseal Dysplasia; Silfverskiöld Syndrome.

Classification:

Type A: Morquio Syndrome A; Galactosamine-4-Sulfatase (GALNS) Deficiency

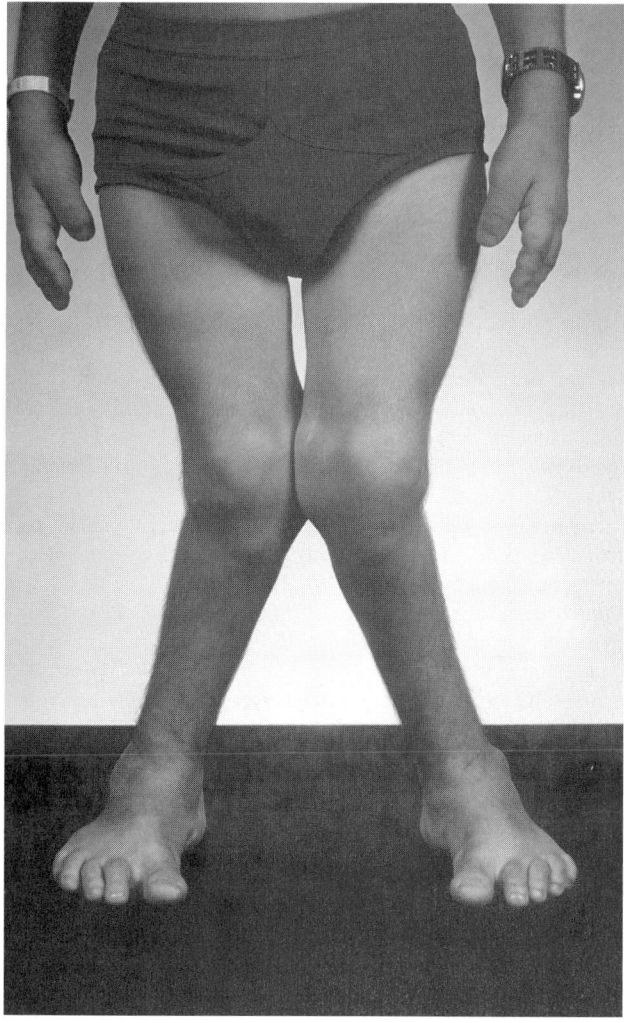

Morquio syndrome Short stature and marked varus gonarthrosis (knock knees) in a patient with Morquio syndrome.

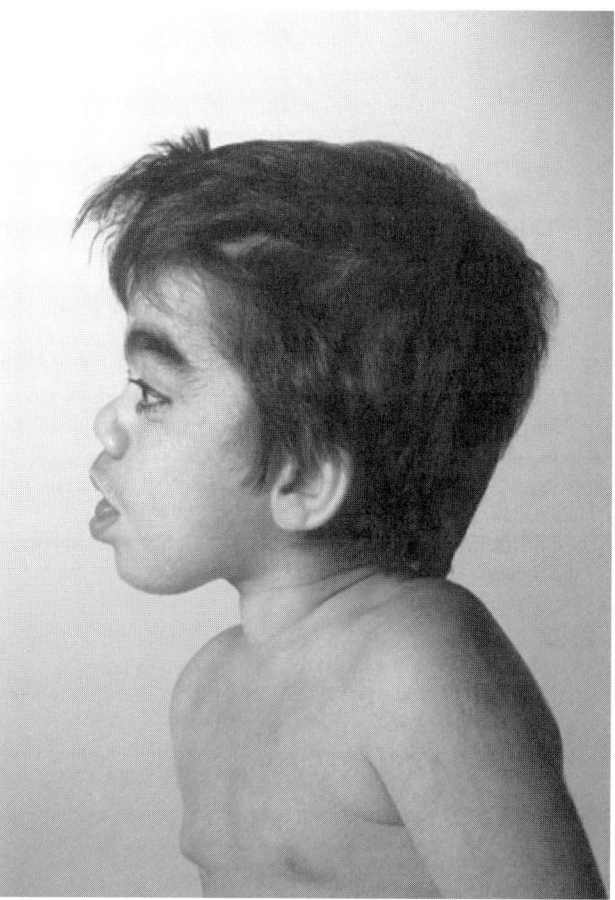

Morquio syndrome Characteristic facies with mild coarsening, midface hypoplasia, and macroglossia in a young boy with Morquio syndrome.

Type B: Morquio Syndrome B; Morquio-Like Syndrome; β-Galactosidase Deficiency

History: First described by L. Morquio, a Uruguayan pediatrician, in 1929 while living in Montevideo, Uruguay. He observed the disease in four sibs in a Swedish family. It is also suggested that J. F. Brailsford, a British pediatrician from Birmingham, England, simultaneously described the disease.

Incidence: It is estimated between 1:40,000 and less than 1:200,000 live births. In the United States, it is estimated that 1 in 25,000 births results in some form of mucopolysacchidosis.

Genetic inheritance: Autosomal recessive.

Pathophysiology: Deficiency of N-acetylgalactosamine-6-sulfate sulfatase (type A) or β-galactosidase (type B) leads to storage of keratan sulfate in tissues.

Diagnosis: Two types lead to identical phenotype. Keratan sulfate in urine. Specific enzyme assay diagnostic.

Clinical aspects: Affected children have normal mental development but severe physical manifestations. Short trunk, lax joints, short neck, corneal clouding, midface hypoplasia with mild coarsening of the facies. Progressive kyphoscoliosis leads to cardiorespiratory failure with death from cor pulmonale in third or fourth decade. May have aortic insufficiency. Hypoplasia of the odontoid is common, causing atlantoaxial subluxation and cord compression. Platyspondyly. Tracheal collapse with flexion of the neck reported. Very thin teeth enamel in type A. Progressive hearing loss.

Precautions before anesthesia: Assess cardiorespiratory status carefully and obtain appropriate investigations, for example, echocardiogram. Assess airway carefully. Obtain radiographs of cervical spine. Sleep apnea syndrome caused by hypertrophied tonsils and adenoids in a reduced pharyngeal space should be ruled out by polysomnography or night oximetry.

Anesthetic considerations: Airway management is frequently problematic, with direct laryngoscopy and tracheal intubation reported as difficult in half of cases. Laryngeal mask airway and fiberoptic laryngoscope should be ready for use. May require an endotracheal tube that is smaller than predicted by age because of the mucopolysaccharide deposits. Cervical spine abnormalities are common and manipulation of the spine during tracheal intubation should be minimized. Manual in-line stabilization may be used during intubation. Some patients may require surgical fusion of the cervical spine. In a report of two children affected with the condition, it is suggested that regional anesthesia (e.g., spinal anesthesia) can be used safely.

Pharmacological implications: Sedatives and opiates must be used cautiously in the postoperative period because of potential airway problems.

REFERENCES:

Morgan KA, Rehman MA, Schwartz RE: Morquio's syndrome and its anaesthetic considerations. *Paediatr Anaesth* 12:614, 2002.

Tobias JD: Anesthetic care for the child with morquio syndrome: General versus regional anesthesia. *J Clin Anesth* 11:242, 1999.

Walker RWM, Darowski M, Morris P, et al: Anesthesia and mucopolysaccharidoses. A review of airway problems in children. *Anesthesia* 49:1078, 1994.

Mount Reback Syndrome

At a glance: Hereditary familial disease characterized by attacks of choreoathetosis and torsion without loss of consciousness, each episode lasting from a few minutes to several hours. Alcoholic beverages, coffee, hunger, fatigue, emotional stress, and tobacco are the precipitating factors. The presence of an atypical Kayser-Fleischer ring is the principal ocular feature.

Synonyms: Mount Syndrome; Paroxysmal Nonkinesigenic Dyskinesia (PNKD); Paroxysmal Dystonic Choreoathetosis (PDC).

History: First described in 1940 by Lester A Mount, an American physician, and Stan Reback, also an American physician, in a family with many members over five generations affected with paroxysmal choreoathetosis.

Incidence: There are no epidemiological studies establishing the incidence or prevalence. Only few cases have been reported in the literature.

Genetic inheritance: Autosomal dominant. Gene locus is 2q33-2q35.

Pathophysiology: Unknown; has been suggested it could be an anomaly of the sodium channel even though it is not a seizure disorder.

Diagnosis: Movement disorder can be recognized in the first week of life. Usually, attacks of choreoathetosis lasting only a few minutes and occurring several times per day are not associated with loss of consciousness. The attacks never occur during sleep and at their height are similar to those occurring in Huntington chorea. Attacks are precipitated by fatigue, hunger, alcohol, tobacco, or coffee, but not by movement, contrary to kinesigenic choreoathetosis. Attacks are usually preceded by an aura. The presence of an atypical Kayser-Fleischer ring is the principal ocular feature.

Clinical aspects: Usually discovered during the first week of life. Patients are automatically place on benzodiazepine (diazepam or clonazepam) therapy to decrease the incidence of crisis and risk.

Precautions before anesthesia: Administration of benzodiazepines must be continued up to the operation.

Anesthetic considerations: No specific anesthetic experience reported. No specific medication regimen required; surgery usually performed under general anesthesia. Bradycardias following small doses of opiates respond to atropine at normal doses. Monitoring of the level of neuromuscular blockade is helpful. Maintain normothermia by adequately warming up the room and infused fluids to prevent shivering. If preoperative or postoperative sedation is needed, use benzodiazepines. Remember this is not a seizure disorder.

Pharmacological implications: No specific drug required or to be avoided. However, benzodiazepines are part of the normal therapy.

Other condition to be considered:

☞**HUNTINGTON CHOREA:** An inherited disease characterized by choreiform movements and progressive dementia. First described in 1872 by George Huntington, a long island physician. The most famous patient was folk singer Woody Guthrie.

REFERENCE:

Hofele K, Benecke R, Auburger G: Gene locus of dystonic Mount Reback-type of autosomal dominant paroxysmal choreoathetosis. *Neurology* 49:1252, 1997.

Mowat-Wilson Syndrome

At a glance: Autosomal dominant complex developmental disorder characterized by short stature, microcephaly, severe mental retardation, delayed motor development, epilepsy, and a wide spectrum of clinically heterogeneous features suggestive of neurocristopathies at the cephalic, cardiac, and vagal nerve levels.

Synonyms: Hirschsprung Disease Syndrome; Hirschsprung Disease-Mental Retardation Syndrome.

Incidence and genetic inheritance: Autosomal dominant pattern. It is believed to be caused by a mutation in the SMAD-interacting protein 1 gene (SMAD1P1).

Clinical aspects: Patients present with short stature, microcephaly, hypertelorism and iris coloboma, ptosis, convergent strabismus, and wide nasal bridge. The cardiovascular system is always affected and involves a patent ductus arteriosus and ventricular septal defect. Neurologically, the presence of severe mental retardation and seizure activities must be noted. Most patients are affected with muscle hypotonia. Abdominal distension, megacolon, and vomiting are frequent features. Barium enema shows transition zone between aganglionic contracted segment and dilated proximal bowel.

Anesthetic considerations: Preoperatively, complete assessment of the cardiac function must be done. Use of antibiotic for cardiac protection is mandatory. Myoclonic seizures are frequent, and oral antiepileptic therapy must be evaluated carefully and possibly replaced by intravenous medications. The presence of hypotonia must be taken into consideration if muscle relaxation is indicated. No pharmacological contraindications are associated with this syndrome.

Other condition to be considered:

MIETENS-WEBER SYNDROME: Autosomal recessive pattern characterized by severe mental retardation, corneal opacity, nystagmus, strabismus, small pinched nose, flexion contracture of the elbows, dislocation of head of radius, abnormally short ulna and radius, and clinodactyly.

REFERENCES:

Cerruti Mainardi P, Pastore G, Zweier C, et al: Mowat-Wilson syndrome and mutation in the zinc finger homeo box 1B gene: A well defined clinical entity. *J Med Genet* 41:E16, 2004.

Mowat DR, Wilson MJ, Goossens M: Mowat-Wilson syndrome. *J Med Genet* 40:305, 2003.

Moyamoya Syndrome

At a glance: Progressive disease that affects the cerebrovascular circulation. Characterized by narrowing and/or complete obstruction of the carotids. Clinically, may cause paralysis. Headaches, various vision problems, mental retardation, and psychiatric problems may occur. Cerebral hemorrhage (subarachnoid), cerebral infarction, severe headaches, speech disorders, and sudden onset of recurrent paralysis are part of the presentation but most often occur in juvenile moyamoya patients. Children may have convulsions or involuntary movements. Hemianopia, diplopia, bilateral decreased visual acuity, and inability to recognize objects are clinical symptoms.

Synonyms: Nishimoto-Takeuchi-Kudo-Suzuki Disease; Puff-of-Smoke Disease.

Incidence: The estimated prevalence is undetermined and considered rare. Approximately 7% of all moyamoya cases are familial in Greece. The sex distribution is reported to be a female-to-male ratio of 1.8:1.

Genetic inheritance: Sporadic; however, for the 7 to 10% that are familial cases, 24% of which are mother-sibling inherited, autosomal recessive. Gene map locus is 3-p24.2-p26. Although it may

occur at any age, the age of onset tends to determine the various symptoms.

Pathophysiology: Moyamoya disease is a result of progressive stenosis of cerebral arteries located at the base of the brain. It affects the intracerebral part of the internal carotids and causes a secondary collateral network that produces a radiologic image of a "puff of smoke" during cerebral angiography ("moyamoya" in Japanese). This aspect may be idiopathic or secondary to a known cause (drepanocytic anemia, radiotherapy, tuberculous meningitis, or in some patients affected by neurofibromatosis type I or William syndrome). It is caused by fibrocellular thickening of the intima and disorganization of the lamina elastica of the affected arteries. The collateral network consists of small- or medium-size penetrating arteries, mainly at the base of the skull, and results in hemodynamic implications different from atherosclerotic cerebrovascular disease of the elderly patient.

Diagnosis: Diagnosis is suggested by brain scans and magnetic resonance images showing multiple ischemic accidents of different ages, possibly hemorrhage and abnormal vessels at the base of the brain. Conventional angiography ascertains the diagnosis and assesses the stage of the disease.

Clinical aspects: In 50% of cases, the disease starts before age 10 years. It usually presents with transient motor disturbances resulting from transient brain ischemia. Progression may be insidious with headaches, epileptic seizures, language disorders, and upper cerebral dysfunctioning. More often signs are acute and focal, the most common being hemiplegia, sometimes hemichorea. The usual picture is alternating hemiplegia because of repeated deficiencies. Episodes are precipitated by hyperventilation (crying, blowing balloons) and emotions. Adults usually present with intracranial hemorrhage. Surgical treatment by creation of extracranial anastomosis (e.g., EDAS [encephaloduroarteriosynangiosis]).

Precautions before anesthesia: Document full neurologic history and examination. Check if exercise tolerance can be tolerated without neurologic symptoms. Usual preoperative investigations. Ensure that seizure medication is maintained and check recent control of convulsions.

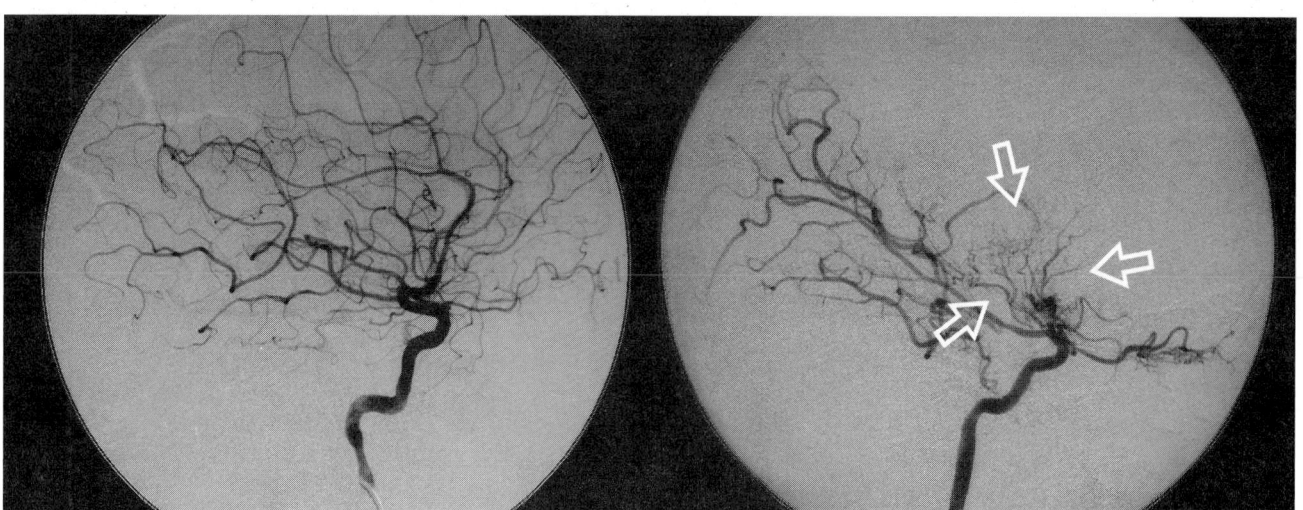

Moyamoya disease   Left: Normal lateral cerebral angiogram. Right: Typical findings of moyamoya disease in a 6-year-old boy. Characteristic "puff-of-smoke" sign *(arrows)* above the carotid syphon, with mainly preserved perfusion in the area of the anterior and the posterior cerebral artery.

Anesthetic considerations: Patients have a precarious cerebral circulation where the collateral vessels in the ischemic hemisphere are maximally dilated. Their management requires maintenance of adequate cerebral blood flow, normalization of intracranial pressure, and avoidance of both cerebral vasoconstriction and vasodilation. Cerebral blood flow is decreased with hypocapnia, and hypercapnia may reduce collateral flow by intracerebral steal effect; normocapnia is preferred. Placement of invasive arterial monitoring allowing frequent control of arterial CO_2 is mandatory. Regional cortical blood flow is decreased by inhaled anesthesia in patients with Moyamoya, and such an anesthetic may provoke intracerebral steal. Total intravenous anesthesia lacks these effects and therefore may be safer. Depth of anesthesia must be appropriate to prevent sudden changes in hemodynamics and intracerebral hemorrhage. Regional anesthesia is useful, especially in obstetric practice. Adequate postoperative pain relief is essential to prevent postoperative intracerebral hemorrhage secondary to pain. Avoid hypothermia. The priority is to maintain cerebral perfusion pressure.

Pharmacological implications: Beware of both hypoventilation and hyperventilation, and titrate adequate pain relief. Chronic administration of phenytoin increases nondepolarizing neuromuscular blocker requirements, produces gingival hyperplasia and bleeding, and may cause hepatic dysfunction. Ketamine, enflurane, and methohexital are relatively contraindicated.

Other conditions to be considered: May be secondary to ☞Sickle Cell Anemia, ☞Neurofibromatosis Type I, or ☞William Syndrome. It is also present in some children with ☞Alagille Syndrome.

REFERENCES:

Baykan N, Özgen S, Ustalar ZS, et al: Moyamoya disease and anesthesia. *Pediatr Anaesth* 15:1111, 2005.

Bingham RM, Wilkinson DJ: Anaesthetic management in moyamoya disease. *Anaesthesia* 40:1198, 1985.

Kurehara K, Ohnishi H, Touho H, et al: Cortical blood flow response to hypercapnia during anaesthesia in moyamoya disease. *Can J Anaesth* 40:709, 1993.

Soriano SG, Setha NF, Scott RM: Anaesthetic management of children with moyamoya disease. *Anesth Analg* 77:1066, 1993.

Moynahan Alopecia Syndrome

At a glance: Syndrome consisting of alopecia or hypotrichosis, oligophrenia, microcephaly, seizures, and mental retardation.

Synonyms: Alopecia-Epilepsy-Oligophrenia Syndrome; Alopecia-Mental Retardation-Epilepsy-Microcephaly Syndrome; Epilepsy-Oligophrenia Syndrome of Moynahan.

Classification: Three types of this disorder are suggested:

Type I: Total alopecia and mental retardation, the main features, in association with microcephaly

Type II: Subtotal alopecia and mental retardation with or without epilepsy

Type III: Subtotal alopecia and psychomotor retardation with microcephaly and epilepsy

History: First described in 1962 by E.J. Moynahan, an British dermatologist practicing in London.

Incidence: The incidence remains unknown.

Genetic inheritance: Familial with parental consanguinity; autosomal recessive trait.

Pathophysiology: Unknown.

Diagnosis: Microcephaly, alopecia or hypertrichosis, and epilepsy (grand mal seizures).

Clinical aspects: Sparse or absent scalp hair, microcephaly, seizures, short stature; hypogonadism with late puberty. Poor musculature. Sometimes sensorineural deafness.

Precautions before anesthesia: No literature on anesthesia in this condition. However, full neurologic history and examination, epileptic history, especially of control and medications, and associated anomalies resulting from microcephaly must be reviewed.

Anesthetic considerations: Epileptic control is essential; usual medications should be maintained until the morning of surgery wherever possible and appropriate nontriggering anesthetic agents used. Psychomotor retardation with poor speech skills may lead to a uncooperative patient.

Pharmacological implications: Note potential for interaction with antiepileptic drugs. Chronic phenytoin administration increases nondepolarizing neuromuscular blocker requirements, produces gingival hyperplasia and bleeding, and may cause hepatic dysfunction. Ketamine, enflurane, and methohexital are relatively contraindicated. High concentration (greater than 5–6%) of sevoflurane at induction might trigger epilepsy.

REFERENCES:

Baraitser M, Carter CO, Brett EM: A new alopecia/mental retardation syndrome. *J Med Genet* 20:64, 1983.

Moynahan EJ: Familial congenital alopecia, epilepsy, mental retardation with unusual electroencephalogram. *Proc R Soc Med* 55:411, 1962.

Perniola T, Krajewska G, Carnevale F, et al: Congenital alopecia, psychomotor retardation, convulsions in two sibs of a consanguineous marriage. *J Inherit Metab Dis* 3:49, 1980.

Muckle-Wells Syndrome

At a glance: Very rare genetic disorder diagnosed in infancy and characterized by deafness (adolescence), nonpruritic urticaria, and renal amyloidosis type AA. Other clinical features include arthralgias and/or conjunctivitis.

Synonym: Urticaria-Deafness-Amyloidosis Syndrome.

Incidence and genetic inheritance: Fewer than 150 cases reported since the first description in 1962. Autosomal dominant with variable penetrance.

Clinical aspects: Most patients present with some or all of the following manifestations: chronic urticaria, sensorineural deafness, periodic arthritis, "aguey bouts." "Aguey bouts" are composed of (a) chills, rigors, and malaise; (b) aching pains in distal limbs and large joints; and (c) urticarial rash over the whole body. Associated findings may include renal amyloidosis (and renal insufficiency), aminoaciduria, conjunctivitis, abdominal pain, angioedema, meningitis, and aphthous ulceration of the buccal mucosa. Hyperglycinuria, and renal stones, as well as renal amyloidosis, have been reported, but neither is required for the diagnosis.

Anesthetic considerations: Evaluation of renal function if indicated. Because attacks may be induced by cold, hypothermia should be prevented. Renal function must be considered in the selection of anesthetic agents.

REFERENCES:

Berthelot J, Maugars Y, Robillard N, et al: Autosomal dominant Muckle-Wells syndrome associated with cystinuria, ichthyosis, and aphthosis in a four-generation family. *Am J Med Genet* 53:72, 1994.

Muckle TJ: The "Muckle-Wells" syndrome. *Br J Dermatol* 87:87, 1979.

Mucolipidosis

Type I: Sialidosis type II (see *Sialidosis*)
Type II: Leroy I-cell syndrome (see *I-Cell Syndrome*)
Type III: Pseudo-Hurler polydystrophy (see *Pseudo-Hurler Polydystrophy*)

Mucopolysaccharidosis (MPS)

At a glance: Metabolic storage disease with multiorgan involvement.

Synonyms and classification: MPS.

MPS I H: ☞Hurler Syndrome (Hurler-Pfaundler Syndrome; Johnie McL Syndrome; Thompson Syndrome; Hurler-Scheie Syndrome; Mucopolysaccharide Storage Disease I; α-L-Iduronidase Deficiency Syndrome; Dysostosis Multiplex; Dysostotic Idiocy; Hurler-Pfaundler Syndrome; Gargoylism; Lipochondrodystrophy; Pfaundler-Hurler Syndrome)

MPS I S: Scheie Syndrome

MPS I H/S: Hurler-Scheie Syndrome

MPS II: ☞Hunter Syndrome (Hurler-Hunter Disease; Mucopolysaccharide Storage Disease II)

MPS III: Sanfilippo Syndrome (Mucopolysaccharide Storage Disease III; Heparitinuria; HS-Mucopolysaccharidosis; Polydystrophic Oligophrenia)

Type A: Sanfilippo Syndrome A (Heparan Sulfate Sulfatase Deficiency)
Type B: Sanfilippo Syndrome B (N-Acetyl-Alpha-D-Glucosaminidase [NAG] Deficiency)
Type C: Sanfilippo Syndrome C (Acetyl-Coa:Alpha-Glucosamide N-Acetyltransferase Deficiency)
Type D: Sanfilippo Syndrome D (N-Acetylglucosamine-6-Sulfate Sulfatase Deficiency)

MPS IV: ☞Morquio Syndrome (Mucopolysaccharide Storage Disease IV; Morquio-Brailsford Syndrome; Morquio-Ullrich Syndrome; Atypical Chondrodystrophy; Dysotosis Enchondralis Metaepiphysaria; Eccentrochondrodysplasia; Eccentro-Osteochondrodysplasia; Familial Osseous Dystrophy; Hereditary Chondrodysplasia; Hereditary Osteochondrodystrophy; Hereditary Polytopic Enchondral Dysostosis; Keratansulfaturia; KS Mucopolysaccharidosis; Osteochondrodystrophia Deformans; Osteochondrodystrophy; Spondylo-Epiphyseal Dysplasia; Silfverskiold Syndrome; Morquio-Silfverskiold Syndrome)

Type A: Morquio Syndrome A (Galactosamine-4-Sulfatase [GALNS] Deficiency)
Type B: Morquio Syndrome B (Morquio-Like Syndrome; β-Galactosidase Deficiency)

MPS V: Obsolete, previously known Ellis-Sheldon Syndrome
MPS VI: Maroteaux-Lamy Syndrome (Mucopolysaccharide Storage Disease VI; Arylsulfatase B [ARSB] Deficiency; N-Acetylgalactosamine-4-Sulfatase Deficiency; Polydystrophic Dwarfism; Pyknodysostosis of Maroteaux-Lamy)

MPS VII: Sly Syndrome (Mucopolysaccharide Storage Disease VII; Beta-Glucuronidase Deficiency; Beta-Glucuronidase Deficiency Mucopolysaccharidosis; GUSB Deficiency)

MPS VIII: ☞Di Ferrante Syndrome.

> *NB:* Di Ferrante Syndrome should not be used as a term to describe MPS VIII because it has been proved that the author committed fraud based on observation obtained from only one patient.

MPS F: ☞Fucosidosis (Mucopolysaccharide Storage Disease F; α-L-Fucosidase [FUCA] Deficiency)

Incidence: The incidence of MPS is estimated at 0.04–0.3% of living births and considered 1.5% of all congenital disorders. The average surviving for these patients is around 20–30 years and cardiac failure or infections to the gastrointestinal tract cause death. The instability to the atlantoaxial joint is also implicated as cause of death.

Genetic inheritance: MPS I and III are autosomal recessive; MPS II is X-linked with locus at Xq27-q28; MPS IV is autosomal recessive and located on chromosome 16 long-arm; MPS VI is autosomal recessive; MPS VII is autosomal recessive, with GUSB locus on long arm of chromosome 7; fucosidosis is an autosomal recessive trait with occasional parental consanguinity, located on the short arm of chromosomes 1 and 2.

Pathophysiology: *MPS I:* Inborn error of mucopolysaccharide metabolism with α-L-iduronidase deficiency in leucocytes and fibroblasts and abnormal mucopolysaccharide incorporation and degradation by fibroblasts. Three types are recognized. All three types have similar laboratory findings, except the fibroblasts differ.

MPS I-H (Hurler Syndrome): Most severe of the three types with coarse (gargyloid) facies, accelerated growth from infancy followed by progressive decline in rate of development, mental retardation, dysostosis multiplex, corneal clouding, and death before age 10 years as a consequence of pneumonia and heart failure. Some symptoms (hernia, macrocephaly, respiratory infections, and limited hip abduction) become apparent early in infancy, but the complete clinical picture develops during the second year of life.

MPS I-S (Scheie Syndrome): More moderate autosomal recessive form caused by deficiency of α-L-iduronidase leading to accumulation of dermatan sulfate in tissues. It is marked by corneal opacities, clawhand, aortic valve disease, normal stature, mild or absent intellectual impairment, and nearly normal lifespan, depending on cardiac complications. The condition is seldom recognized during infancy or early childhood.

MPS H/S (Hurler-Scheie Syndrome): Intermediate form between the previous two variants, which includes short stature, dysostosis multiplex, hepatosplenomegaly, corneal clouding, umbilical or inguinal hernia, generally normal mental development with psychotic symptoms later in life, and death by age 25 years caused by acute or chronic cardiac failure (cor pulmonale). Symptoms are usually apparent by age 2 years.

Diagnosis: Clinical characteristics and demonstration of α-L-iduronidase deficiency, abnormal deposits of mucopolysaccharides, and increasing urinary heparan sulfate and dermatan sulfate.

Clinical aspects: Coarse (gargyloid) facies, macrocephaly with frontal bulging, scaphoidocephaly, premature closure of sagittal and metopic sutures, J-shaped sella turcica, full cheeks, and prominent nasolabial fold. Thick earlobes. Prominent lower eyelids, shallow orbits, corneal opacity, glaucoma, and synophrys. Flat philtrum, wide and anteverted nares, broad tip and depressed bridge of nose. Wide mouth with protruding tongue, big lips, and widely spaced teeth. Short neck. Stiff rib cage with pectus excavatum or carinatum. Prominent abdomen with hernia. Stiff fingers with clawhand. Joint contractures, long bone deformities, genu valgum, and hip deformities. Kyphosis, dysplastic (hook-shaped) vertebral bodies, lumbar lordosis. May have hypoplastic odontoid with at-lantoaxial subluxation. Dysostosis multiplex. Dry, pale, coarse skin with hypertrichosis. Hydrocephalus. Arteriosclerosis with coronary artery narrowing, valvular defects, mainly mitral valve thickening. Hepatosplenomegaly. Recurrent chest infections. Early accelerated growth followed by failure with mental and motor retardation. Poor gag and swallowing reflexes, rhinorrhea, noisy respiration, and sleep apnea syndrome, deafness (sensorineural and conductive), blindness, and psychosis.

Precautions before anesthesia: Full motor and mental milestones as well as medical history. Note respiratory status, arterial blood gases where indicated, and chest radiographs; pulmonary function tests where possible; treat infection before anesthesia. C1-C2 subluxation is frequent so neck instability must be ruled out. Spinal cord compression may occur as a consequence of thickening of the dura and odontoid hypoplasia, so preoperative MRI of the spinal cord is suggested. Cardiac investigation (echocardiography) is necessary to evaluate cardiac involvement: valves, myocardial function, coronary arteries. Rule out sleep apnea syndrome with polysomnography or night oximetry: sleep apnea syndrome, if present, should be treated preoperatively (i.e., nasal continuous positive airway pressure).

Anesthetic considerations: There are copious oral secretions: anticholinergic premedication is very helpful. A standard facial mask might be difficult to fit to the patient's face because of facial deformities; try placing the mask upside-down. Thickening of the tongue and oropharyngeal soft tissues, the presence of a short neck, and the limited mobility of the cervical spine and temporomandibular joint make direct laryngoscopy and tracheal intubation extremely difficult. A laryngeal mask airway and a fiberoptic laryngoscope should be ready for use. A nasopharyngeal airway can be useful but might be difficult to insert because of choanal narrowing by accumulation of mucopolysaccharide deposits; moreover, it might induce bleeding. An oral airway is often difficult to insert and can displace the tip of epiglottis downward. Poor gag and swallowing reflexes are present so a rapid-sequence induction is theoretically necessary, but careful inhalational induction or awake fiberoptic intubation in a cooperative patient is the safest option. Stiff chest wall with prominent abdomen could lead to difficulty with ventilation. Mental retardation, psychosis, and short stature with contractures may make IV access and patient control difficult. Hydrocephalus cases have raised intracranial pressure, so appropriate precautions are essential. Anesthetic management should take into account the presence of coronary and/or valvular disease.

Pharmacological implications: Although there are no specific pharmacological implications, each condition might have specific limitations. For instance, the use of sedative medications in the Hunter and Hurler patient may lead to airway obstruction. In the presence of cardiac anomalies, the pharmacological implications are those associated with the anomaly. Antibiotic prophylaxis in case of valvular involvement.

SPECIFIC DESCRIPTION OF MUCOPOLYSACCHARIDOSIS TYPES I THROUGH IX:

Mucopolysaccharidosis I: Characterized by a wide range of phenotypic involvement with three major recognized clinical entities: *Hurler (MPS IH), Scheie (MPS IS),* and *Hurler-Scheie (MPS IH/S) syndromes.* All three variants are caused by a deficiency of α-L-iduronidase. Hurler and Scheie syndromes represent phenotypes at the severe and mild ends of the MPS I clinical spectrum, respectively, and Hurler-Scheie syndrome is intermediate in phenotypic expression. MPS I is more frequent than MPS II (Hunter syndrome), which has no corneal clouding and pursues a slower course. The clinical characteristics are discussed under *Mucopolysaccharidoses.*

MPS II (Hunter Syndrome): Caused by a deficiency of iduronate sulfatase with storage of dermatan sulfate and heparan sulfate in many tissues. It is similar to MPS I, except for the absence of corneal clouding and slower progression of the course of the disease and central nervous system deterioration. Two types are recognized, both of which are normal at birth: *severe (MPS IIA),* which is characterized mainly by mental retardation and progressive physical deterioration and early death, and a *mild form (MPS IIB),* in which patients may survive into adulthood. Onset of MPS IIA occurs between 2 and 4 years of age; deterioration, chronic diarrhea, recurrent ear infections, hearing impairment, and communicating hydrocephalus with increased intracranial pressure are progressive features, with death occurring between the ages of 10 and 15 years. Obstructive airway disease caused by hypertrophied adenoids and tonsils. Cardiac valvular dysfunction, myocardial thickening, pulmonary hypertension, coronary disease, and myocardial dysfunction may complicate the illness. MPS IIB is milder without mental retardation. Symptoms include hearing impairment, carpal tunnel syndrome, joint stiffness, discrete corneal opacities, and papilledema. Death may occur in young adulthood and can be caused by airway obstruction or cardiac failure. Laryngoscopy and tracheal intubation are usually very difficult.

MPS III (Sanfilippo Syndrome): Autosomal recessive inheritance inborn error of metabolism with a deficiency of the intralysosomal enzymes involved in heparan sulfate (HS) degradation. Affected infants appear normal at birth, with slowing of development taking place at about 1 to 2 years of age, occasionally not becoming apparent until early school age. Behavioral disorders, mental deterioration, and loss of motor skills are the principal features, with hirsutism, macrocephaly, and limited joint movements. *Four biochemically distinct types,* each with a different enzyme deficiency, are recognized: *A, B, C,* and *D.* The phenotype is similar in all four types and consists mainly of some facial coarsening with dull appearance, slightly sunken nasal bridge, and abundant scalp hair. Early development is usually normal, followed between the ages of 2 and 6 years by mainly behavioral disorders with progressive loss of mental and motor skills with spastic diplegia. The patient eventually becomes bedridden. Death usually occurs between 10 and 20 years of age. *Type A* has the most severe course with the earliest onset and mortality. Type A is caused by heparan sulfatase (EC 3.10.1.1) deficiency. *Type B* is caused by N-acetyl-alpha-D-glucosaminidase (EC 3.2.1.50) deficiency. *Type C* is caused by acetyl-CoA:alpha-glucosamide N-acetyltransferase (EC 2.3.13) deficiency. *Type D* is caused by N-acetylglucosamine-6-sulfate sulfatase (EC 3.1.6.14) deficiency. Behavioral problems can make induction and awakening from anesthesia problematic. Even though the incidence of difficult tracheal intubation is much less than in the other mucopolysaccharidoses, it is still very important to assess the airway carefully. Assess cardiorespiratory status carefully. Younger children with Sanfilippo syndrome often have only mild physical abnormalities. Severe mental retardation and aggressive behavior may cause problems during induction of anesthesia, and the presence of a parent may be helpful. Difficulty with airway management is less likely than in other forms of mucopolysaccharidosis.

MPS IV (Morquio Syndrome): Inborn error of metabolism characterized by faulty degradation of keratan sulfate in cartilage and lysosomal accumulation. Clinical features include short trunk dwarfism, dysostosis multiplex, progressive spinal deformity, short neck, pectus carinatum, genu valgum, pes planus, and odontoid hypoplasia with varying degrees of severity. Mental development is usually normal, but progressive intellectual deterioration is reported in type B. Two types are recognized according to the enzymes involved. *Type A* is caused by galactosamine-6-sulfate sulfatase (EC 3.16.4) and is more severe than type B. It is marked by shortness and hyperextension of the neck causing the head to appear as if it were resting directly on the shoulders; short trunk; long extremities with excessive joint mobility; kyphosis or kyphoscoliosis; pectus carinatum; the sternum extending from clavicular junction and angling downward in midsection; spinal cord compression associated with atlantoaxial dislocation (they often require posterior cervical fusion at a young age) and thoracolumbar gibbus; protruding abdomen; and clouding of the cornea. Aortic valve insufficiency is common late in the disease. *Type B* is caused by β-galactosidase (EC 3.2.1.23) deficiency and is marked a milder phenotype consisting of dysostosis multiplex, pectus carinatum, odontoid hypoplasia, kyphosis, genua valga, platyspondyly, and corneal clouding. Direct laryngoscopy and intubation are usually very difficult because of cervical spine instability or previous fusion. Endotracheal tube size may be smaller than predicted.

MPS V (Scheie Syndrome, now MPS I-S): Autosomal recessively inherited disease that presents with the same deficient enzyme as observed in Hurler syndrome, but in this case it is specific for dermatan sulfate. The clinical manifestations are milder than in Hurler syndrome and do not appear until age 5 years. Patients have normal intelligence with mild facial coarsening and skeletal abnormalities. Corneal clouding leads to visual impairment. Aortic insufficiency is common. Patients reach normal height and have a near-normal life expectancy. Assess airway for evidence of aortic regurgitation. These children are less severely affected than are children with Hurler syndrome but may still present difficulty with airway management. Obstructive sleep apnea has been reported. Children with cardiac valve abnormalities should receive antibiotic prophylaxis for endocarditis.

MPS VI (Maroteaux-Lamy Syndrome): Inborn error of metabolism characterized by arylsulfatase B (EC 3.1.6.12) deficiency preventing degradation of mucopolysaccharides, with their accumulation in soft tissues causing obstruction and compression of the blood vessels, trachea, and peripheral nerves, and disruption of normal bone development. It is associated with the phenotype similar to that in MPS I, but generally patients are of normal intelligence (mental retardation has been reported in a few isolated cases). Three basic types are recognized. The *mild type* (type B) is marked by usually normal childhood until approximately 6 years of age, when short stature, Legg-Perthes–like changes of the hips, aortic stenosis, spinal deformities, and corneal clouding begin to appear; survival is into adulthood. The *intermediate type* has a phenotype similar to that in mucolipidosis III with coarse Hurler-like facies, stiff joints with decreased mobility, and short

stature. The *severe type* (sometimes designated Maroteaux-Lamy syndrome type A) is usually associated with onset of symptoms in early childhood, a rapidly progressive course, and death in adolescence. Short stature, coarse facies, hyperextended head, corneal clouding, defective hearing, heart abnormalities, and musculoskeletal anomalies are the main characteristics. Direct laryngoscopy and tracheal intubation are usually very difficult. Beware of cardiac involvement.

MPS VII (Sly syndrome): Autosomal recessive inborn error of metabolism characterized by beta-glucuronidase (EC 3.2.1.31) deficiency leading to accumulation of chondroitin 4/6 sulfate, with abnormal storage of mucopolysaccharides in various tissues. The phenotype consists mainly of short stature, hepatosplenomegaly, dysostosis multiplex, and mild mental retardation. *Type I* is the most severe, with hydrops fetalis, coarse facies with hypertelorism and depressed nasal bridge, cloudy cornea, and onset of symptoms at birth. *Type II* has a less severe course, with moderate Hurler facies and hypertelorism, and onset at age 2 to 3 years. *Type III* has the mildest symptoms, with onset during adolescence. Mitral and aortic valve involvement. Intubation may be difficult. Assess cardiorespiratory status carefully and obtain appropriate investigations (e.g., chest radiograph, echocardiogram). Assess airway and cervical spine. Check history for evidence of obstructive sleep apnea. Difficulty with airway management should be anticipated in more severely affected patients. Spontaneous respiration should be preserved until the airway is secure.

MPS VIII: Inborn error of mucopolysaccharide metabolism with glucosamine-6-sulfate sulfatase deficiency and characteristics similar to those of mucopolysaccharidosis II and IV. Delayed physical and mental development, hypertrichosis, hepatosplenomegaly, dysostosis multiplex, and mild deafness are the main symptoms.

Fucosidosis: Lysosome storage disease caused by α-L-fucosidase (EC 3.2.1.51) deficiency in leukocytes manifested by abnormal accumulation in tissues and urinary excretion of partially catabolized oligosaccharides, glycoasparagines, and glycolipids with α-linked fucose at the nonreducing end of the glycogen chain. The phenotype is variable and may include delayed growth and mental development, progressive neurologic deterioration, Hurler-like (mucopolysaccharidosis I-H) coarse facies, recurrent infections, visceromegaly, skeletal abnormalities, joint contractures, deafness, and angiokeratoma corporis diffusum. Several types are recognized by different researchers. The form exhibiting a longer survival, mild neurologic manifestations, and angiokeratoma is sometimes referred to as *fucosidosis type II.* In a different scheme, three different types are recognized according to their age of onset. *Types I and II* are the most severe, with onset at 10 and 18 months, respectively, with a life expectancy of 6 years. *Type III* is a juvenile form marked by a milder expression of psychomotor retardation and a slower deterioration of neurologic activities. Hurler-like gargyloid facies occurs mainly in types I and II and is less common in type III (for further information see *Fucosidosis*).

REFERENCES:

Beck M, Glossl J, Grubisic A, et al: Heterogeneity of Morquio disease. *Clin Genet* 29:325, 1986.

Broadhead PM, Kirk JM, Burt AJ, et al: Full expression of Hunter's disease in a female with X-chromosome deletion leading to a nonrandom inactivation. *Clin Genet* 30:392, 1986.

Chan YL, Lin SP, Man TT, et al: Clinical experience in anesthetic management for children with mucopolysaccharidoses. Report of ten cases. *Acta Paediatr Taiwan* 42:306, 2001.

Danks DM, Campbell PE, Cartwright E, et al: The Sanfilippo syndrome: Clinical, biochemical, radiological, haematological, and pathological features of nine cases. *Austral Paediatr J* 8:174, 1972.

de Kremer RD, Givogri I, Argarana CE, et al: Mucopolysaccharidosis type VI (beta-glucuronidase deficiency): A chronic variant with an oligosymptomatic severe skeletal dysplasia. *Am J Med Genet* 44:145, 1992.

Diaz JH, Belani KG: Perioperative management of children with mucopolysaccharidoses. *Anesth Analg* 77:1261, 1993.

Moores C, Rogers JG, McKenzie IM, et al: Anaesthesia for children with mucopolysaccharidoses. *Anaesth Intensive Care* 24:459, 1996.

Morgan KA, Rehman MA, Schwartz RE: Morquio's syndrome and its anesthetic considerations. *Paediatr Anaesth* 12:641, 2002.

Walker RWM, Darowski M, Morris P, et al: Anesthesia and mucopolysaccharidoses. A review of airway problems in children. *Anesthesia* 49:1078, 1994.

Yuichiro T, Mamoru T, Kiyoshi M, et al: Complete heart block during anesthetic management in a patient with mucopolysaccharidosis type VII. *Anesthesiology* 95:1035, 2001.

Mucoviscidosis

At a glance: Congenital multiorgan disease affecting mainly the lungs, liver, and pancreas. Frequent lung infections, hemoptysis, intolerance to exercise, presence of clubbing fingers suggesting pulmonary hypertension, rectal prolapse, and nasal polyps.

Synonym: Cystic Fibrosis (CF).

Incidence: In the United States, CF is the most common lethal disease inherited in the white population. In America and Northern European origin, the prevalence is estimated at 1:3000. In African Americans, the prevalence is 1:15,000 whereas in hispanics, it is estimated at 1 case per 9200. In Asian Americans, the prevalence is reported at 1 case per 31,000.

Genetic inheritance: Autosomal recessive. More than 1000 mutations have been described on the long arm of chromosome 7 (7q21.3-7q22.1); the most frequent is ΔF508, which results in a defect of the CF transmembrane regulator protein called CFTR.

Pathophysiology: Malfunction of the gene coding for the CF transmembrane conductance regulator (CFTR) protein causes defective cAMP-dependent chloride secretion from the epithelium of different exocrine tissues, leading to thick viscous and difficult-to-clear secretions in lungs, sinuses, pancreas, intestine, liver, and reproductive tract. In addition, the CFTR-mediated regulation of sodium channel activity may fail, leading to increased sodium absorption from the airways, which contributes to the fluidity and mobilization of the airway secretions. Also, hyperplastic airway epithelium with areas of erosion and squamous metaplasia of the submucosal glands leads to plug of mucoid material and subsequently to the release of inflammatory cells. Eventually, grossly dilated airways with purulent secretions are observed and severely congested parenchyma develops. Radiologic findings reflect the pathologic changes in the airways. Although the lungs of infants born with CF are structurally normal at birth, respiratory symptoms are usually the first sign of CF.

Diagnosis: Difficult in children. Depends on the clinical history and a high index of suspicion together with a family history of the disease; a high sweat sodium concentration greater than 60 mmol/l, or abnormal in vivo nasal potential difference. A normal nasal potential difference value is 0.9–24.7 mV, whereas an abnormal measurement is 1.8–53 mV (difference of potential voltage difference between the nasal mucosa and a reference electrode into the forearm). Absent vas deferens and epididymis in the male. Immunoreactive trypsin.

Clinical aspects: CF is now the most common cause of recurrent bronchopulmonary infection in childhood and is an important cause in early adult life. Finger clubbing is almost universal, hemoptysis is frequent, and breathlessness occurs in the later stages as airflow limitation develops. Older children may develop nasal polyps. Gastroesophageal reflux is often present. Puberty and skeletal maturity are delayed in most patients with the disease. Males are always infertile as a result of failure of development of the vas deferens and epididymis. Females are able to reproduce, but often develop secondary amenorrhea as the disease progresses. Approximately 85% of patients have symptomatic steatorrhea because of pancreatic dysfunction. Children may be born with meconium ileus because of the viscoid consistency of meconium in CF and later in life develop the meconium equivalent (MIE) syndrome, an important cause of small bowel obstruction unique to CF. Cholesterol gallstones appear to occur with increased frequency, and biliary cirrhosis with portal hypertension develops in approximately 5 to 10% of older patients. Diabetes mellitus occurs in 20% of adults. Risk of spontaneous pneumothorax increases with age; pleurodesis is sometimes necessary. Ventilation/perfusion inequality is prominent as the disease progresses.

Precautions before anesthesia: Many of these children become severely emotionally upset. They require careful attention and much reassurance. Assess the patient's condition carefully: clinical examination (dyspnea, productive cough, hepatosplenomegaly), pulse oximetry while breathing room air (and arterial blood gases if hypoxemia; check $PaCO_2$), chest radiograph (emphysema, bubbles, infection), blood glucose and electrolytes, and renal and liver function tests. Chronic respiratory disease may result in cor pulmonale. Do not give opiates as premedication. Give benzodiazepines cautiously if indicated to counter anxiety. Ensure optimal hydration; fluids must not be withheld for long periods of time. Order chest physiotherapy immediately before anesthesia and postoperatively. Strongly suspect chronic colonization of lungs with antibiotic-resistant *Pseudomonas* or *Staphylococcus* species, or even *Aspergillus*.

Anesthetic considerations: Copious, extremely viscous secretions in the respiratory tract; nebulization of recombinant human DNAse is very helpful in decreasing their viscosity. Hypoxia may develop rapidly because of V/Q disturbances, and induction of anesthesia is prolonged. Lung compliance is reduced. In severe advanced cases, very high airway pressure may be required to provide adequate ventilation and prevent hypoxemia. Therefore, use a cuffed endotracheal tube whenever possible. Use local or regional anesthesia wherever possible. If general anesthesia is given, administer 100% O_2 for at least 5 minutes, then intravenous induction. Tracheal intubation; use cuffed tube; suction as often as necessary to prevent blocking by thick plugs, and use as high an FiO_2 (fraction of inspired oxygen) as necessary (may need 100%). Prevent hyperventilation and be aware of the risk of gas trapping. High risk for bronchial hyperreactivity and pneumothorax. Avoid long-acting opioids for postoperative pain relief, but effective analgesia is mandatory to allow chest physiotherapy. Use regional anesthesia for postoperative pain relief if possible. Aim for early postoperative emergence from anesthesia. Note the importance of postoperative fluids and a humid environment, as well as of physiotherapy. Encourage the patient to cough. Long postoperative ileus or even subocclusive episodes possible even in the absence of surgical complication.

Pharmacological implications: Use of anticholinergic agents is controversial (risk of inspissated secretions), and ketamine is best avoided (increased bronchial secretions). Malnutrition and underweight for age are common as a result of chronic infection or malabsorption therefore, drug dosages must be adjusted accordingly. Mild liver dysfunction is not unusual. Drug dosages should be adapted accordingly.

Other conditions to be considered:

Lubani Al Saleh Teebi Syndrome: Cystic fibrosis with *Helicobacter pylori* gastritis, megaloblastic anemia, and subnormal mentality.

☞Alpha₁-Antitrypsin Deficiency: Relatively common inherited disorder; primarily presents with early-onset panacinar lung emphysema and in a minority of the patients also with liver cirrhosis. Cardiac arrest in association with general anesthesia has been described.

☞Kartagener Syndrome: Genetically transmitted polymalformative syndrome characterized by bronchiectasis, situs inversus, and chronic sinusitis.

REFERENCES:

Cameron AJ, Skinner TA: Management of a parturient with respiratory failure secondary to cystic fibrosis. *Anaesthesia* 60:77, 2005.

Walsh TS, Young CH: Anaesthesia and cystic fibrosis. *Anaesthesia* 50:614, 1995.

Weeks AM, Buckland MR: Anaesthesia for adults with cystic fibrosis. *Anaesth Intensive Care* 23:332, 1995.

Precautions before anesthesia: Only in relation with the underlying disease leading to the operation.

Anesthetic considerations: No specific measures must be undertaken in the anesthetic care of these individuals.

Pharmacological implications: No known pharmacological implications. However, patients receiving radiotherapy or chemotherapy will require special review of the medication used and the potential implications with anesthesia.

Other conditions to be considered:

☞Epidermal Nevus Syndrome: Characterized by the presence of linear nevus sebaceus of the midline of the face associated with epilepsy, seizures, and mental retardation. Other clinical features include alopecia, hypoplastic sebaceous glands, verrucous lesions with hyperplastic sebaceous glands developing during adolescence, and benign or malignant tumors developing in the later stage.

Familial Presenile Sebaceous Gland Hyperplasia: Occurs frequently in men older than 50 years. The clinical presentation includes a solitary or several elevated, soft, yellow papules with central umbilication on the face, particularly the forehead. The lesions may spread to the neck and upper part of the thorax.

REFERENCES:

Esche C, Kruse R, Lamberti C, et al: Muir-Torre syndrome: Clinical features and molecular genetic analysis. *Br J Dermatol* 136:913, 1997.

Schwartz RA, Torre DP: The Muir-Torre syndrome: A 25-year retrospect. *J Am Acad Dermatol* 33:90, 1995.

Muir-Torre Syndrome (MTS)

At a glance: Multiple cutaneous tumors, including sebaceous neoplasms and visceral malignancies. A familial cancer syndrome that combines at least one sebaceous neoplasm (sebaceous adenoma, sebaceous epithelioma, or sebaceous carcinoma) and at least one visceral malignancy (usually gastrointestinal or genitourinary carcinomas).

Synonyms: Cutaneous Sebaceous Neoplasms and Keratoacanthomas, Multiple with Gastrointestinal and Other Carcinomas; Lynch Cancer Family Syndrome II.

Classification: A subgroup of this syndrome is part of the Lynch cancer family syndrome II, which has been related to mutation in the MSH2 gene located on 2p. Mutations in the MLH1 gene located in 3p also cause the syndrome.

History: G.G. Muir and D. Torre first described this syndrome in 1967.

Incidence: In 1995, 147 cases were described. Patients ranged in age from 37 to 89 years at diagnosis; female-to-male ratio is 2:3.

Genetic inheritance: Autosomal dominant.

Diagnosis: Keratoacanthoma can be considered a marker for this syndrome in only two circumstances: (a) if they are multiple and are associated with two or more low-grade visceral malignancies in a patient with a family history of the syndrome, or (b) when a keratoacanthoma displays sebaceous differentiation histologically.

Clinical aspects: Any sebaceous neoplasm except sebaceous hyperplasia and nevus sebaceous of Jadassohn should signal the possibility of MTS. Because visceral malignancies in MTS are low grade, surgical removal of primary tumor(s), even metastatic ones, may prove valuable and at times appears curative.

Mulibrey Nanism Syndrome

At a glance: Mulibrey is an acronym for *mu*scle, *li*ver, *br*ain, and *ey*e. An extremely rare inherited disorder characterized by dwarfism and distinctive abnormalities of the muscles, liver, brain, and eyes. Characteristic symptoms include low birth weight, short stature, muscle hypotonia, hepatomegaly, and hydrocephalus. Infants typically have yellow discolorations in their eyes, amblyopia, and choriocapillaris hypoplasia. A serious consequence is the presence of constrictive pericarditis in infancy. Pulmonary effusion and ascites are present.

Synonyms: Perheentupa Syndrome; Constrictive Pericarditis-Dwarfism Syndrome; Dwarfism-Pericarditis Syndrome; Growth Failure-Pericardial Constriction Syndrome; Nanism-Constrictive Pericarditis Syndrome; Pericardial Constriction-Growth Failure Syndrome.

Incidence and genetic inheritance: Rare, familial, autosomal recessive trait. Most reported cases are from Finland.

Clinical aspects: Prenatal-onset growth retardation associated with muscle, liver, brain, and eye abnormalities. Hypotonia; congestive pericarditis with elevated venous pressure; triangular face, often with hydrocephaloid skull; long and shallow sella turcica; yellowish dots and pigment dispersion in the fundus oculi; and borderline mental deficiency. There is a depressed and broad bridge of nose, delayed tooth eruption, malocclusion, hypodontia, and small tongue. Thin and short limbs and cystic dysplasia of the tibia and hypotonia are present. Nevus flammeus are present on the skin. Obstructive pericarditis, elevated venous pressure, prominent left atrium and/or right ventricle, dilated neck veins, and congestive heart failure. Hepatomegaly and abnormalities of kidneys and ureters are present.

Neonatal pituitary insufficiency and neonatal hypoglycemia. There are growth and mental retardation and variable pubertal development with characteristic high-pitched voice and hyperopia.

Precautions before anesthesia: Check cardiac function (thick adherent pericardium with constrictive pericarditis), pleural effusion, and neurologic status (increased intracranial pressure as a consequence of hydrocephalus).

Anesthetic considerations: Patients may have raised intracranial pressure as a consequence of hydrocephalus. They have a large head with prominent occiput and facial abnormalities, which may make direct laryngoscopy and tracheal intubation difficult. Obstructive pericarditis is likely, with elevated venous pressure, prominent left atrium or right ventricle, dilated neck veins, and congestive heart failure. Central venous and arterial pressure measurements are essential, with either pulmonary artery catheter or transesophageal echocardiography as needed. Pituitary disease may be associated with raised intracranial pressure; it also may have implications for thyroid and adrenal function. Possibility of diabetes insipidus. Fragile teeth.

Pharmacological implications: No specific pharmacological implication unless the affected patient presents with constrictive pericarditis, in which case any cardiopressive anesthetic agents must be avoided.

REFERENCES:

Balg S, Stengel-Rutkowski S, Dohlemann C, et al: Mulibrey nanism. *Clin Dysmorphol* 4:63, 1995.

Lapunzina P: Mulibrey nanism: Three additional patients and a review of 39 patients. *Am J Med Genet* 55:349, 1995.

Linpsayen-Nyman M, Perheentvpa J, Rapola J, et al: Mulibrey heart disease. Clinical manifestations, long term course and results of pericardiectomy in a series of 49 patients born before 1985. *Circulation* 107:2810, 2003.

Muller Barth Menger Syndrome

At a glance: Genetic disease characterized by multiple cerebral malformation, seizures, hypertrichosis, distinct face, clawhands, and overlapping fingers.

History: First described in 1993 in a brother and sister, the offspring of first-cousin Kurdish parents.

Incidence: Only two infants have been described. The karyotype was normal in both sibs. The brother died in a tonic extension spasm at age 4 months.

Genetic inheritance: Autosomal recessive inheritance (very frequently).

Pathophysiology: Multiple malformation syndrome of cerebral malformation, seizures, hypertrichosis, distinct face, clawhands, and overlapping fingers.

Clinical aspects: The clinical features described are hydrocephaly, macrocephaly, cerebellar agenesis/hypoplasia, hyperreflexia, corpus callosum/pellucidum agenesis, hypotonia/spasticity/rigidity, camptodactyly, simian crease, coarse/thick hair, overlapping fingers, seizures (any type), pharyngeal abnormality, abnormally placed nipples, and undescended/ectopic testes. Dolichocephaly/scaphocephaly, sutural synostosis (multiple), laryngeal abnormality, synophrys, posterior angulation of and low-set ears with or without anomaly (shape/structure), long philtrum, megaesophagus, microphthalmos, broad nasal root, long/thick lashes, abnor-

mal cry/voice, increased body hair, depressed nasal bridge, deep-set eyes/enophthalmos, and ulnar deviation of fingers can also be associated.

Precautions before anesthesia: Ascertain adequacy of seizure medication and recent control of convulsions. Special reference should be made to finding any signs of pharyngeal or laryngeal abnormality: stridor (inspiratory/expiratory), wheeze, breathlessness, or strange sounding cry/altered voice. An anesthetic consultation should be obtained.

Anesthetic considerations: The position of the head during induction of anesthesia may be difficult to stabilize and may complicate attempts to ventilate and/or intubate the trachea. Pharyngeal or laryngeal abnormalities where present may make tracheal intubation or ventilation impossible. Raised intracranial pressure is a potential hazard, and the presence of a ventriculoperitoneal shunt requires antibiotic prophylaxis. Regional anesthesia should be used where possible.

Pharmacological implications: Chronic phenytoin administration increases nondepolarizing muscle relaxant and fentanyl requirements, produces gingival hyperplasia and bleeding, and may cause hepatic dysfunction. Ketamine, enflurane, and methohexital are relatively contraindicated. Use of high concentrations of sevoflurane during induction should be avoided because of the risk of triggering seizure activity.

REFERENCE:

Muller FM, Barth GM, Menger H, et al: Cerebral malformation, seizures, hypertrichosis, distinct face, claw hands and overlapping fingers in sibs of both sexes. *Am J Med Genet* 47:698, 1993.

Multicore Myopathy

At a glance: Congenital muscular disease. Muscle weakness is generally mild and nonprogressive. Cardiac involvement has been described; the cardiomyopathy can be congestive, hypertrophic, or restrictive. Muscle hypotonia begins in infancy ("floppy baby") and is usually affecting mainly the proximal musculature leading to decreased muscle bulk. Ptosis and oculomotor palsy are sometimes observed.

Synonym: Minicore Myopathy.

Incidence: Rare; 80 cases have been described.

Genetic inheritance: Most cases seem sporadic, but an autosomal recessive inheritance pattern is sometimes found.

Pathophysiology: Accumulation of desmin in both skeletal muscle and myocardium.

Diagnosis: Muscular biopsy shows increased variation in fiber size and a predominance of type 1 fibers. Multiple circumscribed small lesions (cores) are seen within each involved fiber. Both type 1 and type 2 fibers are affected. Histologically, the core of the muscles are areas characterized by loss and/or disorganization of the myofibrillar structure and by absence or severe reduction of mitochondria.

Clinical aspects: Muscular weakness is generally mild and nonprogressive, but cardiac involvement has been described in some patients. The cardiomyopathy can be congestive, hypertrophic, or restrictive, sometimes requiring cardiac transplantation. Muscle weakness that begins in infancy ("floppy baby") is usually proximal, with hypotonia and decreased muscle bulk. Ptosis and oculomotor palsy are sometimes observed. Motor development is delayed, but intelligence is normal. Diaphragmatic involvement can lead to hypoventilation during sleep.

Precautions before anesthesia: As in any child presenting with a muscular disorder, thorough cardiac evaluation (ECG, echocardiography) is mandatory; respiratory involvement should be assessed both in the awake and the sleeping state (polysomnography). For elective surgical procedure, it is recommended to obtain an anesthesiology consultation.

Anesthetic considerations: By analogy with central core disease, malignant hyperthermia-triggering agents should be avoided in these patients. One case of unexplained fever and death has been described in a 30-month-old boy with this disease a few hours after cardiac catheterization with meperidine, hydroxyzine, and intravenous ketamine.

Pharmacological implications: Careful titration of nondepolarizing muscle relaxants if needed; succinylcholine should be avoided for fear of rhabdomyolysis and hyperkalemia or even malignant hyperthermia crisis.

REFERENCES:

Gordon CP, Litz S: Multicore myopathy in a patient with anhidrotic ectodermal dysplasia. *Can J Anesth* 39:966, 1992.

Koch BM, Bertolini TE, Eng GD, et al: Severe multicore disease associated with reaction to anesthesia. *Arch Neurol* 42:1204, 1985.

Willemsen MAAP, van Oort AM, ter Laak HJ, et al: Multicore myopathy with restrictive cardiomyopathy. *Acta Paediatr* 86:1271, 1997.

Multiple Carboxylase Deficiency

At a glance: Inborn error of metabolism present in the neonatal period and characterized by tachypnea or Kussmaul breathing, hypotonia, and seizures. Severe metabolic acidosis with ketosis and hyperammonemia. If present during infancy and childhood, lethargy, hypotonia, seizures ataxia; apnea/hyperventilation, and frequent stridor are characteristic. Usually corrected with oral biotin.

Synonyms: Biotinidase Deficiency; Holocarboxylase Synthetase Deficiency.

History: First described in 1971 by Wolf et al. It was immediately observed that biotin administration was curative.

Incidence: 1:112,000–129,000 live births (biotinidase deficiency).

Genetic inheritance: Autosomal recessive; more than 40 different mutations have been described. Gene locus on chromosome 3p25 (biotinidase) or 21q22.1 (holocarboxylase).

Pathophysiology: Biotinidase is essential for generation of free biotin from endogenous recycling or protein-bound biotin found in diet. Holocarboxylase synthetase is required to catalyze binding of biotin to carboxylases. Biotin is required as a cofactor for carboxylases within the body, which are involved in the metabolic pathways for a number of amino acids, gluconeogenesis, and fatty acid synthesis. Defects in either enzyme lead to organic acidosis.

Diagnosis: Clinical features, particularly skin rash and alopecia, but variability of symptoms according to importance of deficiency and amount of free biotin intake. Organic aciduria. Deficiency of specific enzyme measured in plasma. Included in neonatal screening programs in many countries.

Clinical aspects: *Deficiency of holocarboxylase synthetase* presents in more than 50% of cases in the neonatal period with tachypnea or Kussmaul breathing, hypotonia, and seizures. Severe

metabolic acidosis with ketosis and hyperammonemia. Untreated patients and those with less severe defects present with mental retardation, hair loss, and skin lesions (erythematous rash often with superinfection with *Candida*). *Deficiency of biotinidase* presents later in infancy or childhood. Lethargy, hypotonia, seizures, ataxia; respiratory problems (apnea/hyperventilation, frequent stridor). Skin manifestations such as periorificial eczematoid dermatitis and alopecia are less common. Intermittent organic aciduria. Immune deficiency leads to recurrent infections. If untreated, psychomotor delay and permanent neurologic deficit (hearing loss, optic atrophy).

Treatment: In both conditions there is a dramatic response to biotin, with resolution of clinical and biochemical abnormalities but not fixed neurologic sequelae. The dose of biotin varies from 2.5 to 5 mg/week (partial deficiency in biotinidase) to 2.5 to 10 mg/day (profound deficiency in biotinidase) or even more; 10 to 20 mg/day in case of holocarboxylase deficiency.

Precautions before anesthesia: Patient should be receiving his or her usual biotin supplements until the morning of surgery. However, if the patient has not received biotin supplementation, a complete evaluation of the cardiovascular, respiratory, and muscle functions should be done. Seizure medications should be continued until the morning of surgery.

Anesthetic considerations: Anesthesia management in this condition has not been described. Patients who are receiving adequate supplementation with biotin may be free of clinical and biochemical abnormalities. Intravenous administration of biotin may be necessary in the perioperative period. Perioperative monitoring of glycemia, lactates, and ammonium (NH_4). If the patient has not received his or her medication, then cardiovascular, respiratory, and muscular considerations dictate the anesthetic preparation.

Pharmacological implications: No agents are specifically contraindicated if the patient has been treated. If not treated, seizure medications should be used pre- or intraoperatively. Avoid cardiovascular depressant medications. Judicious use of muscle relaxant should be considered. Use of succinylcholine might be inappropriate in the presence of severe muscle weakness and atrophy. Use of narcotic for postoperative analgesia should be carefully administered in the presence of severe respiratory depression and limitations.

Other condition to be considered:

ACQUIRED BIOTIN DEFICIENCY: Very rare condition caused by malabsorption as a consequence of short-bowel syndrome, long-term total parenteral therapy, hemodialysis with biotin supplementation, or excessive intake of raw egg white.

REFERENCE:

Baumgartner ER, Suormala T: Biotin-responsive multiple carboxylase deficiency, in Fernandes J, Saudubray J-M, Van den Bergh G (eds): *Inborn Metabolic Diseases*. 3rd ed. Berlin, Springer, 2000, p 277.

Multiple Endocrine Neoplasia (MEN)

At a glance: Multiple endocrine neoplasia consists of benign, and sometimes malignant, tumors (often multiple in a tissue) of the parathyroids, enteropancreatic neuroendocrine system, anterior pituitary, and other tissues. Skin angiofibromas and skin collagenomas are common. Typically, tumors begin two decades earlier than sporadic tumors.

Synonyms and classification: Multiple Endocrine Adeno-matoses.

MEN Type I (☞Wermer Syndrome): Autosomal dominant disorder characterized by a high frequency of peptic ulcer disease and primary endocrine abnormalities involving the pituitary, parathyroid, and pancreas.

MEN Type II A (Sipple Syndrome): Autosomal dominant syndrome including medullary thyroid carcinoma, pheochromocytoma, and parathyroid adenomas.

MEN Type IIB (Wagenmann-Froboese Syndrome; Mucosal Neuroma Syndrome): Characterized by multiple true nervous neuromas, pheochromocytoma, and thyroid carcinoma without parathyroid adenomas. The thyroid cancer is a medullary type, as in MEN IIA. Although the association of pheochromocytoma with neurofibromatosis is well known, the nervous tumor reported in the MEN IIB is a true neuroma, consisting only of nerve cells.

History: MEN type 1 was the first condition described. In 1954, Wermer was instrumental in the presentation of this medical associative condition as a distinct clinical entity.

Incidence: *MEN type I* prevalence is estimated at 0.02–0.2:1000 persons; no racial predilection; both sexes are affected equally. *MEN type II* has an overall frequency of 1:30,000–50,000 persons in the United States. In both types, data in children are not available.

Genetic inheritance: In 1988, pedigree testing first linked the MEN I gene to chromosome 11q13. *MEN I* is an autosomal dominant inherited disease characterized by variable penetrance for tumors of the parathyroids, enteropancreatic neuroendocrine system, and anterior pituitary and less commonly by tumors in other tissues. The "multiple" designation refers both to the occurrence of multiple tumors in the involved endocrine organ (e.g., multiple pancreatic islet tumors) and to the occurrence of tumors in multiple endocrine organs (e.g., parathyroid tumor plus pancreatic islet tumor).

Type I disease must be distinguished from type II disease, another autosomal dominant inherited tumor syndrome. *MEN II* is characterized by bilateral medullary carcinoma of the thyroid, pheochromocytomas (often bilateral), and, in the most common variant, parathyroid tumors. All MEN II subtypes are inherited in an autosomal dominant manner. The probability of a new gene mutation is 5% or less in index cases with MEN IIA and 50% in index cases with MEN IIB. Offspring of affected individuals have a 50% chance of inheriting the mutant gene. Prenatal testing is possible. DNA testing of the RET gene (chromosomal locus 10q11) identifies disease-causing mutations in 95% of individuals with MEN IIA and MEN IIB and in approximately 85% of families with familial medullary thyroid carcinoma.

Pathophysiology: It has been suggested that MEN I, like many hereditary cancer syndromes, is caused by a mutation in a tumor suppressor gene that contributes to neoplasia when both gene copies in a tumor precursor cell have been sequentially inactivated ("two-hit" oncogenesis mechanism). Germline MEN I mutations were found in most families with MEN I and in most cases of sporadic MEN I. In addition, the MEN I gene was the gene most likely to show acquired mutation in several sporadic or nonhereditary tumors—parathyroid adenomas, gastrinomas, insulinomas, and bronchial carcinoids. Two categories of genes contribute to tumorigenesis. First, oncogenes, such as RAS, MYC, and RET, normally act to stimulate cell proliferation but when inappropriately activated or overexpressed permit a cell growth advantage. Second, tumor suppressor genes, such as p53 (mutation of which causes the Li-Fraumeni syndrome) and FAP (mutation of which causes familial adenomatous polyposis of the

colon), normally act as "brakes" on cell proliferation and, when inactivated, permit a cell growth advantage. MEN II is classified into three subtypes: MEN IIA, FMTC (familial medullary thyroid carcinoma), and MEN IIB. All three subtypes have a high risk for development of medullary carcinoma of the thyroid (MTC); MEN IIA and MEN IIB have an increased risk for pheochromocytoma; MEN IIA has an increased risk for parathyroid adenoma or hyperplasia. Additional features in MEN IIB include mucosal neuromas of the lips and tongue, distinctive facies with enlarged lips, ganglioneuromatosis of the gastrointestinal tract, and an asthenic marfanoid body habitus. The onset of MTC is in early childhood in MEN IIB, early adulthood in MEN IIA, and middle age in FMTC.

Diagnosis: Clinical diagnosis of *MEN I* is based on finding tumors in two or more of the three principal organs typically affected in the syndrome. A family history of MEN I-related tumor strengthens the diagnosis. Parathyroid tumors are multiple and often asymmetrical, this population is further enriched for hyperparathyroidism, the most highly penetrant and usually the first expression of MEN I. Enteropancreatic neuroendocrine tumors were identified in 66% of the patients. Gastrinomas of the duodenum and pancreas (with the Zollinger-Ellison syndrome) occurred in 47%. Insulinoma, occurring in 12% of patients, was generally a solitary, benign lesion. Rarely, a clinical syndrome associated with glucagonoma, VIPoma (vasoactive intestinal peptide), or somatostatinoma was seen. Nonfunctioning islet tumors detected by routine radiographic screening (CT and MRI scans) are probably underreported in MEN I because of the variable use and limited sensitivity of these techniques. Pituitary tumors were seen in 47% of patients, and prolactinomas accounted for more than half of those tumors. The reported prevalence of pituitary tumors in MEN I is 16 to 65%. Nonfunctioning pituitary adenomas, ACTH-secreting adenomas, and acromegaly are rarer.

MEN IIA is diagnosed clinically by the occurrence of two or more specific endocrine tumors, in a single individual or in close relatives. The endocrine disorders observed in MEN II are medullary thyroid carcinoma and/or its precursor C-cell hyperplasia, pheochromocytoma, and parathyroid adenomas or hyperplasia. Bilateral or multifocal areas of MTC and C-cell hyperplasia are usually observed at the time of thyroidectomy in patients undergoing prophylactic thyroidectomy. Metastatic spread to regional lymph nodes, i.e., parathyroid, paratracheal, jugular chain, and upper mediastinum or to distant sites, such as the liver, is common and often has occurred in patients with a palpable thyroid mass or diarrhea. Although pheochromocytomas rarely metastasize, they can be lethal because of intractable hypertension or anesthesia-induced hypertensive crises. Parathyroid abnormalities can range from benign parathyroid adenomas to clinically evident hyperparathyroidism with hypercalcemia and renal stones.

Classifying a patient or family by MEN II subtype is useful for determining prognosis and management. *MEN IIB* is diagnosed clinically by the presence of mucosal neuromas of the lips and tongue, as well as medullated corneal nerve fibers, distinctive facies with enlarged lips, an asthenic marfanoid body habitus, and MTC. DNA-based testing of the RET gene (chromosomal locus 10q11) identifies disease-causing mutations in 95% of individuals with MEN IIA and MEN IIB and in approximately 85% of families with FMTC. Such testing is available clinically and is used primarily for presymptomatic identification of at-risk individuals in order to reduce morbidity and mortality through early surgery.

Clinical aspects: Clinical manifestations of *MEN I* include functional effects of hormone hypersecretion, such as hypercalcemia or hypoglycemia, mass effects secondary to tumor growth (particularly in the pituitary), and malignant neoplasm (particularly with malignant gastrinoma).

The *MEN IIA subtype (Sipple syndrome)* makes up approximately 60 to 90% of MEN II cases. The MEN IIA subtype was initially called Sipple syndrome. Since genetic testing for RET mutations has become available, it has become apparent that 95% of individuals with MEN IIA develop MTC, approximately 50% develop pheochromocytoma, and approximately 20 to 30% develop hyperparathyroidism. MTC is generally the first manifestation of MEN IIA. In asymptomatic young individuals, provocative testing may reveal elevated plasma calcitonin levels and the presence of C-cell hyperplasia or MTC. In families with MEN IIA, the biochemical manifestations of MTC generally appear between the ages of 5 and 25 years (mean age is 15 years). MTC typically presents as a neck mass or neck pain between ages 15 and 20 years. However, more than 50% of such patients already have cervical lymph node metastases. Diarrhea, the most frequent systemic symptom, occurs in patients with a plasma calcitonin level greater than 10 ng/ml and implies a poor prognosis. Up to 30% of patients with MTC present with diarrhea and advanced disease. Pheochromocytomas usually present after MTC and typically present with intractable hypertension. They are often bilateral. Sudden death from anesthesia-induced hypertensive crisis has been described in patients with MEN IIA and unsuspected pheochromocytoma. Malignant transformation occurs in approximately 4% of cases. A small number of families with MEN IIA have pruritic cutaneous lichen amyloidosis, also known as cutaneous lichen amyloidosis. This is a lichenoid skin lesion located over the upper portion of the back that may appear before the onset of MTC. In one study, 7 of 44 families (16%) had cosegregation of MEN IIA and HSCR1. The probability that individuals in a family with MEN IIA and an exon 10 Cys mutation would manifest HSCR1 was estimated to be 6% in one series.

The *FMTC subtype* makes up approximately 5 to 35% of MEN II cases. In this subtype of MEN II, MTC is the only clinical manifestation.

The *MEN II B subtype* makes up approximately 5% of MEN II cases. The MEN IIB subtype initially was called *mucosal neuroma syndrome* or *Wagenmann-Froboese syndrome*. MEN IIB is characterized by the early development of an aggressive form of MTC in all patients. Patients with MEN IIB who do not undergo thyroidectomy at an early age (approximately 1 year) are likely to develop metastatic MTC at an early age. Prior to intervention with early prophylactic thyroidectomy, the average age at death in patients with MEN IIB was 21 years. Pheochromocytomas occur in 50% of MEN IIB cases; about half are multiple and often bilateral. Patients with undiagnosed pheochromocytoma may die of a cardiovascular crisis perioperatively. Parathyroid disease is very uncommon. Patients with MEN IIB may be identified in infancy or early childhood by the early presence of mucosal neuromas on the anterior dorsal surface of the tongue, the palate, or pharynx, and a distinctive facial appearance. The lips become prominent (or "blubbery") over time, and submucosal nodules may be present on the vermilion border of the lips. Neuromas of the eyelids may cause thickening and eversion of the upper eyelid margins. Prominent thickened corneal nerves may be seen by slitlamp examination. Approximately 40% of patients have diffuse ganglioneuromatosis of the gastrointestinal tract. Associated symptoms include abdominal distension, megacolon, constipation, and diarrhea. Approximately 75% of patients have a marfanoid habitus, often with kyphoscoliosis or lordosis, joint laxity, and decreased subcutaneous fat. Proximal muscle wasting and weakness can be seen. On rare occasion, individuals with MEN IIB and the M918T mutation have been found to have HSCR1.

Other Subtypes: The International RET Mutation Consortium classified MEN II into six separate phenotypes for the purpose of correlating specific mutations with clinical expression. They specified three forms of MEN IIA—MEN IIA(1), MEN IIA(2), MEN IIA(3)—and single forms of MEN IIB, FMTC, and Other, which included families that did not conform to the other phenotypes. The clinical usefulness of these additional subtypes for MEN IIA has not been demonstrated. Treatment is according to subtype.

Precautions before anesthesia: It is highly recommended to seek an anesthesiology consultation for all elective surgical and/or invasive procedures requiring anesthesia. Complete medical history and physical examination with chart review and patient and parental questioning. All symptoms and investigations, as well as ongoing follow-up and suspected disease, must be ascertained. First, it is essential to categorize which type of MEN the patient has, because there are very different implications to each disease. However, there can be an overlap of these clinically distinct diseases in that sometimes MEN I can manifest pheochromocytoma and other MEN II stigmata. Clinical manifestations of MEN I include functional effects of hormone hypersecretion, such as hypercalcemia or hypoglycemia, mass effects secondary to tumor growth (particularly in the pituitary), and malignant neoplasm (particularly with malignant gastrinoma). Therefore, careful control of blood sugar level perioperatively is essential. Carcinoid tumors of the bronchial tree are common and may have wide-ranging hemodynamic effects.

In MEN II, pheochromocytoma is the most frequent killer under anesthesia. This condition must be sought and appropriately treated before surgery is contemplated. Symptoms in children include headache, nausea, and vomiting, with sustained or, less commonly, episodic hypertension. Abdominal pain may occur. If undiagnosed it might prompt potentially fatal exploratory operation in an unprepared patient. The diagnosis is confirmed by finding increased catecholamines in the urine (or their metabolites). Sustained hypertension with vasoconstriction contracts the intravascular volume and elevates the hematocrit. Careful preoperative preparation with alpha blockers and, if necessary, beta blockers is mandatory.

Check thyroid function, particularly if early thyroidectomy was performed. Levels of electrolytes and blood sugar should be checked, particularly if diarrhea is present. Calcium levels should be checked.

Anesthetic considerations: MEN I requires tight blood sugar control. Beware of hypercalcemia. Thyroid function; adrenal function; raised intracranial pressure; airway compromise secondary to bronchial carcinoid. Kyphoscoliosis may complicate attempts at tracheal intubation and mechanical ventilation. Pheochromocytoma is the biggest risk, but the other elements possibly manifested by the syndrome should not be forgotten. The main problems are related to difficult blood pressure management, with volume status difficult to ascertain. Major blood loss may occur with extensive surgery to locate and remove multiple tumors.

Pharmacological implications: In MEN I care must be taken with drugs excreted by the kidneys. In pheochromocytoma, avoid drugs that might increase the release of catecholamines (e.g., pancuronium, ketamine) or that might sensitize the heart to these substances (e.g., halothane, desflurane). Pancuronium or droperidol may cause a hypertensive crisis. Drugs that release histamine should be avoided (e.g., D-tubocurarine, atracurium).

Other conditions to be considered:

☞**HIRSCHSPRUNG DISEASE:** Disorder of the enteric plexus of the bowel that typically results in its enlargement and constipation or obstipation in neonates; observed in a small number of individuals with MEN IIA. Approximately 20 to 40% of all Hirschsprung disease cases are caused by germline mutations in the RET protooncogene and are designated HSCR1. Some of these RET mutations are located in codons that lead to development of MEN IIA (i.e., codon 609 in exon 10 and codon 620 in exon 11). Other mutations lie in codons that lead to development of MTC (i.e., 618 and 620).

SPORADIC MEDULLARY THYROID CARCINOMA: MTC accounts for 5 to 10% of new cases of thyroid cancer diagnosed annually in the United States. The total number of new cases of MTC diagnosed annually, therefore, is between 1000 and 1200. Approximately 75 to 80% of MTC cases are sporadic. The peak incidence of the sporadic form is in the fifth and sixth decades of life. The major issue is distinguishing patients who have MEN II from patients with isolated (nonsyndromic, nonfamilial) MTC. This is particularly relevant for patients who present with multifocal MTC with a negative family history. DNA analysis of MTC tissue has revealed an approximately 30 to 67% incidence of somatic mutations of codon 918 in the absence of a germline mutation. Tumors with a somatic codon 918 mutation appear to be more aggressive. In contrast, between 1% and 24% of individuals with sporadic medullary thyroid carcinoma have disease-causing germline mutations in the RET gene. Thus, some experts recommend germline RET gene testing for all cases of MTC.

C-CELL HYPERPLASIA: C-cell hyperplasia associated with a positive calcitonin stimulation test occurs in approximately 5% of the general population. Thus, plasma calcitonin responses to stimulation do not always distinguish C-cell hyperplasia from small MTC.

☞**PHEOCHROMOCYTOMA:** Finding an individual with pheochromocytoma and no family history of endocrine tumors who has MEN IIA or a disease-causing mutation in the RET gene is unusual. Pheochromocytomas are occasionally observed in neurofibromatosis type 1 (NF1). Rarely, patients with MEN I have pituitary adenomas and pheochromocytomas, which has led to the hypothesis of an "overlap" syndrome with MEN II. A small number of families with MEN IIA have pruritic cutaneous lichen amyloidosis, also known as cutaneous lichen amyloidosis. This is a lichenoid skin lesion located over the upper portion of the back that might appear before the onset of MTC.

☞**VON HIPPEL-LINDAU SYNDROME (VHL):** Considered a diagnostic possibility for any patient presenting with a pheochromocytoma. This autosomal dominant cancer syndrome is caused by mutations in the VHL gene (chromosomal locus 3p25). It is characterized by pheochromocytoma, renal cell carcinoma, cerebellar and spinal hemangioblastoma, and retinal angioma. Some families with apparent autosomal dominant pheochromocytoma have VHL gene mutations in the absence of other clinical manifestations of VHL. In contrast, unilateral sporadic pheochromocytoma is very unlikely to be caused by VHL.

REFERENCES:

Learoyd DL, Twigg SM, Marsh DJ, et al: The practical management of multiple endocrine neoplasia. *Trends Endocrinol Metab* 6:273, 1995.

Luo A, Guo X, Ren H, et al: Clinical features and anesthetic management of multiple endocrine neoplasia associated with pheochromocytoma. *Clin Med J (Engl)* 116:208, 2003.

Niruthsiard S, Chatrkaw P, Laornual S, et al: Anesthesia for one-stage bilateral pheochromocytoma resection in a patient with MEN type IIA: Attenuation of hypertensive crisis by magnesium sulfate. *J Med Assoc Thai* 85:125, 2002.

Schimke RN: Multiple endocrine neoplasia: How many syndromes? *Am J Med Genet* 37:375, 1990.

Multiple Epiphyseal Dysplasia (MED)

At a glance: Very rare genetic disorder characterized by irregular epiphyseal growth, skeletal deformities, short-limb dwarfism, pain, and stiffness of affected joints. The main clinical features include a waddling gait, reduced height in adults with limbs relatively short in comparison to the trunk, and normal intelligence. Several types of MED have been described but two are important to mention. They are a *mild form* or *Ribbing type*, and a *severe form* or *Fairbank type*. In the mild form, the hands and wrists are usually normal, whereas in the severe form, the hands and feet are short and stubby.

Synonyms and classification: *MED Type I* (Fairbank Epiphyseal Dysplasia; Beighton Goldberg Hoff Syndrome; Ribbing Epiphyseal Dysplasia): Severe osteoarthritis of the hips and changes in the distal tibia develop in early adulthood. A deficiency in the lateral part of the distal tibial ossification center is seen in children. Short stature and brachydactyly are features.

MED Type II: Affected individuals typically presented at age 2.5 to 6 years age with pain in the knees. Knee and ankle pain was present throughout childhood. Bilateral osteotomies were required for gross varus deformities of the knees in some individuals. Hands were mildly short and joints prominent. There were no abnormalities of the spine or chest. Examination of radiographs revealed flattened, irregular epiphyses in most joints, particularly the knees. Childhood radiographs showed small epiphyses with a large physeal space. The vertebrae appeared normal in adulthood, but there were some anterior defects at earlier ages.

MED Type III (Multiple Epiphyseal Dysplasia with Myopathy): Typically present during childhood and adolescence, with waddling gait and stiffness and/or pain in the knees. Few patients experience involvement of other joints, such as the elbow, wrist, or ankle, short stature, and stubby hands. There are no spine abnormalities, and the radiographs show flattened, irregular epiphyses, varus or valgus deformity of the knees, and precocious osteoarthritis of the hips requiring early hip replacement.

MED Type IV (Ribbing type; Autosomal Recessive Multiple Epiphyseal Dysplasia; Multiple Epiphyseal Dysplasia with Clubfoot; Multiple Epiphyseal Dysplasia with Bilayered Patellae): Characterized by bilateral clubfoot and bilateral double-layered patellae.

MED Type V (Multiple Epiphyseal Dysplasia MATN3-related): Characterized by normal birth length and adult height around the third percentile 150 to 165 cm; however, patients complained of knee and hip pain after exercise during early childhood. Radiographs at or after the age of puberty showed a normal spine but persisting epiphyseal dysplasia of the hips and knees.

Incidence: The estimated incidence for MED is believed to be about 10-15:1,000,000 population.

Genetic inheritance: Autosomal dominant with variable expression. Chromosomes 1p32 coding for gene COL9A2 and 19p13.1 coding for gene COMP seem to be linked to this disorder.

Mutations are also indicated and account for 35% of affected individuals. A mutation of the COMP gene on chromosome 19. Fifteen percent have mutations in other undetermined genes. However, in 50%, a mutation cannot be identified.

Pathophysiology: Unknown; possible anomaly of the α_2 chain of type IX collagen.

Diagnosis: Based on the presence of the main features characterizing the disease and on radiologic findings.

Clinical aspects: Short stature, mainly as a consequence of a short lower segment, waddling gait, brachydactyly; patients can have involvement of the hands and feet manifesting as striking shortness. Bone age can be delayed in many cases. Osteoarthritis occurs early in many large joints as a consequence of loss of articular cartilage. This can produce progressive pain and stiffness in joints, particularly the hips, in patients as young as 5 years. Radiologic studies can show platyspondyly, irregularities of the femoral head and neck, loss of definition of the acetabulum, and epiphyseal and metaphyseal irregularities of the tubular bones of the hands and feet. Double-layered patellae often dislocate laterally. In some cases, there may be a more evident shortness of the fourth metatarsal bone.

Precautions before anesthesia: In patient receiving nonsteroidal analgesics for chronic pain from degenerative joint disease, a coagulation profile should be obtained. Ensure that chronic corticosteroid therapy is not used. If it was the case steroid supplementation will be needed preoperatively.

Anesthetic considerations: There are few anesthetic considerations relevant to this disease. Tracheal intubation should not be problematic because the dwarfism is mainly a result of a short lower segment. Careful positioning is necessary for patients with joint pain and stiffness.

Pharmacological implications: No known pharmacological implications. However, if patient has been treated with chronic administration of corticosteroids, intraoperative administration is indicated.

Other conditions to be considered:

☞**LEGG-CALVE-PERTHES DISEASE** is a group of disorders known as the osteochondroses. It is believed to be due to unexplained interruption of the blood supply to the capital femoral epiphysis resulting in avascular necrosis. Clinically, this disease is characterized by limp with or without pain in the hip, knee, thigh, and groin.

☞**PSEUDOACHONDROPLASTIC DYSPLASIA** is a rare inherited disorder characterized by skeletal malformations resulting in short-limbed dwarfism. Affected individuals present brachydactyly, genu varum, and genu valgum. In addition, affected individuals may have lumbar lordosis and kyphosis. Cases of pseudoachondroplastic dysplasia are due to mutations of the COMP gene, meaning that this disorder is allelic to some cases of multiple epiphyseal dysplasia.

REFERENCES:

Ballo R, Briggs MD, Cohn DH, et al: Multiple epiphyseal dysplasia, Ribbing type: A novel mutation in the COMP gene in a South African family. *Am J Med Genet* 68;396, 1997.

Jones KL: Multiple epiphyseal dysplasia, in Jones KL (ed): *Smith's Recognizable Patterns of Human Malformation.* Philadelphia, WB Saunders, 1997, p 380.

Stanescu R, Stanescu V, Muriel M-P, et al: Multiple epiphyseal dysplasia, Fairbank type: Morphologic and biochemical study of cartilage. *Am J Med Genet* 45:501, 1993.

Multiple Synostoses Syndrome

At a glance: Synostosis of many small joints.

Synonyms: Polysynostoses Syndrome; Synostosis Multiplex.

Genetic inheritance: Familial; autosomal dominant inheritance. Chromosome 17q 21-22 has been linked to the disease.

Pathophysiology: Symphalangism, synostoses of the tarsal and carpal bones, and other abnormalities, including orofacial defects and delayed mental development, occurring alone or as a component of other syndromes.

Diagnosis: Numerous skeletal deformities should evoke the diagnosis.

Clinical aspects: Hand abnormalities include synostoses of the carpal bones, radial head subluxation, hypoplasia of the middle phalanges, and metacarpophalangeal synostoses; short and broad first metacarpal bones, disturbances in bone modeling of the metacarpal bones and phalanges, and agenesis of the middle phalanges. Foot abnormalities include synostoses of the tarsal bones, synostoses of the tarsal and metatarsal bones, agenesis of the middle and distal phalanges, and disturbance in bone modeling of the phalanges. Hypoplasia of the alae nasi. Short upper lip. Cubitus valgus, limited extension of the forearm, and limited hip motion. Variable fusion of middle ear ossicles. Moderate mental retardation.

Precautions before anesthesia: Complete neurologic and motor examination encompassing milestones, parental information, and chart information. Determine if another syndrome is associated and its implications. If the patient receives chronic corticosteroid treatment, preoperative supplementation is indicated.

Anesthetic considerations: Difficult vascular access; potentially uncooperative patient. In presence of orofacial anomalies, the possibility of difficult direct laryngoscopy and tracheal intubation must be suspected. Nasal intubation probably problematic.

Pharmacological implications: No known implications for this disease.

Other conditions to be considered:

☞**LEGG-CALVÉ-PERTHES DISEASE:** Group of disorders known as the osteochondroses. Believed to be caused by unexplained interruption of the blood supply to the capital femoral epiphysis resulting in avascular necrosis. Clinically, this disease is characterized by limp with or without pain in the hip, knee, thigh, and groin.

☞**PSEUDOACHONDROPLASTIC DYSPLASIA:** Rare inherited disorder characterized by skeletal malformations resulting in short-limbed dwarfism. Affected individuals present brachydactyly, genu varum, and genu valgum. In addition, affected individuals may have lumbar lordosis and kyphosis. Cases of pseudoachondroplastic dysplasia are the result of mutations of the COMP gene, indicating this disorder is allelic to some cases of multiple epiphyseal dysplasia.

REFERENCES:

da-Silva EO, Filho SM, de Albuquerque SC: Multiple synostosis syndrome: Study of a large Brazilian kindred. *Am J Med Genet* 18:237, 1984.

Jones KL: Multiple synostosis syndrome, in Jones KL (ed): *Smith's Recognizable Patterns of Human Malformation.* Philadelphia, WB Saunders, 1997, p 432.

Krakow D, Reinker K, Powell B, et al: Localization of a multiple synostoses syndrome disease gene to chromosome 17q 21-22. *Am J Hum Genet* 63:120, 1998.

Shiraishi M, Minami K: Anesthesia for a child with Antley-Bixler Syndrome. *Can J Anaesth* 48:828, 2001.

MURCS Association

At a glance: MURCS is an acronym for *mü*llerian duct aplasia, *r*enal aplasia, *c*ervicothoracic *s*omite dysplasia. Very rare disorder that affects only females. Characterized by absence of the uterus, cervix, and upper part of the vagina; kidney agenesia or ectopia; and malformations of the radial ray (phocomelia), ribs, and cervicothoracic spine. Urogenital abnormalities include müllerian duct agenesis. In some cases, neural tube defects, such as occipital encephalocele, can be present. Some affected females exhibit craniofacial malformations.

Synonyms: DK-Phocomelia Syndrome; von Voss-Cherstvoy Syndrome; Müllerian Duct-Renal-Cervicothoracic-Upper Limb Defect Syndrome; Müllerian Duct and Renal Agenesis with Upper Limb and Rib Anomalies; Müllerian-Renal-Cervicothoracic Somite Abnormalities.

History: The name DK-Phocomelia originates from the initials of the last names of the two first-described patients. E. Cherstvoy was the first to report this medical condition in 1980.

Incidence: It is estimated as 1:4000–5000 female newborns and 1:20,000 female visits at a gynecological hospital.

Genetic inheritance: Although most of the cases seem to occur sporadically, autosomal recessive transmission has been reported.

Pathophysiology: The malformations are compatible with a defect in the arrangement of the paraxial mesoderm giving rise to the occipital, cervical, and thoracic somites and the adjoining intermediate mesoderm. These structures contribute to the genesis of occipital bone, cervical spine, upper limbs, and urogenital system.

Clinical aspects: The major findings are the presence of kidney (unilateral or bilateral agenesis, horseshoe kidney) and genital anomalies (müllerian duct agenesis, absence of the cranial two thirds of the vagina, hypoplasia of the uterus). However, affected females usually have normal sexual development because of (most often) normal ovarian function. Other defects may include occipital encephalocele, cerebral cysts, cerebellar hypoplasia, seizures, congenital heart disease (absent papillary muscle of tricuspid leaflet, abnormal coronaries), abnormal lobation of the lungs, and diaphragmatic agenesis. Orthopedic features include phocomelia, radial ray, finger, and vertebral anomalies (approximately 80% have cervicothoracic anomalies, particularly from C5 to T1) and may include Sprengel deformity, cervical fusion vertebrae, single or multiple hemivertebra(e), and scoliosis. Short stature is common for these patients. Furthermore, hemifacial microsomia, small mandible, cleft palate, short, webbed neck, unilateral adrenal and ovarial agenesis, and thrombocytopenia have all been reported.

Precautions before anesthesia: Obtain baseline renal function tests. Thorough examination of the cardiac system including ECG and echocardiogram, if deemed necessary. Complete blood count (thrombocytopenia) and chest and cervical radiographs. Carefully assess the airway (micrognathia) and cervical range of motion.

Anesthetic considerations: Airway management may be difficult because of micrognathia (often mild) and vertebral anomalies with a short neck. Neuraxial anesthesia is not recommended because of thrombocytopenia, vertebral anomalies, and encephalocele/cerebral cysts. Anesthetic management is dictated by the cardiac disease. Anomalies of the arm may render vascular access and placement of blood pressure cuff and tourniquets difficult.

Pharmacological implications: In the presence of renal anomalies with decreased renal function, avoid drugs eliminated mainly by the kidney or adjust the dosage accordingly (e.g., neuromuscular relaxants and antibiotics). In the presence of a seizure disorder, potentially epileptogenic drugs, such as methohexital, ketamine, enflurane, sevoflurane, atracurium, *cis*-atracurium, and meperidine (applies to the latter three only if given in large quantities because of their metabolites laudanosine and normeperidine, respectively), should be avoided. Chronic antiseizure medication can lead to induction of hepatic enzymes, accelerating the metabolism of predominantly hepatic-eliminated drugs. If congenital heart disease is present, subacute bacterial endocarditis prophylaxis may be warranted. Any heart medications must be maintained peroperatively.

Other conditions to be considered:

☞**VACTERL ASSOCIATION:** Rare disorder occurring equally in males and females. Acronym for *v*ertebral dysgenesis, *a*nal atresia, *c*ardiac disease, *t*racheo*e*sophageal fistula, *r*enal anomalies, radial dysplasia, and other *l*imb defects.

WINTER SYNDROME: Extremely rare disorder that affects only females. Characterized by vaginal atresia, unilateral renal hypoplasia or agenesis, and/or ear malformations. In some cases, the fallopian tubes, ovaries, and uterus are normal; however, some affected females exhibit internal genital abnormalities in addition to vaginal atresia.

☞**KLIPPEL-FEIL SYNDROME:** Rare skeletal disorder that affects both males and females. Cervical vertebrae are either missing and/or fused. Other features include scoliosis or kyphoscoliosis, spina bifida occulta, and unilateral renal agenesis.

SPRENGEL DEFORMITY: Rare birth defect characterized by elevation and/or underdevelopment of the scapula, limited movement of the arm on the affected side, hypoplasia of shoulder muscles, scoliosis, fused vertebrae, hemivertebrae, and spina bifida occulta. Occurs sporadically. May be inherited as an autosomal dominant genetic trait.

☞**GOLDENHAR SYNDROME:** Common birth defect of vascular origin involving first and second branchial arch derivatives. Hemifacial microsomia associated with congenital heart defects such as VSD, PDA, tetralogy of Fallot, and aortic coarctation.

☞**MAYER-VON ROKITANSKY-KUSTER-HAUSER SYNDROME:** Characterized by the congenital absence of the vagina, in presence of a female with normal secondary sexual characteristics. The uterus is rudimentary in the form of bilateral and noncanaliculated muscular buds. However, normal tubes and ovaries are present. The endocrine functions are normal and the cytogenetic evaluation does not suggest any anomalies. Primary amenorrhea is often the first reason for evaluation. There is evidence of female-limited autosomal dominant inheritance.

ROKITANSKY SEQUENCE: Characterized by a clinical association with the facioauriculovertebral sequence, also called Goldenhar syndrome. Other features of the Rokitansky sequence include bilateral femoral hypoplasia (proximal femoral focal deficiency). Patients usually have normal kidneys.

REFERENCE:
Mahajan P, Kher A, Khungar A, et al: MURCS association—A review of 7 cases. *J Postgrad Med* 38:109, 1992.

Myasthenia Gravis

At a glance: Neuromuscular disorder characterized by muscle weakness and rapid muscle fatigue. Usually apparent during adulthood; onset may occur at any age. Most individuals present eyelid ptosis, diplopia, and excessive muscle fatigue following exercise. Other clinical features commonly include dysarthria, dysphagia, and proximal limb weakness. Approximately 10% may develop potentially life-threatening complications as a consequence of severe respiratory depression (myasthenic crisis).

Synonyms: Goldflam-Erb Disease; Erb Syndrome; Erb-Goldflam Disease; Erb-Oppenheim-Goldflam Syndrome; Hoppe-Goldflam Syndrome; Hoppe-Goldflam Syndrome Complex; Asthenic Bulbar Paralysis; Bulbospinal Paralysis; Myasthenia Gravis Pseudoparalytica.

Classification:

> Classic Generalized Myasthenia Gravis
> Ocular Myasthenia Gravis
> Transitory Neonatal Myasthenia Gravis
> Juvenile Myasthenia Gravis
> Congenital Myasthenia Gravis
> Familial Infantile Myasthenia Gravis
> Congenital Endplate Acetylcholinesterase Deficiency
> Slow Channel Syndrome
> Fast Channel Syndrome

History: The first written description of myasthenia gravis is granted to Thomas Willis (1621–1675), an English physician, who published a book in 1672 entitled: *De anima brutorum* in which he wrote about "a woman who temporarily lost her power of speech and became 'mute as a fish.'" This was subsequently interpreted as myasthenia gravis. Thomas Willis was born in Great Bedwin, a Wiltshire village in England. He graduated from Oxford University Legion with a Bachelor of Medicine in 1646. In 1660 he was appointed Sedleian Professor of Natural Philosophy at Oxford and given the diploma of MD. The earliest description of the disease was done by Samuel Wilks, an English physician, in 1877 which was reported in *Guy's Hospital Reports* 22:7. However, it seems that it was a case of "bulbar paralysis." Aleksei Kozhevnikov, a Russian physician, described a "progressive familial spastic diplegia" and wrote on the neuropathology of nuclear ophtalmoplegia, myasthenia, and bulbar paralysis. His textbook on nervous diseases was a popular manual because of its brevity and lucidity. He was born in Ryazan and entered the University of Moscow in 1853 and received his MD in 1860. He later studied abroad in Germany, England, Switzerland, and France. Wilhem Heinrich Erb (1840–1921), a German neurologist, was responsible (in part) for the delineation of myasthenia gravis (called Erb-Goldflam-Oppenheim disease at the time). Finally, the use of physostigmine in the treatment of myasthenia gravis is granted to Mary Broadfoot Walker (1896–1974), a salaried Assistant Medical Officer in "Poor Law Service" at St. Alfege's Hospital, Greenwich, England, who introduced it in 1934.

Incidence: Prevalence in general population is 50 to 125:1 million.

Genetic inheritance: Sporadic for acquired cases.

Pathophysiology: In *acquired cases,* there is a decrease in the number of acetylcholine receptors (AChR) at the neuromuscular junction. This decrease is secondary to circulating antibodies against AChR, which increase the rate of degradation of AChR and decrease its rate of synthesis. These antibodies are present in 80 to 90% of the classic and juvenile forms of myasthenia; their production occurs in the thymus. The thymus is abnormal in 80 to 90% of those patients: thymic follicular hyperplasia (65–75%), thymoma (10%, only in adults), and thymic atrophy (10–20%). In *congenital myasthenic*

syndromes, the symptoms are caused by an impaired safety margin of neuromuscular transmission caused by presynaptic, synaptic, or postsynaptic congenital anomalies (see Table M-3).

Diagnosis: Clinical, EMG, presence of AChR antibodies (except for *Congenital Myasthenic Syndromes*), improvement of symptoms after intravenous injection of edrophonium (except in conditions such as *Congenital Endplate Acetylcholinesterase Deficiency* and *Slow Channel Syndrome*).

Clinical aspects: *Classic Generalized Myasthenia Gravis:* Ptosis and diplopia occur early in most patients. Muscle weakness remains localized to extraocular and eyelid muscles in 15% of cases. Bulbar muscle weakness is common and produces dysphagia, aspiration pneumonia, and slurred nasal speech. Laryngeal muscle weakness may cause abduction of the vocal cords and stridor; those symptoms vary considerably from hour to hour and are typically aggravated by exercise. Sometimes dramatic presentation with sudden onset of respiratory failure. Possible cardiac manifestations are atrial fibrillation and atrioventricular block. A staging classification based on the severity of the disease is used:

> Type I = Ocular signs and symptoms only
> Type IIA = Generalized mild weakness
> Type IIB = Generalized moderate weakness
> Type III = Acute fulminating presentation, respiratory
>   dysfunction, or both
> Type IV = Late severe, generalized myasthenia

The primary medical therapy is the administration of cholinesterase inhibitors such as pyridostigmine. Medical control is delicate because overdose produces symptoms of "cholinergic crisis"—abdominal cramping, diarrhea, hypersalivation—and increased muscle weakness. The starting dose of pyridostigmine is 1 mg/kg every 4 hours. Thymectomy is effective and recommended in adults. Immunosuppressive therapy with corticosteroids, azathioprine, and cyclosporine is used when myasthenia is not adequately controlled by anticholinesterase drugs. Short-term immunotherapies include plasmapheresis and administration of IV immunoglobulins.

Transitory Neonatal Myasthenia Gravis: Results from placental transfer of AChR antibodies from a myasthenic mother to her newborn. It occurs in 8 to 15% of such births. Onset is within 72 hours of birth with ptosis, poor cry, hypotonia, and difficult feeding. The condition usually resolves after a few weeks and responds to anticholinesterase treatment.

Juvenile Myasthenia Gravis: Onset is in children older than 1 year, predominantly in girls; clinical features are similar to the adult form, but muscles of the neck and proximal limb muscle are often the most involved (so-called spinal form of myasthenia). The disease is sometimes limited to the oculomotor musculature. It can be associated with other autoimmune diseases such as thyroiditis or diabetes mellitus. Fluctuating evolution with periods of remission and exacerbations can be caused by viral infection, surgery, and pregnancy.

Congenital Myasthenic Syndromes: Caused by structural or functional anomalies of the neuromuscular junction (see Table M-3).

Familial Infantile Myasthenia: Autosomal recessive condition (gene FIM on chromosome 17pter) associated with synaptic vesicles of reduced size. It presents in early infancy with ocular, bulbar, and respiratory features. Anticholinesterase treatment is lifesaving.

Congenital Endplate Acetylcholinesterase Deficiency: Very rare condition caused by total absence of acetylcholinesterases at the

Table M-3   Clinical Features of the Congenital Myasthenic Syndromes

Syndrome	Clinical Picture	Treatment
Presynaptic		
Familial infantile myasthenia	Onset: Infancy	Anticholinesterase!
Synaptic	Severe respiratory and bulbar difficulties	
Acetylcholinesterase deficiency	Onset: Neonate	Anticholinesterase not effective
Postsynaptic		
AChR deficiency	Onset: Neonate or infancy	Anticholinesterase helpful
Slow channel	Onset: Child or adult Slow progress	Quinidine helpful, anticholinesterase worsens!
Fast channel	Onset: Neonatal	Anticholinesterase helpful

neuromuscular junction; the endplate potential remains above threshold for a long time and can cause repeated muscle action potentials. It is refractory to anticholinesterase treatment.

Slow Channel Syndrome: Autosomal dominant condition. Three different genes have been identified: CHRNE coding for the AChR ε subunit on chromosome 17p13, CHRNA coding for the AChR α-subunit on chromosome 2q24-q32, and CHRNB1 coding for the AChR β-subunit on chromosome 17p11-p12. The AChR ion channel has a prolonged open time, leading to desensitization of the postsynaptic membrane; variable age of onset, severity, and muscle distribution. It usually has intermittent exacerbations and long periods of remission. It is refractory to anticholinesterase treatment.

Fast Channel Syndrome: Autosomal dominant condition; gene CHRNE coding for the AChR ε-subunit on chromosome 17p13; neonatal onset. The ion channel opens and closes too rapidly.

Congenital Endplate AChR Deficiency: Autosomal recessive condition; gene CHRNE coding for the AChR ε-subunit on chromosome 17p13. It is extremely rare. The number of AChR is reduced. Onset of symptoms is in the neonatal period. Anticholinesterase treatment is helpful.

Precautions before anesthesia: Check severity and extension of the disease: ocular symptoms, bulbar signs, respiratory problems. Anticholinergic treatment should be adapted in consultation with the neurologist in charge of the patient in order to give the last dose as close as possible to the induction time and to restart therapy as soon as possible after anesthesia. A complete history and physical examination to eliminate any associated anomalies are essential (especially with the classic type)

Anesthetic considerations: When possible, consider delaying procedure in case of recent evolutive crisis. High risk of aspiration because of pharyngeal dysfunction. Strict asepsis is needed considering frequent immunodeficiency associated with disease or its treatment. Postoperative respiratory physiotherapy and monitoring are necessary because of possibility of respiratory insufficiency. The need for postoperative mechanical ventilation must be anticipated. Locoregional anesthetic techniques are very useful. Perioperative electrolyte (Na, K, Mg) must be maintained in the normal range at all times.

Pharmacological implications: Patients are extremely sensitive to nondepolarizing muscle relaxants. If curarization is necessary,

it should be achieved with short-acting drugs such as atracurium, and the dose should be titrated to effect using monitoring of the neuromuscular junction (e.g., train of four). If rapid tracheal intubation is necessary, succinylcholine 0.5 to 1 mg/kg can be used safely. All intravenous and inhalational anesthetic agents have been used safely in these patients, but halogenated agents have been suspected of worsening signs and should be avoided. Antibiotics that decrease production of ACh (e.g., streptomycin, kanamycin, neomycin, and gentamicin) and drugs that affect membrane electric equilibrium (e.g., quinidine, quinine, and diphenylhydantoin) can precipitate a myasthenic crisis. The interactions with immunosuppressive therapy should be taken into account. Narcotics do not directly interfere with neuromuscular transmission in myasthenia, but they should be used with caution in patients who have respiratory insufficiency from myasthenia gravis because of their own action on respiratory function that can make potentiation of ventilatory insufficiency.

Other conditions to be considered:

EATON-LAMBERT SYNDROME (Lambert-Eaton Myasthenic Syndrome): Rare autoimmune disorder of adulthood characterized by muscle weakness and fatigue, particularly of the hip and thigh muscles. Affected individuals frequently present with malignancies, especially lung cancer.

☞**AMYOTROPHIC LATERAL SCLEROSIS:** Degenerative motor neuron disease evolving to progressive muscle weakness, resulting in paralysis.

☞**DERMATOMYOSITIS AND POLYMYOSITIS:** Both diseases belong to a group of connective tissue disorders known as idiopathic inflammatory myopathies. They are a multisystem disease characterized by necrotizing inflammatory myopathy of striated muscles and a skin rash, both of unknown etiology.

REFERENCES:

Bouaggad A, Bouderka MA, Abassi O: Total intravenous anaesthesia with propofol for myasthenic patients. *Eur J Anaesthesiol* 22:393, 2005.

Brown TCK, Gebert R, Meretoja OA, et al: Myasthenia gravis in children and its anaesthetic implications. *Anaesth Intensive Care* 18:466, 1990.

Dillon FX: Anesthesia issues in the perioperative management of myasthenia gravis. *Semin Neurol* 24:83, 2004.

Elder BF, Beal H, Dewald W, et al: Exacerbation of subclinical myasthenia by occupational exposure to an anesthetic. *Anesth Analg* 50:383, 1971.

Goldflam SV: Über einen scheinbar heilbaren bulbärparalytischen Symptomenkomplex mit Beteiligung der Extremitäten. *Dtsch Zeitschr Nervenheilk* 4:312, 1893.

White MC, Stoddart PA: Anesthesia for thymectomy in children with myasthenia gravis. *Paediatr Anaesth* 14:625, 2004.

Myoadenylate Deaminase Deficiency

At a glance: Inherited or secondarily acquired disorder of muscle purine nucleotide metabolism. The clinical manifestations include exercise-induced myopathy, postexertional muscle weakness or cramping, prolonged fatigue after exertion, and limping infant caused by benign congenital hypotonia. Generalized muscle pair is often manifested.

Synonyms: Muscle Adenosine Monophosphate Deaminase Deficiency; MADA Deficiency; AMP Deaminase.

Incidence: This defect is specific to skeletal muscle and may be one of the commonest genetic defects. The heterozygosity is believed to be 1 in 5. It is found in 2% of muscle biopsies of patient presenting with muscle weakness or poor exercise tolerance. It has equal sex distribution.

Genetic inheritance: The *primary deficiency* is transmitted as autosomal dominant. The AMPD1 gene encoding for muscle adenosine monophosphate deaminase (MADM) is located on chromosome 1. The mutant allele is frequent in white people. In *secondary cases*, the defect could be caused by a limitation in AMPD1 transcript availability. In those cases, the participation of the MADM deficit to the patient's phenotype is unclear.

Pathophysiology: MADM is one of the three enzymes of the purine cycle. In the muscle, this cycle removes adenosine monophosphate (AMP) formed during exercise to favor formation of ATP from adenosine diphosphate (ADP), releases ammonia (NH_3) and inosine monophosphate, stimulators of glycolysis and thus energy production, and produces fumarate, an intermediate of the citric acid cycle. This impaired muscular energy production during exercise seems to be the cause of the muscular dysfunction.

Diagnosis: Absence of elevation of plasma ammonia following exercise (as in normal subjects); activity of MADM is lower than 2% in inherited cases and between 2% and 15% in secondary cases. Onset is in childhood or adolescence in nearly 50% of cases.

Clinical aspects: In case of primary defect, postexercise symptoms are the main manifestations: early fatigue, cramps, or myalgias sometimes accompanied by myoglobinuria and increased creatine kinase following moderate to vigorous exercise. Administration of oral ribose could improve muscle strength and endurance.

Precautions before anesthesia: In primary defects, check muscle strength and creatine kinase level; exclude any associated cardiomyopathy by echocardiography. In secondary defects, follow the same precautions as for the associated disease (myopathy, collagen vascular disease, periodic paralysis).

Anesthetic considerations: Muscle energy depends on glucose availability—prevent hypoglycemia and prolonged use of a tourniquet leading to ischemia. As in many other muscular disorders, it is safer to avoid succinylcholine.

Pharmacological implications: Do not use succinylcholine to avoid rhabdomyolysis, hyperkalemia, and cardiac arrhythmias.

REFERENCE:

Van den Bergh G, Vincent M-F, Marie S: Disorders of purine and pyrimidine metabolism, in Fernandes J, Saudubray J-M, Van den Bergh G (eds): *Inborn Metabolic Diseases*. 3rd ed. Berlin, Springer, 2000, p 355.

Myocerebellar Disorder

At a glance: Patients show cerebellar ataxia accompanied by pancytopenia, hypoplastic anemia, acute myelomonocytic leukemia, or decreased bone marrow mitotic activity.

Synonym: Ataxia-Pancytopenia Syndrome.

Incidence: Unknown, only a few cases have been described in the literature.

Genetic inheritance: Autosomal dominant.

Pathophysiology: Progressive expansion of clone of cells with monosomy 7 has been shown, but sensitivity to bleomycin suggests this may also be a chromosomal instability disorder.

Diagnosis: Red cell, platelet, and leukocytes abnormalities. There may be lymphomas or leukemias. Radiologic investigation shows cerebellar atrophy on CT scan. Laboratory investigations show monosomy 7 mosaicism, and electromyographic studies show reduced nerve conduction velocities.

Clinical aspects: Patients may show pancytopenia, hypoplastic anemia, acute myelomonocytic leukemia, or decreased bone marrow mitotic activity. On examination, cerebellar ataxia, brisk deep tendon reflexes, bilateral Babinski reflexes, diminished vibratory sensation in the legs, and unsteady gait can be found. Purpura may be present, and some cases show telangiectasia or angiokeratomata of the skin. Nystagmus and dysmetria are often present (cerebellar signs). Patients usually die of hypoplastic anemia or leukemia.

Precautions before anesthesia: Complete workup, including neurologic and motor milestones, family history, and previous problems. Blood tests are necessary because of marrow involvement, blood count, and clotting profile. Because of potential for defective immunity, the patient may have recurrent pulmonary, sinus, or urinary tract infections. Severe anemia may be present from an early age.

Anesthetic considerations: Check hemoglobin, hematocrit, and pulmonary function as indicated. Treat anemia if severe. Ensure sterile technique for venipuncture (reverse isolation).

Pharmacological implications: Antibiotics may be required.

REFERENCES:

Daghistani D, Curless R, Toledano SR, et al: Ataxia-pancytopenia and monosomy 7 syndrome. *J Pediatr* 115:108, 1989.

Gonzalez-del Angel A, Cervera M, Gomez L, et al: Ataxia-pancytopenia syndrome. *Am J Med Genet* 90:252, 2000.

Myopathy, Distal, Welander Type

At a glance: Genetic disorder characterized by distal, late-onset myopathy. The presenting feature is in 89% of cases weakness and wasting of the small muscle of the hands. Myotonia and sensory changes are not present. Does not involve the heart.

Synonyms: Swedish Distal Myopathy type; Welander Muscular Atrophy.

Incidence: Welander distal myopathy is observed almost exclusively in Sweden, where it was first described; more than 250 cases have been described.

Genetic inheritance: Autosomal dominant inheritance. The gene causing Welander myopathy has not yet been identified but is restricted to a region of 2.4 cM on chromosome 2 (2p13).

Pathophysiology: Unknown, but the gene locus region overlaps with those of Miyoshi myopathy and limb-girdle muscular dystrophy IIB, both of which result from mutation in the dysferlin gene.

Diagnosis: Levels of creatine kinase are normal to slightly increased. The most prominent finding on light microscopy is that of rimmed vacuoles and tubulofilamentous inclusions evidenced by ultrastructural examination.

Clinical aspects: Distal myopathy with late onset (after age 40 years). The first symptom is clumsiness in performing fine motor skills with the index finger and thumb. The weakness subsequently progresses to all the finger extensor muscles, and atrophy of intrinsic hand muscles becomes manifest after several years' duration. The weakness later extends to the anterior muscles of the legs with inability to raise the forefoot appropriately. No proximal weakness and no cardiomyopathy. Progression is slow and does not affect life expectancy.

Precautions before anesthesia: No literature about this condition and anesthesia, but certain considerations must be made. Obtain complete workup, including neurologic and motor milestones, family history, and previous problems. Cardiac function should be assessed in light of cardiomyopathic potential of other distal myopathy. ECG, echocardiography, and/or cardiac catheterization may be appropriate. Other syndromic features should be sought.

Anesthetic considerations: Cardiomyopathic cases (Welander/Swedish type) in general have greater implications for anesthesia. Patients manifesting cardiomyopathy require cardiac monitoring depending on the degree of disease.

Pharmacological implications: Use extreme caution with thiopentone and muscle relaxants; avoid respiratory depressant drugs.

Other conditions to be considered:

DISTAL MYOPATHY TYPE I (MPD I): Late distal myopathy with small hand muscle weakness and wasting. Also associated with a very slow progressive cardiomyopathy. It is inherited as an autosomal dominant pattern.

MIYOSHI MYOPATHY (Late-Onset Distal Muscular Dystrophy): Characterized by onset between 16 and 20 years in 80% of cases, with muscular involvement of lower legs and forearms; small muscles of the feet and hands are relatively spared.

☞INCLUSION BODY MYOPATHY: Characterized by muscular dystrophy, especially of the anterior tibial muscles. Although the hamstring and tibialis anterior muscles are affected severely by early adulthood, the quadriceps muscles are spared even in a late stage of the disorder.

☞LIMB-GIRDLE MUSCULAR DYSTROPHIES: Genetically heterogeneous group of inherited progressive muscular disorders that affect mainly the proximal musculature (hip and shoulder). Several different types have been identified; at least eight have autosomal recessive inheritance and three others are transmitted as an autosomal dominant trait. In most individuals, associated symptoms and findings become apparent during childhood; however, the disease may also present itself during adolescence or adulthood. The muscle weakness may spread from the lower limbs to the upper limbs or vice versa. Although the disorder typically progresses slowly, some affected individuals experience rapid disease progression.

REFERENCE:

Laing NG, Laing BA, Meredith C, et al: Autosomal dominant distal myopathy: Linkage to chromosome 14. *Am J Hum Genet* 56:422, 1995.

Myotonia Congenita

At a glance: Rare genetic disorder characterized by myotonia, muscle stiffness, and abnormal muscle hypertrophy that gives the impression of Herculean or "bodybuilder-like" appearance. Two main forms of myotonia congenita have been described: Thomsen disease and Becker disease. In Thomsen disease, symptoms and findings are usually apparent from infancy to approximately 2 to 3 years of age. In many cases, muscles of the eyelids, hands, and legs are most affected. In Becker disease, symptoms most commonly become apparent between the ages of 4 and 12 years. Affected individuals develop progressive myotonia; however, muscle rigidity and hypertrophy tend to be more severe.

Classification:

- Becker type: Typically manifests between the age of 4 and 12 years. Rarely, it has been reported that the onset may occur as late as approximately 18 years of age. Symptoms are more severe in this type.

- Thomsen type: The onset of the disease may because apparent in infancy but most often by age 2 to 3 years of age. Symptoms stabilize after onset and do not progress.

History: First described in 1876 by Thomas Thomsen in Schleswig, Denmark. Thomsen was himself affected with the condition. In 1971, P.F. Bécker, a German physician, described the more severe variant of myotonia congenita.

Incidence: Epidemiological studies have estimated the incidence internationally at 6:100,000 population. Five hundred persons are affected in Sweden alone. Becker's myotonia congenita is about twice as common as Thomson's disease.

Genetic inheritance: The mutation in both Becker disease and Thomsen disease resides in the muscle chloride channel gene CLCN1, whose locus is on chromosome 7q35. Transmission is autosomal dominant for Thomsen disease and recessive for Becker disease.

Pathophysiology: Decreased conductance of the muscle chloride channel. There is a reduction in Cl^- ions entering the cell; it remains relatively depolarized, resulting in spontaneous oscillations in membrane potential and clinical myotonia. The symptoms may respond to class I antiarrhythmic drugs such as mexiletine.

Diagnosis: Action (e.g., inability to release a handshake) and percussion (e.g., sustained contraction after stimulation of a tendon reflex) myotonia. Attacks of muscle stiffness are usually painless and relieved by exercise (warm-up effect). Enhancement of myotonia by cold. Typical electromyographic tracing; myotonic discharge when a needle is inserted in the muscle. Muscle biopsy shows no signs of dystrophy. Creatine kinase level mildly elevated.

Clinical aspects: The onset of disease is in early infancy in Thomsen disease and later in Becker disease. The child shows decreased ability to relax muscles after contraction; blepharospasm (myotonia of the eyelids); and diffuse hypertrophy of muscles (buttocks, neck, back, shoulders). The disease affects mainly the lower limbs in Becker disease. No cardiac involvement, unlike in myotonic dystrophy. Heiman-Patterson et al. (1988) described two sisters with myotonia congenita who, on halothane contracture testing of skeletal muscle in vitro, had findings consistent with susceptibility to malignant hyperthermia. This could be a nonspecific abnormal response to the test caused by myotonia itself. Other case reports of diffuse muscle rigidity with no signs of rhabdomyolysis following succinylcholine have been published. There is one fatal case report of hyperthermia with muscle rigidity and metabolic acidosis in a 5-year-old boy a few hours after an anesthetic without malignant hyperthermia–triggering agents (Haberer, 1989).

Precautions before anesthesia: Check creatine kinase level and usual treatment (mexiletine, quinidine). Check family history for malignant hyperthermia.

Anesthetic considerations: Prevention of hypothermia. If propofol is used, prevention of pain on injection is mandatory because pain can induce a myotonic reaction of the limb or even of the whole body. Neither regional anesthesia nor muscle relaxation can control myotonic contractions. Succinylcholine should not be used (generalized myotonia), but the response to nondepolarizing agents is normal. There is a possible but poorly documented risk of malignant hyperthermia. If muscle biopsy is to be performed, dantrolene must not be given before because it will affect the test results. Familiarity with malignant hyperthermia protocol and drug placement are essential before attempting any suspected case. Maintain normothermia to prevent shivering and a myotonic response.

Pharmacological implications: Do not use succinylcholine to avoid provoking severe generalized myotonia and malignant hyperthermia. Although the response to nondepolarizing agents is normal, it should be administered with caution and monitored constantly.

Other conditions to be considered:

PARAMYOTONIA CONGENITA: Rare, genetic, nonprogressive disorder that is apparent during infancy. Characterized by myotonia triggered or aggravated by exposure to cold and alleviated by warm temperatures. The myotonia is sometimes described as "paradoxic" because it tends to become more severe rather than improve with exercise. Episodes of weakness or paresis that do not necessarily coincide with exposure to cold temperatures or myotonia may occur. Weakness may be induced by administration of potassium. The disorder is not associated with muscle wasting or hypertrophy. Paramyotonia congenita is a sodium channel disease (sodium channelopathy).

☞PERIODIC PARALYSIS (Hyperkaliemic): Rare genetic disorder that is usually apparent during infancy or childhood. Characterized by periodic episodes of muscle weakness that tend to occur during the daytime. Severe hyperkalemia may occur during episodes as a result of leakage from muscle. Reports suggest that such attacks may be triggered by exposure to cold temperatures (paramyotonia), rest, hunger, or administration of potassium. Hyperkalemic periodic paralysis is transmitted as an autosomal dominant trait and is caused by mutations in the sodium channel gene SCN4A on chromosome 17.

RIPPLING MUSCLE DISEASE: Rare genetic disorder in which mechanically triggered contractions of skeletal muscle spread to adjacent muscle fibers, potentially causing visible "rippling" moving over the muscle. Affected individuals experience myotonia, muscle rigidity, and pain within affected muscles, particularly during exercise in hypertrophic muscle. The disorder is transmitted as an autosomal dominant trait.

REFERENCES:

Binnaz A, Gercek A, Dogan V, et al: Pyoloromyotoms in a patient with paramyotonia congenita. *Anesth Analg* 98:68, 2004.

Farbu E, Softeland F, Bindoff LA: Anaesthetic complications associated with myotonia congenita: Case study and comparison with other myotonic disorders. *Acta Anaesthesiol Scand* 47:630, 2003.

Haberer JP, Fabre F, Rose E: Malignant hyperthermia and myotonia congenita (Thomsen's disease) [letter]. *Anaesthesia* 44:166, 1989.

Heiman-Patterson T, Martino C, Rosenberg H, et al: Malignant hyperthermia in myotonia congenita. *Neurology* 38:810, 1988.

Koch MC, Ricker K, Otto M, et al: Evidence for genetic homogeneity in autosomal recessive generalised myotonia (Becker). *J Med Genet* 30:914, 1993.

Myotonic Dystrophy

At a glance: Congenital anomaly of an ionic channel resulting in a multisystemic disease with anomalies of skeletal, smooth, and cardiac muscles. May cause mental deficiency and loss of hair. The more obvious features are muscle rigidity and lack of muscle relaxation after contraction. Onset occurs during early adulthood. However, it may occur at any age and is extremely variable in degree of severity. Progression of the disease is slow, sometimes evolving over 50 to 60 years. There appear to be at least two forms.

Synonyms: Myotonia Dystrophica; Dystrophia Myotonica; Steinert Disease; Curschmann-Steinert Disease; Curschmann-Batten-Steinert Disease.

Classification:

- Myotonic dystrophy, Type I: Characterized by a multisystem disorder that affects skeletal and smooth muscle, including the eyes, heart, endocrine system, and central nervous system. The clinical expression varies according to three phenotypes: mild, classic, and congenital. *Mild* myotonic dystrophy is characterized by cataract and mild sustained muscle contraction. The life span is normal. *Classic* myotonic dystrophy is characterized by muscle weakness and wasting, myotonia, cataract, and often by cardiac conduction abnormalities. Adults may become physically disabled and the life span can be significantly reduced. *Congenital* myotonic dystrophy is characterized by hypotonia and severe generalized weakness at birth, often with respiratory insufficiency and early death. Mental retardation is common.

- Myotonic dystrophy, Type II: Characterized by progressive muscle weakness, prolonged myotonia, cataracts, cardiac abnormalities, balding, and infertility. Increased sweating, particularly of the hands and trunk, is common in type II myotonic dystrophy. It typically appears in adulthood. It tends to be milder than Type I.

Incidence: Prevalence is 1:8000–10,000 general population. An estimated 98% of people with myotonic dystrophy have type I; the others have the milder form type II.

Genetic inheritance: Myotonic dystrophy is inherited as an autosomal dominant manner; the responsible gene is located on chromosome 19q13.

Pathophysiology: DMPK (myotonin protein kinase) is the myotonic dystrophy gene. The effect of the CTG repeating remains complex, and many unclarified issues remain. Normal CTG repeat is between 5 and 35. The effects of an expanded CTG repeat may be via abnormal RNA transcript processing. The phenomenon of anticipation is typical for myotonic dystrophy: cataracts at first generation, classic form at second generation, and neonatal form at third generation. Myotonic dystrophy is an ion channel disease: Cl⁻conductance is reduced and there are anomalies in the control of the refractory period of Na⁺ channels. This results in larger Na⁺ currents and altered muscle excitability.

Diagnosis: Diagnosis of myotonic dystrophy is suspected in individuals with muscle weakness and atrophy, especially of the distal leg, hand, neck, and face; myotonia (sustained muscle contraction), which often manifests as the inability to quickly release a hand grip and which can be demonstrated by tapping with a reflex hammer on, for example, the thenar muscle group; and cataracts, which requires slitlamp examination for early detection. Myotonic dystrophy is suspected in neonates with some combination of hypotonia, facial muscle weakness, generalized weakness, clubfoot, and respiratory insufficiency or failure. It is confirmed by detection of an expansion of the CTG trinucleotide repeat in the DMPK gene (chromosomal locus 19q13). A CTG repeat length exceeding 37 repeats is abnormal. DNA-based testing is essentially 100% sensitive and is widely available. Typical EMG tracing shows myotonic discharge when a needle is inserted in the muscle.

Clinical aspects: Myotonic dystrophy is a multisystem disorder that affects skeletal muscle and smooth muscle, as well as the eye, heart, endocrine system, and central nervous system. The clinical findings, which span a continuum from mild to severe, have been categorized into three somewhat overlapping phenotypes: mild, classic, and congenital. Degree of muscle disability can be rated using the Muscular Disability Rating Scale.

Grade I: Asymptomatic; the diagnosis of myotonic dystrophy is made by EMG, ophthalmic examination, or DNA analysis

Grade II: Facial weakness, ptosis, nasal speech, temporal atrophy, and weakness of sternocleidomastoids without limb weakness

Grade III: Distal muscle weakness in upper and lower limbs

Grade IV: Proximal and distal muscle weakness in upper and lower limbs

Grade V: Severe proximal muscle weakness with confinement to wheelchair for short or long distances

Mild Myotonic Dystrophy (50–150 CTG Repeats): Persons with mild myotonic dystrophy may have only cataract, mild myotonia, or diabetes mellitus. They may have fully active lives and a normal or minimally shortened lifespan. They are often unaware of having myotonic dystrophy and may be diagnosed only in the course of evaluation of a more severely affected family member. This often occurs when an asymptomatic mother having a CTG repeat size less than 100 gives birth to an infant with congenital myotonic dystrophy with a CTG repeat length in the thousands.

Classic Myotonic Dystrophy (~100 to ~1500 CTG Repeats): Within this range of CTG repeat size, only a rough correlation with severity of symptoms exists. These patients usually develop classic myotonic dystrophy with muscle weakness and wasting, myotonia, cataracts, and, often, cardiac conduction abnormalities. The age of onset for classic myotonic dystrophy is typically in the 20s and 30s, less commonly after age 40 years. However, classic myotonic dystrophy may be evident in childhood, when subtle signs such as myotonic facies and myotonia are observed. In classic myotonic dystrophy, the predominant symptom is distal muscle weakness, leading to foot drop/gait disturbance and difficulty with performing tasks requiring fine dexterity of the hands. The typical facies is mainly a result of weakness of the facial and levator palpebrae muscles. Some patients have ophthalmoplegia; others have dysarthria with nasal speech. Myotonia may interfere with daily activities such as using tools, household equipment, or doorknobs. Smooth muscle involvement may produce dysphagia, constipation, or diarrhea. Cataracts can eventually be observed by slitlamp examination in nearly all patients. The cataracts are often scintillating, iridescent, and multicolored in the early stages. Cardiac conduction defects of varying degrees of severity are common. In one series, 90% of patients had conduction defects. These defects are a significant cause of early mortality in patients with myotonic dystrophy. Less commonly, cardiomyopathy may occur. Minor intellectual deficits are present in some individuals, but in others intelligence is incorrectly assumed to be reduced because of the dull facial expression. Avoidant, obsessive-compulsive, and passive-aggressive personality features have been reported. Gallstones occur as a result of increased tone of the gallbladder sphincter. Hypersomnia and sleep apnea are other well-recognized, although later, manifestations of the disease. Endocrinopathies including hyperinsulinism, testicular atrophy, and possibly abnormalities in growth hormone secretion can be observed, although they are rarely clinically significant. Pilomatricomas and epitheliomas can occur. Rarely, after several decades of disease, myotonic dystrophy progresses such that the patient is confined to a wheelchair. Weakness/myotonia of the diaphragm and a susceptibility to aspiration increase the risk for respiratory compromise, usually in patients with advanced disease. Several studies have evaluated lifespan and mortality in myotonic dystrophy. The most frequent causes of death are pneumonia/respiratory failure, cardiovascular, sudden death/arrhythmia, and neoplasms. In the De Die-Smulders study, half the patients were either partially or totally wheelchair bound shortly before death. Women with myotonic dystrophy are at risk for complications during pregnancy, including increased spontaneous abortion rate, prolonged labor, retained placenta, and postpartum hemorrhage. Complications related to the presence of congenital myotonic dystrophy in the fetus include reduced fetal movements and polyhydramnios.

Congenital Myotonic Dystrophy (>1000 and often >2000 CTG Repeats): Infants with congenital myotonic dystrophy nearly always inherit the expanded DMPK allele from the mother, but inheritance from the father is possible. Most infants with congenital myotonic dystrophy have more than 1000 CTG repeats. Congenital myotonic dystrophy often presents before birth as polyhydramnios and reduced fetal movement. After delivery, the main features are severe generalized weakness, hypotonia, and respiratory compromise. Typically, affected infants have a characteristic inverted "V" shape of the upper lip (also referred to as tented or "fish"-shaped mouth), which is characteristic of significant facial diplegia (weakness). Mortality from respiratory failure is high, but surviving infants experience gradual improvement in motor function. Myotonia appears after age 2 years. Affected children are usually able to walk; however, a progressive myopathy eventually occurs, as in the classic form. Mental retardation is present in 50 to 60% of patients. The cause of mental retardation is unclear, but the brains of children with congenital myotonic dystrophy often show atrophy and ventricular dilation at birth. Mental retardation may result from a combination of early respiratory failure and a direct effect of the myotonic dystrophy mutation on the brain.

Precautions before anesthesia: Check muscle function: weakness and myotonia; eyelid ptosis. Check cardiac function: ECG (conduction defects) and echocardiography (mitral valve prolapse, cardiomyopathy); there is little correlation between severity of muscle disease and severity of cardiac disease. Check respiratory function (restrictive syndrome, cough) and chest radiograph (silent aspiration). Check blood sugar level (diabetes mellitus).

Anesthetic considerations: Because of dysphagia, swallowing problems, and gastric distension, the patient is at risk for perioperative aspiration: cricoid pressure during induction and gastric suction during the postoperative period until bowel transit back to normal. Easy fatigue of respiratory muscles increases the risk of postoperative respiratory failure. Neither regional anesthesia nor muscle relaxation can control myotonic contractions. Prevent hypothermia to avoid shivering and myotonic crises. Beware of postoperative intestinal pseudoocclusion syndrome.

Pharmacological implications: Respiratory drive is very sensitive to all intravenous agents, including propofol, thiopentone, benzodiazepines and opioids—a very small dose can have dramatic and prolonged effects. If propofol is used, prevention of pain on injection is mandatory because pain can induce a myotonic reaction of the limb or even of the whole body. Propofol is otherwise a safe anesthetic agent in this condition. Succinylcholine should not be used (generalized myotonia in some patients, but uneventful use before diagnosis in many); however, the response to nondepolarizing agents is normal.

Other conditions to be considered:

☞**Myotonia Congenita:** Congenital anomaly of muscular chloride channel resulting in prolonged contraction of skeletal muscles.

Proximal Myopathy with Myotonia (PROMM): Clinical presentation is similar to myotonic dystrophy with myotonia, cataracts, and muscle weakness, but only proximal muscles are affected and the facial muscles are relatively spared. There seem to be fewer cardiac problems than in congenital myotonic dystrophy; there are no expanded repeats of CTG. The gene is located on chromosome 3q27.

REFERENCES:

Ashizawa T: Myotonic dystrophy as a brain disorder [editorial; comment]. *Arch Neurol* 55:291-3, 1998.

Bennun M, Goldstein B, Finkelstein Y, et al: Continuous propofol anaesthesia for patients with myotonic dystrophy. *Br J Anaesth* 85:407, 2002.

de Die-Smulders CE, Howeler CJ, Thijs C, et al: Age and causes of death in adult-onset myotonic dystrophy. *Brain* 121:1557, 1998.

Imison AR: Anaesthesia and myotonia: An Australian experience. *Anaesth Intensive Care* 29:34, 2001.

Mathieu J, Allard P, Gobeil G, et al: Anesthetic and surgical complications in 219 cases of myotonic dystrophy. *J Neurol* 49:1646, 1997.

Sakai A, Nakagama I, Ninai H: Propofol anesthesia for a patients with congenital myotonic dystrophy. *Masui* 48:1030, 2000.

Myotubular Myopathy

At a glance: Congenital muscle disease characterized by generalized hypotonia, muscle weakness, and central nuclei on muscle biopsy (myotube-like aspect).

Synonyms: XMTM; X-Linked Myotubular Myopathy; XLMTM; Centronuclear Myopathy.

Incidence: 1:50,000 males births.

Genetic inheritance: Three types of myotubular myopathy are recognized based on the mode of inheritance: X-linked, autosomal recessive, and autosomal dominant. For the neonatal form, the gene has been localized on chromosome Xq28.

Pathophysiology: The myotubular or centronuclear myopathies are a group of inherited myopathies defined by the presence of central nuclei in affected skeletal muscle. Males with XLMTM with identifiable mutations in MTM1 can be said to have MTM1. Typically, X-linked myotubular myopathy is the most severe form, presenting with hypotonia and respiratory distress in affected newborn males. It is associated with high neonatal mortality. Surviving patients typically have prolonged ventilator dependence and grossly delayed motor milestones. Female carriers of XLMTM are generally asymptomatic, although rare manifesting heterozygotes have been described. The autosomal dominant (or adult) form has a later onset and a milder course. The course and severity of the autosomal recessive (or infantile) form is intermediate between the X-linked and the autosomal dominant form. Intelligence is usually within the normal range.

Diagnosis: Creatine kinase level is normal or slightly increased. The diagnosis of XLMTM has traditionally relied upon the presence of characteristic pathology in muscle samples: atrophy predominantly of type I muscle fibers, which have centrally placed myofiber nuclei. The central areas of muscle fibers are devoid of myofibrils, with aggregation of mitochondria. Resemblance to fetal myotubes is thought to reflect an arrest in morphogenesis of the muscle fibers. The diagnosis of XLMTM should be considered in any male with significant neonatal hypotonia and/or muscle weakness. A positive family history suggestive of X-linked inheritance, found in approximately 30% of reported cases, provides further evidence for XLMTM. Although clinical features such as a length and head circumference greater than 90th percentile, cryptorchidism, and/or long fingers and toes are common, none is diagnostic of XLMTM. With the advent of molecular genetic testing, males with milder clinical phenotypes have been found to have mutations in the MTM1 gene.

Clinical aspects: *Neonatal Form:* In males with the classic, severe, neonatal presentation, polyhydramnios with decreased fetal movement is often present. Hypotonia in the neonatal period appears to be a universal finding and, in the US series of Herman et al. (1999), 80% of patients required endotracheal intubation and ventilatory support at birth. Patients often have typical myopathic facies with dolichocephaly, a high forehead, long face with midface hypoplasia, and a narrow, high-arched palate with subsequent severe malocclusion. Additional features in the US series included length greater than 90th percentile with a proportionately lower weight (60%), long fingers and/or toes (43%), cryptorchidism (>50%), contractures including clubfeet (30%), and areflexia (60%). Many patients succumb during infancy to complications of the disorder or as a result of withdrawal of life support. For surviving patients in the United States, the average length of initial hospitalization is approximately 90 days. Most surviving males in the United States are discharged home on 24-hour ventilatory support via tracheostomy and gastrostomy (G-tube) feedings. With the isolation of the MTM1 gene in 1996, it became apparent that some males with a much milder phenotype have mutations in MTM1. A clinical classification for this broader phenotype (termed MTM1) was described by Herman et al. (1999). Neonates were classified as severe, moderate, or mild:

Severe (Classic): Characteristic facies, chronic ventilator dependence, grossly delayed motor milestones, nonambulatory, or death in infancy.

Moderate: More rapid achievement of motor milestones than patients with the severe form; prolonged periods of decreased ventilatory support.

Mild: Ambulatory with minimally delayed motor milestones, lack of chronic ventilatory support beyond the newborn period, lack of typical myopathic facies.

Despite having a chronic illness and prolonged ventilator dependence, many patients with MTM1 have linear growth above the 50th percentile; some patients in the US series achieved greater than 90th percentile for height. An advanced bone age and/or premature adrenarche have been documented in several boys, suggesting some disturbance of endocrine regulation; however, results of endocrinologic studies performed in several patients have been normal. Puberty has occurred normally in the few patients who have reached adulthood, although reproduction by an affected male has not been documented. Cognitive development in the majority of patients is normal if no significant hypoxic episodes have occurred. The muscle disease is not progressive, and muscle strength improves slowly over time. Medical complications related to the underlying myopathy are ophthalmoplegia, ptosis, severe myopia, dental malocclusion (requiring orthodontic care), and scoliosis. Scoliosis often develops in later childhood and may require surgical intervention. Scoliosis can exacerbate respiratory insufficiency and can cause some ventilator-independent boys to become ventilator dependent again as the condition progresses. With more aggressive supportive care and longer survival of some patients with MTM1, medical complications unrelated to the muscle disorder have occurred; these complications include pyloric stenosis, a mild form of spherocytosis, gallstones, kidney stones, nephrocalcinosis, a vitamin K-responsive bleeding diathesis, and liver dysfunction manifested by pruritus and elevated serum transaminases. Several patients have died following prolonged liver hemorrhage or hemorrhage into the peritoneal cavity. In three patients, peliosis hepatis, a rare vascular lesion characterized by the presence of multiple blood-filled cysts within the liver, was noted. Authors are aware of several additional unreported cases of boys with MTM1 and liver dysfunction, peliosis, or hemorrhage into the peritoneum. The pathogenetic mechanisms for these complications are not understood, but their lack of occurrence in other congenital myopathies and neuromuscular disorders, such as spinal muscular atrophy, strongly suggests that they are related to abnormal function of or absence of myotubularin.

Infantile Form: Delayed walking and mild proximal nonprogressive muscles weakness—most patients die or are wheelchair-bound by the second or third decade of life; the myocardium is often involved; scoliosis with restrictive lung disease. Seizures or some degree of mental retardation may be observed.

Adult Form: Stable and slow course; pregnancy worsens the muscle weakness; muscle disease usually becomes apparent by the third decade of life; patients often are wheelchair-bound by the sixth decade of life; cardiomyopathy not unusual.

Precautions before anesthesia: As in any child presenting with a muscular disorder, thorough cardiac evaluation (ECG, echocardiography) is mandatory. Note respiratory status, arterial blood gases where indicated, chest radiograph (scoliosis, infection), and pulmonary function tests where possible. Ensure optimal hydration. Order chest physiotherapy before anesthesia and postoperatively. Postoperative mechanical ventilation might be needed in patients who are not already ventilator dependent. Check blood clotting profile and liver profile, and consider liver scan. Prophylactic vitamin K may be indicated preoperatively.

Anesthetic considerations: Tracheal intubation, where necessary, is likely to be complicated by the facies, high-arched palate, and dental defects. Wherever possible, use local or regional anesthesia and aim for early postoperative emergence from anesthesia. Total intravenous anesthesia has been successfully used in some cases. Regional anesthesia for postoperative pain relief if possible. Although there are no reports of malignant hyperthermia in patients affected with this disorder, inhalational anesthesia agents should be used with caution or avoided.

Pharmacological implications: Malnutrition and underweight for age are common as a result of chronic infection or malabsorption; consequently, drug dosages should be reduced accordingly. By analogy with central core disease, it is probably safer to avoid malignant hyperthermia-triggering agents and succinylcholine. If possible, avoid neuromuscular blocking agents because they produce unreliable effects and may potentiate muscle weakness.

Other conditions to be considered:

☞**CENTRAL CORE DISEASE:** Congenital myopathy with a specific histologic pattern and high susceptibility to malignant hyperthermia.

☞**CONGENITAL MYOPATHY WITH FIBER-TYPE DISPROPORTION:** Rare genetic myopathy presenting at birth with hypotonia, muscle weakness, and high-arched palate. Findings occurring later include short stature, progressive scoliosis, hip dislocation, and deformities of the feet.

☞**NEMALINE ROD MYOPATHY:** Rare congenital and slowly progressive inherited neuromuscular disease usually apparent at birth and characterized by extreme hypotonia.

REFERENCES:

Breslin D, Reid J, Hayes A, Mirakhur RK: Anaesthesia in myotubular (centronuclear) myopathy. *Anaesthesia* 55:471, 2000.

Costi D, van der Walt JH: General anesthesia in an infant with X-linked myotubular myopathy. *Paediatr Anaesth* 14:964, 2004.

Herman GE, Finegold M, Zhao W, et al: Medical complications in long-term survivors with X-linked myotubular myopathy. *J Pediatr* 134:206, 1999.

Price SR, Currie J: Anesthesia for a child with centronuclear myopathy. *Paediatr Anaesth* 5:267, 1995.

Myhre Syndrome

At a glance: Syndrome characterized by mental retardation, short stature, maxillary hypoplasia, prognathism, short palpebral fissures, short philtrum, small mouth, generalized muscle hypertrophy, decreased joint mobility, cryptorchidism, cardiac anomaly, and sensorineural deafness.

Synonym: Growth-Mental Deficiency Syndrome of Myhre.

History: First described by Selma A. Myhre, an American pediatrician, in 1981.

Incidence: Remains unknown.

Genetic inheritance: Autosomal dominant.

Clinical aspects: Maxillary hypoplasia, prognathism, and thick calvaria. Short palpebral fissures and blepharophimosis. Large nose with prominent root and short philtrum is present, with a small mouth and thin upper lip. The thorax has large flat vertebrae with large pedicles. Other bone abnormalities include hypoplastic iliac wings, brachydactyly, and limited joint mobility of short tubular bones. Muscles are hypertrophied. Abnormal EEG and congenital heart defects. Cryptorchidism. Prenatal and postnatal growth deficiency with mental retardation. Early-onset mixed conductive and sensory-type deafness occurs. Radiologically, several particularities are reported and include thickened calvaria, broad ribs, hypoplastic iliac wings, shortened long and tubular bones, and large, flattened vertebrae with large pedicles.

Anesthetic considerations: Requires complete assessment of the neurologic and psychomotor development, family history, and previous problems. The cardiac system should be investigated because of the potential association of congenital heart defect. ECG and echocardiography should be considered before anesthesia. The potential risk for difficult direct laryngoscopy and tracheal intubation should be borne in mind. The presence of maxillary hypoplasia with severe prognathism and a small mouth must be evaluated. No known reports of specific pharmacological implications with this disorder. However, the presence of cardiac anomalies requiring ongoing treatment influences the selection of anesthetic agents during induction and maintenance of anesthesia.

Other condition to be considered:

☞**GOMBO Syndrome (Myhre Gombo Syndrome):** An acronym that stands for *g*rowth retardation, *o*cular abnormalities, *m*icrocephaly, *b*rachydactyly, *o*ligophrenia syndrome. It is characterized clinically by severe microcephaly, microphthalmia, prominent nose, mandibular prognathism, dental anomalies, brachydactyly with clinodactyly V, premature aging of the skin, and severe mental retardation. Other clinical features include waddling gait, motor retardation, narrow pelvis, broad shoulders, and a significant incidence of diaphragmatic hernia at birth. Transmission is familial and believed to be an autosomal recessive trait.

REFERENCES:

Bottani A, Verloes A: Myhre-GOMBO syndrome: Possible lumping of two "old" new syndromes [letter]? *Am J Med Genet* 59:523, 1995.

Myhre SA, Ruvalcaba RHA, Graham CB: A new growth deficiency syndrome. *Clin Genet* 20:1, 1981.

N

N Syndrome

At a glance: Congenital association of ocular and ear anomalies with spasticity of the limbs, mental retardation, cryptorchidism, hypospadias, and a high risk of leukemia.

Synonym: Opitz "N" Syndrome.

History: The term *N Syndrome* is taken from the first letter of the name of the affected family.

Incidence: Unknown.

Genetic inheritance: Autosomal recessive or sex-linked inheritance. It has also been suggested that the N syndrome is X-linked recessive.

Pathophysiology: It has been suggested that N syndrome is caused by a mutation affecting the region of the X chromosome (Xp22-3 p21-1) where the gene for DNA polymerase alpha is located. The high risk of T-cell leukemia observed in the hemizygote is a result of this DNA repair defect.

Diagnosis: The association of impaired hearing and visual problems with genital anomalies in a male infant should be suggestive. Laboratory investigation is useful.

Clinical aspects: Features include a long face with telorism, microretrognathia, arachnodactyly, and a short stature. Visual impairment, sensorineural deafness, laterally overlapping upper eyelids, nystagmus, large corneas, abnormal auricles, cryptorchidism, hypospadias, and spasticity. Anodontia or oligodontia are frequent features. Multiple pigmented nevi can be observed. Sometimes the patient presents with abnormal vertebrae and moderate-to-severe mental retardation. Patients may develop lymphoblastic leukemia with a mediastinal mass and leukemic infiltration of tissues.

Precautions before anesthesia: Check teeth and dental care. The presence of a parent at induction and in the recovery room might be helpful, considering the child's handicaps with communication. An anesthesiology consultation is highly recommended for elective surgery. A CT Scan and echocardiogram must be obtained to eliminate the presence of a mediastinal mass.

Anesthetic considerations: Spasticity may make IV line placement difficult. It may also interfere during direct laryngoscopy and tracheal intubation. In case of microretrognathia, alternative methods for tracheal intubation may be necessary and should be readily available. The presence of a mediastinal mass affecting the cardiovascular function (e.g., preload) will dictate the anesthetic technique. Combined to a difficult airway management and the potential for tracheobronchial extrinsic compression, it is mandatory to maintain spontaneous ventilation at all times.

Pharmacological implications: No specific pharmacological implications.

REFERENCES:

Floy KM, Hess RO, Meisner LF: DNA polymerase alpha defect in the N syndrome. *Am J Med Genet* 35:301, 1990.

Hess RO, Hafez G-R, Meisner LF: Updating the N syndrome: Occurrence of lymphoid malignancy and possible association with an increased rate of chromosome breakage. *Am J Med Genet Suppl* 3:383, 1987.

Hess RO, Kaveggia EG, Opitz JM: The N syndrome, a "new" multiple congenital anomaly-mental retardation syndrome. *Clin Genet* 6:237, 1974.

N-Acetylglutamate Synthetase Deficiency

At a glance: Congenital mitochondrial disorder of the metabolism of ammonium (hyperammonemia) leading to an anomaly in the urea cycle.

Synonym: NAGS Deficiency.

Incidence: Very rare; 37 cases from 24 families since 1981.

Genetic inheritance: Autosomal recessive.

Pathophysiology: N-acetylglutamate is synthesized from acetyl-CoA and L-glutamate by mitochondrial N-acetylglutamate synthetase (NAGS) in the liver. Its role is to activate carbamoylphosphate synthetase, one of the enzymes of the urea cycle. Impairment of the urea cycle produces hyperammonemia.

Diagnosis: Elevated blood ammonium (NH_4) level in a lethargic or comatose patient. A liver needle biopsy is necessary to confirm the diagnosis.

Clinical aspects: Two clinical presentations, depending on complete or partial lack of NAGS.

Neonatal Presentation: Starting within the first 4 days of life: refusal to drink, irritability, persistent vomiting, and mild respiratory alkalosis, followed rapidly by neurologic deterioration leading to coma, convulsions, and hypotonia.

Late-Onset Presentation: Long history of chronic hepatogastric symptoms, such as recurrent episodes of vomiting, failure to thrive, and hepatomegaly. Others present a neurologic picture of chronic encephalopathy, behavioral disorders (agitation, delirium, irritability), or Reye-like syndrome following valproate therapy for seizures. Death may occur during a metabolic crisis precipitated by an infection, surgery, increased catabolism, or a protein-rich diet. In case of seizures, sodium valproate should not be used because it may precipitate acute metabolic decompensation. Liver transplantation is curative. The basic treatment is a low-protein diet carefully calculated and adapted to the child's needs and metabolic tolerance. N-carbamyl glutamate can be given orally at a dose of 100 to 300 mg/kg/day divided into three to six doses, usually before feedings. In case of hyperammonemia:

- Stop protein intake and restrict fluid volume if there is any concern about cerebral edema. Provide a high-energy intake orally or intravenous (IV) (glucose 10–20%).
- Use alternative pathways for nitrogen elimination: give sodium benzoate up to 500 mg/kg/day, sodium phenylbutyrate up to 600 mg/kg/day, and L-arginine 300 mg/kg/day orally or IV. These drugs lead to significant potassium losses, so potassium blood levels should be monitored. Treat sepsis and convulsions aggressively.

Precautions before anesthesia: Check blood glucose and NH_4 levels. Make sure sodium benzoate, sodium phenylbutyrate, and L-arginine are available for emergency treatment of hyperammonemia.

Anesthetic considerations: Prolonged fasting should be avoided; intravenous glucose (5 or 10% solution) should be administered to prevent protein catabolism; monitor blood glucose, ammonium, and lactates level on regular basis. Hypovolemia must be avoided, especially in patients with altered renal function. If there is risk of nasal, pharyngeal, or gastric bleeding, a gastric tube should be inserted to remove swallowed blood, which may provide a protein load that may trigger acute metabolic decompensation. Prolonged postoperative metabolic monitoring for early diagnosis of acute decompensation.

Pharmacological implications: This sort of pathology should be borne in mind when dealing with a supposedly "normal" child who does not wake up after uneventful anesthesia. In case of fever, ibuprofen is preferred over acetaminophen; valproate and haloperidol can unmask a previously undiagnosed urea cycle defect.

Other conditions to be considered:

☞**ARGININEMIA:** Urea cycle disorder that leads to hyperammonemia and neurologic symptoms, which are less severe than reported in other forms of urea cycle abnormalities.

☞**CITRULLINEMIA:** Syndrome arising from argininosuccinate synthetase deficiency leading to hyperammonemia and neurologic consequences.

☞**HHH SYNDROME:** Genetically transmitted inborn error of metabolism resulting from a defect in the transport of ornithine into the mitochondrial matrix; clinically characterized by early growth retardation, learning disabilities, periodic confusion, and ataxia.

☞**METHYLMALONIC ACIDEMIA:** Heterogeneous inborn error of metabolism leading to metabolic acidosis and accumulation of methylmalonic acid and its by-products.

☞**ORNITHINE CARBAMOYLTRANSFERASE DEFICIENCY:** Rare genetic disorder characterized by complete or partial lack of the enzyme ornithine transcarbamylase. Lack of this enzyme results in excessive hyperammonemia, which is a known neurotoxin. Clinically, these patients present with vomiting, refusal to eat, progressive lethargy, and coma.

☞**PROPIONIC ACIDEMIA:** Inborn error of metabolism affecting the mitochondrial catabolism of valine and isoleucine. Untreated, this results in ketoacidosis, lethargy, coma, and eventually death.

REFERENCE:

Leonard JV: Disorders of the urea cycle, in Fernandes J, Saudubray J-M, van den Berghe (eds): *Inborn Metabolic Diseases.* 3rd ed. Berlin, Springer, 2000, p 214.

Nager Syndrome

At a glance: Rare condition characterized by malar hypoplasia, maxillary and mandibular hypoplasia, cleft lip or palate, retroplaced tongue, radial defects (preaxial limb deficiency), downward-slanting palpebral fissures, absent eyelashes (medial third of lower lids), dysplastic ears and conduction deafness, trismus, and respiratory problem in neonates. There may be underdevelopment or absence of the thumb, shortened forearms, and poor movement in the elbow.

Synonyms: Acrofacial Dysostosis 1; Treacher Collins Mandibulofacial Dysostosis Type with Limb Anomalies; Split-Hand Deformity Mandibulofacial Dysostosis.

History: Nager and de Reynier recognized this condition as a specific entity in 1948. Opitz (1987) suggested that Nager acrofacial dysostosis (AFD) represents an "anomaly" rather than a syndrome because of its apparent causal heterogeneity.

Incidence: Rare malformation, of which several syndromic associations have been reported.

Genetic inheritance: No clear genetic background and no molecular data. Most cases have been sporadic. However, it has also been suggested that a dominant mutation was possible. In 1987, the presentation of a father and child consistent with Nager syndrome supported an autosomal dominant inheritance, but no further investigations were able to sustain this observation. It has been reported that a deletion of the heterochromatic block and adjacent euchromatin of chromosome 1q was possible. In this situation, the affected child also presented with severe aortic stenosis and right pulmonary bronchial stenosis. This association with a deletion of chromosome 1q may suggest that this gene region contains crucial information for normal limb, craniofacial, and/or cardiopulmonary development. The association with chromosome 9 has been reported. An infant with Nager syndrome and a chromatid gap within band 3p14 was reported, but there remains no indication that this disease is genetic rather than sporadic. Opitz (1987) suggested that Nager AFD represents an "anomaly" rather than a syndrome because of its apparent causal heterogeneity.

Pathophysiology: No known pathophysiologic explanation for this medical condition.

Diagnosis: The diagnosis seems mostly clinical and radiologic. The limb deformities consist of absence of radius, radioulnar synostosis, and hypoplasia or absence of the thumbs. The mandibulofacial dysostosis is characterized mainly by severe micrognathia and malar hypoplasia. They suggested that ptosis of the lower lids, hypoplasia of the lower lid eyelashes, and cartilaginous pegs between the antitragus and lobule are minimal expressions of the syndrome. At birth, the diagnosis is suspected based on the clinical aspect, characterized by varying severities of mandibulofacial dysostosis with preaxial and/or postaxial limb abnormalities.

Clinical aspects: In the predominant facial form, called *Nager acrofacial dysostosis,* the facial changes resemble strikingly those of the Treacher Collins syndrome: malar hypoplasia, maxillomandibular hypoplasia, cleft lip or palate, conductive hearing loss, and radial limb hypoplasia. Neonates may present respiratory or feeding problems because of severe mandibular hypoplasia. Upper limb malformation is a constant feature of Nager syndrome and ranges from thumb hypoplasia to the absence of the radial ray. Intelligence is usually normal. *Neurologic:* Hydrocephalus, agenesis of corpus callosum, polymicrogyria, and spinal cord defects are reported. *Airway:* Absence of zygomatic arches associated with hypoplastic malar region and frequent hypoplasia of the larynx and epiglottis may contribute to the respiratory distress often observed in these infants. *Cardiac:* Association with congenital heart defect is rare. *Musculoskeletal:* Short stature, hypoplastic or aplastic radius, radioulnar synostosis. Limited elbow extension. The presence of a hypoplastic or aplastic thumb is almost characteristic of this condition. Other features include syndactyly, clinodactyly, or camptodactyly. The humeri are often shortened. Cervical vertebral deformities are frequent. *Visceral:* Association with Hirschsprung disease has been suggested.

Precautions before anesthesia: In neonates, the presence of severe respiratory depression might require placement of a preventive tracheostomy, which requires proper airway evaluation. Complete evaluation of the upper airway must include opening of the mouth, severity of micrognathia, and presence of laryngeal hypoplasia and/or absence of epiglottis. The potential for associated abnormalities of the heart, brain, kidney, or urogenital tract must be evaluated carefully prior to anesthesia. Vertebral body malformations, especially cervical, must be assessed carefully. Evaluate and anticipate the airway obstruction and difficult intubation.

Anesthetic considerations: The need for urgent tracheostomy, most often immediately after birth, can be performed under local anesthetics and controlled sedation. Maintaining spontaneous lung ventilation and oxygenation is highly recommended. Tracheal intubation via a laryngeal mask airway or retrograde technique has been reported. If the patient's trachea is intubated, the child must be carefully assessed postoperatively and extubated while fully awake. Venous access may be difficult in view of the limb deformities. The indication for invasive monitoring, such as radial artery access, can be difficult because of radial aplasia or hypoplasia.

Pharmacological implications: Muscle relaxants and opioids should be avoided before tracheal intubation is achieved and lung ventilation confirmed. Sedative agents should be used with great caution in the preoperative period, especially in the younger patient.

Other conditions to be considered: Six forms of AFD have been described: AFD syndrome of Kelly, Rodriguez or Madrid form, Reynolds or Idaho form, Arens or Tel Aviv type, presumed AFD syndrome of Richieri-Costa, and AFD Patterson-Stevenson-Fontaine syndrome. These disorders have been distinguished based on limb anomalies into preaxial, postaxial, lethal, and atypical forms.

☞**WEYERS II SYNDROME:** Syndrome in which hexadactyly is associated with fusion of the fifth and sixth metacarpal bones and of the proximal phalanges of the fifth and sixth toes. The tooth anomaly involves particularly the lower incisors, which are peg-shaped, small or missing, and widely spaced. A bony cleft of the mandibular symphysis may occur because of delayed ossification.

RODRIGUEZ LETHAL ACROFACIAL DYSOSTOSIS (Acrofacial Dysostosis Syndrome of Rodriguez; Madrid AFD Form): Characterized by severe mandibular hypoplasia, phocomelia and oligodactyly of the upper limbs, absence of fibulas, microtia, cleft palate, internal organ anomalies including arrhinencephaly and abnormal lung lobulation, and early lethality. All patients die of respiratory complications resulting from severe mandibular hypoplasia in the neonatal period. The limb deficiencies are predominantly preaxial (include severe hypoplasia of the shoulder and pelvic girdles), and the postaxial limb anomalies are rare types. Most patients present with cardiac and central nervous system malformations. An autosomal recessive mode of inheritance has been suggested. It has been suggested that the principal disorders that must be differentiated are Genee-Wiedemann syndrome and Nager syndrome.

☞**MILLER SYNDROME (Postaxial Acrofacial Dysostosis; Genee-Widemann Syndrome):** Characterized by the presence of postaxial limb deficiency, cup-shaped ears, and malar hypoplasia. Coloboma of the eyelids and accessory nipples are not present in this medical condition. Micrognathia is the rule and tends to improve with age. Cleft palate has been reported in all patients, whereas a cleft lip is present in only 20% of cases. Other features include bilateral absence of the fifth digit, including the fifth metacarpal, or unilateral aplasia or hypoplasia of the fifth digit. Shortened forearms and radiologic evidence of ulnar hypoplasia. Intelligence appears to be normal. Autosomal recessive inheritance has been suggested. Possible.

☞**TREACHER COLLINS SYNDROME:** Characterized by malar and mandibular hypoplasia, slanted eyes, notching of lower eyelids, and micrognathism. Severe respiratory problems can be seen in the neonatal period because of hypoplastic mandible. The pinna and the external auditory meatus bilaterally may be malformed. The tympanic membrane may be absent. Other facial features include a beak-like nose and acute deafness.

☞**GOLDENHAR SYNDROME:** Rare congenital disorder that involves unusual facial characteristics, such as partial absence of the upper eyelid or an unusual slant of the eyelid, skull asymmetry, prominent forehead, absence of nostrils, cleft palate, and micrognathism. Unilateral paralysis of the eye muscles may occur. Unusual cysts and fatty tissue can be observed at the edge of the eye, and skin tags are often present around the ears. Congenital heart defects are usually present.

☞**ORAL-FACIAL-DIGITAL SYNDROME:** Rare genetic disorder characterized by episodes of neuromuscular disturbances. It is associated with a split tongue, splits in the jaw, midline cleft lip, overgrowth of the frenulum, a broad-based nose, and epicanthic folds. Polysyndactyly and clinosyndactyly are frequent.

☞**JUBERG-HAYWARD SYNDROME:** Rare hereditary disorder characterized by cleft lip and palate, microcephaly, deformities of the thumbs and toes, and growth hormone deficiency resulting in short stature.

HEMIFACIAL MICROSOMIA (HFM): Syndrome that affects 1:5000 births. Although it is often mistaken for Treacher Collins syndrome, this condition is not genetic. Furthermore, some patients present with abnormalities on both sides of the face, whereas both sides of the face appear equally affected in Treacher Collins syndrome. The facial nerve is frequently paralyzed in hemifacial microsomia. Other features include micrognathism, unilateral facial tilting, microtia, facial nerve weakness (40%), macrostomia, and underdevelopment of the cheek and eye on the affected side of the face. Other abnormalities may include fatty tumors over the eye, vertebral body anomalies, ribs deformities, and cleft lip/palate. The association with congenital heart defects and kidney abnormalities has been reported and should be considered.

REFERENCES:

Opitz JM, Mollica F, Sorge G, et al: Acrofacial dysostoses: Review and report of a previously undescribed condition: The autosomal or X-linked dominant Catania form of acrofacial dysostosis. *Am J Med Genet* 47:660, 1993.

Opitz JM: Nager "syndrome" versus "anomaly" and its nosology with the postaxial acrofacial dysostosis syndrome of Genee and Wiedemann. *Am J Med Genet* 27: 959, 1987.

Walker JS, Dorian RS, Marsh NJ: Anesthetic management of a child with Nager's syndrome. *Anesth Analg* 79:1025, 1994.

Nail-Patella Syndrome

At a glance: Rare genetic disorder usually apparent at birth or during infancy. Characterized by dysplasia of the fingernails and toenails, aplasia or hypoplasia of the patellae, webbing of skin at the elbow(s), and abnormal bilateral projections of the iliac superior crest. Other features include glaucoma (open-angle glaucoma) and "cloverleaf-shaped iris" (Lester iris). Approximately 30 to 40% of patients may also develop nephropathy, which is usually apparent during childhood or later in life.

Synonyms: Hereditary Osteo-Onycho-Dysplasia; HOOD Syndrome; Turner-Kieser Syndrome; Fong Disease.

Incidence: Estimated incidence internationally is 1:50,000 live births. Both sexes are affected equally. No racial predilection. Individuals of any age can be affected.

History: First reported clinically by Chatelain in 1820, whereas its hereditary nature was defined by Little in 1897.

Genetic inheritance: This genodermatosis is an autosomal dominant trait with variable expressivity and a high degree of penetrance.

The nail-patella locus is linked to the COL5A1 gene at the 9q34.1 chromosome locus. This suggests that the syndrome is a connective tissue disease because the gene codes for a portion of the type V collagen molecule. In addition, the nail-patella locus and the ABO blood group locus are linked. The gene involved is located on the long arm of chromosome 9.

Pathophysiology: It has been proposed that mutations in the COL5A1 gene may be involved in the pathogenesis of the nail-patella syndrome.

Diagnosis: Electron microscopy shows characteristic ultrastructural changes in the glomerulus where many collagen fibrils are present in the thickened basement membranes and in mesangial matrix of otherwise normal glomeruli; this process is also known as *collagenation of glomerular basement membrane.* Radiologic examination of the pelvis and elbows differentiates this disorder from other causes of micronychia during childhood.

Clinical aspects: Nail deformities are recognized at birth and do not progress: nails are hypoplastic, discolored, and have poorly formed lunulae and/or splitting, most commonly of the thumbnail. Skeletal involvement usually presents with knee dislocation, pain, or gait disturbance. Hypoplasia of first ribs, malformed sternum, spina bifida, dislocation of the head of radius, scoliosis are also seen. Both elbow and knee dysplasia may lead to permanent restrictive deformities (incomplete extension). Cloverleaf pigmentation of the inner margin of the iris in 50% of patients. Nephropathy is commonly presented as proteinuria (50% of patients). The majority of patients with renal involvement have no associated mortality; however, in approximately 20%, slow progression to renal failure occurs within 5 to 25 years. Associated systemic abnormalities include cleft lip and palate, mental retardation, sensorineural hearing loss, hypoplasia or aplasia of some muscles (pectoralis minor, triceps, quadriceps), cataract, and ptosis.

Precautions before anesthesia: Evaluate airway for potential difficulty with direct laryngoscopy and tracheal intubation in the presence of cleft lip/palate. Assess the extent of renal involvement and any drug therapy associated with it (antihypertensives, diuretics, and steroids). If renal impairment is present, optimize volume state and blood pressure control. Investigations include hemoglobin, Na, K, creatinine, chest radiography, ECG, coagulation status. If neuraxial locoregional anesthesia is foreseen, radiography of the spine to exclude spina bifida occulta and to evaluate scoliosis.

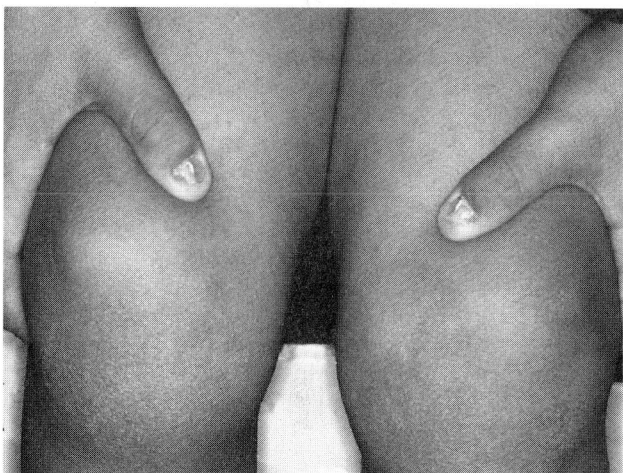

Nail-Patella syndrome   Onychodystrophy of the thumbs and dysplastic patellae in a patient with nail-patella syndrome.

Anesthetic considerations: Conventional anesthetic technique can be used in patients with minimal renal involvement. Cooperation may be difficult in patients with mental retardation. Difficult positioning may be expected if there are joint deformities. Direct laryngoscopy and tracheal intubation may be potentially difficult in patients with cleft lip/palate. In patients with severe renal dysfunction, practice precautions and care as for any such patients.

Pharmacological implications: Hypoalbuminemia results in a higher concentration of free drugs. Therefore, reduce dose of drugs that are normally highly bound to protein. Avoid succinylcholine if serum potassium level is greater than 5 mmol/l or in the presence of glaucoma. Atracurium and *cis*-atracurium may be preferred because of their independence of renal metabolism and excretion.

Other conditions to be considered:

☞**ALPORT SYNDROME:** Characterized by kidney disease, sensorineural hearing loss, glomerulonephritis, hematuria, proteinuria, and cataracts. The mode of genetic transmission has not been clearly defined but is suggested to be autosomal dominant, recessive, or X-linked genetic.

ANONYCHIA-ONYCHODYSTROPHY: Characterized by similar abnormalities observed with the Nail-Patella syndrome. Individuals affected with this medical condition have absent and/or underdeveloped fingernails and toenails. The presence of spontaneous dislocation of the hips at birth is frequent. It is inherited as an autosomal dominant genetic trait.

REFERENCES:

Dreyer SD, Zhou G, Baldini A, et al: Mutations in LMX1B cause abnormal skeletal patterning and renal dysplasia in nail patella syndrome. *Nat Genet* 19:47, 1998.

Silverman R: Nail and appendageal abnormalities, in Schachner LA, Hansen RC (eds): *Pediatric Dermatology.* 2nd ed. New York, Churchill Livingston, 1995, p 630.

Nance-Horan Syndrome

At a glance: Very rare congenital inherited disorder that combines cataract and dental anomalies.

Synonyms: Mesiodens-Cataract Syndrome; Cataract-Dental Syndrome; X-Linked Cataract-Hutchinsonian Theet Syndrome.

Incidence: Several kindreds have been described since this condition was defined in 1974. It is fully expressed in Wales only.

Genetic inheritance: Transmitted as an X-linked trait with tentative mapping to the short arm of chromosome X (Xp21.1-p22.3, Xp22.3-p21.1, and Xp22.3-p22.2).

Pathophysiology: Congenital cataracts with impaired vision, extra incisors, anteverted pinnae, short fourth metacarpals, and variable anomalies. Mental deficiency is present in some patients.

Diagnosis: Typical features of the disease are cataracts and dental anomalies; worse in related males than in females.

Clinical aspects: Males have dense nuclear cataracts and microcorneas, whereas heterozygous females have posterior Y-sutural cataracts, small corneas, and only slightly reduced vision. Teeth show nonsyphilitic hutchinsonian incisors, supernumerary teeth, irregular diastema, and cone-shaped incisors. Dolichocephaly and mandibular prognathism occur, with a high nasal bridge, prominent, anteverted pinnae, and short metacarpals. Developmental delay may be seen. Patients have a marfanoid habitus, and males are often blind.

Precautions before anesthesia: No literature about this condition and anesthesia. Patients may be blind or mentally handicapped.

Anesthetic considerations: Dentition may lead to difficulties in direct laryngoscopy and tracheal intubation, as may oral anomalies. Blind and/or mentally handicapped children need much reassurance. The presence of a parent and/or premedication may help when airway difficulties are not expected.

Pharmacological implications: No specific interactions.

REFERENCES:

Walpole IR, Hockey A, Nicoll A: The Nance-Horan syndrome. *J Med Genet* 27:632, 1990.

Zhu D, Alcorn DM, Antonarakis SE, et al: Assignment of the Nance-Horan syndrome to the distal short arm of the X chromosome. *Hum Genet* 86:54, 1990.

NARP Syndrome

At a glance: Mitochondrial disease. NARP is an acronym for *n*europathy, *a*taxia, and *r*etinitis *p*igmentosa. Other features include corticospinal tract atrophy, developmental delay, dementia, seizures, cerebellar ataxia, sensory neuropathy, and proximal neurogenic muscle weakness.

Incidence: Unknown. Prevalence is estimated at 1:12,000 population.

Genetic inheritance: NARP syndrome is maternally transmitted. A T-to-G point mutation at the base pair nucleotide 8963 of mitochondrial DNA is suspected. This MT ATP6 encodes for subunit 6 of mitochondrial adenosine triphosphatase.

Pathophysiology: Defect of complex V of the respiratory chain enzymes, with progressive loss of mitochondrial bioenergetic capacity.

Diagnosis: Clinical and laboratory confirmation of elevated pyruvate and lactate. Muscular biopsy shows ragged-red muscle fibers, and the biochemical defect is often segmental on histochemistry. On ophthalmoscopy, the retina reveals salt-and-pepper retinopathy.

Clinical aspects: Association of neuropathy, ataxia, and retinitis pigmentosa leading progressively to blindness. Other clinical features include mental retardation, progressive deafness, muscle weakness, developmental delay, and sluggish pupils. Onset in young adulthood, with normal development and language problems.

Precautions before anesthesia: Diagnosis of mitochondrial disease should be considered in any child with a multisystem neurologic disorder or who is being investigated for hypotonia. Anesthesia-related morbidity and mortality risk is essentially linked to the preoperative status of the child, that is, the number and extent of organ dysfunction. The presence of a mitochondrial disease is not considered a risk for malignant hyperthermia. Avoid any elective anesthesia/surgery in the presence of infection or temperature because the increase in cytokines (mainly tumor necrosis factor) inhibits some complex of the respiratory chain. The following should be checked: central nervous system (CNS) (seizures, myoclonus, strokes, swallowing problems; usual venous or arterial concentration of lactates and glucose); *muscles* (hypotonia, contractures, scoliosis); *heart* (even if the child is asymptomatic, ECG and echocardiography to exclude conduction disorders and cardiomyopathy, respectively; check functioning of pacemaker, if present); *respiratory* (frequent infections, chronic lung aspiration, pulse oximetry breathing room air should be obtained, obstructive and/or central

apnea; reduced ventilatory drive is common, and many patients have an abnormal response to both hypoxia and hypercarbia. Deaths have been reported following sedation with chloral hydrate or diazepam). Other organ involvement include: *hepatic* and *renal function*; *nutritional status* and *diet* (glucose and/or lipid rich; tolerance to fasting and treatment [carnitine, vitamin Q, antiepileptic drugs]).

Anesthetic considerations: Usual treatment up to the day of surgery. Preoperative fasting must be as short as possible. If fasting is usually poorly tolerated, a glucose-containing solution should be started when the fasting period begins. A sedative premedication is best avoided because of the possible abnormal response to hypoxia/hypercarbia. *Induction:* According to the anesthesiologist's choice. Sevoflurane is the best choice for inhalation induction; propofol seems the best choice for IV induction, but a 2% solution should be used to lessen the lipid load. *Opiates:* Dose should be carefully titrated according to the patient's needs. *Muscle Relaxant:* Published data are contradictory. Even in the absence of clinical myopathy, the patient's muscular response to nerve stimulation should be measured before administering a muscle relaxant. Atracurium and *cis*-atracurium are the best choices because of their spontaneous degradation. In case of myopathy, succinylcholine should not be used to avoid producing rhabdomyolysis. *Intraoperative Fluids:* Avoid infusion containing lactates such as Ringer lactate or Hartmann solution and Stocker: however, the patient should receive a glucose solution (5 or 10% dextrose according to blood sugar level). Aim for normoglycemia because hyperglycemia can increase lactate production. Monitor frequently (arterial or venous) blood gases and lactate levels. In case of severe lactic acidosis, use dichloroacetate 50 mg/kg intravenously (IV) over 30 minutes to stimulate pyruvate dehydrogenase to metabolize lactate in pyruvate. Perimedullar locoregional anesthesia can be used, but its cost-to-benefit ratio should be evaluated, taking into account the presence of severe scoliosis or degenerative lesions in the spinal cord. Some patients with mitochondrial disease present with axonal neuropathy of peripheral nerves; the possible effects of local anesthetics on these nerves are unknown. Prevention of hypothermia is important to avoid shivering and increased oxygen consumption at awakening.

Pharmacological implications: Patients with mitochondrial disease are very sensitive to the respiratory effects of sedatives. It also seems, according to BIS measurement, that children with an anomaly of complex I of the respiratory chain are much more sensitive to the hypnotic effects of sevoflurane. Most studies performed on isolated mitochondria use doses of anesthetic agents far in excess of those used in daily practice; thus their clinical relevance is often dubious.

Other conditions to be considered:

☞**REFSUM DISEASE:** Autosomal recessive genetic disorder characterized by the accumulation of phytanic acid. The clinical manifestations appear around age 15 years and consist of hemeralopia (loss of vision in the dark), distal motor polyneuropathy, perceptive deafness, cerebellar ataxia, and severe mental retardation. Ichthyosis, polyepiphyseal dysplasia, myocardiopathy, elevated protein in cerebrospinal fluid, and retinitis pigmentosa may be present. Diagnosis is based on biologic evidence of phytanic acid in plasma and urine. Phytanic acid comes exclusively from food (green vegetables and herbivore animals).

☞**COCKAYNE SYNDROME:** Rare autosomal recessive inherited condition that develops between the ages of 1 and 2 years and presents with poikiloderma, dwarfism, mental retardation, retinitis pigmentosa, blindness, and conduction deafness.

☞**ABETALIPROTEINEMIA:** Autosomal recessive inherited metabolic disorder resulting from a mutation in a subunit of the microsomal triglyceride transfer protein (MTP) on chromosome 4q22-q24. The neurologic symptoms are directly associated with a deficiency in vitamin E. The clinical manifestations include a malabsorption syndrome, retinitis pigmentosa degeneration, and progressive ataxic neuropathy. Acanthocytosis is characteristic. Total cholesterol is low (<70 mg/dl) and triglycerides are almost undetectable. A lipoprotein profile shows absent low-density and very-low-density lipoproteins.

☞**USHER SYNDROME:** Defined as a genetically heterogeneous condition comprising 12 independent loci, with three presenting with clinically well-defined entities (USH1, USH2, USH3) corresponding to the development of retinitis pigmentosa, auditory and vestibular, profound sensorineural hearing loss, and absent vestibular function. The age of onset is variable. The prevalence is estimated at 3–4:100,000 in European-based populations.

REFERENCES:

Maslow A, Lisbon A: Anesthetic consideration in patients with mitochondrial dysfunction. *Anesth Analg* 76:884, 1993.

Naguib M, Dawlathy AA, Ashour M, et al: Sensitivity to mivacurium in a patient with mitochondrial myopathy. *Anesthesiology* 84:1506, 1996.

Santorelli FM, Tessa A: Neuropathy, ataxia and retinitis pigmentosa (NARP) syndrome. *Orphanet* April 2004.

Wallace JJ, Perndt H, Skinner M: Anesthesia and mitochondrial disease. *Paediatr Anaesth* 8:249, 1998.

Nélaton Syndrome

At a glance: Paraneoplastic autonomic neuropathic syndrome occurring in association with several primary neoplasias, characterized by antibodies directed against a cellular nuclear component expressed in nearly all nervous tissues.

Synonyms: Paraneoplastic Autonomic Neuropathy; Anti-Hu Syndrome; Denny-Brown Neuronopathy; Subacute Paraneoplastic Sensory Neuropathy; Autoimmune Paraneoplastic Neurologic Syndrome; Paraneoplastic Sensory Neuropathy.

Incidence: Clinically a rare disease, but antibodies can be found in up to 10% of pulmonary small cell tumors.

Genetic inheritance: Acquired autoimmune disease. Not linked to a particular genotype.

Pathophysiology: Autoantibodies directed against a nuclear component of nervous system cells called *Hu*. This antigen is expressed in the central and peripheral nervous systems but can also be expressed by neoplastic cells. It may play a role in nervous system development. Loss of ganglion cells in sacral and lumbar dorsal root ganglia.

Diagnosis: Clinical expression of a subacute mainly sensory neuronopathy, with demonstration of polyclonal anti-Hu antibodies in the plasma. Axons and neuromuscular junctions appear normal on electrophysiologic studies.

Clinical aspects: Mainly found in conjunction with pulmonary small cells tumors but may be encountered with other types of tumors. The sensory neuronopathy can be found up to 1 year before clinical discovery of the tumor. Clinically, there is a subacute neuronopathy, sometimes associated with central limbic symptomatology. It may be misdiagnosed as "herpetic encephali-

tis." Immunosuppression and plasmapheresis have not shown any benefit.

Precautions before anesthesia: Usually, patients present for surgical treatment of the underlying tumor. It is judicious to request a complete neurologic evaluation before and after the procedure to confirm maintenance of neurologic status. In this setting, general anesthesia is preferable, and central neuraxial blockade techniques are not recommended. Look for signs of autonomic dysfunction before induction.

Anesthetic considerations: Anesthetic considerations are those associated with the surgical procedure and not the patient's condition. However, in the presence of neuronopathy, use of anesthetic agent associated with rapid elimination might be appropriate. Usually uneventful recovery.

Pharmacological implications: No specific implications; however, it is believed that the response to local anesthetics is poorly managed.

REFERENCE:

Lovblad KO, Boucraut J, Steck AJ: Paraneoplastic subacute sensory Denny-Brown neuronopathy or anti-Hu syndrome: A classical paraneoplastic syndrome. *Rev Med Suisse Romande* 115:421, 1995.

Nemaline Rod Myopathy

At a glance: Rare, congenital, slowly progressive inherited neuromuscular disease that usually is apparent at birth; characterized by extreme hypotonia.

Synonym: Nemaline Myopathy.

Classification: Nemaline myopathy has been classified into four major subtypes:

Severe neonatal form: Characterized by severe muscle hypotonia with little spontaneous movements, severe dysphagia and absence of sucking ability, and respiratory problems that are considered life-threatening during the first weeks or months of life. A *fetal form ("fetal akinesia sequence")* has been suggested but is still considered part of this entity. It is associated with large quantity of amniotic fluid, abnormal muscle growth, and underdevelopment of the lung.

Mild congenital or "classic" form: Age at onset between birth and the first years of life. It is characterized by extreme muscle weakness, feeding difficulties, delayed motor development (e.g., walking difficulties, speech abnormalities), and respiratory complications that are not considered as severe at the neonatal form. The evolution of the disease is often static or very slowly progressive. Most affected individuals can have an active life; others may experience deterioration during the period of rapid growth before puberty.

Childhood-onset form: Age at onset between 10 and 20 years. The apparition of muscle weakness is slowly progressive and allows motor development to be considered normal. The clinical symptoms typically progress during childhood, but exercises that increase muscle development and strength may offset the progression of the disease.

Late-onset or *adult-onset form:* Characterized by the absence of family history or symptomatology before the apparition of the muscle weakness, which is mostly apparent in the extremities and the trunk.

Incidence: Affects females more than males; estimated incidence is 2:10,000 live births.

Genetic inheritance: Two clinically indistinguishable types are described. *Type I* is autosomal dominant with incomplete penetrance and is caused by a defect in the gene TPM3 (or NEM1) located on chromosome 1q21-q23 and encoding for tropomyosin-3. *Type II* is autosomal recessive and is caused by a mutation of the gene NEM2 located on chromosome 2q21.2-q22 and encoding for nebulin.

Pathophysiology: All muscles, including the diaphragm, may be affected. The disease is nonprogressive or slowly progressive. Cardiac involvement is rare, but cases of cardiomyopathy in adults have been described.

Diagnosis: Serum creatine kinase levels are usually, but not always, normal. Muscle biopsy shows disproportion of type I muscles fibers and subsarcolemmal rod-like structures made of excessive Z-band material.

Clinical aspects: In the neonatal period, hypotonia and muscle weakness produce swallowing problems and weak cry; severe cases progressing rapidly to respiratory failure are described. Motor development (walking) is delayed. Muscle mass is thin; truncal and proximal muscles are most affected, but distal limb, pharyngeal, and facial muscles can be involved. The face is usually long with a high-arched palate, malocclusion, prognathism, or micrognathia. Abnormal gait. Normal intelligence. Scoliosis and intercostal muscle weakness produce severe restrictive lung disease. Congenital heart disease or cardiomyopathy may be rarely present.

Precautions before anesthesia: Check pulmonary function: ability to cough, pulmonary function if the patient is old enough to cooperate. Pulse oximetry while breathing room air should be obtained. Nocturnal oximetry can be useful because hypoxemia during sleep caused by diaphragmatic fatigue has been described. Echocardiography to exclude congenital heart diseases or cardiomyopathy must be performed.

Anesthetic considerations: Malignant hyperthermia has not been reported in patients with nemaline myopathy. The narrow face with malocclusion and micrognathia can make direct laryngoscopy and tracheal intubation difficult. Patients are at risk for postoperative complications. The use of postoperative mechanical ventilation may be indicated to allow good analgesia and chest physiotherapy.

Pharmacological implications: Although some resistance to succinylcholine and a normal response to pancuronium have been observed in one case, it probably is safer to avoid succinylcholine as in any myopathy; if muscle relaxation is necessary, use a short-acting muscle relaxant while assessing the patient's response with neuromuscular monitoring.

Other conditions to be considered:

☞**CENTRAL CORE DISEASE:** Rare inherited neuromuscular disorder that is milder and less progressive than nemaline myopathy. Characterized by hypotonia, especially of the arms and legs. Symptoms begin during the first year of life. Infants with central core disease may have difficulty learning to sit and walk. Other features include joint hypermobility and scoliosis.

☞**WERDNIG-HOFFMAN DISEASE:** Rare, inherited, childhood neuromuscular disorder characterized by degenerative changes in the spinal cord. Early symptoms include generalized muscle hypotonia, hypermobility of joints, and absent tendon reflexes. Other features include dysphagia and problems with breathing and the kidneys.

☞**MYOTUBULAR MYOPATHY:** Rare muscle-wasting disorder that occurs in three forms. The most severe form is present at birth and presents with severe respiratory muscle weakness. A less severe form is present at birth or early childhood and progresses slowly. The least severe form presents between the first and third decades of life and is slowly progressive. Clinically, weakness of the upper eyelid, jaw, tongue, lips, mouth, throat, and neck may be present.

Scoliosis becomes apparent in adolescence. Seizures may be present.

☞**LIMB-GIRDLE MUSCULAR DYSTROPHY:** Rare inherited muscular disorder that may begin at birth or during adulthood. Infants present with generalized muscle weakness, poor sucking ability, and dysphagia. Other features include a high-arched palate, thin face, ptosis, and scoliosis. Adults have a clumsy walk and general hypotonia of the hips and shoulders.

☞**CONGENITAL MYOPATHY WITH FIBER TYPE DISPROPORTION:** Rare inherited muscle disease that affects the growth of type I muscle fibers. Newborn infants usually have generalized hypotonia. Other features include scoliosis, dislocated hip joints, foot deformities, and a high-arched palate. Symptoms tend to improve with age.

BENIGN CONGENITAL HYPOTONIA: Nonprogressive neuromuscular disorder present at birth; characterized by a generalized muscle weakness or "floppiness" (hypotonia). Infants appear weak and listless.

BATTEN TURNER TYPE CONGENITAL MYOPATHY: Extremely rare inherited muscle disorder characterized by lack of muscle tone or severe hypotonia (floppiness) at birth. Slowly progressive during infancy and childhood; this disorder is not progressive in adulthood.

☞**CANAVAN SYNDROME:** Rare inherited disorder characterized by progressive degeneration of the central nervous system, appearing in infancy. Early symptoms include a general lack of energy, floppiness, and loss of previously acquired motor skills. Other features include seizure-like movement of the arms and legs, poor head control, and deafness.

REFERENCES:

Heard SO, Kaplan RF: Neuromuscular blockade in a patient with nemaline myopathy. *Anesthesiology* 59:588, 1983.

Shenkman Z, Sheffer O, Erez I, et al: Spinal anesthesia for gastrostomy in an infant with nemaline myopathy. *Anesth Analg* 91:858, 2000.

Neonatal Lupus Erythematosus

At a glance: Syndrome in newborns characterized by congenital heart block and/or cutaneous lupus erythematosus in the presence of maternal autoantibodies.

Incidence: Estimated to be 1:12,500 live births. An infant born of an anti-Ro(SSA) antibody–positive mother has a 1:20 chance of developing a neonatal lupus syndrome.

Genetic inheritance: No racial or sexual predilection, but there is an increased frequency of the HLA-DR3 phenotype in mothers of infants with neonatal lupus.

Pathophysiology: Believed to be caused by transplacental passage of specific autoantibodies (primarily anti-Ro/SSA and anti-La/SSB) from the mother with systemic lupus erythematosus to the fetus. These autoantibodies bind to fetal Ro and La autoantigens and induce an inflammatory infiltrate in the skin or heart. The latter results in scarring with fibrosis and calcification, causing complete congenital heart block.

Diagnosis: Characteristic skin lesions and/or congenital complete heart block with positive maternal anti-Ro and anti-Ra antibodies.

Clinical aspects: Approximately 50% of infants with neonatal lupus have characteristic skin lesions, with predilection for involvement around the eyes—"raccoon eyes" appearance. In the other 50% of affected infants, cardiac lesions predominate. In approximately

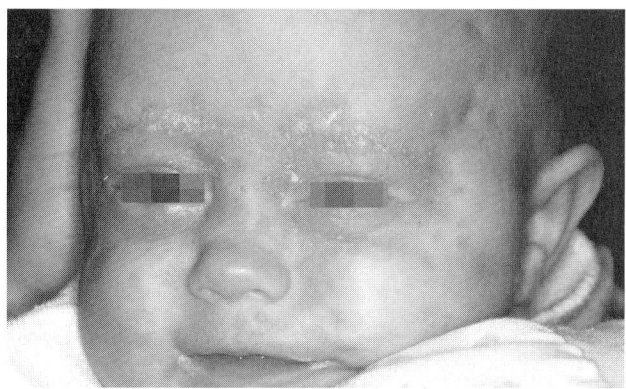

Neonatal lupus erythematosus   Characteristic "raccoon-eyes" in an infant with neonatal lupus erythematosus.

10%, both cutaneous and cardiac lesions are present. The skin lesions (generalized, erythematous, nonscaling, sharply demarcated) develop in the first month or later in life, and they generally disappear by 6 months, which corresponds to the disappearance of the maternal IgG antibodies from the infant's serum. Neonatal lupus dermatitis responds to topical steroids. Avoidance of sunlight exposure is recommended because exacerbation and induction of skin lesions follow ultraviolet light exposure. Congenital abnormalities include patent ductus arteriosus, ventricular septal defect, transposition of the great arteries, atrial septal defect, coarctation of the aorta, and tetralogy of Fallot. The first cause of mortality (15–35%) and morbidity of neonates affected with lupus is complete congenital heart block. A pacemaker is required in one third of infants. Thrombocytopenia and liver involvement occur but are normally mild and transient.

Precautions before anesthesia: Check drug history (steroids, cardiac drugs). Investigations include ECG, echocardiography, chest radiography, arterial blood gases, and levels of electrolytes, urea, creatinine, and hemoglobin. In patients with preexisting permanent pacemaker, ascertain pacemaker function according to institution protocol. A magnet or reprogramming device and expertise that can be used to convert the pacemaker to asynchronous mode should be available. In patients without preexisting permanent pacemaker, measures and expertise for temporary pacing (cardiologist, transcutaneous pacing, transesophageal pacing, transvenous pacing) should be available prior to induction of anesthesia. Chronotropic drugs (atropine, isoprenaline) should be available.

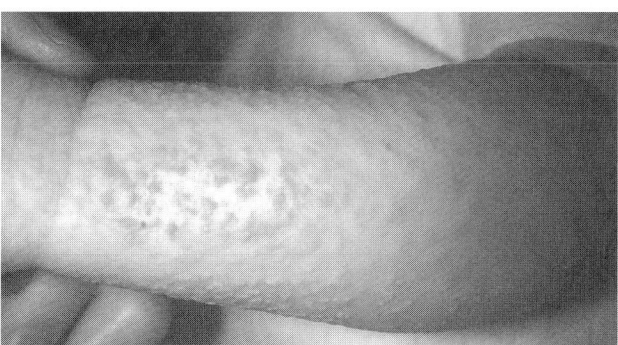

Neonatal lupus erythematosus   Erythematous, nonscaling skin lesions on the forearm of an infant with neonatal lupus erythematosus.

Anesthetic considerations: When transporting and positioning patients with temporary pacing devices, take care to prevent accidental dislodgment of the leads. Acute acid-base or electrolyte imbalance (K^+, $PaCO_2$, glucose, PaO_2) that can increase pacing thresholds should be prevented. Hypothermia also increases pacing threshold, so normothermia should be maintained for optimal pacemaker function. Intraoperative and postoperative normothermia should minimize the development of postanesthetic shivering, which may cause pacemaker failure. Anesthetic considerations specific for the congenital heart defect present should be adapted for clinical management.

Pharmacological implications: Suxamethonium-induced fasciculations may cause physiologic rate-responsive pacemaker failure and should be avoided. If necessary, precurarization with a nondepolarizing agent may be used. Halothane should be avoided because it slows the heart rate and sensitizes the myocardium to arrhythmias more so than isoflurane or sevoflurane. Anesthetic agents with effects on heart conduction and contractility should be avoided.

REFERENCE:

Silverman ED, Laxer RM: Neonatal lupus erythematosus. *Rheum Dis Clin North Am* 23:599, 1997.

Netherton Syndrome

At a glance: Congenital disorder that involves production of abnormal bamboo (brittle) hair (diagnostic marker) and associated with onychodystrophy, cataracts, mental retardation, skin sensitivity to light, and ichthyosis.

Synonyms: Psoriasiform Ichthyosis; Trichothiodystrophy; Ichthyosis Linearis Circumflexa; Trichorrhexis Invaginata; Còmel-Netherton Syndrome.

History: Association between hair shaft bamboo node defects and ichthyosiform erythroderma was described by Albert Touraine, a French dermatologist, and Gabriel Solente, a French physician, in 1937. E.W. Netherton, an American physician, described a young girl with generalized scaly dermatitis in 1958.

Incidence: Frequency is unknown; affects almost only females.

Genetic inheritance: Most likely an autosomal recessive inherited inborn error of metabolism; most often occurs in females.

Pathophysiology: Microscopically, the hairs have a squashed oval shape in cross-section and irregular diameter, mostly caused by a reduction in the content of hair sulfur and cysteine. Studies suggest that the protein gene involved in xeroderma pigmentosum group D (XPD) protein gene can lead to trichothiodystrophy.

Diagnosis: Generalized erythroderma and scaling present within the first week following birth.

Clinical aspects: Affected children present with erythroderma within 1 to 6 weeks of birth. Bamboo hair, atopic diathesis, congenital ichthyosiform erythroderma. Hypogammaglobulinemia. May be confused with atopic dermatitis but does not respond to topical corticosteroid treatment.

Precautions before anesthesia: Evaluate the severity of hypogammaglobulinemia. Ensure that no topical steroids are used (risk of depression of the adrenocortical production of steroids and of perioperative addisonian-like crisis).

Anesthetic considerations: The high risk of infection as a result of immunodeficiency must be considered. Pay special attention to the skin when positioning and securing the intravenous

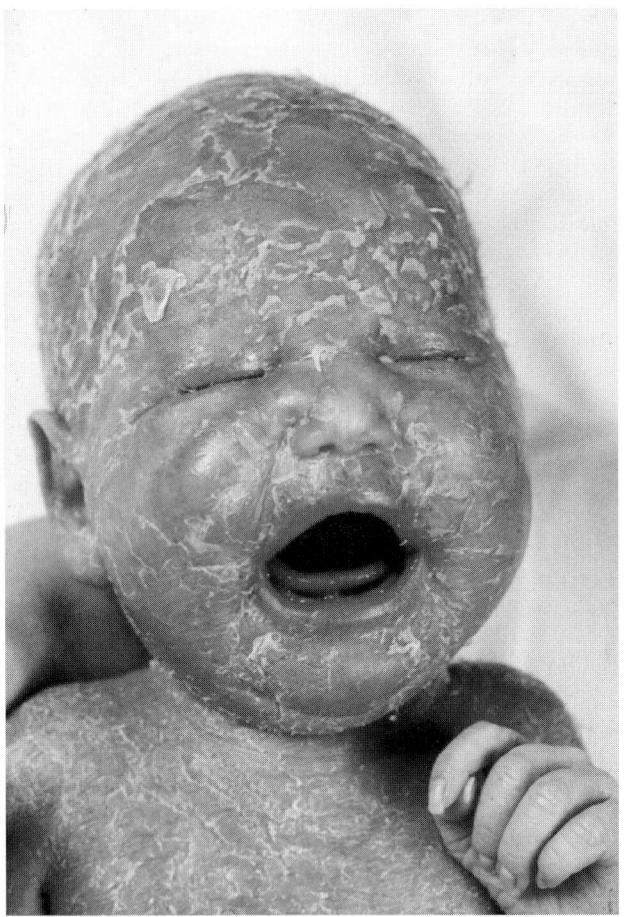

Netherton syndrome Generalized scaling of the skin of a newborn girl with Netherton syndrome.

access and monitoring devices. Temperature regulation management is essential intraoperatively. Fluid and electrolyte management must be very intensive because of excessive skin loss.

Pharmacological implications: No medications are described as harmful. However, it is recommended to avoid thiopentone in the very severe bullous form.

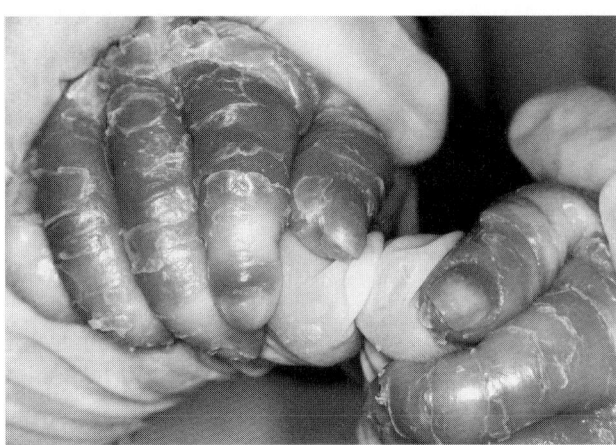

Netherton syndrome Scaling skin lesion affecting the hands of an infant with Netherton syndrome.

Other conditions to be considered:

☞**COLLODION BABY:** Inherited syndrome apparent at birth and present throughout life. The newborn is born encased in a collodion membrane that sheds within 2 weeks, revealing generalized scaling with variable redness of the skin. The clinical consequences are frequently life-threatening sepsis and dehydration by protein and electrolyte loss.

☞**X-LINKED ICHTHYOSIS (Steroid Sulfatase Deficiency Syndrome; Placental Steroid Sulfatase Deficiency Syndrome):** Characterized by onset at birth. It is defined by striking scaling more prominent on the abdomen than on the back, with an extension of scaling down the front of the leg onto the dorsum of the foot. Histologically the epidermis is atrophic in ichthyosis vulgaris and hypertrophic in the X-linked variety.

☞**SJÖGREN-LARSSON SYNDROME:** Rare inborn error of lipid metabolism, characterized by congenital ichthyosis, mental retardation, and spasticity.

☞**REFSUM SYNDROME:** Autosomal recessive genetic disorder characterized by accumulation of phytanic acid. The clinical manifestations appear around age 15 years and consist of hemeralopia (loss of vision in the dark), distal motor polyneuropathy, perceptive deafness, cerebellar ataxia, and severe mental retardation. Ichthyosis, polyepiphyseal dysplasia, myocardiopathy, elevated protein in cerebrospinal fluid, and retinitis pigmentosa may be present. Diagnosis is based on biologic evidence of phytanic acid in plasma and urine. Phytanic acid comes exclusively from food (green vegetables and herbivore animals).

☞**TRIGLYCERIDE STORAGE TYPE III:** Rare hereditary disorder characterized by severe neonatal ichthyosis, myopathy, and presence of vacuoles filled with lipids.

REFERENCE:
Kassis V, Nielsen JM, Klem-Thomsen H, et al: Familial Netherton's disease. *Cutis* 38:175, 1986.

Neurocutaneous Melanosis

At a glance: Rare skin (nevi) and meningeal pigmentation with a high risk of cutaneous or neural malignant degeneration.

Incidence: Only a few cases have been described since 1987.

Genetic inheritance: Sporadic.

Pathophysiology: Probably a developmental problem in the neural crest cells that ultimately form the skin and meninges.

Diagnosis: At birth, large pigmented nevi, usually on the trunk, buttocks, or perineum. Cerebral MRI should be done before age 4 months to detect central nervous system (CNS) involvement.

Clinical aspects: Large pigmented nevi, usually on the trunk, buttocks, or perineum. CNS function may be normal at birth, but MRI examination is necessary to exclude brain or spinal cord involvement. If the CNS is involved, thickening and pigmentation of the meninges with focal accumulation of melanotic cells or brainstem lesions is observed. Progressive pigmentation and thickening of the meninges lead to cerebral deterioration, increased intracranial pressure, mental retardation, seizures, hydrocephalus, cranial nerve palsies, and spinal cord compression.

Precautions before anesthesia: CNS involvement (especially presence of increased intracranial pressure, brainstem lesions) should be excluded by MRI and/or eye fundus examination. If neuraxial blockade is foreseen for postoperative pain management, spinal cord involvement should be excluded. In case of excision surgery, large blood loss should be foreseen.

Anesthetic considerations: In the presence of hydrocephalus, usual precautions to prevent any increase in intracranial pressure must be provided. If a spinal or epidural block is performed, the needle should not be inserted through a pigmented lesion to avoid skin coring and possible perimedullar implantation of melanocytes.

Pharmacological implications: As for any neonatal anesthesia. Patients may require repeated general anesthesia or deep sedation for dressing changes. Patients with seizure activity should have medication optimized prior to surgery or receive intraoperative intravenous supplementation.

Other condition to be considered:

GIANT NEONATAL NEVUS WITH NO CNS INVOLVEMENT: Sporadic; seems to be more frequent in Asian populations; early excision or laser therapy is performed by many medicosurgical teams for fear of malignant transformation.

REFERENCE:

Cruz MA, Cho ES, Schwartz RA, et al: Congenital neurocutaneous melanosis. *Cutis* 60:178, 1997.

Neurofibromatosis Generalisata

At a glance: Neurofibromatosis (NF) type I (NF-I), also called von Recklinghausen disease, is a rare genetic disorder characterized by the development of multiple neurofibromas of the nerves and skin. The presence of café-au-lait spots on the skin of the trunk and other regions, as well as freckling, particularly in the axillary region and in the inguinal area is characteristic of this medical condition. Often evident by age 1 year, the café-au-lait spots tend to increase in size and number over time. At birth or early childhood, plexiform neurofibromas may be present. Benign tumor-like nodules of the colored regions of the eyes (Lisch nodules) may be present. Other features include macrocephaly, seizures, scoliosis, and bowing of the lower legs.

Synonyms: *Type I:* Neurofibromatosis von Recklinghausen; Fibromatosis Molluscum Multiplex; Elephantiasis Neuromatoses.

Classification: Neurofibromatosis is more a spectrum of disorders classified as follows:

NF-I, or *peripheral NF,* is best known as von Recklinghausen neurofibromatosis (VRNF).

NF-II, or *central NF,* is bilateral acoustic neuroma NF (BANF).

NF-III appears to combine at least some features of types I and II.

NF-IV also represents a heterogeneous category (Lisch nodules in the iris are absent).

NF-V, or *segmental NF,* is restricted in its involvement of the body.

NF-VI manifests primarily as café-au-lait spots without neurofibromas.

NF-VII is a late-onset variety.

NF-NOS represents forms of NF that do not appear to fit into categories I to VII.

In a review article published in *JAMA* in 1997, Gutmann et al. seem to categorize forms other than NF-I and NF-II as *mosaic NF.* These individuals may require more detailed counseling than patients with the usual presentation.

Incidence: Approximately 1:3000 in the general population. One million patients estimated in 1987 worldwide. NF-I = 1:4000, NF-II = 1:50,000 in the general population.

Genetic inheritance: Usually autosomal dominant but heterogenic (half of probands represent new mutations). The NF-I defect is on chromosome 17q11.2, and NF-II is caused by a change in the long arm of chromosome 22. NF-I gene produces neurofibromin, which is considered a tumor suppressor gene controlling cell proliferation, differentiation, and interaction. NF-II gene produces merlin or schwannomin.

Differential diagnosis is difficult. NF-I may be associated with ☞Ehlers-Danlos syndrome, which is also situated on chromosome 17. The neurofibromatosis-Noonan syndrome is related and associated with chromosome 22 damage, as is the ☞Watson syndrome. Differential diagnosis also should be made with the proteus syndrome, ☞McCune-Albright syndrome, and multiple endocrine neoplasia type IIB.

Café-au-lait spots may appear in syndromes as different as Bannayan-Riley-Ruvalcaba, Jaffe-Campanacci, ☞LEOPARD (*l*entigines, *e*lectrocardiographic conduction abnormalities, *o*cular hypertelorism, *p*ulmonary stenosis, *a*bnormal genitalia, growth *r*etardation, and *d*eafness), and ☞Tuberous Sclerosis.

Diagnosis:

NF-I patients should have two or more of the following criteria: (A) six or more patchy hyperpigmented skin lesions called café-au-lait spots larger than 5 mm in prepuberty or larger than 15 mm after puberty; (B) two or more neurofibromas of any type or one or more plexiform neurofibromas; (C) skin-fold freckling in the axilla or groin; (D) optic pathway tumor; (E) two or more iris Lisch nodules (benign iris hamartomas); (F) a characteristic bony lesion (dysplasia of the sphenoid bone, dysplasia or thinning of long bone cortex); (G) a first-degree relative with NF-I.

NF-II patients should have (A) bilateral vestibular schwannomas visualized by MRI or (B) a parent, sibling, or child with NF-II, plus (1) unilateral vestibular schwannoma detected before age 30 years or (2) any two of the following: meningioma, glioma, schwannoma, juvenile posterior subcapsular lenticular opacity.

Clinical aspects:

NF-I presents with café-au-lait spots, multiple cutaneous or subcutaneous neurofibromas, or iris Lisch nodules, which are rare in children younger than 3 years. Nodular plexiform neurofibromas are similar to subcutaneous neurofibromas but involve nerve plexuses or dorsal nerve roots; they may grow in the mediastinum. Diffuse plexiform neurofibromas involve all skin levels and are usually hyperpigmented. Neurofibromas may appear anywhere and grow with age. They all carry a risk of functional or anatomical complication by compression or invasion. Other common findings are the following. *Skeletal anomalies:* Sphenoid wing dysplasia, early-onset and rapidly progressive thoracic scoliosis (in 10%) with kyphosis; patients with kyphoscoliosis are at high risk for cervical vertebral anomalies (e.g., dysplasia with or without paraspinal neurofibromas), which can be asymptomatic. *Vascular Anomalies:* Systemic hypertension is very frequent and caused by renal artery stenosis, pheochromocytoma, or catecholamine-secreting nodular plexiform neurofibromas. *Pheochromocytoma:* 5% of patients. *Optic Gliomas:* In 15% of patients with NF-I but only one third become symptomatic and require treatment. *Seizures:* Usually caused by a brain tumor or hydrocephalus, but no anatomical cause is found in 6% of patients. *Learning disabilities* caused by developmental delay: motor problems, hypotonia. *Pseudarthrosis* (usually of the tibia) or pathologic limb fracture in 2% of patients with NF-I. *Congenital glaucoma* is present in 0.5% of neonates with NF-I. *Increased risk* of developing certain types of malignancy: juvenile chronic myelogenous leukemia, Wilms tumor, rhabdomyosarcoma. *Short stature.* Enlarged spinal canal on CT scans is not uncommon with or without diastematomyelia. Secondary involvement of the spinal cord occurs in a variety of ways: compression by adjacent neurofibromas, vertebral collapse from neurofibroma-associated erosions, and compression from severe untreated kyphoscoliosis. Neurofibrosarcomas can occur anywhere; already established neurofibromas develop, probably most often in the large plexiform variety. Visceral nerves are also involved, and the large bowel may demonstrate a nonneurofibroma hyperganglionosis that is functionally similar to Hirschsprung disease.

NF-II is characterized by bilateral acoustic neuromas in at least 90% of patients. Café-au-lait spots are likely to be pale but larger, and usually are fewer in number than in NF-I. Neurofibromas are minimal on the skin but numerous around the vertebras. Meningiomas (intracranial and paraspinal) are frequent, unlike in NF-I, in which they are very rare. The illness may not be obvious until the second or even the fourth decade of life.

NF-III is a mixed form with the cutaneous finding of NF-I, but there is a definite and high risk for intracranial and paraspinal tumors as in NF-II (more likely schwannomas, acoustic neuromas,

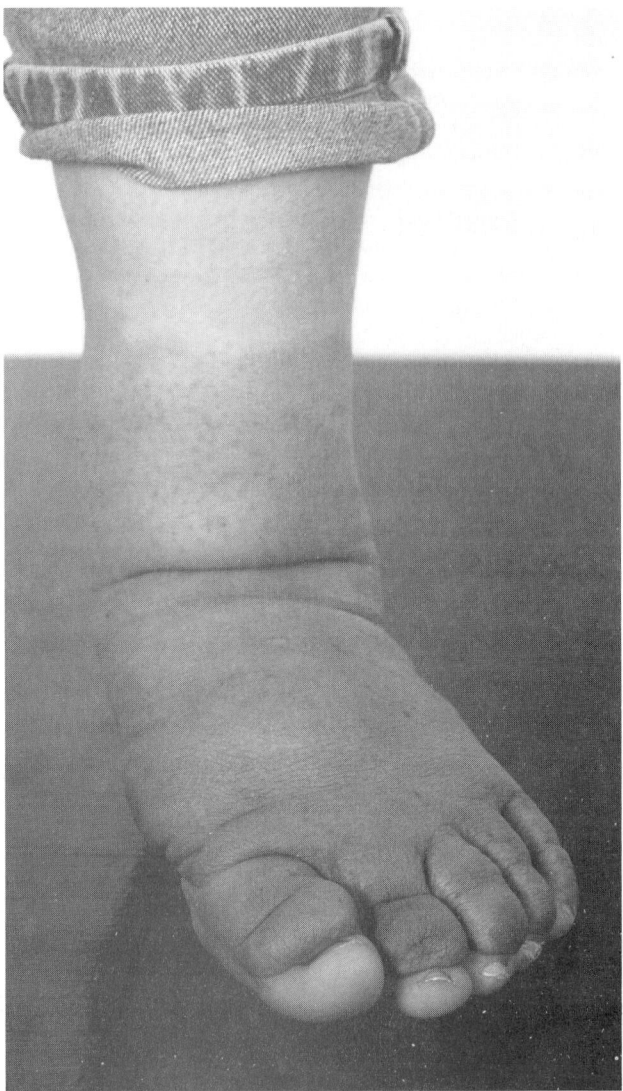

Plexiform neurofibroma   Diffuse plexiform neurofibroma with hyperpigmentation on the foot of a 12-year-old boy.

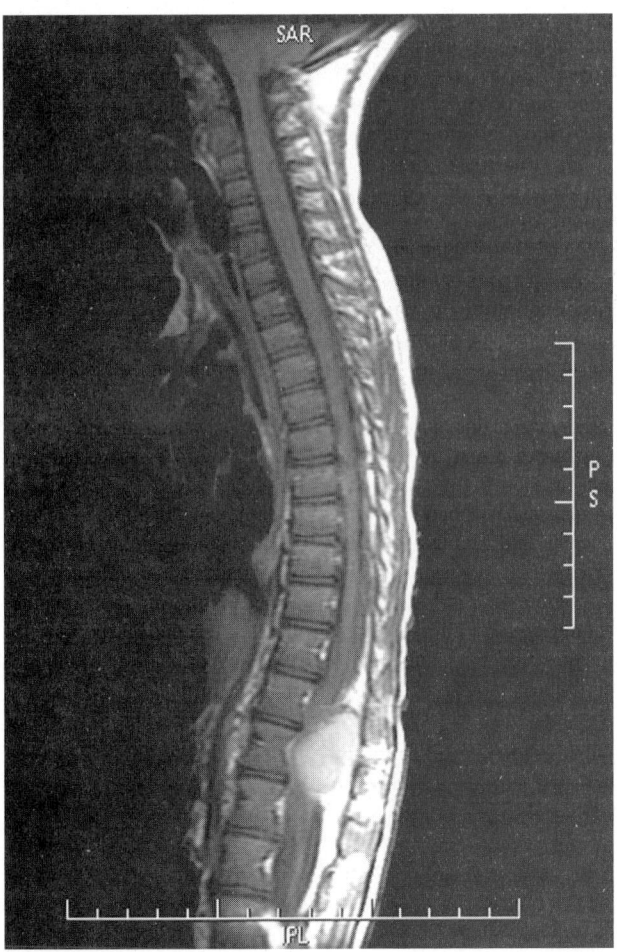

Neurofibromatosis MRI   Lumbar neurofibroma with local destruction and compression of the spinal cord in a patient with neurofibromatosis.

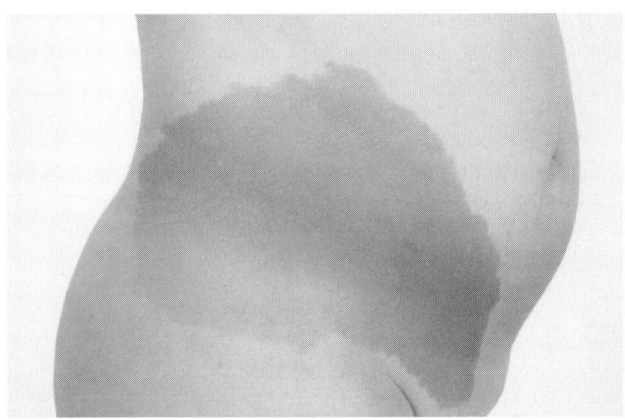

Plexiform neurofibroma   Big café-au-lait spot in an 8-year-old boy with neurofibromatosis.

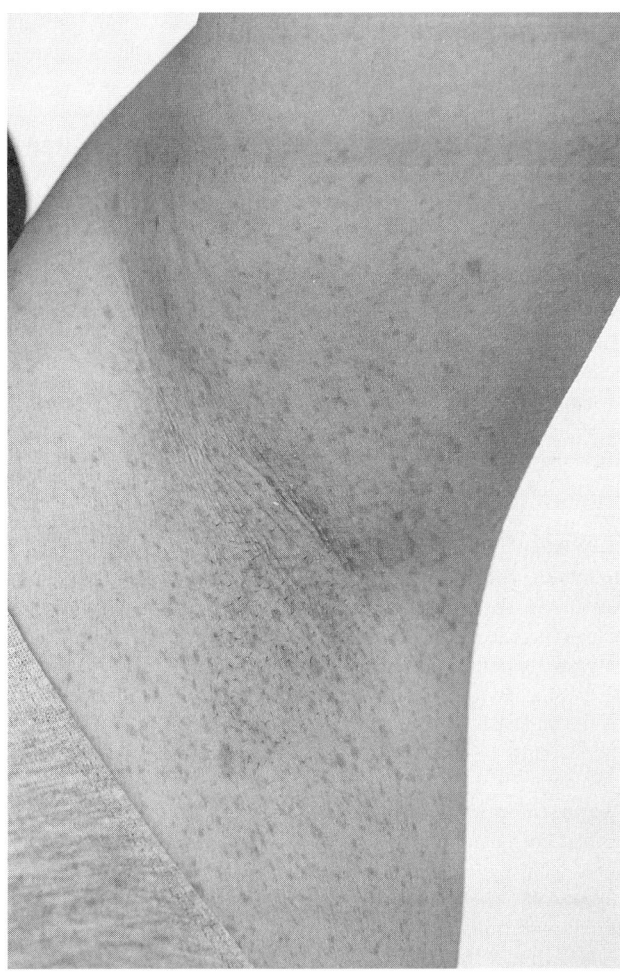

Plexiform neurofibroma   Axillary freckling in a young woman with neurofibromatosis.

and meningiomas). Iris Lisch nodules are absent. Palmar neurofibromas are characteristic for the NF-IIIa type, and the intestinal manifestations are more common in the NF-IIIb type.

Precautions before anesthesia: Prior to anesthesia, the stability of the cervical spine and the integrity of the spinal cord should be assessed to eliminate compression neuromas. Blood pressure measurements should be obtained to assess the association of a pheochromocytoma (☞Multiple Endocrine Neoplasm (MEN) IIb). Development of significant scoliosis may cause severe restrictive lung disease. Presymptomatic screening by CT scan of the brain is advocated for NF-I. MRI is more difficult to assess because 30 to 60% of NF-I patients demonstrate high-signal-intensity lesions in the basal ganglia, thalamus, cerebellum, and brainstem; however, their clinical relevance is still a matter of debate. Presymptomatic screening by MRI of the brain and cervical spine is better for patients with NF-II to search for acoustic neurofibromas, meningiomas, and glials tumors as ependymomas. Cervical spine involvement is frequent. Radiography of the chest (especially in the newborn) must be obtained to exclude the presence of a mediastinal mass. In presence of hypertension, investigate the cause (pheochromocytoma, abdominal of thoracic coarctation, renal arteries stenosis).

Anesthetic considerations: Problems with the airway in the presence of some laryngeal or pharyngeal neurofibromas have been described; face-mask ventilation, direct laryngoscopy and tracheal in-

tubation may be difficult. During direct laryngoscopy, one must remember that neck extension could lead to the possibility of cervical spine compression by intramedullary neuromas. Given the high incidence of spinal cord involvement, spinal or epidural techniques should be used only when neuroimaging has shown the absence of compressing lesions. Neuromuscular monitoring is mandatory. In case of sudden intraoperative hypertension, the presence of a pheochromocytoma should be suspected, blood sample drawn for further analysis, and therapy started as if catecholamine discharge was present.

Pharmacological implications: Some controversy exists about use of muscle relaxants because responses have been described as increased, decreased, or normal. The retrospective article by Richardson et al. suggests no dosing alterations of either succinylcholine or nondepolarizing agents.

Other conditions to be considered:

☞**MᴄCᴜɴᴇ-Aʟʙʀɪɢʜᴛ Sʏɴᴅʀᴏᴍᴇ:** Characterized by bone dysplasia and spontaneous fractures, increasing pain, and limited mobility. Other clinical features include early puberty and café-au-lait spots, hyperthyroidism, and other endocrine abnormalities.

☞**Tᴜʙᴇʀᴏᴜs Sᴄʟᴇʀᴏsɪs:** Characterized by seizures, mental retardation, developmental delays, ocular and skin lesions, and brain tumors. Onset is during infancy or early childhood. Approximately 60 to 90% of infants have café-au-lait or white hypomelanotic spots on the skin at birth. Seizures and myoclonic jerks are the most consistent symptoms and affect more than 80% of affected children. Benign periungual or subungual fibromas may be present.

☞**Pʀᴏᴛᴇᴜs Sʏɴᴅʀᴏᴍᴇ:** Characterized by abnormal and asymmetrical growth in any system of the body. Hypertrophic abnormalities of the skin, face, eyes, ears, lungs, skeletal muscles, and nerves occur. The clinical manifestations are usually present during the first year of life and may include large nevi, hemangiomas, lipomas, and lymphangiomas. Mental impairment, seizures, visual abnormalities, and pulmonary cysts are part of this medical condition.

☞**Nᴏᴏɴᴀɴ Sʏɴᴅʀᴏᴍᴇ:** Characterized by distinctive craniofacial anomalies (e.g., ocular hypertelorism, ptosis, prominent low-set ears), pterygium colli, dwarfism, characteristic abnormalities of the sternum, cryptorchidism and/or congenital heart defects (e.g., pulmonary stenosis, atrial septal defects). Other features include improper development of certain blood or lymph vessels, coagulation disorders and platelet dysfunction, and/or mental retardation. Nevi, skin lentigines, and/or café-au-lait spots help make the diagnosis. It is inherited as an autosomal dominant trait.

☞**Wᴀᴛsᴏɴ Sʏɴᴅʀᴏᴍᴇ:** Extremely rare inherited disorder characterized by café-au-lait spots, lentigines, dwarfism, pulmonary stenosis, and developmental delay. In some cases, the association of macrocephaly, limited movements of the ankles and knees, neurofibromata in certain areas of the body, and/or iris Lisch nodules must be considered. Watson syndrome has been often confused with NF-I. It results from a genetic mutation in the NF-1 gene located on the long arm of chromosome 17 (17q11.2). It is inherited as an autosomal dominant.

Nᴇᴜʀᴏꜰɪʙʀᴏᴍᴀᴛᴏsɪs-Nᴏᴏɴᴀɴ Sʏɴᴅʀᴏᴍᴇ (Quattrin McPherson Syndrome): Association of NF-I and the clinical manifestations of Noonan syndrome. Clinical features include multiple benign tumors of the nerves and skin, dwarfism, pterygium colli, muscle weakness, and/or cognitive disabilities. Congenital heart defects often seen in Noonan syndrome may be present (e.g., pulmonary valve stenosis, atrial septal defect). Whether neurofibromatosis-Noonan syndrome is a rare variant of NF-I is unclear.

REFERENCES:

Gutmann DH, Aylsworth A, Carey JC, et al: The diagnostic evaluation and multidisciplinary management of neurofibromatosis 1 and neurofibromatosis 2. *JAMA* 278:51, 1997.

Hirsch NP, Murphy A, Radcliffe JJ: Neurofibromatosis: Clinical presentations and anesthetic implications. *Br J Anaesth* 86:555, 2001.

Richardson MG, Setty GK, Rawwof SA: Responses to nondepolarizing neuromuscular blockers and succinylcholine in von Recklinghausen neurofibromatosis. *Anesth Analg* 82:382, 1996.

Neuronal Ceroid Lipofuscinoses

At a glance: Hereditary progressive neurodegenerative disorders with mental retardation, visual loss (retinitis pigmentosa), and seizures. Neuronal ceroid lipofuscinoses are probably the most common class of neurodegenerative disease in children.

Synonyms and classification: Four types of neuronal ceroid lipofuscinoses are described in the literature. They are characterized by intralysosomal accumulations of autofluorescent lipopigment in various tissues.

Type I: Infantile Neuronal Ceroid Lipofuscinosis (Finnish Infantile Neuronal Ceroid Lipofuscinosis Type; Infantile Neuronal Ceroid Lipofuscinoses; Santavuori Disease; Santavuori-Haltia Disease)

Type II: Late Infantile Neuronal Ceroid Lipofuscinosis (Jansky-Bielschowsky Disease; Late Infantile Type of Amaurotic Idiocy; Late Infantile Batten Disease): A few variants of this form of neuronal ceroid lipofuscinosis are determined by the mutation on the gene map locus 15q21-q23. Three variants have been described: (A) *neuronal ceroid lipofuscinosis variant 6,* which corresponds to mutations in the CLN6 gene; (B) *Turkish neuronal ceroid lipofuscinosis variant 8* (also called northern progressive epilepsy with mental retardation syndrome), which is caused by mutation in the CLN8 gene; and (C) *Finnish neuronal ceroid lipofuscinosis variant 5,* which is caused by mutation in the CLN5 gene.

Type III: Juvenile Neuronal Ceroid Lipofuscinosis (Infantile Batten Disease; Vogt-Spielmeyer Disease; Amaurotic Familial Idiocy of the Juvenile Type): One genetic variant of the Batten juvenile form of neuronal ceroid lipofuscinosis has been described and consists of the presence of granular osmiophilic deposits (GROD) and the absence of fingerprint curvilinear bodies. Clinically, these patients demonstrate learning disabilities beginning at ages 6 and 10 years but visual failure is delayed until age 14 years.

Type IV: Adult Neuronal Ceroid Lipofuscinosis (Kufs Disease; Autosomal Recessive Kufs Disease): Autosomal dominant form has been described for the Kufs disease and is characterized by progressive neurodegenerative diseases but absence of ocular involvement.

Incidence: 1:20,000 in the general population of Finland for early infantile and juvenile forms to 1:150,000 in the general population.

Genetic inheritance: All neuronal ceroid lipofuscinoses are autosomal recessive and are genetically independent.

Pathophysiology: Precise pathogenesis and etiology of this group of diseases are elusive. The common defect underlying all neuronal ceroid lipofuscinoses affects lysosomal function characterized by intralysosomal accumulation of an autofluorescent lipopigment in the perikaryon of different neuronal cell types in granula, curvilinear, or fingerprint patterns. Clinically, this results in a profound degenera-

tive impact on the central nervous system. In addition to the diseases outlined, numerous atypical variants indicated in the classification of neuronal ceroid lipofuscinoses account for approximately 10 to 20% of patients. Several eponymous names are associated with these disorders, which are sometimes collectively known as *Batten disease.*

Diagnosis: Young patients with gradual onset of blindness and neurologic signs, retinitis pigmentosa, and epilepsy should be examined for neuronal ceroid lipofuscinosis. Urinary dolichol level is raised, and biopsy of the skin or conjunctiva demonstrates characteristic lipofuscin storage.

Clinical aspects: The early juvenile form results in death within the first decade of life. The later-onset forms are associated with dementia and a slower decline.

Precautions before anesthesia: Thorough history and physical examination should reveal the extent of the disorder. Of particular note to the anesthesiologist is the presence of epilepsy. A thorough history of medication use is necessary because these patients may be on long-term anticonvulsant therapy or psychotropic medication.

Anesthetic considerations: No specific indications or contraindications for specific anesthetic techniques. However, in the face of neurointellectual impairment, awake regional techniques may be inappropriate. The presence of microcephaly with history of developmental delay or regression of neurologic development should indicate need to reduce anesthetic doses. Seizure medications must be supplemented intravenously during the surgical procedure.

Pharmacological implications: Carefully select anticonvulsant agents. Proconvulsant agents probably are contraindicated for patients with this condition, whether or not they have a history of convulsions. The use of sevoflurane should be done cautiously.

Other conditions to be considered:

☞**ALPERS DISEASE:** Usually characterized by a clinical triad of psychomotor retardation and mental deterioration; intractable epilepsy; and liver failure in infants and young children. The illness usually begins in early life with severe convulsions unresponsive to anticonvulsant drug therapy (intractable epilepsy). Progressive neurologic disorder characterized by spasticity, myoclonus, and dementia. Status epilepticus is often the terminating development. Definitive diagnosis is shown by postmortem examination of the brain and liver.

☞**RETT SYNDROME:** Rare progressive neurologic disorder that occurs only in females. Affected children appear to develop normally until approximately 6 to 18 months of age, at which time a dramatic change in development is noticeable, even signs of regression become obvious. Other clinical features include a stop of calvarium and brain development leading to microcephaly by age 1 year. As the disorder progresses, stereotypical hand movements (e.g., rubbing and "hand washing") are characteristic of this medical condition. Hyperventilation, seizure episodes, and progressive loss of additional motor abilities can be present.

☞**GANGLIOSIDOSIS TYPE II:** Heritable lysosomal storage disorder with ganglioside accumulation leading to severe neurologic impairment and premature death.

☞**LEIGH SYNDROME:** Severe progressive necrotizing encephalopathy caused by a mitochondrial disorder impeding oxidative phosphorylation.

VARIANT JANSKI BIELSCHOWSKI SYNDROME (Lake and Cavanagh Disease): Onset is between 4 and 5 years of age, with mild motor rand mental problems; myoclonias, seizures, and visual loss occur before age 10 years. Death after 20 years.

REFERENCES:

Goebel HH: The neuronal ceroid-lipofuscinoses. *J Child Neurol* 10:424, 1995.

Mole SE: Recent advances in the molecular genetics of the neuronal ceroid lipofuscinoses. *J Inherit Metab Dis* 19:269, 1996.

Description of individual types of neuronal ceroid lipofuscinoses:

HALTIA-SANTAVUORI SYNDROME

At a glance: Hypotonia, seizures, and visual loss beginning between 3 and 18 months of age.

Genetic inheritance: Gene maps on locus 1p32, coding for the lysosomal glycoprotein palmitoyl-thioesterase.

Clinical aspects: Onset between 3 and 18 months of age, with hypotonia, microcephaly, myoclonic seizures, intellectual and psychomotor retardation, and progressive loss of vision caused by macular degeneration before age 2 years. Stereotyped movements of the hands. Cerebellar ataxia is prominent. Electroencephalogram (EEG) tracing rapidly becomes isoelectric ("vanishing EEG"). Cerebral and cerebellar atrophy and thalamic hypodensity on MRI. Death between 5 and 10 years of age.

JANSKI BIELSCHOWSKI SYNDROME

At a glance: Dementia, seizures, and visual loss beginning between the ages of 2 and 4 years.

Incidence and genetic inheritance: Most common in Newfoundland, Canada. Gene map locus is 11p15.5, coding for a lysosomal peptidase.

Clinical aspects: Onset between the ages of 2 and 4 years, presenting with myoclonic seizures, rapid mental deterioration, quadriparesis, dementia, and ataxia. Cerebellar dysfunction is more severe than in Vogt-Spielmeyer syndrome. Retinal degeneration in these patients is most pronounced in the area of the macula but also affects the rest of the retina, resulting in blindness. Optic nerve atrophy is remarkable.

REFERENCES:

Andermann E, Jakob JS, Carpenter S, et al: The Newfoundland aggregate of neuronal ceroid-lipofuscinosis. *Am J Med Genet* 5(suppl):111, 1988.

Haines JL, Boustany RMN, Alroy J, et al: Chromosomal localization of two genes underlying late infantile neuronal ceroid lipofuscinosis. *Neurogenetics* 1:217, 1998.

VOGT-SPIELMEYER SYNDROME

At a glance: Rapid, progressive deterioration of vision and a slower but progressive deterioration of the intellect. Lack of motor control, psychotic behavior, and seizures develop later, with onset at about 10 years of age.

Genetic inheritance: Gene map locus is 16p12.1-11.2.

Clinical aspects: Compared to the other forms, onset is later, at around 10 years of age. It is characterized by rapid and progressive deterioration of vision (because of tapetoretinal degeneration with retinal atrophy) and slower and progressive intellectual deterioration (progressive dementia, cerebellar disturbances, seizures, psychomotor regression, psychosis, and brain atrophy). Prenatal diagnosis on chorionic villus samples is possible. Accumulation of an autofluorescent lipopigment has been found not only in the perikaryon of different neuronal cell types but also in extraneuronal

cells. Vacuolization of lymphocytes is another finding in these patients, affecting up to two thirds of lymphocytes. Myoclonic fitting is less prominent in the later-onset group, but dystonic posturing and antisocial activity are more pronounced features.

REFERENCES:

Kimura S, Goebel HH: Light and electron microscopic study of juvenile neuronal ceroid-lipofuscinosis lymphocytes. *Pediatr Neurol* 4:148, 1988.

Wisnieswski KE, Kida E, Patxot OF, et al: Variability in the clinical and pathological findings in the neuronal ceroid lipofuscinoses: Review of data and observations. *Am J Med Genet* 42:525, 1992.

KUFS DISEASE

At a glance: Very rare disorder marked initially by progressive muscle weakness with ataxia, generalized seizures, chorea athetosis, and rarely blindness. It is linked to excess accumulations of lipofuscins throughout the central nervous system.

Incidence: Estimated to be 2–4:100,000 live births in the United States. The prevalence of this medical condition appears more frequently in northern Europe (Finland, Sweden) than in other international regions.

Genetic inheritance: Inherited disorder; either autosomal recessive (Kufs disease) or autosomal dominant form often known as a variant of Kufs disease and called Parry disease. Recessive form is more serious than the dominant form.

Pathophysiology: This medical entity is often considered a variant of the juvenile neuronal ceroid lipofuscinosis. However, it is known to have an onset age between 20 and 32 years. Symptoms are the result of excessive accumulation of lipofuscins in the brains.

Clinical aspects: Confusion, stupor, or psychotic behavior may be the initial symptoms manifested by the individual. Mental retardation and generalized convulsions follow. Patients affected with this medical entity also present ichthyosis vulgaris that results from excess production and/or retention of keratin.

REFERENCES:

Chou SM, Thomson HG: Electron microscopy of storage cytosomes in Kuf's disease. *Arch Neurol* 23:489, 1970.

Kufs H: Ueber eine Spätform der amaurotischen Idiotie und ihre heredofamiliären Grundlagen. *Z Ges Neurol Psychiat* 95:169, 1925.

Nezelof Syndrome

At a glance: Extremely rare severe immune deficiency disorder characterized by T-cell deficiency with little or no abnormality of γ-globulin. Clinical features include failure to thrive, recurrent lung infections, and metaphyseal dysostosis.

Synonyms: Immune Defect Resulting from Absence of Thymus; Severe Combined Immunodeficiency, Nezelof Type.

History: Genetic disorder first reported by C. Nezelof, a French pediatrician, in 1964.

Genetic inheritance: Autosomal recessive inheritance; some X-linked reports.

Pathophysiology: Abnormal expression of CD44 (an adhesion molecule, interacting with the matrix ligands hyaluronan and fibronectin) could interfere with normal thymocyte and thymic epithelial interaction, leading to abnormal thymocyte differentiation.

Diagnosis: Clinically evocated in patients with recurrent infections and normal humoral immunity.

Clinical aspects: Failure to thrive is common. Main clinical features can include metaphyseal dysostosis, chronic diarrhea, hepatosplenomegaly, eczematoid rash, and pyoderma. Recurrent pseudomonas and monilia infections are frequent, particularly bronchopulmonary infections. Bronchiectasis and emphysema are often observed. Susceptibility to viral infections. Immunologic features are remarkable: absent thymus, T-cell deficiency, impaired antibody synthesis, cellular immune defect, decreased lymphoid tissue while plasma cells are present, impaired delayed hypersensitivity with poor skin graft rejection. Humoral immunity is normal, as is the immunoglobulin level. Lymphopenia is observed.

Precautions before anesthesia: Evaluate immunologic status (obtain full, documented history of infection, complete immunologic status evaluation). Evaluate respiratory function (clinical, chest radiographs/CT, pulmonary function test, arterial blood gas analysis). Evaluate hydration and renal function in case of severe chronic diarrhea (clinical, laboratory tests, including urea and creatinine levels and electrolytes). Preoperative full blood count is recommended.

Anesthetic considerations: Strict asepsis is needed considering the immunity defect. Preoperative hydration correction might be necessary preoperatively. Perioperative respiratory monitoring and physiotherapy can be useful, and postoperative mechanical ventilatory support may be anticipated if necessary.

Pharmacological implications: Prophylactic antibiotics may be adapted to immunologic status and previous infections.

Other conditions to be considered:

BRUTON AGAMMAGLOBULINEMIA TYROSINE KINASE X-LINKED: Tonsillar system is absent.

SWISS-TYPE AGAMMAGLOBULINEMIA: Thymus and tonsillar system are absent.

☞DiGEORGE SYNDROME: Parathyroids and thymus are absent.

REFERENCES:

Knutsen AP, Wall D, Mueller KR, et al: Abnormal in vitro thymocyte differentiation in a patient with severe combined immunodeficiency—Nezelof's syndrome. *J Clin Immunol* 16:151, 1996.

Nezelof C, Jammet M-L, Lortholary P, et al: L'hypoplasie hereditaire du thymus: sa place et sa responsabilite dans une observation d'aplasie lymphocytaire, normoplasmocytaire et normoglobulinemique du nourrisson. *Arch Fr Pediatr* 21:897, 1964.

Niemann-Pick Disease

At a glance: Group of rare inherited disorders of fat metabolism. Clinical features include jaundice, progressive loss of motor skills, feeding difficulties, learning disabilities, and hepatosplenomegaly. Lysosomal storage disorder caused by a defect in sphingolipid metabolism and involving brain and/or viscera. There are five types of Newman-Pick disease.

Synonyms: Lipid Histiocytosis; Sphingomyelinase Deficiency.

Classification: Disorders of sphingomyelin storage were initially grouped together under the eponym Niemann-Pick disease and classified as A, B, C, D, E, and F. However, only types A and B are deficient in sphingomyelinase; types C and D are biochemically and genetically different. Types E and F are not well described. A new nomenclature has been proposed that groups types A and B as type I

and types C and D as type II, but this is not yet universally adopted. *Types A and B:* Deficiency in sphingomyelinase. *Types C and D:* Basic defect not yet identified.

Genetic inheritance: Autosomal recessive.

Types A and B: The gene for lysosomal sphingomyelinase is located on chromosome 11p15.1-p15.4. Three mutations have been identified in Ashkenazi Jews carrying type A. Other mutations cause type B phenotype and are found in southern Europe and in the Mediterranean region.

Types C and D: The NPC1 gene on chromosome 18q11-12 is Niemann-Pick disease type C1 gene (found worldwide) and mutated in type D (called Nova Scotia variant because of the high incidence in the province of Nova Scotia, Canada); another gene, NPC2, has been identified.

Pathophysiology: *Types A and B:* Sphingomyelin accumulates in the brain, viscera, and reticuloendothelial system. *Types C and D:* Still unknown but there is accumulation of unesterified cholesterol and glucosylceramide in lysosomes. Sphingomyelinase activity is normal in most tissues but is partially deficient in fibroblasts. In the brain, this anomaly leads to swelling of the proximal neurite segment in the cerebral cortex and accumulation of paired helical filaments, as reported in Alzheimer disease.

Diagnosis: Sphingomyelinase assay in leukocytes or in fibroblasts shows residual activity that tends to be higher in type B than in type A. Cultured fibroblasts obtained from skin biopsy allow staining with filipin to demonstrate accumulated cholesterol.

Clinical aspects:

Type A: Infantile type. Sphingomyelin accumulates mainly in the brain. Starts with feeding difficulties, hepatomegaly. Respiratory infections are common, with a chest radiograph similar to that seen in miliary tuberculosis. Neurologic deterioration in the second part of the first year of life, with loss of contact, hypotonia, and spastic paresis. In 50% of cases, a cherry-red spot is seen in the macula; it is a normal macula surrounded with grayish-colored retina caused by storage compounds. Vacuolized lymphocytes are found in the blood, and foam cells are present in the bone marrow. Anemia and thrombocytopenia are late signs. Death usually occurs by age 3 years. No treatment available.

Type B: Chronic form. Unlike type A, sphingomyelin accumulates mainly in the viscera and reticuloendothelial system. It presents as hepatosplenomegaly or splenomegaly after the infancy period. Liver involvement may lead to cirrhosis and hypersplenism to pancytopenia. Chronic pulmonary involvement as a result of macrophage infiltration in alveolar septa leads to impairment of gas diffusion and eventually cor pulmonale. Hypercholesterolemia is often present. Ataxia, retinal problems, and mild mental retardation may appear in childhood, adolescence, or adulthood.

Type C: Neonatal conjugated hyperbilirubinemia in half of the cases; sometimes a clinical picture of acute fatal hepatitis. Onset of neurologic symptoms may occur at any time during childhood. Early onset, during the second year of life, is characteristic of the severe form, which also presents with hepatosplenomegaly. In the juvenile form, early onset of upward and downward paralysis of the gaze and cataplexy (sudden loss of tone associated with laughter). Seizures. Cerebellar ataxia, dementia, dystonia. Death usually occurs in the second decade of life. Experimental treatment with hypocholesterolemic agents are investigated. Foam cells and specific sea-blue cells in the bone marrow.

Type D: Neonatal hyperbilirubinemia. Neurologic signs start during the second half of the first decade of life.

Precautions before anesthesia: Check blood count and platelets to exclude pancytopenia; check liver function tests; check radiographs and oxygen saturation while breathing room air for pulmonary involvement. Maintain anticonvulsant therapy up to day of surgery. Whether early atheromatosis is present is not known.

Anesthetic considerations: Hepatosplenomegaly may impair gastric emptying; the child should be considered as a full stomach situation. Hepatosplenomegaly can be severe enough to impair ventilation, especially in the young patient.

Pharmacological implications: No specific implications except in case of hepatic failure or cirrhosis.

Other conditions to be considered:

☞**SEA-BLUE HISTIOCYTOSIS SYNDROME:** Characterized by the presence of sea-blue histiocytes in the bone marrow and a cholesterol ester storage disease. Cirrhosis, hepatomegaly, and macular degeneration are associated features. However, impairment of the central venous system is minimal.

☞**GAUCHER DISEASE:** Rare inherited lipid storage disease characterized by bone deterioration, hepatosplenomegaly, and anemia. Most often presents with abdominal distention caused by enlargement of the internal organs. Type II Gaucher disease presents with catatonia.

☞**REFSUM SYNDROME:** Slowly progressive rare disorder of fat metabolism, characterized by retinitis pigmentosa, peripheral neuropathy, ataxia, and increased cerebrospinal fluid protein concentration.

TAY-SACHS DISEASE (☞**Gangliosidosis Type II):** Rare inherited disorder resulting in progressive destruction of the central nervous system. Caused by the absence of the enzyme hexosaminidase A. Generally found in children of Eastern European Jewish heritage. Clinical symptoms include abnormal startle reflex, hypotonia, restlessness, and nystagmus.

REFERENCES:

Barth PG: Disorders of sphingolipid metabolism, in Fernades J, Saudubray J-M, van den Berghe G (eds): *Inborn Metabolic Diseases.* 3rd ed. Berlin, Springer, 2000, p 400.

Bujok L-S, Bujok G, Knapik P: Niemann-Pick disease: Rare problem in anaesthesiological practice. *Paediatr Anaesth* 12:806, 2002.

Nonketotic Hyperglycinemia

At a glance: Inborn error of metabolism that leads to isolated hyperglycinemia.

Synonyms: Glycine Encephalopathy; Glycinemia.

Incidence: 1:250,000 live births; most cases are from Finland (1:12,000 live births).

Genetic inheritance: Autosomal recessive.

Pathophysiology: Defect in enzymes of the hepatic glycine cleavage system leads to accumulation of glycine. The system is composed of four mitochondrial proteins known as P, H, T, and L, and catalyzes the transformation of glycine in CO_2, ammonia, and hydroxymethyltetrahydrofolic acid. Elevation of glycine levels in the brain is thought to be responsible for the clinical symptoms of the disease: glycine is an inhibitory neurotransmitter at the level of the brainstem and spinal cord but has excitatory effects on the cerebral cortex.

Diagnosis: Elevated levels of glycine in plasma, cerebrospinal fluid, and urine with no ketosis. Defect of enzyme system may be demonstrated in liver biopsy specimen or prenatally in cultured chorionic villi.

Clinical aspects: Three clinical presentations exist.

Neonatal Type: Most common presentation. After a few days (rarely more than 48 hours), the neonate presents with rapidly progressing neurologic symptoms: hypotonia, apneic attacks, seizures, lethargy, or coma. Seizures range from myoclonic to grand mal convulsions and are often accompanied by hiccup. A characteristic burst-suppression pattern is seen on electroencephalogram (EEG) during the first month and is later replaced by hypsarrhythmia. Death frequently occurs during infancy or childhood. Survivors have mental retardation, myoclonus, seizures, and microcephaly.

Late-Inset Type: Nonspecific neurologic symptoms develop during infancy to adolescence.

Transient Neonatal Type: High neonatal plasma and cerebrospinal fluid (CSF) levels of glycine return to normal after a few weeks. Immaturity of one of the components of the glycine cleavage system is postulated to be the cause of this transient disease.

There is no effective treatment. Antagonists of N-methyl-D-aspartate (NMDA) receptors, such as oral ketamine (8 mg/kg/day) or dextromethorphan, have been used with some success. Oral benzoate (500–750 mg/kg/day) complexes with glycine to form hippuric acid, which undergoes renal elimination. Benzodiazepines are indicated for seizures.

Precautions before anesthesia: Ensure adequate hydration and calorific intake. Assess neurologic status.

Anesthetic considerations: Surgery may be associated with acute deterioration. Adequate hydration and caloric input should be maintained perioperatively.

Pharmacological implications: Ketamine appears to be a good choice because of its NMDA receptor antagonist properties.

Other condition to be considered:

OHTAHARA SYNDROME: Congenital epileptiform encephalopathy with typical EEG pattern of burst-break suppression awake and asleep. Onset in the first month of life; frequent tonic seizures and severe developmental delay; poor prognosis; usual evolution to infantile spasms.

REFERENCES:

Sami KA: Non-ketotic hyperglycinaemias. *Can Anaesth Soc J* 27:79, 1980.

Tada K: Nonketotic hyperglycinemia, in Fernades J, Saudubray J-M, van den Berghe G (eds): *Inborn Metabolic Diseases.* 3rd ed. Berlin, Springer, 2000, p 254.

Noonan Syndrome

At a glance: Rare genetic disorder present at birth. Characterized by distinctive facial appearance, broad or webbed neck, low hairline in the back of the head, and short stature. Micrognathia, kyphosis and/or scoliosis, and cardiac defects (pulmonary valvular stenosis) are present. Other features include coagulation disorders, platelet deficiencies, mild mental retardation, and cryptorchidism in the first year of life.

Synonym: Turner-like Syndrome.

Nature: Rare genetic disorder. Noonan syndrome is phenotypically similar to Turner syndrome; however, the karyotype in Noonan syndrome is normal.

Incidence: 1:1000–2500 live births.

Genetic inheritance: Autosomal dominant with variable phenotypic expression. Genes have been identified on loci 12q22-qter and 12q24. Sporadic cases arise as a result of sporadic mutations.

Pathophysiology: Unknown. An abnormality of tissue migration in utero is suggested, and the presence of cystic hygromas and lymphedema is cited as evidence supporting this hypothesis.

Diagnosis: Clinical features of Turner syndrome associated with pulmonary valve dysplasia and a normal karyotype.

Clinical aspects: *Neonate:* Marked edema with excess nuchal skin; *Infancy:* Hypotonia, poor feeding.

Features of the Noonan phenotype are webbed neck with low posterior hairline, pterygium colli, flattened midface, cystic hygroma, pectus carinatum or excavatum, short stature (50%), high-arched palate, ptosis, hypertelorism, down-slanting palpebral fissures, dental malocclusion, micrognathia, strabismus, cryptorchidism, mental retardation (25%), kyphoscoliosis, and several skeletal abnormalities (spina bifida occulta, hemivertebra, narrow spinal canal, cubitus valgus). Approximately 50% of patients have a cardiac problem. The most common cardiac anomalies are pulmonary stenosis, hypertrophic cardiomyopathy, atrial septal defect, tetralogy of Fallot, atrioventricular canal anomaly, and coarctation of the aorta. Stature is short. Lymphedema may occur. Coagulopathy is frequent and most commonly caused by factor XI deficiency, although thrombocytopenia and deficiencies of factors XII and VIII are well described.

Precautions before anesthesia: Careful history to evaluate cardiac and respiratory function. Careful airway assessment for potentially difficult laryngoscopy and tracheal intubation. Electroencephalogram, and echocardiography to assess cardiac function/anatomy must be obtained. Cervical spine radiography to exclude atlantoaxial instability and any other anomaly is highly recommended. Lumbosacral spine radiograph if a neuraxial block is foreseen must be done to exclude vertebral anomalies. Consider chest radiograph and pulmonary function tests in presence of severe kyphoscoliosis. Laboratory investigation for coagulopathy is mandatory if regional techniques are under consideration. Continue perioperative medications, especially if taking beta-blocker for hypertrophic obstructive cardiomyopathy.

Anesthetic considerations: Short or webbed neck, micrognathia, and dental malocclusion may make direct laryngoscopy and tracheal intubation difficult. Anesthetic management according to cardiac malformation. Regional techniques have been used but require careful assessment of cardiac function, coagulation, and vertebral anatomy.

Pharmacological implications: Isoflurane may cause undesirable tachycardia. Esmolol may be useful in the presence of hypertrophic obstructive cardiomyopathy.

Other conditions to be considered:

☞**WATSON SYNDROME:** Rare disease combining pulmonary valvular stenosis with café-au-lait spots, dull intelligence, and short stature. Other features include macrocephaly and iris Lisch nodules in most cases, a condition that overlaps those of neurofibromatosis and the Noonan syndrome.

☞**LEOPARD SYNDROME:** Complex congenital dysmorphogenetic disorder associating mainly skin lesions (*l*entigines, multiple), *e*lectrocardiographic conduction abnormalities, *o*cular hypertelorism, *p*ulmonary stenosis, *a*bnormal genitalia, *r*etardation of growth, and *d*eafness (sensorineural).

☞**COSTELLO SYNDROME:** Syndrome characterized by postnatal growth deficiency, coarse facies, redundant skin on the neck, acanthosis nigricans, developmental delay, and papillomata.

☞**REYNOLDS NERI HERMANN SYNDROME:** Characterized by unusually sparse, brittle, curly hair, macrocephaly, prominent forehead with abnormal narrowing of the sides of the forehead (temporal constriction), mental retardation, failure to thrive, congenital heart defect, short stature, and ectodermal abnormalities.

NOONAN-LIKE MULTIPLE GIANT CELL LESION SYNDROME: Rare disorder characterized by giant cells lesions within bone and soft tissue of the jaw; the presence of "freckle-like" spots on the skin (lentigines), pulmonary valve stenosis, and dwarfism. Other features include ocular hypertelorism, abnormally prominent, improperly positioned ears, pterygium colli, and cubitus valgus. Occurs sporadically as a consequence of new genetic mutations.

QUATTRIN MCPHERSON SYNDROME (Neurofibromatosis Noonan Syndrome): Same clinical features as reported for Noonan syndrome, except with characteristic facial appearance (macrosomia), developmental delay, and dysmorphism in presence of neurofibromatosis. Rare. First reported in 1987.

REFERENCES:

Campbell A, Bousfield J: Anesthesia in a patient with Noonan's syndrome and cardiomyopathy. *Anesthesia* 47:131, 1992.

Grange C, Heid R, Lucas S, et al: Anesthesia in a parturient with Noonan's syndrome. *Can J Anaesth* 45:332, 1998.

Lee CK, Chang BS, Hong YM, et al: Spinal deformities in Noonan syndrome. A clinical review of sixty cases. *J Bone Joint Surg Am* 83:1495, 2001.

Norrie Disease

At a glance: Rare inherited neurodevelopmental disorder characterized by congenital bilateral blindness. Other features can include mental retardation, mild-to-profound hearing loss, and cataracts during early infancy. Phthisis bulbi (shrinking of the eye) has been reported.

Synonyms: Anderson-Warburg Syndrome; Fetal Iritis Syndrome; Whitnall-Norman Syndrome; Atrophia Bulborum Hereditaria; Congenital Progressive Oculo-Acoustico-Cerebral Degeneration; Norrie-Warburg Syndrome; Norrie Syndrome; Episkopi Blindness.

History: Norrie disease has been described in patients of various ethnical backgrounds (White, Hispanic, Sri Lankan, Asian, and Canadian Indian).

Incidence: One hundred cases have been described. Clinical expression almost exclusively in males.

Genetic inheritance: X-linked recessive disorder. Rare reports of presumed manifesting heterozygote females exist. The Norrie disease gene is located on the short arm of chromosome X (Xp11.4). It consists of three exons and encodes for a protein named norrin.

Pathophysiology: Unknown.

Diagnosis: Based on clinical features, mode of inheritance, and genetic testing.

Clinical aspects: Characterized by microphthalmia with bilateral degeneration of the retina and vitreous humor leading to early blindness, usually within the first weeks of life. Characteristic ocular findings include retinal detachment, vitreous hemorrhage, and formation of retrolental masses. Pupils are dilated with no light reflex. Cataracts. Phthisis bulbi (shrinkage of the eyeball) develops over the first decade of life. In approximately one third of Norrie disease patients, progressive sensorineural hearing loss occurs, with age at onset varying from a few months of life to adulthood. Some degree of mental retardation is frequent (up to 50% of patients), although many individuals have normal intellectual capabilities. Several individuals with complex syndromic anomalies have been described in whom Norrie disease was part of the clinical findings. Associated anomalies in these cases included hypogonadism, increased susceptibility to infections, skeletal malformations, and a combination of facial features, including hypotelorism, narrow nasal bridge, thin upper lip, and large ears.

Precautions before anesthesia: No literature describing anesthetic experiences in Norrie disease patients. However, adequate anxiolysis is particularly important in patients with deafness and mental retardation.

Anesthetic considerations: Known features of Norrie disease do not suggest an increased risk of anesthesia.

Pharmacological implications: Submicroscopic deletions in the monoamine oxidase (MAO) loci have been described in Norrie disease patients. Although some of these individuals had normal MAO activities, a few were shown to have reduced to nondetectable MAO activity. It seems prudent to minimize drugs associated with an increased risk of adverse reactions when combined with MAO inhibitors such as meperidine.

Other conditions to be considered:

X-linked Familial Exudative Vitreoretinopathy (FEVR): Disorder linked to mutations on the Norrie disease gene. Unlike Norrie disease, FEVR is not associated with hearing loss or mental retardation.

☞**Coat Disease:** Extremely rare disorder characterized by dilation of the retinal blood vessels resulting in vitreous hemorrhages. Retinal detachment has been reported. Leukokoria (white membrane or mass behind the lens) may develop.

☞**Usher Syndrome:** Characterized by hearing loss, retinitis pigmentosa, and progressive blindness.

REFERENCES:

Collins FA, Murphy DL, Reiss AL, et al: Clinical, biochemical, and neuropsychiatric evaluation of a patient with contiguous gene syndrome due to a microdeletion Xp11.3 including the Norrie disease locus and monoamine oxidase (MAOA and MAOB) genes. *Am J Med Genet* 42:127, 1992.

Goodyear HM, Sonsken PM, McConachie H: Norrie's disease: A prospective study of development. *Arch Dis Child* 64:1587, 1989.

Shastry BS, Hiraoka M, Trese DC, et al: Norrie Disease and exudative vitreoretinopathy in families with affected female carriers. *Eur J Ophthalmol* 9:238, 1999.

Nyssen-van Bogaert Syndrome

At a glance: Rare genetic disorder with blindness, deafness, developmental delay, and spasticity.

Synonyms: Nyssen-Van Bogaert-Meyer Syndrome; Opticocochleodentate Degeneration.

Incidence and genetic inheritance: Fewer than 20 cases reported; most likely an autosomal recessive transmitted disease.

Clinical aspects: Dentate nucleus and medial lemniscal structures degenerate, and the patients present in infancy with muscular hypotonia or atonia, which changes in childhood to rigidity and spasticity quadriplegia. Patients are mentally retarded. Blindness occurs secondary to optic nerve atrophy and sensorineural deafness secondary to cochlear degeneration. Death usually occurs before age 10 years.

Anesthetic considerations: Communication with these patients may be difficult (blind, deaf, mentally retarded) and behavioral compliance decreased. Consequently, anxiolytic premedication may be helpful. However, presence of the primary caregiver at the bedside during induction of anesthesia may be even more helpful. Chest radiograph should be obtained preoperatively because recurrent pneumonias secondary to aspiration are common.

Pharmacological implications: Succinylcholine should not be used to avoid a hyperkalemic response.

REFERENCES:

Meyer JE: Über eine kombinierte Systemerkrankung in Klein-Mittel- und Endhirn. *Arch Psychiat Nervenkr* 182:731, 1949.

Nyssen R, van Bogaert L: La dégénérescence systématisée optico-cochléo-dentelée. *Rev Neurol* 2:321, 1934.

O

Oculocerebral with Hypopigmentation Syndrome

At a glance: Extremely rare inherited disorder that may be apparent at birth (congenital) or during early infancy. It is characterized by hypopigmentation of the skin, silvery-gray hair, and abnormalities of the central nervous system that affect the eyes (microphthalmia) and the oculocerebral functional areas.

Synonyms: Cross Syndrome; Kramer Syndrome; Depigmentation-Gingival Fibromatosis-Microphthalmia Syndrome.

Incidence and genetic inheritance: Believed to be inherited as an autosomal recessive genetic trait. Affects males and females equally. However, fewer than 15 cases have been reported in the medical literature. Most of the observed cases occurred within families.

Clinical aspects: Abnormally small eyes, lack of skin and characteristic hair color are usually congenital and therefore apparent at birth. The skin is usually very light and may be extremely sensitive to exposure to the sun. The hair is often silvery or silvery-gray at birth. In addition, infants may be abnormally sensitive to light (photosensitivity). Later during infancy, neurologic abnormalities (e.g., athetoid movements, ataxia, movement of the head beyond the normal range of motion [hyperextension], and increased muscle rigidity or spasticity) may become apparent after age 3 months. In more severe cases, children may experience lack of voluntary movements of the arms and legs (spastic tetraplegia). Other neurologic symptoms may include exaggerated reflexes and/or joint immobility. The legs, arms, shoulders, and hips are most often involved. Affected individuals may have a high-pitched cry or make constant sucking sounds. Patients may exhibit mental retardation and growth retardation, and psychomotor development is often delayed (e.g., holding up the head, sitting, walking). Infants may present severe microphthalmia (unilateral or bilateral) associated with microcornea. The presence of corneal opacity, glaucoma, and horizontal nystagmus can be noted. Ectropion palpebral conjunctivae, cataracts, and optic nerve atrophy have been reported. Such eye abnormalities may result in varying degrees of visual impairment or blindness. Some affected infants exhibit gingival fibromatosis when the first teeth emerge at age 6 months to 3 years. Other symptoms (e.g., developmental delays, mental retardation) may become apparent later during infancy or childhood.

Anesthetic considerations: No specific anesthetic considerations or implications with this syndrome, except in the presence of open glaucoma.

Other conditions to be considered:

☞**CHEDIAK-HIGASHI SYNDROME:** Rare inherited disorder characterized by oculocutaneous albinism, visual difficulties, and immune system deficiencies. The hair is typically blond or light brown with a silvery tint. Affected infants may exhibit photosensitivity, nystagmus, and ataxia. It is inherited as an autosomal recessive genetic trait.

☞**HERMANSKY-PUDLAK SYNDROME:** Rare inherited disorder characterized by albinism, platelet dysfunction with prolonged bleeding time, visual impairment, and abnormal storage of a fatty-like substance in various tissues of the body. The skin, hair, and eyes may vary in color from very pale to almost normal coloring. Other symptoms include easy bruising, bleeding gingivae, and excessive bleeding after surgery or trauma. It is inherited as an autosomal recessive genetic trait.

☞**ALBINISM:** Group of rare inherited disorders characterized by hypopigmentation or complete depigmentation of the skin, hair, and eyes at birth. Patients manifest severe photosensitivity, nystagmus, and myopia.

☞**MENKES DISEASE:** Rare genetic disorder of copper metabolism beginning before birth. Copper accumulates in excessive amounts in the liver and is deficient in most other tissues of the body. Structural changes occur in the hair, brain, bones, liver and arteries. Physical characteristics include poorly pigmented, frail hair, and hypopigmentation.

REFERENCES:

Cross HE, McKusick VA, Breen W: A new oculocerebral syndrome with hypopigmentation. *J Pediatr* 70:398, 1967.

Tezcan I, Demir E, Asan E, et al: A new case of oculocerebral hypopigmentation syndrome (Cross Syndrome) with additional findings. *Clin Genet* 51:118, 1997.

Oculodentodigital Syndrome

At a glance: Very rare form of bone dysplasia characterized by microphthalmia, microsomia, large jaw, and hypoplasia of the dental enamel. Other possible features are syndactyly or clinodactyly and glaucoma.

Synonyms: Oculo-Dento-Osseous Dysplasia; ODOD Syndrome.

Incidence: Only a few cases reported.

History: First described in 1964 by F.D. Gillepsie in a brother and sister.

Genetic inheritance: Two modes of transmission: autosomal dominant for the common form and autosomal recessive for the severe form. The gene responsible for the disease is mapped to the long arm of chromosome 6.

Pathophysiology: Unknown.

Diagnosis: On radiographs the skull shows enlargement of the mandible and osteosclerosis of the skull. The orbits and basal ganglia may exhibit calcification. Other findings include widening of the metaphyses and cortical thickening of the tubular bones. Based on clinical picture and family history; however, many cases are new mutations.

Clinical aspects: *Facial Appearance:* Long, thin nose with hypoplasia of alae nasi and anteverted nostrils; may have cleft lip or palate. *Ocular Anomalies:* Microphthalmia, short palpebral fissures, epicanthal folds and microcornea. The presence of open-angle glaucoma has been reported as a late complication in 20% of patients. *Dental:* Enamel dysplasia with loose or brittle teeth. *Limb Anomalies:* Syndactyly, camptodactyly. *Skeletal:* Widespread osseous anomalies; mandibular overgrowth or micrognathia; broad clavicles and long bones. *Central Nervous System:* Intelligence is usually normal, but patients may have dysarthria, ataxia, or paraparesis. In the *autosomal recessive type,* calcification of basal ganglia, dilated ventricles, and the presence of more severe skeletal involvement (e.g., spinal cord compression from enlarged C1 vertebra) has been reported.

Precautions before anesthesia: It is recommended to check the teeth condition. In case of severe skeletal involvement, CT scan of the brain and cervical spine should be obtained. An ophthalmologic examination to exclude glaucoma must be performed.

Anesthetic considerations: Teeth are very fragile and may be easily broken or avulsed during direct laryngoscopy. Laryngoscopy and tracheal intubation can be difficult because of mandibular overgrowth or microretrognathia. The presence of a small nose can make nasotracheal intubation difficult.

Pharmacological implications: None, except in the presence of open-angle glaucoma.

REFERENCE:

Colreavy F, Colbert S, Dunphy J: Oculodento-osseous dysplasia: Review of anaesthetic problems. *Paediatr Anaesth* 4;4:179, 1994.

Oculogastrointestinal Muscular Dystrophy

At a glance: Very rare form of muscular dystrophy that affects females more often than males. Clinically, patients present with ptosis, external ophthalmoplegia, and absence of intestinal peristalsis, leading to abdominal pain, diarrhea, constipation, malabsorption, and progressive intestinal pseudoobstruction.

Synonym: Intestinal Pseudoobstruction with External Ophthalmoplegia Syndrome; Familial Visceral Myopathy with Ophthalmoplegia.

History: Described for the first time in 1983 by V. Ionasescu and S. Anuras.

Incidence: Rare.

Genetic inheritance: Autosomal recessive.

Pathophysiology: Primary myopathic lesions affect the smooth muscles (musculi propria) of the stomach, jejunum, and colon, while the neurogenic structures (vagus nerve and myenteric plexus) are intact. This disorder leads to progressive intestinal pseudoobstruction with malnutrition. Ocular manifestations, such as ptosis and ophthalmoplegia, are associated with the disorder because of occasional myopathic changes (atrophy) of the striated muscles and involvement of the peripheral nerves and central nervous system, characterized by demyelinating and axonal neuropathy and focal spongiform degeneration of the posterior columns.

Diagnosis: Early onset is characterized by ptosis and ophthalmoplegia during childhood, gastrointestinal symptoms in teenage and early adulthood years; death occurs before age 30 years. Late onset has a milder course with ocular and gastrointestinal manifestations during the fourth and fifth decades of life. Jejunal manometry, gastrointestinal contrast roentgenograms (gastric atony with delayed gastric emptying, hypomotility and dilatation of the small bowel with jejunal and ileal diverticula, megaduodenum, possibly megacolon), and gastrointestinal biopsy (degeneration and fibrosis of the intestinal muscle involving mainly the longitudinal layer) contribute to the final diagnosis. In cases of associated muscular weakness, electromyography shows delayed motor nerve conduction velocities, and sural nerve biopsy may reveal loss of large myelinated fibers and axonal loss. Striated muscle biopsies show myopathic changes involving both fiber types. Creatine kinase levels are often normal.

Clinical aspects: Bilateral ptosis and external ophthalmoplegia (limitation of eye movements in all directions) are associated with gastrointestinal manifestations of chronic diarrhea and symptoms of chronic intestinal pseudoobstruction leading to malnutrition. Some cases of associated neuromuscular impairment (facial, proximal, and distal limbs weakness with decreased deep tendon reflexes, limb hypesthesia) have been described. Mitral valve prolapse may coexist. The main differential diagnosis is oculopharyngeal muscular dystrophy, which consists of an autosomal dominant transmission, ptosis, and ophthalmoplegia. The digestive tract involvement consists only of difficulty in swallowing (no gastrojejunal lesions) or a mitochondrial disease-like myopathy with peripheral neuropathy, encephalopathy, and gastrointestinal disease (*MNGIE* Syndrome).

Precautions before anesthesia: Obtain a full history of gastrointestinal symptoms, "early" versus "late" onset of the disease, associated neuromuscular manifestations, and/or mitral valve prolapse (echocardiogram). Evaluate patient's volume status, electrolyte levels, and obtain a hemoglobin level. If on total parenteral nutrition (TPN), evaluate albumin, glucose, phosphate, calcium, and magnesium levels as well as liver function tests. Muscular weakness seems to affect mainly the limbs (no respiratory muscle weakness reported).

Anesthetic considerations: Optimization of fluid status must be achieved. High risk of pulmonary aspiration mandates a rapid-sequence induction (if associated myopathy, use nondepolarizing muscle relaxant). The intraoperative blood glucose levels must be obtained regularly if the patient is on TPN. Mitral valve prolapse rarely causes significant hemodynamic instability. No indications of increased risk for malignant hyperthermia with this condition; however, must be kept in mind in presence of bilateral ptosis.

Pharmacological implications: In the presence of associated myopathy, avoid succinylcholine. Nondepolarizing muscle relaxants can be used under the control of peripheral nerve stimulator. In presence of associated severe malnutrition or depressed renal and hepatic function secondary to complications of TPN, titrate carefully all anesthetic drugs (low protein levels cause decreased drug binding and higher free drug level).

Other conditions to be considered:

OCULOPHARYNGEAL MUSCULAR DYSTROPHY: Rare disorder with onset during the fourth to eighth decades and inherited as an autosomal dominant trait. Clinical features include ptosis, ophtalmoplegia, progressive dysphagia, weakness of the pharyngeal muscles and, eventually, of the muscles of the shoulder and pelvic girdles. Oculopharyngeal muscular dystrophy affects males and females equally.

OPHTHALMOPLEGIA, PROGRESSIVE EXTERNAL: Rare condition characterized by bilateral ptosis and ophthalmoplegia. Patients eventually develop a backward tilt of the head in order to compensate for the eye problems. Other features include diabetes mellitus, hypoparathyroidism, hyperaldosteronism, thyroid disease, ataxia, spasticity, and retinal degeneration. It is considered a symptom of another disorder; however it can also be inherited.

REFERENCES:

Anuras S, Mitros FA, Nowak TV, et al: A familial visceral myopathy with external ophthalmoplegia and autosomal recessive transmission. *Gastroenterology* 84:346, 1983.

Ionasescu V: Oculogastrointestinal muscular dystrophy. *Am J Med Genet* 3;15:103, 1983.

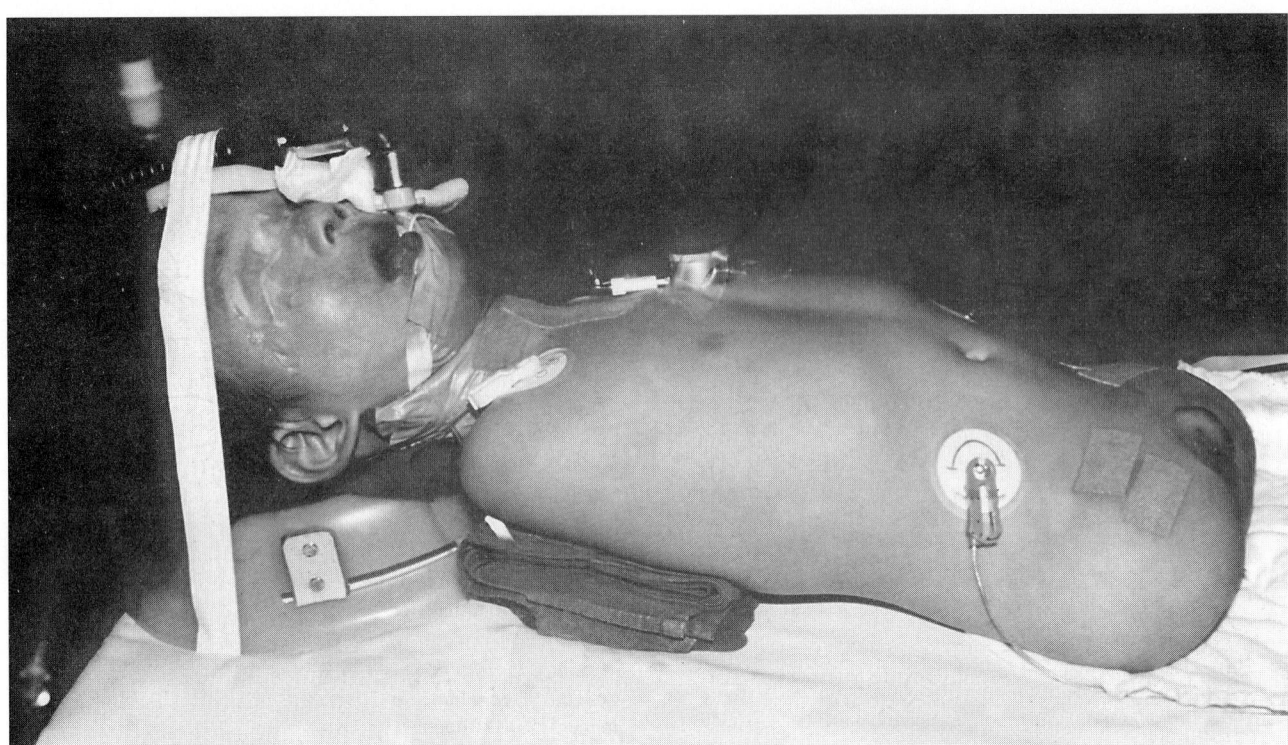

Odontotrichomelic syndrome Almost 2-year-old boy presenting tetramelia as part of odontotrichomelic syndrome, although his ears and nipples do not show any obvious dysplasia. However, hypogonadism is present, and a cleft lip/palate had been surgically repaired earlier.

Odontotrichomelic Syndrome

At a glance: Very rare disorder characterized by severe absence deformities of all four limbs (tetraamelia), hypotrichosis, abnormal teeth, hypoplastic nipples and areolae, and deformed auricles. Consistent features include hypogonadism, thyroid enlargement, incomplete cleft lip, mental retardation, and electrocardiographic (ECG) and electroencephalographic (EEG) abnormalities.

Synonyms: Odontotrichomelic Hypohidrotic Dysplasia; Freire-Maia Syndrome; Tetramelic Deficiency Syndrome.

Incidence and genetic inheritance: Extremely rare disorder most probably inherited as an autosomal recessive pattern.

Clinical aspects: Presents most often with severe absence deformities of all four extremities, abnormal teeth, hypoplastic nipples, malformation of the ears, absent or decreased eyelashes and eyebrows, and hypotrichosis. Other less frequent signs include nail anomalies, hypogonadism, thyroid enlargement and dysfunction, cleft lip, ECG and EEG abnormalities, and growth and mental retardation. Increased concentrations of tyrosine and/or tryptophane in the urine have been reported. Decreased sweating is a feature.

Anesthetic considerations: Preoperative echocardiography to assess cardiac function is recommended. In case of decreased sweating, atropine should not be used and hyperthermia must be prevented. Thyroid function should be evaluated preoperatively. Vascular access may be difficult because of limb anomalies. Parental consanguinity is suspected to be responsible for this disorder, which is often lethal in infancy or early childhood.

REFERENCES:

Cat I, Costa O, Freire-Maia N: Odontotrichomelic hypohidrotic dysplasia: A clinical reappraisal. *Hum Hered* 22:91, 1972.

Freire-Maia N: A newly recognized genetic syndrome of tetramelic deficiencies, ectodermal dysplasia, deformed ears, and other abnormalities. *Am J Hum Genet* 22:370, 1970.

Ogilvie Syndrome

At a glance: Acute colonic pseudoobstruction (ACPO) characterized by clinical signs, symptoms, and radiographic appearance of an acute large-bowel obstruction with no evidence of distal colonic obstruction. The colon may become massively dilated. If not decompressed, the patient risks perforation, peritonitis, and death.

Synonyms: Acute Colonic Pseudoobstruction Syndrome; Nontoxic Megacolon; Adult Hirschsprung Disease.

History: First described in 1948 by Sir Heneage Ogilvie, a British physician, in two patients with signs and symptoms of colonic obstruction but no evidence of organic obstruction to intestinal flow. An imbalance in the autonomic nervous system with sympathetic deprivation to the colon was hypothesized. In 1958, Dudley et al. used the term *pseudoobstruction* to describe the clinical appearance of a mechanical obstruction with no evidence of organic disease during laparotomy. An acquired condition that occurs almost exclusively in adults.

Incidence: Uncommon. No reliable data exist in the United States and internationally. Possible male predominance ratio of 1.5:1.

Genetic inheritance: None.

Pathophysiology: Acute large-bowel obstruction in the absence of an obvious mechanical cause. Colonic dysmotility probably results, in part, from an imbalance in the autonomic innervation of the colon. This syndrome most commonly follows pelvic surgery, trauma, normal pregnancy, or cesarean section, but it has also been described in association with many conditions, including myocardial or mesenteric ischemia, most types of surgery, intraabdominal sepsis, pneumonia, metabolic disturbances, drugs (e.g., antidepressants), and multiple sclerosis. Marked dilatation of the colon may cause localized ischemia of the serosa, resulting in splitting of the serosa, herniation of the mucosa, and ultimately bowel perforation.

Diagnosis: Acute colonic obstruction in the absence of a mechanical cause confirmed clinically and radiologically.

Clinical aspects: Ogilvie syndrome almost invariably occurs in adults (males affected more than females) who are often ill as a result of any of the conditions mentioned in *Pathophysiology*. Patients are frequently hospitalized and complain of colicky abdominal pain and distension. Constipation, nausea, and vomiting are common, and fever may be present in patients with ischemic or perforated bowel. Examination reveals a markedly distended abdomen that may not be as tender as anticipated until ischemia occurs. Plain abdominal radiographs are suggestive of a distal colonic obstruction with proximal large-bowel dilatation. Free air is noted in the presence of perforation. The pseudoobstruction is usually self-limited (3–6 days) and is managed conservatively with nasogastric drainage, correction of fluid and electrolyte disturbances, and removal of pharmacologic agents that might be implicated (e.g., opioids or anticholinergic drugs). Sympathetic blockade caused by an epidural anesthesia may be useful in the management of this acute problem. Colonoscopic decompression is a well-accepted form of therapy, and CT-guided needle decompression has been described. Surgical intervention is reserved for cases in which conservative therapy has failed or in the presence of impending or suspected bowel perforation. Surgical intervention carries a mortality rate of up to 40%, compared with 15% in patients managed conservatively.

Precautions before anesthesia: Patients are frequently ill as a result of their underlying conditions. Fluid and electrolyte status must be carefully evaluated and corrected prior to surgical intervention. When surgical intervention is considered, bowel ischemia/perforation is usually present and may be accompanied by systemic sepsis, major intravascular shift, large third space, and hemodynamic instability.

Anesthetic considerations: Patients must be considered to have a full stomach, and rapid sequence must be considered for tracheal intubation. Fluid and electrolyte status must be corrected prior to administration of anesthesia.

Pharmacological implications: No specific considerations except those associated with the general condition.

REFERENCES:

Crass J, Simmons R, Frick M, et al: Percutaneous decompression of the colon using CT guidance in Ogilvie syndrome. *Am J Roentgenol* 144:475, 1985.

Dorudi S, Berry AR, Kettlewell MGW: Acute colonic pseudo-obstruction. *Br J Surg* 79:99, 1992.

Omenn Syndrome

At a glance: Form of severe combined immunodeficiency (SCID) characterized by erythroderma, desquamation, chronic diarrhea, failure to thrive, lymphadenopathy, and hepatosplenomegaly. Clinically, patients develop fungal, bacterial, and viral infections typical of SCID.

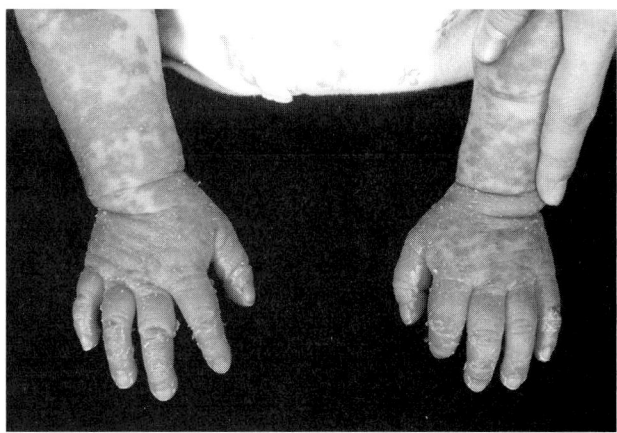

Omenn syndrome Erythroderma and desquamation of the skin on the arms and hands of a 14-month-old patient with Omenn Syndrome.

Synonym: Familial Reticuloendotheliosis Syndrome; Erythroderma Desquamation Syndrome.

Incidence: Frequency in the United States is difficult to ascertain; however, the prevalence of all forms of SCID is estimated to be 1:50,000 population. Although this disorder has been reported throughout the world, it occurs mainly in North America and Europe.

Genetic inheritance: Autosomal recessive transmission.

Pathophysiology: Immunodeficiency secondary to defective T lymphocytes and lack of B cells. Treatment often includes steroids, immunosuppressants, and interferon. This disease is uniformly fatal without bone marrow transplantation. It could be caused by a defect in an ectoenzyme 5′-nucleotidase. Lymphocytosis results from expansion of an oligoclonal population of activated and antigen-stimulated T-helper type 2 (Th2) cells that produce elevated levels of interleukin (IL)-4 and IL-5. The latter cytokines mediate eosinophilia and elevated immunoglobulin E (IgE) levels.

Diagnosis: Diagnosis based on clinical and immunologic criteria, including erythema, pachyderma, alopecia, failure to thrive, elevated T-cell counts (in contrast to other SCIDs), increased IgE,

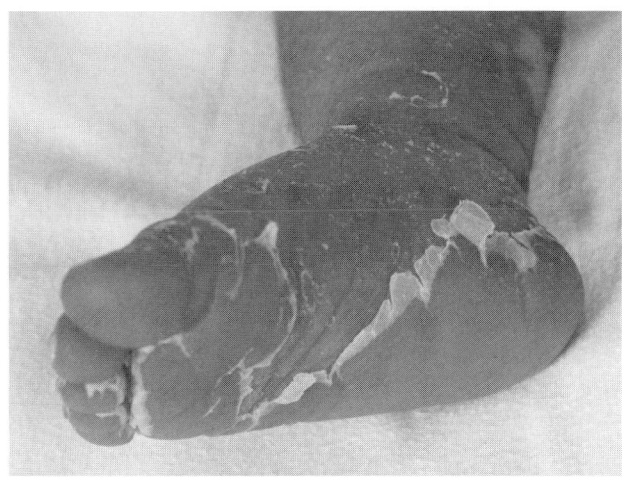

Omenn syndrome Omenn syndrome can also affect the feet, as seen in this infant with extensive desquamation of the skin.

eosinophilia, and DNA or HLA typing confirming that T cells are of host origin.

Clinical aspects: Early presentation (approximately 4 months of age). It is characterized by pulmonary infections, skin eruption (maculopapular rash and severe seborrhea with histiocytic infiltration). Hepatosplenomegaly, lymphadenopathy, diarrhea (66%), lung infections (41%), opportunistic infections (23%), candidiasis (16%), fever (16%), sepsis (16%) have been reported.

Precautions before anesthesia: Check blood counts, chest radiograph, and fluid and electrolyte status must be obtained. All blood products should be irradiated to prevent graft-versus-host disease transmission.

Anesthetic considerations: Aseptic technique. Use only irradiated blood to prevent lethal graft-versus-host disease reaction. Consider the use of leukocyte depletion filters. Temperature regulation and monitoring are mandatory.

Pharmacological implications: Administration of preoperative steroid must be considered. Any anesthetic medication resulting in histamine release should be used judiciously.

REFERENCE:

Stephan JL: Severe combined immunodeficiency: A retrospective single-center study of clinical presentation and outcome in 117 patients. *J Pediatrics* 123:564, 1993.

Omodysplasia

At a glance: Very rare rhizomelic dwarfism disorder characterized by short humeri, hypoplastic everted humeral condyle, proximal radioulnar diastasis, anterolateral radial head dislocation, depressed nasal bridge, broad base of nose, and long philtrum.

Classification and synonyms:

Recessive Form: Autosomal recessive omodysplasia; generalized omodysplasia.

Dominant Form: Omodysplasia.

History: First described in three cases by P. Maroteaux in 1989. Etymologically omodysplasia is defined as shoulder (*omo*– Greek for shoulder) dysplasia.

Incidence: Fewer than 30 cases described until 2004.

Genetic inheritance: Autosomal recessive. Many patients are of Hungarian Gypsy origin. Autosomal dominant form affects only the upper limbs.

Pathophysiology: Pathologic characteristics of this medical condition are the presence of omodysplastic diaphyseal plates showing an expanded zone of proliferating cartilage and an increased number of closely packed small chondrocytes. A functional deficiency of diaphyseal cells is partially replaced by a large number of small chondrocytes in the proliferating zone of the diaphyseal plate. However, the replacement is considered inefficient and leads to weakness of the bone structure. Possible male predominance.

Diagnosis: Clinical appearance and bone radiographs show short humeri, radioulnar diastasis at the elbows, short radii and ulnae, short femora with club-shaped upper end. In some cases, a long bone may be missing.

Clinical aspects: Dwarfism with short limbs and dysmorphic features: flat face with prominent forehead; large tongue; short, upturned nose; brachycephaly; small mandible; large, low-set ears; short neck. Mental retardation and congenital heart disease (patent ductus arteriosus, atrial septal defect, coarctation of aorta, mitral valve prolapse) may be associated. Midline hemangiomas are often present in infants.

Precautions before anesthesia: Check for congenital heart disease (echocardiography), atlantoaxial joint instability, and presence of sleep apnea syndrome (night oximetry) as for any form of dwarfism. Stenosis of the spinal canal can produce paraparesis, and scoliosis with pectus carinatum can cause restrictive lung disease.

Anesthetic considerations: Direct laryngoscopy and tracheal intubation can be difficult because of the presence of macroglossia, micrognathia, and short neck; a laryngeal mask airway and equipment for difficult intubation should be ready for use (e.g., fiberoptic, Bullard laryngoscope, retrograde technique). In case of sleep apnea syndrome, use of a nasopharyngeal airway is recommended during the first hours (and night) after general anesthesia. In case of C1-C2 subluxation, the neck should be stabilized during intubation and positioning of the patient. Special attention to the cervical spine during positioning. Confirm the absence of spinal cord compression before induction of anesthesia or consider somatosensory evoked potentials intraoperatively.

Pharmacological implications: No specific implications.

Other condition to be considered:

☞**ROBINOW SYNDROME:** Extremely rare autosomal dominant disorder characterized by mild-to-moderate short stature (postnatal growth retardation) and distinctive craniofacial anomalies resembling those of an 8-week-old fetus, called the "fetal face." Other features include macrocephaly with frontal bossing, ocular hypertelorism (abnormally prominent), anteverted nose, and sunken nasal bridge. May include forearm brachymelia, abnormally short fingers and toes, clinodactyly, unusually small hands with broad thumbs, scoliosis, and thoracic hemivertebrae.

REFERENCES:

Di Luca BJ, Mitchell A: Anaesthesia in a child with autosomal recessive omodysplasia. *Anaesth Intensive Care* 29:71, 2001.

Masel JP, Kozlowski K, Kiss P: Autosomal recessive omodysplasia, three case reports. *Pediatr Radiol* 28:608, 1998.

Ondine Syndrome

At a glance: Rare congenital failure of autonomic control of breathing during sleep. Other features include Hirschsprung disease and reduced esophageal motility.

Synonyms: Congenital Central Hypoventilation Syndrome (CCHS); Ondine-Hirschsprung Disease; Ondine Curse.

History: The name of this syndrome originates from Old German mythology about the water nymph Ondine (Undine). Nymphs are known to be very beautiful, and Ondine was certainly no exception. Nevertheless, she was very wary of men because they are a threat to a nymph's immortality. Whenever a nymph falls in love with a man, she loses her immortality and begins to age and eventually dies. However, all this was forgotten when Ondine discovered Sir Huldbrecht, a young knight, near her lily pond. Sir Huldbrecht, too, was captured by Ondine's beauty, and soon the two fell in love and married. From this very moment, however, Ondine started to age. Her stunning beauty slowly fading away, Sir Huldbrecht soon found himself looking for a younger and prettier woman. One afternoon, Ondine caught Sir Huldbrecht happily in the arms of a young woman. Having sacrificed her immortality for this man who had sworn love and faithfulness to her, Ondine demanded retaliation. With her magic still powerful enough for vengeance, she cursed Sir Huldbrecht: "As long as you are awake, you shall have your breath, however, as soon as you fall asleep, your breath will be taken from you!" It didn't take long until Sir Huldbrecht fell asleep from exhaustion and died shortly thereafter. This myth illustrates the problem of the patient suffering from congenital central hypoventilation.

Genetic inheritance: Autosomal recessive or autosomal dominant with reduced penetrance (or paternal gonadal mosaicism).

Pathophysiology: Probable anomaly of integration in the central nervous system (CNS) of afferent stimuli from peripheral chemoreceptors. The resulting hypoventilation is most pronounced during sleep, with relative insensitivity to hypercarbia and a lesser insensitivity to hypoxia. The frequent association of CCHS with Hirschsprung disease led to the hypothesis that it could be a form of neural crest disease.

Diagnosis: Polysomnographic recordings show decreased minute ventilation during sleep with hypoxemia and hypercarbia. Acquired causes of alveolar hypoventilation should be excluded: CNS infection, metabolic disease, cerebral or brainstem malformation, myotonic dystrophy.

Clinical aspects: Breathing is usually normal when awake but marked hypoventilation occurs during sleep: respiratory rate slows down to 8 to 10 breaths per minute with long pauses. Onset is usually in the first days or weeks after birth, but precise diagnosis is often delayed. Frequent association with Hirschsprung disease (13–26%), ocular anomalies (66%), or anomalies of the autonomic cardiac control (44%). May have distinctive facies: low-set ears, small nose, triangular mouth, down-slanting palpebral fissures. Inappropriate secretion of antidiuretic hormone (ADH) has been described in a few cases. The incidence of neuroblastoma or ganglioneuroma is higher than in a control population. Pulmonary hypertension and cor pulmonale occur if sleep-induced hypoventilation is not corrected. Treatment occurs at home with positive-pressure ventilation during sleep via a tracheostomy during infancy and childhood, and a face mask afterward. Phrenic nerve pacing is being tried.

Precautions before anesthesia: Check for the presence of cor pulmonale with echocardiography. The size of the tracheostomy tube must be noted. It is recommended not to use sedative premedication unless close monitoring is available. In case of association with Hirschsprung disease, the presence of a neuroblastoma or ganglioneuroma should be excluded (abdominal ultrasonography, urine catecholamines). The child's own ventilator should be present in the recovery room in case of respiratory depression or residual sedation.

Anesthetic considerations: The central nervous system respiratory response to CO_2 is blunted. Perioperative O_2 supplementation may exacerbate hypoventilation. Tracheal extubation must be performed when patient is fully awake. Locoregional anesthesia is recommended if appropriate for the surgical procedure. Esophageal motility could be decreased, so the risk of pulmonary aspiration is increased. Cases of inappropriate ADH secretion have been described; postoperative fluid requirements should be adapted to the patient's needs.

Pharmacological implications: Increased sensitivity to the respiratory effect of opiates is probable.

Other condition to be considered:

HADDAD SYNDROME: Association of Hirschsprung disease (especially total colonic aganglionosis) with congenital central hypoventilation. Neuroblastoma or ganglioneuroma is found in nearly 20% of the cases. Other associated anomalies are ocular problems, sensorineural deafness, and disturbances of gastrointestinal motility.

REFERENCES:

Croaker GDH, Shi E, Simpson E, et al: Congenital central hypoventilation syndrome and Hirschsprung's disease. *Arch Dis Child* 78:316, 1998.

Gozal D, Gaultier C: Proceedings from the 1st International Symposium on the Congenital Central Hypoventilation Syndrome, New Orleans, 11 May 1996. *Pediatr Pulmonol* 23:133, 1997.

Mather JS: Ondine's curse and the anaesthetist. *Anaesthesia* 42:394, 1987.

Opitz-Frias Syndrome

At a glance: Genetic disorder characterized by craniofacial anomalies, ocular hypertelorism, cleft lip and palate, epicanthal folds, and a wide, flat nasal bridge. Affected males present cryptorchidism, bifid scrotum, and/or hypospadias. The most significant anomalies are the presence of cleft in the larynx and trachea, pulmonary hypoplasia, dysphagia, and respiratory obstruction. Hypoplasia or agenesis of the corpus callosum, kidney abnormalities, cardiac defects, and mental retardation have been reported.

Synonyms: G Syndrome; X-Linked Opitz G/BBB Syndrome; X-Linked Opitz Syndrome; Opitz-G Syndrome Type I; Opitz BBBG Syndrome Type I; Hypertelorism-Hypospadias Syndrome; Telecanthus-Hypospadias Syndrome.

Incidence: Rare; however, a number of families have been reported.

Genetic inheritance: X-linked recessive type is based on various defects in the midline 1 (MID1) gene located on Xp22.3, and an autosomal dominant form with variable penetrance has been mapped to chromosome 22q11.2.

Pathophysiology: MID1 encodes for a protein named midin, which is believed to play a role in anchoring the cellular microtubules that form the cytoskeleton.

Diagnosis: Based on clinical features, family history, and genetic testing.

Clinical aspects: Originally described as distinct syndromes, the G and BBB syndromes are now summarized as a single disorder characterized by hypertelorism, hypospadias. and other midline defects. In particular, congenital heart defects are frequent and include patent ductus arteriosus, atrial septal defect, ventricular septal defect, coarctation of the aorta, and complex malformations, such as tetralogy of Fallot and double-outlet right ventricle (conotruncal anomalies). A variety of genitourinary defects other than hypospadias, such as cryptorchidism, bifid scrotum, and imperforate anus, also belong to the phenotypic spectrum of Opitz syndrome. Other facial anomalies include cleft lip and palate, a broad, flat nasal bridge, micrognathia, and up-slanting or down-slanting palpebral fissures with epicanthal folds. Frequent anomalies are laryngeal malformation (or cleft) and a high carina or tracheoesophageal fistula. Dysphagia associated with recurrent aspiration is common. Achalasia of the esophagus and/or hiatus hernia. MRI may show absent or hypoplastic corpus callosum, or cortical atrophy with ventriculomegaly. Mild-to-moderate mental deficiency with hypotonia.

Precautions before anesthesia: Careful airway evaluation must be performed. If time allows, consultation with an otorhinolaryngologist must be considered to stage the laryngeal cleft. History of aspiration or the presence of cough during swallowing must be explored during questioning. Dysphagia is a frequent symptom, and

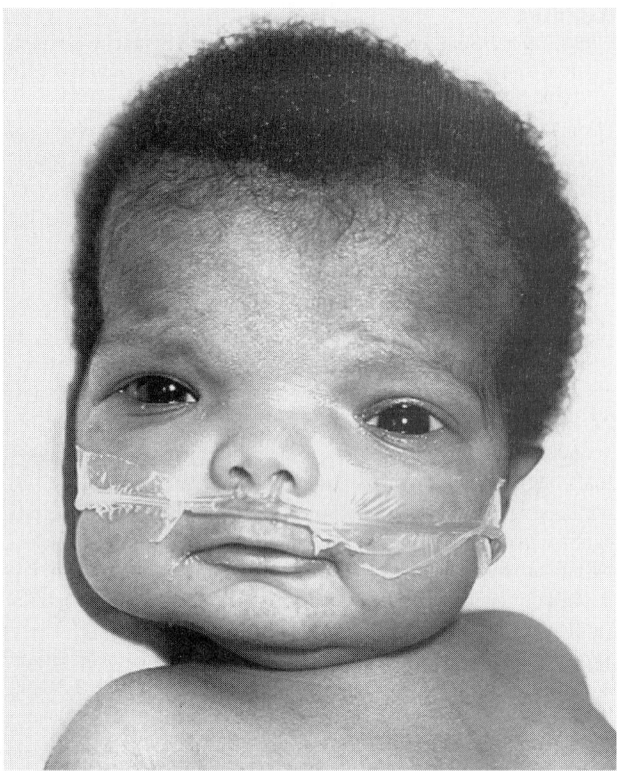

Opitz-Frias syndrome Micrognathia and a broad and flat nasal bridge with marked hypertelorism in a neonate with Opitz-Frias syndrome. He underwent successful cardiac surgery for repair of coarctation of the aorta.

recurrent aspirations are not uncommon. Therefore, a chest radiograph should be routine prior to general anesthesia in individuals at risk. Cardiac examination, including echocardiogram, must be performed.

Anesthetic considerations: Expect difficult tracheal intubation from facial and laryngotracheal malformations. Maintain spontaneous ventilation until the airway has been secured and gas exchange confirmed. Patients are at risk for aspiration during induction and recovery. May require an endotracheal tube smaller than foreseen by age-based formulas. Recurrent aspiration or lung hypoplasia may limit pulmonary reserve. The further anesthetic approach is determined mainly by the underlying cardiac defect.

Pharmacological implications: Depending on the cardiac function, agents with a potential for myocardial depression should be used with caution.

Other conditions to be considered:

☞**DIGEORGE SYNDROME (DG):** Genetic defect leading to a wide range of phenotypic presentations, mainly developmental defects in the outflow tract of the heart, hypoparathyroidism with hypocalcemia, and thymic hypoplasia/aplasia with immune defects.

☞**VELOCARDIOFACIAL (VCF) SYNDROME:** Syndrome includes typical facies and cardiac anomalies. Many other malformations can be associated (endocrine and ophthalmic). Anesthetic implications are frequent (intubation, cardiac, infectious). Some patients with Opitz syndrome were found to have deletions on 22q11.2, which are the underlying genetic defects in DG/VCF. However, several findings are distinctive enough to separate Opitz syndrome from DG/VCF.

☞**EASTMAN-BIXLER SYNDROME:** Characterized by a classic facies (malar hypoplasia, prominent antegonial notch of the mandible), horseshoe kidney, congenital heart defects, muscular hypoplasia, mental retardation, and delayed physical development.

REFERENCES:

Bissonnette B: Opitz-Frias syndrome: Anesthesia management, in Roizen MF, Fleischer LA (eds): *Essence of Anesthesia Practice.* 2nd ed. Philadelphia, WB Saunders, 2001.

Jacobson Z, Glickstein J, Hensle T, et al: Further delineation of the Opitz G/BBB syndrome: Report of an infant with complex congenital heart disease and bladder exstrophy, and review of the literature. *Am J Med Genet* 78:294, 1998.

Robin NH, Opitz JM, Muenke M: Opitz G/BBB syndrome: Clinical comparisons of families linked to Xp22 and 22q, and a review of the literature. *Am J Med Genet* 62:305, 1996.

Oral-Facial-Digital Syndrome (OFD)

At a glance: Group of disorders characterized by frequent episodic neuromuscular disturbances, congenital malformations such as cleft palate, malformation of the hands and feet, shortened limbs, and differing degrees of mental retardation. At least nine types of oral-facial-digital syndrome have been identified.

Classification:

OFD Type I (Psaume Syndrome; Papillon-Leage-Psaume Syndrome): Characterized by malformations of the face, thickened alveolar ridges and abnormal dentition, including absent lateral incisors, polycystic kidney disease, and digital malformations. The central nervous system may be involved in as many as 40% of cases. It is transmitted as an X-linked dominant condition with lethality in males. OFD I can be easily distinguished from the other OFD types by its X-linked dominant inheritance pattern and by the association with polycystic kidney disease, which seems to be specific to type I.

OFD Type II (Mohr Syndrome): Autosomal recessive or X-linked (weak possibility) transmitted disorder with polydactyly, syndactyly, brachydactyly, lobate tongue with papilliform protuberances, cranial vault (sutures) exostosis, and neuromuscular disturbances. Laryngeal anomalies are reported. Does not have the skin and hair changes of the X-linked OFD type I but presents with conductive hearing loss. Tachypnea is frequent.

OFD Type III (Sugarman Syndrome): Autosomal recessive transmitted disorder; postaxial polydactyly, bulbous nose with extra small teeth; macular red spots associated with myoclonic jerks and/or winking of the jaw and eyelids.

OFD Type IV (Burn-Baraister Syndrome): Autosomal recessive transmitted disorder with short stature, preaxial and postaxial polydactyly of hands and feet, and cerebral atrophy with porencephaly. Short tibias and, hence, short limbs.

OFD Type V (Thurston Syndrome): Autosomal recessive transmitted disorder with midline cleft lip and postaxial polydactyly of hands and feet.

OFD Type VI (Varadi-Papp Syndrome): Autosomal recessive transmitted disorder with preaxial polydactyly of toes and postaxial polydactyly in fingers; cerebellar anomalies (Dandy-Walker anomaly, hypoplasia of vermis).

OFD Type VII (Whelan Syndrome): OFD with congenital hydronephrosis and kidney abnormalities, facial asymmetry, and preauricular tags. Occurred in one family.

OFD Type VIII (Edwards Syndrome): X-linked recessive transmitted disorder presenting with retinal abnormalities (atrophic areas); bifid and hamartomatous tongue and multiple frenula.

OFD Type IX (Orofaciodigital Syndrome with retinal anomalities): Autosomal recessive or X-linked transmitted disorder. Occurred in three males. OFD with retinal anomalies (atrophic areas), median cleft upper lip, and multiple oral frenula.

OFD Type X (Orofaciodigital Syndrome with Fibula aplasia): Similar to OFD type IX except that the retinal abnormalities are associated with severe brain atrophy.

OFD Type XI (Toriello Syndrome): Characterized by multiple hamartomas of the oral cavity, lobulated tongue, alveolar frenula, small median cleft of the upper lip, atrophy of the frontal and parietal cerebral lobes, and broad big toes. Autosomal recessive.

Genetic inheritance: All modes of transmission are reported, with mode depending on the type (see *Classification*). However, in the majority of affected males, it is X-linked dominant with lethality.

Pathophysiology: Unknown.

Diagnosis: Based on the clinical aspects and family history.

Clinical aspects: *Face:* Hypoplastic alae nasi; lateral placement of inner canthi, choanal atresia; occasional hypoplastic mandibular ramus. *Oral:* Multiple and/or hyperplastic frenula between buccal mucosae and alveolar ridge; median cleft lip; lobated or bifid tongue; cleft of alveolar ridge; cleft palate; dental caries and anomalous anterior teeth. *Digits:* Asymmetric shortening of digits with clinodactyly, syndactyly of hands and unilateral polydactyly of feet. *Other:* Variable mental deficiency; spotty alopecia; brain malformation with absence of corpus callosum, and heterotopia of gray matter in 20% of patients.

Precautions before anesthesia: Check teeth; check renal function in case of polycystic renal disease; exclude presence of associated brain anomaly.

Anesthetic considerations: In case of choanal atresia, an orotracheal tube must be inserted to prevent respiratory complications. Do not attempt intubation or insertion of a nasogastric tube.

Pharmacological implications: No specific implications.

Other conditions to be considered:

☞**SHORT RIB POLYSYNDACTYLY SYNDROME TYPE II (Majewski Syndrome):** Polydactyly with neonatal chondrodystrophy. Epiglottis and laryngeal anomalies. Short limbs and ribs. Lethal in the perinatal period in most cases.

☞**JUBERG-HAYWARD SYNDROME:** Rare hereditary disorder characterized by cleft lip and palate, microcephaly, deformities of the thumbs and toes, and short stature.

☞**ACROFACIAL DYSOSTOSIS NAGER TYPE:** Rare hereditary disorder marked by abnormal facial development (mandibulofacial dysostosis). Other features include cleft lip and palate, defective development of bones of the jaw and arms, and smaller than normal thumbs.

☞**JOUBERT SYNDROME:** Very rare hereditary neurologic disorder affecting the cerebellar functions. Neuromuscular and eye movement disturbances similar to those of oral-facial-digital syndrome occur. Additionally, psychomotor retardation and respiratory problems may develop. Some symptoms may decrease with age.

REFERENCES:

Holub M, Potocki L, Bodamer OA: Central nervous system malformations in oral-facial-digital syndrome. *Am J Med Genet A* 136(2):218, 2005.

Silengo MC, Bell GL, Biagiolo M: Oro-facial-digital syndrome II. Transitional type between the Mohr and the Majewski syndromes: Report of two new cases. *Clin Genet* 31:331, 1987.

Toriello HV: Oral-facial-digital syndromes, 1992. *Clin Dysmorphol* 2:95, 1993.

Ornithine Carbamoyltransferase Deficiency (OTCD)

At a glance: Rare genetic disorder characterized by complete or partial lack of the enzyme ornithine transcarbamylase (OTC). Lack of the enzyme results in excessive hyperammonemia, which is known as a neurotoxin. Clinically, patients present vomiting, refusal to eat, progressive lethargy, and coma.

Synonym: Ornithine Transcarbamylase Deficiency.

Nature: The urea cycle disorders are a group of rare disorders that affect the urea cycle, a series of biochemical processes in which nitrogen is converted into urea and removed from the body through the urine. Nitrogen is a waste product of protein metabolism. Failure to break down nitrogen results in the abnormal accumulation of nitrogen, in the form of ammonia, in the blood.

Incidence: Approximately 1:80,000 live births. Estimated prevalence for disorders of urea cycle is approximately 1:30,000 population.

Genetic inheritance: Partially dominant X-linked (Xp21.1). The phenotype of heterozygote females cannot be predicted because of random inactivation of the X chromosome. Some female carriers present clinical symptoms a few weeks after delivery, at the time of uterine involution.

Pathophysiology: Ornithine carbamoyltransferase is one of six enzymes that play a role in the breakdown and removal of nitrogen in the body, a process known as the *urea cycle.* The entire urea cycle resides exclusively in periportal hepatocytes. It is an essential pathway for waste nitrogen excretion. It is involved in a cascade of six enzymatic transformations converting toxic ammonia to nontoxic water-soluble urea.

Diagnosis: Elevated blood NH_4 level in a lethargic or comatose patient; liver biopsy; increased urinary orotic acid levels.

Clinical aspects: *Neonatal Presentation:* Starts within the first 4 days of life: refusal to feed, irritability, persistent vomiting, mild respiratory alkalosis, followed rapidly by neurologic signs with coma, convulsions, hypotonia.

Late-Onset Presentation: Long history of chronic hepatogastric symptoms such as recurrent episodes of vomiting, failure to thrive, and hepatomegaly. Others present a neurologic picture of chronic encephalopathy; behavioral disorders such as agitation, delirium, and irritability; or Reye-like syndrome following sodium valproate therapy for seizures. Some patients spontaneously avoid protein-rich food and remain relatively asymptomatic. Death may occur during a metabolic crisis precipitated by infection, surgery, increased catabolism, or a protein-rich diet.

In case of seizures, sodium valproate should not be used because it may precipitate acute metabolic decompensation. Liver transplantation is curative.

Basic treatment is a low-protein diet carefully adapted to the child's needs and metabolic tolerance and administration of ammonia-scavenging drugs (Na-benzoate, Na-phenylbutyrate, L-arginine) three to four times per day. Their administration should be linked to meals to maximize their effect.

In case of hyperammonemia:

- Stop protein intake and restrict fluid volume if there is any concern about cerebral edema. Provide a high-energy intake orally or IV (glucose 10–20%).
- Use alternative pathways for nitrogen elimination: give Na-benzoate up to 500 mg/kg/day, Na-phenylbutyrate up to 600 mg/kg/day, and L-arginine 300 mg/kg/day orally or IV. Because these drugs lead to K wasting, K blood levels should be monitored.
- Treat sepsis and convulsions.

Precautions before anesthesia: Check blood glucose and NH_4 levels. Ensure Na-benzoate, Na-phenylbutyrate, and L-arginine are available for emergency treatment of hyperammonemia. Seizure medication must be maintained. Check fluid and electrolyte status, especially in presence of renal dysfunction.

Anesthetic considerations: Prolonged fasting should be avoided. Intravenous glucose (5 or 10% solution) should be used to avoid protein catabolism. Monitoring of blood glucose, ammonium, and lactate levels must be done regularly. Prevention of hypovolemia at all times, especially if altered renal function. If there is a risk of nasal, pharyngeal, or gastric bleeding, a gastric tube should be inserted to remove swallowed blood, which provides a protein load that may trigger acute metabolic decompensation. Prolonged postoperative metabolic monitoring must be provided for early diagnosis of acute decompensation.

Pharmacological implications: Pathology of the urea cycle should be borne in mind when dealing with a supposed "normal" child who does not wake up after uneventful anesthesia. In case of fever, ibuprofen is preferred over acetaminophen; sodium valproate and haloperidol can unmask a previously undiagnosed urea cycle defect.

Other conditions to be considered:

UREA CYCLE DISORDERS: Group of rare disorders characterized by accumulation of hyperammonemia and clinically presenting with a lack of appetite, vomiting, drowsiness, seizures, and/or coma. Other features include hepatomegaly and cerebral dysfunction caused by the urea level. Life-threatening complications may result. In addition to OTCD, carbamyl phosphate synthetase (CPS) deficiency, citrullinemia (argininosuccinate synthetase deficiency), argininosuccinate lyase deficiency, argininemia, and N-acetylglutamate synthetase (NAGS) deficiency must be considered in individuals affected with these symptoms.

☞**REYE SYNDROME:** Rare childhood disease characterized by liver failure, encephalopathy, hypoglycemia, and hyperammonemia. It can be triggered by use of aspirin in children recovering from chickenpox or influenza (viral infection). Deficiencies of the urea cycle enzymes have been suggested as a possible mechanism in the development of Reye syndrome. Clinical features include vomiting, diarrhea, rapid breathing, irritability, fatigue, and behavioral changes. Neurologic symptoms may be life-threatening and include generalized seizures, stupor, and coma.

ORGANIC ACIDEMIAS: Group of rare inherited metabolic disorders characterized by the presence of hyperammonemia, hyperacidemia, thrombocytopenia, and muscle weakness.

☞**ARGININEMIA:** Urea cycle disorder that leads to hyperammonemia and neurologic symptoms that are less severe than in other forms of urea cycle abnormalities.

☞**CITRULLINEMIA:** Syndrome arising from argininosuccinate synthetase deficiency leading to hyperammonemia and neurologic consequences.

☞**HHH SYNDROME:** Genetically transmitted inborn error of metabolism resulting from a defect in the transport of ornithine into the mitochondrial matrix, clinically characterized by early growth retardation, learning disabilities, periodic confusion, and ataxia.

☞**METHYLMALONIC ACIDEMIA:** Heterogeneous inborn error of metabolism leading to metabolic acidosis and accumulation of methylmalonic acid and its by-products.

☞**N-ACETYLGLUTAMATE SYNTHETASE DEFICIENCY:** Congenital mitochondrial disorder affecting the metabolism of ammonium and results in hyperammonemia.

☞**PROPIONIC ACIDEMIA:** Inborn error of metabolism affecting the mitochondrial catabolism of valine and isoleucine. Untreated, this results in ketoacidosis, lethargy, coma, and finally death.

REFERENCES:

Leonard JV: Disorders of the urea cycle, in Fernandes J, Saudubray J-M, van den Berghe G (eds): *Inborn Metabolic Diseases.* 3rd ed. Berlin, Springer, 2000, p 214.

Schultz REH, Salo MK: Underrecognition of late onset ornithine transcarbamylase deficiency. *Arch Dis Child* 82:390, 2000.

Ornithine Delta-Aminotransferase Deficiency

At a glance: Rare genetic disorder affecting mitochondrial metabolism of ornithine. It is characterized by the presence of gyrate atrophy of the retina leading to night blindness that begins in late childhood, accompanied by sharply demarcated circular areas of chorioretinal atrophy. The areas of atrophy enlarge during the second and third decades. Posterior subcapsular cataracts have been associated by the end of the second decade. Computed tomography and magnetic resonance imaging (MRI) studies demonstrated the presence of type II muscle fiber changes in large muscle groups because of hyperornithinemia-induced deficiency of high-energy creatine phosphate. Brain MRI revealed degenerative lesions in the white matter in 50% of the gyrate atrophy patients, and 70% present premature atrophic changes. Early degenerative, atrophic brain changes and abnormal EEG are features of gyrate atrophy, in addition to the well-characterized eye and muscle manifestations.

Synonyms: OAT Deficiency; Hyperornithinemia Gyrate Atrophy of the Choroid and Retina.

Nature: Genetic disorder leading to visual disturbances caused by progressive chorioretinal atrophy.

Genetic inheritance: Autosomal recessive transmission; high incidence in the Finnish population. The gene has been mapped on chromosome 10.

Pathophysiology: OAT is a mitochondrial enzyme requiring pyridoxal phosphate. In the neonatal period, the role of OAT reaction is to synthesize ornithine to produce arginine via citrulline; later, the role of OAT is to catabolize excess ornithine generated from dietary arginine. The cause of chorioretinal degeneration could be insufficient proline synthesis from ornithine in the retinal pigment epithelium.

Diagnosis: Plasma ornithine levels more than 10 to 20 times normal. Diagnosis usually established by specialized ophthalmologic examination.

Clinical aspects: Night blindness and myopia in early childhood are the first symptoms. Retinopathy can be detected at electroretinography before visual disturbances are obvious. Chorioretinal atrophy can be detected at funduscopy. Considerable differences in severity of the disease. Subcapsular cataracts at the end of the second decade of life. Blindness caused by chorioretinal atrophy between 40 and 50 years of age in patients unresponsive to pyridoxine. Muscle pathology with type II fiber atrophy and tubular aggregates in some patients. Treatment consists of pharmacological doses of pyridoxine (vitamin B_6) and/or a low-arginine diet.

Precautions before anesthesia: No specific precautions before anesthesia except for the surgical procedure involved.

Anesthetic considerations: Individual affected might be visually impaired or blind. Bright operating room will provide reassurance. The presence of muscle atrophy or dysfunction should be considered when using neuromuscular blocking agents.

Pharmacological implications: No known implication between anesthesia medication and administration of large doses of vitamin B_6.

Other condition to be considered:

☞**HHH Syndrome:** Resembles ornithinemia with gyrate atrophy except there are no visual problems or fundus changes. The pathophysiology involves diminished ornithine transport into mitochondria, resulting in ornithine accumulation in the cytoplasm and reduced ability to clear carbamoyl phosphate and ammonia loads. Autosomal recessive inheritance has been suggested.

REFERENCE:

Shih VE, Stöckler-Ipsiroglu S: Disorders of ornithine and creatine metabolism, in Fernandes J, Saudubray J-M, van den Berghe G (eds): *Inborn Metabolic Diseases.* 3rd ed. Berlin, Springer, 2000, p 232.

verts orotic acid into orotidine monophosphate; the second, catalyzed by orotidine decarboxylase, transforms orotidine monophosphate into uridine monophosphate. The classic type I disease is caused by diminished activity of both enzymes; type II disease could be caused by diminished activity of orotidine decarboxylase only.

Diagnosis: Urinalysis shows massive oversecretion of orotic acid (up to 1.5 g/day) and crystalluria. However, orotic aciduria can also result from some urea cycle defects, parenteral nutrition, or essential amino acid deficiency. The enzymatic diagnosis can be performed on red blood cells. A deficiency of orotidylic acid pyrophosphorylase and/or decarboxylase activities in leukocytes, erythrocytes, hepatic cells, and cultured skin fibroblasts is characteristic. The presence in the *serum* of megaloblastic anemia is typical.

Clinical aspects: Megaloblastic anemia with anisocytosis and hypochromia appearing a few weeks or months after birth is the first manifestation. It does not respond to iron, folic acid, or vitamin B_{12}. If the disorder is unrecognized, failure to thrive with growth and developmental retardation ensues. Urinary obstruction (renal, ureteral, or urethral) from orotic acid crystals has been reported. For treatment, the enzymatic defect can be bypassed by the administration of uridine, which is converted into uridine monophosphate by uridine kinase. The hematologic response is quick. The dosage is adapted in order to achieve the lowest possible urinary output of orotic acid.

Precautions before anesthesia: Check hemoglobin level.

Anesthetic considerations: Perioperative hydration should be sufficient to maintain a high urine output to prevent increasing the urinary concentration of orotic acid and the ensuing risk of urinary stones.

Pharmacological implications: No specific implications.

REFERENCE:

Van den Berghe G, Vincent M-F, Marie S: Disorders of purine and pyrimidine metabolism, in Fernandes J, Saudubray J-M, van den Berghe G (eds): *Inborn Metabolic Diseases.* 3rd ed. Berlin, Springer, 2000, p 355.

Orotic Aciduria

At a glance: Very rare congenital disorder characterized by an inborn error of pyrimidine metabolism resulting in hematologic (megaloblastic anemia unresponsive to vitamin C, vitamin B_{12}, or folic acid) and neurologic (growth and mental retardation) manifestations. Onset in childhood.

Synonyms: Hereditary Orotic Aciduria; Uridine Monophosphate Synthase Deficiency.

Classification: There are two clinical types: *type I,* which is a deficiency of the OMP-PP portion of uridine monophosphate synthetase, and *type II,* which is a deficiency of the OMP-DC portion of uridine monophosphate synthetase.

Genetic inheritance: Autosomal recessive. Genetic defect is described as a deficiency of OMP-PP and/or OMP-DC activities, accumulation of orotic acid, plus interference with RNA and DNA synthesis, leading to hematologic manifestations because vigorous synthesis of RNA and DNA is necessary for normal hematopoiesis.

Pathophysiology: Uridine monophosphate synthase is a bifunctional enzyme involved in the de novo synthesis of pyrimidines. A first reaction catalyzed by orotate phosphoribosyltransferase con-

Osgood-Schlatter Disease

At a glance: Benign inflammation of the tibial tuberosity characterized by abnormal bone and cartilage formation in the tibia. Clinically, patients may experience pain, swelling, and tenderness of the knee and ankle.

Synonyms: Schlatter Disease.

Pathophysiology: Pain is caused by osteochondritis of the tibial tuberosity at the point of insertion of the tendon of the patella or by a small stress fracture.

Diagnosis: Swelling and tenderness over the tibial tuberosity.

Clinical aspects: Pain over the tibial tuberosity that is exacerbated by running or jumping. Common pain syndrome in growing children and adolescents.

Precautions before anesthesia: No specific precautions. Coagulation profile should be obtained if the patient is taking antiinflammatory medication.

Anesthetic considerations: Chronic administration of steroids must be considered. Peroperative coverage needed. The use of regional anesthesia might be advantageous if feasible.

Pharmacological implications: Patient may be on nonsteroidal antiinflammatory drug therapy.

Other conditions to be considered:

KEINBOECK DISEASE: Acquired bone disorder affecting the wrist, particularly the lunate bone following an injury or inflammation. Recurrent pain and stiffness occur in conjunction with thickening, swelling, and tenderness. The range of motion in the wrist is most often limited.

☞**LEGG-CALVÉ-PERTHES DISEASE:** Rare disease affecting the hip joint. Abnormalities in bone growth early in life may result in permanent deformity of the hip joint several years later.

REFERENCE:

Rosenberg ZS, Kawelblum M, Cheung YY, et al: Osgood-Schlatter lesion: Fracture or tendonitis? Scintigraphic, CT and MR imaging features. *Radiology* 185:853, 1992.

Osteogenesis Imperfecta

At a glance: Group of rare disorders affecting the connective tissue and characterized by extremely fragile bones that break or fracture easily during the antenatal and postnatal periods (brittle bones). The severity of osteogenesis imperfecta varies greatly, even among individuals of the same family. Four main types have been identified. *Type I* is the most common and the mildest form of the disorder. *Type II* is the most severe form.

Synonyms: Brittle Bone Disease; Ekman-Lobstein Syndrome; Lobstein Disease; Fragilitas Ossium.

Classification: There are four types of osteogenesis imperfecta. Subdivision types A and IB are based on the absence or presence of dentinogenesis imperfecta within each condition.

Type I (Osteogenesis Imperfecta Tarda; Osteogenesis Imperfecta with Blue Sclerae): Dominantly inherited, generalized connective tissue disorder characterized mainly by bone fragility and blue sclerae.

Type II (Osteogenesis Imperfecta Congenita; Neonatal Lethal Form Osteogenesis Imperfecta; Vrolik Osteogenesis Imperfecta Syndrome): Autosomal dominant characterized by spontaneous fractures, generalized osteoporosis, and wormian bones in the area of the lambdoidal sutures. Blue sclerae and deafness are not present. Mucoid changes in the connective tissue of the heart valves and aorta lead to congestive heart failure and death.

Type III (Osteogenesis Imperfecta Progressively Deforming with Normal Sclerae): Believed to be about one eighth as frequent as dominantly inherited osteogenesis imperfecta with blue sclerae. In this type, dentinogenesis imperfecta is particularly striking, especially in the primary dentition. Severe kyphoscoliosis and multiple limb deformities are reported.

Type IV (Osteogenesis Imperfecta with Normal Sclerae): Autosomal dominant characterized by short stature, often below 5th percentile, hearing loss and otosclerosis, normal-grayish sclerae, and presence of dentinogenesis imperfecta. The skull presents wormian bones. Onset is in the newborn period, with fractures occurring in utero, during labor and delivery, or shortly after birth.

Incidence: 2.2:10,000 live births.

Genetic inheritance: Autosomal dominant (can also be recessive for type II and III).

Pathophysiology: Osteogenesis imperfecta results from genetic defect that affects the body's production of collagen. Caused by mutation in either the collagen I, alpha-1 gene (COL1A1) or the collagen I, alpha-2 gene (COL1A2), located on17q21.31-q22, 7q22.1.

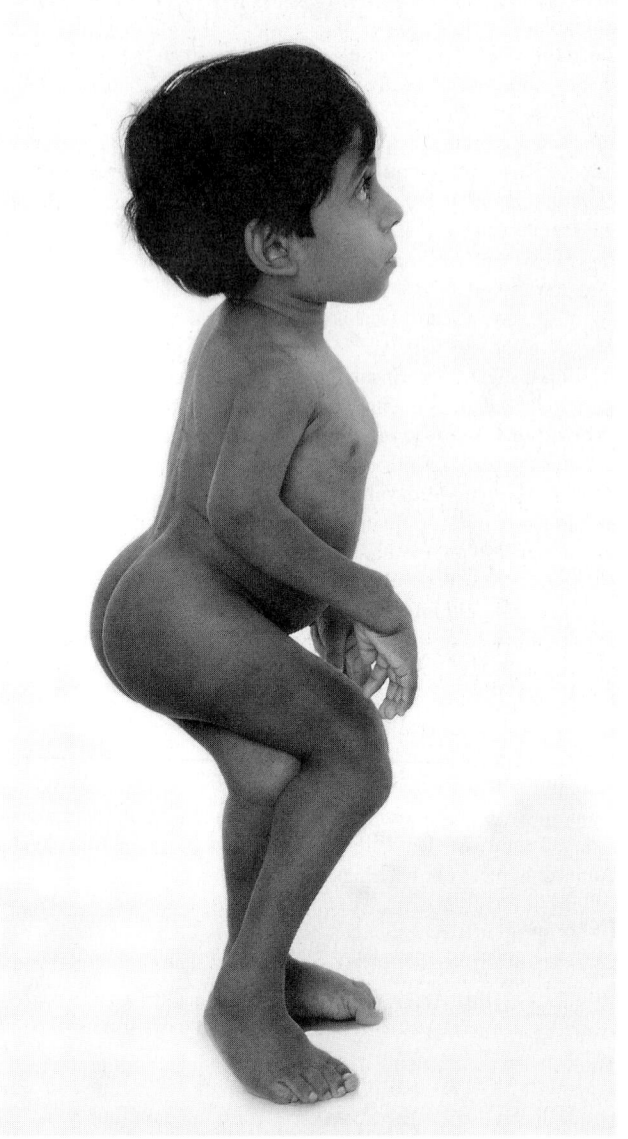

Osteogenesis imperfecta   Boy with scoliosis and short stature suffers from osteogenesis imperfecta type III.

Diagnosis: Characteristic features of osteogenesis imperfecta can greatly vary. Intelligence is normal. Diagnosis is clinically evocated on multiple bone fractures, short stature, blue sclerae, and abnormal teeth color. It has been suggested that antenatal echography can be contributive in some cases. Diagnosis confirmed by genetic testing and biochemical analysis of collagen.

Clinical aspects: There are multiple clinical manifestations. The commonly used clinical classification of Sillence divides the condition into four major types.

Type I: Mutations in COL1A1. The most common and usually the mildest form. It is characterized by multiple bone fractures usually occurring during childhood through puberty. Fractures during the neonatal period are rare. The frequency of fractures usually declines after puberty. Repeated fractures may result in bowing of the tibia and femur. A distinguishing feature associated with osteogenesis imperfecta type I is blue sclera that does not fade with age, the presence of a normal mitral valve, and normal teeth. In

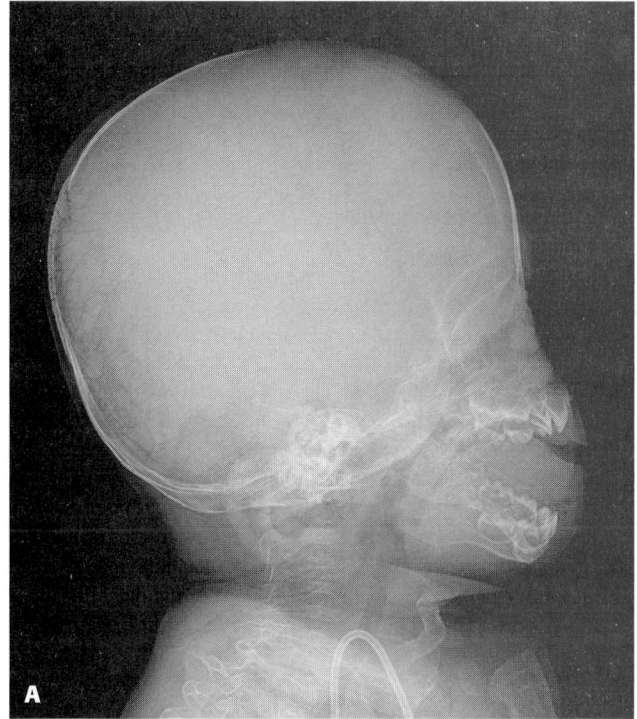
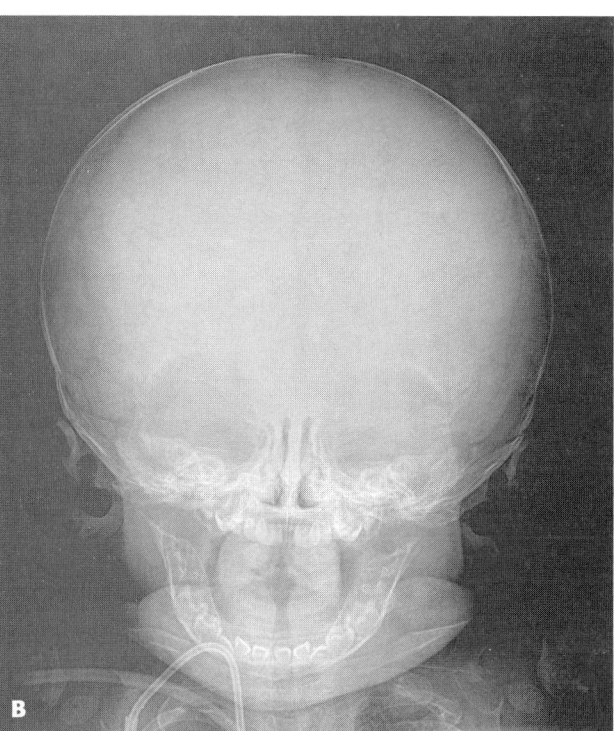

Osteogenesis imperfecta   Head radiographs of a 6-month-old child with osteogenesis imperfecta congenita show an enlarged skull with multiple wormian bones.

some cases, hearing impairment (conductive and/or sensorineural) has been associated with osteosclerosis and occurs most often in the third decade of life. However, it can occur as early as the second decade or as late as the seventh decade. Individuals may have a triangular facial appearance, macrocephaly, postnatal growth deficiency, and scoliosis or kyphosis. Hyperextensible joints, hypotonia,

and easy bruising (capillary fragility and platelet dysfunction). Hyperthyroidism has been associated. Unexplained postoperative fever has been observed (malignant hyperthermia test negative).

Type II: Mutations in COL1A1 and COL1A2. The most severe type of osteogenesis imperfecta. Affected infants often experience life-threatening complications at, or shortly after, birth. Often lethal as a result of cardiac failure and respiratory insufficiency because of underdeveloped lungs, an abnormally small thorax, and congestive heart failure. Infants have low birth weight, abnormally short limbs, and blue sclera. Infants usually present with extremely

Osteogenesis imperfecta   Multiple and bilateral rib fractures with healing callus formation can be identified on the chest radiograph (same patient as in previous pictures).

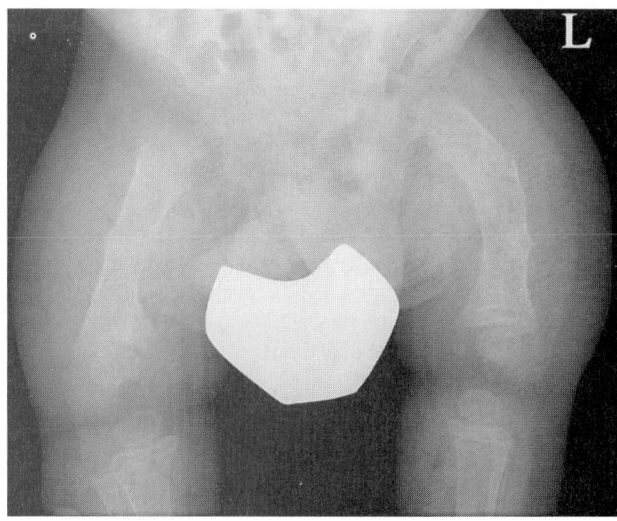

Osteogenesis imperfecta   Deformation and buckling fractures of the femora bilaterally (same patient as in previous pictures).

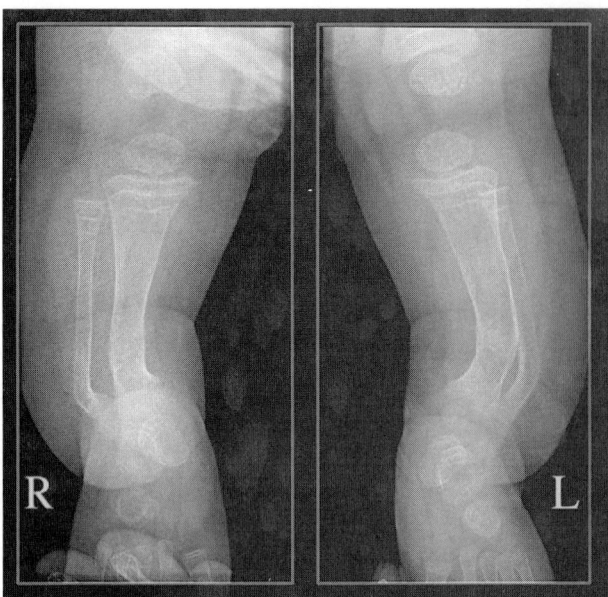

Osteogenesis imperfecta Severe deformity of tibia and fibula with buckling fractures on both sides in the same child with osteogenesis imperfecta congenita. Growth retardation lines can be identified on the proximal diaphysis of tibia and fibula.

fragile bones and numerous fractures at birth. Other features include a small, narrow nose, micrognathia, and abnormally soft calvaria with abnormally large fontanelle. Abnormally thin and fragile skin and hypotonia are present. Osteogenesis imperfecta type II has been subdivided into three subgroups (A, B, and C) based upon small differences in bone formation seen only on radiographs. Premature birth with low weight and multiple antenatal fractures is common. Other characteristics include flattened vertebrae, bowed femur, humerus, and tibia, soft calvaria, and antenatal fractures. Antenatal diagnosis is possible at 17 weeks.

Type III: Mutations in COL1A1 and COL1A2. Characterized by extremely fragile bones, multiple fractures, and malformed bones. Multiple fractures are often present at birth. Fractures and malformation of various bones (most often the ribs and long bones) may lead to progressive malformation as affected infants and children age. Other features include short stature (adult size <1 m [39.4 inches]), scoliosis and kyphosis, and malformation of the occipital bone and basilar impression. Some patients develop pulmonary insufficiency and respiratory problems. Infants may have blue sclerae at birth, which tend to fade during the first year of life. Infants may have a triangular facial appearance as a result of abnormally prominent frontal bossing and significant micrognathia. Hearing impairment and brittle discolored teeth (dentinogenesis imperfecta), severe osteoporosis, hydrocephalus, macrocephaly, and pulmonary hypertension are frequent.

Type IV: Patients have fragile bones, and fractures are more common before puberty. Affected individuals experience mild-to-moderate bone malformation and are usually of short stature. Patients present with scoliosis and kyphosis. Other features include a triangular facial appearance. In most cases, the sclerae are normal or pale blue during infancy. As an affected infant ages, the pale blue discoloration of the sclerae fades. Affected individuals may experience hearing impairment and brittle discolored teeth (dentinogenesis imperfecta).

Types III and IV are less frequent.

Unclassified Osteogenesis Imperfecta: Many cases of individuals with the bone abnormalities characteristic of osteogenesis imperfecta have been reported in the medical literature. However, these cases have additional symptoms that prevent them from being classified under one of the four main types of osteogenesis imperfecta. These cases may be subgroups of one of the four main types of osteogenesis imperfecta, an additional type of osteogenesis imperfecta (e.g., osteogenesis imperfecta type V), or separate disorders.

Precautions before anesthesia: Evaluate cardiac function (type II) (clinical, chest radiograph, echography). Evaluate respiratory function because scoliosis can cause restrictive respiratory insufficiency (clinical chest radiograph, pulmonary function test, arterial blood gas analysis). Laboratory investigation should include levels of phosphorus and calcium, blood and urinary balance, platelet count, and hemostasis study. Evaluate thyroid function (type I).

Anesthetic considerations: High risks of bone fracture are present and necessitate careful intraoperative positioning. Because tourniquet and blood pressure cuff can cause fractures, an arterial line may be used as alternative (especially type II). Severe kyphoscoliosis can make positioning difficult. Regional anesthesia is not contraindicated but can be difficult to achieve. Medullar anesthesia should be avoided in case of severe deformities and/or platelet anomalies. Direct laryngoscopy and tracheal intubation can be difficult because of micrognathia, severe dental anomalies, and flattened vertebrae (type III) and are always dangerous because of bone fragility. Laryngeal mask airway or fiberoptic intubation can be useful. However, direct laryngoscopy must be performed with great care.

Pharmacological implications: Succinylcholine should be avoided because the intensity of fasciculations may cause fractures. Prophylactic antibiotics as indicated in case of cardiac lesion.

Other conditions to be considered:

BRUCK SYNDROME (Osteogenesis Imperfecta and Congenital Joint Contractures): Characterized by severe joint contractures. Autosomal recessive gene on chromosome 17p12.

☞**COLE CARPENTER SYNDROME:** Extremely rare disorder characterized by very fragile bones and multiple fractures. Affected infants may show blue sclerae, craniosynostosis, frontal bossing, micrognathia, and proptosis. Affected infants may experience growth failure and severe ophthalmologic anomalies (blindness, vitreous hyperplasia, corneal opacity, secondary glaucoma). Approximately five cases of this disorder have been reported in the medical literature. Cole-Carpenter syndrome is inherited as an autosomal dominant trait on a gene located on 11q13.4, 11q12-q13.

DENTINOGENESIS IMPERFECTA (Opalescent Dentin, Opalescent Teeth Without Osteogenesis): Characterized by the presence of blue-yellow, small, misshapen teeth resulting from a defect in synthesis of Type 1 collagen. Not associated with bone fragility. Autosomal dominant (4q13-q21).

☞**ACHONDROPLASIA:** Inherited disorder characterized by short-limbed dwarfism, macrocephaly, frontal bossing, low nasal bridge, and/or midface hypoplasia. Skeletal malformations may include brachydactyly, lordosis, genu varum, and/or stenosis of the spine. Additional abnormalities may include limited extension of the elbows and hips, hypotonia, and frequent otitis media. Usually appears sporadically.

☞**HYPOPHOSPHATASIA:** Rare disorder characterized by defective bone mineralization resulting in fragile bones. The long bones of the arms and legs may be abnormally thick, short, and bowed. Other features include microcephaly and short stature. Inherited as an autosomal recessive trait.

☞**PYKNODYSOSTOSIS:** Rare disorder characterized by osteosclerosis, short stature, underdeveloped mandible, and dental abnormalities. Affected individuals often have fragile bones and may be prone to stress fractures. Inherited as an autosomal recessive trait.

☞**OSTEOPETROSIS:** Rare disorder marked by increased bone density, brittle bones, and skeletal abnormalities. The adult type of osteopetrosis is milder than the malignant infantile and intermediate types of osteopetrosis and may not be diagnosed until adolescence or adulthood, when symptoms first appear. More serious complications occur in the malignant infantile and intermediate types of osteopetrosis.

REFERENCES:

Barros F: Caudal block in a child with osteogenesis imperfecta, type II. *Paediatr Anaesth* 5:202, 1995.

Karabiyik L, Parpucu M, Kurtipek O: Total intravenous anaesthesia and the use of an intubating laryngeal mask in a patient with osteogenesis imperfecta. *Acta Anaesthesiol Scand* 46:618, 2002.

Silence DO, Rimoin DL: Classification of osteogenesis imperfecta. *Lancet* 13(1):1041, 1978.

Vogel TM, Ratner EF, Thomas RC Jr, et al: Pregnancy complicated by severe osteogenesis imperfecta: A report of two cases. *Anesth Analg* 94:1315, 2002.

Osteopetrosis

At a glance: Heterogenous genetic disorder resulting in increased bone mass as a consequence of defective bone resorption. Depending on the mode of inheritance, its course can be either uniformly fatal with pancytopenia, recurrent pathologic fractures, blindness, and other neurologic symptoms, or it can exist in a much milder form with later manifestation and favorable prognosis.

Synonyms and classification:

Dominant Osteopetrosis Type I

Dominant Autosomal Osteopetrosis Type II (Albers-Schonberg Disease; Autosomal Dominant Marble Bones; Osteosclerosis Fragilis Generalisata)

Mild Autosomal Osteopetrosis (Osteopetrosis Renal Tubular Acidosis; Osteopetrosis Resulting from Carbonic Anhydrase II Deficiency)

Autosomal Recessive Osteopetrosis (Malignant Osteopetrosis; Autosomal Recessive Marble Bones; Autosomal Recessive Albers-Schonberg Disease)

Incidence: 1:100,000–500,000 live births for the autosomal dominant form and 1:200,000 live births for the autosomal recessive form.

Genetic inheritance: Exists in both autosomal recessive form (infantile or malignant osteopetrosis) and autosomal dominant form (benign osteopetrosis). The responsible mutations have been mapped to several gene loci: for the autosomal recessive form they are 16p13 (chloride channel 7 gene), 11q13.4-q13.5 (T-cell immunoregulator 1 gene), and 6q21 (spontaneous mouse gray lethal

mutation). For the autosomal dominant form, the gene has also been mapped to 11q12-13 and to 16p13 (chloride channel 7 gene). The frequency of the two forms is about equal.

Pathophysiology: On the one hand, the increased skeletal mass is the result of defective bone resorption, which is caused by failure of the (morphologically and numerically normal) osteoclasts to resorb the calcified cartilage during bone development. On the other hand, bone formation and enchondral ossification continue. This combination results in the typical dense radiologic appearance of the sclerotic bones. The microscopic finding of persistent primary spongiosa, which consists of calcified cartilage bars within the sclerotic bone, is considered pathognomonic. This process can occupy the majority of the medullary cavity and thereby affect bone marrow function and lead to extramedullary hematopoiesis with hepatosplenomegaly. The increased fragility of the bones is caused by deficient remodeling presenting as an inability to replace the woven bone by lamellar, mechanically more competent bone.

Diagnosis: Based on radiographic findings and laboratory investigations revealing low serum calcium and elevated serum phosphate and alkaline phosphatase concentrations.

Clinical aspects: Different forms of osteopetrosis have been described.

Autosomal Recessive or Malignant or Infantile Osteopetrosis: Symptoms may be present in fetal life (with risk of stillbirth and spontaneous abortion) or manifest in early infancy. Initial presenting symptoms are failure to thrive with growth retardation and a chronically stuffed nose. Later on, the most common signs are predisposition to pathologic fractures, macrocephaly, progressive blindness and deafness, and hepatosplenomegaly. Hematologic complications are present in more than 70% of these infants and are caused by marked reduction in the volume of bone marrow cavities throughout the body, resulting in severe anemia, thrombocytopenia, and leukoerythroblastosis. Hypersplenism may occur and lead to thrombocytopenia, leukopenia, and hemolytic anemia as a result of extracorpuscular destruction. High levels of fetal hemoglobin (HbF) are possible. Deafness, blindness, optic nerve atrophy, extraocular muscle paralysis, and facial paralysis are thought to represent cranial nerve entrapments caused by bony encroachment to the foramina resulting in compression and ischemia of nerves and nerve roots. Increased intracranial pressure may result from encroachment of the cranial vault, and brainstem compression may occur when the foramen magnum is affected. Seizures have been described but are most often caused by hypocalcemia (tetany). Upper respiratory tract infections are more frequent in these infants, with a higher risk of airway obstruction, most likely because of bony encroachment of the nasal turbinates, mandibular enlargement or hypoplasia, and head and neck anomalies. Frontal bossing, hypertelorism, proptosis, high-arched palate, and diminished mobility in the temporomandibular joints are other facial features. Teeth eruption is delayed or absent, and distorted molars and cavities are common. Hepatosplenomegaly because of extramedullary hematopoiesis leads to cranial displacement of the diaphragm with reduced lung volume (functional residual lung capacity) and atelectases, putting these infants at risk for profound arterial desaturation, particularly during induction and emergence of anesthesia. Untreated, this form of osteopetrosis is invariably fatal during early childhood. Several treatment plans have been attempted. An increasing number of these patients are undergoing HLA-identical allogenic bone marrow transplant, with 5-year survival rates up to almost 80%. However, long-term prognosis still is not favorable for these patients. Severe hypercalcemia has been reported during recovery of osteoclast function in patients with successful engraftment.

Autosomal Dominant or Benign or Adult Osteopetrosis: Usually diagnosed in adolescence or early adulthood; about half of patients are asymptomatic and diagnosed only by accident or based on the family history. A majority of patients complain about bone pain. Recurrent fractures (in almost half of patients) and osteomyelitis (typically in the mandible) are the leading reasons for seeking medical attention. Patients suffer from cranial nerve entrapment and other compression neuropathies (e.g., carpal tunnel syndrome), but in general the symptoms are significantly milder than in the neonatal form. Bone marrow function in these patients is normal. Visual impairment can occur, but in contrast to the neonatal form it seems not to be caused by nerve entrapment but by retinal degeneration. Psychomotor retardation has been described. The autosomal dominant form is divided into two types (I and II), which mainly differ in their distribution of the osteopetrotic changes. Furthermore, type II patients have an increased risk of pathologic fractures, whereas type I patients seem to have normal bone strength. Age and gender are not significantly different for the two groups.

Autosomal Dominant or Benign Osteopetrosis Type I: Although there is generalized osteosclerosis, the most significant changes affect the cranial vault. Patients may suffer from bone pain and hearing loss (nerve entrapment) but can also be asymptomatic with a low risk of fractures. No signs of spinal osteosclerosis. "Bone-in-bone" changes (endobones) in the pelvis and long bones are absent, as is the transverse banding of metaphyses. Serum acid phosphatase concentrations are normal, and serum phosphate levels are lower than in type II.

Autosomal Dominant or Benign Osteopetrosis Type II: Osteosclerosis is generally more pronounced, and cranial sclerosis mainly affects the skull base. The spine is significantly affected with osteosclerosis of the endplates and reduced density between them, resulting in "sandwich vertebrae" or "rugger-jersey spine" appearance on radiography. The finding of endobones in the pelvis and long bones is typical. Pathologic fractures (in up to 80% of patients) with delayed healing and dental abscess are leading complications. Approximately 25% of patients develop osteoarthropathy, of which 50% require hip arthroplasty. Serum acid phosphatase and creatinine kinase BB isoenzyme concentrations are significantly elevated.

Precautions before anesthesia:

Infantile Form of Osteopetrosis: Evaluate for possible difficult airway management, especially in the presence of significant frontal bossing or facial narrowing. Obtain complete blood count with differentiation, serum electrolytes, including calcium, phosphate, and magnesium preoperatively. Need coagulation profile. Patients are at risk for cardiac conduction abnormalities and cardiovascular instability with hypocalcemia, hypophosphatemia, and hypomagnesemia. Preoperative correction of electrolyte and hematologic abnormalities is recommended. Erythropoietin, colony-stimulating factor, γ-interferon, and steroids have been used to correct hematologic abnormalities and immune function. Obtain a 12-lead ECG to evaluate conduction anomalies secondary to electrolyte disturbances (i.e., calcium and phosphate). Consider endocrinology and hematology consultations preoperatively. Assess neurologic function and physical examination to evaluate cranial nerve palsies and tetany and to exclude increased intracranial pressure. Obtain cervical spine flexion-extension radiographs if cervical spine stability is questionable. A full

set of body radiographs can be necessary to identify pathologic fractures.

Adult Form of Osteopetrosis: In general, these patients have a significantly lower anesthetic risk than individuals with infantile osteopetrosis. Check for signs of entrapment of cranial and other nerves. Evaluate the range of motion in the cervical spine with regard to airway management. Check serum electrolytes. Central neuraxial blockade may be challenging because of vertebral changes and difficulty in positioning the patient properly.

Anesthetic considerations:

Infantile Form of Osteopetrosis: Airway management has been described as difficult in 17% of patients and tracheal intubation difficult in 14%. The difficulty can be explained by mandibular hypoplasia or overgrowth, decreased mobility in the temporomandibular joints, blocked nasal passage, and decreased range of motion in the cervical spine. Perioperative morbidity but also mortality resulting from pulmonary complications (at least partly anesthesia-related) have been reported. Bony encroachment of the nasal turbinates either demands a smaller endotracheal tube than expected or makes nasal intubation impossible. Beware of profuse hemorrhage caused by forceful trials of nasal intubation in the presence of uncorrected thrombocytopenia. Exercise caution when positioning these patients because they are prone to pathologic fractures. Patients are at risk for tetany in the postoperative period. Inherent defects of the immune system (leukocyte and macrophage dysfunction) predispose these patients to infections and require strict aseptic technique for all interventional procedures.

Adult Form of Osteopetrosis: Anesthetic management is not expected to be significantly different from that of a healthy patient undergoing the same procedure. Nevertheless, careful positioning to prevent fractures is recommended for these patients. Psychomotor retardation and hearing and visual impairment can make cooperation difficult. Sedative and anxiolytic sedation and the presence of the primary caregiver during induction may be helpful.

Pharmacological implications: Patients may be receiving calcium and calcitonin supplementation preoperatively. Volatile anesthetics, propofol, midazolam, ketamine, opioids, and depolarizing, as well as nondepolarizing, neuromuscular blockers have all been used successfully in these patients without adverse effects attributed to the drug used. Patients receiving chronic steroid administration must receive peroperative supplementation.

Other conditions to be considered:

☞**CRANIODIAPHYSEAL DYSPLASIA:** Bone disorder characterized by marked hyperostosis of the craniofacial bones and diaphyseal expansion of the tubular bones resulting in significant clinical complications.

☞**DYSOSTEOSCLEROSIS:** Genetic disorder with unfavorable prognosis manifesting as blindness, mental retardation, and characteristic skeletal changes.

REFERENCES:

Benichou OD, Laredo JD, De Vernejoul MC: Type II autosomal dominant osteopetrosis (Albers-Schönberg disease): Clinical and radiological manifestations in 42 patients. *Bone* 26:87, 2000.

Burt N, Haynes GR, Bailey MK: Patients with malignant osteopetrosis are at high risk of anesthetic morbidity and mortality. *Anesth Analg* 88:1292, 1999.

Felix R, Hofstetter W, Cecchini MG: Recent developments in the understanding of the pathophysiology of osteopetrosis. *Eur J Endocrinol* 134:143, 1996.

Otopalatodigital (OPD) Syndrome Type I

At a glance: Rare congenital association characterized by hypertelorism, prominent supraorbital ridges, abnormal pinnae, broad nasal bridge with small nose and mouth, and downward-slanting palpebral fissures. Brachydactyly with cone-shaped epiphyses, cutaneous syndactyly, flattened tip of thumbs, splayed "frog" feet with a short hallux and a large gap between the first and second toes, and lateral curvature of the toes (clinodactyly on the fifth fingers and broad big toes). Other features include coarse facies, posterior cleft palate, and conduction deafness. The skull and limb are most often abnormal.

Synonym: Taybi Syndrome.

Genetic inheritance: X-linked transmission with intermediate expression in females and complete expression in males; the altered gene has been mapped to chromosome Xq28.

Pathophysiology: Unknown.

Diagnosis: Based on clinical aspect and radiography; female carriers present mild clinical expression (short nails, clinodactyly of toes, radiograph of anomalies in limbs and skull). A secondary ossification center at the base of the second metacarpal and metatarsal is characteristic.

Clinical aspects: Small stature (<10th percentile for age); mild mental deficiency with moderate conductive deafness. Facial bone hypoplasia with hypertelorism, small nose and mouth are present. The presence of a broad nasal root gives the affected individual a pugilistic appearance. Partial anodontia; cleft soft palate. Thickened base of skull and frontal bone with frontal and occipital prominence; failure of fusion of the posterior aspects of the spine. Absent frontal and sphenoid sinuses. Pectus excavatum. Broad thumbs and great toes; short nails, clinodactyly, limited elbow extension with dislocation of radial head. Small iliac crests.

Precautions before anesthesia: Check teeth for caries and fragility. It is recommended to obtain a radiograph of the spine to rule out cervical instability (especially C1-C2 junction) and/or risk of brainstem compression during head flexion or extension. Severe pectus excavatum may result in restrictive pulmonary disease. Facial bone hypoplasia with small nose places the patient at risk for obstructive sleep apnea.

Anesthetic considerations: Possible difficult direct laryngoscopy and tracheal intubation. Postoperative brainstem compression secondary to thickened base of the skull has been reported.

Pharmacological implications: No specific implications.

REFERENCES:

Clark JR, Smith LJ, Kendall BE, et al: Unexpected brainstem compression following routine surgery in a child with oto-palato-digital syndrome. *Anaesthesia* 50:641, 1995.

Pazzaglia UE, Beluffi G: Oto-palato-digital syndrome in four generations of a large family. *Clin Genet* 30:338, 1986.

Otopalatodigital (OPD) Syndrome Type II

At a glance: Genetic disorder involving the craniofacial, oral, and osseous structures, characterized by short stature, unusual facies, cleft palate, and multiple skeletal malformations. Usually psychomotor development is normal, but some affected individuals are mentally retarded. Affected males show a very high incidence of neonatal and infancy death.

Synonyms: Crarioorodigital Syndrome; Faciopalatoosseous Syndrome; FPO.

Incidence: Approximately 20 cases reported in the literature.

Genetic inheritance: As in otopalatodigital syndrome type I, X-linked transmission with intermediate expression in females and complete expression in males. The gene for OPD II could be allelic with the gene for OPD I.

Pathophysiology: Unknown.

Diagnosis: Clinical based on the association of a characteristic facies and limb defects that can be confirmed radiologically. The presence of other affected male relatives in the maternal family makes diagnosis easier. Female carriers may present some milder features of the syndrome.

Clinical aspects: Affected patients have a characteristic facies with severe micrognathia, microstomia, cleft palate, posteriorly rotated ears, prominent forehead, hypertelorism, and midfacial hypoplasia. They also present skeletal anomalies consisting of broad and short thumbs and halluces associated with short first and second metacarpals/metatarsals on the radiographs, bowing of the long bones, subluxation of many joints in the upper and lower limb, flexed overlapping fingers, clinodactyly, syndactyly of digits 3 and 4, and syndactyly of toes 2 to 5. Other features have been described, such as conductive deafness, growth failure, omphalocele, and other midline defects. Possible anomalies of the cervical spine. In affected boys, death often occurs before age 5 months as a consequence of respiratory insufficiency induced by recurrent aspiration and infection.

Precautions before anesthesia: Chest radiograph to rule out pulmonary infection. Radiograph of the spine to rule out cervical anomalies. Perform careful evaluation of the airway.

Anesthetic considerations: Patients present multiple craniofacial features that may render direct laryngoscopy and tracheal intubation difficult, so different intubating devices should be readily available.

Pharmacological implications: No known implications.

Other conditions to be considered: The similarity of these conditions has suggested this is a "family" or spectrum of skeletal dysplasias with a common biochemical and/or genetic etiology in their pathogenesis.

☞**LARSEN SYNDROME:** Genetic syndrome characterized by special facial features, multiple joint dislocations, finger and foot deformities, and airway and cardiac abnormalities.

☞**BOOMERANG DYSPLASIA:** Genetic disorder characterized by a form of lethal neonatal dwarfism in which the long bones have a boomerang shape, resulting in skeletal dysplasia.

☞**DIASTROPHIC DYSPLASIA:** Rare disorder present at birth. Characterized by short stature and short-limbed dwarfism, skeletal dysplasia, joint dysplasia, scoliosis and/or kyphosis, abnormal tissue changes of the outer visible portions of the ears (pinnae), and craniofacial anomalies.

☞**MELNICK-NEEDLES SYNDROME:** Lethal male form is a genetic disorder characterized by abnormal bone development. Bowing of the bones in the arms and legs is characteristic. Particular facial appearance includes hypertelorism, full cheeks, small facial bones, and severe micrognathia. Other features include a relatively small chest cavity with irregular ribbon-like ribs, short clavicle, short stature, and narrow shoulders. Pectus excavatum is often present. Dislocation of the hip occurs occasionally. May present with hydronephrosis caused by urinary retention as a result of small ureters.

REFERENCES:

Holder SE, Winter RM: Otopalatodigital syndrome type II. *J Med Genet* 30:310, 1993.

Young K, Barth CK, Moore C, et al: Otopalatodigital syndrome type II associated with omphalocele: Report of three cases. *Am J Med Genet* 45;481, 1993.

Otospondylomegaepiphyseal Dysplasia

At a glance: Disease with peculiar facies and severe degenerative joint disease of the osteoarthritis type affecting predominantly the hips, knees, elbows, and shoulders.

Synonyms: Nance Insley Syndrome; Nance Sweeny Chondrodysplasia; Chondrodystrophy with Sensorineural Deafness; OSMED.

Incidence: Unknown.

Genetic inheritance: Autosomal recessive and dominant forms exist. The responsible gene is located on 6p21.3.

Pathophysiology: Otospondylomegaepiphyseal dysplasia (OSMED) is a type XI collagenopathy with mutations in the procollagen XI genes (COL11A1 and COL11A2). However, the exact pathomechanism remains unclear.

Diagnosis: Based on the clinical association of peculiar facies (hypoplastic midface with short, upturned nose having depressed nasal bridge, prominent eyes, and prominent supraorbital ridges), progressive sensorineural deafness, and severe degenerative joint disease of the osteoarthritis type predominantly affecting the hips, knees, elbows, and shoulders.

Clinical aspects: Can involve *head* and *neck* (mandibular hypoplasia, Pierre-Robin sequence [micrognathia, glossoptosis, cleft palate/uvula], flattened nose and cheek bones, anteverted nares), *limbs* (shortening of the long bones, short fingers, and metacarpals, fusion of the carpal bones, restricted joint mobility, metaphyseal flaring, large tarsal bones, prominent interphalangeal joints), and *axial skeleton* (enlarged odontoid in childhood, platyspondyly, anterior vertebral wedging, coronal vertebral clefts, kyphosis, scoliosis, square iliac wings,). Other features may include ventricular septal defect, recurrent lower respiratory tract infections, hemangiomas, and lacrimal duct abnormalities.

Precautions before anesthesia: If cardiac disease is suspected, evaluate cardiac function (clinically, ECG, echocardiogram). Assess for signs of difficult airway management. If kyphosis/scoliosis is severe, obtain lung function tests and chest radiograph.

Anesthetic considerations: Features of the disease suggest that direct laryngoscopy and tracheal intubation may be difficult. Special precautions against corneal injury should be taken in the presence of prominent eyes and lacrimal duct abnormalities. Patient may have ventricular septal defect, which requires specific anesthesia precautions. Vascular access and patient positioning may be difficult because of joint contractures.

Pharmacological implications: Avoid neuromuscular blockers and maintain spontaneous ventilation until the airway has been secured. Subacute bacterial endocarditis prophylaxis may be indicated in the presence of a cardiac lesion.

Other conditions to be considered: OSMED is allelic with Stickler syndrome and Weissenbacher-Zweymüller syndrome.

☞**STICKLER SYNDROME:** Autosomal dominant inherited disorder most often caused by mutation in the COL2A1 gene; mutations in the COL11A1 and COL11A2 are less common. The pathognomonic feature is an vitreous gel architecture, which is associated with high, congenital, and nonprogressive myopia and a significantly increased risk of rhegmatogenous (associated with retinal tears) retinal detachment. Other signs include midface hypoplasia, flat nasal bridge, short nose with anteverted nares, micrognathia, and cleft palate. Joint hypermobility usually improves with age, whereas degenerative osteoarthritic symptoms (mainly hip and knee) are progressive and become manifest in the third or fourth decade of life. Conductive (secondary to cleft palate with chronic otitis media) but predominantly sensorineural hearing loss is common. Patients are most often mentally normal and of normal height. Mitral valve prolapse syndrome (☞Barlow Syndrome) has been reported to be a common finding (patients may require subacute bacterial endocarditis prophylaxis if thickened leaflets or signs of regurgitation are present).

WEISSENBACHER-ZWEYMÜLLER SYNDROME (Pierre-Robin Syndrome with Fetal Chondrodysplasia): Micrognathia and rhizomelic chondrodysplasia with enlargement of the epiphyses and metaphyses of the long bones resulting in a typical dumbbell shape (especially of humeri and femora) are the hallmarks of this autosomal recessive inherited syndrome. However, the overall changes are milder than those observed in OSMED and tend to resolve with increasing age, with impressive catch-up growth finally resulting in normal adult height. Midface hypoplasia, eye (optic nerve hypoplasia, severe myopia, retinal detachment) and ear (sensorineural hearing loss) anomalies, vertebral coronal clefts, and meningoceles/encephaloceles have been described in some patients. Psychomotor development is often delayed.

☞**MARSHALL SYNDROME:** Autosomal dominant inherited disorder characterized by cataracts, myopia, abnormal vitreous, hypertelorism, midfacial hypoplasia, and congenital deafness. Some researchers consider Stickler and Marshall syndromes to be distinct entities, whereas others believe they are basically the same disease. This issue has not been resolved. Cleft palate is not as common in Marshall syndrome as in Stickler syndrome. In Marshall syndrome, the midface is described as flat with an upturned nose and large eyes; in Stickler syndrome, the face is rather long and flat with depressed nasal bridge.

☞**WAGNER SYNDROME:** Characterized by several optical malformations (e.g., ensheathed retinal vessels, retinal pigmentation, circular membranes in a liquefied vitreous, choroidal atrophy) with progressive clinical course ending with optic atrophy and blindness. In contrast to Stickler syndrome, retinal detachment is not a typical finding.

REFERENCES:

Denton R: Anaesthetic problems in the Nance Insley syndrome. *Anaesthesia* 51:100, 1996.

Nance WE, Sweeney A: A recessively inherited chondrodystrophy. *Birth Defects Orig Art Ser* VI:25, 1970.

Van Steensel MA, Buma P, de Waal Malefijt MC: Oto-spondylomegaepiphyseal dysplasia (OSMED): Clinical description of three patients homozygous for a missense mutation in the COL11A2 gene. *Am J Med Genet* 70: 315, 1997.

P

Pachydermoperiostosis (PDP)

At a glance: Characterized by hypertrophic osteoarthropathy, digital clubbing, and subperiosteal new bone formation leading to pain, cutis verticis gyrata, seborrhea, and hyperhidrosis.

Synonyms: Hypertrophic Osteoarthropathy Primary or Idiopathic; Touraine-Solente-Gole Syndrome.

History: First described by Friedreich in 1868.

Incidence: It is associated with more than 5% of all cases of hypertrophic osteoarthropathy. The male-to-female case ratio is approximately 7:1. It is more common in African Americans than whites. In the United States, PDP is a rare disorder and the precise incidence is unknown.

Genetic inheritance: Autosomal dominant pattern with variable penetrance; autosomal recessive forms have been reported.

Pathophysiology: Unknown.

Diagnosis: Clinically with appearance during childhood and slowly progression. Although the evolution of the disease typically stops after 10 years, significant morbidity can be seen. Severe kyphosis, restricted motion, and neurologic manifestations are often significant. Life expectancy is normal except for individuals presenting severe mental impairment. Three forms have been described:

- Complete form with pachydermia (thickening of the facial skin and/or scalp) and periostitis;
- Incomplete form with evidence of bone abnormalities but lacking pachydermia;
- Form fruste with prominent pachydermia and minimal to absent skeletal changes.

Clinical aspects: Features include *skin anomalies* (thick skin, hypoplastic hyperconvex fingernails, cutis gyrata, hyperhidrosis) and *limb malformations* (epiphyseal and cortical anomalies, terminal broadening fingers, arthrosis). Lordosis, dislocated hip, genu varum, osteolysis, and osteoporosis may occur. Acromegaloid facial features have been described.

Precautions before anesthesia: Evaluate the airway in case of severe pachydermic and acromegaloid changes (clinical, radiographs). The thyroid gland should be checked.

Anesthetic considerations: Direct laryngoscopy and tracheal intubation can be difficult and might require adapted anesthetic management. Digital pulse oximetry sensors can be of poor reliability because of fingernail deformations. Careful intraoperative positioning is needed because of skeletal involvement. Vascular access can be difficult because of skin thickening.

Pharmacological implications: Avoid muscle relaxants until tracheal intubation is achieved and lung ventilation confirmed.

Other condition to be considered:

ROSENFELD-KLOEPFER SYNDROME: Characterized by an enlargement of the mandible and/or the maxilla; large hands, feet, nose, lips, and tongue. Other features include prominence of the upper part of the forehead; cutis verticis gyrata, and corneal leukoma. It is known as a variant of PDP.

REFERENCES:

Friedreich N: Hyperostose des gesammten Skelettes. *Arch Pathol Anat* 43:83, 1868.

Jajic Z, Jajic I, Nemcic T: Primary hypertrophic osteoarthropathy: Clinical, radiologic, and scintigraphic characteristics. *Arch Med Res* 32:136, 2001.

Sinha GP, Curtis P, Haigh D, et al: Pachydermoperiostosis in childhood. *Br J Rheumatol* 36:1224, 1997.

PAGOD Syndrome

At a glance: The disorder is called PAGOD syndrome for *P*ulmonary Hypoplasia, Hypoplasia of the Pulmonary *A*rtery, *Ag*onadism, *O*mphalocele/Diaphragmatic Defect, and *D*extrocardia. Other multiple internal organ malformations are also reported.

Synonyms: Agonadism with Multiple Internal Malformations; Kennerbrecht Sorgo Oberhoffer Syndrome.

History: First described by Kennerbrecht in 1993.

Incidence: Unknown; eight cases worldwide.

Genetic inheritance: Autosomal recessive syndrome.

Pathophysiology: Secondary regression of midline structures, including wolffian and müllerian structures, has been evocated to explain pathogenesis (considering mesodermal structures malformations and association of 46,XX constitution with agonadism and intact urogenital tract).

Diagnosis: Signs association does not exist in any other described syndrome and may evocate the diagnosis.

Clinical aspects: Genital abnormalities are always observed with abnormal ovaries, small or atrophic testis, uterine and vaginal malformations. Cardiopulmonary disorders can include hypoplastic lungs, pulmonary artery hypoplasia, cardiac septal defect, coarctation of the aorta, and patent ductus arteriosus. Gastrointestinal tract malformations concern exomphalos and malrotation of the colon. Diaphragmatic hernia is present. Cleft palate, short stature, and mental retardation were observed in two cases.

Precautions before anesthesia: Precise medical evaluation has to be done before any surgical or interventional procedure. Evaluate cardiac function (ECG, echocardiography); pulmonary function (chest radiograph, arterial blood gas analysis, CT, pulmonary function test in old-enough patients). Search for and evaluate other malformative associations (digestive, facial, genital).

Anesthetic considerations: Significant incidence of anesthesia consideration because of cardiac and pulmonary disorders. Hemodynamic systemic variables must be improved before induction of anesthesia. In newborns, the presence of lung hypoplasia and its ongoing management should delay elective surgery.

Pharmacological implications: Drugs with cardiac depressive effects have to be used carefully. Use prophylactic antibiotics.

Other condition to be considered:

☞KENNERBRECHT VOGEL SYNDROME: Characterized by a normal female external genitalia, and absence of gonadal tissue. Except for omphalocele, right renal agenesis, and malrotation of the colon, internal organs tend to be normal. Mental retardation, dwarfism, and markedly retarded bone age are reported. Other minor anomalies include peculiar face, hypodontia, short neck, inverted nipples, thoracolumbar scoliosis, "dysplastic" hips, and partial clino-/syndactyly of the toes. It represents a new autosomal recessive syndrome with a normal 46,XY chromosomal constitution.

REFERENCES:

Kennerknecht I, Sorgo W, Oberhoffer R, et al: Familial occurrence of agonadism and multiple internal malformations in phenotypically normal girls with 46,XY and 46,XX karyotypes, respectively: A new autosomal recessive syndrome. *Am J Med Genet* 47:1166, 1993.

Macayran JF, Doroshow RW, Phillips J, et al: PAGOD syndrome: Eighth case and comparison to animal models of congenital vitamin A deficiency. *Am J Med Genet* 108(3):229, 2002.

Silengo M, Del Monaco A, Linari A, et al: Low birth-weight, microcephalic malformation syndrome in a 46,XX girl and her 46,XY sister with agonadism: Third report of the Kennerknecht syndrome or autosomal recessive Seckel-like syndrome with previously undescribed genital anomalies. *Am J Med Genet* 101:275, 2001.

Pallister-Hall Syndrome

At a glance: Congenital syndrome characterized by hypothalamic hamartoblastoma with panhypopituitarism. Other features include craniofacial abnormalities, polydactyly, endocrine, cardiac, and renal defects. Laryngeal cleft and epiglottis dysplasia are common. Mild retardation is most often present.

Synonyms: CAVE (Cerebro-Acro-Visceral Early Lethality) Complex; Hall-Pallister Syndrome; Congenital Hypothalamic Hamartoblastoma, Hypopituitarism, Imperforate Anus, and Postaxial Polydactyly Syndrome.

History: This medical condition was described in 1980 by Judith G. Hall, an American geneticist, after observing these anomalies in six children. Philip D. Pallister, an American pediatrician and human geneticist, contributed to the genetic determination before his retirement in 1981.

Incidence: Prevalence estimated to fewer than 1000 patients.

Genetic inheritance: Associated with mutations in the GLI3 gene (short arm chromosome 7), a gene regulating other genes in early fetal development; most cases are sporadic, but cases of autosomal dominant inheritance have been observed.

Pathophysiology: Unknown.

Diagnosis: Hormonal deficiencies; hypothalamic hamartoblastoma on MRI: it extends from the optic chiasma to the interpeduncular fossa, thus replacing the hypothalamus and nuclei originating from the embryogenic hypothalamic plate. Other associated cerebral anomalies may be present, including occipital encephalocele and Dandy-Walker malformation.

Clinical aspects: *At birth:* variable syndactyly and postaxial polydactyly with imperforate anus or variable degrees of rectal atresia; flat midface and nasal bridge; short nose with anteverted nares; external ears anomalies (absent auditory canals, malformed pinnae); micrognathia. Laryngeal cleft and dysplastic epiglottis are common. Bifid epiglottis is present in more than 40% of patients. Congenital heart disease: atrial septal defect, ventricular septal defect, patent ductus arteriosus, coarctation of aorta. Patients present with kidney dysplasia, testicular hypoplasia, micropenis, and cryptorchidism. Severely affected infants have impaired pituitary function: growth hormone deficiency and hypothyroidism are common; hypocortisolemia and diabetes insipidus are rarer. Hypoplastic adrenal glands. Some cases with precocious puberty. Bifid, hypoplastic, or absent epiglottis at laryngoscopy. Cases of laryngeal cleft have been described. Abnormal tracheal cartilage and anomalies of pulmonary lobation and lung hypoplasia or dysplasia is frequent. The major-

ity of patients described have died by 3 years of age, the major cause of neonatal death being hypoadrenalism. Long-term survivors are on hormonal therapy from birth or early infancy. Headaches are common. Some patients have seizures. Intelligence is usually normal.

Precautions before anesthesia: Check hormonal treatment: it should be continued up to the day of surgery and adapted with the help of the child's endocrinologist; echocardiography to exclude the presence of a congenital heart defect. A proper evaluation of the airway must be done to eliminate the presence of a laryngeal cleft. The medical history for seizure and antiepileptic medication must be reviewed.

Anesthetic considerations: Tracheal intubation may be difficult in case of microretrognathia and in the presence of an anomalous epiglottis; anomalies of the larynx or trachea may require an endotracheal tube a size smaller than predicted by age. In the presence of a laryngeal cleft, the maintenance of spontaneous respiration is highly recommended. The anesthetic conduct is dictated by the presence of cardiac anomaly.

Pharmacological implications: Antibioprophylaxis in case of cardiac defect.

Other conditions to be considered:

☞**GREIG CEPHALOPOLYSYNDACTYLY SYNDROME:** Characterized by polydactyly, syndactyly, craniofacial malformations frontal bossing, an abnormally broad nasal bridge, and ocular hypertelorism. It is suggested that the inheritance is an autosomal dominant pattern.

☞**ORAL-FACIAL-DIGITAL SYNDROME:** A rare condition categorized into types I to IV. Symptoms common to all four types include neuromuscular disturbances, overgrowth of the frenulum, epicanthus, broad-based nose, polydactyly and syndactyly, extra cranial plate divisions, and clefts of the tongue, jaw, and/or lip. Other clinical features include mental disturbances, dental anomalies, and exotropia.

☞**HOLT-ORAM SYNDROME:** Characterized by distinctive malformations of the bones of the thumbs and upper limbs and/or congenital heart defects. The thumbs may be absent or hypoplastic or triphalangic. Hypoplasia of the scaphoid bones, metacarpals, and upper limb (radius, ulna, and humerus) bones. The congenital heart defects include ventricular and atrial septal defect.

☞**McKUSICK-KAUFMAN SYNDROME:** Characterized by hydrometrocolpos. It develops in females and is associated with anomalies of the limbs (postaxial polydactyly) and congenital heart malformation. The same presentation associated with urogenital anomalies (e.g., hypospadias, prominent scrotal raphe) has been reported in male.

HYDROLETHALUS SYNDROME: Characterized by severe central nervous system malformations (brain and spine) and polydactyly of the hands and toes. Two great toes on each foot, hypoplastic eyes, micrognathia, and poorly formed nose are common features. The presence of macrocephaly with frontal and occipital protuberances, postaxial hexadactyly, and duplicated hallux are characteristics. The association with lung and heart abnormalities is reported in more than 50% of cases. They consist of a large aortic valve (AV) communis defect, stenosis of the airway, and abnormal lobation of the lungs.

☞**SMITH-LEMLI-OPITZ SYNDROME:** A rare inherited disorder of lipid metabolism consisting of a deficiency of the 7-dehydrocholesterol reductase. In type II, the severe form, infants may not survive the newborn period. A less severe clinical expression (type I) may include a small, abnormally long and narrow head, eye abnormalities, a broad nasal tip with anteverted nostrils, broad lateral ridges in the roof of the mouth, and microglossia. Other features include simian creases, syndactyly, unusual fingertip skin patterns, and genital abnormalities. The incidence occurs in relatively high frequency: approximately 1 in 20,000 to 30,000 births in populations of northern and central European background.

REFERENCES:

Biesecker LG, Abbott M, Allen J, et al: Report from the workshop on Pallister-Hall syndrome and related phenotypes. *Am J Med Genet* 65:76–81, 1996.

Stevens CA, Ledbetter JC: Significance of bifid epiglottis. *Am J Med Genet* 134:447, 2005.

Papillon-Lefèvre Syndrome

At a glance: Congenital hyperkeratosis of palms and soles appearing within first 4 years of life. Usually diffuse type, seldom punctate type, and generally not severe. Other features include severe periodontal disease and calcification of the choroid plexus and tentorium.

Synonyms: Keratosis Palmoplantaris with Periodontopathy; Palmoplantar Ectodermal Dysplasia type IV.

History: First described by M.M. Papillon and P. Lefèvre, French dermatologists, in 1924.

Incidence: Four cases per 1 million live births.

Genetic inheritance: Autosomal recessive, maps to the long arm of chromosome 11

Classification: Belongs to the very large group of palmoplantar keratoses, which comprises a number of different clinical entities with both hereditary and acquired forms.

Diagnosis: The periodontosis is the main aspect of this illness with the association of palmoplantar keratoses. May be present at birth but become obvious after 6 months of age. The genetic determination is the only accurate diagnostic.

Clinical aspects: Periodontosis, premature loss of primary and adult teeth, hypodontia. Hyperkeratosis palmoplantaris with transgression onto the elbows and the knees, as well as other areas, hypotrichosis, nail fragility, ectopic intracranial (essentially dura mater) calcifications, eyelid cysts. May be associated with mental retardation, deafness, retardation of skeletal maturation, osteoporosis, arachnodactyly, and, rarely, acroosteolysis. The periodontosis is associated with an elevated rate of cutaneous abscesses and pyogenic infections of internal organs (liver, spleen mainly). No constant association has been found with immunologic disorders. Patients affected with autosomal dominant palmoplantar keratosis often present with malignancies of the esophagus and/or other malignancies (lymphomas, pancreas, breast, etc.). This feature may be associated with severe stricture of the esophagus in childhood. In the absence of genetic differential diagnosis, palmoplantar keratosis must be considered. Aggressive dental treatment and retinoid medication helps to keep definitive denture.

Precautions before anesthesia: Evaluate the gravity of periodontosis and the stability of the residual dentition. Check the infectious status to eliminate the clinical evidence of pyogenic infection (white blood cell count, fever, tenderness of the abdomen, abscesses in the mouth). Estimate the importance of acroosteolysis, if present. A careful evaluation of the medication taken by the patient must be obtained, because the use of retinoid drugs may lead to hypervitaminose A and potential neurological and liver complications.

Anesthetic considerations: A special attention must be given during airway management (insertion of oral airway or laryngeal mask airway, endotracheal intubation) because of the fragility of the teeth and the periodontosis. Because some cases involve the dorsal part of the hand and the feet with poor healing of the skin, it would be better to avoid intravenous access placement in these locations.

Pharmacological implications: These patients are often being treated with retinoid compounds and may present typical status of hypervitaminosis A. No interactions are known with anesthetic products however, neurological and liver side-effects are possible.

Other condition to be considered:

Mal de Meleda (Maleda Syndrome; Keratosis Extremitatum Hereditaria Trangrediens et Progrediens Syndrome): This is a rare medical condition with a prevalence of 1 case in 100,000 population. It is characterized by diffuse, thick keratoderma with a prominent erythematous border that spreads onto the dorsa of the hands and the feet, constricting bands around digits resulting in spontaneous amputation. Other clinical features may include well-circumscribed psoriasis-like plaques or lichenoid patches on the knees and the elbows, hyperhidrosis, periorbital erythema and hyperkeratosis, nail changes (koilonychia, subungual hyperkeratosis), and lingua plicata, syndactyly, hair on the palms and the soles, high-arched palate, and left-handedness.

REFERENCES:

Lucker GPH, Van De Kerkhof PC, Steijlen PM: The hereditary palmoplantar keratoses: An updated review and classification. *Br J Dermatol* 131:1, 1994.

Silvermann AK, Ellis CN, Voorhees JJ, et al: Hypervitaminosis A syndrome: A paradigm of retinoid side effects. *J Am Acad Dermatol* 16:1027, 1987.

Stevens HP, Kelsell DP, Bryant SP, et al: Linkage of an American pedigree with palmoplantar keratoderma and malignancy (palmoplantar ectodermal dysplasia type III) to 17q24: Literature survey and proposed updated classification of the keratodermas. *Arch Dermatol* 132:640, 1996.

Parana Hard Skin Syndrome

At a glance: A very rare syndrome, often lethal in childhood and characterized by a total skin thickening leading to restricted joint mobility and respiratory insufficiency that may lead to death.

Synonym: Hard Skin Syndrome, Parana type.

Incidence and genetic inheritance: Very rare syndrome with geographical influence (Southern Parana region in Brazil). Probable autosomal recessive inheritance.

Clinical aspects: Onset in the first months of life. Generalized thickening of skin and severe growth retardation are the main features. Other signs involve *skin and hair* (hyperkeratosis, increased pigmentation, increased body hair, bushy eyebrows), *face* (round face with down-turned mouth), *musculoskeletal* (abnormal gait, restricted joint mobility, osteoporosis, tapered fingers), and *chest* (pectus carinatum, abnormally placed nipples, respiratory distress).

Anesthetic considerations: Movement limitations because of skin thickening affect whole body and necessitate, probably, a preoperative evaluation of the airway (difficulty of neck extension) and respiratory function (clinical, radiographs, pulmonary function test with arterial blood gases analysis). Postoperative ventilatory support might be necessary. Both venous access and regional anesthesia can be difficult because of skin thickening. Careful intraoperative positioning is needed but can be difficult to realize.

Other conditions to be considered:

STIFF SKIN SYNDROME: Characterized by thickened and indurated skin of the entire body and limitation of joint mobility with flexion contractures. Flexion deformities of fingers and toes, limited motion of several other joints and the vertebral column, sclerodermatoid changes of the skin, and underdeveloped muscles.

SYNDESMODYSPLASIC DWARFISM: Characterized by severe dwarfism and progressive stiff joints, including spine and hips. The skin is, however, considered normal. It has been reported in Berber people of northern Algeria.

REFERENCES:

Cat I, Rodrigues-Magdalena NI, Parolin-Marinoni L, et al: Parana hard-skin syndrome: Study of seven families. *Lancet* I:215, 1974.

Mau U, Kendziorra H, Kaiser P, et al: Restrictive dermopathy: Report and review. *Am J Med Genet* 71(2):179, 1997.

Paroxysmal Cold Hemoglobinuria

At a glance: Paroxysmal Cold Hemoglobinuria (PCH) is characterized by a sudden onset of hemoglobinuria either spontaneously or after exposure to cold. It is considered as one type of Cryopathic Hemolytic Syndrome, which includes two types of autoimmune hemolytic anemias because of cold-reacting autoantibodies.

Synonyms: Donath-Landsteiner Syndrome; Cryopathic Hemolytic Syndrome.

Incidence: Accounts for up to 5% of autoimmune hemolytic anemia. It may be responsible for more than 40% of autoimmune hemolytic anemias in children younger than 5 years. There is no race and sex predilection.

Genetic inheritance: None.

Pathophysiology: Infections, both bacterial and viral, induce the formation of "Donald-Landsteiner" antibodies that are specific for the human P blood group antigen. The P antigen is a glycosphingolipid that is similar to glycolipids in many microorganisms. The Donald-Landsteiner autoantibody is a biphasic hemolysin capable of causing severe hemolysis. These antibodies bind to red cells upon exposure to cold and dissociate at 37°C (98.6°F). However, prior to dissociation, they fix complement and cause hemolysis. Why infections stimulate these antibodies is unknown. During the early 1900s, syphilis was the leading etiology, although today it is more commonly viral.

Diagnosis: The biphasic Donald-Landsteiner test, which consists of mixing the patient's serum with RBCs at 4°C (39.2°F), then heating them to 37°C (98.6°F) and assessing for hemolysis.

Clinical aspects: Fatigue, dyspnea, jaundice, dark urine, and cold urticaria are frequent. Usually self-limited, although occasional fulminant hemolysis requires transfusion. The acute transient form is more common in children than adults.

Precautions before anesthesia: Check hematocrit. Check blood bank availability of P antigen-negative. Transfusion of P-positive RBCs is usually necessary, as the incidence of P antigen-positive blood is about 1:200,000 in general population but can be done safely.

Anesthetic considerations: Avoid hypothermia. Use fluid and blood warmers. Use P antigen-negative blood if available, though P-positive blood is acceptable in urgent situations.

REFERENCE:

Jeffries LC: Transfusion therapy in autoimmune hemolytic anemia. *Hematol Oncol Clin North Am* 8:1087, 1994.

Paroxysmal Nocturnal Hemolytic (PNH) Anemia

At a glance: A rare, acquired hemolytic stem cell disorder.

Synonym: Immune Hemolytic Anemia.

Incidence: PNH is an uncommon disorder of unknown frequency both in the United States and worldwide. It is estimated that it is observed 5–10 times less than with aplastic anemia. It may be more frequent in Southeast Asia and the Far East. The disease process is insidious and has a chronic course, with a median survival of about 10 years. The morbidity is influenced by the importance of the hemolysis, bone marrow failure, and thrombophilia. Men and women are affected equally and the onset begins in childhood (<2 years of age) to adulthood (as old as 85 years of age). Other complications include infections and thrombosis.

Pathophysiology: Hemopoietic stem cell disorder leads to the production of defective platelets, granulocytes, and RBCs. The hemolysis might be triggered by acidosis during sleep. The RBCs have increased sensitivity to complement-mediated hemolysis as a result of deficient decay-accelerated factor. Platelets, too, are more sensitive to complement activation.

Diagnosis: Laboratory diagnosis is based on the Ham test, which mixes affected RBCs with slightly acidified, but otherwise normal, serum. This leads to complement-mediated hemolysis.

Clinical aspects: Chronic hemolysis, anemia, pancytopenia, potentially life-threatening thrombosis secondary to platelet activation, low serum haptoglobin, elevated lactate dehydrogenase, hemosiderinuria, intermittent hemoglobinuria, especially when urine is concentrated, and normal peripheral smear, ± steroids.

Precautions before anesthesia: Check hematocrit, anticipate need for transfusion. Check prothrombin time if the administration of anticoagulant is considered against thrombosis.

Anesthetic considerations: Maintain oxygen-carrying capacity. Avoid regional anesthesia if the patient is anticoagulated or if thrombocytopenia is present.

Pharmacological implication: Steroid supplementation is highly recommended.

REFERENCES:

Kjaer K, Comerford M, Godalla F: General anesthesia for cesarean delivery in a patient with paroxysmal nocturnal hemoglobinuria and thrombocytopenia. *Anesth Analog* 98:1471, 2004.

Tabbara IA: Hemolytic anemias diagnosis and management. *Med Clin North Am* 76(3);649, 1992.

Parry-Romberg Syndrome

At a glance: Progressive facial hemiatrophy characterized by unilateral atrophy of the skin including the subcutaneous tissue and underlying bone or cartilage. In contrast to "sclérodermie en coup de sabre," this form more often affects the lower half of the face (but is not limited to it) with cutaneous sclerosis and possible involvement of tongue, developing teeth, lips, and salivary glands. Seizures and trigeminal-like pain have been reported.

Synonyms: Facial Hemiatrophy; Progressive Hemifacial Atrophy; Romberg Syndrome.

Incidence: Very rare.

History: It was described in the last century (1825) by Parry and Henoch and subsequently in 1846 by Romberg.

Genetic inheritance: Most cases are sporadic; mendelian inheritance with autosomal dominance has been evocated.

Pathophysiology: Unknown; autoimmunity is evocated.

Diagnosis: Characterized by progressive atrophy of some or all tissues on one side of the face, occasionally extending to other parts of the body.

Clinical aspects: Onset occurs most often before puberty or during adolescence. There is no sexual predominance. The process may be bilateral in 5 to 10% of cases, with preferential left-sided involvement. In most affected individuals, hemifacial atrophy typically progresses over approximately 3 to 5 years and then ceases. All

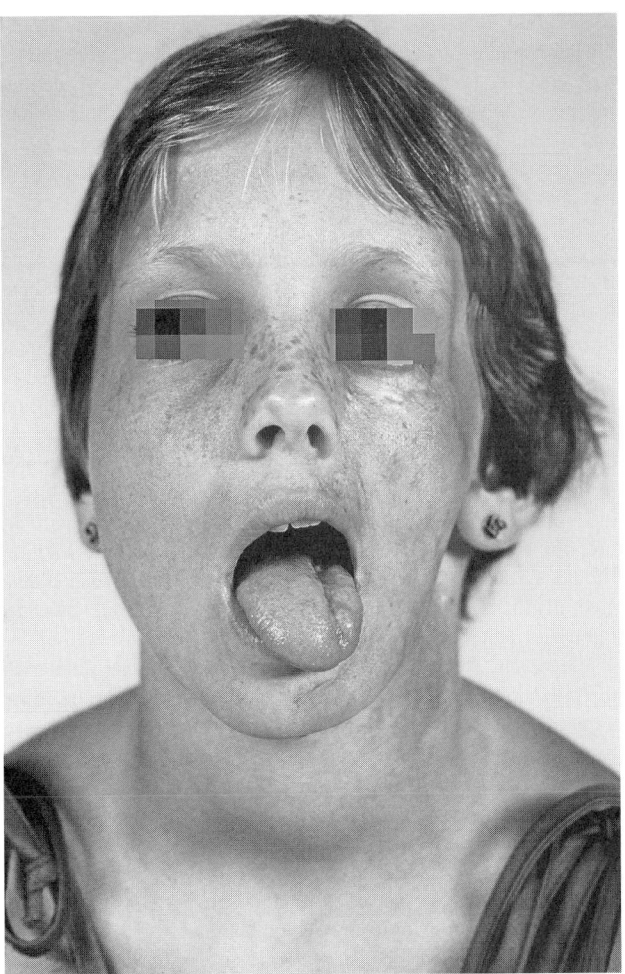

Parry-Romberg syndrome This adolescent girl with Parry-Romberg syndrome presents with a severe form of left-sided hemifacial atrophy involving the skin, subcutaneous tissue, and the osseous structures. This results in left-sided enophthalmos (not shown) and profound atrophy of the skin and the left side of the tongue.

tissues of the face can be involved, including skin (circumscribed cicatricial alopecia, poliosis, increased patchy skin pigmentation), tongue, lip, gingiva, soft palate, cartilage of the nose, ear, subcutaneous fat, larynx, muscle (facial muscle atrophy), eye (enophthalmos, lagophthalmos, ptosis, blepharoptosis, blepharophimosis, loss of periorbital fat, mixed coloring of iris), and bone (basilar kyphosis short body and ramus of mandible). Delayed teeth eruption on ipsilateral side, which leads to malocclusion is frequent. Neurological signs are associated: Horner syndrome, trigeminal neuralgia, ataxia, migraine, and seizures (contralateral Jacksonian epilepsy).

Precautions before anesthesia: Evaluate neurological function (clinical, history, CT scan, EEG); vision (clinical); airway (clinical, radiographs).

Anesthetic considerations: Direct laryngoscopy and tracheal intubation may be difficult because of tongue atrophy and mandibular anomalies. Tracheal intubation may also be difficult because of laryngeal muscles atrophy. Extubation should probably be overseen for the same reasons. Ventilation with facial mask can be difficult because of hemifacial atrophy. Spontaneous respiration must be maintained until the trachea has been secured and lung ventilation confirmed. A laryngeal mask airway should be immediately available. Ocular protection is imperative.

Pharmacological implications: Consider interaction between antiepileptic agent and anesthetic drugs.

Other condition to be considered:

☞**CREST Syndrome:** An autoimmune connective tissue disorder associated with anticentromere antibodies. A form of scleroderma associated with esophageal dysmotility.

REFERENCES:

Lewkonia RM, Lowry RB: Progressive hemifacial atrophy (Parry-Romberg syndrome): Report with review of genetics and nosology. *Am J Med Genet* 14:385, 1983.

Parry CH: Facial hemiatrophy, in *Collections from the Unpublished Medical Writings of the Late Caleb Hillier Parry.* Vol. I. London, Underwood, 1825, p 478.

Stone J: Parry-Romberg syndrome: a global survey of 205 patients using the Internet. *Neurology* 61:674, 2003.

Patterson Pseudo-Leprechaunism Syndrome

At a glance: An extremely rare hyperpigmentation, endocrine anomalies, and mental retardation syndrome.

Diagnosis: Patterson and Watkins originally described a 10-month-old boy who they thought had leprechaunism. However, in view of the normal birth weight (rather than the usual severe intrauterine growth retardation in leprechaunism) and marked cutis gyrata of hands and feet, as well as a generalized skeletal disorder, they suggested the disorder is distinct from leprechaunism. Since then the syndrome is characterized by skeletal dysplasia, hyperpigmentation, cutis laxa, endocrine abnormalities, and mental impairment. The boy also had hyperadrenocorticism and diabetes mellitus. There is no insight as to the genetics or other etiology of this disorder.

Clinical aspects: Children are usually of normal birth weight. They may have generalized skeletal abnormalities, hyperadrenocorticism, and diabetes mellitus. In addition they have cutis gyrata of the hands and feet. Case reports have noted bladder diverticula and marked enlargement of the adrenal glands, especially of the zona fasciculata.

Anesthetic considerations: Obtain full history and examination. Recent blood glucose and evaluation of sodium, potassium, and water balance in view of possible hyperadrenocorticism. May have undiagnosed hypertension.

REFERENCE:
David TJ, Webb BW, Gordon IRS: The Patterson syndrome, leprechaunism, and pseudoleprechaunism. *J Med Genet* 18:294, 1981.

Pearson Syndrome

At a glance: Mitochondrial Cytopathy Disease presenting in infancy as sideroblastic anemia, pancytopenia, defective oxidative phosphorylation, exocrine pancreatic insufficiency, and variable hepatic, renal, and endocrine failure. Death often occurs in infancy as a consequence of infection or metabolic crisis. Those who survive the first year of life present with ☞Kearns-Sayre Syndrome (progressive mitochondrial disorder characterized by progressive external ophthalmoplegia and weakness of skeletal muscle).

Synonym: Pearson Marrow-Pancreas Syndrome.

History: Originally described by Pearson et al. in 1979, the disorder involves the hematopoietic system (sideroblastic anemia with vacuolization of marrow precursors) and exocrine pancreatic dysfunction, as well as liver and kidney dysfunction.

Incidence: Unknown; isolated case reports only.

Genetic inheritance: The existence of an autosomal dominant mitochondrial DNA breakage syndrome is well established. There is mitochondrial DNA (mtDNA) deletion in a lymphoblastoid cell line in patients with Pearson Syndrome. Both sexes are affected.

Pathophysiology: This disease results from a defect of oxidative phosphorylation associated with deletions of the mitochondrial DNA. Severe, transfusion-dependent, macrocytic anemia starting in infancy may be associated with variable degree of neutropenia and thrombopenia. In addition there may be defects in liver (hepatic failure), kidney (proximal tubulopathy), gut (watery diarrhea), and skin (patchy erythematous lesions). High lactate/pyruvate molar ratios in plasma.

Diagnosis: Pearson Syndrome resembles the Shwachman Syndrome in some ways in that bone marrow dysplasia and exocrine pancreas failure also occurs. However, the disorders differ in bone marrow morphology and Shwachman Syndrome also includes metaphysical chondrodysplasia. The bone marrow in patients with Pearson Syndrome is characterized by marked vacuolization of myeloid precursors and ringed sideroblasts and reduction in the size and number of the islets, fibrosis, and acinar atrophy of the pancreas. In addition, there is vacuolation of renal tubules, glomerulosclerosis, and "ragged red" fibers of skeletal muscles. mtDNA deletion is present in liver and skeletal muscle biopsies. In 1992, Gibson et al. detected 3-methylglutaconicaciduria in four patients with Pearson Syndrome and suggested that this finding may be a useful marker for Pearson Syndrome and more specific than other organic acids identified in this disorder. This disorder is fatal and few patients survive beyond a few years.

Clinical aspects: Typical hematologic symptoms (transfusion-dependent severe macrocytic anemia, neutropenia, thrombocytopenia) in early infancy. Insulin-dependent diabetes mellitus may develop during the course of the illness. There is failure to thrive

secondary to exocrine pancreatic dysfunction and malabsorption. A few neonates with Pearson Syndrome have been reported to present with lactic acidosis. The tissue distribution and relative proportions of abnormal mtDNA molecules determine the phenotype and the clinical course. In general, the clinical course is progressive and death occurs in infancy. Some surviving patients later developed features of Kearns-Sayre Syndrome (another mtDNA deletion disorder with retinopathy, myopathy, and cardiac involvement), depending on the distribution of deleted mtDNA.

Precautions before anesthesia: The diagnosis of mitochondrial disease should be considered in any child with a multisystem neurological disorder or who is being investigated for hypotonia. Anesthesia-related morbidity and mortality risk is essentially linked to the preoperative status of the child, that is, the number and extent of organ dysfunction. The presence of a mitochondrial disease is not considered a risk for malignant hyperthermia. Avoid any elective anesthesia/surgery in the presence of infection or temperature because cytokines (mainly tumor necrosis factor) inhibit some complex of the respiratory chain. The following should be checked: *CNS:* seizures, myoclonus, strokes, swallowing problems; *metabolic:* usual venous or arterial concentration of lactates and glucose; *muscles:* hypotonia, contractures, scoliosis; *cardiac:* even if the child is asymptomatic, ECG and echocardiography to exclude for conduction disorders and cardiomyopathy, respectively; if a pacemaker has been inserted, check it to be sure that it is functioning properly; *pulmonary:* frequent infections, chronic aspiration, pulse oximetry breathing room air, obstructive and/or central apnea; reduced ventilatory drive is common and many patients have an abnormal response to both hypoxia and hypercarbia; deaths have been reported following sedation with chloral hydrate or diazepam; *hepatic* and *renal* function must be evaluated; *nutritional status* and *diet* (glucose and/or lipid rich), tolerance to fasting and treatment (carnitine, vitamin Q, antiepileptic drugs).

Anesthetic considerations: Usual treatment up to the day of surgery. Preoperative fasting for as short a time as possible; if fasting is usually poorly tolerated, a glucose-containing solution should be started when fasting period starts. A sedative premedication is best avoided because of the possible abnormal response to hypoxia/hypercarbia. *Induction:* according to the anesthesiologist's choice; sevoflurane is the best choice for inhalation induction; propofol seems the best choice for IV induction but a 2% solution should be used to lessen the lipid load. *Opiates:* The dose should be carefully titrated according to the patient's needs. *Muscle relaxant:* Published data are often contradictory. Even in the absence of clinical myopathy, the patient's muscular response to nerve stimulation (e.g., tetralogy of Fallot) should be measured before administering a muscle relaxant. Atracurium or *cis*-atracurium is the best choice because of their spontaneous degradation. In case of myopathy, succinylcholine should not be used so as to avoid producing rhabdomyolysis. *Intraoperative fluids:* avoid infusion containing lactates such as Ringer lactate or Hartmann solution, but give the patient a glucose (5 or 10% according to blood sugar level) solution. Aim for normoglycemia because hyperglycemia can also increase lactate production. Monitor (arterial or venous) blood gases and lactate levels: in case of severe lactic acidosis use dichloroacetate 50 mg/kg IV over 30 minutes to stimulate pyruvate dehydrogenase to metabolize lactate in pyruvate. Perimedullar locoregional anesthesia can be used, but its cost:benefit ratio should be evaluated taking into account the presence of severe scoliosis or of degenerative lesions in the spinal cord. Some patients with mitochondrial disease also present with axonal neuropathy of peripheral nerves; the possible effects of local anesthetics on these nerves are unknown. Prevention of hypothermia is important to avoid shivering and increased oxygen consumption at awakening.

Pharmacological implications: Patients with mitochondrial disease are very sensitive to the respiratory effects of sedatives. It also seems, according to BIS measurement, that children with an anomaly of complex I of the respiratory chain are much more sensitive to the hypnotic effects of sevoflurane. Most studies performed on isolated mitochondria use doses of anesthetic agents far in excess of those used in daily practice and their clinical relevance is thus often dubious.

Other conditions to be considered:

☞SHWACHMAN-DIAMOND SYNDROME is characterized primarily by exocrine pancreatic insufficiency, hematologic abnormalities, increased risk of malignant transformation, and skeletal abnormalities (metaphyseal dysostosis type). The most frequent hematological abnormality is neutropenia (88%); however, leukopenia, thrombocytopenia, and anemia are also frequently encountered. Pancytopenia can be seen in these patients. Individuals affected with Shwachman-Diamond Syndrome are predisposed to hematologic malignancies similar to those that occur with Fanconi anemia. The exocrine pancreas is replaced by fat, whereas the islets of Langerhans are normal.

☞KEARNS-SAYRE SYNDROME: Characterized by a mitochondrial encephalomyopathy leading to external ophthalmoplegia, a typical retinitis pigmentosa, and cardiomyopathy.

REFERENCES:

Pearson HA, Lobel JS, Kocoshis SA, et al: A new syndrome of refractory sideroblastic anemia with vacuolization of marrow precursors and exocrine pancreatic dysfunction. *J Pediatr* 95(6):976, 1979.

Rotig A, Cormier V, Blanche S, et al: Pearson's marrow-pancreas syndrome: A multisystem mitochondrial disorder in infancy. *J Clin Invest* 86:1601, 1990.

Rotig A, Cormier V, Koll F, et al: Site-specific deletions of the mitochondrial genome in the Pearson marrow-pancreas syndrome. *Genomics* 10:502, 1991.

Pectus Excavatum

At a glance: Abnormal formation of the rib cage leading to a depression deformity of the lower part of the sternum, resulting in a sunken chest appearance. Most often associated with a large range of disorders where pectus excavatum is a prominent feature.

Synonym: Familial Congenital Funnel Chest.

Incidence: Pectus excavatum occurs in an estimated 1 in 300–400 births in the United States, with male predominance (male-to-female ratio of 3:1). It is typically noticed at birth, and more than 90% are confirmed within the first year of life. No specific data are available in relation to the international frequency; however, it is probably the same as that reported for the United States. Pectus excavatum appears to be most prevalent in the white population. Clinical observation indicates that treating African Americans with pectus excavatum is unusual. The male-to-female ratio is 3:1. Despite such observation, no known genetic factor linked to the X or Y chromosome exists.

Genetic inheritance: Usually sporadic. Familial occurrence has also been reported as an autosomal dominant trait.

Pathophysiology: The condition may be congenital or acquired. The acquired form may be secondary, caused by chronic airway obstruction in infancy secondary to enlarged tonsil and adenoids, laryngomalacia, or external pressure applied to the anterior surface of the chest. Familial Congenital Funnel Chest has also been described with an autosomal dominant inheritance. This condition may result in a restrictive lung pattern defect. Occasionally, the heart may be shifted leftward, which rarely may adversely cardiac function.

Diagnosis: Characteristic morphologic deformities. The superior manubrium is normal. The sharp slope inward and toward the vertebral column begins at the manubrioglabior junction. The depth of the concavity varies from a shallow depression to near contact with the vertebral column. Chest radiography confirms the diagnosis.

Clinical aspects: It is usually an isolated skeletal anomaly. The deformity at birth may be minimal or extensive, and may progress, regress, or remain stationary. With time, there is restricted growth of the thorax in the anteroposterior direction but lateral development is unrestricted. In the newborn, the pliable sternum may move paradoxically with respiration but is otherwise asymptomatic. In the older child, there may be decreased effort tolerance, chest pain, wheezing, stridor, and repeated upper respiratory tract infections. The narrowing of the thoracic cavity may lead to restrictive lung disease. It may be associated with segmental bronchomalacia, especially involving the left main stem bronchus. Cardiac dysfunction, especially the right side of the heart, may occur in some patients. Mitral valve prolapse has been reported in 20–60% of cases. Exercise tolerance is usually normal. The Ravitch-Sutherland procedure, and, more recently, a minimally invasive method, is usually performed to correct respiratory and/or cardiac functional impairment caused by the malformation or mainly for cosmetic reasons. Good functional and cosmetic long-term results are obtained.

Precautions before anesthesia: Preoperative abnormalities of ECG are common (incomplete right bundle-branch block, left atrium enlargement, and sinus arrhythmia); usually a result of displacement rather than intrinsic heart disease. Pulmonary function is restricted in patients with severe pectus excavatum and repeated chest infections. The tracheobronchial tree should be assessed with tomography or CT scan in those patients with severe pectus excavatum. Assess for other syndromes. Important to have a detailed postoperative pain plan.

Anesthetic considerations: General anesthesia with controlled ventilation is employed. Invasive arterial pressure monitoring is not necessary unless there is significant underlying cardiopulmonary disease. Abnormal thoracic configuration can cause respiratory distress secondary to severe compression of the central airways. A fiberoptic bronchoscopic examination may be necessary in these patients to ensure that the endotracheal tube is below the obstructed area to optimize intraoperative ventilation. Possibility of pneumothorax during surgical correction. Massive bleeding from the internal thoracic artery has also been reported. Most patients can be extubated at the end of the surgery. Supplemental oxygen therapy is often necessary in the postoperative period. Postoperative pain leads to splinting of the chest, which can cause atelectasis and/or pneumonia. Epidural anesthesia have been shown to reduce severe postoperative pulmonary complications. Other common postoperative complications include residual pneumothorax and pleural effusions.

Pharmacological implications: No particular anesthetic agent is indicated or contraindicated. Some would recommend that nitrous oxide be avoided in view of the possibility of pneumothorax development intraoperatively.

Other conditions to be considered: A pectus excavatum is considered a prominent feature of the following conditions: Marfan Syndrome; Ehlers-Danlos Syndrome; Homocystinuria; Osteogenesis Imperfecta; Down Syndrome; Turner Syndrome; Noonan Syndrome; Rett Syndrome; Cutis Laxa, X-Linked; Beals Syndrome; Shprintzen-Goldberg Craniosynostosis Syndrome; Camptodactyly Syndrome.

REFERENCES:

Canovas Martinez L, Dominguez Garcia M, Fernandez Gil N, et al: Thoracic epidural analgesia in the postoperative period of pediatric surgery for the repair of pectus excavatum and pectus carinatum. *Rev Esp Anesthesiol Reanim* 45:148, 1998.

Leung AKC, Hoo JJ: Familial congenital funnel chest. *Am J Med Genet* 26:887, 1987.

Nuss D, Kelly RE, Croitoru DP, et al: A 10-year review of a minimally invasive technique for the correction of pectus excavatum. *J Pediatr Surg* 33:545, 1998.

Pelizaeus-Merzbacher Syndrome

At a glance: A very rare, slowly progressive dysmyelinating disease affecting, in a diffuse pattern, the cerebrum, cerebellum, brainstem, and spinal cord. Two types are described: X-linked (infantile form) and the autosomal dominant (preadulthood form). Clinical features also include stridor, muscle spasticity, and nystagmus. Often fatal in the first year of life from respiratory complications.

Synonyms: Perinatal Sudanophilic Leukodystrophy Acute Infantile form; Connatal Pelizaeus-Merzbacher Syndrome; Seitelberger type of Pelizaeus-Merzbacher Syndrome.

History: Described in 1908 by F. Palizaeus, a German neurologist, and L. Merzbacher, a German psychiatrist.

Incidence: In the United States and internationally, prevalence is estimated to be about 1:100,000 to 1:1 million. There are no reports of African descent published; however, African American cases do exist. Also present in Asia and Europe.

Genetic inheritance: X-linked recessive (infantile form) affects boys. Female heterozygotes can be clinically affected. Autosomal dominant (preadulthood form). Caused by a mutation of PLP on the X chromosome. PLP encodes two products—PLP and a smaller protein DM20. Approximately 60 to 70% of cases result from duplication of the X chromosome that contains the PLP protein.

Pathophysiology: There is a loss of myelin with intact axons because of an anomaly in the gene for proteolipid protein located on chromosome X-q22; this makes oligodendrocytes unable to produce myelin. Severe Pelizaeus-Merzbacher disease is often fatal in the first year of life, typically from respiratory complications. Patients with classic Pelizaeus-Merzbacher disease may survive until the sixth decade. Patients affected with the Spastic Paraplegia type II (SPG II) generally have a normal life span.

Diagnosis: Only men are affected. Diagnosis is based on the clinical constellation. CT scan and MRI are normal in the early stages, but may show ventricular enlargement. Evoked potentials are usually normal but may show delayed latencies.

Clinical aspects: Group of diseases characterized by progressive mental retardation and abnormal movements; there are three forms of clinical presentation.

Infantile form (fast progression): Also called the connatal Pelizaeus-Merzbacher disease. During the first 2 weeks of life the infant presents with severe head shaking with nystagmus and roving eye movements. Poor airway tone with stridor and respiratory complications, severe hypotonia. Motor function is very severely limited. Choreoathetotic movements and spasticity. Developmental milestones are delayed. Acquired microcephaly. Optic atrophy and facial weakness develop later. Seizures are possible. Death usually occurs before 5 to 7 years of age.

Infantile form (slow progression): The signs of the disease appear later and the evolution is slower. The nystagmus is weaker but stridor, dystonia, and pyramidal signs are present. Seizures and cerebellar ataxia are possible. Dysarthria and difficult swallowing develop later. Acquired microcephaly. These children never walk and are unable to sit without support. Death usually occurs in the second to third decade.

Preadulthood form: Nystagmus may not be present or mild. Limb spasticity that is much worse in the legs, ataxia that affects speech, hyperreflexia, and Babinski signs are present. Mild distal sensory loss.

Precautions before anesthesia: Check for antiepileptic medication. Premedication should improve gastric emptying and reduce secretions (atropine).

Anesthetic considerations: Continue preoperative antiepileptic medication until anesthesia and continue it—by parenteral route if necessary—immediately postoperatively. Check for possible perioperative seizures. Children are at risk of aspiration as a consequence of gastroesophageal reflux. Clean the copious oral secretions. Extubate only when fully awake; there are airway complications because of poor pharyngeal muscle control.

Pharmacological implications: Succinylcholine is not recommended when ataxia and spasticity is severe. Dopaminergic-blocking drugs (metoclopramide, butyrophenones) may exacerbate movement disorders. Avoid any drug with proconvulsant activity. No reported problems with nondepolarizing neuromuscular blockers.

Other conditions to be considered: (An overview table can be found under ☞Leukodystrophies)

☞**ALEXANDER SYNDROME:** A degenerative and progressive disorder of the nervous system caused by leukodystrophy. Affects mainly males and usually begins at about 6 months of age. Symptoms include mental and physical retardation, enlargement of the brain and head, spasticity (arms and legs), and seizures.

☞**CANAVAN SYNDROME:** A progressive leukodystrophy caused by spongy degeneration of the central nervous system. It is uniformly fatal within 18 months after onset of symptoms.

☞**METACHROMATIC LEUKODYSTROPHY:** An inherited disorder of myelin metabolism with progressive loss of white matter in the central and peripheral nervous system.

☞**X-LINKED ADRENOLEUKODYSTROPHY:** A disorder characterized by progressive demyelinization of the central nervous system and peripheral adrenal insufficiency.

☞**SCHILDER SYNDROME:** A rare, progressive and lethal disease of the central nervous system that affects mostly children and is characterized by adrenal atrophy and diffuse central demyelination. Presents with progressive dementia, spasticity, cortical blindness, deafness, hemiplegia, quadriplegia, ataxia, pyramidal signs, retrobulbar neuritis, and pseudobulbar palsy. Seizures. Onset in late childhood. Most die within a few months after onset.

☞**ZELLWEGER SYNDROME:** A disorder characterized by the congenital absence of functioning peroxisomes (the cellular structures that are responsible for the elimination of toxic substances) resulting in a cerebrohepatorenal syndrome. The disease affects brain development, particularly myelination. Most important features include hepatomegaly, polycystic kidney disease, visual disturbances, and high plasma levels of iron and copper. Other features include muscular hypotonia already noticeable at birth, mental retardation, seizures, coagulopathy, and dysphagia with recurrent aspiration. Congenital heart defects have been described. Life expectancy is approximately 6 months.

☞**COCKAYNE SYNDROME:** A complex congenital genetic disorder characterized by the association of dwarfism, deafness, microcephaly, facies similar to progeria syndrome, ataxia, photosensitivity and eye malformations, retinal atrophy, and renal insufficiency with premature aging and atherosclerosis.

KRABBE LEUKODYSTROPHY SYNDROME: A rare, progressive and lethal disease of the central nervous system leading to sudanophilic cerebral sclerosis, metachromatic leukodystrophy, and adrenoleukodystrophy. Affects mostly children and characterized by adrenal atrophy and diffuse central demyelination. Presents with progressive dementia, spasticity, cortical blindness, deafness, hemiplegia, quadriplegia, ataxia, pyramidal signs, retrobulbar neuritis, and pseudobulbar palsy. Seizures. Onset in late childhood. Most die within a few months after onset.

REFERENCE:
Tobias JD: Anaesthetic considerations for a child with leukodystrophy. *Can J Anaesth* 39:394, 1992.

Pemphigoid

At a glance: Chronic nonhereditary blistering disease of the skin or mucosae. Usually considered an autoimmune disease.

Synonym: Bullous Pemphigoid Brunsting-Perry type.

Classification: Bullous pemphigoid affects the skin; cicatricial pemphigoid affects the mucosal surfaces of the body and, occasionally, the skin.

Diagnosis: Clinical appearance of the eruption and skin biopsy.

Clinical aspects:

Bullous pemphigoid: Multiple tense bullae arising from large, irregular urticarial plaques; lesions occur most typically on the flexion surfaces of the extremities or lower torso but may be generalized in severe cases. It may occur at any age, but is most common in the elderly. Clinical course of exacerbations and remissions.

Cicatricial pemphigoid: Bullous eruptions involving mainly the oropharynx, conjunctiva, larynx, esophagus, genitalia, and anus. The scarring of the mucosal surface as a consequence of the recurrent blistering can result in blindness, nasal or laryngeal obstruction, or esophageal stenosis.

It is often associated with dermatitis herpetiformis, also with multiple sclerosis (with no involvement of mucous membrane, but with an early onset). It is described as associated with autoimmune thrombocytopenia, nephropathy, and ulcerative colitis.

Precautions before anesthesia: History of the associated disease: renal, ulcerative colitis, multiple sclerosis. History of medications, usually high-dose corticosteroids, dapsone, azathioprine, and/or other immunosuppressive agents such as cyclosporin.

Anesthetic considerations: The same considerations as for the other blistering diseases: difficult venous access, friction of the skin or mucosae may cause blistering; careful padding; avoid tapes; use petroleum jelly gauze; lubricate blade and tubes well. In case of cicatricial pemphigoid, airway instrumentation should be avoided if possible.

Pharmacological implications: Many medications can induce pemphigoid; the more common are furosemide, ibuprofen, D-penicillamine, α-aminobenzylpenicillin, penicillin G, sulfasalazine, 5-fluorouracil, 8-methoxypsoralen; it is best to avoid these medications if possible.

Other condition to be considered:

CHRONIC BENIGN BULLOUS DERMATOSIS OF CHILDHOOD: Large tense bullae of the skin, resembling bullous pemphigoid, occurring in preschool-age children. Spontaneous remission usually occurs within 2 or 3 years. Therapy: corticosteroids, sulfa drugs.

REFERENCE:
Fellner MJ: Drug-induced bullous pemphigoid. *Clin Dermatol* 11:515, 1993.

Pemphigus

At a glance: A rare, blistering autoimmune disease that affects the skin and mucous membranes. Patients have circulating antibodies to an intercellular cement substance of the basal membrane.

Incidence: It affects males and females in equal numbers and is most common in middle-aged and elderly people. Few cases have been reported in children. All ethnic groups and races can be affected; however it is believed to be more common in Jewish or Mediterranean descent. It occurs once in 100,000 people in the United States.

Classification: Large family of rare blistering disease.

Pemphigus Vulgaris: The most common familial pemphigus vulgaris. Occurs predominantly in Jewish or Mediterranean peoples. It usually appears as painful nonhealing oral ulcers, which may be the only evidence of the disease for weeks or months. The typical lesions are small, flaccid bullae arising from normal skin; they rupture rapidly, leaving nonhealing painful erosions. Patients often complain of burning and pain. Lesions may be present in the esophagus and nasal cavity. The blister is intraepidermal; autoantibodies directed to desmoglein 3 (a keratinocyte surface antigen) are present. Untreated, the disease normally progresses to loss of most

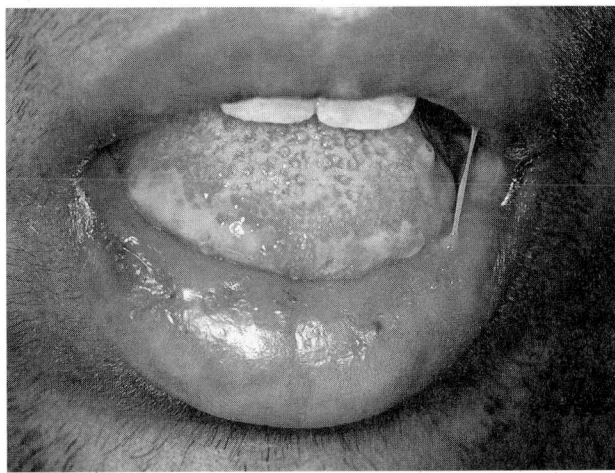

Pemphigus Enoral ulcerations in young man with pemphigus vulgaris.

of the epidermis and death. It can appear antenatally from women who have an active pemphigus or who are in remission. The outcome of the fetus is very poor, including demise.

Pemphigus Foliaceus: This is extremely rare, and presents as small crusted lesions on the scalp, face, chest, and back. The site of cleavage is high in the epidermis. Autoantibodies directed to desmoglein 1 are present. It often resembles seborrheic dermatitis.

Hailey-Hailey Disease (Benign Familial Pemphigus; Benign Chronic Pemphigus): This is an autosomal dominant disease. The recurrent eruption of bullae and vesicles involves predominantly the neck, groin, and axillary areas. The acantholysis is suprabasal. There could be some overlap between Darier and Hailey-Hailey disease.

Pemphigus Erythematosus (Senear-Usher Syndrome): Pemphigus is an autoimmune bullous skin disease with acantholysis in the epidermis. The cutaneous lesions often consist of well-marginated plaques that are erythematous, scaly, hyperkeratotic, and crusted. The lesions have a seborrheic distribution and are often present in a butterfly pattern over the malar area.

Genetic inheritance: Most forms of pemphigus are generally considered to be autoimmune-related. However, *Benign Familial Pemphigus (Hailey-Hailey Disease)* is inherited as an autosomal dominant transmission. The gene responsible is chromosome 3 (3q21-q24). *Fogo Selvagem (Brazilian Pemphigus Foliaceus)* is an autoimmune blistering disorder transmitted through the bite of blackflies. *Pemphigus* may also occur following x-ray exposure or adverse reaction to drugs such as D-penicillamine or rifampin.

Pathophysiology: Blisters in the outer layer of the skin are common to all types of pemphigus (epidermal acantholysis). Deposits of IgG in the epidermal cells are called keratinocytes. Antiepidermal antibodies directed against skin cells are typically present in the fluid of the blisters (biopsy).

Diagnosis: Based on the appearance of the lesions and confirmed by skin biopsy. The diagnosis of pemphigus requires microscopic examination of cells in the blisters as well as detection of the IgG antibodies that characterize this disease.

Clinical aspects: Flaccid blisters occur on the neck, scalp, mucous membranes, axillary areas, and the inguinal areas.

Pemphigus Vulgaris is the most common form and begins with isolated blisters on the scalp and the mouth. They may persist for several months. Blistering of the esophagus, nose, rectum, and conjunctivae are reported. The blisters are soft. They rupture easily and heal poorly. Pressure on the borders of blisters causes them to spread. The Nikolsky sign, pressure applied on normal skin, may make it blister. Untreated, it may cause life-threatening complications.

Pemphigus Vegetans is a variation of *Pemphigus Vulgaris.* The blisters are fast-growing and hypertrophic lesions in the inguinal and axillary areas.

Pemphigus Foliaceus is less severe and less common. Soft blisters typically occur close to the surface of the skin and when they rupture, they ooze and become crusty, scaly, and susceptible to infection. Blisters may occur on the scalp, face, upper chest, and back. The mucous membranes are usually not affected. Small, horny plugs attached to the undersurface of the affected skin also may be seen.

Pemphigus Foliaceus occurs in South America, particularly Brazil and Colombia, and is called *Fogo Selvagem.* Individuals affected present with symptoms of both *Pemphigus Foliaceus* and systemic lupus erythematosus; they are said to have *Pemphigus Erythematosus.*

Pemphigus may also occur as a result of an adverse reaction to certain drugs such as D-penicillamine and rifampin; symptoms usually resemble those of *Pemphigus Foliaceus* rather than *Pemphigus Vulgaris.*

Pemphigus Herpetiformis is a subtle form of pemphigus with its own characteristic blisters. However, blisters that form during a relapse may resemble those of *Pemphigus Foliaceus.*

Benign Familial Pemphigus (Hailey-Hailey Disease) is characterized clinically with recurrent blisters on the neck, groin, and axillae. Blisters may recur because of sweating, skin infections, and exposure to extreme heat and/or ultraviolet light.

Precautions before anesthesia: Careful history of the medication, because most patients are under corticosteroid, methotrexate, cyclosporine, or dapsone therapy. Tetracycline and niacinamide seem to be the more appropriate drugs for treatment.

Anesthetic considerations: Very careful positioning and padding. Avoid the sticky tape, use petroleum jelly gauze, and lubricate the blade and the tube well. If the back is not involved, use of neuraxial regional anesthesia is possible.

Pharmacological implications: A rare complication of dapsone is methemoglobinemia.

Other conditions to be considered:

BULLOUS PEMPHIGOID: Chronic nonhereditary blistering disease of the skin or mucosae. Usually considered an autoimmune disease. The mucous membranes are rarely affected by bullous pemphigoid.

☞DARIER-WHITE DISEASE: A progressive inherited skin disorder characterized by elevated lesions (papules) on the skin and mucous membranes, finger, and toe nail changes in appearance. A sensation of itching or burning on the skin, especially the scalp, forehead, face, neck, and back, is the first manifestation. The symptoms tend to become more severe during periods of emotional stress or with exposure to sunlight.

EPIDERMOLYTIC HYPERKERATOSIS (Bullous Type): Characterized by hyperkeratosis and erythroderma. The symptoms are present at birth and may range from mild to severe. The skin may appear "warty," blistered, and thick over most of the body, particularly in the skin creases over joints.

☞ERYTHEMA MULTIFORME: An allergic inflammatory skin disorder characterized by erythematous macules or papules that may grow into larger blisters. Affected areas generally include the hands, forearms, feet, and/or mucous membranes of the mouth, nose, and/or genitals. The skin lesions and blisters tend to heal in approximately 2 to 6 weeks. Other clinical features may also cause fever, joint pain, cough, and a sore throat.

☞EPIDERMOLYSIS BULLOSA: Represents a group of inherited bullous disorders characterized by blister formation in response to mechanical trauma.

EPIDERMOLYSIS BULLOSA ACQUISTA: A rare autoimmune disorder of the skin that typically affects middle-aged and elderly people. Trauma may cause blisters on the skin of the elbows, knees, pelvis, buttocks, and scalp. Increased levels of IgG are usually found around the blisters; scars usually remain after healing.

REFERENCES:

Abdus SA, Kaye AD: Pemphigus and anesthesia. *Surv Anesthesiol* 46:113, 2002.

Rabinowitz LG, Esterly NB: Inflammatory bullous diseases in children. *Dermatol Clin* 11(3):565, 1993.

Szeremeta W, Dohar JE: Dapsone-induced methemoglobinemia: An anesthetic risk. *Int J Pediatr Otorhinolaryngol* 33(1):75, 1995.

Pena-Shokeir Syndrome Type I

At a glance: Early lethal syndrome involving multiple joint contractures, camptodactyly, facial anomalies, and pulmonary hypoplasia.

Synonyms: Fetal Akinesia/Hypokinesia Sequence; Fetal Akinesia Deformation Syndrome (FADS).

History: First described by S.D.J. Pena and W.H.K. Shokeir in 1974.

Incidence: Rare; more than 30 cases reported. First identified in 1974. F = M.

Genetic inheritance: Autosomal recessive in more than half the cases. Etiology heterogeneous. Risk of recurrence has been estimated between 10 and 15% unless there is maternal myasthenia gravis (several cases), in which case recurrence is high. Thought to represent a lesser degree of clinical expressivity of the same mutation.

Pathophysiology: The clinical phenotype is probably caused by decreased in utero movement, whatever the cause (muscular, spinal, or cerebral). This results in ankylosis of multiple joints, absence of breathing in association with pulmonary hypoplasia, absence of swallowing resulting in polyhydramnios, and absence of facial muscle movements leading to craniofacial anomalies.

Diagnosis: Clinical based on the multiple features of disease. Approximately 30% are stillborn and those that reach term are small for dates. Antenatal ultrasonography shows lack of fetal movement and polyhydramnios. Confirmation is with muscle histology or at postmortem examination.

Clinical aspects: *Neurological:* muscle atrophy, generalized hypotonia, and hyporeflexia/areflexia. *Musculoskeletal:* arthrogryposis of multiple joints, multiple ankyloses, camptodactyly, rocker-bottom feet, short neck. *Craniofacial:* expressionless faces, hypertelorism, micrognathia, cleft palate. *Pulmonary:* hypoplasia. *Cardiac:* cardiac hypoplasia, arrhythmias, congenital defects. *Endocrine:* adrenal hypoplasia, failure to thrive. Death usually occurs in the neonatal period as a consequence of lung hypoplasia and there have been no survivors after 1 year in babies.

Precautions before anesthesia: It is unlikely that anesthesia will be required in these babies. Full assessment of the severity of the syndrome is needed. It is likely that the babies will be ventilated initially.

Anesthetic considerations: Micrognathia may make direct laryngoscopy difficult. May have significant pulmonary hypoplasia.

Pharmacological implications: Adrenal hypoplasia may require steroid supplementation.

REFERENCES:

Jones KL: *Smith's Recognisable Patterns of Human Malformations.* 5th ed. WB Saunders, Philadelphia 1997, p 174.

Katzenstein M, Goodman R: Pre- and postnatal findings in Pena-Shokeir 1 syndrome: Case report and review of the literature. *J Craniofac Genet Dev Biol* 8(2):11, 1988.

Takada E, Koyama N, Ogawa Y et al: Neuropathology of infant with Pena-Shokeir 1 syndrome. *Pediatr Neurol* 10(3):241, 1994.

Pena-Shokeir Syndrome Type II

At a glance: Rapidly progressive neurological disorder leading to brain atrophy with intracerebral calcifications, cataracts, microcornea, optic atrophy, progressive joint contractures, and growth failure.

Synonyms: Cerebro-Oculo-Facio-Skeletal Syndrome; COFS Syndrome.

History: First described by S.D.J. Pena and W.K.H. Shokeir in 1974.

Incidence: Very rare. The original reports are mainly from the Manitoba aboriginal population in Canada.

Genetic inheritance: Autosomal recessive.

Pathophysiology: Pena-Shokeir Syndrome type II is caused by mutations in complementation genes 2 and 6. Death usually occurs by the age of 5 years but patients with milder forms may survive beyond childhood. Genes are located on 19q13.2-q13.3, 13q33, and 10q11.

Clinical aspects: Clinically evocated by association of arthrogryposis, ocular signs, and growth failure. Many features are apparent at birth. The disease involves *head and neck* (microcephaly, micrognathia/retrognathia, upper lip overlaps the lower lip, sloping forehead, long philtrum and prominent nasal root, large ear pinnae), *CNS* (mental retardation, hemiparesis, hypoplasia of the optic tract, focal microgyria, corpus callosum agenesis, seizures, infantile spasm, hypotonia, third ventricle subependymal focal gliosis, cerebellar hypoplasia), *eyes* (cataracts, blepharophimosis, microphthalmia, deep-set eyes, and nystagmus), *skeleton* (osteoporosis, vertebral segmentation defects, kyphoscoliosis, coxa valga, shallow acetabular angle, elbow and knee flexion contractures, camptodactyly, vertical talus, rocker-bottom feet, longitudinal groove on the soles, posterior placement of the second metatarsal). Other inconstant features can include widely spaced nipples, insulin resistance, hirsutism, and heart defects. Early death, associated with feeding difficulties and pneumonia, often occurs.

Precautions before anesthesia: Active respiratory tract infections should be sought and treated. Evaluate tracheal intubation (clinical, radiographs, fiberoptic) because of facial malformations and evaluate neurological function (clinical, EEG, CT/MRI).

Anesthetic considerations: Anesthesia care has not been described in the literature. The features of the disease suggest that tracheal intubation may be difficult. Patient positioning and intravascular access may be difficult because of contractures. Patients are prone to seizures.

Pharmacological implications: Chronic use of anticonvulsants may alter the metabolism of some anesthetic agents.

Other conditions to be considered:

NEU-LAXOVA SYNDROME: An autosomal recessive condition characterized by multiple abnormalities at birth such as microcephaly and abnormal limbs, skin, external genitals, and placenta.

☞POTTER SYNDROME: Characterized by an excess of skin dehydrated looking, a flattened face with a "parrot-beak" nose, eyelid anomalies, micrognathism, and low-set ears. A kidney may be absent or underdeveloped. Skeletal abnormalities include clubfeet and contracted joints occur frequently in infants.

☞SECKEL SYNDROME: Characterized by low birth weight, microcephaly, mental retardation, large eyes, a beak-like nose, a narrow face, and micrognathia. Other features include an underdeveloped thumb, femoral dislocation, clubfoot, scoliosis, and GI abnormalities. It is transmitted as an autosomal recessive genetic disorder.

☞COCKAYNE SYNDROME: A rare form of dwarfism, characterized by the presence of three signs (1) dwarfism, (2) photosensitivity, and (3) progeria. Other features include deafness, microcephaly, ataxia, eyes malformations, retinal atrophy, atherosclerosis, and renal insufficiency.

REFERENCES:

Del Bigio MR, Greenberg CR, Rorke LB, et al: Neuropathological findings in eight children with cerebro-oculo-facio-skeletal (COFS) syndrome. *J Neuropathol Exp Neurol* 56:1147, 1997.

Meira LB, Graham JM Jr, Greenberg CR, et al: Manitoba aboriginal
kindred with original cerebro-oculo-facio-skeletal syndrome has a
mutation in the Cockayne syndrome group B (CSB) gene. *Am J Hum
Genet* 66:1221, 2000.

Pena SDJ, Shokeir MHK: Autosomal recessive cerebro-oculo-facio-
skeletal (COFS) syndrome. *Clin Genet* 5:285, 1974.

Pendred Syndrome

At a glance: A genetic association that accounts for as much as
10% of sensorineural deafness. Associated with a thyroid goiter but
only occasionally hypothyroid. However, the hypothyroidism may
be severe enough to cause mental and physical impairment. Age of
onset is in infancy. It is not considered progressive, and it usually
involves both ears.

Synonyms: Goiter-Deafness Syndrome; Goiter Sensorineural
Deafness Syndrome.

History: First described by Pendred, in 1896, in two deaf sisters
with goiter.

Incidence: 7:100,000 live births; M = F. Risk factors are familial.

Genetic inheritance: Autosomal recessive with variable expression, involving the Pendrin (protein related to sulphate transport)
gene, locus on chromosome 7q22-31.1

Pathophysiology: Gene mutation affects sulfate transport resulting in defective sulfated proteins in the thyroid, including thyroglobulin. Role of pendrin in cochlear development is not clear.

Diagnosis: Clinical features; biochemical (normal or low T_4 levels, high thyroid-stimulating hormone [TSH] levels, perchlorate discharge test positive, indicating defective organic binding of iodine
in the thyroid gland, exaggerated response to thyrotropin-releasing
hormone [TRH]).

Clinical aspects: Sensorineural hearing loss caused by cochlear
malformation, is present at birth or detected in early infancy, and
accounts for 10% of all childhood deafness. May have impaired
vestibular dysfunction because of widened vestibular aqueduct. Goiter usually appears in middle or late childhood but can present in the
newborn, causing airway obstruction and respiratory distress. The
goiter is usually euthyroid but occasionally hypothyroidism may be
severe. There is a very small risk of malignant neoplasm. Mental
retardation has also been reported. Normal life span can be expected.

Precautions before anesthesia: Thyroid function should be evaluated (TSH, T_4 = high TSH and low T_4 would confirm the presence
of hypothyroidism). A perchlorate test should be performed to determine the extent of the thyroid dysfunction. However, it is not
consistently positive in affected individuals. A medical consultation with the endocrine service is essential before any elective and
emergency (if possible) surgical procedures.

Anesthetic considerations: The presence of hypothyroidism
should be an indication to postpone elective surgery until corrected.
Deafness and vestibular dysfunction contributes to a patient's anxiety. Preoperative evaluation of thyroid function and correction of
hypothyroidism is necessary. Airway assessment is mandatory in
the presence of large or long-standing goiter. Airway obstruction
and respiratory distress in neonatal goiter may require emergency
airway access. Possibility of postoperative tracheomalacia after excision of long-standing goiter.

Pharmacological implications: Delayed metabolism of anesthetic drugs and opioids in case of hypothyroidism.

REFERENCES:

Everett LA, Glaser B, Beck JC, et al: Pendred syndrome is caused by
mutations in a putative sulphate transporter gene (PDS). *Nat Genet*
17:411, 1997.

Wintle RV, Choong YF, Laws DE: Unilateral corneal anesthesia and ulceration following squint surgery in a child with Pendred Syndrome
and bilateral sixth nerve palsy. *B J Ophthalmol* 87:1192, 2003.

Penta X Syndrome

At a glance: A rare chromosomal disorder manifested by the presence of five X chromosomes leading to short stature, mental retardation, fifth finger clinodactyly, short neck, microcephaly, cardiac
anomalies (ventricular septal defect, atrial septal defect, patent ductus arteriosus), and horseshoe kidneys. Onset is during childhood.

Synonyms: XXXXX Syndrome; Pentasomy X; 49XXXXX
Syndrome.

History: First described by Kesaree and Wooley in 1963.

Genetic inheritance: The X chromosomes are of maternal origin.
Risk factors for females only. The incidence is rare, about 25 cases
reported. The pathogenesis is believed to be a result of successive
nondisjunctive meiotic divisions within the mother.

Diagnosis: Chromosomal analysis.

Clinical aspects: Prenatal onset growth deficiency with failure to
thrive and short stature. Microcephaly with upward slant of palpebral fissures and hypertelorism. Seizure activity has been reported in
20% of patients without abnormal brain function (MRI and EEG).
Low nasal bridge, short neck. Small hands with clinodactyly of
the fifth finger. Forty percent of patients are known to have congenital heart defect: ventricular septal defect, conotruncal or patent
ductus arteriosus. Premature loss of deciduous teeth. Moderate to
severe mental retardation. Occasional findings include coloboma of
the iris, myopia, micropthalmus, and optic nerve hypoplasia (15%).
Macroglossia, cleft palate, micrognathia, low-set ears, club feet,
multiple joint dislocation, renal dysplasia, and horseshoe kidney
(10%). Usually associated with equinovarus, overlapping toes, multiple joint dislocations (shoulder, elbow, hip, wrist, and finger), and
radioulnar synostosis.

Precautions before anesthesia: Check renal function and cardiac anatomy. A cardiac echocardiography might be indicated.

Anesthetic considerations: The association of micrognathia with
macroglossia could lead to difficult airway management. Careful
positioning to avoid joint dislocation. Specific considerations will
be dictated by the cardiac and renal anomalies.

Pharmacological implications: Antibioprophylaxy may be indicated in case of cardiac defect.

REFERENCE:

Linden MG, Bender BG, Robinson A: Sex chromosome tetrasomy and
pentasomy. *Pediatrics* 96:672, 1995.

Pentalogy of Cantrell

At a glance: Congenital defects of the supraumbilical abdominal
wall leading to defect of the lower part of the sternum and involving
the sternum, diaphragm, pericardium, and heart.

Synonyms: Thoraco Abdominal Syndrome; Cantrell-Haller-Ravitsch Syndrome; Cantrell Syndrome; Peritoneo Pericardial Diaphragmatic Hernia; Thoracoabdominal Ectopia Cordis.

History: Congenital disorder of midline fusion resulting in multiple congenital anomalies; the full pentalogy of Cantrell is thought to represent the extreme end of the spectrum of ventral midline anomalies.

Incidence: Unknown. Pentalogy of Cantrell (sporadic mutation) estimated at 5.5:1 million live births.

Genetic inheritance: X-linked (Xq25-q26.1), with dominant expression.

Pathophysiology: The existence of this syndrome is thought to support the theory of an X-linked midline developmental field. The defects are determined by 16 to 18 days in utero life, resulting from failed fusion of the mesoderm. This results in defects of diaphragm, heart, sternum, abdominal wall, and/or neural tube (encephalocele most commonly).

Diagnosis: Prenatal ultrasonography, clinical presentation (mild forms only).

Clinical aspects: Ectopia cordis represents one end of the spectrum of anomalies, close examination of such patients often reveals further features of the pentalogy of Cantrell. Pentalogy of Cantrell is comprised of (1) midline supra-umbilical abdominal defect, (2) sternal fusion defects, (3) deficiency or absence of the diaphragmatic pericardium, (4) deficiency of the anterior diaphragm, and (5) congenital cardiac disease (atrial septal defect [ASD], ventricular septal defect [VSD], tetralogy of Fallot). Mildly hypoplastic lungs are a common finding. Additional malformations may include hydrocephalus, anencephaly, cleft lip/palate, cystic hygroma, transposition of the great vessels, patent ductus arteriosus, ventral hernia, omphalocele, renal agenesis, and hypospadias.

Precautions before anesthesia: Anesthesia care will be influenced by the nature of the surgical intervention and the degree of organ dysfunctions. The potential for multiple organ abnormalities warrants a comprehensive evaluation of cardiovascular, respiratory, and renal function. Fully define abnormalities by clinical examination. Obtain a chest radiograph to assess the degree of lung hypoplasia and compression by intra-abdominal organs. Obtain an ECG and echocardiography to define cardiac abnormalities. Cardiac catheterization may be indicated in the early neonatal period. Laboratory investigations should include a cell blood count, electrolytes, and parameters of renal function (creatinine, blood urea nitrogen). Ensure adequate fluid resuscitation in the presence of large ventral hernias or omphalocele. Prolonged ventilation and organ support may be required postoperatively.

Anesthetic considerations: The cardiac anatomy and the presence of systemic to pulmonary shunts may dictate the anesthetic technique. These patients may have bronchopulmonary dysplasia secondary to prolonged neonatal ventilation. Careful positioning is needed to avoid pressure over the sternal defect (decreased cardiac output), or abdominal defect (compression of lungs leading to hypoxia). The threshold for invasive hemodynamic monitoring should be low. Large fluid losses are likely during the repair of ventral hernias, omphaloceles, and neural tube defects. Caudal analgesia has been used successfully for inguinal hernia repair in these patients and the place of subarachnoid anesthesia is open to debate.

Pharmacological implications: Specific indications and contraindications are primarily determined by the underlying cardiac anomaly.

REFERENCES:

Cantrell JR, Haller JA, Ravitsch MM: A syndrome of congenital defects involving the abdominal wall, sternum, diaphragm, pericardium and heart. *Surg Gynec Obstet* 107:602, 1958.

Carmi R, Boughman J: Pentalogy of Cantrell and associated midline anomalies. A possible ventral midline developmental field. *Am J Med Genet* 42:90, 1992.

Laloyaux P, Veyckemans F, Van Dyck M: Anaesthetic management of a prematurely born infant with Cantrell's pentalogy. *Paediatr Anesth* 8:163, 1998.

Saito T, Suzuki A, Takahata O, et al: Anesthetic management of a patient with Cantrell's pentalogy diagnosed prenatally. *Can J Anesth* 51:946, 2004.

Pentosuria

At a glance: Disorder of carbohydrate metabolism. Benign anomaly of the metabolism of glucuronic acid.

Synonyms: Essential Pentosuria; L-Xylulosuria; Xylitol Dehydrogenase Deficiency; L-Xylulose Reductase Deficiency.

History: Inborn error of metabolism in which 1.0 to 4 g L-xylulose is excreted in the urine each day. It is a benign metabolic disturbance, which occurs almost exclusively in Ashkenazim of Polish-Russian extraction.

Incidence: 1:40,000 to 1:50,000 in the U.S. population; the frequency in Ashkenazim may be as high as 1:2500 and is 1:5000 in Israeli Jews. In the vast majority of cases, antecedents have been traced to Eastern Europe.

Genetic inheritance: Autosomal recessive.

Pathophysiology: Essential pentosuria is the result of a partial deficiency of L-xylulose reductase in the glucuronic acid oxidation pathway. The basic fault concerns nicotinamide adenine dinucleotide phosphate (NADP)-linked xylitol dehydrogenase.

Diagnosis: L-Xylose dehydrogenase converts L-xylose to xylitol. Xylitol is converted to D-xylose, which becomes D-xylose-5-phosphate and enters the pentose phosphate shunt. Deficiency of this enzyme leads to increased concentration of L-xylose in the blood and urine. No therapy is required. Red cells from pentosuric patients contain only the minor L-xylulose reductases isozyme (normally major and minor).

Clinical aspects: Affected individuals cannot degrade L-xylulose derived from glucuronic acid. It is a benign condition that is of clinical significance only when confused with diabetes mellitus. Blood sugar is normal. The pentose (urine) does not react with glucose oxidase test papers.

Anesthetic considerations: There are no considerations for this pathology, only those associated with the surgical procedure involved.

Other condition to be considered:

ALIMENTARY PENTOSURIA: Arabinose or xylose is found in the urine of normal people following the ingestion of very large quantities of fruits such as cherries, grapes, and fruit juices. Large quantities of D-ribose may be found in the urine of some patients with muscular dystrophy, probably as a result of breakdown of ribose-containing nucleotides in degenerating muscle.

REFERENCES:

Khachadurian AK: Essential pentosuria. *Am J Hum Genet* 14:249, 1962.

Lane AB, Jenkins T: Human L-xylulose reductase variation: Family and population studies. *Ann Hum Genet* 49:227, 1985.

PEP Syndrome

At a glance: A plasma cell dyscrasia (bone marrow disorder) that causes multisystem disorders, including neuropathy, organ overgrowth, endocrine dysfunctions, and skin changes. PEP is an acronym that stands for **P**lasma Cell Dyscrasia, **E**ndocrinopathy, **P**olyneuropathy.

Synonyms: Polyneuropathy Organomegaly Endocrine Monoclonal Protein Skin Lesions Syndrome; POEMS Syndrome; Osteosclerotic Myeloma.

Incidence: Mainly affects adults in the 45- to 65-year-old age range.

Genetic inheritance: No genetic inheritance demonstrated. Probably an inflammatory disease.

Pathophysiology: Pathophysiology is not fully elucidated. Chronic inflammatory process with high circulating cytokines (interleukin [IL]-1, IL-6, tumor necrosis factor) and coagulation activator levels. Parainflammatory axonal demyelinization with polyneuropathy.

Diagnosis: Association of polyneuropathy, organomegaly, endocrinopathy, monoclonal protein plasma cell dyscrasia, and skin changes. Diagnosis based on monoclonal plasma cell demonstration in bone marrow biopsy.

Clinical aspects: The clinical picture is dominated by a demyelinating polyneuropathy with motor disability and sclerotic skeletal lesions. Cranial nerves and autonomic nervous system usually unaffected. Hepatomegaly and sometimes splenomegaly and lymph node enlargement. Endocrine involvement mainly affects gonadotrophins and androgens. Hemostasis studies shows procoagulant activity and thrombocytosis. Rarely associated with fractures and renal involvement. If localized sclerotic lesions are found, radiotherapy may improve systemic polyneuropathy and if widespread chemotherapy (melphalan and steroids) is helpful. Survival at 5 years is 60%.

Precautions before anesthesia: Mainly dominated by a potentially severe pulmonary hypertension and recurrent cerebrovascular insults. Check coagulation tests before and define anticoagulation strategy. Check plasma calcium. Obtain preoperative neurologic evaluation.

Anesthetic considerations: Because of vascular abnormalities and potential organ ischemia, avoid hypotension. Specific considerations in presence of severe pulmonary hypertension must apply.

Pharmacological implications: Interaction between anesthetic medications and cerebroinvasive and antihypertensive medications will be considered.

REFERENCE:

Lesprit P, Godeau B, Authier FJ, et al: Pulmonary hypertension in POEMS syndrome: A new feature mediated by cytokines. *Am J Respir Crit Care Med* 157:907, 1998.

Periodic Paralysis (PP)

At a glance: Genetic disorder involving ion channels of the cellular membrane and affecting electrolyte conductance leading to episodic muscle weakness. It is characterized by episodes of flaccid muscle weakness occuring at irregular intervals. Most of the conditions are hereditary.

Synonyms: Familial Periodic Paralysis, Hypokalemia, Hyperkalemia, Myotonia, Paramyotonia Congenita, Potassium-aggravated Myotonia; Becker Myotonia Congenita; Thomsen Myotonia Congenita; Adynamia Episodica Hereditaria with or without Myotonia; Gamstorp Disease; Thyrotoxic Periodic Paralysis.

Classifications: Primary periodic paralysis can be classified according to the membrane electrolyte defect:

   Sodium Channel: Hyperkalemic PP; Paramyotonia Congenita; Potassium-aggravated myotonia

   Calcium Channel: Hypokalemic PP; Thyrotoxic PP (secondary form)

   Chloride Channel: Normokalemic PP; Becker Myotonia Congenita; Thomsen Myotonia Congenita

Incidence: In the United States, the frequency for all forms of PP remains unknown. Hypokalemic periodic paralysis form is the most common. It has a prevalence of 1 per 100,000 population. Becker myotonia congenita has a reported prevalence of 1 per 50,000, whereas Thomsen myotonia congenita seems significantly rarer. Internationally, the incidence for this medical condition has not been established. Thyrotoxic periodic paralysis is more common in males (85%) of Asian descent, leading to a frequency of approximately 2%.

Genetic inheritance: All are autosomal dominant but penetrance seems to be variable in female carriers. Hypokalemic periodic paralysis is caused by a mutation in the alpha-1 unit of the dihydropyridine-sensitive calcium channel CACNL1A3; the gene is located on chromosome 1q31-32. Hyperkalemic periodic paralysis is caused by a mutation in the alpha subunit of the Na channel SCN4A; the gene is located on chromosome 17q13.1-q13.3. It is the same gene as paramyotonia congenita. The gene of normokalemic periodic paralysis is still unknown—whether it is a separate entity or a subgroup of the hyperkalemic form is a subject of debate.

Pathophysiology: The physiopathologic basis of flaccid muscle weakness is inexcitability of the muscle membrane, i.e., the sarcolemma. In the hypokalemic form, potassium (K) outflow is diminished by altered calcium homeostasis in the muscle fibers; in the hyperkalemic form, the muscle fibers remain depolarized and their membranes are inexcitable.

Diagnosis: Based on history, clinical examination, and measurement of serum electrolytes during the attacks.

Clinical aspects:

Hypokalemic form: Onset rarely occurs before the second decade of life. Attacks of muscle weakness typically occur at night or in the early morning. They are triggered by increased physical exercise, stress, cold, or a large carbohydrate intake. Paralysis is flaccid, affects mainly the girdle of the lower limbs, and spares the respiratory muscles as well as the muscles supplied by the cranial nerves. The attack usually lasts 6 to 24 hours. ECG signs of hypokalemia can be observed. Treatment: Oral KCl in case of attack but electrolytes should be monitored as rebound hyperkalemia is frequent; prophylaxis with acetazolamide or spironolactone. Thyrotoxic periodic paralysis is the most common hypokalemic PP. It is most common in adults 20–40 years of age. Hyperinsulinemia, carbohydrate load, and exercise may all cause PP attacks. When severe, it may involve respiratory and bulbar muscles. Attacks last hours to days. The prevalence of thyrotoxicosis PP in patients affected with thyrotoxicosis is 0.2% in caucasians and 13–14% in Chinese. Ninety-five percent are sporadic.

Hyperkalemic form: Onset usually occurs in the first decade of life but cases starting in infancy have been observed. Attacks are triggered by rest after exercise, cold, hunger, stress, and ingestion of K. Paralysis affects mainly the spinal muscles and rarely the neck and facial muscles; in severe forms, intercostal muscles are affected too. The attack is often heralded by peribuccal or limb paresthesia. An attack lasts typically 30 to 120 minutes. A myotonic response to muscle percussion (mainly the tongue and the eyelids) is often observed during and between attacks. ECG signs of hyperkalemia can be observed. Treatment: acetazolamide, thiazide-like diuretics; a carbohydrate-rich and potassium-poor diet is recommended.

Normokalemic form: Onset usually occurs in early childhood. The attacks are severe with loss of the cough reflex; they last a few days and can be accompanied by multifocal ectopic beats. K administration decreases the arrhythmia but worsens the weakness. Treatment: Large doses of Na to correct or prevent paralysis and cardiac arrhythmia are recommended; fluorohydrocortisone and acetazolamide can be used for prophylaxis.

Precautions before anesthesia: Monitor serum electrolytes; appropriate premedication to avoid preoperative stress. *Hypokalemic form:* usual acetazolamide or spironolactone dose. *Hyperkalemic form:* prolonged preoperative fasting and K-containing IV fluids should be avoided; start a glucose-containing solution at the beginning of fasting time. *Normokalemic form:* Na loading and avoidance of prolonged preoperative fasting.

Anesthetic considerations: Avoidance of hypothermia (heating blanket, forced warm air) maintaining K level and acid–base status in the normal range, continuous ECG monitoring and as follows. *Hypokalemic form:* A case of malignant hyperthermia has been described but the response to in vitro muscle testing was equivocal; there seems to be no association between hypokalemic periodic paralysis and malignant hyperthermia but because of the dysregulation of muscular calcium metabolism, a hypermetabolic state mimicking malignant hyperthermia without hyperkalemia and muscular rigidity is possible. Avoid infusion of glucose-containing solutions except in case of documented hypoglycemia, when you should provide K in the IV infusion. Monitor muscle relaxation at the facial nerve because it is usually spared during attacks. *Hyperkalemic form:* In case of hyperkalemic attack, administer glucose and insulin, calcium gluconate or chloride, or beta-agonists. *Normokalemic form:* In case of paralysis, administer a large dose of NaCl.

Pharmacological implications: Avoid using succinylcholine, as in any muscle disease; although the response to nondepolarizing muscle relaxants seems to be normal, careful titration of muscle relaxants using teratology of Fallot monitoring; atracurium or *cis*-atracurium are the first choice.

Other conditions to be considered:

THYROTOXIC HYPOKALEMIC PERIODIC PARALYSIS: Acquired hypokalemic periodic paralysis in which the drop in serum K is greater than in the congenital form. It occurs in association with hyperthyroidism, more often in males, and its prevalence is much higher in Asians. Treatment involves beta blockade and administering KCl.

☞ANDERSEN CARDIODYSRHYTHMIC PERIODIC PARALYSIS SYNDROME: This disorder is characterized by the clinical triad of potassium-sensitive periodic paralysis (either low, normal, or high potassium levels), ventricular arrhythmias (bigeminy, long-QT interval, ectopy, and bidirectional ventricular tachycardia), and dysmorphic facial features. Sudden death has been reported. Andersen syndrome must not be confused with Andersen disease (glycogen storage disease type IV).

REFERENCES:

Ashwood EM, Russell WJ, Burrow DD: Hyperkalaemic periodic paralysis and anaesthesia. *Anaesthesia* 47:579, 1992.

Lambert C, Blanloeil Y, Krivosic-Horber R, et al: Malignant hyperthermia in a patient with hypokalemic periodic paralysis. *Anesth Analg* 79:1012, 1994.

Walsh F, Kelly D: Anaesthetic management of a patient with familial normokalaemic periodic paralysis. *Can J Anaesth* 43:684, 1996.

Weller JF, Richard E, Pronovost PJ: Spiral anesthesia for a patient with familial periodic paralysis. *Anesthesiology* 97:259, 2002.

Wong GW-K, Leung TF, AF-C Lo, et al: Thyrotoxic periodic paralysis in a 14-year-old boy. *Eur J Pediatr* 159:935, 2000.

Perlman Syndrome

At a glance: Neonatal gigantism accompanied with visceromegaly (especially renal dysplasia or tumour) and at risk for hypoglycemia. This condition is comprised of nephromegaly, renal dysplasia, Wilms tumor, macrosomia, hypotonia, cryptorchidism, and multiple facial dysmorphism (round full face, micrognathia, macrosomia).

Synonyms: Gigantism Renal Dysplasia Syndrome; Fetal Gigantism, Renal Hamartomas and Nephroblastomatosis Syndrome; Fetal Ascites, Macrosomia, Wilms Tumor, and Nephroblastomatosis Syndrome.

History: Described by Max Perlman, an Australian Pediatrician.

Incidence: Twelve cases have been reported, with five cases from Yemenite Jewish families. Fetal and neonatal mortality is more than 60% and survivors have a high incidence of neurodevelopmental delay.

Genetic inheritance: Autosomal recessive.

Pathophysiology: Unclear but it has been postulated that dysplastic medullary parenchyma in preterm infants develops into nephroblastoma and hamartoma, and eventually into Wilms tumor. No chromosomal abnormalities have been reported. Survival was poor with most children dying within 1 year. Children may have multiple defects in several organ systems.

Diagnosis: In utero presentation with polyhydramnios, ascites, and visceromegaly. The facies is characteristic: macrocephaly, high forehead, depressed nasal bridge, epicanthal folds, low-set ears, anteverted upper lip, high-arched palate, and micrognathia.

Clinical aspects: A high perinatal mortality rate, with 6 of the 12 documented patients dying in the first 4 days of life. Mental retardation is present. Features include macrosomia, visceromegaly, and pancreatic islet hyperplasia. Hypoglycemia from hyperinsulinism is an important feature and may be a preventable cause of death. Isolated cardiac anomalies (interrupted aortic arch, anomalous left coronary artery), diaphragmatic hernia, and cerebral anomalies (cysts, white matter hypoplasia, gray matter heteropsia) have been reported. Renal involvement includes hydronephrosis, renal dysplasia, hamartomas, and nephroblastomatosis. Wilms tumor developed in almost 50% of patients. These tumors usually present in the first year of life and are often bilateral. Ultrasonography screening for Wilms tumor is performed every 3 months. Wilms tumor is treated by surgical resection, radiation, and chemotherapy.

Precautions before anesthesia: Assessment of difficulty in tracheal intubation (high-arched palate and micrognathia). Correct anemia and electrolyte imbalance resulting from Wilms tumor. Assess cardiac anatomy and function—dysfunction may be present as a result of hypertension and chemotherapy. *Investigations:* complete cell blood count, coagulation tests, urea and creatinine levels, serum electrolytes, chest radiograph, ECG, echocardiography, blood sugar level.

Anesthetic considerations: The presence of micrognathia and macrosomia might contribute to render the direct laryngoscopy and tracheal intubation difficult. If there is a large intraabdominal tumor, the infant is prone to regurgitation on induction and a rapid sequence induction is mandatory. Ventilation may be impaired by the size of the tumor, surgical retraction, and metastases to the lungs. Blood loss may be massive and adequate venous access is required. Resection of the extension of the tumour into the inferior vena cava may result in tumor embolism. Both the arterial and central venous lines are useful to monitor rapid changes in the hemodynamics and acid–base status. Close monitoring of the blood sugar level should be performed perioperatively.

Pharmacological implications: Anesthetic drugs that are excreted through the kidneys should be used with caution or avoided in patients with severe renal impairment (e.g., pancuronium, vecuronium). In patients with cardiac dysfunction, drugs with negative inotropic effect should be used with care.

Other conditions to be considered:

☞BECKWITH-WIEDEMANN SYNDROME: Most often occurs sporadically and is characterized by exomphalos, macroglossia, gigantism, and hypoglycemia because of hyperinsulinism. Because of the overlapping of clinical features between this medical condition and the Perlman syndrome, the findings of a cytogenetic abnormality of chromosome 11 is of interest.

REFERENCES:

Fahmy J, Kaminsk CK, Parisi MT: Perlman syndrome: A case report emphasizing its similarity to and distinction from Beckwith-Wiedemann and prune-belly syndromes. *Pediatr Radiol* 28:179, 1998.

Henneveld HT, van Lingen RA, Hamel BC, et al: Perlman syndrome: Four additional cases and review. *Am J Med Genet* 86:439, 1999.

Perlman M, Levin M, Wittels B: Syndrome of fetal gigantism, renal hamartomas and nephroblastomatosis with Wilms' tumour. *Cancer* 35:1212, 1975.

Picaone M, Cecconi M, Giuffre M, et el: Perlman syndrome: Clinical report and nine-year follow-up. *Am J Med Genet* 138:410, 2005.

Pernicious Anemia

At a glance: Vitamin B_{12} deficiency resulting from decreased production and availability of intrinsic factor secondary to autoimmune-induced gastric mucosa atrophy.

Synonyms: Biermer-Erhlich Anemia; Hunter-Addison Anemia; Lederer Anemia; Macrocytic Achylic Anemia; Biermer Anemia; Addison-Biermer Anemia.

Incidence: It affects males and females equally. The most common form, *Adult Onset Pernicious Anemia*, affects people after the age of 35 years. Studies suggest that about 1% of the elderly population is affected. *Congenital Pernicious Anemia* is very rare and has an onset of age between 4 and 28 months. *Juvenile Pernicious Anemia* has symptoms similar to the adult-onset type, seems to occur between the ages of 4 and 20 years. North America and in Europe among people of Scandinavian, English, or Irish descent has the higher prevalence. It is extremely rare among Asians. Approximately 1.9%

of cases may go undiagnosed. Pernicious anemia shows a 10-fold increase in patients with multiple myeloma and a 250-fold increase in adults with immunoglobulin deficiency.

Genetic inheritance: Autosomal dominant inheritance with incomplete penetrance.

Pathophysiology: Autoantibodies against gastric parietal cells account for the defect in intrinsic factor production and availability. The resultant vitamin B_{12} deficiency produces megaloblastic changes in red cells and neuropathies. The latter result from demyelination with the accumulation of odd-chain fatty acids secondary to impaired cobalamin-dependent degradation of methylmalonyl coenzyme A to succinyl-CoA.

Diagnosis: Decreased oral absorption of cobalt-60–labeled vitamin B_{12}.

Clinical aspects: Usual symptoms of anemia. Sore tongue. Patients may present with symptoms and signs of lateral and posterior spinal column involvement with progression to paraplegia and bowel/bladder dysfunction if left untreated.

Precautions before anesthesia: Patients with anemia should have the red cell indices examined to exclude megaloblastic changes. Document preexisting neurologic deficits. *Investigations:* CBC, red cell indices.

Anesthetic considerations: Avoid nitrous oxide administration in patients with increased mean corpuscular volume or in patients with documented vitamin B_{12} deficiency. Regional anesthesia may be relatively contraindicated in patients with preexisting neurologic deficits.

Pharmacological implications: Irreversible oxidation of coenzyme B_{12} and methionine synthase by N_2O. It has been shown that patients with preexisting B_{12} deficiencies can develop megaloblastic anemia and neurologic deficits after 2 hours or less of nitrous oxide exposure. The neurologic deficits developed 2 to 6 weeks postoperatively and improved with B_{12} therapy.

Other conditions to be considered:

CONGENITAL TRANSCOBALAMIN II DEFICIENCY (Transcobalamine II Deficiency): Retinal degeneration and megaloblastic anemia in early infancy that is caused by impairment of cobalamin utilization.

ACQUIRED VITAMIN B_{12} DEFICIENCY: This can occur in infants breast-fed by a vegetarian mother, in vegetarian children, and in children who have undergone large resection of the small bowel (ileum) and who do not receive supplemental vitamin B_{12}. Infection with the fish tapeworm *Diphyllobothrium latum* is nowadays a rare cause of pernicious anemia.

REFERENCES:

Marie RM, Le Biez E, Bisson P, et al: Nitrous oxide anesthesia-associated myelopathy. *Arch Neurol* 57:380, 2000.

McNeely JK, Buczulinski B, Rosner DR: Severe neurological impairment in an infant after nitrous oxide anesthesia. *Anesthesiology* 93:1459, 2000.

Toh BH, van Driel IR, Gleeson PA: Pernicious anemia. *N Engl J Med* 337(20):1441, 1997.

Perrault Syndrome

At a glance: A genetic disorder leading to congenital sensorineural deafness with ovarian dysgenesis. Right bundle branch block and mental retardation are also features.

Synonyms: XX-type Gonadal Dysgenesis with Deafness; Ovarian Dysgenesis with Sensorineural Deafness.

History: First described by M. Perrault in 1951.

Incidence: Rare; only 11 families (28 persons) have been described in the literature. However, it has been suggested that this medical entity might not be so uncommon, most cases being unrecognized.

Genetic inheritance: Autosomal recessive with gonadal dysgenesis and neurosensory hearing loss in females but only isolated neurosensory hearing loss in brothers.

Clinical aspects: Female patient with gonadal dysgenesis and severe neurosensory hearing loss. There may be developmental delay, with the hearing loss diagnosed during the toddler years. Cognitive function may be impaired. Progressive nervous system involvement has been observed. It includes severe sensory and motor neuropathy. Abnormal neurologic findings and signs of cerebellar dysfunction are common (ataxia, hypotonia, abnormal extraocular muscle movement, and chorea). Touch and proprioception are normal. Secondary sexual development is absent in the females and primary amenorrhea may be a presenting complaint. In conjunction with gonadal dysgenesis and deafness, there have been additional reports of patients having short stature, nystagmus, limited extraocular movement, and pes equinovarus.

Precautions before anesthesia: Document neurological abnormalities and assess adequacy of respiratory muscle function. Obtain an ECG to eliminate the presence of a right bundle branch block. Preoperative sedation is contraindicated in case of preexisting hypotonia.

Anesthetic considerations: There are no previous reports of anesthesia in this group of patients. However, special considerations must be given to the neurological dysfunction and the presence of right bundle branch block.

Pharmacological implications: The choice of muscle relaxant should take into account the preexisting hypotonia. Special attention to anesthetic medication with negative inotropic effects.

REFERENCES:

Fiumara A, Sorge G, Toscano A, et al: Perrault syndrome: Evidence of progressive nervous system involvement. *Am J Med Genet* 128:246, 2004.

Gottschalk ME, Coker SB, Fox LA: Neurologic anomalies of Perrault syndrome. *Am J Med Genet* 65(4):274, 1996.

Nishi Y, Hamamoto K, Kajiyama M, et al: The Perrault syndrome: Clinical report and review. *Am J Med Genet* 31:62, 1988.

Pettigrew Syndrome

At a glance: Congenital mental retardation with Dandy-Walker malformation of the cerebellum and fourth ventricle. Associated with basal ganglia disease and seizures.

Synonyms: Dandy-Walker Malformation with Mental Retardation; Basal Ganglia Disease and Seizures; X-Linked Mental Retardation Syndromic-5 with Dandy-Walker Malformation.

Nature: One of the nonspecific X-linked mental retardation syndromes.

Incidence: Four-generation family of Dutch descent. The incidence of X-linked mental retardation is estimated to be 1:546 live male births, with a carrier frequency of 1:410 female births.

Genetic inheritance: X-linked transmission. This disease gene map locus is at Xq25-q27.

Pathophysiology: Unknown.

Diagnosis: Clinical features (mental retardation, abnormal neurological signs) together with radiological findings of dilatation of the fourth ventricle. Necropsy demonstrates iron accumulation in the basal ganglia with neuroaxonal dystrophy.

Clinical aspects: The major symptom is mental retardation. The phenotypic features are variable and nonspecific. Other key manifestations include early hypotonia with progression to spasticity and contractures, choreoathetosis, seizures, a long, narrow face with coarse features, cystic enlargement of the fourth ventricle with cerebellar hypoplasia (Dandy-Walker Malformation).

Precautions before anesthesia: The patient's history should be evaluated in relation to seizures and, in particular, current anticonvulsant therapy and complications resulting from the therapy. In patients with raised intracranial pressure, no sedative premedication should be administered.

Anesthetic considerations: Unwillingness or inability to cooperate because of fear, anxiety, and incapacity to communicate in addition to the degree of mental retardation.

Pharmacological implications: Pharmacological triggers that potentiate occurrence of seizures are to be avoided (enflurane with hypocapnia, methohexital, ketamine). Drugs that potentially cause or exacerbate extrapyramidal symptoms (e.g., phenothiazines, butyrophenone derivatives including droperidol, and metoclopramide) should be avoided. Ketamine has been shown to be effective as a monotherapy in hypotonic children for minor surgical procedures.

REFERENCE:

Pettigrew AL, Jackson LG, Ledbetter DH: New X-linked mental retardation disorder with Dandy-Walker malformation, basal ganglia disease, and seizures. *Am J Med Genet* 38(2–3):200, 1991.

Peutz-Jeghers Syndrome

At a glance: A genetic disorder leading to congenital hamartomas of the gastrointestinal tract associated with perioral melanin spots.

Synonyms: Familial Hamartomatous Polyposis Syndrome; Jegher Syndrome; Hutchinson-Weber-Peutz Syndrome; Lentigio-Polypose-Digestive Syndrome.

Incidence: 1:100,000 in the United States.

Genetic inheritance: Autosomal dominant with high degree of penetrance. Mutation in the serine threonine kinase (SK11) gene on chromosome 19p13.3.

Pathophysiology: Hamartomatous muscularis mucosae polyps are present in the esophagus, stomach, small bowel, and colon. They are usually multiple but not premalignant. There is, however, an increased risk for adenomas and adenocarcinomas of the gastrointestinal (GI) tract. Polyps may also be present in the nasopharynx, bronchial mucosa, bladder, and ureter.

Diagnosis: Polyps may occur in any part of the GI tract, but jejunal polyps are a consistent feature. Melanin spots (also called lentigines) on the lips, buccal mucosa, and digits, and around the anus: they are dark brown to black and round to oval. They are present in infancy and childhood, but may fade with age.

Clinical aspects: Intussusception, colicky abdominal pain, and bleeding are the usual symptoms. Approximately 50% of patients develop an intestinal or extraintestinal cancer: bronchogenic carcinoma, benign or malignant thyroid disease; breast, pancreatic, or reproductive tract cancer. Affected females are prone to develop

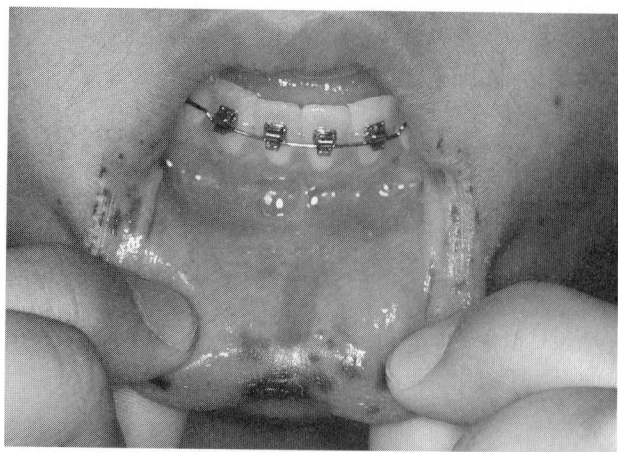

Peutz-Jeghers syndrome Lentigines on the lips and oral mucosa in a child with Peutz-Jeghers syndrome.

benign ovarian tumor; testicular tumors are described in boys 4 to 6 years old with gynecomastia.

Precautions before anesthesia: Check hemoglobin level because anemia caused by chronic intestinal bleeding is frequent. Check renal function if there is a history of hematuria.

Anesthetic considerations: The presence of nasal polyps should be excluded before inserting nasal tubes or catheters.

Other conditions to be considered:

FAMILIAL POLYPOSIS: A gastrointestinal system disorder characterized by adenomatous polyps leading to diarrhea and bleeding. Other clinical features include abdominal pain, cramps, and weight loss. Left untreated, intestinal malignancy may develop between the ages of 30 and 40 years.

GARDNER SYNDROME (Intestinal Polyposis, Type III): Known to affect the colon. It is also associated with supernumerary dentition, dysplasia of the skull and jaw, multiple fibrous tumors, and epithelial cysts. Other clinical features include bleeding, diarrhea or constipation, abdominal pain, and weight loss.

CRONKHITE-CANADA DISEASE (Allergic Granulomatous Angiitis): An extremely rare gastrointestinal disorder characterized by polyps, alopecia, skin hyperpigmentation, and the loss of nails from the fingers and toes. Other clinical features include abdominal pain, cramping, and diarrhea. Very few cases have been reported and all have been sporadic in apparition. There is no evidence that it may be hereditary.

☞TURCOT SYNDROME: Characterized by familial polyposis and tumors of the central nervous system (i.e., medulloblastoma, glioblastoma, or ependymoma). Other clinical features include diarrhea, intestinal bleeding, abdominal discomfort, ataxia, and speech problems. Neurological symptoms vary greatly and depend on the type and location of the brain tumor.

REFERENCES:

Flageole H, Raptis S, Trudel JL, et al: Progression toward malignancy of hamartomas in a patient with Peutz-Jeghers syndrome: Case report and literature review. *Can J Surg* 37(3):231, 1994.

Jolly DT, McKin JC, Corrin MH: A family with intussusception and malignant hyperthermia *Can. Med Assoc J* 127:737, 1982.

Uchiyama M, Iwafuchi M, Yagi M, et al: Fiberoptic colonoscopic polypectomy in children: Report and review of cases. *Pediatr Int* 43:259, 2001.

PHACE Syndrome

At a glance: PHACE is a neurocutaneous syndrome and an acronym that stands for: *P*osterior Fossa Brain Malformations, *H*emangiomas of the Face, *A*rterial Anomalies, *C*ardiac anomalies, and *E*ye Abnormalities. The addition of an S to the PHACE Syndrome becomes PHACES Association and refers to the association of ventral developmental defects, such as *S*ternal clefting or *S*upraumbilical raphe.

Synonym: PHACES Association.

Incidence: Rare; 120 cases described up to 2001. It has been suggested that the disorder may be X-linked with lethality in males.

Genetic inheritance: Unknown, but 87% of patients are female.

Pathophysiology: Unknown; possibly a developmental error between the sixth and eighth week of gestation.

Diagnosis: This syndrome should be considered in any infant presenting with a large, segmental, plaque-type facial hemangioma; careful cardiac, neurologic, and ocular examination is mandatory.

Clinical aspects: Seventy percent of patients have only one extracutaneous manifestation of the syndrome. *Hemangioma:* facial, usually unilateral, with a "plaque" morphology, most commonly involving the V1 trigeminal dermatome. *Extracutaneous hemangiomas:* occur in 22% of patients; the subglottic area is then the most common location. *Brain and cerebrovascular abnormalities:* Dandy-Walker malformation occurs in 33% of patients; hypoplasia or agenesis of cerebellum or cerebellar vermis. Aneurysmal dilatations and anomalous branches of the carotid artery occur in 50% of patients; arteriovenous or angiomatous malformations of the cerebral vessels. Neurologic sequelae (seizures, developmental delay, cerebral infarction, hemiparesis) are frequent if those anomalies are present. *Cardiac and/or aortic abnormalities:* occur in more than 33% of patients; coarctation of the aorta is the most frequent; patent ductus arteriosus, atrial septal defect, ventricular septal defect. Aberrant origin of subclavian artery, malformations of the aortic arch. *Ophthalmic abnormalities:* These are ipsilateral to the facial hemangioma; increased retinal vascularity, Horner syndrome, microphthalmia, cataracts.

Precautions before anesthesia: Careful cardiac, neurologic, and ocular examination to evaluate possible associated anomalies. In case of stridor, the presence of a subglottic hemangioma should be suspected. These children often receive steroid therapy to try reducing the size of the facial hemangioma.

Anesthetic considerations: The anesthetic strategy should be adapted to the extracutaneous manifestations of the syndrome, especially the cerebral, cerebrovascular, and cardiac manifestations.

Pharmacological implications: Steroid coverage in case of steroid therapy.

Other condition to be considered: PHACE syndrome is the same spectrum of anomalies as are associated with ventral development defects such as partial or complete sternal clefting or supraumbilical raphe.

☞STURGE-WEBER SYNDROME: Characterized by the association of three major manifestations: leptomeningeal angiomas often combined with calcium accumulation in the brain, seizures, and unilateral facial nevus flammeus. Angiomas similar to those found in the brain can develop inside the eye, often with secondary glaucoma.

REFERENCE:

Metry DW, Dowd CF, Barkovich AJ, et al: The many faces of PHACE. *J Pediatr* 139:117, 2001.

Phenylketonuria

At a glance: Inborn error of phenylalanine metabolism. Results in severe irreversible mental retardation at infancy.

Incidence: 1:10,000 to 12,000 live births in North America; considerable geographic variability.

Genetic inheritance: Autosomal recessive.

Pathophysiology: Deficiency of the liver enzyme phenylalanine hydroxylase, which converts phenylalanine to tyrosine; it leads to accumulation of phenylalanine and abnormal metabolites thereof.

Diagnosis: Neonatal screening programs for phenylketonuria (PKU) are established in many countries (Guthrie test). Elevated plasma levels of phenylalanine are seen in affected infants after protein feeding.

Clinical aspects: Affected infants are normal at birth. Untreated children develop severe mental retardation with movement disorders. They typically have pale, dry skin and blue eyes. Severe vomiting, mimicking infantile pyloric stenosis, may be the presenting feature. Typical mousy pungent odor caused by the excretion of phenylacetic acid. Perirectal eczema-like or scleroderma-like skin rash. Treatment consists of a diet low in phenylalanine.

Precautions before anesthesia: Ensure patient is receiving appropriate diet.

Anesthetic considerations: There should be no difficulties with anesthetic management of children who are receiving appropriate dietary manipulation.

Pharmacological implications: There are no specific implications.

Other conditions to be considered:

Tetrahydrobiopterin (BH$_4$) Deficiency: Of children with phenylketonuria, 1 to 2% have a defect in the gene coding for that cofactor of phenylalanine hydroxylase instead of a deficiency in the enzyme itself. BH$_4$ deficiency also causes decreased synthesis of L-dopa, 5 hydroxytryptophan, and nitric oxide (NO). Without treatment, the most severe form leads to microcephaly, developmental delay, and progressive neurological deterioration with parkinsonian symptoms. Treatment includes the daily administration of L-dopa (up to 10 to 12 mg/kg/d) and 5-hydroxytryptophan (up to 8–10 mg/kg/d).

References:

Dal D, Celiker V: Anesthetic management of a strabismus patient with phenylketonuria *Paediatr Anaesth* 13:740, 2003.

Rezvani I: Defects in metabolism of amino acids, in Behrman RE, Kliegman RM, Arvin AM (eds): *Nelson Textbook of Pediatrics.* 15th ed. Philadelphia, WB Saunders, 329–333, 1995.

Pheochromocytoma

At a glance: Tumor of chromaffin tissue (neuroectodermal origin), most commonly affecting the adrenal medulla (90% of patients), but may occur in any tissue derived embryologically from the neuroectoderm, including any sympathetic ganglia, the GI tract, bladder, and thorax. Catecholamine-secreting tumor.

Synonym: Chromaffin Tumors.

Incidence: Total incidence: 2 to 8 cases per 1 million people of which 10% occur in children. It is the cause of 1 to 2% of systemic hypertension cases in the pediatric population. Compared to adults, children are more likely to present tumors that are bilateral, multiple, or extraadrenal in origin. Familial cases are also more common in children and adolescents. It is more frequent in boys than in girls.

Genetic inheritance: Autosomal dominant. Mutation of RET protooncogene that is located on chromosome 10. Pheochromocytoma can be associated with Neurofibromatosis type I, von Hippel-Lindau Disease, Multiple Endocrine Neoplasia type IIa (Sipple syndrome), Tuberous Sclerosis (Bourneville disease), Sturge-Weber Disease, or Carney triad (gastric leiomyosarcoma, pulmonary chondroma, and extraadrenal pheochromocytoma).

Pathophysiology: Ninety percent of tumors are benign; multiple sites occur in approximately 35% of children and in 8% of adults. Epinephrine can only arise from the adrenal medulla, norepinephrine can arise from any sympathetic tissue. Elevated catecholamines cause an increase supraventricular rhythm, hypertension, increased cardiac contractility, and rate. Hyperglycemia may result from alpha-2 antagonism of insulin secretion. The catecholamines are metabolized by monoamine oxidase and catechol-O-methyltransferase, 5% of norepinephrine being excreted unchanged; urinary levels reflect plasma levels.

Diagnosis: History and examination, especially finding of paroxysmal or sustained hypertension at a young age. Demonstration of elevated urine catecholamine levels.

Clinical aspects: Symptoms include sweating, palpitations, headache, pallor, vomiting, weight loss, polyuria, polydipsia, and chest pain, which may be cardiac in origin. Examination reveals hypertension, which may be sustained or paroxysmal tachycardia, hypertensive retinopathy, and possibly signs of ventricular failure caused by dilated cardiomyopathy. The ECG may reveal dysrhythmia. In childhood, other catecholamine-secreting tumors, such as neuroblastoma, ganglioneuroblastoma, and ganglioneuroma, should be considered in the differential diagnosis. The tumor may be defined by ultrasonography, CT scan, or MRI scan. Laboratory investigations may reveal a raised hematocrit. Urinary vanillylmandelic acid (VMA) and metanephrines are elevated, as are plasma catecholamine levels. Extraadrenal sites of tumor should be excluded by [131]metaiodobenzylguanidine (MIBG) uptake scan. In children, norepinephrine is usually the predominant catecholamine. In case of metastatic malignant tumor, therapeutic doses of ^{131}I-MIBG are administered.

Precautions before anesthesia: *History:* Inquire for symptoms of dysrhythmia or ventricular dysfunction. Catecholamine-induced cardiomyopathy is present in approximately 58% of patients. *Cardiovascular assessment:* ECG, echocardiography. Start alpha blockade. Competitive alpha-antagonists (e.g., phentolamine, prazosin) have been used but do not give the same stability as noncompetitive blockade (phenoxybenzamine). Beta blockade may be started after alpha blockade to control dysrhythmias. The minimum duration for alpha blockade is 36 hours, although the optimal period is not defined. End points used for adequate blockade have included a 5% drop in hematocrit or the maximum dose of phenoxybenzamine at which the side effects are tolerated by the individuals. *Respiratory assessment:* Chest radiograph to exclude pulmonary congestion. *Renal function:* Check renal function; hypertensive nephropathy may be present and nephrectomy is occasionally necessary to achieve tumor excision. *Metabolic factors:* Check blood glucose (insulin rarely needed); exclude hypercalcemia.

Anesthetic considerations: Premedication may be desirable. Invasive monitoring, central venous pressure, arterial blood pressure are essential. Swan-Ganz catheter can be useful. Induction of anesthesia and tracheal intubation can be a period of major cardiovascular instability. Surgery is performed by laparotomy or laparoscopy.

There may be a place for pulmonary artery catheter use in select patients. Careful attention to patient positioning. Prepare a vasodilator such as sodium nitroprusside to control surges in blood pressure during tumor manipulation. According to the local team experience, other vasodilators may be used (e.g., phentolamine and calcium antagonists such as nicardipine, magnesium sulfate). Esmolol is probably the beta blockade of choice to control dysrhythmias. Hypotension following tumor excision or clamping of its venous drainage should initially be treated with volume loading but a transient infusion of the catecholamine secreted by the removed tumor is sometimes necessary. Communication with the surgeon is mandatory to enable stopping the vasodilator infusion just before tumor excision or venous clamping. Epidural supplementation of general anesthesia is reported but is probably only of use for postoperative analgesia because its intraoperative use may complicate the anesthetic. Postoperatively monitor for hypotension, hypertension, and hypoglycemia in a critical care setting.

Pharmacological implications: Haloperidol, pancuronium, and desflurane are contraindicated. Atropine should be used with caution. The use of magnesium sulfate is recommended to control symptoms and signs of sudden release of catecholamines.

Other condition to be considered:

PARAGANGLIOMA: This is an extraadrenal pheochromocytoma-like tumor. It is thoracic (posterior mediastinum) in 15% of cases and rarely can secrete catecholamines. It is also located within the bladder.

REFERENCES:

Chiu M, Crosby ET, Yelle JD: Anesthesia for laparoscopic adrenalectomy (pheochromocytoma) in an anemic adult Jehovah's witness. *Can J Anesth* 47:556, 2000.

Dubois R, Chappuis JP: Pheochromocytoma in the pediatric age group. *Arch Pediatr* 4:1217, 1997.

Hack HA: The perioperative management of children with phaeochromocytoma. *Paediatr Anaesth* 10:463, 2000.

James MF, Cronjé L: Pheochromocytoma crisis: The use of magnesium sulfate. *Anesth Analg* 99:680, 2004.

Minami T, Adachi T, Fukuda K: An effective us of magnesium sulfate for intraoperative management of laparoscopic adrenalectomy for pheochromocytoma in a pediatric patient. *Anesth Analg* 95:1243, 2002.

Phosphoenolpyruvate Carboxykinase Deficiency

At a glance: Congenital metabolic disease leading to defect of gluconeogenesis and severe acidemia. Other clinical features include hypotonia, hypoglycemia, hepatomegaly, and growth delay.

Synonym: PEPCK Mitochondrial Deficiency.

Incidence: Extremely rare (four patients up to 2002).

Genetic inheritance: Phosphoenolpyruvate carboxykinase (PEPCK) is encoded by two genes PCK1 (cytosolic form, located on chromosome 20) and PCK2 (mitochondrial form), and its expression is limited to the liver, kidney, and adipose tissue. Mode of inheritance is suspected as an autosomal recessive trait.

Pathophysiology: PEPCK is the rate-controlling enzyme of gluconeogenesis in the liver and kidney; it converts pyruvate, lactate, alanine, and intermediates of the tricarboxylic acid cycle to glucose.

Diagnosis: Hypoglycemia associated with lactic acidosis; measurement of PEPCK activity on fresh liver biopsy. *Caution:* PEPCK

activity is physiologically depressed in hyperinsulinar states and might be a secondary phenomenon in case of respiratory chain dysfunction.

Clinical aspects: Major manifestation is fasting hypoglycemia with lactic acidosis; multisystem involvement may be present with neuromuscular deficits, hepatic damage, renal tubular acidosis. Hepatomegaly with lethargy and hypotonia are common. Patients do not survive longer than 36 months.

Precautions before anesthesia: A glucose-containing IV solution should be started at the beginning of the preoperative fasting period.

Anesthetic considerations: Avoidance of hypoglycemia; monitoring of lactacidemia.

Pharmacological implications: There are no specific implications.

Other conditions to be considered:

KORSAKOFF SYNDROME (Wernicke-Korsakoff Syndrome; Transketolase Defect Syndrome; Alcohol-induced Encephalopathy Syndrome): Characterized by acute encephalopathy followed by chronic impairment of short-term memory. Early treatment with high doses of thiamine stabilizes the disease, yet thiamine deficiency is not sufficient to cause the syndrome. It is a deficiency of vitamin B-1 (thiamine) caused by absorption problems and causing cardiovascular, CNS disturbances, including peripheral nerve manifestations. It is common in the Orient where excessive milling of rice reduces its thiamine content. Beriberi is caused by lack of dietary thiamine and its symptoms include myocardial failure, reversible by thiamine treatment.

☞LEIGH SYNDROME: An early-onset progressive neurodegenerative disorder with a characteristic neuropathology consisting of focal, bilateral lesions in one or more areas of the central nervous system, including the brain stem, thalamus, basal ganglia, cerebellum, and spinal cord. The lesions are areas of demyelination, gliosis, necrosis, spongiosis, or capillary proliferation. Clinical symptoms depend on which areas of the CNS are involved. The most common underlying cause is a defect in oxidative phosphorylation. Other clinical features include lesions of the optic nerve, heart, and breathing system. Symptoms during infancy include failure to thrive, tremors, and skin changes. It is suggested that it is inherited as an autosomal recessive trait.

☞PYRUVATE CARBOXYLASE DEFICIENCY: A rare metabolic disorder characterized by severe lactic acidemia, CNS deterioration, vomiting, irritability, electrolyte imbalances, inactivity, hypotonia, abnormal eye movements, and seizures. The course of this disorder is progressive. It is inherited as an autosomal recessive trait.

REFERENCES:

Kerr DS, Wexler ID, Zinn AB: Disorders of pyruvate metabolism and the tricarboxylic acid cycle, in Fernandes J, Saudubray J-M, van den Berghe G (eds): *Inborn Metabolic Diseases*. 3rd ed. Berlin, Springer, 2000, p 126.

Leonard JV, Hyland K, Furukawa N, et al: Mitochondrial phosphoenolpyruvate carboxykinase deficiency. *Eur J Pediatr* 150:195, 1991.

Phosphoglycerate Kinase Deficiency

At a glance: A rare congenital enzymatic defect in glycolysis process, mainly located in the muscles and red blood cells.

Synonym: Glycogenosis type X.

Genetic inheritance: X-linked disorder. The enzyme is encoded by a gene located on Xq13.

Pathophysiology: This enzyme catalyzes the interconversion of 3-phosphoglycerate and 1,3-diphosphoglycerate with the production of adenosine triphosphate (ATP). There are several variants of the disease with variable involvement of red cells, muscle, and central nervous system (CNS). This could be a result of organ-specific isoenzymes being affected differently by the mutation(s).

Diagnosis: Chronic hemolytic anemia, occasional hemoglobinuria; phosphoglycerokinase activity low (<5%) in muscle cells or RBCs. Normal muscle biopsy.

Clinical aspects: Hemolytic anemia, mental retardation, and myopathy may coexist or manifest in various combinations. *Neonatal period:* nonimmune hydrops, jaundice, hepatomegaly, hemolytic anemia. *Childhood:* mild mental retardation (delayed language), behavioral problems, seizures. *Adolescence and Adulthood:* nonspherocytic hemolytic anemia; exercise-induced cramps, myalgia, and rhabdomyolysis; myoglobinuria after vigorous exercise.

Precautions before anesthesia: Check hemoglobin level; a long preoperative fasting time should be avoided.

Anesthetic considerations: Monitor blood glucose level; in case of rhabdomyolysis, ensure increased diuresis with IV mannitol and intravascular fluid.

Pharmacological implications: Avoidance of succinylcholine because of the risk of rhabdomyolysis.

REFERENCE:

Aasly J, van Diggelen OP, Boer AM, et al: Phosphoglycerate kinase deficiency in two brothers with McArdle-like clinical symptoms. *Eur J Neurol* 7:111, 2000.

Phytosterolemia

At a glance: A rare inherited disorder characterized by congenital hypercholesterolemia, presenting clinically with tendon xanthomas, premature coronary artery disease, and premature atherosclerosis.

Synonym: Sitosterolemia.

History: First described in 1974 by Battacharyya and Connor in two sisters.

Incidence: As of year 2000, in the United States approximately 50 patients have been identified. The incidence is suggested at 1:1,000,000 population. No ethnic predilection.

Genetic inheritance: Autosomal recessive. The gene defect in sitosterolemia remains to be elucidated.

Pathophysiology: The nature of the primary defect is unknown at the molecular level, although enhanced intestinal absorption and reduced excretion of plant sterols appear to be the abnormality. Affected homozygote individuals show an enhanced absorption of both cholesterol and sitosterol from the diet, and decreased bile clearance of these sterols and their metabolites, resulting in markedly expanded whole-body cholesterol and sitosterol pools. Increased content of sitosterol in red cells may be responsible for the fragility of the RBCs and results in chronic hemolytic anemia.

Diagnosis: Sitosterolemic homozygotes show elevation of plasma plant sterol (sitosterol and campesterol) concentrations.

Clinical aspects: Absorption of sitosterol in affected patients is 20 to 30%, as compared to 5% in normal individuals. The plasma concentrations of sitosterol in affected patients varies between 15 and 27% of the total sterol content and increased concentrations are found in cell membranes, xanthomas, and atherosclerotic plaques. Tendon and tuberous xanthomas developed at an early age, as with early development of atherosclerosis, and episodes of hemolysis and painful arthritis are features. Coronary atherosclerosis is common. Phytosterols can cause cholestasis in susceptible infants. Extramedullary sitosterolemic xanthomas have been reported to result in spinal cord compression. Episodic hemolysis and chronic hemolytic anemia may be present.

Precautions before anesthesia: Detailed cardiovascular assessment. Where indicated, not only should the global ventricular function be assessed by echocardiography, but angiography with angioplasty may improve coronary flow prior to elective surgery. Elective surgery should be postponed until at least 6 months from any myocardial infarction. Current congestive heart failure also carries higher risk of another perioperative cardiac event. Obtain drug history (nitrates, beta blockers, calcium channel blockers, antiplatelet agents, digoxin). Patients with painful arthritis may be on long-term nonsteroidal anti-inflammatory drugs (NSAIDs). The signs and symptoms of anemia must be sought. Anemia is poorly tolerated in patients with coronary artery disease and every effort should be made to correct the deficit preoperatively. *Investigations:* cell blood count, ECG, chest radiograph, coagulation studies, and bleeding time if the patient is on antiplatelet agents and/or heparin. Premedication with adequate sedation to reduce anxiety, continue medical therapy, and administer oxygen therapy during transport to the operating theatre.

Anesthetic considerations: The conduct of anesthesia and the choice of monitors depend primarily on the underlying cardiac status of the patient, and the type and extent of the proposed surgery. Aim to maintain optimal myocardial oxygen supply–demand balance (avoid hypoxemia, sympathetic stimulation, pain, and tachycardia). A central neuraxial block (spinal, epidural) is relatively contraindicated in those patients on aspirin or other antiplatelet agents.

Pharmacological implications: Considerations must be given to the effects of the anesthetic medications and the cardiovascular problems.

Other conditions to be considered:

☞**APOLIPOPROTEIN C-II DEFICIENCY:** An inborn error of metabolism characterized by the deficiency in a necessary cofactor for the activation of lipoprotein lipase. Diabetes mellitus, pancreatitis, epigastric pain, does not exclude the possibility of angina in early age and congestive heart failure.

☞**BERARDINELLI-SEIP SYNDROME:** Inherited disorder with hyperinsulinemia because of insulin-resistance combined with lipodystrophy and acromegaloid features.

☞**FAMILIAL HYPERLIPOPROTEINEMIA TYPE I:** Inherited inborn error of metabolism characterized by a massive accumulation of chylomicrons and triglycerides in plasma resulting in recurrent abdominal pain and hepatosplenomegaly.

☞**FAMILIAL HYPERLIPIDEMIA TYPE IIA:** A genetic disorder of lipid metabolism causing accumulation of cholesterol and thus increasing the risk of cardiovascular diseases. Hypercholesterolemia, Low Density Lipoprotein – LDL – Receptor Disorder

☞**KOBBERLING DUNNIGAN SYNDROME:** Genetically transmitted metabolic disorder characterized by partial lipodystrophy, insulin resistance leading to glucose intolerance and hypertriglyceridemia. Affects children and young adults. Onset is slow, manifested by progressive loss of subcutaneous fat. Other features include: hypocomplementemia, glomerulonephritis, autoimmune disorders. Affecting mostly women.

REFERENCE:
Berger GM, Pegoraro RJ, Patel SB, et al: HMG-CoA reductase is not the site of the primary defect in phytosterolemia. *J Lipid Res* 39:1046, 1998.

Pickwickian Syndrome

At a glance: Acquired obesity-associated sleep apnea, cyanosis, somnolence, muscle twitching, and periodic breathing.

Synonyms: Obesity-Hypoventilation Syndrome; Syndrome de Pickwick (French appellation).

History: Named after the fat boy Joe, in Charles Dickens's *Pickwick Papers*. This disorder is characterized by morbid obesity, cyanosis, somnolence, muscular twitching, and periodic breathing.

Incidence: In the United States, it is observed in 20–27% of obese children and adolescents. Higher mortality and morbidity is reported in this group of patients. During the second decade of life, females are more affected than males; 80% of teenagers with obesity will remain affected in adulthood.

Pathophysiology: Reduction in lung volumes including expiratory reserve volume, vital capacity, and functional residual capacity. Closing capacity is increased, leading to airway closure in the dependent areas of the lung and V/Q mismatch, reduced chest and diaphragmatic excursions, decreased alveolar ventilation, and diminished sensitivity of the respiratory center to hypoxia and hypercarbia—all contributing to hypoxia and hypercarbia. Intermittent upper airway obstruction and hypoxia during sleep with resultant chronic sleep deprivation and daytime somnolence; severe and chronic hypoxia leading to polycythemia, pulmonary hypertension, right ventricular hypertrophy, and failure.

Diagnosis: Clinical features; biochemical (polycythemia, hypoxia, hypercarbia); lung function tests (reduced lung volumes including total lung capacity, functional residual capacity, vital capacity, and expiratory reserve volume); ECG (right axis deviation); chest radiography or echocardiography (cardiomegaly); sleep studies (obstructive sleep apnea).

Clinical aspects: Morbidly obese, lethargy, drowsiness, headache, and muscle twitching; may develop mental retardation; exertional dyspnea, cyanosis, and periodic breathing, particularly marked during sleep, enuresis; hypertension and later signs of chronic cor pulmonale (distended neck veins, enlarged heart and liver, peripheral edema). Major improvement is usual following nasal continuous positive airway pressure at night: daytime sleepiness and behavioral problems regress, and a better quality of sleep allows enhanced physical activity and favors weight loss.

Precautions before anesthesia: Detailed preoperative cardiac and respiratory assessment is required; some weight loss might be advisable prior to elective surgery.

Anesthetic considerations: Difficulty in maintaining patent airway during mask ventilation and difficult tracheal intubations common; arterial desaturation usually rapid because of reduced functional residual capacity; intraoperative hypertension, arrhythmias and heart failure may occur; tolerates hypovolemia poorly because of reduced blood volume per unit body weight; reliable indirect blood pressure monitoring is difficult to achieve because of large arm size; difficult venous access; identification of landmarks for regional blocks and invasive lines difficult; increased incidence of postoperative respiratory complications; supine position is associated with a drop in PaO_2 and is to be avoided postoperatively; nasal continuous positive airway pressure or continuous positive airway pressure mask recommended for obstructive sleep apnea; polycythemia may predispose to deep venous thrombosis, although pulmonary embolism is extremely rare in children.

Pharmacological implications: Use of prophylaxis against gastric aspiration recommended; require lower drug doses on a per kilogram basis; increased sensitivity to respiratory depressants, including opioids.

Other condition to be considered:

☞PRADER-LABHART-WILLI SYNDROME: Disorder characterized by morbid obesity, cyanosis, excessive daytime sleepiness, shortness of breath, elevated arterial partial pressure of carbon dioxide, flushed face, high blood pressure, polycythemic, muscular twitching, and periodic breathing. Most patients present with sleep apnea syndrome.

REFERENCES:
Chung F: Sleep apnea syndrome and anesthesia. *Can J Anaesth* 29: 439–45, 1982.

Falsetti HL, Hanson JS, Tabakin BS: Obesity-hypoventilation syndrome in siblings. *Am Rev Resp Dis* 90:105, 1964.

Newmann GG, Baldwin CC, Petrini AJ et al: Perioperative management of a 430-kilogram (946 pound) patient with Pickwickian syndrome. *Anesth Analg* 65:985–87, 1986.

Werner RJ, Pierson DJ. The Pickwickian syndrome: Special challenge for the anesthetist. *AANA J* 45:57, 1997.

Pierre Robin Syndrome

At a glance: Very frequent syndrome with multiple etiologies resulting from mandibular aplasia. Characterized by association of cleft palate, glossoptosis, and micrognathia.

Synonyms: Robin Sequence; Pierre-Robin Sequence.

Incidence: This heterogenous birth defect has a prevalence of approximately 1 per 8500 live births. The male-to-female ratio is 1:1, except in the X-linked form.

Genetic inheritance: The Pierre Robin Syndrome is qualified as a sequence—the possibility of its being mendelian cannot be excluded. Association of Pierre Robin sequence with deletion 2q32.3-q33.2 has been demonstrated and mapped to a chromosome region previously shown to have a nonrandom association with cleft palate. An X-linked form and an association with trisomy 18 and other syndromes have also been evocated.

Pathophysiology: Hypoplasia of the mandibular area prior to 9 weeks in utero causes a posterior position of the tongue that prevents palatal shelves from closing on the midline.

Diagnosis: Glossoptosis, micrognathia, and cleft soft palate must evocate diagnosis. Mandible grows during the first few months so that normal mandibular profile is common at the age of 4 to 6 years old.

Clinical aspects: In addition to the three classical signs that make the diagnosis, this syndrome can also include cardiovascular (cor pulmonale, vagal hyperactivity) and neuromuscular dysfunctions (brainstem dysfunction, central apnea). Facial abnormalities can provide obstructive apnea and respiratory distress in neonatal period. Prone position is often used to prevent the tongue from falling back. Nasopharyngeal airway can be useful and if necessary suture of the tongue to the lip or even tracheostomy. Feeding difficulties can be observed because of facial malformation and/or neurological swallowing problems.

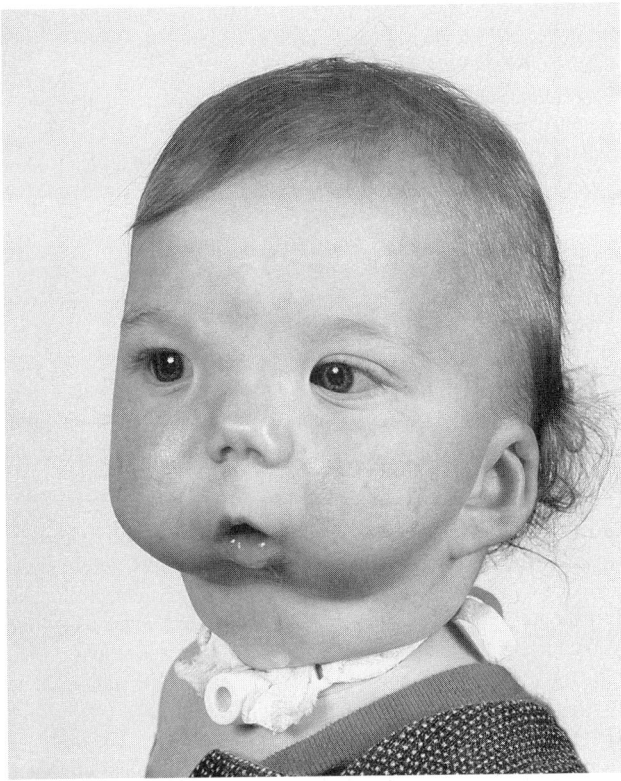

Pierre Robin syndrome Severe mandibular hypoplasia and microstomia in a 15-month-old boy with Pierre Robin syndrome. Because of the severity of the findings associated with airway obstruction and the difficulties in airway management, the boy underwent tracheotomy.

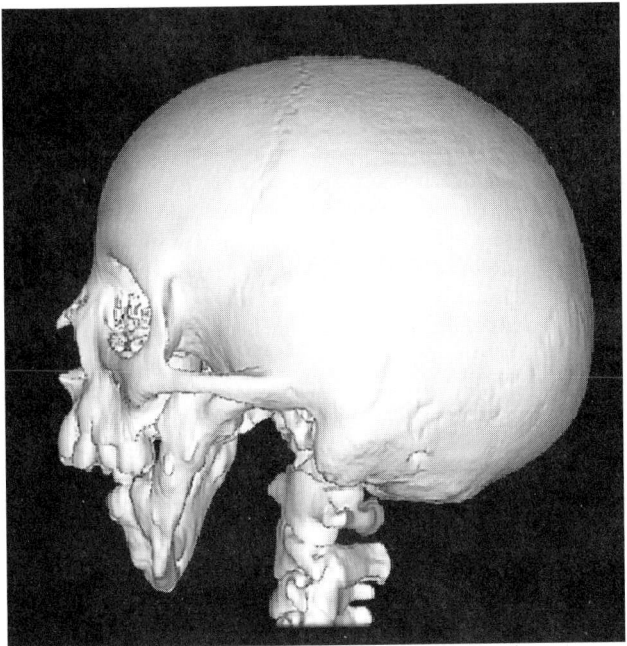

Pierre Robin syndrome This three-dimensional reconstruction of the head CT scan of a patient with Pierre Robin syndrome shows marked mandibular hypoplasia.

Precautions before anesthesia: Obtain full history of apnea (central and/or obstructive), respiratory complications, hospital stays, protracted intubation, tracheotomy, feeding, growth, and development. Evidence of facial signs will help to precisely evaluate the airway management possibilities. Evaluate for difficult tracheal intubation and lung ventilation. The most obstructive apnea is severe, the most tracheal intubation and ventilation by facial mask is difficult. Evaluate for tracheomalacia and stenosis after intubation or tracheotomy: chest radiograph. Evaluate for cardiac defects: echocardiography. Vagal hyperreflexia is common: vagolytic premedication is useful both to counteract it and to avoid the presence of excessive oral secretions. Previous surgical procedure and tracheal intubation provide precious information but cleft palate repair can provide new laryngoscopic difficulties. Obtain full personal medical history and search for existence of apnea. Evaluate other factors of respiratory distress: coexistence of central apnea, tonsil hypertrophy, cardiopathy. Evaluate for present infection in the orolaryngotracheal area and within the lungs from recurrent pulmonary aspiration. Evaluate for esophageal reflux.

Anesthetic considerations: The complication rate is high because of difficult airway management. Direct laryngoscopy and tracheal intubation can be extremely difficult especially in the very young patient. However, the difficulty decreases with age. Intravenous access prior to anesthesia induction has to be considered and difficult airway management procedures have to be clearly planned. Different techniques have been successfully used in such patients: fiberoptic intubation, laryngeal mask airway, Bullard laryngoscope, retrograde tracheal intubation, digitally assisted intubation, and blind nasal intubation in prone position with hyperextension of the neck. In all cases, well-controlled and light anesthesia induction allowing preservation of spontaneous ventilation must be used. Halothane or sevoflurane can be used for this purpose. The possibility of manually assisted ventilation using a face mask has to be verified prior to any attempt of direct laryngoscopy. Close postoperative observation is necessary to detect any apnea. Prone position can be used for patients with swallowing problems, or in a case of postoperative pharyngeal bleeding, to avoid pulmonary inhalation. Muscle relaxants are contraindicated until confirmation of maintenance of face-mask ventilation and/or direct laryngoscopy and tracheal intubation can be performed. The major concern is difficult or impossible ventilation by face mask. Spontaneous ventilation must be preserved during laryngoscopy and tracheal intubation attempts. Possibility for reintubation must be considered before tracheal extubation. Postoperative stay in a pediatric intensive care unit may be required in patients with considerable airway obstruction.

Pharmacological implications: Whatever the anesthetic medication used, muscle relaxation increases during induction of anesthesia and may affect the maintenance of the airway. Benzodiazepines have to be used with extreme caution. Muscles relaxants should be avoided until tracheal intubation is performed.

Other conditions to be considered: Multiple related syndromes have been described.

☞**Cerebrocostomandibular Syndrome:** An extremely rare disorder characterized by micrognathia, cleft palate, glossoptosis, and rib dysplasia leading to pulmonary insufficiency in early infancy. Other features include mental retardation and congenital brain anomalies. Autosomal dominant inheritance reported but most cases known as sporadic expression. Diagnosis established radiologically by the presence of gaps in the posterior rib shafts as a result of replacement of normal rib by cartilaginous or fibrous tissue. Combine the sequence with mental retardation, short size, ventricular septal defect, osseous abnormalities (hip, foot, clavicle, vertebrae) and severe tracheal and thoracic abnormalities (gaps in ribs, bell-shaped thorax) that lead often to respiratory insufficiency.

☞**CATEL-MANZKE SYNDROME:** An X-linked recessive disorder characterized by micrognathia, high-arched palate, cleft palate and lip, Robin anomaly, glossoptosis, malformed ears, and short neck. Other features include cardiovascular anomalies (ventricular septal defect, aortic coarctation, dextrocardia), pectus carinatum or excavatum, seizures, joint laxity and dislocations, hyperphalangy of index finger, fifth finger clinodactyly, single transverse palmar crease, and talipes equinovarus.

☞**STICKLER SYNDROME:** Hereditary (autosomal dominant), arthroophthalmopathy with a neonatal form that combined Pierre Robin syndrome with fetal chondrodysplasia, flat facies with marfanoid appearance, joint hyperlaxity, frequent mitral valve prolapse, and severe ophthalmic abnormalities.

☞**TORIELLO-CAREY SYNDROME:** Multiple congenital anomalies consisting of agenesis of corpus callosum, telecanthus, short palpebral fissures, small nose with anteverted nares, Robin sequence, malformed ears, redundant neck skin, macrocephaly, micrognathia, laryngeal and sublaryngeal abnormalities, heart defect (pulmonic stenosis and atrial septal defect), muscular hypotonia, occasional Hirschsprung disease, and moderate to severe developmental delay.

ARNOLD STICKLER BOURNE SYNDROME (Corneal Crystals Myopathy Nephropathy Syndrome): Arthroophthalmopathy that requires caution with muscle relaxants and the avoiding of succinylcholine. Characterized by corneal crystals, retinal pigment epithelial mottling, oropharyngeal and hand weakness and/or atrophy, proteinuria, and hypertension.

PIERRE ROBIN SYNDROME WITH CONGENITAL HEART MALFORMATION AND CLUBFOOT: Recessive X-linked transmission. Similar presentation than Pierre Robin syndrome but associated with congenital heart defect, club foot, and cleft palate.

CHITAYAT MEUNIER HODGKINSON SYNDROME: Pierre Robin sequence with faciodigital anomaly: cleft palate, micro/retrognathia, microdontia, glossoptosis, broad nose, and high forehead with frontal bossing and long philtrum. Flat cheekbones and supraorbital ridges. Exophthalmos. Limbs. Clinodactyly of the fifth finger. Triphalangeal thumb. Syndactyly of the toes. Terminal hypoplasia of the fingers. Hypoplastic nails and sparse scalp hair. Anesthesia has not been described in this condition; however, the features suggest that face-mask ventilation, direct laryngoscopy, and tracheal intubation might be challenging. Particular attention should be paid to eye care in the presence of exophthalmos.

MARTSOLF REED HUNTER SYNDROME (Pierre Robin Syndrome Oligodactyly): Pierre Robin syndrome with skeletal dysplasia polydactylia.

FRANCESCHETTI SYNDROME: Mandibulofacial dysostosis presenting at birth with cyanotic spells. Fishlike facial characteristics, hypoplasia of the mandible, receding chin, considerable overbite, high-arched palate, macrostomia, low-set ears. An autosomal dominant inheritance. The difference with Treacher Collins is believed to be the absence of flattening of the molar bones.

REFERENCES:

Chadd GD, Crane DL, Phillips RM, et al: Extubation and reintubation guided by the laryngeal mask airway in a child with the Pierre-Robin syndrome. *Anesthesiology* 76(4):640, 1992.

Chadha IA, Chadha A, Vakil SD: Pierre Robin Syndrome: Obstructive airway and anesthetic management. *J Anaesth* 18:91, 2002.

Jones SE, Derrick GM: Difficult intubation in an infant with Pierre Robin syndrome and concomitant tongue tie. *Paediatr Anaesth* 8(6):510, 1998.

Rasch DK, Browder F, Barr M, et al: Anaesthesia for Treacher Collins and Pierre Robin syndromes: A report of three cases. *Can Anaesth Soc J* 33(3 pt 1):364, 1986.

Pilomatrixoma

At a glance: A benign skin appendage tumor frequently involving the skin of the head, neck, and upper extremities in young children.

Synonyms: Epithelioma Calcificans of Malherbe; Pilomatricoma Malherbe Epithelioma; Malherbe Tumor; Calcifying Epitheliomia of Malherbe.

Incidence: Isolated lesions are not rare in children with antecedent trauma, which has been described in 30% of cases. Pilomatrical neoplasms are considered the most common solid cutaneous tumors in patients 20 years of age or younger. In the United Kingdom, pilomatrixomas account for 1 in 500 histologic specimens. Cases have been reported in Japan (37), Turkey (15) and France (33) up to year 2000. The female-to-male ratio is 1.5:1.

Genetic inheritance: Isolated lesions are sporadic. The presence of multiple lesions may be suggestive of an autosomal dominant transmission. In this case, it may be associated with myotonic dystrophy.

Pathophysiology: The tumor arises from hair matrix cells. The cause has been suggested as the result of a mutation in the beta-catenin gene.

Diagnosis: Pathologically, the tumors were situated in the dermis or subcutaneous tissue. The histopathologic findings of viable basaloid cells in the periphery, shadow cells in the central part, and foci of calcification are characteristic of pilomatrixoma. Computed tomography scans clearly demonstrated a well-defined, subcutaneous mass with amorphous calcifications. Lesions are most often discovered in the first 2 years of life.

Clinical aspects: This benign lesion is a firm, circumscribed tumor, 1 to 2 cm (0.4 to 0.8 inches) in diameter, usually in the head and neck area, attached to the subcutaneous tissue and overlying skin. Usually it is an asymptomatic superficial mass that increased slowly in size. Multiple lesions occur in 2 to 3% of reported series, in some cases in association with myotonic dystrophy. Complete surgical excision is the best management.

Precautions before anesthesia: Presence of myotonic dystrophy should be sought in any patient with more than one pilomatrixoma and in any patient with a family history of pilomatrixoma.

Anesthetic considerations: The presence of myotonic dystrophy dictates the choice and conduct of the anesthesia. Isolated pilomatrixoma does not have any special anesthetic or pharmacological implications.

Pharmacological implications: The use of neuromuscular blocking agents should be used with cautions.

REFERENCES:

Baltogiannis N, Faviou E, Cigliano B, et al: Diagnosis of pilomatrixoma in childhood. *Plast Reconst Surg* 115:1783, 2005.

Demircan M, Balik E: Pilomatricoma in children: A prospective study. *Pediatr Dermatol* 14:430, 1997.

Wells NJ, Blair GK, Magee JF, Whiteman DM: Pilomatrixoma: A common, benign childhood skin tumour. *Can J Surg* 7:483, 1994.

Pitt-Rogers-Danks Syndrome

At a glance: Intrauterine growth retardation with subsequent dwarfism, prominent slanting eyes, telecanthus, short upper lip, microcephaly, and mental retardation

Synonyms: Unusual Facies-Mental-Retardation-Intrauterine Growth Retardation Syndrome; Pitt syndrome.

History: First described in 1984 by D.M. Danks, D.B. Pitt, and J.G. Rogers, all three Australian physicians.

Incidence: Very rare; fewer than 20 patients.

Genetic inheritance: Initially thought to be autosomal recessive transmission but recent studies question this mode of inheritance. Deletion of the short arm of chromosome 4(4P-) and duplication of the long arm of chromosome II are reported in some cases.

Pathophysiology: The molecular defects associated with both the Pitt-Rogers-Danks Syndrome (PRDS) and another multiple congenital malformation syndrome, the Wolf-Hirschhorn Syndrome (WHS), show considerable amount of overlap; both of these conditions result from the deletion in the same region of 4p16.3 and the clinical differences observed between these two syndromes are likely the result of allelic variation in the remaining homologue.

Diagnosis: Intrauterine growth retardation, subsequent dwarfism, and unusual characteristic facies (classical "Greek warrior helmet"). Chromosomal analysis demonstrates found microdeletions of the 4p16.3 segment. Fetal ultrasonography may diagnosis proportionate dwarfism in utero.

Clinical aspects: Pre- and postnatal growth retardation with proportionate dwarfism, mental retardation (moderate to severe), seizures, characteristic facies (microcephaly with prominent glabella, hypertelorism, large mouth, beaked nose, prominent slanting eyes with short upper lip, hypoplastic maxilla), and ocular abnormalities. Clinically, Pitt-Rogers-Danks patients tend to be less severely affected than WHS patients, with no early mortality reported. Many patients show defects in midline closure, such as cleft lip and palate, iris coloboma, hypospadias, sacral dimple.

Precautions before anesthesia: The patient's history should be evaluated in relation to epilepsy and the anticonvulsant therapy (type and any resultant complications). Anticonvulsant therapy should be continued up to and including the day of surgery. Assess the patient for any known abnormalities associated with proportionate dwarfism: atlantoaxial instability—via history and clinical examination (progressive weakness, hypotonia, spasticity, hyperreflexia, clonus), difficult airway in view of facial dysmorphism and hypoplastic maxilla, and thoracic dystrophy with consequent cardiorespiratory involvement. *Investigations:* cell blood count, electrolytes, chest radiograph, arterial blood gas, or pulmonary function test, if appropriate.

Anesthetic considerations: No previous anesthetic reports in these patients. Patients with severe mental retardation may not be cooperative. Triggers known to exacerbate seizures perioperatively should be avoided (hypocapnia, electrolyte derangement, etc.). Regional anesthesia (spinal and epidural) has been used successfully in dwarfs; however, because of the potential for development of neurologic problems as a result of spinal stenosis and vertebral misalignment, as well as the need for patient cooperation, a central

neuraxial block is usually reserved for those patients for whom the benefits of the technique far outweigh those of the risks of general anesthesia. For patients with thoracic dystrophy, positive-pressure ventilation should be carefully instituted to prevent barotrauma. One important note is that there are two case reports of malignant hyperthermia in patients with WHS, another 4p-deletion syndrome. Because of the genetic and clinical similarities between the two syndromes, close monitoring for early signs of the development of malignant hyperthermia is mandatory. Means to institute cooling should be available.

Pharmacological implications: Malignant hyperthermia triggers must be avoided. Dantrolene should be available.

Other condition to be considered:

☞WOLF-HIRSCHHORN SYNDROME (WHS): A syndrome characterized by severe muscular hypotrophy with prenatal onset and a distinctive facial dysmorphism resembling a "Greek warrior's helmet," microcephaly, micrognathia, gastroesophageal reflux, hydrocephalus, seizures, and severe mental retardation. Malignant hyperthermia is a potential complication. Cardiac malformation (atrial and ventricular septal defects) is observed in half the cases. Mental retardation is usually severe.

REFERENCES:

Chen JC, Jen RK, Hsu YW, et al: 4P– syndrome (Wolf-Hirschhorn syndrome) complicated with delay onset of malignant hyperthermia: A case report. *Acta Anaesthesiol Sin* 32:275, 1994.

Wright TJ, Clemens M, Quarrell O, et al: Wolf-Hirschhorn and Pitt-Rogers-Danks syndromes caused by overlapping 4p deletions. *Am J Med Genet* 75:345, 1998.

Pitt-Williams Brachydactyly Syndrome

At a glance: An autosomal dominant disorder characterized by brachydactyly, short metacarpals, hypoplastic ulnar side hand distal phalanges, and normal stature.

Synonyms: Brachydactyly, Combined types B and E. Brachydactyly Ballard type.

Incidence and genetic inheritance: One family with dominant inheritance of this subtype of brachydactyly described 12 members of 4 generations. The syndrome is named after the affected family.

Clinical aspects: Members of this family have shortened metacarpals and metatarsals IV and V. In addition, broadened thumbs were described in some family members, as well as distorted fingernails on the affected fingers. Hypoplasia of the distal phalanges of the ulnar side is also seen. There were no other abnormalities.

Anesthetic considerations: No anesthetic implications arise from the described features. However, the presence of brachydactyly is significant because of its association with other syndromes, such as Albright hereditary osteodystrophy and Turner syndrome. Thus, if brachydactyly is found, a thorough clinical examination looking for other malformations, which might have specific implications for anesthesia, is warranted.

REFERENCE:

Pitt P, Williams I: A new brachydactyly syndrome with similarities to Julia Bell types B and E. *J Med Genet* 22:202, 1985.

Pituitary Dwarfism

At a glance: Deficiency in growth hormone that is either isolated or combined with deficiency in other anterior pituitary hormones.

Synonyms and classifications: There are four types of pituitary dwarfism:

Pituitary Dwarfism type I: (Primordial Dwarfism; Sexual Ateleiotic Dwarfism; Isolated Autosomal Recessive Growth Hormone Deficiency Dwarfism) is characterized by sexual ateleiotic dwarfism, hypoglycemia, puppet (baby doll) facies, antibodies to administered growth hormone. It is inherited as an autosomal recessive trait.

Pituitary Dwarfism type II: (Laron Dwarfism type I; ☞Laron Syndrome; Growth Hormone Receptor Deficiency Syndrome; Growth Hormone Insensitivity Syndrome) is characterized by marked short stature and short limbs. Clinical hyposomatotropism. However, the body proportions in childhood appear normal. In the adult period, the body proportions are childlike. Interestingly, the body proportions are more marked in the stature than head size. There is increased resistance to the action of growth hormone (GH). Occasionally blue sclerae. Other clinical features include hip degeneration, limited elbow extensibility, acrohypoplasia, and high-pitched voice. Distorted sex ratio (19F:2M) in Loja province Ecuador cases. Markedly advanced osseous maturation for height and age. It is believed to be cause by a failure to generate somatomedin (or insulin-like growth factor, IGF1) in response to GH. Normal or increased levels of GH. Growth hormone receptor (GHR) defect. Low IGF1 despite normal or increased levels of GH. It is inherited as an autosomal recessive trait.

Pituitary Dwarfism type III: (Panhypopituitarism; Ateliotic Dwarfism with Hypogonadism Syndrome; Hanhart Dwarfism; Rigid Cervical Spine Pituitary Hormone Deficiency Syndrome) is characterized by ateliotic dwarfism, multiple endocrine anomalies (hypothyroidism, hypoadrenalism, hypogonadism and panhypopituitarism), neonatal hypoglycemia, and hypoglycemic seizures. Laboratory investigation reveals the presence of sequential loss of anterior pituitary tropic hormones, GH, gonadotropin, thyroid-stimulating hormone (TSH), adrenocorticotropic hormone (ACTH), and prolactin deficiency. It is inherited as an autosomal recessive trait.

Pituitary Dwarfism type IV: (Normal Immunoreactive Growth Hormone and Low Somatomedin Pituitary Dwarfism Syndrome; Biodefective Growth Hormone Syndrome; Kowarski Syndrome) is characterized by growth retardation, pituitary dwarfism, and delayed bone age. Normal immunoreactive GH after stimulation, low somatomedin, exogenous human GH responsive, structural abnormality of GH molecule confirmed the diagnosis. It is inherited as an autosomal recessive trait.

Incidence: The incidence of types I and II pituitary dwarfism are not known, but panhypopituitary dwarfism is not excessively rare; there are probably 7000 to 10,000 cases in the United States alone.

Genetic inheritance: Both types I and II pituitary dwarfism are inherited autosomal recessively. The human GHR gene is mapped to 5p13.1-p12. Many cases of panhypopituitary dwarfism are caused by craniopharyngioma and other nongenetic causes. The form inherited as an autosomal recessive or X-linked form is rare.

Pathophysiology: There is a defect in the gene encoding GH resulting in either biodefective GH, GH deficiency, or GHR deficiency. The isolated GH deficiency in type I dwarfism may be the result of a defect in hypothalamic releasing factor. Laron syndrome is caused by target resistance to the action of GH.

Diagnosis: Laron type I syndrome is characterized by (a) clinical signs of GH deficiency (short stature, decreased growth velocity and delayed bone age) despite normal or increased plasma GH levels; (b) low IGF1 levels that are unresponsive to exogenous GH; and often by (c) low GH-binding protein levels.

Clinical aspects: In types I and II, dwarfism with child-like body proportions and small facies in adult period. In types III and IV, the clinical picture depends on the age of loss of pituitary function. In type I pituitary dwarfism, the dwarfism is more extreme than in other cases, hypoglycemia is a conspicuous feature, and the puppet facies ("baby doll facies") is exaggerated. In addition, development of anti-GH antibodies occurs when exogenous GH is administered. Laron syndrome has a very similar clinical appearance to those with isolated GH deficiency. Laron syndrome is characterized by clinical hyposomatotropism manifested by short stature, delayed bone age, and, occasionally, blue sclerae, and hip degeneration. Instability of the odonto-atlantoid joint has been described. The stimulation of growth by IGF1 treatment is prescribed, although the long-term effects have not been documented. Delayed puberty and high-pitched voice. In panhypopituitary dwarfism, the patients show sequential loss of anterior pituitary tropic hormones usually in the order of GH, gonadotropin, TSH, and adrenocorticotropic hormone (hypoglycemia, hypogonadism, hypothyroidism, hypoadrenalism).

Precautions before anesthesia: Avoid prolonged preoperative fasting because these patients are prone to hypoglycemia. Blood sugar levels should be monitored regularly. In patients with panhypopituitary dwarfism, thyroid function should be assessed both clinically and biochemically, and any replacement thyroxine therapy optimized prior to elective surgery. Ensure supplementation of mineralocorticoids and glucocorticoids in the presence of hypoadrenalism. In a case of Laron syndrome, check odonto-atlantoid joint by cervical radiograph.

Anesthetic considerations: Pituitary dwarfism patients have a proportionately smaller airway without anatomic difficulties. A range of laryngoscope blades, handles, and airways appropriate for a smaller patient should be available. The endotracheal tube size could be estimated from the patient's height, in a fashion similar to that of a child of normal height.

Pharmacological implications: Hypothyroidism may cause increased sensitivity to centrally depressant drugs such as opioids, volatile anesthetics, and intravenous anesthetic agents. It may also reduce drug metabolism and excretion.

REFERENCES:

Desai M, Colaco MP, Samuel AM, et al: Pituitary dwarfism. *Indian Pediatr* 22(1):13, 1985.

Ratner EF, Hamilton CL: Anesthesia for caesarean section in a pituitary dwarf. *Anesthesiology* 89:253, 1998.

Plott Syndrome

At a glance: Congenital X-linked laryngeal abductor paralysis associated with psychomotor retardation.

Synonyms: Familial Vocal Cord Dysfunction; Laryngeal Abductor Paralysis.

History: First described by D. Plott, an American neurologist, in 1964. A congenital laryngeal abductor anomaly was seen in three brothers.

Incidence: Very rare condition. Ten patients have been diagnosed up to 2000.

Genetic inheritance: X-linked recessive disorder. Familial genetic disorder; clinical expression in male children only.

Pathophysiology: Abnormal development of nerve nuclei is thought to be involved in the pathophysiology of this disease; medullar nucleus ambiguus abnormalities can explain laryngeal dysfunction by total dysfunction of the posterior cricoarytenoid that provides a midline adducted position of the vocal cords at rest and a complete adduction when crying. Ninth, tenth, and twelve cranial nerve nuclei can also be involved.

Diagnosis: This syndrome belongs to a larger group of congenital laryngeal abductor paralysis but is often associated with mental, growth, speech, and motor retardation.

Clinical aspects: Inspiratory stridor, laryngomalacia, respiratory distress, and swallowing difficulty can occur as a consequence of laryngeal abnormalities; neonatal death has been suspected. It is also possible to observe hypotonia, blank facies, and, more rarely, blindness, nystagmus, optical nerve atrophia, and hearing deficiency.

Precautions before anesthesia: Evaluate mental and motor retardation. Evaluate severity of the laryngeal abnormalities through patient history (frequency of dysphonia, stridor, or asphyxia). Evaluate pulmonary consequences by chest radiograph, arterial blood gas analysis, and 24-hour SaO_2 record. Evaluate swallowing difficulty by barium swallow.

Anesthetic considerations: No difficult tracheal intubations have been reported in this syndrome. Postoperative stridor can be observed and pulmonary inhalation has to be considered for food reintroducing. Postoperative SpO_2 monitoring is recommended.

Pharmacological implications: Drugs used to premedicate must avoid respiratory depression. When muscle relaxants are used, monitoring is imperative. Locoregional anesthesia rather than opioids is preferred for postoperative pain relief so as to avoid hypoxemic risk.

Other conditions to be considered:

BARBIERI SYNDROME **(Laryngeal Abductor Paralysis with Cerebellar Ataxia and Motor Neuropathy Syndrome):** Characterized by late-onset and slowly progressive cerebellar ataxia and severe dysphonia because of laryngeal abductor paralysis. Other clinical features include urinary incontinence, dysphagia, diffuse limb fasciculations with mild distal muscular wasting. It is most likely transmitted as an autosomal recessive trait.

☞ERYTHROMELALGIA: Characterized by neonatal stridor, vocal cord paralysis, laryngeal abductor paralysis, mental retardation, infantile swallowing difficulty, and microcephaly. It is also considered a familial vocal cord dysfunction with mental retardation. It is most likely inherited as an autosomal dominant trait with variable expression but may also be X-linked.

REFERENCES:
McDonald D: Anesthetic management of a patient with Plott's syndrome. *Paediatr Anaesth* 8:155, 1998.

Plott D: Congenital laryngeal-abductor paralysis due to nucleus ambiguus dysgenesis in three brothers. *N Engl J Med* 271:593, 1964.

Poland Syndrome

At a glance: Unilateral hypoplasia or aplasia of the chest wall muscles, mainly pectoralis major and cutaneous syndactyly of the ipsilateral hand.

Synonyms: Poland Sequence; Poland Syndactyly; Poland Anomaly.

History: Named after Sir Alfred Poland who, in 1841, described a chest wall anomaly while still a medical student studying dissection on cadaver. His observations were reported in the Guy's Hospital Gazette. He specifically noted the absence of the sternocostal portion of the pectoralis muscle, absence of the pectoralis minor, hypoplastic serratus, but the presence of an intact clavicular origin.

Incidence: Estimated in one review at 1:30,000 to 40,000 live births.

Genetic inheritance: Sporadic but some cases may show autosomal dominant inheritance.

Pathophysiology: Unknown, but it has been suggested that there may be an interruption of early embryonic blood supply in the subclavian arteries, the vertebral arteries, and/or their branches, resulting in unilateral upper limb deformities and unilateral or, very rarely, bilateral chest wall deformities. The term subclavian artery supply disruption sequence (SASDS) has been suggested for a group of birth defects—Poland, Moebius, and Klippel-Feil sequences— possibly caused by it.

Clinical aspects: There may be aplasia of the sternal head of pectoralis major, of serratus anterior, and of latissimus dorsi. Unilateral symbrachydactyly may occur and there may be patchy absence of axillary hair. Unilateral breast aplasia occurs in females. Chest wall defects are variable and may include rudimentary development or absence of the anterior portions of the second to fifth ribs. Absence of bone or muscle from the chest wall may cause paradoxical respiratory movements. The anomaly may be associated with dextrocardia, atrial septal defect, contralateral syndactyly, club foot, toe syndactyly, hemivertebrae, and scoliosis. Renal aplasia, hypospadias, and inguinal hernia may also occur. Situs inversus has been reported with this syndrome.

Precautions before anesthesia: Ensure full cardiac investigations, including echocardiography, if there is suspicion of any cardiac lesion. Chest radiograph to elucidate extent of bony defect in chest wall. Blood examination: urea, creatinine, and electrolytes if renal abnormalities are present.

Anesthetic considerations: Because paradoxical chest movement during spontaneous ventilation may result in inadequate ventilation,

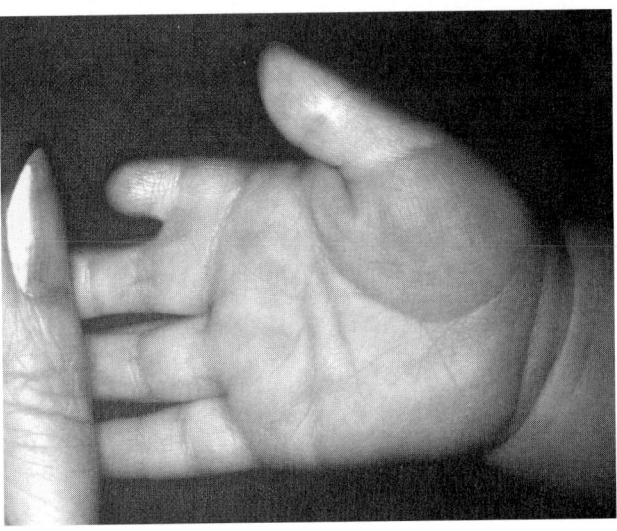

Poland syndrome Brachydactyly of the index finger in an infant with Poland syndrome.

mechanical ventilation is recommended. Antibiotic prophylaxis may be required for invasive procedures in the presence of cardiac defects. Renal aplasia requires care with fluid balance and administration of renally excreted drugs.

Pharmacological implications: Atracurium, *cis*-atracurium, or mivacurium are suitable muscle relaxants if renal aplasia exists. Suxamethonium should be avoided, especially if associated with Moebius syndrome. If there is compromised respiratory function, then care should be taken with the administration of opioids and benzodiazepines.

Other conditions to be considered:

☞**POLAND-MOEBIUS SYNDROME:** Both the Poland and the Moebius syndromes are well-described malformations. The Moebius syndrome is characterized by multiple cranial nerve palsies, orofacial malformations, and limb anomalies. The association probably represents a formal genesis malformation syndrome of unknown etiology. Moebius syndrome is inherited autosomal dominantly with the gene map locus localized to 13q12.2-q13. A "mask-like facies" is present, with the child not smiling or moving its facial muscles on crying. Moebius syndrome consists of bilateral palsies of cranial nerves VI and VII, but occasionally also cranial nerves V, X, XI, and XII, resulting in difficulties with chewing, swallowing, and coughing, often leading to aspiration with respiratory complications.

☞**ADAMS-OLIVER SYNDROME:** A very rare inherited disorder characterized by defects of the scalp associated with multiple scarred and hairless areas that usually have dilated blood vessels directly under the skin. Scalp defects are already present at birth. The extremities are either short (hypoplastic fingers and toes) or characterized by absent hands and lower legs. Congenital heart defect must be ruled out.

REFERENCES:

Kupper HJ: Anesthesia in Poland Syndrome. *Can J Anesth* 46:513, 1999.

Sethuraman R, Kannan S, Bala I, Sharma RK: Anesthesia in Poland syndrome [see comments *Can J Anaesth* 46:513, 1999]. *Can J Anaesth* 45:277, 1998.

Poland-Moebius Syndrome

At a glance: Both the Poland and the Moebius syndromes are well-described malformations. The Moebius syndrome is characterized by multiple cranial nerve palsies, orofacial malformations, and limb anomalies. The Poland syndrome consists of unilateral symbrachydactyly and ipsilateral aplasia of the sternal head of the pectoralis major muscle. The association probably represents a formal genesis malformation syndrome of unknown etiology.

History: Moebius syndrome, anomalies first described by Henry Thomas in 1898. The Poland disorder was first described by Sir Alfred Poland in 1841.

Incidence: 1:32,000 to 1:87,550 live births for Poland syndrome.

Genetic inheritance: Most patients with Poland syndrome are the result of mutation or sporadic with rarely familial (autosomal dominant) reports. Moebius syndrome is inherited as an autosomal dominant trait with the gene map locus localized to 13q12.2-q13. Alternately, all three genetic conditions may belong to the spectrum of the same syndrome; perhaps both syndromes are expressions of the same gene.

Pathophysiology: Poland syndrome and Moebius syndrome are each the result of interruption of the early embryonic blood supply in the subclavian arteries, the vertebral arteries and/or their branches. The term subclavian artery supply disruption sequence (SASDS) was suggested for this group of birth defects.

Diagnosis: The Poland syndrome consists of usually unilateral absence of the pectoralis muscle, syndactyly, brachydactyly, and hypoplasia of the hand. Absence of ribs may result in paradoxical chest wall movement. Classically, lung herniation through the chest defect may be seen during crying or a Valsalva maneuver. Patients with Moebius syndrome are usually diagnosed soon after birth because of incomplete closure of eyelids during sleep, drooling, and difficulties in sucking. A "mask-like facies" is present, with the child not smiling or moving its facial muscles on crying. Moebius syndrome consists of bilateral palsies of cranial nerves VI and VII, but occasionally also cranial nerves V, X, XI, and XII, resulting in difficulties with chewing, swallowing, and coughing, often leading to aspiration with respiratory complications. Arthrogryposis, limb deficiencies, contractures of the fingers, and strabismus may also occur with this condition.

Clinical aspects: Patients with Poland syndrome do not often have any functional disability and can present either for diagnostic radiological procedures or for cosmetic breast reconstructive surgery. Associated anomalies may include cardiovascular (dextrocardia, atrial septal defect), musculoskeletal (scoliosis), genitourinary (renal aplasia, hypospadias, inguinal hernia), gastrointestinal (extension of liver through chest), and hematological (lymphoma, leukemia). Patients with Moebius syndrome have congenital paralysis of the sixth and seventh cranial nerves, resulting in esotropia and facial paralysis. Occasionally, cranial nerves V, X, XI, and XII are also involved, resulting in chewing, swallowing, and coughing, and repeated aspiration with respiratory complications. Patients with Moebius syndrome have a high incidence of other anomalies, including congenital cardiac disease, spinal anomalies, corneal abrasions, and peripheral neuropathies, and a careful preoperative assessment is essential. Affected children most commonly present for anesthesia for correction of strabismus, or for orthopedic procedures to improve limb function.

Precautions before anesthesia: The presence of associated anomalies should be determined in patients and appropriate investigations ordered. Concomitant respiratory infections in patients with Moebius syndrome should be optimally treated prior to elective surgery. *Investigations:* arterial blood gas, chest radiograph, ECG, serum urea and electrolytes, cell blood count. Antisialagogue premedication to decrease pharyngeal secretions. Ensure full cardiac investigations, including echocardiography, if there is suspicion of any cardiac lesion. Ensure respiratory function is optimized and infections treated with appropriate antibiotics and physiotherapy. Chest radiograph to elucidate acute or chronic lung changes and/or chest wall deformity. *Blood examination:* urea, creatinine, and electrolytes if renal abnormalities are present. Arterial blood gas analysis if indicated by respiratory status.

Anesthetic considerations: Problems can arise during anesthesia for children with Moebius syndrome; there is a high incidence of difficult or failed tracheal intubation. The use of a face mask or laryngeal mask airway and spontaneous breathing technique is reported to be safe, although laryngospasm may occur from the accumulation of pharyngeal secretions and special attention should be given to this eventuality. The potential for problems with aspiration of oral secretions should be remembered and the use of antisialagogue premedication is recommended. In the Poland syndrome, unilateral absence of ribs leads to poor development of subatmospheric pressure in the thorax and paradoxical respiration, and may cause inadequate pulmonary ventilation and hypoxia. Positive-pressure ventilation is recommended to maintain ventilation during surgery. The anesthetic technique and the need for invasive monitoring is influenced by, among other factors, the presence and severity of cardiovascular disease and respiratory impairment secondary to the spinal anomalies. Ophthalmic ointments should be applied and the eyes taped closed to prevent further ocular complications in those patients with corneal injuries. Where a regional anesthetic technique is to be used, careful documentation of existing neuropathies should be done. Recurrent aspiration may cause acute and chronic pulmonary changes and increased oxygen requirement. Paradoxical chest movement during spontaneous ventilation may result in inadequate ventilation; therefore mechanical ventilation is recommended. A period of postoperative mechanical ventilation may be required to facilitate bronchial toilet in these patients. Antibiotic prophylaxis may be required for invasive procedures in the presence of cardiac defects. Renal aplasia requires care with fluid balance and administration of renally excreted drugs.

Pharmacological implications: Antisialagogues such as atropine and glycopyrrolate are recommended to reduce upper airway secretions. Atracurium, *cis*-atracurium, and mivacurium are suitable muscle relaxants if renal aplasia exists. Suxamethonium should be avoided. If there is compromised respiratory function, extreme care should be taken with the administration of opioids and benzodiazepines.

REFERENCES:

Ferguson S: Moebius syndrome: A review of the anesthetic implications. *Paediatr Anaesth* 6:51, 1996.

Parker DL, Mitchell PR, Holmes GL: Poland-Mobius syndrome. *J Med Genet* 18:317, 1981.

Sethuraman R, Kannan S, Bala I, Sharma RK: Anaesthesia in Poland syndrome. *Can J Anaesth* 45:277, 1998.

POLIP Syndrome

At a glance: POLIP is an acronym that stands for: *P*olyneuropathy, *O*phthalmoplegia, *L*eukoencephalopathy, and Chronic *I*ntestinal *P*seudoobstruction and consider a mitochondrial myopathy characterized by a tetrad of progressive sensorimotor peripheral nerve disease. Other clinical features include myopathy, diffuse leukoencephalopathy, and ptosis.

Synonym: Myoneuro-Gastrointestinal Encephalopathy Syndrome; MNGIE Syndrome.

Incidence: Very rare; 33 patients up to 1997.

Genetic inheritance: There were suggestions that this disorder is an autosomal recessive trait with pathology of the nuclear genome, probably involving the control of the mitochondrial DNA replication (multiple deletions of mitochondrial DNA). Sporadic cases were also reported. Recent report of the MNGIE (mitochondrial neurogastrointestinal encephalomyopathy) locus at 22q13.32-qter.

Pathophysiology: The precise etiology and pathophysiologic significance of the mitochondrial DNA (mtDNA) deletions and the heterogeneity of the modifications of the mtDNA remain unknown. A mutation in the gene encoding thymidine phosphorylase possibly results in a defect of cytochrome *c* oxidase in liver and muscle.

Diagnosis: MRI and CT scans are consistent with leukodystrophy involving the cerebral and cerebellar white matter. Histology shows widespread endoneurial fibrosis and demyelination in the peripheral nervous system. Muscle biopsy with histologic features of mitochondrial myopathy (ragged red fibers, muscle fibers with increased succinate dehydrogenase stain or ultrastructurally abnormal mitochondria). Biochemical examination of the liver and muscle tissues reveals defect of cytochrome *c* oxidase (complex IV of the respiratory chain). Nerve conduction and electromyographic (EMG) studies are compatible with a sensorimotor neuropathy; quantitative EMG may show a myogenic process. Southern blot analysis reveals multiple deletions of mtDNA.

Clinical aspects: Symptoms begin before age of 20 years. The first signs are gastrointestinal symptoms (recurrent nausea, vomiting, or diarrhea with intestinal dysmotility) in the majority of cases, or an ophthalmoparesis in some cases. The neurologic manifestations are predominantly outside the central nervous system (CNS); gastrointestinal (GI) dysmotility is a result of severe visceral neuropathy. Gastrostomy or jejunostomy tube feeding may fail because of dysmotility. Malabsorption with intermittent diarrhea and chronic malnutrition ensues. Parenteral alimentation is often necessary. Lactic acidosis after moderate glucose loads may occur. Prokinetic agents, including erythromycin and cisapride, are unsuccessful in improving intestinal motility. Visual disturbances may manifest as blepharoptosis and ophthalmoparesis. Proximal muscle weakness and mild ataxia is common. Neurosensory hearing loss, proximal myopathy with marked muscle atrophy, polyneuropathy, and encephalopathy (with hypodense areas in the white matter on MRI examination) are present. In addition, there also may be an autonomic neuropathy. Electrocardiography may show cardiac conduction abnormalities. Respiratory function may be severely affected. The prognosis is poor because of a severe weight loss bordering on cachexia, with a mean survival age of 28.5 years. The prognosis seems to be worsened by a young age of onset.

Precautions before anesthesia: The diagnosis of mitochondrial disease should be considered in any child with a multisystem neurological disorder or who is being investigated for hypotonia. Anesthesia-related morbidity and mortality risk is essentially linked to the preoperative status of the child, that is, the number and extent of organ dysfunction. Avoid any elective anesthesia/surgery in the presence of infection or temperature because cytokines (mainly tumor necrosis factor) inhibit some complex of the respiratory chain. The following should be carefully evaluated: *CNS:* seizures, myoclonus, strokes, swallowing problems; *metabolic:* usual venous or arterial concentration of lactates and glucose; *muscles:* hypotonia, contractures, scoliosis; *cardiac:* even if the child is asymptomatic, ECG and echocardiography to exclude for conduction disorders and cardiomyopathy, respectively; if a pacemaker has been inserted, check it to be sure that it is functioning properly; *pulmonary:* frequent infections, chronic aspiration, pulse oximetry breathing room air, obstructive and/or central apnea; reduced ventilatory drive is common and many patients have an abnormal response to both hypoxia and hypercarbia; deaths have been reported following sedation with chloral hydrate or diazepam; *hepatic* and *renal* function must be evaluated; *nutritional status* and *diet* (glucose and/or lipid rich), tolerance to fasting and treatment (carnitine, vitamin Q, antiepileptic drugs).

Anesthetic considerations: Usual treatment must be maintained until the morning of surgery. Preoperative fasting must be kept as short as possible; if fasting is usually poorly tolerated, a glucose-containing solution should be started when fasting period begins. A sedative premedication is best avoided because of the possible abnormal response to hypoxia/hypercarbia. *Induction:* according to the anesthesiologist's choice; sevoflurane is the best choice for inhalation induction; propofol seems the best choice for IV induction but a 2% solution should be used to lessen the lipid load. *Opiates:* The dose should be carefully titrated according to the patient's needs. *Muscle relaxant:* Published data are often contradictory. Even in the absence of clinical myopathy, the patient's muscular response to nerve stimulation should be measured before administering a muscle relaxant. Atracurium or *cis*-atracurium are the best choice because of their spontaneous degradation. In case of myopathy, succinylcholine should not be used so as to avoid producing rhabdomyolysis. There is no evidence of an increased risk of malignant hyperthermia; however, one should be careful in the presence of confirmed myopathy. *Intraoperative fluids:* Avoid infusion containing lactates such as Ringer lactate or Hartmann solution, but give the patient a glucose (5 or 10% according to blood sugar level) solution. Aim for normoglycemia because hyperglycemia can also increase lactate production. Monitor (arterial or venous) blood gases and lactate levels; in case of severe lactic acidosis use dichloroacetate 50 mg/kg IV over 30 minutes to stimulate pyruvate dehydrogenase to metabolize lactate in pyruvate. Perimedullar locoregional anesthesia can be used, but its cost:benefit ratio should be evaluated, taking into account the presence of severe scoliosis or of degenerative lesions in the spinal cord. Some patients with mitochondrial disease also present with axonal neuropathy of peripheral nerves; the possible effects of local anesthetics on these nerves are unknown. Prevention of hypothermia is important to avoid shivering and to increase oxygen consumption upon awakening.

Pharmacological implications: Patients with mitochondrial disease are very sensitive to the respiratory effects of sedatives. It also seems, according to BIS measurement, that children with an anomaly of complex I of the respiratory chain are much more sensitive to the hypnotic effects of sevoflurane. Most studies performed on isolated mitochondria use doses of anesthetic agents far in excess of those used in daily practice and their clinical relevance is thus often dubious.

REFERENCES:

Hirano M, Silvestri G, Blake DM, et al: Mitochondrial neurogastrointestinal encephalomyopathy (MNGIE): Clinical, biochemical, and genetic features of an autosomal recessive mitochondrial disorder. *Neurology* 44(4):721, 1994.

Simon LT, Horoupian DS, Dorfman LJ, et al: Polyneuropathy, ophthalmoplegia, leukoencephalopathy, and intestinal pseudo-obstruction: POLIP syndrome. *Ann Neurol* 28:349, 1990.

Pollitt Syndrome

At a glance: Inherited syndrome characterized by trichorrhexis nodosa, psychomotor retardation, microcephaly, and the deficiency of high-sulfur protein in the hair.

Synonyms: Trichorrhexis Nodosa Syndrome; Trichothiodystrophy-Neurocutaneous Syndrome; Neurotrichocutaneous Syndrome.

History: First described in 1968 by R.J. Pollitt, a British physician.

Incidence and genetic inheritance: Extremely rare. Most likely autosomal recessive inheritance. More common in females than in males.

Clinical aspects: Psychomotor developmental delay and trichorrhexis nodosa. Mental retardation is secondary to an abnormal cortical cell layer pattern in the brain and marked microcephaly. The hair defect results from a reduced content in sulfur matrix protein (mainly because of a half-normal cystine content), hence the alternative term "trichothiodystrophy" was suggested for this disease (although this expression is also used to name the whole group of diseases with this type of hair defect associated with other ectodermal and neuroectodermal disorders). Microscopically, the hair defect is characterized by trichoschisis (transverse fractures of the hair); using polarized light reveals the typical alternation of dark and bright regions, producing a tiger-tail pattern. In the two children described by King et al. from unrelated Scottish parents, the head circumference, length, and weight were below the third percentile at the age of 6 months, which was associated with developmental delay. Facial features included stubby eyebrows, protruding ears, and retrognathia. Neurologically, jerky eye movements, spastic diplegia, and either absent or hyperactive deep tendon reflexes were noted. Microcephaly with a short skull and small cranial vault, small and bridged sella turcica (radiological) complete the neurological defect. The ectodermal changes included ichthyosis, severe flexural eczema, and brittle, hypoplastic nails with koilonychia. By the age of 4 years, photosensitivity of the skin was also reported, whereas all the other manifestations remained basically unchanged. One patient also developed bilateral cataracts.

Anesthetic considerations: No reports exist about anesthesia in these patients. However, the presence of retrognathia could make airway management difficult. Most likely, a smaller endotracheal tube than calculated for the age is required. Endotracheal tube and IV-line fixation, as well as vascular access in the presence of ichthyosis, may be difficult. These patients may benefit from preoperative anxiolysis and sedation.

Other conditions to be considered:

☞**BRITTLE HAIR AND MENTAL DEFICIT SYNDROME:** Genetic disorder characterized by abnormal hair fibers and mental deficiency.

☞**AMISH HAIR-BRAIN SYNDROME:** Inherited syndrome in Amish people with mild psychomotor retardation, hypogonadism, short stature, and brittle hair.

☞**NETHERTON SYNDROME:** This most likely autosomal recessive transmitted inborn error of metabolism manifests with bamboo hair, atopic diathesis, congenital ichthyosiform erythroderma, and hypogamma-globulinemia.

☞**MENKES DISEASE:** A genetic disorder of copper metabolism beginning before birth. Copper accumulates in excessive amounts in the liver, and is deficient in most other tissues of the body. Structural changes occur in the hair, brain, bones, liver, and arteries. Other features include spontaneous hypothermia, severe developmental delay, loss of early development skills, and seizures.

REFERENCES:

King MD, Gummer CL, Stephenson JB: Trichothiodystrophy-neurotricho-cutaneous syndrome of Pollitt: A report of two unrelated cases. *J Med Genet* 21:286, 1984.

Pollitt RJ, Jenner FA, Davies M: Sibs with mental and physical retardation and trichorrhexis nodosa with abnormal amino acid composition of the hair. *Arch Dis Child* 43:211, 1968.

Pollitt RJ, Stonier PD: Proteins of normal hair and of cystine-deficient hair from mentally retarded siblings. *Biochem J* 122:433, 1971.

Polyarteritis Nodosa (PAN)

At a glance: Systemic necrotizing vasculitis affecting medium-sized arteries. The cutaneous form of PAN is associated with streptococcal infection and seems to be a little more frequent in children.

Synonym: Periarteritis Nodosa; Kussmaul's Disease; Necrotizing Arteritis Syndrome.

History: First described in 1866 by Kussmaul and Meier. They identified a condition that consisted of "focal, inflammatory, artery nodules".

Incidence: Onset is generally between the ages of 40 and 50 but may also occur at any age. The male-to-female ratio is 3:1. The cause and the true incidence remain unknown.

Pathophysiology: The cause remains unknown; however, the variety of pathologic features suggests multiple pathogenic mechanisms. Spontaneously occurring polyarteritis nodosa occurs in hyperimmunized human volunteers, in animals with experimental serum sickness, and in patients developing hypersensitivity reactions. Drugs (e.g., sulfonamides, penicillin, iodide, thiouracil, bismuth, thiazides, guanethidine, methamphetamine), vaccines, bacterial infections (e.g., streptococcal, staphylococcal), and viral infections (e.g., serum hepatitis, influenza, HIV) have been associated with disease onset. Segmental, necrotizing inflammation of media and adventitia characterizes the lesion. The pathologic process most commonly occurs at points of vessel bifurcation, beginning in the media and extending into the intima and adventitia of medium-sized arteries, often disrupting the internal elastic lamellae. Early endothelial lesions contain polymorphonuclears and occasionally eosinophils; later lymphocytes and plasma cells can be seen. Immunoglobulin, complement components, and fibrinogen are deposited in the lesions, but their significance is unclear. Intimal proliferation with secondary thrombosis and occlusion leads to organ and tissue infarction. Weakening of the muscular vessel wall may cause small aneurysms and arterial dissection. Healing can result in nodular fibrosis of the adventitia.

Diagnosis: Histologically, it is a necrotizing angiitis of small- and medium-size vessels whose manifestations are weight loss, fever, asthenia, peripheral neuropathy, renal involvement, musculoskeletal and cutaneous manifestations, hypertension, gastrointestinal (GI) tract involvement, cardiac failure, and cerebral infarcts.

Clinical aspects: Attacks of fever and cutaneous rash that occasionally progress to gangrene and amputation of distal portions of toes and fingers. The cutaneous PAN is usually restricted to the musculoskeletal system and skin. Clinical findings can range from isolated cutaneous findings to widespread multisystemic involvement (kidney, heart, liver). The illness may present as ischemic colitis. Cardiac failure may be caused by pericardial thickening or by histological changes of the myocardium and atrioventricular valves, or by myocardial infarction. Cardiac involvement may lead to cerebral infarction coming from the lesions of the endocardium or the valves. Often associated with hypertension and eosinophilia. The unique coexistence of polyarteritis nodosa, antiphospholipid antibodies (aPL), and perinuclear antineutrophil cytoplasmic antibodies (p-ANCA) is described. Disseminated intravascular coagulation may complicate the illness. Treatment includes high-dose corticosteroids, often in combination with cytotoxic or immunosuppressive agents such as cyclophosphamide or azathioprine.

Precautions before anesthesia: In acute phase, check carefully the cardiac and renal function. Check complete cell blood count for eosinophilia, hemoglobin, and platelets (effects of treatment, GI tract may bleed). The brain must be carefully assessed (MRI if the neurological exam is abnormal). Ensure intraoperative steroid coverage.

Anesthetic considerations: All techniques that could enhance the peripheral blood supply should be considered. Because of the associated myopathy, these patients should be carefully monitored when muscle relaxants are used. The cerebral involvement may lead to acute encephalitis so these patients should be considered at high risk for cerebral edema and raised intracranial pressure.

Pharmacological implications: Succinylcholine should be avoided in these cases where massive muscle loss and myopathy symptoms are present.

Other condition to be considered:

COGAN SYNDROME: This disorder affects more often young adults, but occasionally also elderly persons. Presents with a sudden onset of a painful uni- or bilateral interstitial keratitis resulting

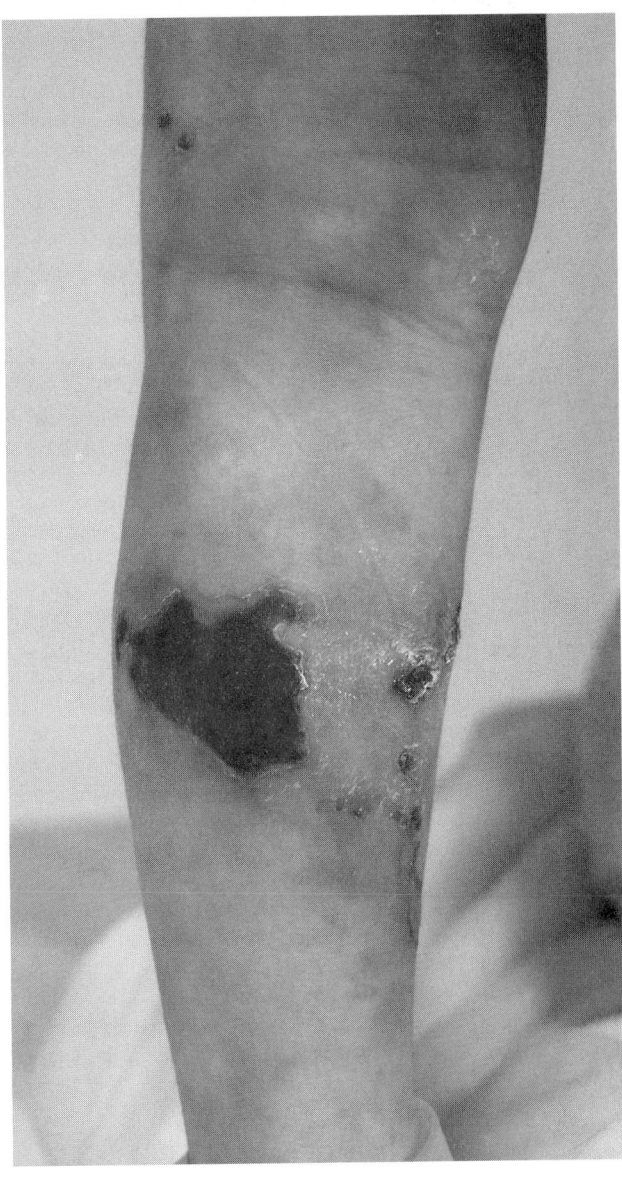

Polyarteritis nodosa Ulcerations and necrosis of the skin in a patient with polyarteritis nodosa.

in blurred vision, lacrimation, blepharospasm, and photophobia. It is followed by bilateral audiovestibular symptoms manifesting as vertigo, nausea, and tinnitus, which rapidly progresses to deafness. The cause of this syndrome is unknown; however, in about half the patients an underlying systemic disease, most commonly polyarteritis nodosa, can be diagnosed.

REFERENCES:

Maes K, Billiet J, Haerens M: Massive bilateral renal and perirenal hemorrhage due to polyarteritis nodosa: A life-threatening condition. *Eur Urol* 38:349, 2000.

Provenzale JM, Allen NB: Neuroradiologic findings in polyarteritis nodosa. *Am J Neuroradiol* 17(6):119, 1996.

Siberry GK, Cohen BA, Johnson B: Cutaneous polyarteritis nodosa (reports of two cases in children and review of the literature). *Arch Dermatol* 140:884, 1994.

Polycystic Kidney Disease (PKD)

At a glance: Genetic disorder frequently producing renal failure in childhood. It is the most common genetically determined childhood cystic disease of the kidneys. Congenital malformation of the collecting tubules.

Synonym: PCKD.

Classification: A polycystic kidney disease classification has been described by E.L. Potter in 1964 (see Table P-1).

Incidence: 1:10,000 to 1:40,000 live births. The age distribution of cases has two peaks, one at birth and one between the ages of 30 and 60 years.

Genetic inheritance: Autosomal recessive PKD is a neonatal disease that has been associated to a gene map locus at 6p21.1-p12. The later form is believed to be a familial pattern of an autosomal dominant inheritance. Both sexes are affected. There is also a form of renal cystic disease not inherited and described as the acquired cystic kidney disease, which develops in those individuals with long-term kidney problems.

Pathophysiology: There is distention of the renal collecting tubules caused by localized proliferation and aberrant secretion of epithelial cells. The expanding structures develop into cysts that are filled with fluid containing biologically active ligands for the epidermal growth factor receptor (EGFR), such as epidermal growth factor and transforming growth factor-alpha. The EGFR, normally localized at the basolateral surfaces of the collecting tubule epithelium, becomes mislocalized to the apical surface on the cells lining cystic structures. This mislocalization of EGFR is a common end point associated with several different forms of PKD that are initiated by mutations in different genes.

Diagnosis: Ultrasonography is the best diagnostic tool, and in late pregnancy can allow presumptive in utero diagnosis in most cases (increased echogenicity and renal enlargement). The feasibility and reliability of DNA obtained by amniocentesis or chorionic villus sampling during prenatal testing is being examined. Hepatic involvement is invariable with generalized portal and interlobular fibrosis, and bile duct proliferation. The remainder of the hepatic parenchyma is normal.

Clinical aspects: One of the notable features is the variability of the phenotype, with respect to both disease progression and extrarenal manifestations. While a significant component of this variance is probably a result of genetic heterogeneity, marked variability

of clinical disease, even within kindreds, is documented. The clinical presentation varies with age.

Perinatal and neonatal form: "Potter's face" ("squashed" nose, micrognathia, large, floppy, low-set ears) is present in most or all. The Potter face resembles that of a child with his face pressed to a window pane. Severely affected neonates commonly have pulmonary hypoplasia secondary to the in utero effects of renal dysfunction. Stillbirth is common, as is neonatal renal failure and respiratory insufficiency in survivors. These infants often die in the first few days or weeks of life. Less severely affected neonates have a protuberant abdomen with huge, firm, smooth-surfaced, symmetric kidneys and hepatomegaly.

Infantile form: Infants who survive the first few years show progressive renal failure. Renal function is decreased in more than two-thirds of the patients, while 10% develop end-stage renal failure. Hypertension is present in 70% of cases. Growth retardation is present. Generally, those first presenting in early childhood show mainly renal-related symptoms (e.g., pain, hematuria, urinary tract infection, systemic hypertension, nephrolithiasis), whereas those first presenting as adolescents show mainly hepatic-related symptoms.

Juvenile form: Signs of portal hypertension may appear (esophageal and gastric varices, hypersplenism) between the ages of 5 and 10 years. In those individuals in whom the initial symptomatology becomes obvious in adolescence, nephromegaly is less marked. Renal insufficiency may be mild to moderate. The major symptoms are related to progressive hepatic fibrosis (portal hypertension, gastric and esophageal varices, hepatic insufficiency, and hypersplenism). The prognosis is limited, whether hepatic or renal dysfunction predominates. Treatment is supportive and aimed at preserving renal function: adequate fluid and salt supplementation, sodium bicarbonate, and antibiotic therapy for urinary or biliary infection. Its seems that caffeine-containing products enlarge the renal cysts. To prevent damage or rupture of enlarged abdominal organs, contact sports are best avoided. Portacaval or splenorenal shunts have been successful in reducing morbidity but not mortality. Combined renal–hepatic transplantation is successful.

Adult form: An autosomal dominant inheritance, representing the most common form, is responsible for approximately 90% of all cases. It manifests itself between the ages of 30 and 40 years. However, it can sometimes appear during adolescence.

Precautions before anesthesia: Note drug history. Systematic review of cardiovascular status is indicated. Improve a most often poor nutritional status. Note method and timing of last dialysis. Examine for signs of dehydration or fluid overload. Note site of any arteriovenous fistula. Depending on the surgical procedure, have adequate supplies of cross-matched blood available. The need for platelets and fresh-frozen plasma should be anticipated. *Investigations:* complete cell blood count (anemia, hypersplenism), clotting times, urea, creatinine and electrolytes, liver function tests, ECG, chest radiograph. In case of portal hypertension, the presence of a hepatopulmonary syndrome (orthodeoxia) should be excluded. Sedative premedication should be adapted to the level of renal and/or hepatic insufficiency.

Anesthetic considerations: Adequate preoxygenation is necessary as rapid desaturation may occur during induction because of reduced functional residual capacity as a result of the distended abdomen. Avoid using intravenous access that may compromise future surgical arteriovenous fistulae formation for dialysis. Fluid balance and electrolytes should be monitored carefully. The use of a central venous line for this purpose will be dictated by the

*Table P-1   Potter's Classification of Polycystic Kidney Disease**

Type	Name	Inheritance	Symptoms
Type I	Recessive Polycystic Kidney Disease (RPKD)	Autosomal recessive pattern	Pulmonary hypoplasia; oligohydramnios; kidneys are affected bilaterally; cysts 1-2 mm on average; congenital hepatic fibrosis on autopsy
Type II	Multicystic Renal Dysplasia	Sporadic	Most common form of inherited cystic disease; the cysts are variable sizes (1 mm to 1 cm), filled with clear fluid; no recognizable glomeruli and tubules. The hallmark is the presence of "primitive ducts" in pathology (associated with Meckel-Gruber syndrome)
Type IIa	Large Multicystic Renal Dysplasia	Sporadic	Affected kidney is large
Type IIb	Small Multicystic Renal Dysplasia	Sporadic	Hypodysplasia kidney or "quite small."
Type III	Dominant Polycystic Kidney Disease (DPKD)	Autosomal dominant	Middle-aged to older adults; progressive renal failure as the cysts become larger; rarely seen prenatally or in children; patients are prone to have berry aneurysms of the cerebral arteries
Type IV	Cystic Change with Obstruction (Hallmark: cortical microcysts)	No genetic involvement	In the fetus and newborn with urinary tract obstruction; in addition to hydroureter, hydronephrosis, and bladder dilation; urethral valves (males) or atresia (females); oligohydramnios, pulmonary hypoplasia
Type V	Miscellaneous Cystic Renal Changes in Adults	No genetic involvement	The most common cystic change of all is the appearance of one or more "simple renal cysts" in adults; may reach 10 cm or more; present renal failure leading to long-term dialysis

*Described by Edith Louise Potter in 1964.

patient's underlying cardiovascular status and the surgery. Tracheal intubation and intermittent positive-pressure ventilation must be used for all surgical procedures. Care must be taken when passing a nasogastric tube in the presence of esophageal varices. There are no contraindications to the use of regional anesthesia as long as there is no coagulopathy or thrombocytopenia. Elective postoperative mechanical ventilation may be required for patients who had undergone a prolonged surgery, or who had severe blood loss.

Pharmacological implications: Nonsteroidal anti-inflammatory drugs (NSAIDs) should not be used for fear of precipitating acute renal failure. Atracurium, *cis*-atracurium, and mivacurium are preferred for neuromuscular blockade because of their rapid elimination, which is independent of renal and hepatic functions. Isoflurane and desflurane are preferred over halothane (hepatic toxicity), enflurane, or sevoflurane.

REFERENCE:

Zerres K, Mucher G, Becker J, et al: Autosomal recessive polycystic kidney disease. *Contrib Nephrol* 122:10, 1997.

Polycystic Liver Disease

At a glance: A form of hepatobiliary fibropolycystic disease characterized by an overgrowth of biliary epithelium and supportive connective tissue. Multiple cysts are present in the liver parenchyma. The condition is usually associated with polycystic kidney disease and congenital biliary duct disease.

Synonym: PCLD.

Incidence: Of patients referred for ultrasonographic examination of the abdomen, 2 to 5% have hepatic cysts, of which fewer than one-third are multiple with one to three cysts. Hepatic cysts are exceptionally rare in children; frequency increases from 0% in first two decades of life to 7% in the eighth decade of life.

Genetic inheritance: Autosomal dominant. Polycystic liver disease occurs either alone or in association with autosomal dominant polycystic kidney disease.

Pathophysiology: Alterations in the development and differentiation of bile ducts and intralobular bile ductules with development of biliary microhamartomas and cysts. Cystic dilatation of peribiliary glands around the large intrahepatic bile ducts may also give rise to the cysts.

Diagnosis: Magnetic resonance imaging may be the most sensitive method to differentiate a complicated cyst from an uncomplicated one.

Clinical aspects: Despite the great differences in the number and size of the cysts, the volume of the noncystic liver parenchyma remains normal; therefore, most patients with polycystic liver disease are asymptomatic and have normal liver function tests. Symptoms may be caused by complicated hepatic cysts, by the mass effect of one or several cysts, or by a massively enlarged liver. Hemorrhage or rupture of the hepatic cysts are rare complications that present as an acute abdomen. Infection of hepatic cyst may be indistinguishable from acute cholecystitis. Percutaneous drainage of the infected cyst is usually effective and safe and surgical drainage is reserved for patients with relapses. Mass effects of large cysts include symptoms related to the increased intraabdominal pressure, obstruction of the hepatic veins, inferior vena cava, and obstruction of the bile ducts. When indicated, surgical treatment for polycystic liver disease is directed at reducing the volume of the cystic tissue. Cystic aspiration followed by instillation of a sclerosing agent may be performed for symptomatic cysts that are strategically located. Superficial cysts may be treated by laparoscopic fenestration. Combined hepatic resection and fenestration have met with limited success. In those patients incapacitated by severe hepatomegaly secondary to massive cystic replacement without areas of parenchymal sparing, liver transplantation is a therapeutic option.

Precautions before anesthesia: Concomitant renal evaluation is mandatory to exclude polycystic kidney disease. Complex hemostatic abnormalities may be present. H_2 antagonists can be given to reduce the risk of gastrointestinal bleeding and to reduce the risk of aspiration of gastric contents from the delay of gastric motility and hyperacidity. *Investigations:* Complete cell blood count, coagulation studies, ECG, chest radiograph, electrolytes, urea, and creatinine levels. Check for the presence of portal hypertension and ascites.

Anesthetic considerations: Passage of nasogastric tubes should be done with care in patients with esophageal varices. If coagulation function is compromised, particular care should be paid to insertion of invasive lines and intubation. Regional techniques are worth considering if there is no coagulopathy. Otherwise, intubation and controlled ventilation should be employed, especially in patients with ascites or pleural effusion, and to minimize the risk for pulmonary aspiration. Patients with significant hepatic impairment and hyperbilirubinemia (>180 mmol/L) are at higher risk for renal failure; these patients should be adequately hydrated (guided by central venous pressure if necessary), and maintenance of diuresis before, during, and after operation with fluid loading, mannitol, or furosemide. Partial hepatectomy is usually associated with massive blood loss, with subsequent massive blood transfusion and its attendant complications. Close monitoring of blood loss is necessary, as is the need to maintain adequate venous access, normothermia, electrolytes, and acid–base balance.

Pharmacological implications: Choice of anesthetic drugs according to the presence and importance of liver fibrosis, portal hypertension, cirrhosis, and/or renal insufficiency. Isoflurane has the least effect on the liver circulation.

Other condition to be considered:

☞**CAROLI SYNDROME:** Congenital cystic dilatation of the intrahepatic biliary tree associated with periportal fibrosis, portal hypertension, and, eventually, liver failure. Associated with polycystic kidneys in 40 to 50% of cases.

REFERENCES:

Conn M: Preoperative evaluation of the patient with liver disease. *Mt Sinai J Med* 58(1):75, 1991.

Torres VE: Polycystic liver disease. *Contrib Nephrol* 115:44, 1995.

Polyostotic Osteolytic Dysplasia

At a glance: A disorder characterized by congenital fibrous bone remodeling leading to painful, disabling bone deformity, early conductive hearing loss, early dentition loss, and tendency to pathological bone fracture.

Synonyms: Hereditary Expansile Osteolysis; McCabe Disease; Familial Expansile Osteolysis.

History: An inherited bone dysplasia first described in 1989 by Wallace and Osterberg. It has some histologic similarity to Paget disease.

Incidence: Rare; only a few kindreds have been reported in people of Northern Irish, German, or American ancestry.

Genetic inheritance: An autosomal dominant inheritance. The gene is mapped to 18q21.1-q22. The gene TNFRSF11A encodes the receptor activator of nuclear factor-kappa-B (RANK), which is essential for osteoclast formation.

Pathophysiology: The primary feature is one of active remodeling. The bone matrix is abundant and dense in the early stages, but with increased numbers of osteoblasts lining the bone trabeculae and focal collections of multinucleated osteoclasts at areas of active resorption. As the disease progresses, the matrix becomes scantier with osteoblastic activity becoming intense in advanced cases. Subsequently, there is a reduction in the amount of bone matrix associated with an increasingly disorganized arrangement of bone trabeculae. There is a corresponding increase in the prominence of fibrous tissue with more extensive vascularity. In the end stage of the disease, there is almost complete fatty replacement of the bone, with few remaining features of the original nature of the tissue.

Diagnosis: Bone biopsies obtained from affected patients show focal concentrations of multinuclear osteoclasts containing virallike microcylindrical inclusions. The radiographic features are distinctive. Generalized features are either altered trabecular pattern or modeling abnormalities. Focal features comprise lytic areas that progressively enlarge, producing expansion of the bone and its eventual disintegration because of fibrous and, finally, fatty replacement of the normal medulla. Almost 90% of these lesions occur in the appendicular skeleton. The radiographic features in combination with the histopathology render the condition unique. The serum alkaline phosphatase and urinary hydroxyproline are elevated to a variable degree.

Clinical aspects: The initial symptom may be early-onset hearing loss in the first decade, which is typically conductive in nature, but may progress to a mixed type. Skeletal changes manifest in the second decade of life and are predominantly distributed in the extremities as severe bone pain, deformity, and pathologic fractures. There are also dental abnormalities with bizarre and extensive resorption of the cervical region of the teeth and the root apex resulting in loss of dentition. There is an initial rapid but nonsustained biochemical response to parenteral dichloromethylene-diphosphonate. Current treatment is based on the drugs used in the treatment of Paget disease (calcitonin, etidronate sodium). None has had any significant sustained effect.

Precautions before anesthesia: Airway assessment should be done in those patients with craniofacial involvement. Assess dentition condition and note presence of loose teeth. If a central neuraxial anesthetic technique is planned, carefully document the presence of any vertebral fractures. Patients taking nonsteroidal anti-inflammatory drugs (NSAIDs) or salicylates should have the platelet function assessed. Appropriate perioperative steroid coverage should be given to those on corticosteroid therapy. *Investigations:* cell blood count, bleeding time.

Anesthetic considerations: Careful movement and positioning of the patient is necessary because fractures occur with even mild trauma. Padding of all pressure areas is recommended. Direct laryngoscopy and tracheal intubation must be performed gently to avoid mandibular fractures. In addition, care must be taken to avoid further dentition damage. Patients with extensive craniofacial involvement may have difficult airway management. Fiberoptic-assisted intubation may be necessary. The use of a laryngeal mask airway can also be useful. No particular anesthetic technique is recommended. Spinal or epidural anesthesia may be difficult in patients with vertebral involvement.

Pharmacological implications: There are no specific implications.

REFERENCES:

Osterberg PH, Wallace RG, Adams DA, et al: Familial expansile osteolysis. A new dysplasia. *J Bone Joint Surg Br* 70(2):255, 1988.

Wallace RG, Barr RJ, Osterberg PH, et al: Familial expansile osteolysis. *Clin Orthop* 248:265, 1989.

Porokeratosis of Mibelli

At a glance: Congenital or acquired genodermatosis disorder of keratinization. Clinically, presents one or more atrophic patches surrounded by a distinctive ridge-like border called the cornoid lamella. There are five variants and the disseminated superficial actinic porokeratosis is relatively common.

Synonym: Mibelli Porokeratosis.

Classification:

Porokeratosis of Mibelli: It is a rare keratoatrophoderma characterized by cutaneous centrifugally spreading patches. The lesions are surrounded by narrow horny ridges and with central atrophy and appear as crater-like formations.

Porokeratosis Actinic Disseminated Superficial type I (DSAP I): It is characterized by the existence of photosensitivity developing after the age of 16 years and complete clinical manifestation during the fourth decade. It is much more frequent than the porokeratosis of Mibelli from which it must be distinguished.

Porokeratosis Actinic Disseminated Superficial type II (DSAP II): Similar to the DSAP1 in clinical presentation. However, a hereditary condition only reported in a Chinese family.

Porokeratosis Plantaris et Disseminata: A type of porokeratosis most probably distinct from both the Mibelli and disseminated superficial actinic types. The clinical features include lesions that appear first on the palms and soles during the late teens and early twenties. It is a chronic progressive disorder of keratinization with annular or gyrate plaques showing elevated borders. It is consistent with either an autosomal or X-linked dominant inheritance.

Porokeratosis Punctata Palmaris et Plantaris (PPPP; Keratoderma Palmoplantar Punctate Type II): A disease characterized by spinous keratoses on the volar aspects of the hands and feet that appear in the early twenties. The nails, teeth, and sweating system are normal. Histologically, studies show columnar parakeratosis that resembled the cornoid lamella of porokeratosis. This condition can be classified as type II punctate PPK, type I being the Buschke-Fischer-Brauer disorder and type III being acrokeratoelastoidosis. It is considered a hereditary disorder transmitted as an autosomal dominant pattern.

History: The prefix "poro" comes from the Greek for "callus."

Incidence: Isolated cases. The DSAP form is relatively common, whereas the others are rare. The DSAP affects women 3 times more often than men.

Genetic inheritance: Autosomal dominant inheritance, probably with some reduction in penetrance in females. Sporadic occurrence may occur in which a later onset is usual.

Pathophysiology: Histogenesis thought to be a clonal expansion of abnormal epidermal cells, which in susceptible individuals may be triggered by sunlight, irradiation, trauma, infection, or immunosuppression. Recent evidence showed a chromosomal abnormality with preferential involvement of chromosome 3, region 3p14-p12 being involved. In turn, the chromosomal instability may predispose to malignancy. The development of porokeratosis in immunosuppressed patients may be caused by allogenic inhibition of normal epidermal cells by immunosuppression, allowing phenotypic expression of porokeratosis in genetically predisposed individuals.

Diagnosis: Distinctive "crater-like" plaques characterized by narrow horny ridges with central atrophy. The histopathological hallmark is a circumferential cornoid lamella, a parakeratotic horn arising from a cell in the epidermis.

Clinical aspects: Skin eruption usually begins in childhood (although it can appear at any age), with asymptomatic porokeratotic lesions on sun-exposed skin. Individual lesions begin as keratotic papules that slowly enlarge to form characteristic annular plaques. The central portion is usually hairless, slightly atrophic, and hypopigmented, although hypertrophy and hyperpigmentation may occur. A raised border may occur and can be up to 1 cm (0.4 inches) in height. Lesions have been reported on the face and on the oral mucosa. They appear most often on the limbs and show a tendency to centrifugal spread. The face, genitalia, oral mucosa, and cornea may be affected. Approximately 7% of patients eventually develop skin cancer (squamous cell and basal cell carcinomas), usually on the extremities. Quiescent lesions become active and extensive after immunosuppression for heart or renal transplantation. Various treatment modalities were used, with no one method being more superior to another. Patients should be advised to avoid excessive sunlight, to use sunscreen, and to have periodic examinations by a dermatologist with a view to close skin malignancy surveillance. There are no other associated anomalies.

Precautions before anesthesia: Determine if the porokeratosis developed as a result of immunosuppressive therapy given post-transplantation. Further systemic evaluation depends on the type of organ transplantation. The immunosuppressive agents should also be considered. In particular, cyclosporine is nephro- and hepatotoxic and detailed evaluation of these organ functions is necessary. Patients on azathioprine should have an appropriate hematologic evaluation. Cardiac function should be assessed to eliminate any effects of immunosuppressive agents (echocardiograph).

Anesthetic considerations: There is no reported anesthetic experience in patients with this condition. The main anesthetic consideration lies in the proper evaluation of patients who developed this dermatosis as a result of either renal or cardiac transplantation. Theoretical possibility that lesions affecting the face may cause difficulty in maintaining a seal during face-mask anesthesia. **Pharmacological implications:** The immunosuppressive agents should also be considered.

REFERENCE:
Schamroth JM, Zlotogorski A, Gilead L: Porokeratosis of Mibelli: Overview and review of the literature. *Acta Derm Venereol* 77:207, 1997.

Porphyrias

At a glance: Inherited disorder of heme biosynthesis.
Classification: See Table P-2.
Nature: Inherited enzymatic defects of heme biosynthesis. The heme molecule is thereafter included in the biosynthesis of hemoproteins such as hemoglobin, myoglobin, microsomal cytochrome P450, peroxidase, and cyclooxygenase. They are classified as erythropoietic or hepatic depending on the primary organ in which excess production of porphyrins or precursors occurs (see Table P-2).
Incidence: Acute intermittent porphyria (AIP) 1:20,000 in Europe, 1:10,000 in Sweden; variegate porphyria (VP) 1:250 to 1:500 in white South Africans; erythropoietic protoporphyria (EPP) 1:35,000 live births.
Genetic inheritance: See the classification Table P-2.
Pathophysiology: Overproduction of specific heme precursors occurs upstream the characteristic enzymatic defect. This leads to increased baseline aminolevulinic acid (ALA) synthetase activity. The first and last three enzymes involved in heme synthesis are located in the mitochondria. The others are in the cytosol. Disease manifestations may be a result of increased ALA synthetase activity, increased porphyrin accumulation, or decreased heme production. Porphyrins are highly reactive oxidants, and skin accumulation causes photosensitivity. Neuronal damage throughout the central and peripheral nervous system also occurs, though the mechanism of this severe neuropathy is unknown.

Diagnosis: Difficult in the latent stage, but diagnosis is possible by DNA analysis. The presence of urine that becomes dark or port-wine reddish color after staying should prompt a diagnosis workup. During a porphyric crisis, measurement of urine porphyrin and porphyrinogen precursors is indicated and will confirm the diagnosis.
Clinical aspects:

Acute attacks occur in AIP, hereditary coproporphyria (HCP), *VP, and Doss porphyria (DP)*. These attacks are often triggered by certain drugs, although these drugs (see *Pharmacological Implications* and Table P-4 below) do not always trigger attacks, as well as by fasting, alcohol intake, or infection. Although hepatic porphyrias are rarely symptomatic before puberty, latent carriers such as prepubertal children, may have an acute attack following exposure to a triggering drug. Classic signs and symptoms include severe abdominal pain, vomiting, anxiety, autonomic dysfunction (hypertension and tachycardia), dark urine, dehydration, and electrolyte disturbances (hyponatremia, hypokalemia, and hypocalcemia). Neurologic dysfunction of both the sympathetic and parasympathetic systems is a hallmark, although the central nervous system (CNS) (bulbar symptoms, seizures, coma) and peripheral nervous system are also affected. Paralysis may occur, and may cause death if affecting the respiratory system.

Treatment of an attack of acute porphyria (AIP, HCP, VP, DP):

1. As soon as the diagnosis is established, carefully search for any precipitating factor: drugs, infection, hypocaloric diet, alcohol.
2. Symptomatic treatment: Pain often requires opiates. Agitation is usually controlled with chlorpromazine.
3. Specific treatment: Adequate intravenous administration of glucose and of hematin (3 mg/kg/d for 4 days). Hematin is a solution of human hemin arginate (it contains some ethanol). Possible side effects of hematin are local phlebitis (frequent) and coagulopathy (rare). Hemin acts by refurbishing the depleted heme pool and decreasing the synthesis of ALA synthase.

It is important to monitor for bulbar dysfunction, because this is a harbinger of respiratory failure. Mortality during acute attacks is 10%, usually secondary to respiratory failure or arrhythmias, but may be as high as 40% in parturients. Variegate porphyria and

Table P-2   Classification of the Inherited Human Porphyrias

Classification	Inheritance	Deficient Enzyme	Symptoms
Hepatic			
Acute Intermittent Porphyria	Autos D	Porphobilinogen deaminase	Neurologic
Hereditary Coproporphyria (HC)	Autos D	Coproporphyrinogen oxidase	Neuro + Cut
Variegate Porphyria (VP)	Autos D	Protoporphyrinogen oxidase	Neuro + Cut
Doss Porphyria (DP)	Autos R	ALA dehydratase	Neurologic
Porphyria Cutanea Tarda (PCT)	Autos D	Uroporphyrinogen decarboxylase	Cutaneous
Erythropoietic			
Günther Disease or Congenital Erythropoietic Porphyria (CEP)	Autos R	Uroporphyrinogen III synthetase	Cut + Hemato
Hepato Erythropoietic Porphyria (HEP)	Autos R	Uroporphyrinogen decarboxylase	Cut + Hemato
☞Erythropoietic Protoporphyria (EPP)	Autos D	Ferrochelatase	Cutaneous

ABBREVIATIONS: Autos: autosomal; Neuro: neurologic; Cut: cutaneous; Hemato: hematologic; ALA: delta-aminolevulinic acid; Doss: named after the author who described this new type of porphyria-delta-aminolevulinate dehydratase deficiency.

Table P-3 *Pathophysiology of Porphyrias and Enzyme Defects*

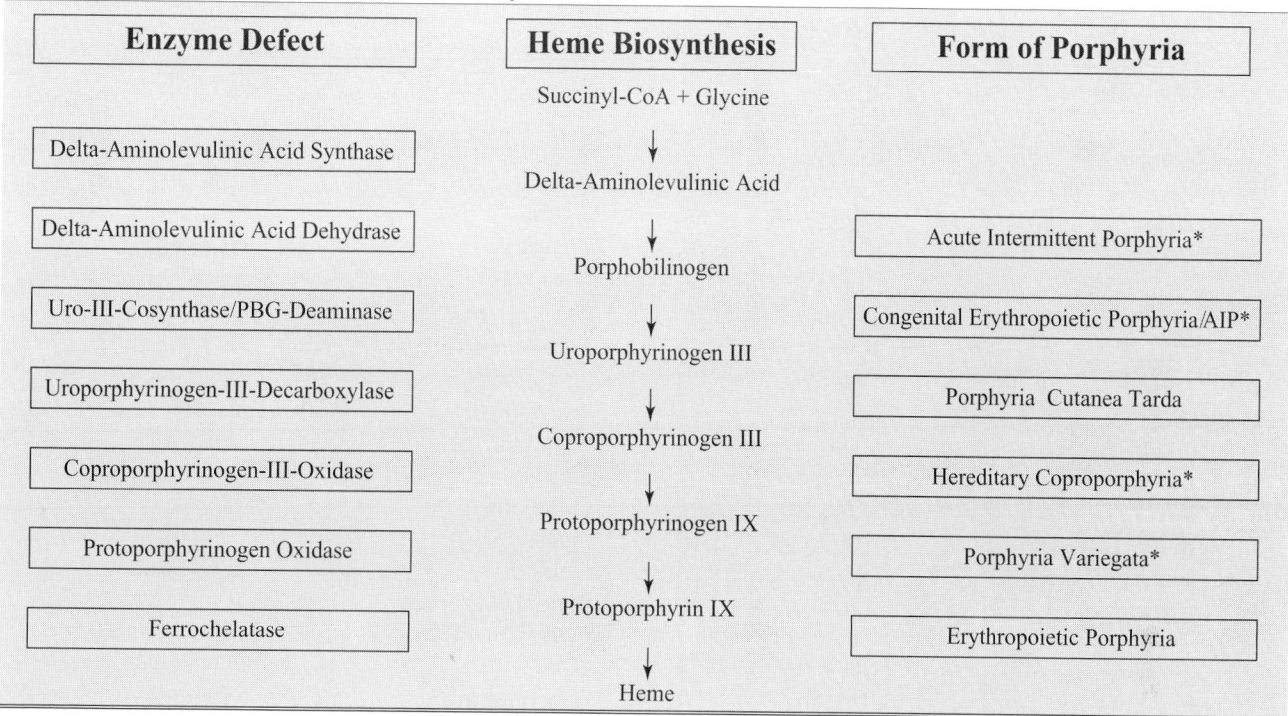

*Hepatic porphyrias: Uro-III Cosynthase = uroporphyrinogen-III-cosynthase; PBG-Deaminase = porphobilinogen deaminase; AIP = acute intermittent porphyria.

hereditary coproporphyria are inducible by triggering drugs and may also present with skin lesions caused by cutaneous photosensitivity: bullae, hyperpigmentation, and hypertrichosis.

Porphyria Cutanea Tarda (PCT) is not inducible with drugs, and is associated with hepatic, not neurologic, disease. Vesicles and bullae develop on sun-exposed areas. The sun-exposed skin is friable and minor trauma may lead to bullae or denudation of the skin. Liver dysfunction is common and the risk of hepatocellular carcinoma is increased. The preferred treatment is a course of phlebotomies at 1- to 2-week intervals because it leads to remission of the disease; if phlebotomies are contraindicated, low-dose chloroquine therapy can be tried.

CEP and HEP: severe cutaneous photosensitivity with formation of bullae. Scarring with hyperpigmentation. Hemolytic anemia with hypersplenism and cirrhosis.

Erythropoietic Protoporphyria (EPP) causes extreme skin photosensitivity, but lacks neurologic sequelae or drug inducibility. Pain, burning, or itching of light-exposed skin, with some redness and swelling. Some patients develop bullae or areas of increased pigmentation and thickening of the skin. Symptoms start in childhood. Hemolysis leading to biliary protoporphyrin-containing stones. Possible cirrhosis (late). Use of protective clothing and opaque sunscreens is useful. In all porphyrias with cutaneous symptoms photosensitivity is triggered at wavelengths near 400 nM.

Precautions before anesthesia: The precise diagnosis should be known; baseline neurologic examination must be obtained preoperatively and noted. Check fluid and electrolyte status. Premedicate to avoid stress-induced porphyria attack.

Anesthetic considerations: Regional anesthesia relatively contraindicated in case of neuropathy, and during acute attacks; avoid triggering agents (see *Pharmacological Implications* below); treat

autonomic dysfunction with propranolol; use invasive monitors during acute attacks; postoperative monitoring for acute attacks (delayed up to 5 days). In case of erythropoietic porphyria (CEP, HEP, or mainly EPP), yellow acrylate filters should be used in the operating room to eliminate light transmitted at wavelengths <530 nM from the usual operating room light sources. Fragile skin in case of PCT, CEP, HEP, and EPP.

Pharmacological implications: Medications believed safe or unsafe are listed in Table P-4.

For many drugs the actual status is uncertain. While one source considers a drug safe, another source rates the same drug unsafe. This can have several pharmacological reasons. However, it usually means that there are not enough data to support either rating. The following web sites may be consulted for further or updated information:

1- http://www.porphyria-europe.com/
2- http://bnf.org/bnf/bnf/current/doc/34979.htm
3- http://www.cs.nsw.gov.au/csls/RPAH/porphyria/druglist1.htm

REFERENCES:

Asokumar B, Kierney C, James TW, et al: Anaesthetic management of a patient with erythropoietic protoporphyria for ventricular septal defect closure. *Paediatr Anaesth* 9:356, 1999.

Durmus M, Turkoz A, Togal T, et al: Remifentanil and acute intermittent porphyria. *Eur J Anaesthesiol* 19:839, 2002.

Jensen NF: Anesthetic considerations in porphyrias. *Anesth Analg* 80:591, 1995.

Messmer M, Gerheuser F, Forst H: Desflurane in acute intermittent porphyria. *Anaesthetist* 53:244, 2004.

Nordmann Y, Puy H, Deybach JC: The porphyrias. *J Hepatol* 30:12, 1999.

Table P-4   *Medications Safe and Unsafe in Patients Affected with Porphyria*

Safe Drugs	Safe Drugs	Unsafe Drugs	Unsafe Drugs
Acebutolol	Insulin	Acetaminophen/paracetamol	Methylergometrin
Acetazolamide	Isoflurane	Allopurinol	Metronidazole
Acetylsalicylic acid	Labetalol	Amiodarone	Nifedipine
Acyclovir	Lisinopril	Amphetamine	Nitrazepam
Adrenaline/epinephrine	Loperamide	Androgens	Ondansetron
Alfentanil	Lorazepam	Baclofen	Paracetamol/
Amitryptiline/amoxicillin	Meperidine/pethidine	Barbiturates	acetaminophen
Amphotericin B	Methotrexate	Bromocriptine	Pentamidine
Atenolol	Metoclopramide	Bupivacaine (except	Pentazocine
Atracurium	Metoprolol	for epidural use)	Phenobarbital
Atropine	Midazolam	Busulfan	Phenoxybenzamine
Azathioprine	Minoxidil	Captopril	Phenytoin
Beclomycin	Morphine	Carbamazepine	Pravastatine
Bromazepam	Naloxone	Clobazam	Prilocaine
Bupivacaine (epidural	Naproxen	Clofibrate	Primidone
administration only)	Nitroprusside	Clonidine	Probenecid
Buprenorphine	Noradrenaline/	Cyclophosphamide	Progesterone
Chloralhydrate	norepinephrine	Cyclosporin A	Pyrazolones
Chlorprocaine	Norfloxacin	Diazepam	Ranitidine
Chlorpromazine	Nystatin	Dimenhydrinate	Rifampin/rifampicin
Cimetidine	Ofloxacin	Disopyramide	Ropivacaine
Clomipramine	Omeprazole	Econazole	Simvastatin
Clonazepam	Oxazepam	Enalapril	Spironolactone
Codeine	Oxytocin	Enflurane	Sulfonamides
Corticosteroids	Pancuronium	Ergotamines	Sulfonylureas
Diazoxide	Paraldehyde	Erythromycin	Sumatriptan
Diclofenac	Penicillin	Estrogens	Tamoxifen
Dicoumarol	Pethidine/meperidine	Ethanol	Tetrazepam
Digitoxin	Piroxicam	Ethosuximide	Theophylline
Digoxin	Prazosin	Etidocaine	Thiopental
Diltiazem	Procainamide	Etomidate	Ticlopidine
Diphenhydramine	Procaine	Famotidine	Tolbutamide
Dipyridamole	Promethazine	Fenofibrate	Topiramate
Domperidone	Propofol	Ferric chloride	Tramadol
Doxycycline	Propranolol	Fluconazole	Triazolam
Droperidol	Rocuronium	Flunarizine	Trimethoprim
Epinephrine/adrenaline	Salbutamol	Flurbiprofen	Trimipramine
Fentanyl	Succinylcholine	Halothane	Urapidil
Flumazenil	Sufentanil	Hydralazine	Valproic acid
Flunitrazepam	Terbutaline	Ibuprofen	Vigabatrin
Fluoxetine	Tetracaine	Ketamine	Zolpidem
Furosemide	Thyroxine	Ketoconazole	
Gabapentin	Timolol	Ketorolac	
Gentamicin	Tranexamic acid	Lamotrigine	
Glucagon	Vaccinations (all)	Lidocaine	
Haloperidol	Vecuronium	Mefenamic acid	
Heparin	Verapamil	Mepivacaine	
Hydrochlorothiazide	Vitamins (all)	Meprobamate	
Indomethacin		Methohexital	

Rigal JC, Blanloeil Y: Anaesthesia and porphyria. *Minerva Anesthesiol* 68:326, 2002.

Sheppard L, Dorman T: Anesthesia in a child with homozygous porphobilinogen deaminase deficiency: A severe form of acute intermittent porphyria. *Paediatr Anaesth* 15:426, 2005.

Potter Syndrome

At a glance: A possible genetic disorder characterized by oligohydramnios secondary to renal diseases such as bilateral renal agenesis. Other possible renal defects include obstructive uropathy, autosomal recessive polycystic kidney disease, medullary dysplastic kidney, and renal hypoplasia. Clinical features include Potter facies (i.e., flattened nose, recessed chin), pulmonary hypoplasia, skeletal anomalies, and congenital heart defects.

Synonyms: Oligohydramnios Sequence; Potter Sequence. Potter's disease; Potter facies.

Incidence: Renal agenesis occurs in 1:3000 live births and is responsible for 20% of Potter cases. Males have an increased incidence.

Genetic inheritance: Unclear. Different reports suggests an autosomal recessive, autosomal dominant or X-linked recessive. Male:female ratio of 2.5:1.

Pathophysiology: The possible mechanism of renal agenesis or hypoplasia may be failure of the ureteric bud formation, failure of the bud to reach the metanephric blastema, or failure of the bud and the metanephric blastema to influence each other. The ensuing decreased or absent intrauterine urine production results in oligo- or anhydramnios. This results in compression of the fetus and the typical anomalies found. Other causes of oligohydramnios (obstructive uropathy, polycystic kidneys, chronic leakage of amniotic fluid) produce a similar spectrum of anomalies.

Diagnosis: Based on ultrasonographic evidence of renal agenesis in addition to the typical clinical picture. Prenatal diagnosis of renal agenesis or hypoplasia is possible after 18 weeks of gestation.

Clinical aspects: *Potter facies:* mild hypertelorism, prominent inner canthus, flattened nose, mild micrognathia, large low-set ears. *Lungs:* severe pulmonary hypoplasia similar to that of congenital diaphragmatic hernia. *Skeletal:* malformation of spine, bowing of legs, club feet, large hands. *Cardiovascular:* Ventricular septal defects, tetralogy of fallot, patent ductus arteriosus, endocardial cushion defect. Prognosis is very poor. Death usually shortly after birth as a consequence of pulmonary hypoplasia.

Precautions before anesthesia: Unlikely to present for surgery in view of poor prognosis. Assess pulmonary status. Evaluate renal function: absent in case of renal agenesis or hypoplasia, variable in other causes of oligohydramnios.

Anesthetic considerations: Severe pulmonary hypoplasia requiring special techniques of mechanical ventilation. Endotracheal intubation may be difficult because of micrognathia. Renal agenesis may affect management. The association of cardiovascular malformations will influence the anesthetic management.

Pharmacological implications: According to renal function.

References:

Jones K: Oligohydramnios sequence, in Jones KL (ed): *Smith's Recognizable Patterns of Human Malformation.* 5th ed. WB Saunders, Philadelphia, 1997, p 632.

Zerres K, Völpel M, Weiss H: Cystic kidneys: Genetics, pathologic anatomy, clinical picture, and prenatal diagnosis. *Hum Genet* 68:104, 1984.

Powell Venencie Gordon Syndrome

At a glance: A rare keratodermal syndrome where nail dystrophies are associated with axonal neuropathy and sometimes respiratory insufficiency.

Synonym: Palmoplantar Keratoderma with Nail Dystrophy and Hereditary Motor-Sensory Neuropathy Syndrome; Axonal Neuropathy with Palmoplantar Keratoderma; Charcot-Marie-Tooth Disease with Palmoplantar Keratoderma and Nail Dystrophy Syndrome.

History: First described by J.L. Thonie in 1988.

Incidence: Very rare; unknown precisely.

Genetic inheritance: Autosomal dominant heterogeneous.

Pathophysiology: The cause remains unknown. The concurrence of the lesions can be interpreted to mean either that the keratoderma and the paraplegia are the pleiotropic effects of the same mutant gene or, less likely, that they are the manifestations of two different autosomal mutations.

Diagnosis: Must be evoked by association of signs. No certitude.

Clinical aspects: Nail dystrophy affects both toes and fingers; it can be present at birth or developed during early childhood. Palmoplantar keratoderma becomes apparent in later childhood. Clinical (abnormal gait, hypertonia, spasticity, rigidity, paraparesis, quadriparesis) or electrophysiological evidence of axonal neuropathy with muscular atrophia are observed. Muscle histological lesions can be present. Respiratory insufficiency can occur.

Precautions before anesthesia: Evaluate severity of the neurological and muscular lesions (clinical, electromyography, somatosensory, and motor evoked potentials). Evaluate respiratory function (chest radiograph, pulmonary function test, arterial blood gas analysis).

Anesthetic considerations: Intraoperative positioning must be careful. Pulse oximetry signal can be difficult to obtain because of nail dystrophy and its reliability has to be evaluated. Perioperative respiratory function survey if necessary.

Pharmacological implications: Muscles relaxants are not contraindicated but have to be used with caution and with a monitoring device. Succinylcholine must be avoided in case of acute exacerbation of the neurological signs (risk of hyperkaliemia). Opioids could be used with caution in spontaneously breathing patients. Regional anesthetic techniques, when applicable, might be preferable even though there are no data in this pathology.

Other conditions to be considered:

Venencie Powell Winkelmann Syndrome: In this syndrome multiple orthopedic malformations are associated including scoliosis and brachydactyly. A particular face is observed (narrow nose, prematurely aged face).

Fitzsimmons Syndrome: Mental retardation with spastic paraplegia and palmoplantar hyperkeratosis. The spasticity affects all four limbs (spastic paraplegia), pes cavus deformity with abnormal gait, and skin changes. It was described in four brothers in 1983 by J.B. Fitzsimmons, a British physician.

Reference:

Powell FC, Venencie PY, Gordon H, et al: Keratoderma and spastic paralysis. *Br J Dermatol* 109:589, 1983.

Prader-Labhart-Willi Syndrome

At a glance: Infantile hypotonia, early childhood-onset obesity, hypogonadism, and mental retardation.

Synonyms: Prader-Willi Syndrome; Willi-Prader Syndrome.

History: First described in 1956 by A. Prader, A. Labhart, and H. Willi, all three Swiss pediatricians and internists, on the basis of observation obtained from nine children with the tetrad of short stature, mental retardation, severe obesity, and small hands and feet. In 1961, muscle hypotonia in infancy was added to the phenotype. Diabetes mellitus usually develops in childhood.

Incidence: In the United States, most cases are sporadic in occurrence. Rate of prevalence is reported to be 1:16,062 live births by Burd et al., whereas Butler et al. reports a prevalence of 1:25,000 live births. Internationally, the reported prevalence range from 1:8,000 in rural Sweden to 1:16,000 in western Japan.

Genetic inheritance: Syndrome results from the loss of the paternal copy of chromosome 15q11.2-13. It is described as a microdeletion/disomy disorder. However, most cases arise sporadically. More than 70% of patients have a deletion of the paternal copy. Approximately 25% of patients have maternal uniparental disomy for chromosome 15. The remainder present with translocation or other structural aberration in chromosome 15.

Pathophysiology: Reduction in lung volumes, including expiratory reserve volume, vital capacity, and functional residual capacity; closing capacity is increased, leading to airway closure in the dependent areas of the lung and V/Q mismatch; reduced chest and diaphragmatic excursions; decreased alveolar ventilation; diminished sensitivity of the respiratory center to hypoxia and hypercarbia—all contributing to hypoxia and hypercarbia. Intermittent upper airway obstruction and hypoxia during sleep with resultant chronic sleep deprivation and daytime somnolence; severe and chronic hypoxia leading to polycythemia, pulmonary hypertension, right ventricular hypertrophy, and failure.

Diagnosis: Neonatal hypotonia is one hallmark feature of this disorder and is a valuable clue to initiate diagnostic testing. Clinical features; biochemical (polycythemia, hypoxia, hypercarbia); lung function tests (reduced lung volumes including total lung capacity, functional residual capacity, vital capacity, and expiratory reserve volume); ECG (right axis deviation); chest radiograph or echocardiography (cardiomegaly); sleep studies (obstructive sleep apnea).

Clinical aspects: The syndrome is biphasic; initially the picture is one of hypotonia and later changes to hyperphagia leading to obesity.

Antenatal: delayed onset and reduced fetal activity during pregnancy; often breech presentation at birth.

Neonatal and infancy: low birth weight, infantile hypotonia ("floppy infant"), neonatal asphyxia, poor feeding, and failure to thrive; gross motor developmental delay, weak cry and cough, hypogonadism with genital hypoplasia. Neonates may require tube feeding for 3 to 4 months, although this usually improves by 6 months and by 12 to 18 months, uncontrollable hyperphagia occurs.

Childhood: endocrine (polyphagia, insatiable hunger, hypoglycemia, rapid weight gain after 1 year of age, morbid obesity, short stature, hypogenitalism, and hypogonadism); craniofacial (narrow bitemporal head dimension, almond-shaped eyes with strabismus and myopia, thin upper lips with down-turned corners, dental enamel hypoplasia and early caries, viscous saliva); neurological (global de-

velopmental delay, skin picking, high pain threshold, behavioral and personality problems, sleep disturbances, speech problems, hyporeflexia, seizures); musculoskeletal (small hands and feet with tapered fingers, hypermobile joints, scoliosis, kyphosis); respiratory (poor cough, hypoventilation, sleep apnea, restrictive lung disease, recurrent chest infections, hypoxia); cardiovascular system (pulmonary hypertension and cor pulmonale secondary to chronic hypoxia, cardiac failure and arrhythmias, primarily premature ventricular contractions); other (skin hypopigmentation, defective temperature regulation, ischemic gastroenteritis, and gastric dilatation). Diabetes mellitus most often is diagnosed at that time because of high calorie intake.

Adolescence: delayed puberty, alimentary diabetes because of high caloric intake, emotional lability (temper tantrums and obsessive-compulsive behavior), poor gross motor and cognitive skills, signs of cardiac failure. Ventilatory control: abnormal responses to hyperoxia, hypoxia, and hypercarbia whether awake or asleep. Because growth hormone therapy seems to increase respiratory drive in these patients, both a peripheral (nearly absent

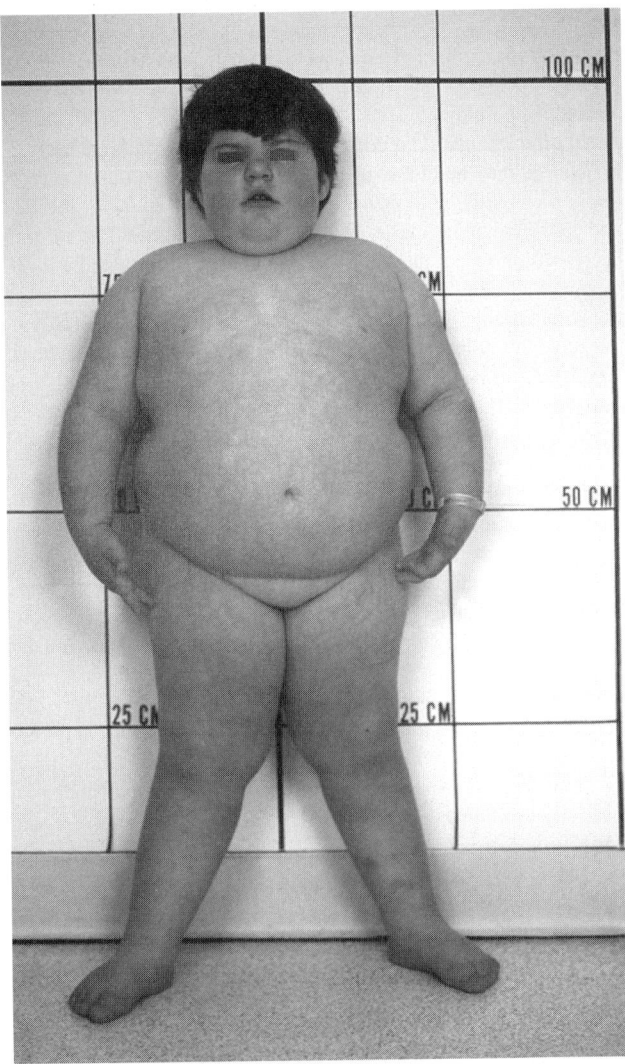

Prader-Labhart-Willi syndrome This 7-year-old boy with obesity, short stature, characteristic shape of the mouth, acromicria, genua valgum, and hypogonadism has Prader-Labhart-Willi syndrome.

chemoreceptor activity) and a central mechanism (hypothalamus) must be involved. Arrhythmias, conduction abnormalities, hypertension, and cardiac failure may occur. Truncal obesity may result in a restrictive defect in pulmonary function and there may also be a respiratory muscle weakness. Type II diabetes mellitus is common. Sleep apnea, thermoregulatory disturbance, and convulsions may occur. There may be abnormally thick, viscous saliva. Death usually occurs in the third decade of life from complications of diabetes, respiratory failure, and cardiac failure.

Precautions before anesthesia: Detailed preoperative cardiac and respiratory assessment is required; although weight loss might be advisable prior to elective surgery. It is most often impossible to achieve for the patient. *Infancy:* history relating to episodes of neonatal aspiration, severe hypotonia, and associated pneumonia. *Childhood and adolescence:* history relating to sleep apnea. Evaluate respiratory function tests. Obtain full cardiac history with attention to ECG, hypertension, and signs of cardiac failure (echocardiography to rule out cor pulmonale). Ensure appropriate perioperative blood glucose control if diabetic. The recommendations from the patient's endocrinologist must be followed. Strict consideration for feeding guidelines must be assessed. Make sure the patient has no access to food, otherwise nil per os instructions will not be followed.

Anesthetic considerations: Difficult child because of behavioral problems and mental retardation. Because of obesity, venous access and identification of landmarks for regional anesthesia may be difficult. Difficulty in maintaining patent airway during face-mask ventilation. Direct laryngoscopy and tracheal intubations could be difficult because of morbid obesity. The risk of gastric aspiration is increased because of obesity, gastric dilatation, rumination, and/or stealing of food. The stomach should never be considered empty. Airway obstruction during induction and awakening; reduced functional residual capacity and higher closing capacity result in poor respiratory reserve with rapid oxygen desaturation. High risk of postoperative hypoventilation and obstructive sleep apnea. Intraoperative hypertension and arrhythmias may require specific management. Close perioperative monitoring of blood glucose levels is mandatory and patients may need glucose-containing intravenous fluids. Intraoperative temperature monitoring is mandatory because hypothermia or hyperthermia may occur. Obese patients require lower drug doses on a per-kilogram basis. Succinylcholine has been used without complications but must be used only if face-mask positive-pressure ventilation is confirmed. Cautious use of respiratory depressants is advisable. Preoperative premedication may not be advisable in most patients. Postoperative apnea monitoring is required. Supine position is associated with a drop in PaO_2 and is to be avoided postoperatively; nasal continuous positive airway pressure or continuous positive airway pressure mask recommended for obstructive sleep apnea. Polycythemia may predispose to deep venous thrombosis in the postoperative period, although pulmonary embolism is extremely rare in children.

Pharmacological implications: Preoperative sedation should be avoided because of the risk of hypoventilation and apnea. Use of prophylaxis against gastric aspiration recommended; require lower drug doses on a per-kilogram basis; increased sensitivity to respiratory depressants, including opioids; increased incidence of postoperative respiratory complications.

Other conditions to be considered:

☞**BARDET-BIEDL SYNDROME:** Mental retardation, pigmentary retinopathy, polydactyly, obesity, renal anomalies, and hypogenitalism.

☞**ALBRIGHT HEREDITARY OSTEODYSTROPHY:** Round face, short stature and neck, and obesity. Intracranial and subcutaneous calcification; neuromuscular problems such as fatigue and muscle cramps; seizures; pseudohypoparathyroidism and hypocalcemia; hypertension. Correction of chronic hypocalcemia is treated by oral calcium and vitamin D. Avoid respiratory or metabolic alkalosis. If surgery cannot be delayed, intravenous calcium therapy must be given with continuous ECG monitoring.

☞**CHUDLEY MENTAL RETARDATION SYNDROME:** Extremely rare disorder characterized by mental retardation, distinctive mouth, obesity, and hypogonadism.

REFERENCES:

Falsetti HL, Hanson JS, Tabakin BS: Obesity-hypoventilation syndrome in siblings. *Am Rev Resp Dis* 90:105, 1964.

Olefsky JM: Obesity, in Petersdorf RG, Adams RD, Braunwald E et al: *Harrison's Principles of Internal Medicine.* 10th ed. New York, McGraw-Hill, 1985, p 443.

West JB: Disorders of ventilation, in Petersdorf, Adams RD, Braunwald E et al: *Harrison's Principles of Internal Medicine.* 10th ed. New York, McGraw-Hill, 1985, p 1589.

Precocious Puberty

At a glance: Premature onset of pubertal changes.

History: So-called isosexual precocious puberty is usually defined as onset of menarche in the female before age 8.5 years or pubertal changes in the male before age 10 years. Schedewie et al. (1981) and Rosenthal et al. (1983) also described a syndrome of sexual precocity in boys, characterized by a sex-limited autosomal dominant inheritance pattern and extremely rapid virilization, where increased gonadal testosterone secretion appears to be gonadotropin-independent (male-limited precocious puberty or familial male precocious puberty).

Genetic inheritance: In 80 to 90% of girls and approximately 50% of boys with precocious puberty, no causative factor can be found. Precocious puberty is a more frequent occurrence in females than in males, but familial occurrence seems rarer in females. In males, sex-limited autosomal dominant inheritance was postulated, with the trait transmitted only by affected males to half their sons. In the syndrome of male-limited precocious puberty, the disorder is caused by constitutively activating mutations of the luteinizing hormone receptor gene.

Pathophysiology: There is a premature activation of the hypothalamic–pituitary–gonadal axis as shown by increased secretion of luteinizing hormone and follicle-stimulating hormone. In male-limited precocious puberty, testicular Leydig cell hyperplasia is observed and the resultant virilization results from increased secretion rather than decreased clearance of gonadal testosterone.

Diagnosis: Levels of plasma follicle-stimulating hormone and luteinizing hormone are elevated for the age of the patient. Plasma testosterone (in boys) and estradiol (in girls) are usually elevated to levels consistent with the stage of puberty and osseous maturation. In the syndrome of male-limited precocious puberty, both basal and gonadotropin-releasing hormone-induced secretion of luteinizing hormone is low and there are no suppressive effects of potent gonadotropin-releasing hormone analogues. Advanced spermatogenesis is confirmed on testicular biopsy.

Clinical aspects: Extremely variable clinical course. Puberty may occur before 3 years of age. Affected children may complete sexual maturation rapidly or slowly. Adult height is reduced as the increased rate of ossification results in early closure of the epiphyses. Dental age and mental development are usually compatible with chronologic age. Hypothyroidism is occasionally accompanied by precocious puberty and thyroid function should be checked and if it is the case, treatment should be administered in these patients. Otherwise, treatment consists mainly of psychological support of the patient and family. Sexual precocity, fibrous dysplasia, and patchy pigmentation occur in McCune-Albright syndrome where hyperthyroidism is common. Precocious puberty may also result from organic brain lesions such as hypothalamic hamartomas. Signs of increased intracranial pressure may surface years later. Computed tomography scan of the head is indicated in all boys with true precocious puberty when no specific cause can be found. In boys, other causes of the precocity should be evaluated, including adrenogenital syndrome, Leydig cell tumor, and gonadotropin-producing hepatoma.

Precautions before anesthesia: In patients in whom precocity arises as the result of intracranial lesions, examine for signs of increased intracranial pressure. Determine thyroid function status; patients on thyroxine replacement for hypothyroidism should have the therapy continued until the morning of the surgery. While physical attributes may be advanced, the mental and emotional age is compatible with the chronologic age. A sedative premedicant commensurate to children of the same chronologic age is recommended. Sedative premedicant is to be avoided in symptomatic hypothyroid patients.

Anesthetic considerations: There are no specific considerations for patients with signs of sexual precocity. Patients with underlying thyroid function derangements or cerebral lesions should have the anesthetic technique tailored according to the degree of the abnormalities.

Pharmacological implications: There are no specific implications except if the patient is taking thyroid medication and steroid supplementation. If it is the case, preoperative administration of thyroid medication and steroid supplementation must be done.

REFERENCES:

Garibaldi L: The endocrine system: Precocious puberty, in Behrman RE, Kliegman RM, Jenson HB (eds): *Nelson Textbook of Pediatrics.* 15th ed. WB Saunders, Philadelphia, 1997.

Lincoln EA, Zuber TJ: Management of precocious puberty. *Hosp Pract (Off Ed)* 33(4):173, 1998.

Primary Immunodeficiencies

At a glance: A heterogenous group of genetic disorders characterized by a congenital deficit in humoral or cellular immunity.

Synonym/Classification: Prototypes include: X-linked Agammaglobulinemia (☞Bruton Agammaglobulinemia; XLA); Hyper-IgM Syndrome (☞Jobs Syndrome); Common; Variable Immunodeficiency (CVI); Severe Combined Immunodeficiency (☞SCI); defects in the expression of the major histocompatibility complex (MHC) (☞Bare Lymphocyte Syndrome); ☞Wiskott-Aldrich Syndrome.

Incidence and genetic inheritance: *XLA:* recessive inheritance, based on mutations in the btk gene (Bruton, or B-cell, tyrosine kinase) on chromosome Xq21.1-22. *Hyper-IgM:* X-linked recessive (Xq26) in 70% of patients, unclear in 30%. *CVI:* autosomal dominant, autosomal recessive, and X-linked. Most common primary immunodeficiency among persons of European descent. *SCI:* 50 to

60% of patients have an X-linked inheritance mapped to Xq13, thus the overall male predominance in SCI. Inheritance in the remainder is autosomal recessive. *Isolated MCH class I* defects are very rare. MCH class II deficiency is inherited autosomal recessively, and is seen mostly in North African kindreds. *Wiskott-Aldrich syndrome* inheritance is X-linked recessive, mapped to Xp11.23.

Pathophysiology: In *XLA,* the defect is in cytoplasmic signal-transducing molecule. *Hyper-IgM* reflects the defective immune globulin class switching from IgM to IgG production in the course of a humoral immune response as a result of a defective CD40 ligand on T$_H$ cells. *CVI* pathogenesis is unclear, evidence hints at a defective T-cell and B-cell interaction. Interleukin receptor defects play a role in X-linked *SCI,* with a defective purine metabolism in the autosomal recessive forms. In *MHC class II deficiency,* the transcription of these molecules is defective.

Diagnosis: Clinical picture and in *XLA:* agammaglobulinemia with absent antibody formation to vaccines; *Hyper-IgM:* elevated IgM and IgD, and further immunologic workup; *CVI:* exclusion of other causes of hypogammaglobulinemia; *CVI and MHC deficiencies:* complex immunologic workup; *Wiskott-Aldrich syndrome:* triad of thrombocytopenia, eczema, and susceptibility to infections, as well as immunologic workup.

Clinical aspects: The clinical picture is generally dependent on the underlying defect.

X-linked agammaglobulinemia: Once passive immunity from maternal antibodies subsides, affected boys suffer from recurrent pyogenic infections, mainly from *Staphylococcus aureus,* *Haemophilus influenzae,* and *Streptococcus pyogenes.* Regular intravenous immune globulin (IVIG) therapy is effective in preventing infections and formation of bronchiectasis. Female carriers are asymptomatic because of nonrandom inactivation of the mutant X chromosome.

Hyper-IgM syndrome: In addition to the susceptibility to pyogenic infections, male patients are prone to *Pneumocystis carinii* infections and autoimmune diseases, mainly directed against blood cells (hemolytic anemia, thrombocytopenia, and neutropenia). Neutropenia responds to IVIG and granulocyte colony-stimulating factor (G-CSF). Proliferation of IgM-producing plasma cells may lead to infiltration of GI organs, and there is an increased risk for abdominal cancers.

Common variable immunodeficiency: Heterogeneous group of antibody deficiency syndromes, usually presenting in adolescence and young adulthood. These patients are prone to pyogenic (sinopulmonary) infections (with formation of bronchiectasis), gastrointestinal infections (e.g., *Giardia lamblia*), malignancy (e.g., high risk for gastric carcinoma and lymphoma), autoimmune disorders (usually involving blood cells), and inflammatory bowel disease. Lymphadenopathy and splenomegaly is frequent, and granuloma formation can be found. Baseline treatment consists of regular IVIG administration.

Severe combined immunodeficiency: Onset of manifestation is usually around 3 months of age, most commonly thrush and (diaper) rashes. Other common features include chronic diarrhea, *Pneumocystis carinii,* and severe viral infections. Failure to thrive is common. The only curative treatment is bone marrow transplantation. Female carriers in the X-linked form are asymptomatic because of nonrandom inactivation of the mutant X chromosome.

Defects in the expression of the major histocompatibility complex (MHC): Isolated MHC class I deficiency is associated with recurrent, severe pulmonary infections. MHC class II deficiency manifests with severe protracted diarrhea, fungal infections, and failure to thrive. Other features include frequent pneumonias and sclerosing cholangitis. Bone marrow transplantation is the only curative treatment in this otherwise fatal condition.

Wiskott-Aldrich syndrome: Early onset of profound thrombocytopenia with small platelets, eczema, and opportunistic infections. In the past, death occurred in the first decade from bleeding, infection, or malignancies. Treatment options include splenectomy, IVIG, and bone marrow transplantation. Female carriers are asymptomatic because of nonrandom inactivation of the mutant X chromosome.

Precautions before anesthesia: No particular organ malformations are associated with the various primary immunodeficiencies. Preanesthetic assessment should establish whether there is active infection, autoimmune anemia, or thrombocytopenia. Physiotherapy has a place in patients with significant bronchiectasis.

Anesthetic considerations: Expect significant oxygenation failure especially in *P. carinii* pneumonia. Special attention to aseptic technique during mobilization and/or contact with the patient.

Pharmacological implications: If applicable, drugs with a potential for myeloic suppression (e.g., nitrous oxide) should be avoided. Strict aseptic technique during all the anesthetic procedures (insertion of lines, intubation, etc.).

References:

Cooper MA, Pommering TL, Koranyi K: Primary immunodeficiencies. *Am Fam Physician* 68:2001, 2003 (review).

Rosen FS, Cooper MD, Wedgewood RJP: The primary immunodeficiencies. *N Engl J Med* 333:431, 1995.

Sorensen RU, Moore C: Antibody deficiency syndromes. *Pediatr Clin North Am* 47:1225, 2000.

Primary Pulmonary Hypertension (PPH)

At a glance: Primary Pulmonary Hypertension (PPH) is a progressive disease characterized by raised pulmonary vascular resistance, which results in impaired right-heart function as a consequence of the increased right ventricular afterload and occurring in the absence of an identifiable cause.

Synonyms: Idiopathic Pulmonary Hypertension (IPAH); pulmonary hypertension (PHT). It is also termed precapillary pulmonary hypertension.

History: First described clinically and hemodynamically in 1951 by D.T. Dresdale and colleagues.

Incidence: Approximately 1–3:1,000,000 population per year in the United States and internationally.

Genetic inheritance: Autosomal dominant inheritance with incomplete penetrance and a 2.5:1 female predilection. The PPH1 gene was mapped to chromosome 2q31-q32. A worsening of the disease occurs in successive generations.

Pathophysiology: Current theories on pathogenesis focus on abnormalities in interaction between endothelial and smooth-muscle cells. Endothelial-cell injury may result in an imbalance in endothelium-derived mediators, favoring vasoconstriction. Defects in ion-channel activity in smooth-muscle cells in the pulmonary artery may contribute to vasoconstriction and vascular proliferation. Inflammatory oxidant mechanisms and deficiency in nitric oxide (NO) have also been implicated in the pathogenesis of pulmonary hypertension. In addition, the findings of frequent monoclonal endothelial cell proliferation in PPH also suggest that a somatic genetic alteration similar to that present in neoplastic processes might be responsible for the pathogenesis of PPH.

Diagnosis: On chest radiography, the width of the pulmonary arteries is increased and the peripheral lung fields are clear. The electrocardiogram demonstrates right ventricular hypertrophy, as does echocardiography. Cardiac catheterization with measurement of pulmonary artery pressures demonstrates elevation of systolic pulmonary artery pressure >35 mmHg or mean pulmonary artery pressure >25 mmHg. Histology shows extension of muscle layers into small pulmonary arteries that are normally nonmuscular. The cross-sectional area of the pulmonary vascular bed is also decreased. Histopathology shows plexiform lesions composed of proliferating endothelial cells present in 20 to 80% of cases of primary pulmonary hypertension. Other diagnostic testing primarily excludes secondary causes.

Clinical aspects: Neonatal pulmonary hypertension results in right-to-left shunting via the foramen ovale, or ductus arteriosus, or both. Right-heart failure is inevitably present. It is usually lethal. In older children or adults, the predominant symptoms include exertional dyspnea and fatigue, which result from fixed cardiac output in response to exertion. PPH occurs most commonly in young and middle-age women; mean survival from onset of symptoms is 2 to 3 years. Primary pulmonary hypertension is progressive, and there is no specific treatment. The terminal event may be related to right-heart failure and is often sudden, possibly related to arrhythmias.

Precautions before anesthesia: Catheterization is necessary to assess hemodynamics and to evaluate vasoreactivity during acute drug challenge. Decrease in pulmonary vascular resistance in response to acute vasodilator challenge (intravenous epoprostenol or inhaled NO) occurs in approximately 30% of patients, and predicts a good response to chronic therapy with oral calcium-channel blockers (nifedipine, diltiazem, amlodipine). Determination of the presence of cor pulmonale. Prophylaxis of infective endocarditis.

Anesthetic considerations: The principal consideration is to prevent increases in pulmonary hypertension that may result in right-heart failure. Continuous monitoring of arterial and central venous pressure, electrocardiography, and pulse oximetry are recommended for every anesthetic procedure. The use of a pulmonary artery catheter is controversial. Transesophageal echocardiography is useful. The choice of anesthetic technique and drugs per se is of secondary importance and should be governed by individual preferences. Avoid known factors that may exacerbate pulmonary hypertension—hypoxemia, hypercarbia, acidosis, high airway pressures, positive end-expiratory pressure, stress, and pain. Tracheal intubation increases positive airway pressure and causes right-heart strain. A "stress-free" anesthetic with controlled ventilation, gentle intubation, and continuous hemodynamic monitoring would provide ideal conditions. An appropriate regional anesthetic technique performed with care to avoid any hemodynamic disturbances, and with deafferentation of all noxious input is equally satisfactory.

Pharmacological implications: Nitrous oxide causes considerable increases in pulmonary vascular resistance patients with pulmonary hypertension. Ketamine may increase vascular resistance and should be avoided. A continuous intravenous infusion of epoprostenol (prostacyclin [PGI$_2$]) may be used to improve hemodynamics. Inhaled nitric oxide (iNO) has been used as a selective pulmonary vasodilator with variable success in the treatment of persistent pulmonary hypertension.

REFERENCES:

Burrows FA, Klinck JR, Rabinovitch M, et al: Pulmonary hypertension in children: Perioperative management. *Can Anaesth Soc J* 33:606, 1986.

Gaine SP, Rubin LJ: Primary pulmonary hypertension. *Lancet* 352:719, 1998.

Harsoor SS, Suyajna J. Anaesthetic management of parturient with primary pulmonary hypertension posted for caesarean section-A case report. *Ind J Anaesth* 49(3):223, 2005.

Hohn L, Schweizer A, Morel D, et al. Circulatory failure after anesthesia induction in a patient with severe primary pulmonary hypertension. *Anesthesiology* 91(6):1943, 1999.

Primary Torsion Dystonia

At a glance: A movement disorder that manifests in childhood and advances to total incapacitation within a few years.

Synonyms: Primary Dystonia; Idiopathic Torsion Dystonia; Dystonia Musculorum Deformans (Early Onset Primary Torsion Dystonia); Ziehen-Oppenheim Disease; Ziehen-Schwalbe-Oppenheim Syndrome.

History: First described in 1908 by S. Schwalbe in a Jewish family and in 1911, Oppenheim termed this condition as dystonia musculorum deformans (DMD).

Incidence: About 10 to 15:100,000 live births. A female predilection has been reported for focal and segmental primary torsion dystonia. Primary Torsion Dystonia is more common among the Ashkenazi Jewish population.

Genetic inheritance: For both early-onset and late-onset primary torsion dystonia, transmission is autosomal dominant with a low penetrance; for the early form, it is 30 to 40% penetrance, and for late-onset primary torsion dystonia, it is even lower at 10 to 15% penetrance. Negative family history does not exclude the diagnosis. The mutation for the early form has been mapped to 9q34, identified as a GAG deletion and called DYT1 gene. The resulting protein, torsinA, is an ATP-binding protein with some similarities to the heat-shock protein superfamily. The mutation of the late-onset primary torsion dystonia has been mapped to 8p21-q22 (DYT 6 gene) and to 18p (DYT 7 gene).

Pathophysiology: Unknown. However, it has been hypothesized that the dystonic movements originate from a functional disturbance of the basal ganglia (most likely because of an increased striatal inhibition on globus pallidum and substantia nigra) in combination with a severely altered pattern of normal spontaneous neuronal activity. This may affect the thalamic control on planning and execution of movements, as well as brainstem and spinal inhibitory reflexes, and result in the dystonic pattern of pathological cocontraction of agonist and antagonist muscles with abnormal recruitment of more extraneous muscle groups (as seen in the EMG).

Diagnosis: The diagnosis is mainly based on clinical findings of involuntary movements. So far, neuroimaging studies (CT, MRI scans), postmortem examinations, and laboratory studies have not revealed any pathological findings in primary torsion dystonia. Perinatal asphyxia is the most common cause for secondary dystonia in children, and among other causes with similar symptoms such as encephalitis, traumatic brain injury, neurotoxins, and drugs, has to be ruled out. Its onset is usually—but not always—in the first 3 years of life. In primary torsion dystonia, most patients are and re-main mentally normal; however, patients with severe developmental delay have also been described.

Clinical aspects: The hallmark of primary torsion dystonia is sustained muscle contractions that often result in twisting, repetitive movements, and/or abnormal postures. Depending on the anatomical sites that are affected by the dystonic movements, primary dystonia can be divided in focal (only one anatomical site, e.g., neck, eyelids, mouth, larynx, hand), multifocal (several, noncontiguous anatomical sites), segmental (contiguous anatomical sites), hemidystonic (limited to one body side), and generalized (leg in combination with other body sites) primary torsion dystonia. Generalized primary torsion dystonia is the most common form in children, whereas the focal and the segmental forms (e.g., spasmodic torticollis) are rare in the general population. The muscles show resistance to passive motion attempts by the examiner and tend to go back to the original position after forceful deflection. The dystonic movements do not occur during sleep. More than 10 different forms of dystonia have been described, but our focus is on the two most important ones.

Early-onset Primary Torsion Dystonia: The first symptoms of this disease occur between the ages of 4 and 16 years and commonly consist of a plantar flexion and inversion of the foot. Initially, this occurs only intermittently and more often under stress, but becomes more and more constant over time and finally spreads to other body parts. Typically, these are the wrist (writer's cramp), the neck (torticollis), and the trunk. Dystonic movements may also affect the face (problems with speech and swallowing) or visceral musculature (paroxysmal dyspnea). Whereas dystonic movements in the beginning need a trigger (most often motion of other body parts, stress), this comes down to dystonic movements even at rest without any obvious trigger as the disease progresses. Finally, affected body parts may assume a fixed, abnormal position, with intermittent signs of athetosis superimposed. As the disease progresses further, patients present with incoordinated movements, spastic dystonia of the extremities, neck, and trunk, lordotic arching of the axial musculature, athetosis of fingers and toes, and uncontrolled rotatory flailing of their extremities, which can even lead to fractures, and, finally, to deforming contractures (expressed by the synonymous name "dystrophia musculorum deformans"). Those patients are usually confined to a wheelchair within a few years after the onset of the disease.

Late-onset Primary Torsion Dystonia: (Late refers to onset after the age of 26 years.) This form is also called focal or cervicocranial primary torsion dystonia. In patients with the DYT 6 mutation, the symptoms usually occur at a mean age of around 40 to 45 years, whereas in patients with the DYT 7 mutation the mean age of onset is about 18 to 20 years. Cranial or cervical muscle involvement is common (spasmodic torticollis, spasmodic dysphonia) and the symptoms may either primarily start here or secondary spread from the limbs (e.g., writer's cramp) to this area. Only rarely, though, are the symptoms confined to the cervicocranial site.

Surgical treatment used to consist of bilateral thalamotomy, but there was a high complication rate (ataxia, spasticity, hemiparesis, dysarthria, dysphagia) associated with unsatisfactory results in many cases. A new treatment option for intractable dystonia consists of simultaneous, bilateral posteroventral pallidotomy and has proven to be more effective with a lower incidence of complications and side effects.

Precautions before anesthesia: Evaluate the involved anatomical sites, particularly the head and neck, to get an impression about potential difficulties with airway management and limitations for positioning during the procedure. Check the preoperative medications and check their side effects. In case of developmental delay, sedative or anxiolytic premedication might be helpful.

Anesthetic considerations: Positioning may be difficult in the presence of contractures. Benzodiazepines and propofol have been used with variable success to reduce the muscle spasms. Inhalational anesthetics, however, seem to work more reliably in that perspective, and the same applies for neuromuscular blockers. Opisthotonus and torticollis can be very severe and can make mask ventilation difficult until a sufficiently high concentration of the inhalational anesthetic has been reached or neuromuscular blockers have been administered. However, there is a risk that once muscle contractures have become chronic, they may not respond well—or at all—any more to these anesthetic drugs.

Pharmacological implications: Preoperatively, some patients may be on medical treatment with anticholinergic drugs (e.g., trihexyphenidyl, benztropine, procyclidine, diphenhydramine), which can be associated with autonomic side effects. Thus, you must be either prepared to deal with the side effects or make sure these medications have been discontinued for a sufficient period of time before surgery. However, keep in mind that fast weaning can precipitate profound cholinergic symptoms. As this disorder is primarily of neurological nature, malignant hyperthermia is not expected to have a higher incidence in these patients; however, a hyperkalemic response to succinylcholine is possible.

Other conditions to be considered: Exclude secondary forms of dystonia, which can be caused by central nervous system diseases (e.g., trauma, tumors, infections), drugs (e.g., chemotherapy, antihistamines, tricyclic antidepressants, phenytoin, lithium, ketamine), and other diseases (e.g., glutaric acidemia, leukodystrophy, neuronal ceroid lipofuscinoses, and Wilson disease).

REFERENCES:

Bressman SB: Dystonia. *Curr Opin Neurol* 11;363, 1998.

Marsden CD, Harrison MJ: Idiopathic torsion dystonia (dystonia musculorum deformans)—A review of forty-two patients. *Brain* 97:793, 1974.

Menkes JH: Heredodegenerative diseases, in Menkes JH, Sarnat HB (eds): *Child Neurology*. 6th ed. Philadelphia, Lippincott, Williams and Wilkins, 2000, p 345.

Progeria Syndrome

At a glance: A sporadic syndrome of premature aging with characteristic facies, severe cardiac lesions (including myocardial infarction), and various orthopedic and otorhinolaryngologic lesions.

Synonyms: Hutchinson-Gilford Progeria Syndrome; Gilford Syndrome; Premature Senility Syndrome.

History: Rare genetic disease characterized by premature aging. First described by Jonathan Hutchinson in 1886.

Incidence: Sporadic cases. Fewer than 100 cases reported in the literature. Progeria affects between 1:4 million (estimated actual) and 1:8 million (reported) live births.

Genetic inheritance: In most patients, the syndrome is caused by random genetic changes occurring for unknown reasons. Because it occurs sporadically, it is believed to be an autosomal recessive disorder. However, these mutations might be transmitted as an autosomal dominant trait. Male:female ratio is 1.5:1. Whites account for 97% of all reported cases.

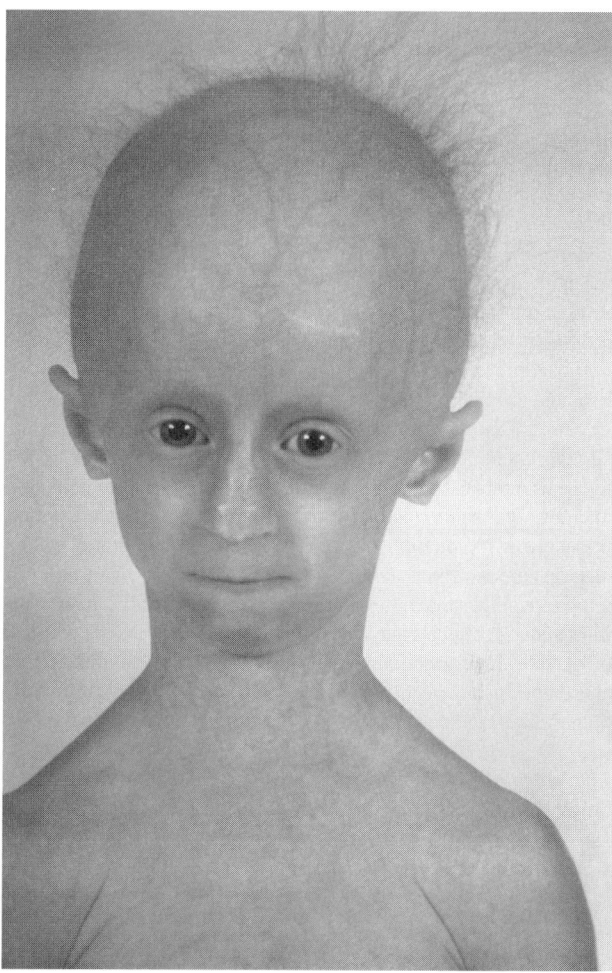

Progeria This 6-year-old boy with alopecia, thin skin, and hypoplastic ear lobes has progeria.

Pathophysiology: A reduction in the amount of cell DNA repair activity has been demonstrated and postulated as a cause of the premature aging. The genes controlling cell division and DNA or RNA synthesis and processing commonly are downregulated in elderly people and in progeria (15 genes involved). This suggests that abnormal regulation of the separation of the chromosomes during cell division occurs. There are characteristic changes in expression of *actin-binding proteins* (caldesmons), which are involved in cell cycle–dependent reorganization of the cytoskeleton, *desmoplakin I,* which plays a role in intercellular adhesive junctions, and *autotaxins,* which are involved in cellular chemotaxis. On the other hand, transforming growth factor-β (TGF-β) is highly upregulated in patients with progeria, thus yielding tissue fibrosis.

Diagnosis: No firm diagnostic criteria have been described in patients with premature aging of postnatal onset, including characteristic facies, musculoskeletal abnormalities, and early death caused by atherosclerosis and/or myocardial ischemia.

Clinical aspects: Clinical manifestations are evident by the first or second year of life. The appearance includes facial hypoplasia with micrognathia, thin skin, alopecia, dental late eruption, ophthalmic abnormality (microphthalmia, exophthalmia, cataract), ear abnormality (hypoplastic lobe, conductive hearing loss), and a high-pitched voice. Cardiovascular lesions are severe and frequent, characterized by a progressive atherosclerosis (coronary, aortic, and cerebral artery). Hypertension, myocardial infarction, or congenital heart failure often cause premature death. There is no mental retardation. Orthopedic modifications are numerous: hip dislocation, early osteoporosis, dwarfism, restricted joint mobility, clavicle anomalies, and large fontanel. Hypoplastic toe nails are frequent. Hypogonadism and diabetes can be observed.

Precautions before anesthesia: Obtain full personal history to find existence of symptomatic vascular or CNS disorders. Cardiovascular evaluation is needed (ECG, chest radiograph, echography, coronarography, and even radionuclide imaging to eliminate the possibility of advanced ischemic disease). Evaluate tracheal intubation conditions by cautious clinical examination and radiography. Evaluate the extent of osteoporosis and diabetes.

Anesthetic considerations: Cautious patient positioning is imperative to avoid pathological fractures. Direct laryngoscopy and tracheal intubation could be difficult because of facial abnormalities and micrognathia. Loss of teeth occurs more often. Spontaneous ventilation must be maintained, and gentle manipulations are necessary to avoid neck injury during a difficult intubation. Fiberoptic intubation can be proposed in this case. Central venous access by the subclavian vein must be avoided in case of clavicle malformation. Cardiovascular status would influence anesthetic management; avoid hypotension and tachycardia. Hypothermia is frequent because of the thin skin and subcutaneous fat.

Pharmacological implications: Avoid cardiovascular depressive drugs; avoid succinylcholine (fasciculation can cause pathological fracture in patient with severe osteoporosis).

Other conditions to be considered:

Ruvalcaba Churesigaew Myhre Syndrome (**Progeria Variant Syndrome Ruvalcaba Type**): A progeria variant that includes kyphosis, mental retardation, and amyotrophy.

Mulvihill Smith Syndrome (**Progeria Short Stature Pigmented Nevi**): A progeria variant that includes multiple pigmented nevi and mental retardation.

Pseudoprogeria Syndrome (**Halberg Rudolph Syndrome**): Autosomal recessive transmission with mental retardation, seizure, progressive spastic quadriplegia, and glaucoma.

☞Werner Syndrome: Autosomal recessive, located on 8p12. The disorder first begins during adolescence. It is rare in Europe, more frequent in northern Japan (1:500,000 live births). Characteristic features include scleroderma-like skin changes, especially in the extremities, prematurely aged facies, cataract, subcutaneous calcification, premature atherosclerosis, diabetes mellitus, an increase in malignancies (10% of patients), and retinal degeneration.

☞Wiedemann Rautenstrauch Syndrome: Autosomal recessive transmission. Characteristic features of this disorder include prognathism, general absence of subcutaneous fat but paradoxical, fat accumulation at flanks, buttocks, and anogenital area, psychomotor development deficiency, pseudohydrocephalus, macrocephaly, dysphagia, congenital heart defect, and sudanophilic leukodystrophies.

☞Cockayne Syndrome: An autosomal recessive disease caused by mutations in the excision–repair cross-complementing group 6 gene with premature aging, poikiloderma, dwarfism, mental retardation, pigmentary retinopathy, blindness, and conduction hearing loss. Photoprotection of eyes and skin is crucial because of an important deficiency in DNA repair after exposure to the sun.

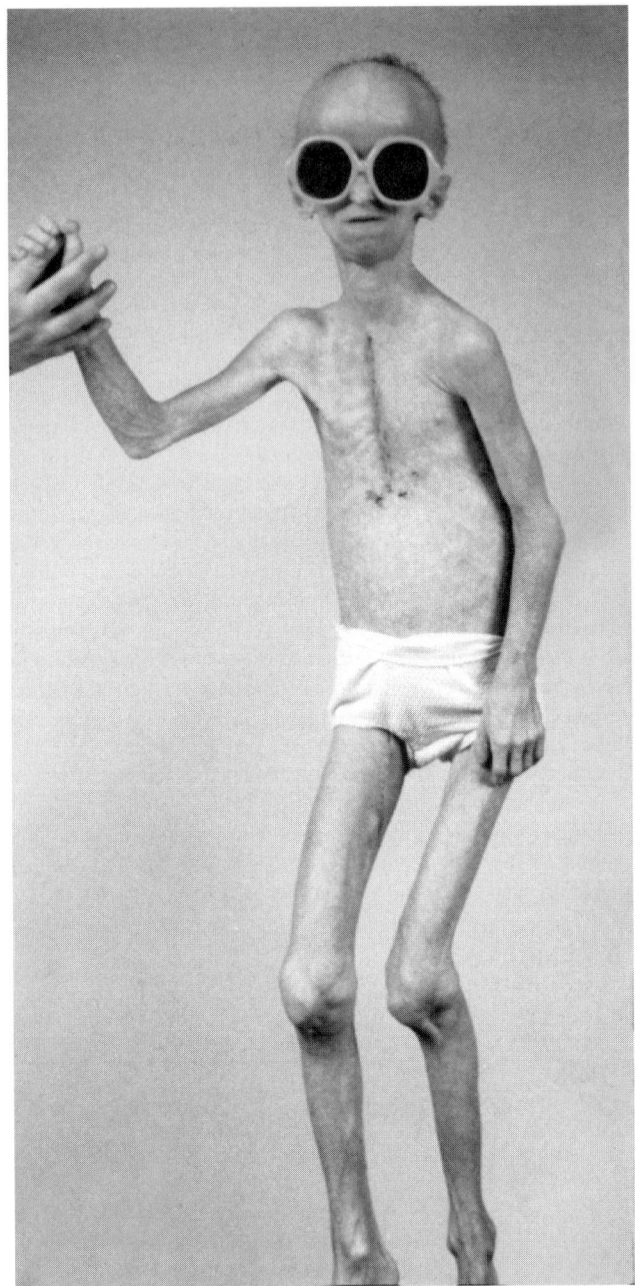

Progeria This 6-year-old boy with progeria is wearing his (funny) sunglasses because of his light photosensitivity and cataracts. Aside from the obvious features of progeria, note the sternotomy scar resulting from coronary artery bypass grafting secondary to severe coronary sclerosis.

Progeroid Syndrome Petty Type (**Petty Laxová Wiedemann Syndrome**): Prematurely aged face, prognathism, brittle hair, increased body hair, and loose skin.

Souques-Charcot-Geroderma (**Geroderma Infantilis**): Features loose, shiny, dry skin, subcutaneous atrophy, eunuchoid habitus, and intellectual deficiency.

☞Geroderma Osteodysplastica Syndrome: Connective-tissue disease resulting in early aging processes of the skin and generalized osteopenia with predisposition to fractures.

Other features include joint hyperlaxity, muscle hypotonia, hip dislocation, sunken eyes, microcorneas, and failure to thrive. Inheritance is X-linked recessive with occasional manifestations in females. Less severe in female heterozygotes.

PANGERIA: Premature generalized aging appearance beginning between 15 and 30 years of age. Clinical features include hypogonadism, beak-shaped nose, high-pitched voice, sclerodermous skin and ulcers, severe arteriosclerosis.

REFERENCES:

Chapin JW, Kahre J: Progeria and anesthesia. *Anesth Analg* 58:424, 1979.

Liessmann CD: Anaesthesia in a child with Hutchinson-Gildford progeria. *Paediatr Anaesth* 11:611, 2001.

Nguyen NH, Mayhew JF: Anaesthesia for a child with progeria. *Paediatr Anaesth* 11:370, 2001.

Progressive Bulbar Palsy of Childhood

At a glance: A very rare inherited condition characterized by progressive degeneration of bulbar nuclei and anterior horn cells of the cranial nerves with little or no involvement of the spinal cord. Clinical features include significant atrophy of muscles innervated by cranial nerves and corticobulbar tracts, dysphagia, ptosis, bilateral facial weakness, absent gag reflex, and hyperreflexia.

Synonym: Fazio-Londe Syndrome/Disease.

History: The original description was first reported in 1894 by Paul F.L. Londe, a French neurologist, and E. Fazio, an Italian Physician.

Incidence: Depends on the genetic type. Very rare to frequent.

Genetic inheritance: Three forms: a very rare autosomal dominant form, as described by Fazio, and both an early-onset and a late-onset autosomal recessive form.

Pathophysiology: Mechanism and/or cause unknown. Clinically it is the result of degeneration of motor neurons arising from bulbar nuclei. Upper motor neurons are normal. The denervation injury is associated with reinnervation from adjacent motor unit, making giant motor units. This degenerative mechanism seems to begin in fetal life and progressing in infancy and childhood.

Diagnosis: Mainly clinical with a bulbar motor neuronopathy, preserved pyramidal tracts. Muscle biopsy and EMG may be helpful. Brainstem auditory evoked potentials.

Clinical aspects: Usually a child presents with difficulties in swallowing, facial weakness, immobile vocal cords, and ptosis. There is an absent gag reflex and generalized hyperreflexia. Death occurs between the ages of 3 and 10 years from swallowing and feeding difficulties and recurrent aspiration pneumonia. Auditory involvement is usually not present in progressive bulbar palsy.

Precautions before anesthesia: Obtain complete medical history, particularly about muscle wasting, previous complications, especially aspiration pneumonia, respiratory failure, or anesthesia-related complications. Assess airway control and importance of bulbar palsy.

Anesthetic considerations: Should always be considered a high-risk candidate for gastric content regurgitation and pulmonary aspiration. Because of poor airway control and weak ventilatory muscles, extubate the trachea only when the patient is fully awake.

Postoperative mechanical ventilatory support is mandatory after major surgery.

Pharmacological implications: As with other lower motor neuron disease it is recommended to avoid succinylcholine (hyperkalemic cardiac arrest). The sensitivity and duration of action of nondepolarizing drugs is markedly increased and proper neuromuscular monitoring is indicated.

Other conditions to be considered:

☞**BROWN-VIALETTO-VAN LAERE SYNDROME:** Progressive pontobulbar palsy associated with sensorineural deafness; it starts in late childhood or adolescence with progressive deafness.

CONGENITAL FOIX-CHAVANY-MARIE SYNDROME: Suprabulbar (pseudobulbar) palsy caused by bilateral anterior opercular lesions; it is present from birth and characterized by dysphagia, dysarthria, and facial diplegia; it can be associated with mental retardation.

☞**KENNEDY DISEASE:** Progressive X-linked spinobulbar muscular atrophy with proximal muscle weakness and fasciculations, caused by an abnormality in the gene for the androgen receptor (chromosome locus Xq11-q12). Clinical features include gynecomastia, testicular atrophy, and reduced fertility.

CONGENITAL BILATERAL PERISYLVIAN SYNDROME (Bilateral Opercular Syndrome): A structural malformation of the brain consisting of polymicrogyria, i.e., the development of small and prominent convolutions separated by shallow and enlarged sulci. MRI scan shows irregular thickening and a lumpy aspect of the brain. Clinically characterized by paralysis of the face, tongue, and hypopharynx, with dysarthria and severe drooling. Most patients present seizures (onset age is 4 to 12 years; seizures are poorly controlled in 60% of cases) and severe cognitive deficit. Most seizures are atypical absences, tonic or atonic drop attacks. Tonic–clonic seizures (e.g., Lennox-Gastaut syndrome) are also present. Arthrogryposis has been described.

WORSTER-DROUGHT SYNDROME: Upper motor neuron bulbar palsy leading to "cerebral palsy-like syndrome" involving only the muscle of the mouth, tongue, and pharynx. The signs and symptoms include difficulties with voluntary lip, tongue, and palate movements, with a brisk jaw jerk.

BIPARIETAL POLYMICROGYRIA SYNDROME: A malformation of the cerebral cortex, giving the surface of the brain a lumpy aspect. Possibly a variant of the bilateral perisylvian syndrome in which the radiologic features include a longitudinal extension of the sylvian fissure, involvement of the posterior insular cortices, and dysmorphic cerebral ventricles.

REFERENCE:

McShane MA, Boyd S, Harding B et al: Progressive bulbar paralysis of childhood: A reappraisal of Fazio-Londe disease. *Brain* 115:1889, 1992.

Progressive Familial Intrahepatic Cholestasis (PFIC)

At a glance: Rare and severe type of cholestasis liver disease, beginning in infancy and progressing to cirrhosis before adolescence.

Classification and synonyms:

Cholestasis Progressive Familial Intrahepatic type I (PFIC I; Byler Disease; Fatal Intrahepatic Cholestasis): with low level of gamma-glutamyl transferase (GGT); gene ATP8B1 (previously termed FIC 1) mapped on 18q21.

Cholestasis Progressive Familial Intrahepatic type II (PFIC II): with a low level of GGT; gene ABCB11 (previously termed BSEP) mapped on 2q24.

Cholestasis Progressive Familial Intrahepatic type III (PFIC III; MDR 3 Deficiency; Progressive Intrahepatic Cholestasis with Elevated Serum Gamma-Glutamyltransferase Syndrome): with a high level of GGT; gene MDR3 mapped on 7q21.1.

Cholestasis Progressive Familial Intrahepatic type IV

History: First described by Clayton, in 1965, in an Amish descendant of Jacob Byler.

Incidence: The exact frequency is unknown in the United States and internationally. Fewer than 200 patients have been reported for the low-GGT PFIC, whereas less than 20 are known in the high-GGT PFIC type. It is a lethal medical condition in childhood if not treated. Males and females are affected equally.

Genetic inheritance: Autosomal recessive (majority of patients), also autosomal dominant with variable penetrance, or sporadic. Type II is found in the Middle East, Greenland, and Sweden.

Pathophysiology: Type I seems to be caused by a defect in bile salt synthesis. Type II seems to be caused by defective bile salt secretion. Type III is caused by a mutation in MDR3 protein, which mediates the translocation of phosphatidylcholine across the canalicular membrane of the hepatocyte.

Diagnosis: Symptoms of cholestasis (pruritus and jaundice) appear in the first few months of life. Serum GGT activity is low to normal in type I and type II, and elevated in type III. Cholesterol serum is normal. Cholangiography shows normal morphology of intra- and extrahepatic ducts. Liver biopsy in type I and type II is characterized by the absence of true proliferation of ducts within the liver and only periportal biliary metaplasia of hepatocytes. In type III, liver histology is characterized by ductular proliferation and inflammatory infiltrate.

Clinical aspects: Initially, episodes of severe cholestasis followed by intervals of good health. Pruritus is typically severe (more than the degree of bilirubinemia). Evolution is characterized by growth retardation, hepatomegaly, and then cirrhosis, hepatic failure, and death early during the childhood if not treated. Hepatocellular carcinoma may be present at age 2 years. Consequences of cholestasis (neurological anomalies caused by vitamin E deficiency, skin excoriations because of pruritus, rickets because of vitamin D deficiency, epistaxis as a result of coagulopathy or thrombocythemia). Pancreatic anomalies in type II may be present. In type III, symptoms appear later with a slower evolution. Jaundice is less visible and pruritus less intense.

Precautions before anesthesia: Obtain a complete medical history of cholestatic episodes and their frequency and clinical consequences: if of prolonged duration, inquire about parenteral fat-soluble vitamins supplementation (deficiency of vitamin D: rickets, osteomalacia; vitamin K: coagulation disorders; vitamin E: ataxia, peripheral neuropathy; vitamin A: retinopathy). *Serum levels:* bilirubin, bile acids, alkaline phosphatase, transaminases. *Coagulation profile:* if prolonged, prothrombin time (PT); parenteral vitamin K should be given several days prior to surgery.

Anesthetic considerations: During prolonged cholestatic episodes, in cases of vitamin K deficiency, regional anesthesia is inadvisable until correction of the PT by administration of fresh-frozen plasma (FFP). With vitamin D deficiency, patients are more susceptible to fractures, thus careful positioning and padding is required. High bilirubin levels may be associated with increased risk of postoperative renal failure and generous pre- and intraoperative hydration is recommended.

Pharmacological implications: During cholestatic episodes, albumin and alpha-1 acid glycoprotein levels remain within normal range. Phase I and phase II hepatic metabolic reactions are not significantly affected, but the use of anesthetic agents with minimal hepatotoxicity is advisable. Morphine should be titrated cautiously (morphine glucuronide may cumulate, particularly in case of postoperative renal insufficiency, because of inadequate hydration, as mentioned previously).

Other conditions to be considered:

☞**CRIGLER-NAJJAR SYNDROME:** Inherited disorder of bilirubin metabolism, in which the bilirubin cannot be converted into its water-soluble form, bilirubin glucuronide, because of a lack of the functional enzyme bilirubin glucuronyltransferase; this causes jaundice and multiple organ malfunctions. Clinically, neonates have jaundice and neurological manifestations, including severe brain and nerve damage, seizures, and death from bilirubin toxicity.

☞**GILBERT SYNDROME:** Benign inherited disorder (allelic to Crigler-Najjar syndrome) characterized by chronic jaundice (unconjugated hyperbilirubinemia) but that does not lead to particular complications and is not a progressive disorder.

HANOT DISEASE: Chronic mesenchymatous hepatitis with perilobar cholestasis as a result of bile duct obstruction by giant peripheral lymphoid follicles.

BENIGN RECURRENT INTRAHEPATIC CHOLESTASIS: Caused by mutations in ATP8B1, never cirrhosis. The hallmark of this medical condition is cholestasis, elevated bilirubin, bile acids, and alkaline phosphatase. Patients present with severe pruritus.

INTRAHEPATIC CHOLESTASIS OF PREGNANCY: Caused by an impairment of bile secretion in the liver. As the bile backs up in the liver, the level of bile acids increases in the bloodstream. These bile acids are deposited in the skin causing the intensive itching. Chomesterol, triglyceride, and bilirubin levels are also increased.

REFERENCES:

Muller G, Veyckemans F, Calier M, et al: Anaesthetic considerations in progressive familial intrahepatic cholestasis (Byler's disease). *Can J Anaesth* 42(12):1126, 1995.

Wang L, Soroka CJ, Boyer JL: The role of bile salt export pump mutations in progressive familial intrahepatic cholestasis type II. *J Clin Invest* 110:965, 2002.

Prolidase Deficiency

At a glance: A rare congenital disorder of the small peptides metabolism (imidazoles dipeptides). It is characterized by mild to severe skin lesions affecting mostly the face, palms, lower legs, and soles. These recalcitrant ulcerations respond partially to treatment and steroids.

Synonyms: Imidodipeptidase; Peptidase D; Proline Dipeptidase.

Genetic inheritance: Autosomal recessive; the PEPD gene maps to chromosome 19p13.2; prolidase deficiency seems to be a risk factor for the development of systemic lupus erythematosus.

Pathophysiology: The deficiency in exopeptidase prolidase (or peptidase C) produces massive excretion of imidopeptides (i.e., dipeptides with a proline or hydroxyproline *N*-terminal).

Diagnosis: Hyperiminopeptiduria; low or absent prolidase activity in leukocytes or fibroblasts.

Clinical aspects: First symptoms appear between birth and 22 years of age; prognosis, age of onset, and severity of the lesions are highly variable: *skin lesions:* rash with diffuse telangiectasia, ecchymosis, difficult to cure leg ulcers; *characteristic facies:* prominent skull sutures, ptosis and proptosis; *recurrent infections* of the skin, chronic ear and sinus infections; *impaired motor or cognitive* development may be present. *Treatment:* oral ascorbate or manganese is useful for the treatment of skin lesions.

Precautions before anesthesia: Presence of foci of chronic infection.

Anesthetic considerations: Careful positioning because of fragile skin and the presence of ulcers.

Pharmacological implications: There are no known pharmacological implications.

REFERENCE:

Larsson A, Jaeken J: Disorders in the metabolism of glutathione and imidazole peptides, in Fernandes J, Saudubray J-M, Van den Bergh G (eds): *Inborn Metabolic Diseases.* 3rd ed. Berlin, Springer, 2000, p 312.

Propionic Acidemia

At a glance: Inborn error of metabolism affecting the mitochondrial catabolism of valine and isoleucine untreated resulting in ketoacidosis, lethargy, coma, and, finally, death.

Synonyms: Propionic Aciduria; Ketotic Hyperglycinemia; Hyperglycinemia with Ketoacidosis and Leukopenia; Propionyl-CoA Carboxylase Deficiency.

History: First described in 1961 by B. Childs, an American pediatrician.

Incidence: Approximately 1:100,000 live births with both genders equally affected. Incidences as high as 1:2000 to 1:5000 live births have been reported from Saudi Arabia.

Genetic inheritance: Autosomal recessive. The enzyme is composed of two independently encoded enzyme subunits, an α subunit encoded on chromosome 13 and a β subunit encoded on chromosome 3. Biotin is a cofactor and binds to the α subunit. Two distinct genotypes can be identified by cell complementation: PCCA (propionyl-CoA carboxylase A) resulting in a defect of the α subunit and PCCB (propionyl-CoA carboxylase B) in a defect of the β subunit. A defect in the synthesis or function of biotin (deficiency of biotinidase, which is responsible for the cleaving of biotin from biocytin), or a deficiency of holocarboxylase synthetase (biotin-methylcrotonyl-CoA-carboxylase ligase), which catalyzes the incorporation of biotin into apo-carboxylases) can, however, lead to a similar clinical picture.

Pathophysiology: The mutation results in a defect in the mitochondrial enzyme propionyl-CoA carboxylase. This enzyme is responsible for the generation of methylmalonyl-CoA from propionyl-CoA, which derives from the catabolism of essential amino acids such as isoleucine, valine, methionine, and threonine, as well as from odd-chain fatty acids and cholesterol. Accumulation of propionyl-CoA results in inhibitory effects on various pathways of intermediary mitochondrial metabolism and secondary carnitine deficiency. The appearance of increased levels of long, odd-chain fatty acids may be related to the increased concentration of propionyl-CoA, which is a primer for these compounds. Ketoacidosis develops secondary to inhibition of the citric acid cycle enzymes by propionic acid. Propionyl-CoA is split in coenzyme-A and propionic acid, which contributes to the metabolic acidosis. Decreased ureagenesis and hyperammonemia seem to be secondary to inhibition of

mitochondrial carbamyl phosphate synthetase (CPS) by intramitochondrial accumulation of organic acids and CoA-esters caused by the defect in propionyl-CoA carboxylase. Furthermore, increased concentration of propionate results in decreased levels of hepatic *N*-acetyl-glutamate, which is an allosteric effector for CPS. In contrast, hyperglycinemia may be nonspecific because it can also be found in other conditions in children with negative nitrogen balance. Moreover, anaerobic fermentation of odd-chain fatty acids in the GI tract also yields propionic acid.

Diagnosis: Made by clinical presentation and organic aciduria with high levels of propionic acid, methylcitrate, and tiglylglycine. Tiglylglycine is an intermediate product of the catabolism of isoleucine. It is a potential marker of disorders of the respiratory chains. Cultured fibroblasts are used to analyze the enzyme activity. However, propionyl-CoA carboxylase activity does not necessarily correlate with the clinical picture, because there are (unexplained) case reports with almost absent enzyme activity but no clinical symptoms. Measuring propionyl-CoA carboxylase activity in cultured amniotic cells or chorionic villous biopsies allows for prenatal diagnosis. Alternatively, methylcitrate concentration in the amniotic fluid can be used.

Clinical aspects: There are three different clinical presentations.

Severe neonatal-onset form: Onset is within the first hours to weeks of life (often coincides with weaning from breast milk, which has a relatively low protein concentration) and symptoms include protein intolerance, poor feeding, vomiting, failure to thrive, profound metabolic acidosis, increased plasma levels of lactate and ammonia, lethargy progressing to unexplained coma with signs of cerebral edema, and characteristic muscle movements, such as hypertonic episodes with opisthotonus, boxing, or pedaling movements, axial hypotonia with limb hypertonia, and myoclonic jerks. Anemia, neutropenia, and thrombocytopenia are common and most likely reflect bone marrow suppression by toxic metabolites. Recurrent attacks with severe metabolic ketoacidosis are usually precipitated by intercurrent infections, excessive protein intake, or constipation. Osteopenia and pancreatitis are other known complications.

Acute, intermittent, late-onset form: Onset is after a symptom-free period of more than 1 year (sometimes occurring in adolescence or adulthood). These children may be entirely normal between attacks, which follow acute catabolic stress (infection) or increased protein intake. The most frequent presentation is lethargy or coma with ketoacidosis and hyperammonemia. A "Reye syndrome-like" picture with coma, acute liver dysfunction, hyperammonemia, and fatty infiltration of the liver has been reported in some of these patients. Neutropenia and thrombocytopenia are not uncommon.

Chronic progressive form: this form has two variants:

- *Digestive form,* which presents with anorexia, failure to thrive, recurrent vomiting, and osteoporosis. It is easily misdiagnosed in infancy as gastroesophageal reflux and/or intolerance to milk.

- *Neurologic form,* which manifests with developmental delay, severe hypotonia, and muscle weakness, and which may result in respiratory failure.

Adequate lifelong dietary control usually prevents major complications, which may include delayed cerebral myelinization and acute or progressive extrapyramidal symptoms as a result of bilateral necrosis of the basal ganglia, renal tubular acidosis with hyperuricemia, interstitial nephritis slowly progressing to renal failure, psoriasiform eruption and desquamation of the skin, alopecia, and corneal ulcerations. Acute cardiac failure secondary to cardiomyopathy may occur as part of the presenting illness or during metabolic decompensation.

The basic treatment consists of a carefully calculated low-protein diet adapted to the child's needs and metabolic tolerance. Special mixtures of amino acids selectively reduced in isoleucine, valine, methionine, and threonine (i.e., propionate-producing amino acids) are available to prevent protein deficiency. Continuous gastric tube feeding at night is often needed during infancy and childhood to minimize protein catabolism. Chronic oral administration of L-carnitine prevents carnitine depletion and also functions as a scavenger of propionic acid, and favors its excretion in form of propionyl-carnitine in the urine. Large quantities of carbohydrates are required to meet these patients' metabolic demands, which may be reflected in hypoglycemic episodes. Metronidazole is used to inhibit formation of propionic acid by anaerobic colonic flora. This is reflected in an approximately 35% reduction in the urinary excretion of propionate metabolites. Administration once daily for 10 days per month is effective and limits the side effects of this therapy (gastrointestinal and neurological symptoms, carcinogenic effect). Biotin, a cofactor for propionyl-CoA carboxylase, is often part of the medical treatment. In order to avoid—or at least to limit—brain damage from refractory hyperammonemia, peritoneal dialysis, or even hemodialysis, may be requested. In acute intercurrent decompensation (infection, trauma, anesthesia, surgery), the underlying cause should be treated if possible (antibiotics), protein intake reduced or even halted, and rehydration started with dextrose- and bicarbonate-containing solutions. Intravenous rehydration for 24 hours is often sufficient; however, total parenteral nutrition may sometimes be required. Although less-severe courses have now been described, the prognosis is still guarded and significant brain damage is common.

Precautions before anesthesia: Check developmental level, muscle tone, gastrointestinal function, hydration, nutritional status, and medical treatment. Preoperative lab studies should include complete blood count (bone marrow suppression), electrolytes, acid–base status, and serum levels of glucose, ammonium, lactate, and protein. Check renal function. In case of elective surgery, reduce protein intake 48 hours prior to surgery. Elective surgery needs to be postponed until all variables have been optimized as much as possible. The preoperative administration of an intravenous 10% dextrose-, bicarbonate- (to provide the patients usual daily bicarbonate dose), and, if possible, L-carnitine–containing infusion should prevent protein catabolism and acidosis during prolonged fasting. Prolonged postoperative mechanical ventilation has been described as a consequence of general hypotonia and the inability to clear secretions effectively. Potential admission to the intensive care unit should therefore be arranged preoperatively.

Anesthetic considerations: Dehydration, arterial hypotension, hypoxia, inappropriate caloric intake (catabolism, high-protein diet), and inadequate anesthesia technique can result in severe metabolic acidosis. Lactate-containing solutions (Hartmann or Stocker [Swiss lactated ringer with increased sodium concentration]) should be avoided, because they may not be metabolized appropriately in the presence of dysfunctional mitochondria and therefore contribute to the acid load. The regular bicarbonate requirements of the patients should be replaced intravenously in the perioperative period. A rapid-sequence induction is recommended for patients with reflux or vomiting. Depending on the length of the procedure, an arterial line may be inserted to facilitate mandatory perioperative monitoring of acid–base status, blood glucose, ammonia, and lactate levels. Often, these patients already show lethargy

and muscle hypotonia preoperatively. Careful titration of opioids and other central nervous system–depressant drugs is therefore recommended. If there is a risk of nasal, pharyngeal, or gastric bleeding, a gastric tube should be inserted to remove swallowed blood, which may otherwise provide a significant protein load and trigger an acute metabolic decompensation. Perioperative gastroduodenal ulcus prophylaxis with an H_2-antagonist or proton pump inhibitor may be indicated. Osteoporosis (secondary to malnutrition because of a low-protein diet) requires careful positioning. Prolonged postoperative metabolic monitoring for early diagnosis of an acute decompensation is recommended. Lubrication of the eyes and taping of the eyelids help prevent corneal ulcers.

Pharmacological implications: Drugs containing or metabolized to propionic acid, odd-chain organic acids, odd-chain fatty acids, odd-chain alcohols, and acrylic acids must be avoided because they can be metabolized to propionic acid, inhibit citric acid cycle enzymes, and result in ketoacidosis. These drugs include muscle relaxants metabolized by ester hydrolysis (succinylcholine, atracurium, *cis*-atracurium, mivacurium). Furthermore, propionic acid-derived NSAIDs (e.g., naproxen, ketoprofen, ibuprofen) should also be avoided. Propofol contains polyunsaturated fat (soybean oil) and should therefore not be used.

Other conditions to be considered: Propionyl-CoA can also accumulate in the following disorders.

☞**MULTIPLE CARBOXYLASE DEFICIENCY (MCCD):** Inborn error of metabolism characterized by defective activity of all biotin-dependent carboxylases. Clinically, it is characterized by seizures, developmental delay, eczema and progressive hearing loss leading to deafness.

☞**METHYLMALONIC ACIDEMIA:** A heterogeneous inborn error of metabolism affecting amino acid metabolism leading to metabolic acidosis and accumulation of methylmalonic acid and its by-products. Clinical features include poor feeding, vomiting, progressive lethargy, hypotonia, and floppiness in a previously healthy newborn.

☞**MAPLE SYRUP DISEASE:** This autosomal recessive transmitted inborn error of metabolism is caused by a defect in the branched-chain α-ketoacid dehydrogenase resulting in the characteristic smell of the urine. Untreated, this disorder leads to mental retardation, seizures, and, usually, death.

☞**ARGININEMIA:** A urea cycle disorder that leads to the triad of hyperammonemia, encephalopathy, and respiratory alkalosis, which are less severe than in other forms of urea cycle abnormalities. Characterized by severe mental retardation, athetosis, and spasticity.

☞**CITRULLINEMIA:** A syndrome arising from argininosuccinate synthetase deficiency leading to hyperammonemia and neurological consequences. Symptoms include enuresis, mental retardation, nocturnal sweats and terrors, and recurrent vomiting.

☞**HHH SYNDROME:** A genetically transmitted inborn error of metabolism because of a defect in the transport of ornithine into the mitochondrial matrix, clinically characterized by early growth retardation, learning disabilities, periodic confusion, and ataxia.

☞**N-ACETYLGLUTAMATE SYNTHETASE DEFICIENCY:** Congenital mitochondrial disorder affecting the metabolism of ammonium and results in hyperammonemia. A lethal condition in the neonatal period.

☞**ORNITHINE CARBAMOYLTRANSFERASE DEFICIENCY:** A rare genetic disorder characterized by complete or partial lack of the enzyme ornithine transcarbamylase. The lack of this enzyme results in excessive hyperammonemia, which is a known neurotoxin.

Clinically, these patients present with vomiting, refusal to eat, progressive lethargy, and coma.

☞**CARNITINE DEFICIENCY:** A disorder because of decreased carnitine concentrations in plasma and tissues preventing mitochondria from adequate beta oxidation. Primary and secondary defects have been described. The manifestations are cardiomyopathy, encephalopathy, and myopathy.

☞**ISOVALERIC ACIDEMIA:** A genetic disorder affecting the branched-chain organic acids, the most frequent form of leucine metabolism disorders. It results in accumulation of isovaleric acid (and its metabolites), leading to vomiting, dehydration, severe metabolic acidosis, and neurological manifestations.

REFERENCES:

Fenton WA, Gravel RA, Rosenblatt DS: Disorders of propionate and methylmalonate metabolism, in Scriver CR, Beaudet AL, Sly WS, et al. (eds): *The Metabolic and Molecular Bases of Inherited Disease.* 8th ed. New York, McGraw Hill, 2001, p 2165.

Harker HE, Emhardt JD, Hainline BE: Propionic acidemia in a four-month-old male: A case study and anesthetic implications. *Anesth Analg* 91:309, 2000.

Ogier de Baulny H, Saudubray JM: Branched-chain organic acidurias, in Fernandes J, Saudubray JM, Van den Bergh G (eds): *Inborn Metabolic Diseases.* 3rd ed. Berlin, Springer Verlag, 2000, p 196.

Turpin B, Tobias JD: Perioperative management of a child with short-chain acyl-CoA dehydrogenase deficiency. *Paediatr Anaesth* 15:771, 2005.

Protein C Deficiency

At a glance: Congenital or acquired control of the clotting mechanism resulting in a widespread thrombotic tendency. Protein C is a vitamin K-dependent serine protease zymogen that selectively inhibits factors Va and VIII:C in human plasma, and thus has an important anticoagulant role. It is associated with an increased tendency to thrombosis. It is either inherited or acquired: bacterial sepsis (especially of meningococcal origin), hepatic disease, disseminated intravascular coagulation, L-asparaginase therapy, nephrotic syndrome, conditioning therapy in bone marrow transplantation, warfarin-induced skin lesions.

Synonyms: Congenital Thrombotic Protein C Deficiency; Hereditary Thrombophilia; PC Deficiency; ProC Deficiency.

History: The addition of Protein C deficiency in the list of thrombotic diseases was suggested by J.H. Griffin in 1981.

Incidence: Inherited forms: 1:200 to 1:300 for heterozygotes; 1:200,000 for homozygotes.

Genetic inheritance: Autosomal dominant trait with variable expressivity. Gene map locus: 2q13-q14.

Pathophysiology: Inherited thrombophilia has been associated with abnormalities of antithrombin III, fibrinogen, and plasminogen. Protein C is a vitamin K-dependent serine protease anticoagulant factor. It has several roles: (a) it is converted on site and on demand during the coagulation activation into activated protein C; its anticoagulant activity is related to inactivation of factors Va and VIIIa; the presence of protein S as a nonenzymatic cofactor is necessary for those reactions; (b) it promotes fibrinolysis by binding plasminogen activator inhibitor I; (c) it prevents the proinflammatory consequences of local thrombin formation, for example, release of vasoactive proinflammatory factors (tumor necrosis factor

(TNF)-α, interleukin (IL)-1β, etc.), and an increase of endothelial permeability. Consequently, a deficiency in protein C results in defective control of the clotting mechanism with a widespread thrombotic tendency. Heterozygotes show an increased thrombotic tendency, whereas homozygotes present with severe thrombotic sequelae in the neonatal period. Most cases of protein C deficiency have had a quantitative defect in the protein C molecule. Protein C deficiency with a mutation that causes diminished synthesis of protein has been referred to as type I and that with synthesis of a dysfunctional molecule as type II.

Diagnosis: Positive family history and a significant history of thrombosis or gangrene (skin, retinal, etc.). Severe symptoms typically develop when the serum protein C level is below 20 to 25% of normal (4 μg/mL). Specific laboratory tests and assays are needed to exclude other causes of disseminated intravascular coagulation.

Clinical aspects: *Heterozygotes for Protein C Deficiency* (serum concentrations 40 to 60% of normal) usually presents in adolescence with recurrent thrombophlebitis, deep venous thrombosis, and pulmonary thromboembolism. There is also an increased risk of thrombotic renal and cerebral disease and an increased risk of myocardial infarction.

Homozygotes manifest fatal thromboses in the neonatal period—massive subcutaneous thrombosis (neonatal purpura fulminans) with cutaneous necrosis, gangrene, and widespread venous thrombosis, which usually starts in the first 24 hours of life. Severe bilateral vitreous hemorrhages, gangrene, and widespread venous thrombosis have been reported. Bilateral adrenal hemorrhage may lead to abdominal pain, hypotension, and hyponatremia. Hypertension and congestive cardiac failure commonly result from renal involvement. Treatment with heparin, antiplatelet drugs, or both is not effective. The only successful treatment is protein C replacement using protein C human concentrate, fresh-frozen plasma, or factor IX concentrate.

In case of portal hypertension with normal or near-normal liver function (e.g., in case of portal cavernoma), reestablishing portal flow through the liver restores normal serum protein C levels. Availability of a human protein C concentrate purified by monoclonal antibody allows specific replacement of protein C; the initial dose is 60 to 80 IU/kg.

Precautions before anesthesia: Protein C Deficiency does not cause abnormalities in the routine screening coagulation tests; a high index of suspicion is necessary in case of familial or personal history of thrombotic events at a young age, and in patients at risk for acquired protein S deficiency (e.g., nephrotic syndrome, asparaginase therapy). Detailed systemic review, particularly of the cardiovascular and renal systems, and the CNS. Optimize antihypertensive therapy and continue all medications until the day of surgery. *Investigations:* CBC, urea and creatinine, serum electrolytes, coagulation studies, ECG. Fresh-frozen plasma and/or protein C human concentrate should be available to manage the hypercoagulability state in such patients. Adrenal hormone supplementation may be required. Hypertension may also require specific management. Ensure adequate protein C levels by human protein C concentrate, or fresh-frozen plasma administration.

Anesthetic considerations: Thrombosis may be triggered by endothelial damage, immobility, and blood stasis—all common occurrences during surgery and anesthesia. Some authors advocate avoidance of endotracheal intubation because airway trauma may result in oral and tracheal submucosal thrombosis and necrosis. Regional anesthesia should be considered as an alternative to general anesthesia. Pad pressure and bony points adequately to avoid pressure necrosis. Hypovolemia and hypotension should be avoided.

Antiembolism stockings and subcutaneous low-molecular-weight heparin therapy might be appropriate.

Pharmacological implications: Care should be taken with drugs that are excreted via the kidneys especially if there is impairment of renal function.

REFERENCES:

Delalande JP, Sauvanaud D, Abgrall JF, et al: Disclosure of protein C deficiency with pulmonary embolism followed by cardiac arrest during the recovery period. *Ann Fr Anesth Reanim* 11:96, 1992.

Kogure S, Makita K, Saitoh Y, et al: Anesthetic management of a patient with protein C deficiency associated with pulmonary thromboembolism. *Masui* 47:831, 1998.

Kumagai K, Nishiwaki K, Sato K, et al: Perioperative management of a patient with purpura fulminans syndrome due to protein C deficiency. *Can J Anesth* 49:1070, 2001.

Wetzel RC, Marsh BR, Yaster M, et al: Anesthetic implications of protein C deficiency. *Anesth Analg* 65:982, 1986.

Protein S Deficiency

At a glance: Congenital or acquired control of the clotting mechanism resulting in a widespread thrombotic tendency. Protein S is a nonenzymatic, vitamin K-dependent cofactor of activated protein C. It is either inherited or acquired and leads to liver disease, nephrotic syndrome, systemic lupus erythematosus, pregnancy, and disseminated intravascular coagulation.

Synonyms: Protein S alpha Deficiency; Protein S Pseudogene; Purpura fulminans.

Classification: Three types of protein S deficiency are described:

Type I: reduced production
Type II: abnormality of C4bBP
Type III: functionally abnormal Protein S.

History: Protein S deficiency was first identified in 1979 in Seattle, United States, and arbitrarily named after the city of this discovery.

Incidence: Unknown; one study found 8% of 179 patients with a positive family history or who had spontaneous thrombosis to be deficient in protein S.

Genetic inheritance: Autosomal dominant inheritance with male-to-male transmission observed. Gene map locus is 3p11.1-q11.2. Additional factors are necessary to precipitate thrombosis because some family members of the affected are asymptomatic even though they have equally low levels of protein S and because there are instances of a skipped generation.

Pathophysiology: Protein S is a vitamin K-dependent plasma protein that inhibits blood clotting by serving as a cofactor for activated protein C. Deficiency of protein S causes thrombotic disease. Protein S exists in two forms in plasma: the free, functionally active form (40%) and the inactive form complexed with C4b-binding protein (C4bBP).

Diagnosis: Familial history of thromboembolic events at a young age. Low plasma protein S levels.

Clinical aspects: Deficiency of protein S manifests as severe recurrent thromboembolic disease (leg vein thrombosis, pulmonary embolism, superficial thrombophlebitis, and thrombosis in uncommon sites—axillary, mesenteric, and cerebral veins). While patients with homozygous deficiency present as neonatal purpura fulminans, those with heterozygous forms (30 to 60% of normal) manifest later with venous and, more rarely, arterial thrombosis.

Precautions before anesthesia: Protein S deficiency does not cause abnormalities in the routine screening coagulation tests; a high index of suspicion is necessary in case of familial or personal history of thrombotic events at a young age and in patients at risk for acquired protein S deficiency (e.g., nephrotic syndrome). Preventive measures, such as low-molecular-weight heparin to prevent deep venous thrombosis, should be instituted before operation and continued postoperatively until the patient is ambulant. Initiation of oral anticoagulation therapy without antecedent heparin therapy is fraught with risks of worsening of thrombotic tendencies. Detailed evaluation of the cardiac and cerebrovascular systems. *Investigations:* complete blood count, clotting studies including thromboelastography, protein S levels.

Anesthetic considerations: If a locoregional anesthetic technique is used, the timing of its performance (and of the withdrawal of the catheter) should be adapted to the timing of low-molecular-weight heparin therapy. Use heparin-bonded central venous catheter to reduce the risk of central venous thrombosis. Arterial catheters should be removed as soon as possible.

Pharmacological implications: The use of antifibrinolytics (e.g., ε-aminocaproic acid) is contraindicated because they would exacerbate any deficiency in endogenous antifibrinolysis. The effect of aprotinin is still unclear.

REFERENCES:

Borgel D, Gandrille S, Aiach M: Protein S deficiency. *Thromb Haemost* 78:351, 1997.

Grocott HP, Clements F, Landolfo K: Coronary artery bypass graft surgery in a patient with hereditary protein S deficiency. *J Cardiothorac Vasc Anesth* 10:915, 1996.

Gupta B, Prakash S, Gujral K: Anaesthetic management of the parturient with protein S deficiency and lumboperitoneal shunt. *Anaest Intensive Care* 31:573, 2003.

Zimmerman AA, Watson RS, Williams JK: Protein S deficiency presenting as an acute postoperative arterial thrombosis in a four-year-old child. *Anesth Analg* 88:535, 1999.

Proteus Syndrome

At a glance: A rare congenital hamartomatous disorder characterized by multiple, diverse, somatic manifestations: partial bilateral gigantism of hands and feet, nevi, hemihypertrophy, subcutaneous tumors, macrocephaly with cranial hyperostoses.

Synonyms: Elattoproteus Syndrome; Wiedemann Syndrome; Partial Gigantism of Hands and Feet Syndrome; Nevi Hemihypertrophy Macrocephaly Syndrome; Encephalocraniocutaneous Lipomatosis Syndrome; Hamartomas Disorder, Multifarious Mesodermal Malformation, Plurifocal Overgrowth.

History: It is named after the Greek god Proteus, "the polymorphous," who could change his shape at will to avoid capture. Proteus lived on the Island of Pharos, close to the mouth of the Nile or in the caves of the island of Karpatos, between Crete and Rhodos. It was described by Hans-Rudolf Wiedemann, a German pediatrician, in 1983. Joseph Merrick, known as the "elephant man" is now, in retrospect, believed to have been affected by Proteus syndrome.

Incidence: Internationally, it is estimated that approximately 200 individuals are affected with this medical condition. The prevalence

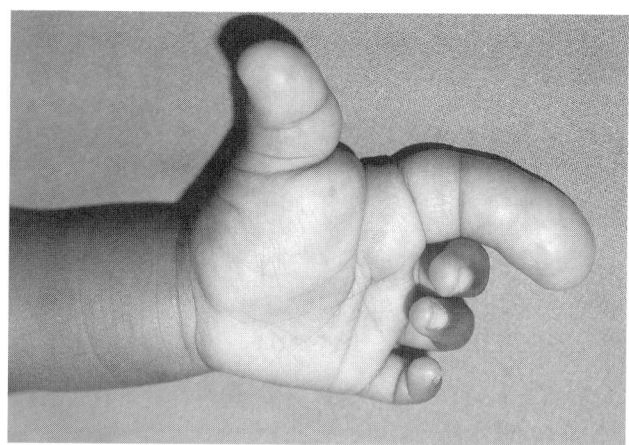

Proteus syndrome   Digital gigantism in an infant with Proteus syndrome.

is believed to be less than 1 per 1,000,000 live births. There is no predilection for any race and sex. All cases are sporadic. At least, some of the abnormalities are present at birth, or they appear within the first year of life. This medical condition usually progresses until puberty.

Genetic inheritance: Postulated to be genetic although cases are mainly sporadic. Few cases with autosomal inheritance reported. The cause may be a dominant lethal gene, with survival by somatic mosaicism.

Pathophysiology: May involve abnormal secretion of a growth factor or abnormal tissue or tissue response to a growth factor.

Diagnosis: The diagnostic criteria of Proteus syndrome include regional generalized tissue hyperplasia (such as digital gigantism, macrocephaly, hemihypertrophy), skin lesions (e.g., hypo- or hyperpigmented, thickened skin creases), and mesodermal hamartomas (such as lipoma, lymphangioma, hemangioma, exostosis, or fibroma). There is unique marked hypertrophy of the skin of the soles—"moccasin sole"—with light microscopic findings of elongation of the cytoplasm of basal cells. Histologic examination of subcutaneous masses has identified a variety of lipomatous, hamartomatous, and angiomatous tumors.

Clinical aspects: The disease appears soon after birth and progresses at a variable rate leading to gross deformity in later childhood. Some patients are born with large, complex, mixed vascular malformations. Overgrowth, usually digital, is noted during infancy. In childhood, patients may also develop linear epidermal nevi. The skeletal system is mainly affected with hemihypertrophy, macrodactyly, scoliosis, and exostoses over the skull. Intelligence is usually normal. Spinal compromise may develop in Proteus syndrome from vertebral anomalies (e.g., angular kyphoscoliosis) or tumor infiltration. There may be associated pulmonary involvement (rapidly progressive diffuse cystic emphysematous pulmonary disease that is potentially fatal, secondary chronic restrictive pulmonary disease from scoliosis). Pulmonary hypertension is often a feature of this syndrome. Anomalies of the cervical spine (vertebral enlargement, hemivertebrae, dysplastic vertebrae, dystrophic intervertebral diseases) are common and may predispose to airway obstruction. The prognosis is unknown. Surgical removal of lymphatic, fatty, or hemangiomatous elements is difficult and results in unsightly scars and keloids. A predisposition to tumors exists, especially cystadenomas of the ovary and mesothelioma. Thrombosis is a frequent complication and more frequent in males.

Precautions before anesthesia: Scoliosis is common, as is cystic emphysematous pulmonary disease and restrictive pulmonary disease. Their presence requires a detailed respiratory assessment, including pulmonary function tests. A difficult tracheal intubation may be anticipated in patients with cervical spine anomalies and prominent carious teeth. An antisialogogue should be given if a fiberoptic scope-assisted intubation is to be attempted. Patients on anticonvulsant therapy should have the appropriate drug levels checked and the seizure control optimized prior to surgery. *Investigations:* full blood count, serum electrolytes, anticonvulsant level, chest radiograph, arterial blood gas, lung function test, cervical spine radiograph.

Anesthetic considerations: Preparation for a difficult direct laryngoscopy and tracheal intubation should be done. The presence of severe spinal deformities may make positioning difficult and predispose the patient to pressure sores. A regional anesthetic technique may also be difficult in the presence of spinal deformity. Intermittent positive-pressure ventilation should be used with care in patients with cystic lung changes. These patients are at risk for deep venous thrombosis, pulmonary embolism, and pulmonary hypertension.

Pharmacological implications: The presence of cystic changes in the lungs contraindicates the use of nitrous oxide.

Other conditions to be considered:

☞**KLIPPEL-TRENAUNAY SYNDROME:** A vascular malformation involving the lower or upper limbs, but usually, only one limb is affected. The vascular (i.e., capillary, lymphatic, and venous) malformations always exist in combination. Unilateral overgrowth is present at birth. This medical entity is considered more severe than the vascular malformations reported in the Proteus syndrome. However, Klippel-Trenaunay syndrome lacks subcutaneous tumors, palmar and/or plantar cerebriform hyperplasia, and cranial exostoses, which usually are found in Proteus syndrome.

PARKES-WEBER SYNDROME: A vascular malformation involving the upper and lower limbs. It is characterized by a diffuse capillary blushing, warmth, and underlying arteriovenous shunts.

☞**MAFFUCCI SYNDROME:** Characterized by hemangiomas and enchondromas.

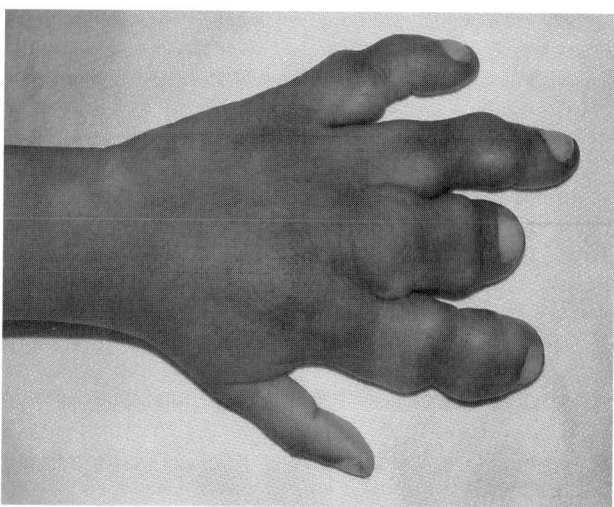

Proteus syndrome   Digital gigantism involving digits II-V in a 6-year-old girl with Proteus syndrome.

☞**NEUROFIBROMATOSIS TYPE I:** Characterized by the presence of café-au-lait macules, axillary freckling, Lisch nodules, and neurofibromas, rather than epidermal nevi and hamartomas.

☞**BANNAYAN ZONANA SYNDROME:** Characterized by macrocephaly, lipomas, capillary malformations, and polyposis of the colon and rectum. It does not cause asymmetric growth, cranial exostoses, epidermal nevi, palmar, or plantar changes.

HEMIHYPERPLASIA LIPOMATOSIS SYNDROME: Lacks the progressive overgrowth seen in patients with Proteus syndrome.

ENCEPHALOCRANIOCUTANEOUS LIPOMATOSIS: It is considered to be a circumscribed form of Proteus syndrome. However, it is believed by most authors that both conditions are different. This disease is a congenital hamartomatous disorder characterized by partial gigantism (hands and feet, macrodactyly), hemihypertrophy, macrocephaly, scoliosis, exostoses, and nevi.

☞**COWDEN SYNDROME:** A rare syndrome characterized by multiple hamartomas (small flesh-colored bumps on the skin involving a hair follicle and small wart-like growths) and a risk of breast, thyroid, and uterine neoplasias.

☞**RILEY-SMITH SYNDROME:** A rare syndrome very similar to the Bannayan-Zonana syndrome characterized by macrocephaly, pseudopapillema, hemangiomata, and multiples lipomas. Subcutaneous hemangioma may be present at birth or appear later in childhood.

REFERENCES:

Biesecker LG, Happle R, Mulliken JB, et al: Proteus syndrome: Diagnostic criteria, differential diagnosis, and patient evaluation. *Am J Med Genet* 84:389, 1999.

Cekmen N, Kordan AZ, Tuncer B, et al: Anesthesia for Proteus syndrome. *Paediatr Anaesth* 14:689, 2004.

Pennant JH, Harris MF: Anesthesia for Proteus syndrome. *Anesthesia* 46:126, 1991.

Pradhan A, Sen I, Batra YK, et al: Proteus syndrome: A concern for the anesthesiologist. *Anesth Analg* 96:915, 2003.

Proximal Muscular Dystrophy

At a glance: Inherited symmetric muscular weakness, initially of the lower limbs, with slow progression and associated cardiac anomalies. This term includes: Limb-Girdle Muscular Dystrophy; Leyden-Möbius Muscular Dystrophy; Pelvofemoral Muscular Dystrophy; Scapulohumeral Muscular Dystrophy.

History: The earliest description of the proximal muscular dystrophy is described to Leyden and Möbius in 1876 and 1879, respectively. They described adult patients with pelvic and femoral distribution of weakness and atrophy with a benign course. At that time, the differentiation between the spinal muscular atrophies and weakness associated with central nervous system (CNS) disorders and primary muscle disease had not been established.

Incidence: Exact figures are not available. The frequency in the general population because of the heterogenous nature of this disease. There is no racial predilection and it affects either sex equally.

Genetic inheritance: The mutation for this disease is located on the long arm of chromosome 1 and inheritance is most often autosomal dominant, although an autosomal recessive variant may exist as well. Recent genetic research demonstrated that Emery-Dreifuss and proximal muscular dystrophy are allelic disorders.

Pathophysiology: The pathophysiology of the proximal muscular dystrophies depends on the specific genetic defect of each associated condition and is discussed with each individually in this book.

Diagnosis: Of the various muscular dystrophies, the dystrophinopathies are the most common, accounting for the majority of male disease and 10% of female patients presenting for muscular dystrophy or persistent high serum creatine kinase.

Clinical aspects: Symmetric muscular weakness starts proximal in the lower extremities usually before the age of 20 years. Slow progression over the next 10 to 20 years results also in weakness of the upper limb. In contrast to Bethlem myopathy and Emery-Dreifuss muscular dystrophy, contractures of the elbows and the Achilles tendon are absent or subtle. Cardiologic abnormalities (atrioventricular conduction defects with arrhythmias and risk of sudden death) occur in almost two-thirds of these patients. Rarely, dilated cardiomyopathy may be present. In general, neuromuscular symptoms precede cardiac abnormalities. Serum creatine phosphokinase levels are either normal or only moderately elevated.

Anesthetic considerations: Cardiac evaluation with ECG and echocardiography is recommended. If the patient already has a pacemaker, ensure proper function. Although congenital myopathies have been associated with malignant hyperthermia, the evidence supporting this causal relationship is poor. No case reports of malignant hyperthermia reaction in proximal muscular dystrophy have been published. Nevertheless, caution should be exercised when using known trigger agents and full monitoring (including core and peripheral temperature) should be used in the perioperative period.

Pharmacological implications: Avoidance of known trigger agents may be advisable until more information about the condition is available. If nondepolarizing muscle relaxants are to be used, they should be titrated to effect by using a peripheral nerve stimulator. *Cis*-atracurium can be used and seems to offer good neuromuscular blockade without prolongation of recovery. However, a delayed onset of action is possible. The benign myopathy associated with this condition, which makes it unique amongst the other congenital myopathies, suggests that an exaggerated response to these agents is unlikely. Anticholinergic premedication is recommended if fiberoptic intubation is planned.

Other conditions to be considered:

☞**BETHLEM MYOPATHY:** An autosomal dominant medical disorder presenting with an onset in early infancy, slow progression, moderate weakness, and muscular atrophy of the trunk and limbs. The proximal muscles are more affected than the distal muscles and the extensors more than the flexors. Early flexion contractures of the elbow and interphalangeal joints of the last four fingers and plantar flexion contractures of the ankles are constant features.

☞**EMERY-DREIFUSS MUSCULAR DYSTROPHY (EDMD):** An X-linked degenerative myopathy characterized by weakness and atrophy of muscle without involvement of the CNS. The onset for the flexion deformities of the elbows is in early childhood. Other clinical features include mild pectus excavatum, cardiac anomalies, absence of muscle pseudohypertrophy, forearm muscles involvement, and mental retardation. The cardiac conduction defect in EDMD patients is the most serious and life-threatening clinical manifestation of the disease. Cardiac defects have been described in female carriers in the absence of any skeletal muscle abnormality, suggesting a prominent role in cardiac conduction for emerin. There are two Emery-Dreifuss syndromes caused by mutation in the laminin A/C gene: one displays similar features to EDMD and is autosomal dominant and the other appears to lack cardiac features and is autosomal recessive.

BECKER MUSCULAR DYSTROPHY: An inherited disease with a male distribution pattern and clinical picture similar to that of Duchenne muscular dystrophy (DMD); however, it is generally considered milder than DMD, and the onset of symptoms usually occurs later. The muscle weakness is less severe, allowing the patient to be ambulatory until the age of 15 to 20 years. The incidence is estimated at 1:30,000 male births, compared to incidence for DMD of 1:3,500 male births. The international incidence probably is similar to that in the United States.

REFERENCES:

Bonnemann CG, Finkel RS: Sarcolemmal proteins and the spectrum of limb-girdle muscular dystrophies. *Semin Pediatr Neurol* 9:81, 2002.

Caron MJ, Girard F, Girard DC, et al: Cisatracurium pharmacodynamics in patients with oculopharyngeal muscular dystrophy. *Anesth Analg* 100:393, 2005.

Mathieu J, Allard P, Gobeil G, et al: Anesthetic and surgical complications in 219 cases of myotonic dystrophy. *J Neurol* 49:1646, 1997.

Muchir A, Bonne G, van der Kooi AJ, et al: Identifications of mutations in the gene encoding lamins A/C in autosomal dominant limb girdle muscular dystrophy with atrioventricular conduction disturbances (LGMD1B). *Hum Mol Genet* 9:1453, 2000.

van der Kooi AJ, van Meegen M, Ledderhof TM, et al: Genetic localization of a newly recognized autosomal dominant limb-girdle muscular dystrophy with cardiac involvement (LGMD1B) to chromosome 1q11-21. *Am J Hum Genet* 60:891, 1997.

Prune Belly Syndrome

At a glance: Congenital absence of abdominal musculature leading to urinary and respiratory problems. The major prognostic factor is the degree of dilation of the urinary tract; 20% of patients are stillborn, 30% die of renal failure or urosepsis within the first 2 years of life, and the remaining 50% have varying degrees of urinary pathology requiring numerous surgical procedures.

Synonyms: Eagle-Barrett Syndrome; Abdominal Muscular Deficiency Syndrome; Triad Syndrome; Fröhlich Syndrome.

History: First described in 1839 by F. Fröhlich and the name "prune-belly syndrome" was given by W. Osler in 1901. It was fully described by W. Obrinsky in 1949. G.S. Barrett and J.F. Eagle, Jr., American urologists, popularized this medical condition. The pathogenesis is not clearly understood. The triad (see *Diagnosis*) may arise simply from the effects of early urethral obstruction and distended bladder, or, alternatively, from a basic defect of the mesoderm. The full syndrome probably occurs only in males.

Incidence: 1:40,000 live births; male:female ratio of 20:1 (95% in males).

Genetic inheritance: Autosomal recessive inheritance with sex-limited expression that partially mimics autosomal dominant X-linkage has been suggested, but not proven.

Pathophysiology: In 1903, Strumme proposed that the syndrome may be caused by in utero obstruction of the bladder, stating that dilation of the urinary tract in utero leads to secondary pressure atrophy of the abdominal wall and the subsequent clinical findings. The prevailing theory is the theory of mesodermal arrest, which would explain the involvement of the genitourinary tract, the testes, and the abdominal wall. A noxious insult would have to occur between the sixth and tenth weeks of gestation. It has been suggested that

the embryogenesis of this disorder resides in the 3 weeks of development which could also explain the prostatic hypoplasia and poor glandular development. The mesodermal arrest theory is supported by the histologic findings in the abdominal wall, the urinary tract, and the male genital system. Today, the etiology of prune belly syndrome remains a mystery. The thinned abdominal wall has been attributed to hydronephrosis and the distended urinary system to interfering with normal descent of the testes. However, other patients with severe hydronephrosis may not show the same abdominal wall disorder.

Diagnosis: Based on the triad of (a) deficient abdominal wall musculature, (b) urinary tract dilatation, and (c) cryptorchidism.

Clinical aspects: There is an absence of the muscles in the lower central and medial part of the abdominal wall. The abdominal wall is lax and thin, and there may be a visible intestinal pattern. The abdominal skin is wrinkled, giving rise to the "prune belly" appearance. The syndrome is always accompanied by urinary tract anomalies, although their severity varies (distended bladder, fetal urinary tract obstruction, posterior urethral valves, hydronephrosis, hydroureter,

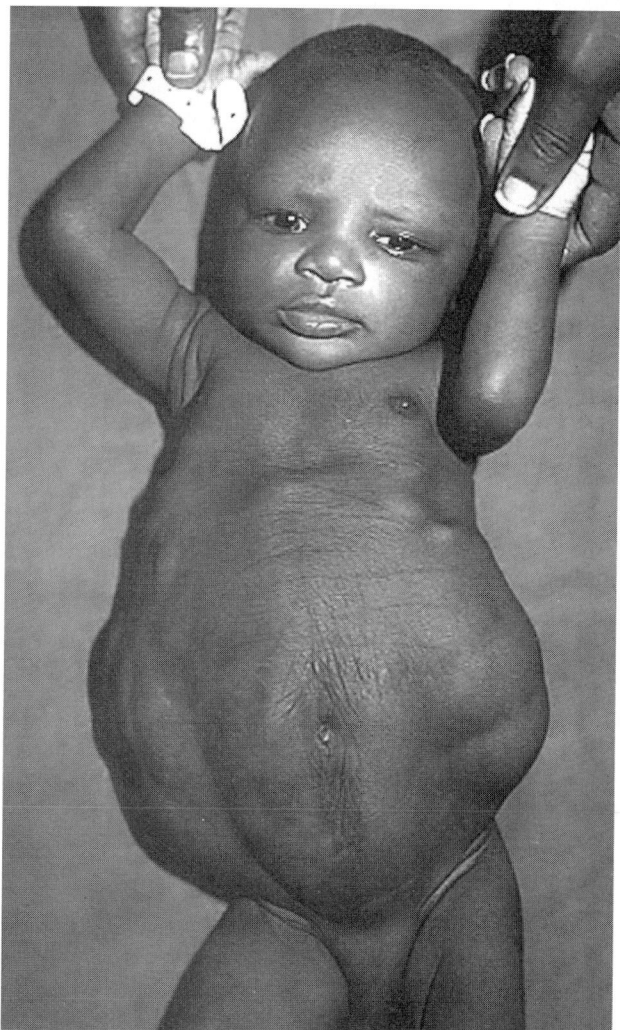

Prune belly syndrome (Eagle-Barrett syndrome)   The absence of the abdominal muscles in a newborn with Eagle-Barrett syndrome results in the visibility of the contours of the bowel loops, explaining the synonym prune belly syndrome.

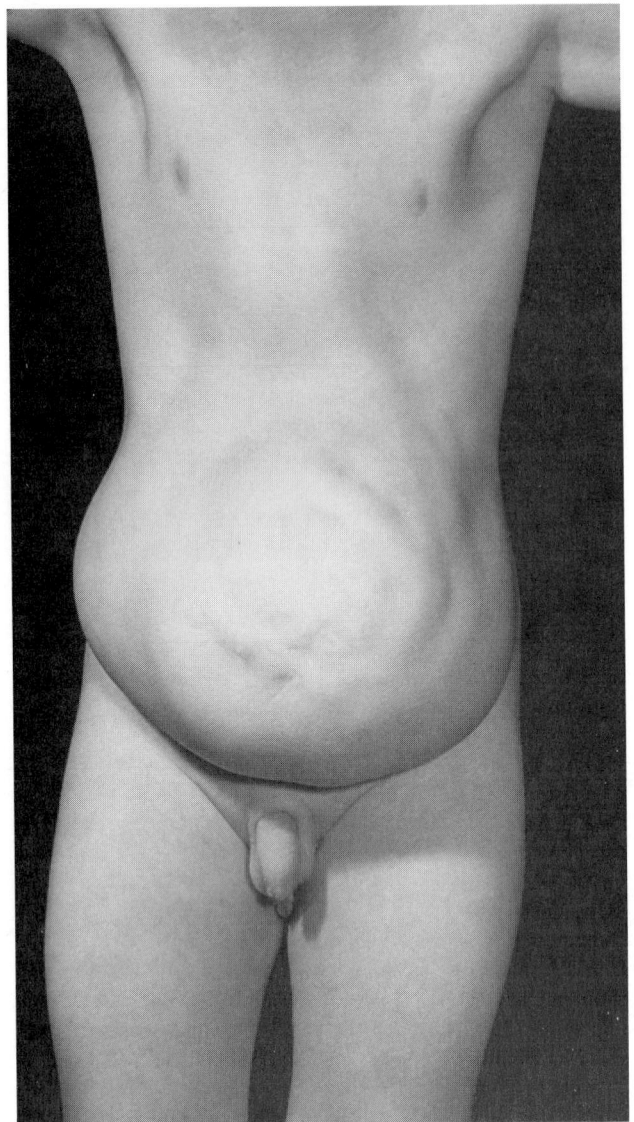

Prune belly syndrome (Eagle-Barrett syndrome)   Eagle-Barrett syndrome in a 9-year-old boy.

and cryptorchidism). Chronic renal failure may develop in those with the most severe urinary tract abnormalities, as well as in those with recurrent urinary tract infections. The most severe forms result in stillbirth or neonatal death, usually from uremia or pulmonary hypoplasia. The musculoskeletal abnormalities include marked abnormality of the hip with congenital dislocation (typically resistant to conventional treatment), scoliosis, pectus excavatum, flared ribs, and talipes equinovarus (clubfoot). Some association with oligohydramnios, cleft lip, imperforate anus, gut malrotation, omphalocele, and congenital muscular dystrophy has been reported. Recurrent respiratory tract infections are common as a consequence of retention of secretions and reduced ability to cough because of the absence of abdominal musculature. When respiratory function is evaluated, either gas trapping (caused by poor expiratory effort) or restrictive lung disease (secondary to musculoskeletal anomalies) is observed. There is a 10% incidence of patent ductus arteriosus or other congenital heart defect (atrial septal defect, ventricular septal defect, tetralogy of Fallot).

Precautions before anesthesia: Evaluate renal function, including plasma urea, creatinine, and electrolytes. Ensure full assessment of respiratory function and include chest radiograph and pulmonary function tests if the child is cooperative. Preoperative chest physiotherapy is indicated. Full evaluation of cardiovascular system for congenital lesions. Echocardiography may be indicated.

Anesthetic considerations: There is no indication of difficult airway management with this medical condition. Lack of abdominal musculature may lead to respiratory difficulties both intraoperatively and postoperatively. Any existing respiratory infection should be treated aggressively with appropriate antibiotics. Active physiotherapy is recommended both pre- and postoperatively.

Pharmacological implications: It is safer to avoid succinylcholine because of the possible association with a congenital muscular dystrophy. Caution should be exercised with the use of opioid analgesics and benzodiazepines and any other drugs known to produce respiratory depression. The utilization of regional anesthesia is highly recommended perioperatively and for postoperative pain management.

REFERENCES:

Baris S, Karayaka O, Ustun E, et al: Complicated airway management in a child with prune belly syndrome. *Paediatr Anaesth* 13:557, 2003.

Ewig JM, Griscom NT, Wohl ME: The effect of the absence of abdominal muscles on pulmonary function and exercise. *Am J Respir Crit Care Med* 53(pt 1):1314, 1996.

Henderson AM, Vallis CJ, Sumner E: Anaesthesia in the prune-belly syndrome. A review of 36 cases. *Anaesthesia* 42:54, 1987.

Leyten QH, Renier WO, Gabreels FJ, et al: Association of congenital muscular dystrophy with hypoplasia of the lateral abdominal wall musculature and hypoplasia of the external genitalia. *Neuropediatrics* 27:108, 1996.

Ushijima K, Matsuyama K, Ezaki K, et al: General anesthesia for a case of abdominal musculature deficiency prune belly, syndrome. *J Anesth* 5:294, 1991.

Psaume Syndrome

At a glance: A congenital X-linked syndrome lethal for males. It is characterized by orofacial and digital defects associated with renal failure.

Synonyms: Gorlin-Psaume Syndrome; Papillon-Léage Syndrome; Digito-Orofacial Syndrome I; Orofaciodigital Syndrome I; Gorlin Syndrome I; Papillon-Léage-Psaume Syndrome.

History: Genetic disorder that was first described by Psaume (1962) and known worldwide because of Gorlin's works. First described in 1954 by E. Papillon-Léage, a French dentist, and J. Psaume, also a French dentist. R. J. Gorlin, an American oral pathologist and geneticist, made this condition internationally known.

Incidence: 1:250,000 live births.

Genetic inheritance: X-linked dominant.

Pathophysiology: Caused by mutations in the CXORF5 gene mapped on Xp22.3-p22.2. One hypothesis is that the OFD1 protein may have widespread influence on organogenesis and be essential for fetal survival.

Diagnosis: Clinically evocated in females with characteristic facies, multiple digits anomalies, and renal failure.

Clinical aspects: Features involve *head and neck* (microcephaly or macrocephaly, micrognathia, frontal bossing, zygomatic hypoplasia, increased cranial base angle, hypertelorism, telecanthus, choroid coloboma, hypoplastic alar cartilage, broad nasal root, short upper lip, median cleft lip, cleft palate, palatal grooves, alveolar notching, hyperplastic oral frenula, lobulated/bifid tongue, tongue hamartomas, missing incisor teeth, supernumerary teeth, periodontal diseases, malocclusion), *digits* (brachydactyly, clinodactyly, syndactyly), *skin* (dry scalp, sparse hair, alopecia), central nervous system (hydrocephaly, hydranencephaly, porencephaly, partial agenesis of the corpus callosum, hamartoma of the hypothalamus, gray matter heterotopias, conductive deafness), and *kidneys* (renal failure, polycystic kidneys). Mild mental retardation and irritability occur in 50% of cases. Seizures, precocious puberty, and short stature can be associated.

Precautions before anesthesia: Evaluate tracheal intubation (clinical, radiographs), neurological function (clinical, CT/MRI scans, EEG), and renal function (clinical, echography, laboratory).

Anesthetic considerations: Tracheal intubation can be difficult and may require adapted anesthetic management. Increase in intracranial pressure is possible and makes spinal anesthesia not recommended.

Pharmacological implications: Consider interaction between antiepileptic treatment and anesthetic drugs. Intraoperative fluid regimen and anesthetic drugs choice should consider renal function.

REFERENCES:

Ferrante MI, Giorgio G, Feather SA, et al: Identification of the gene for oral-facial-digital type I syndrome. *Am J Hum Genet* 68:569, 2001.

Papillon-Léage E, Psaume J: Une malformation héréditaire de la muqueuse buccale, brides et freins anormaux: Généralities. *Rev Stomatol* 55:209, 1954.

Pseudo-Achondroplastic Dysplasia

At a glance: A heterogeneous inherited chondrodystrophic growth disorder associated with disproportionate short stature and limbs, marked joint deformities, and early-onset osteoarthritis.

Synonyms: Pseudo-Achondroplasia; Pseudo-Achondroplastic Spondyloepiphyseal Dysplasia.

History: In 1969, Hall and Dorst suggested a classification into four types: two dominant (formerly designated types I and III) and two recessive (formerly designated II and IV).

Incidence: 4:1,000,000 live births; one of the most frequent of the skeletal dysplasias.

Genetic inheritance: Both autosomal dominant of gonadal mosaicism and autosomal recessive inheritance has been reported. Gene map locus is 19p13.1.

Pathophysiology: It results as T mutations in the gene for cartilage oligomeric matrix protein (COMP). COMP produces soft cartilage, which deforms markedly under stress. Accumulation of a noncollagenous protein in the rough endoplasmic reticulum of chondrocytes and the absence of a proteoglycan "population" from the cartilage suggest that an abnormally synthesized or processed protein core is not properly transferred to the Golgi system. The structurally abnormal COMP is expressed in tendon explains the loose joints that are a consistent feature of pseudoachondroplasia.

Diagnosis: Clinically characterized by marked shortening of the limbs with a normal head and face (which makes the difference with achondroplasia). Radiologically, all long bones are short with widened metaphyses and fragmentation, and irregularities of the developing epiphyses. In childhood, platyspondyly is characteristic, with anterior tonguing as a result of delayed ossification of the annular epiphyses; after puberty, the vertebrae become more normal in appearance. Cytoplasmic metachromasia of fibroblasts is seen under microscopy.

Clinical aspects: Patients appear normal at birth and growth retardation is seldom recognized until the second year of life when the body proportions may resemble classical achondroplasia. Skeletal lesions occur as a result of stresses on soft epiphyseal cartilage. Thus, at sites such as the anterior vertebral margins, and the wrists, ankles, and knee joints, there may be severe cartilaginous deformity. Sites not subjected to excessive stress, such as the base of skull, face, sacrum, and central portions of the vertebrae, appear relatively normal. Unlike achondroplasia, head size is normal for age and the face appears normal. Intelligence is not affected. Lumbar lordosis, kyphosis, and scoliosis may all occur. Waddling gait. There may be atlantoaxial dislocation and odontoid hypoplasia. The fingers are hyperlax and short, and do not show the trident configuration typical of achondroplasia. Ligamentous laxity contributes to the leg deformities (from genu varum to genu valgum). Chronic compression myelopathy of the cervical cord as a consequence of chronic atlantoaxial dislocation has been reported. Extraskeletal complications are uncommon. Adult height ranges from 80 to 130 cm (31.5 to 51.2 inches).

Precautions before anesthesia: Evaluation of the stability of the atlantoaxial joint should be made (history, neurologic examination, radiographic examination including flexion/extension views, CT, MRI). Document any preoperative neurologic deficit. Thoracic dystrophy and kyphoscoliosis are present and a detailed cardiopulmonary assessment should be made (chest radiograph, echocardiography, and lung function tests).

Anesthetic considerations: Careful positioning of the patient is important to prevent injury to the lax joints. If atlantoaxial instability is present, procedures to ensure protection of the spinal cord must be used. Tracheal intubation with a fiberoptic bronchoscope may be preferred. Regional anesthesia had been used with success but is recommended only for those patients for whom the advantages offered by this technique outweigh those of a general anesthetic because of the potential for development of neurologic problems as a result of spinal stenosis and vertebral misalignment. Endotracheal tube size will be half to one size smaller than would be predicted for the patient's age. Postoperative ventilatory support is required for those with significant thoracic dystrophy.

Pharmacological implications: Care should be taken with the use of opioids and benzodiazepines if there is any respiratory compromise.

Other conditions to be considered:

☞**LEGG-CALVE-PERTHES DISEASE:** A group of disorders known as the osteochondroses. It is believe to be because of unexplained interruption of the blood supply to the capital femoral epiphysis resulting in avascular necrosis. Clinically, this disease is characterized by limp with or without pain in the hip, knee, thigh, and groin. Most cases occur sporadically. Other cases are thought to be inherited as an autosomal dominant genetic trait.

☞**MULTIPLE EPIPHYSEAL DYSPLASIA:** A very rare genetic disorder characterized by irregular epiphyseal growth, skeletal deformities, short limb dwarfism, pain and stiffness of affected joints. There are two types of MED, a mild form or Ribbing type, and a severe form or Fairbank type. In the mild form, the hands and wrists are usually normal, whereas in the severe form, the hands and feet are short and stubby.

REFERENCE:

Khungar A, Mahajan P, Gupte G, et al: Pseudoachondroplastic dysplasia. *J Postgrad Med* 39:91, 1993.

Pseudohypoparathyroidism

At a glance: A very rare disorder characterized by renal and/or bony anomalies caused by their insensitivity to parathyroid hormone.

Classification: Pseudohypoparathyroidism (PHP) is a group of diseases in which target cells (renal tubular or osseous) are insensitive to parathyroid hormone.

Type I (PHP I) is caused by the inability of parathyroid hormone to activate renal cell adenylcyclase.

Type Ia (☞Albright Hereditary Osteodystrophy) is the most frequent, is because of a defect in the α subunit of the membrane-bound stimulatory G protein.

Type Ib (PHP IB) is probably caused by abnormalities at the parathyroid hormone receptor.

Type II (PHP II) is because of the inability of cAMP to initiate the metabolic events caused by stimulation of the parathyroid hormone receptor.

Genetic inheritance: PHP type Ia and pseudopseudohypoparathyroidism are caused by heterogenous mutations in the Gsα encoding exons of GNAS1 (chromosome 20q13.3); PHP type Ia occurs only if the mutation is inherited from a female carrier.

Pseudopseudohypoparathyroidism occurs if the mutation is inherited from a male carrier. *PHP type Ib* has the same pattern of inheritance as is observed as for PHP type Ia but the mutation has not been identified yet.

Pathophysiology: The skeletal and developmental features of type Ia are those of the classic Albright hereditary osteodystrophy. Because the stimulatory G protein involved in type Ia is required for responsiveness to other hormones, hypothyroidism and gonadal dysfunction are common in this type of PHP.

Diagnosis: Hypocalcemia, hyperphosphatemia, and elevated parathyroid hormone levels.

Clinical aspects: Children with PHP type Ia present with the classic Albright hereditary osteodystrophy appearance: small stature with moderate obesity, mild mental deficiency, rounded face with short neck, dental aplasia or enamel dysplasia, and subcapsular cataracts. Radiography shows osteoporosis, short metacarpal bones, and cone-shaped epiphyses. Cervical vertebral anomalies may be present. Cutaneous or subcutaneous calcifications. Hypocalcemia, which usually develops in the first years of life, may lead to tetany, muscle cramps, or seizures. Children with PHP types Ib and II have a normal physical appearance. PHP type I or II is treated with vitamin D and oral phosphate binders. Spontaneous amelioration of hypocalcemia may occur with time.

Precautions before anesthesia: Check calcium and phosphate blood levels and correct them as required; in a case of PHP type Ia, assess the presence of other endocrinopathies (mainly hypothyroidism).

Anesthetic considerations: Hypocalcemia may lead to prolonged QT, tetany, and laryngospasm. Hyperventilation should be avoided.

In type Ia, obesity may make venous access, mask ventilation, and laryngoscopy difficult.

Pharmacological implications: Beware of hypocalcemia if there is rapid administration of blood or fresh-frozen plasma.

Other conditions to be considered:

    PSEUDOPSEUDOHYPOPARATHYROIDISM: The patient has the phenotype of Albright hereditary osteodystrophy but has normal calcium and phosphate levels. It represents a variant of PHP type Ia.

    PSEUDOHYPOHYPERPARATHYROIDISM: Resistance to parathyroid hormone is limited to the renal tubules; the bony response to elevated parathyroid hormone levels is thus normal, leading to subperiosteal resorption and osteitis fibrosa cystica.

REFERENCES:

Breslau NA: Pseudohypoparathyroidism: Current concepts. *Am J Med Sci* 298:130, 1989.

Wilson LC, Trembath RC: Albright's hereditary osteodystrophy. *J Med Genet* 31:779, 1994.

Pterygium Syndrome

At a glance: Association of multiple pterygia with facial anomalies, and orthopedic and genitourinary malformations. It is characterized by short stature, webbing of the neck, antecubital, digital, popliteal, and intercural areas. Joint contractures, vertebral fusion defects, and rocker-bottom feet are usually associated.

Synonyms: Multiple Pterygium Syndrome; Escobar Syndrome; Pterygium Universale; Pterygium Colli Syndrome.

History: First described in 1978 by V. Escobar, an American physician.

Incidence: Remains unknown; however, several cases have been described.

Genetic inheritance: Autosomal recessive inheritance in many cases, autosomal dominant determination in others. Some cases have been reported as sporadic occurrence.

Pathophysiology: Neuromuscular disorder has been evocated as underlying pathogenesis of this disease.

Diagnosis: On the association of multiple pterygia, syndactyly, cleft palate, and micrognathia.

Clinical aspects: Facial anomalies are frequent (severe micro- or retrognathia, ptosis, telecanthus, microcephaly, spoonlike shape of the tongue (lingua cochlearis), cleft hard palate, ankyloglossia, deafness), normal intelligence, cardiac defect can be present, muscle weakness, myopathy, multiple orthopedic modifications (scoliosis, symphalangy, webbed neck, webbing of joints, talipes varus/valgus, syndactyly of fingers, short stature, vertebral segmentation abnormality and fusion), genitourinary tract malformation, and occasional diaphragmatic hernia. Joint contractures and rocker-bottom feet are frequently seen.

Precautions before anesthesia: Evaluate carefully the airway (clinical, radiograph, and even endoscopy) because of facial anomalies and webbed neck. Evaluate pulmonary function (chest radiograph, pulmonary function test, arterial blood gas analysis) because of the high rate of restrictive lung disease that is observed. Search for congenital heart defect or cardiomyopathy (clinical, echography). Laboratory test should include creatine phosphokinase because of the association in one case of malignant hyperthermia (no certitude).

Anesthetic considerations: There is a high rate of tracheal intubation difficulties because of anatomical status; laryngeal mask airways have been successfully used. Fiberoptic intubation can be useful. Caution with intraoperative patient positioning (pterygia, fixed joints). Close perioperative respiratory observation in case of respiratory insufficiency. Perimedullar anesthesia is not contraindicated but could be difficult to perform because of vertebral fusion and kyphoscoliosis. In presence of cardiac defects, the anesthetic management should be tailored according.

Pharmacological implications: Antibiotic prophylaxis in case of cardiac anomalies. Avoid succinylcholine (joint contractures, malignant hyperthermia status not clear). Muscle relaxant should be used with careful monitoring (muscle weakness, myopathy) and only after airway is secured. Postoperative opioids are not contraindicated but should be used with care in patients with respiratory insufficiency and spontaneous breathing.

Other conditions to be considered:

MULTIPLE PTERYGIUM SYNDROME, LETHAL TYPE: Autosomal recessive as well as an X-linked form (multiple pterygia, dysmorphic facies, hypoplastic lungs, hypoplastic heart, jugular lymphatic obstruction sequence, generalized amyoplasia).

POPLITEAL PTERYGIUM SYNDROME (Faciogenital Popliteal Syndrome): Autosomal dominant (cleft lip/palate, paramedian mucous cysts of the lower lip, popliteal pterygium, digital and genital anomalies).

POPLITEAL PTERYGIUM SYNDROME, LETHAL TYPE: Autosomal recessive (Bartsocas-Papas syndrome) with cleft lip, neonatal/infantile death, and severe limb malformation;

PTERYGIA MENTAL RETARDATION FACIAL DYSMORPHISM (Haspeslagh Fryns Muelenaere Syndrome): Autosomal dominant with multiple pterygia, trigonocephaly, bulging forehead, muscle agenesis, mental retardation, and congenital cardiac anomaly.

☞**KHALIFA GRAHAM SYNDROME:** X-linked dominant versus autosomal dominant (pterygium colli, mental retardation, edema of the dorsum of hands and feet, proximally displaced small thumbs, widened interphalangeal joints, broad terminal phalanges, webbed neck).

PTERYGIUM SYNDROME ANTECUBITAL: Autosomal dominant, antecubital posterior subluxation of radial head ulnar and radius absent/abnormal, maldevelopment of radioulnar joint, limited elbow extension webbing.

REFERENCES:

Fryns JP, Moerman P: Popliteal pterygium and multiple pterygium syndromes. *Am J Med Genet* 100:81, 2001.

Kuzma PJ, Calkins MD, Kline MD, et al: The anesthetic management of patients with multiple pterygium syndrome. *Anesth Analg* 83:430, 1996.

Pulmonary Alveolar Microlithiasis

At a glance: Pulmonary Alveolar Microlithiasis (PAM) is characterized by deposition of calcium phosphate within the alveolar airspaces (calcospherites).

Incidence: Approximately 300 patients with this disorder have been reported worldwide.

Genetic inheritance: The high rate of familial occurrence ($>50\%$) led to the suggestion of an inborn error of metabolism with autosomal recessive transmission.

Pathophysiology: Mechanism or cause unknown. Microliths or calcospherites are intraalveolar and interstitial deposits of calcified granules with a diameter of 0.05 to 3.0 mm, consisting of laminated calcium and phosphate complexes in a ratio similar to hydroxyapatite in bone. Groups of multinucleated osteoclast-like macrophages surround the microliths, which are sometimes completely embedded in woven bone or lamellar structured bone containing osteocytes. Apoptotic bodies can be found in the nuclear chromatin and cytoplasm of modified type II alveolar pneumocytes. Microliths seem to act like autologous osteoconductive material when implanted in pulmonary parenchyma and serve as a substrate on which bone can easily be formed. PAM has also been described in association with mitral stenosis; however, the microliths are more uneven and bosselated. Interstitial pulmonary fibrosis is common and pulmonary arterial hypertension may develop.

Diagnosis: The radiographic appearance with apical bullae and diffuse micronodular shadows (representing multiple minute calcifications located in the alveoli) is pathognomonic and results in a "sandstorm" or "snowstorm" picture in the chest radiograph. Most of the lesions occur in the posterior part of the lung bases. Heart border and diaphragm often appear obliterated. Bronchoalveolar lavage, transbronchial or open lung biopsy, or sputum analysis are used to confirm the diagnosis. The discrepancy between impressive radiological findings and the lack of clinical symptoms can be striking.

Clinical aspects: Children with the disease are usually asymptomatic or present either with chronic cough or gradually decreasing exercise tolerance. The physical examination is usually unremarkable. The disease has already been described in premature twins; however, the reduction in pulmonary function usually starts in adulthood and progresses until death results from pulmonary failure in early or mid-adult life. Hitherto, no effective therapy exists to stop the relentless course toward progressive respiratory failure. Lung transplantation may be an option for those with end-stage disease. Until then, inotropic and diuretic drugs, as well as oxygen, are administered for symptomatic relief.

Precautions before anesthesia: Evaluation of respiratory function should include a chest radiograph and pulmonary function tests. An arterial blood gas analysis is recommended. Appropriate antibiotic therapy and chest physiotherapy may be required for respiratory tract infections. Assess cardiac function including ECG and echocardiography for signs of pulmonary hypertension and right-ventricle stains. Look for evidence of cor pulmonale and optimize cardiac function where possible (diuretics, vasodilators). Laboratory investigations should include a cell blood count, electrolytes, blood urea nitrogen, and creatinine. Sedative premedication should be avoided in the presence of significant respiratory impairment. Postoperative respiratory support may be required and should be arranged preoperatively.

Anesthetic considerations: There are no special considerations for patients with a mild form of the disease. However, patients with significant respiratory impairment and concomitant pulmonary arterial hypertension and cor pulmonale have a high anesthetic risk. The extent of invasive monitoring should be determined by the planned procedure and the presence and severity of the underlying cardiac and respiratory dysfunction. Chronically cyanotic patients are often polycythemic and may present with coagulation disorders. Phlebotomy and hemodilution may be beneficial. A ventilator appropriate for patients with severe forms of lung disease should be available (adjustable respiratory-cycle waveforms, high levels of positive end-expiratory pressure, etc.). High airway pressure, acidosis, hypercapnia, and hypoxia should all be avoided (pulmonary arterial hypertension). A respiration rate higher than normal with reduced tidal volumes may be necessary to succeed. Regional anesthesia techniques should be preferred whenever appropriate, either alone or in conjunction with general anesthesia, because good analgesia permits optimal postoperative chest physiotherapy.

Pharmacological implications: Caution should be exercised with the use of opioids and benzodiazepines if respiratory function is compromised.

Other condition to be considered:

☞**PULMONARY ALVEOLAR PROTEINOSIS:** In this disorder, the alveoli are filled with periodic acid–Schiff (PAS)-positive proteinaceous material that is chemically similar to surfactant. Major anesthetic implications.

REFERENCES:

Barbolini G, Rossi G, Bisetti A: Pulmonary alveolar microlithiasis. *N Engl J Med* 347:69, 2002.

Edelman JD, Bavaria J, Kaiser LR, et al: Bilateral sequential lung transplantation for pulmonary alveolar microlithiasis. *Chest* 112:1140, 1997.

Volle E, Kaufmann HJ: Pulmonary alveolar microlithiasis in pediatric patients—Review of the world literature and two new observations. *Pediatr Radiol* 17:439, 1987.

Pulmonary Alveolar Proteinosis

At a glance: In this disorder, the alveoli are filled with periodic acid–Schiff (PAS)-positive proteinaceous material that is chemically similar to surfactant. Significant respiratory problems leading to severe hypoxemia, recurrent pulmonary infections, and cardiac problems.

Synonyms: Alveolar Lipoproteinosis; Alveolar Phospholipidosis; Pulmonary Alveolar Phospholipoproteinosis.

History: First described in 1958. Two forms were recognized: (1) primary or idiopathic and (2) secondary to lung infections, hematologic malignancies, inflammation from mineral dusts such as silica, titanium oxide, aluminum, and insecticides.

Incidence: Approximately 410 patients have been described. In the United States, the estimated prevalence is established at 1 case per 100,000. Mortality rates can be as high as 30% in the secondary PAP form, depending on the underlying cause is less than 10% in the primary form. There is a male predominance (2.6:1) in adults, but not in children.

Genetic inheritance: The congenital form seems to be transmitted in an autosomal recessive way and the mutation most commonly responsible is a frameshift mutation in the surfactant protein B (SP-B) gene and maps to 22q12.2-q13.1. The late-onset form is usually idiopathic or associated with lymphoproliferative disorders or infection (HIV, tuberculosis). The male:female ratio is 3:1.

Pathophysiology: The cause of the congenital form of pulmonary alveolar proteinosis could be an inborn error of surfactant metabolism. There is evidence that the disease is caused by a mutation in pulmonary surfactant–associated protein-B (SP-B), resulting in deficiency or absence of this protein, which is also involved in the formation of tubular myelin (surfactant is initially stored in lamellar bodies after its synthesis, to then be secreted as tubular myelin, which is required to form the surfactant film in the alveoli). Another theory focuses on a congenital or acquired defect in the β chain of the GM-CSF (granulocyte-macrophage colony-stimulating factor) receptor (this β chain is common to GM-CSF-2-RB [granulocyte-macrophage colony-stimulating factor receptor beta], CSF-2-, interleukin-3-, and interleukin-5-receptors). This results in defective activation of alveolar macrophages by GM-CSF and decreased local recycling of surfactant proteins. The net result is an imbalance in the homeostasis between production of surfactant and its clearance by alveolar macrophages and the mucociliary elevator.

Diagnosis: Confirmed by bronchoalveolar lavage and/or lung biopsy that shows alveoli filled with PAS-positive proteinaceous material. The bronchoalveolar lavage material looks cloudy or milky and the cytologic examination shows foamy macrophages, reactive pulmonary pneumocytes, and cholesterol crystals. The alveolar architecture and intralobular septae are usually well preserved and the conductive airways unaffected. The congenital form is characterized by absent surfactant protein B. The chest radiograph shows bilateral pulmonary infiltrates (ground-glass aspect) with hilar prominence (bat-wing shape) and progression to fibrosis and a "honeycomb" appearance.

Clinical aspects: *Neonatal-onset form:* The neonate presents with acute respiratory distress with marked hypoxemia shortly after birth. Initially, the symptoms are indistinguishable from hyaline membrane disease (neonatal respiratory distress syndrome). Slow resolution of the initial illness, pneumonia, or persistence of atelectases result in prolonged ventilator dependence. All reported infants with congenital alveolar proteinosis died within the first year of life despite maximal medical therapy. Administration of GM-CSF or exogenous surfactant does not influence outcome.

Later-onset form: Onset is insidious with mild cough and progressive dyspnea (shortness of breath initially on exertion only). Symptoms of upper respiratory tract infection occur more and more frequently and may be associated with dyspnea, cyanosis, and finger clubbing. The median age at onset is 4 months (range: 2 months to 7 years). The chances of survival are higher in these children, but they often require treatment with repeated whole-lung lavage. Prolonged oxygen dependence, dyspnea, chronic cough, and failure to gain weight are other symptoms. Almost two-thirds of the patients who survive show ongoing symptoms of dyspnea, wheezing, cough, and chest pain. Administration of GM-CSF has no effect in the congenital forms of pulmonary alveolar proteinosis. In these cases, alveolar proteinosis is a nonspecific injury pattern caused by or associated with intolerance to dibasic proteins (anomaly of the metabolism of arginine, lysine, and ornithine), altered cellular immunity (congenital or acquired), underlying malignancy (mainly acute myeloid leukemia and lymphoma), opportunistic infections (*Pneumocystis carinii*, *Histoplasma*, *Nocardia*, fungus), or sideroblastic anemia. Often, these children have poor appetite and delayed weight and height gain. Although not common, a pneumothorax should always be excluded when an acute exacerbation of these patients occurs. The only effective treatment is lung transplantation; however, a few case reports of recurrence of pulmonary alveolar proteinosis in the graft exist.

Adult form: Pulmonary alveolar proteinosis in adults typically presents between 20 and 50 years of age (mean: 39 years for males, 35 years for females) with dyspnea and cough, and can be caused by industrial exposure to mineral dusts (e.g., cement dust, aluminum dust, titanium dioxide, nitrogen dioxide), fibrous insulation material, or silicone dioxide. Smoking is common in these patients and physical examination is usually otherwise normal with nonspecific laboratory findings. Lung function tests reveal the restrictive pneumopathy with a decrease in lung volumes, compliance, and diffusing capacity. The chest radiograph shows an alveolar infiltration pattern. The risk for pulmonary infections is increased. Spontaneous resolution of the disease occurs in 30% of patients. Half of the remaining group needs whole-lung lavage (usually only one) to relieve their symptoms (shortness of breath, severe hypoxemia, intractable cough), while the other half suffers from progressive disease with pulmonary fibrosis despite maximal medical treatment including whole-lung lavage. Hypoxia may be severe and result in clinical and ECG evidence of cor pulmonale. Subcutaneous administration of GM-CSF has been tried with some success in up to 50% of the patients. Up to 80% of adults report a mild, usually dry, cough and dyspnea.

Precautions before anesthesia: Baseline lung function tests, chest radiograph, and arterial blood gas analysis should be obtained. Cyanotic patients are often polycythemic.

Anesthetic considerations: Preoxygenation is mandatory, as the risk of hypoxemia during induction of anesthesia is significant (decreased functional residual capacity and increased intrapulmonary shunt). An arterial line is placed, preferably prior to induction. Appropriate antibiotic therapy and chest physiotherapy may be required for intercurrent respiratory tract infection. Most often these patients present for whole-lung lavage and require single-lung ventilation. The operating room temperature and the irrigating fluids should be kept warm.

Pharmacological implications: Extreme care must be exercised with the use of benzodiazepines and opioids.

REFERENCES:

Lippmann M, Mok MS: Anesthetic management of pulmonary lavage in adults. *Anesth Analg* 56:661, 1977.

Seymour JF, Presneill JJ: Pulmonary alveolar proteinosis. Progress in the first 44 years. *Am J Respir Crit Care Med* 166:215, 2002.

Troje C, Mounsaveng S, Dubois MC, et al: Therapeutic bronchoalveolar lavage for pulmonary alveolar proteinosis in an infant. *Paediatr Anaesth* 4:123, 1994.

Vazquez-Fidalgo AM, Vazquez-Perez MJ, Baldomir-Pan E, et al: Massive bronchial lavage under general anesthesia in pulmonary alveolar proteinosis. *Rev Esp Anestesiol Reanim* 44(8):336, 1999.

Pulmonary Arteriovenous Malformation

At a glance: Pulmonary Arteriovenous Malformation (PAVM) is a direct communication between branches of the pulmonary arterial and venous vessels representing right-to-left shunting and therefore not participating in pulmonary gas exchange. Usually congenital (70% are associated with Osler-Rendu-Weber Disease), less commonly acquired (hepatic cirrhosis, mitral stenosis, trauma, actinomycosis, Fanconi Syndrome).

Synonym: Pulmonary Arteriovenous Fistula; PAVM; Rendu-Osler-Weber Syndrome; Osler's disease.

History: First described in 1896 by Henry Jules Rendu after his description of telangiectasia and epistaxis. Sir William Osler reported a family known to have hereditary hemorrhagic telangiectasia in 1897. In 1907, Federick Weber described the other manifestations.

Incidence: Unknown, but very rare. Approximately 10% of the cases are identified during infancy and childhood, with a gradual increase through the fifth and sixth decades. Only about 20 cases have been described in neonates. Frequency in United States, 1:39,216 persons. In some regions of France, 1:2351 persons has been reported.

Genetic inheritance: Unknown. Male predominance during the neonatal period, but female preponderance (2:1) in adults.

Pathophysiology: The exact pathogenesis of PAVM still unknown. Pulmonary lesions function as right-to-left shunts and may cause hypoxemia or paradoxical embolization. Histologically, there is endothelial and smooth-muscle cell degeneration, defects in the endothelial junctions, and weakness of the perivascular connective tissue. Weakness of the vessel walls may predispose to hemorrhage despite normal coagulation and platelet functions. Autopsy results show that 75% of patients had unilateral disease, 35% had multiple lesions, and about half of the latter had bilateral lesions. The PAVM can be classified as simple (those with a single feeding segmental artery and a single draining vein) and complex (two or more feeding arteries or veins). The pulmonary artery pressure is normal or low in nearly all patients with PAVM.

Diagnosis: The diagnosis is usually suspected from the clinical history. The classical radiological sign on a chest radiograph is that of a round or oval mass of uniform density, frequently lobulated, but sharply defined, found most often in the lower lobes. Shunt fraction measurement in 100% oxygen is a sensitive and reasonably specific diagnostic test for PAVM. The presence of a PAVM can be further evaluated via contrast echocardiography, radionuclide perfusion lung scan, 3D helical CT scan, or MRI. However, pulmonary angiography remains the standard criterion in the diagnosis of PAVM.

Clinical aspects: Symptoms vary from being totally asymptomatic to severe with presentation in childhood with cyanosis and shortness of breath on exertion, congestive heart failure, or respiratory failure. Murmurs or bruits over the site of the PAVM may be present in half the patients and louder during inspiration. Increased FiO_2 (fraction of inspired oxygen) may not significantly improve oxygenation. Secondary polycythemia is present and the degree depends on the severity of cyanosis. The condition is associated with hereditary hemorrhagic telangiectasia (Rendu-Osler-Weber syndrome) in 60 to 70% of patients; conversely, 15 to 30% of patients with hereditary hemorrhagic telangiectasia have PAVM. Hemoptysis from rupture of the lesions may occur. Thrombosis may occur within the fistula with systemic embolization leading to neurological complications (transient ischemic attacks, hemiplegia, brain abscesses, or seizures) in about one-third of the patients. Hemothorax and/or hemoptysis are often lethal complications of arteriovenous fistulae. Because mortality is high in symptomatic patients, surgical resection of the involved lung segment is often performed. However, embolotherapy based on occlusion of the feeding arteries of the PAVM is currently the treatment of choice.

Precautions before anesthesia: Evaluate the site and involvement of the pulmonary arteriovenous fistula, including chest radiograph, CT scan, and/or MRI of the thorax. Pulmonary angiography enables visualization of the lesions and guides surgical or radiological management. Exclude concomitant cerebral arteriovenous malformation or abscess by neuroimaging studies. Check cardiac function and look for signs of high-output congestive heart failure, because a big PAVM may lead to increased cardiac output. Laboratory investigations should include a CBC and arterial blood gas analysis.

Anesthetic considerations: Systemic desaturation from intrapulmonary shunt is little influenced by supplemental oxygen therapy. Cardiac output should be maintained to avoid further desaturation. Nasal intubation and insertion of a nasogastric tube carry a high risk of bleeding in hereditary hemorrhagic telangiectasia patients and should be avoided. Maneuvers that reduce blood flow through the fistula improve oxygenation (fistula in nondependent position, avoidance of positive end-expiratory pressure, lowering of pulmonary vascular resistance). Venous lines should be meticulously checked and cleared from air bubbles to prevent systemic embolization. Polycythemia may result in neurologic deficits and should be controlled perioperatively. Tracheal intubation should be performed with care to prevent bleeding from telangiectatic airway lesions. Blood loss may be considerable during resection of the PAVM; therefore large-bore intravenous access and replacement blood should be available. Lung separation via a double-lumen tube or bronchial blocker should be used to protect the dependent lung from possible endobronchial bleeding.

Pharmacological implications: There are no known pharmacological implications.

Other condition to be considered:

☞**HEREDITARY TELANGIECTASIA:** Autosomal dominant transmitted mucocutaneous and visceral fibrovascular dysplasia with telangiectasia, arteriovenous malformations, and aneurysms, often widely distributed throughout the cardiovascular system. It is usually recognized as a "triad" of telangiectasia, recurrent epistaxis, and a family history of the disorder.

REFERENCES:

Alfirevic AJ, Mossad E, Niezgoda J: Unexpected ST segment changes in children—a case report. *Paediatr Anesth* 15:63, 2005.

Gossage JR, Kanj G: Pulmonary arteriovenous malformations. A state-of-the-art review. *Am J Respir Crit Care Med* 158:643, 1998.

Pulmonary Hypoplasia

At a glance: Failure of the lung to develop to its normal size. Primary isolated pulmonary hypoplasia is rare. Secondary pulmonary hypoplasia is more common and occurs in association with congenital diaphragmatic hernia, oligohydramnios (mostly related to renal dysfunction), skeletal dysplasias, fetal hydrops, malformations of the central nervous system, and neuromuscular diseases.

Incidence: Isolated primary pulmonary hypoplasia is very rare. However, conditions such as congenital diaphragmatic hernia are more common and inevitably associated with pulmonary hypoplasia.

Genetic inheritance: Possibility of autosomal recessive transmission in the isolated form has been described.

Pathophysiology: There is a decrease in lung volume and weight and there is a commensurate decrease in pulmonary function. Microscopic examination may reveal absent or reduced development of the lungs with a deficit in any combination of tubular bronchioles, acini, or alveoli, incapable of significant gas exchange or reduced airway generation, with fewer and smaller alveoli.

Diagnosis: Based on measurement of lung volumes (e.g., whole-body plethysmography or inert gas dilution method) and the exclusion of other pathologies that may cause tachypnea. Oligohydramnios is a well-known risk factor. Chest CT scan or ante- and postnatal MRI are presently the diagnostic tools of choice.

Clinical aspects: The symptoms depend on the severity of the hypoplasia. Pulmonary hypoplasia is a (milder) form of pulmonary agenesis and can occur unilaterally or bilaterally. Whereas unilateral pulmonary hypoplasia has the same frequency for each side, left-sided lesions have a much better prognosis. Secondary pulmonary hypoplasia describes a decrease in intrathoracic volume as a result of extrathoracic compression (e.g., oligohydramnios secondary to renal agenesis or dysplasia, congenital thoracic or skeletal dysplasia causing thoracic constriction and leading to limited lung development with bilateral pulmonary hypoplasia) or intrathoracic compression (e.g., congenital diaphragmatic hernia, polycystic kidney disease [secondary to the large abdominal mass], tumors, congenital cystic adenomatoid malformation, or large pleural effusions). Furthermore, there is an association with malformations of the central nervous system (e.g., anencephaly) and neuromuscular diseases (affecting respiratory muscles/diaphragm). In a few cases, abnormalities of the face (hemifacial microsomia, dysplastic ears, torticollis) or jaw (unilateral mandibulofacial dysostosis) ipsilateral to the side of the pulmonary lesion (if unilateral) have been described. Anomalies of the extremities (in the majority of cases, the arm ipsilateral to the lesion) are not uncommon and include ulnar, radial, and thumb anomalies. Thoracic asymmetry may be associated with vertebral anomalies. The diaphragm may be high riding on the affected side, but in contrast to hemidiaphragmatic paralysis, it is not paralyzed and functions normally. Unilateral pulmonary hypoplasia must be differentiated from other conditions potentially resulting in mediastinal shift, such as cystic adenomatoid malformation, diaphragmatic hernia, or bronchopulmonary sequestration.

Precautions before anesthesia: The presence of other associated anomalies should be excluded and the involved system assessed. Facial dysmorphism and jaw anomalies may result in difficult airway management and make preoperative airway assessment mandatory. Laboratory investigations should include a complete blood cell count and arterial blood gas analysis. A preoperative chest radiograph is strongly recommended and echocardiography should be performed to rule out any coexisting congenital cardiac lesions. Postoperative mechanical ventilatory support is almost always required and arrangements for it should be made in advance.

Anesthetic considerations: The anesthetic management depends on the severity of the pulmonary hypoplasia and on any other significant malformations present. Intermittent positive-pressure ventilation should be used with caution because the compliance of the hypoplastic lung is poor and the risk of barotrauma is high with the use of positive pressure. Always keep in mind that sudden hemodynamic signs of cardiovascular collapse can be associated with a pneumothorax under tension. Pulmonary hypertension is common and nitric oxide therapy has been successfully used in some cases. Acidosis, hypercarbia, and hypoxia should all be avoided because they increase pulmonary vascular resistance further. Gas exchange is impaired as a result of the reduced surface area of the lung, requiring a high respiration rate with lower tidal volumes. While low levels of positive end-expiratory pressure may be beneficial, high positive end-expiratory pressure values should be avoided since this can easily result in increased pulmonary vascular resistance.

Pharmacological implications: These are dictated by the cause of lung hypoplasia. Nitrous oxide should be avoided in the presence of marked pulmonary hypertension; the influence of ketamine is still controversial.

Other conditions to be considered:

☞**JEUNE SYNDROME:** A rare form of chondrodysplasia that often leads to death in infancy from respiratory insufficiency as a consequence of severe thoracic restrictive deformation. Common association with multiple skeletal malformations, liver, renal, and retinal dysfunction.

☞**OSTEOGENESIS IMPERFECTA:** An autosomal dominant disorder with multiple bone fractures (post- and antenatal). Four major types have been described and type I is the one most frequently encountered in anesthesia. Multiple anesthetic implications (position, intubation, cardiac, and respiratory failure).

☞**PENA-SHOKEIR SYNDROME, TYPE I:** An autosomal recessive syndrome characterized by multiple ankyloses, camptodactyly, facial abnormalities, pulmonary hypoplasia, and short-bowel syndrome. Neurologic involvement includes hydrocephalus, microgyria, and cerebellar hypoplasia.

☞**THANATOPHORIC DWARFISM:** A severe form of micromelic dwarfism with narrow thorax. Death generally occurs in the first hours of life.

REFERENCES:

Frey B, Fleischhauer A, Gersbach M: Familial isolated pulmonary hypoplasia: A case report, suggesting autosomal recessive inheritance. *Eur J Pediatr* 153:460, 1994.

Guruswamy V, Roberts S, Arnold P, et al: Anaesthetic management of a neonate with congenital cyst adenoid malformation. *Br J Anaesth* 95:240, 2005.

Langer R, Kaufmann HJ: Primary (isolated) bilateral pulmonary hypoplasia: A comparative study of radiologic findings and autopsy results. *Pediatr Radiol* 16:175, 1986.

Purine Nucleoside Phosphorylase Deficiency

At a glance: Inherited disease of the purine catabolism resulting in deficient T-cell immunity, and often in neurologic symptoms as well.

Incidence: Fewer than 50 patients have been described.

Genetic inheritance: Autosomal recessive, which explains the increased risk in consanguineous parents. The mutation has been mapped to 14q13.1.

Pathophysiology: Purine nucleoside phosphorylase (PNP) is a protein trimer of approximately 90 kDa and present in almost all tissues, but the highest concentration is found in lymphoid tissues. This fact explains why PNP deficiency predominantly affects the lymphatic system. The enzyme is part of the purine salvage pathway and required to catalyze the degradation of (deoxy)inosine and (deoxy)guanosine to hypoxanthine and guanine and, finally, to uric acid. The lack of PNP results in accumulation of deoxyguanosine and deoxyinosine, predominantly in lymphocytes. These two compounds block the enzyme ribonucleotide reductase in T cells, which is used for DNA synthesis (deoxynucleotides), thereby inhibiting the normal T-cell proliferation required for an appropriate immune response. This manifests as defective T-cell immunity and as some degree of B-cell dysfunction.

Diagnosis: The combination of neurological defects or recurrent viral infections with undetectable, or extremely low, blood and urine concentrations of uric acid in a child is suggestive of PNP deficiency. In these patients, normally extremely low or even undetectable plasma concentrations of inosine, guanosine, deoxyinosine, and deoxyguanosine are grossly elevated and the same compounds are excreted in excessive amounts in the urine. In severe cases,

markedly decreased or even undetectable serum levels of uric acid have been found. The finding of decreased PNP activity in erythrocytes, lymphocytes, or fibroblasts finally confirms the diagnosis. Although heterozygotes show intermediate levels of PNP activity, they appear clinically normal. T-cell function may be normal at birth, but then decreases progressively, although T-cell function may vary to some degree through time.

The thymus is significantly reduced in size and histologic examination reveals depletion of thymocytes. In contrast to severe combined immunodeficiency syndrome, Hassall corpuscles in the thymus are present, but they are not well defined. Lymphoid tissue examination shows abnormalities predominantly in T-cell–dependent areas (paracortical zone). Prenatal diagnosis is possible.

Clinical aspects: Generally, neurologic symptoms or recurrent or severe viral (e.g., varicella, measles), but also bacterial, fungal (oral candidiasis), mycobacterial, or protozoal infections, with potentially fatal outcome start between the ages of 1 and 5 years. However, symptoms may already occur in the first months of life and include irritability, failure to thrive, hypotonia, lymphopenia, and deficient T-cell–mediated immunity. The B-cell count may be low; however, immunoglobulin levels are often normal, although they may also be decreased or even elevated. About two-thirds of the patients show neurologic symptoms (mental retardation, spastic para- or tetraparesis, ataxia, and tremor). There is an increased incidence of autoimmune hemolytic anemia (in about one-third of the patients) or immune thrombocytopenia, neutropenia, thyroiditis, systemic lupus erythematosus, and B-cell lymphoma. Graft-versus-host disease has been observed in undiagnosed patients receiving transfusion of nonirradiated blood. Immunization with live vaccines in children prior to their diagnosis may result in severe infections. PNP deficiency also is associated with neurologic symptoms, including mental retardation and muscle spasticity, in 67% of patients. Intermittent blood transfusions may be required to supply adequate exogenous enzyme activity. Bone marrow transplantation has been used successfully to cure the immunologic defect in some patients, but does not improve the neurological symptoms. No other satisfactory therapy has yet been found. Severely affected patients invariably die within the first 5 years of life. Long-term survivors show residual PNP activity and only mild or no neurological involvement.

Precautions before anesthesia: Obtain a CBC (anemia in 30%, thrombo- and neutropenia). Blood cells have to be irradiated prior to transfusion to prevent graft-versus-host disease. This also applies for patients after bone marrow transplantation until they have engrafted. Some patients with mental retardation are better off with sedative or anxiolytic premedication.

Anesthetic considerations: Strict aseptic technique is mandatory in the care for these patients. Spasticity may make positioning and vascular access challenging.

Pharmacological implications: Vaccination with attenuated, living viruses must be avoided, because these patients may otherwise suffer from a severe infection.

Other conditions to be considered:

☞**ADENOSINE DEAMINASE DEFICIENCY:** A heterogeneous and systemic disorder caused by the deficiency of adenosine deaminase resulting primarily in severe combined (cellar and humoral) immunodeficiency, but also systemic abnormalities.

☞**NEZELOF SYNDROME:** A genetic form of hypoplasia of the thymus resulting in a lack of competent T cells. It may also include some abnormalities in humoral immunity (i.e., affecting B lymphocytes).

☞**DiGeorge Syndrome** is a genetic defect leading to a wide range of phenotypic presentations, mainly developmental defects in the outflow tract of the heart, hypoparathyroidism with hypocalcemia, and thymic hypoplasia or aplasia with immune defects.

REFERENCES:

Baguette C, Vermylen C, Brichard B, et al: Persistent developmental delay despite successful bone marrow transplantation for purine nucleoside phosphorylase deficiency. *J Pediatr Hematol Oncol* 24:69, 2002.

van den Berghe G, Vincent MF, Marie S: Disorders of purine and pyrimidine metabolism, in Fernandes J, Saudubray J-M, Van den Berghe G (eds): *Inborn Metabolic Diseases*. 3rd ed. Berlin, Springer-Verlag, 2000, p 354.

Purtscher Disease

At a glance: This is an acquired form of retinopathy associated with a variety of thromboembolic events. It is the consequence of hemorrhagic and vasoocclusive vasculopathy.

Synonym: Purtscher Angiopathic Retinopathy.

History: First described in 1910 by O. Purtscher as a syndrome of sudden blindness associated with seveve head trauma. These patients presented with multiple white retinal patches and retinal hemorrhages associated with seveve vision loss.

Incidence and genetic Inheritance: There is no reported incidence. Variable depending on the underlying pathology. Acquired disease.

Clinical aspects: The clinical findings have traditionally been associated with severe crush injuries. However, Purtscher retinopathy has also been reported in association with pancreatitis, thrombocytopenic purpura, hemolytic uremic syndrome, systemic lupus erythematosus, dermatomyositis, scleroderma, and amniotic fluid embolism. The ophthalmoscopic findings associated with this syndrome are peripapillary cotton-wool spots, intraretinal hemorrhages, asymmetrical venous engorgement, and retinal whitening. Obviously, the circumstances in which Purtscher retinopathy develops determine the whole clinical picture.

Anesthetic considerations: The anesthetic management needs to take into consideration the different causes of the underlying pathology. To avoid sudden increases in intraocular pressure, medication susceptible to affect it such as succinylcholine and ketamine should be avoided if possible. Moderate hyperventilation can contribute to reduce intraocular pressure.

REFERENCE:

Power MH, Regillo CD, Custis PH: Thrombocytopenic purpura associated with Purtscher's retinopathy. *Arch Ophthalmol* 115:128, 1997.

Pyknodysostosis

At a glance: Dwarfism with osteosclerosis. Congenital sclerosing osteodysplasia.

Synonym: Toulouse-Lautrec Disease.

History: The disease is named after the French painter Henri de Toulouse-Lautrec, since Maroteaux and Lamy, the first describers of pyknodysostosis, concluded from complaints found in letters to his friends and relatives that he was suffering from pyknodysostosis, although this has been the subject of vivid debate.

NB: Some authors consider pyknodysostosis synonymous with Maroteaux-Lamy Syndrome. Although it is true that these two French physicians were the first to describe and name pyknodysostosis, the name Maroteaux-Lamy Syndrome (which is used for at least four different syndromes) most often refers to mucopolysaccharidosis type VI.

Incidence: Nearly 150 cases have been reported.

Genetic inheritance: Autosomal recessive with parental consanguinity being a known risk factor. The mutation has been mapped to 1q21.

Pathophysiology: Pyknodysostosis results from a gene defect affecting cathepsin K, the only lysosomal cysteine protease with high expression in osteoclasts. This fact, in combination with the highest type I collagenolytic, elastinolytic, and gelatinolytic activities of all cysteine proteases, suggests that cathepsin K plays a key function in bone matrix resorption. Pyknodysostosis can therefore be considered a skeletal dysplasia secondary to cathepsin K deficiency, which makes it a lysosomal disease. The principal site of action for cathepsin K is the subosteoclastic space into which the enzyme is secreted for bone matrix degradation. The process of bone resorption is characterized by solubilization of inorganic mineral and subsequent proteolytic degradation of the organic matrix, primarily type I collagen. The osteoclast number in pyknodysostosis is normal, but the area of demineralization surrounding each individual osteoclast is enlarged. Ultrastructural examination of these osteoclasts shows big, abnormal intracytoplasmic vacuoles filled with collagen fibrils from bone. It seems therefore that step one (demineralization) of normal bone resorption is intact, whereas step two (degradation of the organic matrix) is defective. The inadequate resorption and remodeling of bones in pyknodysostosis leads to abnormally dense and brittle bones.

Diagnosis: Clinical features and radiologic appearance of bones (osteosclerosis, increased thickness of the trabecular bone as a result of increased density).

Clinical aspects: Short stature (adult height usually less than 150 cm [59 inches] for males) caused by short limbs, large, disproportionate head with frontal and occipital bossing, delayed suture closure and prolonged persistence of fontanels, and lack of frontal sinuses. The midface is hypoplastic with a prominent nose, grooved palate, and hypoplasia of the mandibular angles, making these patients prone to obstructive sleep apnea. The clavicles are affected by partial or complete aplasia. Progressive acro-osteolytic dysplasia affects the distal phalanges of fingers and toes with dystrophic, flattened, grooved, and brittle nails. Spondylolysis may occur at the L4-L5 level and scoliosis is a common finding. Dentition anomalies include delayed eruption and irregularities of the permanent teeth, with or without partial anodontia. The brittle bone results in fractures secondary to minimal trauma and the sometimes blue appearance of the sclera may initially result in the diagnosis of osteogenesis imperfecta. The intelligence is usually normal for the chronologic age but mild mental retardation has been reported in some cases. Rarely, hyperostosis can lead to the development of hematological complications (pancytopenia) similar to those found in osteopetrosis. A low concentration of insulin-like growth factor-1 has been reported for many patients suffering from pycnodysostosis. Therapy with exogenous growth hormone showed improvement in the linear growth. A significant abnormality of the hypothalamic–pituitary, thyroid, or adrenal axis in these patients is generally not found.

Precautions before anesthesia: Check mouth opening and other signs predictive for difficult airway management. Assessment of obstructive sleep apnea should include a polysomnographic study or, at least, continuous sleep pulse oximetry. If obstructive sleep apnea is present, its consequences on the cardiovascular system (cor pulmonale) should be evaluated and nasal continuous positive airway pressure therapy started prior to elective surgery. The teeth are generally in poor condition and need to be assessed. Laboratory investigations should include at least a CBC (anemia or even pancytopenia) and an arterial blood gas analysis (together with a chest radiograph) in the presence of scoliosis.

Anesthetic considerations: Careful positioning is mandatory because of increased bone fragility. Although not reported, direct laryngoscopy and tracheal intubation could be difficult secondary to midface hypoplasia and anomalies of the mandible and the clavicles. In the presence of obstructive sleep apnea, nasal continuous positive airway pressure should be resumed in the recovery room and close postoperative monitoring for apnea is recommended. Neuraxial blockade may turn out to be difficult because of scoliosis and a radiograph of the lumbar spine might be helpful. Infraclavicular approach for brachial plexus anesthesia and puncture of the subclavian vein may be difficult because of partial aplasia of the clavicles.

Pharmacological implications: Avoidance or at least careful titration of opioids and benzodiazepines is recommended if obstructive sleep apnea is suspected.

Other conditions to be considered:

☞**CLEIDOCRANIAL DYSPLASIA:** Generalized skeletal dysplasia resulting in defects in the development of skull, clavicles, pelvis and dental abnormalities.

☞**OSTEOPETROSIS:** A heterogenous genetic disorder resulting in increased bone mass caused by defective bone resorption. Depending on the mode of inheritance, its course can be either uniformly fatal with pancytopenia, recurrent pathological fractures, blindness, and other neurological symptoms, or exist in a much milder form with later manifestation and favorable prognosis.

☞**DYSOSTEOSCLEROSIS:** Genetic disorder with unfavorable prognosis manifesting with blindness, mental retardation, and characteristic skeletal changes.

☞**OSTEOGENESIS IMPERFECTA:** An autosomal dominant disorder with multiple bone fractures (post- and antenatal). Four major types are known. Type I is the one most frequently encountered in anesthesia.

REFERENCES:

Edelson JG, Obad S, Geiger R, et al: Pycnodysostosis: Orthopedic aspects with a description of 14 new cases. *Clin Orthop* 280:263, 1992.

Gelb BD, Shi GP, Chapman HA, et al: Pycnodysostosis, a lysosomal disease caused by cathepsin K deficiency. *Science* 273:1236, 1996.

Hunt NP, Cunningham SJ, Adnan N, et al: The dental, craniofacial, and biochemical features of pyknodysostosis: A report of three cases. *J Oral Maxillofac Surg* 56:497, 1998.

Pyle Disease

At a glance: Inherited bone dysplasia affecting the enchondral growth of long bones, which results in failure of modeling and causes increased circumference of the ends of the shafts.

Synonyms: Pyle Metaphyseal Dysplasia; Familial Metaphyseal Dysplasia. If the cranial features are significant, the disease is also called craniometaphyseal dysplasia.

NB: Metaphyseal dysplasia and metaphyseal chondrodysplasia are *not* the same disease.

History: First described by E. Pyle, an American orthopedic surgeon.

Incidence: About 25 cases have been reported.

Genetic inheritance: Autosomal recessive.

Pathophysiology: The mechanism or cause remain unknown; however, abnormal tubulation of the bone may play a role.

Diagnosis: Made by clinical features and radiographic studies. Symmetrical expansion of the metaphyses of long bones results in the so-called "Erlenmeyer flask deformity," describing the flaring of long bones (mainly of distal femur and proximal tibia) in combination with cortical thinning in affected areas. This sign is typical, but not pathognomonic, because it can also be seen in osteopetrosis, Niemann-Pick, and Gaucher diseases. Osteoporosis of the long bones with an increased risk for fractures is common.

Clinical aspects: The patient may be clinically asymptomatic. The patients are almost always tall as a result of increased limb length (especially femur and tibia). The most frequent clinical feature is genu valgum, which is usually mild but may predispose to fractures. The elbows may not fully extend, the proximal humerus is abnormally wide, as are the distal radius and ulna. The widening of the lower end of the femurs may be palpable. There is a gross defect in metaphyseal modeling. Radiologic examination of the spine may reveal platyspondyly, which could be attributed to either the same defect in modeling seen in the metaphyses of the long bones or to pathological fractures as a result of osteoporosis. Scoliosis has been reported in some patients. The head is enlarged with diffuse hyperostosis of the entire cranial vault, bony encroachment on the cranial foramina (potentially resulting in nerve compression with visual and hearing impairment/loss), absent or poorly pneumatized paranasal sinus, significantly thickened bone in the area of the glabella with hypertelorism, and often obstructed nasal breathing (breathing difficulties during upper airway infections have been described). Inconsistently, the presence of deciduous teeth is prolonged with marked cavities and prognathia may be present. Intelligence and general health are normal.

Precautions before anesthesia: Assess airway and loose teeth. Visual and hearing impairment could make communication difficult. Sedative and anxiolytic premedication, as well as the presence of the primary caregiver, for induction could be helpful.

Anesthetic considerations: Airway management could be difficult secondary to the potentially grotesque facial features. Careful positioning is recommended because of an increased risk for fractures secondary to osteoporosis.

Pharmacological implications: There are no specific pharmacological implications.

Other conditions to be considered:

☞**NIEMANN-PICK DISEASE:** Lysosomal storage disorder caused by a defect in sphingolipid metabolism and involving brain and/or viscera.

☞**GAUCHER DISEASE:** Most common form of inherited lipid storage disease, particularly common in Ashkenazi Jewish people (Eastern European ancestry). Accumulation of glucocerebrosides (derived from RBCs) in many tissues, especially the macrophages in the bone marrow, resulting in impairment of their function.

☞**OSTEOPETROSIS:** A heterogenous genetic disorder resulting in increased bone mass as a result of defective bone resorption. Depending on the mode of inheritance, its course can be either uniformly fatal with pancytopenia, recurrent pathological fractures, blindness, and other neurological symptoms, or exist in a much milder form with later manifestation and favorable prognosis.

☞METAPHYSEAL CHONDRODYSPLASIA: A heterogenous group of moderate to severe dwarfism with joint dysfunction and in some forms hypercalcemia.

REFERENCES:

Beighton P: Pyle disease (metaphyseal dysplasia). *J Med Genet* 24:321, 1987.

Ross MW, Altman DH: Familial metaphyseal dysplasia. Review of the clinical and radiologic feature of Pyle's disease. *Clin Peadiatr (Phila)* 6:143, 1967.

Turra S, Gigante C, Pavanini G, et al: Spinal involvement in Pyle's disease. *Pediatr Radiol* 30:25, 2000.

Pyruvate Carboxylase Deficiency

At a glance: Mitochondrial disease impairing synthetic pathways and leading to hypoglycemia and severe lactic acidosis. Clinically characterized by seizures, neuromuscular incoordination, abnormal eye movements, and poor response to visual stimuli. Other clinical features include lethargy, vomiting, and poor feeding. Apnea, dyspnea and/or respiratory depression complete the presentation.

Incidence: Approximately 1:250,000 newborns. In North America, a high incidence has been found in the linguistic group of Algonquian-speaking Native Americans (Manitoba, Saskatchewan, and Nova Scotia, Canada).

Genetic inheritance: Autosomal recessive; the gene has been mapped to 11q13.4-q13.5.

Pathophysiology: Pyruvate carboxylase (PC) is a biotin-dependent mitochondrial enzyme that converts pyruvate and CO_2 to oxaloacetate, one of two essential substrates (beside acetyl-CoA) in the production of citrate. As a result of this enzyme defect, the citric acid cycle cannot start because its first substrate (oxaloacetate) is missing or available only in low concentrations. The accumulation of pyruvate, the metabolite proximal to the enzyme defect, results in activation of alternate pyruvate pathways with increased production of lactic acid and acetyl-CoA, which then is converted into ketones because the tricarboxylic acid cycle pathway is closed. Glucose production is affected because the now lacking oxaloacetate is also involved in gluconeogenesis, which puts patients at risk for hypoglycemia during fasting periods. Because the tricarboxylic acid cycle is not available, energy delivery is entirely dependent on glycolysis. Compared to the tricarboxylic acid cycle, however, glycolysis is highly inefficient and results in the depletion of glucose. Oxaloacetate is also involved in the generation of aspartate, which is required for the synthesis of argininosuccinate, an intermediate metabolite in the urea cycle. This results in decreased urea production and hyperammonemia. Furthermore, oxaloacetate also participates in the malate–aspartate shuttle, which represents the principal mechanism for the transport of reducing equivalents from the cytoplasm into the mitochondria. The reduction of oxaloacetate to malate by cytoplasmic malate dehydrogenase also results in oxidation of the reduced form of nicotinamide adenine dinucleotide (NADH) to nicotinamide adenine dinucleotidase (NAD^+). Malate (carrying the electrons) then enters the mitochondria, where mitochondrial malate dehydrogenase reverses the previous action, resulting in conversion of malate to mitochondrial oxaloacetate. During oxidative phosphorylation in the mitochondria, these electrons of NADH get coupled to the ATP production. PC is also involved in lipogenesis and the formation of some nonessential amino acids (aspartate, glutamate).

Diagnosis: To be considered in any infant presenting with severe lactic acidosis with increased blood lactate/pyruvate ratio, ketosis, hyperammonemia, and neurologic anomalies. Lactic acidosis improves following ingestion of carbohydrate. The measurement of amino acids and organic acids in the urine has been used for screening. The deficiency in PC can be confirmed by measuring the enzyme activity in fibroblasts or other tissues.

Clinical aspects: The clinical presentation is highly variable; however, three distinct clinical presentations have been described.

Severe neonatal ("French") type: Total absence of PC activity leads to severe, progressive, lactic acidosis and ketosis, hypoglycemia, hepatomegaly with steatosis, and neurologic dysfunction (seizures, coma, abnormal muscle tone). The lactate/pyruvate ratio is increased and postprandial hyperketonemia may be observed. Impairment of the urea cycle leads to hyperammonemia. Furthermore, citrullinemia and hyperlysinemia have also been reported. Death usually results in the first 3 months of life.

Less severe ("American") type: Residual PC activity is about 2% of normal values. Onset is in infancy with failure to thrive, psychomotor retardation, seizures, spasticity, and, in some cases, renal tubular acidosis. It can be a cause of sudden infant death syndrome or Leigh disease. Hepatomegaly, poor myelinization with ventricular enlargement, and periventricular cysts.

Benign type: This is the rarest form. It is characterized by recurrent attacks of lactic acidosis, either without or with only mild neurologic deficits.

Treatment focuses on avoidance of prolonged fasting and some patients even need continuous intravenous administration of 10% glucose. Supplementation of citrate provides the required substrate for the tricarboxylic cycle and results in decreased acidosis. Aspartic acid supplementation allows urea cycle function and reduces the ammonia level.

Precautions before anesthesia: Medical history must focus on the respiratory function and feeding habits. A glucose-containing IV solution should always be started already at the beginning of the preoperative fasting period. Proper evaluation of persistent acidosis and electrolyte imbalance must be performed. Evaluate the electrolyte and fluid status.

Anesthetic considerations: Monitor serum glucose and lactic acid levels; see *mitochondrial diseases*, but there is no clinical cardiac or muscular involvement. Postoperative special attention to high risk of apnea must be considered.

Pharmacological implications: Sedative and narcotic drugs should be used with caution because these patients can be very sensitive to the effects of these drugs.

Other conditions to be considered:

☞LEIGH DISEASE: Severe, progressive, necrotizing encephalopathy caused by a mitochondrial disorder impeding oxidative phosphorylation.

☞PYRUVATE DEHYDROGENASE COMPLEX DEFICIENCY: This is a mitochondrial disease that leads to lactic acidosis without hypoglycemia.

REFERENCES:

De Meirleir D: Defects of pyruvate metabolism and the Krebs cycle. *J Child Neurol* 17:3S26, 2002.

Kerr DS, Wexler ID, Zinn AB: Disorders of pyruvate metabolism and the tricarboxylic acid cycle, in Fernandes J, Saudubray JM, Van den

Berghe G (eds): *Inborn Metabolic Diseases.* 3rd ed. Berlin, Springer-Verlag, 2000, p 128.

Pyruvate Dehydrogenase Complex Deficiency

At a glance: Pyruvate Dehydrogenase Complex Deficiency (PDHCD) is a mitochondrial disease that leads to lactic acidosis without hypoglycemia.

Synonym: Pyruvate Dehydrogenase Deficiency.

Incidence: The exact incidence is unknown, but several hundred cases have been described.

Genetic inheritance: All the components of the pyruvate dehydrogenase complex are encoded by nuclear genes and are synthesized in the cytoplasm before being transported into the mitochondria. Most of these genes are autosomal, but the E1α subunit gene has been mapped to Xp22.3. Hence, most cases of pyruvate dehydrogenase complex deficiency are X-linked with more severe consequences in males than in heterozygous females; the frequency, however, is the same for both genders.

Pathophysiology: Pyruvate dehydrogenase (PDH) is an enzyme complex consisting of three catalytic subunits, pyruvate dehydrogenase (E1, a tetramer), dihydrolipoamide acyltransferase (E2, a monomer), and dihydrolipoamide dehydrogenase (E3, a dimer), and two cofactors, thiamine pyrophosphate and lipoic acid. A sixth component, previously named X-protein and recently renamed E3-binding protein (E3-BP), has been found to be mutated in a few patients. The enzyme complex converts pyruvate—after it enters the mitochondria—into acetyl-CoA, one of two essential substrates (oxaloacetate being the other) in the production of citrate. PDHCD therefore leads to a limited production of citrate and because citrate is the first substrate in the tricarboxylic acid (citric acid or Krebs) cycle, the cycle is blocked and other metabolic pathways need to be stimulated to produce acetyl-CoA. Nevertheless, the decreased level of energy substrates (ATP) primarily affects the CNS, because brain acetyl-CoA is synthesized almost exclusively from pyruvate. The most common deficiency involves the E1 subunit, a heterotetramer consisting of two alpha and two beta subunits with the defect located on the alpha subunit (E1alpha), which contains several serine phosphorylation sites and seems to be involved in the regulation of the whole complex. Mutations in E2, E3, and E3-BP are less often the cause for PDHCD. The enzyme defect causes more pyruvate to be metabolized to lactate and leads to lactic acidosis.

Diagnosis: The combination of an otherwise unexplained lactic acidosis with early-onset neurological disease and structural brain anomalies should always include PDHCD in the differential diagnosis. In addition to pyruvate carboxylase deficiency, defects in the mitochondrial chain of electron transport or in gluconeogenesis should be considered. However, lactic acidosis in the absence of hypoglycemia does not match with a defect in gluconeogenesis, whereas a defect in the mitochondrial respiratory chain would also affect other organ systems, such as muscle, heart, liver, and kidneys. In contrast to a respiratory chain defect, the blood lactate/pyruvate ratio in PDHCD is normal and both lactate and pyruvate decrease after fasting. Specific enzyme assays are available to measure the total PDH activity, as well as that of the individual components of the enzyme complex. However, measured residual enzyme activity does not always correlate with the clinical picture.

Clinical aspects: The range of clinical expression is wide and has four different ways of presentation: fatal infantile lactic acidosis, psychomotor retardation, progressive neurological deterioration (Leigh disease), and carbohydrate-sensitive ataxia.

Fatal infantile lactic acidosis: These patients (most often boys) have very low levels of residual enzyme activity (approximately 15% of the norm value) and present in the neonatal period with brain anomalies (agenesis of the corpus callosum, cystic brain lesions) and severe, chronic, lactic acidosis refractory to treatment, most often resulting in death in the first 6 months of life.

Psychomotor retardation: Although these children (more often girls than boys) suffer from mild to moderate lactic acidosis, significant acid–base changes only occur intermittently, usually related by an intercurrent infection, prolonged fasting, or stimulation of gluconeogenesis. Hypotonia, confusion, and coma may occur. The residual activity of PDH is about 28% of the norm. It is not unusual that these patients go undetected until developmental delay has been diagnosed. MRI and/or CT scanning of the head may reveal cortical atrophy, basal ganglia defects, and internal hydrocephalus.

Leigh Disease (Cytochrome Oxydase Deficiency Disease; Progressive Neurological Deterioration): These children develop the typical signs of Leigh disease within the first 5 years of life, which is characterized by developmental delay, seizures, ataxia, episodic weakness, progressive neuropathy, and basal ganglia and brainstem dysfunction (e.g., loss of respiratory control) caused by cystic lesions and necrosis in these areas. The residual activity of PDH is about 22% of the norm.

Carbohydrate-Sensitive Ataxia: These patients are all male, are without significantly elevated lactate serum levels, and suffer from either episodic or chronic ataxia. Ataxia is often carbohydrate-induced and can be controlled by ketogenic diet (i.e., the dietary caloric intake is composed of 65 to 80% from fat, and carbohydrates and proteins are restricted to less than 5% and 15%, respectively). The residual activity of PDH is about 30% of the norm.

About one-third of patients with PDHCD suffer from facial anomalies quite similar to fetal alcohol syndrome (i.e., thin upper lip, long philtrum, microcephaly, broad nasal bridge, anteverted nostrils, frontal bossing, short palpebral fissures, maxillary hypoplasia, cleft lip or palate). Cardiac defects (ventricular septal defect), hydronephrosis, and short neck have been described in a few cases.

Precautions before anesthesia: Obtain a complete history focused on neurological symptoms, metabolic exacerbations, and their triggers. Ask about the diet and tolerance to fasting. During the fasting period, it is strongly recommended to give to these patients (except the subgroup with carbohydrate-sensitive ataxia) on a dextrose-containing intravenous solution to provide glucose at a rate of 8 to 10 mg/kg/min. Laboratory investigations should include a complete blood count, serum electrolytes, glucose and lactate levels, and a venous or arterial blood gas analysis. Anesthesia-related morbidity and mortality is linked to the preoperative status of the child. Elective procedures should be canceled in the presence of decompensated acid–base status, infections, or fever. These patients may have an abnormal response to both hypoxia and hypercarbia, and may require postoperative mechanical ventilation. Because lactate levels are already elevated in these patients, lactate-containing intravenous solutions must be avoided. Assess the facial dysmorphism for features predictive of difficult airway management. Patients with psychomotor retardation may be better off with sedative or anxiolytic premedication; however, the abnormal respiratory drive requires careful titration and monitoring.

Anesthetic considerations: Because the hypothalamus and the brainstem is often involved in the disease process, meticulous care should be devoted to perioperative maintenance of temperature and control of respiration (if the maintenance of spontaneous breathing is an option). Hypocapnia should be avoided because it inhibits pyruvate decarboxylase and further increases lactate levels. Avoid hypothermia, because rewarming hypermetabolism can result in decompensated metabolic acidosis and hypoglycemia. Maintain normal blood glucose levels by providing perioperative dextrose supplements and repeatedly check blood glucose and lactate concentrations. A stress-free anesthesia decreases the metabolic response to surgery, as well as lactate production. Maintain normovolemia and adequate pre- and afterload to prevent lactic acidosis secondary to inappropriate tissue perfusion. The use of regional anesthesia is recommended when applicable.

Pharmacological implications: The presence of a mitochondrial disease is not considered as a risk factor for malignant hyperthermia.

Other conditions to be considered:

☞Leigh Disease: Severe, progressive, necrotizing encephalopathy caused by a mitochondrial disorder impeding oxidative phosphorylation.

☞Pyruvate Carboxylase Deficiency: Mitochondrial disease impairing synthetic pathways and leading to hypoglycemia and severe lactic acidosis.

References:

Acharya D, Dearlove OR: Anaesthesia in pyruvate dehydrogenase deficiency. *Anaesthesia* 56:799, 2001.

Cooper MA, Fox R: Anesthesia for corrective spinal surgery in a patient with Leigh's disease. *Anesth Analg* 97:1539, 2003.

De Meirleir D: Defects of pyruvate metabolism and the Krebs cycle. *J Child Neurol* 17:3S26, 2002.

Dierdorf SF, McNiece WL: Anaesthesia and pyruvate dehydrogenase deficiency. *Can Anaesth Soc J* 30:413, 1983.

Kerr DS, Wexler ID, Zinn AB: Disorders of pyruvate metabolism and the tricarboxylic acid cycle, in Fernandes J, Saudubray J-M, Van den Berghe G (eds): *Inborn Metabolic Diseases*. 3rd ed. Berlin, Springer-Verlag, 2000, p 132.

Pyruvate Kinase Deficiency (PKD)

At a glance: This is the most common enzyme defect. It results in hereditary, nonspherocytic hemolytic anemia.

Synonyms: Pyruvate Kinase Deficiency of Erythrocytes; Pyruvate Kinase Liver type Deficiency.

History: First described in 1952 by J.V. Dacies et al. in patients with congenital hemolytic anemia who presented with hereditary spherocytosis. However, in the more recently described anemia, it is shown that the osmotic fragility is normal and spherocytes not encountered.

Incidence: The prevalence rate of a heterozygous carrier is approximately 1 to 3% and the prevalence of confirmed cases has been estimated at about 1:300,000 live births. Pyruvate kinase deficiency (PKD) affects both genders equally and occurs in all races (a high incidence has been reported in Amish people from Pennsylvania). Internationally, PKD has been reported in Northern Europe and Japan. The prevalance in Germany is reported at 1% and Hong Kong 3%. In the United Kingdom, the prevalence is 3.2 cases per million population.

Genetic inheritance: Autosomal recessive. It is caused by mutations in the PKLR gene (pyruvate kinase expressed in liver and red blood cells (RBCs), which has been mapped to 1q21 and encodes the L (liver) and R (red cells) pyruvate kinase isozymes.

Pathophysiology: The mature erythrocytes have neither a nucleus nor mitochondria, and therefore depend entirely on anaerobic glycolysis as a source of energy. Pyruvate kinase (PK) catalyzes the conversion of phosphoenolpyruvate to pyruvate and is one of three rate-limiting kinases (together with hexokinase and phosphofructokinase) in the Embden-Meyerhof pathway, which is responsible for adenosine triphosphate (ATP) production by anaerobic glycolysis. On the one hand, this defect results in accumulation of intermediate and various glycolytic metabolites in the erythrocyte upstream of the enzymatic block; on the other hand, these RBCs lack the products downstream in the pathway (lactate and ATP). ATP is required to maintain erythrocyte transmembranous electrolyte concentration gradients (mainly potassium) across the cellular membrane, hydration, and flexibility of the RBC. Consequently, the lack of ATP results in loss of potassium, dehydration, and rigidity of the cellular membrane, and, finally, in premature destruction of the erythrocytes in spleen and liver. A shunt in the glycolytic pathway unique to the erythrocyte (Rapoport-Luebering shunt) is responsible for the two- to threefold increase in intracellular 2,3-DPG concentration, and hence a marked right shift in the oxygen dissociation curve of hemoglobin with decreased affinity of hemoglobin for oxygen. Two different PK genes (PKLR and PKM) encode for four PK isozymes: L in liver, R in RBCs, M1 in muscles, and M2 in leukocytes and platelets.

Diagnosis: In the absence of blood loss, a chronic normochromic, normocytic, or macrocytic anemia (usually with hemoglobin concentrations between 60 and 120 g/L) in combination with marked reticulocytosis (5 to 15%) is suggestive of hemolysis. Enzyme assays (with residual PK activity of 5 to 25% in homozygotes and approximately 50% [wide range] in heterozygous carriers) and polymerase chain reaction for DNA analysis are available to confirm not only the diagnosis, but also a carrier status. Careful removal of leukocytes and platelets is required before the enzyme assay is done, because these cell lines contain high concentrations of PK and would lead to false-negative results. After splenectomy, reticulocyte counts as high as 70% have been reported (despite reduced hemolysis), which is a result of the now prolonged survival of the reticulocytes.

Clinical aspects: There is a wide range in clinical expression. The age at onset usually correlates with the severity. In the most severe cases, the fetus dies in utero. Severely affected patients present as newborns with anemia requiring transfusions, hepatosplenomegaly, and jaundice, occasionally complicated by kernicterus. However, most affected persons with PKD are detected during childhood, whereas mildly affected patients may go undetected until late adulthood. Although the severity of the disease often decreases with age, splenectomy may be necessary in severely affected patients who otherwise require repeated transfusions. Because of the increased 2,3-DPG levels, these patients tolerate their anemia surprisingly well. Gallstones are found with increasing frequency in adolescence and thereafter, and regular screening ultrasonographic examinations of the gallbladder are recommended to prevent acute biliary pancreatitis. Indirect hyperbilirubinemia can be used to assess the severity of the hemolytic process. Iron overload is a potential complication and is not limited to patients frequently transfused. Chronic leg ulcers and splenic abscesses are other reported complications. In severe cases, frontal bossing secondary to increased hematopoiesis in the cranial bone marrow occurs. In older patients, infections and pregnancy may require sporadic blood transfusions. Intermittent aplastic crises with a precipitous drop in hemoglobin concentration have been described and are typically associated with a parvovirus B19 infection (which replicates in erythroid progenitors cells [reticulocytes], lasts for about 1 week, and leads to erythema infectiosum following the aplastic crisis). In general, these patients are otherwise healthy with normal physical and mental development. Some medical conditions (e.g., acute leukemia, complications arising from chemotherapy) may lead to acquired PKD. However, the clinical course of this form is milder.

Precautions before anesthesia: Check hemoglobin, liver function, and bilirubin levels. Iron overload, or even secondary hemochromatosis in severe cases, most often (but not exclusively) caused by frequent transfusions, has been described and should prompt the anesthetist to search for and assess associated abnormalities (arrhythmias and congestive heart failure, gray or bronze skin pigmentation, cirrhosis of the liver, liver cancer, diabetes mellitus [pancreas fibrosis], hypopituitarism, decreased thyroidal, adrenal, and gonadal function) that could significantly affect the anesthetic management.

Anesthetic considerations: Usually these patients present for splenectomy or cholecystectomy. The main problem is the hemolytic anemia. However, because of the chronic nature of the anemia, these patients are well adapted to the lower hemoglobin concentrations and transfusion to normal hemoglobin values preoperatively is—although depending on the planned procedure—generally unnecessary.

Pharmacological implications: Succinylcholine has been used without adverse side effects.

Other condition to be considered:

☞**GLUCOSE PHOSPHATE ISOMERASE DEFICIENCY:** This autosomal disease is caused by a deficiency in the enzyme glucose phosphate isomerase and is clinically characterized by nonspherotic hemolytic anemia and spontaneous hemolytic crises.

REFERENCES:

Glader BE, Lukens JN: Hereditary hemolytic anemias associated with abnormalities of erythrocyte glycolysis and nucleotide metabolism, in Lee RG, Foerster J, Lukens N, et al. (eds): *Wintrobe's Clinical Hematology.* 10th ed. Philadelphia, Lippincott, Williams and Wilkins, 1999, p 1160.

Hirono A, Kanno H, Miwa S, et al: Pyruvate kinase deficiency and other enzymopathies of the erythrocyte, in Scriver CR, Beaudet AL, Sly WS, et al. (eds): *The Metabolic and Molecular Bases of Inherited Disease.* 8th ed. New York, McGraw Hill, 2001, p 4637.

Stirt JA: Succinylcholine in congenital pyruvate kinase deficiency. *Anesth Analg* 61;620, 1982.

Q

Qazi Markouizos Syndrome

At a glance: Mental retardation associated with myopathy, facial malformation, and seizures.

Synonym: Puerto Rican Infant Hypotonia Syndrome.

Incidence and genetic inheritance: Three cases have been described; genetic inheritance unknown.

Clinical aspects: Features include myopathy, (congenital fiber type disproportion, i.e., type I muscle fibers are significantly smaller than type II fibers (normally about the same size), and a predominance of type I fibers by numbers (normally about equal)), nonprogressive hypotonia, facial malformations (hypertelorism, broad nasal root, long philtrum, mouth held open, high-arched and narrow palate, microdontia), delayed bone age with abnormal ossification, pectus excavatum, seizures, and mental retardation.

Anesthetic considerations: Direct laryngoscopy and tracheal intubation could be difficult because of facial malformations. Avoid anesthetic muscle relaxants until the airway has been secured. Evaluate neurological function (clinical, history, CT/MRI, EEG). Consider interaction between antiepileptic treatment and anesthetic drugs. Evaluate myopathy (history, clinical, creatine phosphokinase); avoid succinylcholine and halogenated drugs. Reduce neuromuscular blocking agent doses because of hypotonia and use a peripheral nerve stimulator.

REFERENCE:

Qazi QH, Markouizos D, Rao C, et al: A syndrome of hypotonia, psychomotor retardation, seizures, delayed and dysharmonic skeletal maturation, and congenital fibre type disproportion. *J Med Genet* 31(5):405, 1994.

(De) Quervain Thyroiditis

At a glance: Most common cause of a painful thyroid gland. It is caused by transient nonbacterial inflammation. Hyperthyroidism often occurs initially and can be followed by hypothyroidism.

Synonyms: Granulomatous Giant Cell Thyroiditis; De Quervain Subacute Struma; Quervain Syndrome; Subacute Painful Thyroiditis.

History: An acquired disease that was first described by Fritz de Quervain, (1868–1940), a Swiss surgeon, in 1904.

Incidence: Five percent of all patients with thyroid pathology. Peak incidence in the fourth and fifth decade of life; sex ratio female:male 3.5:1. Most common during summer and fall. High incidence of HLA-B35 positivity.

Table Q-1   Characteristic Course of de Quervain Thyroiditis

Stage	1	2	3	4
Symptoms	Hyperthyroid	Euthyroid	Hypothyroid	Euthyroid (recovery)
T4, T3	Elevated	Normal	Decreased	Normal
TSH	Decreased	Normal	Elevated	Normal

Pathophysiology: Presumably caused by a viral infection or postviral inflammatory response. A proposed mechanism is that a viral antigen binds to HLA-B35 molecules and that the complex activates cytotoxic T lymphocytes that damage thyroid follicular cells because of their similarity with the infection-related antigen. Destruction of follicular epithelium involves the release of thyroid-binding globulin into blood. T3 and T4 concentration in serum is increased and thyroid-stimulating hormone secretion is suppressed. The thyroid follicles then regenerate and thyroid hormone synthesis and secretion resume.

Diagnosis: Made on clinical grounds (history, pain, symptom of hyperthyroidism), ultrasound; thyroid-stimulating hormone and free T4 measurement to determine the cause of hyperthyroidism; serum thyroglobulin (elevated) and erythrocyte sedimentation rate (>50 mm/h). Thyroid biopsy shows characteristic giant cell inflammation.

Clinical aspects: Features include gradual onset of pain in the region of the thyroid gland (aggravated with swallowing and head movement), dysphagia, fever, weakness, and fatigue. Weight loss and diarrhea may occur. Symptoms of moderate hyperthyroidism (palpitations, tremor, heat intolerance, nervousness, sweating, skeletal muscle weakening) appear in the initial phase, usually over 3 to 6 weeks. The initial phase is followed by the transient asymptomatic phase over the next 1 to 3 weeks. In 50% of patients, symptoms of hypothyroidism occur in the late phase. It may become permanent in 5 to 10% of patients. Acute complications (severe hyperthyroidism, pancreatitis) are exceptional.

Precautions before anesthesia: Evaluate thyroid function (clinical, thyroid-stimulating hormone, T3, free T4). Laboratory investigations should include serum levels of calcium, phosphate and amylase. Preoperative ECG is recommended. Evaluate tracheal intubation in case of voluminous thyroid (clinical, CT, fiberoptic). Evaluate hydration in case of diarrhea and fever (clinical, electrolytes).

Anesthetic considerations: Nonurgent surgery should be postponed until the clinical situation has stabilized. Tracheal intubation can (rarely) be difficult. An adapted anesthetic management for thyroid imbalance may be required. Perioperative invasive blood pressure and cardiac monitoring are recommended.

Pharmacological implications: Adapt doses to increased metabolism. Use beta-sympathetic blocker in case of tachycardia. Avoid anticholinergic drugs.

REFERENCES:

Duininck TM, van Heerden JA, Fatourechi V, et al: de Quervain's thyroiditis: Surgical experience. *Endoc Pract* 8:255, 2002.

Kramer AB, Roozendaal C, Dullaart RP: Familial occurrence of subacute thyroiditis associated with human leukocyte antigen B 35. *Thyroid* 14:544, 2004.

Sheu SY, Schmid KW: [Inflammatory disease of the thyroid gland. Epidemiology, symptoms and morphology.] *Pathologe* 24:339, 2003.

Quincke Edema

At a glance: Acquired Angioneurotic Edema (AAE) is characterized by profound swelling of the dermis associated with abdominal pain. Edema is usually painless, nonpruritic, nonurticarial, and nonpitting. Edema of the larynx and other portions of the airways is the most fearsome feature of this disorder and can be life-threatening.

Synonyms: Acquired Angioneurotic Edema (AAE); Bannister Disease/Syndrome; Milton Urticaria; Milton-Quincke Syndrome; Quincke Disease/Syndrome.

History: The German internist Heinrich Iranaeus Quincke (1842–1922) was by no means the first to report the disease. This honor goes to the Italian physician Marcello Donati, who described a young count with sensitivity to eggs. Quincke however was the first to publish a review (without referencing earlier descriptions of the disease) in 1882.

Incidence: Varies with etiology; hereditary angioneurotic edema (HAE) is found in 1:10,000 to 1:150,000 persons. AAE has been reported in fewer than 50 cases. Angioedema following use of angiotensin-converting enzyme (ACE) inhibitors is found in 1 to 2 cases per 1000 persons. Other forms of angioedema (not secondary to HAE or AAE) will affect 10 to 20% of the population at some time in their lives.

Classification: Angioedema is associated with the following disorders: 1) acquired C1-esterase inhibitor deficiency and 2) hereditary C1-esterase inhibitor deficiency. Traditionally two types of HAE have been described. HAE type I, which accounts for approximately 85% of patients is the result of decreased C1-esterase inhibitor production. The remainder 15% of patients suffer from HAE type II, which is characterized by normal or even elevated levels of a functionally impaired C1-esterase inhibitor. (An HAE type III has recently been assigned to a possibly X-linked inherited form of HAE.)

ACE-induced angioedema is *idiopathic*.

Allergic (IgE-mediated) may be caused by inhalants (ethylene-glycol), bites and stings, drugs (morphine, codeine, iodine-dye, aspirin, or nonsteroidal anti-inflammatory drugs) and sera, foods and food additives, physical induction (cold, exercise, pressure, vibration, facial piercing), parasitic infections, paraneoplastic or autoimmune disorders.

Genetic inheritance: The hereditary form is autosomal dominant transmitted and caused by a mutation in the C1 inhibitor gene (C1-esterase inhibitor) located on chromosome 11p11.2-q13.1. Male:female ratio is 0.85, but 20% are de novo mutations. The acquired form is often associated with B-cell lymphoproliferative disorders.

Pathophysiology: C1, the first component of the classical pathway of the complement system is a complex macromolecule. Activation leads to cleavage producing the C1 esterase, which may now act on C4 and C2. C1-esterase inhibitor is the control protein that inhibits the spontaneous activation. It is also able to inhibit the Hageman factor (XIIa), plasma thromboplastin (XIa), and kallikrein.

Diagnosis: Clinical (mildly or nonpruritic, relapsing edema that does not respond to antiallergic treatment). Diagnosis of hereditary form is difficult; precise criteria have been validated by the European study group on HAE ("Oedème Angioneurotique", OAN). One major clinical sign is either a) limited subcutaneous angioedema, not associated with urticaria, lasting at least 12 hours and relapsing frequently; or b) recurrent idiopathic abdominal pain lasting at least 6 hours; or c) recurrent laryngeal edema and one biological sign being either a) C1-esterase inhibitor concentration below 50% of the normal value in two distinct samples; or b) C1-esterase inhibitor functional activity below 50% of the normal value; or c) detection of a C1-esterase inhibitor mutation altering the gene product synthesis and/or function must be present.

Clinical aspects: The two major features are subcutaneous or submucosal, white, soft, nonpruritic edema (occurring episodically and lasting 3 to 5 days). Most commonly, the edema affects the skin, respiratory and gastrointestinal tract. These edemas do not respond to treatment with corticosteroids or antihistamines. Rarely, seizures and hemiparesis may accompany HAE attacks and are thought to represent cerebral edema and hypoperfusion. Triggering events can be present (trauma [even minor], stress, and certain times of the female hormonal cycle). The onset may be precipitated by mononucleosis. The laboratory findings most commonly show a low level of C1-esterase inhibitor, a low level of C4, and a normal level of C1, and often leukocytosis. Abdominal pain may be the only clinical manifestation and simulate a surgical emergency (ileus). Angioedema caused by acquired C1-inhibitor deficiency is associated with benign or malignant B-cell lymphoproliferative disorders; one case has been caused by IgA paraprotein. The patients with chronic urticaria and angioedema have an increased frequency of autoimmune thyroiditis. HAE attacks precipitate disseminated intravascular coagulation or multiple organ failure in elderly people, causing a profound decrease in antithrombin-III activity.

Precautions before anesthesia: Careful history of the illness to assess the quality of long-term treatment, the severity of illness, and the need for the specific C1-esterase inhibitor serum treatment. Ask about the use of ACE inhibitors. Obtain full history. For all patients that have suffered from Quincke Edema, the key is to avoid any triggering events.

Anesthetic considerations: The decision to perform tracheal intubation should be carefully evaluated against the risk (benefit ratio). If considered necessary, prophylactic edema treatment (e.g., steroids) should be administered. Be careful with all the hemodilutional techniques that lower the plasma level of C1-esterase inhibitor. During periods of acute clinical manifestations, the potential for significant swelling within the airway suggests that it might be appropriate to secure the airway early by using an endotracheal tube. The progression can be so severe that even tracheostomy may be ineffective in providing a patent airway. C1-esterase inhibitor-specific serum is the definite treatment (fresh-frozen plasma only if the former is not available). Warm the patient (some studies show that when the core temperature is raised by 0.7°C, that the anaphylaxis part of the syndrome does not appear). Treatment for airway access and anaphylactic reactions are supportive.

Pharmacological implications: The existence of HAE does not influence drug choices for the induction of either general or regional anesthesia, or for the use of muscle relaxants, including succinylcholine. Prophylaxis with *antifibrinolytic agents* produces better results in the acquired form than in the inherited form, in which androgen derivatives are more effective. *Epsilon-aminocaproic acid* (EACA) was once thought to be useful in long-term therapy. However, it is not often used because of the side effects. It seems to work by limiting the formation of plasmin, which can activate C1. *Tranexamic acid* may limit the activation of C1, but it too, is rarely used. Prophylaxis with testosterone is effective so the use of *danazol* is frequent; currently, *stanozolol* is the therapeutic mainstay. Both act by increasing the synthesis of C1-esterase inhibitor in the liver. This drug also raises the level of the deficient protein in α_1-antitrypsin deficiency and in hemophilias A and B. It seems to be effective even in the treatment of severe acute attacks. Fresh-frozen plasma contains C1-esterase inhibitor as well as the kinins and substrate I, including uncleaved C2 and C4, that may trigger complement activation. It is the emergency treatment for associated disseminated intravascular coagulation or if specific serum is not available. *Purified vapor heated C1-esterase inhibitor* concentrate is the therapy of choice. After infusion, C1-esterase inhibitor concentrate can be effective within 30 minutes (in about two thirds of patients), while within 4 hours 95% of patients respond to treatment. This treatment may be protective for approximately 2 days. In some countries, this concentrate has not been licensed, yet.

REFERENCES:

Donati M: *De Medica Historia Mirabili.* Mantuae, per Fr. Osanam, 1586.

Jensen NF, Weiler JM: C1 esterase inhibitor deficiency, airway compromise, and anesthesia. *Anesth Analg* 87:480, 1998.

Nzeako UC, Frigas E, Tremaine WJ: Hereditary angioedema: A broad review for clinicians. *Arch Intern Med* 161:2417, 2001.

R

Rabson-Mendenhall Syndrome

At a glance: An extremely rare genetic disorder characterized by severe insulin resistance and craniofacial anomalies, abnormalities of the teeth and nails, and acanthosis nigricans (hyperpigmentation and hyperkeratosis), particularly of the neck, groin, and underarms.

History: In 1956, S.M. Rabson and E.N. Mendenhall described this familial syndrome comprising insulin-resistant diabetes, pineal hyperplasia, and various somatic anomalies.

Genetic inheritance: Autosomal recessive. A genetic deficiency of insulin receptors. Gene locus at 19p13.3-p.13.2.

Pathophysiology: The causative mutation(s) reside in the insulin receptor gene with the defect between synthesis of the receptor precursor and insertion of it into the membrane. The severely impaired insulin-binding capacity results in highly insulin-resistant diabetes mellitus.

Diagnosis: Dental and skin abnormalities (acanthosis nigricans, truncal hypertrichosis, malpositioned teeth), short stature, coarse facial features with prognathism, abdominal distension, and phallic enlargement. Highly insulin-resistant diabetes mellitus. The pineal body is hyperplastic. Studies of melatonin state show raised melatonin metabolite excretion in the urine, as might be expected with disordered pineal function.

Clinical aspects: Somatic anomalies present at birth. Diabetes manifests during childhood or adolescence and may result in ketoacidosis and intercurrent infections. Mortality from ketoacidotic coma has been reported. Acanthosis usually decreases in intensity and extent over time. Hypophysectomy has been of short-term benefit, but the problems of insulin resistance persist.

Precautions before anesthesia: Optimization of blood sugar control via tight monitoring and institution of appropriate insulin therapy. An appropriate assessment and management of coexisting disease is mandatory. *Investigations:* blood sugar levels, electrolytes, CBC, ECG, chest radiograph. Other investigations will be necessary to evaluate various end-organ function and should be ordered as directed by clinical findings.

Anesthetic considerations: Regional techniques, where appropriate, are preferable to general anesthesia, because they usually allow an earlier return to a normal feeding pattern. The stress response to surgery may also be partially obtunded.

Pharmacological implications: There are no known specific implications for this condition.

REFERENCES:

Hirsch IB, McGill JB, Cryer PE et al: Perioperative management of surgical patient with diabetes mellitus. *Anesthesiology* 74:346, 1991.

Rabson SM, Mendenhall EN: Familial hypertrophy of pineal body, hyperplasia of adrenal cortex and diabetes mellitus. *Am J Clin Pathol* 26:283-90, 1956.

Radial Aplasia Syndrome

At a glance: Very rare X-linked syndrome with radial aplasia, anogenital anomalies, and sometimes hydrocephalus.

Synonym: Radial Aplasia and Anogenital Anomalies.

Incidence and genetic inheritance: Very rare. X-linked genetic inheritance.

Clinical aspects: Radial aplasia with normal legs, hydrocephalus, hypospadias, imperforate anus.

Anesthetic considerations: Perioperative positioning must prevent extrinsic compression of upper limb arteries. Avoid radial artery catheterization. Evaluate neurological status.

Other conditions to be considered: Radial aplasia can be observed in many syndromes, including the following:

WILMS TUMOR RADIAL BILATERAL APLASIA NEPHROBLASTOMA: Metacarpal anomalies, radius absent or abnormal lower limb deficiency, terminal hypoplasia fingers, and chromosomal rearrangement.

BALLER-GEROLD SYNDROME: Autosomal recessive, characterized by short stature, absent or hypoplastic radii, craniosynostosis, congenital cardiopathy, and various other anomalies such as turribrachycephaly, low-set, posteriorly rotated ears with conductive hearing loss; down-slanting palpebral fissures and epicanthal folds. Other features include hypertelorism; microstomia; perineal fistula; anteriorly placed anus; imperforate anus; renal anomalies; rectovaginal fistula; vertebral anomalies; fused carpal bones; mental retardation; absent or hypoplastic thumbs; absent carpals; metacarpals; and phalanges.

REFERENCE:

Gibson CC, Genest DR, Bieber FR, et al: X-linked phenotype of absent radius and anogenital anomalies. *Am J Med Genet* 45:743, 1993.

Radio-Ulnar Synostosis

At a glance: An anomaly, consisting of longitudinal segmentation, resulting in forearm shortening with fixed pronation because of radioulnar synostosis.

History: First described by G.B. Davenport, in 1924.

Genetic inheritance: Usually sporadic; however, autosomal dominant with variable expression has also been suggested.

Pathophysiology: Can occur as the only abnormality. Often associated with other chromosomal constellation abnormalities including XXXY syndrome and 48,XYYY syndrome. Upper limb bud arises at 26 days of age. The defect in longitudinal segmentation occurs at the seventh week of development when, for a time, the proximal radius and ulna are united and share a common perichondrium. It is possible that abnormal genetic or teratogenic factors operating at this time would interfere with proximal radioulnar joint morphogenesis. Radioulnar synostosis occurs bilaterally in 60% of cases.

Diagnosis: Clinically evocated by family history and the presence of an average fixed flexion contracture, forearm shortening, hypermobility of wrist, and fixed pronation. Confirm by radiological features showing synostosis from proximal fibrous union to total synostosis of radius and ulna. Chromosomal study normal in isolated radioulnar synostosis.

Clinical aspects: There are two types described. In *type I*, there is a proximal, smooth fusion of 2 to 6 cm (0.8 to 2.4 inches) between radius and ulnar, and absent radial head. In *type II*, there is a fusion just distal to the proximal radial epiphysis in association with congenital dislocation of the radial head. Both types result in a limitation of pronation and supination of the forearm, and in type II, there is also limited extension of the elbow. Common associated abnormalities are mental retardation, hypotonia, and abnormal facies.

Precautions before anesthesia: Document function of limbs.

Anesthetic considerations: None in isolated radioulnar synostosis. Proper care should be taken in positioning limb. Regional anesthesia is not contraindicated; however, radial nerve blockade at the elbow is best avoided, particularly in type II.

Pharmacological implications: There are no specific implications for this condition.

REFERENCES:

Bauer M, Jonsson K: Congenital radioulnar synostosis. *Scand J Plast Reconst Surg* 22:251, 1988.

Davenport CB, Taylor HL, Nelson LA: Radio-ulnar synostosis. *Arch Surg* 8:705, 1924.

Ramban-Hasharon Syndrome

At a glance: A rare defect of fucose metabolism leading to a syndrome that combines neutrophil adhesion deficiency with severe neurological impairment, psychomotor retardation and short stature.

Synonyms: Leukocyte Adhesion Deficiency type II; Congenital Disorder of Glycosylation type IIc.

History: First described in 1992 in two unrelated boys, both offspring of consanguineous parents in Israel.

Genetic inheritance: Autosomal recessive.

Pathophysiology: Inborn deficiency of several fucosylated glycoproteins. Caused by mutation in the gene encoding guanosine diphosphate (GDP)-fucose transporter-1 (FUCT1) located on chromosome 11. Lack of CD15, a cell-surface glycoprotein, leads to marked decrease in neutrophil motility. Lack of H antigen, a precursor to ABO antigen, leads to Bombay blood type (hh).

Diagnosis: Clinically evocated in patients with unusual facial appearance, severe mental retardation, microcephaly, cortical atrophy, seizures, hypotonia, dwarfism, and recurrent infections with neutrophilia. Blood typing, leukocyte function test, and chromosomal study will confirm diagnosis. Can be diagnosed prenatally with cordocentesis for blood typing in suspected fetus.

Clinical aspects: Five cardinal manifestations can be defined: (a) *Unusual facial appearance:* microcephaly, coarse features, flat face, hypertelorism, anteverted nostrils, long upper lip, large protruding tongue, narrow palate, mandible may be small and retracted. (b) central nervous system: severe mental retardation, seizure, hypotonia, cerebral cortical atrophy. (c) *Short stature:* dwarfism. (d) *Defective neutrophil motility:* recurrent bacterial infection with neutrophilia common, particularly pneumonia, periodontitis, otitis media, and localized cellulitis with pus formation. (e) *Bombay blood phenotype.*

Absence of pus formation at site of infection is common. Frequency of infections decreases generally after age of 3 years.

Precautions before anesthesia: Assess for evidence of concurrent infection, particularly pneumonia. Assess neurological function, including seizure control (clinical, EEG, CT). Assess airway for possible difficult tracheal intubation (clinical, radiographs). Ensure availability of blood if transfusion is anticipated.

Anesthetic considerations: Strict asepsis is needed because of neutrophil function alteration. No known particular risk with anesthesia. In view of the abnormal facies, should prepare for airway difficulties if they appear likely in the preoperative assessment. Careful intraoperative positioning is needed.

Pharmacological implications: Consider interaction between antiepileptic treatment and anesthetic drugs. Muscle relaxants should be avoided until airway is secured. Consider prophylactic antibiotics as in immunodeficient patients.

REFERENCES:

Etzioni A, Sturla L, Antonellis A, et al: Leukocyte adhesion deficiency (LAD) type II/carbohydrate deficient glycoprotein (CDG) IIc founder effect and genotype/phenotype correlation. *Am J Med Genet* 110:131–135, 2002.

Frydman M, Etzioni A, Eidlitz-Markus T, et al: Ramban-Hasharon syndrome of psychomotor retardation, short stature, defective neutrophil motility and Bombay phenotype. *Am J Med Genet* 44:297, 1992.

Hidalgo A, Ma S, Peired AJ, et al: Insights into leukocyte adhesion deficiency type 2 from a novel mutation in the GDP-fucose transporter gene. *Blood* 101(5):1705, 2003.

Ramon Syndrome

At a glance: A syndrome characterized by mental deficiency, epilepsy, cherubism, and stunted growth.

Synonyms: Cherubism Gingival Fibromatosis Epilepsy Mental Deficiency Syndrome; Gingival Fibromatosis Hypertrichosis Cherubism Mental Retardation Epilepsy Syndrome.

Genetic inheritance: Autosomal recessive.

Diagnosis: The diagnosis is a clinical one based on the presence of cherubism, mental retardation, and short stature.

Clinical aspects: The affected individuals have a characteristic cherubic facies as a result of fibrous dysplasia of the mandible associated with gingival fibromatosis and overgrowth that leads to inability to close the mouth. Other features include epilepsy, mental retardation, hypertrichosis, and small stature. Some of the reported cases had clinical and radiological signs of juvenile rheumatoid arthritis. Other patients present with ocular involvement (anterior and posterior segment ocular abnormalities, including Axenfeld anomaly, retinopathy, and pale anomalous optic discs). Finally, other manifestations have been described, such as diabetes mellitus, telangiectasia, sensorineural deafness, and changes in the retina.

Precautions before anesthesia: If juvenile rheumatoid arthritis is present and severe, obtain cervical spine radiograph to rule out atlantoaxial instability. Evaluate tracheal intubation (clinical, radiographs). Evaluate neurological function (clinically, electroencephalographic), including seizure medications.

Anesthetic considerations: Because of the gingival and mandibular overgrowth and dysplasia, tracheal intubation may be difficult. Avoid teeth trauma. If the patient presents with juvenile rheumatoid arthritis, vascular access and positioning might be more difficult.

Pharmacological implications: Muscle relaxants should be avoided until airway is secured. Consider interaction between antiepileptic treatment and anesthetic drugs.

REFERENCES:

de Pina-Neto JM, Moreno AFC, Silva LR, et al: Cherubism, gingival fibromatosis, epilepsy, and mental deficiency (Ramon syndrome) with juvenile rheumatoid arthritis. *Am J Med Genet* 25:433, 1986.

Parkin B, Law C: Axenfeld anomaly and retinal changes in Ramon syndrome: Follow-up of two sibs. *Am J Med Genet* 104:131, 2001.

Ramon Y, Berman W, Bubis JJ: Gingival fibromatosis combined with cherubism. *Oral Surg* 24:436, 1967.

Ramsay Hunt Syndrome Type I

At a glance: A very rare genetic disorder characterized by predominant neurological syndrome with alteration of cerebellum and globus pallidus. Muscular functions can also be affected.

Synonym: Myoclonus and Ataxia Syndrome.

Genetic inheritance: Autosomal dominant, heterogeneous.

Pathophysiology: Neurological lesions or anomalies are often observed (cerebellar dentate nucleus, degeneration of globus pallidus, elevated cerebrospinal fluid uric acid); muscle biopsy shows the presence of ragged red fibers that probably are caused by mitochondrial abnormalities, which could explain the pathophysiology of this syndrome. Controversy exists about considering Ramsay Hunt Syndrome as a specific entity.

Diagnosis: Association of myoclonus ataxia and occasional seizures.

Clinical aspects: Neurological signs are isolated. No other association is known. Myoclonus, cerebellar ataxia, intention tremor, and occasional tonic–clonic seizures are the only symptoms.

Precautions before anesthesia: Evaluate the neurological repercussion. Evaluate muscular status especially for the presence of myoclonic tone. Verify ability of patients to use patient-controlled analgesia if necessary.

Anesthetic considerations: The presence of epilepsy must be considered and medication known to stimulate convulsions (e.g., sevoflurane) should be avoided.

Pharmacological implications: The antiepileptic medication must be continued until the morning of surgery. Avoid succinylcholine in presence of muscular abnormalities and potential risk (undocumented) of hyperkalemic response. Avoid enflurane, methohexital, and hypnomidate because of seizure.

Other conditions to be considered:

☞**PARALYSIS AGITANS JUVENILE OF HUNT:** Autosomal dominant. This syndrome is characterized by mask-like facies, parkinsonism, tremor, bradykinesia, dysarthria, rigidity, gait disturbance, and flexion dystonia of fingers. Progression is slow. Onset in teens or earlier.

DYSSYNERGIA CEREBELLARIS MYOCLONICA OF HUNT (Cerebelloparenchymal Disorder V, Spinodentate Atrophy): Autosomal recessive with ataxia, myoclonic jerks, dentate neuron loss superior, and cerebellar peduncle fiber loss.

REFERENCE:

Bomont P, Watanabe M, Gershoni-Barush R, et al: Homozygosity mapping of spinocerebellar ataxia with cerebellar atrophy and peripheral neuropathy to 9q33-34, and with hearing impairment and optic atrophy to 6p21-23. *Eur J Hum Genet* 8(12):986, 2000.

Ramsay Hunt Syndrome Type II

At a glance: A very rare and progressive cerebellar dyssynergia with intention tremor first localized to one extremity, convulsions, and myoclonic epileptic jerks. Ragged red fibers are seen on muscle biopsies.

Synonyms: Dentate Cerebellar Ataxia; Dentatorubral Atrophy; Primary Dentatum Atrophy.

History: First described by James Ramsay Hunt, an American neurologist in 1921.

Genetic inheritance: Autosomal dominant with reduced penetrance.

Pathophysiology: Neurological lesions or anomalies are often observed (cerebellar dentate nucleus, degeneration of globus pallidus, elevated cerebrospinal fluid [CSF] uric acid); muscle biopsy shows presence of ragged red fibers that probably are caused by mitochondrial abnormalities, which could explain the pathophysiology of this syndrome. Controversy exists about considering Ramsay Hunt syndrome as a specific entity.

Diagnosis: Association of myoclonus ataxia and occasional seizures.

Clinical aspects: Neurological signs are isolated. No other association is known. Myoclonus, cerebellar ataxia, intention tremor, and occasional tonic–clonic seizures are the only symptoms.

Precautions before anesthesia: Evaluate the neurological repercussion (clinical, EEG, CT) and muscular status.

Anesthetic considerations: Patients should be considered epileptic and the use of anesthetic agents inducing seizures (e.g., enflurane, sevoflurane) should be avoided.

Pharmacological implications: The antiepileptic medication(s) should be continued until the morning of surgery. Because of the presence of muscular abnormalities and risk (undocumented) of hyperkalemic response it is recommended to avoid succinylcholine. Consider interaction between antiepileptic treatment and anesthetic drugs.

Other conditions to be considered:

☞**JUVENILE PARALYSIS AGITANS OF HUNT:** Autosomal dominant, this syndrome is characterized by mask-like facies, parkinsonism, tremor, bradykinesia, dysarthria, rigidity, gait disturbance, and flexion dystonia of fingers. Progression is slow. Onset in teens or earlier.

DYSSYNERGIA CEREBELLARIS MYOCLONICA OF HUNT (Cerebelloparenchymal Disorder V, Spinodentate Atrophy): Autosomal recessive with ataxia, myoclonic jerks, dentate neuron loss superior, and cerebellar peduncle fiber loss.

REFERENCES:

Hunt JR: Dyssynergia cerebellaris myoclonica—Primary atrophy of the dentate system: A contribution to the pathology and symptomatology of the cerebellum. *Brain* 44:490, 1921.

Marsden CD, Obeso JA: Viewpoints on the Ramsay Hunt syndrome: 1. The Ramsay Hunt syndrome is a useful clinical entity. *Move Disord* 4:6, 1989.

Raynaud Syndrome

At a glance: Short duration vasospasms of the small arteries of the arms and legs, hands and feet. Usually diagnosed before age 40 years.

Synonyms: Raynaud Disease; Raynaud Phenomenon; Acrocyanosis Chronica Anesthetica; Symmetric Asphyxia.

Classification: *Raynaud Disease* refers to the familial (genetic) part. *Raynaud Syndrome or Phenomenon* refers to the acquired symptoms that are often associated with underlying diseases.

Disorders associated with Raynaud Phenomenon include the following:

- Neurovascular compression (thoracic outlet syndromes, crutch pressure carpal tunnel syndrome)
- Arterial diseases (thromboangiitis obliterans, thromboembolism, arteriosclerosis)
- Blood abnormalities (cryoglobulinemia, cryofibrinogenemia, cold hemagglutinins, monoclonal gammopathy, polycythemia)
- Occupational (percussion and vibratory tool workers, traumatic occlusive arterial disease, vinyl chloride workers)
- Drugs and toxins (ergot, methylsergide, beta-blocker drugs, chemotherapy, epinephrine)
- Connective-tissue diseases (systemic sclerosis, systemic lupus erythematosus, mixed connective-tissue disease, rheumatoid arthritis, dermatomyositis, polymyositis)
- Miscellaneous (complex regional pain syndrome—reflex sympathetic dystrophy, hypothyroidism, pheochromocytoma, neoplasm, primary pulmonary hypertension, variant angina)

History: First described by A.G. Maurice Raynaud, French Physician, in 1862.

Incidence: Not known because of the confusion between the acquired form and familial illness; however, reported to range from 0.06 to 30 from 0.006 to 30% in the general population. Primary disease may vary from 15 to 75% in this population. Male:female ratio is 1:5. Most common in young women and 60 to 90% of reported cases are idiopathic.

Genetic inheritance: No evidence of genetic inheritance.

Pathophysiology: Unknown.

Diagnosis: Clinically evocated by characteristic attack of distal vasospasm with whitening of the extremities.

Clinical aspects: Intermittent attacks of numb and white fingers. The classic description includes three phases. *First,* vasospasm leads to pallor of the fingers and toes. Usually bilateral and involves all fingers. Occasionally, it may involve ears and nose. *Second,* capillaries dilate after a few minutes, but the digital arteries still are in spasm. The fingers get blue and the numbness and pain appear. *Finally,* the vessels dilate with redness of the fingers with a feeling of warmth and itching and tingling. In long-standing cases, atrophy and resorption of the fingertips with or without painful areas of necrosis may appear.

Precautions before anesthesia: Assess the presence and the severity of the underlying diseases.

Anesthetic considerations: Special attention to avoid cold exposure.

Pharmacological implications: Avoid methylsergide and ergot derivatives. Minimize the use of beta-blocking drugs, and, if possible, catecholamines, especially the more potent alpha-vasoconstrictive ones. If absolutely necessary, consider regional sympathetic blockade for the extremities.

Other conditions to be considered:

☞**CREST SYNDROME:** An autoimmune connective tissue disorder associated with anticentromere antibodies. A form of scleroderma associated with esophageal dysmotility.

☞**ERYTHROMELALGIA:** A disorder characterized by vasodilatation associated with paroxysmal, intense burning pain, and episodic reddening of the extremities (mainly feet). The symptoms of redness, heat, pain, and swelling, when not associated with organic disease, constitute the primary form, which has also been termed "erythermalgia" because of the significance of the heat.

The secondary or acquired form is related to underlying medical conditions.

REFERENCES:

Bedforth NM, Lockey DJ: Raynaud's syndrome following intravenous induction of anaesthesia. *Anaesthesia* 50(3):248, 1995.

Kone-Paut I, Olivar E, Elbhar C, et al: Raynaud's syndrome in children. Study of 23 cases. *Arch Pediatr* 9(4):365, 2002.

Raynaud AGM: De l'asphyxie locale et de la gangrène symétrique des extrémités. Doctoral thesis, published February 25, 1862.

REAR Syndrome

At a glance: A very rare syndrome that can also be associated with cardiac and neurological anomalies. REAR is an acronym that stands for: **R**enal-**E**ar-**A**nal-**R**adial.

Synonyms: Townes-Brocks Syndrome; Imperforate Anus, Hand, Foot, and Ear Anomalies; Sensorineural Deafness with Imperforate Anus and Hypoplastic Thumbs Syndrome; Branchiootorenal-like Syndrome.

Genetic inheritance: Autosomal dominant, total penetrance, variable expressivity. The gene (SALL1) is mapped on chromosome 16 (16q12.1).

Pathophysiology: Caused by consequence of a mutation in a gene coding for a transcription factor.

Diagnosis: Association of four signs: anorectal malformations (80%), hand and feet deformities (50%), external ear abnormalities (65%), sensorineural deafness (40%).

Clinical aspects: Features include *gastrointestinal* signs (duodenal atresia, imperforate anus, anal stenosis, anterior placement of anus, rectovaginal/rectoperineal fistula), *abnormality of the extremity* (radial ray deformities, broad thumb, bifid thumb, triphalangeal thumb, preaxial polydactyly, syndactyly, fusion of metatarsals, absent/hypoplastic third toe, fifth toe clinodactyly, pseudoepiphysis of second metacarpal), *ear deformations* (overfolding of superior helix, large ears, preauricular tags, preauricular pits, microtia satyr ear, sensorineural hearing), *cardiovascular anomalies* (e.g., tetralogy of Fallot or ventricular septal defect), *microcephaly* (with some cases of mental retardation), and multiple *genitourinary deformations* (hypospadias, bifid scrotum, prominent midline perineal raphe, hypoplastic kidneys, vesicoureteral reflux, urethral valves, multicystic kidneys, dysplastic kidneys, renal failure).

Precautions before anesthesia: Evaluate cardiac function (clinical, ECG, echocardiography, radionuclide imaging if necessary); renal function (blood analysis: kaliemia, creatinine, sodium, abdominal echography, eventually CT scan).

Anesthetic considerations: Anesthetic management will be adapted to both cardiopathy and renal status. Venous access and pulse oximetry can be more difficult because of extremity deformities. Fluid regimen must be adapted to renal status. Prophylactic antibiotics must be done in case of cardiopathy.

Pharmacological implications: Avoid cardiac-depressive drugs; prefer drugs with hepatic or plasmatic metabolism. Aminoglycosides are not contraindicated but must be adapted to renal clearance and benefit has to be clearly evaluated in case of renal insufficiency and incomplete deafness. Prophylactic antibiotics in case of cardiopathy as indicated.

Other conditions to be considered:

☞**HOLT-ORAM SYNDROME:** Characterized by thumb anomaly and atrial septal defect, although abnormality of the upper extremities can be more extensive in some cases. The thumb may be absent or may be a triphalangeal, nonopposable, finger-like digit. Upper extremity phocomelia and ventricular septal defect have been reported in few patients.

IMPERFORATE ANUS: A rare abnormality that can occur alone or as an anomaly of another disorder.

☞**VATER ASSOCIATION** is an acronym for (V)ertebral anomalies, (A)nal atresia, (T)racheo(E)sophageal fistula and (R)enal anomalies. Abnormalities are present at birth. This syndrome is different than the REAR Syndrome.

REFERENCES:

Devriendt K, Fryns JP, Lemmens F, et al: Somatic mosaicism and variable expression of Townes-Brocks syndrome. *Am J Med Genet* 111(2):230, 2002.

Powell CM, Michaelis RC: Townes-Brocks syndrome. *J Med Genet* 36:89, 1999.

Surka WS, Kohlhase J, Neunert CE, et al: Unique family with Townes-Brocks syndrome, SALL1 mutation, and cardiac defects. *Am J Med Genet* 102:250, 2001.

Reardon Wilson Cavanagh Syndrome

At a glance: A very rare neurological disorder, first described by Reardon, comprised of ataxia, deafness, and mental retardation.

Synonyms: Ataxia Deafness Reardon type; Ataxia-Deafness-Retardation (ADR) Syndrome.

Incidence and genetic inheritance: Fewer than 20 cases worldwide. Autosomal recessive.

Diagnosis: Diagnosis is clinical on the association of the ataxia, mental retardation, progressive sensorineural deafness. In addition to the three principal signs that make diagnosis, hypotonia and abnormal gate can also be observed.

Anesthetic considerations: Evaluate the significance of the muscle weakness and the degree of deafness. Careful intraoperative positioning should be used because of hypotonia. Previous knowledge of gait abnormality intensity is necessary before authorizing board discharge in day surgery. Aminoglycosides should be used with great caution because of the progressive deafness.

REFERENCE:

Reardon W, Wilson J, Cavanagh N, et al: A new form of familial ataxia, deafness, and mental retardation. *J Med Genet* 30:694, 1993.

Recombinant Chromosome 8 Syndrome

At a glance: Chromosomal disorder found in individuals of Hispanic descent with ancestry from the San Luis Valley in the Southwest of the United States. The association of mental retardation, congenital heart defects, seizures, a characteristic facial appearance, and urogenital anomalies characterizes the syndrome.

Synonym: San Luis Valley Syndrome; Rec 8 Syndrome.

History: First described by A. Fujimoto in 1975.

Incidence: Rare; mostly seen in Hispanic children born in the southwestern United States.

Genetic inheritance: Because of an unbalanced recombinant chromosome 8 with partial duplication of the long arm of the maternal pericentric inversion (inv 8p23.1q22.1). There is an approximately 6% risk that an inv(8) carrier will have an offspring with Recombinant Chromosome 8 Syndrome.

Pathophysiology: Recombinant 8 genotype has a duplication 8q(q22->qter) and deficiency 8p(p23->pter), resulting in rec8 (8qter->8q22.1:8p23.1->8qter). The rec8 phenotype consists of a characteristic set of minor facial anomalies, cardiovascular and other major malformations, and moderate to severe mental retardation.

Diagnosis: Clinical based on the characteristic facies and the presence of mental retardation, cardiac, and urogenital malformations. Chromosomal study.

Clinical aspects: Features involve *head* (brachycephaly, wide face, midface hypoplasia, infraorbital creases, hypertelorism, anteverted nares, thin upper lip, thick lower lip, downturn mouth, gingival hyperplasia, micrognathia, strabismus, nystagmus, low-set ears, hearing loss with frequent otitis media), *heart* (conotruncal defect and tetralogy of Fallot are most common), central nervous system (CNS) (moderate to severe mental retardation, seizure, abnormal muscle tone with either hypertonia or hypotonia, scoliosis common from neuromuscular origin), *urogenital system* (cryptorchidism, hypoplastic scrotum, other urinary tract anomalies, impairment of renal function).

Precautions before anesthesia: Full cardiac evaluation including ECG, chest radiograph, echocardiogram, and cardiac catheterization must be obtained because it is the major cause of mortality. Depending on the severity of the facial anomalies, a careful evaluation of the airway must be conducted (clinical, radiographic). Renal function tests must include renal ultrasonography, intravenous pyelogram, routine electrolytes, urea, and creatinine. Neurological test includes clinical, EEG, CT, and MRI.

Anesthetic considerations: Techniques should be tailored to the cardiac defect present and the procedure planned. Measures to prevent air embolism must be taken. Adequate intravascular hydration must be ensured. The presence of macroglossia and micrognathia may contribute to difficult laryngoscopy and tracheal intubation. A laryngeal mask should always be available. Positioning may be difficult if contracture occurred from hypertonia. The risk of pressure necrosis must be considered.

Pharmacological implications: May consider avoiding suxamethonium if there is evidence of delayed myelination in CNS. Consider interaction between antiepileptic medication and anesthetic drugs. Endocarditis prophylaxis as indicated. Avoid muscle relaxants until airway is secured.

REFERENCES:

Fujimoto A, Wilson MG, Towner JW: Familial inversion of chromosome no. 8: An affected child and a carrier fetus. *Humangenetik* 27:67, 1975.

Gelb B, Towbin J, McCabe E, et al: San Luis Valley recombinant chromosome 8 and tetralogy of Fallot: A review of chromosome 8 anomalies and congenital heart disease. *Am J Med Genet* 40:471, 1991.

Smith ACM, Spuhler K, Williams TM, et al: Genetic risk for recombinant 8 syndrome and the transmission rate of balanced inversion 8 in the Hispanic population of the southwestern United States. *Am J Hum Genet* 41: 1083, 1987.

Sujansky E, Smith A, Prescott K, et al: Natural history of the recombinant (8) syndrome. *Am J Med Genet* 47:512, 1993.

Refetoff Syndrome

At a glance: Inherited condition resulting in clinical euthyroidism or hypothyroidism in the presence of elevated serum thyroxine levels. End-organ unresponsiveness to thyroid hormone. Other features include congenital deafness, goiter, and exophthalmos.

Synonyms: Thyroid Hormone Unresponsiveness; Thyroid Hormone Resistance.

Genetic inheritance: It has been suggested that both autosomal dominant and recessive forms exist because of different mutations in the same gene. However, mutations that affect the TH receptors are called dominant-negative mutations.

Pathophysiology: Thyroid Hormone Resistance Syndromes may be classified as Generalized Thyroid Hormone Resistance (GTHR) or Pituitary Thyroid Hormone Resistance (PTHR). Although both GTHR and PTHR result from similar mutations, PTHR is selective in that only the pituitary gland is affected. Mutation of the c-erbA beta gene results in a beta-thyroid hormone receptor that is dominant and has an inhibitory effect on normal beta and alpha thyroid hormone receptors, rendering affected tissues refractory to the effects of thyroxine. The molecular mechanisms of this inhibitory effect are currently under investigation. GTHR is usually heterozygous (one mutant beta allele) The GTHR phenotype is variable and may reflect variable expression of mutant alleles or the presence of other genetic regulatory factors as yet undefined. Refetoff syndrome is caused by complete absence of the beta receptor. A variant in which patients are homozygous for the mutant beta allele (two dominant negative alleles expressed) is also described.

Diagnosis: Elevated serum T_4 and T_3. Normal or moderately elevated serum thyroid-stimulating hormone, which is inappropriate in context of the elevated T_4 and T_3. Clinically euthyroid or hypothyroid. In PTHR, the clinical picture is of hyperthyroidism.

Clinical aspects: Goiter is common in GTHR. Delayed speech development, mental retardation, and delayed skeletal maturation represent subtle signs of hypothyroidism. Florid clinical signs and symptoms of hypothyroidism are unusual. Attention deficit disorder is commonly associated with GTHR. GTHR has been erroneously diagnosed as thyrotoxicosis on the basis of laboratory investigations; however, GTHR does not demonstrate depression of thyroid-stimulating hormone levels as is seen in thyrotoxicosis. Treatment is not required for GTHR except in the presence of growth retardation or delayed skeletal maturation. PTHR results in loss of negative feedback to the pituitary with normal peripheral tissue response to thyroxine causing clinical hyperthyroidism which has been treated successfully with D-thyroxine. The condition should be distinguished from a primary pituitary thyroid-stimulating hormone-secreting tumor.

Precautions before anesthesia: Examine for signs of clinical hypothyroidism (GTHR) and hyperthyroidism (PTHR). Consider ECG in presence of bradycardia or history suggestive of dysrhythmia. Review and continue current drug therapy perioperatively. Review thyroid function.

Anesthetic considerations: Euthyroid patients should not cause great concern; however, the possibility of differential resistance to thyroxine between tissues exists. The occurrence of tachydysrhythmias under anesthesia may represent hyperthyroid effects on cardiac muscle requiring beta blockade. Overt clinical hypothyroidism (or hyperthyroidism) should be controlled in consultation with an endocrinologist prior to anesthesia. Regional anesthesia may be useful when the procedure permits.

Pharmacological implications: Esmolol is probably the perioperative beta blocker of choice if signs of hyperthyroidism develop.

REFERENCE:
Usala S: Resistance to thyroid hormone in children. *Curr Opin Pediatr* 6:468, 1994.

Refsum Syndrome

At a glance: A rare disorder of lipid metabolism characterized by peripheral neuropathy, ataxia, retinitis pigmentosa, and bone and skin changes. Other features include cutaneous ichthyosis and cardiac failure.

Synonyms: Phytanic Acid Oxidase Deficiency; Heredopathia Atactica Polyneuritiformis; Hereditary Motor and Sensory Neuropathy IV.

Genetic inheritance: Autosomal recessive. This slowly progressive disorder is most common in children and young adults of Scandinavian heritage.

Pathophysiology: Phytanic acid is derived from the metabolism of chlorophyll. Refsum disease is caused by mutations in the gene encoding phytanoyl-CoA hydroxylase (PAHX or PHYH) or the gene encoding peroxin-7 (PEX7), resulting in accumulation of exogenous phytanic acid (milk, fat of cows and sheep) in blood plasma and tissues. It belongs to the pathological group of leukodystrophy that affects growth of the myelin. Genes are located on 6q22-q24 and 10pter-p11.2.

Diagnosis: Usually evocated and diagnosed during childhood or young adulthood on the association of retinitis pigmentosa, chronic polyneuropathy, and cerebellar signs. It can be confirmed by laboratory investigations: phytanic acid oxidase deficiency and 3,7,11,15-tetramethyl-hexadecanic acid in serum and tissue deposits. Histological analysis shows interstitial hypertrophic polyneuritis and degeneration of nuclei and fiber tracts in brainstem.

Clinical aspects: Congenital skeletal abnormalities can occur: multiple epiphyseal dysplasia, and bilateral fourth metatarsal shortening. Progressive problems appear secondarily: *ocular* (retinitis pigmentosa, myosis, ptosis, cataract, nystagmus), *neurological* (chronic polyneuritis, cerebellar signs, ataxia, anosmia, nerve deafness, hypotonia, hemiparesis), *cardiac* (electrocardiographic changes, congestive heart failure), and *cutaneous* (ichthyosis). Other features include renal failure, amyotrophy, and respiratory distress.

Precautions before anesthesia: A complete evaluation of the cardiac function (echography, ECG, radionuclide imaging if necessary); renal function (kalemia, urea, creatinine); respiratory function (chest radiograph, arterial blood gas analysis, pulmonary function test) must be obtained. A review of the neuropathy evolution and muscular weakness is essential.

Anesthetic considerations: Exacerbation of this disease has been observed with surgery and pregnancy. Perioperative fluid management should be realized in case of renal dysfunction. Careful perioperative positioning is necessary to avoid nerve compression in these patients with neuropathy. Cardiac perioperative monitoring is necessary because of the risk of ECG change.

Pharmacological implications: Avoid cardiodepressive, ototoxic, and nephrotoxic drugs. Aminoglycosides can be used, but real interest has to be evaluated in the presence of incomplete deafness or renal dysfunction. Avoid succinylcholine in patients with neuropathy (risk of hyperkalemia). Local anesthetics are not contraindicated; however, the interest should be evaluated in consideration for an evolutive neuropathic disease. Clear information has to be given and understood by the patient.

Other conditions to be considered:

REFSUM INFANTILE FORM (**Infantile Phytanic Acid Storage Disease**): Autosomal recessive. Caused by mutations in peroxisomal membrane protein-3 (35 kDa); gene located on 8q21.1, 7q21-q22. Clinical features include early onset, mental retardation, minor facial dysmorphism, retinitis pigmentosa, sensorineural hearing deficit, hepatomegaly, osteoporosis, failure to thrive, and hypocholesterolemia.

REFSUM DISEASE WITH INCREASED PIPECOLIC ACIDEMIA (**RDPA**): Autosomal recessive. Gene located on 10pter-p11.2. Characterized by accumulation of L-pipecolic acid and clinically by rapidly progressing neurological deteriorations.

> *Note:* Refsum Disease can be confused with other similar disorders, including Bassen-Kornzweig Disease and Kearns-Sayre Syndrome. (See each description in the book)

REFERENCES:

Jansen GA, Ofman R, Ferdinandusse S, et al: Refsum disease is caused by mutations in the phytanoyl-CoA hydroxylase gene. *Nat Genet* 17:190, 1997.

van den Brink DM, Brites P, Haasjes J, et al: Identification of PEX7 as the second gene involved in Refsum disease. *Am J Hum Genet* 72(2):471, 2003.

Wierzbicki AS, Lloyd MD, Schofield CJ, et al: Refsum's disease: A peroxisomal disorder affecting phytanic acid alpha-oxidation. *J Neurochem* 80(5):727, 2002.

Reifenstein Syndrome

At a glance: A syndrome characterized by hypogonadism as a result of a defect in androgen receptor. Often described as the male pseudohermaphrodism, presenting with hypospadias, gynecomastia, normal XY karyotype, and a pattern X-linked recessive inheritance.

Synonyms: Partial Androgen Insensitivity; Gynecomastia-Hypospadias Syndrome; Hereditary Familial Hypogonadism; Male Pseudohermaphroditism.

Classification: Two types have been suggested: Type I refers to the familial incomplete male pseudohermaphrodism and Type II is the autosomal recessive.

Incidence: Undetermined; however, it is certainly common because of its often mild and variable features.

Genetic inheritance: X-linked recessive.

Pathophysiology: Underlying defect is the partial deficiency of androgen receptors (AR), causing partial androgen resistance, and not because of a lack of androgen synthesis.

Diagnosis: Clinical features (hypogonadism); family history; elevated plasma luteinizing hormone and testosterone levels; oligospermia or azoospermia; testis biopsy show normal Leydig and Sertoli cells but immature germinal cells and no spermatozoa; cultured fibroblast from genital skin show reduced levels of androgen receptor present with decreased cytoplasmic dihydrotestosterone binding capacity. The normal chromosomal study (46,XY) and normal testos-

terone conversion enzyme study (particularly 5-reductase level) exclude other causes of androgen resistance.

Clinical aspects: The phenotype is quite variable as a consequence of the partial sensitivity of the androgen receptors. In its mildest form, the man is infertile but otherwise normal. In its most severe form, the male pseudohermaphrodite may have hypospadias, cryptorchism, bifid scrotum, microphallus, atrophic ectopic testes, pseudovagina, gynecomastia, and absent vas deferens. Axillary and pubic hair is usually normal but chest and facial hair are minimal. Temporal recession of hairline is minimal and the voice is prepubertal in character. Azoospermia is common and occasionally accompanied by hypoplasia of vas deferens. Most have a male psychological development. Germ cell malignancies can occur.

Anesthetic considerations: There are no reported consideration for this disorder. However, supplemental steroid administration perioperatively might be indicated.

Other conditions to be considered:

17-BETA HYDROXYSTEROID DEHYDROGENASE DEFICIENCY (**17-Ketosteroid Reductase Deficiency; 17-Beta HSD**) presents clinically as male pseudohermaphroditism associated with significant enlargement of the adrenal glands and production of steroids impaired. It is inherited as either autosomal recessive or X-linked recessive.

17-ALPHA HYDROXYLASE DEFICIENCY presents in adolescence because of failure of the adrenal gland and testes to produce androgens. Because males are not exposed to androgens during fetal development they are born with female external genitalia. Failure to menstruate or to develop secondary sexual traits such as breasts or body hair, hypertension, and hypokalemia are characteristic.

3-BETA HYDROXYSTEROID DEHYDROGENASE DEFICIENCY (**3-Beta-HSD**) is present at birth and leads to death within the first few hours. Glucocorticoids and mineralocorticoids are not produced. Boys are born with female or ambiguous external genitalia. A few patients with incomplete forms of this disorder may only be detected later in childhood or adulthood. Menstruation may occur between the ages of 4 and 8, the clitoris is enlarged, acne and advanced maturation of the skeleton may be seen in young children as well as hirsutism.

☞KLINEFELTER SYNDROME is a disorder resulting from an excess of X chromosomes. It affects males only and is characterized by small testes, lack of sperm, enlarged mammary glands, and an abnormally small penis. An absence of facial and body hair, lack of muscular development, and a high-pitched voice are characteristic.

☞ROSEWATER SYNDROME is characterized by the presence of gynecomastia with hypogonadism occurring only in males in a pattern consistent with X-linked or autosomal dominant inheritance. It differs from the Reifenstein syndrome by the absence of hypospadias. However, the presence of hypogonadism enter the differential diagnosis of male hypogonadism. It has been suggested that this condition is the mildest expression of incomplete male pseudohermaphroditism, type I.

REFERENCES:

Amrhein J, Klingensmith G, Walsh P, et al: Partial androgen insensitivity: The Reifenstein syndrome revisited. *N Engl J Med* 297(7):350, 1977.

Gottlieb B, Pinsky L, Beitel LK, et al: Androgen insensitivity. *Am J Med Genet* 89(4):210, 1999.

Griffin J, Wilson J: The syndrome of androgen resistance. *N Engl J Med* 302(4):198, 1980.

Renal-Coloboma Syndrome

At a glance: A rare familial syndrome combining ocular, renal and neurological signs.

Synonyms: Papillorenal Syndrome; Optic Nerve Coloboma with Renal Disease; Optic Coloboma, Vesicoureteral Reflux, and Renal Anomalies Syndrome; Coloboma-Ureteral-Renal Syndrome.

Incidence and genetic inheritance: Unknown incidence. Autosomal dominant because of mutation in the PAX2 gene (a transcription factor known to play a critical role in embryogenesis and to be expressed in the developing eye, ear, kidney, ureteric bud, and midbrain/hindbrain) located on 10q24.3-q25.1.

Clinical aspects: Ophthalmic and renal anomalies of this syndrome are most often bilateral, but highly variable. The mutations in the PAX2 gene lead to colobomatous eye defects. Developmental abnormalities of the optic fissure result in a group of defects including orbital cysts, microphthalmia, optic disc dysplasia, and colobomas of the optic nerve (sometimes referred to as "Morning Glory Disc Anomaly") and retina at the posterior pole of the globe. (Iris colobomas have not been observed in patients with mutations in PAX2). Optic nerve colobomas involve the optic nerve head or optic papilla, and also result in thinning of the surrounding retinal epithelium, causing congenital blindness or loss of visual acuity, although not all patients with optic nerve colobomas have visual defects. Progressive deterioration of visual acuity over several decades has been described. The kidneys often appear small. The degree of renal disease is very variable, but the disease is usually progressive and often requires dialysis and/or renal transplant (although the age at end-stage renal disease is very variable). Patients with basically normal renal function have also been described. Renal biopsies may demonstrate mesangial fibrosis, glomerulosclerosis, glomerular hyalinization, hyperplastic glomeruli, tubular atrophy, and an overall rarefaction of glomeruli. Pathological examination of kidneys may find cortical thinning, hypoplastic papillae, a decreased number of glomeruli in the cortex and collecting ducts in the papilla, consistent with renal hypoplasia. Vesicoureteral reflux (VUR) is common in these children; however, it is not known to which extent VUR is responsible for the kidney changes described above. Some of these patients may also suffer from high-frequency hearing loss, central nervous system anomalies (seizure disorder, ☞Arnold Chiari Syndrome Type I), joint laxity, and genital anomalies (cryptorchidism).

Anesthetic considerations: Preoperative laboratory investigations should include a complete cell blood count (CBC) (renal anemia), serum electrolytes, serum albumin (proteinuria), creatinine, and blood urea nitrogen. In case of end-stage renal disease, ask about the date of the last hemodialysis, residual urine production, and the daily maximal allowable amount to drink. Avoid potassium-containing intravenous solutions in these patients. Chronic antiepileptic treatment may interfere with the metabolism and elimination of anesthetic drugs.

Other conditions to be considered:

☞**CHARGE Syndrome:** A life-threatening, congenital syndrome of multiple abnormalities, consisting of coloboma, heart disease, choanal atresia, mental and growth retardation, genital and urinary anomalies, and ear anomalies with deafness. The prognosis worsens if the disorder is associated with concomitant cyanotic congenital heart disease, central nervous system anomalies, and esophageal atresia.

☞**COACH Syndrome:** An inherited syndrome characterized by the combination of hepatic fibrosis, early-onset ataxia, cerebellar aplasia, oligophrenia, and coloboma.

☞**Joubert Syndrome:** A genetic disorder characterized by cerebral malformations (vermis and brainstem) resulting in severe coordination (ataxia) and breathing (sleep apnea, hyperpnea) disorders.

☞**Loken Senior Syndrome:** Inherited disorder characterized by rapidly progressive renal insufficiency (nephronophthisis) and eye disease (retinitis pigmentosa).

REFERENCES:

Eccles MR, Schimmenti LA: Renal-coloboma syndrome: A multisystem developmental disorder caused by PAX2 mutations. *Clin Genet* 56:1, 1999.

Ford B, Rupps R, Lirenman D, et al: Renal-coloboma syndrome: Prenatal detection and clinical spectrum in a large family. *Am J Med Genet* 99:137, 2001.

Renal Tubular Dysgenesis

At a glance: A very rare familial disorder characterized by incompletely or abnormally developed cortical tubules. Similar renal pathology is seen in infants born of women who had taken angiotensin-converting enzyme (ACE) inhibitors during pregnancy. Prognosis is poor.

Synonym: Primitive Renal Tubule Syndrome.

History: First described by J.E. Allanson in 1992.

Genetic inheritance: Autosomal recessive inheritance.

Pathophysiology: Probably related to ischemia or hypoperfusion of renal parenchyma with resultant hypoxia affecting those organs requiring a high oxygen tension for normal growth. Another postulation attributed to a lack of angiotensin II growth stimulation, as is found in ACE-inhibitor fetopathy.

Diagnosis: Nephromegaly with characteristic histological appearance whereby the cortical tubules lack normal features of the proximal or distal convolutions. The tubules are short and straight, primitive, and reminiscent of collecting tubules. The glomeruli are crowded with the medullary pyramids smaller than usual. Late second-trimester sonographic demonstration of oligohydramnios, with structurally normal kidneys, should suggest the diagnosis. Associated skull abnormalities may help in suggesting the diagnosis.

Clinical aspects: Gestations are complicated by late-onset oligohydramnios. Liveborns are anuric and develop renal failure. A number of the affected children have skull abnormalities (calvarial hypoplasia, microcephaly, underdeveloped cranial bones, or widely patent fontanelles) with characteristic Potter facies. Hypotonia may occur; respiratory failure, too.

Precautions before anesthesia: Assess intravascular volume and electrolyte imbalances, especially potassium. Correct all anomalies preoperatively. Systematic review of cardiovascular and respiratory status (clinical, ECG, chest radiographs, echocardiography, arterial blood gas analysis). *Investigations:* CBC (note severity of anemia), clotting times, urea, creatinine, and electrolytes, liver function tests. The effects of sedative drugs for premedication are unpredictable because of the changes in plasma protein levels and the altered pH.

Anesthetic considerations: Fluid balance and electrolytes should be monitored carefully. The use of a regional anesthetic technique may be considered, provided there is no coagulopathy or thrombocytopenia. Postoperative ventilatory support can be necessary in case of respiratory failure.

Pharmacological implications: Use barbiturates in lower doses and with caution because the free drug percentage is increased as a consequence of hypoalbuminemia. Avoid suxamethonium if the serum potassium levels >4 mmol/L or if there is presence or suspicion of peripheral neuropathy. Atracurium, *cis*-atracurium, and mivacurium are preferred for neuromuscular blockade because of their rapid elimination that is independent of renal and hepatic functions. Remifentanil would probably also be preferred for the same reason. Morphine and pethidine should be used with caution, because their metabolites tend to accumulate. Aminoglycosides should be used with great caution and doses adapted to renal function.

Other condition to be considered:

ALLANSON PANZAR MCLEOD SYNDROME (Primitive Renal Tubule Syndrome; Renovascular Dysgenesis Syndrome): An autosomal recessive medical condition characterized by renotubular dysgenesis, Potter facies, pulmonary hypoplasia and oligohydramnios. It is usually lethal at birth. Pathological studies reveal the absence, or abnormal form of, proximal convoluted tubules resembling collecting tubules.

REFERENCES:

Allanson JE, Hunter AGW, Mettler GS, et al: Renal tubular dysgenesis: A not uncommon autosomal recessive syndrome: A review. *Am J Med Genet* 43:811, 1992.

McFadden DE, Pantzar JT, Van Allen MI, et al: Renal tubular dysgenesis with calvarial hypoplasia: Report of two additional cases and review. *J Med Genet* 34:846, 1997.

Reticular Dysgenesia

At a glance: One of the rarest and most severe forms of combined immunodeficiency characterized by congenital agranulocytosis, lymphopenia, and lymphoid and thymic hypoplasia with absent cellular and humoral immunity functions. Prognosis is generally poor in the first weeks of life.

Synonyms: Reticular Dysgenesis; De Vaal Disease; Congenital Aleukia; Severe Combined Immunodeficiency with Leukopenia; Hematopoietic Hypoplasia Syndrome.

History: First described by O.M. de Vaal and V. Seynhaeve in 1959.

Genetic inheritance: Autosomal recessive.

Pathophysiology: An abnormality, yet undefined, interferes with normal growth and maturation of immune cells along lymphoid and myelomonocytic pathway, resulting in absent cellular and humoral immunity function.

Diagnosis: Blood cell count shows normal erythrocytes and platelets but no leukocytes. Bone marrow shows absent myeloid elements; myeloid lineage has a characteristic maturation arrest at the stage of promyelocyte. Thymus is small and without Hassall corpuscles. Lymph nodes and spleen are hypoplastic and histologically devoid of lymphocytes.

Clinical aspects: Nearly all affected cases died from overwhelming infections within a few days or weeks of birth. One child survived for 17 weeks in an isolated sterile environment. One case was reported to have bone marrow transplant from an HLA-identical brother and survived with full hematological and immunological reconstitution to 3 years of age.

Precautions before anesthesia: Maintain sterility in all procedures. These individual should be isolated at all time.

Anesthetic considerations: No known experience because of the severity and the very early mortality associated with this condition. Anesthetic considerations are related to a very high risk of infections.

Pharmacological implications: Prophylactic antibiotics as indicated for immunodeficient patients.

REFERENCES:

de Vaal O, Seynhaeve V: Reticular dysgenesia. *Lancet* II:1123, 1959.

Levinsky R, Tiedeman K: Successful bone-marrow transplantation for reticular dysgenesis. *Lancet* I:671, 1983.

Retinoblastoma

At a glance: A familial malignant ocular embryonic tumor develops in the retina because of a defect in a regulatory gene. Prognosis is good. Association with other primary malignancies is frequent.

Synonym: RB.

Incidence: Estimated at 1:16,000 to 23,000 live births in the United States. Over 90% are diagnosed before the age of 5 years. Nonwhite individuals present with a prevalence four times greater than whites. Bilateral cases occur in 20%.

Genetic inheritance: In general, 5 to 10% of cases are inherited, 20 to 30% are new germinal mutations, and 60 to 70% are sporadic (unilateral mainly). Most (90%) bilateral cases are familial. Retinoblastoma gene (Rb) gene is located at 13q14.1-q14.2.

Pathophysiology: Usually develop in posterior portion of retina with multiple foci. Typically invade locally and grow forward into vitreous or backward into optic nerve. Rarely metastasize until very late. Rb gene is thought to have a suppressor function. Retinoblastoma would occur by loss or inactivation of both alleles of this gene. There is a high incidence of second primary tumors, suggesting a key role in the etiology of several other primary malignancies (osteogenic sarcoma, pinealoma, leukemia, lymphoma, and Ewing sarcoma).

Diagnosis: Clinical features and careful ophthalmologic examination. CT and MRI assessment of the eye and orbit is also recommended. Median age at diagnosis is 11 months for bilateral disease and 23 months for unilateral disease.

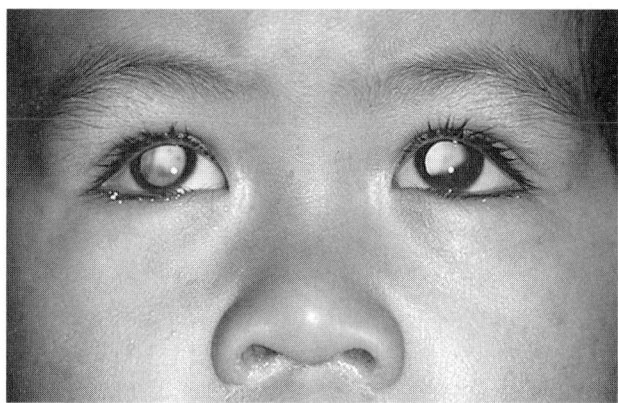

Retinoblastoma This 2-year-old boy with bilateral retinoblastoma shows typical leukocoria (white "cat's eye" reflex).

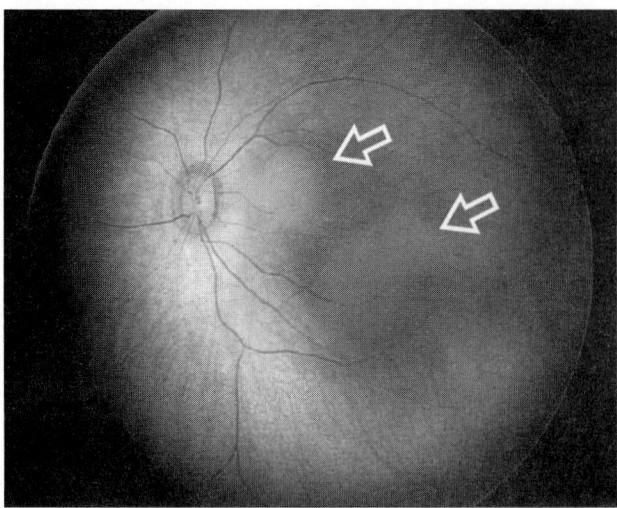

Retinoblastoma The funduscopy in a preterm baby reveals two small retinoblastomas.

Clinical aspects: Early presenting feature is leukocoria (white "cat's eye" reflex), a yellowish-white reflex in the pupil caused by tumor behind the lens. Other common findings include diminishing or absent vision and strabismus. In more advanced disease, there may be pupillary irregularity, hyphema, and pain. Severe disease may have ptosis, raised intracranial pressure, and bone metastasis. Treatment includes cryotherapy, laser ablation, local radiation, and, finally, enucleation. Overall survival is greater than 90%. There is a high risk of other malignancies, particularly osteogenic sarcoma and other germ cell tumors. Retinoblastoma may occur in association with other "13q-syndromes," which are typically characterized by growth delay, mental retardation, and minor facial anomalies.

Precautions before anesthesia: These patients often come to the operating room for examination, laser therapy, cryotherapy, radiotherapy, or staging. A review of the chemotherapy and steroid administration must be obtained. Overall, medical condition must be reviewed.

Anesthetic considerations: There are no specific considerations in isolated form. With multiple and frequent general anesthesia, good rapport with patient and family is important. If laser ablation is used, considerations include laser safety and immobility during laser use. All anesthesia considerations associated to radiotherapy treatment must be applied.

Pharmacological implications: Probably avoid anesthetic drugs with increased intraocular pressure effects in case of vitreous hemorrhage. Prophylactic antibiotics as indicated in immunodeficient patients.

REFERENCES:

Lee WH, Bookstein R, Hong F, et al: Human retinoblastoma susceptibility gene: Cloning, identification, and sequence. *Science* 235:1394, 1987.

Warburg M: Retinoblastoma, in Goldberg M (ed): *Genetic and Metabolic Eye Disease*. Boston, Little, Brown, 1974, p 447.

Watts P, Westall C, Hean E, et al: Visual results in children treated for macular retinoblastoma. *Eye* 16(1):75, 2002.

Wu L, de Bruin A, Saavedra HI, et al: Extra-embryonic function of Rb is essential for embryonic development and viability. *Nature* 421:942, 2003.

Retino-Hepato-Endocrinologic Syndrome

At a glance: A familial syndrome combining peculiar facies, retinal anomalies (progressive cone dystrophy without pigmentation) with degenerative liver disease and endocrine dysfunction (hypothyroidism, diabetes, infertility).

Synonyms: RHE Syndrome; Hansen-Larsen-Berg Syndrome.

History: First described in 1976 by Egill Hansen, Norwegian ophthalmologist, Kare Ingmar Berg, Norwegian geneticist and Ingered Froyshov Larsen, Norwegian internist.

Genetic inheritance: Autosomal recessive.

Pathophysiology: Unknown.

Diagnosis: Clinically evocated by apparition of total colorblindness from progressive cone dystrophy with endocrine involvement. Family history and characteristic fundal examination findings are essential to establish the diagnosis. Blood chemistry shows elevated creatine phosphokinase in all cases.

Clinical aspects: Features include *eyes* (total color blindness from progressive cone dystrophy; no photopic function but scotopic function is well-preserved; fundi examination shows retinal atrophy with no pigmentation, attenuated retinal vessels, and disc pallor), *liver* (degenerative liver disease), *endocrine system* (hypothyroidism, "maturity-onset diabetes of the young," infertility, or repeated abortions). Intelligence and life span are normal.

Precautions before anesthesia: Assess liver function by examination and laboratory investigations, including liver function tests and coagulation profile. Check blood sugar level and if required, begin an insulin regimen. An infusion of dextrose solution should be initiated if necessary. Assess thyroid function by history, examination, and laboratory results. Preoperative laboratory investigations should include creatine phosphokinase levels.

Anesthetic considerations: No reported complications. Blood sugar level should be monitored throughout the perioperative period. Antihypoglycemic drugs and insulin regimen should be tailored to the severity of the disease, the length of fasting, and the type of procedure performed. Severe liver disease is uncommon but coagulation abnormalities, if present, should be corrected prior to major procedure. Perimedullar blockade should be avoided in case of coagulopathy.

Pharmacological implications: If liver dysfunction is present, the use of halothane and muscle relaxants with liver metabolism should be avoided. Succinylcholine is not contraindicated but is best avoided, particularly when abnormal creatine phosphokinase levels are observed.

REFERENCES:

Froyshov Larsen I, Hansen E, Berg K: Familial syndrome of progressive cone dystrophy, degenerative liver disease, and endocrine dysfunction II: Clinical and metabolic studies. *Clin Genet* 13:176, 1978.

Hansen E, Froyshov Larsen I, Berg K: A familial syndrome of progressive cone dystrophy, degenerative liver disease, endocrine dysfunction and hearing defect. I. Ophthalmological findings. *Acta Ophthalmol* 54:129, 1976.

Rett Syndrome

At a glance: A severe and global developmental disorder affecting the central nervous system (CNS) characterized by autism, dementia, ataxia, and loss of purposeful use of the hand. It is known as a uniform and striking progressive encephalopathy. Evolution in four phases after diagnosis is typical. Cardiac, respiratory, and gastrointestinal (GI) signs are associated.

Synonyms: RTS; Autism Dementia Ataxia and Loss of Purposeful Hand Use Syndrome.

History: First described by Andreas Rett, Austrian pediatrician in 1966; Hagberg in 1983 report 35 patients from France, Portugal, and Sweden.

Incidence: Only females are affected; incidence estimated at 1:15,000 to 1:20,000 in the general population. However, it has been suggested that the prevalence is about 1 in 10,000 to 15,000 female newborns in the United States but most are not reported or misdiagnosed.

Genetic inheritance: Probably X-linked dominant with 100% antenatal lethality in hemizygous male. All cases should be new mutations explicable on the basis of gonadal mosaicism or X-autosomal translocation in the mother.

Pathophysiology: Caused by mutation in the gene encoding methyl-CpG-binding protein-2 (MECP2) located on Xq28. Exact physiopathology is still unknown, but several reports have shown elevated endorphin levels in cerebrospinal fluid (CSF) and respiratory pattern is improved with opioid antagonists. The loss of function of MECP2 protein might intervene at the level of neurotransmitters and lead to cerebral hypoperfusion.

Diagnosis: Clinically evocated. Essential criteria are abnormal prenatal and perinatal period; an apparently normal psychomotor development until 6 months of age; a deceleration of head growth (between 5 months and 4 years of age); a loss of acquired purposeful hand skills with development of severely impaired speech associated with severe psychomotor retardation, stereotypic hand movements, and gait and truncal apraxia.

Clinical aspects: Usually normal development until age 1 year followed by regression of language milestones, with appearance of fine tremor of the hands, ataxic gait, and loss of purposeful movement of the hands, which may not appear until the girl is 2 to 3 years old. Autistic behavior becomes evident at this stage. Rupture of head growth becomes evident and is known as "acquired" microcephalia. The disease is also marked with generalized tonic–clonic seizures that are well-controlled by antiepileptic drugs, peculiar sighing respiration, and periods of apnea. There are associated vasomotor disturbances of the legs. After the initial neurological degradation phase, the disease appears to plateau (between 6 and 18 months of age) followed by a rapid regression that stays for a few weeks to a few months. It is followed by stabilization for a few years and, finally, by a long phase of motor deterioration with loss of ambulation. Clinical features can also involved *heart* (prolonged QT interval and T-wave abnormalities), *respiratory system* (periodic apnea while awake or hyperventilation, breath holding), *GI* (constipation, gastroesophageal reflux, cachexia), *muscles and skeleton* (scoliosis, kyphosis, small feet, vasomotor disturbance with cold feet, muscle wasting).

Precautions before anesthesia: A thorough evaluation of the neurological function (clinical, EEG, CT/MRI); cardiac function (clinical, ECG); respiratory function because of scoliosis and breathing dysfunction (clinical, chest radiographs, pulmonary function test if possible, and arterial blood gas analysis); and gastroesophageal reflux (clinical, endoscopy, manometry) is essential. Preoperative laboratory investigations should include electrolytes because of prolonged QT interval.

Anesthetic considerations: Careful intraoperative positioning is needed. A rapid sequence induction is recommended considering the increased risk of pulmonary aspiration because of gastroesophageal reflux. Delayed recovery is common after anesthesia. Postoperative intensive care admission is advised because of poor respiratory control. The need for mechanical ventilation is highly probable. Postoperative analgesia must take into account the already elevated endorphin levels and poor respiratory control. A case report of sudden death occurring 4 weeks after anesthesia is reported. Loco-regional anesthesia techniques have not been reported, but should be considered given the respiratory system involvement and the reduction in opioid use. However, patient compliance is most likely poor and sedation will be required.

Pharmacological implications: Continue antiepileptic medication up to the operation and resume them afterwards as soon as possible. In case of prolonged surgical procedure, the administration of intraoperative Dilantin or phenobarbital must be considered to avoid undetected seizure activities. Consider the interaction between antiepileptic and anesthetic drugs. Avoid sedatives in the preoperative period since these patients may be very sensitive to their respiratory depressive effect. Careful titration of opioids is recommended. No problems have been reported with neuromuscular blocking agents.

REFERENCES:

Dearlove OR, Walker RW: Anesthesia for Rett syndrome. *Paediatr Anaesth* 6:155, 1996.

Konarzewski WH, Misso S: Rett syndrome and delayed recovery from anesthesia. *Anesthesia* 49:357, 1994.

Zeev BB, Yaron Y, Schanen NC, et al: Rett syndrome: Clinical manifestations in males with MECP2 mutations. *J Child Neurol* 17:20, 2002.

Reye Syndrome

At a glance: Possible life-threatening multifactorial syndrome resulting from a previous viral infection treated by aspirin and a genetic sensibility. Dehydration, intracranial hypertension, and liver insufficiency must be considered. Presentation includes seizures, vomiting, lethargy, irrational behavior, and delirium. Tachypnea, jaundice, fever, and coma suggest end-stage of disease. Reye Syndrome appears usually 3 to 5 days after the onset of chickenpox rash.

Synonyms: Fatty Liver with Encephalopathy; Reye-Johnson Syndrome.

Incidence: Rare (1:1,000,000 in the general population); incidence has decreased since 1993.

Genetic inheritance: There is no known genetic association with this condition.

Pathophysiology: Reye Syndrome is a two-phase illness because it is almost always associated with a previous viral infection, such as influenza, cold, or chickenpox. It tends to appear with greatest frequency during January, February, and March. It has been proposed that Reye syndrome develops from the interaction of a viral illness, genetic susceptibility to the disease, and exposure to chemicals, such as salicylates, pesticides, and aflatoxin. Abnormal accumulations of fat begin to develop in the liver and other organs of the body, which can cause a severe increase of intracranial pressure. Unless diagnosed and treated successfully, death is common, often within a few days.

Diagnosis: Syndrome occurs in children and teens (96%). Diagnosis is made by clinical signs (persistent or recurrent vomiting, listlessness, personality changes present during or soon after a viral illness) and by elimination of other diagnoses such as metabolic illness, meningitis, encephalitis, diabetes, drug overdose, sudden infant death, toxic ingestion, head trauma, renal or hepatic failure poisoning, that could imitate Reye Syndrome.

Clinical aspects: Persistent or continuous vomiting; signs of brain dysfunction; listlessness, loss of pep and energy; drowsiness can be observed first and then irritability, aggressive behavior, disorientation, confusion, irrational behavior delirium, convulsions, coma. Beyond these neurological signs, it is possible to observe respiratory disturbances such as hyperventilation. Anemic episodes and hypoglycemia are common;

Precautions before anesthesia: Evaluate liver function (echography, CT, laboratory tests: coagulation, serum glutamic-oxaloacetic transferase [SGOT] and serum glutamic-pyruvic transaminase [SGPT] [increase generally], albumin); respiratory function (clinical, chest radiograph, arterial blood gas analysis); hydration status of the patient (clinical, electrolytes values, urea, creatinine); neurological function (clinical, CT).

Anesthetic considerations: Indication of anesthesia during the evolution of a Reye Syndrome has to be exceptional. Steady state should be raised before starting. Careful monitoring of respiratory function should be done (SpO$_2$ [arterial oxyhemoglobin saturation], etCO$_2$ [end-tidal carbon dioxide concentration], arterial blood gas analysis) in case of respiratory disturbance, since normo- or mild hypocapnia are important, considering the risk of high intracranial pressure. Fluid regimen also needs to be adapted to the existence of dehydration and of high intracranial pressure. It is necessary to measure regularly blood levels for hypoglycemia and hypokalemia.

Pharmacological implications: Avoid succinylcholine because of the possibility of severe raise in intracranial pressure. Avoid drugs with known hepatotoxic effect and metabolism because of common cytolytic hepatitis. Choice of anesthetic drugs should consider their action on intracranial pressure. Regional anesthesia is not contraindicated but it is recommended to check the coagulation profile and bleeding time because of salicylates absorption.

REFERENCES:

Prandota J: Important role of prodromal viral infections responsible for inhibition of xenobiotic metabolizing enzymes in the pathomechanism of idiopathic Reye's syndrome, Stevens-Johnson syndrome, autoimmune hepatitis, and hepatotoxicity of the therapeutic doses of acetaminophen used in genetically predisposed persons. *Am J Ther* 9(2):149, 2002.

Thabet F, Durand P, Chevret L, et al: Severe Reye syndrome: Report of 14 cases managed in a pediatric intensive care unit over 11 years. *Arch Pediatr* 9(6):581, 2002.

Reynolds Neri Hermann Syndrome

At a glance: A rare syndrome characterized by postnatal short stature with cardiac defect (atrial septal defect, pulmonic stenosis) and craniofacial anomalies (facial features similar to Noonan syndrome). Other features include relative macrocephaly, micrognathia, high-arched palate, splenomegaly, hypotonia, hypertonia, hydrocephalus and raised intracranial pressure, and brainstem atrophy (gait ataxia).

Synonyms: Cardio-Facio-Cutaneous Syndrome; CFC syndrome; Facio-Cardio-Cutaneous Syndrome.

History: First described in 1986 by James F. Reynolds, American geneticist, Giovanni Neri, Italian geneticist, and Jürgen Herrmann, German physician.

Incidence: One hundred patients have been presented in the medical literature.

Genetic inheritance: Autosomal dominant, sporadic. Gene map locus at 12q24.1; however, most cases reported are considered sporadic. Associated with advance paternal age.

Diagnosis: Clinical. The manifestations include congenital heart defects, characteristic facial appearance, ectodermal abnormalities, and growth failure.

Clinical aspects: This short-stature patient can present with *cardiac lesions* (78% of cases, pulmonary valve/artery stenosis, congenital cardiac anomaly, atrial septal defect), *cephalic malformations* (ptosis, short neck, brittle hair, microcephaly, epicanthic folds helix, high forehead, bitemporal constriction, thickened/depressed nasal bridge, micrognathia, sparse/absent scalp hair, nystagmus, palate deformations), *orthopedic deformations* (hyperextensible fingers, multiple palmar creases, multiple plantar creases), *cutaneous lesions* (severe atopic dermatitis, ichthyosis, hyperkeratosis, hypohidrosis), and *neurological disturbance* (mild to moderate mental retardation, seizures, hypotonia, hypertonia, hydrocephalus, cortical atrophy, frontal lobe hypoplasia, brainstem atrophy). Hepatosplenomegaly and ectopic testes can also occur.

Precautions before anesthesia: Evaluate cardiac lesion (chest radiograph, echocardiography, ECG, radionuclide imaging if necessary); neurological function (clinical, EEG, somatosensory evoked potentials, CT).

Anesthetic considerations: Careful intraoperative positioning is needed; in case of cardiopathy, perioperative cardiac monitoring should be used and adapted anesthetic technique for the cardiac anomaly. Direct laryngoscopy and tracheal intubation can be difficult because of facial deformation. Fiberoptic intubation may be required. Avoid hyperthermia because of hypohidrosis. Perimedullar anesthesia is not contraindicated but one must consider the risk because of the neuroectodermal origin of most lesions.

Pharmacological implications: Prophylactic antibiotics must be considered as indicated in case of cardiopathy. Antiepileptic and cardiac drugs must be continued until the day of the surgery. Consider interaction between antiepileptic treatment and anesthetic drugs. Avoid muscle relaxants until airway is secured.

Other conditions to be considered:

☞**NOONAN SYNDROME:** Characterized by a distinctive facial appearance similar to the CFC syndrome. The clinical features include webbing of the neck, short stature, characteristic abnormalities of the chest (pectus carinatum and/or pectus excavatum), congenital heart defects (pulmonary stenosis), and/or other abnormalities of which the most relevant are thrombocytopenia and coagulation factor deficiencies. Abnormally large and/or present in unusual places bruising and bleeding are common. It is inherited as an autosomal dominant transmission. There is disagreement in the medical literature whether Noonan and CFC syndromes are distinct medical conditions.

☞**COSTELLO SYNDROME:** Characterized by short stature, distinctive facial characteristics (excessive loose skin on the neck, palms of the hands, fingers, and soles of the feet), perioral papillomata and mental retardation. Macrocephaly, depressed nasal bridge, abnormally wide nostrils, low-set ears with large, thick lobes, palmoplantar hyperkeratosis, and the potential for congenital heart defects. Most cases occur sporadically with no family history of the disorder. Such cases are thought to represent new dominant gene mutations.

REFERENCES:

Bottani A, Hammerer I, Schinzel A: The cardio-facio-cutaneous syndrome: Report of a patient and review of the literature. *Eur J Pediatr* 150:486, 1991.

Kavamura MI, Peres CA, Alchorne MMA, et al: CFC index for the diagnosis of cardiofaciocutaneous syndrome. *Am J Med Genet* 112:12, 2002.

Reynolds JF, Neri G, Herrmann JP, et al: New multiple congenital anomalies/mental retardation syndrome with cardio-facio-cutaneous involvement—the CFC syndrome. *Am J Med Genet* 25:413, 1986.

Rhizomelic Chondrodysplasia Punctata Type I

At a glance: Peroxisomal disorder belonging to the chondrodysplasia punctata group. Punctate calcifications and rhizomelia, congenital cataract, and progressive mental retardation are the main features. Poor prognosis.

Synonyms: RCDPI; Chondrodystrophia Calcificans Punctata.

Incidence: Rare; 1:100,000 live births.

Genetic inheritance: Autosomal recessive.

Pathophysiology: Caused by defective peroxisome metabolism as a result of a mutation in the PEX7 gene, which encodes the peroxisomal type 2 targeting signal (PTS2) receptor gene located in 6q22-q24.

Diagnosis: The combination of punctate calcifications, rhizomelia, and biochemical abnormalities (deficient red cell plasmalogens, increased concentration of phytanic acid) is pathognomic. Antenatal diagnosis by identifying peroxisome enzymes in fetal blood is possible.

Clinical aspects: Features involve *skeleton* (scoliosis, punctate epiphysis, metaphyseal anomaly, rhizomelic micromelia, short stature, spina bifida occulta, restricted joint mobility), *head* (microcephaly; congenital bilateral and symmetric cataract; flat face; epicanthic folds; micrognathia; cleft palate; high forehead; small, upturned nose; long, flat philtrum), central nervous system (CNS) (sensorineural deafness, mental retardation, seizures developed between 18 months and 5 years of age), and *skin* (ichthyosis, alopecia). Dislocated hips and shoulder and cardiac malformations (atrial defect, mitral valve prolapse) have been described. Respiratory infections are frequent as a consequence of aspiration; 60% of patients die during the first year of life, and all die before reaching the teen years.

Precautions before anesthesia: Evaluate pulmonary function (clinical, chest radiographs, pulmonary function test if necessary, arterial blood gas analysis); neurological function (clinical, history, EEG, CT/MRI); cardiac function (clinical, ECG, echography); and tracheal intubation (clinical, radiographs).

Anesthetic considerations: Perioperative physiotherapy is needed to avoid pulmonary superinfection. Airway management can be difficult because of cleft palate and micrognathia. Careful intraoperative positioning is needed because of skeletal defect. Regional anesthesia is not contraindicated but can be difficult to perform. Rapid sequence induction should be considered because of the high risk of pulmonary aspiration.

Pharmacological implications: Consider interaction between antiepileptic treatment and anesthetic drugs. Prophylactic antibiotics in case of cardiopathy as indicated. Muscle relaxants should be avoided until airway is secured.

Other condition to be considered: Other chondrodysplasia punctata, as well as the following:

RHIZOMELIC CHONDRODYSPLASIA TYPE II (RCDPII): RCDP caused by dihydroxyacetone phosphate acyltransferase deficiency. Clinical features are identical to the RCDPI.

REFERENCES:

Raymond GV: Peroxisomal disorders. *Curr Opin Pediatr* 11(6):572, 1999.

White AL, Modaff P, Holland-Morris F, et al: Natural history of rhizomelic chondrodysplasia punctata. *Am J Med Genet* 118A(4):332, 2003.

Richards Rundle Syndrome

At a glance: A rare syndrome with association of mental retardation, ataxia, and deafness. Ketoaciduria is present and various neurological and muscular anomalies (peripheral muscle wasting) can be observed.

Synonym: Ketoaciduria Mental Deficiency with Ataxia and Deafness Syndrome.

Genetic inheritance: Autosomal recessive.

Pathophysiology: Unknown.

Diagnosis: Progressive onset of clinical signs in childhood with normal life duration. Diagnosis is made based on the association of mental retardation, ataxia, and deafness. Laboratory investigation shows ketoaciduria.

Clinical aspects: In addition to the three principal signs, abnormal gait, hypogonadism, amyotrophy or muscle agenesis, hyperreflexia, hypertonia or spasticity, osteoporosis, and restricted joint mobility can be observed. Metabolism anomalies and nystagmus can also occur.

Precautions before anesthesia: Evaluate muscular weakness (clinical); deafness; and respiratory function (chest radiograph, pulmonary function test, arterial blood gas analysis). Laboratory investigation should include creatine phosphokinase and renal and liver function.

Anesthetic considerations: Careful intraoperative positioning because of hypertonia, limited joint mobility, and muscular weakness. Perioperative respiratory monitoring should be used such as pulse oximetry in the postoperative period for 12 hours. The potential for sustained mechanical ventilation postoperatively following significant surgical procedure must be considered.

Pharmacological implications: Aminoglycosides should be used carefully in presence of progressive deafness and renal dysfunction. Avoid succinylcholine in patients with muscular weakness, hypotonia, and osteoporosis because of the risk of hyperkalemia and pathologic fractures, respectively. Sensibility to anesthetic drugs has to be evaluated because of the presence of metabolism disorder.

REFERENCES:

Fehlow P, Walther F: Richards-Rundle syndrome. *Klin Padiatr* 203(3): 184, 1991.

Richards BW, Rundle AT: A familial hormonal disorder associated with mental deficiency, deaf mutism and ataxia. *J Ment Defic Res* 3:33, 1959.

Riley-Smith Syndrome

At a glance: A rare form of PTEN-MATCHS (phosphatase and tensin homologue–macrocephaly, autosomal dominant, thyroid disease, cancer, hamartomata, skin abnormalities) Syndrome. Close to Bannayan-Zonana Syndrome and characterized by macrocephaly, pseudopapilledema, hemangiomata, and multiple lipomas. Subcutaneous hemangioma may be present at birth or appear later in childhood. Multiple signs can be associated (head, chest, abdominal, and genital).

Synonyms: Macrocephaly Multiple Lipomas and Hemangiomata Syndrome; Macrocephaly, Pseudopapilledema and Multiple Hemangiomata Syndrome; Rovsing Syndrome.

History: First described in 1986 as a different disease. It has been proposed recently that three medical conditions, i.e., the Bannayan-Zonana Syndrome, the Riley-Smith Syndrome, and the Ruvalbaca-Myhre-Smith Syndrome are similar entities and should be most appropriately represented as the Bannayan-Riley-Ruvalbaca Syndrome.

Genetic inheritance: Autosomal dominant.

Incidence: Not known. Male predominance. However, females can be affected, although in a milder form which explains why it remains mostly undiagnosed.

Pathophysiology: Results from mutations in the phosphatase and tensin homologue (PTEN) gene. Gene map location is 10q23.3. The homologies displayed by the structure of PTEN suggested to the investigators that it may suppress tumor cell growth by antagonizing protein tyrosine kinases and that it may regulate tumor cell invasion and metastasis through interactions at focal adhesions.

Diagnosis: Clinical. It is based on the association of macrocephaly, multiple lipomas, intestinal hamartomatous polyps, vascular malformations, and abnormal pigmentation of the penis. The definite diagnosis is determined genetically.

Clinical aspects: Multiple signs can be observed with relative frequencies: *head anomalies* (macrocephaly, scaphocephaly, down-slanting palpebral fissures, strabismus, amblyopia, prominent Schwalbe lines, hypertelorism, exotropia, pseudopapilledema tongue, polyps, high-arched palate), *chest anomalies* (pectus excavatum, supernumerary nipples), *genital anomalies* (enlarged penis, enlarged testis), *abdominal anomalies* (ileal hamartomatous polyps, colonic hamartomatous polyps, intussusceptions, rectal bleeding), *neurological anomalies* (hypotonia, seizures, thick corpus callosum, intracranial hemangioma), *orthopedic anomalies* (scoliosis, joint hyperextensibility, macrodactyly), and *dermatological lesions* (tan macules on the glans and the shaft of the penis, acanthosis nigricans, angiokeratoma, café-au-lait spots, lipomas, hemangiomas, cutis marmorata). The lipomas spontaneously regress with age. Motor and speech development are delayed, mild mental retardation, and incoordination are lifelong features. A myopathy caused by abnormal lipid storage can occur with proved muscle carnitine deficiency. Patients may have an increased risk of intracranial tumors. An increased incidence of Hashimoto thyroiditis has been suggested.

Precautions before anesthesia: The presence of brain edema and raised intracranial pressure must be assumed until proven otherwise. Proper evaluation of the neurological functions, including CT scan must be obtained before anesthesia. It is essential to check the hemoglobin level and coagulation profile because of the risk of bleeding from the hemangioma. The association with arteriovenous malformations may impact the heart and lead to high output cardiac failure, even in the small infant, it is imperative to assess carefully the cardiac function and obtain an ECG and echocardiogram before induction of anesthesia. The severity of the muscle involvement (myopathy) must be evaluated as well as the respiratory function. Because the thyroid gland can be involved in this process, thyroid hormone level must be measured and appropriate treatment provided before anesthesia.

Anesthetic considerations: Difficult direct laryngoscopy and tracheal intubation must be expected in the presence of a high-arched palate. Spontaneous ventilation must be maintained until confirmation that face-mask ventilation can be provided. A laryngeal mask airway should be available in case of a failure to intubate the trachea. Fiberoptic technique for the most difficult cases might be a good alternative. One must be careful with intraoperative positioning (because of the presence of hypotonia, myopathy, and orthopedic deformations). Special precautions have to be provided for the protection of the protruding eyes. Locoregional anesthesia should be carefully discussed with the patient and/or parents because of the presence of an arterivenous malformation (possibly intracranial) which could influence the hemodynamic response. The association with spinal and epidural hemangiomas makes regional anesthesia relatively contraindicated.

Pharmacological implications: It is recommended to avoid the use of succinylcholine because of the association of hypotonia and myotonia. The antiepileptic treatment should be continued to the day of the surgery.

Other conditions to be considered:

☞**COWDEN DISEASE:** An autosomal dominant condition with variable expression that results from a mutation in the PTEN gene on the chromosome arm 10q. Associated with hamartomatous neoplasms of the skin and mucosa, gastrointestinal tracts, bones, central nervous system, eyes, and genitourinary tract. The skin is involved in 90 to 100% of cases, the thyroid gland in 66% of cases. It is associated with several types of malignancy, including a marked increase in the incidence of breast and thyroid cancer.

☞**BANNAYAN ZONANA SYNDROME:** Closely related to Cowden Disease. An autosomal dominant condition characterized with multiple hamartomas (especially multiple angiomas and multiple encapsulated lipomas), macrocephaly, developmental delay, and hypotonia. However, the incidence of malignancy transformation is very low when compared to Cowden Disease.

REFERENCES:

Ahmed SF, Marsh DJ, Weremowicz S, et al: Balanced translocation of 10q and 13q, including the PTEN gene, in a boy with a human chorionic gonadotropin-secreting tumor and the Bannayan-Riley-Ruvalcaba Syndrome. *J Clin Endocr Metab* 84:4665, 1999.

Riley HD Jr, Smith WR: Macrocephaly, pseudopapilledema and multiple hemangiomata: A previously undescribed heredofamilial syndrome. *Pediatrics* 26:293, 1960.

Ruvalcaba RHA, Myhre S, Smith DW: Sotos syndrome with intestinal polyposis and pigmentary changes of the genitalia. *Clin Genet* 18:413, 1980.

Ritscher-Schinzel Syndrome

At a glance: A syndrome combining an atrioventricular septal defect with a Dandy-Walker–like malformation and craniofacial malformations.

Synonyms: 3C Syndrome (Cranio-Cerebello-Cardiac Dysplasia Syndrome); Dandy-Walker–like Malformation with Atrioventricular Septal Defect Syndrome.

Nature: Congenital genetic disorder first reported by D. Ritscher and A. Schinzel in 1987.

Incidence: Very rare (fewer than 30 cases worldwide). It seems to be more frequent in Canadian Native Americans.

Genetic inheritance: Autosomal recessive.

Pathophysiology: May result from a 3C mutant gene and/or an environmental teratogen.

Diagnosis: Clinically evocated by the association of cardiac malformations, cerebellar hypoplasia, and cranial dysmorphism. The association with immunoglobulin deficiency (IgG$_2$ and IgG$_4$) was reported in one patient. Chest radiographs may show multiple ossification defects.

Clinical aspects: Clinical features include *head* (macrocephaly, hypertelorism, prominent forehead and occiput, down-slanting palpebral fissure, depressed nasal bridge, low-set ears, narrow palate, short neck), central nervous system (hydrocephalus, hypoplastic cerebellar vermis, posterior fossa cyst/dilated fourth ventricle [Dandy-Walker malformation], cranial nerve palsies, nystagmus, truncal ataxia and mild to moderate growth and psychomotor retardation), *heart* (wide range of anomalies from cleft mitral valve to complete atrioventricular defect), and *skeleton* (first rib aplasia, camptodactyly of fingers, hip dislocation, hemivertebra, hypoplasia of terminal phalanges, micronychia). Other clinical signs include hypospadias, coloboma of the iris and/or retina, congenital glaucoma, optic nerve atrophy, malrotation of the gut, anal atresia, hydronephrosis, and immunodeficiency.

Precautions before anesthesia: It is recommended to review carefully the neurological history (motor/mental milestones) and any complications that might have happened during the administration of previous anesthesia. Assess neurological function, particularly the cranial nerves and the cerebellar function. Also, the potential for raised intracranial pressure (clinical, EEG, CT sacn) must be carefully evaluated. A complete cardiac evaluation, including ECG, chest radiographs, echocardiogram, and cardiac catheterization is highly suggested because of several reports of early death due to the severity of the cardiac defect. Assess airway for difficulty with ventilation and tracheal intubation.

Anesthetic considerations: Techniques should be tailored according to the cardiac defect present and the surgical procedure planned. Antibiotic prophylaxis for endocarditis and prevention of air embolism with adequate intravascular hydration are mandatory. Patient may be uncooperative as a consequence of mild mental retardation. Difficult airway may be anticipated with abnormal facial appearance, enlarged occiput, and short neck. Possible risk of pulmonary aspiration must be kept in mind. The presence of cranial nerve palsy increases the risk. Caution must be used with supraclavicular brachial nerve block because of the possible aplasia of the first rib. Ophthalmologic examination must be obtained to eliminate the presence of glaucoma.

Pharmacological implications: Depends on the underlying cardiac defect and the possibility of raised intracranial pressure from hydrocephalus. Muscle relaxants should be avoided until airway is secured and ventilation confirmed. Prophylactic antibiotics in case of cardiopathy as indicated. Avoid medications that can increase ocular pressure in case of glaucoma (e.g., succinylcholine).

REFERENCES:

Hoo J, Kreiter M, Halverson N, et al: 3C (cranio-cerebello-cardiac) syndrome: A recently delineated and easily recognizable congenital malformation syndrome. *Am J Med Genet* 52:66, 1994.

Leonardi ML, Pai GS, Wilkes B, et al: Ritscher-Schinzel cranio-cerebello-cardiac (3C) syndrome: Report of four new cases and review. *Am J Med Genet* 102:237, 2001.

Zankl A, Gungor T, Schinzel A: Cranio-cerebello-cardiac (3C) syndrome: Follow-up study of the original patient. *Am J Med Genet* 118A(1):55, 2003.

Roberts Syndrome

At a glance: Phocomelia-like syndrome associated with mental retardation and craniofacial abnormalities, including exophthalmia. Multiple other malformations can be observed such as urogenital (cryptorchidism, enlargement of the phallus and clitoris), cardiac (atrial septal defect, ventricular septal defect), and microcephaly.

Synonyms: Long Bone Deficiencies Associated with Cleft Lip-Palate; Tetraphocomelia-Cleft Lip-Palate Syndrome.

History: A form of dwarfism first described by John Bingham Roberts, an American surgeon, in 1919.

Genetic inheritance: Autosomal recessive trait. Affect males and females equally.

Pathophysiology: Premature separation of centromeric heterochromatin of many chromosomes is found in half of patients and has been evocated as a possible cause of the disease. Maternal ingestion of clonidine has also been suggested.

Diagnosis: Clinical: association of symmetric phocomelia-like limb defects similar to those seen in thalidomide embryopathy, craniofacial abnormalities, growth retardation, and mental deficiency.

Clinical aspects: Important clinical signs can be observed at birth. This complex severe multiple congenital anomaly syndrome leads often to premature birth. There is intrauterine growth retardation (birth length <40 cm [15.7 inches], birth weight <1.5 kg [3.3 lb]). Microcephaly and mental retardation can be associated with other *craniofacial anomalies* (craniosynostosis hydrocephalus, encephalocele, blue sclerae, exophthalmia, and cleft palate and lip). *Limb deformities* include talipes varus or valgus, and symmetrical absence or hypoplasia of the radius, ulna, tibia, fibula, and femur. The joints exhibit flexion contractures, especially the knees and elbows. There may be delayed ossification of the carpal bones. *Urogenital signs* (enlarged penis and clitoris, cryptorchism, ambiguous genitalia, hypospadias, enlarged or cleft labia minora, septate vagina, bicornuate uterus, polycystic or horseshoe kidneys, hydronephrosis, and ureteral stenosis) may be associated with gallbladder anomalies, accessory spleen, and *cardiac anomalies* (atrial septal defect, ventricular septal defect, patent ductus arteriosus). Other features usually involve the skin, nails, and hair.

Precautions before anesthesia: Evaluate cardiac function (clinical, ECG, echocardiography); neurological status (clinical, CT, transfontanellar echography, EEG); airway (clinical, radiographs); renal function (echography, biology); and spleen (echography). Laboratory investigation should include urea, kalemia, calcemia, creatinine because of renal anomalies; serum glutamic-oxaloacetic transaminase, serum glutamic-pyruvic transaminase, coagulation, bilirubin because of biliary anomalies, and platelet count because of thrombocythemia.

Anesthetic considerations: Direct laryngoscopy and tracheal intubation can be difficult. Maintenance of spontaneous ventilation until the trachea is intubated and ventilation confirmed is recommended. A laryngeal mask airway and fiberoptic equipment might be required. Careful intraoperative positioning is necessary because of significant malformations. Venous and arterial access can be a challenge because of the shortened and abnormal limbs. Regional anesthesia can be difficult. Platelet count should be measured before any procedures.

Pharmacological implications: Prophylactic antibiotics should be used in a case of cardiac defect. Choice of anesthetic drugs should consider renal and hepatic functions. Muscle relaxants should be avoided until airway is secured and ventilation has been confirmed.

Other condition to be considered:

☞**TAR SYNDROME:** Characterized by severe thrombocytopenia and absence or underdevelopment of the radius bones. The underdevelopment of the ulna, associated with defects of the hands, legs, and/or feet may also occur.

REFERENCES:

Bates AW: Autopsy on a case of Roberts syndrome reported in 1672: The earliest description? *Am J Med Genet* 117A(1):92, 2003.

Hwang K, Lee DK, Lee SI, et al: Roberts syndrome, normal cell division, and normal intelligence. *J Craniofac Surg* 13(3):390, 2002.

McDaniel LD, Prueitt R, Probst LC, et al: Novel assay for Roberts syndrome assigns variable phenotypes to one complementation group. *Am J Med Genet* 31;93(3):223, 2000.

Robinow Syndrome

At a glance: A form of dwarfism characterized by short limbs with abnormal morphogenesis of the face and external genitalia.

Synonyms and classification:

Recessive form: Costovertebral Segmentation Defect with Mesomelia (COVESDEM) Syndrome.

Dominant form: Robinow Dwarfism; Fetal Face Syndrome; Acral Dysostosis with Facial and Genital Abnormalities Syndrome.

Genetic inheritance: Recessive forms caused by mutation in the ROR2 gene located on 9q22 (allelic to brachydactyly type B); autosomal dominant forms exist.

Diagnosis: Characteristic *facial* features include macrocephaly; dolichocephaly; bulging forehead; micrognathia; hypertelorism; wide palpebral fissures; S-shaped lower eyelids; down-slanting palpebral fissures; short, upturned nose with anteverted nostrils and long philtrum; V-shaped or tented upper lip; triangular mouth; crowded teeth; gingival enlargement; and ankyloglossia. They are combined with mesomelic shortening of the forearm and hypoplastic genitalia.

Clinical aspects: Features can also involve *head and neck* (large anterior fontanel, posteriorly rotated ears, absent uvula, crowded teeth, prominent eyes), *heart* (right ventricular outlet obstruction), *genitourinary* (renal duplication, hydronephrosis, small penis, small clitoris, small labia majora), *gastrointestinal (GI)* (abnormal umbilicus, umbilical hernia cryptorchism), and *skeleton* (scoliosis, ribcage, hand and foot abnormalities, small stature, developmental delay).

The main discriminating feature is the occurrence of multiple rib and vertebral anomalies in the recessive form.

Precautions before anesthesia: Evaluate cardiac function (clinical, ECG, echocardiography, radionuclide imaging, and cardiac catheterization if necessary); renal function (clinical, echography, laboratory); airway (clinical, radiographs); and respiratory function if scoliosis is important (clinical, chest radiographs, pulmonary function test, arterial blood gas analysis).

Anesthetic considerations: Direct laryngoscopy and tracheal intubation can be difficult. Spontaneous respiration must be maintained until the airway is secured and ventilation confirmed. Tracheal intubation can be difficult. A laryngeal mask and fiberoptic equipment for tracheal intubation may be required. Perioperative cardiac and respiratory monitoring should be considered. Careful intraoperative positioning is needed because of skeletal anomalies. Regional anesthesia is not contraindicated however, the presence of vertebral anomalies should be considered.

Pharmacological implications: Fluid regimen and anesthetic drugs should be adapted to renal function. Muscle relaxants should be avoided until airway is secured and ventilation confirmed.

REFERENCES:

Butler MG, Hayes BG, Hathaway MM et al: Specific genetic diseases at risk for sedation/anesthesia complications. *Anesth Analg* 91(4):837, 2000.

Macdonald I, Dearlove OR: Anaesthesia and Robinow syndrome. *Anaesthesia* 50(12):1097, 1995.

Patton MA, Afzal AR: Robinow syndrome. *J Med Genet* 39(5):305, 2002.

Rogers Syndrome

At a glance: A rare medical condition caused by a defect in a transporter of thiamine, which results in anemia, diabetes, puffiness, deafness. Situs inversus viscerum totalis is also characteristic.

Synonyms: Thiamine-Responsive Anemia Syndrome; Thiamine-Responsive Myelodysplasia; Thiamine-Responsive Megaloblastic Anemia Combined with Diabetes Mellitus and Sensorineural Deafness.

History: First described by L.E. Rogers in 1969.

Genetic inheritance: Autosomal recessive; caused by a defect in a thiamine transporter protein (SLC19A2) located on 1q23.2-q23.3.

Pathophysiology: It is unclear but there is some evidence of decreased uptake of thiamine into some cell types causing a thiamine-dependent state, leading to similar features observed in "thiamine-deficiency beriberi of childhood." The thiamine reserve and synthesis are normal, however the patients require high-dose thiamine therapy for treatment and for maintaining normal function. Relapse can recur on discontinuation of thiamine therapy.

Diagnosis: Clinical features include generalized puffiness, diabetes mellitus, sensorineural deafness. Blood cell count shows megaloblastic anemia or, occasionally, pancytopenia. Bone marrow aspirate shows megaloblastic erythropoiesis and ringed sideroblasts. Urinary sample showed aminoaciduria in one patient. Blood transketolase activity must be obtained to assess thiamine status. Responsiveness to thiamine supplement is often immediate and dramatic. Age of diagnosis is usually within first few years of life.

Clinical aspects: Characterized by megaloblastic anemia responsive only to thiamine administration, diabetes mellitus, and sensorineural deafness. Other clinical features of "beriberi" may be evident and include generalized puffiness, hoarseness, cardiac failure, and neurological disturbances. Most signs and symptoms are resolved on administration of high doses of thiamine, however the presence of diabetes melitus may persist. Other occasionally reported features include cardiac septal defects, progressive optic atrophy, and situs inversus viscerum totalis.

Precautions before anesthesia: Complete history and physical assessment with further investigation depending on findings. Ensure the correction of the hematological, neurological and cardiovascular symptoms by administration of a high dose of thiamine. Fulminant "beriberi" symptoms are a contraindication for anesthesia. Preoperative fasting and antidiabetic medications should be tailored according to the severity of the diabetic status and to the surgical procedure planned. Check blood sugar level pre- and postoperatively. Evaluate cardiac function (clinical, chest radiographs, echocardiography).

Anesthetic considerations: There are no specific risks when the patient has been treated. Thiamine administration should be continued during the perioperative period. The glycemia should be monitored frequently and treated accordingly. The placement of central venous catheter could be difficult because of anatomical anomalies as a consequence of situs inversus.

Pharmacological implications: Prophylactic antibiotics in case of cardiac defect.

REFERENCES:

Bazarbachi A, Muakkit S, Ayas M, et al: Thiamine-responsive myelodysplasia. *Br J Haematol* 102:1098, 1998.

Neufeld EJ, Fleming JC, Tartaglini E, et al: Thiamine-responsive megaloblastic anemia syndrome: A disorder of high-affinity thiamine transport. *Blood Cells Mol Dis* 27(1):135, 2001.

Rogers L, Porter F, Sidbury J: Thiamine-responsive megaloblastic anemia. *J Pediatr* 74:494, 1969.

Rolland-Desbuquois Syndrome

At a glance: A lethal neonatal syndrome characterized by chondrodystrophy, micromelic dyssegmental dwarfism, vertebral and metaphyseal abnormalities, advanced carpotarsal ossification, dislocation of the patellae and hips, glaucoma, and mental deficiency. Prognosis is poor.

Synonyms: Dyssegmental Dwarfism Rolland-Desbuquois type; Dyssegmental Dysplasia Rolland-Desbuquois type; Anisospondylic Campto-Micro-Melic Dwarfism.

Genetic inheritance: Autosomal recessive transmission.

Pathophysiology: Evidence for possible deficiency of alpha-1 chain in collagen peptides. This may be responsible for increased cross-linking and abnormal collagen stiffness.

Diagnosis: Clinical features (micromelia, limited joint mobility associated with cardiac and neurological anomalies) and radiological features (symmetrical short extremities, shortened trunk length, and narrow thorax). Gel electrophoresis shows abnormal collagen pattern. Chromosomal study is usually normal.

Clinical aspects: Clinical features can involve *skeleton* (short, thick, bowed long bones; marked metaphyseal flaring and cupping; abnormal vertebrae with different sizes, thicknesses, and widths that may consist of two or more separate ossified masses; narrow thorax with horizontal ribs; reduced joint motility), and *CNS* (hydrocephalus, occipital encephalocele). Other occasionally reported features include hydronephrosis, hypertrichosis, and congenital heart defect in one case. In severe cases (also classified as Silverman-Handmarker Syndrome), death usually occurs within few days or weeks of birth. Even in milder form, survival beyond the first year of life is rare. Cause of death is usually respiratory related.

Precautions before anesthesia: Evaluate the airway for potential difficult tracheal intubation (clinical, radiographs). Assess respiratory function (clinical, chest radiograph, arterial blood gas), oxygen, and ventilatory requirement. Assess neurological status, which might include clinical and CT scan for possible hydrocephalus and raised intracranial pressure.

Anesthetic considerations: No reported experience. The potential for difficult airway management is present because of the flat face, small mouth, and short neck. There is a significant risk for difficult lung ventilation because of the narrow thorax and poor lung compliance. The requirement for postoperative ventilatory monitoring or support may be indicated. Intravenous access may be difficult because of the skin condition. Poor joint motility may be prone to pressure necrosis and require careful intraoperative positioning.

Pharmacological implications: Muscle relaxants should be avoided until airway is secured and lung ventilation confirmed. Prophylactic antibiotics are indicated in case of cardiopathy. Opioids should be used carefully because of the increased respiratory risk. Avoid succinylcholine in the presence of glaucoma.

Other condition to be considered:

SILVERMAN-HANDMAKER SYNDROME (Dyssegmental Dysplasia): Lethal form of neonatal short-limbed dwarfism. Clinical and radiological features include chondrodysplasia with dyssegmental ossification of the spine. The term "dyssegmental dysplasia" refers to differences in size and shape of the vertebral bodies (anisuspondyly).

REFERENCES:

Aleck K, Grix A, Clericuzio C: Dyssegmental dwarfism: Clinical, radiographic and morphologic evidence of heterogeneity. *Am J Med Genet* 27:295, 1987.

Gruhn J, Gorlin R, Langer L: Dyssegmental dwarfism: A lethal anisospondylic camptomicromelic dwarfism. *Am J Dis Child* 132:382, 1978.

Rombo Syndrome

At a glance: Genetic disorder characterized by facial follicular skin atrophy, milia, telangiectasias, absent eyelashes and eyebrows, and basal cell carcinomas later on in life.

Incidence and genetic inheritance: Unknown incidence; inheritance seems to be autosomal dominant.

Clinical aspects: The skin changes usually start between the ages of 7 and 10 years with follicular atrophy (so-called atrophoderma vermiculatum), particularly on the cheeks, and with discoloration of the lips and hands (cyanosis-like). Milia-like papules with telangiectasias develop in adulthood, and basal cell carcinomas are a frequent complication of this syndrome, but appear later in life than in Bazex Syndrome. Basal cell carcinomas with milia and coarse, sparse hair syndrome or congenital hypotrichosis with milia syndrome. Microscopically, a widespread lack of elastin in many skin areas with clumping of elastic components in other areas can be identified. Dermal collagen fibrils may have signs of hyalinization and vacuolization. Skin can get the aspect of solar elastosis. The eyebrows and eyelashes may either show an irregular, patchy distribution with distorted and maldirected growth, or may be missing completely.

Anesthetic considerations: No anesthetic complications are expected to arise from this syndrome, and no literature is available.

Other conditions to be considered:

☞**BAZEX SYNDROME:** Characterized by lesions suggesting "multiple ice-pick marks" on the dorsum of the hands and elbows dating from early infancy. Basal cell carcinomas may developed on the face between ages 15 and 26 years. Hypotrichosis is identical to the skin lesions seen in Conradi Disease and in Basal Cell Nevus Syndrome. It is considered X-linked dominant and presents similar features to the Rombo Syndrome. Other features include the presence of a "pinched" nose with hypoplastic alae and prominent columella. This medical condition has been reported mainly in France and all patients were Caucasians.

REFERENCES:

Michaelsson G, Olsson E, Westermark P: The Rombo syndrome: A familial disorder with vermiculate atrophoderma, milia, hypotrichosis, trichoepitheliomas, basal cell carcinomas and peripheral vasodilation with cyanosis. *Acta Derm Venerol* 61:497, 1981.

Van Steensel, MA, Jaspers, NG, Steijlen PM: A case of Rombo syndrome. *Br J Dermatol* 144:1215, 2001.

Rosenberg-Chutorian Syndrome

At a glance: A very rare neurodegenerative disorder. Clinical features include deafness, polyneuropathy, and optic atrophy. The distal muscular atrophy resembles those observed in Charcot-Marie-Tooth Disease.

Synonym: Optic Atrophy Polyneuropathy and Deafness Syndrome.

Incidence and genetic inheritance: Very rare; inheritance not fully elucidated. X-linked semi-dominant; however, autosomal dominant and autosomal recessive forms of Charcot-Marie-Tooth disease with deafness have also been reported.

Clinical aspects: Diagnosis is based on clinical criteria, including a rapidly progressive polyneuropathy with distal muscular atrophy associated with blindness caused by optic nerve atrophy and neurosensorial deafness. Paraparesis is frequent.

Anesthetic considerations: Check respiratory function (clinical, chest radiographs, arterial blood gas analysis); postoperative ventilatory support may be necessary. Normal response to neuromuscular blocking agents (atracurium and mivacurium tested). Succinylcholine is best avoided considering muscle anomalies.

Other conditions to be considered:

☞**CHARCOT-MARIE-TOOTH DISEASE:** Characterized by muscle weakness and atrophy, most prominent in the legs and the small muscles of the hands. Patients may remain active and have a normal life span. Segmental demyelination of peripheral nervous system including the axons represent classic features of this medical condition. Symptoms usually begin gradually between middle childhood and age 30 years. The most incapacitating symptom is "foot drop," producing a slapping gait and the associated paresthesias. A decrease in vibration, pain, and thermal sensation in the hand, foot, and lower part of the leg that manifest following a distribution pattern of glove and stocking shape. The disease is slowly progressive, but may arrest spontaneously.

REFERENCES:

Antognini JF: Anesthesia for Charcot-Marie-Tooth disease: A review of 86 cases. *Can J Anaesth* 39:398, 1992.

Hirsch NP: Respiratory insufficiency in Charcot-Marie-Tooth disease. *Anesthesia* 53:1034, 1998.

Rosenberg RN, Chutorian A: Familial opticoacoustic nerve degeneration and polyneuropathy. *Neurology* 17:827, 1967.

Rosenthal-Kloepfer Syndrome

At a glance: A rare syndrome where affected patients are tall with large extremities corneal leukoma, and skin modifications.

Synonym: Acromegaloid Changes, Cutis Verticis Gyrata, and Corneal Leukoma Syndrome.

Incidence and genetic inheritance: Autosomal dominant. Very rare.

Clinical aspects: Features involve *eyes* (corneal leukoma usually presents in first decade, progressing to total blindness), *skin* (excessive skin undulation on face, typically in coronal direction [cutis verticis gyrata]; skin on the hand is usually soft with abnormal dermal "split ridges" palm), and *skeleton* (acromegaloid changes with progressive enlargement, hand, feet, and chin, large and unusually tall). No evidence of pituitary dysfunction. Affected individuals have normal daily function and expectancy. Skull radiograph shows enlarged jaw, normal sella turcica.

Anesthetic considerations: Vascular access can be difficult because of skin changes.

REFERENCE:

Rosenthal J, Kloepfer H: An acromegaloid, cutis verticis gyrata, corneal leukoma syndrome: A new medical entity. *Arch Ophthalmol* 68:722, 1962.

Rosewater Syndrome

At a glance: A rare form of gynecomastia with hypogonadism. Similar to the Reifenstein syndrome but without hypospadias.

Synonym: Familial Gynecomastia.

History: First described by S. Rosewater in 1965.

Genetic inheritance: X-linked or autosomal dominant.

Pathophysiology: Unclear; resistance to androgen action suggested. Masculinization by monthly administration of testosterone has been demonstrated.

Diagnosis: Clinical features (gynecomastia with hypogonadism); biochemical (increased levels of testosterone and estrogen, but with low levels of luteinizing hormones); histology (decreased Leydig cells on testicular biopsy).

Clinical aspects: Gynecomastia, hypogonadism, sterility.

Anesthetic considerations: Endocrine dysfunction appears to be limited to the reproductive system. Psychological attention must be given to patients affected with this conditions because of the embarrassment caused by the gynecomastia.

Other condition to be considered:

☞**REIFENSTEIN SYNDROME:** Characterized by male pseudohermaphroditism, which means that the individual has testes but presents clinically with the secondary sexual characters both male and female. The severity of androgen insensitivity determines the clinical presentation.

REFERENCE:

Rosewater S, Gwinup G, Hamwi SJ: Familial gynaecomastia. *Ann Intern Med* 63:377, 1965.

Rosseli-Gulienetti Syndrome

At a glance: A controversial form of cleft lip/palate-ectodermal dysplasia syndrome combining anhidrosis, hypotrichosis, microdontia, cleft lip and palate, hand and foot deformity, and mental retardation.

Incidence and genetic inheritance: Autosomal recessive. Very rare.

Clinical aspects: Features involve *head* (oval face, cleft lip and palate, anteverted ears, hypodontia), *skin* (short sparse "kinky" hair, sparse eyebrows, desquamation of the skin of the face, palmar and plantar hyperkeratosis, hypotrichosis or anhydrosis, hypoplastic dermatoglyphic, onychodysplasia, popliteal and perineal pterygium), and *skeleton* (syndactyly, aplasia or hypoplasia of the thumbs). Other features include mental retardation, genitourinary anomaly, deafness, and accessory nipple. Affected adults have normal daily function and expectancy. Early death in the neonatal or childhood period has been reported; however, the cause of death is unknown.

Anesthetic considerations: Excessive environmental heat and the administration of cholinergic drugs are best avoided because of the anhydrosis.

Other conditions to be considered:

ZLOTOGORA-OGUR SYNDROME (Cleft Lip/Palate-Ectodermal Dysplasia Syndrome; Ectodermal Dysplasia Cleft Lip/Palate Mental Retardation Syndactyly Syndrome): Characterized by the presence of bilateral cleft lip/palate ectodermal dysplasia, sparse scalp hair, malformed protruding ears, and partial syndactyly of the fingers and toes. Mental retardation, pili torti, and renal abnormalities have been reported.

REFERENCES:

Rosseli D, Gulienetti R: Ectodermal dysplasia. *Br J Plast Surg* 14:190, 1961.

Zlotogora J: Syndactyly, ectodermal dysplasia and cleft lip/palate. *J Med Genet* 31:957, 1994.

Rothmann Makai Syndrome

At a glance: A very rare variant of lobular panniculitis, presenting with numerous large subcutaneous lesions, affecting children and occurring within the first 12 months of age.

Synonym: Lipogranulomatosis Subcutanea.

History: First described by M. Rothman, a German pathologist, and E. Makai, a Hungarian surgeon, in 1900.

Incidence and genetic inheritance: Very rare. Belongs to the group of panniculitis. The differential diagnosis between Weber-Christian disease, Rothmann-Makai, and lipophagic panniculitis is only made histologically.

Clinical aspects: In the Rothmann-Makai type, the nodules are small and multiple and seem to be self-limited with no severe systemic involvement. Histologically, the lesions are most marked in the fat. There are dermal changes with foci of small round cells and macrophages around blood vessels and appendages. Presence of granulomata composed of macrophages, fibroblasts, multinucleate cells, and polymorphs. There is absence of caseation. The panniculitis is an inflammation of subcutaneous fat responsible for fairly uniform clinical features including nodules and plaques, or swelling located in the subcutaneous tissue, occasionally progressing to at-

rophy of subcutaneous fat. The hypothesis of an abnormal fragility of adipose tissue or of a failure in the mechanisms of protection against lipophagia has been raised.

Anesthetic considerations: The differential diagnosis with the ☞Weber-Christian Syndrome should be evaluated. In case of doubt, the patient should be treated as having Weber-Christian Disease. Intraoperative proper pressure point padding and positioning of the patient should be meticulous because interruption of vascular and oxygen supply seems to be a trigger. Vascular access placement and fixation can be very difficult because of skin lesions.

Other condition to be considered:

☞WEBER-CHRISTIAN DISEASE: Rare skin disorders characterized by single or multiple, tender or painful subcutaneous nodules (1 to 2 cm) leading to the development of panniculitis. The legs and feet are most often affected; however, it can also erupt under the arms, abdomen, and face. It is associated with fever, generalized malaise, myalgia, and abdominal pain. The clinical presentation is variable and may subside after a short period of a few days or weeks and recur months or years later to become chronic.

REFERENCES:

Burford JC, Clarke DM: Lipogranulomatosis subcutanea of Rothman-Maki. *Aust J Dermatol* 13(3):117, 1972.

Winkelmann RK, Mc Evoy MT, Peters MS: Lipophagic panniculitis of childhood [review]. *J Am Acad Dermatol* 21:971, 1989.

Rothmund-Thomson Syndrome

At a glance: Rare recessive syndrome with bullous extensive skin anomalies, juvenile cataract skeletal disorders, and malignancy predisposition (skin and osseous). Trisomy 8 mosaicism is frequent. Trisomy 8 occurs in 2.5% of the peripheral lymphocytes. This low incidence could be overlooked in routine karyotyping. Maintaining hydration is a major concern.

Synonyms: Poikiloderma Atrophicans and Cataract; Poikiloderma Congenitale.

Incidence: Fewer than 100 cases described.

Genetic inheritance: Autosomal recessive; variable phenotype; mutations in a recQ helicase gene (RECQL4) at locus 8q24.3 in several patients.

Pathophysiology: The DNA helicase gene RECQL4 is involved in this syndrome. In vivo clonal chromosomal re-arrangements causing an acquired somatic mosaicism have been evocated to explain this pathology.

Diagnosis: Clinical, evocated by the association of skin abnormalities (starting in infancy), skeletal disorders, juvenile cataract, and predisposition to malignancy and characteristic rash. Karyotype may show abnormalities of chromosome 8 in a minority of patients.

Clinical aspects: The skin changes begin within the first year of life in 89% of patients. These are defined as erythematous patches or red edematous plaques, sometimes accompanied by blistering. Characteristically, these begin on the cheek and spread to the forehead, ears, and neck. Usually by this time, erythema has also appeared on the dorsal aspects of the hands, extensor aspects of the arms and forearms, and the legs and buttocks. Poikiloderma is a feature of atrophy, areas of hyper- and hypopigmentation, and telangiectases. Skin, nails, and hair are primarily involved: erythematous or bullous skin lesions, poikiloderma (atrophic plaques with telangiectasia), telangiectasia, skin atrophy, sun sensitivity (35%),

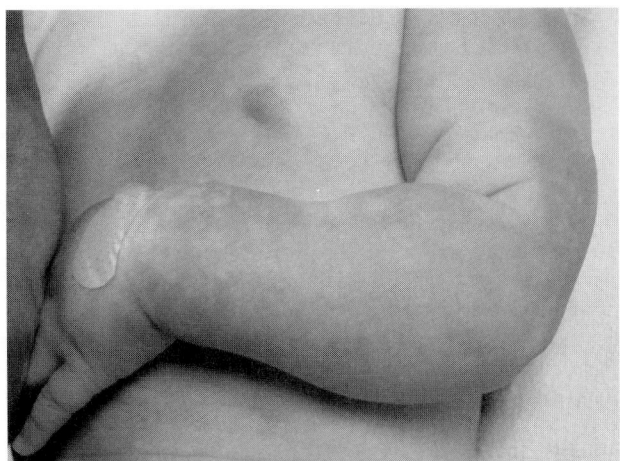

Rothmund-Thomson syndrome These erythematous skin changes are caused by photosensitivity in this infant with Rothmund-Thomson syndrome. See color plates.

abnormal scar formation, atrophic nails (24%), sparse hair, alopecia. Premature graying of hair can frequently be observed and may be associated with short stature (54%), mental retardation, and facial deformation: frontal bossing, prognathism, small saddle nose, dental and ocular anomalies (juvenile zonular cataracts [52%], microphthalmia, microcornea, strabismus, glaucoma). Skeletal repercussions also concern limbs with osteoporosis, forearm reduction defects, absence of patella joint, contractures, thumb hypoplasia, small hands, and small and club feet. Other clinical features are occasional and can affect digestive area (annular pancreas, anterior positioning of the anus, duodenal stenosis) and genitourinary structures (hypogonadism, cryptorchidism nephritis or nephropathy with vascular hypertension). Anemia, growth hormone deficiency, and immunoglobulin abnormality have also been reported. There is an increased risk of basal cell carcinoma, squamous cell carcinoma, and osteogenic sarcoma. Treatment includes constant use of sunscreen and avoidance of sun exposure. Regular ophthalmic screening and evaluation of any bone pain are mandatory. One case was described with Addison disease and one case was described with growth hormone deficiency.

Precautions before anesthesia: Good medical history and physical examination must be obtained to exclude obvious Addison disease. Look carefully at the future emplacement of the intravascular infusion lines. Special attention to the teeth (implantation and looseness). Creatinine and urea levels are useful in the presence of hypertension. Check preoperative hemoglobin. A complete evaluation of intravascular volemia and electrolytes status (risk of dehydration as a consequence of skin lesions and nephropathy) and high blood pressure consequences (ECG, echocardiography, renal echography). Laboratory investigations should include natremia, kalemia, calcemia, urea, creatinine, growth hormone, and hematocrit.

Anesthetic considerations: Careful intraoperative positioning and skin protection is necessary. Consider a smaller endotracheal tube than expected because of the presence of short stature and delayed physical development. The presence of loose teeth will require special attention during direct laryngoscopy for tracheal intubation. Also, special attention will be needed even for placement of a laryngeal mask airway where dislodgment of a tooth or teeth

could be catastrophic. Vascular access placement can be difficult because of the presence of skin lesions. Proper pressure point and padding, careful positioning is essential and avoiding the use of sticky tapes is important. Blood pressure cuff should be padded to limit chances of provoking skin lesions. Intraoperative fluid regimen should be controlled carefully because of the association of nephropathy (over-hydration) and the risk of dehydration (hypo- or anhydrosis).

Pharmacological implications: Prophylactic antibiotics should be used because of the high incidence of immunodeficiency in these patients, leading to a high risk of infection. Avoid parasympatholytic drugs (dyshidrosis). Avoid succinylcholine in the presence of glaucoma.

Other conditions to be considered:

☞**WERNER SYNDROME:** Progressive disorder characterized by progeria-like appearance. Although the age of onset is the third or fourth decades of life, certain clinical features can be present during childhood, adolescence, and early adulthood. Children often appear unusually small for age because of an abnormally slow growth rate. By the mid-20s, affected individuals have alopecia. Bilateral senile cataracts, osteoporosis, hypogonadism, diabetes mellitus type II, and generalized atherosclerosis. It is inherited as an autosomal recessive trait.

☞**COCKAYNE SYNDROME:** Characterized by dwarfism, distinctive skin abnormalities and craniofacial malformations, and a progeria-like appearance. Other clinical features include optic nerve atrophy, retinal degeneration, and cataracts. The skin may be abnormally sensitive to sunlight, leading to scarring, abnormal pigmentation, and atrophy of affected areas. Characteristic facial abnormalities include a thin nose, sunken eyes, and prognathism. It is inherited as an autosomal recessive trait.

☞**ECTODERMAL DYSPLASIAS:** Skin rashes, impaired healing of the skin, sparse or absent hair, dental defects, craniofacial malformations, ocular abnormalities, dwarfism, can also be considered similar to those associated with Rothmund-Thomson Syndrome.

☞**BLOOM SYNDROME:** Characterized by dwarfism and distinctive skin abnormalities of the facial area. The facial lesions are described as abnormally red, inflamed areas resembling erythema (sunburn), photosensitivity, and telangiectasia (typically, referred to as "butterfly" pattern across the cheeks and the nose). Other craniofacial features include malar hypoplasia, mandible hypoplasia, a prominent nose. Leukemia is believed to be more frequent.

REFERENCES:

Wang LL, Levy ML, Lewis RA, et al: Clinical manifestations in a cohort of 41 Rothmund-Thomson syndrome patients. *Am J Med Genet* 22;102(1):11, 2001.

Wang LL, Worley K, Gannavarapu A, et al: Intron-size constraint as a mutational mechanism in Rothmund-Thomson syndrome. *Am J Hum Genet* 71(1):165, 2002.

Rotor Syndrome

At a glance: A benign form of mixed jaundice with conjugated (50%) and unconjugated (50%) bilirubin. Normal hepatic function and histology probably related to a defective binding and storage protein for bilirubin in liver cells.

Synonym: Hyperbilirubinemia Rotor type.

Genetic inheritance: Autosomal recessive.

Pathophysiology: Benign, familial, unconjugated, nonhemolytic hyperbilirubinemia. Jaundice caused by impaired excretion or storage of conjugated bilirubin.

Diagnosis: Routine blood tests reveal conjugated hyperbilirubinemia. Albumin, transaminases, alkaline phosphatase, and prothrombin time are normal. Gross and microscopic examination of the liver are normal. Bromosulphthalein transport is reduced. Elevated urinary coproporphyrin is present.

Clinical aspects: Benign hyperbilirubinemia of no clinical importance. No identified precipitating factors. No specific treatment.

Anesthetic considerations: Avoid halothane and drugs that can displace bilirubin from albumin (e.g., cephalosporin).

Other conditions to be considered: The hereditary hyperbilirubinemias include firstly those predominantly unconjugated hyperbilirubinemia, i.e., Gilbert or Arias Syndrome, Crigler-Najjar Syndrome type I, and Crigler-Najjar Syndrome type II, and secondly those resulting in predominantly conjugated hyperbilirubinemia: Dubin-Johnson Syndrome, Rotor Syndrome, and several forms of Intrahepatic Cholestasis.

☞**GILBERT SYNDROME:** Characterized by normal liver function tests of the usual type, normal liver histology, delayed clearance of bilirubin from the blood, and mild jaundice that tends to fluctuate in severity, particularly after fasting. This disorder is difficult to distinguish from prolonged posthepatic hyperbilirubinemia. Gilbert Syndrome is distinguished by the lack of morbidity in patients and by a lower total serum bilirubin level, ranging from 1 to 6 mg/dL.

☞**CRIGLER-NAJJAR SYNDROME** presents in two forms: **Type I** and **Type II.** *Type I* is characterized by a deficiency in hepatic glucuronyltransferase activity. Hyperbilirubinemia is severe, with total serum bilirubin levels ranging from 20 to 45 mg/dL most often associated with kernicterus. Type I patients do not respond to phenobarbital treatment and only traces of bilirubin glucuronides can be found in their bile. It is inherited by autosomal recessive transmission. In *type II*, total serum bilirubin ranges from 6 to 20 mg/dL and phenobarbital treatment lowers serum bilirubin levels by more than 30%. Bilirubin glucuronides are present in bile. Type II is less severe than type I.

☞**DUBIN-JOHNSON SYNDROME:** Characterized by hyperbilirubinemia, deposition of melanin-like pigment leading to hepatomegaly and abdominal pain, prolonged retention of sulfobromophthalein (which may show a higher concentration at 60 to 90 minutes than at 45 minutes), and otherwise normal liver function. The incidence is reported for the Iranian Jews to 1 per 1,300. Age at onset for the jaundice varied from 10 weeks to 56 years. Penetrance is reduced in females. Sixty-four of all cases reported were Iranian Jews. The inheritance is consistent with autosomal recessive with reduced penetrance. Urinary coproporphyrin I is a good indicator of the homozygote and heterozygote states in the Dubin-Johnson Syndrome. Normal individuals excreted 24.8% of urinary coproporphyrin as coproporphyrin I, whereas homozygotes and heterozygotes excreted 88.9 and 31.6%, respectively. Factor VII deficiency has been suggested in Japanese cases that were diagnosed in the neonatal period.

DHUMEAUX BERTHELOT SYNDROME (Hyperbilirubinemia Type III): Characterized by the presence of conjugated hyperbilirubinemia presumably distinct from either the Rotor form or the Dubin-Johnson form.

REFERENCES:

Chowdry J, Wolkoff A, Chowdry N, et al: Hereditary jaundice and disorders of bilirubin metabolism, in Scriver C, Beaudet A, Sly W, Valle

D (eds): *The Metabolic and Molecular Bases of Inherited Disease.* 7th ed. New York, McGraw-Hill, 1995, p 2187.

Lidofsky S, Scharschmidt B: Jaundice, in Feldman M, Sleisenger M, Scharschmidt B (eds): *Sleisenger & Fordtran's Gastrointestinal and Liver Disease: Pathophysiology/Diagnosis/Management.* 6th ed. Philadelphia, WB Saunders, 1998, p 16.

Roussy-Levy Syndrome

At a glance: Autosomal dominant spinocerebellar degeneration. Appears in early childhood and progresses slowly.

Synonyms: Roussy-Levy Hereditary Areflexic Dystasia; Lévy-Roussy Syndrome; Symonds-Shaw Syndrome; Abortive type of Friedreich Disease; Familial Claw-Foot with Absent Tendon Jerks; Hereditary Areflexic Dystasia; Hereditary Ataxia-Muscular Atrophy Syndrome.

Genetic inheritance: Autosomal dominant.

Pathophysiology: Not exactly known; spinocerebellar degeneration.

Diagnosis: Association of truncal ataxia, lower limb muscular atrophy, bilateral pes cavus, and loss of deep reflexes.

Clinical aspects: Symptoms first appear in early childhood and progress slowly throughout life with moderate disability. Beyond ataxia, loss of reflexes, and muscular atrophy, clinical features can include scoliosis, absent leg tendon jerks, distal sensory loss, static hand tremor, abnormal gait, and slow peripheral nerve conduction velocity. Absence of cerebellar signs, speech disturbances, Babinski sign, and nystagmus.

Precautions before anesthesia: Evaluate muscular weakness (clinical) and neurological function (clinical, EMG, somatosensory evoked potentials, nervous conduction speed).

Anesthetic considerations: Careful intraoperative monitoring. Regional anesthesia is not contraindicated; however, complete information about the risks involved has to be clearly expressed by the physician and understood by the patient/parents. Similar to most cases of Friedreich Ataxia, somatosensory evoked potential intraoperative monitoring during scoliosis surgery should be impossible.

Pharmacological implications: Avoid succinylcholine because of the risk of hyperkalemia as a consequence of muscle denervation.

Other conditions to be considered:

☞**FRIEDREICH ATAXIA (FRDA):** A genetic disorder characterized by a progressive dysfunction of the posterior spinal cord, the cerebellum (ataxia, nystagmus), and peripheral nerves. It typically becomes apparent by adolescence. Clinical features include unsteady posture, frequent falling, progressive ataxia characterized by foot deformities, increasing incoordination of the arms and hands, dysarthria, and nystagmus. It may also be associated with cardiomyopathy, chest pain, arrythmias, and diabetes mellitus. All patients have normal intelligence.

☞**CHARCOT MARIE TOOTH DISEASE:** A hereditary polyneuropathy condition presenting with distal weakness and muscular atrophy (myopathy). The most common complaint is distal leg weakness, which manifests as frequent tripping and muscle atrophy. Hand involvement follows in most cases. Pregnancy may exacerbate a preexisting weakness in 50% of patients with early-onset disease.

REFERENCES:

Auer-Grumbach M, Strasser-Fuchs S, Wagner K, et al: Roussy-Levy syndrome is a phenotypic variant of Charcot-Marie-Tooth syndrome

IA associated with a duplication on chromosome 17p11.2. *J Neurol Sci* 154:72, 1998.

Roussy G, Lévy G: Sept cas d'une maladie familiale particulière: Troubles de la marche, pieds bots et aréflexie tendineuse généralisée, avec, accessoirement, légère maladresse des mains. *Rev Neurol (Paris)* 1:427, 1926.

Rubinstein-Taybi Syndrome

At a glance: A rare syndrome with craniofacial anomalies and complex multiple malformations, including cardiac, digestive, and respiratory malformations.

Synonyms: Rubinstein Syndrome; Broad Thumbs and Great Toes, Characteristic Facies, and Mental Retardation Syndrome; Broad Thumbs-Hallux Syndrome.

History: First described in 1963 by Jack Herbert Rubinstein, an American pediatrician and Hooshang Taybi, an American pediatric radiologist.

Incidence: Rare (less than 600 cases have been described); usually sporadic; 1:125,000 live births. More frequent in patients with mental retardation.

Genetic inheritance: Autosomal dominant; however, most cases are sporadic.

Pathophysiology: Caused by mutation in the gene encoding the transcriptional coactivator CREB-binding protein located on 16p13.3. Involved in transcription regulation, chromatin remodeling, and the integration of several signal transduction pathways.

Diagnosis: Clinical: association of mental retardation (100%), characteristic facies (100%), broad thumbs (100%), hallux (50%), and other malformations.

Clinical aspects: Progressive onset of the disease is usual and characteristic facies is observed later in infancy. Other clinical features include short stature (94%), microcephaly (84%) with micrognathia (100%), and various defects: *cranial* (frontal bossing, large fontanel, narrow mouth and palate, choanal atresia), *ear* (low-set ears, hearing loss), *eyes* (heavy eyebrows, long eyelashes, ptosis, glaucoma, coloboma, cataract epicanthal folds), *heart* (33%) (patent ductus arteriosus, atrial or ventricular defect), *genitourinary* (cryptorchism, hypospadias and renal defect), *skin* (keloid scars, hemangioma, café-au-lait spots, hirsutism, nevus flammeus), *neurological* (corpus callosum agenesis, hypotonia, hyperreflexia, seizures), and *orthopedic* (scoliosis, spina occulta, pes planus, patellar dislocation, clinodactyly, syndactyly). Swallowing troubles and feeding difficulties are frequent, as are respiratory infection and asthma. There is an increased risk of tumor, mainly of neurological origin (neuroblastoma, meningioma).

Precautions before anesthesia: Evaluate cardiac function (clinical, chest radiograph, echocardiography) and airway for the potential of difficult tracheal intubation (clinical, radiograph).

Anesthetic considerations: Pulmonary aspiration risks are significant as a consequence of gastrointestinal anomalies. Direct laryngoscopy and tracheal intubation may be difficult because of facial malformations. It is recommended to maintain spontaneous ventilation until the trachea is intubated and lung ventilation confirmed. A laryngeal mask airway and fiberoptic equipment might be required. Careful intraoperative positioning is necessary because of skeletal deformation. Nasal intubation and nasogastric tube should be performed with caution because of the presence of choanal atresia. Specific consideration will be directed by the cardiorespiratory problems.

Pharmacological implications: Avoid cardiodepressive drugs and use prophylactic antibiotics in case of cardiopathy. Avoid parasympatholytic medications in patient with glaucoma. Aminoglycoside agents can be used, however the dose must be calculated according to the renal function. Various problems have been described with anesthetic drugs such as atropine, neostigmine, succinylcholine (arrhythmias), propofol, and isoflurane (delayed awakening). However, these problems are isolated cases.

Other conditions to be considered:

☞**Trisomy 13 syndrome:** Characterized by central nervous system and craniofacial abnormalities, polydactyly, severe mental retardation, and congenital heart defects. Some clinical features include microcephaly, forehead bossing, microphthalmia, cleft lip/palate, camptodactyly, and capillary hemangiomas. Eighty percent of individual affected with this medical condition present with congenital heart defects.

☞**Brachman de Lange syndrome:** Recognized on the basis of characteristic facies (low anterior hairline, synophrys, anteverted nares, maxillary prognathism, long philtrum, "carp" mouth) in association with prenatal and postnatal growth retardation, mental retardation and, in many cases, upper limb anomalies. Other clinical features include dyspnea, hypertonia, and hyperthermia. Muscle biopsy showed severe distortion of the mitochondrial architecture. The ophthalmologic findings include ptosis, nystagmus and high myopia, poor macula reflex, hypertropia and nasolacrimal duct fistula.

☞**Saethre-Chotzen syndrome:** Characterized by severe brachycephaly, hypertelorism, maxillary hypoplasia with a narrow palate, lacrimal duct abnormalities, and ptosis. Craniosynostosis can also be present. Other features include brachydactyly, clinodactyly, abnormally broad great toes, and syndactyly.

REFERENCES:

Critchley LA, Gin T, Stuart JC: Anaesthesia in an infant with Rubinstein-Taybi syndrome. *Anaesthesia* 50(1):37, 1995.

Dearlove OR, Perkins R: Anaesthesia in an adult with Rubinstein-Taybi syndrome. *Br J Anaesth* 90(3):399, 2003.

Hanauer D, Argilla M, Wallerstein R: Rubinstein-Taybi syndrome and hypoplastic left heart. *Am J Med Genet* 112(1):109, 2002.

Rud Syndrome

At a glance: A syndrome characterized by ichthyosis, mental retardation with seizures, short stature, retinitis pigmentosa, polyneuropathy, and hypogonadism.

Synonyms: Dwarfism-Ichthyosiform Erythroderma-Mental Deficiency Syndrome; Ichthyosis and Male Hypogonadism Syndrome.

Nature: Belongs to the neuroichthyosis group with a difficult differential diagnosis among all medical conditions involved: (CHIME [*C*oloboma, *H*eart Defects, *I*chthyosiform Dermatosis, *M*ental Retardation, *E*ar Defects] Syndrome, Refsum Disease, Sjögren-Larsson Syndrome, Netherton Syndrome, KID [*K*eratitis, *I*chthyosis, and *D*eafness] Syndrome, and IBIDS [*I*chthyosis, *B*rittle Hair, *I*mpaired Intelligence, *D*ecreased Fertility, and *S*hort Stature] Syndrome).

> *N.B.:* Controversies exist about whether Rud Syndrome is a distinct entity.

Genetic inheritance: X-Linked (continuous gene syndrome) or recessive.

Incidence: About 30 cases have been described with a ratio female:male of 1:2.

Pathophysiology: Unknown; however, defects in the steroid sulfatase and the Kallmann loci on the X chromosome have been identified.

Diagnosis: Congenital or neonatal ichthyosis of the skin. The presence of poorly developed secondary sexual characteristics, associated with mental retardation and polyneuropathy completes the clinical presentation.

Clinical aspects: Features can involve *skin* (ichthyosis, acanthosis nigricans, and alopecia), *skeleton* (short stature, arachnodactyly, hypoplastic or absent teeth, and structural abnormalities of the hands and the feet), *CNS* (seizures, anosmia, and hypertrophic polyneuropathy), and *genitourinary* (hypogonadism, primary or hypogonadotrophic in origin). Cerebral atrophy may be seen, and in some cases is associated with steroid sulfatase deficiency. Hyperchromic macrocytic anemia and low pituitary gonadotropic hormones are frequent.

Precautions before anesthesia: It is very important to check the level of anemia. During the very exudative and inflammatory phase of ichthyosis, the patient's heat and water losses may be considerable. Evaluate for significant intravascular hypovolemia. Evaluate neurological function (clinical, EEG, CT).

Anesthetic considerations: Particular attention should be given to proper preoperative padding and protection against heat loss. Hydration is also very important. According to the degree of anemia and the surgical procedure involved, proper blood cross-matched is essential. The anemia should be corrected.

Pharmacological implications: Consider interaction between antiepileptic treatment and anesthetic drugs.

REFERENCES:

Larbrisseau A, Carpenter S: Rud syndrome: Congenital ichthyosis, hypogonadism, mental retardation, retinitis pigmentosa and hypertrophic polyneuropathy. *Neuropediatrics* 13(2):95, 1982.

Munke M, Kruse K, Goos M, et al: Genetic heterogeneity of the ichthyosis, hypogonadism, mental retardation, and epilepsy syndrome: Clinical and biochemical investigations on two patients with Rud syndrome and review of the literature. *Eur J Pediatr* 141:8, 1983.

Stoll C, Eyer D: A syndrome of congenital ichthyosis, hypogonadism, small stature, facial dysmorphism, scoliosis and myogenic dystrophy. *Ann Genet* 42(1):45, 1999.

Rukavina Type Amyloid Polyneuropathy

At a glance: A very rare form of amyloid polyneuropathy. Cardiomyopathy has also been reported with this disorder.

Synonyms: Amyloid Polyneuropathy Indiana type; Hereditary Neuropathic Amyloidosis II; Prealbumin-84 Amyloidosis Type II; Senile Systemic Amyloidosis Syndrome; Dysprealbuminemic Hyperthyroxinemia.

History: First described by J.G. Rukavina in 1956.

Genetic inheritance: Autosomal dominant; gene located on 18q11.2-q12.1. It is allelic to transthyretin.

Pathophysiology: Mutation in the transthyretin (prealbumin) protein. This protein maintains normal levels of thyroid hormone, retinol, alpha-1-Antitrypsin and retinol-binding protein in the circulation.

Diagnosis: Demonstration of amyloid deposition in various tissues. The specific amyloidosis type is based on the genetic demonstration of a mutation in the prealbumin protein (substitution of serine for isoleucine at position 84). Onset is usually in the fifth decade of life. Neuropathic manifestations begin and predominate in the upper limbs. Carpal tunnel syndrome is characteristic.

Clinical aspects: The disease is milder in females, appearing in adult age and progressing slowly, with a 20-year survival time. Autonomic dysfunction is an early finding with orthostatic hypotension. Vitreous opacities and visceral manifestations (cardiac and renal amyloidosis) are milder than in amyloidosis I.

Precautions before anesthesia: Proper medical history and physical examination for cardiac involvement of amyloidosis (diastolic cardiac dysfunction, cardiac failure) and conduction problems (clinical, ECG, Holter, echocardiography, radionuclide imaging if necessary) must be obtained. If the patient is carrying a permanent pacemaker, a preoperative pacemaker check is advised. Evaluate renal function (clinical, echocardiography, laboratory) and thyroid hormones and function (free thyroxin and thyroid-stimulating hormone levels). A thorough assessment for signs of severe autonomic dysfunction such as orthostatic hypotension must be obtained.

Anesthetic considerations: Be prepared for a high degree of cardiac conduction block. A transcutaneous pacing device must be available in the operating room. If the patient is equipped with a pacemaker, the usual precautions are applicable during the intraoperative period (e.g., magnet). Watch for hemodynamic instability caused by autonomic dysfunction. Consider the existence and severity of the polyneuropathy and autonomic dysfunction before using regional anesthesia (lumbar epidural anesthesia described).

Pharmacological implications: Since alpha-1-antitrypsin level can be affected, precautions must be taken with anesthetic indications having affinity with this protein. Premedication or induction should include atropine; avoid conduction-blocking agents or parasympathomimetic effects. When making anesthetic drug choice and dose, consider renal status.

REFERENCES:

Eriksson P, Boman K, Jacobsson B, et al: Cardiac arrhythmias in familial amyloid polyneuropathy during anesthesia. *Acta Anaesthesiol Scand* 30:317, 1986.

Rukavina JG, Block WD, Jackson CE, et al: Primary systemic amyloidosis: A review and an experimental, genetic and clinical study of 29 cases with particular emphasis on the familial form. *Medicine (Baltimore)* 35:239, 1956.

Rundles-Falls Syndrome

At a glance: Congenital anemia usually appearing after the age of 12 years. Hemorrhagic risk and consequences of anemia must be considered before anesthesia. Without treatment, pyridoxine deficiency can also be observed.

Synonyms: Hereditary Iron-Loading Anemia Syndrome; Pyridoxine-Responsive Anemia; Sideroblastic Anemia Syndrome.

History: First described by the American physicians Ralph Wayne Rundles and Harold Francis Falls, in 1946.

Genetic inheritance: Always female transmission, but some cases of X-linked inheritance.

Diagnosis: Clinical and biological: usually occurs after patient is 12 years old; characterized by red cell abnormalities, enlargement of the spleen, and responsiveness to pyridoxine without signs of pyridoxine deficiency.

Clinical aspects: Other clinical features include weakness, fatigue, occasionally leg pain and paresthesias of the feet, pallor, hepatomegaly and splenomegaly. Pretibial edema and skin pigmentation may occur. Females usually have erythrocyte abnormalities without anemia and an enlarged spleen.

Precautions before anesthesia: Evaluate degree of anemia (clinical, hematocrit) and splenomegaly (echography).

Anesthetic considerations: Large-size venous access is preferred because of the significant risk of hemorrhagic complications and transfusion possibility. Perioperative invasive monitoring (and transfusion) is recommended in case of severe anemia. Preoperatively cross-matched blood must be available before any surgical procedure presenting even minimal risk of bleeding normally.

Pharmacological implications: Regional anesthesia is not contraindicated but the risk has to be clearly explained to patient because of paresthesia that can occur during the evolution of the disease.

Other condition to be considered:

FABER SYNDROME (Faber Anemia; Achylanemia; Achylia Gastrica with Anemia; Achylic Achloranemia; Anemia Achlorhydrica Simplex; Chronic Hypochromic Anemia): Caused by deficient intake absorption or metabolism of iron. Characterized by small, pale-red erythrocytes and associated with achlorhydria, glossalgia, koilonychia, pallor fatigability, and premature graying of the hair; occurs more often in women than in men in the third to fifth decades.

REFERENCE:

Rundles RW, Falls HF: Hereditary (sex-linked) anemia. *Am J Med Sci* 211:641, 1946.

Russell Weaver Bull Syndrome

At a glance: Complex multiple anomalies syndrome resulting from blastogenesis defect with association of neonatal surgical defects and neurological and orthopedic anomalies. Cardiac and pulmonary lesions can also occur.

Synonym: Axial Mesodermal Dysplasia Spectrum Blastogenesis Defect.

History: First described by L.J. Russell, D.D. Weaver, and M.J. Bull in 1981.

Diagnosis: This polydysmorphic syndrome is often lethal. Evocation of the diagnosis on the clinical signs present at birth (facial deformations associated with multiple malformations).

Clinical aspects: Features of both the Goldenhar and the Caudal Regression Syndromes are observed. Antenatal period anomalies are frequent and often associated with oligoamnios and prematurity. Patients present with short stature and neurological anomalies (cerebral cortex atrophy, hydrocephalus). Neonatal lesions can include diaphragmatic hernia, omphalocele, and tracheoesophageal fistula. Orthopedic features are multiple: scoliosis, short neck, skeletal, vertebral and joint anomalies, sacrococcyx agenesia, talipes varus or valgus. Facial deformations are also frequent with micrognathia, facial structural asymmetry, preauricular tags, and thickened gingivae. Other signs concern digestive organs (hiatal hernia, anus, spleen, liver, biliary and gastrointestinal tract anomalies), and genitourinary structures (abnormal bladder and genitalia ectopic, horseshoe-shaped or fused kidney, megaureter). Hypoplas-

tic lungs and ventricular septal defects are also present in some cases.

Precautions before anesthesia: Evaluate cardiac and respiratory function (clinical, ECG, echocardiography, arterial blood gas analysis, chest radiograph, and, if necessary, CT scan). Airway (clinical, fiberoptic, radiography); and liver and renal status (echography, CT, laboratory investigation: serum glutamic-oxaloacetic transaminase, serum glutamic-pyruvic transaminase, bilirubin, coagulation, kaliemia, natremia, calcemia, urea).

Anesthetic considerations: Direct laryngoscopy and tracheal intubation can be very difficult because of facial and vertebral (cervical spine) anomalies. Aspiration risks exist because of digestive malformations. Cardiac anomalies will dictate management and proper monitoring. Perioperative fluid management should be carefully evaluated considering renal function. Perimedullar anesthesia should be avoided in cases of vertebral anomaly.

Pharmacological implications: Prophylactic antibiotics should be used in cases of cardiopathy. Anesthetic drug choice should consider renal and hepatic functions.

REFERENCE:

Russell LJ, Weaver DD, Bull MJ: The axial mesodermal dysplasia spectrum. *Pediatrics* 67(2):176, 1981.

Russell-Silver Syndrome

At a glance: A genetic disorder characterized by a severe form of asymmetric dwarfism with growth retardation, peculiar facies, and frequent hypoglycemia.

Synonyms: Silver-Russell Dwarfism; Silver Syndrome; Silver-Russell Syndrome.

Incidence: Rare; more than 150 cases have been described.

Genetic inheritance: Autosomal recessive. Most cases are sporadic. No established mendelian or chromosomal basis, with new dominant mutation or X-linked dominant inheritance possible. Gene map locus at 17q25.

In 1985, Partington proposed an X-linked inheritance for this syndrome, but described children with no asymmetry and a pigmentary anomaly quite different from the café-au-lait spots. This syndrome is sometimes called Russell-Silver X-linked or Partington syndrome, but should not be confused with the true Partington syndrome, which is characterized by the association of mental retardation, X-linked transmission, dystonic movements, ataxia, and seizures.

Diagnosis: The two main features are low birth weight dwarfism and lateral asymmetry.

Clinical aspects: The first feature is extreme intrauterine growth retardation with normal head circumference, sometimes referred as pseudohydrocephalus. The characteristic *facial* features are craniofacial disproportion, delayed fontanel closure, triangular facies, turned-down mouth corners, and micrognathia. Asymmetry of arms and/or legs causes hemihypertrophy and lateral asymmetry. Fifth finger clinodactyly and syndactyly of toes are observed. The radiology findings are usually fifth finger middle or distal phalangeal hypoplasia, ivory epiphyses, second metacarpal pseudoepiphysis, vertebral abnormalities, absent sacrum, and absent coccyx. Hypoglycemia at birth and even after is common. Café-au-lait spots, precocious sexual development, and cryptorchism are frequent. Cardiac defects can be observed. Gastrointestinal manifestations are now known to be a part of the disease (gastroesophageal reflux, esophagitis, food aversion, and failure to thrive). Susceptibility to malignancies is higher. Normal intelligence is the rule with some delay in the early motor milestones because of the decreased muscle bulk and relatively large head. The children remain thin with a lack of subcutaneous fat. Therapeutic trials with growth hormone have not corrected the growth pattern.

Precautions before anesthesia: The airway must be carefully assessed (clinical, radiographs). Search for cardiac defect (clinical, echocardiography). Evaluate hypoglycemic risk (clinical, history, glucose level). Search for gastroesophageal reflux (clinical, endoscopy, manometry).

Anesthetic considerations: The potential for difficult direct laryngoscopy and tracheal intubation is common because of facial malformations. In case of difficult airway or suspicion of difficulty, it is recommended to maintain spontaneous ventilation until the trachea is secured and lung ventilation confirmed. A laryngeal mask airway and fiberoptic equipment must be available. Pay special attention to the glucose need because of the easily depleted glycogen storages and severe hypoglycemia intraoperatively. Preoperative fasting may be minimal or preoperative glucose infusion realized. Careful intraoperative positioning is needed because of skeletal malformations. Regional anesthesia is not contraindicated but can be difficult to realize as a result of anatomical modifications and may also require intraoperative glucose monitoring because of the suppression of adrenergic response to surgical stress that is induced by these techniques. Rapid induction sequence is needed in cases of gastroesophageal reflux.

Pharmacological implications: Avoid muscle relaxants until airway is secured. Prophylactic antibiotic in cases of cardiopathy. Drugs should be adapted to body area more than to body weight.

Other conditions to be considered:

☞**THREE M SYNDROME:** Rare inherited disorder characterized by low birth weight, dwarfism, triangular-shaped face, frontal bossing, and dolichocephaly. Other clinical features include clinodactyly, and hypospadias. Skeletal abnormalities include unusually thin diaphyses of the long bones of the arms and legs, abnormally long vertebrae, and distinctive malformations of scapulae.

☞**FLOATING-HARBOR SYNDROME:** Characterized by dwarfism, a triangular face, wide downturned mouth with thin lips and large bullous rounded nose. Other clinical features include clinodactyly, brachydactyly, posteriorly rotated ears, and speech and psychomotor development delay. Congenital heart defects have been reported in some cases and consisted of atrial/ventricular septal defects. The original cases were reported at the Boston Floating Hospital and Harbor General Hospital, Torrance, California, hence the name Floating-Harbor syndrome. It is probably inherited as an autosomal dominant.

☞**SHORT SYNDROME:** An acronym that stands for (S)hort stature, (H)yperextensibility, (O)cular depression, (R)ieger anomaly, and (T)eething delays. Individual affected presents a triangular-shaped face, downturned corners of the mouth, sunken eyes, and Rieger anomaly (gray or white ring in the margin of the cornea) and glaucoma. Other clinical features include clinodactyly, lipoatrophy, dental abnormalities, a high incidence of inguinal hernia. It has been suggested that an autosomal recessive transmission was most probable.

☞**MULIBREY NANISM SYNDROME:** Based on the acronym "MULIBREY" that stands for (MU)scles, (LI)ver, (BR)ain, and (EY)es. Infants usually have low birth weight and failure to thrive leading to growth delays and dwarfism. Other clinical features include hepatomegaly, craniofacial anomalies, a triangular-shaped face, and hydrocephalus. It might be inherited as an autosomal recessive pattern.

REFERENCES:

Anderson J, Viskochil D, O'Gorman M, et al: Gastrointestinal complications of Russell-Silver syndrome: A pilot study. *Am J Med Genet* 113:15, 2002.

Dinner M, Goldin EZ, Ward R, et al: Silver syndrome: Anesthetic implications. *Anesth Analg* 78(6):1197, 1994.

Monk D, Bentley L, Hitchins M, et al: Chromosome 7p disruptions in Silver Russell syndrome: Delineating an imprinted candidate gene region. *Hum Genet* 111:376, 2002.

Rutledge Lethal Multiple Congenital Anomaly Syndrome

At a glance: A lethal form of mesomelic dwarfism associated with severe multiple cardiac, respiratory, and skeletal malformations. It is also known as the polydactyly, sex reversal, renal hypoplasia, and unilobular lung disease.

Synonyms: Smith-Lemli-Opitz Syndrome type II; Lethal Acro-Dysgenital Syndrome; Lethal Multiple Congenital Anomaly Syndrome.

History: First described by J.C. Rutledge in 1984.

Genetic inheritance: Autosomal recessive; allelic to Smith-Lemli-Opitz syndrome type I.

Pathophysiology: Possible primary fetal adrenal defect, resulting in multiple congenital abnormalities. May be linked to mutations in delta-7-dehydrocholesterol reductase; gene located at 11q12-q13.

Diagnosis: Clinical features (mesomelic dwarfism, micrognathia, V-shaped upper lip, ambiguous genitalia, clubfeet, fused fontanelles, inclusion cysts of the tongue, widely spaced nipples, and digital anomalies). Prenatal diagnosis by ultrasonography and analysis of cholesterol level from amniocentesis is possible.

Clinical aspects: Features include mesomelic dwarfism, *craniofacial deformations* (fused fontanelles, low-set ears, micrognathia, V-shaped upper lip, thick alveolar ridges, high-arched palate or cleft palate, abnormal tongue, cataract), *cardiac and respiratory malformations* (severe congenital heart defect, pulmonary hypoplasia, unilobar lungs, laryngeal hypoplasia), *genitourinary signs* (ambiguous genitalia, oligopapillary, renal hypoplasia), *gastrointestinal* (gallbladder hypoplasia, pancreatic islet cell hyperplasia, megacolon), and *orthopedic malformations* (polydactyly, syndactyly, clubfoot, joint contractures). Cerebellar hypoplasia is associated. Affected patients usually die within a few hours or days of birth.

Precautions before anesthesia: Complete examination and full assessment of cardiac, respiratory, and renal function (clinical, radiographs, echography, arterial blood gas analysis). Complete biochemistry evaluation should be obtained. Volemia should be assessed because of renal anomalies. Because of the possibility of laryngeal hypoplasia, proper evaluation must be sought.

Anesthetic considerations: No reported experience because of the rarity and very early lethality of the syndrome. Direct laryngoscopy and tracheal intubation could probably be difficult because of facial anomalies. Postoperative ventilatory support may be necessary.

Pharmacological implications: Perioperative fluid regimen and drugs doses should be adapted to renal function. Cardiac prophylactic antibiotics as indicated.

REFERENCES:

Curry CJR, Carey JC, Holland JS, et al: Smith-Lemli-Opitz syndrome-type II: Multiple congenital anomalies with male pseudohermaphroditism and frequent early lethality. *Am J Med Genet* 26:45, 1987.

Rutledge JC, Friedman JM, Harrod MJE, et al: A "new" lethal multiple congenital anomaly syndrome: Joint contractures, cerebellar hypoplasia, renal hypoplasia, urogenital anomalies, tongue cysts, shortness of limbs, eye abnormalities, defects of the heart, gallbladder agenesis, and ear malformations. *Am J Med Genet* 19:255, 1984.

Ruvalcaba Syndrome

At a glance: Syndrome characterized by microcephalia, mental retardation, dwarfism, and urogenital and skeleton anomalies.

Synonyms: Ruvalcaba-Reichert-Smith Syndrome; Osseous Dysplasia with Mental Retardation Ruvalcaba type.

History: First described in 1971 by Rogelio H.A. Ruvalcaba, David Weyhe Smith, American pediatricians and A. Reichert, American physician.

Genetic inheritance: Uncertain; autosomal dominant; semidominant X-linked inheritance has also been suggested.

Pathophysiology: Unknown.

Diagnosis: Based on typical clinical findings and the familial nature of the syndrome. No specific genetic or biochemical investigation has been described.

Clinical aspects: Features involve *head* (microcephalia; small, narrow, beak-shaped nose; thin lips and down-slanting palpebral fissures; hypoplastic maxilla; and pointed mandible), *musculoskeletal system* (short stature; clinodactyly; osteochondritis of the vertebral column and Scheuermann disease [anterior fragmentation of the vertebrae]; narrow trunk; pectus carinatum; kyphosis or scoliosis; short extremities with widening of the epiphyses; limitation of joint extension), *urogenital* (delayed puberty, hypoplastic testicles, cryptorchism, malrotation, megaureter, and hydronephrosis), and *skin* (typical hypoplastic "onion skin"). Varying degrees of mental retardation.

Precautions before anesthesia: One must obtain a complete history particularly related to neurological development. The presence of renal anomalies must be excluded. The association of congenital hydrocephalus and Dandy-Walker anomaly must be eliminated.

Anesthetic considerations: Mental retardation may affect cooperation during induction of anesthesia and premedication may be necessary. No anesthetic experience has been reported but the possibility of a difficult tracheal intubation must be considered in the presence of a hypoplastic maxilla and narrow arch. Careful intraoperative positioning is necessary because of skeletal deformation. Possible association with raised intracranial pressure.

Pharmacological implications: Muscle relaxants should be avoided until airway is secured.

Other conditions to be considered:

HUNTER-MCALPINE CRANIOSYNOSTOSIS SYNDROME: Inherited as an autosomal dominant disorder and characterized by craniosynostosis, mental deficiency, microcephaly, almond-shaped palpebral fissures, oval-shaped face, blunt nose, downturned mouth or small mouth, mild acral-skeletal anomalies, unusually small hands and dwarfism.

☞TRICHORHINOPHALANGEAL SYNDROME TYPE III (TRPS III; Sugio-Kajii Syndrome): Characterized by the presence of sparse hair, beaked nose, long upper lip, and severe metacarpophalangeal shortening. Although it was suggested to be an example of Ruvalcaba Syndrome, it is differentiated by the absence of mental retardation and microcephaly. The abnormalities of the hands and feet are more severe. The sparse hair, "pear-shaped nose" and radiological cone-shaped epiphyses are also present as features of TRPS types I and II. However, the presence of severe generalized shortening of all phalanges and metacarpals (brachydactyly) differentiated the condition from TRPSI and the absence of mental deficiency and exostoses from TRPSII.

REFERENCES:

Bianchi E, Livieri C, Arico M, et al: Ruvalcaba syndrome: A case report. *Eur J Pediatr* 142:301, 1984.

Ruvalcaba RHA, Reichert A, Smith DW: A new familial syndrome with osseus dysplasia and mental deficiency. *J Pediatr* 79:450, 1971.

Sugio Y, Kajii T: Ruvalcaba syndrome: Autosomal dominant inheritance. *Am J Med Genet* 19:741, 1984.

S

Sabin-Feldman Syndrome

At a glance: An infective disorder, sporadic in nature, that leads to chorioretinitis and cerebral calcification. Transplacental infection may occur with devastating results for fetal development.

Synonyms: *Toxoplasma gondii; T. gondii;* Chorioretinitis-Toxoplasmosis Syndrome.

Incidence: Many adults demonstrate antibodies to *Toxoplasma gondii,* the causative organism; consequently, subclinical infection is probably common. In the United States, it is demonstrated that 3–70% of healthy adults are serologically positive for *T. gondii.* In general, the incidence of the infection varies with the population group and the geographical area studied. *T. gondii* infection affects more than 3500 newborns in the United States each year. *T. gondii* seropositivity rates among HIV-infected patients vary from 10–45%. Toxoplasmic encephalitis (TE) has been reported in 1–5% of AIDS patients. Internationally, the seropositivity prevalence rate is as high as 75% by the fourth decade of life, in countries such as France and El Salvador. As many as 90% of adults in Paris are seropositive. Approximately 50% of the adult population in Germany is infected. Women of childbearing age in much of Western Europe, Africa, and South and Central America have seroprevalence rates of greater than 50%.

History: This syndrome was described by A.B. Sabin and H.A. Feldman, American epidemiologists.

Pathophysiology: *T. gondii* oocysts are shed in animal feces and may be ingested in dust form by humans.

Diagnosis: Fever, headache, lymphadenopathy, myalgia, anorexia, and arthralgia are the most common presenting features in adults and children infected with toxoplasmosis. A minority of patients develop visual symptoms, however about half of patients show characteristic lesions in the retina on ophthalmoscopy.

Precautions before anesthesia: Patients with toxoplasmosis should be treated as potentially contagious to the operating room personnel. In view of the serious consequences of transplacental spread, patient contact with pregnant personnel must be avoided. Patients should be assessed to determine the degree of involvement. Dehydration may be a feature of the acute illness. As these patients are infected, arrangements must be made to use disposable anesthetic and surgical equipment or to protect nondisposable equipment from bacterial contamination.

Anesthetic considerations: There are no reports of anesthesia with this medical condition. The presence of cerebral calcification might be associated with seizures and potentially a change in the intracranial dynamic, i.e., intracranial pressure. The antiepileptic medications must be continued until the morning of surgery. Antibiotic must be given before anesthesia and elective surgical procedures should be delayed in patients with active infections.

Pharmacological implications: No agents are indicated or contraindicated, except in the presence of seizure activities, triggering anesthetic agents should be avoided. In the case of ophthalmic disease occurring subsequent to acute infection, treatment may involve steroid administration and preoperative steroid stress doses may be necessary. Antibiotics may be administered and any possible drug interaction should be considered.

REFERENCE:
Teutsch SM, Juranek DD, Sulzer M et al: Epidemic toxoplasmosis associated with infected cats. *N Engl J Med* 300:695, 1979.

Salt-Depletion Syndrome

At a glance: Adrenal crisis or salt-losing signs most often associated with genital anomalies. Adaptation of steroid therapy, fluid management, and blood pressure monitoring are imperative.

Synonyms: Salt-Losing Syndrome; Fibiger-Debré Von Gierke Syndrome; De Crecchio Syndrome; Fibiger-Debré Syndrome; Gallais Syndrome; Pirie Syndrome; Adrenal Virilizing Syndrome; Female Pseudohermaphroditism; Macrogenitosomia Praecox; Pseudosexual Precocity; Suprarenal Genital Syndrome; Suprarenal Pseudohermaphroditism-Virilism-Hirsutism Syndrome; Virilizing Adrenocortical Hyperplasia.

Incidence: Congenital Adrenal Hyperplasia has an incidence about 1:5000 live births; Salt-Losing Syndrome incidence has been evaluated at 1:26,292 live births.

Genetic inheritance: Autosomal recessive.

Pathophysiology: The gene is located on 6p21.3. The disease is closely linked to HLA and results from deficiency in one or another of the enzymes involved in the cortisol biosynthesis. In approximately 95% of cases, 21-hydroxylation is impaired in the zona fasciculata of the adrenal cortex which prevent the conversion to 11-deoxycortisol, resulting in overproduction of adrenocorticotropic hormone (ACTH) and cortisol precursors. Three principal biochemically distinct types have been described: virilizing adrenal hyperplasia, mixed adrenal hyperplasia, and nonvirilizing adrenal hyperplasia. A fourth one, often defined as acquired, is sometime considered. Of these children, 75% have salt-losing syndrome.

Diagnosis: Evocated shortly after birth in cases of salt-losing signs (vomiting, dehydration, electrolyte changes, cardiac arrhythmias, and even adrenal crisis) or virilization signs. Biological signs include elevated urinary 17-ketosteroids, normal or decreased urinary 17-hydroxycorticosteroids, elevated 17-OH progesterone in blood, elevated serum dehydroepiandrosterone (DHEA) sulfate, and abnormal blood and urinary sodium levels.

Clinical aspects: Salt-losing signs can be associated with hypertension, recurrent fever, and hypoglycemia. Adrenal crisis can occur spontaneously in patients affected with severe adrenal hyperplasia. It includes various signs (headache, weakness, vomiting, low blood pressure, dehydration, fever, coma, tachycardia, joint and abdominal pain, weight loss, tachypnea) and can lead to death. Clinical features can also include genital signs (hypospadias, masculinizing female sexual characteristics, testicular tumors in adults, virilization, gynecomastia in adults). Growth is accelerated but adult stature is often short.

Precautions before anesthesia: Evaluate salt-loss severity (clinical, history, weight, blood and urinary electrolytes, urea, creatinine) and cardiac implications (clinical, iterative cardiac blood measurement, ECG, echocardiography). Laboratory investigations should include glycemia, cortisol, and blood gas analysis.

Anesthetic considerations: Electrolyte balance should be obtained before surgery. Blood pressure should be closely supervised during the perioperative period. An indwelling arterial catheter is recommended for major procedures or in case of emergency. Strict asepsis is necessary in patients with steroid therapy. Glycemia and electrolytes should be regularly measured during the perioperative period.

Pharmacological implications: Steroid therapy must be adapted to the importance of the surgical stress and consist in the administration of hydrocortisone 2 mg/kg. Prophylactic antibiotics are indicated in immunodeficient patients. Hypnomidate is contraindicated because of its effect on the adrenal gland. Succinylcholine should be avoided in patients presenting electrolytes instability (risk of hyperkalemia). Adrenal crisis can require vasoactive drugs (to support low blood pressure), supplementary hydrocortisone, and appropriate fluid regiment with extra sodium.

Other conditions to be considered:

WILKINS DISEASE: Individuals affected with this medical condition present with pseudospasm of the pylorus, vomiting, severe dehydration, and death.

3β-HYDROXYSTEROID DEHYDROGENASE DEFICIENCY: Characterized by the evidence of less virilization but more severe salt wasting.

17ALPHA-HYDROXYLASE DEFICIENCY: Characterized by similar symptomalogy previously described and in addition, the association with significant hypertension and hypochloremic, hypokalemic alkalosis.

REFERENCES:

Abel M, von Petrykowski W: Perioperative substitution therapy in congenital adrenogenital syndrome with salt loss. *Anaesthesist* 33(8):374, 1984.

Gordon MT, Conway DI, Anderson DC: Genetics and biochemical variability of variants of 21-hydroxylase deficiency. *J Med Genet* 22:354, 1985.

Sandifer Syndrome

At a glance: Association of torsional dystonia, mainly involving the neck and upper extremities, with either esophageal reflux or hiatus hernia. During paroxysmal dystonic posture crisis, opisthotonos may be present.

Synonym: Sandifer Complex.

Incidence: Incidence is unknown, although there is some suggestion that it occurs in less than 1% of children with gastroesophageal reflux.

Clinical aspects: Torsional dystonia occurs shortly after feeding for 1 to 3 minutes (commonly mistaken for seizures). A relationship with feeding may suggest a diagnosis of Sandifer syndrome.

Anesthetic considerations: No particular anesthetic consideration is known, however the disorder should be known because of its possible confusion with seizures. Rapid sequence induction is recommended for these patients because of gastric reflux. Postoperative administration of antacid medication is useful.

REFERENCE:

Puntis JW, Smith HL, Buick RG, et al: Effect of dystonic movements on oesophageal peristalsis in Sandifer's syndrome. *Arch Dis Child* 64(9):1311, 1989.

Sandrow Syndrome

At a glance: A rare disorder characterized by ulnar and fibula dimelia associated with polysyndactyly and peculiar facies.

Synonyms: Laurin-Sandrow Syndrome; Sandrow Sullivan Steel Syndrome; Duplication of Fibula and Ulna with Absence of Tibia and Radius; Mirror Hands and Feet with Nasal Defects; Tetrameic Mirror-Image Polydactyly; Mirror-Image Polydactyly.

History: First described by Laurin in 1964 and subsequently by Sandrow in 1970.

Genetic inheritance: Autosomal dominant.

Pathophysiology: Causal mechanism seems to be a gene that may determine anterior–posterior pattern in early developing (MIPOLI: mirror-image Polydactyly gene). It has been located on chromosome 14 (14q13).

Diagnosis: Clinical, at birth. Association of polydactyly, absent tibia and radius, nasal defect (hypoplastic nasal alae, grooved columella). The presence of mirror-image polydactyly usually confirms the diagnosis.

Clinical aspects: This polymalformative syndrome can be associated with other orthopedic abnormalities: tarsal fusion, wrist anomalies, joint dislocation, syndactyly of toes and fingers, talipes varus/valgus, restricted joint mobility, claw hand/camptodactyly of all fingers, genu valgum, genu recurvatum. Other clinical features are less frequent and can include capillary hemangioma ectopic testes.

Precautions before anesthesia: Evaluate orthopedic functional status (clinical).

Anesthetic considerations: Intraoperative positioning should be achieved carefully and can be difficult because of deformation and restricted mobility. Blood pressure measurement and venous and arterial access can be difficult because of multiple limb deformations. Regional anesthesia is not contraindicated but can be difficult in presence of skeletal anomalies, especially with neuraxial blockade.

Pharmacological implications: There are no known specific implications with this condition.

REFERENCES:

Kantaputra PN: Laurin-Sandrow syndrome with additional associated manifestations. *Am J Med Genet* 98:210, 2001.

Laurin CA, Favreau JC, Labelle P: Bilateral absence of the radius and tibia with bilateral reduplication of the ulna and fibula: A case report. *J Bone Joint Surg Am* 46A:137, 1964.

Sandrow RE, Sullivan PD, Steel HH: Hereditary ulnar and fibular dimelia with peculiar facies: A case report. *J Bone Joint Surg Am* 52A:367, 1970.

Sanjad-Sakati Syndrome

At a glance: Genetically transmitted polymalformative syndrome characterized by hypoparathyroidism, growth retardation, developmental delay, seizures, and facial dysmorphism (e.g., micrognathia).

Synonyms: Hypoparathyroidism with Short Stature, Mental Retardation, and Seizures; Kalam Hafeez Syndrome.

Genetic inheritance: Autosomal recessive. The genetic locus is on the short arm of chromosome 1 at position 42-43 (1q42-q43).

Pathophysiology: Virtually undetectable levels of parathyroid hormone resulting in hypocalcemia associated with hypophosphatemia. Growth hormone and insulin-like growth factor levels were also found to be low in affected children. Treatment with human growth hormone produced a rapid increase in the height and weight of one affected 5-year-old child. It was speculated that the hypothalamus plays a role in the regulation of both parathyroid hormone and growth hormone.

Diagnosis: Clinical features plus the onset of hypocalcemia with very low parathyroid hormone levels, usually in the newborn period. Usually consanguineous parents.

Clinical aspects: Early onset hypocalcemia, which may be asymptomatic, associated with hyperphosphatemia. Very low parathyroid hormone levels, and possibly low growth hormone and insulin-like growth factor. Consequently, patients have retarded growth (more than 2 SD [standard deviations] below the mean). Facial dysmorphism is very consistent, especially within families with more than one affected child: microcephaly, deep-set eyes, depressed nasal bridge with beaked nose, long philtrum, thin upper lip, micrognathia, and large, floppy ear lobes. Most children have skeletal defects, such as medullary stenosis. Developmental delay is usual. Seizures may occur. Reduced numbers of some T-cell subsets have been detected in some patients, but immunological function seems normal.

Precautions before anesthesia: An anesthesiology consultation is recommended before elective surgery. Detect and treat hypocalcemia/hyperphosphatemia. Evaluate the patient carefully for potential difficult tracheal intubation.

Anesthetic considerations: A difficult direct laryngoscopy and tracheal intubation may be expected, especially in patients with micrognathia. If so, spontaneous respiration should be maintained until the airway is secured and lung ventilation confirmed. Considerations of uncorrected hypocalcemia: long QT interval and associated dysrhythmias, hypotension caused by peripheral vasodilation and ventricular dysfunction, seizures, and increased neuromuscular irritability (prone to laryngospasm). Respiratory or metabolic acidosis can further decrease ionized calcium by increasing protein binding, and thus increase the likelihood of the above-mentioned considerations. Affected patients may be more sensitive to nondepolarizing muscle relaxants. Older children may be uncooperative as a result of developmental delay.

Pharmacological implications: Increased sensitivity to muscle relaxants.

Other conditions to be considered:

☞**DiGeorge Syndrome:** Recurrent infections, defective thymus functions, heart defects, and characteristic facial features caused by a deletion in chromosome 22.

☞**Kenny-Caffey Syndrome:** Congenital hypoparathyroidism associated with short stature, mental retardation, seizures, and a characteristic physiognomy. Cortical thickening of bones (osteosclerosis) and hypocalcemia. Autosomal recessive, which maps to the same region (1q42-q43); probably allelic to Sanjad-Sakati syndrome.

References:

Kalam MA, Hafeez W: Congenital hypoparathyroidism, seizure, extreme growth failure with developmental delay and dysmorphic features—Another case of this new syndrome. *Clin Genet* 42:110, 1992.

Kelly TE, Blanton S, Saif R, et al: Confirmation of the assignment of the Sanjad-Sakati (congenital hypoparathyroidism) syndrome (OMIM 241410) locus to chromosome 1q42-43. *J Med Genet* 37:63, 2000.

Marsden D, Nyhan WL, Sakati NO: Syndrome of hypoparathyroidism, growth hormone deficiency, and multiple minor anomalies. *Am J Med Genet* 52:334, 1994.

Sarcoidosis

At a glance: An inflammatory disease characterized by the presence of granulomas (small areas of inflamed cells) that usually affects the lungs. Pulmonary sarcoidosis usually leads to restrictive pulmonary disease with significant loss of lung tissue. However, all organs can be affected and the nodule can be seen as sores if the skin is involved.

Synonyms: Boeck Sarcoid; Besnier-Boeck-Schaumann Disease; Schaumann Disease.

Nature: May have a nongenetic basis but presents a familial predisposition. Seems to be more likely to present with class I HLA A1, B8, and DR3.

Incidence: Worldwide, affecting persons of all races, both sexes, and all ages. Interestingly, cases present most commonly in the winter and early spring months. About 1 to 40 cases per 1,000,000 population. More frequent in blacks than in whites.

Diagnosis: Systemic disorder of unknown cause characterized by noncaseating granulomas. Most typically, sarcoidosis is an interstitial lung disorder involving alveoli, blood vessels, and bronchioles, and producing clinical findings of dry rales, restricted lung volumes, and abnormalities in gas exchange.

Clinical aspects: Bilateral hilar adenopathy, pulmonary infiltration. Erythema nodosum, maculopapular rash, enlarged lacrimal glands, iridocyclitis, glaucoma, and chorioretinitis. Enlarged salivary glands. Bone cysts. Associated with inflammatory bowel disease, especially Crohn disease. Hyperglobulinemia, multisystem granulomatous disease with positive Kveim test. Neurosarcoidosis can mimic more common disease processes, such as meningioma, glioma, or metastases. The granulomas are frequently present in multiple organs, including the liver. Serious cardiac dysfunction is detected in 5 to 10% of patients. Sudden deaths are described. The main clinical feature with cardiac sarcoidosis is the recording of ECG abnormalities in terms of rhythm, conduction, and repolarization. Some have papillary muscle dysfunction, infiltrative cardiomyopathy with congestive heart failure, and pericarditis.

Precautions before anesthesia: It is highly recommended to obtain an anesthesiology consultation before any elective surgical procedures. Because all organs can be involved, perform a complete cell blood count, electrolytes (sodium, potassium and calcium), creatinine, liver function tests, ECG, and chest radiography. In an acute case, echocardiography can be helpful. The serial pulmonary function tests and chest radiography are the best predictive values in long term.

Anesthetic considerations: Coincidentally or not, the complete heart block cases reported during anesthesia are described with enflurane anesthesia. Airway complications caused by laryngeal involvement and bronchial stenosis have also been described.

Pharmacological implications: Because these patients are chronically on steroid therapy, they will need to receive steroid supplementation during the perioperative stress period. Sometimes the musculoskeletal involvement responds better to methotrexate. Avoid succinylcholine and other drugs that may increase intraocular pressure in the presence of glaucoma.

References:

Newman LS, Rose CS, Maier LA: Sarcoidosis. *N Engl J Med* 336:1224, 1997.

Thomnas DW, Mason RA: Complete heart block during anesthesia in a patient with sarcoidosis. *Anesthesia* 43(7):578, 1988.

Sarcosinemia

At a glance: Autosomal recessive disease characterized by sarcosine dehydrogenase deficiency. Controversies about clinical repercussion exist.

Synonyms: SAR; Hypersarcosinemia; Complex Deficiency of Sarcosine Dehydrogenase; SARD Deficiency; SARDH Deficiency.

Incidence: 1:28,000 to 1:350,000 live births (screening programs).

Genetic inheritance: Autosomal recessive.

Pathophysiology: Caused by mutations in the gene for sarcosine dehydrogenase located on 9q33-q34. Mutation causes deficient activity of sarcosine dehydrogenase and then accumulation of sarcosine, which could explain clinical manifestations.

Diagnosis: Increased concentration of sarcosine in plasma and urine as a result of sarcosine dehydrogenase deficiency.

Clinical aspects: Usually a benign metabolic state that produces no clinical disease. Multiple symptoms have been reported in sarcosinemia such as mental retardation, growth failure, hepatomegaly, craniostenosis, syndactyly, and cardiomyopathy. There is large number of patients with a high level of sarcosine in plasma who do not present any symptoms. Reported association with clinical symptoms could be as a result of an ascertainment bias.

Precautions before anesthesia: Evaluate cardiac function (clinical, ECG, echocardiography).

Anesthetic considerations: Prophylactic antibiotics should be considered in case of cardiopathy.

Pharmacological implications: There are no known specific implications with this condition.

REFERENCES:

Brunialti ALB, Harding CO, Wolff JA, et al: The mouse mutation sarcosinemia (SAR) maps to chromosome 2 in a region homologous to human 9q33-q34. *Genomics* 36:182, 1996.

Eschenbrenner M, Jorns MS: Cloning and mapping of the cDNA for human sarcosine dehydrogenase, a flavoenzyme defective in patients with sarcosinemia. *Genomics* 59:300, 1999.

Gerritsen T, Waisman HA: Hypersarcosinemia: An inborn error of metabolism. *N Engl J Med* 275:66, 1966.

SC Phocomelia Syndrome

At a glance: A very rare, autosomal recessive, severe, polymalformative disease in which skeletal anomalies can involve the whole body.

Synonyms: Hypomelia-Hypotrichosis-Facial Hemangioma Syndrome; SC-Pseudothalidomide Syndrome; SC Syndrome.

History: Genetic disorder that is likely allelic with Roberts syndrome.

Incidence: Unknown

Genetic inheritance: Autosomal recessive inheritance.

Pathophysiology: Chromosome studies reported premature centromere separation, splaying the Y-chromosome heterochromatin and repulsing the short arms of the acrocentric chromosomes.

Diagnosis: Association of nearly symmetrical reductive malformations of the limbs (resembling phocomelia), flexion contractures of various joints, multiple minor anomalies, intrauterine and extrauterine growth retardation, and mental retardation.

Clinical aspects: This severe polymalformative syndrome involves skeletal signs that can affect the whole body. Micrognathia

and microbrachycephalic skull with wormian bones in the occipital region may occur. Hand abnormalities can include absence of the thumb, shortening of the first metacarpal bone, hypoplasia of the first digit, fusion of the fourth and fifth metacarpals, clinodactyly of the second and fifth digits, and hypoplasia of the middle phalanges, with symmetric reduction deformity (upper limbs being more severely affected than the lower ones) and flexion contractures of the joints. Other clinical features concern hypotrichosis with scanty silvery blond hair, growth and occasional mental retardation, seizures, aortic stenosis, and cloudy cornea.

Precautions before anesthesia: Evaluate cardiac function (clinical, chest radiograph, echocardiography), neurological function (maintenance of seizure therapy), and airway (clinical, radiography).

Anesthetic considerations: Arterial and venous access because blood pressure can be difficult to manage as a consequence of the limb deformities. Direct laryngoscopy and tracheal intubation can be difficult because of micrognathia and skull deformation. In these conditions, it is highly recommended to maintain spontaneous respiration until trachea is intubated and lung ventilation confirmed.

Pharmacological implications: Prophylactic antibiotics should be used in cases of cardiopathy. Antiepileptic treatment should be continued on day of surgery; consider interaction between epileptic and anesthetic drugs.

Other conditions to be considered:

☞HOLT-ORAM SYNDROME: Characterized by thumb anomaly and atrial septal defect, although abnormality of the upper extremities can be more extensive in some cases. The thumb may be absent or may be a triphalangeal, nonopposable, finger-like digit. This syndrome was first clearly described in 1960 by Holt and Oram who observed atrial septal defect in members of four generations of a family. Upper extremity phocomelia and ventricular septal defect have been reported in few patients.

BALLER-GEROLD SYNDROME (Craniosynostosis with Radial Defects; Craniosynostosis-Radial Aplasia Syndrome): Characterized by the presence of craniosynostosis with radial defects. The radial anomalies consist of radial aplasia and slight ulnar hypoplasia. Other clinical features include bilateral conductive hearing loss, malformation or absence of some carpals and metacarpals, and absent or hypoplastic thumbs and other skeletal anomalies of the spine and pelvis. Short stature is always present. Anteriorly placed and imperforate anus is often present with either perineal fistula or rectovaginal fistula. Anomalies of the heart and urogenital system and mental and/or motor retardation have been noted.

REFERENCES:

Feingold M: History of C-patient with SC-Roberts/pseudothalidomide syndrome [letter]. *Am J Med Genet* 43:898, 1992.

Hermann J, Feingold M, Tuffi GA et al: A familial dysmorphogenic syndrome of limb deformities, characteristic facial appearance and associated anomalies: The "pseudothalidomide" or "SC-Syndrome." *Birth Defects* 5(3):81, 1969.

Schilder Syndrome

At a glance: A rare, progressive, and lethal disease of the central nervous system that affects mostly children and characterized by adrenal atrophy and diffuse central demyelination. Presents with progressive dementia, spasticity, cortical blindness, deafness, hemiplegia, quadriplegia, ataxia, pyramidal signs, retrobulbar neuritis, and pseudobulbar palsy. Seizures. Onset in late childhood. Most patients die within few months after onset.

Synonyms: Flatau-Schilder Syndrome; Heubner-Schilder Syndrome; Schilder-Addison Syndrome (could be a misnomer); Addison-Schilder Syndrome; Scholz type of Diffuse Cerebral Sclerosis; Encephalitis Periaxialis Diffusa; Diffuse Periaxial Encephalitis; Scholz type of Metachromatic Leukodystrophy; Myelinoclastic Diffuse Sclerosis.

History: First described by Paul Schilder (1886–1940), an Austrian neurologist.

Incidence: In the United States, the frequency is considered very rare (5:100,000 children). There are no international epidemiological studies large enough to determine the incidence.

Genetic inheritance: X-linked.

Diagnosis: Based on clinical features. May be confirmed by familial history and the finding of striking metachromasia on brain histology.

Clinical aspects: Onset during the first decade and characterized by neural degeneration, including deafness, blindness, weakness, and spasticity of the lower legs. Poor pharyngeal control with aspiration pneumonia. Adrenal insufficiency (Addison-Schilder syndrome).

Precautions before anesthesia: Upper motor neuron disease with peripheral degeneration producing a giant motor unit. Paraplegia with poor autonomic control. High prevalence of seizure disorder. Gastric reflux with an elevated risk of pulmonary aspiration. Relevant airway complications related to poor pharyngeal muscle control complicated by the presence of copious oral secretions. Adrenal involvement is frequent: check adrenal function and serum electrolytes.

Anesthetic considerations: Hemodynamic instability may be present as a result of neural degeneration. Most patients show a poor airway control which necessitates that the tracheal extubation be performed when the patient is fully awake. Recovery should be conducted with the patient lying on the side.

Pharmacological implications: The use of succinylcholine should be avoided because of the risk of hyperkaliemia (nerve denervation). In addition, because of adrenal involvement, steroid hormone supplementation may be necessary intra- and postoperatively.

Other conditions to be considered:

KRABBE DISEASE: Similar neurochemistry disorder and presentation as Schilder disease but leads to sudanophilic cerebral sclerosis, metachromatic leukodystrophy, and adrenoleukodystrophy.

MULTIPLE SCLEROSIS: An inflammatory disease of the central nervous system (CNS) affecting mostly the white matter and leading to patches of neural tissue damage called myelin plaques. Central demyelination leading to spasticity, cortical blindness, motor nerve dysfunction with potential to hemiplegia, quadriplegia, ataxia, pyramidal signs, retrobulbar neuritis, and pseudobulbar palsy is often associated.

☞**ALEXANDER SYNDROME:** A degenerative and progressive disorder of the central nervous system caused by leukodystrophy. Affects mainly males and usually begins at about 6 months of age. Symptoms include mental and physical retardation, enlargement of the brain and head, spasticity (arms and legs), and seizures.

☞**CANAVAN SYNDROME:** A progressive leukodystrophy caused by spongy degeneration of the CNS. It is uniformly fatal within 18 months after onset of symptoms.

☞**METACHROMATIC LEUKODYSTROPHY:** An inherited disorder of myelin metabolism with progressive loss of white matter in the central and peripheral nervous system.

☞**PELIZAEUS-MERZBACHER SYNDROME:** A very rare slowly progressive dysmyelinating disease affecting in a diffuse pattern the cerebrum, cerebellum, brainstem, and spinal cord. Two types are described: X-linked (Infantile form) and the autosomal dominant (preadulthood form). Clinical features also include: stridor, muscle spasticity, nystagmus. Often fatal in the first year of life from respiratory complications.

☞**X-LINKED ADRENOLEUKODYSTROPHY:** A disorder characterized by progressive demyelinization of the CNS and peripheral adrenal insufficiency.

☞**ZELLWEGER SYNDROME:** A disorder characterized by the congenital absence of functioning peroxisomes (the cellular structures that are responsible for the elimination of toxic substances) resulting in a cerebrohepatorenal syndrome. The disease affects brain development, particularly myelination. Most important features include hepatomegaly, polycystic kidney disease, visual disturbances, and high plasma levels of iron and copper. Other features include muscular hypotonia already noticeable at birth, mental retardation, seizures, coagulopathy, and dysphagia with recurrent aspiration. Congenital heart defects have been described. Life expectancy is approximately 6 months.

REFERENCE:

Tobias JD: Anaesthetic considerations for the child with leukodystrophy. *Can J Anaesth* 39:394, 1992.

Schindler Disease

At a glance: A very rare autosomal recessive disease characterized by accumulation of glycosphingolipids in many tissues, which lead to neurological and ophthalmic lesions and to frequent, severe, pulmonary infections.

Synonyms: N-acetyl-α-D-Galactosaminidase (NAGA); Kanzaki Disease (Schindler Disease adult form).

Incidence: Very rare (10 cases reported).

Genetic inheritance: Autosomal recessive.

Pathophysiology: Caused by mutation of gene α-N-acetylgalactosaminidase (α-GalNAc) located on 22q11. In individuals with Schindler disease, deficiency of the α-NAGA enzyme leads to an abnormal accumulation of certain complex compounds (glycosphingolipids) in many tissues of the body. It is classified among oligosaccharidoses or glycoproteinoses.

Diagnosis: Clinical evocation is difficult because the disorder is clinically heterogeneous. The *infantile form of Schindler Disease*, in which onset occurs by the end of the first year, is characterized by progressive hypotonia, extrapyramidal signs, and rapid psychomotor regression (as a result of abnormal lipid storage in nervous system). Death occurs within the first decade. In the *adult form*, angiokeratomas (abnormal lipid storage in the vessels) and moderate mental retardation are observed. Certitude diagnosis is biological: characteristic profile on the chromatography of urinary oligosaccharides, confirmed by the measurement of the α-N-acetylgalactosaminidase activity in leukocytes, fibroblasts, amniocytes, or trophoblasts.

Clinical aspects: In the *infantile form* there is increasing neurological impairment, with progressive hypotonia, spasticity, no voluntary movements, decorticating posture, symmetric hyper-reflexia, profound psychomotor retardation, and seizures by the age of 3 to 4 years. Other clinical features include ophthalmologic manifestations: bilateral optic atrophy, cortical blindness, nystagmus, and strabismus. Severe respiratory infections occur.

Precautions before anesthesia: Evaluate neurological status (clinical, CT/MRI, EEG, somatosensory evoked potentials) and muscular atrophy caused by nerve denervation (clinical). Assess respiratory function with chest radiograph.

Anesthetic considerations: Intraoperative positioning must be done carefully because of the severe spasticity. Patients affected with active pulmonary infections must be postponed when possible. The presence of residual respiratory tract infection should not be disregarded because the perioperative incidence of complications is very high.

Pharmacological implications: Avoid succinylcholine because of the association of nerve demyclination and amyotrophic changes. The risk of hyperkalemia and sudden cardiac arrest is significant. Epileptic treatment has to be given the day of anesthesia. Consider anesthetic and antiepileptic drugs interactions.

Other conditions to be considered:

☞**SEITELBERGER SYNDROME:** A rare inherited disorder characterized by the progressive degeneration of the central nervous system. Individuals affected with this disorder develop normally within the first 6 months to 2 years of age, at which time their psychomotor development slows and individuals begin to lose previously acquired skills. Clinically, this condition is characterized by severe nystagmus and strabismus, optic nerve atrophy and loss of vision, hypotonia, muscle spasticity, and/or deafness. Later on, children may exhibit dementia and neurological decerebration. It is inherited as an autosomal recessive genetic trait.

☞**HALLERVORDEN-SPATZ DISEASE:** A rare neurological movement disorder characterized by the progressive degeneration of the central nervous system and abnormal accumulation of iron pigment in certain areas of the brain. It typically develops during childhood and occasionally may begin during adulthood. The most common neuromuscular symptoms may include dystonia, rigidity, spasticity, and/or ataxia. Neurological symptoms may include progressive confusion, disorientation, and/or dementia. It is inherited as an autosomal recessive genetic trait.

☞**FABRY DISEASE:** A rare inherited disorder of lipid metabolism characterized by a deficiency of the enzyme alpha-galactosidase A. It consists of abnormal accumulation of fatty material and carbohydrates, i.e., glycolipids such as glycosphingolipid in various organs of the body, particularly blood vessels and the eyes. The clinical features include angiokeratomas, as seen in Schindler Disease, Type II. Abdominal pain and/or visual impairment have been reported. Kidney failure, heart problems, and/or neurological symptoms may lead to serious complications. It is inherited as an X-linked recessive genetic trait, primarily affecting males. A milder form of the disease has been identified in females.

REFERENCES:

Bakker HD, de Sonnaville ML, Vreken P, et al: Human alpha-*N*-acetylgalactosaminidase (alpha-NAGA) deficiency? No association with neuroaxonal dystrophy? *Eur J Hum Genet* 9:91, 2001.

Kanzaki T, Yokota M, Irie F, et al: Angiokeratoma corporis diffusum with glycopeptiduria due to deficient lysosomal alpha-*N*-

acetylgalactosaminidase activity: Clinical, morphologic, and biochemical studies. *Arch Dermatol* 129:460, 1993.

Schindler D, Bishop DF, Wallace S, et al: Characterization of alpha-*N*-acetylgalactosaminidase deficiency: A new neurodegenerative lysosomal disease [abstract]. *Pediatr Res* 23:333A, 1988.

Schinzel Syndrome

At a glance: A very rare autosomal dominant syndrome, characterized by bone malformations and apocrine deficiency.

Synonyms: Ulnar Mammary Syndrome; Ulnar Mammary Syndrome of Pallister; UMS.

Genetic inheritance: Autosomal dominant.

Pathophysiology: Mutations in the T-Box 3 (TBX3) gene, located on 12q24.1, are responsible for Schinzel syndrome.

Diagnosis: Characterized by skeletal abnormalities affecting the bones of the forearms and hands. Underdevelopment and dysfunction of certain sweat glands and/or the breast is also observed.

Clinical aspects: The syndrome is associated with multiple signs: short stature, obesity, and complex skeletal malformations that can include skeletal abnormalities affecting the hands and/or forearms (hypoplasia, complete absence of the bone on the outer aspect of the forearm [ulna] and third, fourth and fifth fingers). Additionally, affected infants may have additional finger malformations with or without ulnar and/or digital abnormalities on the other side of the body. Other abnormalities associated with Schinzel syndrome include absent or incorrectly positioned (ectopic) teeth, delayed growth, uterine and vaginal abnormalities, hypogenitalism (delayed puberty), subglottic stenosis, inguinal hernia, anal atresia, pyloric stenosis, and kidney agenesis or ectopy.

Precautions before anesthesia: It is essential to assess the condition of the apocrine system (clinical, historical); airway (clinical, fiberoptic endoscopy); and renal function (electrolytes, urea, creatinine, echography, CT scan, radionuclide imaging if necessary).

Anesthetic considerations: Direct laryngoscopy and tracheal intubation can be difficult because of mouth malformation and the presence of tracheal substenosis. Preserving spontaneous ventilation should be preferable until the trachea is secured and lung ventilation confirmed. The availability of a laryngeal mask airway and/or fiberoptic intubating equipment is highly recommended. Venous, arterial access, as well as blood pressure and SpO_2 (arterial oxyhemoglobin saturation) measurement, can be difficult to obtain because of limb malformation. Regional anesthesia is not contraindicated but can be difficult to realize. Hyperthermia should be prevented because of apocrine gland deficiency.

Pharmacological implications: Avoid parasympatholytic drugs because of a dysfunction in the sweat response. Avoid nephrotoxic drugs in cases of renal dysfunction.

Other conditions to be considered:

ABSENCE OF ULNA AND FIBULA WITH SEVERE LIMB DEFICIT (Al Awadi Teebi Farag Syndrome; Limb/Pelvis-Hypoplasia/Aplasia Syndrome; Al-Awadi Raas-Rothschild Syndrome; Schinzel Phocomelia Syndrome): Autosomal recessive with severe deficiency of all four limbs, including absent feet, hypoplastic femora, absent ulnae, absent fibulae, thoracic dystrophy, and pelvic deformity.

☞**ADULT SYNDROME:** An acronym that stands for Acro-Dermo-Ungueal-Lacrimal-Tooth. The main findings are hypodontia, very brittle and/or premature loss of permanent teeth, and ectrodactyly (split hands and feet). There is no evident impairment of general health in patients with ADULT Syndrome.

☞**ECTRODACTYLY-ECTODERMAL DYSPLASIA AND CLEFTING SYNDROME:** Autosomal dominant inherited syndrome with maxillary hypoplasia, mild malar hypoplasia, cleft lip and palate, choanal atresia, hearing loss, photophobia and blepharophimosis, dacryocystitis, cryptorchidism, hypogonadotropic hypogonadism renal agenesis or dysplasia, hydronephrosis, occasionally mental retardation, central diabetes insipidus.

LIMB MAMMARY SYNDROME (LMS): This very rare syndrome is characterized by severe anomalies of the hands and feet in combination with hypoplasia or aplasia of the mammary gland and nipple. As in ADULT Syndrome, the lacrimal duct can be atretic or obstructed, the nails may be thickened and dystrophic. Hypodontia and cleft palate have been described. A newer study placed the ADULT syndrome gene locus in the same chromosome region as the LMS locus, thereby suggesting that these two conditions are allelic.

☞**AEC SYNDROME:** A disorder characterized by cleft lip and/or palate, uni- or bilateral fusion of the eyelids, hair anomalies, onychodystrophy, hypohidrosis, and dental anomalies. The mutation has been mapped to 3q27, like all the other disorders mentioned above.

REFERENCES:

Bamshad M, Lin RC, Law DJ, et al: Mutations in human TBX3 alter limb, apocrine and genital development in ulnar-mammary syndrome. *Nat Genet* 16:311, 1997.

Olney RS, Hoyme HE, Roche F, et al: Limb/pelvis hypoplasia/aplasia with skull defect (Schinzel phocomelia): Distinctive features and prenatal detection. *Am J Med Genet* 103:295, 2001.

Schinzel A: Ulnar-mammary syndrome. *J Med Genet* 24:778, 1987.

Schinzel-Giedion Syndrome

At a glance: A distinct dysmorphic syndrome of congenital hydronephrosis, skeletal dysplasia (open cranial sutures, steep short skull, wide occipital synchondrosis) and severe developmental retardation. Coarse facies characterized by midface retraction, bulging forehead, facial hemangiomas, short nose with anteverted nostrils, protruding large tongue, and hypertelorism. Patient usually dies during infancy.

Synonym: Schinzel-Giedion Midface-Retraction Syndrome.

Genetic inheritance: Probably autosomal recessive.

Clinical aspects: *Craniofacial:* midface retraction, large fontanelles, hypertelorism, low-set ears, choanal stenosis, macroglossia, short, broad neck; *hair:* hypertrichosis; *skin:* facial telangiectasia, dermal ridge hypoplasia, narrow nails; *cardiac:* atrial septal defect, other cardiac defects; *neurological:* seizure, spasticity, developmental delay, cerebral atrophy; *renal:* hydronephrosis, hydroureter; *skeletal:* hypoplastic ribs and broad ribs, postaxial polydactyly, mesomelic brachymelia, hypoplastic distal phalanges, hyperdense long tubular bone, broad ribs, clubbed feet, polysyndactyly; *growth:* growth retardation. Affected patients usually die in early neonatal or infancy period.

Precautions before anesthesia: Assess for potential airway difficulty with presence of choanal stenosis, midface retraction, large tongue, short neck. The cardiac function must be assessed for possible congenital heart defect with the aid of physical examination,

ECG, chest radiograph, and echocardiogram. A complete evaluation of the respiratory function for evidence of respiratory failure must be obtained through a complete physical, chest radiograph, and blood gas analysis if indicated.

Anesthetic considerations: There are no anesthesia reports because of the early lethality. The airway should be assessed for difficult tracheal intubation and ventilation. Avoid nasal intubation if choanal stenosis is suspected. Nasal or facial surgery may lead to further upper airway compromise. Respiratory complication is frequent with pneumonia and upper airway obstruction. Intravenous access may be difficult with abnormal joint position.

Pharmacological implications: Anticonvulsant drugs should be continued throughout perioperative period. Drugs used should be tailored according to the cardiac and respiratory functions. Precautions for cardiac defect should include prophylactic antibiotics, avoidance of air embolism, and adequate rehydration.

Other conditions to be considered:

☞**AICARDI SYNDROME:** A rare disorder characterized by partial or complete agenesis of the corpus callosum, infantile spasms (spasm-like epilepsy), mental retardation, and an ocular abnormality called lacunae of the retina. Often associated with other features such as microcephaly and porencephalic cysts. The onset is generally between the age of 3 and 5 months. The disorder affects only females.

☞**WEST SYNDROME:** A disorder characterized by the triad of infantile spasms, an interictal EEG pattern termed hypsarrhythmia, and mental retardation. This severe epilepsy syndrome is an age-dependent expression of a significantly damaged brain. It was the English physician W.J. West in 1841 who provided the first description of this bizarre epilepsy pattern, which he found in his own child. He described the pattern as "bobbings" causing a complete heaving of the head forward and toward the knees, then followed by immediate relaxation into the upright position. Repetitive in few seconds, 10 to 20 times at each attack, however continuing for no more than 2 to 3 minutes, 3 or more times a day.

☞**LENNOX-GASTAUT SYNDROME:** Severe form of epilepsy resulting in significant learning disabilities and impaired organization of movements.

PALLISTER SYNDROME(Ulna-Mammary Syndrome type Pallister): A syndrome of abnormal development of the ulna, forearms, mammary glands, axillary apocrine glands, teeth, palate, and vertebral and urogenital systems. Absence of body odor and axillary sweating, absence of breast tissue, and hypoplasia of nipples and areolas. Both sexes affected equally. Autosomal dominant inheritance.

REFERENCES:

Al-Gazali L, Farndon P, Burn J, et al: The Schinzel-Giedion syndrome. *J Med Genet* 27:42, 1990.

Schinzel A, Giedion A: A syndrome of severe midface retraction, multiple skull anomalies, clubfeet, and cardiac and renal malformation in sibs. *Am J Med Genet* 1:361, 1978.

Schinzel Acrocallosal Syndrome

At a glance: A very rare, autosomal recessive, complex, polymalformative disease characterized by predominant neurological and skeletal anomalies.

Synonyms: Hallux Duplication, Postaxial Polydactyly, and Absence of Corpus Callosum; Acrocallosal Syndrome.

History: Described in 1979 by Albert AGL Schinzel, an Austrian human geneticist, in Vienna.

Incidence: A rare condition reported in Austria, Switzerland and Turkey.

Genetic inheritance: Autosomal recessive (consanguinity frequent).

Pathophysiology: Unknown; gene located at 12p13.3-p11.2.

Diagnosis: Association of mental retardation, peculiar facies, absence of the corpus callosum, and polydactyly.

Clinical aspects: Global syndrome constitutes a complex polymalformative disease characterized by macrocephaly, large anterior fontanel, epicanthal folds, prominent occiput, and bulging forehead. Agenesis of corpus callosum, seizures, hyperreflexia, anencephaly occurs in some cases. Facial deformations can include low-set posteriorly rotated ears, down-slanting palpebral fissures, exotropia, protruding eyeballs, hypertelorism, broad and short nose, anteverted nostrils, short upper lip, and high-arched cleft palate. Skeletal deformations are also observed: postaxial polydactyly of the fingers and toes, bifid terminal phalanges of the thumbs, duplicated halluces, and tapered fingers. Umbilical and inguinal hernia, light curly hair, hypospadias, hypogonadism, and cardiac defects can occur.

Precautions before anesthesia: The airway must be carefully evaluated (clinical, radiography) because of craniofacial anomalies. Cardiac function (clinical, chest radiograph, echocardiography); neurological function (clinical, EEG, CT, MRI) must be obtained. One must ensure that the seizure therapy is optimal (history, clinical, biology).

Anesthetic considerations: Direct laryngoscopy and tracheal intubation may be difficult and may require fiberoptic intubation because of malformations. The availability of a laryngeal mask airway is recommended.

Pharmacological implications: Prophylactic antibiotics must be considered in presence of cardiac defect. Avoid cardiodepressive drugs. Antiepileptic treatment should be continued on day of surgery; consider interaction between antiepileptic and anesthetic drugs.

REFERENCES:

Koenig R, Bach A, Woelki U, et al: Spectrum of the acrocallosal syndrome. *Am J Med Genet* 108:7, 2002.

Schinzel A: Postaxial polydactyly, hallux duplication, absence of the corpus callosum, macrencephaly and severe mental retardation: A new syndrome. *Helv Paediatr Acta* 34:141, 1979.

Scholz-Greenfield Syndrome

At a glance: A severe and fatal form of metachromatic leukodystrophy that begins around the age of 18 months.

Synonyms: Leukodystrophy Metachromatic; Arylsulfatase A Deficiency; Greenfield Syndrome; Henneberg Disease; Scholtz Disease; Scholz-Bielschowsky-Henneberg Syndrome; Greenfield Disease.

Incidence: Metachromatic Leukodystrophy has a global incidence in general population of 1:100,000; Scholz-Greenfield syndrome represents 60% of all Metachromatic Leukodystrophy.

Genetic inheritance: Autosomal recessive; arylsulfatase A (ARSA) gene located at 22q13.31-qter.

Pathophysiology: Arylsulfatase A is a lysosomal enzyme that catalyzes the hydrolysis of the 3-*O*-sulfate linkages of cerebroside sulfate to form galactocerebroside. The deficiency of this enzyme involves accumulation of sulfatides, which results in the progressive breakdown of membranes of the myelin sheath. A small concentration of sulfatide is stored in the kidneys, gallbladder, and other visceral organs.

Diagnosis: Characterized by normal infancy followed by locomotive disorders between the ages of 12 and 18 months (never walk or difficulty in walking, hypotonia, weakness, and loss of reflexes). Diagnosis is confirmed by deficiency of arylsulfatase A activity in leukocytes and cultured skin fibroblasts. Antenatal diagnosis is possible and a deficiency of enzyme activity in cultured chorionic villi or amniocytes can be measured.

Clinical aspects: Death occurs within the first decade of life (2 to 4 years after diagnosis). Clinical features are dominated by neurological ones (ataxia, spasticity, progressive hypotonia and motor weakness, absent deep tendon reflexes, peripheral neuropathy with decreased conduction speed, dysarthria and aphasia, mental regression, dysphagia with bulbar and pseudobulbar palsies, and myoclonic seizures). Other clinical features concern the eyes (nystagmus and optic atrophy), digestive organs (gastroesophageal reflux, excessive salivation, megacolon, undernutrition, gallbladder dysfunction), orthopedics (frequent genu recurvatum and possibility of hip dislocation), and muscle anomalies.

Precautions before anesthesia: Evaluate neurological status (clinical, full history, MRI, electromyography, EEG, somatosensory evoked potentials) and digestive function (clinical, pH-metry).

Anesthetic considerations: Careful intraoperative positioning is needed because of nervous and orthopedic impairment. Reflux, dysphagia, and hypersalivation increase the patient's risk of pulmonary aspiration and require postoperative care and survey. Particular attention has to be given to postoperative pain relief because of the potential trigger effect of pain on seizures. Regional anesthesia is not contraindicated, but nervous pathological lesion can lead to difficult predictable effects. Benefit has to be evaluated and explained to patient (if possible) and family.

Pharmacological implications: Antiepileptic treatment must be maintained until the morning of surgery and interaction with anesthetic drugs must be considered. Use of preoperative atropine should be recommended to dry excessive oral secretions. Succinylcholine should probably be avoided because of muscle anomalies and the risk of hyperkalemic response to the presence of nerve denervation.

Other condition to be considered:

☞**Nyssen-Van Bogaert Syndrome (van Bogaert-Nyssen-Pfeiffer Syndrome):** Adult form with similar clinical features and the psychiatric presentation of presenile dementia.

REFERENCES:

Greenfield JGA: A form of progressive cerebral sclerosis in infants associated with primary degeneration of the interfascicular glia. *J Neurol Psychopathol (London)* 13:289, 1933.

Quader MA, Healy TE: Muscle fibrillation following thiopentone and pancuronium bromide. An association with metachromatic leukodystrophy. *Anaesthesia* 32(7):644, 1977.

Tobias JD: Anaesthetic considerations for the child with leukodystrophy. *Can J Anaesth* 39(4):394, 1992.

Schönlein-Henoch Purpura Syndrome

At a glance: A form of anaphylactoid or nonthrombopenic purpura that is the most common connective tissue disorder in children. This syndrome is an allergic reaction to a β-hemolytic streptococci. It usually presents 1 to 3 weeks after an upper respiratory tract infection. Characterized by a purpuric rash, painful swollen joints, abdominal pain with vomiting. Onset in preschool age with peak in spring and fall, occurring more often in males than females.

Synonyms: Anaphylactoid Purpura; Allergic Nonthrombocy-topenic Purpura; Allergic Purpura-Arthralgia-Gastrointestinal Symptoms; Peliosis Rheumatica; Purpura Abdominalis; Purpura Infectiosa Acuta.

Incidence: The most common vasculitis in children, usually occurring beyond age 2 years until adolescence. Idiopathic; male:female ratio = 3:2.

Pathophysiology: Leukoclastic vasculitis of small vessels, with the potential for necrotizing vasculitis of the kidney and gastrointestinal tract. IgA and C3 deposition is found in the small vessels of the skin and the glomeruli. Etiology is unknown, although it occurs following exposure to infection and drugs.

Diagnosis: Based on clinical findings of rash over the lower extremities and buttocks, arthritis, and colicky abdominal pain. Fifty percent of patients have fever and palpable purpura. IgA deposition may also be found in the skin, and serum titers may also be elevated.

Clinical aspects: Rash over lower extremities and buttocks, arthritis, abdominal pain that may mimic an acute abdomen, intussusception, renal disease (10 to 40%), although usually resolves over the long term. Less frequent clinical features include: pulmonary hemorrhage, convulsions, hemiparesis, mononeuropathies, scrotal vasculitis, and pancreatitis. No specific treatment, although acute attacks may be treated with hydration, non-steroidal antiinflammatory

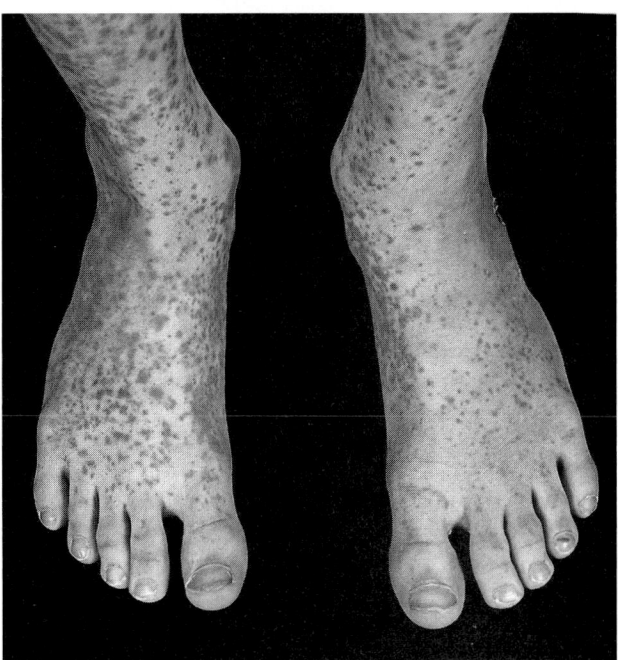

Schönlein-Henoch purpura Purpuric rash in an adult patient with Schönlein-Henoch purpura.

drugs (NSAIDs), and steroids. Prognosis favors recovery in weeks to months.

Precautions before anesthesia: Check a complete cell blood count (CBC) and electrolytes. Query for pulmonary involvement.

Anesthetic considerations: Consider renal dysfunction when choosing drugs. Regional anesthesia is not contraindicated with normal platelet counts or lack of bleeding diathesis.

Pharmacological implications: The administration of anesthetic agents or other medications dependent on renal elimination must be avoided. Any medication with potential renal toxic by-products must be avoided in the presence of renal dysfunction.

REFERENCE:
Athreya BH: Vasculitis in children. *Pediatr Clin North Am* 42:1239, 1995.

Schopf-Schulz-Passarge Syndrome

At a glance: Keratosis palmoplantaris with cystic eyelids, hypodontia, and hypotrichosis. Eccrine tumors with ectodermal dysplasia are part of this medical condition.

Synonyms: Keratosis Palmoplantaris with Cystic Eyelids, Hypodontia and Hypotrichosis; Eccrine Tumors with Ectodermal Dysplasia Syndrome.

Genetic inheritance: Autosomal recessive inheritance

Pathophysiology: A comprehensive classification of the primary palmoplantar keratodermas was suggested by Stevens et al. in 1996. The term "palmoplantar ectodermal dysplasia" was used where more than a single ectodermal structure was involved to emphasize the generalized nature of the disorder. They further identified a total of 19 subtypes and the Schopf-Schultz-Passarge syndrome was determined to be Type XXIX. Cause unknown. Chromosomal study normal.

Diagnosis: Clinical features characterized by a disorder of hair, nail, teeth, and sweat glands in various combinations. The eyelid cysts are considered expansion of the glands of Moll.

Clinical aspects: Hypotrichosis: fine, sparse head hair; sparse eyelash and eyebrows. Hypodontia: early loss of decidual teeth; few permanent teeth. Eyes: epidermal cysts of eyelids are characteristic. Skin changes: plantar and palmar keratosis; nail dystrophy. Exocrine gland tumor may occur on hands and feet. Affected individuals have normal lifespan and function.

Anesthetic considerations: There are no specific anesthesia considerations associated with this condition. Any considerations will be related to the surgical procedure only.

Other conditions to be considered:

☞**PAPILLON-LEFEVRE:** An extremely rare genetic disorder that typically becomes apparent during the first 5 years of life. It is characterized by palmar-plantar hyperkeratosis in association with periodontium. The deciduous teeth are lost by age 5 years. Without treatment, most of the permanent teeth may also be lost by approximately age 17 years. Other clinical features include frequent pyogenic skin infections, nail dystrophy, and hyperhidrosis. It is transmitted as an autosomal recessive trait.

☞**HAIM-MUNK SYNDROME:** Characterized by palmoplantar hyperkeratosis and onychogryphosis. Pes planus, arachnodactyly, and/or acroosteolysis have been reported. Periodontosis may also be present. It is inherited as an autosomal recessive trait. Some researchers believe the disorder may be a variant of Papillon-Lefevre Syndrome.

MELEDA DISEASE (Mal de Meleda): An extremely rare disorder characterized by the slow progressive development of palmoplantar hyperkeratosis. Affected skin may be unusually red and become abnormally thick. Affected children may exhibit abnormalities of the nails, hyperhidrosis with unpleasant odor, and/or lichenoid plaques. In addition, cardiac abnormalities and cardiomegaly have been reported. It is inherited as an autosomal recessive trait.

☞**SJÖGREN-LARSSON SYNDROME:** A rare inherited disorder characterized by ichthyosis, palmoplantar hyperkeratosis, and ecchymosis. Affected infants may show mental retardation, spastic paraplegia, seizures, and eye abnormalities. It is inherited as an autosomal recessive trait.

FITZSIMMONS SYNDROME: An extremely rare inherited disorder characterized by slow progressive development of palmoplantar keratosis, mental retardation, and spastic paraplegia. Children may show an abnormally high pes cavus. It is thought to be inherited as an X-linked genetic transmission.

REFERENCES:

Craifen W, Levy M, Lewis R: Schopf-Schulz-Passarge syndrome with an unusual pattern of inheritance. *Am J Med Genet* 71:186–188, 1997.

Stevens HP, Kelsell DP, Bryant SP et al: Linkage of an American pedigree with palmoplantar keratoderma and malignancy (palmoplantar ectodermal dysplasia type III) to 17q24: Literature survey and proposed updated classification of the keratodermas. *Arch Derm* 132: 640–651, 1996.

Schwartz-Jampel Syndrome

At a glance: A very rare autosomal recessive condition manifested by a combination of muscle stiffness (hypertrophied muscle) and mild, largely nonprogressive muscle weakness (myotonia). Onset age is during the first year of life. Other clinical features include mostly ophthalmological anomalies and a pectus carinatum.

Synonyms: Catel-Schwartz-Jampel Syndrome; Schwartz-Jampel-Aberfeld Syndrome; Chondrodystrophia Myotonia.

Genetic inheritance: Autosomal recessive.

Pathophysiology: Three types are recognized. *Type Ia* is usually recognized in childhood and is associated with moderate bone dysplasia. *Type IB* is recognized at birth and is associated with more pronounced bone dysplasia. *Type II* is recognized at birth and is associated with increased mortality. The *SJS-I* locus (1p34-p36) maps to a region that contains the gene encoding perlecan (HSPG2). This heparan sulphate proteoglycan is highly expressed in cartilage and basement membranes. Three mutations in this gene have been described in families with this syndrome. Contractures are most severe by mid-adolescence.

Diagnosis: Problems with the motor development become evident during the first year of life. The characteristic dysmorphic features lead to an early diagnosis.

Clinical aspects: Features include *facial malformations* (microstomia, micrognathia, retrognathia, blepharophimosis, short palpebral fissures, telecanthus, sad "fixed" facies, low-set ears, short neck), and *musculoskeletal signs* (myopathy, myotonia, muscular hypertrophy, restricted joint mobility, osteoporosis, dislocated hip, delayed bone age, epiphyseal anomaly, kyphosis, scoliosis, pectus carinatum, abnormal vertebral size/shape, anterior bowing of the long bones). Mental retardation (20%) and areflexia/hyporeflexia are described. Short stature, intrauterine growth retardation, myopia, cataract, umbilical hernia, generalized hirsutism, feeding and swallowing difficulties, and recurrent hyperthermia may be observed.

Precautions before anesthesia: An anesthesiology consultation is highly recommended before elective surgery. Detailed examination of the airway. Evaluate the extent of the myopathy.

Anesthetic considerations: The airway features suggest that face-mask ventilation, direct laryngoscopy and tracheal intubation may be difficult. Until confirmation that proper lung ventilation can be maintained, either with face-mask or following tracheal intubation, spontaneous respiration should be maintained. Vascular access and positioning may be difficult because of joint contractures.

Pharmacological implications: Succinylcholine should be used with caution or simply avoided in the presence of a myopathy because of the risk of hyperkaliemia and malignant hyperpyrexia.

Other conditions to be considered:

STUVE-WIEDMANN SYNDROME (Schwartz-Jampel Syndrome type II; Schwartz-Jampel Syndrome Neonatal form; Stuve-Wiedmann-Schwartz-Jampel Syndrome): Characterized by congenital bowing of the long bones, short stature, camptodactyly with ulnar deviation and contractures of the elbows and fingers. Radiographically the long bones were short and thick with large metaphyses, a broad coracoid process bilaterally, long scapulae, relatively thin ribs, pubic and ischial bones broad and the ilia relatively small. Other features include susceptibility to respiratory problems and hyperthermia (suspicion of malignant hyperthermia).

☞**MARDEN-WALKER SYNDROME:** A rare connective tissue disorder that is inherited as an autosomal recessive transmission. The clinical features include craniofacial anomalies (mask-like face), micrognathia, ptosis, blepharophimosis, cleft palate, and cleft lip. In addition, joint contractures, kyphoscoliosis and pectus carinatum have been reported.

☞**KING-DENBOROUGH SYNDROME:** An extremely rare disorder and a form of Malignant Hyperthermia. Clinical characteristics include craniofacial anomalies, midface hypoplasia and low-set ears. In addition, ptosis, palpebral fissures, skeletal abnormalities, kyphoscoliosis, abnormally short stature, and pectus carinatum have been reported. Mild muscle weakness may be present as well as joint contractures. It is sporadic, however it has been suggested that an autosomal recessive transmission could not be excluded.

VAN DYKE-HANSON SYNDROME: A rare inherited neuromuscular disorder presenting with congenital joint contractures. During early childhood, the presence of periodic ataxia affecting the trunk leading to titubation of the head is characteristics of this disorder. Short, spontaneous spasms and contractions within groups of muscle fibers (myokymia) in the face, arms, and legs are characteristic. It is inherited as an autosomal dominant genetic trait.

REFERENCES:

Nicole S, Davoine CS, Topaloglu H, et al: Perlecan, the major proteoglycan of basement membranes, is altered in patients with Schwartz-Jampel syndrome (chondrodystrophic myotonia). *Nat Genet* 26:480, 2000.

Ray S, Rubin AP: Anaesthesia in a child with Schwartz-Jampel syndrome. *Anaesthesia* 49(7):600, 1994.

Theroux MC, Kettrick RG, Khine HH: Laryngeal mask airway and fiberoptic endoscopy in an infant with Schwartz-Jampel syndrome. *Anesthesiology* 82:605, 1995.

Viljoen D, Beighton P: Schwartz-Jampel syndrome (chondrodystrophic myotonia). *J Med Genet* 29(1):58, 1992.

SCIDS (Severe Combined Immunodeficient Syndrome)

At a glance: The World Health Organization recognizes approximately 70 primary immune deficiencies including X-Linked Agammaglobulinemia, Common Variable Immune Deficiency (Hypogammaglobulinemia), Selective IgA Deficiency and Severe Combined Immune deficiency. SCID leads to severe T- and B-cell dysfunction. It is generally considered to be the most serious of the primary immunodeficiency diseases. Without intervention, death in children occurs by age 2 years.

Classification:

SCIDS X-Linked form:
  –SCIDX
Autosomal Recessive SCID (Swiss type Agammaglobulinemia):
  –Janus Associated Kinase 3 Deficiency (JAK 3 Deficiency)
  ☞Adenosine Deaminase Deficiency (ADA Deficiency)
  ☞Purine Nucleoside Phosphorylase Deficiency (PNP Deficiency)
Bare Lymphocyte Syndrome
IL-2 Deficiency
ZAP-70 Protein Tyrosine Kinase Deficiency (ZAP-70 PTK Deficiency)
  ☞Reticular Dysgenesia
  ☞Omenn Syndrome

Incidence: 1:100,000 live births. Higher incidence recently reported (1:50,000 to 1:75,000 live births), probably because of better identification of affected subjects.

Genetic inheritance: Of all SCID cases, 50% are X-linked (gene mapped to Xq13) and 50% are various forms of autosomal recessive. Approximately 25% of the patients with an autosomal recessive SCID are Janus-associated kinase 3 (JAK3) deficient and 40% are adenosine deaminase (ADA) deficient. Gene mapped to 8q11, 5p13.

Pathophysiology: The pathophysiology and molecular biology vary according to the type of immunodeficiency. However, the lack of T- and B-cell function is the common endpoint in all forms of SCIDS.

X-Linked form: Mutation of the common gamma chain of the interleukin (IL-2R, IL-4R, IL-7R, IL-9R, IL-15R) resulting in loss of cytokine function. Loss of IL-2R function leads to the loss of a lymphocyte proliferation signal. Loss of IL-4R function leads to the inability of B cells to class switch. Loss of IL-7R function leads to the loss of an antiapoptotic signal, resulting in a loss of T-cell selection in the thymus. Loss of IL-7R function is also associated with the loss of a T-cell receptor (TCR) rearrangement. Loss of IL-15R function leads to the ablation of NK cell development. Lymphopenia occurs primarily from the absence of CD3+ and NK cells. Variable levels of B cells occur, which do not make functional antibodies.

Autosomal recessive SCID includes different types.

- Janus-Associated Kinase 3 (JAK3) Deficiency: JAK3 is a protein tyrosine kinase (PTK) that associates with the common gamma chain of the IL receptors. Lymphopenia occurs primarily from the absence of T cells (CD3+) and NK cells. Normal or high levels of B cells occur, which do not make functional antibodies.
- Adenosine Deaminase (ADA) Deficiency: Lymphopenia occurs from the death of T and B cells secondary to the accumulation

of toxic metabolites in the purine salvage pathway. Functional antibodies are decreased or absent.

- Purine Nucleoside Phosphorylase (PNP) Deficiency: Same as ADA deficiency with circulating B cells normal in number. B-cell function is poor, as evidenced by the lack of antibody formation.
- Bare Lymphocyte Syndrome: This is a deficiency of major histocompatibility complex (MHC). The lymphocyte count is normal or mildly reduced, the CD4+ are decreased, and the CD8+ are normal or mildly increased. The B-cell numbers are normal or mildly decreased, but the ability to make antibodies is decreased.
- IL-2 Deficiency: The exact molecular defect is unknown, but it is often associated with other cytokine production defects. Normal numbers of T cells exist (both CD4+ and CD8+). The production of functional antibody is decreased.
- ZAP-70 Protein Tyrosine Kinase (PTK) Deficiency: A mutation occurs in the gene coding for this tyrosine kinase, which is important in T-cell signaling. Lymphopenia occurs because of the absence of CD8+. Functional antibodies are decreased or absent.
- Reticular Dysgenesis: Lymphopenia occurs from the absence of myeloid cells in the bone marrow. RBCs and platelets are present and functioning.
- Omenn Syndrome: A mutation that impairs the function of Ig and TCR recombinase genes. Normal or elevated T-cell numbers are present, but these are of maternal not fetal origin. The B cells are usually undetectable, NK cells are present, and the total Ig level is markedly low with poor antibody production. Eosinophils and serum IgE level are elevated.

Diagnosis: Clinically evocated in infants with severe infections secondary to the lack of T-cell function.

Clinical aspects: Features include failure to thrive, dehydration from chronic diarrhea, eczema from graft-versus-host disease (Omenn syndrome), lymphadenopathy and hepatosplenomegaly (Omenn syndrome or Bare Lymphocyte syndrome), neurological sequelae, and developmental regression (not caused by infections but genetic in PNP deficiency). Main causes of infections are Pneumocystis carinii, atypical mycobacterium, herpes viruses (generalized herpetic infections), Candida (and other systemic fungal infections), Cryptosporidium, and Pneumococcus.

Precautions before anesthesia: An anesthesiology consultation is highly recommended before elective surgical procedures. A complete medical history and physical examination must be obtained. The state of infection (systemic or local) must be evaluated carefully (clinical, chest radiographs, documented infectious history). Other important considerations include, hydration (clinical, electrolytes, renal function), and respiratory function in cases of recurrent lung infections (clinical, chest radiographs/CT, pulmonary function test, arterial blood gas analysis).

Anesthetic considerations: Strict asepsis is needed. Blood products must be irradiated to avoid graft-versus-host reaction. Regional anesthesia is best avoided in this infectious context.

Pharmacological implications: These patients are immunodeficient and the choice of prophylactic antibiotics should be made on the basis of both their infectious history and their immunological status.

Other conditions to be considered:

PRIMARY AGAMMAGLOBULINEMIAS (X-Linked Immunodeficiency): A group of inherited immune deficiencies characterized by insufficient antibodies. Some children with Primary Agamma-globulinemias experience joint swelling and pain.

☞**DiGeorge Syndrome:** A very rare immune deficiency that results from developmental defects in the thymus and parathyroid glands. Infantile seizures is often associated with the presence of abnormal function of the parathyroid gland. These infants cannot resist infections from viruses, fungi, and other bacteria. Chronic nasal infections, diarrhea, oral candidiasis, and *Pneumocystis* pneumonia are frequent.

☞**Nezelof Syndrome:** A rare immune deficiency disorder characterized by the impairment of cellular immunity in response to infections. Oral candidiasis, diarrhea, skin infections, septicemia, urinary tract infections, measles, and pulmonary infections are frequent clinical presentations.

☞**Wiskott-Aldrich Syndrome:** A rare X-linked inherited disorder characterized by an immune deficiency primarily affecting B lymphocytes. The symptoms generally begin during infancy. Excessive bleeding may happen during circumcision or minor trauma because of thrombocytopenia. Otitis media, pneumonia, meningitis, and sepsis are most often life-threatening for these infants.

REFERENCES:

Bonilla FA, Geha RS: Primary immunodeficiency diseases. *J Allergy Clin Immunol* 111(2 suppl):S571, 2003.

Buckley RH: Treatment options for genetically determined immunodeficiency. *Lancet* 361(9357):553, 2003.

Scimitar Syndrome

At a glance: Congenital anomalous venous drainage of the right pulmonary veins into the inferior vena cava, associated with hypoplasia or aplasia of one or more lobes of the right lung.

History: The name *scimitar syndrome* originates from the anomalous pulmonary vein on the right side, which drains into the inferior vena cava. This vein is sometimes visible on the radiograph of the chest resulting in a curvilinear shadow just above the right diaphragm. The shape of this shadow resembles a scimitar, a saber typically used by Arabs and Turks.

Incidence: 1:300,000 live births.

Pathophysiology: Anomalous venous drainage of the right lung into the inferior vena cava represents a large left-to-right shunt. If an atrial septal defect is present and is not restrictive, right-to-left shunting occurs at the atrial level and compensates for the shunt caused by the anomalous pulmonary venous drainage. The left side of the heart is volume underloaded while the right side has an increased load. The scimitar syndrome is associated with pulmonary artery hypoplasia or atresia, predisposing to right ventricular failure. Obstruction of the anomalous venous drainage may occur at the level of the diaphragm or at insertion into the inferior vena cava, resulting in pulmonary venous congestion and pulmonary hypertension.

Diagnosis: Cyanotic heart disease in presence of 'scimitar sign' on chest radiograph. Echocardiography is nonspecific. Anomalous venous drainage confirmed by cardiac catheterization.

Clinical aspects: Failure to thrive, cyanosis, tachycardia, signs and symptoms of right ventricular failure. Auscultation may reveal fixed, wide splitting of the second heart sound, a diastolic murmur of tricuspid origin, and a pulmonary ejection murmur in the presence of pulmonary hypoplasia. Presentation may be delayed in the presence

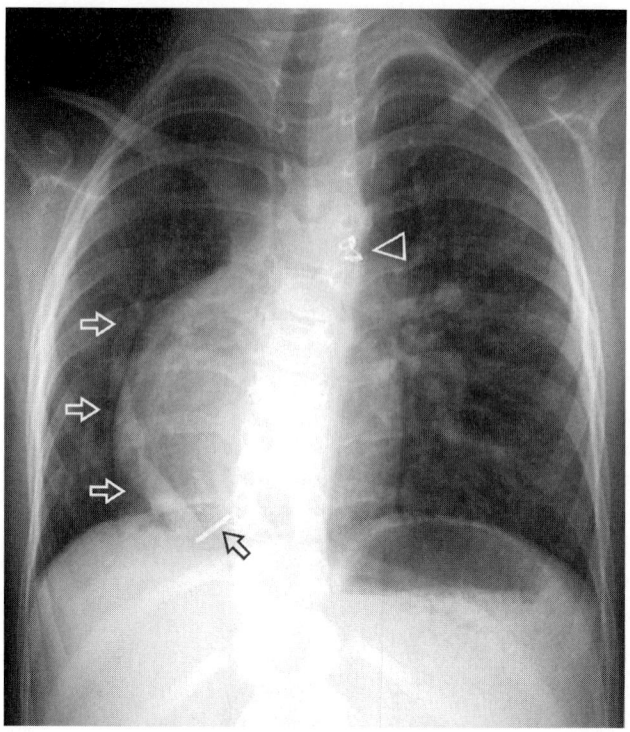

Scimitar syndrome Mild to moderate hypoplasia of the right lung results in displacement of the heart to the right side in a 6-year-old girl with scimitar syndrome. Right ventricular enlargement is seen. There is an anomalous pulmonary vein on the right side (because of its shape called scimitar vein (see text, white arrows) draining into the inferior vena cava. This vein has been surgically clipped (black arrow). Furthermore, the persistent ductus arteriosus had to be coiled (triangle).

of a nonrestrictive atrial septal defect until growth results in the atrial septal defect becoming restrictive causing a fall in arterial oxygen pressure (PaO_2). The ECG shows right axis deviation and signs of right ventricular strain. The anomalous vein(s) cause a vertical scimitar shape on chest radiograph.

Precautions before anesthesia: Take a history and examine to assess cardiac function, systemic perfusion, and oxygenation. Respiratory assessment: chest radiograph to examine for pulmonary edema and evidence of lung hypoplasia; measure oxygen saturation and arterial blood gases. Cardiovascular assessment: review the ECG, echocardiography, and cardiac catheter data. Metabolic investigations: investigate for signs of organ failure and metabolic acidosis secondary to hypoperfusion.

Anesthetic considerations: Invasive monitoring should be considered for all except minor procedures. High concentrations of volatile agents may not be well tolerated because of poor ventricular function. Positive pressure ventilation may improve oxygenation by overcoming hypoxic pulmonary vasoconstriction.

Pharmacological implications: Minimize use of agents that cause myocardial depression.

REFERENCE:

Lake CL: Anomalies of the systemic and pulmonary venous returns, in Lake CL (ed): *Pediatric Cardiac Anesthesia*. 3rd ed. Connecticut, Appleton and Lange, 1998, p 353.

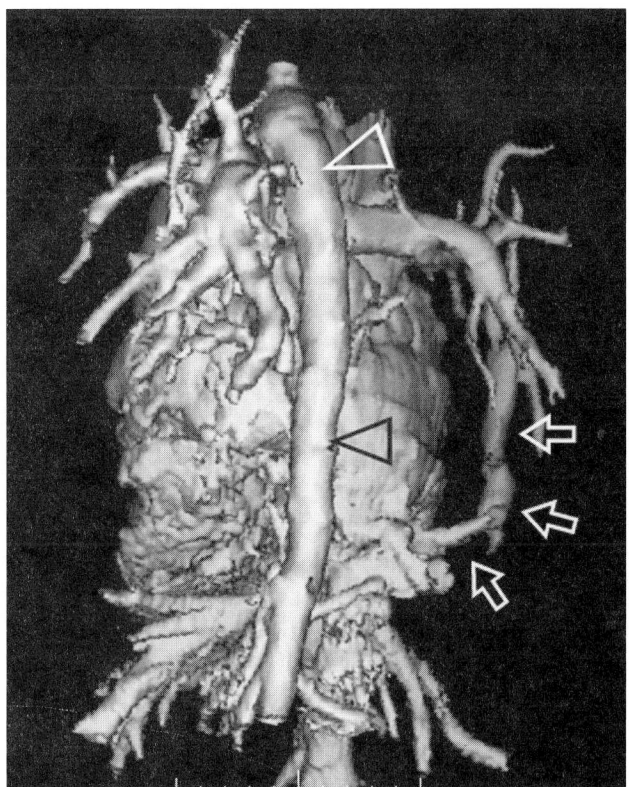

Scimitar syndrome   In this posterior view of the three dimensional reconstruction of the chest CT scan of the same patient, the scimitar vein can easily be identified (white arrows) draining into the inferior vena cava. The triangles indicate the aorta.

Sclerema Neonatorum

At a glance: Half of affected infants are premature. They are often of low birth weight (<2500 g), cyanotic, and with low Apgar scores. Physical findings appear suddenly, first on thighs and buttocks and spreading rapidly to all parts of the body except hands, soles, and genitalia. The skin is firm to hard and purplish in color. Skin cannot be pitted or picked up. Temperature instability, restricted respiration, difficulty in feeding, and decreased spontaneous movement are characteristics.

History: The classic description of this clinical entity is credited to Underwood, who described it in 1784 and appropriately termed it *Skinbound Disease.*

Incidence: A rare disorder limited to the newborn during the first weeks of life.

Classification: The differential diagnosis in patients with subcutaneous fat necrosis, early scleroderma, Transient Hyperammonemia of the Newborn (THAN) is often difficult but of almost importance because of the different prognosis of these illnesses.

Diagnosis: Diffuse hardening of the subcutaneous adipose tissue in the newborn.

Clinical aspects: Sclerema neonatorum generally presents in gravely ill, often preterm, infants with diffuse yellowish-white woody induration. The affected skin is cold, nonpitting, and immobile, given an appearance of tight, shiny, bound-down skin with herniation of the usually spared nipple area. Beginning on the but-

tocks, thighs, or calves, the process extends rapidly and symmetrically to involve nearly the entire body surface. Sclerema appear frequently in premature newborn, with associated diseases as sepsis, congenital heart disease, respiratory distress. Sclerema is not specific of THAN, but an observation has been made that sclerema neonatorum may be an early manifestation of THAN; consequently, it is recommended that the blood ammonia concentration be determined in any infant with this clinical sign. THAN infants have an excellent chance of survival, if recognized early.

Precautions before anesthesia: Consider that it is a septic, usually dehydrated, newborn with incomplete diagnosis (high incidence of congenital heart failure). Check ammonia blood level, glucose, urea. Check temperature (they are less able than the normal newborn to keep homeothermic). Consider long-term ventilatory assistance (the thickening of the subcutaneous fat and the tense of the skin limit the excursion of the rib cage and the abdomen).

Anesthetic considerations: Difficult intravenous access. Direct laryngoscopy might be difficult because of reduced mouth opening (skin limitation). Subjected to temperature instability during anesthesia, especially severe hypothermia. All anesthetic considerations of anesthesia for the premature must also be applied.

Pharmacological implications: Newborn with immature pathways, especially in the urea cycle.

REFERENCES:
Heilbron B, Saxe N: Scleredema in an infant. *Arch Dermatol* 122(12):1417, 1986.
Lindenberg JA, Milstein JM, Cox KL: Sclerema neonatorum: A sign of transient hyperammonemia of the newborn. *J Pediatr Gastroenterol Nutr* 6(3):474, 1987.

Scurvy Syndrome

At a glance: A vitamin C deficiency characterized by tooth and gum bleeding and decay, hemorrhages, and increased susceptibility to infection.

Synonyms: Hypoascorbemia; Vitamin C Deficiency.

Incidence: Not known. Uncommon in developed countries but increasing incidence in certain populations, including alcoholics, institutionalized elderly, and those with postsurgical malabsorption syndrome.

Pathophysiology: Scurvy arises from the deficiency of ascorbic acid (vitamin C), which is often the result of prolonged lack of fresh fruit or vegetables in diet, historically common among the sailors on long sea voyages. Humans, unlike most other animals, do not possess the enzyme L-gulonolactone oxidase and thus are unable to synthesize ascorbic acid from the glucuronic acid or galactonic acid derived from glucose. Recommended daily allowance for ascorbic acid is 35 mg in infants, 45 to 50 mg for children, and 60 mg for adults. Ascorbic acid accelerates the hydroxylation reactions in a number of biosynthetic pathways. If ascorbic acid is replaced by other reductants, most of the enzymes in these pathways are still functional but not at optimal activity. It is best known for its essential role in the hydroxylation of proline and lysine to enable cross-linking and stabilization of collagen.

Diagnosis: Clinical features and laboratory evaluation. Plasma ascorbate level is absent in clinical significant cases. Blood count usually shows anemia, which may be as a result of poor iron and/or folate absorption. Coagulation and biochemistry may also show abnormalities in association with poor nutritional status, including prolonged activated partial thromboplastin time (aPTT) and international normalized ratio (INR), low albumin, low protein, low cholesterol, and low sodium and potassium levels. Skin biopsy may show the characteristic hyperkeratosis of hair follicles and rule out vasculitis.

Clinical aspects: "The four Hs" are the classical manifestations of scurvy: hemorrhagic signs, hyperkeratosis of hair follicles, hypochondriasis, and hematologic abnormalities. The earliest sign is usually petechial hemorrhages, usually in hyperketotic areas such as the anterior forearms. Next to occur are ecchymoses and purpura, usually at sites of pressures, trauma, or irritation. Further depletion brings coiled (corkscrew) and fragmented hair with hyperkeratosis and hemorrhagic gingivitis. In severe cases, other symptoms include lower extremity edema, muscle tenderness, conjunctival and ocular hemorrhages, arthralgias, hemarthroses, gastrointestinal hemorrhage, sicca (dry eye) syndrome, poor wound healing, and peripheral neuropathy. Generalized symptoms are weakness, fatigue, and weight loss. Psychological symptoms include hypochondriasis, emotional lability, depression, and hysteria. Sudden death for unknown reasons has been reported. Treatment is simple, by replacing body stores of vitamin C by oral or intravenous route in severe case.

Precautions before anesthesia: Establish diagnosis from history, examination, and laboratory results. Ensure that treatment is adequate from clinical and biochemical status. Make sure that all hematologic disorders are corrected before elective surgery.

Anesthetic considerations: Few reports have considered anesthesia in cases of scurvy because of its rarity in the last 50 years in developed countries. In principle, no surgery or anesthesia should be considered in cases with clinically significant scurvy because of the systemic manifestations of bleeding diathesis, poor wound healing, and psychological disturbances. Bleeding diathesis would also preclude the use of regional techniques in patients with scurvy.

Pharmacological implications: There are no known implications with this condition.

REFERENCES:

Levine M: New concepts in the biology and biochemistry of ascorbic acid. *N Engl J Med* 314(14):892, 1986.

Oeffinger K: Scurvy: More than historical relevance. *Am Fam Physician* 48(4):609, 1993.

Sea-Blue Histiocytosis Syndrome

At a glance: Genetic and acquired forms of this clinical entity exist. It is associated to the presence of sea-blue histiocytes in the bone marrow and a cholesterol ester storage disease. It is clinically characterized by the presence of splenomegaly, mild thrombocytopenia, and progressive neurological disease (e.g., ataxia, dementia and seizures).

Synonym: Sea-Blue Histiocytosis Disease; Niemann-Pick Disease type F.

Incidence: The incidence is unknown, however, the presence of sea-blue histiocytes is a common abnormality of the bone marrow in myelodysplastic syndromes.

Genetic inheritance: Autosomal recessive.

Pathophysiology: Unknown. Sea-Blue Histiocytosis syndrome is named for its characteristic macrophage. There are densely packed granules that stain blue with Wright-Giemsa stain. This syndrome is associated with abnormal storage of phosphosphingolipid and glycosphingolipid, which occurs mainly in the spleen and liver.

Diagnosis: Bone marrow examination reveals the characteristic cells. Also, an hepatosplenomegaly workup confirms the diagnosis for hepatosplenomegaly.

Clinical aspects: Usually diagnosed before the age of 40 years. Hepatosplenomegaly, thrombocytopenia, macular abnormalities, pulmonary infiltrates on chest radiograph, patchy brownish-gray pigmentation of the upper body, occasional neurologic abnormalities (ataxia, dementia, seizures), predisposition for parasitic infections, and elevated bleeding times in albino patients with normal platelet counts.

Precautions before anesthesia: Check platelet count. Document neurologic abnormalities. Platelet availability.

Anesthetic considerations: Avoid central–neuraxial anesthesia in albino patient even with normal platelet counts (increased bleeding times) and patients with thrombocytopenia. Platelets should be transfused if platelet counts is less than 50,000/mm^3, in presence of active oozing or bleeding and in Albino patients.

Pharmacological implications: There are no specific pharmacological implications.

REFERENCE:

Sawitsky A: The sea-blue histiocyte syndrome, a review: Genetic and biochemical studies. *Semin Hematol* 9(3):285, 1972.

Seckel Syndrome

At a glance: Syndrome involving a form of primordial dwarfism with a characteristic facial-head shape ("bird-headed" appearance) and spongioid microcephaly (called also the Chimpanzee brain). Other clinical features include large ears, sparse hair, joint defects, clubfoot, trident hands and mental retardation.

Synonyms: Bird-Headed Dwarfism; Nanocephalic Dwarfism; Microcephalic Primordial Dwarfism; Harper Syndrome; Seckel Nanism; Virchow-Seckel Syndrome.

History: First described in 1960 by Helmut Paul George Seckel, German pediatrician.

Incidence: Extremely rare; about 40 cases in the literature. Clinical delineation has been inconsistent and probably only one-third of reported cases are truly affected and only seven familial cases have been reported.

Genetic inheritance: Autosomal recessive inheritance. Chromosome instability has been seen in a small subgroup of patients.

Pathophysiology: Seckel syndrome may be caused by a mutation in the gene encoding ataxia-telangiectasia and RAD3-related protein, which maps to chromosome 3q22.1-q24. Another locus for Seckel syndrome has been mapped to chromosome 18p11-q11. Central nervous system anomalies suggest an underlying neuronal migration disorder.

Diagnosis: Clinical supported by imaging of the brain.

Clinical aspects: Dwarfism, low birth weight. Small head, large eyes, beak-like nose, narrow face, and receding mandible. Laryngeal stenosis. Mental retardation, very small brain with agenesis of the corpus callosum, dysgenetic cerebral cortex, cerebral cysts. Pancytopenia.

Precautions before anesthesia: Assessment of airway must be conducted for possible difficult tracheal intubation. The presence of laryngeal stenosis must be eliminated using imaging if indicated. Case report of intraoperative abnormal hypertension suggests that renal examination and imaging must be performed.

Anesthetic considerations: Direct laryngoscopy and tracheal intubation are usually not difficult, however, the potential for laryngeal stenosis requires that smaller than predicted endotracheal tubes must be available. It is recommended to monitor the arterial blood pressure invasively because of the significant risk of severe hypertension.

Pharmacological implications: There are no abnormal responses to drugs reported. Also, patients are not known to have greater sensitivity to narcotics even in presence of severe microcephaly.

Other conditions to be considered:

☞**CEPHALOSKELETAL DYSPLASIA (Osteodysplastic Primordial Dwarfism Type I):** An extremely rare inherited disorder characterized by low birth weight, dwarfism, microcephaly, and "beak-like" protrusion of the nose. Other characteristic facial features include abnormally large eyes, micrognathia, retrognathia, a narrow face, and low-set ears. Affected children may exhibit mental retardation. This condition closely resembles Seckel syndrome, except that, in Cephaloskeletal Dysplasia, the body proportions are abnormal and the limbs are unusually short and bowed. In Seckel syndrome, the proportions are normal. It is suggested that the inheritance is an autosomal recessive trait.

OSTEODYSPLASTIC BIRD-HEADED DWARFISM TYPE II (Osteodysplastic Primordial Dwarfism Type II): An extremely rare inherited disorder characterized by severe dwarfism, microcephaly, "beak-like" nose, and various skeletal abnormalities especially the arms and legs. Low birth weight may be present. Other clinical features include retrognathia, a narrow face, and dysplastic ears. Mental retardation may also be present. It is inherited as an autosomal recessive transmission.

OSTEODYSPLASTIC BIRD-HEADED DWARFISM TYPE III (Osteodysplastic Primordial Dwarfism Type III): Characterized by short stature, microcephaly, and a "beak-like" nose. Retrognathia, a narrow face, receding forehead, and alopecia have been reported. Some affected individuals may exhibit skeletal deformities. It is inherited as an autosomal recessive transmission.

☞**HALLERMANN-STREIFF SYNDROME:** A rare inherited disorder characterized by dwarfism, craniofacial anomalies, a "beak-like" nose, microcephaly that may appear brachycephalic, malar hypoplasia, micrognathia, hypoplasia of the mandible, and cleft lip/palate. The eye abnormalities may include strabismus, nystagmus, cataracts, microphthalmia, and blue sclera. Affected individuals may show sparse hair on the scalp and body (hypotrichosis), dental abnormalities, and skin atrophy, especially on the nose and scalp. Most cases appear to be sporadic.

REFERENCES:

Rajamani A, Kamat V, Murthy J, et al: Anesthesia for cleft lip surgery in a child with Seckel syndrome—a case report. *Paediatr Anaesth* 15:338, 2005.

Shanske A, Caride DG, Menasse-Palmer L et al: Central nervous system anomalies in Seckel syndrome: Report of a new family and review of the literature. *Am J Med Genet* 70(2):155, 1997.

Shiraishi N, Takakuwa K, Yamamoto N et al: Anesthetic management of Seckel syndrome: A case report. *Masui* 44(5):735, 1995.

Segawa Syndrome

At a glance: Described by the presence of jerky movement at the age of 3 months. It is associated with generalized rigidity and no diurnal variability. Evolving rapidly to expressionless face, ptosis, drooling, and tremulous tongue movements. Usually associated with a low concentration of the dopamine metabolite homovanillic acid (HVA) in the cerebrospinal fluid.

Synonyms: Parkinsonism Infantile; Dystonia 5; Dystonia-Parkinsonism with Diurnal Fluctuation; Dopa-Responsive Dystonia; Tyrosine Hydroxylase Deficiency.

Genetic inheritance: Autosomal recessive inheritance. An autosomal dominant form of this clinical entity has also been described. In this case, it is believed to be caused by a mutation in the GCH1 gene. A linkage has been found between Segawa syndrome and a point mutation in exon 11 of the tyrosine hydroxylase (TH) gene resulting in a gin381-to-lys exchange.

Pathophysiology: Evidence of a mutation in the GTP-cyclohydrolase 1 gene, causing limited conversion of GTP to BH4 (tetrahydrobiopterin). BH4 is a cofactor for tyrosine hydroxylase, which is the rate-limiting step in dopamine synthesis. These patients may produce BH4 at a rate that is insufficient to compensate for the normal consumption of the cofactor during the day, leading to aggravation of symptoms toward the evening.

Diagnosis: Historical and clinical features. Measurement of tyrosine hydroxylase and GTP-cyclohydroxylase 1 activity. Genetic mapping for GTP-cyclohydroxlase 1 on chromosome 14q.

Clinical aspects: Predominantly occurs in females. Characterized by postural and motor disturbances with marked diurnal fluctuation. Onset is usually in early childhood presenting with lower limbs and axial dystonia, followed by parkinsonism. Commonly the inversion and plantar flexion of feet can be seen early in association with increasing flexion of the hip and the knee, resulting in a toe-walking gait. Both flexor and extensor posture of the arms may occur. Posture reflex is impaired. Slowly progressive parkinsonian features include slowed movement, muscle rigidity, and balance difficulty. Symptoms are remarkable and are alleviated after sleep and aggravated toward the evening. Response to a small dose of L-dopa is immediate and most often associated with dramatic improvement. The coexistence of parkinsonian features and the dramatic response to L-dopa distinguish this syndrome from other forms of idiopathic torsion dystonia. The sustained nature of L-dopa responsiveness and the lack of complications from therapy (including wearing-off, "on-off" and unpredictable dose response) distinguish it from other causes of childhood-onset parkinsonism.

Precautions before anesthesia: Complete neurological examination and documentation must be obtained in symptomatic patients. The hydration status must be assessed.

Anesthetic considerations: No reported complications. The potential for intraoperative labile blood pressure, particularly with postural changes during surgery, must be carefully monitored. Fluid management must be ensured to prevent the possibility of volume depletion. Care in positioning of patient.

Pharmacological implications: Should continue L-dopa or anticholinergic medication through the perioperative period.

REFERENCES:

Nygaard T, Duvoisin R: Hereditary dystonia-parkinsonism syndrome of juvenile onset. *Neurology* 36:1424, 1986.

Priscu V, Lurie S, Savir I, et al: The choice of anesthesia in Segawa's syndrome. *J Clin Anesth* 10:153, 1998.

Segawa M, Hosaka A, Miyagawa F, et al: Hereditary progressive dystonia with marked diurnal fluctuation. *Adv Neurol* 14:215, 1976.

Seitelberger Syndrome

At a glance: A very rare degenerative encephalopathy with associated visceral malformations. Demyelinating disease with early onset and absence of stainable myelin. The affected child is normal at birth and development is normal until 2 years of age. Motor dysfunction manifests by difficulty standing and walking, progressive deterioration of neurological function and speech, nystagmus, strabismus, blindness, seizures, and areflexia.

Synonym: Infantile Neuroaxonal Dystrophy.

Genetic inheritance: Autosomal recessive but because of the low incidence of carriers, cases may appear as sporadic.

Pathophysiology: Unknown. Investigations show a progressive degenerative encephalopathy, with axonal swelling and spheroid axonal degeneration.

Diagnosis: Usually based on the clinical criteria. At autopsy, spheroid bodies are widely distributed, particularly in the hypothalamus, infundibulum, and neurohypophysis, and in the mesenteric plexus of the colon.

Clinical aspects: Degenerative encephalopathy associated with mental retardation, weakness with hypotonia, generalized seizures, and myoclonic epilepsy. Other clinical signs include a lack of tears with dry keratitis. Endocrine investigations shows hypothalamus–pituitary dysfunction with central hypothyroidism, diabetes insipidus, and central thermoregulation problems. The clinical picture is similar but not identical to Hallervorden-Spatz disease.

Precautions before anesthesia: Check airways and pulmonary function carefully. Because patients present with a decrease in respiratory drive, a complete medical history and observation of breathing pattern must be obtained. Often these patients use myorelaxing medication, such as benzodiazepines. Continue myorelaxing medication until the operation. The use of anticholinergics must be considered to reduce saliva production.

Anesthetic considerations: Because of an unpredictable and potentially difficult airway, it is recommended to maintain spontaneous ventilation. With deep anesthesia, the torticollis, scoliosis, and oromandibular muscular rigidity disappear. However with long-lasting musculoskeletal deformation, bone and joint changes may fix these deformities and prevent the relaxation. Signs of basal ganglias dysfunction (chorea, athetosis, and rigidity) reappear on emergence. Very poor airway control. Aspiration pneumonitis occurs easily. The potential for postoperative mechanical ventilation is high and proper preoperative arrangement must be obtained from the intensive care unit. A disorder in temperature regulation is often present.

Pharmacological implications: Because of diffuse axonal changes and muscular denervation, hyperkalemic cardiac arrest following the administration of succinylcholine is possible. No problems related to inhalational anesthetics have been described. Do not discontinue regular medications, and during the immediate postoperative period, give the medications through a nasogastric tube if needed.

Other conditions to be considered:

☞**Pelizaeus-Merzbacher Syndrome:** Sudanophilic leukodystrophy or leukoencephalopathy, which usually affects only males. It is a chronic disease of the central nervous system with onset early in the infancy period, and which might persist for decades.

It is characterized by rotary nystagmus, ataxia, intention tremor, spasticity, and dementia. Autosomal recessive inheritance. There is a second, congenital, autosomal recessive form with late onset (adulthood) associated with a faster course marked by photosensitivity of the skin, dwarfism, cerebellar ataxia, corticospinal signs, cataracts, deafness, and retinitis pigmentosa.

☞**Hallervorden-Spatz Syndrome:** Progressive degeneration of the globus pallidus, red nucleus, and reticular part of the substantia nigra of the brain. Characterized by progressive Parkinson-like rigidity, athetotic movements and progressive mental and emotional retardation. Onset in late childhood, with death usually occurring within 10 years, but disease courses up to 30 years have been reported. A heredofamilial syndrome, inherited as an autosomal recessive trait.

REFERENCE:

Gaytan-Garcia S, Kaufmann JC, Young GB: Adult onset Hallervorden-Spatz syndrome or Seitelberger's disease with late onset: Variants of the same entity? A clinico-pathological study. *Clin Neuropathol* 9:136, 1990.

Senear-Usher Syndrome

At a glance: Localized pemphigus-like syndrome and lupus erythematous that could be drug-induced and which is frequently associated with autoimmune diseases. Penicillamine is the medication most commonly implicated.

Synonyms: Pemphigus Seborrheic; Pemphigus Erythematosus.

History: Described by E. Senear, an American dermatologist, and B. Usher, a Canadian dermatologist.

Incidence: 0.5 to 3.2:100,000 in general population.

Genetic inheritance: Unknown.

Pathophysiology: Frequency increases with HLA A10 DRW6 A26. In pemphigus vulgaris and pemphigus erythematosus, acantholytic cells and perilesional cells exhibit normal dotted pattern along the cell periphery.

Diagnosis: Occurs in persons 17 to 84 years of age but has been reported in children as young as age 6 years. Pemphigus Erythematosus can often be distinguished on clinical grounds by the restriction of the lesions to the seborrheic areas of the face and trunk. The presence of antinuclear antibodies is also suggestive of pemphigus erythematosus. The diagnosis can often be confirmed by demonstration of immunoglobulin and complement at the dermal–epidermal junction.

Clinical aspects: Facial lesions have a predilection for the malar region and truncal lesions are often confined to the V area of the chest and interscapular region. There are isolated flaccid bullae or erythematous plaques surfaced with vesicles, erosions, or scale. They can be photoactivated. Electrolyte imbalance and loss of temperature control can occur.

Precautions before anesthesia: Pemphigus Erythematosus has been seen in association with autoimmune diseases, including Lupus Erythematosus, Myasthenia Gravis, and Thymoma; look for this association. Laboratory investigation should include anti-DNA antibodies and electrolytes; evaluate adrenal function (treatment usually includes prednisone) and skin subinfection.

Anesthetic considerations: Cardiac monitoring can be difficult in cases of extensive thorax lesions. Central venous access even in healthy skin can be difficult. In presence of Myasthenia Gravis and Thymoma, the anesthetic considerations are those associated with these disorders. Photosensitivity may also be a problem before induction.

Pharmacological implications: Pemphigus Erythematosus may be drug induced. Penicillamine is the medication most commonly implicated. In case of long-time prednisone treatment, hydrocortisone should be given before anesthesia (twice usual dose).

Other conditions to be considered:

HAILEY-HAILEY DISEASE (Familial Benign Chronic Pemphigus [Autosomal Dominant]): A family history usually is present. The onset of age is usually in the fourth and fifth decade. It is characterized by the presence of vesicles and erythemateous plaques with overlying crusts typically in the genital areas, also seen in the chest, neck and axillary regions. Burning and itching most often accompany the eruption, and a malodorous drainage occurs as a result of secondary infection. Symptoms related to staphylococcal and candidal overgrowth are common. The characteristic clinical appearance, as well as biopsy, readily confirms the diagnosis. It has been suggested that Hailey-Hailey disease results from a genetic defect in a calcium pump protein. The gene is localized on chromosome 3. The dotted pattern is lost in acantholysed and perilesional areas and antidesmoplakin I + II-positive proteins are observed diffusely in the cytoplasm.

PEMPHIGOID BULLOUS PACHYDERMOPERIOSTOSIS (Touraine-Solente-Golé Syndrome): This disorder is characterized by cutis verticis gyrata (corrugated overgrowth of the scalp, or "bulldog scalp" lesion).

REFERENCES:

Amerian ML, Ahmed AR: Pemphigus erythematosus: Presentation of four cases and review of the literature. *J Am Acad Dermatol* 16:472, 1987.

Senear FE, Usher B: An unusual type of pemphigus combining features of lupus erythematosus. *Arch Dermatol Syphilol* 13:761, 1926.

Sengers Syndrome

At a glance: Cataract and cardiomyopathy. Considered a mitochondrial disease (complex I).

Synonym: Cataract-Cardiomyopathy Syndrome.

Incidence: Unknown. All previously described families originated from the southeast region of the Netherlands.

Genetic inheritance: Autosomal recessive.

Pathophysiology: Likely caused by nicotinamide adenine dinucleotide (reduced form) (NADH):ubiquinone oxidoreductase (complex 1) deficiency, causing excessive production of hydroxyl radicals and lipid peroxidation. Histologically, abnormality of mitochondria and storage of lipid and glycogen are found in both skeletal and heart muscle.

Diagnosis: Clinical features and measurement of plasmatic levels of lactate obtained at rest and after exercise. A biopsy of the skeletal and cardiac muscle confirms the diagnosis.

Clinical aspects: Patients usually present with congenital cataract and followed by hypertrophic cardiomyopathy, usually a diffuse and symmetrical type. Hypertrophic cardiomyopathy is progressive and by far the main cause of premature death. A distinct feature is the development of marked lactate acidemia on mild exercise. Other features include easy fatigue, muscular hypotonia, and delayed motor development. Significant arrhythmia may occur in later stages of disease.

Precautions before anesthesia: An anesthesiology consultation is highly recommended before elective surgical procedure. A complete cardiac medical history must be obtained, including exercise tolerance and fatigability. Full cardiac evaluation including ECG, chest radiograph, echocardiogram for left ventricular and valvular function, Holter monitoring for arrhythmia, cardiac catheterization, and endocardial biopsy when indicated. Check plasmatic lactate level before, during, and after procedure if possible. Patients receiving cardiotonic medications must continue until the day of surgery. Electrolyte level must be obtained, especially potassium (e.g., patients on digoxin).

Anesthetic considerations: No reported experience. Anesthetic technique should be tailored to the condition of the cardiac function and to the surgical procedure planned. Many of these patients are anesthetized for various ophthalmological procedures without problems. Continuous ECG monitoring is mandatory because of the potential for arrhythmia and coronary ischemia. Premedication to avoid stress and anxiety is recommended. Ensure adequate preload with fluid hydration and avoidance of tachycardia.

Pharmacological implications: Ketamine should be avoided in hypertrophic cardiomyopathy. Avoid positive inotropic and chronotropic drugs if possible. Only a pure alpha-agonist should be used as a vasopressor. Avoid excessive vasodilatation because it could result in reflex tachycardia and consequently a decrease in filling time and cardiac output. Consider halothane as volatile agent of choice if no arrhythmia occurs, because it causes less vasodilatation and more cardiac depression than other volatile agents. Can use suxamethonium because there is no proven association with malignant hyperthermia.

REFERENCES:

Sengers R, ter Haar B, Trijbels J, et al: Congenital cataract and mitochondrial myopathy of skeletal and heart muscle associated with lactic acidosis after exercise. *J Pediatr* 86:873, 1975.

Smith WQ, Abu-Harb M: Undiagnosed cardiomyopathy in a neonate: Significance of low oxygen saturation during anaesthesia, *Br J Anaesth* 86:435, 2001.

Valsson J, Laxdal T, Jonsson A, et al: Congenital cardiomyopathy and cataracts with lactic acidosis. *Am J Cardiol* 61:193, 1988.

Sensenbrenner Syndrome

At a glance: An autosomal recessive disorder characterized by dolichocephaly, sagittal suture synostosis, sparse and slow-growing fine hair, hypertelorism, nystagmus, taurodontia, dental fusion, anteverted nares, brachydactyly, clinodactyly, narrow thorax leading to respiratory problems, and mild mental retardation.

Synonyms: Cranioectodermal Dysplasia; Levin Syndrome I.

Genetic inheritance: Autosomal recessive.

Diagnosis: Clinical and radiological features. Radiological features include generalized osteoporosis with shortening of the ribs and long bones, particularly the humeri and fibulae; distal phalanges are short and broad; the epiphysis of long bones tends to be flattened; the vertebral bodies have convex upper and lower surfaces with short pedicles in lumbar spine area; the skull shows dolichocephaly, in association with premature fusion of sagittal synostosis.

Clinical aspects: *Craniofacial:* dolichocephaly is most characteristic (in some cases, it is caused by sagittal suture synostosis); hypertelorism; epicanthic folds; broad nasal bridge; anteverted nares;

everted lower lip; high-arched palate. *Chest:* narrow thorax, mild pectus excavatum. *Limbs:* short, bowed limbs with rhizomelia (arms more affected); brachydactyly; single palmar crease, short, broad toes. *Ectodermal:* nails are short and stubby; scalp hair is fine, sparse, slow-growing with absence of central pigment core on microscopy; teeth are few, small, and widely spaced. Other reported features include congenital heart disease with cor triatrium in one case. A cor triatum is an anomaly where the pulmonary vein is not attached to the left atrium, but rather empties in an accessory chamber superior to the left atrium, simulating a mitral valve stenosis. Subsequent photophobia and chronic renal failure has also been described in some cases. All patients have normal intellect but growth is mildly retarded. Most of the premature deaths are respiratory related.

Precautions before anesthesia: Patients must be assessed for respiratory function with examination, chest radiography, arterial blood gas analysis, and oxygen requirements (multiple chest infections are frequent). Assess for cardiac defect with examination, chest radiography, ECG, echocardiogram, and cardiac catheterization when suspected. Biochemistry test, including potassium, creatinine, and urea, must be obtained to assess renal function. Abnormal calcium homeostasis has been reported.

Anesthetic considerations: No reported experience. Position head appropriately for tracheal intubation considering the abnormally shaped head, frontal bossing, and occipital protuberance. Potential for ventilation problems in presence of a narrow thorax and frequent respiratory infections. Intravenous access may be difficult with abnormal limbs.

Pharmacological implications: There are no known pharmacological implications with this condition.

REFERENCES:

Levin L, Perrin J, Ose L, et al: A heritable syndrome of craniosynostosis, short thin hair, dental abnormalities, and short limbs: Cranioectodermal dysplasia. *J Pediatr* 90:55, 1977.

Young I: Cranioectodermal dysplasia (Sensenbrenner's syndrome). *J Med Genet* 26:393, 1989.

Serpentine Fibula-Polycystic Kidney Syndrome

At a glance: Elongated serpentine fibulas, bowed lower legs and forearms, bowed radii, polycystic kidneys, small stature, unusual facial appearance, large skull and occipital depression, severe pectus excavatum, hirsutism, and deafness but normal intelligence.

Synonym: SFPKS.

Genetic inheritance: Most likely autosomal recessive; predominance of affected females raises the possibility of X-linked dominance with lethality in hemizygous affected males.

Pathophysiology: Unknown.

Diagnosis: Clinical and radiological features. Most striking radiological feature is the elongated and deformed S-shaped fibulae. Other features include bowing of forearms and lower legs and metatarsus adductus. Abdominal ultrasonography must be used to confirm the presence of polycystic kidney. Chromosomal study is normal.

Clinical aspects: *Unusual facial appearance:* coarse hair, hirsute forehead and neck, marked eyebrows, micrognathia. *Skull:* large skull with occipital depression in one patient. *Thorax:* shield chest; pectus excavatum. *Urology:* polycystic kidney. Other features include short neck, low-set ears, and deafness in some cases. *Cardiac:* atrial septal defect and patent ductus arteriosus in one report. *Growth:* small stature in most cases. Intelligence is normal in all cases. Renal function usually well maintained until late.

Precautions before anesthesia: The cardiac function must be assessed through examination, chest radiography, ECG, and echocardiogram to rule out cardiac defect. Assess the airway for potential difficulty if micrognathia and short neck are present. Biochemistry screen for potassium, creatinine, and urea to assess renal function.

Anesthetic considerations: Potential for difficult airway with abnormal facies.

Pharmacological implications: Considerations for cardiac defect include prophylactic antibiotic, avoidance of air embolism, and adequate rehydration.

Other condition to be considered

☞**MELNICK-NEEDLES SYNDROME:** Characterized by severe typical facies (exophthalmos [frog-like eyes], full red cheeks, high forehead, micrognathia and malalignment of teeth), flaring of the metaphyses of long bones, S-like curvature of bones of legs, irregular constrictions in the ribs, and sclerosis of base of skull. It is caused by mutations in the gene encoding filamin A.

☞**HAJDU CHENEY SYNDROME:** Characterized by acroosteolysis, multiple wormian bones, and hypoplasia of ramus of mandible. The presence of generalized osteoporosis and multiple fractures of the skull, spine and digits, short stature, persistent cranial sutures, early loss of teeth, and joint laxity are reported as features associated in varying degrees. The patients show bathrocephaly (projection of the occipital area and a deep groove at the lambdoidal sutures between the occipital and parietal bones). In addition to micrognathia and narrow high palate, prominent ears may be a feature.

TER HAAR SYNDROME: Characterized by bone changes and facial features (frog-like eyes, micrognathia), bilateral glaucoma, congenital heart defect (ventricular septal defect), delay in closure of the anterior fontanel and sclerosis of the base of the skull and mastoids. It is considered an autosomal recessive disorder. Other features include brachycephaly with flat occiput, large anterior fontanel, hypertelorism, anteverted nostrils, thoracolumbar kyphosis, prominent coccyx with skin fold, short hands and feet, flexion deformity of fingers, and clubfeet.

REFERENCE:

Majewski F, Enders H, Ranke M, et al: Serpentine fibula-polycystic kidney syndrome and Melnick-Needles syndrome are different disorders. *Eur J Pediatr* 152:916, 1993.

Setleis Syndrome

At a glance: Puckered periorbital skin, absent or multiple rows of eyelashes.

Synonyms: Focal Facial Dermal Dysplasia Type II; Bitemporal Forceps Marks Syndrome.

Incidence: First described in eight patients from Puerto Rico. Later reported also from other countries.

Genetic inheritance: Probably in an autosomal dominant fashion with variable expressivity and reduced penetrance.

Pathophysiology: Histological analysis of the skin lesions demonstrates mesodermal dysplasia, characterized by loss of subcutaneous fat and almost complete continuity between the epidermis and underlying skeletal muscle. Areas of skin puckering are caused by hypoplasia of the corium and subcutaneous fat.

Diagnosis: Clinical features and skin biopsy.

Clinical aspects: Setleis syndrome is characterized by an aged, leonine facial appearance, puckered skin around the eyes with periorbital fullness, and absent or multiple rows of eyelashes. Flat nasal bridge, bulbous nasal tip, and big lips. Redundant facial soft tissue. These patients also show characteristic bitemporal skin marks (original description noted similarity to obstetric 'forceps marks'). An association of Setleis syndrome has been suggested with imperforate anus, megaureter, bifid scrotum, and supernumerary nipples has been reported. Initially, these patients were reported to have normal mental development, but now several reports about learning difficulties in these patients exist.

Anesthetic considerations: Reports suggest that the epidermis overlying the lesions may be more susceptible to injury following trauma. Careful padding of the affected regions against pressure and trauma during anesthesia is therefore recommended.

Pharmacological implications: There are no known pharmacological implications with this condition.

Other conditions to be considered:

☞**BRAUER SYNDROME:** The main finding in this autosomal dominant inherited syndrome is a wrinkling or puckering of the skin at the temples. In addition, some patients had guttate areas on the lateral aspects of their forehead and chin. It seems to be more common than Setleis syndrome (FFDD II), existing in three large kindreds (in Australia, Germany, and England).

☞**ADAMS-OLIVER SYNDROME:** A very rare inherited disorder characterized by defects of the scalp associated with multiple scarred and hairless areas that usually have dilated blood vessel directly under the skin. Scalp defects are already present at birth. The extremities are either short (hypoplastic fingers and toes) or characterized by absent hands and lower legs. Congenital heart defect must be ruled out.

☞**APLASIA CUTIS CONGENITA:** A most often inherited disorder with circumscribed or more extensive skin lesions, that may also involve underlying tissues. Neurological and cardiac anomalies have also been described in these patients.

☞**CUTIS MARMORATA TELANGIECTATICA CONGENITA:** Congenital cutaneous disorder with persistent cutis marmorata, telangiectasia, and phlebectasia. Often reported in association with a variety of other congenital anomalies.

☞**DELLEMAN OORTHUYS SYNDROME:** A multiple congenital anomaly syndrome mainly affecting the central nervous system, eyes, and skin.

☞**JOHANSON-BLIZZARD SYNDROME:** Polymalformative syndrome characterized by nasal alar hypoplasia (beak shaped), scalp defects, hypothyroidism, pancreatic achylia, and congenital deafness.

☞**GOLTZ SYNDROME:** A complex meso-ectodermal hereditary disorder characterized by focal dermal atrophy with herniation of fat producing multiple papillomas, in association with a skeletal, dental, ocular, and other anomalies.

REFERENCES:

Brauer A: Hereditärer symmetrischer systematisierter Naevus aplasticus bei 38 Personen. *Derm Wsch* 89:1163, 1929.

McGaughran J, Aftimos S: Setleis syndrome: Three new cases and a review of the literature. *Am J Med Genet* 111:376, 2002.

McGeoch AH, Reed WB: Familial focal facial dermal dysplasia. *Birth Defects Orig Artic Ser* 7:96, 1971.

Sheehan Syndrome

At a glance: Hypopituitarism resulting from an infarct of the pituitary gland following postpartum shock or hemorrhage. Damage to the anterior portion of the pituitary gland causes partial or complete loss of thyroid, adrenocorticoid, and gonadal functions. Very rarely pituitary infarction occurs with diabetic vasculitis, sickle cell anemia, and idiopathic disease (most often called in these conditions as the Simmonds syndrome).

Synonyms: Reye-Sheehan Syndrome; Postpartum Panhypopituitarism Syndrome; Postpartum Hypophyseogenic Myxedema.

History: Described by Harold Leeming Sheehan, English pathologist, in 1937.

Incidence: Incidence is estimated incidence at 1 to 2:10,000 pregnancies in the 1960s. Disorder is rare in modern obstetric practice but the occasional case is still reported every year.

Pathophysiology: Sheehan reported a series of cases of hypopituitarism following intrapartum hypotension. Typically, the patient suffered from massive peripartum hemorrhage and the ensuing hypotension led to ischemia and infarction of the highly vascular pituitary gland in the pregnant patient. In many of the reported cases, postmortem examination demonstrated anterior pituitary necrosis. A case of posterior pituitary damage with clinical evidence of diabetes insipidus has also been reported.

Diagnosis: Clinical features. Laboratory evidence of abnormal adrenal (low urinary steroids and low plasma cortisol), thyroid (low plasma T_3 and T_4) or ovarian (low follicle-stimulating hormone, luteinizing hormone, plasma estrogen, progesterone) function. Also, low growth hormone and low prolactin levels, with growth hormone secretion usually being the first one to fail. Further confirmation by provocative tests including insulin tolerance test, metyrapone, thyrotropin-releasing hormone, or luteinizing hormone-releasing hormone.

Clinical aspects: The cardinal characteristics for diagnosis are loss of sexual function, asthenia, and low basal metabolic rate. Patients usually have lack of lactation and amenorrhea postpartum. There is a characteristic facies, described as waxy white and sallow, as a result of a lack of melatonin. There is a loss of pubic and axillary hair, the skin is dry, the eyebrows thin. The thyroid may be impalpable. Untreated patients may have a low pulse rate with an often low and labile blood pressure. Atypical patient may have maintained menstruation and with subsequent pregnancies, may have much improved symptoms because of the adrenocortical hormones secreted by the placenta. Treatment is by hormone replacement including hydrocortisone and thyroxine, and ovulation may be induced with follicle-stimulating hormone and luteinizing hormone therapy.

Precautions before anesthesia: An anesthesiology consultation is highly recommended before elective surgical procedures. Establish diagnosis by history, clinical examination, and laboratory evidence. Assess fluid and electrolyte status and correct if required. Intravenous hydrocortisone should be available and used if suspected in untreated hypopituitarism before anesthesia commence.

Anesthetic considerations: Hydrocortisone cover should be continued throughout the perioperative period because of the inadequate stress response by the pituitary remnants. Adequate fluid hydration should be given and care should be taken to avoid further stressors such as hypotension, hypoxia, and hypothermia. These patients are reported to have increased sensitivity to barbiturates and opioids, even into the postoperative period. Although not reported, regional techniques would seem beneficial if fluid status is adequately replaced.

Pharmacological implications: Careful titration of doses of intravenous anesthetic drugs, including barbiturates and opioids. Perioperative stress doses of corticoids are necessary.

Other conditions to be considered:

☞SIMMONDS SYNDROME: Hypopituitarism resulting from an infarct of the pituitary gland. Damage to the anterior portion of the pituitary gland causes partial or complete loss of thyroid, adrenocorticoid, and gonadal functions. Very rarely pituitary infarction occurs with diabetic vasculitis, sickle cell anemia, and idiopathic disease. Postpartum hemorrhage and cardiovascular shock is better known as Sheehan syndrome and the other pituitary condition is better known as Simmonds syndrome.

☞AMENORRHEA-GALACTORRHEA SYNDROME TYPE I: One of the three eponymic amenorrhea–galactorrhea syndromes (the other two follow). Persistent lactation, amenorrhea, and atrophy of the uterus and ovaries, lasting months—even years—following childbirth. It is caused by continued secretion of the prolactin and decreased gonadotrophin production. A pituitary adenoma may or may not be present. Mental depression, trunk, back, and head pain. It commences after pregnancy.

☞AMENORRHEA-GALACTORRHEA SYNDROME TYPE II: Amenorrhea–galactorrhea syndrome not associated with pregnancy. There is estrogen deficiency and decreased urinary gonadotrophin levels.

☞AMENORRHEA-GALACTORRHEA SYNDROME TYPE III: Amenorrhea–galactorrhea syndrome caused by a chromophobe prolactin-producing adenoma of the pituitary.

REFERENCES:

Cohen B, Baillie P: Sheehan's syndrome followed by successful pregnancy: A case report. *S Afr Med J* 57:838, 1980.

Wilson A: Anesthesia for Sheehan's syndrome: A case report. *Br J Anaesth* 40:996, 1968.

Shokeir Syndrome

At a glance: A very rare inherited disorder characterized by association of alopecia and seizures.

Synonym: Alopecia Epilepsy Pyorrhea Mental Subnormality Syndrome.

Genetic inheritance: Autosomal dominant.

Diagnosis: Association of alopecia, mental subnormality, and psychomotor epilepsy.

Clinical aspects: Alopecia is congenital, permanent, and universal. Periodontal disease is present in all patients. Pigmented nevi can be observed.

Anesthetic considerations: Evaluate epilepsy treatment efficacy (EEG, history). Direct laryngoscopy should be performed carefully to prevent periodontal bleeding. Epilepsy medications should be given the day of surgery. Consider anesthetic drug interaction with epileptic treatment.

REFERENCE:

Shokeir MHK: Universal permanent alopecia, psychomotor epilepsy, pyorrhea and mental subnormality. *Clin Genet* 11:13, 1977.

Shone Complex or Syndrome

At a glance: Very rare disease characterized by severe and often lethal triple cardiac malformation. It is a series of four obstructive or potentially obstructive left-sided cardiac lesions consisting of supravalvular mitral ring, parachute deformity of the mitral valve, subaortic stenosis, and coarctation of the aorta.

Synonyms: Mitral Stenosis, Aortic Stenosis, Coarctation of the Aorta.

Incidence and genetic inheritance: In the United States, it has been suggested that congenital mitral valve stenosis occurs in 0–5% of patients with congenital heart disease. There is no racial or sex predilection.

Clinical aspects: This syndrome is present at birth. It is an association of multiple levels of left ventricular inflow and outflow obstruction (subvalvar and valvar left ventricular outflow tract obstruction, coarctation of the aorta, and mitral stenosis). Death can occur in first weeks of life.

Anesthetic considerations: Document the level of obstruction (heart catheterization with or without provocative testing). Quantify the severity and anatomy of the obstruction (clinical examination, ECG, chest radiographs, echo-Doppler, transesophageal echocardiography to define precisely the anatomy, MRI to assess associated lesions such as pulmonary artery stenosis or coarctation). Prophylactic antibiotics should be used as indicated. Consider invasive intraoperative blood pressure measurement. Perioperative cardiac monitoring is mandatory.

REFERENCES:

Sekhar KC, Mastan S, Farooqi A, et al: Anaesthetic management of a case of Shone's syndrome. *Ind J Anaesth* 48:212, 2004.

Shone JD, Sellers RD, Anderson RC et al: The developmental complex of "parachute mitral valve," supravalvular ring of left atrium, subaortic stenosis and coarctation of aorta. *Am J Cardiol* 11:714, 1963.

Short-Rib Polysyndactyly Syndrome

At a glance: The Short-Rib Polysyndactyly syndrome is a descriptive category for a group of lethal skeletal dysplasias characterized by a hypoplastic thorax, short ribs, short limbs, polydactyly, and visceral abnormalities.

Classifications and synonyms: The Short-Rib Polysyndactyly Syndrome is subdivided into four types: classified as follow :

Type I: Saldino-Noonan Syndrome (Polysyndactyly with Neonatal Chondrodystrophy type I)

Type II: Majewski Syndrome (Polysyndactyly with Neonatal Chondrodystrophy type II)

Type III: Verma-Naumoff Syndrome (Polysyndactyly with Neonatal Chondrodystrophy type III)

Type IV: ☞Beemer-Langer Syndrome (Short Rib Syndrome, Beemer type).

Genetic inheritance: All variants are believed to be inherited as autosomal recessive pattern. However, because of the frequent phenotypic overlap, there is controversy as to whether the variants are because of variable expression or genetic heterogenity.

Clinical aspects: *Type I or Saldino-Noonan Syndrome* is a lethal condition (dwarfism) in the newborn period. The infant has a hydropic appearance, postaxial polydactyly, severely shortened and flipper-like limbs and striking metaphyseal dysplasia of tubular bones. Severe micromelia is often noted. The cardiac system often presents a transposition of the great vessels. Ossification is defective in the calvaria and vertebrae. It also affects the pelvis and bones of the hand and feet. The pelvis resembles that in the Ellis-van Creveld Syndrome and the Asphyxiating Thoracic Dystrophy Syndrome. The visceral abnormalities involve gastrointestinal (GI) atresia, genitourinary atresia, and polycystic kidneys.

Type II or Majewski Syndrome is a lethal disease in the perinatal period. It is characterized by the presence of median cleft-lip and palate, hypoplastic epiglottis, malformed larynx, and pulmonary hypoplasia. The presence of short ribs and GI atresia may mislead the diagnosis and often it is suggested to be a type I variant. However, the genitourinary system is largely affected with polycystic kidneys, ambiguous genitalia, and glomerular and renal tubular cysts. Neurologically, the presence of a hypoplastic cerebellar vermis and pachygyria is classical to this entity.

Type III or Verma-Naumoff Syndrome: The most important distinguishing features of this type are to be found in the skull: the cranial base is short, the forehead is bulging, the nasal bridge is depressed and the occiput is flat. Another difference resides in the radiologic appearance of the long tubular bones, which show a distinct corticomedullary demarcation, somewhat widened metaphyses and marked longitudinal spurs. The neonatal period is often associated with asphyxiating episodes because of the narrow thorax and very short ribs. In comparison with type II, the genitourinary system does not show as frequent abnormalities.

Type IV or Beemer Langer Syndrome is characterized by short ribs with pulmonary hypoplasia, associated with a variety of other visceral malformations. Short tubular bones, perinatal hydrops and macrocephaly are present in virtually all children. Midline cleft with or without cleft palate, congenital heart disease, central nervous system malformations, GI and urogenital abnormalities are other frequently encountered features. The syndrome is generally lethal with most children dying in utero or during early infancy because of respiratory insufficiency secondary to pulmonary hypoplasia.

Precautions before anesthesia: Because of the dismal prognosis of all variants, these patients are unlikely candidates for anesthesia. If a surgical intervention is indicated, the full extent of craniofacial, cardiac malformations, and pulmonary functions needs to be assessed carefully.

Anesthetic considerations: Anesthetic implications vary according to the type involved. However, most of them present with potentially difficult airway management (especially type II), oxygenation failure on the ventilator, and severe difficulties to wean from the mechanical ventilation. The anesthetic considerations concerning the cardiovascular system depend on the pathophysiology of the underlying cardiac defect.

Pharmacological implications: Depending on the cardiac state, agents causing myocardial depression or resulting in changes of systemic and/or pulmonary vascular resistance should be used cautiously.

Other conditions to be considered:

☞**ELLIS VAN CREVELD SYNDROME:** Polydactyly, and abnormalities of the ectoderm (dystrophy of the fingernails, change in the upper lip variously called "partial hare-lip, " lip-tie, cleft lip and palate) occurs. Micrognathia may be present. Frequent genital anomalies. Presence of cardiac malformations (usually a septal defect and often single atrium) in 60% of affected patients. Respiratory distress is common in the newborn because of pulmonary hypoplasia within a narrow dysplastic thorax with extremely short ribs.

Dandy-Walker malformation, hydrocephalus. Management consists of dental care, orthopedic treatment of polydactyly, and correction of cardiac defects.

☞**JEUNE SYNDROME:** This asphyxiating thoracic dysplasia is a rare autosomal recessive chondrodysplasia that often leads to death in infancy because of a severely constricted thoracic cage and respiratory insufficiency. Most often associated with pulmonary hypoplasia, recurrent respiratory infections leading to respiratory insufficiency. Long, narrow thorax, short, horizontal ribs, handlebar clavicles, and bulbous irregular rib ends. The frequency is 1/100,000 to 1/130,000 live births. The survivors may develop renal failure and hepatic fibrosis, polycystic liver disease, jaundice, and pancreatic fibrosis. Proteinuria and hyperbilirubinemia must be assessed.

REFERENCES:

Elcioglu N, Karatein G, Sezgin B, et al: Short-rib polysyndactyly syndrome in twins: Beemer-Langer type with polydactyly. *Clin Genet* 50:159–163, 1996.

Ho NC, Francomano CA, van Allen M: Jeune asphyxiating thoracic dystrophy and short-rib polysyndactyly syndrome type III (Verna-Naumoff) are variants of the same disorder. *Am J Med Genet* 90: 310–14, 2000.

Sarafoglou K, Funai EF, Fefferman N, et al: Short-rib polysyndactyly syndrome: More evidence of a continuous spectrum. *Clin Genet* 56: 145–148, 1999.

SHORT Syndrome

At a glance: The acronym SHORT stands for *S*hort Stature, *H*yperextensibility of Joints or Hernia or both, *O*cular Depression, *R*ieger Anomaly, and *T*eething Delay. Short stature with loss of fat under the skin (lipoatrophy) of the arms and face are very frequent features. Other distinguishing symptoms include defective development of the anterior chamber of the eye and diabetes mellitus.

Synonyms: Reiger Anomaly-Growth Retardation Syndrome.

Genetic inheritance: Uncertain. Probably an autosomal recessive trait. Individuals affected with this disorder are usually born with a low birth weight. Some reported cases of autosomal dominant inheritance.

Pathophysiology: Unknown.

Diagnosis: Clinical features. Radiological features include delayed bone age. Growth hormone and thyroid function test are normal.

Clinical aspects: *Craniofacial:* distinctive triangular face; broad forehead; down-slanting palpebral fissures; broad nasal bridge; hypoplastic alae; down-turned corners of mouth; mild micrognathia. *Teeth:* delayed dentition; small, stained teeth. *Eyes:* sunken eyes, iridocorneal anomaly, congenital glaucoma. *Ears:* anteverted ears; sensorineural deafness. *Joints:* hyperextensibility; congenital hip dislocation. *Limbs:* clinodactyly. *Abdominal:* inguinal hernia. *Growth:* low birth weight dwarfism; short stature; lipoatrophy. *Neurological:* developmental delay; speech delay. *Endocrinological:* diabetes mellitus. Not all features may be present for the diagnosis.

Precautions before anesthesia: Check blood glucose levels before, during, and after procedure.

Anesthetic considerations: Preoperative fasting and glucose/insulin requirement depends on the presence and the severity of diabetes mellitus. Developmental delay and deafness may cause anxiety and a lack of cooperation. Care with positioning of patient to avoid dislocation of hyperextensible joints.

Pharmacological implications: Avoid succinylcholine and other drugs that may increase intraocular pressure in the presence of glaucoma.

Other conditions to be considered:

AARSKOG OSE PANDE SYNDROME: First described in 1983. Characterized by lipodystrophy especially on the face and buttocks, Reiger anomaly, short stature, insulopenic diabetes mellitus, glucose intolerance, midface hypoplasia, hypotrishosis, and retarded bone age. It has been suggested that this medical condition is distinct from SHORT syndrome because of the absence of joint hypermobility and less extensive lipodystrophy. The diabetes mellitus is usually noted by the fourth decade of life, but the onset may also be variable. The incidence is estimated as high as 1:133,000 Northern European regions, especially in the Lofoten Islands of Norway. An autosomal dominant inheritance trait has been suggested.

RIEGER SYNDROME: A genetically determined syndrome of the anterior chamber of the eyes and the teeth, combining features of the Axenfeld syndrome with oligodontia. An opaque ring at the margin of the cornea, iris adhesion to the Schwalbe ring, hypoplasia of the anterior stroma of the iris, and tooth anomalies. Other features include hypoplasia of the malar bones, broad and flat nose, prognathism, and hypertelorism. Myotonic dystrophy, mental retardation, brachydactyly, clinodactyly, arachnodactyly, and polydactyly have been reported. Autosomal dominant inheritance but sporadic cases are also seen, suggesting a recessive pattern. When occurring without the dental and skeletal defects, it is called the SHORT syndrome.

AXENFELD SYNDROME: Considered a variant of the Rieger syndrome. Defects limited to the peripheral anterior segment of the eye.

REFERENCES:

Sorge G, Ruggieri M, Polizzi A, et al: SHORT syndrome: A new case with probable autosomal dominant inheritance. *Am J Med Genet* 61:178, 1996.

Toriello H, Wakefield S, Komar K, et al: Report of a case and further delineation of the SHORT syndrome. *Am J Med Genet* 22:311, 1985.

Shwachman Syndrome

At a glance: A rare congenital defect characterized by pancreatic insufficiency with neutropenia (60% of cases) and growth retardation. Other features may include recurrent and fatal infections, aplastic anemia, leukemia, skeletal abnormalities (metaphyseal dysostosis, thoracic dystrophy), hepatic failure, and ichthyotic skin changes.

Synonym: Shwachman-Diamond Syndrome.

Incidence: Approximately 1:50,000 live births.

Genetic inheritance: Autosomal recessive but may occur sporadically.

Pathophysiology: A multiorgan condition whose underlying cause is uncertain. Reduction in pancreatic exocrine function that is partly a result of fatty infiltration of the pancreas; evidenced by low or absent amylase, lipase and trypsin activity resulting in malabsorption, and the need for enzyme supplementation. Skin sweat test is normal. Bone marrow has varying degrees of hypoplasia resulting in intermittent neutropenia and thrombocytopenia. Neutrophil chemotaxis is impaired.

Diagnosis: Based on clinical scenario in addition to evidence of pancreatic exocrine insufficiency, intermittent or persistent neutropenia and thrombocytopenia, and abnormal neutrophil chemotaxis. Hypoplastic bone marrow may be present.

Clinical aspects: Initially, neonates may present with failure to thrive, diarrhea, feeding difficulties, and hypotonia. Growth retardation persists into adulthood. Although pancreatic exocrine function is abnormal, endocrine function is normal. Motor and speech development are invariably delayed and intelligence quotient low. Skeletal abnormalities are common and include metaphyseal dysplasia in long bones, knees, wrists, ankles, and vertebrae. Clinodactyly or duplication of the thumb has been described. Ribs are frequently short, resulting in a narrow thoracic cavity. This frequently improves with age. Chest wall compliance is reduced and lung compliance normal. Forced expiratory volume at 1 second (FEV_1) and forced vital capacity (FVC) are usually reduced. Renal tubular dysfunction may be present. Myocardial fibrosis and cardiomegaly have been described and may make patients extremely sensitive to chemotherapy-induced cardiotoxicity. Leukemic transformation has been described in 5 to 33% of patients.

Precautions before anesthesia: *Hematologic:* evaluate for evidence of pancytopenia and correct abnormalities preoperatively. Pulmonary function testing particularly in patients with chest wall abnormalities. *Cardiac function:* particularly echocardiogram following chemotherapy.

Anesthetic considerations: Patient cooperation may be limited as a consequence of developmental delay. Pulmonary function usually is not severely impaired. Consider side effects of steroids and chemotherapeutic agents used in treatment of malignant transformation and bone marrow transplantation.

Pharmacological implications: Cardiac-depressant drugs should be used with care. Corticosteroid coverage following steroid use.

REFERENCES:

Aggett PJ, Cavanagh NPC, Matthew DJ, et al: Shwachman's syndrome: A review of 21 cases. *Arch Dis Child* 55:331, 1980.

Dror Y, Ginzberg H, Dalal I, et al: Immune function in patients with Shwachman-Diamond syndrome. *Br J Haematol* 114:712, 2001.

Okcu F, Roberts W, Chan K: Bone marrow transplantation in Shwachman-Diamond syndrome: Report of two cases and review of the literature. *Bone Marrow Transplant* 21:849, 1998.

Tamhane P, Newton NI, White S: Anaesthetic management of quinsy in a patient with Shwachman-Diamond syndrome. *Anaesthesia* 59:198, 2004.

Shy-Drager Syndrome

At a glance: A progressive disease of the central and autonomic nervous systems in which idiopathic orthostatic hypotension is a major feature. Other features include bladder and bowel incontinence, anhidrosis, iris atrophy, amyotrophy, ataxia and rigidity. It is known as a multiple system atrophy, which helps to distinguish it from syndromes of pure autonomic failure. More common in males.

History: Described in 1960 by G.M. Shy, an American Neurologist, and G.A. Drager, an American physician, in Houston, Texas.

Genetic inheritance: Autosomal dominant.

Pathophysiology: Postmortem examination demonstrates degeneration of autonomic neurons in the intermediolateral columns, putamen, substantia nigra, locus ceruleus, inferior olivary nuclei, and degenerative change in peripheral ganglia. Loss of central sympathetic tone results in inability to vasoconstrict or to mount a tachycardia in response to posture changes causing hypotension. Involvement of the corticospinal, corticocerebellar, and pyramidal tracts later in the disease process gives rise to symptoms of parkinsonism.

Diagnosis: A consensus statement generated by the American Autonomic Society and the American Academy of Neurology, defining the various neurogenic causes of autonomic dysfunction, suggested abandonment of the term 'Shy-Drager' syndrome in 1996. A new classification for the autonomic disorders has been best summarized as follows: (1) *primary or cause unknown*, described as pure autonomic failure (previously called idiopathic orthostatic hypotension or the Bradbury-Eggleston syndrome) and in which no neurologic defects other than autonomic dysfunction are present; and (2) *multiple system atrophy*, a sporadic, progressive, adult-onset disorder characterized by autonomic dysfunction, parkinsonism, and ataxia in any combination. History, demonstration of postural hypotension, and special investigations to demonstrate sympathetic insufficiency. Must exclude all other possible causes of orthostatic hypotension. It usually ends in death 7 to 10 years after the onset of symptoms.

Clinical aspects: Symptoms include dizziness on rising, syncope, and anhydrosis. Sexual dysfunction, urinary incontinence, fecal incontinence, dysphagia, unequal pupils, atrophy of the iris, external ophthalmoplegia, and wasting of distal limb muscles all reflect the degenerative changes within the central nervous system and autonomic ganglia. Nocturnal polyuria and natriuresis are present early in the natural history of the Shy-Drager syndrome and cause relative hypovolemia and exacerbation of hypotension on rising from bed. Central sleep apnea has been demonstrated on rare occasions. Signs and symptoms of bradykinesia, rigidity, and tremor occur following a variable interval (ranging from weeks to years) after development of orthostatic hypotension. An abnormal response to the Valsalva maneuver is easily demonstrated. Special investigations include stress tests to show absent sympathetic response; demonstration of lack of response to atropine; assessment of ability to sweat; infusion of direct-acting sympathomimetic agents, which causes hypertension and tachycardia, in contrast to indirect-acting agents (e.g., ephedrine) that has a limited or no effect. The most useful treatment appears to be 9α-fludrocortisone and compression stockings along with elevation of the head of the bed when sleeping. Amphetamines, monoamine oxidase inhibitors (MAOIs), indomethacin, dihydroergotamine, and propranolol have all been used with varying success.

Precautions before anesthesia: An anesthesiology consultation is highly recommended before elective surgical procedures. A complete clinical examination must be done to assess clinical examination to assess sympathetic function and degree of neurological involvement, including evidence of dysphagia and sleep apnea. Review medication history. Check for electrolyte abnormalities. Ensure normal circulating volume prior to induction.

Anesthetic considerations: Maintenance of normovolemia is essential to the administration of safe general anesthesia in these patients. Regional anesthesia has been used, although extreme caution is needed with the use of vasopressors. Stirt et al. showed that catecholamine release did not occur in a patient anesthetized for laparotomy with 5 μg/kg of fentanyl and 60% nitrous oxide.

Pharmacological implications: Direct-acting sympathomimetics may cause profound hypertension because of denervation hypersensitivity and should be used with caution. It has been reported that the use of norepinephrine was effective for hypotension while dopamine was not. There are suspicion that the pharmacodynamic of some medication such as vecuronium, norepinephrine, and dopamine might be altered in these patients. Succinylcholine is relatively con-

traindicated (especially in the presence of muscle wasting). Potential drug interactions in patients treated with MAOIs.

REFERENCES:

Dewhurst A, Sidebottom P: Anaesthetic management of a patient with multiple system atrophy (Shy-Drager syndrome) for urgent hip surgery. *Hosp Med* 60:611, 1999.

Hutchinson R, Sugden J: Anesthesia for Shy-Drager syndrome. *Anesthesia* 39:1229, 1984.

Konarzewski WH, Knorr C: Spinal anaesthesia and Shy Drager syndrome. *Anaesthesia* 52:1020, 1997.

SIADH

At a glance: SIADH is an acronym that stands for: **S**yndrome of **I**nappropriate of **A**nti**D**iuretic **H**ormone Secretion. The most common cause of euvolemic hyponatremia characterized by hypokalemic, hypochloremic, metabolic alkalosis, and normotensive, hyperreninemic hyperaldosteronism. A state of positive water balance rather than sodium depletion is present. Numerous etiologies have been associated with this manifestation (see the following table).

Synonyms: Schwartz-Bartter Syndrome; Aldosteronism-Normal Blood Pressure Syndrome; Juxtaglomerular Hyperplasia Syndrome.

History: First reported in 1957 by William Benjamin Schwartz, American cardiologist, and Frederic Crosby Bartter, American physician. They described two adult patients with bronchial carcinoma who developed persistent hyponatremia, hypoosmolality, and urinary loss of sodium and chloride.

Pathophysiology: Overproduction of vasopressin from the hypothalamus leads to water retention, urinary sodium loss, and hyponatremia. Results in resultant volume expansion promoting urine flow rate, thus limiting further water retention.

Diagnosis: Clinical features and biochemical (low serum sodium levels and low serum osmolality, increased urine sodium content and osmolality, suppression of plasma renin activity, normal/high serum aldosterone level, high plasma antidiuretic hormone and atrial natriuretic hormone levels). Conditions known to be associated with antidiuretic hormone secretion (normal renal, liver, adrenal, thyroid, and cardiac functions) must be excluded.

Clinical aspects: Symptoms, when present, are caused by acute loss of sodium and are often masked by or mistaken as manifestations of the primary problem (anorexia, confusion, headache, muscle weakness, vomiting, convulsions, and coma). Chronic hyponatremia, lasting longer than 2 to 5 days, usually has minimal or no symptoms. Vascular volume is normal or mildly increased, and peripheral edema is very rare. Blood pressure is normal, even with postural changes; urine output is usually low.

Anesthetic considerations: Hyponatremia may contribute to delayed awakening and postoperative confusion, and potentiates the action of neuromuscular blockers. Symptomatic hyponatremia (serum sodium levels <120 mmol/L) should be corrected slowly at a rate of <1 mmol/L/h until a serum level of approximately 130 mmol/L is reached. Rapid correction of long-standing (>2 days) advanced hyponatremia (<110 mmol/L) to normal levels within less than 20 hours can cause central pontine myelinosis. Treatment consists of water restriction, hypertonic saline, and loop diuretics. Drugs have little or no place in the treatment of SIADH in children.

Table S-1   Causes of SIADH

CNS	Pulmonary	Neoplastic	Pharmacologic

Infection
  –meningitis
  –encephalitis
  –abscess
Subarachnoid hemorrhage
Hypoxia-ischemia
Intraventricular
Hemorrhage of newborn
Trauma
Cerebrovascular accident
Tumor
Psychosis (dipsogenic)
Guillain-Barré syndrome
Vasculitis
VA shunt obstruction
Cavernous sinus
  Thrombosis
Stress
	Infection:
	  –bacterial
	  –mycoplasma
	  –fungal
	  –viral
	  –tuberculosis
	Decreased left atrial
	pressure:
	  –pneumothorax
	  –atelectasis
	  –asthma/bronchiolitis
	  –PDA ligation
	Cystic fibrosis
	Hyaline membrane of
	  newborn
		Bronchogenic carcinoma
		Adenocarcinoma of:
		  –pancreas
		  –prostate
		Carcinoma of:
		  –ureter
		  –prostate
		Thymoma
		ALL
		Lymphoma
		Lymphosarcoma
		Mesothelioma
		Hemophagocytic syndrome
			Increased water
			Permeability of nephron:
			  –vasopressin
			  –desmopressin
			  –oxytocin
			Promote ADH release:
			  –nicotine
			  –barbiturates
			  –narcotics
			  –carbamazepine
			  –colchine
			  –diuretics
			  –isoproterenol
			  –vincristine
			  –vinblastine
			  –amitriptyline
			  –clofibrate
			  –histamine
			Inhibit prostaglandin
			synthesis
			  –salicylates
			  –acetaminophen
			  –NSAIDs
			Potentiate ADH action
			  –chloropramide
			  –cyclophosphamide
			  –tolbutamide
			  –phenformin

ABBREVIATIONS: CNS: central nervous system; VA shunt: ventriculo-atrial shunt; NSAIDs: non-steroidal antiinflammatory drugs; PDA: patent ductus arteriosus; ADH: antidiuretic hormone; ALL: acute lymphocytic leukemia

REFERENCES:

Haycock GB: The syndrome of inappropriate secretion of antidiuretic hormone. *Pediatr Nephrol* 9:375, 1995.

Sternes RH, Riggs JE, Schochet SS Jr: Osmotic demyelination syndrome following correction of hyponatremia. *N Engl J Med* 314:1535, 1986.

Sialidosis

At a glance: A genetic neurodegenerative disease, divided into two types. These conditions are caused by a missing enzyme (sialidase) that results in the accumulation of sialic acid in the nerve cells. Type II is reported in infants and toddlers.

Synonyms and classifications:
  Sialidosis type I: Cherry-Red-Spot, Myoclonus Syndrome
  Sialidosis type II: Mucolipidosis type I; Sialidase Deficiency; Glycoprotein Neuraminidase Deficiency; NEUG Deficiency; Lipomucopolysaccharidosis.

Incidence: Genetic disorder with a 2.5:1 male preponderance.

Genetic inheritance: Autosomal recessive. The majority of type I patients have been Italian. The lysosomal sialidase gene has been mapped to chromosome 6 (6p21.3). Prenatal diagnosis (amniotic fluid cells) is possible.

Pathophysiology: The enzyme lysosomal neuraminidase (sialidase) normally removes the terminal sialyl linkages of several oligosaccharides and glycoproteins. Its deficiency results in excessive accumulation of complex sugars rich in sialic acid.

Diagnosis: Excessive urinary oligosaccharides can be demonstrated. Definitive diagnosis is based on sialidase activity present in tissue samples (e.g., fibroblasts, WBCs).

Clinical aspects: Clinically, sialidosis can have two forms. *Type I (mild form)* presents with a cherry-red spot myoclonus phenotype that is usually associated with isolated neuraminidase deficiency. Nystagmus, ataxia, and seizures are reported. *Type II (severe form)* has abnormal somatic features including coarse faces, broad nasal root, thick lips, deafness, delayed bone age, pectus carinatum, scoliosis, short rib cage, and dysostosis multiplex. Other clinical features include lipidosis, sulfatidosis, macular pigmentary abnormality, movement disorder, dwarfism, speech defect, splenomegaly, and storage liver disease.

Precautions before anesthesia: Chest radiographs and resting oxygen saturation must be obtained in view of frequent respiratory infections/obstructive sleep apnea. Abnormal airway with macroglossia, thickened mucosal folds in oro- and naso-pharynx, together with skeletal deformities. Liver function tests and coagulation profiles if hepatomegaly is present.

Anesthetic considerations: Airway management will be a major challenge with or without endotracheal intubation. Loss of muscle tone after general anesthesia induction results in upper airway obstruction. It is recommended to have a laryngeal mask airway available in case of failure to ventilate with face-mask or intubate the trachea. Patient positioning in the presence of contractures can be difficult. Chronic pulmonary infections and kyphoscoliosis can lead to postoperative respiratory failure.

Pharmacological implications: Avoid the use of muscle relaxants if possible until the trachea is intubated and lung ventilation is confirmed. The use of opioids should also be prudent in the presence of sleep apnea and mental retardation.

Other conditions to be considered: There are three other categories of genetic neurodegenerative disorders that can be distinguished from one another based on head CT scan, head MRI, nerve conduction velocities, visually evoked potentials, auditory evoked potentials, electroretinography, and, to a lesser extent, electroencephalography. The ultimate diagnosis is obtained from skin, conjunctival, and nerve biopsies.

SPHINGOLIPIDOSES: This category includes six specific diseases: Niemann-Pick Disease; Gaucher Disease; Krabbe Disease (Globoid Cell Leukodystrophy) and Metachromatic Leukodystrophy; G_{M1}-Gangliosidosis and G_{M2}-Gangliosidosis. The common features of all these entities is the ability to destroy storage of fats within nerve cells.

☞NEURONAL CEROID LIPOFUSCINOSES: This is a group of inherited, neurodegenerative, lysosomal-storage disorders that are characterized by progressive mental and motor deterioration, seizures, and early death. Visual loss is a feature of most forms. The phenotypes have been classified clinically by age of onset and order of appearance of the clinical features.

ADRENOLEUKODYSTROPHY: A rare genetic disorder characterized by the breakdown or loss of the myelin sheath surrounding the nerve cells in the brain and progressive dysfunction of the adrenal glands. Onset of the classic childhood form, which is the most severe and affects only boys, may occur between the ages of 4 and 10 years. Features include visual loss, severe learning disabilities, seizures, dysarthria, dysphagia and recurrent aspiration, deafness, ataxia and gait disturbances, fatigue, and progressive dementia.

surgical trauma, fibrous, inflammatory, or degenerative infiltration of the sinus node and ischemia.

Diagnosis: Clinical history, ECG with or without Holter monitoring.

Clinical aspects: May remain asymptomatic. Symptoms include dizziness, syncope, palpitations, and chest pain. A 12-lead ECG should be examined for sinus bradycardia, sinus arrest, and junctional escape rhythm; however, a single recording may appear normal. Continuous monitoring may be necessary to demonstrate alternating episodes of bradycardia and tachycardia. Episodes of tachycardia may be controlled with digoxin or beta blockade. If beta blockade is used, cardiac pacing (dual-mode, dual-pacing, dual-sensing) usually becomes necessary to prevent profound bradycardia. Acquired sick sinus syndrome may be caused by lithium and carbamazepine therapy.

Precautions before anesthesia: Obtain a complete medical history of frequency of syncope/palpitations, drug history, and pacemaker details. Attempt to define etiology of the sick sinus syndrome in the individual patient may be impossible. If the syndrome is newly diagnosed, consider temporary pacing. Cardiovascular assessment: review recent ECG(s). Further investigations must be carried on medical grounds. Metabolic considerations: check serum electrolytes.

Anesthetic considerations: Decreased systemic vascular resistance caused by volatile agents or major regional blockade may result in profound hypotension because a reflex tachycardia is not generated. Stroke volume is the primary determinant of cardiac output, therefore myocardial contractility and optimal filling pressures should be maintained. Complete atrioventricular block during anesthesia is also reported.

Pharmacological implications: Atropine will not treat the bradycardia. Chronotropic agents have minimal effect on heart rate.

REFERENCES:

Burt D: The sick sinus syndrome: A complication during anesthesia. *Anesthesia* 37:1108, 1982.

Iinuma Y, Maruyama K, Hara K. Complete atrioventricular block during anesthesia in a patient with sick sinus syndrome under atrial pacing. *J Anesth* 19(1):92, 2005.

Underwood S, Glynn C: Sick sinus syndrome manifest after spinal anesthesia. *Anesthesia* 43:307, 1988.

Zipes DP. Specific arrhythmias: diagnosis and treatment, in Braunwald E (ed): *Heart Disease: A Textbook of Cardiovascular Medicine.* 5th ed. Philadelphia, WB Saunders, 1996, pp. 640–645.

Sick Sinus Syndrome

At a glance: Abnormality of sinoatrial node (SAN) function or atrial conduction.

Genetic inheritance: The syndrome may be acquired or congenital. Between 2 and 6% of cases are familial and inherited as an autosomal dominant trait.

Pathophysiology: Sinoatrial node depolarization is irregular or fails, resulting in bradycardia or sinus arrest. In the presence of sinus arrest or extreme sinus bradycardia, a junctional escape rhythm may develop. Irregular depolarization of the sinus node, however, causes paroxysms of tachycardia (supraventricular tachycardia/atrial fibrillation) between episodes of bradycardia. Acquired causes include

Sickle Cell Anemia

At a glance: An inherited blood disorder characterized by episodes of pain, chronic hemolytic anemia, and severe infections, usually beginning in early childhood. As a result of the vasoocclusive nature of the disease, in the worst situation, patients may present with congestive heart failure, cerebral infarction, kidney damage with bloody urine, splenomegaly, hepatomegaly and jaundice, eye damage, and bone marrow defects.

Classification: There are four different types: Sickle Cell Trait; Hemoglobin SS; Hemoglobin SC Disease; Hemoglobin Sickle Beta-Thalassemia.

Incidence: Sickle Cell Anemia is the most common inherited blood disorder in the United States, affecting 1 in 375 to 500 African

Americans. Eight percent of African Americans are affected. Homozygous HbS disease occurs in 0.2% of African Americans, while heterozygous sickle cell trait occurs in 8%. Globally, a quarter of a million children are born every year with the disease. At least five haplotypes of sickle cell disease are recognized based upon their origin: Senegal, Cameron, Benin, Central African Republic, and India. Among these, patients from the Central African Republic have the most severe disease and those from Senegal the least severe. Other nationalities with sickle cell include Arabs, Greeks, Italians (mostly southern), and Latin Americans.

Genetic inheritance: Autosomal recessive inheritance caused by a point mutation in the hemoglobin beta gene (HBB) found on chromosome 11p15.4.

Pathophysiology: HbS is characterized by the substitution of valine for glutamic acid in the sixth position of the B chain. When deoxygenated, the red cells change conformation, forming a sickle shape that rheologically favors vascular stasis and subsequently ischemia. While the red cells of patients with sickle cell trait have less than 50% HbS, the red cells of homozygotes may have upwards of 70 to 90% HbS. Clinical severity improves with increased levels of fetal hemoglobin (HbF). Other Sickle Cell Diseases include Hemoglobin SC Disease, Sickle Cell Beta-Thalassemia, and Hemoglobin SD Disease. These diseases are often, but not always, milder than Hemoglobin SS Disease. Sickle Trait is usually asymptomatic, although hematuria and inability to concentrate urine may occur.

Diagnosis: *Sickle Cell Trait* suggests a person who carries a sickle hemoglobin-producing gene inherited from one parent with a normal (HbA) and an abnormal (HbS) gene leading to Hb AS on the electrophoresis. This form does not cause HbSS Disease. Fetal diagnosis is via chorionic villus biopsy. Electrophoresis of umbilical cord blood is also indicated to establish the diagnosis in neonates. Peripheral smear with sickled cells, target cells, and reticulocytosis is characteristic. Hydroxyurea, an antitumor, is effective in preventing painful crises because it induces the formation of fetal Hb (HbF), preventing sickling.

Clinical aspects: Vasoocclusive (painful) crises (bones, abdomen, chest) are characteristic of this disease and caused by sickling red cells leading to ischemia. Aplastic crisis (associated with parvovirus B19 infection) can also be seen. Sequestration crisis (usually children, though can affect adults with Hemoglobin SC Disease and Sickle Cell Beta-Thalassemia) is another mode of clinical presentation. Hemolytic crisis, growth retardation, bone defects/osteomyelitis (salmonella), renal papillary necrosis, priapism, splenomegaly/autoinfarction, jaundice/cholelithiasis, acute chest syndrome (potentially fatal pulmonary infarctions), retinopathy and cerebral vascular accidents are clinical features. Predisposition to infections because of blood stasis. Chronic transfusions with alloimmunization are frequent.

Precautions before anesthesia: Check hematocrit and renal function. Avoid preoperative dehydration/overtransfusion which affects the rheologic characteristic of the blood flow. Assess for cor pulmonale. Anticipate difficulty cross-matching blood. A consultation with the hematologist caring for the patient must be obtained to discuss the need for exchange transfusion versus conservative (nonexchange) transfusion. The important studies of the Preoperative Transfusion in Sickle Cell Disease Study Group demonstrate that simple transfusion to a hemoglobin of 10 mg/dL is as effective as aggressive exchange transfusion (defined as HbS level <30%) in preventing perioperative complications, while having fewer transfusion (alloimmunization) complications. However, one must weight

the risk of transfusion in function of the surgical procedure to be performed and the risk of red blood cell sickling. The risks associated with blood transfusion have led some clinicians to question this procedure. Delayed hemolytic reaction from a transfusion given prior to general anesthesia might be a complication. The controversy of red blood cell transfusion in this patient group still persists.

Anesthetic considerations: Avoid conditions that promote sickling (hypoxia, hypovolemia, hypocarbia, and hypothermia). It is essential to maintain proper intravascular volemia. The use of dextran solution might be considered to favor blood pooling in large conductance vessels and reduce potential stasis within capacitance vasculature. Use of cell salvage devices is controversial. An exchange transfusion is unlikely except in extreme conditions (e.g., cardiopulmonary bypass). Surveillance for postoperative complications (especially acute chest syndrome) and peripheral vascular occlusion (whitening of toes, fingers, etc.) must be carefully checked. Positioning is essential to reduce venous stasis and mechanical vascular occlusion. The use of tourniquet during surgery should be avoided although some reports from Latin America have suggested that it is safe to use if maintained for less than 30 minutes.

Pharmacological implications: There are no known specific implication with this condition.

REFERENCES:

Beutler E: The sickle cell diseases and related disorders, in Williams WJ, Beutler E, Erslev AJ, et al. (eds): *Hematology*. 5th ed. New York, McGraw-Hill, 1995, p 616.

Firth PG: Anaesthesia for peculiar cells—a century of sickle cell disease. *Br J Anaesth* 95:287, 2005.

Firth PG, Head CA: Sickle cell disease and anesthesia. *Anesthesiology* 101:766, 2004.

Vichisky EP: A comparison of conservative and aggressive transfusion regimens in the perioperative management of sickle cell disease. *N Engl J Med* 333(4):206, 1995.

Simmonds Syndrome

At a glance: Hypopituitarism resulting from an infarct of the pituitary gland. Damage to the anterior portion of the pituitary gland causes partial or complete loss of thyroid, adrenocorticoid, and gonadal functions. Pituitary infarction can very rarely occur with diabetic vasculitis, sickle cell anemia, and idiopathic disease. Postpartum hemorrhage and cardiovascular shock is better known as Sheehan syndrome whereas this pituitary condition is better known as Simmonds syndrome.

Synonyms: Glinski-Simmonds Syndrome; Simmonds Cachexia; Hypopituitarism Syndrome; Panhypopituitarism Syndrome; Pituitary Cachexia.

History: In 1939, the German Medical Society recommended that anterior pituitary deficiency be called Simmonds Disease, named after Maurice Simmonds, German physician, who, in 1914, described a female patient with chronic pituitary failure following puerperal sepsis. Nowadays, postpartum hypopituitarism is better known as Sheehan syndrome whereas all other pituitary failure are known as Simmonds Disease.

Incidence: Can occur in both sexes but more prevalent in females. The onset usually occurs in the postpubertal period.

Pathophysiology: Hypofunction and atrophy of the anterior pituitary gland can be observed with tumors, infections, surgery, or radiotherapy; occasionally idiopathic; associated with secondary atrophy of the thyroid gland, adrenal glands, and the gonads.

Clinical aspects: Asthenia and weight loss, atrophy of all body tissues; loss of body hair, atrophic skin; genital organ atrophy, loss of libido and potency; hypothermia sensitive; bradycardia and severe postural hypotension; psychic changes are all characteristic of this medical condition.

Diagnosis: History and clinical features; biochemical (low levels of T_3, T_4, thyroid-stimulating hormone, adrenocorticotropic hormone (ACTH), and gonadotropins); anemia; low basal metabolic rate; radiology (pituitary tumor demonstrated by CT scan of brain).

Anesthetic considerations: Preoperative replacement therapy should be undertaken because dramatic improvement can be expected; in the untreated case, the patient will be bradycardic and hemodynamically unstable perioperatively. Slow clearance of drugs renders the patient sensitive to effects of most drugs, including anesthetic drugs, opioids, and neuromuscular blockers; prone to hypothermia intraoperatively.

Pharmacological implications: Careful titration of doses of intravenous anesthetic drugs, including barbiturate and opioids, must be done to avoid hypotension. Adequate hydrocortisone cover before, during, and after anesthesia is essential.

Other condition to be considered:

☞**SHEEHAN SYNDROME:** Hypopituitarism resulting from an infarct of the pituitary gland following postpartum shock or hemorrhage. Damage to the anterior portion of the pituitary gland causes partial or complete loss of thyroid, adrenocorticoid, and gonadal functions.

REFERENCES:

Birch CA: Simmonds disease. Morris Simmonds 1855–1925. *Practitioner* 212(1271):737, 1974.

Magalini IM, Magalini SC: Simmonds, in *Dictionary of Medical Syndromes.* 3rd ed. New York, Lippincott, 1990, p 816.

Simpson-Golabi-Behmel Syndrome

At a glance: A rare entity characterized by prenatal and postnatal overgrowth syndrome. Clinical features include abnormal sacrum, absent nails/claws, cleft palate most often associated with a cleft of the lower lip, coarse facial features, macroglossia, coloboma, congenital heart defects (ventricular septal defect, atrial septal defect), diaphragmatic hernia, hepatomegaly, fusion of cervical vertebra and limited extension, hydronephrosis, intestinal malrotation, kidney failure, macrocephaly, and increased risk of embryonal cancers.

Synonyms: Bulldog Syndrome; Simpson Dysmorphia Syndrome; X-Linked Dysplasia Gigantism Syndrome.

Genetic inheritance: X-linked overgrowth syndrome in relation to the GPC3 coding region. Most families map Xq26; however, one large pedigree maps to Xp22.

Pathophysiology: Mutation in gene for glypican-3 (GPC3) located in the region of Xq26. GPC3 may modulate insulin-like growth factor 2 (IGF-2) in controlling embryonic mesodermal tissue to cause overgrowth syndrome.

Diagnosis: The clinical manifestations include (according to the genetic origin): *Xq26:* coarse facies with mandibular overgrowth, cleft palate, congenital heart defects, hernias, supernumerary nipples, and renal and skeletal abnormalities; *Xp22:* lethal form, multiple organ anomalies, hydrops fetalis, and death within first

8 weeks of life. Radiological findings include flare of iliac wings, narrow sacroiliac notches, and advanced bone age in one series.

Clinical aspects: Wide spectrum of clinical manifestations from mild course with survival to adulthood to severe course with early neonatal death. *Growth:* increased birth weight and height; prenatal/postnatal overgrowth; broad, stocky, "bulldog" appearance. *Craniofacial:* large head; coarse facies; hypertelorism; wide nasal bridge; upturned nasal tip; cup-shaped ears; large mouth; protruding jaw; enlarged tongue; cleft of lower lip; cleft palate. *Eyes:* cataract; retinal detachment. *Trunk:* short neck; pectus excavatum; accessory nipple; coccygeal skin tag and bony appendage. *Cardiac:* ventricular septal defect and pulmonary stenosis; arrhythmia may be common and is a possible cause of the high incidence of sudden death. *Neurology:* normal intelligence; clumsiness. *Limbs:* broad, short hands and fingers; postaxial polydactyly; syndactyly; simian crease. *Gastroenterology:* intestinal malrotation; Merkel diverticulum. *Genitourinary:* cryptorchidism; hypospadias. In one review, a similarity with Beckwith-Wiedemann syndrome was noted, and increased risk of neonatal hypoglycemia and embryonal tumor was suggested. High early perinatal and infant mortality was noted in another series.

Precautions before anesthesia: Full history and examination must be obtained to delineate the clinical features present because of its wide spectrum. Assess cardiac function with examination, ECG, chest radiograph, Holter monitor, echocardiogram, and catheterization if indicated. Assess airway for potential difficulty.

Anesthetic considerations: Anesthetic technique should be tailored to the cardiac status and the procedure planned, including endocarditis prophylaxis, air embolism avoidance, and adequate rehydration. Arrhythmia is reported to be common and should be monitored for during the perioperative period. There is a significant potential for difficult airway maintenance during sedation or face-mask ventilation and possible difficult direct laryngoscopy and tracheal intubation in severe case of macroglossia. Blood sugar level should be monitored and intravenous dextrose may be required to avoid hypoglycemia.

Pharmacological implications: The use of antibiotics for endocarditis prophylaxis must be considered.

Other condition to be considered:

☞**BECKWITH-WIEDEMANN SYNDROME:** Sporadic syndrome characterized by exomphalos, macroglossia, gigantism, and hypoglycemia as a consequence of hyperinsulinism.

REFERENCES:

Neri G, Gurrieri F, Zanni G, et al: Clinical and molecular aspects of the Simpson-Golabi-Behmel syndrome. *Am J Med Genet* 79:279, 1998.

Tsuchiya K, Takahata O, Sengoku K, et al: Anesthetic management in a patient with Simpson-Golabi-Behmel syndrome. *Masui* 50:1106, 2001.

Singleton-Merten Syndrome

At a glance: Heterogenous syndrome characterized by the association of familial aortic stenosis, calcifications of the aorta, aortic and mitral valves anomalies and osteoporosis. There is an increased globulin levels with immunologic disorders.

Synonym: Merten-Singleton Syndrome.

Incidence: No epidemiological studies have been reported for this very rare condition.

Genetic inheritance: Thought to be autosomal dominant.

Pathophysiology: Linear calcification of the ascending aorta and severe calcific mixed aortic valve disease (stenotic and regurgitant). Associated with increased globulin levels, a lambda-chain gammopathy, and increased T4:T8 lymphocyte ratio. Histology shows extensive medial necrosis of the proximal aorta and its branches with secondary plaques of calcium confined to those areas. No evidence of previous inflammation or destructive/reparative processes.

Diagnosis: Clinical findings consistent with aortic stenosis, possibly associated with mild regurgitation and left ventricular hypertrophy. ECG may show left ventricular hypertrophy, left axis deviation, or left bundle branch block. Radiographic examination characteristically shows severe tubular calcification of the ascending aorta and aortic valve. Cases described have not shown aortic dilatation. Echocardiographic and cardiac catheter studies may reveal the aortic stenosis and regurgitation across a tricuspid aortic valve. History, examination, and investigations must exclude other causes of aortitis and aortic calcification, for example, syphilis, arthrosclerosis, rheumatoid arthritis, and ankylosing spondylitis. Immunologic findings as above. The Singleton-Merten syndrome is also described as showing ascending aortic calcification and aortic valve disease developing in childhood, but is characterized by dental dysplasia and osteoporosis.

Clinical aspects: Cardiac murmur detected in first or second decades of life. Features of aortic stenosis and radiographic evidence of calcification seen from second decade. Progressive course with eventual need for aortic valve replacement.

Precautions before anesthesia: Obtain full cardiac history, particularly with regard to heart failure, syncope, and chest pain. Evaluate ECG for evidence of left ventricular hypertrophy and bundle branch block. Review chest radiograph for evidence of aortic calcification, ventricular dilatation, and pulmonary congestion. Echocardiography to assess aortic valve gradient and left ventricular function. Review cardiac catheter studies if available.

Anesthetic considerations: Those pertinent to aortic stenosis and/or regurgitation. Bacterial endocarditis prophylaxis necessary.

Pharmacological implications: Caution with use of intravenous induction agents in presence of decreased cardiac output. Circulation time may be prolonged. Avoid excessive decreases in systemic vascular resistance in presence of relatively fixed cardiac output across a stenotic valve.

Other conditions to be considered:

CALCIFIC AORTIC STENOSIS: A rare complication of aortic sclerosis that occurs as a consequence of aging, affecting approximately 2 to 3% of those older than 75 years of age. Narrowing of the aortic orifice because of calcification of the valvular ring. May occur in an idiopathic form without any predisposing conditions in the elderly. However, because aortic sclerosis is a common problem in the general population, the overall number of patients with calcific aortic stenosis is rather high.

CALCIFIED ASCENDING AORTA: A common complication of familial hypercholesterolemia.

☞WILLIAM SYNDROME: A development disorder affecting vascular, connective tissue, and the central nervous system. Leads to a polymalformative syndrome with elfin-like facies, mental retardation, and supravalvular aortic stenosis. It is caused by a microdeletion in the elastin gene in the long arm of chromosome 7 (7q11.23), and can lead to a partial monosomy 7q11.23 in 26% of patients

REFERENCES:

Tentolouris C, Kontozoglou T, Toutouzas P: Familial calcification of aorta and calcific aortic valve disease associated with immunologic abnormalities. *Am Heart J* 126:904, 1993.

Theman TE, Silver MD, Haust MD, et al: Morphological findings in idiopathic calcification of the ascending aorta and aortic valve disease affecting a young woman. *Histopathology* 3:181, 1979.

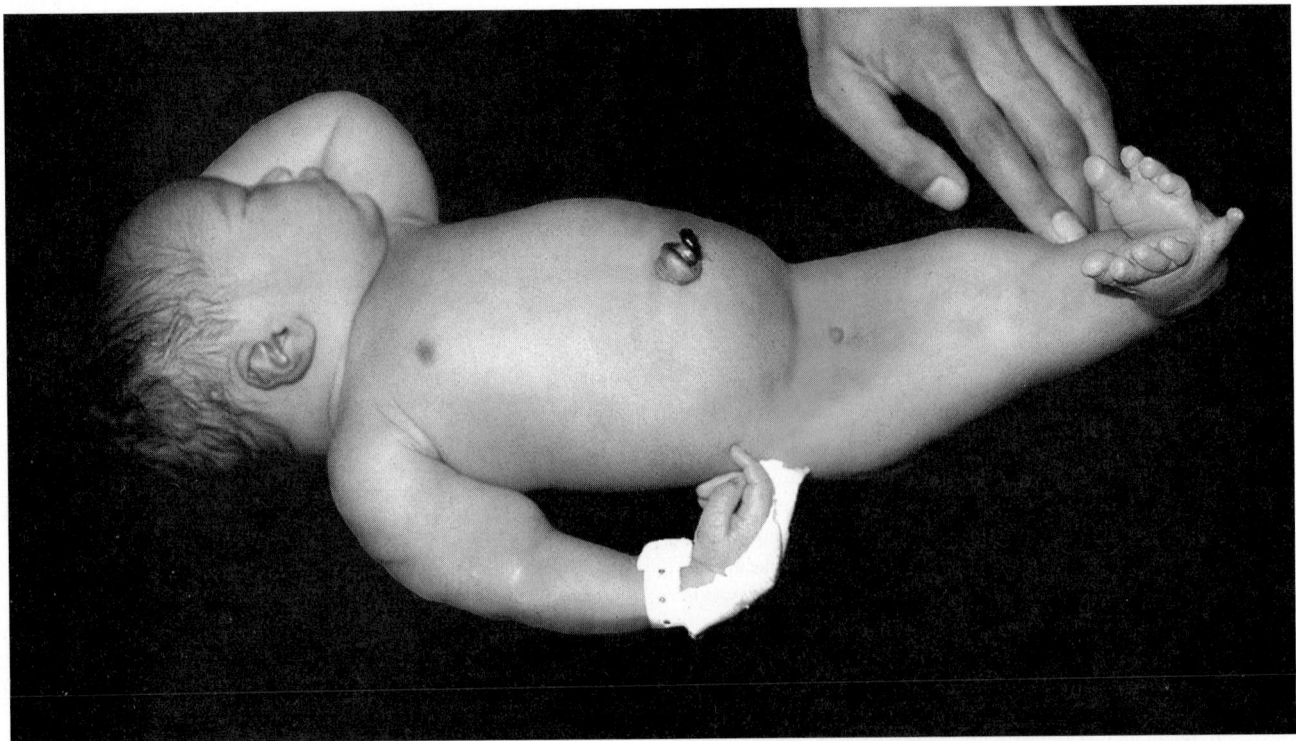

Sirenomelia The anomaly in this newborn with a single, fused, lower extremity is called sirenomelia.

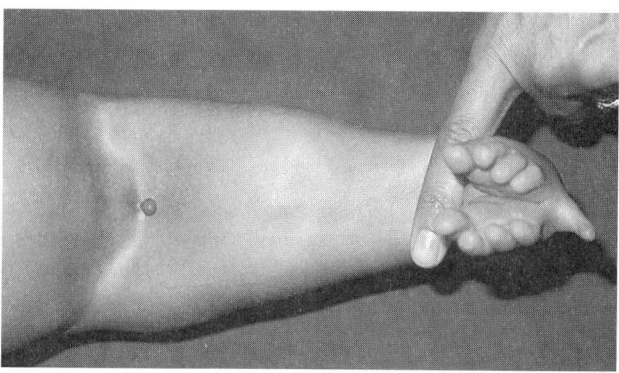

Sirenomelia The pelvis and the lower extremity of the same patient. Note the absence of the external genitalia.

Sirenomelia

At a glance: Congenital disorder characterized by a single lower extremity. Only one case of a living child described.

Synonym: Mermaid Malformation.

Classification: Sirenomelia is classified into three types:
- –*Simpus Apus:* absence of feet, one tibia, one femur
- –*Simpus Unipus:* One foot, two femur, two tibia, two fibula
- –*Simpus Dipus:* two feet and two fused legs (flipper-like), which is called a "mermaid".

Incidence: Sirenomelia has a prevalence of two to three cases per 100,000 births. The male-to-female ratio is 3:1. About 300 cases have been reported in the world literature, eight in india.

Genetic inheritance: Genetic mapping is not known. Incidence is increased in monozygotic twins, making a genetic mechanism possible to discuss.

Pathophysiology: Etiology is unknown, with a male:female ratio of 2.7:1. An aberrant vascular supply, leading to "vitelline artery steal" has been evoked (persistence of the vitelline artery leads to abnormal aortic development with curtailment of blood flow to the lower extremities). Some other theories include posterior axial mesodermal defect, teratogenic effect, axial mesodermal dysplasia sequence, and midline development at field defect. Some of the manifestations have been related to oligohydramnios and vascular insufficiency.

Diagnosis: Sirenomelia sequence is a birth defect in which affected infants are born with a single lower extremity or with two legs that are fused together.

Clinical aspects: In a case of live birth, the treatment is supportive and the prognosis is very poor, with the baby succumbing in the early neonatal period. Common associated malformations include absent external genitalia, imperforate anus, renal agenesis, and lumbosacral, vertebral, and pelvic abnormalities. Sirenomelia with craniorachischisis totalis has also been described.

Anesthetic considerations: Only one debatable case of a living child described. Probably evaluate renal function and ensure proper intraoperative fluid regimen. Renal elimination of administered drugs can be severely affected. Avoid perimedullar blockade.

Other condition to be considered:

Caudal Regression Syndrome (Sacral Agenesis Syndrome): Characterized by an abnormal development of the caudal part of the spine. Clinical features include absence or underdevelopment of the lower vertebrae, pelvis, and coccyx, paralysis or paresis of the legs, anal and urinary problems, hip dislocation and/or fixation, muscle atrophy, clubfoot, polycystic kidneys, and hypospadias in the male. Other less frequent anomalies include hydrocephaly, hypopituitarism, cleft lip/palate, micrognathia, congenital heart defects, and polysyndactyly. Renal function must be evaluated before anesthesia. There are no specific causes that have been determined;

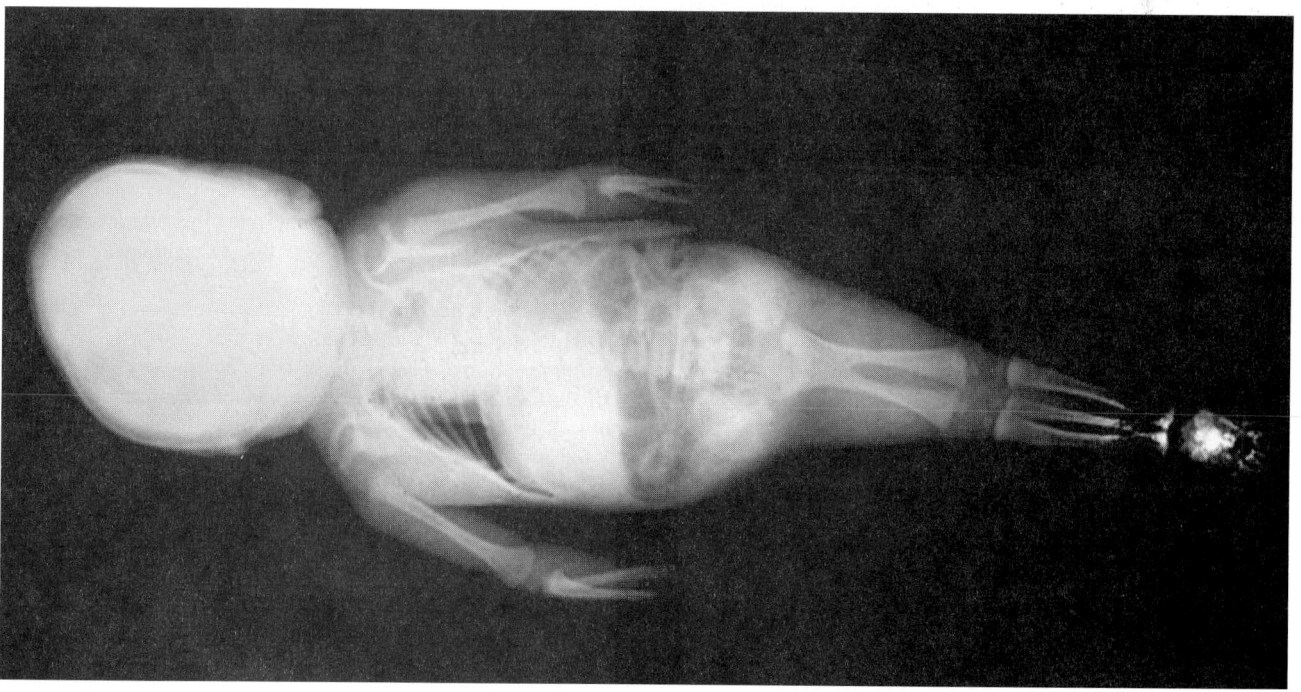

Sirenomelia This whole-body radiograph of the same baby shows partial fusion of the femora in the proximal third, whereas the bones of the lower leg are fused in the distal third.

however, 60% of individuals affected with this disorder had diabetic mothers. An autosomal dominant inheritance has been suggested in few cases.

REFERENCE:
Stevenson RE, Jones KL, Phelan MC, et al: Vascular steal. The pathogenetic mechanism producing sirenomelia and associated defects of viscera and soft tissue. *Pediatrics* 78:451, 1986.

Situs Inversus

At a glance: Congenital condition caused by malrotation of viscera in utero. Can be classified further into situs inversus with dextrocardia or situs inversus with levocardia. The classification is independent of the cardiac apical position. The association of situs inversus and ciliary dyskinesia is known as the Kartagener syndrome.

Incidence: Present in 0.01% of the population. Patients present a normal life expectancy. In the rare instance of cardiac anomalies, the life expectancy is determined by the heart condition and not the presence of a situs inversus. The male:female ratio is 1:1.

Genetic inheritance: Autosomal recessive inheritance and congenital anomalies.

Pathophysiology: Unknown. Abnormal rotation of the viscera in utero results in the orientation of the lungs and abdominal organs being reversed. Dextrocardia may or may not be present. The occurrence of situs inversus viscerum with levocardia is associated with severe congenital heart disease.

Diagnosis: Radiological and echographic demonstration of abnormal orientation of organs with or without dextrocardia.

Clinical aspects: Situs inversus may remain asymptomatic throughout life, with little impact on cardiorespiratory function. Situs inversus is a feature of Kartagener syndrome, asplenia syndrome, and polysplenia syndrome. Clinical features of these medical conditions may therefore be present. Congenital heart disease described with situs inversus includes ventricular septal defect, atrial septal defect, transposition of the great arteries, and conotruncal malformations.

Precautions before anesthesia: Examine for features of Kartagener syndrome (increased risk of pneumonia and perioperative respiratory embarrassment). Consider chest radiograph. Full cardiac evaluation, including history, examination, ECG, and echocardiography if congenital heart disease is present. Cardiac catheter data as indicated clinically.

Anesthetic considerations: Anesthetic technique dictated by presence or absence of cardiac disease. If part of Kartagener syndrome, a technique to maximize ability to clear secretions and early use of physiotherapy postoperatively should be considered.

Pharmacological implications: There are no known specific implications with this condition.

Other conditions to be considered:

SITUS AMBIGUOUS: When the situs orientation cannot be determined, the patient has situs ambiguous or heterotaxy. The liver may be midline, the spleen absent or multiple, the axial morphology unclear, and the bowel malrotated. Two primary subtypes include: right isomerism or asplenia syndrome, and left isomerism or polysplenia syndrome.

☞**KARTAGENER SYNDROME:** The association of situs inversus and ciliary dyskinesia is known as the Kartagener syndrome.

Genetically transmitted polymalformative syndrome characterized by bronchiectasis, situs inversus, and chronic sinusitis. Twenty percent of patients with situs inversus are affected with Kartagener syndrome.

REFERENCES:
Mathew PJ, Sadera GS, Sharafuddin S, Pandit B. Anaesthetic considerations in Kartagener's syndrome—a case report. *Acta Anaesthesiol Scand* 48:518, 2004.
Sahajananda H, Sanjay OP, Thomas J, Daniel B: General anaesthesia for lobectomy in an 8-year-old child with Kartagener's syndrome. *Paediatr Anaesth* 13:714, 2003.

Sjögren Larsson Syndrome (SLS)

At a glance: Rare inborn error of lipid metabolism, characterized by congenital ichthyosis, mental retardation, and spasticity.

Synonyms: Fatty Acid Alcohol Oxidoreductase Deficiency; FAO Deficiency; Fatty Aldehyde Dehydrogenase Deficiency; FALDH Deficiency; SLS.

Incidence: There are no epidemiological studies reported for SLS, however, it has been demonstrated that in regions where there is a significant consanguinity within the population, SLS is much more common (e.g., in the Haliwas of Halifax and Warren Counties in North Carolina). Internationally, the same pattern is reproduced in populations where consanguineous marriages are noted (e.g., Vasterbotten and Norrbotten County in Sweden). In these two regions, it has been discovered that a mutation was introduced around the 13th century. The prevalence of patients with SLS in northern Sweden is 8.3 cases per 100,000 births, whereas the prevalence of heterozygotes is 2% and the gene frequency is 0.01%. The overall incidence in Sweden is estimated to be around 0.6 cases per 100,000 births. A lower incidence (<1 case per 100,000 births) has been observed worldwide. Sjogren Larsson Syndrome is estimated at 1:1000 patients with mental retardation and in 1:2500 pediatric dermatologic patients. It is not a fatal medical condition because most patients do not show a progressive neurodegenerative course. There is no apparent racial predilection as well as no sexual predilection. Onset is in the newborn period, when symptoms usually begin and the first signs of the disease (first ichthyosis, subsequent neurologic symptoms) appear. The latter form of the disease develops in patients aged 4–30 months.

Genetic inheritance: Autosomal recessive; gene mapped on 17p11.2; multiple allelic variants exist.

Pathophysiology: Caused by a deficiency in fatty alcohol oxidoreductase, which catalyzes the oxidation of medium-chain and long-chain fatty acids.

Diagnosis: The disorder begins at birth with generalized ichthyosis and erythroderma. As the child ages, the scale becomes darker without erythema and is more pronounced around the umbilicus, neck, and flexures, typically sparing the face.

Clinical aspects: Clinical features involve *skin* (dry skin, ichthyosis, diffuse increased skin pigmentation, urticaria) and central nervous system (spastic diplegia or tetraplegia, scissor gait, seizures, mental retardation, speech deficits). Kyphosis, pigmentary retinal degeneration, and short stature are frequently associated.

Precautions before anesthesia: Evaluate neurological function (clinical, CT/MRI scan, electroencephalography).

Anesthetic considerations: Regional anesthesia can be difficult because of kyphosis and skin lesions that can be superinfected. Venous access can be achieved generally without difficulty because skin lesions are generally spare on the dorsum of the hands and feet.

Pharmacological implications: Consider interaction between antiepileptic treatment and anesthetic drugs.

REFERENCES:

Fernandez-Vozmediano JM, Armario-Hita JC, Gonzalez-Cabrerizo A: Sjögren-Larsson syndrome: Treatment with topical calcipotriol. *Pediatr Dermatol* 20(2):179, 2003.

Rizzo WB, Carney G, Lin Z: The molecular basis of Sjögren-Larsson syndrome: Mutation analysis of the fatty aldehyde dehydrogenase gene. *Am J Hum Genet* 65:1547, 1999.

Van Mieghem F, Van Goethem JW, Parizel PM, et al: MR of the brain in Sjögren-Larsson syndrome. *AJNR Am J Neuroradiol* 18:1561, 1997.

Willemsen MA, Ijlst L, Steijlen PM, et al: Clinical, biochemical and molecular genetic characteristics of 19 patients with the Sjögren-Larsson syndrome. *Brain* 124(pt 7):1426, 2001.

Sjögren Syndrome

At a glance: Frequent autosomal recessive disorder characterized by dysfunction and destruction of exocrine glands. Neurological and immunological function could be involved. Humidification of mucous membrane must be rigorous during anesthetic procedure.

Synonyms: Sjögren-Gougerot Syndrome; Sicca Syndrome; Gougerot-Houwer-Sjögren Syndrome; Arthro-Oculosalivary Syndrome.

Incidence: 1 to 3% in general population (primary syndrome). Genetic disorder that mostly affects women (female:male ratio is 9:1).

Genetic inheritance: Autosomal recessive.

Pathophysiology: Strong association with HLA-Dw3 and HLA-Dw4. Because of the significant infiltration of the lacrymal and salivary glands with lymphocytes, acetylcholine activation does not lead to eccrine secretion.

Diagnosis: Sjögren syndrome is characterized by dysfunction and destruction of the exocrine glands, associated with lymphocytes infiltrates and immunological hyperreactivity. These include the affirmation of subjective complaints about oral and/or eye dryness, the objective evidence of salivary gland and/or ocular involvement (lymphocytic infiltrative lesions in the salivary glands), as well as of autoimmune reactivity. Presence of serum autoantibodies against Ro and La.

Clinical aspects: Generally, the syndrome has an indolent or slowly progressive course with the disease confined to the exocrine glands. In 30% of patients, general signs occur, which can involve neurological function (abnormal gait, autonomic dysfunction, seizures, movement disorder, ataxia/incoordination, insensitivity to pain, hyperreflexia, and even paraparesis or quadriparesis), immunological disorder (immune system anomalies, dysfunction autoimmunity), pharyngeal abnormality, respiratory tract modification (interstitial-like disease), chronic atrophic gastritis, celiac-like disease, distal renal tubular acidosis, Raynaud phenomenon (35% of cases), and other skin anomalies. Lymphoma and mortality are higher in these patients. All of these general signs are usually moderate. Secondary Sjögren syndrome occurs in 10 to 20% of patients with Rheumatoid Arthritis, Systemic Lupus Erythematosus, and Scleroderma. Various other diseases can imitate this syndrome, including Sarcoidosis, Lipoproteinemia, and Amyloidosis.

Precautions before anesthesia: A complete medical history, i.e., evolution of the disease and symptomatology, as well as a thorough physical examination is important. An abdominal and renal echography, chest radiograph, and laboratory investigation may be indicated.

Anesthetic considerations: Prevent a keratoconjunctivitis with strict ocular protection and regular corneal humidification. Avoid respiratory dryness using humidified fresh gases. The administration of anesthetic agents, hypnotics and local anesthetics must be done slowly and in presence of blood pressure monitoring because of the possibility of autonomic nervous system dysfunction.

Pharmacological implications: Patient receiving chronic therapy must continue the medication until the morning of surgery. Avoid parasympatholytic and anticholinergic drugs because of decrease in gland secretions.

Other conditions to be considered:

MIKULICZ SYNDROME (Mikulicz-Radecki Syndrome; Mikulicz-Sjögren Syndrome; von Mikulicz Syndrome; Mikulicz-Gougerot-Sjögren Syndrome) presents with hypertrophic salivary and lacrimal glands, especially the parotids. The association of lacrimal gland and parotid gland enlargements, dry mouth, and dry eyes are the classic signs of this condition. The tonsils and other glands in the soft tissue of the face and neck may also be involved. It always occurs in association with another underlying disorder such as tuberculosis, leukemia, syphilis, Hodgkin disease, lymphosarcoma, Sjögren syndrome, or lupus erythematous. The incidence for lymphoma is significantly higher in the individuals affected with this disorder. Some patients may experience recurring fevers associated with dry eyes because of diminished tear production, and uveitis. There are suggestions that Mikulicz syndrome should be considered a form of Sjögren syndrome.

DRY EYE SYNDROME (Keratoconjuctivitis Sicca; Xerophthalmia; Keratitis Sicca): Characterized by a persistent dryness of the cornea and conjunctiva because of decreased function of the lacrymal glands. The cornea may be thickened and visual acuity decreased. Dry eye syndrome usually occurs in people who are otherwise healthy. It is more common with older age, because tear production decreases with age. In rare cases, it can be associated with rheumatoid arthritis, lupus erythematosus, and it may also be caused by thermal or chemical burns.

REFERENCES:

Lichtenfeld JL, Kirschner RH, Wiernick PH: Familial Sjögren syndrome with associated primary salivary gland lymphoma. *Am J Med* 60:286, 1976.

Zoukhri D, Kublin CL: Impaired neurotransmitter release from lacrimal and salivary gland nerves of a murine model of Sjögren syndrome. *Invest Ophthalmol Vis Sci* 42:925, 2001.

Smith-Lemli-Opitz Syndrome

At a glance: A syndrome characterized by the inability to make cholesterol. Affects the central nervous system (CNS) (white matter) and characterized by growth retardation, developmental delay, severe dysphagia, microcephaly, micrognathia, cleft palate, cataracts, ptosis, polysyndactyly and syndactyly of the second and third toes, and congenital heart defects (transposition of the great vessels is frequent). Congestive heart failure and liver failure are not uncommon.

Synonyms: RSH Syndrome; SLOS I Syndrome; 7-Dehydrocholesterol Reductase Deficiency.

Incidence: 1:20,000 to 1:60,000 live births in the United States among white people. Smith-Lemli-Opitz syndrome is uncommon in Hispanic population. Carrier frequency for Smith-Lemli-Opitz syndrome is approximately 1 in 30 in individuals of northern European descent, suggesting a disease incidence between 1:5000 and 1:18,000 in Europe. Internationally, Smith-Lemli-Opitz syndrome has been described in patients from the United States, Japan, South America, and Canada.

Genetic inheritance: Results from a mutation in either the DHCR7 (7-dehydrocholesterol-delta7-reductase) gene on chromosome 11 or the SLOS gene on chromosome 7. Autosomal recessive inheritance.

Pathophysiology: The classic paradigm is an inborn error of metabolism, which includes the accumulation of a toxic precursor (7DHC) leading to the deficiency in production of an essential product (cholesterol). The absence in cholesterol can be implicated in the production of all the anomalies described. Cholesterol is required for normal development because of its involvement in cell and mitochondrial membranes, as well as steroid metabolism and myelination.

Diagnosis: As a result of the defect in cholesterol metabolism, serum cholesterol levels are very low and levels of 7-dehydrocholesterol (a cholesterol precursor) are high in serum as well as any other tissue specimens. This biochemical finding associated with the clinical findings confirms the diagnosis of Smith-Lemli-Opitz syndrome. The mortality/morbidity is associated with stillbirths, or spontaneous abortion, or immediately after birth from multiorgan failure (during the first week of life). Causes of death include pneumonia, lethal congenital heart defect (most often transposition of the great vessels), congestive heart failure (not uncommon), and hepatic failure.

Clinical aspects: Prognosis is poor. *Neuromuscular:* initially hypotonia followed later by hypertonia; mental deficiency can be severe (IQ as low as 20); seizures and generalized nerve demyelination. *Cardiovascular:* malformations may be present in up to 44% of cases. The incidence of atrioventricular canal defects and anomalous pulmonary venous drainage is relatively high. *Craniofacial:* microcephaly, strabismus, epicanthic folds, elfin facies, ptosis, low-set ears, and micrognathia may be present. *Genital tract:* Developmental anomalies of the genital tract (particularly male) are common. *Gastrointestinal/Nutrition:* feeding difficulties and failure to thrive; Hirschsprung Disease may be more common.

Precautions before anesthesia: Cardiac evaluation: echocardiogram to rule out congenital heart disease. Neurological assessment to evaluate degree of disability. Careful airway evaluation in view of micrognathia. The presence of frequent vomiting, feeding difficulties, electrolyte disturbances, and failure to thrive requires complete assessment.

Anesthetic considerations: The presence of muscular hypertonia raises the concern of malignant hyperthermia. Generalized muscle rigidity and hyperthermia have been reported following the use of halothane with and without succinylcholine. However, these episodes were not associated with a mesurable plasmatic increase in creatine kinase and dantrolene was not given. Also, the presence of craniofacial anomalies such as micrognathia contribute to make airway management difficult. Until proven otherwise, maintenance of spontaneous ventilation is recommended until trachea is intubated and lung ventilation confirmed. A laryngeal mask airway should be available in case of failure to ventilate or intubate. The association with congenital heart disease must be carefully evaluated and anesthetic management adjusted accordingly. The use of preoperative sedation in older patients may be useful, especially for individuals affected with mental retardation.

Pharmacological implications: Antiepileptic medications must be continued until the morning of surgery. Endocarditis antibiotic prophylaxis must be considered in the presence of congenital heart disease.

Other conditions to be considered:

☞**RUTLEDGE LETHAL MULTIPLE CONGENITAL ANOMALY SYNDROME:** Polydactyly, ambiguous genitalia, renal hypoplasia, and unilobar lung. Includes mesomelic dwarfism, micrognathia, V-shaped upper lip, early fused fontanelles, clubfeet, microglossia, severe congenital heart defects, cerebellar hypoplasia, and laryngeal hypoplasia.

HYDROLETHALUS SYNDROME: Characterized by polydactyly (preaxial in the hands and postaxial in the feet) and CNS malformation leading to severe hydramnios. The intracerebral ventricles are open to the subarachnoid space (encephalocele) leading to external hydrocephalus. The foramen magnum is keyhole shaped. Severe micrognathia and presence of hypoplastic eyes.

☞**PALLISTER-HALL SYNDROME:** A syndrome of hypothalamic hamartoblastoma, craniofacial abnormalities, polydactyly, and endocrine (thyroid and adrenal dysplasia with severe hypoadrenalism and hypothyroidism), cardiac (patent ductus arteriosus, ventricular septal defect, atrial septal defect, mitral and aortic valve defects, coarctation of the aorta), respiratory (lung hypoplasia or dysplasia, laryngeal cleft, dysplastic epiglottis), and renal (kidney dysplasia) defects. Mild mental retardation in some cases.

☞**ULLRICH-FEICHTIGER SYNDROME:** A congenital syndrome characterized by an association of micrognathia, ocular, dental, and genital malformations. Other clinical features include deafness, rudimentary toes, clubfoot, partial atresia of the anus, hypospadias, and mask-like facies. The entity of this syndrome as a variant of Smith-Lemli-Opitz syndrome has been suggested by a number of authors.

☞**MECKEL-GRUBER SYNDROME:** Characterized by polydactyly and CNS malformation (severe hydrocephalus), cystic kidney, and liver failure.

REFERENCES:

Jones KL: Smith-Lemli-Opitz syndrome, in Jones KL (ed): *Smith's Recognizable Patterns of Human Malformation.* 5th ed. Philadelphia, WB Saunders, 1997, p 112.

Lin A, Ardinger H, Ardinger R, et al: Cardiovascular malformations in Smith-Lemli-Opitz syndrome. *Am J Med Genet* 68:270, 1997.

Petersen W, Crouch ER Jr: Anesthesia-induced rigidity, unrelated to succinylcholine, associated with Smith-Lemli-Opitz syndrome and malignant hyperthermia. *Anesth Analg* 80:606, 1995.

Smith-Magenis Syndrome

At a glance: A syndrome of multiple congenital anomalies characterized by midface hypoplasia, broad face, hearing loss (conductive and/or sensorineural), congenital heart defect, hypothyroidism, severe scoliosis, brachydactyly, and decreased pain sensitivity but peripheral neuropathy.

Synonym: SMS.

Incidence: Incidence estimated to be 1:25,000 live births.

Genetic inheritance: Anomaly caused by a chromosomal microdeletion (17p11.2) rather than a mutation. Many of the characteristics of this clinical entity may be a result of a disruption of the RAI1 gene.

Pathophysiology: Twelve genes have been identified within the deleted 17p11.2 region. The significance of the absence of these genes remains to be clarified, although single abnormalities of some of these genes give rise to distinct syndromes. In some series of patients, elevations of low-density lipoproteins are reported, suggesting that deletion of the sterol regulatory element binding protein (SREBF1) may play a role. Because this disorder is because of deletion in the area of chromosome 17, where a form of Charcot-Marie-Tooth maps, it has been suggested that the association of peripheral neuropathy and Smith-Magenis syndrome should be considered a contiguous gene syndrome.

Diagnosis: Diagnosis is based on the clinical phenotype and is confirmed by high-resolution cytogenetic studies.

Clinical aspects: All patients have a characteristic facial appearance (brachycephaly, midface hypoplasia, prominent forehead, broad nasal bridge) and a degree of mental retardation. Delayed speech development, hoarse voice, ocular abnormalities (strabismus, myopia, microcornea, iris anomalies, cataracts, optic nerve hypoplasia, and retinal detachment) and a peripheral neuropathy are common. Sleep disorders become more common during childhood. Decreased or absent rapid eye movement (REM) sleep has been demonstrated by polysomnography. The syndrome is classically associated with aggressive outbursts, attention-deficit, attention-seeking behaviors, and self-harm. However, these patients are eager to please and respond well to adult attention. A history of infantile hypotonia is often present. Scoliosis is common (65% of patients). Less-common findings are congenital heart disease (37% of patients), major urogenital anomalies (35% of patients), hypothyroidism (29% of patients), immunoglobulin deficiencies (23% of patients), and cleft lip/palate (9% of patients). Behavioral and sleep disturbances may respond to treatment with carbamazepine or selective serotonin reuptake inhibitors.

Precautions before anesthesia: Obtain history of developmental milestones, abnormal behavior patterns, and current medical management. Examine for evidence of congenital heart disease, renal disease, and hypothyroidism. Assess severity and extent of the peripheral neuropathy. Carefully assess airway. Cardiovascular assessment, ECG, and echocardiography are essential if congenital heart disease is suspected. Consider formal assessment of lung function and chest radiograph in the presence of severe scoliosis. Laboratory investigations: consider assessing renal function and thyroid function.

Anesthetic considerations: Premedication may be desirable in view of behavioral problems. Excessive skin folds on the arms may make intravenous access difficult. The presence of congenital heart disease dictates the anesthetic technique. If regional anesthesia is considered, the extent of the peripheral neuropathy should be documented preoperatively.

Pharmacological implications: Succinylcholine should be considered relatively contraindicated in the presence of neonatal hypotonia.

REFERENCES:

Chen R, Lupski J, Greenberg F, et al: Ophthalmic manifestations of the Smith-Magenis syndrome. *Ophthalmology* 103(7):732, 1996.

Smith A, Dykens E, Greenberg F: Behavioral phenotype of Smith-Magenis syndrome (del 17p11.2). *Am J Med Genet* 81:179, 1998.

Smith A, Dykens E, Greenberg F: Sleep disturbance in Smith-Magenis syndrome (del 17p11.2). *Am J Med Genet* 81:186, 1998.

Sneddon Syndrome

At a glance: A very rare progressive disorder affecting blood vessels and characterized by multiple cerebrovascular accidents and the presence of idiopathic livedo reticularis.

Synonyms: Livedo Reticularis and Cerebrovascular Accidents; Sneddon-Champion Syndrome.

History: A genetic disorder first described by Ian Bruce Sneddon, British dermatologist in 1965.

Genetic inheritance: Autosomal dominant.

Pathophysiology: May be a particular form of obliterating vasculitis or of an antiphospholipid antibodies syndrome.

Diagnosis: Clinically evocated in patients combining livedo reticularis and neurological signs. Skin biopsies can be contributive (arterial intimal hyperplasia).

Clinical aspects: Onset possible in childhood. A delay from months to years is possible between skin and neurological lesions. Features can involve *skin* (livedo reticularis with no infiltration, and affecting the limbs, trunk, and sometimes the face), central nervous system (cerebrovascular accidents, epilepsy, vertigo, and sometimes pseudobulbar syndrome, chorea, episodes of amnesia, or transient amaurosis), and *cardiovascular system* (occlusive noninflammatory arteriopathy; arteriography can show multiple occlusions in medium-sized arteries; CT scan can show defect corresponding to infarct). Laboratory investigations can find antiphospholipid antibodies, anticardiolipin antibody, lupus anticoagulant.

Precautions before anesthesia: Evaluate neurological function (clinical, history, EEG, CT/MRI scan). The cardiovascular function must be systematically evaluated to eliminate the presence of systemic arteries obliteration that have been described.

Anesthetic considerations: Blood pressure control is necessary and may require invasive monitoring. Regional anesthesia is not contraindicated but benefit (particularly of central blockade) has to be clearly established.

Pharmacological implications: Consider interaction between antiepileptic treatment and anesthetic drugs.

REFERENCES:

Boesch SM, Plorer AL, Auer AJ, et al: The natural course of Sneddon syndrome: Clinical and magnetic resonance imaging findings in a prospective six-year observation study. *J Neurol Neurosurg Psychiatry* 74(4):542, 2003.

Bruyn RPM, van der Veen JPW, Donker AJM, et al: Sneddon's syndrome: Case report and literature review. *J Neurol Sci* 79:243, 1987.

Heesen M, Rossaint R: Anaesthesiological considerations in patients with Sneddon's syndrome. *Paediatr Anaesth* 10(6):678, 2000.

Sotos Syndrome

At a glance: Characterized by excessively rapid growth during the first year of life, acromegalic craniocerebral features (macrocephaly, prominent forehead) and a nonprogressive cerebral disorder with mental retardation. Other clinical features include high-arched palate and prognathism with premature eruption of teeth, hypotonia, hyper- or hypothyroidism, and delayed motor and cognitive development.

Synonym: Cerebral Gigantism Syndrome.

History: First described by Juan Fernandez Sotos, American pediatrician in 1964.

Incidence: Uncommon. About 150 cases reported. Affects males and females equally.

Genetic inheritance: Autosomal dominant—5q35 or 15q22 have been suggested as the gene locus. Occurs also sporadically.

Pathophysiology: Caused by a mutation in the NSD1 gene. Possibly prenatal abnormality or yet unidentified growth-stimulating factor.

Diagnosis: Clinical based on facial gestalt, growth pattern, bone age, and developmental delay. Typical abnormalities of the brain on the MRI scan, including absence of the corpus callosum. The most common abnormalities of the cerebral ventricle are prominence of the trigone (90%), occipital horns (75%), and ventriculomegaly (60%).

Clinical aspects: Prenatal onset of excessive growth. Birth weight and length usually greater than 90th percentile. Large hands and feet at birth. Neonatal problems with feeding and respiration. Rapid early growth, arm span greater than height, and advanced osseous maturation. Normal levels of growth hormone. Scoliosis. Macrocephaly, prominent forehead, strabismus, hypertelorism, high-arched palate, alveolar ridge exostoses, early teeth, and prominent jaw. Developmental and mental retardation, neonatal hypotonia, and seizures. Significant behavioral problems. Abnormal glucose tolerance test; hyper- and hypothyroidism. Normal growth hormone. Congenital cardiac defects; increased risk for tumors.

Precautions before anesthesia: Assessment of severity of syndrome with particular consideration of airway and endocrine abnormalities—all children should have endocrine assessment and exclusion of glucose intolerance and thyroid dysfunction. Assessment of associated abnormalities such as cardiac or scoliosis, including investigations and appropriate referrals.

Anesthetic considerations: A major problem with these children is the high rate of behavioral disorder with hyperactive and aggressive behavior. Premedication is recommended and is well tolerated orally. Parental presence has been required despite premedication to control some of these children for induction. Although there are no reports of difficult tracheal intubation, it should be anticipated because of the presence of significant macroglossia. Spontaneous respiration should be maintained until confirmation that assisted ventilation is possible or tracheal intubation is achieved. Endocrine (thyroid function) and cardiac considerations if appropriate. Patient may require intraoperative glucose monitoring.

Pharmacological implications: Relative resistance to premedication has been reported. If a difficult tracheal intubation is predicted, nondepolarizing agents should not be used for induction. Endocrine management may be required. Prophylactic antibiotics may be indicated.

Other condition to be considered:

☞**CRAMER NIEDERDELLMANN SYNDROME:** A very rare syndrome combining cerebral gigantism and basal cell nevi (pigmented nevi), jaw cysts, macrocephaly, mild hydrocephalus, intracranial calcification, and EEG abnormalities.

REFERENCES:

Adhami EJ, Cancio-Babu CV: Anaesthesia in a child with Sotos syndrome. *Paediatr Anaesth* 13:835, 2003.

Jones KL: Sotos Syndrome, in Jones KL (ed): *Smith's Recognisable Patterns of Human Malformations.* 5th ed. Philadelphia, WB Sauders, 1997, p 128-129.

Suresh D: Posterior spinal fusion in Soto's syndrome. *Br J Anaesth* 66(6):728, 1991.

Varvinski A, McGill FJ, Judd V, Hodzovic I: Sotos' syndrome . . . a rare challenge? *Anaesthesia* 56:809, 2001.

Spastic Diplegia of Infancy

At a glance: A very rare syndrome combining mental retardation and early spastic diplegia.

Incidence and genetic inheritance: Incidence is unknown. Autosomal recessive inheritance.

Clinical aspects: Affected patient presents with spastic diplegia in early infancy. Motor development is slow and there is generalized muscular hypotonia and hyperreflexia. Ataxia is usually absent but gait is often waddling with inward-turning feet. There is mild to moderate mental retardation with slow speech development. Long-term followup has not been reported.

Anesthetic considerations: Assess gait and motor function. Obtain history of previous anesthetics and muscle biopsy result if available. Biochemistry including potassium and creatine phosphokinase level. Careful intraoperative positioning is needed.

REFERENCE:

Gustavson K, Modrzewska K, Erikson A: Hereditary spastic diplegia with mental retardation in two young siblings. *Clin Genet* 36:439, 1989.

Spina Bifida

At a glance: Congenital defect of spine and spinal cord.

Incidence: Approximately 1:1000 live births. Risk in a subsequent sibling is 3 to 4% and up to 10% with two previously affected siblings.

Genetic inheritance: Unclear. Genetic predisposition is clearly seen in the increased incidence among siblings, but nutritional and environmental factors also have a role in the pathogenesis.

Pathophysiology: Arises from the failure of the fetal neural tube to close within the first 3 weeks of gestation. This leads to the incomplete fusion of the posterior lamina and spines of the vertebral column, most commonly in the lumbosacral segments. The underlying spinal cord tissue may also have developmental abnormalities, including syringomyelia, diastematomyelia, and a tethered cord.

Diagnosis: Clinical and radiological features. Investigation of the abnormal spine includes plain radiograph, CT scan, and MRI with or without contrast. CT scan of head is also recommended to assess the presence of hydrocephalus and other neural abnormalities. Prenatal diagnosis can be made by demonstration of the defect on ultrasonography and the detection of alpha-fetoprotein in amniotic fluid. Alpha-fetoprotein in maternal serum is an effective test for screening in high-risk patient.

Clinical aspects: In *Spina Bifida Occulta*, there is a midline defect of the spinal column without protrusion of the spinal cord or meninges. Most affected individuals are asymptomatic and lack neurological signs. In some cases, it may be associated with patches of hair, a lipoma, discoloration of the skin, or a dermal sinus in the midline of the low back. In meningocele, the meninges herniate through the defect, but the spinal cord assumes normal position in the spinal canal. The spinal cord may or may not be normal.

In *Meningomyelocele*, various amounts of neural tissue and meninges herniate through the defect to form a sac-like cystic structure covered by a thin layer of skin tissue that may rupture and leak cerebrospinal fluid. Early repair and closure is recommended to reduce the risk of infection and to preserve neurological function. The extent of the neurological deficit depends greatly on the location of the meningomyelocele; it most commonly occurs in the lumbosacral region. The conus medullaris is usually disrupted and abnormal. Clinical features include flaccid paralysis of the lower limbs, absence of deep tendon reflexes, lack of response to touch and pain, and urinary and fecal incontinence. Lesions above T4 generally result in paraplegia, whereas lesions below S1 allow ambulation. Hydrocephalus in association with a type II Arnold-Chiari Malformation occurs in many of these patients. Postural abnormalities of the lower limbs including clubfeet and subluxation of the hip are also common.

Precautions before anesthesia: Obtain a full history, including perinatal history, previous anesthesia and surgical procedures, and any known allergies. Neurological examination to document the motor, sensory, and autonomic functions and the presence of hydrocephalus. Assess presence of coexisting disease. Assess volume status and rehydrate if required.

Anesthetic considerations: For infants who present for meningomyelocele repair, protect the neural sac during induction by positioning in either the left lateral position or supine with the sac protected by a cushioned ring. Prone position during surgery with attention to securing of endotracheal tube and its connections; position the bolster to avoid impeding ventilation; pad bony areas; and avoid pressure on the eye globes. Potential for hypothermia with exposure of large body surface area. Volume status with large third-space fluid loss from the skin defect. Blood loss is difficult to measure and transfusion may be necessary in complex cases, although transfusion is uncommon. Early awakening and extubation to assess postoperative neurological function is desirable. Consider the possibility of latex allergy in children with spina bifida who had multiple surgical procedures and regular home urinary catheterization.

Pharmacological implications: Succinylcholine can be used safely in infants undergoing meningomyelocele repair. Muscle relaxants are usually avoided after tracheal intubation if neuroelectromonitoring, such as nerve stimulation is required during the surgery.

REFERENCES:

Bracco D, Bissonnette B: Neurosurgery and neurotraumatology: Anesthetic considerations and postoperative management, in Bissonnette B, Dalens BD (eds): *Pediatric Anesthesia: Principles and Practice*. New York, McGraw Hill Co, 2002, p 1120.

Singh CV: Anaesthetic management of meningocele and meningomyelocele. *J Indian Med Assoc* 75:130, 1980.

Schroeder HG, Williams NE: Anesthesia for meningomyelocele surgery: Some problems associated with immediate surgical closure in the neonate. *Anesthesia* 21:57, 1966.

Spinal Muscular Atrophy Syndrome

At a glance: Second most common lethal recessive disease in the white population. Neurological disorder (five types) that leads to severe amyotrophy with respiratory insufficiency has been described. Clinical evolution according to the type involved.

Classifications and synonyms:

- Spinal Muscular Atrophy Type I (Werdnig-Hoffman Disease; SMA Infantile Acute form; Infantile SMA)
- Spinal Muscular Atrophy Type II (Dubowitz Disease; Intermediate type of SMA; Infantile Chronic form of SMA)
- Spinal Muscular Atrophy Type III (Juvenile Muscular Atrophy; Childhood-Onset Proximal SMA; ☞Kugelberg Welander Syndrome; Childhood Isolated SMA; Wohlfart-Kugelberg-Welander Syndrome)
- Spinal Muscular Atrophy Type IV (Distal Hereditary Motor Neuropathy; Adult Spinal Muscular Atrophy)
- Spinal Muscular Atrophy Type V or Adult Onset X-Linked SMA (☞Kennedy Syndrome; Bulbospinal Muscular Atrophy)

Incidence: 1:6000 live births.

Genetic inheritance: Autosomal recessive. However, some forms have been suggested to be inherited as autosomal dominant and occasionally X-linked. In adult onset (type IV), the causal gene is located on chromosome 12 (12q24).

Pathophysiology: The disorder is characterized by degeneration and loss of anterior horn cells in the spinal cord and sometimes also in the brainstem, leading to symmetrical muscle weakness and wasting of voluntary muscles. There is evidence that at least two identifiable genes are associated with the disease: SMN1 (survival motor neurone) and NAIP (neuronal apoptosis inhibitory protein), and possibly a third gene, BTF2p44 (basal transcription factor 2H, subunit p44). The SMN gene is missing in the majority of SMA patients and small, intragenic mutations have also been associated with SMA. Approximately half of the severely affected patients are also missing the NAIP gene, which may affect the severity of the disease.

Diagnosis: Clinical features. CT scan and MRI are used to exclude other pathologies. Electromyography usually shows neurogenic and occasional myogenic pattern. Nerve conduction study is normal. Serum creatine kinase is normal. Muscle biopsy shows a large number of round atrophic fibers and clumps of hypertrophic fibers that are type I by ATPase reaction. DNA testing for SMN and NAIP genes is reliable and confirmatory for the phenotype. Prenatal DNA testing is less reliable because a small percentage of population lack an SMN gene but are not clinically affected.

Clinical aspects: Spinal Muscular Atrophy is the second most common lethal autosomal recessive disease in the white population.

Type I (Werdnig-Hoffman Disease): Early onset and diagnosis (before 3 months), with severe intrauterine growth retardation, polyhydramnios, and tongue fasciculations. Child never sits or walks. There is difficulty with swallowing and feeding. Respiratory function is always severely impaired: diaphragmatic breathing, respiratory infection, and distress. Absent deep tendon reflexes, hypotonia, and weakness, but normal intelligence and no sensory loss are observed. Restricted joint mobility and kyphoscoliosis are also frequent. Death before age of 2 years old is common but does not always occur.

Type II (Dubowitz Disease or Chronic form): Intermediate SMA with onset between the age of 3 and 18 months and survival beyond 4 years (usually until adolescence or later). Child often can sit unsupported but never ambulates. Feeding problems, recurrent pulmonary aspiration and pneumonia, and tongue fasciculations occur less often than in type I, but a fine tremor in the outstretched fingers is common.

Type III (Wohlfart-Kugelberg-Welander Disease; Childhood-Onset Proximal SMA): This is a mild, chronic form with onset after the age of 18 months. Typical presentation includes atrophy and weakness of the proximal limb muscles, primarily in the legs, followed by distal involvement. Neurological testing shows hypotonia, decreased or absent deep tendon reflex, muscle fasciculation, and no sensory loss. However, tongue fasciculations are rarely seen. Joint deformities occur secondary to muscle weakness, often with abducted hips and flexed knees. Progressive loss of pulmonary reserve with frequent pulmonary infections is common and respiratory failure is usually the common mode of death. Presentation after 18 months of age. Individuals develop ability to stand and walk but with abnormal gait. Intracardiac arrhythmia can be observed and may require a pacemaker.

Type IV (Adult Onset): Beginning between the end of the fourth and the sixth decades and showing rapid progression without evidence of cortical spinal tract dysfunction. Death from respiratory failure occurs within 2 years of onset.

Type V or Adult-Onset X-Linked SMA (Kennedy Syndrome; Bulbospinal Muscular Atrophy): Occurs only in men, although 50% of female offspring are carriers. This form of SMA is associated with a mutation in the gene that codes for part of the androgen receptor; male presents with gynecomastia. Tongue and facial muscles movement are present.

Other variant types of SMA have also been described, including the Facioscapulohumeral type and the Ryukyuan type.

Precautions before anesthesia: Evaluate the extent of the muscle weakness (clinical, EMG); impact on the respiratory function (clinical, chest radiograph, respiratory function test, arterial blood gas analysis); cardiac function for SMA type III (ECG, Holter, echocardiography); and malnutrition (clinical, albumin). Check blood electrolytes, particularly serum potassium and creatine kinase.

Anesthetic considerations: Respiratory failure is the main concern in these patients because it is the most common complication and eventual cause of death. Elective surgery under general anesthesia is not indicated if respiratory function is severely reduced (usually forced vital capacity [FVC] <25%, peak expiratory flow rate [PEFR] <30%). Elective intensive care unit admission and mechanical support after general anesthesia should be considered for major procedure and/or for patient with poor respiratory reserve. Bulbar involvement is rare with this disorder but represents a potential cause for pulmonary aspiration if present. Hyperkalemia may occur prior to anesthesia as a consequence of continuing muscle wasting and is likely to rise to a dangerous level with the use of suxamethonium. Central neural blockade for peripheral surgery is not advisable in most cases because it may worsen the clinical picture of the disease. It is unclear if epidural analgesia may improve the respiratory function and facilitate earlier extubation. No clear evidence of an association with malignant hyperthermia. Joint deformities may cause difficulty in obtaining intravenous access and positioning of patient.

Pharmacological implications: There is no evidence of an increase risk of malignant hyperthermia (neurological disorder), however, it seems prudent to avoid succinylcholine because of contractures and bone fragility (risk of hyperkalemia and fractures). Non-depolarizing muscle relaxants can be used but require adequate titration and monitoring. The use of opioid agents is not contraindicated however, when indicated, regional anesthesia should be preferred because of the decrease risk of respiratory depression. Remifentanil can be useful because of its short duration.

Other conditions to be considered:

☞**MYOPATHY DISTAL WELANDER TYPE:** Gene located on 2p13. Onset in the fourth decade with muscle weakness, wast-

ing of the small muscles of the hands, myotonia, and sensory changes.

ARAN-DUCHENNE SMA (Cruveilhier Disease; Duchenne-Aran SMA; Duchenne-Aran Syndrome; Duchenne-Griesinger Disease): Muscular fasciculation, simian hand (eventually becoming "cadaveric hand"), round-shouldered posture, and forward drop of the head, drop foot, steppage gait, and dyspnea.

SMA CONGENITAL NONPROGRESSIVE OF LOWER LIMBS: Characterized by nonprogressive muscular atrophy involving mainly the lower extremities. Onset is in infancy or early childhood. The clinical features include atrophy of the muscles of the lower extremity, mild flexion contractures of the knees, pes equinovarus, and mild weakness of the adductor muscles. There may also be minimal involvement of the jaw muscles and neck flexors, however, it is not considered characteristic of this medical condition. Sensory examination and tendon reflexes are normal. Serum creatine kinase activity may be marginally elevated. This disorder differs from arthrogryposis multiplex congenita because there is usually no involvement of the upper extremities. It differs from other spinal muscular atrophies because it appears early in life and is nonprogressive. Scapuloperoneal SMA is characterized by stridorous breathing in the newborn due to laryngeal palsy, while the presence of progressive lower limb weakness, and contractures appear only in the first or second decade. Autosomal dominant inheritance has been suggested.

PROXIMAL SMA ADULT TYPE (Finkel Late Adult Type Spinoceerebellar Atrophy Syndrome): Characterized by an onset age in the fourth decade (median age of 37 years). It has been estimated that 30% of adult onset cases of SMA are due to an autosomal dominant gene. It has also been suggested that a separate gene may be responsible for the autosomal dominant SMA observed in childhood (birth to 8 years). The clinical features include a slow and progressive spinal muscular atrophy of late onset, which is defined as a slow loss of muscle strength and progressive proximal muscular atrophy. It usually begins in the legs and later involves the arms and is associated with hypoactive or absent deep tendon reflexes and generalized fasciculations.

X-LINKED LETHAL INFANTILE SMA: This congenital form of spinal muscular atrophy is characterized by severe hypotonia, multiple joint contractures, generalized osteopenia, and congenital fractures. The diagnosis is usually confirmed by sural nerve and muscle biopsies consistent with spinal muscular atrophy. Other clinical features may include respiratory difficulty, decreased muscle mass, congenital fractures, and severe osteopenia. Contractures are usually not present.

REFERENCES:

Biros I, Forrest S: Spinal muscular dystrophy: Untangling the knot? *J Med Genet* 36:1, 1999.

Hausmanowa-Petrusewicz I, Zaremba J, Borkowska J: Chronic proximal spinal muscular atrophy of childhood and adolescence: Problems of classification and genetic counselling. *J Med Genet* 22:350, 1985.

Stucke AG, Stuth EA: Use of rapacuronium in a child with spinal muscular atrophy. *Paediatr Anaesth* 11(6):725, 2001.

Spinocerebellar Ataxia (SCA): An Overview

At a glance: The development of ataxia is a neurologic sign that may provide a clue to the nature of the underlying disorder.

Interruption of afferent and efferent connections within the spinocerebellar system results in ataxic gait, scanning dysarthria, explosive speech, intention tremor, dysdiadochokinesia, dysmetria, and abnormalities of eye movements. Many variations are encountered in the clinical phenotype, ranging from findings of pure cerebellar dysfunction to mixed patterns of involvement reflecting extrapyramidal, brainstem, and cerebral cortical involvement. Spinocerebellar Ataxia represents a group of hereditary ataxia of varying inherited degrees of rarity, which is in contrast to a related group of neurological disorders that are acquired following traumatic injuries or other external agents. Until recently, all autosomal dominant ataxias were called Marie Ataxia and all autosomal recessive ataxias were called Friedreich Ataxia. They may be present at almost any time between infancy and adulthood.

Classification: This classification is based on the pattern of inheritance or mode of transmission (i.e., autosomal dominant, autosomal recessive and X-linked). The autosomal dominant ataxias are most often referred to as the Spinocerebellar Ataxias, identified as SCA1 through SCA25. Some ataxias are called "Episodic Ataxias." There is a very rare disorder known as Dentato-Rubro-Pallido-Luysian Atrophy (DRPLA) which is also considered in the classification. Table S-2 reports the autosomal dominant hereditary ataxias and each type is indicated as SCA#. There are fewer autosomal recessive hereditary ataxias than autosomal dominant hereditary ataxias, and X-linked forms of ataxia are very rare.

Autosomal Dominant Cerebellar Ataxias (ADCAs) are a heterogeneous group of disorders in which progressive cerebellar ataxia is the primary feature. In ADCA I, cerebellar ataxia of gait and limbs is invariably associated with supranuclear ophthalmoplegia, pyramidal or extrapyramidal signs, mild dementia, and peripheral neuropathy. In ADCA II, macular and retinal degeneration are added to the features. ADCA III is a pure form of late-onset cerebellar ataxia. ADCA I includes SCA1, SCA2, and SCA3 (Machado-Joseph disease).

History: Early attempts to classify inherited ataxias were based on anatomic localization of pathologic changes (e.g., spinocerebellar, pure cerebellar ataxias). In 1993, Harding introduced another classification in which the ataxias were placed into three categories, congenital, inherited metabolic syndromes with known biochemical defects, and degenerative ataxias of unknown cause. The last category was subdivided further into early-onset (<20 y) and late-onset (>20 y) subtypes.

Genetic inheritance: The molecular genetic explanations for the autosomal-dominant spinocerebellar ataxias rapidly are being unraveled, although the precise pathogenesis is not clearly understood in many of these disorders. The mode of inheritance also varies. Autosomal-dominant, recessive, and nonmendelian inheritance patterns have been described. Nonmendelian inheritance patterns have become increasingly significant in the understanding of the biology of human diseases. The term refers to disorders of inheritance for which the rules of mendelian genetics do not apply. Disorders of triplet repeat expansion and certain mitochondrial defects are examples. For example, the molecular mechanism underlying Friedreich ataxia is because of a triplet repeat expansion, affecting the production of a protein called frataxin. The biochemical defect now is believed to result in impaired mitochondrial function.

Pathophysiology: The spinocerebellar pathways principally are involved in most genetic ataxia syndromes. The pathologic bases of many clinically recognized phenotypes show considerable overlap. However, the genetic molecular and biochemical causes for these disorders are often distinct. The phenotypes may present with pure ataxia or involve multiple levels of the nervous system (including dementia, seizures, disturbance in proprioceptive function, movement disorders, and polymyoclonus).

Clinical aspects: Although ataxia is a prominent feature of all these disorders, the presentation can be variable (static vs progressive, intermittent vs chronic, early vs delayed). Lesions of the midline cerebellar vermis produce truncal and gait ataxia, while involvement of the lateral cerebellar hemispheres produces a limb ataxia. Other features of cerebellar involvement include scanning dysarthria, dysmetria, abnormalities of eye movements, and dysdiadochokinesia.

Anesthetic considerations: General anesthetic considerations for spinocerebellar ataxia include the risk of impaired airway protection due to pharyngeal dysfunction and recurrent pulmonary aspiration. Also, the presence of alveolar hypoventilation from respiratory muscle weakness must be expected in most types of this medical condition. The need for preoperative sedation might be indicated in these patients; however, the risk of respiratory depression and aspiration must be weighed individually. If one elects to administer sedation to the patient, proper vigilance must be provided at all times. The potential complication associated with an impaired airway and breathing is an utmost consideration. The potential need for sustained mechanical ventilation after a surgical procedure must be considered and should be arranged before the beginning of the procedure. Finally, anesthetic management will be otherwise influenced by the specific clinical characteristics present with all different phenotypes of the disease.

Other conditions to be considered:

OLIVOPONTOCEREBELLAR ATROPHY (OPCA): Refers to a group of ataxias characterized by progressive neurological degeneration affecting the cerebellum, the pons, and the inferior olives. The clinical characteristics include upper and lower limbs ataxia, dysarthria, muscle stiffness, spasms and weakness, tremor of the hand or arm, reduction or slowness of movements, declined in psychomotor functions, autonomic nervous system dysfunctions (e.g. bladder), and severe fatigue.

MULTIPLE SYSTEM ATROPHY (MSA): Refers to three slowly progressive neurological disorders consisting of olivopontocerebellar atrophy (OPCA); striatonigral degeneration resembling Parkinson disease and Shy-Drager disease. In all three forms of MSA, the patient can have severe and sudden drops in blood pressure when standing up. Other clinical symptoms include stiffness and rigidity, loss of balance and coordination, impaired speech, breathing and swallowing difficulties, blurred vision, male impotence, and constipation and urinary difficulties.

☞**CHARCOT-MARIE-TOOTH DISEASE:** Characterized by weakness and atrophy, primarily in the legs. Segmental demyelination of peripheral nerves and associated axonal degeneration characterize this disorder.

☞**FRIEDREICH ATAXIA:** A recessive type of hereditary neuromuscular syndrome characterized by slow degenerative changes of the spinal cord, peripheral nerves, and the brain. It usually begins during childhood or the teen years.

☞**LOUIS-BAR SYNDROME:** A progressive cerebellar ataxia that usually begins during infancy. It involves progressive loss of coordination in the limbs, head, and eyes with a below-normal immune response to infections. In later stages, telangiectasias appear in the eyes and skin. Individuals are more susceptible to sinus and lung infections, and to the secondary development of neoplasms.

Table S-2   *Spinocerebellar Ataxia: An Overview of Autosomal Dominant Types*

Type	Age at Onset (Range)	Synonyms and Inclusions	Clinical Aspects	Investigation (Laboratory; MRI; CT Scan; Biopsy; etc.) Physical Examination	Gene Location
SCA 1	30 (20–40)	Spinocerebellar ataxia type I; Spinocerebellar atrophy I Olivopontocerebellar atrophy I (OPCA I); Menzel type OPCA	Involuntary choreiform progressive cerebellar ataxia; Hyperreflexia; explosive speech; Muscle incoordination; Amyotrophy; Slow motor-nerve conduction; Deep tendon reflexes increased; Babinski sign present; 3 major criteria of eye movements (saccade amplitude, saccade velocity, gaze-evoked nystagmus,)	Brain biopsy: markedly reduced aspartic acid and elevated taurine content. 50–60% reduction in platelet glutamate dehydrogenase	6p23
SCA 2	Third decade (1–60) Rarely reported in infant	Spinocerebellar ataxia type II; Spinocerebellar atrophy II; Olivopontocerebellar atrophy II Cuban type spinocerebellar ataxia	Ophthalmoplegia and slow saccades; Nystagmus; Ocular motor apraxia; Retinitis pigmentosa (rare); Progressive cerebellar ataxia; Hyporeflexia; Dysarthria; Dysphagia hypotonia; Myoclonus; Dementia may manifest as "ataxic" phenotype without parkinsonian features or as late-onset "parkinsonian" phenotype without severe ataxic features; Dopamine-responsive parkinsonism; Bradykinesia; Rigidity; Olivopontocerebellar atrophy; Sensory neuropathy;	Caused by expanded CAG trinucleotide repeats in the ataxin-2 gene (ATX2)	12q24
SCA 3	35 (5–70)	☞Machado-Joseph disease; Spinocerebellar ataxia type 3; Spinocerebellar atrophy III; Azorean neurologic disease; Spinopontine atrophy; Nigrospinodentatal degeneration;	Gaze-evoked nystagmus; External and supranuclear ophthalmoplegia; Blepharoptosis; Bulging eyes; Progressive cerebellar ataxia; Spasticity; Pyramidal and extrapyramidal signs; Facial-lingual fasciculations; Parkinsonism; Dysarthria; Rigidity dementia (<20%); Dystonia (<20%); Distal muscular atrophy	Loss of neurons and gliosis in basal ganglia; cranial nerve nuclei, and spinal cord Mild loss of neurons in the cerebellum Sparing of the inferior olives Enlargement of the fourth ventricle on MRI Abnormal electrooculogram	14q24.3–q31

Continued

Table S-2   Continued

Type	Age at Onset (Range)	Synonyms and Inclusions	Clinical Aspects	Investigation (Laboratory; MRI; CT Scan; Biopsy; etc.) Physical Examination	Gene Location
SCA 4	39 (19–59) 4th–5th decade	Spinocerebellar ataxia type 4; Spinocerebellar ataxia with sensory axonal neuropathy; Cerebellar ataxia type IV;	Earliest symptoms: gait disturbances; Progressive cerebellar ataxia; Dysarthria; Hyporeflexia; Areflexia; Extensor plantar responses; Sensory neuropathy; Pyramidal signs;	Length-dependent neuropathy on examination: vibratory and joint position sense loss; 95% minimal pinprick-sensation loss; absent ankle-jerk reflexes; knee-jerk reflexes absent in 85%; complete areflexia seen in 25%.	16q22.1
SCA 5	30 (10–70) 3rd–4th decade	Spinocerebellar ataxia type 5	Progressive "pure" cerebellar ataxia; Mild gait disturbance; Limb incoordination Dysarthria; Cerebellar atrophy; Pyramidal tract dysfunction (juvenile onset); Bulbar dysfunction (juvenile onset);	By linkage to DNA markers	11p11– q121
SCA 6	55 (30–70)	Spinocerebellar ataxia type 6	Mild and slowly progressive "pure" cerebellar ataxia; Progresses over 20–30 years; Dysarthria; Nystagmus; Mild vibratory and proprioceptive sensory loss; Hypotonia; Horizontal gaze nystagmus; Tendon reflexes normal or slightly increased; Absence of extracerebellar symptoms (pyramidal or extrapyramidal tract signs, ophthalmoparesis, or decreased sensation).	The disease is insidious and most patients do not realize they are affected initially	19p13
SCA 7	35 (0–70)	Spinocerebellar ataxia type 7 Olivopontocerebellar atrophy III; OPCA III; OPCA with retinal degeneration; OPCA with macular degeneration and external ophthalmoplegia syndrome	Progressive visual loss; Slow saccades; Optic atrophy; Supranuclear ophthalmoplegia; Progressive cerebellar ataxia; Dysarthria; Dysphagia; Pyramidal signs; Extrapyramidal signs; Chorea; Hyperreflexia; Extensor plantar responses; Spasticity;	Macular degeneration Pigmentary retinal degeneration	3p21.1– p12

Continued

Table S-2   Continued

Type	Age at Onset (Range)	Synonyms and Inclusions	Clinical Aspects	Investigation (Laboratory; MRI; CT Scan; Biopsy; etc.) Physical Examination	Gene Location
SCA 7			Orofacial dyskinesia; Cognitive dysfunction (rare) Dysmetria Olivopontocerebellar degeneration		
SCA 8	Infantile	Spinocerebellar ataxia type 8; ☞Infantile onset spinocerebellar ataxia; OHAHA syndrome; Ophthalmoplegia-Hypotonia-Hypacusis-Athetosis-Ataxia syndrome	Sudden onset of deafness, decrease sense of vibration; ophthalmoplegia with convergence; nystagmus; ataxia and athetosis developing later; normal intelligence but inability to speak; strabismus; keeps mouth open giving impression of stupidity; Muscular hypotonia, athetotic dyskinesia of the face and upper limbs. Polyneuropathy.	Marked decrease in sensory nerve conduction velocities; progressive loss of myelinated fibers in sural nerve biopsies; abnormal EEG with advancing age; neuroradiologic studies show cerebellar atrophy.	13q21
SCA 10	25 (14–44)	Spinocerebellar ataxia type 10	Progressive cerebellar ataxia; Dysarthria; Seizures; Nystagmus; Ocular movement abnormalities; Pyramidal signs; Nerve conduction abnormalities	MRI shows cerebellar atrophy	22q13
SCA 11	25 (15–45)	Spinocerebellar ataxia type 11	Nystagmus; Progressive cerebellar ataxia; Dysarthria; Hyperreflexia; Cerebellar atrophy;	MRI shows cerebellar and cortical atrophy	15q14–q21.3
SCA 12	35 (8–55)	Spinocerebellar ataxia type 12	Progressive cerebellar ataxia; Upper extremity tremor; Head tremor; Dysarthria; Dysmetria; Dysdiadochokinesis; Hyperreflexia; Parkinsonism; Dementia; Ocular movement abnormalities; Depression; Anxiety; Delusions	MRI shows cortical atrophy and cerebellar atrophy	5q31–q33
SCA 13	Child (1–45)	Spinocerebellar ataxia type 13 Autosomal dominant cerebellar ataxia with mental retardation	Progressive cerebellar ataxia; Delayed motor development; Dysarthria; Hyperreflexia; Nystagmus; Mental retardation; Pyramidal signs;	Cerebellar atrophy; MRI shows moderate cerebellar and pontine atrophy.	19q13.3–q13.4

Continued

Table S-2 Continued

Type	Age at Onset (Range)	Synonyms and Inclusions	Clinical Aspects	Investigation (Laboratory; MRI; CT Scan; Biopsy; etc.) Physical Examination	Gene Location
SCA 14	31 (10–50)	Spinocerebellar ataxia type 14	Progressive cerebellar ataxia; Dysarthria; Ocular dysmetria; Hyperreflexia; Slow saccades; Myoclonus (rare); Eye movement abnormalities; Nystagmus;	MRI shows cerebellar atrophy	19q13.4–qter
SCA 15	25 (10–50)	Spinocerebellar ataxia type 15	Progressive cerebellar ataxia; mild degree of gait ataxia;	MRI shows cortical atrophy (vermis)	3p24.2–3pter
SCA 16	40 (20–60)	Spinocerebellar ataxia type 16	Slowly progressive cerebellar ataxia; Benign evolution; Head tremor;	Cerebellar atrophy	8q22.1–q24.1
SCA 17	23 (6–45)	Spinocerebellar ataxia type 17; Huntington disease-like 4; HDLA4	Progressive disorder; Pyramidal signs: Gait ataxia; Limb ataxia; Dysarthria; Dysphagia; Dysmetria; Dystonia; Intention tremor; Bradykinesia; Parkinsonism; Chorea; Dementia; Depression; Hallucinations; Paranoia; Aggression; Mutism; Disorientation; Severe intellectual impairment; Psychiatric symptoms may be the presenting sign	TBP- and 1C2-immunoreactive neuronal inclusions Caused by trinucleotide repeat expansion in the TATA box-binding protein gene Brain biopsy: moderate loss of small neurons with gliosis	6q27
SCA 19	34 (11–45)	Spinocerebellar ataxia type 19	Cerebellar ataxia (mild); Myoclonus; Postural tremor, slow, irregular Cognitive impairment	MRI shows variable degree of cerebellar atrophy Poor performance on the Wisconsin Card Sorting Test	1p21–q21
SCA 20	46 (19–64)	Spinocerebellar ataxia type 20	Onset an average 10 years earlier in the children of affected parents. Dysarthria; Progressive gait ataxia; Upper limb ataxia; mild pyramidal signs, hypermetric saccades; mild nystagmus; palatal tremor; myoclonus	CT scan shows pronounced dentate calcification	? poss.11

Continued

Table S-2   Continued

Type	Age at Onset (Range)	Synonyms and Inclusions	Clinical Aspects	Investigation (Laboratory; MRI; CT Scan; Biopsy; etc.) Physical Examination	Gene Location
SCA 21	18 (6–30)	Spinocerebellar ataxia type 21	Slowly progressive cerebellar ataxia; Limb ataxia and akinesia; Dysarthria; Dysgraphia; hyporeflexia; postural tremor; rigidity resting tremor; eye movements; normal cognitive impairment	MRI shows cerebellar atrophy Poor performance on the Wisconsin Card Sorting Test	7p21.3–p15.1
SCA 22		Spinocerebellar Ataxia type 22 Familial Hyperchylomicronemia	Slowly progressive cerebellar ataxia; Dysarthria; nystagmus; hyporeflexia;	MRI shows cerebellar atrophy Lipoprotein lipase deficiency	6p23
SCA 25	Childhood (1.5–39)	Spinocerebellar Ataxia type 25	Cerebellar ataxia present, variable in intensity and progression. Areflexia of the lower limbs; peripheral sensory neuropathy; decreased touch and pain sensation; nystagmus; decreased visual acuity, facial tics; extensor plantar responses; urinary urgency; GI symptoms	Sural nerve biopsy show loss of myelinated fibers EMG demonstrates sensory conduction deficit. MRI shows cerebellar atrophy.	2p15–21
DRPL A	30 (0–62)	Dentalo-Rubro-Pallido-Luysian Atrophy Myoclonic Epilepsy with Choreoathetosis; Naito-Oyanagi Disease; NOD Allelic to Haw River Syndrome (HRS)	Progressive cerebellar ataxia; Myoclonus; Seizures; Choreoathetosis; difficulty controlling the head; dementia; hyperkinetic movements, involuntary movements	Degeneration of the dentatorubral and pallidoluysian systems Genetic anticipation Phenotypic heterogeneity MRI shows olivopontocerebellar atrophy; cerebral white matter lesions (delayed myelination)	12p13.31
DRPL A-like	30 (0–60)	Haw River Syndrome	Fundamentally the same clinical features as observed with DRPLA except for the absence of myoclonic seizures	MRI shows extensive demyelinization of the subcortical white matter, basal ganglia calcifications, and neuroaxonal dystrophy which are not seen in DRPLA	Possibly the same chromosome
EA1		Episodic Ataxia type 1			12p13
EA2	Childhood	Episodic Ataxia type 2 Episodic Ataxia with nystagmus; Nystagmus-associated cerebellopathy; Hereditary paroxysmal ataxia; Familial paroxysmal	Gaze-evoked nystagmus; Tinnitus; Vertigo; Episodic Ataxia; Myotonia; Dysarthria Migraine headache; Weakness;	EEG with paroxysmal activity; Atrophy of cerebellar vermis; Response to acetazolamide	19p13

Continued

Table S-2 Continued

Type	Age at Onset (Range)	Synonyms and Inclusions	Clinical Aspects	Investigation (Laboratory; MRI; CT Scan; Biopsy; etc.) Physical Examination	Gene Location
EA2		acetazolamide-response hereditary cerebellar ataxia	Paresthesias; Symptoms precipitated by sudden movement, stress, exertion, fatigue Symptoms may subside in later life		
EA3	45 (30–60)	Episodic ataxia type 3; Periodic vestibulocerebellar ataxia	Tinnitus; Diplopia; Oscillopsia; Abnormal smooth pursuits; Inability to suppress vestibuloocular reflex; Gaze-evoked nystagmus; Esophoria GI symptomatology; nausea; Slowly progressive cerebellar ataxia mostly manifested as episodic ataxia; Vertigo; Spasticity Symptoms precipitated by sudden movement, stress, exertion, fatigue	MRI shows vestibulocerebellar atrophy	Not determined

This table was constructed from information obtained from the following sources: Schöls L, Bauer P, Schmidt T, et al: Autosomal dominant cerebellar ataxias: Clinical features, genetics and pathogenesis. *The Lancet Neurology* 3:291–304, 2004.

Bird TD: *The Physician's Guide to Hereditary Ataxia*. NORD:1-10, 2003.

Online Mendelian Inheritance in Man, OMIM. McKusick-Nathans Institute for Genetic Medicine, Johns Hopkins University (Baltimore, Maryland) and National Center for Biotechnology Information, National Library of Medicine (Bethesda, Maryland), 2000. http://www.ncbi. nlm.nih.gov/omim/

Sponastrime Dysplasia

At a glance: Sponastrime is an acronym that stands for: *Spo*ndylar and *Nas*al Alterations with *Stri*ated *Me*taphyses. Short-limb dwarfism with saddle nose, abnormal vertebral bodies with age-dependent changes, severe scoliosis and lumbar lordosis, midface hypoplasia, frontal bossing, and metaphyseal striation. Normal intelligence.

Genetic inheritance: Autosomal recessive.

Diagnosis: Clinical and radiological features. Radiological features may change with age. Radiograph of vertebral spine typically shows abnormal lumbar vertebral bodies with marked variability. These include marked reduced height with anterior part of body taller than posterior part, convex endplate, and central anterior body protuberance. Radiograph of long bones typically shows irregularity of metaphyseal margins and variable density with vertical-oriented striations in metaphyseal regions.

Clinical aspects: Common features are short-limb dwarfism, minor craniofacial anomalies, and normal intelligence. *Growth:* pro-

gressive growth failure, lower limbs more involved than upper limbs. *Craniofacial:* large head, frontal bossing, epicanthal folds, midface hypoplasia, broad and anteverted "saddle" nose is characteristic, mild prognathism. Other occasional reported features include subglottic stenosis, bronchomalacia, avascular necrosis of hip, increased lordosis, scoliosis, progressive infantile coxa vara, and joint deformities.

Precautions before anesthesia: Assess airway for potential difficulty with direct laryngoscopy.

Anesthetic considerations: The potential for difficult direct laryngoscopy and tracheal intubation is present because of the large head, abnormal facies, and mild prognathism. Caution with positioning of head and short limbs with deformed joints.

Pharmacological implications: There are no known specific implications with this condition.

REFERENCE:

Langer L, Beals R, LaFranchi S, et al: Sponastrime dysplasia: Five new cases and review of nine previous published cases. *Am J Med Genet* 63:20–27, 1996.

Spondylocarpotarsal Synostosis Syndrome

At a glance: An autosomal recessive syndrome characterized by anomalies of the hands, feet and, spine. Patients present with short stature and predominantly a very short thorax. Special attention must be given to a high incidence of odontoid hypoplasia and cervical spine instability.

Synonyms: Congenital Synspondylism; Vertebral Fusion with Carpal Coalition Syndrome.

Incidence and genetic inheritance: An autosomal recessive inheritance pattern. However, the responsible genetic marker has been identified.

Clinical aspects: The most characteristic clinical finding is the presence of short stature with a disproportionate short trunk (thorax). The association of odontoid hypoplasia causing cervical spine instability and the failure of normal segmentation of the thoracic vertebrae resulting in fused segment of the spine (unilateral segmented bar) are characteristic of this syndrome. This anatomical problem leads to severe scoliosis or lordosis. The fused spine is difficult to identify in early childhood since the ossification of the vertebrae is not complete. Most patients have a broad and round face, cleft palate, enamel hypoplasia, sensorineural hearing loss, preauricular skin tag, hypertelorism, cataracts, retinal pigmentation, and narrow retinal vessels. Other clinical features include postaxial polydactyly, decreased range of motion of elbows, and the presence of pes planus.

Anesthetic considerations: The presence of odontoid hypoplasia and cervical spine instability requires meticulous attention. Patients may have significant hearing loss. Severe scoliosis may affect ventilation and positioning. There may be an increased risk of postoperative respiratory complications.

REFERENCES:

Honeywell C, Langer L, Allanson J: Spondylocarpotarsal synostosis with epiphyseal dysplasia. *Am J Med Genet* 109(4):318–322, 2002.

Seaver LH, Boyd E: Spondylocarpotarsal synostosis syndrome and cervical instability. *Am J Med Genet* 91(5):340–344, 2000.

Spondylo-Enchondro-Dysplasia

At a glance: Type of dwarfism characterized by enchondromatosis with marked involvement of the spine.

Synonyms: Spondylo-Enchondromatosis; Spondylo-Metaphyseal Dysplasia with Enchondromatous Changes.

Genetic inheritance: Autosomal recessive.

Diagnosis: Clinical and radiological features. Radiograph of vertebral spine typically shows platyspondyly i.e., congenital flattening of the vertebral bodies, which is often accentuated dorsally, and frequently associated with a spina bifida. Radiograph of long bones shows the metaphyses as irregular and slightly widened with varying radiolucent lesions. Radiolucent areas may also be present in diaphyses, epiphyses, iliac crest, scapulae, and sternum.

Clinical aspects: Common clinical features include growth retardation, minor craniofacial anomalies and peculiar enchondromatous changes in skeletal bones. *Growth:* short limbs, short trunk, short stature. *Craniofacial:* dolichocephaly, frontal bossing, mild

midface hypoplasia. *Skeletal:* increased lumbar lordosis; kyphoscoliosis; barrel chest; genu valgum or varus; short, broad hands. *Neurology:* variable mental capacity, ranging from mostly normal intelligence to occasionally moderate retardation. A type 2 has been described with the presence of calcification of basal ganglia on CT scan and associated with progressive spastic quadriparesis. A spina bifida is often present.

Precautions before anesthesia: A careful evaluation of the airway must be conducted to eliminate a potentially difficult airway management.

Anesthetic considerations: No specific consideration. The possibility of difficult airway management must be anticipated because of the craniofacial anomalies, i.e., a large head, midface hypoplasia and cervicothoracic vertebral fusion. Care in positioning of patient must be provided because of the increased lumbar lordosis, large head, and short limbs.

Pharmacological implications: There are no known specific implications with this condition.

REFERENCES:

Frydman M, Bar-Ziv J, Preminger-Shapiro R, et al: Possible heterogeneity in spondyloenchondrodysplasia: Quadriparesis, basal ganglia calcification, and chondrocyte inclusions. *Am J Med Genet* 36:279, 1990.

Menger H, Kruse K, Spranger J: Spondyloenchondrodysplasia. *J Med Genet* 26:93, 1989.

Spondyloepimetaphyseal Dysplasia

At a glance: Spondyloepimetaphyseal Dysplasia (SEMD) describes a group of disorders which have major radiological abnormalities of the spine, epiphyses, and metaphyses in common. Multiple forms exist and the phenotypes, modes of inheritance, and radiographic abnormalities vary considerably.

Synonyms: Spondyloendochromatosis; Camera Stella Syndrome; Leonard Hughes Syndrome.

Classification:

Strudwick type of SEMD (Strudwick Syndrome)
SEMD with Joint Laxity
SEMD with Micromelia
SEMD Iraqi type (Sohat type of SEMD)
SEMD Irapa type
SEMD type II
X-linked type of SEMD
☞Sponastrime Dysplasia
SEDM with Short Limbs and Abnormal Calcifications
SEMD with Multiple Joint Dislocations (Hall type of SEMD)

Incidence: The incidence for spondyloepimetaphyseal dysplasia remains unknown. However, the overall incidence for all skeletal dysplasias is approximately 1 case per 4000–5000 births in the USA. However, some authors have suggested that the true incidence may be twice as high because many skeletal dysplasias do not manifest clinically until the individual is diasgnosed with short stature, joint symptoms, or other complications that arise during childhood. Lethal skeletal dysplasias are estimated to occur in 0.95 per 10,000 live births. The 4 most common skeletal dysplasias are thanatophoric dysplasias, achondroplasia, osteogenesis imperfecta, and achondrogenesis. Thanatophoric dysplasia and achondrogenesis account for

62% of all lethal skeletal dysplasias. Achondroplasia is the most common nonlethal skeletal dysplasia.

Genetic inheritance: Autosomal dominant inheritance is found in Strudwick type of SEMD and SEMD with Multiple Dislocations. Autosomal recessive transmission occurs in SEMD with Joint Laxity, Iraqi type of SEMD, Irapa type of SEMD, Short Limb-Abnormal Calcification type of SEMD, and Sponastrime Dysplasia. X-Linked SEMD is likely to be inherited in an (X-linked) dominant manner. Inheritance in the Micromelic type of SEDM has not been determined, yet.

Pathophysiology: Skeletal dysplasias are characterized by abnormal growth of bone and cartilage. Involvement of both the epiphyses and metaphyses distinguishes the Spondyloepimetaphyseal Dysplasias from the Spondylometaphyseal Dysplasias and the Spondyloepiphyseal Dysplasias.

Diagnosis: Clinical syndromes with characteristic radiological findings. In utero ultrasonography may identify limb abnormalities but is not diagnostic.

Clinical aspects: The clinical features depend on the type of SEMD and the age of the patient.

Strudwick type of SEMD presents at birth with cleft palate, short limbs and trunk, protruding abdomen, and respiratory distress secondary to small chest with short ribs. Other clinical features include hypertelorism and a flat face. Intelligence and life expectancy are normal. Features occurring later on in life include severe coxa vara (with possible dislocation), a waddling gait, lumbar hyperlordosis (platy- and anisospondyly) and myopia with retinal detachment. Before these children reach school age, the characteristic changes in the metaphyses of the long bones become evident, which usually affect the ulna more severely than radius, fibula, or tibia. The disorder manifests as fragmentation of the long bone metaphyses mixed with areas of sclerosis. Lung function tends to remain compromised, even more so if kyphoscoliosis develops. Cervical spine instability may be present because of hypoplasia of C_3 and/or the odontoid process. The genetic defect has been mapped to 12q13, involving the COL2A1 (collagen type II) gene.

SEMD with Joint Laxity is characterized by short stature, mental retardation, joint and ligamentous laxity with dislocations (e.g., hips, radial heads). Kyphoscoliosis is already present at birth, may progress rapidly and lead to significant cardiopulmonary changes (cor pulmonale) and even paraplegia. The face appears oval, often has a long philtrum, and either a high arched palate or a cleft palate. Congenital cardiac lesions (e.g., atrial and/or ventricular septal defects) are common. Ocular features include blue sclerae, myopia, and lens dislocation. This form of SEMD has the highest incidence in South Africa, where it was also first described.

SEMD with Micromelia presents at birth and is characterized with short stature, small thoracic dimensions, and brachydactyly. Mental retardation is common.

SEMD Iraqi type: The name originates from the first family described with this disorder, who was from Iraq. The patients present at birth with short stature, short limbs, and short neck. Generalized joint laxity and varus deformity of the hips and knees are characteristic findings. Hepatosplenomegaly with prominent abdomen is common. The chest is often short and narrow. The vertebrae may be abnormal (platyspondyly, cleft vertebrae), and the interpeduncular distance is decreased.

SEMD Irapa type: This disorder is named after the Indians in Venezuela's Irapa district on the north shore, where it was first detected. Presentation is usually delayed until approximately 5 years

of age, when symptoms of joint pain and walking difficulties occur. There is a limited range of movement in affected joints and premature osteoarthrosis and osteoporosis develop. Generalized platyspondyly, widening and shortening of the tubular bones with anomalies of the metaphyses, shortening and occasionally fusion of the metacarpalia, coxa vara and pelvic anomalies (acetabular dysplasia) are the main skeletal findings.

SEMD type II: Usually presents with skeletal features such as shortened legs with bowing of the femurs and tibia. With the exception of short stature, these modelling defects improve spontaneously by the onset of adolescence.

X-Linked type of SEMD: Short stature is present, but becomes usually not evident before the age of 2 years. Radial dislocation of the hands is a typical feature caused by relative elongation of the ulna. Progressive platyspondyly and predominately lumbar narrowing of the interpeduncular distance define the spinal anomalies. Coxa vara is common.

Sponastrime Dysplasia: Less than 20 patients have been reported. This type of SEMD presents early in infancy with short stature and craniofacial dysmorphism including enlarged head with frontal bossing, midface hypoplasia with a short, upturned nose and depressed nasal root. However, microcephaly and mental retardation have also been described in these patients. Progressive lumbar lordosis and kyphoscoliosis may develop and result in cardiopulmonary changes (restrictive lung disease and cor pulmonale). Striation of the metaphyses refers to the irregular, longitudinal sclerotic changes seen on radiographs, most notably in the distal femur and proximal tibia metaphyses. Coxa vara (with potential dislocation) and avascular necrosis of the capital femoral epiphyses have been described. In contrast to most other forms of SEMD, vertebral body size can be enlarged (despite platyspondyly), resulting in increased interpeduncular distance. Subglottic stenosis and tracheobronchomalacia have been reported.

SEDM with Short Limbs and Abnormal Calcifications characterized by short limbs (including short hands and feet), but in contrast to most other forms of SEDM, the trunk is relatively long. Facial dysmorphic features include hypertelorism, midfacial hypoplasia, depressed and wide nasal bridge, and micrognathia. The chest is narrow, and progressive kyphoscoliosis may lead to cor pulmonale. Ligamentous laxity and anomalies of the odontoid process with subluxation of C_1 and C_2 may cause compression of the cervical cord.

SEMD with Multiple Joint Dislocations: These patients present with short stature, midface hypoplasia, and severe, generalized muscular hypotonia. Almost one-third of these patients has some form of laryngeal stenosis and/or tracheomalacia. Tracheo(s)tomy has been necessary in a few of these children. One patient has been reported with inspiratory stridor secondary to laryngeal stenosis. Joint laxity is progressive and results in dislocations mainly affecting the hips and the knees. The changes in the spine include sacral dysraphism, mild platyspondyly (or other forms of abnormally shaped vertebrae), and decreased interpeduncular distance. Scoliosis may develop, but is usually mild.

Precautions before anesthesia: Preoperative investigations are determined by the specific disease pattern. Pulmonary function testing, echocardiography, and arterial blood gas analysis should be performed in the presence of kyphoscoliosis and/or the narrowing of the chest. Electrocardiography and echocardiography should also be performed if cardiac dysfunction or congenital cardiac lesions are suspected. A detailed neurological evaluation should be performed in disorders associated with cervical instability and in the presence of kyphoscoliosis because of its association with paraplegia. Facial dysmorphisms may indicate difficult airway management. Cervical spine imaging may be required to ascertain bony stability. Renal function should be checked because of occasional renal dysfunction. Regional anesthesia is not contraindicated per se, but central neuraxial blocks may be difficult to perform given the anomalies of the spine (hyperlordosis, kyphoscoliosis, diminished interpeduncular distance). Some patients may be mentally retarded, hence cooperation may be difficult. Anxiolytic and sedative premedication (careful in patients with cardiopulmonary compromise) and the presence of the primary caregiver for induction may be helpful. Kyphoscoliosis with associated respiratory dysfunction increases the risk for postoperative mechanical ventilation, which should be arranged in advance.

Anesthetic considerations: Expect airway management to be difficult. Maintain spontaneous ventilation until the airway has been secured and lung ventilation confirmed. A laryngeal mask airway should be available in case of failure to ventilate and/or intubate. Cervical instability and subluxations require in-line stabilization of the cervical spine during direct laryngoscopy. Primary fiberoptic tracheal intubation may therefore be the approach of choice for these patients. Careful positioning is requested secondary to joint laxity with the risk of dislocations.

Pharmacological implications: Avoid neuromuscular blockers until the airway has been secured.

Other conditions to be considered:

☞**MORQUIO SYNDROME:** An inborn error of metabolism characterized by the deficiency of one of ten specific lysosomal enzymes, resulting in the inability to metabolize complex carbohydrates (mucopolysaccharides) into simpler molecules. May be detected as early as 18 to 24 months of age. The skeletal abnormalities may include macrocephaly, a broad mouth, prominent cheekbones, an unusually small nose, short neck, short barrel chests, disproportionately long arms, enlarged and possibly hyperextensible wrists, stubby hands, and "knock knees." The joint laxity and bony abnormalities of the spine can result in life-threatening spinal cord compression. The presence of thoracic kyphoscoliosis may also contribute to the risk of spinal cord ischemia during positioning. Aortic regurgitation and deafness have also been reported.

REFERENCES:

Anderson CE, Sillence DO, Lachman RS, et al: Spondylometepiphyseal dysplasia, Strudwick type. *Am J Med Genet* 13:243, 1982.

Beighton P: Syndrome of the month: Spondyloepimetaphyseal dysplasia with joint laxity (SEMDJL). *J Med Genet* 31:136, 1994.

Figuera LE, Ramirez-Duenas ML, Gallegos-Arreola MP, et al: Spondyloepimetaphyseal dysplasia (SEMD) Sohat type. *Am J Med Genet* 51:213, 1994.

Hall CM, Elcioglu NH, Shaw DG: A distinct form of spondyloepimetaphyseal dysplasia with multiple dislocations. *J Med Genet* 35:566, 1998.

Holder-Espinasse M, Fayoux P, Morillon S, et al: Spondyloepimetaphyseal dysplasia (Hall type) with laryngeal stenosis: A new diagnostic feature? *Clin Dysmorphol* 13:133, 2004.

Nishimura G, Honma T, Shiihara T, et al: Spondyloepimetaphyseal dysplasia with joint laxity leptodactylic form: Clinical course and phenotypic variations in four patients. *Am J Med Genet* 117A(2):147, 2003.

Shebib SM, Chudley AE, Reed MH: Spondylometepiphyseal dysplasia congenita, Strudwick type. *Pediatr Radiol* 21:298, 1991.

Stargardt Syndrome

At a glance: The most common form of inherited juvenile macular degeneration. Characterized by a reduction of central vision with a preservation of peripheral vision. Onset before the age of 20 years; macula presents yellow-white spots of irregular shapes.

Synonyms: Stargardt Disease; Stargardt Macular Degeneration; Familial Juvenile Macular Degeneration; Juvenile Hereditary Disciform Macular Degeneration; Fundus Flavimaculatus; Central Retinitis Pigmentosa.

Incidence and genetic inheritance: This autosomal recessive transmitted disease with gene map locus 1p21-p13 is the most common cause of juvenile-onset macular degeneration and affects at least 1 in 20,000 children older than the age of 6 years. The disorder is characterized by subretinal deposition of lipofuscin-like material (termed "flecks") around the macular area. There is evidence that the disease is caused by a mutation in the retina-specific ATP-binding cassette transporter (ABCR) gene.

Clinical aspects: In general, the age at manifestation of the disease is between 6 and 20 years with decreased central vision being the first symptom, although some patients do not suffer from any symptoms (loss of color vision, loss of peripheral vision, photophobia, paracentral scotoma, night blindness) until the age of 40 years. Fundus flavimaculatus is the descriptive term for this macular degeneration surrounded by white-yellowish flecks and spots distributed all over the fundus, although some researchers consider fundus flavimaculatus to be an allelic variant of Stargardt disease with differences in age at onset (between 17 and 60 years), severity, and clinical course (more progressive). The rapidly progressive disease occurs usually bilaterally and symmetrically and results in legal blindness in 50% of patients by the age of 50 years. No effective treatment is available.

Anesthetic considerations: Especially in younger patients undergoing ophthalmic examination under general anesthesia, oculocardiac reflex with profound bradycardia should be expected. No other specific anesthetic considerations are expected to arise from this disease.

REFERENCES:

Armstrong J, Meyer D, Xu S, et al: Long-term follow-up of Stargardt's disease and fundus flavimaculatus. *Ophthalmology* 105:448, 1998.

Hadden OB, Gass JD: Fundus flavimaculatus and Stargardt's disease. *Am J Ophthal* 82:527, 1976.

Kaplan J, Gerber S, Larget-Piet D, et al: A gene for Stargardt's disease (fundus flavimaculatus) maps to the short arm of chromosome 1. *Nat Genet* 5:308, 1993.

Stein-Leventhal Syndrome

At a glance: Characterized by amenorrhea, infertility, hirsutism, and enlarged polycystic ovaries.

Synonym: Polycystic Ovary Syndrome (PCOS); Sclerocystic Disease of the Ovaries.

History: Stein and Leventhal first described this entity in 1935.

Incidence: Most authors agree that it is present in 3 to 7% of women worldwide. Approximately 75% of women with irregular menses and/or infertility may have polycystic ovaries. Based on ultrasonographic studies, 50% of women with regular menstrual cycles had polycystic ovaries.

Genetic inheritance: Unknown. Believed to be autosomal dominant.

Pathophysiology: In Stein-Leventhal syndrome patients, the preovulatory follicle in the ovary does not develop. As a result, multiple subcapsular follicles develop. This creates an androgenic ovary, which is usually anovulatory.

Diagnosis: The National Institutes of Health has defined PCOS as a state of hyperandrogenism and chronic anovulation in the absence of other causes, for example, congenital adrenal hyperplasia, hyperprolactinemia, and Cushing syndrome. The diagnosis is made on clinical grounds, in addition to the presence of bilateral polycystic ovaries in 90% of patients. Increased plasma levels of luteinizing hormone but normal or reduced levels of follicle-stimulating hormone. Other biochemical tests are done to exclude other causes.

Clinical aspects: Stein-Leventhal Syndrome is a condition that is usually diagnosed after the expected onset of menstruation. Symptoms can include amenorrhea or menstrual irregularity, hirsutism in androgen-dependent regions (face, chest, lower abdomen), upper body obesity (in 50% of patients), and infertility in patients of childbearing age. Associated with the obesity, patients frequently have insulin resistance resulting in adult-onset diabetes. Treatment may include progestins, oral contraceptives, antiandrogens (including spironolactone), weight reduction, ovulation-inducing medication, and surgery (laparoscopic ovarian cautery or laser vaporization).

Precautions before anesthesia: Fasting blood sugar in older patients (particularly obese patients). Ensure other conditions have been excluded, for example, Cushing Syndrome.

Anesthetic considerations: Consider implications of obesity and glucose intolerance, if present.

Pharmacological implication: There are no known implications with this condition.

REFERENCES:

Goudas V, Dumesic D: Polycystic ovary syndrome. *Endocrinol Metab Clin North Am* 26;4:893–911, 1997.

Legro R: The genetics of polycystic ovary syndrome. *Am J Med* 98(suppl 1A):9S, 1995.

Stickler Syndrome

At a glance: Stickler syndrome is an autosomal dominant hereditary progressive arthro-ophthalmology condition characterized by congenital abnormalities of the eye, micrognathia, and a cleft palate. Other clinical features include flat midface, intracranial calcifications, and deafness. More than 50% of patients affected with this condition have a mitral valve prolapse and authors have suggested that in the presence of an autosomal dominant inherited mitral valve prolapse, a Stickler syndrome should be suspected until proven otherwise.

Classification: There are three types of Stickler syndrome:

Stickler syndrome type I (Stickler Syndrome Vitreous type I; Stickler Syndrome Membranous Vitreous Type; Progressive Hereditary Arthro-Ophthalmopathy Syndrome) is characterized by progressive myopia with an onset of age within the first 10 years, resulting in retinal detachment and blindness. Individuals affected with this type also present premature degenerative changes in various joints with abnormal epiphyseal development and slight hypermobility.

Stickler Syndrome type II (Stickler Syndrome Vitreous type II; Beaded Vitreous Stickler Syndrome type II) is characterized by the usual clinical characteristic of ocular, auditory, and orofacial features seen in Stickler syndrome but with the architecture of an abnormal vitreous. This sign is a hallmark of this syndrome and is a prerequisite for the diagnosis.

Stickler Syndrome type III (Stickler Syndrome Monocular type) is characterized by the usual features of Stickler Syndrome, however, the ocular signs observed with the other types (high myopia, vitreoretinal degeneration, and retinal detachment) are absent.

Genetic inheritance: Autosomal dominant.

Diagnosis: Evocated by myopia in the first years of life.

Clinical aspects: *Eye findings:* high myopia, congenital but deteriorating in the first years of life. Total, sudden retinal detachment associated with no trauma in first decade of life. Dense, complicated cataract formation, uveitis keratopathy, and secondary glaucoma developing after retinal detachment. *Joint manifestations:* bony enlargement of joints at birth, especially ankles, knees, and elbows. Soreness of joints in early childhood. Progressive arthritis in early adult life. Joints mostly wrists, elbows, knees, hips, and ankles. Hypermobility of joints, particularly fingers. Pierre Robin syndrome and sensorineural deafness associated in 10% of cases.

Precautions before anesthesia: Although neck involvement in the arthropathy is not typical, it would be prudent to carefully examine neck movements to anticipate problems during direct laryngoscopy and tracheal intubation. A careful history reveals positions in which the patient is uncomfortable and consideration should be given to this when positioning the patient for surgery.

Anesthetic considerations: It may be feasible for the patient to position himself for surgery to prevent damage to arthritic joints. Regional techniques may well be appropriate in this group of patients. Intellectual function is normal, although blindness is common. There are no specific recommendations for the conduct of anesthesia.

Pharmacological implications: Avoid succinylcholine and other drugs that may increase intraocular pressure in the presence of glaucoma. No other specific indications or contraindications exist for anesthetic agents.

Other conditions to be considered:

☞**MARSHALL SYNDROME:** This autosomal dominant inherited disorder is characterized by cataracts, myopia, abnormal vitreous, hypertelorism, midfacial hypoplasia, and congenital deafness. While some researchers consider Stickler and Marshall syndrome to be distinct entities, others think that they are basically the same disease. Hitherto, this issue has not been resolved. Cleft palate in Marshall syndrome patients is not as common as in Stickler syndrome. The midface is described as flat with an upturned nose and large eyes, in Stickler syndrome, the face is rather long and flat with depressed nasal bridge.

☞**WAGNER SYNDROME:** An autosomal dominant disorder characterized by changes in the peripheral fundus with narrowed and ensheathed retinal vessels, retinal pigmentation, and circular membranes in a liquefied vitreous attached to the retina.

☞**OTOSPONDYLOMEGAEPIPHYSEAL DYSPLASIA:** A disease with peculiar facies and severe degenerative joint disease of the osteoarthritis type affecting predominantly the hips, knees, elbows, and shoulders.

WEISSENBACHER-ZWEYMÜLLER SYNDROME (Pierre Robin Syndrome with Fetal Chondrodysplasia): Micrognathia, and rhizomelic chondrodysplasia with enlargement of the epi- and metaphyses of the long bones resulting in a typical dumbbell-shape (especially of humeri and femora) are the hallmarks of this autosomal recessive inherited syndrome. However, the overall changes are milder than in OSMED and they tend to resolve with increasing age with impressive catch-up growth finally resulting in normal adult height. Midface hypoplasia, eye (optic nerve hypoplasia, severe myopia, retinal detachment) and ear (sensorineural hearing loss) anomalies, vertebral coronal clefts, and meningoceles/encephaloceles have also been described in some of these patients. Psychomotor development is often delayed.

REFERENCE:
Stickler GB, Belau PG, Farrell FJ, et al: Hereditary progressive arthro-ophthalmopathy. *Mayo Clin Proc* 40:433, 1965.

Stiff Baby Syndrome

At a glance: A rare neurological disease characterized by the occurrence of hypertonia at birth that progressively decreases over the first year of life. However, attacks of hypertonia heightened by the slightest physical stimulus often occur and are responsible for apnea, respiratory depression, severe cyanosis, and death.

Synonyms: Essential Startle Disease; Exaggerated Startle Reaction; Hyperekplexia Kok Disease; Familial Startle Disease.

History: First described in 1962 by O. Kok.

Genetic inheritance: Autosomal dominant. There is evidence that the disease is caused by a mutation of the gene for the alpha-1 subunit of the inhibitory glycine receptor on chromosome 5q33.2-5q33.3. The defective receptor causes disruption of the normal inhibitory pathway, descending to the spinal cord to modulate reflexes.

Pathophysiology: A condition that inhibits the production and release of central gamma-aminobutyric acid (GABA). The pathophysiology of hypertonia and the exaggerated startle response remains unclear but several hypothesis have been proposed. One hypothesis is that there are hyperactive long-loop reflexes acting as the physiologic basis for the startle disease, suggesting increased cortical neuronal excitability. Electroencephalography is normal, whereas electromyography shows persistent muscle activity (even during sleep); rarely associated with electric quietness. The nerve conduction is normal.

Diagnosis: The diagnosis is a clinical one and is more easily made when other members of the family are affected. The recognition of this entity is important to avoid an erroneous diagnosis of epilepsy and consequent treatment with anticonvulsants. It is also important to distinguish the stiff baby syndrome from other neurological diseases. Electroencephalography (EEG) and electromyography (EMG) are normal while awake and asleep. Low cerebrospinal fluid (CSF) GABA level was demonstrated. Responsiveness to diazepam and clonazepam therapy.

Clinical aspects: Onset occurs from birth with hypertonia, hypokinesia, flexed posture, and a peculiar staccato cry. Neonates suffering from the disease are at risk of sudden death from apnea or aspiration if they undergo a prolonged period of rigidity. Later in childhood, individuals may show an exaggerated startle response during waking state with acute generalized hypertonia and loss of voluntary muscle control, resulting in "falling like a log." The startle can be easily elicited by a loud, unexpected noise or by touching the nose. Marked nocturnal myoclonic jerks are also characteristic. Intelligence is normal. Inguinal/umbilical hernias and congenital dislocation of hip are common. Symptoms are exacerbated by stress, fatigue, cold, and rainy weather.

Precautions before anesthesia: It is important to mention that affected patients may fall as a consequence of the startle response and injure themselves, i.e., causing bone fractures or even subdural hematomas. Thus, a careful clinical examination and history are recommended prior to an anesthesia to rule out major associated injuries.

Anesthetic considerations: No reported experience in the literature although many of these patients had undergone several procedures. In the operating theater, avoid loud noise so as not to produce a hypertonic crisis. Good preoperative communication and premedication may help to allay anxiety. Keep patient warm throughout the perioperative period. Adequate depth of anesthesia and analgesia helps to reduce the perioperative stress. Regional technique is recommended if indicated.

Pharmacological implications: The neuromuscular response to volatile anesthetic agents and succinylcholine might be abnormal; consequently, even if there are no reports of such complications, intraoperative neuromuscular monitoring is recommended. If the patient is on clonazepam, the patient's regular dose should be given on the day of surgery.

Other conditions to be considered: In addition to the disorders discussed below, conditions that can produce an increase in muscle tonicity include Encephalomyelitis, Creutzfeldt-Jakob Disease, metoclopramide, strychnine poisoning, and Myoclonic Epilepsy.

☞**GILLES DE LA TOURETTE SYNDROME:** Neurological syndrome characterized by repeated and involuntary stereotyped motor movement (spasmodic twitchings and startling reactions) or vocalization (tics).

☞**ISAACS-MERTENS SYNDROME:** Characterized as a peripheral motor neuron disorder leading to muscular stiffness and cramping, particularly in the limbs. Continuous fine vibrating muscle movement (myokymia) can be observed. Muscle relaxation is most often impossible, especially after physical activity. Hypertonia with fasciculations occurs around the age of 30 years; however, neonatal forms have been reported.

☞**JUMPING FRENCHMAN OF MAINE SYNDROME:** Neurological disease characterized by exaggerated startle reflexes produced by the slightest stimulus. Violent startles associated with echolalia and echopraxia.

STIFF MAN SYNDROME (Moersch-Wolman Syndrome): Characterized by a neuromuscular condition in which a hyperactive startle reflex results in contraction of muscles causing violent spasms. These spasms are capable of slamming the victim into walls and furniture, causing injuries. An autoimmune disorder has been suggested. Age of onset is around 40 to 50 years.

REFERENCES:
Murphy C, Shorten G: Train of four fade in a child with stiff baby syndrome. *Paediatr Anaesth* 10:567, 2000.

Praveen V, Patole SK, Whitehall JS: Hyperekplexia in neonates. *Postgrad Med J* 77:570, 2001.

Ryan SG, Sherman SL, Terry JC, et al: Startle disease, or hyperekplexia: Response to clonazepam and assignment of the gene (STHE) to chromosome 5q by linkage analysis. *Ann Neurol* 31:663, 1992.

Stiff Heart Syndrome

At a glance: Acquired cardiomyopathy caused by cardiac deposition of amyloid leading to decreased heart function (especially contractility).

Synonym: Cardiac Amyloidosis.

Genetic inheritance: Commonly acquired secondary to multiple myeloma. Familial forms of amyloidosis are usually inherited by an autosomal mode resulting in mutations of transthyretin (prealbumin); 40 variants have been described.

Pathophysiology: Deposition of amyloid occurs in the myocardium, epicardium, and pericardium. Echocardiography classically shows a normal diastolic volume, slow ventricular filling throughout diastole, minimal shortening during systole, and high systolic volumes, resulting in a reduced stroke volume and low cardiac output state. The left ventricle is poorly compliant and left ventricular end-diastolic pressure is elevated. Consequently, endocardial perfusion is dependent on maintaining diastolic blood pressure. Localized septal deposition of amyloid protein may present clinically as hypertrophic obstructive cardiomyopathy. Infiltration of the conduction system may cause dysrhythmias and bundle branch block. Other forms of restrictive cardiomyopathy may be distinguished from cardiac amyloidosis by rapid ventricular filling early in diastole.

Diagnosis: Clinical history and signs of cardiomyopathy. Echocardiographic findings and demonstration of amyloid on rectal or endocardial biopsy.

Clinical aspects: Evidence of cardiac amyloid is present in up to 90% of cases of primary and multiple myeloma-associated amyloidosis. Cardiac amyloidosis is also found in association with lymphoma, rheumatoid arthritis, tuberculosis, osteomyelitis, and bronchiectasis. The predominant clinical features are those of cardiac failure, tachypnea, orthopnea, decreased exercise tolerance, elevated jugular venous pressure, pulmonary edema, and hepatic distension. The ECG may show bundle branch block or rhythm abnormalities. The chest radiograph may show cardiomegaly (secondary to a pericardial effusion) or pleural effusions. The ventricular failure is often refractory to medical management.

Precautions before anesthesia: Full medical history and physical examination to evaluate cardiac function and significance of any associated disorders. Proper evaluation of the restrictive nature of the cardiomyopathy must be obtained. Respiratory assessment and chest radiograph are mandatory. Cardiovascular assessment, ECG, and echocardiography should be performed prior to anesthesia. Ensure optimal control of cardiac function prior to induction of anesthesia.

Anesthetic considerations: Technique aimed to maintain ventricular preload, avoid further depression of myocardial contractility, maintain diastolic blood pressure, maintain sinus rhythm, and avoid tachycardia/bradycardia. Use of invasive monitoring should be strongly considered, although pulmonary artery catheters may be misleading because of the altered left ventricular compliance.

Pharmacological implications: Cardiac depressant anesthetic medications must be used judiciously. The induction of significant tachycardia must be prevented (e.g., pancuronium is relatively contraindicated).

REFERENCES:

Arora S, Arora A, Makkar RP, Monga A: Stiff heart syndrome. *CMAJ* 168:1690, 2003.

Chew C, Ziady G, Raphael M et al: The functional defect in amyloid heart disease. The stiff heart syndrome. *Am J Cardiol* 36:438–444, 1975.

Kushwaha S, Fallon J, Fuster V: Restrictive cardiomyopathy. *N Engl J Med* 336:267, 1997.

Stimmler Syndrome

At a glance: Microcephaly at birth, low birth weight, severe mental retardation, and dwarfism. Diabetes mellitus is associated.

Synonym: Alaninuria with Microcephaly, Dwarfism, Enamel Hypoplasia, and Diabetes Mellitus.

Genetic inheritance: Autosomal recessive.

Clinical aspects: Dwarfism, microcephaly, hypoplastic enamel of teeth, diabetes mellitus. Excessive quantities of alanine in urine.

Anesthetic considerations: Ensure proper control of diabetes and insulin requirements. Check blood gas analysis and blood lactate level because of the potential association with chronic lactic acidosis. Mental retardation may cause the patient to be uncooperative at induction of anesthesia and the benefit of a premedication must be weighed against the severity of the clinical condition. It is essential to ensure proper perioperative control of diabetes mellitus. Chronic lactic acidosis may be present and should be treated accordingly before any elective surgical procedures.

REFERENCE:

Stimmler L, Jensen N, Toseland P: Alaninuria, associated with microcephaly, dwarfism, enamel hypoplasia, and diabetes mellitus in two sisters. *Arch Dis Child* 45:682, 1970.

Streeter Anomaly

At a glance: Constricting amniotic bands leading to amputation with scarring, distal syndactyly, cleft lip and palate, anencephaly, encephalocele, hydrocephaly, omphalocele, and gastroschisis. Other internal anomalies involve the head, heart, lungs, diaphragm, kidneys, and gonads. Although the peripheral defect is often minimal, a thorough examination is mandatory.

Synonyms: Congenital Constricting Bands; Amniotic Band Sequence or Disruption; Streeter Dysplasia Syndrome; ADAM Complex; Terminal Transverse Defects of Arm.

Incidence: Reported as 1:1200 live births in some populations.

Genetic inheritance: Possibly autosomal recessive, but in general the cause of amnion disruption is unknown.

Pathophysiology: Unknown. Various theories include these mechanisms: vascular, mechanical, genetic disruption, or germ disc disruption (Streeter's hypothesis). The amniotic band so formed disrupts early embryonic growth and results in unusual fetal malformations. It has also been suggested that the defect occurs prior to 26 days postconception and before the establishment of effective embryonic circulation (because of the involvement of several internal organs).

Clinical aspects: Wide case-to-case variation. Typically include amputation of digits and limbs from ring-like band constriction in most cases. The described ADAM Complex (Amniotic Deformity, Adhesions, and Mutilation) includes amniotic deformity, cleft lip and palate, and other facial malformations. The described LBWD

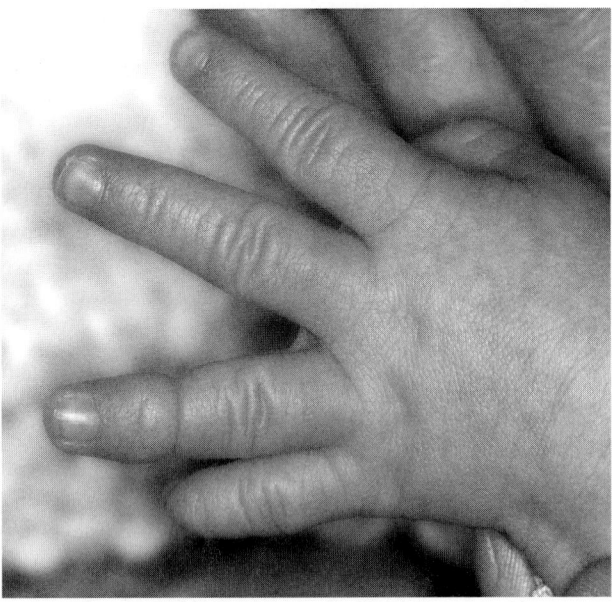

Streeter anomaly Amniotic bands led to partial amputation of the end phalanx of the fifth finger and stricture of the fourth finger in this child with Streeter anomaly.

(Limb and Body Wall Defect) Complex occurs in severe cases with hypoplasia of all major internal organs, major limb defects, and death soon after birth.

Precautions before anesthesia: Assess for clinical associated features such as cardiac, neurological, and respiratory abnormalities. Assess the airway for potential difficulty with direct laryngoscopy and tracheal intubation.

Anesthetic considerations: Difficult peripheral intravenous access may be encountered because of the self-mutilation. Special attention must be given to positioning because of vascular compromise in the extremities. In the presence of facial malformations, the potential for difficult airway management must be anticipated.

Other conditions to be considered:

☞**ADAMS-OLIVER SYNDROME:** A very rare inherited disorder characterized by defects of the scalp and associated with multiple scars and hairless areas that usually have dilated blood vessel directly under the skin. Scalp defects are already present at birth. The extremities are either short (hypoplastic fingers and toes) or characterized by absent hands and lower legs. Congenital heart defect must be ruled out.

☞**AINHUM:** A narrow strip of hardened skin, a constricting ring formation on the little toe at the level of digitoplantar fold leading progressively to spontaneous amputation.

REFERENCE:

Bamforth J: Amniotic band sequence: Streeter's hypothesis re-examined. *Am J Med Genet* 44:280, 1992.

Lubinsky M, Sujansky E, Sanger W, et al: Familial amniotic bands. *Am J Med Genet* 14:81, 1983.

Stanek J, de Courten-Myers G, Spaulding AG, et al: Case of complex craniofacial anomalies, bilateral nasal proboscides, palatal pituitary, upper limbs reduction, and amnion rupture sequence: Disorganization phenotype? *Pediatr Dev Pathol* 4:192, 2001.

Sturge-Weber Syndrome

At a glance: A neurocutaneous syndrome characterized by the presence of vascular tumors of the face (facial hemangioma and nevus flammeus, usually called "port-wine stain"), ipsilateral vascular anomalies (angioma of the meninges and choroid), and intracranial calcifications. Other clinical features include contralateral hemiparesis, hemianopia, and severe seizures. This nevus flammeus of the face corresponds to the ophthalmic division of the trigeminal nerve. All organs can be involved.

Synonyms: Fourth Phacomatosis Syndrome; Dimitri Disease; Jahnke Syndrome; Kalischer Syndrome; Lawford Syndrome; Müller Syndrome; Parkes Weber Syndrome; Parkes, Weber, and Dimitri Syndrome; Schirmer Syndrome; Sturge Disease; Sturge Syndrome; Sturge-Kalischer-Weber Syndrome; Sturge-Weber Angiomatosis; Sturge-Weber-Dimitri Syndrome; Sturge-Weber-Krabbe Syndrome; Weber Syndrome; Weber-Dimitri Syndrome.

History: First described by the English physician William Allen Sturge, English physician in 1879. Frederick Parkes Weber, also an English physician, deserves credit for the description of intracranial calcifications in 1922. Vincente Dimitri, Austrian dermatologist, and S. Kalischer, German physician, provided further insights in the disease.

Incidence: 1:50,000 live births; male:female ratio is equal. The facial nevus is present at birth, and the age of onset for seizures is younger than 1 year.

Genetic inheritance: Unknown (autosomal dominant inheritance has been evocated). Almost all incidences are sporadic cases.

Pathophysiology: Unknown. It is likely that an acquired vascular abnormality arises early in development. The localization of aberrant vasculature in the meninges, facial skin, and eyes is consistent with a defect arising in a limited part of the cephalic neural crest, with cells migrating to the pia mater, choroid, and supraocular dermis. The basic lesion consists of ipsilateral angiomas. The distribution of the leptomeningeal vascular anomalies is in the following order: occipital > parietal > temporal > frontal regions. The sluggish flow of blood in these affected regions may lead to anoxic injury in the underlying cortex, mental retardation, hemiparesis, and hemianopia.

Diagnosis: Clinical; characterized by nevus flammeus of the face and angioma of the meninges. Presence of a port-wine stain on the face in the appropriate distribution is supported by imaging on CT scan and MRI of angiomas. Radiography shows intracranial calcifications in 90% of cases (railroad track pattern) by late childhood. The radiological characteristic of the calcifications is described as a "railroad track pattern" (curvilinear, parallel configuration). The facial nevus distribution corresponds to V1 (upper face, superior eyelid, and supraorbital region) but may also involve V2 and V3 and cross the midline. May cause hypertrophy of the involved areas and the nasopharynx (bleeding).

Clinical aspects: This syndrome involves *brain* (seizures, macrocephaly, cerebral cortex atrophy, paraparesis or quadriparesis, mental retardation, intracranial calcifications), *skin* (hemangioma-capillary, hemangioma-cavernous), and *eyes* (coloboma of iris, glaucoma, and choroids calcification with buphthalmos). Coarctation of the aorta, visceral angiomatosis and intraoral angiomatosis on the buccal mucosa and lips, macrocheilia, occasional involvement of palate and tongue can also occur. Cutaneous hemangiomata are present at birth and seizure onset may begin in the first 2 to 7 months of life. Hemangiomata in the trigeminal distribution, facial

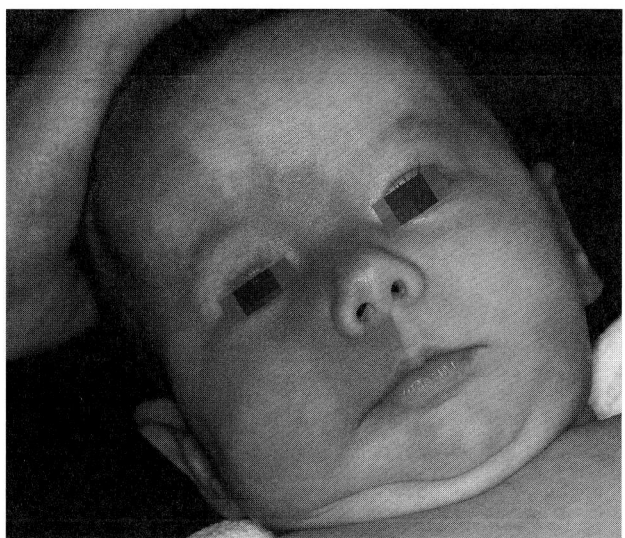

Sturge-Weber syndrome Unilateral nevus flammeus in an infant with Sturge-Weber syndrome.

hemangiomata (56% of patients) may involve nasopharynx. Arachnoid hemangiomata (98% of patients): occipital > parietal > temporal > frontal.

Precautions before anesthesia: Evaluate neurological function (clinical, EEG, CT scan); cardiac function must be evaluated for malformation and signs of cardiac failure as a result of shunt that can be caused by the hemangioma (clinical, echocardiography, radionuclide imaging if necessary); and airway (oropharyngolaryngeal hemangioma). Preoperative laboratory investigation should include hematocrit, coagulation test, and platelet count because of frequency of thrombosis and/or bleeding. A complete review of the seizure history must be obtained and antiepileptic medications continued until the morning of the surgical procedure.

Anesthetic considerations: Avoid nasal intubation because of the possible involvement of the nasopharynx and risk of excessive bleeding. The eyes must be carefully protected with lubrication and taping. Direct laryngoscopy and tracheal intubation can be a challenge because of pharyngeal and laryngeal angioma. Bleeding can complicate the attempt. Facial mask ventilation can also be difficult because of facial deformation. A laryngeal mask airway should be available in case of failure to ventilate; however, one must keep in mind that it may not help in the presence of a large laryngeal angioma. Spontaneous respiration must be maintained at all times in case of doubts. Avoid regional anesthesia particularly medullar blockades because of meningeal hemangioma. Pulse oximetry can be difficult because of capillary anomalies.

Pharmacological implications Perioperative blood pressure should be controlled because of abnormal vessel regulation. Neurological medications should be taken for as long as possible. Consider interaction between anesthetic drugs and anticonvulsive medication. Avoid, if possible, anesthetic drugs that could activate seizures (methohexital, enflurane). Parasympatholytic drugs should be also avoided because of glaucoma. Use of succinylcholine is possible if there is a proven absence of denervation lesion and no glaucoma.

Other conditions to be considered:

☞**NEUROFIBROMATOSIS (NF):** A genetically determined disorder with highly variable symptoms that can be generalized. Onset usually occurs in childhood but the disease becomes more active at puberty, during pregnancy, and at menopause. The classical features include the presence of subcutaneous tumors resulting in disfigurement and other complications such as the airway and spinal cord compression.

☞**TUBEROUS SCLEROSIS:** Presents with benign brain tumors (often compressive), skin lesions, and occasional involvement of other internal organs. Epileptic seizures and varying degrees of mental retardation are characteristic of this disorder.

☞**VON HIPPEL-LINDAU SYNDROME:** A possibly hereditary disorder characterized by angioma of the retina associated with a benign tumor. Hemangioma in the central nervous system is characteristic.

☞**KLIPPEL-TRENAUNAY SYNDROME:** Characterized by the presence of cutaneous hemangiomata with hypertrophy of the related bones and soft tissues. The disorder resembles, clinically and in its lack of definite genetic basis, the Sturge-Weber syndrome.

REFERENCE:

Batra RK, Gulaya V, Madan R, et al: Anaesthesia and the Sturge-Weber syndrome. *Can J Anaesth* 41:133, 1994.

Ceyhan A, Cakan T, Basar H, et al: Anaesthesia for Sturge-Weber syndrome. *Eur J Anaesthesiol* 16:339, 1999.

De Leon-Casasola OA, Lema MJ: Anesthesia for patients with the Sturge-Weber disease and the Klippel-Trenaunay syndrome. *J Clin Anesth* 3:409, 1991.

Sturge WA: A case of partial epilepsy, apparently because of a lesion of one of the vasomotor centres of the brain. *Trans Clin Soc Lond* 12:162, 1879.

Succinyl-CoA:3-Ketoacid CoA-Transferase Deficiency

At a glance: Inherited metabolic disorder resulting in ketoacidotic episodes.

Synonym: Succinyl-CoA:3-Oxoacid CoA-Transferase (SCOT) Deficiency.

Incidence and genetic inheritance: Extremely rare disorder (fewer than 20 patients described) with autosomal recessive transmission and chromosomal mapping to 5p13.

Pathophysiology: SCOT is an extrahepatic, mitochondrial matrix protein necessary for the synthesis of acetoacetyl-CoA from succinyl-CoA and acetoacetate. Acetoacetyl-CoA is then cleaved by mitochondrial acetyl-CoA thiolase and enters the tricarboxylic acid cycle. Of three different acetyl-CoA thiolases (a peroxisomal, a cytoplasmic, and a mitochondrial form), only the mitochondrial one needs to be considered here.

Clinical aspects: The disorder usually manifests as a severe ketoacidosis in the first week of life with tachypnea (caused by severe metabolic acidosis) being the most prominent sign (later onset has been described). Usually pyruvate, lactate, ammonia, and blood glucose levels are normal during the ketoacidotic event; however, hypoglycemia does not rule out SCOT deficiency. Similar to acylcoenzyme A cholesterol acyltransferase (ACAT) deficiency, the treatment of the ketoacidotic attacks consists of dextrose-containing fluid replacement therapy (keep blood glucose in the high normal range to suppress ketogenesis) and sodium bicarbonate. Common triggers of an attack are usually fever and/or infections, and the attacks tend to present more often with lethargy and coma after the neonatal period. Between these episodes the patients are free of symptoms, although elevated concentrations of ketone bodies in the urine can also be found during that time. Mildly restricted protein and fat intake should help to control ketogenesis. Some patients are on a carbohydrate-rich diet with oral sodium bicarbonate supplements.

Anesthetic considerations: Cardiomegaly and congestive heart failure have been described in some of these patients. The maintenance of high glucose level is mandatory to prevent ketoacidosis.

Other condition to be considered:

☞**Mitochondrial Acetoacetyl-CoA Thiolase Deficiency:** Inherited mitochondrial disease affecting isoleucine catabolism resulting in recurrent episodes of ketoacidosis.

Reference:

Kassovska-Bratinoba S, Fukao T, Song XQ, et al: Succinyl CoA:3-oxoacid CoA transferase (SCOT): Human cDNA cloning, human chromosomal mapping to 5p13, and mutation detection in a SCOT-deficient patient. *Am J Hum Genet* 59:519, 1996.

Synderman SE, Sansaricq C, Middleton B: Succinyl-CoA:3-ketoacid CoA transferase deficiency. *Pediatrics* 101:709, 1998.

Tildon JT, Cornblath M: Succinyl-CoA:3-ketoacid CoA transferase deficiency: A cause for ketoacidosis in infancy. *J Clin Invest* 51:493, 1972.

Sudden Infant Death Syndrome (SIDS)

At a glance: The sudden death of an apparently healthy infant, who is younger than 1 year of age, which is unexpected by history and which remains unexplained after a thorough postmortem investigation (autopsy), and where examination of the death scene failed to demonstrate an adequate cause for death.

Synonyms: SIDS; Crib Death Syndrome.

Incidence: In most countries, it is <1 per 1000 live births in the last few years following the "Back to Sleep" programs. In the United States alone, the incidence has been reduced (1998) to 0.53 per 1000 live births. Previously, it was nearly 2 per 1000 live births.

Pathophysiology: Uncertain; probably multifactorial, involving subtle cardiac, respiratory, and neurological abnormalities and precipitating environmental factors. Current theories include prolonged apnea secondary to immature neurorespiratory control, combined with fatigue secondary to relative lack of type 1 fibers in the respiratory muscle, and sudden arrhythmia secondary to prolonged QT interval on ECG. A higher risk has been demonstrated in infants placed in a sleeping position to which they were unaccustomed.

Diagnosis: Diagnosed by exclusion only where cause of death remains unexplained and should be considered after an adequate postmortem examination that includes (a) an autopsy, (b) investigation of the scene and circumstance of the death, and (c) exploration of the medical history of the infant and the family.

Clinical aspects: A common scenario is that of a previously well infant being put into a crib for a nap and then found dead some time later by the parents. Cause of death remains unexplained after investigation. From epidemiological studies, risk of SIDS is found to be increased with a variety of factors. Demographic factors include the age of the infant (2 to 4 months), male predominance, high birth

order, lower socioeconomic status, and younger maternal age. Antenatal factors include low birth weight, low gestational age, multiple pregnancies, maternal smoking, and substance-abusing mother. Postnatal factors include parental smoking, prone sleeping position, overheating of bedroom, soft mattress with excessive wrappings, and recent respiratory tract infections. Beast-feeding appears to have a protective effect from SIDS. By far, the most significant factor in the last few years has been the avoidance of a prone sleeping position, which has led to the reduction in the incidence of SIDS in many countries.

Precautions before anesthesia: Obtain full perinatal medical history of "apneic spells" in near-SIDS or SIDS siblings.

Anesthetic considerations: In case of near-SIDS or SIDS siblings (particularly a SIDS twin), the risk of SIDS is unknown but presumed to be increased after anesthesia. Therefore, the patient should have cardiorespiratory monitoring for a 24-hour postoperative period or longer, particularly if an opioid-based analgesia regimen is further utilized. It is uncertain whether regional anesthesia techniques may lessen the risk of SIDS postoperatively. There is the potential for an increased risk of apnea during spontaneously breathing techniques, but this increase has not been documented. The patient should be nursed in back position as much as possible postoperatively. There are also recent suggestions that the use of the BIS monitor may help to monitor these patients postoperatively. As an indicator of the level of consciousness in these babies, it may help to prevent sudden infant death syndrome.

Pharmacological implications: Aminophylline and caffeine citrate have been used in some centers to decrease the incidence of apneas in near-SIDS infants postoperatively.

Reference:

Dwyer T, Ponsonby A: SIDS epidemiology and incidence. *Pediatr Ann* 24(7):350, 1995.

Fifer WP, Myers MM, Sahni R, et al: Interactions between sleeping position and feeding on cardiorespiratory activity in preterm infants. *Dev Psychobiol* 47:288, 2005.

Lucey J: Comments on a sudden infant death article in another journal. *Pediatrics* 103(4):812, 1999.

Schwartz P, Stramba-Badiale M, Segantini A, et al: Prolongation of the QT interval and the sudden infant death syndrome. *N Engl J Med* 338(24):1709, 1998.

Uezono S, Kamata A, Nagata O, et al: Intraoperative awareness and the depth of anesthesia in children: a perspective from pediatric anesthesia. *Sleep Med* 3 Suppl 2:S67, 2002.

Sulfocysteinuria

At a glance: An inborn error of metabolism leading to fatal neurologic disease, severe development delay, and ectopia lentis in children. Infants often present with acute hemiplegia. Clinically manifested by ataxic gait, generalized dystonia, and choreoathetosis. Confirmed by the presence of sulfite in the urine ("strip-test").

Synonym: Sulfite Oxidase Deficiency.

Genetic inheritance: Autosomal recessive inheritance.

Pathophysiology: Genetic defect in sulfite oxidase, the enzyme converting sulfite to sulfate, resulting in the accumulation of sulfite and decreased secretion of inorganic sulfate. The excess sulfite is partially converted to thiosulfate and to *S*-sulfocysteine, and also combined with the aldehyde groups. This may lead to poor cross-linking of collagen and elastin.

Diagnosis: Clinical and biochemical features. Blood sulfite level is low. Urine collection shows increased sulfite and decreased sulfate excretion. Cultured fibroblast enzyme study shows decreased sulfite oxidase activity.

Clinical aspects: Patient usually presents in early infancy with infantile acute hemiplegia, hypotonia, hypertonia, generalized dystonia, seizure, progressive choreoathetoid movement, ataxia, myoclonus, and progressive cerebral palsy. The finding of dislocated lens on ophthalmological examination is highly suspicious. Course of disease usually follows a rapid deterioration and is often fatal in early childhood, although a milder course has also been described.

Precautions before anesthesia: Assess neurological function from medical history and physical examination. The respiratory status should be assessed because there is a potential risk of aspiration and pneumonia. General history, examination, chest radiograph, and arterial blood gas analysis should be obtained.

Anesthetic considerations: No reported case. Patient may not be cooperative because of the mental retardation. Potential risk of aspiration pneumonia in severe cases.

Pharmacological implications: There are no known implications.

REFERENCE:

Shih V, Abrams I, Johnson JL, et al: Sulfite oxidase deficiency: Biochemical and clinical investigations of a hereditary metabolic disorder in sulfur metabolism. *N Engl J Med* 297:1022, 1977.

Summerskill Syndrome

At a glance: Intermittent cholestasis with spontaneous resolution.

Synonyms: Benign Recurrent Intrahepatic Cholestasis (BRIC); Summerskill-Walshe-Tygstrup Syndrome.

Incidence and genetic inheritance: Often autosomal recessive (caused by mutations in a gene designated ATP8B1 on 18q21). Autosomal dominant forms exist. The disease is perhaps allelic with Byler Disease (Intrahepatic Cholestasis Syndrome).

Clinical aspects: Characterized by intermittent episodes of cholestasis without extrahepatic bile duct obstruction. Initial elevation of serum bile acids is followed by cholestatic jaundice; spontaneous resolution in a few weeks or months. Biliary cirrhosis and intrahepatic cholestasis can occur.

Anesthetic considerations: No specification with other hepatobiliary diseases. Evaluate severity of liver lesion (clinical, echography, CT scan, MRI). Laboratory investigations should include coagulation test with factor V, bilirubin, serum glutamic-oxaloacetic transaminase (SGOT), serum glutamic-pyruvic transaminase (SGPT), and albumin. Anesthesia drugs requiring hepatic metabolism should be avoided.

Other condition to be considered:

BYLER DISEASE (☞Progressive Familial Intrahepatic Cholestasis Syndrome; Fatal Intrahepatic Cholestasis Syndrome): Characterized by a variety of intrahepatic cholestasis that lead to death in the first decade of life. It is has been reported in the Old Order Amish. The clinical features include an early onset of loose, foul-smelling stools, post-infection "attacks" of jaundice,

hepatosplenomegaly, dwarfism, and death between the first year and 8 years of age.

REFERENCES:

Floreani A, Molaro M, Mottes M, et al: Autosomal dominant benign recurrent intrahepatic cholestasis (BRIC) unlinked to 18q21 and 2q24. *Am J Med Genet* 95:450, 2000.

Summerskill WHJ, Walshe JM: Benign recurrent intrahepatic "obstructive" jaundice. *Lancet* 2:686, 1959.

Superior Mesenteric Artery Syndrome (SMAS)

At a glance: Inherited syndrome associated with vomiting because of compression of the third part of the duodenum by the superior mesenteric artery.

Synonym: Cast Syndrome.

Incidence and genetic inheritance: Acquired, the exact incidence is unknown, but is probably higher than previously thought.

Clinical aspects: Occasionally, this disorder is seen after body casting or corrective spinal surgery. It presents with clinical features of upper gastrointestinal obstruction and is attributed to extrinsic compression of the third part of the duodenum between the aorta (posteriorly) and the superior mesenteric artery (anteriorly) (decrease in aortomesenteric angle). Symptoms of persistent vomiting with abdominal distention, epigastric tenderness, and tympanic percussion note usually beginning 6 to 8 days after surgery or the application of a body casting, but may occur up to 40 days thereafter. In contrast to postoperative ileus, bowel sounds are usually present in Superior Mesenteric Artery Syndrome (SMAS). It is thought to be more common in the second decade of life when increased spinal flexibility and truncal casting increase lordosis and subsequently alter the anatomic relationship between the superior mesenteric artery, the aorta, and the duodenum. The combination of surgery to correct spinal deformities (most often scoliosis) and generalized weight loss are known risk factors for duodenal obstruction. It is most frequently seen in patients after spinal or pelvic surgery, but has also been described after femoral fractures. Patients with acute SMAS may be severely dehydrated and have profound electrolyte abnormalities. Close monitoring of hydration and serum electrolytes is therefore mandatory, since fatal outcome secondary to severe metabolic alkalosis and electrolyte disturbances has been described. Furthermore, duodenal obstruction has resulted in death from gastric perforation. Contrast radiography is used to demonstrate an abrupt cutoff in the third part of the duodenum representing the external compression by the superior mesenteric artery. A nasojejunal feeding tube (distal to the obstruction) has been used successfully to provide feeds and favoring weight gain, which seems to have a positive effect on SMAS. Alternatively, total parenteral nutrition has been used; however, the enteral way is usually preferred. The left lateral and/or prone position and/or adjusting the body cast may alleviate the symptoms; however, surgery may be necessary in up to half of the patients to resolve the compression (duodenal mobilization with division of the ligament of Treitz or bypass procedures such as duodenojejunostomy or gastrojejunostomy have been used).

Anesthetic considerations: Assess and correct hydration, serum electrolyte, and acid-base imbalances preoperatively. A rapid sequence induction technique is recommended, because of the increased risk of gastroduodenal content regurgitation and pulmonary aspiration.

REFERENCES:

Crowther MA, Webb PJ, Eyre-Brook IA: Superior mesenteric artery syndrome following surgery for scoliosis. *Spine* 27:E528, 2002.

Kepros JP: Superior mesenteric artery syndrome after multiple trauma. *J Trauma* 53:1028, 2002.

Shah MA, Albright MB, Vogt MT, et al: Superior mesenteric artery syndrome in scoliosis surgery: Weight percentile for height as an indicator of risk. *J Pediatr Orthop* 23:665, 2003.

Sweet Syndrome

At a glance: A syndrome characterized by the abrupt onset of fever; arthritis; raised painful plaques on the limbs, face, and neck; neutrophilic leukocytosis; and dense dermal infiltration with mature neutrophilic polymorphs. Evolution can be favorable or recurrent. Associated diseases are frequent.

Synonyms: Acute Febrile Neutrophilic Dermatosis; Sweet Disease; Gomm-Button Disease.

Classification: There are four groups of Sweet Syndrome:

Classic/Idiopathic
Parainflammatory
Paraneoplastic
Pregnancy Associated

The malignant form represents 20% of cases. Pediatric cases account for 8%.

History: First described by Robert Douglas Sweet, an English dermatologist, in 1964.

Incidence: Hundreds of cases have been described.

Pathophysiology: Unclear; Sweet Syndrome seems to be in some cases a response to systemic factors (hematological disease, infection, or drug exposure to granulocyte colony-stimulating factor, minocycline, Bactrim, lithium, furosemide, hydralazine, carbamazepine, and levonorgestrel/ethinyl estradiol). There is a neutrophil mediation, associated neutrophilia, and response to medications that impact neutrophil activity. Tumor necrosis factor is thought to be implicated, as well as type 1 helper T cells.

Diagnosis: Clinically evocated by abrupt fever associated with nodules followed by headache; myalgias and arthralgias are common.

Clinical aspects: *Skin lesions* characteristically affect primarily the face and the extremities in an asymmetric distribution: reddish blue or violaceous papules, plaques that can coalesce into circinate or arcuate plaques, nodules, subepidermal edema pustules. Ulcers and bullae are more common in malignancy-associated disease. A pathergy phenomenon is often associated. Lesions could be *mucosal* (conjunctivitis), *pulmonary* (chronic cough or pulmonary infiltrates on chest radiographs), *renal* (proteinuria, hematuria, and decreased creatinine clearance), *skeletal* (sterile chronic recurrent multifocal osteomyelitis), or central nervous system (CNS) (cerebrospinal fluid pleocytosis). Other clinical features can include splenomegaly, storage liver disease, thrombocytopenia, and anemia. Associated diseases are frequent: malignancies (myelodysplasia, chronic myelogenous leukemia, acute myeloid leukemia, lymphoma, genitourinary cancers) and systemic disorders (Crohn Disease, Ulcerative Colitis, Sjögren Syndrome, Behçet Disease, Lupus Erythemato-

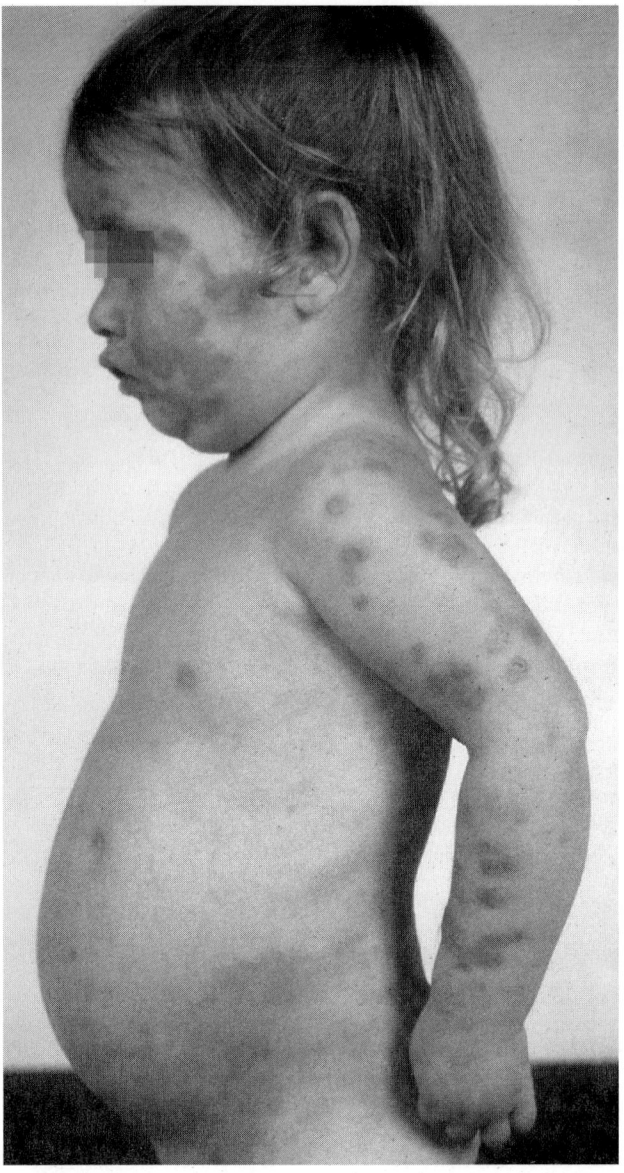

Sweet syndrome This young girl with painful skin lesions, mainly on her face (coalescent) and arm, suffers from Sweet syndrome.

sus, Rheumatoid Arthritis, and undifferentiated connective-tissue disease).

Precautions before anesthesia: Evaluate pulmonary function (clinical, chest radiographs, pulmonary function test if necessary); renal function (clinical, echography); and hepatic function (clinical, biochemical, coagulation, echography). Preoperative laboratory investigations should include full blood count, electrolytes, serum glutamic-oxaloacetic transaminase (SGOT), serum glutamic-pyruvic transaminase (SGPT), urea, and creatinine. Evaluate associated diseases.

Anesthetic considerations: Tolerance of anemia has to be evaluated preoperatively and should require transfusion. Regional anesthesia is not contraindicated but platelet count should be obtained preoperatively and pathergy, i.e., all associated allergic morbid manifestations, should be considered.

Pharmacological implications: Perioperative fluid regimen and anesthetic drugs dosages should be adapted to renal function.

Preoperative stress doses of steroid should be given if necessary. Avoid drugs that trigger Sweet Syndrome.

Other conditions to be considered:

☞**BEHÇET DISEASE OR SYNDROME:** Characterized by four major symptoms: oral aphthous ulcers, skin lesions, ocular symptoms, and genital ulcerations, and occasionally by inflammation in tissues and organs throughout the body, including the gastrointestinal tract, central nervous system, vascular system, lungs, and kidneys. Viral and autoimmune etiologies had been suggested. Other reported clinical features include alopecia areata, Raynaud disease, and rheumatoid arthritis suggestive of autoimmune disease. Behçet Syndrome and Sweet Syndrome have overlapping symptoms, including eye lesions, oral aphthae, genital ulcers, and skin lesions. The incidence of Behçet Syndrome is very high in Japan (1:15,000), although no cases of Sweet Syndrome with Behçet Syndrome had been reported outside Japan, several Japanese patients with Behçet Syndrome also had features of Sweet Syndrome.

REFERENCES:

Cohen PR, Kurzrock R: Sweet's syndrome: A review of current treatment options. *Am J Clin Dermatol* 3(2):117, 2002.

James WD: Newer neutrophilic dermatoses. *Arch Dermatol* 139(1):101, 2003.

von den Driesch P: Sweet's syndrome (acute febrile neutrophilic dermatosis). *J Am Acad Dermatol* 31(4):535, 1994.

Swyer Syndrome

At a glance: A condition that affects the development of reproductive and genital organs. Patients present with a functioning Y chromosome but without internal female organs because of an abnormality on the X chromosome that renders the body completely or partially incapable of recognizing the androgens produced.

Synonym: Gonadal Dysgenesis XY-Female type.

Genetic inheritance: Sporadic in most cases but may be X-linked in some cases.

Pathophysiology: There is evidence that most cases are caused by point mutation or deletion of the SRY (sex-reversed, Y) gene on the Y chromosome, which may actually be the TDF (testis-determining factor) gene. Some cases may also be caused by a mutation on the X chromosome in the region of Xp22.3-p21, termed SRVX (sex-reversed, X) locus.

Diagnosis: Clinical features. The finding of "streak gonads" at exploratory laparotomy is pathognomonic. Chromosomal study shows 46 XY karyotype. Sex chromatin study is negative.

Clinical aspects: Patients appear to be normal female phenotype from birth. However, they do not develop secondary sexual characteristics at puberty, do not menstruate, and have "streak gonads." Most have normal or above-average stature and eunuchoidal proportion. Intelligence is normal. The streak gonads have a high incidence of becoming malignant (gonadoblastoma or germinoma), particularly in association with presence of H-Y gene on the Y chromosome.

Anesthetic considerations: There are no specific anesthetic considerations.

REFERENCES:

Berta P, Hawkins J, Sinclair A, et al: Genetic evidence equating SRY and the testis-determining factor. *Nature* 348:448, 1990.

Chenke J, Carmichael R, Stewart J, et al: Familial XY gonadal dysgenesis. *J Med Genet* 7:105, 1970.

Swyer-James-Macleod Syndrome

At a glance: A rare acquired syndrome characterized by a probable manifestation of postinfectious obliterative bronchiolitis leading to a smaller, radiologically hyperlucent, affected lung.

Synonyms: Hyperlucent Lung Syndrome; MacLeod Syndrome.

Genetic inheritance: No genetic inheritance.

Pathophysiology: Lung grows by progressive alveolarization, generally before the age of 8 years. Following an infectious syndrome, a reduced pulmonary perfusion that leads to an arrest of progressive growth and alveolarization of the lung. Swyer-James-Macleod Syndrome generally follows a severe bronchiolitis but has also been described following infection by *Mycoplasma pneumoniae* and *Streptococcus pneumoniae*.

Diagnosis: Evocated a few months or years after an infection in a child with respiratory symptoms and eventually an asymmetric chest, or on a systematic chest radiograph with a hyperlucent lateralized aspect.

Clinical aspects: Involves only respiratory function with hyperlucency, air trapping upon expiration, wheezing, and abnormal time-attenuation curves during inspiration and forced expiration.

Precautions before anesthesia: Evaluate respiratory function (clinical, pulmonary function test with arterial blood gas analysis, CT scan).

Anesthetic considerations: The use of positive pressure ventilation support must be done carefully and the potential for sudden pneumothorax must be kept in mind in pesence of hemodynamic instability. Perioperative physiotherapy is needed to avoid pulmonary superinfection.

Pharmacological implications: Probably best to avoid nitrous oxide because it can increase the risk of pneumothorax.

REFERENCES:

Braunschweig M, Gal I: Swyer-James syndrome. *JBR-BTR* 84(2):57, 2001.

Fregonese L, Girosi D, Battistini E, et al: Physiologic and roentgenographic changes after pneumonectomy in a boy with Macleod/Swyer-James syndrome and bronchiectasis. *Pediatr Pulmonol* 34(5):412, 2002.

Sylvian Syndrome

At a glance: Syndrome is characterized by pseudobulbar palsy, epilepsy, cognitive deficits, and bilateral perisylvian malformations on imaging.

Synonym: Congenital Bilateral Perisylvian Syndrome.

Incidence: Unknown. Recently recognized following advances in neuroimaging techniques as a distinct syndrome.

Genetic inheritance: Autosomal recessive; male:female ratio is equal.

Pathophysiology: Unknown. Disorder of neuronal migration.

Diagnosis: Suspected by clinical picture and supported by classical MRI findings. These are radiological indications of bilateral perisylvian cortical malformations consistent with polymicrogyria involving the sylvian fissure and opercular cortex.

Clinical aspects: Pseudobulbar palsy, dysarthria, mental retardation (85% of patients) and cognitive deficits, and seizures (87% of patients) that are atypical and difficult to control by medication (55% of patients). Infantile spasms in the first 6 months of life are often the presenting seizure type. Hypotonia, hemiparesis, apneas. Pharyngeal and masticatory muscle diplegia, especially tongue. Micrognathia, arthrogryposis.

Precautions before anesthesia: Full assessment of the airway, oromotor function, and degree of pseudobulbar palsy is essential. Preparation for prolonged intubation should be made if appropriate. Seizure type, frequency, and control needs to be reviewed by neurology and optimized. Medication should be continued preoperatively. Assessment of other neurological deficits should be documented. Evidence of acute and chronic effects of aspiration should be looked for and a chest radiograph performed.

Anesthetic considerations: The potential for gastric regurgitation, recurrent pulmonary aspiration and irritation with ventilation (restrictive disease) must be considered. Mouth opening and tongue movement are likely to be significantly impaired. Use of an antisialagogue to reduce secretions is helpful preinduction. Induction of anesthesia should be either by spontaneous ventilating inhalational technique or rapid sequence induction with cricoid pressure once face-mask ventilation has been established. Seizures should be considered as a cause of delay in emergence. Extubation should only occur once the child is fully awake; the child may need intubation until fully recovered. Apneas are more frequent postoperatively and appropriate monitoring should be used. The need for sustained mechanical ventilation postoperatively must be considered because of the pseudobulbar palsy.

Pharmacological implications: Use of nondepolarizing agents should be delayed until the airway has been secured and lung ventilation confirmed. Avoid drugs that may trigger seizures, such as enflurane and sevoflurane, and consider interactions with antiseizure medication. Caution with opioids if there is a history of apnea.

REFERENCES:

Kuzniecky R, Andermann F, Guerrini R: Congenital bilateral perisylvian syndrome: Study of 31 patients. The CBPS Multicenter Collaborative Study. *Lancet* 341(8845):608, 1993.

Kuzniecky R, Andermann F, Guerrini R: Infantile spasms: An early epileptic manifestation in some patients with the congenital bilateral perisylvian syndrome. *J Child Neurol* 9(4):420, 1994.

Gropman AL, Barkovich AJ, Vezina LG et al: Pediatric congenital bilateral perisylvian syndrome: Clinical and MRI features in 12 patients. *Neuropediatrics* 28(4):198, 1997.

Syringomyelia

At a glance: Autosomal dominant syndrome characterized by spinal cyst formation. Frequent association with Arnold-Chiari Malformation. Characteristic suspended loss of pain and temperature sensation.

Synonym: Morvan Disease.

Incidence: Prevalence is 8.4:100,000 in general population.

Genetic inheritance: Autosomal dominant. It has also been reported after traumatic injury (acquired disorder).

Pathophysiology: Chronic syndrome characterized by cavitations and gliosis of the spinal cord (usually cervical or thoracic), the medulla, or both. An obstacle to cerebrospinal fluid circulation in

the fourth ventricle toward the subarachnoid space has been evocated to explain the syndrome. It seems similar to a craniocervical junction malformation such as Chiari type I and the Arnold-Chiari, which is associated in 84% of cases (intramedullary tumors and hydrocephalus have been also observed). The cavity, for unknown reasons, often expands during adolescence or the young adult years.

Diagnosis: Clinical (back pain; headaches; stiffness or weakness of shoulders, arms, or legs; loss of the ability to feel extremes of hot or cold). Radiography, CT scan, and particularly MRI make diagnosis.

Clinical aspects: Onset most commonly occurs between the ages of 25 and 40 years, but it can be earlier. First sign is usually paresthesias in the upper limbs; then loss of pain and temperature sensation in a characteristic distribution, usually "suspended," involving arms and trunk but not legs (because of lesion to the posterior horns and the fascicle of Lissauer sensory fibers). The progression is very slow. Other clinical features can be observed that involve neurological function: autonomic pathways such as Horner Syndrome, skin trophic changes, neurogenic bladder, reduced or absent reflex in arms, and bilateral Babinski signs. Spastic paraparesis can occur. Scoliosis is frequent.

Precautions before anesthesia: Evaluate neurological function with a precise clinical examination. Locate intramedullary cysts (MRI).

Anesthetic considerations: Careful positioning is needed, particularly in the case of an association with Arnold-Chiari Malformation. Perimedullar anesthesia should be avoided and is contraindicated at the level of the cyst because of the size diminution of epidural space. Somatosensory evoked potential monitoring can be difficult in a case of scoliosis surgery. There should be no concerns with the intracranial pressure.

Pharmacological implications: Probably best to avoid succinylcholine because of the increase in intracranial pressure.

Other condition to be considered:

CONGENITAL MUSCULAR DYSTROPHY WITH SYRINGOMYELIA: Disorder with myopathy, mental retardation and multiple skeletal malformations.

REFERENCES:

Sarnat HB: Embryology and dysgenesis of the posterior fossa, in Batzdorf U (ed): *Syringomyelia: Current Concepts in Diagnosis and Treatment.* Baltimore, Williams & Wilkins, 1991, p 3.

Systemic Lupus Erythematosus (SLE)

At a glance: A chronic and potentially fatal autoimmune (antinuclear antibodies) disease characterized by unpredictable exacerbation and remission of inflammatory multisystemic disorder of connective tissue. The circulation of immune complexes and activation of the complement leads to involvement of the skin, joints, kidneys, serosal membranes, lungs, gastrointestinal tract, and heart.

Classification: There are four types of lupus erythematous.

Systemic Lupus Erythematosus type I (Discoid or Cutaneous Lupus) affects only the skin. Round skin lesions may be scaly, raised, violet, or red occur. The distribution of the skin lesions is mainly the face, neck, scalp, ears, arms, and sometimes the chest. The skin manifestation is often worse when the person is exposed to sunlight. Most people affected with this type of lupus do not present

Table S-3 Medications Associated with Drug-Induced Lupus

ACE inhibitors (captopril, lisinopril).
Procainamide hydrochloride
Hydralazine hydrochloride
Isoniazid
Hydantoins
Chlorpromazine hydrochloride
Methyldopa
Minocycline
Interferon-alfa
D-penicillamine
Trimethoprim (Bactrim)
Sulfa

ACE, angiotensin-converting enzyme.

systemic symptomatology. Cutaneous lupus is sometimes confused with psoriasis.

Systemic Lupus Erythematosus type II (Subacute Cutaneous Lupus): This type of lupus often causes a more widespread skin rash than type I. The skin lesion begins as small, reddened, raised areas that turn into raised, scaly patches or ringlike patches. The shoulders, forearms, neck, and upper torso are most likely to be affected. This form of lupus does not cause scarring or thinning of the skin. Individuals affected with this type present with systemic symptoms involving muscle or joint pain, fatigue, or low-grade fever.

Systemic Lupus Erythematosus type III (Drug-Induced Lupus and possible drug triggers of systemic lupus): Medications can cause temporary symptoms and signs of lupus. Most often, the symptoms disappear when the medication is stopped, generally within a few weeks. Symptoms are usually milder than in classical lupus, and the kidneys and central nervous system (CNS) are rarely affected. Most often, the administration of medication for the control of seizure in children may cause a lupus-like condition similar the type seen in adults. Medications that have been associated with drug-induced lupus include those shown in Table S-3.

☞*Neonatal Lupus:* A rare condition presenting in infants born to mothers who have lupus. The skin lesions develop when the neonate is exposed to ultraviolet light. It usually clears up within 6 months.

Incidence: The disorder is three times more common in African American blacks than in American whites. It is also more common in Asians and in China alone, it may be more common than rheumatoid arthritis. The ethnic group at greatest risk is African Caribbean blacks. The annual incidence is 35 new cases per 100,000 population per year. The prevalence in the United States is estimated at 250,000 to 500,000. A recent study indicated a prevalence of 500 per 100,000 (1:200) in women residing in the areas surrounding Birmingham, Alabama. The prognosis has greatly improved over the last few decades with at least 90% survival at 10 years.

Genetic inheritance: Twin studies that showed higher concordance for clinical and serologic abnormality supported a significant genetic factor. Occurs three to four times more frequently in blacks than in whites, and there is also a female preponderance. Using a gene marker, the likely locus is chromosome 1q23.

Pathophysiology: Although the etiology is still unknown, lupus erythematosus is thought to represent a failure of the regulatory mechanisms of the autoimmune system. The origin of SLE appears to be multifactorial—diet, drugs, toxins, infection, environment,

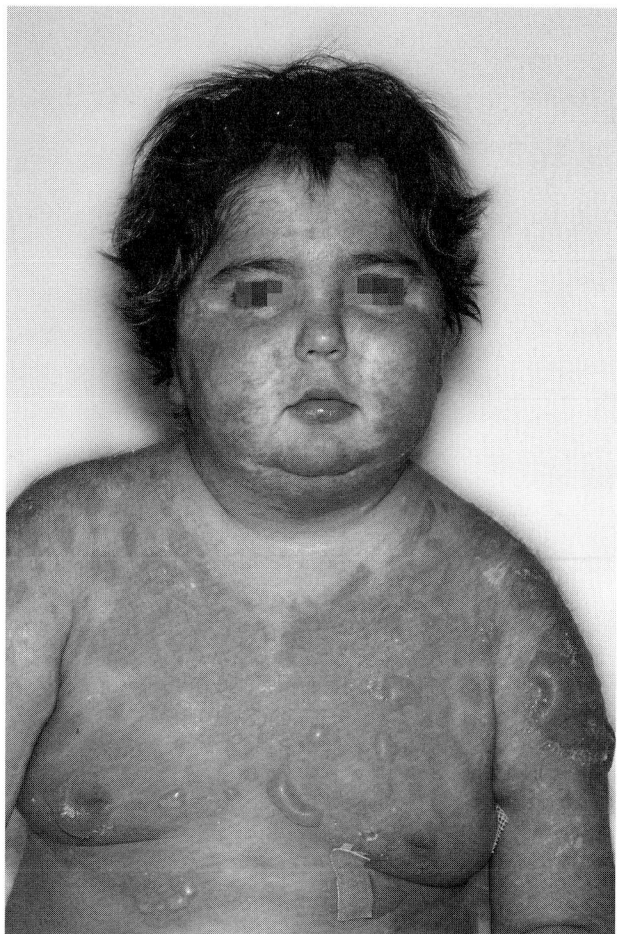

Systemic lupus erythematosus   A young girl with severe cutaneous manifestation of systemic lupus erythematosus.

hormones, and genetics, among other things, all seem to play a part. Recent evidence shows that an increased oxidative activity may generate a chemical change in the endogenous DNA in vivo and therefore may be a primary event in the pathogenesis of autoimmunity in some patients with SLE.

Diagnosis: Onset of the disease between puberty and the fourth decade of life with a female:male ratio of 9:1; clinical and serologic abnormalities (serum antinuclear antibody, anti-RNA antibodies).

Clinical aspects: SLE is more common in females than in males (9:1). Usual onset is in the third and fourth decades of life. Periods of prolonged remission are punctuated by life-threatening exacerbations. Involvement of the cardiac (myocarditis [15% of cases], pericarditis [60% of cases], endocarditis [25% of cases]), respiratory (pleural effusion [25% of cases], interstitial fibrosis, pneumonitis [20% of cases]), and renal (renal hypertension [50% of cases], glomerulonephritis) systems are common. Lupus anticoagulant (30% of patients) prolongs the activated partial thromboplastin time and increases the risk of arterial and venous thromboses formation. Treatment is usually approached with a combination of nonsteroidal antiinflammatory drugs (NSAIDs), antimalarial agents, corticosteroids, and immunosuppressants. Plasmapheresis is also used.

Precautions before anesthesia: Assess the extent of the illness. Determine if the patient is in remission or has acute exacerbation, because the perioperative risk is much higher with the latter. Assess systemic involvement: *cardiovascular* (heart failure, valve lesions, pericardial effusion); *respiratory* (effusion, pneumonitis, interstitial fibrosis); *renal* (failure, hypertension); *CNS* (peripheral neuropathy, cerebrovascular accident); and *Raynaud phenomenon*. Check drug history (NSAIDs, antimalarials, steroids, immunosuppressants, cardiac drugs) and plasmapheresis. *Investigations:* ECG; echocardiography; chest radiography; arterial blood gases; electrolytes; urea and creatinine; hemoglobin; white cell count; platelet count; coagulation screen; lung function tests; plasma cholinesterase levels (reduced by plasmapheresis); and lupus anticoagulant status. Preoperative optimization of cardiovascular and respiratory functions. In particular check control of hypertension, treatment of angina, arrhythmias, heart failure, drainage of significant effusions (pericardial and pleural), and treatment of pneumonia. Take antithrombotic measures in patients with positive anticardiolipin antibodies and lupus anticoagulant (antiembolic stocking, avoid dehydration, subcutaneous heparin). Assess joint mobility of the neck and temporomandibular joints. Examine oral cavity for erosive ulcers of the mucosa that may make the placement of an oral airway difficult. Antibiotic coverage should be given in those with history of endocarditis. Most patients will be on chronic steroid coverage and will require the administration preoperatively of a supplementation to cover the intraoperative stress responses.

Anesthetic considerations: Because of the potential presence of cardiovascular instability, it is recommended at induction to avoid drugs and techniques likely to cause tachycardia, hypertension, hypotension, or reduced myocardial contractility (e.g., ketamine, thiopentone). Cricoarytenoid arthritis resulting in a narrowed airway has been reported. Recent plasmapheresis may prolong the duration of ester drugs (e.g., suxamethonium). In the presence of renal impairment, maintain fluid balance and avoid drugs that are renally metabolized or excreted. Avoid vasoconstrictors and radial artery cannulation in Raynaud Disease. Neuromuscular monitoring is essential if cyclophosphamide or plasmapheresis is used. Check the coagulation status before using a regional anesthetic technique. Document existing neurologic deficits prior to the use of regional techniques. The presence of lupus anticoagulant and a history of thrombotic events signify an increased predisposition to thrombosis formation so that coagulation status should be monitored and heparin given if necessary. Those patients with Sjögren Syndrome should have their eyes protected by an ophthalmic ointment.

Pharmacological implications: Perioperative steroid cover is needed for patients who are receiving steroids. Use of cyclophosphamide may prolong the duration of ester drugs (e.g., suxamethonium and mivacurium). Avoid or reduce dose of pancuronium and vecuronium. Hypoalbuminemia in nephrotic syndrome affects drug distribution. The use of anticholinergic agents is discouraged in Sjögren Syndrome.

REFERENCE:

Smith GB: Systemic lupus erythematosus, in Goldstone JC, Pollard RB (eds): *Handbook of Clinical Anesthesia*. New York, Churchill Livingston, 1996, p 234.

T

Takayasu Disease

At a glance: An inflammatory chronic progressive panendarteritis of the aorta that occludes one or more of the large branches of the aortic arch, leading to hypoperfusion of major peripheral organs, including the brain and the spinal cord. Also known as the "pulseless women disease." Symptoms consist of aphasia, transient hemiparesis, unilateral transient amblyopia or persistent blindness, headache, vertigo, and syncopal attacks. Progressive evolution with poor prognosis. Autoimmune in origin. Affects mostly young women.

Synonyms: Martorell Syndrome; Martorell-Fabré Syndrome; Reader-Harbitz Syndrome; Takayasu Arteritis; Takayasu-Martorell-Fabré Syndrome; Takayasu-Onishi Syndrome; Aortic Arch Arteritis; Maladie des Femmes sans Pouls (French appellation).

History: First described by Mikito Takayasu, a Japanese ophthalmologist, in 1908.

Incidence: 1.2 to 2.5:1,000,000 population per year in whites; higher in Asian populations. Affects young women less than 30 years in 80 to 90% of cases. The female-to-male ratio is 8:1. In the United States, it is suggested that Takayasu arteritis affects approximately 1 person per 1000 in the general population. Internationally it afflicts 6 person per 1000. The mortality is usually caused by vascular complications such as hypertension, stroke and aortic insufficiency.

Genetic inheritance: None; probably autoimmune.

Pathophysiology: Histology demonstrates granulomatous infiltration of the adventitia and media of arteries with lymphocytes, plasma cells, histiocytes, and giant cells. Following the acute phase of inflammation, a chronic sclerotic phase develops. Immune complexes have been demonstrated; however, an immune complex-mediated etiology has never been confirmed. Antiendothelial antibodies have been demonstrated by a number of workers, but elevated levels are not specific to Takayasu arteritis.

Diagnosis: Age of onset, clinical history, and examination. The diagnosis is confirmed by arteriography to assess degree of vascular involvement. Four types of late-phase are described:

- Type I is the classic pulseless form that involves the brachiocephalic vascular region, the carotid arteries, and the subclavian arteries.
- Type II is a combination of type I and III.
- Type III is represented by an atypical coarctation of the thoracic and abdominal portion of the aorta, distal to the arch and major branches.
- Type IV affects the aorta in its entire length, causing an extensive dilatation. The major arterial branches of the aorta are also affected.

The most common type is in 65% of patients, type III. The most common vessel involved is the subclavian artery (50%).

Clinical aspects: Onset occurs at younger than 40 years of age. Clinical findings include limb claudication, multiple vascular bruits (carotid and aortic in 70% of patients), and less frequently the femoral and subclavian artery manifestations. Asymmetric pulse between limbs; vertebrobasilar insufficiency secondary to vessel stenosis; arthralgia and myalgia. Up to 30% of patients report visual disturbance, including amaurosis and diplopia. Funduscopy may reveal microaneurysms, venous beading, and in the later stages of the disease, hemorrhagic arteriovenous anastomoses, optic atrophy, or retinal detachment. Cardiovascular findings include main coronary artery stenoses, aortic regurgitation, cardiac failure, aneurysm formation, arterial stenosis, and hypertension. Although not always clinically evident, pulmonary hypertension is present in 50% of patients. Disease activity can be monitored by measurement of the erythrocyte sedimentation rate. Takayasu arteritis is associated with autoimmune diseases such as connective-tissue disorders, glomerulonephritis, and endocrine abnormalities. Treatment is with high-dose steroids, immunosuppressant drugs being used occasionally. Anticoagulants have not been proven to be of use.

Precautions before anesthesia: Full clinical assessment of respiratory and cardiovascular systems. Assess for signs of hypo- and hyperthyroidism. Note blood pressure discrepancies between limbs. Review arteriograms to define sites of arterial stenoses. Cardiovascular assessment, 12-lead ECG to exclude myocardial ischemia, echocardiography to assess left ventricle and aortic valve function. Assess renal function (renal artery stenosis is a common occurrence). Consider thyroid function testing. Ensure active inflammation has resolved or is well controlled by medical therapy by reviewing serial erythrocyte sedimentation rate measurements.

Anesthetic considerations: Anesthesia for patients with Takayasu arteritis is complicated by severe uncontrolled hypertension, end-organ dysfunction resulting from hypertension, stenosis of major blood vessels affecting regional circulation, and difficulties encountered in monitoring arterial blood pressure. Consider sites for blood pressure measurement, the radial arteries may be occluded and not suitable for invasive monitoring. Invasive monitoring as indicated by preoperative assessment and procedure, although threshold for such monitors should be low in light of cardiac involvement and prevalence of pulmonary hypertension. Regional anesthesia is relatively contraindicated in the presence of aortic regurgitation or evidence of spinal cord hypoperfusion.

Pharmacological implications: Provide adequate steroid cover for procedure.

Other conditions to be considered:

☞**HORTON SYNDROME:** A generalized vascular disorder characterized by inflammation of the arteries resulting from the accumulation of granular tissue. It affects the large arterial branches of the aortic arch, principally the temporal arteries. The clinical features include symptoms that appear suddenly or in a more gradual onset of low-grade fever, arthritis, and muscle weakness. Throbbing headache and scalp tenderness have been reported.

POLYMYALGIA RHEUMATICA SYNDROME: A rare inflammatory disorder characterized by muscle pain, stiffness, fatigue, and fever. Nonsteroidal antiinflammatory drugs have been used efficiently. Clinically, it starts abruptly with pain and stiffness in the neck, shoulders, upper arms, hips, and/or legs. Other clinical features include anorexia, muscle weakness, and/or nervous depression.

POLYMYALGIA NODOSA SYNDROME (PAN): Characterized by the presence of granular nodules following the distribution of small and medium-sized arteries. Fever, chills, fatigue, and/or weight loss are early sign of the disease. Abdominal pain, peripheral neuropathy, skin eruptions, joint pain, and/or generalized muscle pain have also been observed. Organ ischemia because of reduce arterial flow and the presence of blood clots is possible.

REFERENCES:

Hall S, Buchbinder R: Takayasu's arteritis. *Rheum Dis Clin North Am* 16:411, 1990.

Karaca S, Akgun I: Epidural anaesthesia for arthroscopic knee surgery in a patient with Takayasu's arteritis. *Eur J Anaesthesiol* 19:528, 2002.

Kathirvel S, Chavan S, Arya VK, et al: Anesthetic management of patients with Takayasu's arteritis: A case series and review. *Anesth Analg* 93:60, 2001.

Tangier Disease

At a glance: A genetic disorder of cholesterol transport named for the secluded island of Tangier, off the coast of Virginia. Characteristically, patients present orange tonsils, very low levels of high-density lipoprotein (HDL), and enlarged liver and spleen.

Synonyms: High-Density Lipoprotein (HDL) Deficiency; Analphalipoproteinemia.

Genetic inheritance: Although the molecular basis remains unknown, a mutation in the ABC1 (ATP-binding cassette) gene on chromosome 9q31 has been reported. ABC1 codes for a protein that helps rid cells of excess cholesterol. Autosomal codominant disorder. Heterozygotes do not have any clinical manifestations.

Pathophysiology: The primary problem appears to be a defect in cell signaling and in mobilization of cellular lipids, leading to intracellular cholesterol esters accumulation. This defect is compounded by a low plasma concentration of apolipoprotein A-I (an essential component of HDL) caused by a pathologically rapid catabolism. This results in a low level of HDL in plasma, making it unable to scavenge cholesterol from tissues. Tissues that accumulate excessive cholesterol include tonsils, liver, spleen, lymph nodes, thymus, intestines, and peripheral nerves. Histology reveals deposits of cholesterol esters outside of lysosomes in the cytoplasm.

Diagnosis: Homozygotes have a marked deficiency of HDL cholesterol and apolipoprotein (apo) A-I levels (both <10 mg/dL), decreased low-density lipoprotein (LDL) cholesterol levels (about 40% of normal), and mild hypertriglyceridemia.

Clinical aspects: Large orange tonsils, splenomegaly, neuropathy, and rectal mucosal changes (orange-brown spots). Neuropathy may include demyelination (mononeuropathic or polyneuropathic) and axonal degeneration with a syringomyelic (dissociative) picture. Sensory loss may lead to global anesthesia but autonomic neuropathy has not been described. Unlike earlier beliefs, it is now known that the risk of atherosclerosis is increased in older patients. Mitral and pulmonary valve abnormalities have been reported. Loss of vision, incomplete eyelid closure. May have abnormal platelet function. The possibility of an association with cerebellar dysgenesis, cardiac defects and renal anomalies has been reported. Also, few case reports of annual pancreatic defect have been suggested. There is no specific treatment, although dietary fat restrictions are recommended.

Precautions before anesthesia: Anemia and hemolysis, thrombocytopenia (prolonged bleeding time correctable with desmopressin acetate). Sleep apnea (airway obstruction). Liver function tests, electrolytes (malabsorption). ECG, echocardiogram, stress test/coronary angiography if ischemia suspected. Evaluate extent of neurological deficit, cranial nerve palsy (upper airway reflexes).

Anesthetic considerations: Rapid sequence induction is recommended if upper airway reflexes are lost. Complete airway obstruction is possible if tonsils are "kissing" (use nasopharyngeal airway to relieve). Meticulous positioning with adequate padding during surgery and recovery. Regional techniques are relatively contraindicated in the presence of neuropathy. Management depends upon systemic manifestations of the disease, such as ischemic heart disease. The presence of neuropathies or muscle weakness requires cautious use of muscle relaxants and patient positioning. Regional techniques should be avoided in the presence of neuropathy or platelet dysfunction. Care should be taken to protect the eyes.

Pharmacological implications: Avoid succinylcholine if neuropathy is present (risk of hyperkalemia). Reduce the dosage of nondepolarizing muscle-relaxant drugs in patients with extensive neuropathy or muscle weakness. Use of muscle relaxants should be guided by neuromuscular monitoring. If sleep apnea is present, short-acting agents allow for rapid recovery (especially opioids).

Other conditions to be considered:

☞**ABETALIPOPROTEINEMIA:** An autosomal recessive inheritance disorder, most often observed in cosanguineous population. It is characterized by the absence of low-density lipoproteins and steatorrhea. Other clinical features include acanthocytosis, retinitis pigmentosa, ataxia, and mental retardation because of the reduced or absence of absorption of fat-based vitamins and other derivatives. Therefore, neurological complications are often delayed by the administration of large quantities of vitamins E and A.

REFERENCES:

Mentis SW: Tangier disease. *Anesth Analg* 83(2):427, 1996.

Serfaty-Lacrosniere C, Civeira F, Lanzberg A, et al: Homozygous Tangier disease and cardiovascular disease. *Atherosclerosis* 107(1):85, 1994.

TAR Syndrome

At a glance: TAR is an acronym that stands for *T*hrombocytopenia, *A*bsent *R*adius. This is a rare condition that is most severe in the neonatal period and early infancy and which is associated with thrombocytopenia and bilateral radial aplasia. It was first described in 1951. An autosomal recessive inheritance disorder that presents with abnormalities in skeletal, gastrointestinal, hematologic, and cardiac systems. Pancytopenia similar to Fanconi. The major cause of mortality is hemorrhage. The incidence of hemorrhage is limited to the first 14 months of life.

Incidence: The frequency is 0.42 cases per 100,000 live births in Spain. Male:female ratio is equal. This medical condition is very rare in the United States.

Genetic inheritance: Autosomal recessive.

Pathophysiology: Unknown. It is suggested that the "TAR gene" probably exerts its effect between gestation weeks 4 and 8 because this would explain the association of limb deformity and congenital heart disease found in this syndrome.

Diagnosis: Finding of bilateral absence of the radius and thrombocytopenia.

Clinical aspects: Skeletal anomalies in addition to absent radii include ulnar hypoplasia, humeral hypoplasia, shoulder girdle hypoplasia, various hand anomalies, and lower limb dysplasias. Mandibular and maxillary hypoplasia are occasional findings. Congenital cardiac disease occurs in 30% of patients, most commonly tetralogy of Fallot and atrial septal defect. Additional findings may include hepatosplenomegaly and renal abnormalities. Symptomatic thrombocytopenia occurs in 50% of patients by the age of 1 week, although it may not occur until early adult life. Purpura, petechiae, epistaxis, gastrointestinal hemorrhage, and hematuria are common modes of presentation. Patients presenting outside the neonatal period may give a history of easy bruising. Thrombocytopenia may be episodic and is commonly precipitated by infection. In those patients surviving to adult life, the thrombocytopenia tends to be less severe and may be asymptomatic. Laboratory investigations may reveal a normal or low platelet count and eosinophilia. During episodes of thrombocytopenia, a leukocytosis with left shift is common. Anemia is usually secondary to blood loss rather than marrow aplasia. Megakaryocytes are not seen on examination of the bone marrow. The thrombocytopenia has been treated by steroids and splenectomy.

Precautions before anesthesia: Careful assessment of airway for maxillary/mandibular hypoplasia. Cardiovascular assessment: examine for evidence of cardiac disease; consider ECG and echocardiography. Cardiac catheterization as indicated by proposed procedure and cardiac status. Laboratory investigations: full blood cell count, electrolytes, urea, and creatinine. Correct anemia secondary to blood loss; administer platelets preoperatively in presence of ongoing hemorrhage or if the platelet count is less than $50,000/mm^3$.

Anesthetic considerations: Presence of cardiac disease may dictate specific technique, risk of paradoxical air embolism should be considered in all these patients. Intravenous access may be difficult because of limb malformation, and central venous cannulation may be difficult because of shoulder girdle hypoplasia. The radial artery is usually present but may be abnormally positioned if intraarterial pressure monitoring is indicated. Ensure platelets are available for the perioperative period. Regional anesthesia is relatively contraindicated even in the absence of cardiac disease.

Pharmacological implications: Nonsteroidal antiinflammatory drugs are contraindicated. Antibioprophylaxis in case of cardiac defect.

REFERENCES:
Hall JG, Levin J, Kuhn JP, et al: Thrombocytopenia with absent radius (TAR). *Medicine* 48(6):411, 1969.

Menghsol SC, Harris RD, Omvold K: Thrombocytopenia and absent rodii, TAR syndrome: Report of cerebral dysgenesis and newly identified cardiac and renal anomalies. *Am J Med Genet A* 123:193, 2003.

Sola MC, Slayton WB, Rimsza LM, et al: A neonate with severe thrombocytopenia and radio-ulnar synostosis. *J Perinatol* 25:296, 2005.

Tel Hashomer Camptodactyly Syndrome

At a glance: Genetic disorder with muscular hypoplasia, skeletal anomalies, increased creatine phosphokinase levels, and abnormal electromyogram.

Synonym: Camptodactyly with Muscular Hypoplasia, Skeletal Dysplasia, and Abnormal Palmar Creases Syndrome.

Incidence and genetic inheritance: This is an extremely rare syndrome with autosomal recessive inheritance.

Clinical aspects: Skeletal dysplasia, muscle hypoplasia, camptodactyly, and an abnormal dermatoglyphic pattern are the characteristics of this syndrome. Additional features may include spina bifida at C1, hypertelorism, long philtrum, and underdevelopment of the thenar and hypothenar eminences. Increased creatine kinase, abnormal electromyogram, and muscle biopsy resulted in the proposition that this condition may primarily be a myopathy. The presence of mitral valve prolapse has been reported but is not considered a constant feature of this disorder.

Anesthetic considerations: One must consider the possibility of cervical spina bifida (avoid hyperextension of the neck) and the underlying myopathy. Although no reports exist, it is recommended to administer a malignant hyperthermia-trigger-free general anesthetic or a locoregional anesthesia where possible. In presence of mitral valve prolapse, antibiotics might have to be considered depending on the surgical procedure.

REFERENCES:
Pagnan NA, Gollop TR, Lederman H: The Tel Hashomer camptodactyly syndrome: Report of a new case and review of the literature. *Am J Med Genet* 29:411, 1988.

Patton MA, McDermot KD, Lake BD, et al: Tel Hashomer camptodactyly syndrome: Report of a case with myopathic features. *J Med Genet* 23:268, 1986.

Temtamy Syndrome

At a glance: Craniofacial dysmorphism with iris coloboma, agenesis of the corpus callosum, and aortic arch dilatation with aortic valve regurgitation. Patients present with moderate mental retardation.

History: Congenital disorder. First described by S. Temtamy et al. in 1991.

Genetic inheritance: Autosomal recessive.

Pathophysiology: Unknown. A connective-tissue abnormality has been shown on electron microscopy with wide intercellular spaces and thickening of collagen fibers.

Diagnosis: Demonstration of clinical features of the syndrome, that is, craniofacial dysmorphism with ocular coloboma, absent corpus callosum, and aortic dilatation.

Clinical aspects: Facial features described include macrodolichocephaly, arched eyebrows, antimongoloid eye slant, beaked nose, low-set ears, lop ears, long philtrum, short upper lip, micrognathia, and hypertelorism. Coloboma of the iris ("keyhole" appearance), retina, and choroid are present, and lens dislocation may occur. Mental retardation is present and the absence of the corpus callosum can be demonstrated radiographically. Connective-tissue dysplasia is a feature of the syndrome and results in aortic dilatation and aortic regurgitation.

Precautions before anesthesia: Careful airway assessment and planning for a potentially difficult airway. Cardiovascular assessment is very important and must include an ECG, echocardiogram, and eventually a catheterization. Examine for signs of aortic regurgitation and ventricular impairment. Laboratory investigations as indicated by procedure and current drug therapy.

Anesthetic considerations: Potentially difficult airway. Mental retardation may result in behavioral problems during induction of anesthesia and premedication may be helpful. Aortic regurgitation and impaired ventricular function are the main concerns. Aim to maintain sinus rhythm, minimize myocardial depression, maintain left ventricular filling, and reduce systemic vascular resistance. Invasive monitoring should be considered. The place of regional anesthesia is controversial, especially if ventricular function is impaired.

Pharmacological implications: Ketamine is relatively contraindicated.

REFERENCE:

Temtamy S, Salam M, Aboul-Ezz E, et al: New autosomal recessive multiple congenital abnormalities/mental retardation syndrome with craniofacial dysmorphism absent corpus callosum, iris colobomas, and connective tissue dysplasia. *Clin Dysmorphol* 5(3):231, 1996.

Tethered Spinal Cord Syndrome

At a glance: A syndrome resulting from abnormal development of the filum terminale resulting in persistent anchoring of the spinal cord conus medullaris at or below the L2 level.

Genetic inheritance: Occurs as part of inherited syndromes but has not been described in isolation.

Pathophysiology: Normal regression of the distal embryonic spinal cord produces a thread-like filum terminale attached to the coccyx when differential growth of the conus medullaris occurs in the child. When this regression is abnormal, it results in a thick rope-like filum that anchors the conus at or below L2 level instead of the usual final L1 level. Usually associated with spina bifida. This may coexist with diastematomyelia and Arnold-Chiari malformation. Neurological signs may develop as a consequence of increased tension on the cord compromising blood supply, particularly with flexion and extension.

Diagnosis: Clinical signs confirmed by CT or MRI scan.

Clinical aspects: May be asymptomatic or present with progressive neurological dysfunction of the lower cord. Asymmetric leg growth, talipes cavus, muscle wasting. Bladder dysfunction, progressive scoliosis. Diffuse pain. Midline skin lesion is usually observed in 70% of patients affected. Hyperpigmentation, hemangioma, lipoma dermal pit are frequent other physical characteristics of this syndrome.

Precautions before anesthesia: Routine preoperative assessments. In the presence of a significant scoliosis, respiratory evaluation, including spirometry, should be obtained.

Anesthetic considerations: Usual considerations for prone position. The use of intraoperative neuromonitoring for tethered cord release contributes significantly to maintain functional integrity and is highly recommended. May require catheterization; care with padding if bladder dysfunction or scoliosis is present. Regional anesthesia is not contraindicated, however, its indication must be assessed carefully for each patient because of the spina bifida often associated.

Pharmacological implications: There are no specific implications with this condition.

Other condition to be considered:

   ☞**DIASTEMATOMYELIA:** Characterized by pain, weakness of legs, and incontinence. Surgical repair during infancy recommended.

REFERENCES:

Ali L, Stocks GM: Spina bifida, tethered cord, and regional anesthesia. *Anaesthesia* 60:1149, 2005.

Haslam R. Tetherd cord syndrome, in Behrman RE, Kliegman RM, Nelson WA, et al. (eds): *Nelson Textbook of Pediatrics.* 14th ed. Philadelphia, WB Saunders, 1992: 1536–1537.

Kothbauer KF, Noval K: Intraoperative monitoring for tethered cord. An update. *Neurosurg Focus* 16:18, 2004 (review).

Rafael M: Tetherd cord. *J Neurosurg* 90:175, 1999.

Tetralogy of Fallot

At a glance: A cause of cyanotic congenital heart disease. The tetralogy is composed of a ventricular septal defect, right ventricular outflow tract (RVOT) obstruction, overriding aorta, and right ventricular hypertrophy.

Incidence: Five to 7% of all congenital heart disease.

Genetic inheritance: Autosomal dominant. Risk for tetralogy of Fallot in a sibling of the proband is 1%; risk for any congenital heart disease in a sibling is approximately 3%.

Pathophysiology: Etiology remains to be defined. The physiological impact of tetralogy is variable, and dependent primarily on the degree of obstruction to right ventricular outflow and the size of the ventricular septal defect (VSD) (usually large). Right ventricular outflow obstruction may occur below the pulmonary valve, at the valve annulus, or distally as far as the pulmonary arteries. This obstruction, together with a nonrestrictive VSD, results in right-to-left shunting of blood and arterial hypoxemia. Hypoxia, hypercarbia, and acidosis increase pulmonary vascular resistance and increase right-to-left shunting; similarly, decreases in systemic vascular resistance increase right-to-left shunting. These factors are important in the development of "TET" spells (episodes of paroxysmal hypercyanosis) as is infundibular spasm of the RVOT. However, the precise etiology of these episodes is unclear.

Diagnosis: Clinical history and presentation in neonatal period or early infancy. Radiographic and echocardiographic findings.

Clinical aspects: Cyanosis is the predominant sign and tends to be most severe in the neonatal period, improving up to 2 years of age. Symptoms include exertional dyspnea; "TET" spells precipitated by crying or feeding and characterized by shortness of breath, restlessness, occasionally syncope, and cyanosis. Examination may reveal cyanosis, clubbing, signs of ventricular failure, a right ventricular heave, a systolic ejection murmur caused by flow across the obstructed right ventricular outflow and a single second valve sound (S2). The chest radiography reveals a boot-shaped cardiac shadow and the ECG shows right axis deviation and right ventricular hypertrophy. Echocardiography is required to define the cardiac anatomy; a right aortic arch is present in 20% of cases. Polycythemia is commonly present and hyperviscosity is a potential problem. Treatment may involve palliative surgery by a Blalock-Taussig (B-T) shunt or by definitive correction in early life (now the most common method). Following repair of the tetralogy, ventricular ectopic beats become more common with time, ventricular dysrhythmia and supraventricular tachycardia are common (up to 70% of patients). Right bundle branch block is common and occurs with left anterior hemiblock in 10% of patients. Right ventricular dysfunction/failure and pulmonary hypertension are common following repair, and may be reflected by decreased exercise tolerance. Patients palliated with a B-T shunt will have an absent or weak right radial pulse, are polycythemic, and are at increased risk of intracerebral abscess, cerebrovascular infarction, and bacterial endocarditis. A 30-year survival rate of 86% following repair was suggested by one series.

Precautions before anesthesia: Full history and examination to elicit frequency and duration of cyanotic episodes; examine for evidence of ventricular failure. If repaired, note type and date of repair and assess for symptoms and signs suggestive of deteriorating ventricular function. Respiratory assessment. Chest radiography, measure oxygen saturation (SaO$_2$) in air, and consider measurement of arterial gases. Cardiovascular assessment. ECG and echocardiography are essential. If available, cardiac catheter data should be evaluated. In patients with repaired tetralogy of Fallot additional investigations that should be considered include 24-hour Holter monitoring (supraventricular tachycardia/ventricular dysrhythmia are prevalent). Consider temporary pacing in presence of right bundle branch and left anterior hemiblock. Laboratory investigations. Full blood count is mandatory to assess for polycythemia. Continue concurrent cardiac medications.

Anesthetic considerations: Neonate/infant, premedication is desirable to decrease likelihood of cyanotic episodes. Aim to minimize or decrease right-to-left shunting, avoid hypoxia, hypercarbia, acidosis, i.e., maintain low pulmonary vascular resistance. This will be more easily achieved with positive-pressure ventilation than with spontaneous respiration. Minimize and treat any decrease in systemic vascular resistance (increase right-to-left shunt). Control stress response to laryngoscopy to avoid infundibular spasm. Ketamine is useful for diagnostic or minor procedures. Inhalational induction will be prolonged by the right-to-left shunt. Invasive monitoring should be strongly considered for major procedures.

Pharmacological implications: Phenylephrine should be available to treat decreases in systemic vascular resistance. Esmolol is probably the beta blocker of choice for treatment of cyanotic episodes associated with infundibular spasm. In the presence of right ventricular dysfunction requiring inotropic support, phosphodiesterase inhibitors such as amrinone should be considered because they decrease pulmonary vascular resistance.

REFERENCES:

Finlow D, Doyle E: Congenital heart disease in adults. *Br J Anaesth* 78:416, 1997.

Samuelson PN, Lell WA: Tetralogy of Fallot, in Lake CL (ed): *Pediatric Cardiac Anesthesia*. 3rd ed. Connecticut, Appleton and Lange, 1997, 303–314.

Thalassemia

At a glance: The most frequent hematological genetic disorder and one that has a large geographic influence. Clinical signs are a result of hemolysis by chronic anemia. Clinical features include hepatosplenomegaly, bone deformations, and cardiac failure. Strict asepsis is needed.

Classification: α-thalassemia, β-thalassemia, and Cooley Anemia (β-thalassemia homozygote).

Incidence: Most frequently occurring genetic disorder, geographic variability (for example, for α-thalassemia in general population: Congo 60%, Laos 35%, Caribbean 30%, South Europe 10%, France 0.1% of the general population). Other geographical distributions include Asia, Filipino, Mediterranean, Middle Eastern, and, less frequently, India.

Genetic inheritance: Autosomal dominant except for major thalassemia, which is autosomal recessive.

Pathophysiology: The disease affects synthesis of either α (gene located at 16p13.33 to 16p13.11) or β chain (gene located at 11p15.5) of the hemoglobin.

Diagnosis: Hemoglobin synthesis normally provides a just balance between the three different chains α, β, and γ. Thalassemia modifies this status and leads to an abnormal presence of β chain (hemoglobin H) and γ chain (hemoglobin Barts). Hemoglobin (Hb) A is preponderant and so a child with α-thalassemia presents at birth with abnormal HbH and Hb Barts levels. Those allow quantifying of the severity of the thalassemia. Fetal hemoglobin, which disappears within a few months after birth by substitution with HbA, will also be higher. This is a quantitative deficit and clinical expression varies according to deficit. In β-thalassemia HbA2 will be higher than normal but signs will appear after a few months. Certitude diagnosis is obtain by high-performance liquid chromatography (HPLC) of hemoglobin.

Clinical aspects: Varies with the severity of the disease.

α-*thalassemia:* Class 1 and class 2 (less than 50% deficit): few signs with anemia; class 3: severe hemolytic anemia with erythroblastopenia, frequent infection, an increased spleen size, and hemosiderosis. Cardiac failure can occur as a consequence of chronic hemolysis. In class 4, generally fetal or neonatal death with anasarca.

β-*thalassemia:* Other clinical features seen in this disease include major hepatosplenomegaly, growth failure, unconjugated hyperbilirubinemia, and bone marrow hyperplasia that lead to skeletal deformation (frontal bossing, prominent maxilla). Transfusions are frequent with their own complications. Folate deficiency is frequent.

Cooley Sideroblastic Anemia: First described by Thomas Benton Cooley, a Detroit pediatrician-hematologist, who also first described thalassemia in a definitive way. Also known as Thalassemia Major or Homozygous β-Thalassemia. The clinical include severe anemia detected first in childhood, growth retardation, hepatosplenomegaly, and jaundice. Facial and skeletal deformity develop later. Hyperferricemia and abundance of siderocytes in peripheral blood after splenectomy have also been described. Death occurs from hemochromatosis at a relatively young age because of cardiac, hepatic, and endocrine dysfunction.

Precautions before anesthesia: Evaluate severity of the disease (clinical, history); anemia (clinical, hematocrit, spleen echography); cardiac function (chest radiograph, ECG, echography). Laboratory investigations should include hematocrit, hemoglobin, bilirubin, erythrocyte volume, reticulocyte, HbH.

Anesthetic considerations: Strict asepsis is needed during procedures. Difficult direct laryngoscopy can occur as a result of skull malformation. Perioperative cardiac monitoring should be necessary in case of heart failure. Precautions have to be taken during cardioplegia because of the risk of hemolysis at temperature lower than 4°C (39.2°F).

Pharmacological implications: These patients should be considered as immunodeficient for antibioprophylaxis (particularly in the case of a splenectomy). In α-thalassemia, oxidant drugs are contraindicated because they can increase hemolysis (prilocaine, aspirin, vitamin K, sulfonamide, nitroprusside). Other drugs, such as sulprostone and iron, should also be avoided.

Other conditions to be considered:

☞**ATR-X SYNDROME:** The acronym ATR-X means alpha-thalassemia, Mental Retardation X-Linked Syndrome. It is characterized by genital abnormalities, microcephaly, midface hypoplasia, severe mental retardation, neuromotor dysfunction, seizures, and hypotonia. Occasionally, the patient might present a ventricular septal defect and gastrointestinal reflux.

☞**SICKLE CELL DISEASE:** Includes a vasoocclusive crisis.

REFERENCES:

Drew SJ, Sachs SA: Management of the thalassemia induced skeletal facial deformities. *J Oral Maxillofac Surg* 55:1331, 1997.

Kattamis C, Tzotzos S, Kanavakis E, et al: Correlation of clinical phenotype to genotype in haemoglobin H disease. *Lancet* 27;442–4, 1988.

Kitoh T, Taraka S, Ono K, et al: Anesthetic management of a patient with beta-thalassemia intermedia undergoing splenectomy. A case report. *J Anesth* 19:252, 2005.

Rowbottom SJ, Sudhaman DA: Haemoglobin H disease and cardiac surgery. *Anaesthesia* 43:1033, 1988.

Thanatophoric Dwarfism

At a glance: A severe form of micromelic dwarfism with narrow thorax with short ribs, severe hydrocephalus, and hydronephrosis. Death generally occurs in the first hours of life.

Synonym: Thanatophoric Dysplasia.

Incidence: 1:10,000 to 1:35,000 live births.

Genetic inheritance: Autosomal dominant inheritance but most cases are de novo mutations.

Pathophysiology: Caused by mutation in the fibroblast growth factor receptor-3 gene (FGFR3, which belongs to the tyrosine kinase receptors) located on 4p13.6. Formation of cysteine residues with disulfide bonds between the extracellular domains of mutant monomers has been reported as resulting from FGFR3 mutation. Perturbation of terminal chondrocyte differentiation could be the final result of this mutation.

Diagnosis: Clinically evocated in a baby with severe shortening of the limbs, narrow thorax, macrocephaly, and normal trunk length. Antenatal diagnosis on ultrasonographic findings is possible.

Clinical aspects: Major skeletal deformations observed involve: *skull* (macrocephaly, frontal bossing, depressed nasal bridge), *limbs* (micromelic dwarfism, brachydactyly, enlarged and bowed diaphysis), and *trunk* (abnormal rib with narrow rib cage, scapula anomaly, intervertebral disk anomaly, abnormal vertebral size, and pelvis anomaly). Other clinical features can include glaucoma, temporal lobe heterotopias, hydrocephalus, profound mental retardation, and hypotonia in survivors. Respiratory insufficiency is frequent because of restrictive thoracic deformations.

Precautions before anesthesia: Because of the early death, it will be extremely rare for an anesthesiologist to provide care for surgery, except for airway and cardiovascular support at birth. If the patient survives, a complete evaluation of neurological function (clinical, EEG, CT) must be obtained. Evaluate respiratory function (clinical, chest radiographs, pulmonary function test, arterial blood gas analysis).

Anesthetic considerations: Careful intraoperative positioning is needed. Both arterial and venous access can be difficult because of limb deformations. Regional anesthesia is not contraindicated but can be difficult to perform. Postoperative physiotherapy is useful. Postoperative mechanical ventilatory support may be necessary.

Pharmacological implications: Avoid atropine and other cholinergic drugs because of glaucoma.

Other conditions to be considered:

THANATOPHORIC DYSPLASIA WITH KLEEBLATTSCHÄDEL (Cloverleaf Skull with Thanatophoric Dwarfism; Thanatophoric Dysplasia type II): Autosomal dominant, lethal micromelic dwarfism with cloverleaf head and small facies; also caused by mutations in FGFR3.

THANATOPHORIC DYSPLASIA, GLASGOW VARIANT (Neonatally Lethal Short-Limb Skeletal Dysplasia, Glasgow type): Autosomal recessive disorder that combines dwarfism with cataracts, anemia, and hepatosplenomegaly.

☞JARCHO-LEVIN SYNDROME: A rare genetic disorder characterized by distinctive malformations including short thorax because of fusion of thoracic vertebrae and ribs. This skeletal problems often leads to respiratory insufficiency, pneumonia resulting in life-threatening complications. Other features include vertebral dysplasia, and hemivertebrae. In addition, abnormalities with the cervical vertebrae may cause shortness of the neck, limited neck motion, and an abnormally low hairline appearance. During the infancy period, the abdomen may be abnormally prominent and the arms and legs may appear unusually long suggesting often a marfanoid appearance. This disorder is thought to be inherited as an autosomal recessive genetic trait.

☞DIASTROPHIC DYSPLASIA: An autosomal recessive inherited form of short-limb dwarfism associated with spine anomalies.

☞CHONDRODYSPLASIA: GIANT CELL TYPE: A lethal form of chondrodysplasia characterized by rhizomelic limb shortening with giant cell chondrodysplasia.

REFERENCES:

Simsek M, Al-Gazali L, Al-Mjeni R, et al: Improved diagnosis of a common mutation (R248C) in the human growth factor receptor 3 (FGFR3) gene that causes type I thanatophoric dysplasia. *Clin Biochem* 36(2):151, 2003.

Wilcox WR, Tavormina PL, Krakow D, et al: Molecular, radiologic, and histopathologic correlations in thanatophoric dysplasia. *Am J Med Genet* 78:274, 1998.

Thanos-Stewart-Zonana Syndrome

At a glance: A very rare syndrome characterized by association of four clinical features, including craniosynostosis, exostoses, nevus, and epibulbar dermoids.

Synonym: Craniosynostosis, Exostoses, Nevus, Epibulbar Dermoids Syndrome.

Clinical aspects: Clinical features include mental retardation, conductive deafness, craniofacial anomalies (frontal bossing, thickened skull, sutural synostosis, facial structural asymmetry, flared nostrils, broad nose), myopia, speech defect, multiple exostoses, pigmented nevi, and epibulbar dermoids.

Anesthetic considerations: Direct laryngoscopy and tracheal intubation can be difficult because of malformation and has to be evaluated carefully (clinical, radiograph). Careful intraoperative positioning is necessary. Aminoglycosides should be used cautiously because of their otologic effects.

Three M Syndrome

At a glance: Congenital disorder that includes dwarfism, low birth weight, and dysmorphic craniofacial features (dolichocephaly, prominent forehead [frontal bossing], triangular-shaped face with pointed chin, large ears, and small mouth). Other features include fragile vertebral column, distinctive malformations of the ribs and scapulae, clinodactyly, short fifth finger, and hyperextensibility of joints.

Synonyms: Dolichospondylic Dysplasia; Three M Slender-Boned Nanism (3-MSBN), Le Merrer Syndrome, Gloomy Face Syndrome, 3M Syndrome.

History: The three M refers to the initials of the authors (McKusick, Miller, and Malvaux) who described this syndrome.

Genetic inheritance: Autosomal recessive trait. It has been suggested that it is located on chromosome 6 (6p21.1).

Clinical aspects: The clinical features are low birth weight dwarfism, short stature, triangular-shaped face (hatchet face), prominent lips, prominent trapezia muscles, grooved anterior thorax, horizontal ribs, winging of the scapulae, hypospadias, spina bifida occulta, and delayed closure of the anterior fontanelle. Radiologically, the vertebral bodies are tall, long bones appear slender, and there is evidence of delayed bone maturation.

Anesthetic considerations: Careful assessment of airway anatomy. Careful assessment of pulmonary function in presence of marked deformity. High incidence of spina bifida occulta. Changes in vertebral bodies may cause difficulty if using regional techniques. Difficult laryngoscopy may be expected because of the small mouth opening and shape.

REFERENCE:

Winter R, Braitser M, Grant D et al: The 3-M syndrome. *J Med Genet* 21:124, 1984.

Thrombotic Thrombocytopenic Purpura (TTP)

At a glance: A genetic disorder affecting mostly adults and associated with pregnancy, HIV, cancer, bacterial infection, and vasculitis. Has also been observed after bone marrow transplantation. Clinical features include seizure, hemiplegia, fatigue, abdominal pain, arthralgias, neurological deficit, and renal insufficiency. Idiopathic presentation with a 60% female preponderance.

Synonyms: Moschowitz Syndrome; Thrombotic Microangiopathic Hemolytic Anemia.

History: First described by Eli Moschcowitz, American pathologist in 1924.

Incidence: More than 75 years ago, the occurrence was 1/1,000,000 in general population. However, the incidence seems to have increased. Ten years ago, the rate was reported at 3.7 cases per 1 million patients. However, the incidence today is much higher because of greater awareness and increasing reports of TTP secondary to other illnesses and drugs. One report indicated a case rate of 1:6000 hospital admissions. The mortality rate was 100% until 1980, but a major drop has been observed with early diagnosis and improvement in therapy with plasma exchange. Untreated, mortality remains high at 95%, whereas survival is 90% if treated. Approximately 60% of patients are female. The female-to-male ratio is 3:2.

Genetic inheritance: Most familial cases are recessive but dominant pedigrees have also been reported. The phenotypes might be identical but mutations in the ADAMTS13 gene are involved for Moschowitz disease; the locus is at 9q34.

Pathophysiology: Characterized by microangiopathic hemolysis and idiopathic platelet aggregation/hyaline thrombi leading to diffuse thrombosis of small blood vessels, with organ ischemia and microangiopathic hemolytic anemia. Platelet transfusion can actually cause deterioration secondary to increased activation and deposition. The thrombi partially occlude the vascular lumina with overlying proliferative endothelial cells. The endothelia of the kidneys and brain are particularly vulnerable to TTP. However, the lungs and liver are affected to a lesser extent. The megakaryocytes and endothelial cells produce and release the ultra-large von Willebrand factor multimer, which favors binding to platelets in the microcirculation. Treatment includes plasmapheresis, which either removes a platelet activator or adds an inhibitor, and immunosuppression. Splenectomy follows failure of medical therapy.

Diagnosis: Based on clinical and laboratory findings, including the hemolytic anemia, consumptive thrombocytopenia, central nervous system (CNS) dysfunction, and petechiae.

Clinical aspects: Peak prevalence in third decade of life, hemolytic anemia, consumptive thrombocytopenia, central nervous system (CNS) dysfunction, and petechiae. Seizure activity (16%), hemiplegia (12%), and paresthesias have been reported. Also the possibility of heart failure and arrhythmias must be borne in mind. Twenty-five percent of patients present with abdominal pain due to gastrointestinal ischemia.

Precautions before anesthesia: The heterogenicity of the patients-adults and children-renders the evaluation difficult. Obtain a full history of the concomitant illnesses (if any) and assess thoroughly the involvement of the kidneys and the CNS. The severity of the infection associated (if any) must be known. Aseptic technique, especially with immunosuppression. Supplemental steroids as needed. Check baseline renal and CNS function and obtain a complete cell blood count. Myopathy/neurotoxicity is possible with vincristine therapy.

Anesthetic considerations: Postpone elective surgery until patient is in remission. Avoid IM injections. Avoid central neuraxial blockade. Judicious sedation with CNS dysfunction. Careful padding. Treat coagulopathy with packed red blood cells and fresh-frozen plasma, not platelets. Consider these patients to be at high risk for bleeding therefore the necessity to place a large bore peripheral venous access. In the presence of neurological signs, standard brain protection must be instituted with moderate hyperventilation, and effort made to minimize the secondary insults. Hemodynamic control to avoid CNS bleeds.

Pharmacological implications: Avoid succinylcholine with myopathy or neurologic deficit. Patients treated for seizures must receive their medications until the morning of surgery. Avoid anesthetic agents known to trigger seizure activities.

Other conditions to be considered:

HEMOLYTIC UREMIC SYNDROME (HUS): A more common disorder in children, characterized by prominent renal involvement. Associated with epidemics of diarrhea caused by verocytotoxin-producing bacteria or of familial origin (caused by mutation in the gene encoding factor H or ADAMTS13).

☞**UPSHAW-SCHULMAN SYNDROME:** A very rare syndrome characterized by congenital microangiopathic hemolytic anemia, thrombotic thrombocytopenic purpura, and response to fresh plasma infusion. Neonatal onset and frequent relapses are typical.

REFERENCES:

Elliott MA, Nichols WL: Thrombotic thrombocytopenic purpura and hemolytic uremic syndrome. *Mayo Clin Proc* 76(11):1154, 2001.

Pivalizza EG: Anesthetic management of a patient with thrombotic thrombocytopenic purpura. *Anesth Analg* 79:1203, 1994.

Thyrotoxic Periodic Paralysis

At a glance: An acquired, sporadic disorder characterized by intermittent episodes of muscle weakness alternating with periods of normal muscular function. Occurring during hyperthyroidism and thyrotoxicosis. During attack, hypokalemia is present. May be precipitated by a low plasma concentration of insulin.

Synonym: Hashitoxic Periodic Paralysis

Incidence: Most common in Chinese and Japanese. The incidence is estimated at 1.9 to 8.8% of hyperthyroid patients. The disorder is rare in non-Asian populations and only 5% of cases occur in women. A few cases have been reported in African Americans, and this disorder may be more frequent in black patients.

Pathophysiology: Exact pathophysiology remains to be defined. The following factors appear to be important in the pathogenesis: (a) hyperthyroidism increases Na/K pump ATPase activity, (b) increased platelet Na/K pump ATPase activity has been demonstrated in patients with thyrotoxic periodic paralysis, as compared with thyrotoxic patients, (c) thyroxine sensitizes beta-adrenergic receptors to the effects of catecholamines (Na/K pump ATPase activity is increased), (d) insulin increases Na/K ATPase activity, which may explain the relationship of acute episodes of paralysis to carbohydrate ingestion. These factors result in an intracellular shift of potassium and reduction of the extracellular potassium, causing membrane hyperpolarization. Some of the changes are present in patients who do not develop thyrotoxic periodic paralysis, therefore a role for Na/K ATPase-independent potassium influx has been suggested and the role of Ca^{2+} gated ion channels is under investigation. The sarcolemmal membrane is thought to be the site of the primary defect. Hypophosphatemia is occasionally found in conjunction with thyrotoxic periodic paralysis and may be synergistic in producing paralysis.

Diagnosis: Demonstration of clinical or subclinical hyperthyroidism associated with muscle weakness or paralysis.

Clinical aspects: Thyrotoxic Periodic Paralysis is uncommon in childhood, with approximately 80% of cases presenting after the age of 20 years. Symptoms include myalgia, fatigue, muscle weakness, and symptoms of hyperthyroidism, although these are often subtle. There may be a history of weakness related to exercise and carbohydrate or alcohol intake. Proximal muscles are more affected than distal muscles, and lower limbs more than upper limbs. Examination commonly reveals a goiter and flaccid paralysis in the affected muscles. Respiratory and bulbar muscles are rarely involved. Cardiac dysrhythmias (atrial fibrillation/flutter, supraventricular tachycardia ventricular extrasystoles) are common. Electrocardiographic changes reflect the hypokalemia (U waves, small T wave, ST depression, long QT interval). Definitive treatment is correction of the hyperthyroidism. Beta$_2$-antagonism with propranolol may prevent paralysis in the face of hypokalemia. Potassium supplementation may be used in the setting of acute paralysis; however, it should be noted that body potassium stores are normal and that hyperkalemia may occur as paralysis resolves.

Precautions before anesthesia: Elective surgery is absolutely contraindicated until the patient is rendered euthyroid; paralysis will not occur in the euthyroid state. Examine for evidence of muscle weakness and decrease reflexes. An ECG is mandatory to exclude dysrhythmia and ECG signs of hypokalemia. Laboratory investigations, measure and correct serum electrolytes (Na^+, K^+, Ca^{2+}, Mg^{2+}), consider measurement of serum phosphate during acute episode. Consider K^+ supplementation and propranolol prior to urgent surgery. Delay of urgent surgery by 4 to 6 hours allows resolution of most episodes of paralysis.

Anesthetic considerations: Consider premedication and measures to attenuate the stress response to laryngoscopy to minimize catecholamine surges. Neuromuscular monitoring should be used

if paralysis is required for surgery. There are no contraindications to regional anesthesia. Avoid large volumes of dextrose-containing fluids.

Pharmacological implications: Use sympathomimetic agents with caution. Drugs contraindicated include potassium-wasting diuretics, cholinesterase inhibitors, and desflurane (relative).

Other conditions to be considered:

☞**PERIODIC PARALYSIS:** An inherited condition not associated with high thyroid hormone levels. Characterized by episodes of flaccid muscle weakness occurring at irregular intervals. Most conditions are hereditary and episodic rather than periodic. There are three conditions defined as hypokaliemic, hyperkaliemic and paramyotonic.

☞**ANDERSEN CARDIODYSRHYTHMIC PERIODIC PARALYSIS SYNDROME:** This disorder is characterized by the clinical triad of potassium-sensitive periodic paralysis (either low, normal, or high potassium levels), ventricular arrhythmias (bigeminy, long QT interval, ectopy, and bidirectional ventricular tachycardia), and dysmorphic facial features. Sudden death has been reported. Andersen Syndrome must not be confused with Andersen Disease (Glycogen Storage Disease Type IV).

REFERENCES:

Brimacombe J, Newell S: Successful anaesthetic management of a patient with thyrotoxic hypokalaemic periodic paralysis for coincidental appendicitis. *Anaesth Intensive Care* 23:109, 1995.

Norris L, Levine B, Ganesan K: Thyrotoxic periodic paralysis associate with hypokalemia and hypophosphatemia. *Am J Kidney Dis* 28(2):270, 1996.

Ober K: Thyrotoxic periodic paralysis in the United States. Report of 7 cases and review of the literature. *Medicine (Baltimore)* 71(3):109, 1992.

Tooth and Nail Syndrome

At a glance: A rare autosomal dominant ectodermal dysplasia characterized by defects of the nail plates of the fingers (onychorrhexis) and toes (koilonychia). Familial hypodontia with normal hair and sweat gland function.

Synonyms: Witkop Syndrome; Dysplasia of Nails with Hypotonia.

Nature: Described by C.J. Witkop in 1965.

Incidence: Condition is frequent among Dutch Mennonites in Canada.

Genetic inheritance: Autosomal dominant. Mapping found linkage in the region of the MSX1 locus.

Pathophysiology: In a model of MSX1-deficient mice, histologic analysis confirmed that the MSX1 expression in mesenchyme of developing nail beds showed thinner nail and tooth development disrupted.

Diagnosis: Nail dysplasia, hypoplastic dentition, normal hair, normal sweat and salivary gland function.

Clinical aspects: A variable number of teeth may be hypoplastic, the permanent incisors and second molars are most commonly affected. Complete adontia is rare. The nails are thin, centrally hollow, and brittle. Bilateral polycystic ovaries have been reported with the syndrome.

Precautions before anesthesia: Inspect dentition for teeth at risk of being dislodged during laryngoscopy and tracheal intubation. Special investigations as indicated by the proposed procedure.

Anesthetic considerations: The presence of hypodontia may be associated with a higher risk of dental damage during direct laryngoscopy. Otherwise, there are no specific considerations other than those relating to the proposed surgery.

Pharmacological implications: There are no known specific implications with this condition.

REFERENCE:

Murdoch-Kinch C, Miles D, Poon C: Hypodontia and nail dysplasia syndrome. *Oral Surg Oral Med Oral Pathol* 75:403, 1993.

TORCH Syndrome

At a glance: An acronymic syndrome referring to a group of fetal infectious malformations. It stands for: *T*oxoplasmis, *O*ther agents, *R*ubella, *C*ytomegalovirus, and *H*erpex Simplex. Common signs involve essentially intracranial anomalies.

Incidence: Unknown (e.g., in cytomegalovirus infection approximately 1% of all newborns are infected but only 10% present symptoms at birth).

Pathophysiology: TORCH Syndrome refers to infection of a developing fetus or newborn by any of a group of infectious agents.

Diagnosis: Association of small size, small brain, enlarged liver and spleen, eye anomalies, jaundice, intracranial calcifications, and high intracranial pressure. Blood screening is possible.

Clinical aspects: May include fever, difficulties feeding, small areas of bleeding under the skin (causing the appearance of small reddish or purplish spots), hearing impairment, abnormalities of the eyes, seizures. Each infectious agent may also result in additional abnormalities.

Precautions before anesthesia: Evaluate neurological function (clinical, CT, MRI, EEG) and liver function (clinical, echography). Laboratory investigation should include bilirubin, serum glutamic-oxaloacetic transaminase (SGOT), serum glutamic-pyruvic transaminase (SGPT), coagulation test, hematocrit, and platelet count.

Anesthetic considerations: Vascular access can be difficult in cases of edema. Because the patient may be more prone to bleeding problems, if a major surgery is planned, be sure to have the required blood products in the operating room.

Pharmacological implications: Avoid succinylcholine and ketamine because they can increase intracranial pressure. Consider interaction between anesthetic drugs and antiepileptic medications. If bilirubin level is very high, it can displace other drugs from albumin, thereby increasing the free fraction and clinical effect of drugs such as muscle relaxants.

Other conditions to be considered:

PSEUDO-TORCH SYNDROME (Intrauterine Infection-Like Syndrome with Microcephaly, Intracranial Calcification, and Central Nervous System Disease; Pseudotoxoplasmosis Syndrome, Microcephaly with Calcification of Cerebral White Matter Syndrome): Characterized by microcephaly, quadriplegia, seizures, developmental delay, marked microphthalmia, congenital cataracts, cerebral and cerebellar hypoplasia, and intracranial calcification. No evidence of intrauterine infection was found. Previous reports of features resembling intrauterine infection and associated with an autosomal recessive inheritance have been reported.

BARAITSER BRETT PIESOWICZ SYNDROME: Microcephaly, intracranial calcification, and central nervous system disease; autosomal recessive with spasticity.

☞CONGENITAL VARICELLA SYNDROME: A rare congenital nongenetic disorder because of maternal transmission of varicella in the first and second trimesters of pregnancy manifesting with cutaneous, neurological, and limb involvement.

☞AICARDI-GOUTTIERES SYNDROME (Encephalopathy, Familial Infantile, with Calcification of Basal Ganglia and Chronic Cerebrospinal Fluid Lymphocytosis, AGS-1): Characterized by progressive familial encephalopathy in infancy, calcification of the basal ganglia and chronic cerebrospinal fluid (CSF) lymphocytosis, evolving rapidly to a vegetative state and early death in infancy. It has been suggested that it is a distinct type of leukodystrophy transmitted as autosomal recessive.

REFERENCES:

Jones CA: Congenital cytomegalovirus infection. *Curr Probl Pediatr Adolesc Health Care* 33(3):70, 2003.

Slee J, Lam G, Walpole I: Syndrome of microcephaly, microphthalmia, cataracts, and intracranial calcification. *Am J Med Genet* 84:330, 1999.

Toriello-Carey Syndrome

At a glance: Multiple congenital anomaly consisting of agenesis of corpus callosum; telecanthus; short palpebral fissures; small nose with anteverted nares; Pierre Robin sequence; malformed ears; redundant neck skin; macrocephaly; micrognathia; laryngeal and sublaryngeal abnormalities; heart defect (pulmonary stenosis and atrial septal defect); muscular hypotonia; occasional Hirschsprung Disease; and moderate to severe developmental delay.

Synonym: Agenesis of the Corpus Callosum with Facial Anomalies and Robin Sequence.

Genetic inheritance: This syndrome is familial and was originally reported as an autosomal recessive trait; however, later findings indicated an X-linked transmission.

Pathophysiology: Unknown.

Diagnosis: Demonstration of corpus callosum agenesis; telecanthus; short palpebral fissures; small nares; Pierre Robin sequence; redundant neck skin; laryngeal anomalies; congenital heart disease; short hands; and hypotonia.

Clinical aspects: Laryngeal hypoplasia is the most common laryngeal anomaly described. Tracheal intubation for respiratory failure as a consequence of hypotonia may be necessary in the neonatal period. Cerebellar and brainstem hypoplasia are described in addition to corpus callosum agenesis. Seizures have been a feature in some patients. Mental retardation may be severe. Congenital heart disease appears to be a common, although inconsistent, finding.

Precautions before anesthesia: Careful airway assessment. Potential difficult direct laryngoscopy; laryngeal hypoplasia may further complicate attempts to intubate the trachea. Examine for signs of intercurrent lung disease, and hypotonia causing respiratory impairment. Careful examination for signs of congenital heart disease, low threshold for preoperative echocardiography and ECG. Cardiac catheterization as indicated by specific cardiac lesion. Continue any antiepileptic drugs during the perioperative period.

Anesthetic considerations: Difficult airway management should be presumed, inhalational induction may be the method of choice. The maintenance of spontaneous respiration is highly recommended until the trachea has been intubated and lung ventilation confirmed.

Prepare a selection endotracheal tubes (smaller than predicted) prior to induction. The availability of proper size laryngeal mask airway and/or fiberoptic equipment is indicated. The specific anesthetic technique will be dictated by the presence of congenital heart disease. Regional techniques may be of use if not contraindicated.

Pharmacological implications: There are no reports of anesthesia for this syndrome, although succinylcholine should probably be avoided in the presence of marked hypotonia.

REFERENCES:

Jespers A, Buntix I, Melis K et al: Two siblings with midline field defects and Hirschsprung disease: Variable expression of Toriello-Carey syndrome or new syndrome? *Am J Med Genet* 47:299, 1993.

Toriello H, Carey J: Corpus callosum agenesis, facial anomalies, Robin sequence, and other anomalies: A new autosomal recessive condition? *Am J Med Genet* 31:17, 1988.

Treacher Collins Syndrome

At a glance: Craniofacial anomaly characterized by an antimongoloid slant of the eyes, coloboma of the lid, micrognathia (can be severe), microtia and other deformity of the ears, hypoplastic zygomatic arches, and macrostomia. Conductive hearing loss and cleft palate are often present.

Synonyms: Treacher-Collins-Franceschetti Syndrome; Berry-Treacher-Collins Syndrome; Mandibulofacial Dysostosis; TCOF-I Syndrome.

Incidence: 1:10,000 live births

Genetic inheritance: An autosomal dominant transmission with high penetrance and variable expressivity. The gene is localized on the long arm of chromosome 5 (in 5q32-q33.1 locus region, also termed TCOF1 locus) and produces a protein called the "treacle" gene.

Pathophysiology: Dysmorphogenesis of the first and second embryonal branchial arch systems. It has been postulated that it results from a defect in a nucleolar trafficking protein that is critically required during human craniofacial development. Interestingly enough, the facial features are strikingly similar to those observed with vitamin A toxicity in both animals and humans born of a mother who took 2000 IU of vitamin A daily as a supplement during pregnancy.

Diagnosis: The diagnosis of these syndromes is based on the clinical features. The radiographic studies may show poorly developed supraorbital ridges, hypoplastic malar bones, hypoplasia of mandible, and flat or aplastic coronoid and condyloid processes. Prenatal diagnosis is possible by ultrasonographic examination (by the 20th week) and by molecular biology on chorionic villus sample (as source of fetal DNA). All the mutations currently reported suggest haploinsufficiency as the molecular mechanism underlying the disorder. Laboratory and radiological findings, which include supraorbital ridges, hypoplastic malar bones, hypoplasia of mandible, aplastic coronoid and condyloid processes, and abnormal cranial base (basilar kyphosis).

Clinical aspects: The *eyes* show several anomalies: antimongoloid obliquity of palpebral fissures, coloboma of outer portion lower lids, with a deficiency of cilia, absence of the lower lacrimal points, microphthalmia. Flattening of the cheeks. *Facial* features: malar hypoplasia; hypoplastic zygomatic arches; antimongoloid slant; lower eyelid coloboma; microphthalmia; vision loss; strabismus; partial absence of lower eyelashes; nystagmus; atresia of external audi-

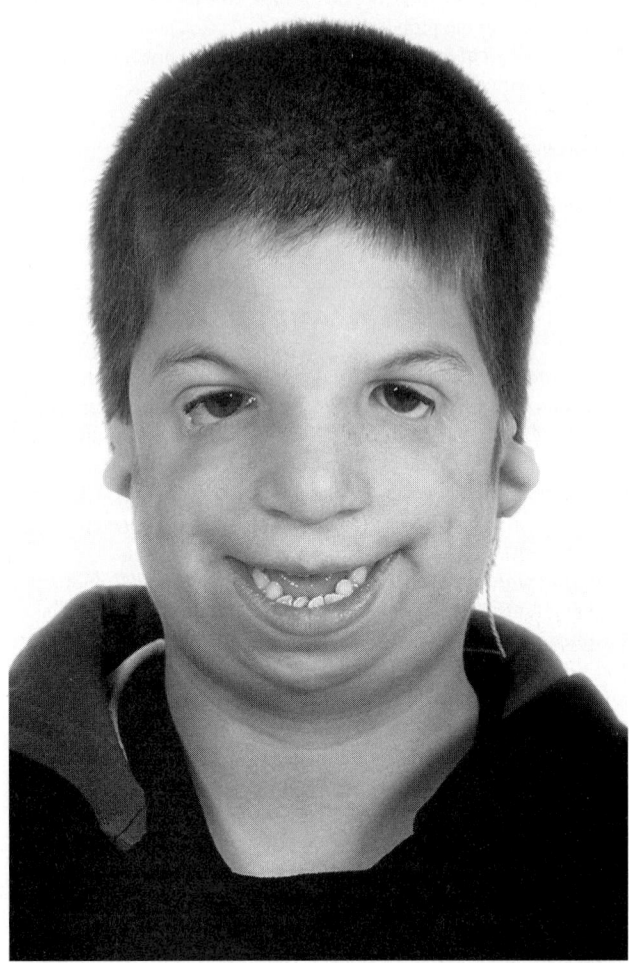

Treacher Collins syndrome This 8-year-old boy shows the characteristic facial features of Treacher Collins syndrome: antimongoloid slanting of the palpebral fissures, lower eyelid coloboma, hypoplastic zygomatic arches, microtia with atresia of the external auditory meatus, and mandibular hypoplasia. The wire behind his left ear connects to an endocochlear implant hearing aid.

tory meatus; microtia; malpositioning or maldevelopment of the pinna. *Mouth:* cleft palate, mandibular hypoplasia, macrostomia, absence of parotid gland. *Other clinical anomalies:* cardiovascular defects; cervical vertebral malformations; renal anomalies; choanal atresia; limb malformations; early failure to thrive; learning disabilities in early life; chronic respiratory insufficiency; cryptorchidism; psychological problems and social stigma as a consequence of facial deformity; sleep apnea syndrome and sudden death; conductive hearing loss; mental retardation.

Precautions before anesthesia: Management of the airway is expected to be difficult. Because of the mandibular retrusion and condylar hypoplasia, tracheal intubation with a fiberoptic laryngoscope is necessary. Sometimes a tracheostomy may be required. Physical examination is directed toward the cardiovascular system, lungs, and upper airway. Laboratory data: blood chemistries, blood group, hemoglobin, and coagulation studies.

Anesthetic considerations: The anesthetic management is a function of the severity of the malformation and of the surgical procedure (oral or nasotracheal intubation). The major problem in anesthesia is the maintenance of a free airway and tracheal intubation. Difficult airway problems must be anticipated and precautions should be taken to manage the patient safely. The maintenance of spontaneous respiration is highly recommended until the trachea has been intubated and lung ventilation confirmed. Use of a laryngeal mask may help. The reason for the demise of the tracheostomy are anesthetic experience, availability of flexible fiberoptic bronchoscope, requirement of a prolonged postoperative endotracheal intubation, and the availability of intensive care facilities (problem may occur in this area such as occlusion of a nasotracheal tube by mucus). Blood loss may be important during craniofacial reconstructive surgery and requires (invasive or noninvasive) monitoring of hemodynamic parameters, estimation of blood loss, arterial blood gas, and electrolyte analysis. Postoperative care often requires transfer to intensive care unit.

Pharmacological implications: Use of muscle relaxants must be avoided until the airway is secure and lung ventilation is confirmed.

Other conditions to be considered:

AKSU STOCKHAUSEN SYNDROME: This autosomal dominant medical condition is defined by the association of brachial arch defects. Characterized by the presence of anotia/microtia, microstomia, preauricular pits, respiratory distress, pharyngeal abnormality, hearing loss, sacral sinus/dimple, hypertonia, spasticity, and muscle rigidity. A proper evaluation of the airway must be done to eliminate the possibility of a difficult airway during face-mask ventilation and tracheal intubation. The potential for hyperkalemia following the administration of succinylcholine must be considered if hypertonia is present.

FRANCESCHETTI SYNDROME (Franceschetti-Zwahlen-Klein Syndrome): Mandibulofacial dysostosis presenting at birth with cyanotic spells. Fish-like facial characteristics, hypoplasia of the mandible, receding chin, considerable overbite, high-arched palate, macrostomia, low-set ears. An autosomal dominant inheritance. The difference between this disorder and Treacher Collins is believed to be the absence of flattening of the malar bones.

☞**GOLDENHAR SYNDROME:** Common birth defect of vascular origin involving first and second branchial arch derivatives, resulting mainly in hemifacial microsomia with absent ear, eye, and vertebral anomalies. Usually associated with cardiovascular anomalies, including ventricular septal defect, atrial septal defect, patent ductus arteriosus, tetralogy of Fallot, and coarctation of the aorta. Arnold-Chiari syndrome and hydrocephalus have been reported. Severe to major anesthetic implications, especially the airway (unilateral hypoplasia of the facial bones and muscles). Epibulbar dermoids. Limited mouth opening, micrognathia, cleft palate.

☞**MILLER SYNDROME:** Postaxial acrofacial dysostosis. Characterized by distinctive major craniofacial malformation (micrognathia, underdeveloped cheekbones, severe LeFort II malformation, and cleft palate) requiring tracheostomy at birth for breathing obstruction. Limb defects include underdevelopment of the ulna and radius (incomplete limb development). Miller syndrome patients are of normal intelligence.

REFERENCES:

Bryden DC, Remington SA, Mason C: Treacher Collins syndrome and difficult intubation. *Br J Hosp Med* 2:53(8):419, 1995.

Dixon MJ: Treacher Collins syndrome. *Hum Mol Genet* 5:1391, 1996.

Nilsson E, Ingvarsson L, Isern E. Treacher Collins syndrome with choanal atresia: One way to handle the airway. *Paediatr Anaesth.* 14:700; 2004.

Takita K, Kobayashi S, Kosu M, et al: Successes and failures with the laryngeal mask airway (LMA) in patients with Treacher Collins Syndrome—a case series. *Can J Anaesth* 50(9):969–70, 2003.

Triad Anomaly

At a glance: Rare association of cranial, cardiac, and genital malformations.

Synonym: Ambiguous Genitalia-Mental Retardation (AGR) Syndrome.

Genetic inheritance: Unknown.

Pathophysiology: Deletion of the short arm of chromosome 11 with a variable phenotype caused in part by a defect in contiguous genes.

Diagnosis: Evocated on the clinical association.

Clinical aspects: Can include multiple anomalies concerning *head* with cranial asymmetry, microcephaly, brachycephaly, prominent forehead, long narrow face, large fontanels, premature synostosis of metopic sutures and biparietal foramina, *face* (prominent bridge, short philtrum, and epicanthal folds), and *eyes* (aniridia, glaucoma, corneal opacity, optic atrophy, strabismus, cataracts, nystagmus, blepharoptosis, and blepharophimosis). High and narrow palate, prominent lower and down-turned upper lip can occur. Urogenital system can present with hypospadias, cryptorchidism, micropenis, fibrous ovaries, gonadal dysgenesis, horseshoe or fused kidneys, duplication of upper urinary tract, kidney aplasia or hypoplasia, and anomalies of urethra. Cardiomyopathy or cardiac defects, vertebral anomalies, and neurological anomalies can also occur. Hemihypertrophia is possible.

Precautions before anesthesia: Evaluate cardiac function in case of cardiomyopathy (chest radiography, echocardiography, ECG); airway (clinical, radiographs); and renal status (echography, creatinine, urea, electrolytes). Look at vertebral anomalies that can make perimedullar anesthesia contraindicated.

Anesthetic considerations: Direct laryngoscopy and tracheal intubation can be difficult because of facial malformation. The availability of proper size laryngeal mask airway and/or fiberoptic equipment may be required.

Pharmacological implications: Avoid parasympatholytic drugs in cases of glaucoma. Consider renal function if necessary to manage intraoperative fluid regimen and the use of nephrotoxic drugs. Cardiac prophylactic antibiotics should be used in cases of cardiac defects.

Other condition to be considered:

☞**WAGR SYNDROME:** An unusual association of Wilms tumor to ocular sign (aniridia) and mental retardation.

REFERENCES:

Gul D, Ogur G, Tunca Y, et al: Third case of WAGR syndrome with severe obesity and constitutional deletion of chromosome (11) (p12p14) [letter]. *Am J Med Genet* 107:70, 2002.

Schmickel RD: Chromosomal deletions and enzyme deficiencies. *J Pediatr* 108:244, 1986.

Tricho-Dento-Osseous (TDO) Syndrome

At a glance: Genetic condition characterized by abnormal development of teeth (enamel hypoplasia), bones (hypocalcification), and curly hair.

Genetic inheritance: Autosomal dominant. It is linked to a mutation on gene locus 17q21.3-q22, which results in altered function of a protein that has an important role in the development of hair (keratin), teeth (enamel), and bone (so-called DLX3 protein).

Pathophysiology: Abnormalities of keratin, enamel, and dentin are described; however, the pathogenesis of the TDO syndrome is unknown at present.

Diagnosis: Presence of "kinky curly hair," enamel hypoplasia, taurodontism (a variation in tooth form characterized by prism-shaped molars with large pulp spaces), and thick cortical bone.

Clinical aspects: Three subtypes or phenotypes for TDO have been suggested.

TDO-I demonstrates a normal calvarium with thickening of the chondrocranium, curly hair, delayed dental eruption with enamel hypoplasia and increased cavities, osteosclerosis, and only occasionally brittle nails. Premature sagittal craniosynostosis results in dolichocephaly. Calvarial thickness and density are normal; however, the chondrocranium may show some thickening.

TDO-II demonstrates more pronounced nail dystrophy (either with laminated splitting of the superficial layers or thick cornification), sparse, curly hair, and thickening and sclerosis of the calvaria. Males may show narrowing of the ear canal. In contrast to TDO-I, not only is dental eruption precocious, but also, in addition to the enamel hypoplasia, the dentin is dysplastic.

TDO-III demonstrates increased calvarial density and macrocephaly. Patients have an increased incidence of dental caries and abscess formation. Sagittal synostosis may result in dolichocephaly. Nails may be brittle or demonstrate increased cornification. There is no facial phenotype associated with the syndrome, although an increase in the length of the body of the mandible has been shown.

Precautions before anesthesia: Assess airway for abnormal anatomy or trismus related to abscess formation. Inspect dentition for teeth at risk during airway manipulation.

Anesthetic considerations: There are no specific considerations other than those relating to poor dentition and potential for difficult airway management in the presence of dental abscesses and trismus. As for other ectodermal dysplasias associated with dental anomalies, laryngoscopy must be performed very carefully to avoid any damages to the teeth.

Pharmacological implications: There are no known specific implications with this condition.

Other conditions to be considered:

☞AMELOGENESIS IMPERFECTA: An inherited condition that affects the enamel of the teeth making them soft and thin. The teeth appear yellow because the dentin is visible through the thin enamel and are easily damaged.

HYPOMATURATION-HYPOPLASIA TYPE WITH TAURODONTISM SYNDROME: The dental findings are apparently identical to those of tricho-dento-osseous syndrome from which it differs only by the lack of changes in the hair and bones. True taurodontism is defined by a change in the mandibular first permanent molar.

REFERENCES:
Hart TC, Bowden DW, Bolyard J: Genetic linkage of the tricho-dento-osseous syndrome to chromosome 17q21. *Hum Mol Genet* 6:2279, 1997.
Wright JT, Kula K, Hall K, et al: Analysis of the tricho-dento-osseous syndrome genotype and phenotype. *Am J Med Genet* 72:197, 1997.

Tricho-Oculo-Dermo-Vertebral Syndrome (TODV Syndrome)

At a glance: An arthrogryposis and unusual ectodermal dysplasia/malformation syndrome, including generalized bronchodysplasia, dry skin with scaling, hyperchromic spots on the limbs, hyperkeratosis (particularly the soles), dermatoglyphic abnormalities, dwarfism, bilateral cataracts, narrow palpebral fissures, and kyphoscoliosis. Other clinical features include microcephaly, brachycephaly, amyotrophy (muscle), and a high incidence of diabetes mellitus.

Synonyms: Alves Syndrome; Arthrogryposis and Ectodermal Dysplasia.

Incidence: Less than twenty cases have been described since its identification in 1981 by A. Alves.

Genetic inheritance: Autosomal recessive.

Diagnosis: Association of ectodermal dysplasia with arthrogryposis.

Clinical aspects: The skin is hyperkeratotic and hypohidrotic and bruises and scars easily after scratching or minor trauma. Onychodysplasia and hyperpigmented areas on the limbs may be present. Eyebrows are absent, palpebral fissures are narrow, and bilateral cataracts may occur. Craniofacial abnormalities include oligodontia, enamel hypoplasia, brachycephaly, microcephaly, and cleft lip/palate. Arthrogryposis may be marked. Other major skeletal abnormalities are kyphoscoliosis and short stature.

Precautions before anesthesia: Assess for airway abnormalities and poor dentition. In the presence of severe kyphoscoliosis, evaluate pulmonary function by chest radiography, lung function tests, and blood gases, as clinically indicated.

Anesthetic considerations: Vascular access may be difficult because of hyperkeratotic skin and arthrogryposis. Regional anesthesia may be technically difficult because of skeletal abnormalities but is not absolutely contraindicated. Severe kyphoscoliosis with impaired lung function may be an indication for elective postoperative ventilation following major surgery.

Pharmacological implications: There are no known specific implications with this condition.

Other condition to be considered:

COTE ADAMOPOULOS PANTELAKIS SYNDROME: Described a 16-year-girl with arthrogryposis and ectodermal dysplasia. The clinical features included the absence of nails and only one hair on the head. Diabetes mellitus was diagnosed at the age of 2 years and well controlled with insulin. At the age of 16 years she was only 120 cm tall. Arthrogryposis was most evident in the hands, but all joints seemed affected. The authors thought that the arthrogryposis, ectodermal dysplasia, growth retardation of prenatal onset, and diabetes mellitus were unlikely to have arisen all independently.

REFERENCE:
Alves AFP, dos Santos PAB, Castelo-Branco-Neto E, et al: An autosomal recessive ectodermal dysplasia syndrome of hypotrichosis, onychodysplasia, hyperkeratosis, kyphoscoliosis, cataract, and other manifestations. *Am J Med Genet* 10:213, 1981.

Tricho-Rhino-Phalangeal Dysplasia Type I

At a glance: Syndrome characterized by facial anomalies (bulbous nose, cone-shaped epiphyses), high-arched palate, and horizontal groove on the chin. Also includes hypoplastic nails and short metatarsal and metacarpals joints.

Synonym: TRPS I.

Incidence: Rare, although more than 30 cases have been identified. First described in 1974. Males affected more often than females.

Genetic inheritance: Autosomal dominant contiguous gene syndrome, probably the result of chromosome 8 deletion. An autosomal recessive trait has also been suggested.

Pathophysiology: It is caused by haploinsufficiency of a specific zinc finger protein that is putative transcription factor (TRPS I).

Diagnosis: Clinical supported by genetic analysis. Long bone radiographs reveal cone-shaped epiphyses.

Clinical aspects: Tendency for bone fracture and variable growth; hyperextensible joints. Scoliosis is also present. Characteristic appearance with bulbous broad nose, bushy eyebrows, sparse scalp hair, dental abnormalities. May present with recurrent pulmonary infections, often associated with pectus carinatum. Neonatal hypotonia has been reported. Micrognathia, prune-belly sequence. Ureteral reflux, persistent cloaca, congenital nephrotic syndrome. Rarely, but suggested, aplasia of epiglottis.

Precautions before anesthesia: Assessment of severity of previous bony problems, which facilitates preoperative positioning. Exclusion of respiratory infection clinically and, if indicated, by chest radiography. Assess airway for micrognathia and epiglottic aplasia.

Anesthetic considerations: Careful positioning and padding because of the tendency to fracture. Direct laryngoscopy and tracheal intubation might be difficult because of the micrognathia and the potential for epiglottic aplasia or laryngeal structure deformity. Spontaneous respiration must be maintained until the trachea has been intubated and lung ventilation is confirmed. The immediate availability of a laryngeal mask airway in case of failure to intubate the trachea is recommended. Fiberoptic equipment may be needed and should be available. The presence of abnormal dentition should also be kept in mind to avoid trauma during laryngoscopy.

Pharmacological implications: Prophylactic antibiotics may be indicated for respiratory or urogenital indications.

Other condition to be considered:

☞**Tricho-Rhino-Phalangeal Dysplasia type III:** Genetic multisystem disorder (ectodermal dysplasia) characterized by mild postnatal growth deficiency with mental retardation, thin hair, unusual facial features, brachydactyly, microencephaly, multiple exostoses, musculoskeletal dysplasia, and redundant skin.

Langer-Giedion Syndrome: Characterized by mental retardation, multiple exostoses, peculiar facies, and loose redundant skin. It is known as one of the few congenital contiguous gene syndromes and is present from birth. The facial features include a bulbous nose with thickened septum and alae, wide prominent philtrum, thin upper lips, and small mandible. During first years of life, patients are subjected to frequent recurrent respiratory infection. Both sexes are affected with similar prevalence.

References:

Carrington PR, Chen H, Altick JA: Trichorhinopharyngeal syndrome, type I. *J Am Acad Dermatol* 31(2 pt 2):331, 1994.

Jones KL: Tricho-Rhino-Phalangeal Syndrome, in Jones KL (ed): *Smith's Recognisable Patterns of Human Malformations.* 5th ed. Philadelphia, WB Saunders, 1997, p 250-1.

Tricho-Rhino-Phalangeal Dysplasia Type II

At a glance: Genetic multisystem disorder (ectodermal dysplasia) characterized by mild postnatal growth deficiency with mental retardation, thin hair, unusual facial features, brachydactyly, and multiple exostoses.

Synonyms: Langer-Giedion Syndrome; Acrodysplasia V; Acrodysplasia Dysostoses Syndrome; Alè-Calò Syndrome; Giedion-Langer Syndrome; Klingmüller Syndrome; Multiple Exostoses-Mental Retardation (MEMR) Syndrome; Trichorhino Auriculophalangeal Multiple Exostoses (TRAMPE) Dysplasia; Trichorhinophalangeal Syndrome with Exostoses.

History: Postnatal growth retardation associated with mild to moderate mental retardation and multiple cartilaginous exostoses described by A. Giedion, a Swiss Radiologist and L. Langer, an American radiologist.

Incidence: Rare. Both sexes affected equally.

Genetic inheritance: Usually sporadic but some cases autosomal dominant. Chromosome deletion extending from 8q24.11 to 8q24.13. One of the contiguous gene syndromes (group of disorders associated with chromosomal microdeletions or microduplications).

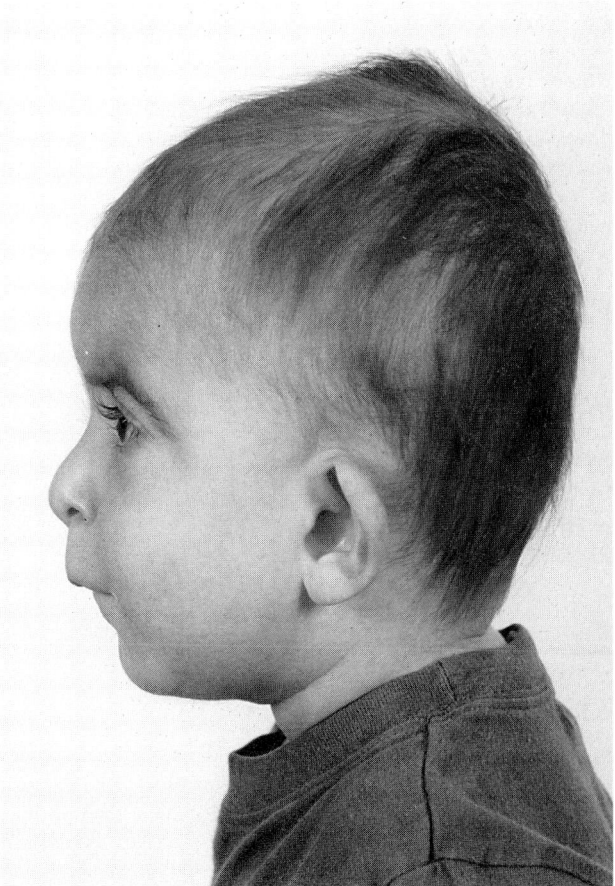

Tricho-Rhino-Phalangeal dysplasia type II This 2-year-old boy with microcephaly, prominent eyebrows, sparse scalp hair, and bulbous nose has tricho-rhino-phalangeal dysplasia type II.

Pathophysiology: Contiguous gene syndrome involving loss of functional copies of TRPS 1 and EXT 1 genes. Deletion of 8q24.13 results in bone exostoses and mental retardation especially when large pieces of 8q are deleted.

Diagnosis: Clinical features supported by genetic analysis. Long bone radiographs reveal cone-shaped epiphyses and the presence of exostoses.

Clinical aspects: Exostoses of bone with tendency for bone fracture and variable growth, hyperextensible joints. Scoliosis may be present. Redundant skin. Microcephaly, characteristic appearance with bulbous broad nose, bushy eyebrows, sparse scalp hair, dental abnormalities. Mental retardation, neonatal hypotonia, delayed speech development, hearing loss. Recurrent respiratory infections. Prune-belly sequence. Ureteral reflux, persistent cloaca, congenital nephrotic syndrome. Aplasia of epiglottis may be present.

Precautions before anesthesia: Assessment of severity of syndrome, previous bony problems, and degree of mental retardation. Exclusion of respiratory infection clinically and, if indicated, by chest radiography. Assessment of genitourinary abnormalities and referral to exclude abnormalities may be indicated. Assessment of rare complications such as prune belly and epiglottic aplasia must be conducted.

Anesthetic considerations: Premedication may be indicated if patient is uncooperative because of mental retardation. Intravenous access may be difficult because of the redundant skin. Careful positioning and padding is highly recommended because of the tendency to spontaneous bone fracture.

Pharmacological implications: Prophylactic antibiotics may be indicated for respiratory or urogenital indications.

Other condition to be considered:

☞Tricho-Rhino-Phalangeal Dysplasia Type I: Syndrome characterized by characteristic facial anomalies (bulbous nose, cone-shaped epiphyses), high-arched palate, and horizontal groove on the chin. Also includes hypoplastic nails and short metatarsal and metacarpal joints. Mental retardation is not associated with this medical condition.

REFERENCES:

Carrington PR, Chen H, Altick JA: Trichorhinopharyngeal syndrome, type 1. *J Am Acad Dermatol* 31(2 pt 2):331, 1994.

Jones KL: Tricho-Rhino-Phalangeal Syndrome, Jones KL (ed): *Smith's Recognisable Patterns of Human Malformations.* 5th ed. Philadelphia, WB Saunders, 1997, p 250–1.

Lu FL, Hou JW, Tsai WS, et al: Tricho-rhino-pharyngeal syndrome type II associated with epiglottic aplasia and congenital nephrotic syndrome. *J Formos Med Assoc* 96(3):217, 1997.

Tricho-Rhino-Phalangeal Dysplasia Type III

At a glance: An extremely rare inherited multisystem disorder characterized by fine, thin light-colored hair, unusual facial features, abnormalities of the fingers and/or toes, and multiple abnormalities of epiphyses leading to skeletal dysplasia. The skeletal dysplasia is mostly observed in the hands and feet.

Synonyms: TRPS III; Sugio-Kajii Syndrome.

Incidence: Extremely rare. Both sexes affected equally. However, of the reported cases, most affected individuals have been female. Approximately 15 cases have been reported in the medical literature

Genetic inheritance: Trichorhinophalangeal Syndrome Type III is suggested as an autosomal dominant genetic transmission.

Pathophysiology: There is evidence suggesting that type III TRPS is caused by mutation in the TRPS1 gene, which is also the site of mutation in type I TRPS.

Diagnosis: This syndrome is characteristically identified by the presence of sparse and thin hair, a beaked nose, long upper lip, and severe metacarpophalangeal shortening visible clinically and confirmed radiologically (e.g., severe shortening of metacarpals, metatarsals, and phalanges) and the abnormal development of the epiphyses of the phalangeal bones (epiphyseal coning). It is different than the Ruvalcaba Syndrome by the absence of mental retardation and microcephaly.

Clinical aspects: This medical condition is characterized by fine, brittled, thin light-colored hair, a beaked nose, and severe brachydactyly. Infants affected with this condition may exhibit several characteristic facial features, including a pear-shaped or rounded nose, hypoplastic alae nasi, an abnormally long, broad philtrum on the upper lip, a protruding upper lip, malar hypoplasia, and/or an abnormally prominent maxilla. Dental anomalies are also considered a frequent occurrence in this syndrome (e.g., malocclusion). The abnormalities of the hands and feet include brachydactyly because of an incomplete development of the metacarpals, metatarsals, and phalanges. Most affected individuals exhibit a clinodactyly (permanent fixation of the fingers). Short stature, osteochondritis, thoracic scoliosis, pectus carinatum, and/or limited movements of certain joints complete the clinical presentation.

Precautions before anesthesia: Assessment of severity of syndrome and previous skeletal problems. Limitation in the range of motion in the hips and various joints must be evaluated. Proper assessment of the upper airway structures must be obtained because of potential limitation during direct laryngoscopy. The severity of the pectus carinatum must be assessed clinically and with chest radiograph if needed. The potential for chronic use of corticosteroids should be considered and assessed prior to surgery.

Anesthetic considerations: Careful positioning and padding must be considered because of the tendency to severe limitation in the range of motion. Unless there is limitation in the maxillomandibular joint and difficult direct laryngoscopy and tracheal intubation expected, the anesthetic considerations in these patients are directly dependent on the surgical procedure to be performed. A laryngeal mask airway should be available in case of failure to ventilate and/or intubate the trachea.

Pharmacological implications: There are no specific pharmacological implications reported.

Other conditions to be considered:

☞Ruvalcaba Syndrome: A rare inherited disorder characterized by short stature, craniofacial abnormalities, mental retardation, skeletal malformations, and/or hypoplastic genitalia. Other clinical features include microcephaly, an abnormally small and narrow nose, and the presence of palpebral fissures. Clinodactyly and/or abnormally short metacarpals and metatarsals resulting in unusually small hands and feet have been reported. Vertebral scoliosis and/or severe pectus carinatum can also be part of the clinical presentation. It has been suggested that an autosomal dominant genetic transmission is responsible for this disorder.

☞Tricho-Rhino-Phalangeal Dysplasia Type I: Characterized by classic facial anomalies (bulbous nose, cone-shaped epiphyses), high-arched palate, horizontal groove on the chin. Also includes hypoplastic nails, and short metatarsal and metacarpals joints. This syndrome differs from Langer-Gideon Syndrome because of the absence of mental retardation, microencephaly, multiple exostoses, musculoskeletal dysplasia, and redundant skin.

☞**Tricho-Rhino-Phalangeal Dysplasia Type II:** An extremely rare inherited multisystem disorder and characterized by fine, thin hair, unusual facial features, dwarfism, brachydactyly, "cone-shaped" epiphyseal ends and/or development of multiple exostoses projecting outward from the surfaces of all bones. Other clinical features include hyperextensible joints, hypotonia, redundant skin, and maculopapular nevi. Mild to severe mental retardation, sensorineural deafness, and delayed speech development have also been reported.

REFERENCES:

Ludecke HJ, Schaper J, Meinecke P: Genotypic and phenotypic spectrum in tricho-rhino-phalangeal syndrome types I and III. *Am J Hum Genet* 68:81, 2001.

Nagai T, Nishimura G, Kasai H: Another family with tricho-rhino-phalangeal syndrome type III (Sugio-Kajii syndrome). *Am J Med Genet* 49:278, 1994.

Sugio Y, Kajii T: Ruvalcaba syndrome: Autosomal dominant inheritance. *Am J Med Genet* 19:741, 1994.

Triglyceride Storage Disease (TSD)

At a glance: A complex group of inherited disorders of lipid metabolism resulting in systemic deposition of triglycerides and, to a lesser extent, cholesterol.

Classification:

TSD type I

TSD type II

TSD type III: Wolman Disease; Lysosomal Acid Lipase Deficiency; Acid Cholesteryl Ester Hydrolase Deficiency, Wolman type; Cholesteryl Ester Storage Disease.

TSD with Impaired Long Chain Fatty Acid Oxydation: Ichthyotic Neutral Lipid Storage Disease; Dorfman-Chanarin Syndrome; Chanarin-Dorfman Syndrome.

Genetic inheritance: TSD type I, unknown. TSD type II, autosomal dominant. TSD type III (Wolman disease), autosomal recessive. TSD with impaired long-chain fatty acid oxidation, autosomal recessive.

Pathophysiology: Normal mobilization of lipids from peripheral tissues requires catecholamine-induced activation of adenyl-cyclase and cAMP, which activate protein kinase. Activated protein kinase, in turn, activates triglyceride lipase, releasing free fatty acids and glycerol from the cell. In type I TSD, a defect of the adenyl-cyclase or catecholamine receptor is postulated. In type II TSD, abnormality of protein kinase is proposed. In type III TSD, a defect of the triglyceride lipase is proposed. Lipogenesis appears normal in all these conditions. The inability or impaired ability to mobilize lipids results in widespread lipid deposition. Classification into myocardial and skin types has been suggested to reflect the predominant tissues of triglyceride deposition, although it is important to note that TSD is a multisystem disorder.

Diagnosis: Clinical history and examination. Laboratory findings include vacuolated granulocytes (Jordan anomaly) and histological evidence of excess triglyceride in adipose tissue. In vitro study of response of tissue adenyl-cyclase to catecholamines may be undertaken.

Clinical aspects: The presentation is variable between and within the subtypes of TSD. *Type I TSD* presents with failure to thrive and emaciation and type II presents with obesity. *Type II TSD* patients are able to mobilize lipids independently of the hormone-sensitive lipase pathway. *Type III TSD (Wolman Disease)* presents in the neonatal period and carries a poor prognosis (death by age 6 months), although less-aggressive forms of type III TSD are described. Signs and symptoms can include cutaneous lipid deposition, ichthyosis, vomiting, diarrhea, steatorrhea, malabsorption, portal hypertension, hepatosplenomegaly, adrenal calcification, and widespread xanthomata. Central nervous system involvement can include developmental delay (especially type III TSD), ptosis, cataracts, nystagmus, ataxia, areflexia, and cranial nerve palsies. Muscle infiltration results in a skeletal myopathy, and cardiac involvement results in a dilated cardiomyopathy. Cardiomyopathy was a common finding in one Japanese cohort. Pulmonary hypertension has been described in one patient with type III TSD. Treatment includes lipid-lowering drugs and careful control of lipid intake.

Precautions before anesthesia: Careful clinical examination for clinical signs of impaired cardiorespiratory reserve, examine for evidence of muscle hypotonia. Cardiovascular assessment. Twelve-lead ECG must be obtained to exclude conduction abnormalities; low threshold for echocardiography must be performed to exclude dilated cardiomyopathy. Chest radiography is indicated if ventricular failure is suspected. Laboratory investigations: check electrolytes and renal function and correct any abnormalities; full blood count; liver function tests including coagulation studies. Consider possibility of hypoadrenalism.

Anesthetic considerations: Premedication may be desirable in the presence of marked developmental delay. Hypotonia may limit the use of spontaneous ventilation under anesthesia and neuromuscular blockade should be monitored by nerve stimulator. The presence of a dilated cardiomyopathy should prompt consideration of invasive monitoring with attention to maintenance of normovolemia and the use of cardiodepressive anesthetic agents. Inhalational anesthetic agents should be used with caution to limit their myocardial depressant effects.

Pharmacological implications: Succinylcholine is relatively contraindicated. Hepatic infiltration may cause a fall in albumin, altering the free fraction of some drugs. Atracurium or *cis*-atracurium may be the muscle relaxant of choice.

REFERENCES:

Galton D, Gilbert C, Reckless J, et al: Triglyceride storage disease. A group of inborn errors of metabolism. *QJM* 43(169):63, 1974.

Takahira T, Utsunomiya T, Ishijima M, et al: Specific myocardial disease caused by multisystemic triglyceride storage in Jordan's anomaly. *Am Heart J* 126(4):995, 1993.

Trimethylaminuria Syndrome

At a glance: An inborn error of metabolism characterized by inability to N-oxidize trimethylamine.

Synonyms: Fish-Odor Syndrome; TMA Syndrome; Flavin Mono-Oxygenase Syndrome; FMO Syndrome.

Incidence: Epidemiologic studies have established the incidence of this condition in Britain at 1:25,000 individuals. Incidence varies with ethnicity. The populations of Ecuador and Papua New Guinea have especially high rates for the disease. The heterozygous carrier state is estimated to be as high as 1% in general population.

Genetic inheritance: Although an autosomal dominant inheritance has been suggested, the possibility of an autosomal recessive trait was suggested by Ayres. Gene locus 1q23-q25. This genetic defect is characterized by the inability of the body to produce the enzyme FMO3 (flavin-containing mono-oxygenase 3), which is needed by the liver to process the protein trimethylamine (TMA). Unprocessed TMA leads to offensive body odor known as the fish-odor syndrome.

Pathophysiology: Trimethylamine is produced by gut flora in the presence of choline- and carnitine-containing foods such as saltwater fish, soya bean, and egg yolk. Trimethylamine is readily absorbed and usually undergoes N-oxidation by hepatic flavin-containing monooxygenases (FMO), which are part of the mixed function oxidase group of enzymes. In trimethylaminuria, the FMO3 isoenzyme is defective, resulting in failure of N-oxidation. Trimethylamine, which has the odor of rotting fish, is subsequently secreted in the saliva, sweat, urine, and other body fluids.

Diagnosis: History of malodor; demonstration of trimethylamine in the urine.

Clinical aspects: Strong and repulsive odor from sweat, urine, and breath is the predominant finding. The implications are predominantly social and have resulted in poor progression at school, anxiety, and clinical depression. Suicide is not uncommon. Menstruation, stress, and pyrexia exacerbate the odor. There is one report of a patient with trimethylaminuria developing hypertension and tachycardia after ingesting tyramine-containing foods and after using ephedrine nasal drops for epistaxis. Management includes dietary restriction of carnitine and choline, and occasional use of neomycin and metronidazole to reduce bacterial production of trimethylamine.

Precautions before anesthesia: Routine anesthetic assessment. Inquire specifically for reaction to tyramine-containing foods and catecholamine-containing medications such as nasal drops. Record drug history.

Anesthetic considerations: Anxiety generated by stress-related body odor may make premedication desirable for the patient.

Pharmacological implications: The effect of abnormal flavin-containing monooxygenases on drug metabolism remains to be determined; however, it is advisable to use catecholamines with extreme caution because of severe hypertensive response. Desflurane should be considered relatively contraindicated.

REFERENCES:

Ayesh R, Mitchell S, Zhang A et al: The fish odour syndrome: Biochemical, familial, and clinical aspects. *BMJ* 307:655, 1993.

Walker V: The fish odour syndrome. *BMJ* 307:639, 1993.

Trisomy 3p

At a glance: Duplication of the short arm of chromosome 3 with severe delay in mental development, craniofacial dysmorphism, urogenital maldevelopement, and various occasional anomalies, including cardiac defects, cleft lip and palate, holoprosencephaly, dermatoglyphic findings, and other malformations.

Synonyms: Chromosome 3p Duplication Syndrome; 3p+ Syndrome; Partial Trisomy 3p.

Incidence: Very rare. More than 50% of children die within the first 2 years of life.

Genetic inheritance: Duplications include dup(3)(pter-p25), dup(3)(pter-p11), dup(3)(pter-p23), and dup(3)(p25-pter). Most reported cases have resulted from paternal or maternal balanced translocation.

Clinical aspects: *Head and neck:* brachycephaly, holoprosencephaly, square face with frontal bossing, flat occiput, temporal indentations, facial clefts and full cheeks. *Ears:* malformed auricles. *Eyes:* hypertelorism, iris coloboma, microphthalmia, cyclopia, down-slanting palpebral fissures. *Mouth and nose:* large mouth, cleft lip and palate, short nose with broad and flat bridge, choanal atresia. *Cardiac defects:* congenital heart defects including tetralogy of Fallot, ventricular septal defect, hypoplastic heart, and transposition of the great vessels. *Central nervous system:* seizures. *Muscles:* severe hypotonia. *Gastrointestinal:* esophageal atresia, atresia of the colon and rectum. *Other features:* short stubby hands and feet, camptodactyly, excessive fingertip whorls are the dermatoglyphic findings, spinal hemivertebrae, hypogonadism, hypospadias, micropenis, cryptorchidism, and kidney hypoplasia.

Precautions before anesthesia: Evaluate cardiac function (clinical, echocardiography, ECG) and renal function (echography, urea, creatinine, electrolytes). Seizure medication should be optimized prior to anesthesia and surgery. Anesthesia consultation should be considered to assess airway condition.

Anesthetic considerations: Careful intraoperative positioning should be done (vertebral anomalies, joint contractures). Direct laryngoscopy and tracheal intubation has, however, not proven to be difficult in the few cases reported. The presence of a large mouth and microstomia seem to facilitate direct laryngoscopy. However, special attention to the possibility of a challenging direct laryngoscopy and tracheal intubation should always be a consideration. Implications of associated cardiovascular congenital anomalies should be treated according to the clinical presentation. Perimedullar anesthesia is often contraindicated or difficult because of vertebral and spine anomalies.

Pharmacological implications: Consider anesthetic drug interactions with antiepileptic medications. Prophylactic antibiotics should be given as indicated in cases of cardiac defect. Maintaining spontaneous ventilation during laryngoscopy might be judicious until direct laryngeal vision is confirmed and tracheal intubation can be performed without problems. Avoid anesthetic drugs with marked cardiovascular effects.

REFERENCES:

Allen DL, Foster RN: Anaesthesia and trisomy 3p syndrome [letter]. *Anaesth Intensive Care* 24:615, 1996.

Kotzot D: De novo direct duplication 3(p25-pter). A previously undescribed chromosomal aberration. *Clin Genet* 50:96, 1996.

Walzer S: A new translocation syndrome (3/B). *N Engl J Med* 275:290, 1966.

Trisomy 4p

At a glance: A rare chromosomal disorder in which all or a portion of the short arm (p) appears three times rather than twice in cells of the body. Clinically characterized by breathing difficulties, craniofacial anomalies, hands and feet abnormalities, and congenital heart defects. Other clinical features include genital anomalies in affected males, skeletal defects, and severe mental retardation.

Synonyms: Chromosome 4, Partial Trisomy; Duplication 4p Syndrome.

Genetic inheritance: Duplication of the short arm of the fourth chromosome (dup(4)) leading to the appearance of three p arm (trisomy).

Clinical aspects: *Head and neck:* microcephaly, square face and flat forehead, prominent supraorbital ridges, short neck. *Ears:* enlarged ears, thickened helix and antihelix. *Eyes:* uveal coloboma, microphthalmia, down-slanting palpebral fissures. *Mouth and nose:* cleft lip and palate, macroglossia, pointed mandible. *Cardiac defects:* congenital heart defects are often associated. *Respiratory system:* absent or additional ribs, recurrent pulmonary aspiration leading to severe respiratory problems, broad chest with aging. *Central nervous system:* mental retardation, agenesis of the corpus callosum, severe seizures. *Neuromuscular:* present with hypertonic responses in the infancy period but becoming severely hypotonic later. *Other clinical features:* clinodactyly of the fifth finger, camptodactyly, hypoplastic nails, preaxial polydactyly, congenital dislocated hips, syndactyly of the second and third toe, joint contractures, vertebral anomalies such as spinal hemivertebrae, hypospadias, micropenis, cryptorchidism, and obesity accompanied with redundant skin.

Precautions before anesthesia: Evaluate cardiac function (clinical, echocardiography, ECG) and assess respiratory function (because of recurrent pulmonary aspiration).

Anesthetic considerations: In presence of severe mental retardation, behavioral problems might affect considerably the preoperative period and anesthesia induction: premedication might be indicated but the potential for a breathing problem may be a limitation. Careful intraoperative positioning should be done (vertebral anomalies, joint contractures and stiffness). Direct laryngoscopy and tracheal intubation can be difficult because of short neck and the presence of micrognathia and macroglossia. It is recommended to maintain spontaneous respiration until tracheal intubation is achieved and lung ventilation confirmed. A laryngeal mask airway must be available. Venous access can be difficult because of the presence of puffy hands (redundant skin). Perimedullar anesthesia is often contraindicated or difficult because of vertebral and spine anomalies.

Pharmacological implications: Consider anesthetic drugs interactions with antiepileptic medications. The use of an intravenous antiepileptic relay must be considered intraoperatively. The chronic use of antiepileptic medications might affect the metabolism of the anesthetic agents. Prophylactic antibiotics should be as indicated in cases of cardiac defect. Preserve spontaneous ventilation before intubation is performed. Avoid anesthetic drugs with marked cardiovascular effects.

REFERENCE:
Patel SV, Dagnew H, Parekh AJ, et al: Clinical manifestations of trisomy 4p syndrome. *Eur J Pediatr* 154:425, 1995.

Trisomy 6q

At a glance: Partial Trisomy 6q is extremely rare. Many affected infants and children have growth retardation, mental retardation, craniofacial anomalies, a short, webbed neck, and joint contractures.

Synonyms: Chromosome 6, Trisomy 6q2; Distal Trisomy 6q; Duplication 6q; Partial Distal Duplication 6q.

Incidence: Extremely rare. Appears to affect males and females equally. Approximately 30 cases have been reported in the medical literature.

Genetic inheritance: Chromosome 6, partial trisomy 6q is the result of a balanced translocation in one of the parents. The duplicated portion of 6q2 begins between bands 6q21 and 6q26 and may extend to the end (or "terminal") of chromosome 6q (qter).

Clinical aspects: Craniofacial abnormalities include microcephaly, an abnormally flat face and occiput, an "almond-shaped," protruding, ocular hypertelorism, and/or downwardly slanting palpebral fissures. Affected individuals may also have a small "bow-shaped" mouth with thin lips, micrognathia, cleft palate, a large, flat nose, malformed ears, and/or thin, arched eyebrows. In some cases, the coronal and sagittal craniosynostosis causing turricephaly has been reported. The neck may be unusually short and wide with abnormal frontolateral webbing, potentially restricting movement of the jaw and neck. The hairline may be abnormally low on the back of the neck (nape). Joint contractures (fingers, wrists, elbows, knees, hips), causing limitation of movement and abnormal postures, are often associated. Polysyndactyly, clubhands and/or clubfeet, scoliosis, reduced diameter of the chest, and widely spaced nipples. Genital abnormalities include, in affected females, hypoplastic labia, and in affected males, micropenis, hypospadias, and cryptorchidism. It may also include cardiac, intestinal, renal, and cerebral abnormalities.

Precautions before anesthesia: Evaluate cardiac function (clinical, echocardiography, ECG) and renal function (echography, urea, creatinine, electrolytes). Anesthesia consultation is indicated to assess the airway and other medical conditions (especially cardiac).

Anesthetic considerations: Careful intraoperative positioning should be done (vertebral anomalies, joint contractures). Direct laryngoscopy and tracheal intubation will be difficult because of short and webbed neck, the presence of micrognathia, a small mouth opening, and retrognathia. Spontaneous respiration must be maintained until the trachea is intubated and lung ventilation confirmed. Venous access can be difficult because of limb anomalies. Perimedullar anesthesia is often contraindicated or difficult because of vertebral and spine anomalies.

Pharmacological implications: Prophylactic antibiotics should be as indicated in cases of cardiac defect. Preserve spontaneous ventilation before and during laryngoscopy until tracheal intubation is secured. Avoid anesthetic drugs with marked cardiovascular effects.

REFERENCES:
Conrad BA, Higgins RR, Pierpont MEM: Duplication 6q22→qter: Definition of the phenotype. *Am J Med Genet* 78:123, 1998.

Dellacasa P: Partial trisomy of the long arm of chromosome 6. A clinical case. *Minerva Pediatr* 45:517, 1993.

Erdel M, Duba HC, Verdorfer I, et al: Comparative genomic hybridization reveals a partial de novo trisomy 6q23-qter in an infant with congenital malformations: Delineation of the phenotype. *Hum Genet* 99:596, 1997.

Trisomy 8

At a glance: Complete Trisomy 8 occurs in 0.8% of spontaneous pregnancy losses. Mosaic trisomy 8 is a well-known syndrome characterized by severe mental retardation, craniofacial dysmorphism,

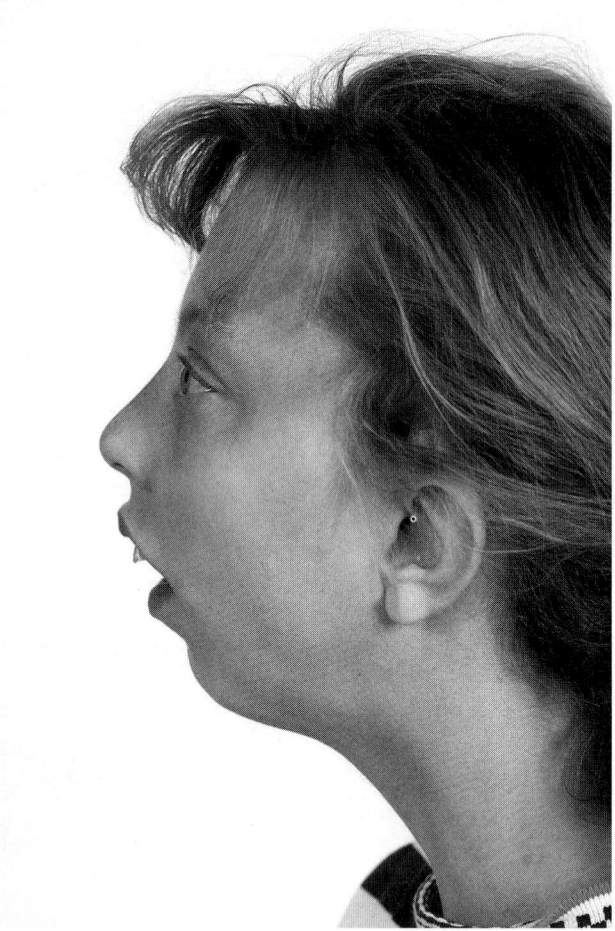

Trisomy 8 This girl with facial dysmorphism (high forehead, hypoplastic mandible) and low-set ears was diagnosed with a trisomy 8 mosaicism.

skeletal anomalies, complex congenital heart defect, and kidney malformations.

Synonyms: Trisomy C; Trisomy 8s.

Genetic inheritance: Mosaicism is less common than what is often referred to as "full" trisomy. A mosaic exists when a person presents with trisomic cells in their body, but in the presence of normal chromosomic cells. The genetic error occurs during the division of cells after fertilization. Trisomy 8 is rarely observed at birth.

Diagnosis: Clinically evocated; patients with trisomy 8 mosaicism present with moderate mental retardation, multiple skeletal anomalies, urogenital malformations, congenital heart defects, deep palmar and plantar furrows, distinct facial dysmorphism, and agenesis of the corpus callosum.

Clinical aspects: Clinical features involve *head and face* (simian crease seizures; expressionless facies; micrognathia; prominent forehead; large dysplastic ears; microphthalmia; strabismus; hypertelorism; corneal opacity; cataract, heterochromia; everted lips; highly arched or cleft palate and stretched) and *skeleton* (short neck; thin, elongated trunk; pectus carinatum; camptodactyly; clinodactyly; short metacarpal and metatarsal bones; absent or dysplastic patellae; multiple joint contractures; coxa valga; abnormal

diaphyses and epiphyses of radial, femoral, and humeral bone; kyphoscoliosis, hemivertebrae; fusion of vertebrae; spina bifida; broad dorsal ribs). *Abdominal and pelvic* organs (hydronephrosis, ureteral reflux, cryptorchidism, malrotation or absence of gallbladder, jejunal duplication, gastric sarcoma) and *thoracic* organs (cardiac septal defects and great vessel anomalies) can present malformations. Deep palmar and plantar furrows are frequent.

Precautions before anesthesia: Evaluate cardiac function (clinical, echocardiography, ECG) and renal function (echography, urea, creatinine, electrolytes).

Anesthetic considerations: Careful intraoperative positioning should be done (vertebral anomalies, joint contractures). Direct laryngoscopy and tracheal intubation can be difficult because of short neck and microretrognathia. Spontaneous respiration must be maintained at all times because face-mask fit may be difficult, and failure to intubate the trachea highly possible. The availability of a laryngeal mask airway and/or fiberoptic equipments is highly recommended. Venous access can be difficult because of limb anomalies. Perimedullar anesthesia is often contraindicated or difficult because of vertebral and spine anomalies.

Pharmacological implications: Consider anesthetic drug interaction with antiepileptic medications. Prophylactic antibiotics should be as indicated in case of cardiac defect. Preserve spontaneous ventilation before intubation is performed. Avoid anesthetic drugs with marked cardiovascular effect.

Other conditions to be considered:

Trisomy 8p: Duplication 8p with craniofacial defects, brevicollis with redundant skin folds, and mental retardation. High, prominent forehead; wide face in infancy; fleshy, everted lower lip; long and poorly defined philtrum with marked macrostomia and gingival hypertrophy; low nasal bridge and antevertebral nostrils; hyperextensibility of the finger joints; and hypoplastic nails. Cardiac malformations (33% of patients) are reported. Agenesis of the corpus callosum with severe epilepsy, spina bifida occulta, and numerous genitourinary anomalies. Phenotypic expression is related to the length of the duplicated segment.

Trisomy 8q: Low birth weight, mental deficiency, prominent forehead, flat occiput, hypertelorism, up-slanting palpebral fissures, ear and nose deformities, thin upper lips, and skeletal defects.

REFERENCES:

Barber JC, James RS, Patch C, et al: Protelomeric sequences are deleted in cases of short arm inverted duplication of chromosome 8. *Am J Med Genet* 50:296, 1994.

Kurytka ZE, Krzykwa B, Piatkowska E, et al: Trisomy 8 mosaicism syndrome. Two cases demonstrating variability in phenotype. *Clin Pediatr (Phila)* 27:557, 1988.

Warkany J, Rubinstein JH, Soukup SW, et al: Mental retardation, absence of patella, other malformations with chromosomal mosaicism. *J Pediatr* 61:803, 1962.

Trisomy 9

At a glance: Chromosomal disorder that can occur in a mosaic or nonmosaic expression, in which all major systems are significantly involved. Clinically characterized by severe gastrointestinal problems, scoliosis and kyphosis, repetitive periods of apnea, complex congenital heart defects, severe immunological disorders, failure to thrive, and severe mental retardation. Death occurs in infancy or early childhood.

Synonym: Chromosome 9 Trisomy Syndrome.

Pathophysiology: Caused by excessive synthesis by an extra chromosome and varies with the characteristic of the trisomy (total or mosaic).

Diagnosis: Clinically evocated by psychomotor retardation and multiple abnormalities of the craniofacial structures, heart, skeletal system, extremities, and other organs; confirm by karyotype studies.

Clinical aspects: This is a severe disease with growth and mental retardation. Death occurs generally in infancy or early childhood. Clinical features involve all major systems. *Cerebral and craniofacial* malformations are constant (Dandy-Walker cyst; subependymal cysts; ventricular dilatation of the brain; microcephaly; prominent occiput micrognathia; wide cranial sutures and fontanels; craniosynostosis; facial cleft and cloverleaf skull; short and up-slanting palpebral fissures; microphthalmia; coloboma; corneal clouding; hypertelorism; deeply set eyes; low-set malformed ears; tongue abnormalities; ankyloglossia; cleft lip/palate). *Skeleton* abnormalities can include short and webbed neck, hip dislocation, abnormally shaped long bones, limitation of joint movement, short limbs, and dysplasia of hands and feet. Other clinical features include *heart* (ventricular septal defect, atrial septal defect, patent ductus arteriosus, valve defects, double-outlet right ventricle, persistent left superior vena cava, endocardial fibroelastosis), *urogenital* system (hydronephrosis, duplication of collecting system, microcystic kidneys, dysplastic kidneys, cryptorchidism, small penis, hypospadias, hypoplastic labia), and *skin* (deep palmar and plantar creases, hyperconvex nails).

Precautions before anesthesia: Evaluate cardiac function (clinical, echocardiography, ECG), renal function (echography, urea, creatinine, electrolytes), and tracheal intubation (clinical, radiography).

Anesthetic considerations: Direct laryngoscopy and tracheal intubation can be difficult because of short neck, ankyloglossia, and microretrognathia, and may require fiberoptic or retrograde intubation. Spontaneous respiration must be maintained until tracheal intubation is achieved and lung ventilation confirmed. A laryngeal mask airway and/or fiberoptic equipments should be readily available. Venous access can be difficult as a result of limb anomalies. Careful intraoperative positioning is necessary considering hip dislocation and joint limitation. Pulse oximetry can be difficult because of nail malformation.

Pharmacological implications: Prophylactic antibiotics should be given as indicated in cases of cardiac defect. Preserve spontaneous ventilation before intubation is performed and avoid anesthetic drugs with marked cardiovascular effects.

Other conditions to be considered:

DUPLICATION 9P PARTIAL **(Trisomy 9p Partial):** Pupillary anomalies, kyphoscoliosis, and gastroesophageal reflux.

DUPLICATION 9Q32 **(Trisomy 9q32):** Chronic inflammatory lung disease, hypotonia, and microstomia.

PARTIAL TRISOMY 9Q **(Chromosome 9q Duplication Syndrome):** Psychomotor retardation, deeply set eyes, microdolichocephaly, beaked nose, and microretrognathia.

REFERENCES:

Cantu ES, Eicher DJ, Pai GS et al: Mosaic vs. nonmosaic trisomy 9: Report of a liveborn infant evaluated by fluorescence in situ hybridization and review of the literature. *Am J Med Genet* 62:230, 1996.

Lopez JJ, Romero DA, et al: Characteristics and dental treatment of partial trisomy 9. *Med Oral* 6:290; 2001.

Roberts DJ, Sandstrom MM, Van Praagh S: Characteristics of structural heart defects in trisomy 9 and their relationship to those in trisomy 13, 18, and 21. *Am Heart J* 125:1681, 1993.

Trisomy 11q

At a glance: Duplication of the long arm of chromosome 11 provides multiple malformations of which variability is related to the size of duplication. Clinically characterized at birth or later by the association of delayed growth and mental development, craniofacial anomalies, musculoskeletal abnormalities, imperforate anus, cryptorchidism, and congenital heart defects.

Synonyms: 11q+ Syndrome; 11q Duplication Syndrome; Chromosome 11q Trisomy Duplication.

Clinical aspects: Malformations can concern *head* (microcephaly, anencephaly, craniorachischisis, and microretrognathia; dysplastic ears and preauricular tags; nystagmus, strabismus, hypertelorism and down-slanting palpebral fissures; short, flat, or broad nose, short septum, long philtrum and epicanthal folds; highly arched palate, cleft palate, cleft lip, macroglossia and retracted lower lip; short neck), *abdomen and pelvis* (abdominal muscle defects, exomphalos, inguinal hernia, imperforate anus, hypoplasia of gallbladder, absent kidneys, bicornis uterus, micropenis, cryptorchidism, and hypoplastic scrotum), *nervous system* (neonatal hypertonia and postnatal hypotonia, seizures, arhinencephaly, agenesis of corpus callosum, and hypoplasia of cerebellar vermis), and *skeleton* (bipartite clavicles, dysplastic and dislocated hips, radioulnar synostosis, clubfoot, and absent thumbs). Congenital heart defects can include ventricular septal defect and abnormal lung lobation. Some patients exhibit symptoms of Cri-Du-Chat Syndrome.

Precautions before anesthesia: Evaluate cardiac function (clinical, echocardiography, ECG), renal function (echography, CT, urea, creatinine, electrolytes), and neurological function (clinical, CT scan, MRI, EEG).

Anesthetic considerations: Direct laryngoscopy and tracheal intubation can be difficult because of malformations and may necessitate to preserve spontaneous ventilation until the trachea is intubated and lung ventilation confirmed. The use of fiberoptic technique, or retrograde approach should be considered. The availability of a laryngeal mask airway is highly recommended. Careful intraoperative positioning is needed but can be difficult because of hip dislocation. Subclavian central venous access can be delicate because of clavicle malformations.

Pharmacological implications: Prophylactic antibiotics should be used in case of cardiac defect as indicated. Avoid nephrotoxic drugs in case of renal failure. Consider interaction between anesthetic drugs and epileptic medications.

REFERENCES:

Characteristics of trisomy 11 in childhood acute leukemia with review of the literature. *Leukemia* 3(10):695–8, 1989.

Noir A, Leroux M, Bresson JL, et al: 11q Trisomy: Apropos of 2 cases. *Pediatrie* 42(6):441, 1987.

Trisomy 13

At a glance: This chromosomal disorder is characterized by specific midline dysmorphic features and organ malformations. Usually leading to death before 6 months of life.

Synonyms: Patau Syndrome; Bartholin-Patau Syndrome; Trisomy D (Trisomy 13s).

History: First described by Thomas Bartholin in 1657, but recognized as a clinical syndrome when the trisomy etiology was discovered by Klaus Patau in 1960.

Incidence: 1:4000 to 1:10,000 live births. Age of onset: newborn. Risk factors include advanced age of mother. Sex distribution is equal.

Genetic inheritance: In 75% of cases, it is manifested by a trisomy of chromosome 13, caused by meiotic nondisjunctions. Translocations (20% of cases) are also present and either associated with de novo or familial translocation with a recurrence rate of 5 to 15%. The presence of mosaicism (5%) is a result of postzygotic (postfertilization) mitotic nondisjunction; however, it is less severe than full trisomy 13, but quite variable.

Pathophysiology: A single defect during the first 3 weeks of development of the prechordal mesoderm can lead to morphologic defects of the midface, eyes, and forebrain, as well as induction defects on the prosencephalon (cerebral hemispheres, diencephalon, hypothalamus, thalamus), leading to holoprosencephaly.

Diagnosis: Diagnosis can be evocated by the characteristic features, including microcephaly, microphthalmia, hypertelorism, cleft lip or palate, polydactyly, cardiovascular, and genitourinary and neurological abnormalities. It is confirmed by karyotype. Death often occurs before 6 months of age.

Clinical aspects: This severe disease is most often associated with midline defects: *mental retardation with head malformations* (microcephaly; cranial asymmetry; arhinencephaly; holoprosencephaly; cerebellar malformations; corpus callosum agenesis; neural tube defects; anencephaly; seizures; sloping forehead; wide sagittal suture and fontanels; cebocephaly; premaxillary agenesis; scalp defects; dysplastic low-set ears; microphthalmia; hypertelorism or hypotelorism; coloboma; retinal dysplasia orbital; cyclopia; choanal agenesis; cleft lip or palate) and *skeleton anomalies* (polydactyly of the fingers and toes, ectrodactyly, valgus deformity, spina bifida, hyperconvex narrow fingernails) are also observed. *Abdomen and pelvis* (Meckel diverticulum; intestinal malrotation; mobile cecum; hypoplastic penis and scrotum; cryptorchidism; bicornis uterus; microcystic and hyperlobulated kidneys; megaureter; hydronephrosis; umbilical hernia; and single umbilical artery) and *thoracic organs* (atrial septal defect, ventricular septal defect, coarctation of the aorta, bicuspid aortic valve, bilobed lung) are also involved. Apnea, feeding difficulty, and deafness are common.

Precautions before anesthesia: Evaluate cardiac function (clinical, echocardiography, ECG), renal function (echography, CT, urea, creatinine, electrolytes), and neurological function (clinical, CT scan, MRI, EEG).

Anesthetic considerations: Direct laryngoscopy and tracheal intubation can be difficult (face, mouth, and neck anomalies); the use of nasal tubes can be impossible because of nose malformations and choanal atresia. Spontaneous respiration must be maintained at all times because face-mask ventilation may be difficult or impossible. A laryngeal mask airway should be available in case of

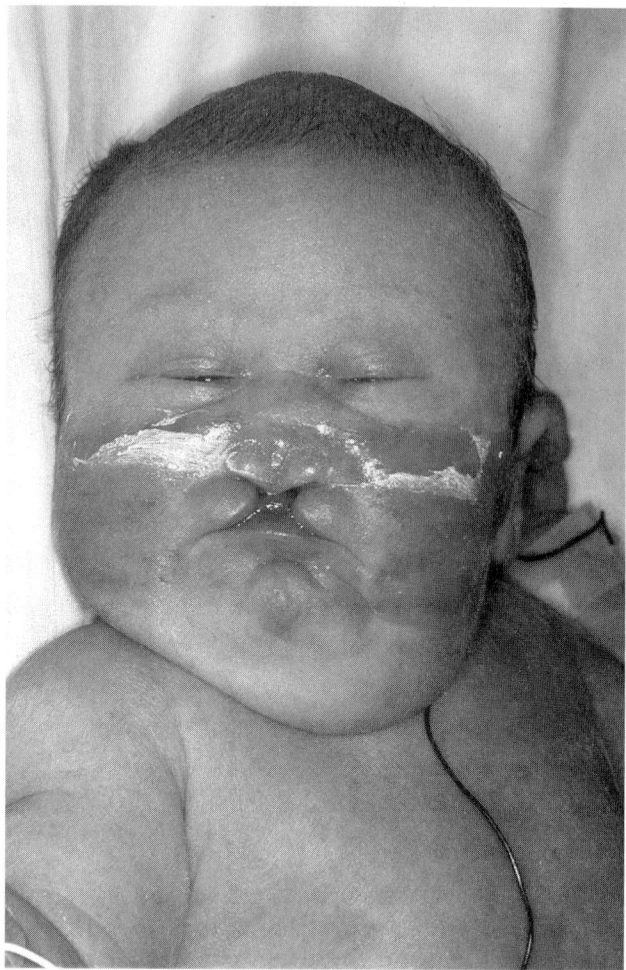

Trisomy 13 Cranial asymmetry, microphthalmia, hypotelorism, and cleft lip and palate in an infant with trisomy 13. The rash in the midface is caused by an allergic reaction to the tape used to secure the endotracheal tube.

failure to ventilate or inability to intubate the trachea. Fiberoptic equipments should be available. Perimedullar anesthesia is contraindicated in cases of neural tube defects. Perioperative cardiorespiratory and blood pressure measurement can be useful because of apnea and cardiac lesions. Pulse oximetry can be difficult (nail anomalies).

Pharmacological implications: Prophylactic antibiotics should be used in cases of cardiac defect as indicated. Avoid nephrotoxic drugs in cases of renal failure. Avoid anesthetic drugs with a marked cardiovascular effect.

REFERENCES:

Martlew RA, Sharples A: Anaesthesia in a child with Patau's syndrome. *Anaesthesia* 50:980, 1995.

Moerman P, Fryns JP, van der Steen K, Kleczkowska A, Lauweryns J: The pathology of trisomy 13 syndrome. A study of 12 cases. *Hum Genet* 32:849, 1988.

Polard RC, Beasley JM: Anaesthesia for patients with trisomy 13 (Patau's syndrome). *Paediatr Anaesth* 6:151, 1996.

Trisomy 18

At a glance: Chromosomal disorder characterized by a broad spectrum of variable dysmorphic features and organ malformations with extremely poor prognosis (90% of patients die before 1 year of age).

Synonyms: Edwards Syndrome; Trisomy E.

History: Chromosomal disorder described simultaneously by Edwards, Patau, and Smith teams in 1960.

Incidence: Incidence is about 1 3,000 to 8,000 live births. Two-thirds of the cases are diagnosed at the time of amniocentesis and are spontaneously aborted before delivery. It is the second most common autosomal aberration and second most common multiple malformation syndrome. Risk factors include advanced maternal age. Girls are approximately 4 times more often affected than boys. The prognosis after delivery is poor with a 10% survival at 1 year, however survival into adulthood has been described. When mosaicism occurs, patients can have a normal intelligence and a mild phenotype.

Genetic inheritance: Mostly sporadic with less than 1% risk of recurrence. Ninety percent are believed to be associated to meiotic nondisjunction (Trisomy 18 presentation). Mosaicism is suspected in 10% of the cases and because of postzygotic mitotic nondisjunction. It leads to partial clinical expression of Trisomy 18 with a longer survival rate. Translocations are very rare.

Diagnosis: The diagnosis is most often already made in utero following an amniocentesis or ultrasound examination. Otherwise a chromosome study after birth confirms the diagnosis if there is clinical suspicion based on the pattern of malformations.

Clinical aspects: More than 130 different abnormalities have been reported in the literature and so only the more common ones will be listed here. Fetal abnormalities consist mainly of polyhydramnios, small placenta with single umbilical artery, and growth deficiency. Neurologically, the patients present with mental deficiency, microcephaly, and hypertonicity. They also have a prominent occiput with a narrow bifrontal diameter. Other craniofacial anomalies consist of low-set, malformed ears, short palpebral fissures, microstomia, narrow palatal arch, and micrognathia. Numerous musculoskeletal abnormalities are present like the characteristic clenched hand with overlapping fingers, short dorsiflexed halluces, short sternum, small pelvis, and limited hip abduction. Cutaneous problems consist of redundancy, mild hirsutism of the forehead and back, and prominent cutis marmorata. Cardiac investigation often finds an atrial or ventricular septal defect, a persistent ductus arteriosus, or coarctation of the aorta. Less frequent anomalies may include malformation or absence of the right lung, diaphragmatic muscle hypoplasia, renal malformations, and cleft lip and palate.

Precautions before anesthesia: These children are very sick and most of them will die in their first year of life as a consequence of the trisomy. If they present for anesthesia, it is imperative to obtain a thorough cardiopulmonary evaluation, including echocardiography, electrocardiogram, and chest radiograph, and an arterial blood gas analysis should be considered. Blood work should include a complete cell blood count and serum concentrations of electrolytes, creatinine, and urea. Evaluate the airway for signs of difficult management.

Anesthetic considerations: Direct laryngoscopy and tracheal intubation may be difficult because of some of the features of the disease such as a prominent occiput, microstomia, narrow palate, and micrognathia. Spontaneous respiration should be maintained until the trachea is intubated and lung ventilation is confirmed. Congenital cardiac lesions require a specific anesthetic approach and should be managed accordingly. These neonates are prone to apnea and desaturations, particularly if there are associated lung or diaphragmatic abnormalities.

Pharmacological implications: In the presence of diminished kidney function, the dose of predominantly renally excreted drugs needs to be adjusted. Depending on the cardiac lesion and the type of surgery, subacute bacterial endocarditis prophylaxis may be required.

Other conditions to be considered:

☞BOWEN CONRADI SYNDROME: A rare genetic disorder that has often been confused with Trisomy 18 Syndrome clinically; however, those with Bowen Hutterite Syndrome have normal chromosomal count. The significant clinical features include low birth weight, failure to thrive, developmental delays, microcephaly, a prominent nose, and micrognathia. Additional features may include skeletal, cardiac, renal, and/or central nervous system abnormalities. This disorder is inherited as an autosomal recessive pattern.

TRISOMY 18-LIKE SYNDROME: This medical condition was described in a newborn infant with first-cousin parents who had a complex congenital heart defect and minor anomalies suggestive of trisomy 18. The clinical characteristics included a broad nasal root, narrow palpebral fissures, telecanthus, deficient alae nasi, malformed low-set ears, preauricular tags, and micrognathia.

REFERENCES:

Collins AL: Further case of trisomy 18 mosaicism with a mild phenotype [letter]. *Am J Med Genet* 56;121, 1995.

Courreges P, Nieuviarts R. Lecoutre D: Anaesthetic management for Edward's syndrome. *Paediatr Anaesth* 13:267; 2003.

Kelly M, Robinson BW, Moore JW: Trisomy 18 in a 20-year-old woman. *Am J Med Genet* 112:397, 2002.

Yoon HR, Park YS, Kim YK: Rapid prenatal detection of Down and Edwards syndromes by fluorescent polymerase chain reaction with short tandem repeat markers. *Yonsei Med J* 43:557, 2002.

Trisomy 21

At a glance: Genetic disorder resulting from trisomy 21. Mosaicism may exist with both trisomic and normal cell lines. Phenotypic expression is variable.

Synonyms: Down Syndrome; Mongolism.

History: First described by the English Physician John Langdon Haydon Down in 1887.

Incidence: It is the most common human chromosomal syndrome. Overall, the incidence is about 1:700 live births. However, it is associated with the parents' age and may affect 1 to 4% of all children born to women older than 40 years. Furthermore, it is estimated that at least half of the affected fetuses are aborted spontaneously in early pregnancy.

Genetic inheritance: Nondisjunction during meiosis I (in more than 90% on the maternal side) ultimately results in three separate copies of chromosome 21 and accounts for 94% of cases. Translocation of the third chromosome to chromosome 14 or 21 accounts for 3.3% of cases. Abnormal mitosis in early fetal development may result in mosaicism with one cell line showing trisomy, the other being of normal karyotype in about 2.4% of cases. The Down syndrome critical region is located at 21q22.

Pathophysiology: Chromosomal analysis has been used to assign the phenotypic features to specific regions of chromosome 21. The region D21S58 to D21S42 is associated with mental retardation and facial features. The D21S55 locus is linked to many of the phenotypic features of the syndrome. However, it remains unlikely that a distinct region of chromosome 21 accounts for all the phenotypic features.

Diagnosis: Can be made antenatally by chorionic villous sampling or by amniocentesis. Postnatally, it is made on the basis of clinical features confirmed by karyotyping.

Clinical aspects: Common features include brachycephaly with a flat occiput, malformed ears, epicanthal folds with up-slanting palpebral folds (mongoloid slanting), strabismus, Brushfield spots on the iris, macroglossia (although most often the tongue is of normal size, but appears too big in the context of midface hypoplasia) with furrowing of the tongue (xerostomia, a consequence of chronic mouth breathing), micrognathia, high-arched palate, small teeth (microdontia) with abnormal roots, a short, broad neck, and occipitoatlantoaxial instability. The hands are short and broad with a single palmar crease, and the middle phalanx of the fifth finger is hypoplastic. The joints are hypermobile, the muscle tonus is decreased with poor response to the Moro reflex, and there is usually a gap between the first and second toes. The angles of the iliac crests and the acetabula are hypoplastic and short stature is common. Respiratory problems include subglottic stenosis, obstructive sleep apnea, and recurrent chest infections. In the presence of uncorrected cardiac defects, pulmonary hypertension should be assumed—the Eisenmenger complex may be present. Up to 40% of these patients suffer from congenital cardiac defects, including endocardial cushion defect (arteriovenous canal abnormalities, atrial septal defect, ventricular septal defect), patent ductus arteriosus, and tetralogy of Fallot. Duodenal atresia, imperforate anus, Hirschsprung disease, and gastroesophageal reflux may occur. Acrocyanosis and cutis marmorata may persist in neonates for a few weeks, even in the absence of cardiac or respiratory disease. The skin is often dry and coarse (xerodermia) with an increased risk for atopic dermatitis. Later in life, hypothyroidism, precocious Alzheimer disease, and conductive hearing loss are more common in these patients than in the general population. Immune deficiency renders patients more susceptible to recurrent infections. Another important feature is the overall 10- to 20-fold increased risk of developing leukemia (acute myelocytic leukemia and acute lymphocytic leukemia); it usually occurs about 3 years earlier than in otherwise healthy children. Congenital leukemia is possible and becomes obvious within the first 3 years of life (most often acute nonlymphocytic leukemias). Transient leukemoid reactions with significantly elevated white cell counts are also possible and either resolve spontaneously or progress to leukemia after initial remission.

Precautions before anesthesia: Careful clinical assessment of current respiratory and cardiac status, with special investigations as indicated. Careful airway assessment is mandatory because airway management can be difficult (as a result of macroglossia, micrognathia, and a narrow hypopharynx). Lateral radiographs of the neck in flexion and extension do not reliably detect occipitoatlantoaxial instability, and it is still controversial as to whether they should be obtained preoperatively. Increased anteroposterior translational motion in the cervical spine, occipitoatlantal and occipitoaxial hypermobility, with the latter only occurring in the presence of atlantoaxial instability, are estimated to exist in up to 20% of Down syndrome patients. A history of abnormal gait, preference for the sitting position, signs of clonus, hyperreflexia, and extensor plantar responses

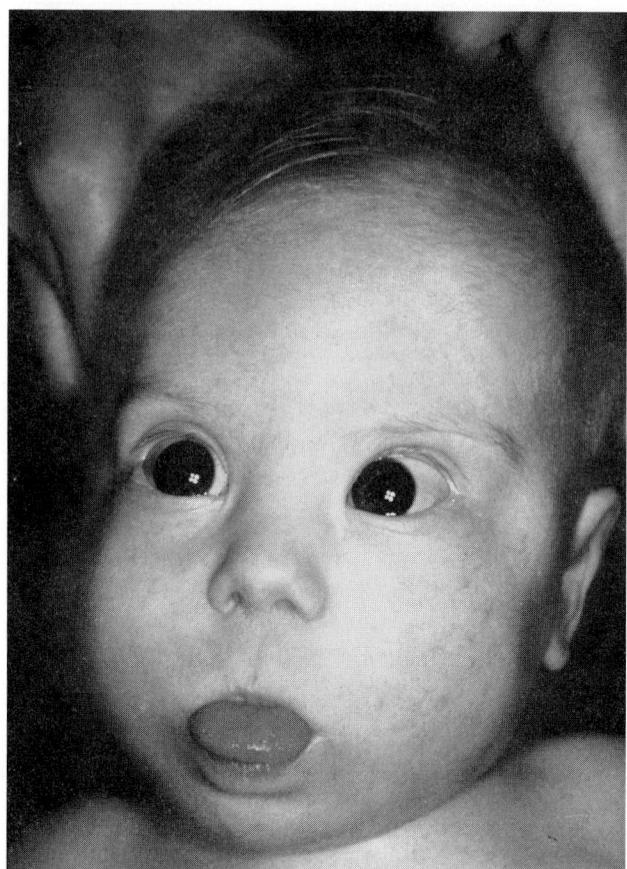

Trisomy 21 Typical facial features in Trisomy 21.

can be suggestive of spinal canal stenosis/cord compression. Check thyroid function.

Anesthetic considerations: Xerodermia and obesity may render vascular access difficult. These patients have a high anesthetic risk in the presence of cardiac disease, particularly when associated with pulmonary hypertension. Cardiac disease dictates the anesthetic technique. Depending on the presence of a cardiac lesion and the kind of procedure, subacute bacterial endocarditis prophylaxis may be required. Avoid forced extension–flexion in the occipitoatlantoaxial joints; either in-line stabilization by a skilled helper or fiberoptic intubation may be necessary. The increased incidence of subglottic stenosis may require a smaller endotracheal tube than predicted. The same also applies for nasal intubation, as the nares are smaller (midface hypoplasia) than in normal children. The roots of the teeth tend to be smaller and conical, which puts them at risk for being damaged during intubation. Use a sterile technique for insertion of all catheters because immune competence is decreased. Macroglossia, hypotonia, and tendency to obstructive sleep apnea necessitate close monitoring in the early postoperative period. The degree of intellectual impairment varies widely in these patients. Anxiolytic and sedative premedication and the presence of the primary caregiver for induction is often helpful.

Pharmacological implications: Increased sensitivity to atropine, with exaggerated mydriasis and increased chronotropic response have been reported; however, atropine has also been used without complications. Vagal blockade may be desirable because of the decreased sympathetic drive associated with the condition.

REFERENCES:

Borland LM, Colligan J, Brandom BW: Frequency of anesthesia-related complications in children with Down syndrome under general anesthesia for noncardiac procedures. *Paediatr Anaesth* 14:733; 2004.

Kobel M, Creighton RE, Steward DJ: Anaesthetic considerations in Down's syndrome: Experience with 100 patients and a review of the literature. *Can Anaesth Soc J* 29:593, 1982.

Meitzner MC, Skurnowicz JA: Anesthetic considerations for patients with Down syndrome. *AANA J* 73:103; 2005.

Mitchell V, Howard R, Facer E: Down's syndrome and anaesthesia. *Paediatr Anaesth* 5:379, 1995.

Uno K, Kataoka O, Shiba R: Occipitoatlantal and occipitoaxial hypermobility in Down syndrome. *Spine* 21:1430, 1996.

Truncus Arteriosus Communis

At a glance: Congenital heart malformation in which one great artery emerges from the heart and subsequently gives origin to the coronary arteries, pulmonary arteries, and systemic arteries.

Incidence: 0.4 to 2.8% of all congenital heart disease.

Genetic inheritance: Autosomal recessive. Gene map locus is at 22q11.

Pathophysiology: Embryologically, truncus arteriosus results from failure of septation of the bulbus cordis, which usually occurs at about 5 weeks' gestation. Failure of conal septation is usually present and results in a ventricular septal defect. Collett and Edwards, and Van Praagh have suggested different classifications for truncus arteriosus based on the origin of the pulmonary arteries and associated anomalies such as hypoplastic aortic arch. Physiologically the pulmonary and systemic circulations are in parallel, with high flow through the low-resistance pulmonary circuit causing left ventricular volume overload and failure. The right ventricle pumps at systemic pressures to maintain truncal flow and is "pressure overloaded." Ventricular function may be compromised further by abnormal coronary anatomy or stenosis, causing ischemia, and by low diastolic pressures as a consequence of excessive flow through the pulmonary circuit, resulting in hypoperfusion of the endocardium. Systemic and pulmonary venous blood mix at the level of the ventricular septal defect, tending to cause desaturation of systemic blood. Continued high pulmonary flow will ultimately result in pulmonary vascular occlusive disease, Eisenmenger syndrome, and death.

Diagnosis: Clinical findings. Echocardiography and angiographic findings.

Clinical aspects: Symptoms are predominantly those of ventricular failure, tachypnea, tachycardia, and feeding difficulties. In older infants, cyanosis and recurrent chest infections become more common. The clinical signs are nonspecific and include various heart murmurs and a collapsing pulse caused by high flow through the low-resistance pulmonary circulation. Facial abnormalities, including micrognathia, may be present as part of the conotruncal anomaly face syndrome. The chest radiograph usually demonstrates increased vascular markings, cardiomegaly, and a "globular or egg-shaped cardiac contour." If one pulmonary artery is absent, there may be hypoplasia of the affected hemithorax. Rarely, left or right main bronchus compression by the abnormal vasculature causes pulmonary collapse. The ECG shows signs of ventricular hypertrophy. Echocardiography and angiocardiography are required to confirm the diagnosis and to define the individual anatomy. Only 18% of affected individuals survive beyond 6 months of age without an op-

eration. Those patients who survive childhood usually die as a result of pulmonary hypertension causing Eisenmenger syndrome in the third decade of life.

Precautions before anesthesia: History and examination for evidence of ventricular failure and respiratory compromise. Examine for possible airway anomalies. Respiratory assessment: chest radiography; consider measurement of arterial blood gases. Cardiovascular assessment: review ECG, echocardiographic, and angiocardiographic data. Continue treatment for ventricular failure preoperatively.

Anesthetic considerations: The major considerations are ventricular failure, parallel pulmonary and systemic circulations, and the risk of myocardial ischemia. Premedication is desirable. Avoid decreases in pulmonary vascular resistance (i.e., avoid hyperoxia and hypocapnia). Moderate reductions in systemic vascular resistance may improve the pulmonary:systemic flow ratio, but may further compromise endocardial perfusion by lowering the diastolic pressure. Balanced anesthesia with opiate, volatile agent, and muscle relaxant allows optimal control of cardiovascular parameters. Invasive monitoring should be considered, depending on the proposed procedure.

Pharmacological implications: Use caution if administering bicarbonate, which can cause hypercarbia and can exacerbate pulmonary hypertension.

REFERENCES:

Calder L, Van Praagh R, Van Praagh S, et al: Truncus arteriosus communis. Clinical, angiocardiographic, and pathological findings in 100 patients. *Am Heart J* 92:23, 1976.

Cheng W, Nichols D, Cameron D: Truncus arteriosus, in Nichols D, Cameron D, et al. (eds): *Critical Heart Disease in Infants and Children,* Mosby, St Louis, 1995, p 797.

Wilson NC, Traber KB, Deschner LS: Anaesthetic management for caesaran section in a patient with uncorrected truncus arteriosus. *Br J Anaesth* 62(4):434–438, 1989.

Tuberous Sclerosis

At a glance: Neurodegenerative syndrome characterized by lesions of the skin, tumor growth, and seizures. Some patients present with mental retardation and autism. Rhabdomyoma of the heart and astrocytoma in the brain are frequent tumoral presentation.

Synonyms: Bourneville Syndrome; Bourneville-Pringle Syndrome.

Incidence: 1:25,000 to 1:30,000 live births. Nearly 1 million people worldwide are known to have tuberous sclerosis, including approximately 50,000 in the United States.

Genetic inheritance: Autosomal dominant with variable penetrance. De novo mutations have been confirmed on gene located on chromosome 9q33-34 and chromosome 16p13. If two or more siblings have tuberous sclerosis, one parent always has at least one skin manifestation of tuberous sclerosis. Sporadic transmission rate varies from 58 to 77%. If both parents are normal, a child with tuberous sclerosis must be a new mutation. It is believed that only 33% of all tuberous scleroses are inherited.

Pathophysiology: Multiorganic disease affecting mainly the brain and skin, but also the heart, lung, kidney, bone, and eye.

Diagnosis: Heterogeneous disease with a wide clinical spectrum. The presence and importance of seizures is variable, as is the importance of mental retardation. In general, the youngest children at the moment of clinical presentation have the worse mental retardation. The diagnosis is based on clinical suspicion and demonstration of typical lesions on the skin or retina. A head MRI or CT scan often confirms the diagnosis. Epilepsy, mental retardation, "salaam" seizures, and angiofibromas of numerous organs with intracranial hamartomatous lesions involving subependymal nodules and cerebral cortical tubers are characteristic of this phacomatosis.

Clinical aspects: Clinical signs appear shortly after birth and worsen with age. Mental retardation and uncontrolled seizures occur in half of the cases. The principal finding is of tuber lesions on the skin or in the brain. *Skin lesions* include adenoma sebaceum (80% of cases), which are rarely present at birth (onset at 4 to 6 years of age), and angiofibromas appearing as pink or red papules in patches or a butterfly-shaped distribution around the nose, cheek, and chin. Ash-leaf spots (90% of patients) are hypopigmented oval- or leaf-shaped spots found on the trunk and limbs in a linear orientation. The Shagreen patches (35% of patients) are isolated, "leathery," raised, and thickened plaques, with an orange-peel consistency that are grayish-green or light brown in color and most often located over the lumbosacral or gluteal region. Usually develop in late infancy or early childhood but may also be present at birth. Café-au-lait spots (7 to 16% of patients) and fibromas are also associated with tuberous sclerosis. Tubers may lead to seizures (90% of patients), which usually present as infantile spasms; 25 to 50% of infants with infantile spasms develop tuberous sclerosis. Older children will develop tonic, clonic, myoclonic, and akinetic Lennox-Gastaut syndrome. Hydrocephalus by obstructing cerebrospinal fluid circulation at the level of the foramen of Monroe. Mental retardation is present in 70% of patients. Tubers are growing tissular lesions that can transform into malignant lesions or calcify. The classical clinical triad is based on epilepsy, mental deficit, and adenomatous lesions. Pathognomonic lesions often appear between 4 and 6 years of age, presenting as thin, red nodules over the face, further enlarging and becoming coalescent. During adolescence, ungual fibroma appear. Other involved organs can include the heart conduction system with ectopic beats and conduction blocks. Heart rhabdomyoma is present in 50% of children with tuberous sclerosis during the neonatal period and may regress. Kidney injury is demonstrated by polycystic kidneys with hamartomas. Fibrous pulmonary changes may lead to pneumothoraces. Mortality is 50% at the age of 20 to 25 years. Abdominal aortic aneurysms have been reported in infants.

Precautions before anesthesia: Epilepsy is often controlled with medication. However, this medication interferes with anesthetic management. Because of potential heart involvement, a preoperative echocardiography and an ECG may be useful. Evaluate renal function (echography, urea, creatinine, electrolytes, CT scan), neurological function (clinical, CT scan, MRI, EEG), airway for the presence of oral and/or laryngeal tumors (clinical, radiography, fiberoptic endoscopy, CT scan), and respiratory function (chest radiograph, CT scan, endoscopy, pulmonary function test, and arterial blood gas analysis).

Anesthetic considerations: Mainly dominated by the fear of epilepsy. For prolong or long or at-risk surgical operations, or if postoperative sedation is planned, a continuous EEG monitoring may be useful to detect subclinical epileptic phenomenon. Direct laryngoscopy and tracheal intubation can be difficult because of oral or laryngeal tumors that may be unknown and asymptomatic at the moment of induction of anesthesia. Adequate procedures and materiel should be available (oral or nasal canula, fiberoptic, laryngeal mask airway, retrograde intubation leader). Anesthetic

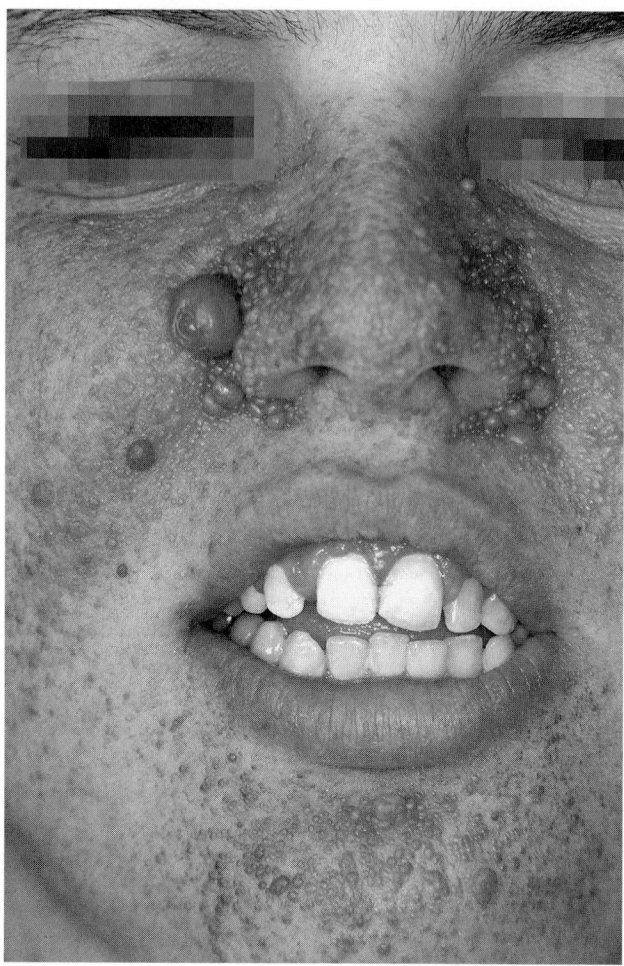

Tuberous sclerosis Characteristic facial adenoma sebaceum in a "butterfly" distribution in the face of a young man with tuberous sclerosis.

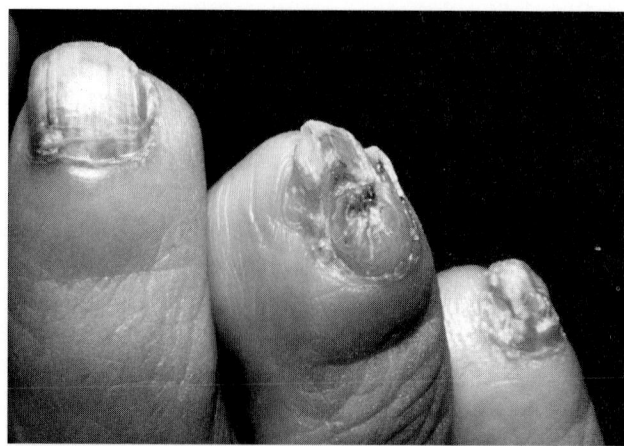

Tuberous sclerosis Subungual fibromas (Koenen tumors) in a patient with tuberous sclerosis.

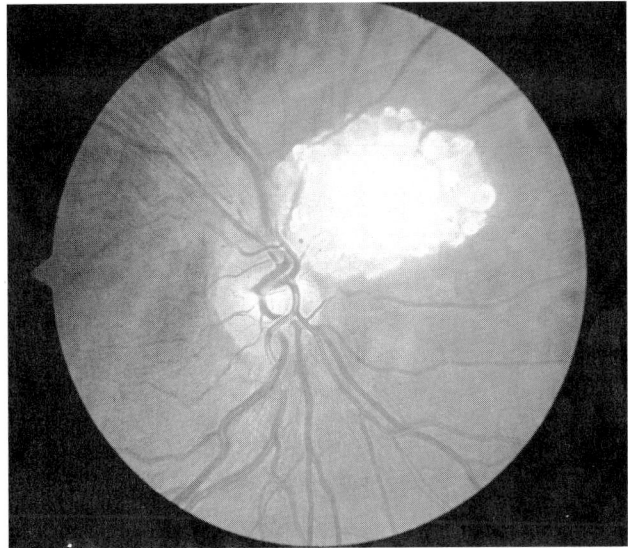

Tuberous sclerosis The funduscopy of the left eye shows an astrocytic hamartoma of the retina with calcifications (Drusen) typical of tuberous sclerosis.

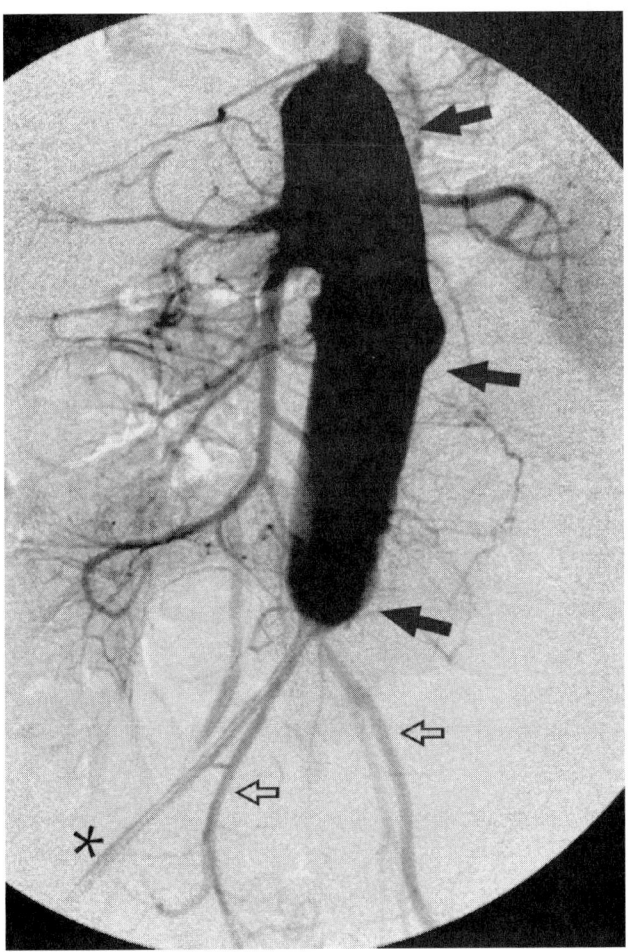

Tuberous sclerosis Large aneurysm of the abdominal aorta in a 2-year-old child with tuberous sclerosis. The aneurysm (solid arrows) extends from the level of the diaphragm all the way down to the aortic bifurcation. The outlined arrows mark the internal iliac arteries, while the catheter (*) is advanced from the femoral artery.

management should preserve spontaneous ventilation until tracheal intubation is realized and lung ventilation confirmed. In case of cardiac tumors, perioperative monitoring is necessary. Intraoperative monitoring should include arterial baseline. Perioperative fluid regimen may consider either cardiomyopathy and renal function. Pulse oximetry can be difficult because of ungual fibroma. Regional anesthesia can be realized but the benefit of medullar blockades should be precisely evaluated in cases of cardiomyopathy or neurological tumors.

Pharmacological implications: Avoid enflurane, ketamine, or other proepileptic drugs. Consider epileptic properties of some anesthetic drugs (e.g., methohexital, enflurane) and interaction with anticonvulsive medications. Avoid nephrotoxic drugs. Catecholamine should be used with caution in cases of cardiomyopathy. In a case of Wolff-Parkinson-White Syndrome, verapamil and digoxin should be avoided. The effects of anesthetic drugs should be considered (isoflurane and sevoflurane have been used successfully).

Other conditions to be considered:

MULBERRY TUMOR: A form of tuberous sclerosis presenting with a characteristic nodular astrocytoma of the retina.

☞LENNOX-GASTAUT SYNDROME: A severe form of epilepsy developing in children between 1 and 8 years of age. Developmental delay and impaired intellectual functioning. This disorder may be the result of brain trauma, infections, or genetic brain diseases (e.g., tuberous sclerosis). The seizures are tonic with severe stiffening of the body involving respiratory patterns and gas exchange, or atonic, leading to brief loss of muscle tone and consciousness, which leads to sudden falls and head trauma. Occasionally, myoclonic seizures may be encountered.

WESTERHOF BEEMER CORMANE SYNDROME (**Macules, Hereditary Congenital Hypopigmented and Hyperpigmented**): Neurocutaneous syndrome. Autosomal dominant with mental retardation, retarded growth, and congenital hypomelanotic and hypermelanotic cutaneous macules.

REFERENCES:

Lee JJ, Imrie M, Taylor V: Anesthesia and tuberous sclerosis. *Br J Anaesth* 73:421, 1994.

Ong EL, Koay CK: Tuberous sclerosis presenting for laparotomy. *Anaesth Intensive Care* 28:94, 2000.

Tsukui A, Noguchi R, Honda T et al: Aortic aneurysm in a four-year-old child with tuberous sclerosis. *Paediatr Anaesth* 5:67, 1995.

Turcot Syndrome

At a glance: A polyposis genetic disorder with an onset in adolescence presenting with gastrointestinal multiple colorectal adenomas and primary central nervous system (CNS) tumors (e.g., supratentorial glioblastoma and cerebellar medulloblastoma). Other clinical features include café-au-lait spots, cutaneous port-wine stain, and focal nodular hyperplasia.

Synonyms: Glioma Polyposis; Familial Polyposis Coli.

Nature: Described by Jacques Turcot (b. 1914), a Canadian physician.

Genetic inheritance: An autosomal recessive inheritance has been proposed for groups I and II (see *Clinical Aspects* below for a discussion of the groups). However, in group III, an autosomal dominant inheritance is strongly supported since this presentation is similar to the familial adenomatous polyposis syndrome. In addition, germ-like mutations in the mismatch repair gene hMLH1 or hPMS2 were found in some families. A mutation in the APC (adenomatous polyposis coli) gene was reported.

Pathophysiology: The relative risk of cerebellar medulloblastoma in patients with familial adenomatous polyposis is 92 times that of the general population. Glioblastoma multiforme is also considered a frequent tumor in association with this syndrome.

Diagnosis: Based on clinical findings; in particular, the presence of multiple adenomatous gastrointestinal polyps is associated with neuroepithelial tumors of the CNS.

Clinical aspects: The Turcot Syndrome has been divided into three groups based on the number and character of the colonic polyps. *Group I* comprises patients with 20 to 100 polyps that are larger than 3 cm in diameter. Malignant transformation usually occurs during the second and third decade of life and occurs in all affected individuals. *Group II* comprises patients with small polyps numbering fewer than 10, whereas *Group III* comprises patients with innumerable small polyps, usually more than 100. *Gastrointestinal:* Usually colonic polyps that may be fewer in number but larger than those found in other familial polyposis syndromes. The polyps are frequently associated with malignant transformation in the second or third decades. Tumors of the stomach, duodenum, and small intestine have also been described. *CNS:* neuroepithelial tumors— glioblastomas, medulloblastomas, and astrocytomas. *Ophthalmic:* congenital hypertrophy of the retinal pigment epithelium. *Others:* thyroid papillary carcinoma, café-au-lait spots.

Precautions before anesthesia: Careful neurologic history to exclude symptoms of CNS tumors. In the presence of central nervous tumor, an assessment for raised intracranial pressure must be conducted, including an eye examination, cell blood count, coagulation profile, and ABO cross-match must be completed for important surgery. The radiological evaluation of all three groups is identical to that of patients with familial adenomatous polyposis syndrome.

Anesthetic considerations: Related to considerations for specific type and site of CNS tumor. The presence of raised intracranial pressure will also dictate the anesthetic technique. Implications associated with major intraabdominal procedures must be applied.

Pharmacological implications: There are no known specific implications with this condition.

Other conditions to be considered:

GARDNER SYNDROME: An autosomal dominant polyposis disorder characterized by gastrointestinal adenomas, mostly colon and periampullary cancer. Other clinical features include soft-tissue lesions, such as sebaceous cysts, fibromas, leiomyomas, and lipomas, as well as bony lesions, such as multiple osteomas, exostoses, bone cortical thickening, and dental abnormalities. Genetically linked to chromosome band 5q21, the adenomatous polyposis coli locus. The wider spectrum of this disease in comparison to the familial adenomatous polyposis syndrome may represent a variable penetrance of a common genetic mutation.

FAMILIAL ADENOMATOUS POLYPOSIS (FAP) SYNDROME: A genetic disorder of colon cancer that is associated with the presence of large numbers of colorectal polyps (even thousands) with significant incidence of cancer transformation. The risk of developing colon cancer with FAP is almost 100% by the age of 40 years. An autosomal dominant inheritance involving the APC gene on chromosome 5.

REFERENCES:

Dirks P, Rutka J: The genetic basis of neurosurgical disorders, in Youmans J (ed): *Neurological Surgery*. 4th ed. Philadelphia, WB Saunders, 1996, p 825.

Itoh H, Ohsato K: Turcot syndrome and its characteristic colonic manifestations. *Dis Colon Rectum* 28:399, 1985.

Munden P, Sobol W, Weingeist T: Ocular findings in Turcot syndrome (glioma-polyposis). *Ophthalmology* 98:111, 1991.

Tyrosinemia

At a glance: Elevated blood tyrosine levels are present in several clinical entities. The term tyrosinemia is used to describe several syndromes. In general, the association of liver and renal failure, marked peripheral edema, epistaxis, and distinctive cabbage-like odor are characteristic of the disease. There are three types of tyrosinemia-related syndromes.

Classification and synonyms:

Tyrosinemia type I: Hepatorenal Tyrosinemia; Fumarylacetoacetase Deficiency; FAH Deficiency.

Tyrosinemia type II: Oculocutaneous Tyrosinemia; Tyrosine Transaminase Deficiency; Tyrosine Aminotransferase Deficiency; Richner-Hanhart Syndrome; Oregon type Tyrosinemia.

Tyrosinemia type III: 4-Hydroxyphenylpyruvic Acid Oxydase Deficiency; 4-Hydroxyphenylpyruvate Dioxygenase Deficiency.

Incidence: In the United States, the estimated incidence is 1:100,000 live births. However, most cases are seen in the French-Canadian population of the Province of Quebec, with an incidence of carriers of a specific mutation in 1:14 of the adult population and symptomatic presentation in 1:1850 newborns.

Genetic inheritance: Autosomal recessive in all cases. The sex distribution is equal.

Pathophysiology: Deficiency of fumarylacetoacetate hydrolase results in a moderate rise in serum tyrosine. Metabolites of tyrosine, including succinylacetone, are thought to be the cause of liver, renal, and neurological damage. Transient tyrosinemia is believed to be the result of delayed enzyme maturation in the tyrosine catabolic pathway. Because it is not caused by a genetic mutation, it does not fall into the category of inborn errors of metabolism. In the hereditary infantile tyrosinemia (type I) form, postmortem examination reveals the presence of severe liver and kidney nodular cirrhosis.

Diagnosis: Succinylacetone and succinylacetoacetate in blood and urine are diagnostic. Enzyme deficiency demonstrable in liver biopsy specimen or cultured fibroblasts.

Clinical aspects: Transient tyrosinemia of the newborn is benign and disappears spontaneously with no sequelae.

Hereditary Infantile Tyrosinemia (type I) is a severe form of tyrosinemia. Patients present with peculiar (cabbage-like) odor, renal tubular dysfunction (Fanconi Syndrome), and have a survival rate of fewer than 12 months of life. Fulminant onset of liver failure occurs in the first few months of life. Occasional cases have a later onset; however, the patient is usually younger than age 6 months. This acute form presents with failure to thrive and severe vomiting. Progressive hepatic failure results in death before 2 years of age.

Richner-Hanhart Syndrome (Tyrosinemia type II) is distinctly different with herpetiform corneal ulcers and hyperkeratotic lesions of the tongue, digits, palms, and soles, as well as mental retardation. Most patients are photophobic in bright light. In this more chronic from, deterioration may not occur after first year of life. Patients fail to thrive and develop liver cirrhosis, renal tubular dysfunction, and vitamin D-resistant rickets. Episodes of polyneuropathy, which often cause severe pain, occur in some patients. Death occurs by age 10 years from hepatic failure or hepatoma. Patients are typically chronically anemic and have a coagulopathy secondary to liver failure. They are most often on protein-restricted diet or phenylalanine-restricted diet.

Tyrosinemia type III is an extremely rare cause of intermittent ataxia without hepatorenal involvement or skin lesions. Treatment consists of a diet low in tyrosine, phenylalanine, and methionine, which results in improvement in some patients. Early liver transplant may also be effective.

Precautions before anesthesia: An anesthesiology consultation is highly recommended before elective surgery. Assess liver and renal function (liver function tests, electrolytes, creatinine). Obtain a complete cell blood count, prothrombin time, and partial thromboplastin time. Avoid prolonged fasting and establish glucose infusion preoperatively. Avoid diet with large amounts of protein.

Anesthetic considerations: Management of anesthesia will be determined by the extent of hepatic and renal dysfunction. The presence of a coagulopathy contraindicates regional techniques and may require correction preoperatively to prevent excessive bleeding intraoperatively. Chronic anemia requires replacement of blood loss with packed red blood cells. Starvation may result in hypoglycemia and intravenous glucose should be provided in the perioperative period.

Pharmacological implications: In the presence of severe hepatic dysfunction, caution should be exercised in the use of opioids and halothane is best avoided. *Cis*-atracurium is the muscle relaxant of choice in the presence of hepatic and renal impairment

REFERENCES:

Bergeron A, Jorquera R, Tanguay RM: Hereditary tyrosinemia: An endoplasmic reticulum stress disorder? *Med Sci* 19:976; 2003.

Rezvani I: Defects in metabolism of amino acids, in Behrman RE, Kliegman RM, Arvin AM (eds): *Nelson Textbook of Pediatrics*. 15th ed. Philadelphia, WB Saunders, 1995.

U

Uhl Anomaly

At a glance: A congenital disease characterized by the absence of a normal development of the myocardial layer of the right ventricle (usually replaced by fibrous or fatty tissue). Because the myocardial layer is dysplastic, the endocardium and epicardium are in apposition, which results in severe dilatation and early congestive cardiac failure. Chest radiography demonstrates marked cardiomegaly and right-sided chamber enlargement. Echocardiography and right-ventricle angiography demonstrate increased right heart volumes, severe diffuse hypokinesis, and tricuspid valve regurgitation.

Synonym: Parchment Right Ventricle.

History: Congenital disorder first described by H.S. Uhl in 1952.

Incidence: Very rare; 80 cases described in the literature.

Genetic inheritance: It is inherited as autosomal dominant with reduced penetrance. Generally sporadic cases caused by mutations or the results of exposure to toxic or infective agents.

Pathophysiology: Not precisely known; may be the result of primary nondevelopment of myocytes or may be a result of selective apoptosis.

Diagnosis: The diagnosis of right ventricular cardiomyopathy is based on the echocardiographic and angiographic documentation of localized or widespread structural and dynamic abnormalities involving mainly or exclusively the right ventricle. The absence of valvular disease, intracardiac shunts, active myocarditis, and/or coronary disease is essential to establish the diagnosis. The performance of endomyocardial biopsy is considered very useful in the differential diagnosis. The prognosis varies greatly from being lethal in the neonatal period to long-term survival in other individuals.

Clinical aspects: The major clinical feature is the presentation of different types of arrhythmias with a left bundle branch block pattern. The most important electrocardiographic abnormalities are T-wave inversion in the right precordial leads and the presence of late potentials in signal averaging ECG. The association with cardiac failure is rare except for those affected with the cardiomegalic form. There is a risk of sudden death and syncopal attacks due to ventricular fibrillation; however, most of the time the arrhythmias are well tolerated. Affected individuals often have good exercise tolerance and do not have a history of previous myocarditis. Congestive cardiac failure is the main sign; it may be associated with massive peripheral edema or massive pleural effusion leading to cardiac tamponade. Pulmonary atresia can be associated.

Precautions before anesthesia: Evaluate the cardiac function (clinical, ECG, echocardiography, chest radiographs), and the extent of the pulmonary involvement (clinical, radiographs, arterial blood gas analysis). Also assess the hepatic function (clinical, laboratory investigation including coagulation test, ultrasound) because of the potential hepatic disturbance secondary to cardiac congestion.

Anesthetic considerations: Elective surgical procedures must be postponed until the cardiovascular function has been corrected. Patients presenting with congestive heart failure should not receive anesthesia for nonurgent procedures. The presence of pericardial and/or pleural effusions should be treated before the administration of anesthesia. Anesthetic agents should be primarily chosen on the basis of their effects on the pulmonary resistance (e.g., nitrous oxide, ketamine, etc.). The pulmonary vascular resistance should be maintained at the lowest possible level. Hypercarbia and hypoxemia should be avoided. Perioperative invasive cardiac monitoring is highly recommended.

Pharmacological implications: Prophylactic antibiotics must be given as indicated. Nitrous oxide should be used with caution because of the effect on the pulmonary vascular resistance.

Other conditions to be considered:

☞**EBSTEIN SYNDROME:** This is a congenital heart defect characterized by displacement of the annulus of the tricuspid valve within the right ventricle (toward the apex of the ventricle) preventing the normal function of the right ventricle. This anomaly leads to loss of some right ventricle muscle mass, which is replaced by fibrous material, affecting contractility. Often associated with the destruction of the bundle of Kent, causing a condition called Wolff-Parkinson-White syndrome.

☞**ARRHYTHMOGENIC RIGHT VENTRICULAR DYSPLASIA:** Autosomal dominant inheritance. Pathologically described by the ventricular myocardial replacement with fat and fibrosis (fibrous elements preferentially involving the right ventricle). Characterized by cardiac failure and arrhythmia are associated.

REFERENCES:

Azhari N, Assaqqat M, Bulbul Z: Successful surgical repair of Uhl's anomaly. *Cardiol Young* 12:192, 2002.

Uhl HS: A previously undescribed congenital malformation of the heart: Lowest or total absence of the myocardium of the right ventricle. *Bull Johns Hopkins Hosp* 91:197, 1952.

Uhl HS: Uhl's anomaly revisited. *Circulation* 93:1483, 1996.

Ullrich Disease

At a glance: A very rare autosomal recessive disorder, characterized by muscular weakness, multiple contractures and orthopedic signs noted at birth or in early infancy. Cellular immunity can be involved.

Synonyms: Ullrich Scleroatonic Muscular Dystrophy; Ullrich Congenital Muscular Dystrophy; Scleroatonic Muscular Dystrophy/Myopathy; Hypotonic Scleroatonic Muscular Dystrophy.

Incidence: Very rare.

Genetic inheritance: Autosomal recessive.

Pathophysiology: Mutations of COL6A2 and COL6A3 (collagen type VI) on chromosome 21q22 are presumed to cause this disease.

Diagnosis: Characterized by the association of nonspecific signs: generalized muscular weakness, contractures of multiple joints, and hyperextensibility in distal joints.

Clinical aspects: Onset at birth. Clinical features include congenital muscular dystrophy, neonatal muscle weakness with orthopedic signs (protrusion of calcaneus, clumsy gait, multiple neonatal proximal joint contractures, limited spine motion, hyperextensible distal joints, hip dislocation). Other signs are less frequent and can include hyperhidrosis and high-arched palate. Insufficient cellular immunity has been reported, which may contribute to the recurrent upper respiratory tract infections and pneumonia often observed.

Precautions before anesthesia: An anesthesiology consultation is highly recommended before elective surgery. The respiratory system must be carefully evaluated in the presence of muscular weakness (clinical, history, chest radiographs, CT, pulmonary function test, arterial blood gas analysis).

Anesthetic considerations: Careful intraoperative positioning is indicated because of joint contractures and spine rigidity. Direct laryngoscopy and tracheal intubation can be difficult because of temporomandibular contractures and palate abnormalities. Perioperative chest physiotherapy can be useful.

Pharmacological implications: Succinylcholine is not contraindicated but is best avoided because of muscular dystrophy and risk of hyperkalemia. Parasympatholytic drugs should be avoided in the presence of hyperhidrosis. If necessary, it is recommended to use glycopyrrolate or scopolamine.

Other conditions to be considered:

☞**BETHLEM MYOPATHY:** This autosomal dominant disorder may be caused by mutation in the COL6A1 gene, COL6A2, or the COL6A3 gene. The onset of age is most often in early infancy, progression may be slow, and most affected individuals may reach an advanced age. Moderate weakness and atrophy of the muscles of the trunk and limbs can be observed. Characteristically the proximal muscles are more involved than the distal muscles, and the extensors are more affected than the flexors. Early flexion contractures of the elbow and interphalangeal joints of the last four fingers can be observed. Plantar flexion contractures of the ankles are constant findings.

☞**EMERY-DREIFUSS MUSCULAR DYSTROPHY:** An X-linked degenerative myopathy characterized by weakness and atrophy of muscle without involvement of the nervous system. Contractures and significant limitations of movement of the neck and spine are often present. Other clinical features include flexion deformities of the elbows beginning in early childhood, mild pectus excavatum, signs of cardiac involvement and absence of muscle pseudohypertrophy, involvement of the forearm muscles, and mental retardation.

REFERENCE:

Demir E, Sabatelli P, Allamand V, et al: Mutations in COL6A3 cause severe and mild phenotypes of Ullrich congenital muscular dystrophy. *Am J Hum Genet* 70:1446, 2002.

Ullrich-Feichtiger Syndrome

At a glance: A congenital syndrome characterized by an association of micrognathia, ocular, dental, and genital malformations. Other features include deafness, rudimentary toes, clubfoot, partial atresia of the anus, hypospadias, and mask-like facies. A number of authors have suggested that this syndrome is a variant of Smith-Lemli-Opitz syndrome.

Synonyms: Anophthalmia-Cleft Lip-Palate-Polydactyly Syndrome; Dyscranio-Pygo-Phalangea Syndrome (German appellation); Micrognathia-Polydactyly-Genital Anomalies Syndrome; Typhus Degenerativus Rostockiensis.

History: This medical condition was described by Otto Ullrich, pediatrician and H. Feichtiger, a German physician, in 1951.

Incidence and genetic inheritance: Rare. Autosomal recessive inheritance. However, sporadic occurrences have been reported.

Clinical aspects: Can include *facial* (micrognathia, dental and ocular malformations, cleft palate), *genital* (hypospadias), *cardiac* (congenital cardiac defects), and *skeletal* anomalies (polydactyly, clubfoot). Renal aplasia could be present.

Anesthetic considerations: Direct laryngoscopy and tracheal intubation may be difficult because of micrognathia, dental malformations, and the presence of a cleft palate. Preoperative evaluation should include clinical examination, radiographs, and fiberoptic intubation, if necessary. Nondepolarizing agents should not be used before the airway is secured and lung ventilation has been confirmed. Evaluate the cardiac function (clinical, echocardiography) and consider the use of prophylactic antibiotics when indicated.

Other condition to be considered:

☞**SMITH-LEMLI-OPITZ SYNDROME:** Characterized by the absence of 7-dehydrocholesterol reductase. It affects the central nervous system (white matter), and leads to growth retardation, developmental delay, microcephaly, micrognathia, cleft palate, severe dysphagia, cataracts, ptosis, polysyndactyly and syndactyly of the second and third toes. Congenital heart defects (often transposition of the great vessels) have been reported. Congestive heart failure and liver failure are not uncommon.

REFERENCES:

Feichtiger H: Ein neuer, typischer, vorwiegend der Akren betreffender Fehlbildungskomplex. Thesis; Rostock, 1943.

Mazur B, Buszman Z: Ullrich-Feichtiger syndrome in a 3-year-old boy. *Pol Tyg Lek* 47(9–10):234, 1992.

Pfeiffer RA, Slavaykoff H: Is there a syndrome of Ullrich and Feichtiger? *Klin Padiatr* 187(2):176, 1975.

Ullrich-Turner Syndrome

At a glance: Chromosomal disorder with a specific aspect (pterygium colli short neck and gonadal insufficiency).

Synonyms: Turner-Varney Syndrome; 45X Syndrome; Bonnevie-Ulrich Syndrome; Monosomy X; XO Syndrome; Turner Syndrome.

Nature: X-linked chromosomal disorder resulting from one functional X chromosome. First described by Henry Hubert Turner, American endocrinologist in 1938, in a patient with sexual infantilism, webbed neck, cubitus valgus, and short stature. The genetic basis was recognized in 1959 by C.E. Ford et al.

Incidence: 1:2500 live births in the female gender.

Pathophysiology: Caused by a defect of one entire chromosome X (50% of patients), mosaicism (20% of patients) or two chromosomes X but one abnormal (30% of patients). Nearly 99% of XO fetuses are aborted. The primary defect is thought to be abnormal development of lymphatic channels in utero, resulting in fetal lymphedema, which prevents normal growth, rotation, and regression of fetal tissues, thus causing the Turner phenotype.

Diagnosis: Small stature, short and broad neck, hypoplasia of the cervical vertebrae, pterygium colli, and gonadal dysgenesis are the most frequent and characteristic signs of the disease. Age of onset is variable according to the presentation: *infant:* lymphedema; *childhood:* short stature; *adolescence:* primary or secondary amenorrhea. Risk factors include advanced paternal age (isochromosome X cases) and mother affected with a mosaic or dilational variant of the Turner syndrome. For certitude, the diagnosis can be confirmed using karyotype studies.

Clinical aspects: Clinical features can concern all systems and part of the bodies: *head* (micrognathia, midfacial hypoplasia, deepening of the posterior cranial fossa, widely spaced mandible, large ears, blepharoptosis strabismus, epicanthal folds, highly arched palate, occasional cleft palate, premature tooth eruption), *skeleton* (thin

ribs, short metacarpal and metatarsal bones, drumstick distal phalanges, pes cavus, Madelung deformity, cubitus valgus, deformed
tibial condyles, hypoplastic and dislocated patellae, faulty fusion
of the epiphyses, scoliosis, osteoporosis), *cardiovascular system*
(coarctation of the aorta, dissecting aortic aneurysm, ventricular septal defect, atrial septal defect, dextrocardia, bicuspid aortic valve,
hypoplastic left heart), *abdomen* (prune belly, telangiectases,
hemangiomas, intestinal bleeding, protein-loosing enteropathy),
genitourinary system (unilateral aplasia or hypoplasia of the kidneys, horseshoe kidneys, malrotation of the kidneys, duplication
dysgenesis, and streak gonads), *endocrinopathy* (hypothyroidism,
Hashimoto disease, diabetes mellitus), and *skin* and *dermatoglyphs*
(puffy hands and feet, pigmented nevi, seborrhea, xerosis, keloid,
nail hypoplasia, low hairline, hirsutism). Abnormally placed nipples are also very frequent. Mental retardation, deafness, blindness,
anorexia nervosa, amenorrhea, and sterility can occur. This complex
polymalformative syndrome benefits of many symptomatic treatments that have greatly improved patients outcome. Features vary
with age of presentation: *newborn:* lymphedema of the hands and
feet, small for age and excessive skin at nape of the neck; *childhood
and adolescence:* short stature (98% of patients), gonadal dysgenesis (95% of patients), high-arched palate (80% of patients), short
neck and low hairline (80% of patients), and broad chest, cubitus
valgus, and nail hypoplasia.

Precautions before anesthesia: Evaluate carefully the cardiac
function (clinical, echocardiography, ECG, radionuclide imaging if
necessary), renal function (ultrasound, urea, creatinine, electrolytes,
CT), airway (clinical, radiographs, fiberoptic endoscopy, CT), and
endocrine function (clinical, echography of thyroid). Laboratory
investigations should include FT_4, T_3, glycemia, and urinary electrolytes.

Anesthetic considerations: Direct laryngoscopy and tracheal
intubation are often difficult because of neck anomalies and
micrognathia (fiberoptic intubation may be required) and necessitate to preserve spontaneous ventilation until tracheal intubation
is confirmed by the presence of end-tidal carbon dioxide. A laryngeal mask airway should be available in case of failure to intubate
the trachea using usual technique. Venous access is sometimes a
challenge because of puffy hands and feet. Careful intraoperative
positioning is necessary. Intraoperative cardiac monitoring will be
adapted according to the existing cardiac anomalies. Pulse oximetry
can be perturbed by nail anomalies. Strict supervision of respiratory
function is needed after extubation in cases of prune belly.

Pharmacological implications: Intraoperative fluid regimen
must take into consideration the renal and cardiac function. Prophylactic antibiotics should be used in cases of cardiac defect.

Other conditions to be considered:

☞**NOONAN SYNDROME:** This syndrome is not a chromosomal
defect, but a genetic disorder involving a gene encoding the non-
receptor protein tyrosine phosphatase SHP2 (maps on 12q24.1).
Noonan syndrome bears a lot of similarities with Turner syndrome.
The principal differences concern sexual characteristics (female and
male in Noonan) and cardiac defects (more often pulmonic stenosis
than left-sided cardiac lesions). Hematologic features are frequently
observed (abnormal platelet, thrombocythemia, von Willebrand disease, and partial deficiency of factors XI:C, XII:C, and XIII:C).

REFERENCES:

Divekar VM, Kothari MD, Kamdar BM: Anaesthesia in Turner's syndrome. *Can Anaesth Soc J* 30(4):417, 1983.

Grange CS, Heid R, Lucas SB, et al: Anaesthesia in a parturient with
   Noonan's syndrome. *Can J Anaesth* 45(4):332, 1998.

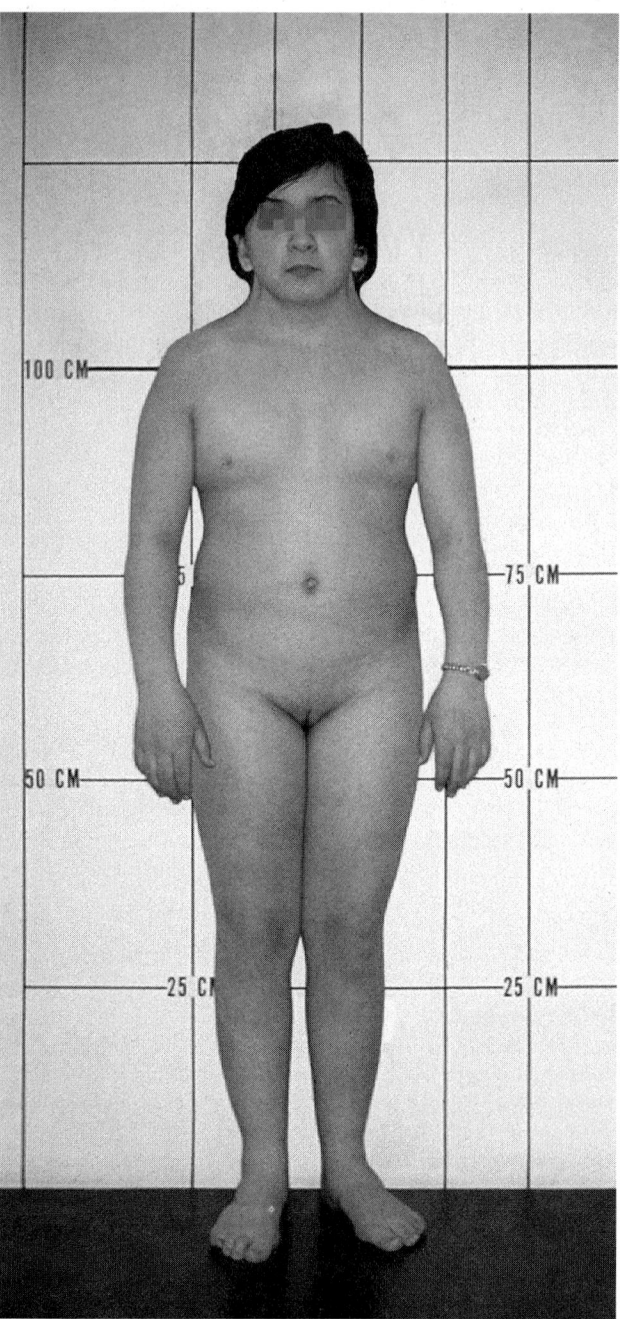

Ullrich-Turner syndrome This 16-year-old girl has Ullrich-Turner
syndrome. The short stature, wide chest, short and webbed neck,
and delayed puberty are characteristic findings.

Schwartz N, Eisenkraft JB: Anesthetic management of a child with
   Noonan's syndrome and idiopathic hypertrophic subaortic stenosis.
   Anesth Analg 74(3):464, 1992.

Upshaw-Schulman Syndrome

At a glance: A very rare syndrome characterized by congenital
microangiopathic hemolytic anemia, thrombotic thrombocytopenic
purpura, and response to fresh plasma infusion. Neonatal onset and
frequent relapses are typical.

Synonyms: Congenital Microangiopathic Hemolytic Anemia; Schulman-Upshaw Syndrome; Deficiency of Upshaw Factor; Familial Thrombotic Thrombocytopenic Purpura.

History: First described by Jefferson D. Upshaw, an American hematologist, in 1978.

Genetic inheritance: Autosomal recessive.

Pathophysiology: Phenotype may be identical to thrombotic thrombocytopenic purpura, which is caused by mutations in the ADAMTS13 gene located on 9q34. Thrombocythemia is caused by a combination of the presence of plasma factor VIII and von Willebrand factor (UL-VWFMs), platelets, and high shear stress generated in the microcirculation. Prostacyclin (PGI_2) may be partly involved.

Diagnosis: Based on congenital Upshaw factor deficiency, distorted and fragmented circulating red cells, and cold insoluble globulin (fibronectin) deficiency.

Clinical aspects: Characterized by frequent episodes of severe thrombocytopenia and severe anemia (microangiopathic hemolytic anemia). It is often in association with a clinically detectable infection or a precipitating stress. A dramatic response to the administration of whole blood or plasma alone. Corticosteroids or splenectomy has no effect. When asymptomatic, patient has a compensated hemolytic state with variable reticulocytosis and low-normal hematocrit levels. Often associated with radioulnar hypoplasia and lobster-claw deformity. Petechial rash may be present with episodic fever and glomerulopathy. Preeclampsia is frequent. Treatment is definitely the administration of plasma and platelet transfusion.

Precautions before anesthesia: A complete cell blood count (especially hemoglobin and platelet count) must be obtained before and after surgery. One must ensure that fresh-frozen plasma is available if blood transfusion is anticipated. Check renal function (glomerulopathy with hematuria and proteinuria is not uncommon).

Anesthetic considerations: Because of the low platelet count, regional anesthesia, particularly perimedullar blockade, should be avoided, as should nasogastric tubes and nasal intubation.

Pharmacological implications: Salicylates are best avoided considering the risk of defective platelets or thrombocytopenia.

REFERENCES:

Konno M, Yoshioka A, Takase T, et al: Partial clinical improvement in Upshaw-Schulman syndrome following prostacyclin infusion. *Acta Paediatr Jpn* 37(1):97, 1995.

Upshaw JD: Congenital deficiency of a factor in normal plasma that reverses microangiopathic hemolysis and thrombocytopenia. *N Engl J Med* 298:1350, 1978.

Yagi H, Konno M, Kinoshita S, et al: Plasma of patients with Upshaw-Schulman syndrome, a congenital deficiency of von Willebrand factor-cleaving protease activity, enhances the aggregation of normal platelets under high shear stress. *Br J Haematol* 115(4):991, 2001.

Urbach-Wiethe Syndrome

At a glance: A congenital lipoid storage disease with multiple tissue infiltrations producing waxiness and thickening of the skin and mucous membranes of the mouth, pharynx, larynx, and hypopharynx. It causes hoarseness and an inability to cry, often from birth. No visceral symptoms or signs are present. Associated disorders

usually consist of grand mal epilepsy, attacks of rage, and mental retardation.

Synonyms: Cutaneomucous Proteinosis; Lipoproteinosis, Hyalinosis Cutis et Mucosae; Lipoid Proteinosis of Urbach and Wiethe; Rössle-Urbach-Wiethe Syndrome.

Nature: Genetic disorder first described in 1929 by Eric Urbach, an Austrian-American allergologist and dermatologist and Camillio Wiethe, an Austrian otologist.

Incidence: Very rare; 300 cases described in the literature. This syndrome is most often seen among people of Dutch or German descent and is rather frequent in South Africa. Both sexes are affected equally. The age of onset is in infancy.

Genetic inheritance: Autosomal recessive inheritance, caused by mutation in the extracellular matrix protein 1. Gene (ECM1) located on 1q21.

Pathophysiology: Not precisely known. An eosinophilic hyaline material is deposited in all affected organs. Controversy exists about the exact origin of the disease (caused primarily by lysosomal disease, abnormality of collagen metabolism, or lipid metabolism disorder).

Diagnosis: Clinically evocated by the association of early hoarseness with an unusual skin eruption. Skin biopsy may help confirm the diagnosis (eosinophilic hyaline thickening of papillary dermal capillaries, hyperkeratosis). The hyaline material stains positively with period acid-Schiff (PAS) and is diastase resistant.

Clinical aspects: All organs can be involved: *skin* (hyalinosis cutis et mucosae, recurrent vesicles, bullae, and hemorrhagic crusts around mucous membranes, papules, plaques, and nodules develop on the face, axillae, and scrotum; patchy area of alopecia, generalized hyperkeratosis can be seen), mouth and pharynx (early hoarseness, papular infiltration of tongue and frenulum, teeth hypoplasia more often lateral incisors and premolars, papular infiltration of larynx and vocal cords), *eyes* (itchy eyes, moniliform blepharitis), and *central nervous system* (seizures, memory impairment, paranoia rage attacks, intracranial calcifications).

Precautions before anesthesia: Evaluate neurological function (history, clinical, radiographs, CT/MRI, EEG) and intubation (clinical, radiographs, CT, fiberoptic).

Anesthetic considerations: When combined with mental retardation, the presence of occasional sudden attacks of rage can affect the preoperative period and induction of anesthesia. There is strong support for premedication and/or presence of parents for induction of anesthesia. Both direct laryngoscopy and tracheal intubation can be difficult because of larynx involvement and may require a smaller tube than predictable. Tracheal wall integrity should be assessed and spontaneous ventilation preserved until airway is secured. Catheter fixation can be difficult because of skin lesions.

Pharmacological implications: Muscle relaxants should be avoided until airway is secured. Consider interaction between anticonvulsant medications and anesthetic drugs.

REFERENCES:

Hamada T, McLean WHI, Ramsay M, et al: Lipoid proteinosis maps to 1q21 and is caused by mutations in the extracellular matrix protein 1 gene (ECM1). *Hum Mol Genet* 11:833, 2002.

Kelly JE, Simpson MT, Jonathan D, et al: Lipoid proteinosis: Urbach-Wiethe disease. *Br J Anaesth* 63(5):609, 1989.

Urbach E, Wiethe C: Lipoidosis cutis et mucosae. *Virchows Archiv für pathologische Anatomie und Physiologie und für klinische Medizin* 273:285, 1929.

Uridine Diphosphate Galactose Epimerase Deficiency

At a glance: A disorder of galactose metabolism characterized by a deficiency of uridylyl diphosphogalactose-4-epimerase activity resulting in benign asymptomatic form (deficiency in blood cells only) and severe forms with hepatic failure, Fanconi syndrome, and neurological impairment.

Synonyms: Galactose Epimerase Deficiency; Gale Deficiency; Galactosemia III. UDP-Galactose-4-Epimerase Deficiency.

Incidence: Very rare medical condition presenting with great variability among populations. A severe form has been described in Japan with an incidence of 1:23,000 live births, whereas it is limited to few cases in England. Benign forms have been reported in African-Americans with a frequency of 1:6,200 live births and 1:64,800 in non-black Americans.

Genetic inheritance: Autosomal recessive.

Pathophysiology: Uridylyl diphosphogalactose-4-epimerase assists in the conversion of galactose-1-phosphate to glucose-1-phosphate by catalyzing the conversion of uridine diphosphate (UDP)-glucose to UDP-galactose. The disease is caused by mutation in the UDP-galactose-4-epimerase gene (GALE) located at 1p36-p35.

Diagnosis: Generally made by the discovery of elevated galactose sugars in newborn screening programs, but associated with a normal level of galactose-1-phosphate uridylyltransferase. Benign forms are associated with a galactose epimerase deficiency in red blood cells and leukocytes, whereas the epimerase activity in the liver, activated lymphocytes and cultured skin fibroblasts is normal.

Clinical aspects: Identical to the classical form of galactosemia involving *gastrointestinal* (vomiting, feeding difficulties, failure to thrive, jaundice, hepatomegaly, hypoglycemia, ascites, splenomegaly, hepatic cirrhosis) and *central nervous system* (sensorineural deafness, lethargy, irritability, hypotonia, mental retardation, language, cognitive, and developmental delay). *Fanconi syndrome* (vomiting, dehydration, weakness, unexplained fever, anorexia, constipation, polydipsia, and polyuria). Cataract can also be present.

Precautions before anesthesia: Evaluate hepatic and renal functions (laboratory investigation, clinical and echography) and neurological function (clinical, EEG, CT scan).

Anesthetic considerations: Few specific considerations; implications are related to renal and cardiac dysfunction.

Pharmacological implications: Perioperative fluid regimen and anesthetic drugs should be adapted in consideration for hepatic and renal functions. Aminoglycosides should be used carefully because of deafness and potential renal dysfunction. Consider interaction between antiepileptic treatment and anesthetic drugs.

REFERENCES:

Maceratesi P, Daude N, Dallapiccola B, et al: Human UDP-galactose 4' epimerase (GALE) gene and identification of five missense mutations in patients with epimerase-deficiency galactosemia. *Mol Genet Metab* 63:26, 1998.

Wohlers TM, Christacos NC, Harreman MT, et al: Identification and characterization of a mutation, in the human UDP-galactose-4-epimerase gene, associated with generalized epimerase-deficiency galactosemia. *Am J Hum Genet* 64:462, 1999.

Urticaria Pigmentosa

At a glance: Localized form of mastocytosis. Degranulation must be avoided during all anesthetic procedures (physiological and psychological stress, drugs).

Synonyms: Urticaria Perstans Hemorrhagica with Pigmentosa; Localized Infantile Mastocytosis; Nettleship E Disease type I; Xanthelasmoidea.

Incidence: Although rare, it is most often seen in children, however it can also occur in adults. Affects males and females equally.

Genetic inheritance: Both autosomal and recessive inheritance have been evocated, however sporadic cases have also been reported.

Pathophysiology: Unknown. When mast cells proliferate, histamine and heparin are released into the skin. Mastocytosis presents with characteristic skin lesions of urticaria and telangiectasis.

Diagnosis: Urticaria pigmentosa is a localized form of mastocytosis. It is generally benign and is usually self-limited. Diagnosis is clinically evocated in a child older than age 2 years with skin lesions affecting the neck, arms, legs, and trunk. The rash consists of reddish-brown spots that turn into hives when they are rubbed hard or scratched. Certitude diagnosis can be obtained with skin biopsy.

Clinical aspects: Skin lesions can also include bullous mastocytosis and telangiectasia macularis eruptiva perstans (multiple hyperpigmented telangiectatic macules, located primarily on the trunk and on the extremities). In the early form, resolution of the condition by adolescence or early adulthood is common. In the form beginning after 5 years of age, the abnormal collections of mast cells sometimes involves other organs. It can affect bone, gastrointestinal tract, lymphatics, spleen, and liver, resulting in clinical signs such as abdominal pain or gastric ulcer. It is even possible to observe an overgrowth of mast cells progressing to a malignant out-of-control process called mast cell leukemia. Mast cells can abruptly release vasoactive mediators, such as histamine, heparin, and prostaglandins, under some physical stresses or in response to drugs. Severe general reaction with shock can occur.

Precautions before anesthesia: Obtain full medical and physical history. One must review the signs and symptoms of previous cardiovascular instability, i.e., hypotension, loss of consciousness, vomiting, and severe flushing and sweating. Evaluate organ involvement (clinical, ultrasound).

Anesthetic considerations: Both regional and general anesthesia can produce life-threatening complications. Avoid mastocyte degranulation (e.g., mild temperature in the operating room), psychological and physical stress. Resuscitation drugs should be present in the operating room. Careful with the insertion of nasal tubes (easy bruising and nose bleeds).

Pharmacological implications: Many drugs have been associated with mast cell degranulation (lidocaine, morphine, oxymorphone, codeine, *d*-tubocurarine, metocurine, acetylsalicylic acid, etomidate, thiopental, succinylcholine, enflurane, isoflurane methylparaben and para-aminobenzoic acid). Consider use of intradermal skin tests to predict which medications may cause problems and those that may be used. Regional anesthesia should be preferred when possible because it restricts the use of several different drugs. (One should prefer amide-type over ester-linked local anesthetics.) Consider preoperative administration of H_1 and H_2 blockers and steroids. Preoperative sedation can be useful (e.g., hydroxyzine) to reduce patient stress. Avoid atropine. Muscle relaxants are not contraindicated but it is recommended to choose those with minimal histamine-liberation. These medications should be administered slowly to prevent a sudden and massive histamine release. Preinduction dose of 25 to 50 mg diphenhydramine intravenously has been suggested to reduce the risk of mastocyte degranulation. Epinephrine should be available at all times to treat general and acute signs of degranulation.

Other conditions to be considered: Other ☞mastocytoses provide more general reaction than urticaria pigmentosa.

REFERENCES:

Auvray L, Letourneau B, Freysz M: Mastocytose: Anesthésie générale par rémifentanil et sévoflurane. *Ann Fr Anesth Reanim* 20:635, 2001.

Coleman MA, Liberthson RR, Crone RK, et al: General anesthesia in a child with urticaria pigmentosa. *Anesth Analg* 59(9):704, 1980.

Greenblatt EP, Chen L: Urticaria pigmentosa: An anesthetic challenge. *J Clin Anesth* 2(2):108, 1990.

Usher Syndrome

At a glance: A genetically heterogeneous condition associating retinitis pigmentosa and deafness. The age of onset varies. Multiple subtypes have been described.

Synonym: Retinitis Pigmentosa-Deafness Syndrome.

Incidence: Prevalence in the general population varies from 1:20,000 to 1:30,000 in Europeans.

History: This medical entity was described by Charles Usher, a British ophthalmologist, in 1914, who emphasized the hereditary nature. However, the earliest description was given by Albrecht von Graefe in 1858, who commented on a relatively high frequency in Jews in Berlin.

Genetic inheritance: Autosomal recessive.

Pathophysiology: Magnetic resonance imaging (MRI) has demonstrated characteristic morphological abnormalities of the central nervous system. These abnormalities vary according to the syndrome subtype. Twelve independent loci with six known genes have been reported.

Diagnosis: The combination of retinitis pigmentosa, sensorineural deafness, abnormal vestibular function, mental retardation, psychosis, and cerebellar ataxia lead to the diagnosis of Usher syndrome. Age of onset of visual disturbance is variable depending on the subtype.

Clinical aspects: It should be emphasized that this is a heterogeneous condition and mental retardation is variable from normal to severe. Vision may be lost in late or early childhood.

Type I (USH I) is characterized by a congenital severe to profound preverbal deafness present at birth, absent vestibular deterioration function, and early onset of retinitis pigmentosa-like deterioration (typically by the age of 5 or 6 years and almost always by the age of 10 years). Different entities of USH I have been described, but cannot be currently differentiated on a clinical basis. It is also known as the French-Acadien ("Cajun") of Louisiana (chromosome 11p) and the French variety (chromosome 11q).

Type II (USH II) has a milder postverbal hearing loss, apparently present from birth and slowly evolutive (some suggests 1 decibel/per decade of life) and a later onset of retinitis pigmentosa-like retinal degeneration (typically between the ages of 10 and 20 years). Vestibular functions are normal and stable.

Type III (USH III) is a controversial form of Usher syndrome. It is more frequent (40% of patients) in eastern Finland, and is distinguished from USH II by its later onset with rapid and progressive hearing loss and retinal degeneration. There is good genetic evidence that the gene for USH III is located on a different chromosome than the genes for USH I and USH II.

Precautions before anesthesia: In view of the variety of presentations, each case has to be treated individually. In all cases, hearing and visual function have to be evaluated.

Anesthetic considerations: Patients may be profoundly deaf and blind, and this combination makes communication potentially very difficult, especially during induction of anesthesia and for the immediate postoperative care. There are no specific anesthetic techniques to recommend.

Pharmacological implications: Consideration must be given to medication, particularly the use of aminoglycosides in patients affected with Usher syndrome types II and III. Psychosis and bipolar affective disorder are common in this group of patients, and many will be receiving psychotropic medication, including major tranquilizers, lithium, or antidepressants. Considerations for potential interactions with anesthetic agents must be reviewed.

REFERENCES:

Fields RR, Zhou G, Huang D, et al: Usher syndrome type III: Revised genomic structure of the USH3 gene and identification of novel mutations. *Am J Hum Genet* 71(3):607, 2002.

Tamayo ML, Maldonado C, Plaza SL, et al: Neuroradiology and clinical aspects of Usher syndrome. *Clin Genet* 50:126, 1996.

Weil D, El-Amraoui A, Masmoudi S, et al: Usher syndrome type I G (USH1G) is caused by mutations in the gene encoding SANS, a protein that associates with the USH1C protein, harmonin. *Hum Mol Genet* 12(5):463, 2003.

VACTERL Association with Hydrocephalus

At a glance: A rare association of neurological lesions, lung and facial anomalies combined in a classical polymalformative syndrome.

Synonyms: Vertebral, Anal, Cardiac, Tracheal, Esophageal, Renal, Limbs with Hydrocephalus; Sujansky Leonard Syndrome; David-O'Callaghan Syndrome; Hunter-MacMurray Syndrome.

Incidence: Very rare syndrome.

Genetic inheritance: Pattern of inheritance is unclear. Both autosomal recessive and X-linked forms may occur. Mutation in the PTEN gene (located on 10q23.31) also has been evocated.

Pathophysiology: VACTERL, like other associations, is causally heterogeneous, reflecting disturbance of a multidimensional developmental process and producing different patterns of anomalies based on the area, timing, magnitude, and nature of the specific insult involved. The hydrocephalus develops secondary to cerebral aqueductal stenosis, distinct from other central nervous system (CNS) malformations.

Diagnosis: At birth, based on clinical features; the diagnosis is one of exclusion of other recognized causes of this phenotype.

Clinical aspects: The acronym emphasizes only the most frequent malformations; a wide variety of other defects, affecting most parts of the body, may be associated including *head* (prominent epicanthus, flat nasal bridge, choanal atresia, micrognathia, low-set malformed ears), *thorax* (spondylocostal dysplasia, hypoplastic lungs, laryngeal stenosis), *heart* (ventricular septal defects, patent ductus arteriosus, tetralogy of Fallot, transposition of the great arteries), *gastrointestinal tract* (anal atresia [controversial], esophageal and duodenal atresia); *urogenital tract* (urethral atresia, renal agenesis, hydronephrocolpos, hydronephrosis, hypospadias), *skeleton* (polydactyly and proximally placed thumbs, humeral hypoplasia, radial aplasia, vertebral dysgenesis, spondylocostal dysplasia, scoliosis, and hemivertebrae), and *CNS* (hydrocephalus, aqueductal stenosis, encephalocele, meningocele, papilledema, and agenesis of corpus callosum). Prognosis is generally poor.

Precautions before anesthesia: Assessment of respiratory function (clinical, chest radiographs, arterial blood gases). Evaluate cardiac function (clinical, ECG, chest radiographs, echocardiography). Vertebral malformations must be sought if regional anesthesia is considered. Evaluate neurological function (clinical, EEG, CT/MRI, transfontanelle ultrasonography) and renal function (echography, laboratory investigations, including urea, creatinine, electrolytes). Preoperative evaluation is often limited by the relative emergency of the surgery.

Anesthetic considerations: Direct laryngoscopy and tracheal intubation can be difficult. High risk of pulmonary aspiration because of the presence of a tracheoesophageal fistula. Meanwhile, preserving spontaneous ventilation is recommended until the trachea is secured. The presence of facial malformations and the tracheoesophageal fistula may lead to unwanted inflation of the stomach during face-mask ventilation. Careful observation of the respiratory function and the presence of any cardiac abnormality must be done at all times. Special attention must be provided with positioning of endotracheal tube because of the presence of the tracheoesophageal fistula. Chest radiography prior to surgery is recommended to assess tube position (just over carina). Arterial catheterization can be difficult to realize in case of radial defect. Postoperative ventilatory support may be considered because of tracheal fistula.

Pharmacological implications: Consider risk of impaired renal function and implications on anesthetic drugs and intraoperative fluid regimen. Antibiotic prophylaxis in cases of cardiac defect. Avoid muscle relaxants until airway is secured and lung ventilation, without stomach insufflation, is confirmed.

Other conditions to be considered:

VACTERL ASSOCIATION WITH HYDROCEPHALUS, X-LINKED: Very rare; features include branchial arch defects.

☞VATER ASSOCIATION: A classical, not so rare, acronymic syndrome that could involve vertebrae, anus, trachea, esophagus and kidney. Cardiac defect can be associated. Anesthetic management must consider cardiac function. Coexisting anomalies must be searched.

REFERENCES:

Evans JA, Stranc LC, Kaplan P, et al: VACTERL with hydrocephalus: Further delineation of the syndrome(s). *Am J Med Genet* 34:177, 1989.

Lomas FE, Dahlstrom JE, Ford JH: VACTERL with hydrocephalus: Family with X-linked VACTERL-H. *Am J Med Genet* 76:74, 1998.

Reardon W, Zhou X-P, Eng C: A novel germ line mutation of the PTEN gene in a patient with macrocephaly, ventricular dilatation, and features of VATER association. *J Med Genet* 38:820, 2001.

VA(C)TER(L) Association

At a glance: Acronym stands for: *V*ertebral Anomalies, *A*nal Atresia, (*C*ardiac Defects), *T*racheo-*E*sophageal Fistula, *R*enal (and *L*imb Anomalies). It already describes the most important defects of this disorder. Other coexisting anomalies must be excluded.

Synonyms: VATERS Association; VACTER Syndrome; Kaufman Syndrome; Quan-Smith Syndrome; Say-Gerald Syndrome; Hydronephrocolpos-Postaxial Polydactyly-Congenital Heart Disease Syndrome.

Nature: Unknown.

Incidence: 1:3,500 to 1.6:10,000 live births.

Genetic inheritance: Sporadic (some are familial, transmitted as an autosomal dominant trait).

Pathophysiology: Unknown; a disruption of blastogenesis seems to be the origin of the association. Multiple exogenous causes have been evocated; familial occurrence has been reported.

Diagnosis: Association can be evocated in the antenatal period. Prematurity is frequent. Diagnosis is evocated on the association of the different signs included in the acronym of VATER or VACTERL: vertebral abnormalities (70% of cases), anal atresia (80% of cases), cardiovascular defects (53% of cases), tracheo-esophageal fistula with esophageal atresia (70% of cases), renal agenesis or dysplasia (53% of cases), and limb abnormalities (65% of cases).

Clinical aspects: The acronyms emphasize only the most frequent malformations and a wide variety of other defects, affecting most parts of the body, may be associated, including *head* (prominent epicanthus, flat nasal bridge, choanal atresia, micrognathia, low-set malformed ears), *thorax* (spondylocostal dysplasia, hypoplastic lungs, laryngeal stenosis, ventricular septal defects, patent ductus arteriosus, tetralogy of Fallot, transposition of the great arteries), *gastrointestinal tract* (absent rectum and anus, duodenal atresia), *urogenital system* (urethral atresia, renal agenesis, hydronephrocolpos, hydronephrosis, hypospadias), and *skeleton* (polydactyly and proximally placed thumbs, humeral hypoplasia, radial aplasia, vertebral dysgenesis, spondylocostal dysplasia, scoliosis, and hemivertebrae).

Precautions before anesthesia: Anesthetic management must consider the emergency of the surgical procedure. Evaluate cardiac function (clinical, chest radiographs, echocardiography, ECG), respiratory function (chest radiographs, arterial blood gas analysis), and renal function (echography, laboratory investigations, including urea, creatinine, electrolytes).

Anesthetic considerations: Various anesthetic management procedures have been described for these patients. Challenge is greater if tracheal fistula ligature is initially closed. Careful intraoperative positioning is necessary but may be difficult. Venous and arterial access can be a challenge in cases of severe limb anomalies. Avoid manual-assisted ventilation to limit aspiration risk. Direct laryngoscopy can be difficult because of micrognathia, and tracheal intubation can be hazardous because of laryngeal stenosis. Consider existence of a tracheoesophageal fistula to determine exact position of tube's end (placement just near a tracheal carina can be useful if fistula is located over the carina). Control chest radiographs or with fiberoptic can be interesting after intubation. Spontaneous ventilation should be preserved until fistula is closed or after confirmation of the position of the tracheal tube past the fistula and absence of gastric air entry. Medullar regional anesthesia should be avoided because of vertebral anomalies. Intraoperative monitoring should include artery, double pulse oximetry or transcutaneous O_2 (one in preductal and the other in postductal).

Pharmacological implications: Anesthetic medications should be chosen to preserve spontaneous ventilation and cardiac function. Prophylactic antibiotics should be used in cases of cardiac defect. Intraoperative fluid regimen must be strict in cases of renal anomalies.

Other conditions to be considered:

☞VACTERL ASSOCIATION WITH HYDROCEPHALUS: Probably autosomal recessive with aqueductal stenosis, hydrocephalus, encephalocele, meningocele, and agenesis of corpus callosum; prognosis is poor.

X-LINKED VACTERL ASSOCIATION WITH HYDROCEPHALUS: X-linked instead of autosomal recessive.

REFERENCES:

Block EC, Filston H: A thin fiberoptic bronchoscope as an aid to occlusion of the fistula in infants with tracheoesophageal fistula. *Anesth Analg* 67:791, 1988.

Corsello G, Maresi E, Corrao AM, et al: VATER/VACTERL association: Clinical variability and expanding phenotype including laryngeal stenosis. *Am J Med Genet* 44(6):813, 1992; erratum in *Am J Med Genet* 47(1):118, 1993.

Reeves ST, Burt N, Smith CD: Is it time to reevaluate the airway management of tracheoesophageal fistula? *Anesth Analg* 81:866, 1995.

Van der Woude Syndrome

At a glance: Inherited developmental disorder characterized by pits of the lower lip and cleft lip or cleft palate. It is the most common cleft lip/palate syndrome.

Synonyms: Cleft Lip and/or Palate with Mucous Cysts of Lower Lip; Lip-Pit Syndrome; Lip-Pit-Cleft Syndrome.

History: Congenital genetic disorder first studied by A. Van der Woude in 1954.

Incidence: 1:70,000 live births.

Genetic inheritance: Autosomal dominant.

Pathophysiology: Caused by mutations in the gene encoding interferon regulatory factor-6 located on 1q32-q41; allelic to popliteal pterygium syndrome. Clinical expression is highly variable from one individual to another.

Diagnosis: Clinically evocated in patients with cleft lip or palate and mucous cysts of lower lip. Lip-Pit Syndrome is the most common manifestation present in 90% of the affected. The cleft of lip and palate occur in 21%.

Clinical aspects: Generally concerns only head with lower lip pits (corresponding to accessory salivary glands), cleft lip, cleft palate, cleft uvula, and hypodontia.

Precautions before anesthesia: Evaluate the airway (clinical, radiographs) and teeth mobility.

Anesthetic considerations: Direct laryngoscopy and tracheal intubation can be difficult because of cleft syndrome. Teeth lesions can occur more frequently.

Pharmacological implications: Avoid muscle relaxants until confirmation that face-mask ventilation is possible or airway is secured.

REFERENCES:

Guner U, Celik N, Ozek C, et al: Van der Woude syndrome. *Scand J Plast Reconstr Surg Hand Surg* 36(2):103, 2002.

Ryns JP, Devriendt K: On the nosology of van der Woude syndrome and popliteal pterygium syndrome: Implications for genetic counseling. *Genet Couns* 11(1):59, 2000.

van der Woude A: Fistula labii inferioris congenita and its association with cleft lip and palate. *Am J Hum Genet* 6:244, 1954.

Van Maldergem Wetzburger Verloes Syndrome

At a glance: Facial abnormalities and malformation of the extremities.

Synonyms: Blepharo-Naso-Facial Syndrome; Pashayan Syndrome; Pashayan-Pruzansky Syndrome; Cerebrofacioarticular Syndrome.

Incidence and genetic inheritance: An extremely rare syndrome of unknown incidence. Transmission is most likely autosomal dominant; however, X-linked dominant inheritance is also possible.

Clinical aspects: Facial abnormalities include midface hypoplasia with broad and flattened nose, large, inverted, W-shaped mouth, and malformed ears. Telecanthus, epicanthus, lateral displacement of the lacrimal puncta, and lacrimal excretory obstruction are characteristic findings. Because of the weakness of the facial muscles, patients have a mask-like appearance. Malformations of the extremities can include camptodactyly, clinodactyly, interdigital webbing, and joint hyperlaxity. Neurological signs comprise torsion dystonia, increased deep tendon reflexes, poor coordination, positive Babinski sign, hearing impairment, and developmental delay.

Anesthetic considerations: Affected patients are otherwise healthy. Hearing impairment may make communication difficult. Careful assessment of the airway is required to rule out difficult airway management because of midface hypoplasia. In general, these patients are not different from healthy children undergoing the same kind of procedure.

Other conditions to be considered:

KLEIN-WAARDENBURG SYNDROME: Autosomal dominant inherited syndrome with congenital sensory hearing loss and pigmentary disturbance of iris and hair, congenital leukoderma, and facial anomalies.

☞FETAL ALCOHOL SYNDROME: Characterized by dysmorphic features (most often midfacial anomalies), intrauterine growth retardation with failure to achieve catch-up growth, and central nervous system involvement with cognitive impairment and learning disabilities.

☞VATER ASSOCIATION: Acronym for vertebral anomalies, anal atresia, cardiac malformations (ventricular septal defects, patent ductus arteriosus, transposition of the great arteries, tetralogy of Fallot), tracheoesophageal fistula, renal anomalies (urethral atresia with hydronephrosis), and radial aplasia (or other limb anomalies such as humeral hypoplasia, hexadactyly, and displaced thumb).

☞MARDEN-WALKER SYNDROME: Autosomal recessive transmitted disease that affects more males than females. Heart and lung anomalies, joint contractures, microcephaly, ocular anomalies, high-arched or cleft palate, mental retardation, muscular hypotonia, and growth retardation.

☞TEL HASHOMER CAMPTODACTYLY SYNDROME: Genetic disorder with muscular hypoplasia, skeletal anomalies, increased creatine phosphokinase levels, and abnormal electromyogram.

REFERENCES:

Pashayan H, Pruzansky S, Putterman A: A family with blepharo-naso-facial malformations. *Am J Dis Child* 125:389, 1973.

Stoll C, Terzic J, Fischbach M: A three generations family with blepharo-naso-facial malformations suggestive of Pashayan syndrome. *Genet Couns* 10:337, 1999.

Van Maldergem L, Wetzburger C, Verloes A, et al: Mental retardation with blepharo-naso-facial abnormalities and hand malformations: A new syndrome? *Clin Genet* 41:22, 1992.

Vaquez-Osler Disease

At a glance: Idiopathic myeloproliferative disease that is rare in childhood. Manifestations are caused by occlusive vascular lesions.

Synonyms: Vaquez Disease; Osler-Vaquez Disease; Vaquez Polycythemia; Polycythemia Vera.

Incidence: 5 to 6:1,000,000 in general population; affects males more often than females.

Diagnosis: Evocated accidentally on routine blood examination. Diagnosis is usually made by the clinical findings of erythrocytosis, leukocytosis, thrombocytosis, and splenomegaly. Also, the association of blood examination and several signs, such as headaches,

weakness, dyspnea, dizziness, or tinnitus, might confirm the diagnosis. However, only two or three of these criteria may be present. Direct determination of red cell mass has also been suggested, but is of uncertain value because of the difficulties in standardization and because of expense. Occasionally reported in childhood, it occurs mostly in middle-age males. Diagnosis can be confirmed by the association of splenomegaly, arterial saturation >92%, and an increased red blood cell (RBC) mass (>36 mL/kg in men and 32 mL/kg in women). Treatment includes phlebotomy and myelosuppression.

Clinical aspects: Insidious onset usually in the sixth decade of life. Erythrocytosis, neutrophilia, thrombocytosis, and splenomegaly are present. Thrombosis (10% with Budd-Chiari syndrome; 50% of patients develop at least one thrombotic complication, which includes cardiovascular accident, myocardial infarction [MI], deep venous thrombosis, and pulmonary embolism). Bleeding and bruising, although usually minor. Pruritus, peptic ulcer disease, gastric varices, angina, MI, congestive heart failure, dizziness. Reports of spinal cord compression from extramedullary hemopoiesis. Gout, secondary to increased urate turnover. Increased perioperative bleeding and thrombosis. Associated with lymphocytic lymphomas. Clinical features can also include headache, mental clouding, facial plethora pruritus, hepatomegaly, high blood pressure, and gout. More severe manifestations, caused by occlusive vascular lesions, can also be observed: transient ischemic attack, digital ischemia, stroke, bleeding (including gastrointestinal tract). Death occurs within 18 months without treatment and within 15 years with appropriate treatment, but there is a 20% incidence of transformation to myelofibrosis and approximately a 5% incidence of transformation to acute leukemia. Vaquez disease is a myeloproliferative disease. Hyperplasia involves all marrow elements and replaces marrow fat. There is increased production and turnover of RBCs, neutrophils, and platelets.

Precautions before anesthesia: Hematology consultation for recommendations regarding phlebotomy. Check complete cell blood count and coagulation status. Postpone elective surgery in presence of myocardial angina and congestive heart failure. Evaluate cardiac function in cases of high blood pressure (clinical, chest radiographs, ECG, echocardiography). Determine toxicity secondary to chemotherapeutics. Evaluate vasoocclusive risk (full history, platelet count, hematocrit, leukocytes) and hepatic function (echocardiography, CT, laboratory investigations, including serum glutamic-oxaloacetic transaminase [SGOT], serum glutamic-pyruvic transaminase [SGPT], bilirubin). Elective surgery should be postponed until the hematocrit is reduced to <42% and platelets to <600,000/μL. Perioperative antithrombotic therapy should be considered.

Anesthetic considerations: Because surgical procedures may be hazardous, elective surgery should be postponed until the hematocrit is reduced to <42% and platelets to <600,000/μL. Normovolemic hemodilution can be useful. Careful intraoperative positioning is necessary. Pulsating boots or elastic stockings placed on the patient's legs can be used to reduce venous blood stasis. Avoid, if possible, the placement of a nasogastric tube in case of bleeding. Avoid regional anesthesia in presence of bleeding disorder. Maintain hydration to decrease viscosity. Avoid esophageal instrumentation in the presence of varices. Deep venous thrombosis prophylaxis is highly recommended.

Pharmacological implications: The full regimen of perioperative antithrombotic therapy, including intravenous heparin, should be reevaluated in patients with recent bleeding episode.

REFERENCES:

Michiels JJ, Thiele J: Clinical and pathological criteria for the diagnosis of essential thrombocythemia, polycythemia vera, and idiopathic myelofibrosis (agnogenic myeloid metaplasia). *Int J Hematol* 76(2):133, 2002.

Schmitt HJ, Becke K, Neidhardt B: Epidural anesthesia for cesarean delivery in a patient with polycythemia rubra vera and preeclampsia. *Anesth Analg* 92(6):1535, 2001.

Sosis MB: Anesthesia for polycythemia vera. *J Clin Anesth* 2(1):31, 1990.

Varadi-Papp Syndrome

At a glance: An orofaciodigital syndrome characterized by the association of metacarpal abnormalities with central polydactyly and cerebellar abnormality.

Synonyms: Oral-Facial-Digital Syndrome type VI; Orofaciodigital Syndrome VI; Polydactyly Cleft Lip/Palate or Lingual Lump and Psychomotor Retardation.

Genetic inheritance: Autosomal recessive.

Pathophysiology: The cerebellar abnormalities are thought to be caused by a primary neuronal or glial cell defect.

Diagnosis: Characteristic malformations generally noted at birth but can also be detected on fetoscopy. Magnetic resonance imaging demonstrates hypoplasia of the cerebellar vermis. Radiography of limb extremities shows polydactyly characterized by a Y-shaped central metacarpal.

Clinical aspects: Reduplicated big toes; hexadactyly; central hand polydactyly; cleft lip; cleft palate; multiple ear abnormalities; lingual nodule; growth retardation; absent olfactory bulbs and tracts; cerebellar signs; congenital heart defect; recurrent episodes of tachypnea and hyperpnea; cryptorchidism; and inguinal hernia are described. Death occurs in neonatal period or early childhood.

Precautions before anesthesia: Assessment of airway. Evaluate cardiac and respiratory function (clinical, chest radiographs, echocardiography, arterial blood gas analysis).

Anesthetic considerations: Possible difficulties with tracheal intubation as a result of facial abnormalities and often the presence of significant lingual nodules, especially the posterior ones. Perioperative cardiac and respiratory monitoring is recommended.

Pharmacological implications: Prophylactic antibiotics must be considered in cases of cardiac defect.

Other conditions to be considered:

☞**ORAL-FACIAL-DIGITAL SYNDROME:** At least nine types of Oral-Facial-Digital Syndrome have been identified. Symptoms common to most include episodic neuromuscular disturbances, split tongue, mandible splits, midline cleft lip, overgrowth frenulum, broad-based nose, epicanthic folds, polysyndactyly, camptodactyly, increased number of calvarial plates.

☞**JUBERG-HAYWARD SYNDROME:** Characterized by cleft lip and palate malformations, microcephaly, deformities of the thumbs and toes, and short stature.

☞**ACROFACIAL DYSOSTOSIS (Nager Type):** Rare hereditary disorder presenting with cleft lip and palate, craniofacial anomalies, micrognathia, and small thumbs.

☞**JOUBERT SYNDROME:** Very rare hereditary neurological disorder characterized by severe ataxia and coordination. The neuromuscular and eye movement disturbances are similar to those of

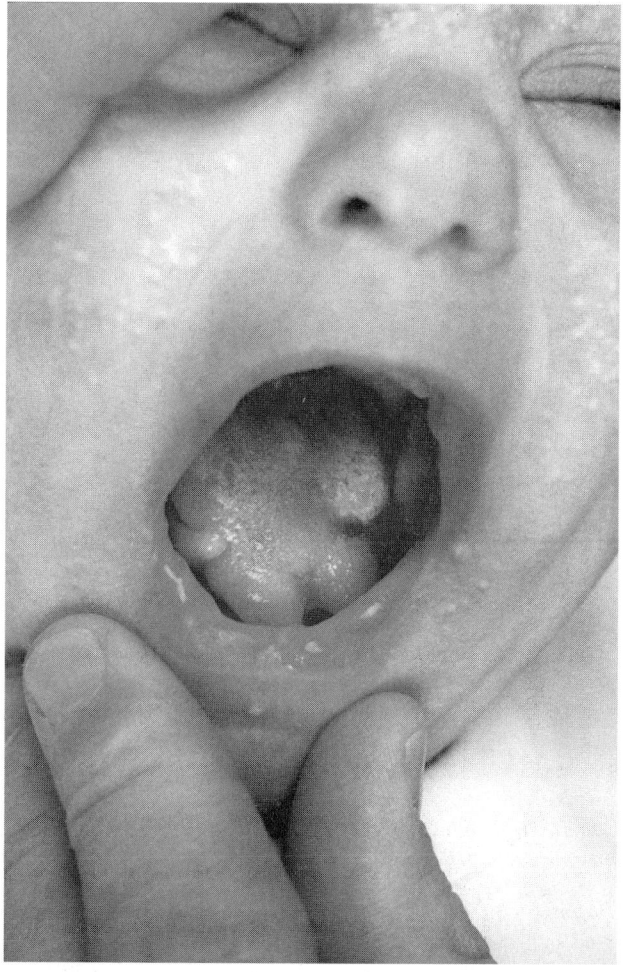

Varadi-Papp syndrome Lingual nodules in a newborn with Varadi-Papp Syndrome.

Oral-Facial-Digital Syndrome. Other clinical features include psychomotor retardation and/or respiratory problems.

REFERENCES:

Doss BJ, Jolly S, Quereshi F, et al: Neuropathologic findings in a case of OFDS type VI (Varadi syndrome). *Am J Med Genet* 77:38, 1998.

Varadi V, Szabo L, Papp Z: Syndrome of polydactyly, cleft lip/palate or lingual lump, and psychomotor retardation in endogamic gypsies. *J Med Genet* 17:119, 1980.

Vasquez Hurst Sotos Syndrome

At a glance: A very rare disorder characterized by the association of obesity, mental retardation, seizures, deafness, microgenitalism, and short stature.

Synonym: X-Linked Hypogonadism Gynecomastia Mental Retardation.

Genetic inheritance: X-linked, recessive. This medical condition is known to affect only males.

Pathophysiology: Unknown.

Diagnosis: X-linked mode of inheritance, distinctive facies, normal-size hands and feet, and gynecomastia are the main characteristics of this syndrome.

Clinical aspects: Patients present with short stature, generalized obesity, hypotonia, mental retardation, abnormal cry, and seizures. Clinical features can include various anomalies, including *craniofacial* (narrow forehead, up-slanted fissures, brachycephaly, microphthalmia, narrow palate, bifid uvula), *orthopedic* (kyphoscoliosis, camptodactyly, genu valgum, proximally set thumb, ulna deviation of fingers, clinodactyly of fifth finger, vertebral segmentation anomaly, increased carrying angle of the elbows), and *genitourinary* (atrophic and ectopic testes, micropenis, hypogonadism, and gynecomastia).

Precautions before anesthesia: Evaluate carefully the airway (clinical, radiographs) and neurological function (clinical, EEG).

Anesthetic considerations: Cautious intraoperative positioning is necessary but difficult because of spine deformities and obesity. Direct laryngoscopy and tracheal intubation can be difficult because of obesity and craniofacial anomalies and may require fiberoptic or retrograde intubation; laryngeal mask airway can be useful and should be available at the time of induction of anesthesia. Venous access (both central and peripheral) can be a real challenge. Regional anesthesia can help decrease opioid use postoperatively. However, regional anesthesia can be difficult to perform because of the presence of skeletal deformities and significant obesity. It may also be dangerous in patients with segmental anomaly.

Pharmacological implications: The use of anesthetic medications allowing the maintenance of spontaneous ventilation is highly recommended until the trachea is secured and lung ventilation is confirmed. Antiepileptic medications must be continued until the morning of the surgical procedure. Anesthetic agents prone to increase seizure activities (e.g., enflurane, sevoflurane) must be used with caution. The use of sedative premedication must be considered. Muscle relaxants are not contraindicated; however, it is recommended to limit their use once the trachea is intubated and ventilation confirmed. Neuromuscular blocking agents doses must be used carefully because the muscle mass can be significantly reduced in these patients.

Other condition to be considered:

☞ **JUBERG-MARSIDI SYNDROME:** An extremely rare X-linked inherited disorder that affects males and is apparent at birth or during the neonatal period. Severe mental retardation and motor development (e.g., crawling, walking), hypotonia, delayed bone growth and severe failure to thrive are the main characteristics of this disorder. Other features include deafness, microgenitalism), craniofacial anomalies, severe microcephaly, a depressed nasal bridge, and ocular abnormalities.

☞ **BORJESON-FORSSMAN-LEHMANN SYNDROME:** An extremely rare inherited disorder characterized by unusual facial features, mental retardation, seizures, short stature, muscle weakness, hypotonia, and/or hypogonadism. Mental retardation may be mild to severe. Other clinical features include microcephaly, prominent supraorbital ridges, ptosis, unusually deep-set eyes, and/or a short neck. An X-linked dominant or recessive genetic trait has been suggested. Although it is fully expressed in males only, heterozygote females may present some of the symptoms.

GUSTAVSON SYNDROME: A very rare inherited disorder believed to be inherited as an X-linked transmission. However, it affects both males and females equally. Mental retardation, microcephaly, impaired vision or blindness, hearing abnormalities, muscle stiffness and uncontrolled involuntary muscle movements,

seizures, and limited large joint movement are features of this condition.

REFERENCES:

Juberg RC, Marsidi I: A new form of X-linked mental retardation with growth retardation, deafness, and microgenitalism. *Am J Hum Genet* 32:714, 1980.

Vasquez SB, Hurst DL, Sotos JF: X-linked hypogonadism, gynecomastia, mental retardation, short stature, and obesity—A new syndrome. *J Pediatr* 94:56, 1979.

Velocardiofacial Syndrome

At a glance: This syndrome includes typical facies and cardiac anomalies. Many other malformations can be associated (endocrine and ophthalmic).

Synonyms: VCS Syndrome; Shprintzen Syndrome; Sedlacková Syndrome.

Incidence: 1:1800 to 1:5000 live births.

Genetic inheritance: Autosomal dominant (de novo: 80% of cases).

Pathophysiology: Observed anomalies result from microdeletion on 22q11.

Diagnosis: Evocated in patients with typical facies (prominent nose and retrognathia, cleft palate), cardiovascular defects, and mental retardation. Proved by resolution banding and fluorescence in situ hybridization, which can find the 22q11 microdeletion (karyotype study is insufficient).

Clinical aspects: Clinical features also include multiple anomalies overlapping those encountered in other 22q11 deletions. Patients have short stature, overabundant hair, elongated face with mandible anomalies as in Pierre Robin syndrome, malformed ears and eyes (inability to close the eyes, narrow palpebral fissures, malformed retinal vessels, blue sclerae, retinal colobomas, cataracts), and basilar impression. Intracranial lesions concern white matter and vermis. Language is slow and behavior disorders are observed. Immunologic and endocrine systems are often involved: adenoids, tonsils, and thymus are absent or small. In many cases, hypothyroidism and hypocalcemia can occur. Cardiovascular anomalies are frequent, including right aortic arch, ventricular septal defect, tetralogy of Fallot, abnormal internal carotid arteries, and left subclavian artery. Other clinical signs supplement the disease: scoliosis, abnormal extremities, inguinal hernia, and anal anomalies.

Precautions before anesthesia: Evaluate patients for the possibility of cardiopathy (clinical, chest radiography, echocardiography) and airway (clinical, radiographs). Perioperative laboratory investigations should include calcemia, FT_4, T_3.

Anesthetic considerations: Direct laryngoscopy and tracheal intubation can be extremely difficult because of orofacial deformations and may require fiberoptic, laryngeal mask airway, or retrograde intubation. Digitally guided intubation in prone position has been proposed for Robin sequence and can be useful. Spontaneous ventilation should be preserved until airway is secured and lung ventilation confirmed. T-cell immunodeficiency requires strict aseptic procedures and specific blood (irradiated). Spine and extremity deformities need careful intraoperative position; regional anesthesia can be difficult to realize. Central venous access can be dangerous because of carotid and subclavian arteries malposition.

Pharmacological implications: Avoid cardiodepressive drugs. Prophylactic antibiotics must be considered in cases of cardiopathy. The possibility of immunodeficiency is also an indication for antibiotics. Muscle relaxants should be avoided until airway is secured and lung ventilation confirmed. Intraoperative fluid administration should be adapted to the cardiac function.

Other condition to be considered:

☞**DiGeorge Syndrome:** Characterized by hypocalcemia arising from parathyroid hypoplasia, thymic hypoplasia, and outflow tract defects of the heart. Disturbance of cervical neural crest migration into the pharyngeal arches and pouches has been suggested as mechanism. Results from the deletion of chromosome 22q11.2.

References:

Shprintzen RJ, Goldberg RB, Young D, et al: The velo-cardio-facial syndrome: A clinical and genetic analysis. *Pediatrics* 67:167, 1981.

Singh VP, Agarwal RC, Sanyal S, et al: Anesthesia for DiGeorge's syndrome. *J Cardiothorac Vasc Anesth* 11(6):81, 1997.

Velo-Facio-Skeletal Syndrome

At a glance: A very rare syndrome characterized by craniofacial and skeletal anomalies.

Clinical aspects: Clinical evocation on short stature associated with facial skeletal anomalies and hypernasality. There is no 22q11 microdeletion. There is no mental retardation. Clinical features involve *orofacial structures* (epicanthal folds, hypertelorism, posteriorly angulated ears, narrow and high-arched palate, broad and high nasal bridge) and *skeleton* (delayed bone age, mesomelic brachymelia, short broad hands, short stubby thumbs, prominent finger pads, small feet, hyperextensible hand joints).

Anesthetic considerations: Careful intraoperative positioning is necessary. Limb anomalies can create difficulties with noninvasive blood pressure measurement, venous access, and regional anesthesia. Direct laryngoscopy and tracheal intubation can be difficult.

Other conditions to be considered:

☞**Robinow Syndrome:** An extremely rare inherited disorder characterized by mild to moderate short stature due to postnatal growth retardation. Distinctive craniofacial abnormalities associated with skeletal malformations and genital anomalies complete the clinical presentation. The facial features of infants with this disorder resemble those of an 8-week-old fetus. The presence of macrocephaly, frontal bossing, severe ocular hypertelorism, anteverted nostril, and depressed nasal bridge are characteristic of the facial features. It is believed to be an autosomal dominant inheritance; however, some individuals present with an autosomal recessive mode of inheritance.

☞**Aarskog Syndrome:** A rare inherited disorder combining facial, skeletal, and genital abnormalities. The clinical features include a disproportionate short stature, broad facial features, short broad hands and feet, an abnormal fold of skin extending around the base of the penis ("shawl" scrotum), and spinal malformations. Mild mental retardation may occur but is not considered a consistent feature of Aarskog Syndrome. It is inherited as an X-linked recessive trait.

Reference:

Teebi AS, Qumsiyeh MB, Meyers-Seifer CH, et al: Velo-facial-skeletal syndrome in a mother and daughter. *Am J Med Genet* 58:8, 1995.

Verner-Morrison Syndrome

At a glance: A very rare syndrome caused by tumoral-inappropriate vasoactive intestinal peptide secretion. Can be associated with multiple endocrine neoplasias. Clinical aspect is a result of intensive diarrhea that can lead to dehydration and severe hypokalemia.

Synonyms: WDHA Syndrome; Water Diarrhea, Hypokalemia, Achlorhydria Syndrome; WDHH Syndrome; Water Diarrhea, Hypokalemia, Hypochlorhydria Syndrome; Diarrheagenic Syndrome; Pancreatic Cholera; Vipoma Syndrome.

History: Described by John U. Verner and Ashton B. Morrison, both American physicians, in 1958.

Incidence: 3:10,000,000 people in the general population.

Pathophysiology: This disease is caused by inappropriate secretion of vasoactive intestinal peptide (VIP), usually secreted from non-beta islet pancreatic cells in response to food containing fat, proteins, and alcohol. It relaxes smooth muscles, resulting in a decrease of lower esophageal sphincter pressure, relaxation of the gastric antrum and body, and inhibition of gallbladder and intestinal circular muscle contraction. Extra secretion of VIP will provide general manifestations such as vasodilatation, positive inotropic action on the heart, increase in intestinal water and electrolyte secretion, inhibition of gastrin and gastric acid secretion, and stimulation of pancreatic secretion.

Diagnosis: Characterized by severe watery diarrhea and dehydration. Diagnosis is confirmed by *biochemistry* (hypokalemia, hypochloremia, metabolic acidosis, high plasma VIP levels; approximately two-thirds of patients have hypercalcemia and 50% are hyperglycemic), *stool analysis* (isotonic, alkaline, cultures negative), and *ultrasonography and CT imaging* (dilated gallbladder, localization of tumors). Prostaglandin E and E_2 hypersecretion can be associated.

Clinical aspects: Hypermotility, watery diarrhea syndromes with hypokalemia and hypochloremia or hyperchloremia, dehydration. Lethargy, muscular weakness, nausea, vomiting, and abdominal pain are frequent. Fluid secretion may exceed 3 to 5 L, with a loss of 200 to 300 mEq of potassium daily. Some cases of VIPoma have included hypercalcemia, flushing, and glucose intolerance. Ectopic primary sites, such as the liver and jejunum, occur in approximately 10% of patients. In children, the VIPoma syndrome is caused by either a ganglioneuroma or ganglioneuroblastoma. In adults, it is caused by bronchiogenic carcinoma, pheochromocytoma, medullar thyroid carcinoma, and retroperitoneal histiocytoma. Multiple endocrine neoplasia type 1 can be associated (in MEN, hypercalcemia is frequent).

Precautions before anesthesia: Evaluate the extent of the diarrhea (history, clinical repercussion, laboratory investigations including natremia, kalemia, calcemia, urea, creatinine, glycemia, arterial blood gas analysis). Also, the tumor repercussion must be assessed because of the risk of obstruction of the duodenum or of the biliary tract and of vascular erosion (radiography, CT, endoscopy). Preoperative ECG should be done in cases of hypokalemia. Evaluate existence and repercussion of flushing episodes (history, clinical, heart rate and blood pressure measurement during flush).

Anesthetic considerations: Preoperative hydration and electrolyte correction is necessary based on the laboratory investigations. Elective surgical procedures must be postponed until electrolytes and the intravascular fluid status have been corrected. Vascular access can be extremely difficult and an emergency route may be used (intraosseous, superior longitudinal sinus). Central venous access using Seldinger technique should be avoided in cases of hypokalemia and cardiac irritability. Glucose levels should be regularly evaluated and fluid regimen adapted. Perioperative blood pressure and cardiac monitoring should be performed. Normocapnic ventilation is recommended to avoid respiratory alkalosis in cases of severe hypokalemia. Removal of tumor will provide fast resolution of symptoms.

Pharmacological implications: Medullar regional anesthesia should probably be avoided because of the risk of potentialization of the vasoplegic effects of VIP release. Muscle relaxants are not contraindicated but their action can be prolonged in presence of uncorrected hypokalemia (monitoring is necessary).

Other conditions to be considered: Other pancreatic endocrine tumors. Clinical features vary based on secretion: insulinoma (insulin); Zollinger-Ellison syndrome (gastrin); glucagonoma (glucagon); Cushing syndrome (adrenocorticotropic hormone); mild hyperglycemia with cholelithiasis (somatostatin).

REFERENCES:

Krejs GJ: VIPoma syndrome. *Am J Med* 82:37, 1987.

Murphy MS, Sibal A, Mann JR: Persistent diarrhoea and occult vipomas in children. *BMJ* 320(7248):1524, 2000.

Rood RP, DeLellis RA, Dayal Y, et al: Pancreatic cholera syndrome due to a vasoactive intestinal polypeptide-producing tumor: Further insights into the pathophysiology. *Gastroenterology* 94(3):813, 1988.

Vogt-Koyanagi-Harada Syndrome

At a glance: A systemic inflammatory disease with probable immunogenetic predisposition that affects the eye (panuveitis) leading to rapid loss of vision. It is also associated to a characteristic spectrum of nonophthalmic features involving particularly the skin, hair (alopecia), and ear. Meningitis and raised intracranial pressure have also been reported.

Synonyms: Alopecia-Poliosis-Uveitis-Vitiligo-Deafness-Cutaneous-Uveo-Oto Syndrome; Harada Syndrome; Harada Disease; Vogt-Koyanagi Syndrome; Yugé Syndrome; Oculocutaneous Syndrome; Uveocutaneous Syndrome; Uveitis-Vitiligo-Alopecia-Poliosis Syndrome; Uveomeningeal Syndrome; Uveomeningitis Syndrome; Uveomeningoencephalitis; Uveoencephalitis.

History: First described in 1906 by Alfred Vogt, Swiss ophthalmologist.

Incidence: Unknown but more common in darker-pigmented races, particularly Orientals and American Indians.

Genetic inheritance: Unknown but strong association with HLA-DR histocompatibility antigens.

Pathophysiology: Immunocytologic findings are compatible with a T-cell–mediated autoimmune reaction to uveal and dermal melanocytes.

Diagnosis: Requires three of the following features: bilateral iridocyclitis, posterior uveitis (including serous retinal detachment or sunset glow fundus), central nervous system manifestations, and cutaneous manifestations.

Clinical aspects: Patients are often of short stature. In addition to uveitis, ophthalmic features can include visual loss, retinal detachment, cataract, and glaucoma. Other features include the central nervous system and cutaneous origin, including deafness (sensorineural), headache, tinnitus, dysacousis, and meningism associated with cerebrospinal fluid pleocytosis. Alopecia, premature graying of hair, and vitiligo are also observed. Onset is generally in postadolescent life, but two case reports exist in children, the youngest being 4 years old. The condition is treated with high-dose steroids.

Precautions before anesthesia: Complete medical history and physical examination pertaining to central nervous system involvement and the use of steroids are important. Evaluate adrenal function (clinical, electrolytes, glycemia).

Anesthetic considerations: Strict asepsis is needed because of immunodeficiency induced by repeated steroid treatment.

Pharmacological implications: Preoperative stress dose of steroids might be required. Atropine and all drugs that can induce glaucoma should be avoided. Succinylcholine should probably be avoided in case of retinal detachment and because of its action on intraocular pressure. Consider benefit of using aminoglycosides in cases of incomplete deafness.

REFERENCES:

Read RW: Vogt-Koyanagi-Harada disease. *Ophthalmol Clin North Am* 15(3):333, 2002.

Vogt A: Frühzeitiges Ergrauen der Zilien und Bemerkungen über den sogenannten plötzlichen Eintritt dieser Veränderung. *Klin Monatsbl Augenheilkd* 44:228, 1906.

Vohwinkel Syndrome

At a glance: Congenital deafness with keratopachyderma and constrictions of fingers and toes. The risk of autoamputation is significantly high, mostly as a result of trauma and infections.

Synonyms: Mutilating Keratoderma; Keratoderma Hereditarium Mutilans; Congenital Deafness with Keratopachyderma and Constriction of Fingers and Toes Syndrome.

History: First described by K.H. Vohwinkel in 1929.

Genetic inheritance: Autosomal dominant.

Pathophysiology: Caused by mutation in the gene encoding connexin-26, a gap-junction protein (GJB2).

Diagnosis: Hyperkeratoses of the palms and soles occurring in infancy or early childhood. Histological examination shows thickening of the granular layer, moderate acanthosis, and a few mononuclear inflammatory cells in the papillary dermis. Radiological investigation demonstrates mild bone rarefaction and osteoporotic changes distal to the constricting bands.

Clinical aspects: Characterized by diffuse hyperkeratosis of the palms and soles, with a "honeycomb" appearance that progresses to "starfish-shaped" keratotic plaques on the dorsa of the hands and feet, and also involving the wrists, forearms, elbows, and knees. Fibrous constricting bands (pseudoainhum) at the interphalangeal joints, which may lead to autoamputation. May also be associated with hearing loss of varying severity, cicatricial alopecia, ichthyosiform dermatosis, nail abnormalities, mental retardation, and spastic paraplegia or myopathy.

Precautions before anesthesia: Evaluate the severity of pseudoainhum.

Anesthetic considerations: Careful perioperative installation is necessary to avoid further constriction and accidental finger amputation. Same remarks concerning use of digital sensor. Venous access on hands can be difficult.

Pharmacological implications: Consider the benefit of using aminoglycosides in cases of incomplete deafness.

Other conditions to be considered:

☞**BART PUMPHREY SYNDROME:** An inherited syndrome featuring knuckle pads, leukonychia, and sensorineural deafness.

MUTILATING KERATODERMA WITH ICHTHYOSIS: This is a variant caused by mutation of the gene for loricrin, a component of the epidermal differentiation complex (EDC). The gene is located at 13q11-q12. Most prevalent during childhood. More than 200 cases have been reported. Characterized by transient, circumscribed, figurate erythematous patches, hyperkeratosis (yellow-brown and thickened plaques).

REFERENCES:

O'Driscoll J, Muston GC, McGrath JA, et al: A recurrent mutation in the loricrin gene underlies the ichthyotic variant of Vohwinkel syndrome. *Clin Exp Dermatol* 27(3):243, 2002.

Peris K, Salvati EF, Torlone G, et al: Keratoderma hereditarium mutilans (Vohwinkel's syndrome) associated with congenital deaf-mutism. *Br J Dermatol* 132:617, 1995.

Vohwinkel KH; Keratoma hereditarium mutilans. *Arch Dermatol Syph* 158:354, 1929.

Anesthetic considerations: Main risk is the development of hypoglycemia and lactic acidosis perioperatively. Establish infusion of dextrose preoperatively to maintain normal carbohydrate intake (may require 20% dextrose concentration). Avoid prolonged fasting with early establishment of enteral feeding postoperatively if possible. Monitor blood glucose and blood gases (place arterial catheter for prolonged surgical procedures). Avoid regional techniques (bleeding tendency). Hepatomegaly may be sufficient to cause respiratory compromise during mask anesthesia.

Pharmacological implications: *Cis*-atracurium is the muscle relaxant of choice (renal dysfunction). Avoid lactate-containing IV fluids. No agents are specifically contraindicated. Consider the benefit of using aminoglycosides in cases of renal dysfunction.

REFERENCES:

Bevan JC: Anesthesia in Von Gierke's disease. Current approach to management. *Anesthesia* 35:699, 1980.

von Gierke E: Hepato-nephromegalia glykogenica (Glykogenspeicherkrankheit der Leber und Nieren). *Beiträge zur pathologischen Anatomie und zur allgemeinen Pathologie* 82:497, 1929.

Von Gierke Disease

At a glance: An inborn error of glycogen metabolism caused by glucose-6-phosphatase (G6P) deficiency. The disease is characterized by hepatomegaly, hypoglycemia, and hyperlacticacidemia. Lethal in infancy or childhood.

Synonyms: ☞Glycogen Storage Disease type Ia; ☞Glucose-6-Phosphatase Deficiency.

Nature: First described in 1929 by Edgar Otto Conrad von Gierke, a German pathologist.

Incidence: Estimated to be approximately 1:100,000 live births.

Genetic inheritance: Autosomal recessive. Located at 17q21.

Pathophysiology: Deficiency of glucose-6-phosphatase in liver and kidneys, leading to increased glycogen concentrations in these organs. No involvement of skeletal or cardiac muscle. Caused by mutations in the glucose-6-phosphatase catalytic gene (G6PC).

Diagnosis: Infant develops hepatomegaly with poor feeding and failure to thrive. Marked hypoglycemia, lactic acidosis, hyperlipidemia, and hyperuricemia are frequently present. Absent hyperglycemic response to glucagon or epinephrine administration.

Clinical aspects: Delayed growth, peculiar "doll-like" facies. Mental development can be normal; however, seizures are frequently caused by neurological impairment or by hypoglycemia. Episodes of profound hypoglycemia and lactic acidosis may be prevented by frequent daytime feeding and continuous enteral feeding at night. Renal and hepatic involvement can be observed (reduced creatinine clearance, focal segmental glomerulosclerosis, renal stones, liver adenomas, hepatocellular carcinoma, hepatomegaly with enlarged liver and kidneys, secondary platelet dysfunction with prolonged bleeding). Osteoporosis, gouty arthritis, and xanthoma are frequent. Hypertension can occur. Survival to adulthood is common with appropriate management.

Precautions before anesthesia: Obtain history of dietary management. Aim to maintain normal intake of carbohydrate as intravenous (IV) glucose infusion during perioperative period. Obtain history of abnormal bleeding. Check platelet count. Check blood glucose, electrolytes, creatinine, blood gases, and liver function regularly. Evaluate neurological function (clinical, EEG, CT).

Von Hippel Lindau Syndrome

At a glance: This syndrome is characterized by multiple clear cell neoplasms in various organs including the retina, central nervous system (CNS) hemangioblastomas (most frequently cerebellar and spinal), renal cell carcinomas, pheochromocytomas, pancreatic endocrine tumors, and cysts.

Classification: Neumann and Wiesler have classified this entity into two different types based on the presence or absence of a pheochromocytoma. Type I (without pheochromocytoma) and type II (with pheochromocytoma). In 1995, Brauch et al. subdivided type II into IIA (with pheochromocytoma) and type IIB (with pheochromocytoma and renal cell carcinoma). Recently, a type IIC was described when patients affected with von Hippel Lindau had an isolated pheochromocytoma without hemangioblastoma or renal cell carcinoma

Incidence: The estimated birth incidence in East Anglia, Norfolk, UK, is believed to be 1:36,000 live births and an estimated prevalence of heterozygotes to be 1 in 53,000. Direct and indirect estimates of the mutation rate were 4.4 per million gametes per generation and 2.32 per million gametes per generation, respectively. There are no significant associations between parental age or birth order and new mutations. In the Freiburg district of Germany, the prevalence has been calculated for this disorder to be 1 in 38,951. In the northwest of England, 83 affected persons were reported in 1996 and the calculated prevalence for this disease was estimated (heterozygotes) in the region to be 1 in 85,000 persons, with an estimated birth incidence of 1 in 45,500 live births. The incidence of the most common lesions are as follows: retinal angiomatosis (57%), cerebellar (55%), medullary (6%), and spinal (14%) hemangioblastomas; pheochromocytoma (19%), renal cysts (14%), renal cell carcinoma (24%), epididymal cystadenoma (17%), pancreatic cysts (14%), pancreatic malignancy (4%).

Genetic inheritance: The gene is a putative tumor suppressor gene responsible for von Hippel Lindau, an autosomal dominant multitumor syndrome. It is also implicated in the development of sporadic tumors including clear cell renal carcinoma and CNS hemangioblastoma. The gene has recently been isolated by positional cloning and the cDNA encodes 852 nucleotides in 3 exons. The von Hippel Lindau (VHL) gene seems to be unrelated to any known gene families.

Pathophysiology: Interfamilial differences in predisposition to pheochromocytoma in VHL reflect allelic heterogeneity such that there is a strong association between missense mutations and risk of pheochromocytoma.

Diagnosis: The presence of visceral cysts of the kidney, pancreas, and epididymis occurs not only as features of VHL but also in the general population; however, the association of those cysts with retinal, CNS hemangioblastoma may represent a more significant association for the disease. The use of markers as presymptomatic diagnosis of VHL in patients with epididymal cysts has been demonstrated to be not suitable as a diagnostic criterion. Similarly, the genetic studies suggested that VHL with or without pheochromocytomas is caused by defects within the same gene may be misleading. Renal cell carcinoma occurs as part of VHL; a second more proximal region of chromosome 3, 3p14.2, is responsible for "pure familial renal cell carcinoma." It has been suggested that the likelihood of VHL being present in an individual showing a single ocular angioma is conditional upon the age of presentation, results of DNA analysis, family history of VHL, and results of systemic screening. The presence of a positive VHL family history can lead to the diagnosis in a patient with at least 1 typical VHL tumor. Typical VHL tumors are retinal, spinal, and cerebellar hemangioblastoma; renal cell carcinoma; and pheochromocytoma. Endolymphatic sac tumors and multiple pancreatic cysts suggest a positive carriership in the presence of a positive VHL family history because they are uncommon in the general population. In contrast, renal and epididymal cysts occur very frequently in the general population and are, as sole manifestations, not reliable indicators for VHL disease. In patients with a negative family history of VHL-associated tumors, a diagnosis of VHL disease can also be made on the basis of two or more hemangioblastomas or a single hemangioblastoma in association with a visceral manifestation (e.g., pheochromocytoma or renal cell carcinoma). The suspicion for VHL can also be raised in a patient with classic VHL disease (meeting clinical diagnostic criteria) and/or first-degree family members; and/or a person from a family in which a germline VHL gene mutation has been identified (presymptomatic test). Also, a VHL-suspected patient, i.e., one with multicentric tumors in one organ, bilateral tumors, two organ systems affected, or one VHL-associated tumor at a young age (less than 50 years for hemangioblastoma and pheochromocytoma or less than 30 years for renal cell carcinoma); or a patient from a family with hemangioblastoma, renal cell carcinoma, or pheochromocytoma only can also be diagnosed.

Clinical aspects: The cardinal features of von Hippel Lindau syndrome are angiomata of the retina and hemangioblastoma of the cerebellum and/or spinal cord. Hemangioma of the spinal cord has also been reported. Pheochromocytoma occurs in some patients and will help in the classification. The combination of hypertension with angioma may lead to subarachnoid hemorrhage and the consequences associated with this clinical presentation. Hypernephroma-like renal tumors occur in some patients. Polycythemia may be due to either the hemangioblastoma of the cerebellum or the hypernephroma. Hemangiomas of the adrenals, lungs, and liver, and multiple cysts of the pancreas and kidneys have been observed in some instances.

Precaution before anesthesia: The possibility of an association with a pheochromocytoma must be eliminated. A complete history providing information about symptomatology with this vascular disease should include: symptoms of dysrhythmia or ventricular dysfunction, sudden and severe headaches, palpitations, night sweating. Catecholamine-induced cardiomyopathy may be present. A complete evaluation of the cardiovascular system must include: ECG, echocardiography, stress test if the patient is old enough. Start alpha blockade. Competitive alpha antagonists (e.g., phentolamine, prazosin) have been used but do not give the same stability as noncompetitive blockade (phenoxybenzamine). Beta blockade may be started after alpha blockade to control dysrhythmias. The minimum duration for alpha blockade is 36 hours, although the optimal period is not defined. End points used for adequate blockade have included a 5% drop in hematocrit or the maximum dose of phenoxybenzamine at which the side effects are tolerated by the individuals. Respiratory assessment: chest radiograph to exclude pulmonary congestion. Renal function: Check renal function, hypertensive nephropathy may be present and nephrectomy is occasionally necessary to achieve tumor excision. Metabolic factors: blood glucose (insulin rarely needed), exclude hypercalcemia. The presence of intracranial hemangiomas must also be evaluated. Raised intracranial pressure must be eliminated. Spinal cord tumors will also require an evaluation, and the use of sensory evoked potential conductivity should be considered prior to anesthesia.

Anesthetic considerations: In the presence of a pheochromocytoma, the anesthesia management should include a premedication, unless the level of consciousness and/or intracranial pressure prevents its administration. Invasive monitoring, central venous pressure (CVP), arterial blood pressure (BP) are mandatory. Induction of anesthesia and intubation can be a period of major cardiovascular instability. Prepare a vasodilator such as sodium nitroprusside to control surges in blood pressure during tumor manipulation. According to the local team experience other vasodilators may be used (phentolamine, calcium antagonists such as nicardipine, magnesium sulfate). Esmolol is probably the beta blockade of choice to control dysrhythmias. Hypotension following tumor excision or clamping of its venous drainage should initially be treated with volume loading but a transient infusion of the catecholamine secreted by the removed tumor is sometimes necessary. Patients with intracranial involvement may have raised intracranial pressure and caution should be taken to avoid further increases in pressure. The presence of spinal cord tumor in the cervical region may be of significant consideration during laryngoscopy and tracheal intubation since compression of the neural tissue may be caused by extension or flexion of the neck. Careful attention to patient positioning. Epidural catheter anesthesia can be used but special attention must be provided when advancing the catheter in place. This technique has been used successfully for cesarean section and neurosurgery, contributing to limit the vasodilatory effects of general anesthetics. Supplementation of general anesthesia is reported but is probably only of use for postoperative analgesia, as its intraoperative use may complicate the anesthetic. Postoperatively monitor for hypotension, hypertension, and hypoglycemia in a critical care setting.

Pharmacological implications: The pharmacological implications will be dictated by the presence or absence of a pheochromocytoma. For instance, pharmacological agents favoring release of catecholamines, histamines, and/or vasoactive agents (e.g., serotonin) must be avoided. Desflurane is contraindicated in VHL. Atropine should be used with caution.

Other conditions to be considered:

☞**PHEOCHROMOCYTOMA:** Tumor of chromaffin tissue (neuroectodermal origin), most commonly affecting the adrenal medulla (90%) but may occur in any tissue derived embryologically from the neuro-ectoderm, including any sympathetic ganglia, the gastrointestinal tract, bladder, and thorax. Catecholamine-secreting tumor.

☞**MULTIPLE ENDOCRINE NEOPLASIA:** Familial multiple endocrine tumors in parathyroid, thyroid, pancreas and or surrenals. MEN type II is the most probable because of its association with pheochromocytoma.

REFERENCES:

Choyke PL, Glenn GM, Walther MM, et al: von Hippel-Lindau disease: Genetic, clinical, and imaging features. *Radiology* 196(2):582, 1995.

Joffe D, Robins R, Benjamin A: Cesarian section and phaeochromocytoma resection in a patient with von Hippel Lindau disease. *Can J Anaesth* 40:870–874, 1993.

Mugawar M, Rajender Y, Purohit AK, et al: Anesthetic management of von Hippel Lindau syndrome for excision of cerebellar hemangioblastoma and pheochromocytoma surgery. *Anesth Analg* 86:673–675, 1998.

von Willebrand-Jüergens Disease

At a glance: A hereditary family of blood-clotting disorders caused by a deficiency of the von Willebrand factor protein and factor VIII protein, and characterized by prolonged bleeding.

Synonyms: Pseudohemophilia; Angiohemophilia; Constitutional Thrombopathy; Minot-Von Willebrand Disease; Vascular Hemophilia; Willebrand-Jüergens Disease.

Nature: Genetic, although a rare, acquired form exists.

Incidence: Prevalence worldwide is estimated at 1%. Acquired forms are much more rare.

Genetic inheritance: Autosomal dominant or recessive inheritance has been suggested as potential genetic transmission mode.

Pathophysiology: von Willebrand disease is the most common inherited bleeding disorder in humans, and is secondary to abnormalities of von Willebrand factor (vWF). There are several subtypes.

Diagnosis: Mucocutaneous bleeding with normal platelet count, elevated bleeding time, decreased ristocetin cofactor activity (ristocetin is an antibiotic that alters normal vWF structure, causing platelet aggregation), decreased vWF antigen (can be normal in type II), decreased factor VIII activity; gel electrophoresis to determine vWF structure.

Clinical aspects: There are several subtypes. *Type I* has a partial quantitative defect with normal structure, comprises 70% of cases, and has mild to moderate bleeding; it is autosomal dominant. *Type II* has both qualitative and quantitative defects. *Type IIA* (10% of cases) has mild to moderate bleeding and a poor response to desmopressin acetate, while *type IIB* (<5% of cases) has mild to moderate

bleeding, thrombocytopenia, and a contraindication to desmopressin acetate. *Type IIM* (reportable) has a variable bleeding disorder with decreased vWF:Ag, vWF activity, and factor VII:C. *Type IIN* (reportable and autosomal recessive) has a variable bleeding disorder that may resemble hemophilia A. *Type III* (severe and rare, may be autosomal recessive) has a complete deficiency of vWF. *Acquired von Willebrand Disease* is associated with myeloproliferative disease, hypothyroidism, B-cell disorders, and cardiovascular defects, resembles type 1 or 2, and has decreased plasma vWF antigen and normal platelet vWF antigen.

Treatment: Desmopressin acetate, which increases the release of vWF, has a favorable response in 80% of type I patients. The response in type II diseases is variable, because an increased release of qualitatively poor vWF is not useful for platelet binding. Desmopressin acetate may be contraindicated in type IIB, because platelet aggregation may exacerbate thrombocytopenia, but this is controversial. Estrogen may also increase production of vWF. Replacement therapy, for failures or contraindications to desmopressin acetate, was formerly with cryoprecipitate. However, virally inactivated concentrates of factor VIII now exist, although the content of vWF varies. The products of choice are Hemate-P and VHP vWF concentrate. Treatment is empiric, although it should be continued for 7 to 10 days after major surgical procedures, and for 3 to 5 days after minor ones; postpartum hemorrhage may require 1 month of therapy. A suggested regimen for Hemate-P in type III von Willebrand disease for major surgery is bolus of 30 to 40 IU/kg followed by 15 to 25 IU/kg q12h × 3d, then 15 to 25 IU/kg daily for 3 to 5 days.

Precautions before anesthesia: Review medical history and physical examination, especially of prior surgeries. Consult hematologist for treatment regimens.

Anesthetic considerations: Avoid regional anesthesia and intramuscular injections. Blood bank support (fresh-frozen plasma and platelets are effective in massive transfusion).

Pharmacological implications: Controversial contraindication to desmopressin acetate in type IIB von Willebrand disease. Avoid aspirin.

REFERENCES:

Menache D: New treatments of von Willebrand disease: Plasma-derived von Willebrand factor concentrates. *Thromb Haemost* 78(1):566, 1997.

Nitu-Whalley IC, Griffioen A, Harrington C, et al: Retrospective review of the management of elective surgery with desmopressin and clotting factor concentrates in patients with von Willebrand disease. *Am J Hematol* 66(4):280, 2001.

Stedeford JC, Pittman JA: Von Willebrand's disease and neuroaxial anaesthesia. *Anaesthesia* 55(12):1228, 2000.

Waardenburg Syndrome

At a glance: An auditory pigmentary syndrome characterized by hypopigmentation of the skin, iris, hair and stria vascularis of the cochlea. Most patients present with two different colored eyes, white forelock and eyelashes, and premature graying of the hair. Moderate acrocephaly, lack of osseous fusion of the short tubular bones, oligodactyly of the feet, short stature, pericardial cysts, rectal prolapse, and deformed ears are reported. Other features include hypoplastic maxilla, asymmetry of hands, deformity of the first phalanx of the head, absence of the first digit of the foot, and bifid distal phalanges of the second and third toes.

Synonyms: Petrus Johannes Waardenburg Syndrome (Dutch ophthalmologist, 1886–1979); WS I.

Incidence: All forms of WS together, estimates are that about 1:40,000 individuals of the general population are affected by this disorder, which may be responsible for up to 3% of patients with congenital deafness. In Kenya, the estimated frequency is reported at 1:20,000 persons. It is also reported at 1:212,000 individuals in the general population of the Netherlands.

Genetic inheritance: (see also "Clinical Aspects") Autosomal dominant inheritance characterizes Waardenburg Syndrome Type 1 (WS 1), which has been mapped to 2q35. If dystopia canthorum (lateral displacement of the inner canthi of the eyes) is absent, the syndrome is called WS Type 2. WS 3 is a severe form of this disorder in which both, heterozygosity and homozygosity of mutations in the *PAX3* gene (paired box gene 3) have been reported.

Pathophysiology: Almost all cases are at least due in part to mutations of the *PAX3* gene (paired box gene 3), which is involved in the formation of the caudal neural crest derivatives and the migration of myoblasts into the extremities. Children with this syndrome have a normal life expectancy.

Diagnosis: Two major or one major plus two minor features must be present for the diagnosis. *Major features:* congenital sensory hearing loss and pigmentary disturbance of the iris with different-colored eyes or segmental heterochromia; hair hypopigmentation; affected first-degree relative. *Minor features:* congenital leukoderma, medial eyebrow flare, high nasal root, nasal alae hypoplasia, premature graying of scalp.

Clinical aspects: Four different types of Waardenburg Syndrome have been defined:

Waardenburg Syndrome Type 1 (WS 1): It was in 1947, when the Dutch ophthalmologist and geneticist Petrus Johannes Waardenburg first presented a patient with sensorineural hearing loss, dystopia canthorum (lateral displacement of the inner canthi of the eyes), hypertrichosis of the medial aspect of the eyebrows, broad nasal bridge, and pigment anomalies of skin (albinism), iris (heterochromia iridis) retina, and hair (white forelock or poliosis) to the Swiss Society of Genetics. After he found several more patients with similar findings, Waardenburg fully described what is now known as WS 1.

Waardenburg Syndrome Type 2 (WS 2): Has all the features of WS 1, except dystopia canthorum. Both WS 1 and WS 2 are transmitted as autosomal dominant conditions with the responsible gene being mapped to 2q35. Mutations in the microphthalmia-associated transcription factor (MITF) gene, located on chromosome band

3p14.1–p12.3, are responsible for some of the cases of WS 2, while others have been linked to band 1p.

Waardenburg syndrome type 3 (WS 3) (Synonym: Klein-Waardenburg Syndrome): Shows, in addition to the findings of WS 1, musculoskeletal abnormalities (e.g., hypoplasia of the musculoskeletal system with severe flexion contractures, spastic paraplegia, winged scapulae, aplasia of the first two ribs, sacral anomalies, carpal bone fusion, and bilateral syndactylies), microcephaly, and mental retardation. WS 3 is also autosomal-dominant transmitted and some of the patients have even been found to be homozygous for the defect. The defect has been mapped to the same locus as WS 1 and WS 2.

Waardenburg syndrome type 4 (WS 4) (Synonym: Waardenburg-Shah Syndrome): In addition to the features of WS 1, this type is associated with Hirschsprung disease. The inheritance is either autosomal recessive or autosomal dominant and the genetic defect seems

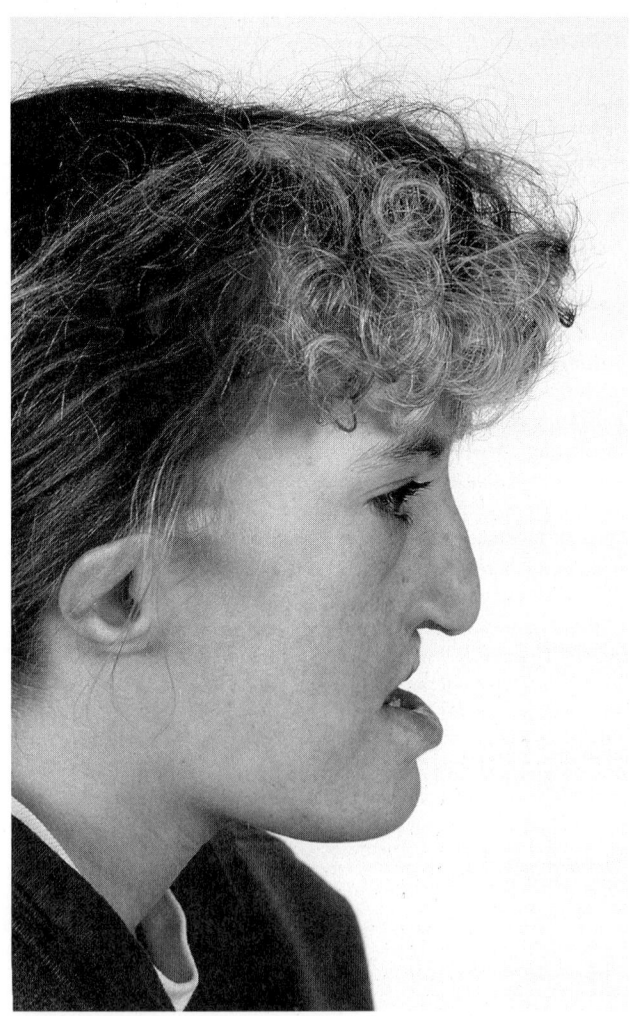

Waardenburg syndrome Hypopigmentation of the hair (white forelock), high nasal root, hypoplasia of the nasal alae, short and retropositioned maxilla, short philtrum, and a dysplastic ear in a 14-year-old girl with sensorineural hearing loss.

to also involve either the endothelin-3 (EDN3) or the endothelin-B receptor (EDNRB) genes and has been mapped to several different gene loci (13q22, 22q13, 20q13.2-q13.3).

Precautions before anesthesia: Depends on the severity of the disease. If there are significant contractures and muscular hypoplasia, then respiratory reserve may be reduced and evaluation with chest radiographs, arterial blood gas, and pulmonary function tests would be of value. The cardiac function should be assessed using echocardiography. The presence of facial abnormalities should be evaluated in preparation for difficult tracheal intubation. Assess the presence of pericardial cysts and cardiovascular compromise. Depending on the surgical procedure prolonged ventilation may be required.

Anesthetic considerations: Mental retardation and hearing deficit may result in poor cooperation at time of induction and premedication may be appropriate. Both direct laryngoscopy and tracheal intubation may be difficult and proper planning should be done. The accessibility to a laryngeal mask airway and/or fiberoptic equipment might be indicated. Intravenous access and positioning on the table may be difficult. Special attention must be provided to reduce pressure point using proper padding. Postoperative analgesia may be uneasy with mental retardation, musculoskeletal abnormalities, and reduced respiratory reserve.

Pharmacological implications: Neuromuscular relaxants may be unnecessary and should be used cautiously. Succinylcholine is relatively contraindicated. Opioids should be used with caution if respiratory reserve is critical. Analgesia using regional techniques should be considered.

REFERENCES:

DeStefano AL, Cupples LA, Arnos KS, et al: Correlation between Waardenburg syndrome phenotype and genotype in a population of individuals with identified PAX3 mutations. *Hum Genet* 102:499, 1998.

Read AP, Newton VE: Waardenburg syndrome. *J Med Genet* 34:656, 1997.

Shah KN, Dalal SJ, Desai MP, et al: White forelock, pigmentary disorder of irides, and long segment Hirschsprung disease: Possible variant of Waardenburg syndrome. *J Paediatr* 99:432, 1981.

Wadia-Swami Syndrome

At a glance: A spinocerebellar degeneration. Abnormal eye movements include absent rapid saccades (scanning) and abnormally slow pursuit (tracking). Lethal within 10 years of onset.

Synonym: Cerebellar Degeneration with Slow Eye Movements.

Incidence and genetic inheritance: Rare disease with autosomal dominant inheritance (also possibly an autosomal recessive form).

Clinical aspects: Slowing of all eye movements thought to be caused by a brainstem lesion of the paramedian pontine reticular formation. Clinical features include an abnormal accompanying movements of head and neck; spinocerebellar degeneration with abnormal gait (ataxia); progressive intellectual impairment, extrapyramidal dysfunction and peripheral neuropathy. Skeletal abnormalities can occur. Muscle biopsy shows nonspecific mitochondrial abnormalities. Magnetic resonance imaging studies of the brain show a significant degree of cerebellar and brainstem atrophy. Death occurs within 10 years of onset.

Anesthetic considerations: It is recommended to evaluate carefully the neurological function (clinical, EEG, CT/MRI) and mus-

cular condition for the presence of myotonia. Careful intraoperative positioning is needed.

REFERENCE:

Najim al-Dim AS, al-kurdi A, Dasouki M, et al: Autosomal recessive ataxia, slow eye movements and psychomotor retardation. *J Neurol Sci* 12(4):61, 1994.

Wadia NH, Swami RK: A new form of heredo-familial spinocerebellar degeneration with slow eye movements. *Brain* 94:359, 1971.

Wagner Syndrome

At a glance: This syndrome is characterized by many optical malformations (e.g., ensheathed retinal vessels, retinal pigmentation, circular membranes in a liquefied vitreous, choroidal atrophy) with a progressive clinical course that ends with optic atrophy and blindness. Often associated with Stickler syndrome.

Synonym: Wagner Vitreoretinal Degeneration; Wagner Haloid Retinal Degeneration Syndrome; Erosive Vitreoretinopathy; Hyaloideoretinal Degeneration of Wagner.

History: First described in 1938 by Hans Wagner, Swiss ophthalmologist.

Genetic inheritance: Autosomal dominant.

Pathophysiology: Unknown. Causal gene is located on chromosome 5 (in the 5q13–q14 area).

Diagnosis: Subnormal electroretinographic response (ERG), retinal detachment associated with poor surgical prognosis, lattice degeneration, retinoschisis, cataract, and glaucoma.

Clinical aspects: *Optical features* include an optically empty vitreous cavity that is pervaded by a few vitreous fibers or membranes, narrow and sheathed retinal vessels, pigment spots in the peripheral fundus or along the retinal vessels, atrophy of the choroids, complicated cataract, myopia, concentric contraction of the visual fields, and, in the advance stage, optic atrophy. Others features involve the *head* (characteristic facies: epicanthus, broad sunken nasal bridge, receding chin associated with micrognathia and cleft palate). Accelerated growth occurs, together with *skeletal* abnormalities such as broad proximal phalanges, broad middle phalanges, and genu valgum.

Precautions before anesthesia: Careful assessment of airway (clinical, radiographs, fiberoptic if necessary).

Anesthetic considerations: Difficult tracheal intubation because of micrognathia, receding chin, and cleft palate must be anticipated. A laryngeal mask airway or fiberoptic equipment should be available. Careful positioning of patient and proper padding of pressure point must be provided because of skeletal abnormalities.

Pharmacological implications: Muscle relaxant should be avoided until airway is secured and lung ventilation confirmed. Medications for glaucoma include the organophosphates such as echothiophate and isofluorphate. These drugs inhibit serum cholinesterase, which is responsible for the hydrolysis and inactivation of succinylcholine and the ester-type local anesthetics (e.g., procaine, chloroprocaine and tetracaine). These ester-type local anesthetics should be avoided in patients treated with eye-drops containing organophosphate. Review current medication in view of glaucoma (avoid atropine and other drugs incriminated). Avoid drugs that may increase intraocular pressure in the presence of glaucoma.

Other conditions to be considered:

☞**O**TOSPONDYLOMEGAEPIPHYSEAL **D**YSPLASIA (OSMED): A disease with peculiar facies and severe degenerative joint disease of the osteoarthritis type affecting predominantly the hips, knees, elbows, and shoulders.

☞**STICKLER SYNDROME:** This autosomal dominant inherited disorder is most often caused by mutation in the COL2A1 gene, while mutations in the COL11A1 and COL11A2 are less common. The pathognomonic feature is the abnormal vitreous gel architecture, which is associated with high, congenital, and nonprogressive myopia and a significantly increased risk of rhegmatogenous (associated with retinal tears) retinal detachment. According to the vitreous gel anomaly, two subtypes of Stickler syndrome can be distinguished (otherwise, the same clinical findings apply). Other signs include midface hypoplasia, flat nasal bridge, short nose with anteverted nares, micrognathia, and cleft palate. Joint hypermobility usually improves with age, while degenerative osteoarthritic symptoms (mainly hip and knee) are progressive and become manifest in the third or fourth decade of life. Conductive (secondary to cleft palate with chronic otitis media), but predominantly sensorineural hearing loss is common. These patients are most often mentally normal and of normal height. Mitral valve prolapse syndrome ☞(Barlow Syndrome) has been reported to be a common finding in these patients (patients may need subacute bacterial endocarditis prophylaxis if thickened leaflets or signs of regurgitation are present.

WEISSENBACHER-ZWEYMÜLLER SYNDROME (Pierre Robin Syndrome with Fetal Chondrodysplasia): Micrognathia, and rhizomelic chondrodysplasia with enlargement of the epi- and metaphyses of the long bones resulting in a typical dumbbell-shape (especially of humeri and femora) are the hallmarks of this autosomal recessive inherited syndrome. However, the overall changes are milder than in OSMED and they tend to resolve with increasing age with impressive catch-up growth finally resulting in normal adult height. Midface hypoplasia, eye (optic nerve hypoplasia, severe myopia, retinal detachment) and ear (sensorineural hearing loss) anomalies, vertebral coronal clefts, and meningoceles/encephaloceles have also been described in some of these patients. Psychomotor development is often delayed.

☞**MARSHALL SYNDROME:** A rare genetic disorder inherited as an autosomal dominant trait. The major clinical features include distinctive flat sunken midface with a typical nose in the form of a saddle, nostrils turned upward, and hypertelorism. The calvaria is significantly thicker than normal and calcium deposits can be found in the skull. Hearing loss may range from slight to severe and is most often the result of sensorineural damage. The eyes often show the presence of cataracts, esotropia, hypertropia, retinal detachment, and glaucoma.

GOLDMANN-FAVRE SYNDROME (Enhanced S-Cone Syndrome; Retinoschisis with Early Hemeralopia; Favre Hyaloideoretinal Degeneration): A hereditary retinal condition that represents a gain in the function of photoreceptors in comparison with other hereditary human retinal degenerative diseases usually affecting the mature photoreceptor topography by reducing the number of cells through neuronal apoptosis, leading to blindness. This disorder is an autosomal recessive retinopathy in which patients have increased sensitivity to blue light; since perception of blue light is mediated by the least populous cone photoreceptor subtype, the S (short wavelength, blue) cones. Individuals suffer early in life from visual loss and night blindness.

CERVENKA SYNDROME: Autosomal dominant hyaloideoretinal degeneration with cleft palate, flattening of the midface and mental retardation.

REFERENCES:

Gupta SK, Leonard BC, Damji KF, et al.: A frame shift mutation in a tissue-specific alternatively spliced exon of collagen 2A1 in Wagner Vitreoretinal Degeneration. *Am J Ophtalmol* 133:203–210, 2002.

Hirose T, Lee KY: Wagner's hereditary vitreoretinal degeneration and retinal detachment. *Arch Ophthalmol* 89:176, 1973.

Perveen R, Hart-Holden N, Dixon MJ, at al: Refined genetic and physical localization of the Wagner Disease (WGN 1) locus and the genes CRTL 1 and CSPG2 to a 2-to 2.5-cM region of chromosome 5q14.3. *Genomics* 57:219–26, 1999.

WAGR Syndrome

At a glance: WAGR is an acronym for *W*ilms tumor, *A*niridia, *G*enitourinary anomalies (e.g., ambiguous genitalia, gonadoblastoma), and mental *R*etardation.

Synonyms: Brusa-Torricelli syndrome; Chromosome 11p Deletion Syndrome; 11p– Syndrome; Chromosome 11p Monosomy; Deletion 11p Syndrome; Monosomy 11p; Partial Monosomy 11p; Aniridia-Wilms Tumor syndrome.

History: First described by the two Italian physicians P. Brusa and C. Torricelli in 1953.

Genetic inheritance: Autosomal dominant; generally sporadic.

Pathophysiology: Patient presents with constitutional deletions at 11p13 and alteration of the WT1 gene (Wilms tumor).

Diagnosis: Characteristic association of aniridia, nephroblastoma, and mental retardation. Affects both sexes. More often in males.

Clinical aspects: Presents with significant phenotypic variability. Clinical features can involve head and neck with microcephaly, cranial asymmetry, brachycephaly, prominent forehead, long, narrow face, large fontanelles, premature synostosis of metopic sutures, biparietal foramina, micrognathia, high and narrow palate, prominent lower lip, and down-turned upper lip. The eyes present with various abnormalities, including aniridia, glaucoma, corneal opacity, optic atrophy, strabismus, cataracts, nystagmus, blepharoptosis, and blepharophimosis; blindness is not uncommon. Ears and nose are often malformed. Genitourinary tract malformations are constant and can be associated with Wilms tumor, hypospadias, micropenis with anomalies of urethra, cryptorchidism, gonadal dysgenesis, horseshoe or fused kidneys, duplication of upper urinary tract, kidney aplasia, or hypoplasia. Various hernias are frequent. Hemihypertrophy of the body, multiple exostoses, kyphoscoliosis, clinodactyly, and abnormal dermatoglyphics have been observed. Cardiomyopathy or ventricular septal defect can be present.

Precautions before anesthesia: Evaluate anatomy in regard to tracheal intubation (clinically, radiography) because of micrognathia; cardiac function (clinically, echocardiography, radionuclide imaging, electrocardiogram); and renal function (ultrasound, scintigraphy, laboratory investigations including creatinine, urea, and electrolytes).

Anesthetic considerations: Direct laryngoscopy can be difficult because of micrognathia and may require adapted anesthetic management. Perioperative fluid regimen should be adapted to renal function. Cautious intraoperative positioning is needed because of skeletal deformation. Central neuraxial anesthesia techniques are not contraindicated, but can be difficult to perform because of kyphoscoliosis and exostosis. Pupillary signs for assessment of depth of anesthesia and neurologic examination are not usable in these patients.

Pharmacological implications: Avoid nephrotoxic drugs. Consider interaction between chemotherapeutics and anesthetic drugs. Prophylactic antibiotics in case of cardiopathy and/or immunosuppression as indicated.

Other conditions to be considered:

☞**DENYS-DRASH SYNDROME:** Gonadal dysgenesis and nephropathy leading to renal failure. Wilms tumor is present in all cases.

☞**BECKWITH-WIEDEMANN SYNDROME:** Organomegaly, hemihypertrophy, renal cyst, adrenal cytomegaly, and Wilms tumor.

WAGRO: WAGR syndrome with severe obesity.

REFERENCES:

Fischbach BV, Trout KL, Lewis J, et al: WAGR syndrome: a clinical review of 54 cases. *Pediatrics* 116:984, 2005.

Yanagidate F, Dohi S, Iizawa A: Anaesthetic management for a patient with WAGR syndrome. *Anaesthesia* 56:1215, 2001.

Waterhouse-Friderichsen Syndrome

At a glance: Fulminant disease associated with bilateral adrenal hemorrhage as a result of coagulopathy associated with severe sepsis, classically meningococcemia (*Neisseria meningitidis* most common), but occasionally with other infections (influenza or colon bacillus). Fatal if not treated immediately.

Synonyms: Friderichsen Syndrome; Friderichsen-Waterhouse Syndrome; Friderichsen-Waterhouse-Bamatter Syndrome; March-and-Waterhouse-Friderichsen Syndrome.

History: Acquired postinfectious disease that was first described by Arthur Francis Voelcker in 1894, and subsequently explained by Carl Friderichsen, Danish pediatrician in 1918.

Incidence: Attack rate of meningococcal disease is highest for children between 6 months and 1 year of age. Another, but lower, incidence has been reported during adolescence; 10 to 20% of patients with generalized meningococcal infection develop the fulminant meningococcemia.

Pathophysiology: Dissemination of meningococci via the blood stream from the primary focus of infection in the nasopharynx, resulting in extensive and acute inflammatory reaction in various organs, particularly the meninges. It is postulated that endotoxin released from the diplococci induces a severe reaction including significant vasomotor disturbance, myocardial failure, disseminated intravascular coagulopathy (DIC), bleeding, and focal necrosis in the adrenal glands and skin.

Diagnosis: Abrupt and rapid deterioration of clinical symptoms; hematological (high polymorphonuclear leukocyte counts, thrombocytopenia, evidence of DIC); biochemical (raised serum urea and creatinine levels, electrolyte disturbances), and clinical (cyanotic pallor, a petechial or purpuric rash, pale with coldness and cyanosis of the extremities as a result of generalized vasoconstriction). Fever is initially moderate but subsequently becomes high.

Clinical aspects: Circulatory collapse, which is characterized by clammy skin, high fever, a rapid, thready pulse, labored respiration, and coma. Other clinical features may include dehydration, vomiting, diarrhea, oliguria, and neck stiffness, and occasionally anuria. Usually occurs in infants or children, occasionally in adults. Death usually occurs after a few hours if not treated. Adrenal insufficiency being the immediate cause. Patients who recover may suffer from extensive sloughing of the skin and loss of digits as a result of gangrene.

Precautions before anesthesia: Evaluate cardiac function (clinical, echography, Swan-Ganz catheter), adrenal function (clinical, electrolytes), coagulation and hemostasis (complete laboratory test including coagulation factors, soluble complexes), and renal and liver functions (clinical, laboratory).

Anesthetic considerations: Surgical indications are strictly limited in such patients. Anesthesia requires aggressive resuscitation using plasma expanders and inotropes, with the aid of invasive hemodynamic monitoring through arterial lines, central venous catheter, and pulmonary arterial catheter, if indicated. Specific antibiotic therapy, preferably high-dose penicillin, should be started as soon as possible because of the natural frequency of meningococcus infectious spread. Corticosteroids may also be indicated if patients remain unresponsive to fluid resuscitation and inotropic therapy. Secure airway immediately in comatose patients; use positive pressure ventilatory support to optimize oxygen delivery. Onset of pulmonary edema or acute respiratory distress syndrome requires the use of positive end-expiratory pressure (PEEP). Avoid nasal intubation with its increased risk of bleeding from the adenoids in patients with DIC. Treatment of elevated intracranial pressure may also be necessary, as well as insertion of devices to monitor intracranial pressure. Patients who survive the first few days of infection remain at risk for arrhythmias, myocarditis, and pericarditis. Regional anesthesia should be avoided, but controversies exist about providing vasodilatation that could help treat peripheral ischemic lesions. Central blockade is a high risk procedure in this indication because of the bleeding risk and because of its potential action on blood pressure; plexus blockade presents a lower risk.

Pharmacological implications: Avoid anesthetic drugs that could affect contractility and cardiac output. Ketamine is a better choice if duration of shock is not prolonged (because of its action via catecholamine release). However, its use must be limited to patients who do not already present with cardiovascular collapse since most endogenous catecholamine reserves may be exhausted and worsening of the collapse may happen. Hypnomidate is best avoided because of its action on the adrenal glands. If regional anesthesia is provided, avoid bupivacaine because of its cardiac toxicity. Neuraxial blockade is not recommended. Peripheral block however may be used to increase peripheral circulation.

Other conditions to be considered:

☞**SCHÖNLEIN-HENOCH PURPURA SYNDROME:** Characterized by purplish or brownish red discolorations on the skin and often associated with internal bleeding in various areas of the body. It affects the joints, gastrointestinal (GI), system, and kidneys. The central nervous system (CNS) can be, very rarely, affected.

RHEUMATIC FEVER: The result of streptococcal infection. This inflammatory syndrome presents initially with moderate fever, sore throat, fatigue and a red rash. Major complications can include cardiovascular complications, severe joint pain and arthritis, dyskinetic movements with characteristic grimaces.

ROCKY MOUNTAIN SPOTTED FEVER: A tick-borne disease presenting after an incubation period of 2 to 12 days. The initial symptoms include the presence of gradual or abrupt rise in body temperature, followed by a characteristic purplish skin rash on the wrists and ankles. The fever and the rash usually become more severe after 7 to 14 days. The diagnosis is confirmed by a blood test.

TOXIC SHOCK SYNDROME: Symptoms appear very suddenly and manifest mostly by severe hyperthermia. The clinical features include headache, sore throat, and conjunctivitis. Other early symptoms include profound lethargy, periods of disorientation, vomiting, severe diarrhea, and a diffuse sunburn-like rash leading to sloughing of skin after several days. In severe cases, the syndrome may progress to cardiovascular shock and circulatory collapse within 48 hours.

INFECTIVE ENDOCARDITIS: Usually very sudden. Low back pain, arthralgia, and/or myalgia are common. Fever, night sweats, chills, headache and loss of appetite may also occur. Hematuria, petechiae, and oval spots on the retina can be observed.

REFERENCES:

Friderichsen C: Nebennierenapoplexie bei kleinen Kindern. *Jahrbuch für Kinderhilkunde* 87:109, 1918.

Willis TM, Hopp RJ, Romero JR, et al: The protective effect of brachial plexus palsy in purpura fulminans. *Pediatr Neurol* 24(5):379, 2001.

Watson Syndrome

At a glance: A rare disease combining pulmonary valvular stenosis with "café-au-lait" spots, dull intelligence and short stature. Other features include macrocephaly and Lisch nodules. In most cases, a condition that overlaps those of neurofibromatosis and the Noonan syndrome.

Synonyms: Neurofibromatosis-Noonan Syndrome; Neurofibromatosis with Noonan Phenotype.

Genetic inheritance: Autosomal dominant (possibly allelic with neurofibromatosis type 1 [NF1]).

Pathophysiology: Possibly caused by a mutation in the NF1 gene located on 17q11.2.

Diagnosis: Characterized by pulmonary valvular stenosis, café-au-lait spots, low-normal intelligence, and short stature.

Clinical aspects: Patients have short stature. Clinical features involve *head and neck* (macrocephaly, short neck, hypertelorism, broad forehead, down-slanted fissures, ptosis, puffy eyelids, triangular face, deeply grooved or flat philtrum, excess nuchal skin, large ears, epicanthic folds), *musculoskeletal system* (limited knee and ankle movement, pectus excavatum, scoliosis kyphosis), central nervous system (CNS) (hypotonia, seizures, mental retardation), and *heart* (ectasia of coronary arteries, pulmonary valve). Other features can include retroperitoneal or visceral neurofibromata, ectopic testes, hypospadias, and inguinal hernia.

Precautions before anesthesia: Evaluate cardiac function (clinical, ECG, echocardiography), neurological function (clinical, CT, EEG) and for potential difficulty during direct laryngoscopy and tracheal intubation because of the possible existence of neurofibromata in the airway (clinical, radiographs, fiberoptic if necessary).

Anesthetic considerations: The anesthetic management will be dictated by the presence of cardiovascular and/or neurological involvement. Care in positioning patient in view of limited knee and ankle movement. The use of regional anesthesia will be limited by the existence of neurofibromata.

Pharmacological implications: Muscle relaxants should be used only after airway is secure and lung ventilation confirmed. Controversies exist about muscle relaxant (both nondepolarizing and depolarizing) action duration in patients affected with neurofibromatosis. Monitoring of the neuromuscular function is necessary. Consider interaction between anesthetic drugs and antiepileptic treatment.

Other conditions to be considered:

☞**NEUROFIBROMATOSIS GENERALISATA:** Rare genetic disorder characterized by neurofibromas and hypo- or hyperpigmentation of the skin.

☞**MCCUNE-ALBRIGHT SYNDROME:** Characterized by café-au-lait spots and very early puberty. The other features include skeletal dysplasia, bone fractures, severe pain, and limited mobility. Hyperthyroidism has been reported.

☞**NOONAN SYNDROME:** A rare genetic disorder characterized by distinctive craniofacial features, including ocular hypertelorism, severe ptosis, prominent low-set ears and pterygium colli. Also, the presence of short stature associated with characteristic abnormalities of the sternum is important in the diagnosis. It is inherited as an autosomal dominant trait.

☞**PROTEUS SYNDROME:** A rare genetic disorder characterized by asymmetric growth of the body usually in the first year of life. Abnormalities of the skin, face, eyes, ears, lungs, skeletal muscles, and nerves occur, usually because one side of the body grows faster than the other. Other clinical features include soft tissue tumors (e.g., hemangiomas, lipomas, and lymphangiomas). Other symptoms may include mental impairment, seizures, visual abnormalities, and cysts in the lungs.

☞**TUBEROUS SCLEROSIS:** A rare inherited neurological disorder characterized by seizures, mental retardation, lesions of the eyes and skin; and brain tumors. The age of onset is usually during infancy or early childhood. Approximately 60 to 90% of infants have café-au-lait spots or hypomelanotic spots at birth. About 80% of affected children have seizures associated with myoclonic jerks as their first symptoms.

REFERENCES:

Allanson JE, Upadhyaya M, Watson GH, et al: Watson syndrome: Is it a subtype of type 1 neurofibromatosis? *J Med Genet* 28:752, 1991.

Hirsch NP, Murphy A, Radcliffe JJ: Neurofibromatosis: Clinical presentations and anaesthetic implications. *Br J Anaesth* 86(4):555, 2001.

Tassabehji M, Strachan T, Sharland M, et al: Tandem duplication within a neurofibromatosis type I (NF1) gene exon in a family with features of Watson syndrome and Noonan syndrome. *Am J Hum Genet* 53:90, 1993.

Weaver Syndrome

At a glance: Rare syndrome of accelerated growth and osseous maturation, unusual craniofacial appearance, hoarse and low-pitched cry, and hypertonia with camptodactyly.

Synonyms: Weaver-Smith Syndrome; WSS.

History: First described in 1974 by David D. Weaver, American physician and David Weyhe Smith, American pediatrician.

Genetic inheritance: Isolated cases. Autosomal dominant inheritance presumed.

Pathophysiology: Caused by mutation in the nuclear receptor-binding Su-var (NSD1 gene), which is located on 5q35.

Diagnosis: Clinically by characteristic facies associated with tall stature, large head, ears, and hands, and a low-pitched voice.

Clinical aspects: Increased prenatal weight and height. Development and speech are delayed; there are mental retardation and behavioral problems. Others features involve *head and neck* (flattened occiput, short broad neck, long philtrum, retrognathia, anterior and cephalad position of the larynx, strabismus, hypertelorism, epicanthal folds, down-slanting palpebral fissures, depressed nasal bridge), *skeleton* (short ribs, disharmonic and advanced bone age, scoliosis, kyphosis, small iliac wings, coxa valga, limited elbow and knee extension, flared metaphyses, camptodactyly, clinodactyly, broad thumbs, feet malformations), genitourinary (GU) (inverted nipples, inguinal hernia, hydrocele, cryptorchism), *skin* (loose skin, thin hair and nails), and central nervous system (CNS) (hypertonia, spasticity, seizures, absent septum pellucidum, lateral ventricle dilatation). Congenital cardiac defects may occur.

Precautions before anesthesia: Evaluate carefully the oropharyngeal anatomy for eventual direct laryngoscopy and tracheal intubation (clinical, radiographs), neurological function (clinical, CT/MRI, EEG), renal function (clinical, echography, lab) and cardiac function (clinical, ECG, echography).

Anesthetic considerations: Tracheal intubation can be difficult because of retrognathia, short broad neck and an anterior and cephalad position of the larynx. It may require adapted anesthetic management. Fiberoptic intubation can be useful. The accessibility to a laryngeal mask airway in case of failed tracheal intubation may also be very useful. Careful intraoperative positioning is needed because of skeletal deformities. Regional anesthesia is not contraindicated but can be difficult to realize because of deformations and spasticity.

Pharmacological implications: Consider interaction between antiepileptic treatment and anesthetic drugs. Avoid muscle relaxants until airway is secured and lung ventilation is confirmed.

Other conditions to be considered:

☞**MARSHALL-SMITH SYNDROME:** Considered similar to the Weaver-Smith syndrome because of the early and rapidly progressive growth and bone maturation. Individuals affected with Marshall-Smith syndrome are underweight in relation to their height and may present with respiratory problems.

☞**McCUNE-ALBRIGHT SYNDROME:** Involves the endocrine and musculo-skeletal systems in children. It is characterized by precocious sexual development, osseous pain caused by alteration of bone integrity, leading to skeleton deformity and disability. Most individuals present with changes in skin pigmentation. Children affected by this disorder present as excessively tall during childhood but smaller during adolescence.

GIGANTISM: Occurs before puberty and is characterized by excessive growth during childhood with relatively normal body proportions and sexual development. Height sometimes reaches 7 or 8 feet.

☞**SOTOS SYNDROME:** A rare hereditary disorder characterized by excessive growth (over the 90th percentile) during the first 4 to 5 years of life. It may affect the CNS, presenting with violent behavior, irritability, clumsiness, an awkward gait, and mental retardation.

REFERENCES:

Celebioglu B, Yener F: Anaesthesia for open-heart surgery in a patient with Weaver's syndrome. *Eur J Anaesthesiol* 19(12):897, 2002.

Crawford MW, Rohan D: The upper airway in Weaver Syndrome. *Paediatr Anaesth* 15(10):893, 2005.

Douglas J, Hanks S, Temple IK, et al: NSD1 mutations are the major cause of Sotos syndrome and occur in some cases of Weaver syndrome but are rare in other overgrowth phenotypes. *Am J Hum Genet* 72(1):132, 2003.

Weaver DD, Graham CB, Thomas IT, et al: A new overgrowth syndrome with accelerated skeletal maturation, unusual facies, and camptodactyly. *J Pediatr* 84:547, 1974.

Weber-Christian Disease

At a glance: A chronic disorder characterized by relapsing febrile episodes and panniculitis. Systemic manifestations as a result of visceral involvement may be present.

Synonyms: Lipophagic Panniculitis; Nodular non-Suppurative Panniculitis; Pfeiffer-Weber-Christian Syndrome.

History: This recurring inflammation in the fat layer of the skin was first described by Victor Pfeiffer, German physician in 1892.

Incidence: Unknown. Some authors think that some of these patients were misdiagnosed for other diseases, for example, for subcutaneous T-cell lymphomas.

Diagnosis: The diagnosis is made on the aspect of the skin and subcutaneous biopsy. Differential diagnosis with the other panniculitis must be made. Weber-Christian Disease (WCD) is usually a diagnosis by default, i.e., being unable to establish an underlying etiology or pathogenesis. The most current misdiagnoses are lupus profundus, all the collagen vascular diseases: alpha-1 antitrypsin deficiency, pancreatic disease, generalized lipodystrophy, paraproteinemia with C-1 inhibitor deficiency, eosinophilic myalgia of fasciitis syndromes and in children, the rare Rothmann-Makay syndrome.

Clinical aspects: It is characterized by recurrent febrile episodes and erythematosus subcutaneous nodules. Recurrent crops of symmetrical, tender lesions, 1 to 2 cm in size, may appear in any area. These nodules rarely suppurate, and spontaneous regression results in a hyperpigmented atrophic scar that is depressed consequent to subcutaneous fat necrosis. Weber-Christian disease implies systemic involvement when the skin lesions are accompanied by arthralgia, myalgias, and abdominal pain. In severe instances, the inflammation can involve the liver, lungs, myocardium, spleen, kidneys, and adrenal glands. Xanthogranuloma of the dura are described.

Precautions before anesthesia: A complete medical history of the severity of the illness must be up to date. Assess for involvement of kidneys, lung, and heart. Evaluate biology (cell blood count, creatinine, liver enzymes). Check for the possibility of congestive heart failure (echocardiography if necessary).

Anesthetic considerations: Xanthogranulomatous masses may appear everywhere within the body including the dura mater. The size of the infiltrates can be microscopic infiltration to 8 cm in diameter. The presence of these nodules should be considered when using a locoregional anesthesia.

Pharmacological implications: The administration of supplemental steroid stress doses must be considered in patients receiving chronic steroid treatment.

Other conditions to be considered:

☞**SWEET SYNDROME:** A rare skin disorder with an unknown genetic or acquired cause. It is characterized by fever, arthritis, and the sudden onset of a severe cutaneous rash. The rash consists of an asymmetric distribution of bluish-red, tender papules that usually occur on the arms, legs, face or neck. In approximately 80% of cases, it is idiopathic and spontaneous. This clinical manifestation can be associated, in 10 to 20% of cases, with hematologic malignancy (leukemia).

ERYTHEMA NODOSUM: Belongs to a group of skin disorders characterized by painful nodules most often affecting the lower extremities. It is often associated with recurring episodes of fever, malaise, fatigue, joint pain and the mechanism remains unknown.

REFERENCES:

Ehman F, Harth M, Spouge AR: Christian disease with severe polyarthritis and polyosteitis. *J Rheumatol* 29(5):1102, 2002.

Lemley DE, Ferrans VJ, Fox LM, et al: Cardiac manifestations of Weber-Christian disease: Report and review of the literature. *J Rheumatol* 18(5):756, 1991.

Winkelmann RK, McEvoy MT, Peter MS: Lipophagic panniculitis of childhood. *J Am Acad Dermatol* 21:971, 1989.

Weill-Marchesani Syndrome

At a glance: Characterized by short stature, brachydactyly, limitation of joint movement, microspherophakia, luxated lenses, glaucoma, and heart malformations (pulmonary stenosis, either valvular or subvalvular, and congestive cardiac failure).

Synonyms: Spherophakia-Brachymorphia Syndrome; Congenital Mesodermal Dysmorphodystrophy; Dystrophia Mesodermalis Congenital Hyperplastica.

Genetic inheritance: Both autosomal dominant and autosomal recessive transmission have been reported. However, the latter is the most probable mode, since there is only a partial expression in heterozygote patients.

Pathophysiology: The pathogenesis is unknown, but the similarities with Marfan syndrome suggest that a disorder of the connective tissue may be responsible.

Diagnosis: Mainly clinical, where ophthalmological findings and a particular somatic morphology leads to the diagnosis of the syndrome. Gene probably located at 19p13.3–p13.2.

Clinical aspects: The *ocular* findings include bilateral microspherophakia and associated lens dislocation. Some patients also present with congenital glaucoma, or may develop in later years. The *musculoskeletal* characteristics are short stature with brachydactyly and joint stiffness, mainly in the elbows, wrists, and hands, but the hips and knees may also be involved. Others features include spina bifida occulta, abnormal vertebral size, cone epiphyses, metaphyseal anomaly, wide rib cage, myopathy, thickened skull with brachycephaly, and short neck. *Cardiac* problems mainly involve pulmonary stenosis, either valvular or subvalvular, that may lead to congestive cardiac failure if undiagnosed and untreated. Intelligence is normal.

Precautions before anesthesia: Obtain an ECG and an echocardiogram if there is a clinical suspicion of cardiac involvement. Evaluate the airway for a potentially difficult tracheal intubation (clinical, radiographs).

Anesthetic considerations: Because of the joint stiffness, positioning might be more problematic and adequate padding is necessary to avoid compression injuries. If the patient has heart disease, the anesthetic should be managed according to the type of lesion.

Pharmacological implications: Antibioprophylaxis given as needed to prevent endocarditis as indicated. Medications for glaucoma include the organophosphates such as echothiophate and isofluorphate. These drugs inhibit serum cholinesterase, which is responsible for the hydrolysis and inactivation of succinylcholine and the ester-type local anesthetics (e.g. procaine, chloroprocaine and tetracaine). These ester-type local anesthetics should be avoided in patients treated with eyedrops containing organophosphate. Review current medication in view of glaucoma (avoid atropine and other drugs incriminated). Muscle relaxants should only be used after airway is secured and lung ventilation confirmed. Succinylcholine should probably be avoided because of myopathy and also in the presence of glaucoma.

Other conditions to be considered:

☞**MARFAN SYNDROME:** An inherited disorder that affects the connective tissue of the cardiovascular system. The musculoskeletal and ocular systems are also affected. Major features include unusual height, large hands and feet, severe lordoscoliosis, and pulmonary dysfunctions. It is inherited as an autosomal dominant trait.

ECTOPIA LENTIS: Characterized by partial or complete displacement of the lens of the eye. It may present as congenital or progressive after birth. It can also be associated as a result of trauma. In such cases, the condition may be present at birth or develop later during life. Simple ectopia lentis is usually inherited as an autosomal dominant trait. In addition to Weill-Marchesani syndrome, ectopia lentis may also occur with Marfan syndrome, and homocystinuria, a metabolic disorder. Individuals affected with this entity present with blurring of vision, diplopia, and iridodonesis.

REFERENCES:
Faivre L, Megarbane A, Alswaid A, et al: Homozygosity mapping of a Weill-Marchesani syndrome locus to chromosome 19p13.3–p13.2. *Hum Genet* 110:366, 2002.

Mégarbané A, Mustapha M, Bleik J, et al: Exclusion of chromosome 15q21.1 in autosomal recessive Weill-Marchesani syndrome in an inbred Lebanese family. *Clin Genet* 58:473, 2000.

Young ID, Fielder AR, Casey TA: Weill-Marchesani syndrome in a mother and son. *Clin Genet* 30:475, 1986.

Weismann-Netter-Stuhl Syndrome

At a glance: A syndrome characterized by dwarfism, bowed legs, saber shins, mental retardation, mild involvement of the arms, and dural calcification.

Synonyms: Anterior Bowing of the Legs with Dwarfism; Toxopachyosteose Diaphysaire Tibio-Peroniere (French).

Incidence: Unknown but rare. A total of 47 cases had been reported in the literature between 1954 and 2000.

Genetic inheritance: Presumed autosomal or X-linked dominant inheritance. Most cases appear to have been sporadic and the relatively small number of familial cases suggests incomplete penetrance.

Pathophysiology: The pathogenesis is unknown. Assumed to be a primary metabolic abnormality of bone.

Diagnosis: Clinical features consistent with the syndrome. Radiological examination is characteristic (anterior bowing of tibiae and fibulae, with cortical hyperostosis on the concave side of the curvature, slight bowing of the radius, ulna and humerus). Inconsistent radiological findings include squaring of the iliac wings, low position of the fifth lumbar vertebra in relation to the ilia, horizontal sacrum, kyphoscoliosis, and dural calcification. Alkaline phosphatase is normal or raised; bone biopsy is normal.

Clinical aspects: Short stature is the most constant manifestation (males averaging 151 cm [59.4 inches] and females 142 cm [56 inches]). Features include anterior bowing of tibiae (saber shins) and lateral bowing of femora (usually bilateral), occasional mild bowing of ulna, radius, and humerus, and delayed ambulation in childhood. Of those affected, 20% have mental retardation of variable severity. Kyphoscoliosis is present in approximately 30% of cases. Age at diagnosis has ranged from 2 weeks to 94 years. The skeletal deformities do not seem to progress during adult life. Normal life expectancy.

Precautions before anesthesia: Detailed clinical history and physical examination must be performed to determine the progression of the syndrome and assess the presence of unrelated medical conditions. Evaluate pulmonary function if kyphoscoliosis present (chest radiography, spirometry, arterial blood gases).

Anesthetic considerations: Careful patient positioning and transfer from the stretcher to the operating room table (patients seem to have an increased propensity to bone fracture following minor trauma). If the kyphoscoliosis is significant, the use of regional anesthetic technique may not be applicable. Technical difficulties may be experienced because of lower spinal abnormalities and the risk of dural puncture is increased. The laryngeal inlet may be smaller than normal for age. A range of endotracheal tubes of sizes smaller than normal should be available.

Pharmacological implications: Sedative premedication may be beneficial in patients with mental retardation. No specific pharmacological considerations.

Other conditions to be considered:

☞**MAFFUCCI SYNDROME:** Rare disorder characterized by skeletal dysplasia. The age of onset can be at birth or not until early childhood. It primarily affects long bones and cartilage. Limb shortening, bowing of the long bones, and/or short stature may occur.

CAMPTOMELIC SYNDROME: A congenital disorder characterized by short stature along with bowing and an unusual angular shape of the legs. The shoulder and the pelvic skeletal structures are often abnormal. Individuals affected with this syndrome usually present with 11 pairs of ribs instead of 12. Two forms have been described: the long-limbed and the short-limbed form. It is inherited as an autosomal recessive trait.

☞**VITAMIN D DEFICIENCY RICKETS:** A rare disorder that appears during infancy and childhood. The clinical features include restlessness, delayed motor development and growth, abnormal development of teeth, and/or bowed legs.

CONGENITAL SYPHILIS: A rare acquired chronic infectious disorder characterized by low birth weight, fever, rash, and/or saber shins. Other clinical features may include hardening of the umbilical cord, hypercholesterolemia in infancy, anemia, hepatosplenomegaly and mental retardation. It is caused by the *Treponema pallidum* bacteria. Fetal syphilis acquired from the mother may be apparent at birth or during early infancy, however, in many individuals, several years may pass before symptoms are recognized.

REFERENCES:

Francis GL, Jelinek JJ, McHale K, et al: The Weismann-Netter syndrome: A cause of bowed legs in childhood. *Pediatrics* 88(2):334, 1991.

Robinow M, Johnson GF: The Weismann-Netter syndrome. *Am J Med Genet* 29:573, 1988.

Tieder M, Manor H, Peshin J, et al: The Weismann-Netter-Stuhl syndrome: A rare pediatric skeletal dysplasia. *Pediatr Radiol* 25(1):37, 1995.

Wermer Syndrome

At a glance: Neoplastic disease, characterized by tumors or hyperplasia of the parathyroid and pituitary glands and the islands of Langerhans, with increased incidence of adrenocortical and thyroid disease. Association with diffuse neuroendocrine tumors in the thymus, bronchi, and duodenopancreas.

Synonym: Multiple Endocrine Neoplasia type I, MEN I.

History: Genetic disorder first reported by Paul Wermer, American internist in 1954, and in 1955 by Robert Milton Zollinger and Edwin Homer Ellison, American surgeons.

Incidence: Both sexes equally affected. It is rare in childhood. Prevalence in general population ranges between 1:20,000 and 1:40,000.

Genetic inheritance: Autosomal dominant. More than 80% of cases caused by inactivating mutations (including nonsense mutations, deletions and insertions) of the *MEN1* gene, MENIN; localized to chromosome 11q13.

Pathophysiology: Precise role of MENIN is unclear. It is likely to be a tumor-suppressor gene. Mutations lead to hyperplasia of the endocrine organs: pancreatic islet cell adenoma (40% of cases, most commonly gastrinomas and insulinomas), parathyroid adenoma (95% of cases), pituitary adenoma (30% of cases), adrenocortical adenoma, prolactinoma, glucagonoma, insulinoma, and vasointestinal peptide tumor. Lesions of nonendocrine organs may also be present: bronchial carcinoma and carcinoids, thymomas and thymic carcinoid, duodenal carcinoid, malignant schwannoma, ovarian tumors, and lipomas.

Diagnosis: Clinical features and the results of biochemical tests according to the presentation (hypoglycemia, hypercalcemia, hyperphosphatemia, anemia, relevant endocrine abnormalities). Also, the addition of radiological information (delineation and localization of peptic ulcers, pituitary tumor, renal stones, bronchial tumors, etc.) is essential.

Clinical aspects: Symptoms and signs associated with the glands involved and the function of adenomas; gastrinoma (intractable peptic ulcer, high incidence of bleeding, perforation and obstruction, ectopic ulcers in esophagus and small intestines, diarrhea, steatorrhea, weight loss); pituitary adenoma (headache, visual field defects; acromegaly; hyperthyroidism; amenorrhea); parathyroid adenoma (hypercalcemia and renal stones); adrenal (Cushing syndrome); insulinoma (hypoglycemia); glucagonoma (hyperglycemia, stomatitis, skin rash); islet cell tumors (can produce glucagon, vasoactive inhibitory polypeptide, prostaglandins, adrenocorticotropic hormone, parathyroid hormone, antidiuretic hormone, serotonin); multiple lipomas; bronchial tumors (cough, hemoptysis, breathlessness).

Precautions before anesthesia: Acid–base balance and electrolyte disturbances must be corrected preoperatively to avoid arrhythmia, hemodynamic instability, and potentiation of action of neuromuscular blockers.

Anesthetic considerations: Emergency surgery may be indicated for complications of peptic ulcer disease. Presence of hypovolemia necessitates perioperative fluid resuscitation, rapid sequence induction, and pharmacological prophylaxis against gastric aspiration (e.g., sodium citrate). Invasive monitoring may be indicated: close perioperative glucose monitoring for hypoglycemia, anesthetic problems associated with acromegaly, Cushing syndrome, and hyperthyroidism. Depending on size and site of bronchial tumor, expect airway compression and ventilatory difficulties; superior vena cava obstruction may impede venous return.

Pharmacological implications: Renal dysfunction may affect clearance of some drugs.

REFERENCES:

Brandi ML, Gagel RF, Angeli A, et al: Guidelines for diagnosis and therapy of MEN type 1 and type 2. *J Clin Endocrinol Metab* 86:5658, 2001.

Thakker RV: Editorial: Multiple endocrine neoplasia—Syndromes of the twentieth century. *J Clin Endocrinol Metab* 83;8:2617, 1998.

Thakker RV: Multiple endocrine neoplasia type 1, in DeGroot LJ (ed): *Endocrinology*. 3rd ed. Philadelphia, WB Saunders, 1995, p 2815.

Werner Syndrome

At a glance: Premature aging disease that begins in adolescence or early adulthood. With short stature, bilateral cataracts, scleroderma-like skin changes, premature graying or loss of hair, and malignancies predisposition. The main risks are associated with cardiovascular and neurological complications because of the atheromatous disease.

Synonyms: Progeria Adultorum; Progeria of the Adult.

History: First described by C.W. Otto Werner, German physician in 1904.

Incidence: 1 to 2 cases per million in general population. More common in Japan and Sardinia than in other geographic areas. As of 2003, about 1000 cases have been reported internationally and 800 of them are in Japan. The mean survival age for these patients is 46 years.

Genetic inheritance: Autosomal recessive.

Pathophysiology: A reduction in the amount of cell DNA repair activity has been demonstrated and postulated as a cause of the premature aging. In addition, these patients are at increased risk of developing malignancies of skin and intestine. Syndrome is caused by mutations in the RecQ protein-like 2 gene located at 8p12–p11.2.

Diagnosis: Characterized by short stature, slender limbs, cataracts, skin hypoplasia, and stocky trunk.

Clinical aspects: Patients with Werner syndrome demonstrate progeria, showing loss of subcutaneous fat, prominent scalp veins, short stature, weight loss, sclerodermoid skin changes, mottled pigmentation, and freckling. Hair loss and premature graying are features. Patients frequently demonstrate premature aging only in their third decade. Development of endocrine disturbance with diabetes and early atherosclerosis occur, as well as osteoporosis, hypofertility, hypogonadism, amyotrophy, and retinal degeneration. Most patients die in their fourth or fifth decade from malignancy (10% of cases; osteosarcoma and meningioma especially).

Precautions before anesthesia: Before anesthesia, patients with this disorder must be thoroughly assessed for evidence of coronary artery disease and other organ dysfunction. Urea and electrolytes, plasma glucose, and, possibly, glucose tolerance tests should be performed. Thyroid function testing should be undertaken. A thorough cardiovascular examination is supplemented by a 12-lead ECG and possibly further investigation of the coronary vascularization.

Anesthetic considerations: A difficult airway and difficulty performing direct laryngoscopy and tracheal intubation is a possibility in these patients because of the skin changes. No specific techniques can be recommended because each of these rare cases must be handled individually.

Pharmacological implications: Anesthetic drugs should be adapted to renal function. Muscle relaxants are not contraindicated but amyotrophic changes may be considered and monitoring is necessary.

Other conditions to be considered:

☞**PROGERIA:** A very rare disorder of childhood. It is characterized by accelerated premature aging, short stature, and charac-

teristic facial features. Severe cardiopulmonary problems (including myocardial infarction in early age) must be carefully considered. Various orthopedic and orthorhinolaryngological problems are reported.

☞**GOTTRON SYNDROME:** A mild, inherited form of progeria which is characterized by abnormally small hands and feet with thin and delicate skin. Children affected by this disorder appear older than their actual age. The skin is unusually thin and very fragile. It has a parchment-like texture on the hands and feet. Unusually prominent veins are visible on the chest. Other important features include the presence of micrognathia. It is inherited as an autosomal recessive trait. Approximately 40 cases have been reported in the medical literature.

DE BARSY-MOENS-DIERCKS SYNDROME (De Barsy Syndrome; Progeroid Syndrome of De Barsy; Corneal Clouding-Cutis Laxa-Mental Retardation Syndrome; Cutis Laxa-Growth Deficiency Syndrome): A rare autosomal recessive disorder. The main characteristics are the severe cutis laxa, athetosis, cloudy corneas of the eyes, large prominent ears, and hypotonia. Other clinical features include hyperextensibility of the joints, frontal bossing, and/or short stature. Significant skin wrinkling is usually present.

☞**WIEDEMANN-RAUTENSTRAUCH SYNDROME:** An extremely rare neonatal genetic disorder characterized by an aged appearance at birth, prenatal and postnatal growth retardation, and subcutaneous lipoatrophy. The skin appears very thin, fragile and excessively wrinkled at birth. Abnormal accumulation of fat is often observed around the buttocks, the anogenital area and body flanks. It is inherited as an autosomal recessive trait.

MULVIHILL-SMITH SYNDROME: An extremely rare inherited condition presenting significant premature aging. Other clinical features include short stature, microcephaly, facial characteristics of early aging, subcutaneous tissue atrophy, multiple nevi, progressive deafness, and/or immunological deficiencies. The age of onset occurs in childhood or adolescence. It has been reported in only four individuals in the medical literature.

STORM SYNDROME (Werner-like Syndrome): An extremely rare inherited disorder combining significant premature aging and severe congenital heart defects. The clinical features during adolescence include the loss of eyebrows and eyelashes and alopecia. The skin over the hands and face is wrinkled in appearance. Arthritis and pain are often manifested.

☞**ROTHMUND-THOMSON SYNDROME:** An inherited skin disorder characterized by abnormal redness of the skin caused by congested and obstructed capillaries associated with small stature, muscle atrophy, photosensitivity and cataracts during adolescence. Other clinical features include underdeveloped teeth and nails, small hands with malformed or missing thumbs, small feet, and/or sparse and prematurely gray hair or baldness.

REFERENCES:

Goto M, Imamura O, Kuromitsu J, et al: Analysis of helicase gene mutations in Japanese Werner's syndrome patients. *Hum Genet* 99:191, 1997.

Motonaga K, Itoh M, Hachiya Y, et al: Age-related expression of Werner's syndrome protein in selected tissues and coexpression of transcription factors. *J Clin Pathol* 55(3):195, 2002.

Pesce JK, Rothe HI: Features of premature aging syndromes. *Clin Dermatol* 14:161, 1996.

West Syndrome

At a glance: A disorder characterized by the triad of infantile spasms, an interictal EEG pattern termed hypsarrhythmia, and mental retardation.

Synonym: Generalized Flexion Epilepsy; Infantile Epileptic Encephalopathy; Infantile Myoclonic Encephalopathy; Jackknife Convulsion; Massive Myoclonia; Salaam Spasms; Infantile Spasms

Incidence and genetic inheritance: Approximately 1.5–5.0 in 10,000 live births are afflicted with this disease that affects both genders equally. There is no genetic basis for the disease, although a positive family history for epilepsy is present in a minority of these patients. However, in a significant number of cases, ☞Tuberous Sclerosis can be found and should therefore be ruled out. Basically any type of brain damage has the potential to result in infantile spasms.

Clinical aspects: Infantile spasms begin in the first year of life, most often around 4 to 7 months of age. Close neurologic examination of the child reveals abnormal mental function with cognitive deficits that are consistent with developmental delay or regression. However, there are no pathognomonic signs for West Syndrome. The symptoms are more likely a reflection of the underlying brain damage. The initial focal signs of brain injury may secondarily involve other sites of the brain resulting in the electroencephalographic picture of hypsarrhythmia. Hypsarrhythmia is characterized by abnormal, random, high voltage slow waves and spikes in cortical areas, which are variable in regard to their duration and location. The electroencephalogram has a chaotic look and is most often nonepisodic. Following a spasm, fast waves and high voltage spikes may be detected. Even though the exact mechanism of action is unknown, therapy with ACTH has long been known to be one of the most effective treatment options and a wide dosage range has been used. It seems that early treatment (usually within a month after onset of infantile spams) improves the therapeutic success rate. Some neurologists combine ACTH with high doses of vitamin B_6, others prefer to use nitrazepam, clonazepam, valproate, vigabatrin or lamotrigine.

Depending on their etiology, infantile spasms are usually classified as symptomatic, cryptogenic, or idiopathic. *Symptomatic* infantile spams are present if a factor responsible for the syndrome can be identified. Theoretically, any form of brain injury (congenital or acquired) can be associated with infantile spasms. Infantile spasms are termed *cryptogenic*, if no cause could be identified, although the seizures are considered to be symptomatic in origin. If psychomotor development was normal prior to the onset of the spasms, but no abnormalities can be found to explain the findings, the term *idiopathic* infantile spasms has been used, although for some neurologist the two terms "cryptogenic" and "idiopathic" are interchangeable. The proportions of cryptogenic and idiopathic infantile spasms therefore varies widely and with diagnostic tools becoming more and more sophisticated, their overall frequency is declining.

Anesthetic considerations: The treatment with ACTH may result in serious side effects including electrolyte imbalance, hypertension, left-ventricular hypertrophy, obesity, osteoporosis, opportunistic infections and behavioral problems. Preoperative work-up should therefore include a complete cell blood count (CBC) and electrolytes serum levels. Some anti-seizure drugs result in induction of microsomal liver enzymes. Similarly metabolized drugs.

Because of mental retardation, cooperation may be difficult and sedative and/or anxiolytic premedication may be helpful. Drugs that are known to have the potential to trigger seizures should be avoided. These patients are usually on chronic antiseizure medication, which may result in induction of microsomal liver enzymes. Consequently, metabolism of similarly metabolized drugs may be accelerated.

Other conditions to be considered:

☞**LENNOX-GASTAUT SYNDROME:** Severe form of epilepsy resulting in significant learning disabilities and impaired organization of movements.

☞**AICARDI SYNDROME:** A rare disorder characterized by partial or complete agenesis of the corpus callosum, infantile spasms (spasm-like epilepsy), mental retardation, and an ocular abnormality called lacunae of the retina. Often associated with other features such as microcephaly and porencephalic cysts. The onset is generally between the age of 3 to 5 months. The disorder affects only females.

☞**TUBEROUS SCLEROSIS:** Neurodegenerative syndrome characterized by lesions of the skin, tumor growth and seizures. Some patients present with mental retardation and autism. Rhabdomyoma of the heart and astrocytoma in the brain are frequent tumoral presentation.

☞**SCHINZEL-GIEDION SYNDROME:** A distinct dysmorphic syndrome of congenital hydronephrosis, skeletal dysplasia (open cranial sutures, steep short skull, wide occipital synchondrosis) and severe developmental retardation. Coarse facies characterized by midface retraction, bulging forehead, facial hemangiomas, short nose with anteverted nostrils, protruding large tongue and hypertelorism. Usually deceased within infancy.

REFERENCES:

Hrachovy RA, Frost JD, Jr: Infantile epileptic encephalopathy with hypsarrhythmia (infantile spasms/West syndrome). *J Clin Neurophysiol.* 20:408. 2003.

Hrachovy RA, Frost JD, Kellaway P. Hypsarrhythmia: variations on the theme. *Epilepsia* 25:317, 1984.

Takuma Y: ACTH therapy for infantile spasms: A combination therapy with high-dose pyridoxal phosphate and low-dose ACTH. *Epilepsia* 39 (Suppl 5):42, 1998.

Weyers Syndrome II

At a glance: Syndrome present from birth, affecting both sexes, and characterized by postaxial polydactyly of the hands and feet, hexadactyly and fusion of fifth and sixth metatarsals and metacarpals, and bony clefts of the mandibular symphysis. Other features include orodental anomalies, hypoplastic and dysplastic nails, short stature, micrognathia, small mouth, and hypoplasia of the larynx. Congenital heart defect may be present.

Synonyms: Acrofacial Dysostosis Weyers type; Acrodental Dysostosis; Curry-Hall Syndrome; Weyers Acrodysplasia.

Nature: Acrofacial dysostoses associated with mandibulofacial dysostosis, limb defects, and various associated anomalies. They represent a heterogeneous group, which supports the hypothesis that the malformations result from polytopic field defects arising during blastogenesis.

Incidence: Rare malformation, of which several syndromic associations have been reported.

Genetic inheritance: No clear genetic background. Clinical data support the hypothesis of autosomal dominant (X-linked inheritance, but also recessive occurrences have been described).

Pathophysiology: Unknown; caused by a mutation in the EVC gene (mutant in Ellis-van Creveld syndrome), located at 4p16.

Diagnosis: At birth, the diagnosis is suspected on the clinical aspect, characterized by varying severities of mandibulofacial dysostosis with pre- and/or postaxial limb abnormalities.

Clinical aspects: In the heterogeneous group of this syndrome with combined defects of craniofacial and limb development, there are several clinical aspects according to the craniofacial and limb malformations, and their association with other visceral or bone abnormalities. In the predominant facial form, called Nager acrofacial dysostosis, the facial changes resemble strikingly those of the Treacher Collins syndrome: malar hypoplasia, maxillomandibular hypoplasia, cleft lip or palate. Neonates may present with respiratory or feeding problems. Upper limb malformation is a constant feature of Nager syndrome and ranges from thumb hypoplasia to the absence of the radial ray.

Precautions before anesthesia: In neonates, make a careful research of associated abnormalities of the heart, brain, kidney, or

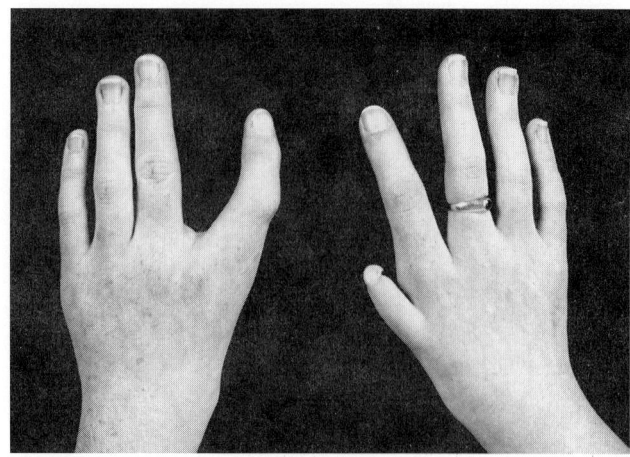

Weyers syndrome II Characteristic anomaly of the hand with shortening of the thumb in an adult with acrofacial dysostosis.

urogenital tract by echography. Vertebral malformations, especially cervical, must be looked for by radiographic exploration. Evaluate and anticipate the airway obstruction and difficult tracheal intubation.

Anesthetic considerations: Refer to ☞Treacher Collins syndrome. The craniofacial abnormalities associated with trismus, retroplaced tongue, and airway obstruction make tracheal intubation difficult and challenging. It is strongly recommended to preserve spontaneous ventilation at all times until the trachea has been intubated and lung ventilation is confirmed. The availability of a laryngeal mask airway in case of failure to intubate the trachea is highly recommended. Fiberoptic equipment will be needed. The child must be carefully assessed postoperatively and extubated when awake. At birth, in cases of life-threatening airway obstruction, use of a laryngeal mask has proved to be successful.

Pharmacological implications: Muscle relaxants and opioids should be avoided before tracheal intubation. Sleep apnea contraindicates any sedation before airway access.

Other conditions to be considered:

☞**ACROFACIAL DYSOSTOSIS NAGER TYPE:** Malar hypoplasia, maxillary and mandibular hypoplasia, cleft lip or palate, retroplaced tongue, radial defects (preaxial limb deficiency), downward slanting palpebral fissures, absent eyelashes (medial third of lower lids), dysplastic ears and conduction deafness, trismus, and respiratory problem in neonates. Inheritance: uncertain.

ACROFACIAL DYSOSTOSIS RICHIERI-COSTA AND PEREIRA FORM: Laryngeal malformations; severe facial and skeletal anomalies; mandibulofacial dysostosis with bilateral radial ray anomalies. Autosomal-recessive inheritance.

☞**MILLER SYNDROME:** Mandibulofacial dysostosis similar to Treacher Collins syndrome, Postaxial limb deficiency.

REFERENCES:

Nagahama H, Suzuki Y, Tateda T, et al: The use of a laryngeal mask in a newborn infant with Nager acrofacial dysostosis. *Masui* 44:1555, 1995.

Opitz JM, Mollica F, Sorge G, et al: Acrofacial dysostoses: Review and report of a previously undescribed condition: The autosomal or X-linked dominant Catania form of acrofacial dysostosis. *Am J Med Genet* 47:660, 1993.

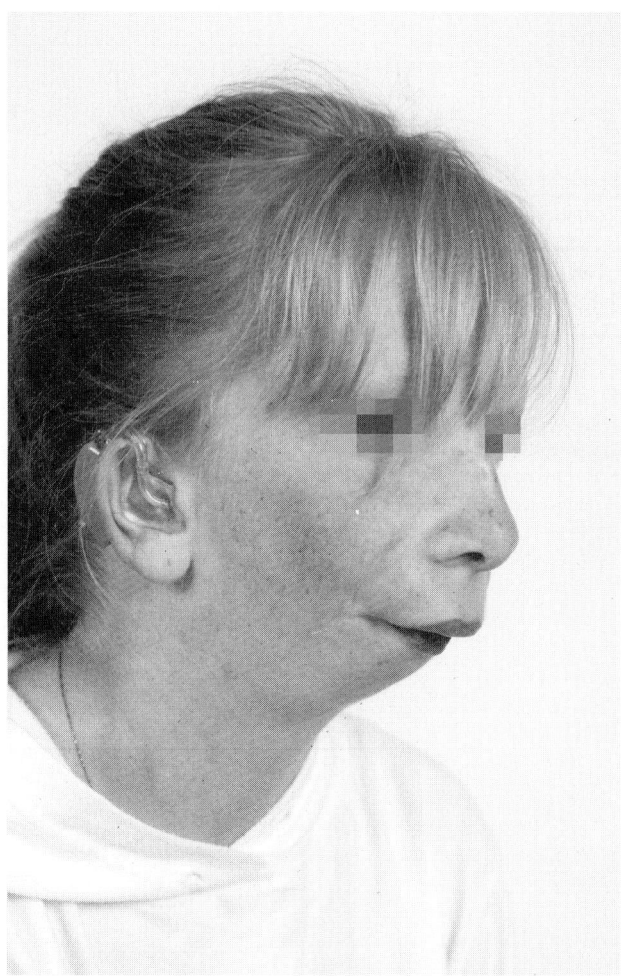

Weyers syndrome II Facial dysmorphism in a 12-year-old girl with acrofacial dysostosis.

Ruiz-Perez VL, Ide SE, Strom TM: Mutations in a new gene in Ellis-van Creveld syndrome and Weyers acrodental dysostosis. *Nat Genet* 24:283, 2000.

Whipple Disease

At a glance: A disease acquired from an infectious agent called *Tropheryma whippelii*, which is closely related to the actinomycetes. It results in a malabsorption syndrome with involvement of small intestine, joints, central nervous system and cardiovascular system. The onset of the disease can be seen at all ages.

Genetic inheritance: Probably no genetic involvement.

Pathophysiology: Invasion of affected tissue by *Tropheryma whippelii* results in local inflammation and organ dysfunction, as well as generalized systemic symptoms. Appears to be associated with the human leukocyte antigen B27 (HLA-B27) haplotype.

Diagnosis: Clinically evocated by arthralgias, arthritis, fever, and diarrhea. Biopsy of duodenum or proximal jejunum reveals infiltration of lamina propria by "foamy" macrophages with granules, which stain positively with the periodic acid-Schiff (PAS) technique. The macrophages contain gram-positive acid-fast negative bacilli—*Tropheryma whippelii*.

Clinical aspects: Can occur at any age (reports range from 3 months to 82 years) but is more common after the fourth decade. More than 70% of patients are male. Although the primary organ system involved is the gastrointestinal (GI) tract, systemic symptoms and those related to involvement of other organ systems frequently precede those attributable to the GI tract. Clinical features can involve *GI system* (diarrhea, steatorrhea, gross or microscopic bleeding, vague abdominal pain and bloating, and anorexia; these may be followed by cachexia, fatigue, hypoalbuminemia, anemia and severe electrolyte disturbances), *articular* (transient, migratory, recurring, and spontaneously resolving arthralgias are common), *neurologic* (dementia, weakness, parkinsonism, cranial nerve symptoms), and *cardiac* (blood culture-negative endocarditis, constrictive pericarditis, myocarditis, conduction abnormalities). Because of the infective nature of the disease, it is amenable to antibiotic therapy, which is often continued for up to 36 months. Ninety percent of patients return to normal, with a small percentage suffering relapses.

Precautions before anesthesia: Evaluate electrolyte status, particularly in patients with ongoing diarrhea. Other blood tests recommended include: serum albumin, hemoglobin. Cardiac evaluation (clinical, ECG, echocardiogram).

Anesthetic considerations: Preoperative correction of electrolyte abnormalities and anemia is mandatory before elective surgical procedures. Adapt anesthetic technique to cardiac involvement, if any. Not a contagious condition.

Pharmacological implications: There are no specific implications with this condition.

REFERENCES:

Durand D, Lecomte C, Cathebras P, et al: Whipple disease: Clinical review of 52 cases. *Medicine (Baltimore)* 76:3:170, 1997.

Silvestry F, Kim B, Pollack B, et al: Cardiac Whipple disease: Identification of Whipple bacillus by electron microscopy in the myocardium of a patient before death. *Ann Intern Med* 126(3):214, 1997.

Swartz MN: Whipple's disease—Past, present, and future [editorial]. *N Engl J Med* 342(9):648, 2000.

Wiedemann-Rautenstrauch Syndrome

At a glance: Characterized by an aged appearance at birth, prenatal and postnatal growth retardation, and subcutaneous lipoatrophy with abnormal deposits of fat around the buttocks, the anogenital area, and the flanks. Characteristic craniofacial abnormalities (frontal and parietal bossing) leading to a pseudohydrocephalus aspect.

Synonyms: Neonatal Progeroid Syndrome; Neonatal Pseudo-Hydrocephalic Progeroid Syndrome of Wiedemann-Rautenstrauch; Rautenstrauch-Wiedemann Syndrome.

History: This medical entity was first described in 1979 by Hans-Rudolf Wiedemann, a German physician and Thomas Rautenstrauch, a German pediatrician, who described two cases of progeria in neonates in 1977.

Genetic inheritance: Autosomal recessive.

Pathophysiology: Unknown.

Diagnosis: Progeroid appearance at birth and during infancy.

Clinical aspects: Patients have premature aging aspect, short stature and a poorly muscled build. Clinical features can involve the central nervous system (CNS) (psychomotor development deficiency, hypotonia, truncal ataxia, intention tremor, and nystagmus), *head and neck* (pseudohydrocephaly and apparent macrocephaly, small face, prognathism, micrognathia, microstoma, low-set ears, high forehead, decreased eyebrows, sparse hair, sparse eyebrows, sparse eyelashes, prominent scalp veins, entropion, greatly widened anterior fontanelles, malar hypoplasia, natal teeth, and beaking of the nose). Other possible features include congenital heart defect, dysphagia, urinary reflux, generalized lipoatrophy, abnormally placed nipples, arachnodactyly, and restricted joint mobility.

Precautions before anesthesia: Assessment of airway must be evaluated in view of craniofacial abnormalities (clinical, radiographs, fiberoptic if necessary). Evaluate congenital heart defect (clinical, ECG, echocardiography). Risk of pulmonary aspiration and respiratory tract infections is significant. Ensure adequate hydration.

Anesthetic considerations: Possible difficulties with direct laryngoscopy and tracheal intubation. Risk of intracranial hemorrhage. Careful temperature control (general absence of subcutaneous fat) and intraoperative positioning (restricted joint mobility) are needed.

Pharmacological implications: Antibiotic prophylaxis in cases of cardiac defect. Muscle relaxants should be used after airway is secured.

Other conditions to be considered:

☞**PROGERIA SYNDROME:** A very rare disorder of childhood. It is characterized by accelerated premature aging, short stature, and characteristic facial features. Severe cardiopulmonary problems (including myocardial infarction in early age) must be carefully considered. Various orthopedic and orthorhinolaryngological problems are reported.

DE BARSY MOENS DIERCKS SYNDROME (De Barsy Syndrome; Progeroid Syndrome of De Barsy; Corneal Clouding Cutis Laxa Mental Retardation Syndrome): A rare autosomal recessive disorder. The main characteristics are the severe cutis laxa, athetosis, cloudy corneas of the eyes, large prominent ears, and hypotonia. Other features include hyperextensibility of the joints, frontal bossing, and/or short stature. Significant skin wrinkling.

☞**WERNER SYNDROME:** Premature aging disease that begins in adolescence or early adulthood. With short stature, bilateral cataracts, scleroderma-like skin changes, premature graying or loss of hair and malignancies predisposition. Main risks are atheroma with cardiovascular and neurological complications.

☞**HALLERMAN-STREIFF SYNDROME:** Characterized by the presence of microcephaly and brachycephaly, frontal bossing, hypoplastic mandible, a "beak-shaped" nose and microstomia. The disorder is also characterized by dwarfism, ocular abnormalities (microphthalmia), congenital cataracts, nystagmus, strabismus, and decreased visual acuity. Dental defects are present. Individuals affected by this disorder typically have a normal intelligence. It is believed to be sporadic, however, in some cases a pattern of autosomal recessive inheritance has been suggested.

☞**COCKAYNE SYNDROME:** A very rare genetic disorder characterized by growth retardation, photosensitivity, and progeroid appearance. In the classical form (Type I), the symptoms are progressive and typically become apparent within the first year of life. In Early Onset form (Type II), associated symptoms and physical findings are apparent at birth. Affected individual presents with microcephaly, sunken eyes, malformed ears, and a thin, beaked nose. The loss of subcutaneous fat is characteristic of this syndrome and gives a prematurely aged appearance. Other clinical features include a short stature, progressive loss of vision because of retinal degeneration, neurological degeneration including progressive mental retardation, movement disturbances, deafness, and dementia have been reported. Arteriosclerosis has been suggested as a potential life-threatening complication. It is inherited as an autosomal recessive.

REFERENCES:

Pivnick EK, Angle B, Kaufman RA, et al: Neonatal progeroid (Wiedemann-Rautenstrauch) syndrome: Report of five new cases and review. *Am J Med Genet* 90:131, 2000.

Toriello HV: Wiedemann-Rautenstrauch syndrome. *J Med Genet* 27:256, 1990.

Williams Syndrome

At a glance: A syndrome characterized by peculiar elfin facies associated with infantile hypercalcemia, cardiac defect and mild mental retardation. High incidence of sudden death.

Synonyms: Williams-Beuren Syndrome; Williams-Barratt Syndrome; Fanconi-Schlesinger Syndrome; Elfin Facies Syndrome; Hypercalcemia-Peculiar Facies-Supravalvular Aortic Stenosis Syndrome.

History: This medical entity was described by J.C.P. Williams, a New Zealand cardiologist.

Incidence: 1:20,000–50,000 live births.

Genetic inheritance: Autosomal dominant with some familial cases, but most seem to be sporadic. Contiguous gene syndrome. Link to chromosome 7 (7q11.23).

Pathophysiology: Because of the transient hypercalcemia occurring during infancy, it has been proposed that Williams syndrome may be caused by an abnormal metabolism of calcium and vitamin D, but this remains to be proven. Mutations (deletions) in the elastin gene (ELM) are responsible, at least in part, for the disorder. The gene for LIM-kinase-1 is also involved in the pathogenesis, and haploinsufficiency of the RFC2 gene has also been postulated as a factor.

Diagnosis: The diagnosis is a clinical one based on the characteristic elfin facies associated with mental retardation, cardiovascular problem, and neonatal hypercalcemia. Diagnosis is established by chromosomal studies (molecular biology). Radiographs may show increased calcification of skull base, periorbital area, and vertebral plates. Angiographic studies evaluate extent and type of vascular lesions.

Clinical aspects: The main features of the *characteristic facies* are epicanthal folds, flat nasal bridge, anteverted nostrils, blue stellate iris, and mandibular hypoplasia associated with dental anomalies and a tendency to keep mouth open. Patients also have a typical hoarse voice. Neonatal hypercalcemia is common and can lead to nephrocalcinosis. The main *cardiovascular* anomaly is supravalvular aortic stenosis, but other anomalies can be present. Sudden death is frequent in patients with coronary artery stenosis or severe biventricular outflow tract obstruction and is a result of myocardial ischemia, decreased cardiac output, and arrhythmia. The overall incidence of sudden death over a 30-year period is reported to be 3%. Patients usually have a friendly personality and normal language skills despite their mental retardation (IQ 40 to 80). During infancy, they may present with hypotonia, which may remain the same or convert to hypertonia at an older age. As the patients grow older, they may develop hypertension, progressive joint limitations, recurrent urinary tract infections, obesity, diverticulosis, and cholelithiasis. Other features include hypoplastic nails, clinodactyly, hallux valgus, pectus excavatum, umbilical hernia, and a small penis.

Precautions before anesthesia: Baseline ECG and echocardiogram should be obtained before surgery and exercise tolerance evaluated, as well as signs of cardiac insufficiency. In infants, hypercalcemia needs to be investigated, because it is more prevalent among this age group. Also, young children present with a feeding problem and frequent vomiting, thus aspiration prophylaxis may be warranted. Evaluate blood chemistries, calcemia (prevention of nephrocalcinosis and deafness), blood group, hemoglobin, and coagulation.

Anesthetic considerations: Tracheal intubation might be problematic because of the hypoplastic mandible and dental anomalies. The main problem associated with anesthesia is the aortic stenosis; those patients with aortic stenosis should be managed in such a fashion as to limit myocardial oxygen demand. In older patients, because of the progressive joint limitation, positioning might be more difficult and the anesthetist must ensure an adequate padding.

Pharmacological implications: Even though this syndrome has not been formally associated with malignant hyperthermia, the two diseases have similar genetic defects. There are two case reports in the literature of abnormally elevated creatinine kinase after general anesthesia in one patient and masseter spasm in the other patient; consequently, it must be kept in mind that these patients might be more susceptible to malignant hyperthermia than the general population. Succinylcholine is best avoided. Nondepolarizing muscle relaxants should be used only after the airway is secure. Prophylactic antibiotics in cases of cardiopathy.

Other conditions to be considered:

☞**NOONAN SYNDROME:** A rare genetic disorder characterized by a wide spectrum of symptoms and physical features that vary greatly in range and severity. In many affected individuals, associated abnormalities include a distinctive facial appearance; a broad or webbed neck; a low hairline in the back of the head; and short stature. Pulmonary valvular stenosis is often present.

IDIOPATHIC INFANTILE HYPERCALCEMIA: Characterized by the idiopathic elevation of blood calcium levels in a newborn. Anorexia, irritability, confusion, weakness, easy fatigability, and/or abdominal and muscle pain are reported. Some studies in the medical literature question whether idiopathic infantile hypercalcemia is a separate disorder from Williams syndrome or simply a variant of the same disease. However, infants with this form of the disease do not have the characteristic facial features or heart defects that are associated with Williams syndrome.

REFERENCES:

Kawahito S, Kitahata H, Kimura H, et al: Anaesthetic management of a patient with Williams syndrome undergoing aortoplasty for supravalvular aortic stenosis. *Can J Anaesth* 45:1203, 1998.

Mammi I, Iles DE, Smeets D, et al: Anesthesiologic problems in Williams syndrome: The CACNL2A locus is not involved. *Hum Genet* 98:317, 1996.

Medley J, Russo P, Tobias JD: Perioperative care of the patient with Williams syndrome. *Paediatr Anaesth* 15:243, 2005.

Patel J, Harrison MJ: Williams syndrome: Masseter spasm during anaesthesia. *Anaesthesia* 46:115, 1991.

Williams-Campbell Syndrome

At a glance: A syndrome caused by a defect of cartilage of the first and second generation bronchi leading to complete collapse during expiration. Respiratory syndromes can be severe. Related syndromes are multiple.

Synonym: Bronchomalacia.

Genetic inheritance: Unknown.

Pathophysiology: Characterized by the absence or markedly diminished cartilage around the bronchi. The exact pathophysiology is still unknown.

Diagnosis: Clinical evocation is difficult; computed tomography (CT) scan and endoscopy can confirm the diagnosis.

Clinical aspects: Chronic respiratory distress in early infancy as a result of bronchial flaccidity. First- and second-generation bronchi almost collapse during expiration. Air trapping and respiratory distress simulate bronchial asthma. Increased frequency of pulmonary infection.

Precautions before anesthesia: Evaluate respiratory status (clinical, CT scan, pulmonary function test, arterial blood gas, bacteriological examination). Evaluate airway dynamic (awake fiberoptic evaluation) and the potential for difficult direct laryngoscopy and tracheal intubation.

Anesthetic considerations: Patients with structural abnormalities of the tracheobronchial tree can be at increased risk for complications when undergoing surgical procedures that impact airway dynamics. Spontaneous ventilation should be preferred when possible; for example, with regional anesthesia. Perioperative physiotherapy is needed to avoid pulmonary superinfection.

Pharmacological implications: Muscle relaxants are not contraindicated but should be avoided to prevent decrease in airway dynamic.

Other conditions to be considered:

MOUNIER-KUHN SYNDROME (Tracheomegaly; Tracheobronchomegaly): Autosomal recessive; death in infancy; musculomembranous tissue projects like corrugations between tracheal cartilaginous rings, composing a congenital tracheobronchomegaly associated with a connective tissue disorder; can also result from parietal fibrosing pulmonary diseases that apply traction to the tracheal walls.

☞**SWYER JAMES MACLEOD SYNDROME:** Generally discovered on chest radiograph. Frequent expiratory adenovirus infections,

decrease exercise tolerance, arterial desaturation and hemoptysis. Frequent pneumothorax may probably contraindicate the use of nitrous oxide.

☞**YELLOW NAIL SYNDROME:** Associates yellow nails (89%), lymphedema (80%), and pleural effusion (36%); dilatation of both visceral and parietal pleural lymphatic with perilymphatic inflammation.

REFERENCES:

Benesch M, Eber E, Pfleger A, et al: Recurrent lower respiratory tract infections in a 14-year-old boy with tracheobronchomegaly (Mounier-Kuhn syndrome). *Pediatr Pulmonol* 29(6):476, 2000.

Jones VF, Eid NS, Franco SM, et al: Familial congenital bronchiectasis: Williams-Campbell syndrome. *Pediatr Pulmonol* 16(4):263, 1993.

Palmer SM Jr, Layish DT, Kussin PS, et al: Lung transplantation for Williams-Campbell syndrome. *Chest* 113:53, 1998.

Wilson Disease

At a glance: An inherited disease of copper metabolism dysfunction characterized by cirrhosis and central nervous system (CNS) findings; fatal if not recognized and treated.

Synonym: Hepatolenticular Degeneration.

History: Genetic disorder most common in Eastern Europeans, Jews, Arabs, Italians, Japanese, Chinese, and Indians.

Incidence: 1:30,000 in general population.

Genetic inheritance: Autosomal recessive. Gene localized to chromosome 13.

Pathophysiology: Caused by mutation in the ATPase, Cu^{2+} transporting, beta-polypeptide gene (ATP7B) located at 13q14.3–q21.1. A defect in copper metabolism leads to decreased incorporation of copper into ceruloplasmin and reduction in biliary excretion of copper. This results in deposition of copper into *liver* (resulting in fatty intracellular accumulations progressing to deposition of collagen, fibrosis, and nodular cirrhosis followed by development of portal hypertension and esophageal and gastric varices), *brain* (particularly basal ganglia, putamen, globus and pallidus, and caudate, resulting in inflammation, gliosis, and eventually loss of neurons), and *kidney* (resulting in Fanconi syndrome, aminoaciduria, glycosuria, phosphaturia, and nephrolithiasis). Other systemic involvement may include hemolytic anemia, osteoporosis, copper deposition in heart, rhabdomyolysis, and hypoparathyroidism.

Diagnosis: Based on clinical course and biochemical findings, including low serum ceruloplasmin, elevated 24-hour urinary copper excretion, and liver biopsy.

Clinical aspects: Characterized by the involvement of several systems. *Hepatic:* a spectrum from fulminant liver failure associated with coagulopathy and encephalopathy (more common in children) to chronic progressive cirrhosis with development of portal hypertension. *Neurologic:* intention tremor, dysarthria, loss of fine motor control, mask-like facies, pseudobulbar involvement, drooling, dysphagia, dystonia, incoordination, difficulty with fine motor tasks, and gait disturbance. *Eyes:* Kayser-Fleischer rings are almost pathognomonic and appear as a brownish deposit at the periphery of the cornea. *Cardiac:* rarely develop cardiomyopathy; rhythm abnormalities and increased autonomic tone are observed. *Renal:* renal complications tend to be functional changes unrelated to identifiable histologic findings. Rarely, patients with Wilson disease develop renal stones and associated symptoms. Renal stones are precipitated by hypercalciuria and poor urine acidification. *Musculoskeletal:* highly variable and includes osteoporosis, osteomalacia, rickets, spontaneous fractures, and polyarthritis. *Skin:* skin pigmentation and a bluish discoloration at the base of the fingernails (azure lunulae). Clinical course depends on presentation. With early diagnosis can be effectively treated with chelating agents, including penicillamine, trientine, and zinc.

Precautions before anesthesia: Clinical evaluation of the hepatic function and neurologic and cardiac status. Evaluate in particular, coagulation status, and the concentration of serum albumin. The correction of any coagulopathy must be done prior to surgery. Cardiac evaluation, including echocardiogram and ECG must be obtained. Blood examination: cell blood count (CBC), renal function. Evaluate for penicillamine side effects.

Anesthetic considerations: Some degree of liver dysfunction is invariably present and should be considered in selection of anesthetic agents. Consider presence of varices and the possibility of gastrointestinal (GI) bleed. Penicillamine may have significant side effects, including leukopenia, thrombocytopenia, aplastic anemia, nephrotic syndrome, and myasthenia-like syndrome.

Pharmacological implications: Anesthetic agents requiring hepatic and, to a lesser extent, renal clearance must be used with care. Caution should be used with neuromuscular blocking agents in the presence of myasthenia-like syndrome.

Other condition to be considered:

☞**CERULOPLASMIN DEFICIENCY:** A group of genetic disorders affecting the expression of the ceruloplasmin gene leading to an iron storage disorder with hepatic failure and progressive dementia.

REFERENCES:

Brewer G, Yuzbasiyan-Gurkan V: Wilson disease. *Medicine (Baltimore)* 71:3:139, 1992.

Cox D, Roberts E: Wilson disease, in Feldman M, Scharschmidt B, Sleisenger M (eds): *Gastrointestinal and Liver Disease.* 6th ed. Philadelphia, WB Saunders, 1998, p 1104.

Forbes JR, Cox DW: Copper-dependent trafficking of Wilson disease mutant ATP7B proteins. *Hum Mol Genet* 9:1927, 2000.

Wilson-Turner Syndrome

At a glance: Mental retardation syndrome affecting mostly males. The phenotype is variable, combining gynecomastia, obesity, speech disability, hypogonadism, and small feet.

Synonyms: X-Linked Mental Retardation Syndromic 6; X-Linked Mental Retardation with Gynecomastia and Obesity.

Incidence and genetic inheritance: Very rare syndrome; X-linked recessive inheritance.

Clinical aspects: Probable developmental anomaly of the central nervous system, dysfunction of the hypothalamic pituitary–gonadal axis, with secondary rather than primary gonadal insufficiency. Principal features are mental retardation, obesity, gynecomastia, speech difficulties, emotional lability, tapering fingers, and small feet. Many other signs have been occasionally described.

Anesthetic considerations: Obesity can make venous access, direct laryngoscopy and tracheal intubation difficult.

REFERENCES:

Gedeon A, Mulley J, Turner G: Gene localisation for Wilson-Turner syndrome (WTS:MIM 309585). *Am J Med Genet* 64:80, 1996.

Wilson M, Mulley J, Gedeon A, et al: New X-linked syndrome of mental retardation, gynecomastia and obesity is linked to DXS255. *Am J Med Genet* 40:406, 1991.

Wiskott-Aldrich Syndrome

At a glance: This syndrome occurs only in males and is characterized by eczema, profound thrombocytopenia, and frequent infections as a result of a defect in both T- and B-cell function. Death frequently occurs during childhood.

Synonyms: Aldrich Syndrome; Eczema-Thrombocytopenia-Immunodeficiency Syndrome; Aldrich-Huntley Syndrome; Aldrich-Dees Syndrome; Aldrich-Wiskott Syndrome; Wiskott Syndrome; Wiskott-Aldrich-Huntley Syndrome; Wiskott-Aldrich-Dees Syndrome.

History: Inherited immune deficiency that was first described by Alfred Wiskott, German pediatrician in 1937, and characterized by Robert Anderson Aldrich, American pediatrician in 1954.

Incidence: 1:200,000 live births.

Genetic inheritance: Transmitted as an X-linked recessive trait.

Pathophysiology: Caused by mutation in the WAS gene located at Xp11.23–p11.22.

Diagnosis: Onset generally occurs before 3 years of age in a boy with hemorrhagic signs, thrombocytopenia with small-size platelets, recurrent infections, and eczema. Early prenatal diagnosis can be made by trophoblast biopsies.

Clinical aspects: Mental retardation is frequent. *Infections* are recurrent and can include the orolaryngotracheal system, the lungs, meningitis, and diarrhea. *Hemorrhagic signs* can involve epistaxis, oral bleeding, hematemesis, melena, petechiae, and purpura; bleeding time is prolonged. *Eczema* is very frequent, nephropathy and signs of autoimmunity are often observed, and there is an increased risk of malignancy (particularly lymphoma). *Laboratory investigations* can show thrombocytopenia (with small-size platelets), anemia (hemolytic, iron deficiency), small and large vessel vasculitis, and sialophorin defectively expressed on surface of blood cells. Immunological patterns concern depressed antibody response to polysaccharide antigens, lymphopenia, abnormal delayed hypersensitivity skin test, absent microvilli on the surface of peripheral blood lymphocytes, increased IgA and IgE levels, decreased IgM levels, raised erythrocyte sedimentation rate and C-reactive protein.

Precautions before anesthesia: It is recommended to obtain an anesthesiology consultation before elective surgical procedures. One must obtain a complete medical history and physical examination. Evaluate pulmonary function because of recurrent lung infections (clinical, chest radiographs, CT scan, pulmonary function test with arterial blood gas analysis), cardiac function because of autoimmune vasculitis that can affect coronary arteries (clinical, ECG, echocardiography if necessary), renal function (clinical, urea, creatinine, electrolytes), neurological function because of the frequent intracranial hemorrhage (clinical, CT), and bleeding risk (clinical, platelet count, bleeding time, red blood cell count).

Anesthetic considerations: Strict asepsis is needed. Avoid all intranasal devices. Perimedullar blockade should be avoided because of the hemorrhagic risk. Benefit of peripheral regional anesthesia has to be established.

Pharmacological implications: Anesthetic drugs and fluid regimens have to be adapted to renal function. Consider these patients

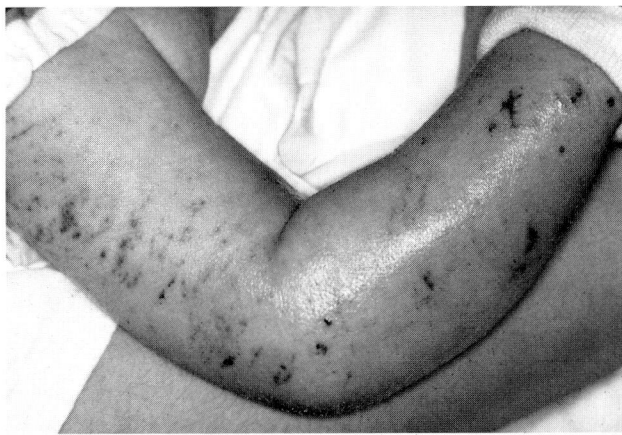

Wiskott-Aldrich syndrome Eczematous and hemorrhagic skin changes in an infant boy with Wiskott-Aldrich syndrome. See color plates.

as immunodeficient when providing prophylactic antibiotherapy. Preoperative steroid stress doses are required in cases of long-term treatment. Blood products must be irradiated to prevent graft versus host reaction.

Other conditions to be considered:

☞**NEZELOF SYNDROME:** A group of rare, inherited disorders characterized by recurrent infections because of the impairment of the T lymphocyte system and, in some cases, the B lymphocyte system. In infancy, severe infections with low-grade or opportunistic microorganisms are often observed. An autosomal recessive or X-linked recessive genetic transmission has been suggested. Males are affected more than females.

☞**IDIOPATHIC THROMBOCYTOPENIA PURPURA:** Characterized by severe thrombocytopenia leading to minor dermal or submucosal hemorrhages (petechia), fever, and splenomegaly. Current evidence supports an immunologic basis. It is believed that females are more affected than males.

X-LINKED AGAMMAGLOBULINEMIA: A rare inherited immune deficiency characterized by defects of the B lymphocyte system and insufficient levels of certain circulating antibodies. Affected individuals experience recurrent bacterial infections during the first year of life. Because this disorder is inherited as an X-linked recessive pattern, only males are affected.

☞**SEVERE COMBINED IMMUNODEFICIENCY (SCID):** A group of rare, inherited disorders characterized by impairment of both the T lymphocyte and B lymphocyte systems ("combined immunodeficiency"), resulting in little or no immune response and severe recurrent infections. Most affected infants present with failure to thrive. It may be inherited as autosomal recessive or X-linked genetic traits. Approximately 80% of individuals with SCID are male.

REFERENCES:

Aldrich RA, Steinberg AG, Campbell DC: Pedigree demonstrating a sex-linked recessive condition characterized by draining ears, eczematoid dermatitis, and bloody diarrhea. *Pediatrics* 13:133, 1954.

Braithwaite K, Abu-Ghosh A, Anderson L, et al: Treatment of severe thrombocytopenia with IL-11 in children with Wiskott-Aldrich syndrome. *J Pediatr Hematol Oncol* 24(4):323, 2002.

Kim AS, Kakalis LT, Abdul-Manan N, et al: Autoinhibition and activation mechanisms of the Wiskott-Aldrich syndrome protein. *Nature* 404:151, 2000.

Wohlfart-Kugelberg-Welander Syndrome

At a glance: Juvenile spinal muscular atrophy, characterized by slowly progressive muscular weakness as a result of degeneration of anterior horn cells (spinal motor neurons). Onset is between the ages of 2 and 17 years. Early symptoms consist of atrophy and weakness of the proximal muscle of the extremities (mainly legs), followed by thoracic muscles. Should not be confused with muscular dystrophy syndromes.

Synonyms: Kugelberg-Welander Syndrome; Juvenile type of Muscular Atrophy Syndrome; Neurogenic Familial Girdle type of Muscular Atrophy, type K-W; Spinal Muscular Atrophy type III; Juvenile Spinal Muscular Atrophy.

Nature: Neurological disorder resulting from degeneration of anterior horn cells. Kugelberg-Welander Spinal Muscular Atrophy is the least severe of the three forms of spinal muscular atrophy.

Incidence: 1:15,000 live births; genetic carrier prevalence is 1:80. Both sexes affected, but more severe in males.

Genetic inheritance: Mostly autosomal recessive; some families with autosomal dominant inheritance; very rarely, X-linked transmission. Gene map location (usually) is 5q13.

Pathophysiology: Degeneration of anterior horn cells.

Diagnosis: Blood DNA analysis, electromyography, and muscle biopsy.

Clinical aspects: Onset at the age of 3 to 4 years, with progressive muscular dystrophy involving, at first, the proximal muscles. Progressive weakness of the axial muscles, pharyngeal control, and swallowing. Decreased or absent tendon reflexes and muscular fasciculations. Progressive respiratory failure as a result of muscular weakness. Cardiac involvement seems to be significant and includes atrial hyperexcitability, atrioventricular blocks, and right-sided heart failure as a result of pulmonary hypertension. Congestive biventricular failure has also been reported.

Precautions before anesthesia: Check pulmonary functions before induction. Numerous postoperative pulmonary infections. Need intensive care unit stay after operation, and may need several days postoperative ventilation. Check ECG for signs of right cardiac overload; echocardiography may be useful. Cardiovascular status and intravascular fluid volume should be evaluated.

Anesthetic considerations: Very poor vascular access. Maintain intravascular volume. Perioperative cardiac monitoring is necessary. Intracardiac stimulation should be available in operating room in case of severe sudden conduction block.

Pharmacological implications: Avoid succinylcholine. Exaggerated response to neuromuscular blockers (complete muscular blockade with 20 to 30% of the usual dose), titration is indicated and the use of neuromuscular monitoring highly recommended. Avoid drugs that could trigger cardiac dysrhythmias.

Other conditions to be considered: Other variants of ☞spinal muscular atrophy including type 1 (Werdnig-Hoffman disease, the most severe form); type 2 (chronic spinal muscular atrophy, juvenile spinal muscular atrophy, or intermediate spinal muscular atrophy); and type 4 (adult spinal muscular atrophy) need to be considered.

REFERENCES:

Fehlings DL, Kirsch S, McComas A, et al: Evaluation of therapeutic electrical stimulation to improve muscle strength and function in children with types II/III spinal muscular atrophy. *Dev Med Child Neurol* 44:741, 2002.

Nicole S, Diaz CC, Frugier T, et al: Spinal muscular atrophy: Recent advances and future prospects. *Muscle Nerve* 26:4, 2002.

Veen A, Molenbuur B, Richardson FJ: Epidural anaesthesia in a child with possible spinal muscular atrophy. *Paediatr Anaesth* 12:556, 2002.

Wolff-Parkinson-White (WPW) Syndrome

At a glance: Ventricular preexcitation associated with a short P-R interval and a wide QRS complex.

Incidence: Incidence 1 to 3:1000 in a general population.

Genetic inheritance: Unclear, an autosomal dominant inheritance is suggested by some kindreds. Can be caused by mutation in the gamma-2 regulatory subunit of AMP-activated protein kinase (PRKAG) located on 7q36.

Pathophysiology: During fetal life, numerous connections link the atria to the ventricles, but they all disappear before birth except for the bundle of His. Sometimes, some of the connections do not disappear. This accessory pathway(s) characterizes the Wolff-Parkinson-White syndrome. An accessory atrioventricular connection (bundle of Kent) bypasses the atrioventricular node, and inserts directly into myocardium (consistent with bypass tracts in Lown-Ganong-Levine syndrome). The accessory bundle may conduct ante- or retrograde. Antegrade conduction causes early commencement of ventricular depolarization, seen as a delta wave on the ECG. Retrograde conduction allows a reentry circuit to develop and is a mechanism for paroxysmal tachycardia generation. The accessory connection may only conduct in a retrograde direction; therefore a delta wave will not appear on ECG. Such a tract is described as concealed. In atrial fibrillation, antegrade conduction along the accessory pathway may result in rapid ventricular rate, which is poorly tolerated.

Diagnosis: History, ECG findings of a short P-R interval, and a delta wave. Electrophysiology studies to define individual pathway anatomy and mechanism for dysrhythmia generation.

Clinical aspects: May be asymptomatic. Symptoms include palpitations (paroxysmal episodes of supraventricular tachycardia or atrial fibrillation), shortness of breath, feeding difficulties in infancy, syncope and chest pain. In infancy, WPW tends to improve in the first year of life and may be associated with Ebstein anomaly. Sudden death secondary to dysrhythmia may occur. *Type A* WPW demonstrates a large R wave in leads V1 and V2. In *type B* WPW, the S or QS waves predominate in leads V1 and V2. Supraventricular tachycardias may be managed by verapamil (potent negative inotrope), beta blockade, amiodarone, adenosine or cardioversion. Adenosine is said to achieve cardioversion in up to 87% of narrow complex tachycardias associated with WPW. Catheter or surgical ablation of pathways or pacemakers may also be indicated.

Precautions before anesthesia: Obtain a history of frequency of dysrhythmia, and current treatment regimen. Continue antidysrhythmic drugs perioperatively. Review results of electrophysiology studies if available. Preoperative ECG mandatory. Pacemaker details if used to control supraventricular tachycardia (atrial overdrive pacing). Correct any electrolyte disturbance (sodium, potassium, and magnesium).

Anesthetic considerations: Minimize perioperative catecholamine surges; premedication may be beneficial. Perioperative beta blockade has been used. Atropine premedication, however,

is relatively contraindicated. Use a technique to minimize risk of hypoxia, hypercarbia, or acidosis, all of which render cardiac muscle membranes unstable and ectopic depolarization more likely.

Pharmacological implications: Enflurane is the volatile agent, which is probably least likely to induce arrhythmia. Halothane should be avoided (proarrhythmogenic, myocardial depressant). Desflurane has a sympathomimetic effect, which is undesirable. Sevoflurane has been used and reported to be appropriate. Propofol has no effect on the refractory period of normal and accessory tissue, thus it is useful for electrophysiology studies and ablation procedures. Pancuronium is relatively contraindicated. Extreme care if administering beta blockade to a patient already taking verapamil (may precipitate heart block). If atrial flutter or fibrillation is the cause of tachycardia, digoxin and verapamil are contraindicated because they may decrease the accessory pathway refractory period and exacerbate the tachydysrhythmia.

REFERENCES:

Chang RK, Wetzel GT, Shannon KM, et al: Age- and anesthesia-related changes in accessory pathway conduction in children with Wolff-Parkinson-White syndrome. *Am J Cardiol* 76(14):1074, 1995.

Sharpe MD, Cuillerier DJ, Lee JK et al: Sevoflurane has no effect on sinoatrial noded function or on normal atrioventricular and accessory pathway conduction in Wolff-Parkinson-White syndrome during alfentanil/midazolam anesthesia. *Anesthesiology* 90:60–65, 1999.

Sharpe M, Dobkowski W, Murkin J, et al: Propofol has no direct effect on sinoatrial node function or on normal atrioventricular and accessory pathway conduction in Wolff-Parkinson-White syndrome during alfentanil/midazolam anesthesia. *Anesthesiology* 82:888, 1995.

Wolf-Hirschhorn Syndrome

At a glance: A syndrome characterized by severe hypotrophy with prenatal onset and a distinctive facial dysmorphism resembling a "Greek warrior's helmet." Cardiac malformation is observed in half the cases. Mental retardation is usually severe.

Synonyms: Deletion 4p; Monosomy 4p.

Genetic inheritance: Caused by partial deletion of the short arm of 1 chromosome 4.

Pathophysiology: The critical zone for development of this disorder is located distal to the Huntington disease-linked G8 (D4S10) marker.

Diagnosis: Clinically evocated by severe growth retardation and mental defect, microcephaly, "Greek helmet" facies, and closure defects. Cytogenetic demonstration of loss of the terminal segment of 4p (4p16.3). Radiological evidence of delayed bone age.

Clinical aspects: Clinical features include severe growth and mental retardation, corpus callosum agenesis, microcephaly, scalp defect, "Greek helmet" facies, severe ocular hypertelorism, prominent glabella, beaked nose, short philtrum, micrognathia, carp-shaped mouth, cleft lip, cleft palate, low-set simple ears, iris coloboma, hypertelorism, downward-slanting palpebral fissures, ventricular septal defect, renal hypoplasia, hypospadias, pulmonary isomerism, hemangioma-capillary, diaphragmatic hernia, sacral dimple, abnormal dermal ridges, common intestinal mesentery, long limbs, and long rib cage. Other clinical features may include absent pubic rami, congenital hip dislocation and scoliosis.

Precautions before anesthesia: Evaluate the airway carefully because of facial abnormalities, including micrognathia (clinical, radiographs, fiberoptic if necessary), cardiac function in cases of cardiopathy (clinical, chest radiographs, ECG, echocardiography), and pulmonary function (clinical, chest, radiographs, pulmonary function test, arterial blood gas analysis).

Anesthetic considerations: Difficult direct laryngoscopy and tracheal intubation may require adequate anesthetic management. Careful intraoperative positioning because of scoliosis. Although, one case report about a child presenting with Wolf-Hirschhorn syndrome developed malignant hyperthermia, there is no evidence to suggest that there is an increased risk of this complication with this medical condition.

Pharmacological implications: Perioperative fluid regimen and anesthetic drug choice should be adapted to the cardiac and renal functions. Muscle relaxant is best used after airway is secured. Antibiotic prophylaxis in cases of cardiopathy.

Other conditions to be considered:

☞**PITT-ROGERS-DANKS SYNDROME:** Prominent eyes, mental retardation, unusual facies, and intrauterine growth retardation, probably involves the deletion of multiple loci on 4p16.3; known as a milder form of the Wolf-Hirschhorn syndrome.

☞**CAT-CRY SYNDROME:** A rare chromosomal disorder that involves a partial deletion of the small arm (p) of chromosome 5. It is clinically similar to the Wolf-Hirschhorn syndrome, especially with the severe ocular hypertelorism, but with one specific additional distinctive high, shrill, mewing, "kitten-like" cry during infancy. This cry becomes less pronounced during late infancy. Other features include failure to thrive, microcephaly, micrognathia, and mental retardation.

REFERENCES:

Iacobucci T, Nanni L, Picoco F, de Francisci G: Anesthesia for a child with Wolf-Hirschhorn syndrome. *Paediatr Anaesth* 14:969, 2004.

Mohiuddin S, Mayhew JF: Anesthesia for children with Wolf-Hirschhorn syndrome: a report and literature review. *Paediatr Anaesth* 15:254, 2005.

Sammartino M, Crea MA, Sbarra GM, et al: Absence of malignant hyperthermia in an infant with Wolf-Hirschhorn syndrome undergoing anesthesia for ophthalmic surgery. *J Pediatr Ophthalmol Strabismus* 36(1):42, 1999.

Shannon NL, Maltby EL, Rigby AS, et al: An epidemiological study of Wolf-Hirschhorn syndrome: Life expectancy and cause of mortality. *J Med Genet* 38:674, 2001.

Thies U, Back E, Wolff G, Schroeder-Kurth T, Hager HD, Schroder K: Clinical, cytogenetic and molecular investigations in three patients with Wolf-Hirschhorn syndrome. *Clin Genet* 42:201, 1992.

Wolfram Syndrome

At a glance: Diabetes mellitus and insipidus with optic nerve atrophy, mental retardation and deafness.

Synonym: Diabetes Insipidus, Diabetes Mellitus, Optic Atrophy and Deafness; DIDMOAD.

History: Genetic syndrome that was first described by D.J. Wolfram in 1938.

Incidence: Unknown; males and females are equally affected.

Genetic inheritance: Autosomal recessive.

Pathophysiology: Caused by a mutation in the gene encoding wolframin (WFS1) on chromosome 4p16.1. Another locus for the disorder has been mapped to 4q (WFS2). Marked atrophy and degener-

ation is seen in the pons, the medullary reticular activating system, substantia nigra, superior and inferior olives, and the cerebellum. Microscopically, neuronal loss and axonal destruction, often accompanied by gliosis, is apparent, together with scattered areas of demyelination in the cerebrum and cerebellum, without inflammatory change.

Diagnosis: A combination of juvenile-onset diabetes mellitus and optic nerve atrophy plus one or more of the following: anosmia, brainstem signs (gaze palsies, nystagmus, dysarthria, dysphagia, primary respiratory failure), deafness, seizures or myoclonus, ataxia, axial rigidity, neuropsychiatric or cognitive abnormalities, neurogenic incontinence or dilated urinary tract, hyporeflexia or areflexia, extensor plantar responses, diabetes insipidus, and family history.

Clinical aspects: Diabetes mellitus, diabetes insipidus, optic nerve atrophy, sensorineural hearing loss, autonomic dysfunction, cardiomyopathy, mental retardation, seizures, nystagmus, hydronephrosis, megaloblastic anemia, sideroblastic anemia, neutropenia, thrombocytopenia.

Precautions before anesthesia: A complete evaluation of the cardiac function (clinical, ECG, echocardiography) must be obtained. Evaluate neurological function (clinical, EEG, CT scan), hematology, and biochemistry.

Anesthetic considerations: Perioperative fluid regimen should be adapted to diabetes insipidus. The use of regional anesthetic technique, especially neuraxial approach, must consider the potential for autonomic dysfunction and hemodynamic instability. A close control of pre- and intraoperative glycemia must be done.

Pharmacological implications: Consider interaction between anesthetic drugs and antiepileptic treatment. Avoid enflurane. Consider renal function and whether beneficial to use aminoglycosides.

Other condition to be considered:

WOLFRAM SYNDROME, MITOCHONDRIAL FORM WITH VASO-PRESSIN DEFICIENCY: Low erythrocyte thiamine pyrophosphate. Low thiamine pyrophosphokinase activity. Heteroplasmic mtDNA deletion. Mild hyperlactatemia.

REFERENCES:

Ajlouni K, Jarrah N, El-Khateeb M, et al: Wolfram syndrome: Identification of a phenotypic and genotypic variant from Jordan. *Am J Med Genet* 115:61, 2002.

El-Shanti H, Lidral AC, Jarrah N, et al: Homozygosity mapping identifies an additional locus for Wolfram syndrome on chromosome 4q. *Am J Hum Genet* 66:1229, 2000.

Minton JA, Rainbow LA, Ricketts C, et al: Wolfram syndrome. *Rev Endocr Metab Disord* 4:53, 2003.

Wyburn Mason Syndrome

At a glance: It is characterized by multiple cerebral arteriovenous shunts leading to intracerebral bleeds and embolic phenomena. The possibility for cardiovascular instability and signs of congestive heart failure must be assessed.

Synonyms: Bonnet-Dechaume-Blanc Syndrome; Cerebroretinal Arteriovenous Aneurysms.

History: This syndrome was first described by P. Bonnet in 1937.

Genetic inheritance: Not probable.

Pathophysiology: Multiple arteriovenous malformations exist; cause is unknown.

Diagnosis: Multiple malformations exist both intracerebrally and elsewhere. Retinal malformations are the most common (81% of cases). Neurological symptoms vary among central nervous system lesions based on location. Diagnosis is confirmed by fluorescein angiography, CT scan, and magnetic resonance imaging (MRI).

Clinical aspects: The presence of intracerebral arteriovenous malformations may lead to intracerebral bleeds and embolic phenomena as the first presenting sign. Alternatively, ophthalmic arteriovenous malformations may cause sudden loss of vision as a result of bleeding. Hemorrhage caused by dental extraction overlying a lesion has been reported. Many of these lesions are now treated by embolization in the radiology department.

Precautions before anesthesia: History and examination must elucidate the location of the lesions.

Anesthetic considerations: Intraoral lesions must be adequately protected at the time of anesthetic induction or intraoral instrumentation. Intracranial arteriovenous malformations are at risk of rupture if subjected to high swings in arterial blood pressure. Intraocular lesions may bleed for similar reasons. Gastrointestinal hemorrhage and hemoptysis have all been described. If very extensive, multiple arteriovenous malformations may lead to a high-output cardiac failure, requiring treatment before anesthesia and surgery. Central regional anesthesia is best avoided because of the risk of associated medullar angioma.

Pharmacological implications: Ketamine and Hypnomidate are best avoided because they can cause high blood pressure that is relatively contraindicated in arteriovenous malformations.

Other conditions to be considered:

☞**Von Hippel-Lindau Syndrome:** Usually begins during young adulthood but may appear during childhood around the age of 8 years. Clinical features include headaches, dizziness and ataxia. Behavior problems may also be present. Cerebroretinal aneurysms may develop. Adrenal gland tumors have been reported.

☞**Sturge-Weber Syndrome:** A hereditary disorder manifested by the presence of large facial port-wine stain angioma and intracranial arteriovenous malformations present at birth. Generalized seizures and an array of neurological symptoms usually occur at the age of 1 or 2 years. The vascular lesions in the brain usually involve the occipital or parieto-occipital regions.

REFERENCES:

Brodsky MC, Hoyt WF: Spontaneous involution of retinal and intracranial arteriovenous malformation in Bonnet-Dechaume-Blanc syndrome. *Br J Ophthalmol* 86(3):360, 2002.

Iizuka Y, Garcia-Monaco R, Alvarez H, et al: Multiple cerebral arteriovenous malformations in children. *Childs Nerv Syst* 8:437, 1992.

Xanthinuria

At a glance: An inherited disorder of purine metabolism that can be asymptomatic or revealed clinically by renal manifestations. Characterized by the excretion of large amounts of xanthine in the urine and tendency to form xanthine stones.

Synonyms: Xanthine Oxidase Deficiency; Xanthic Urolithiasis; Xanthine Dehydrogenase Deficiency.

Incidence: Not exactly known; estimated to be from 1:6000 to 1:60,000 live births. Proportion of each of the two types is 50%.

Genetic inheritance: Autosomal recessive.

Pathophysiology: Deficiency of the enzyme xanthine oxidase, which mediates the oxidation of hypoxanthine to xanthine and of xanthine to uric acid. This leads to an increased urinary excretion of hypoxanthine and xanthine, with a tendency to form xanthine stones. Uric acid is strikingly diminished in the serum and urine. Two distinct forms of xanthinuria are recognized: type I (caused by mutations in the gene encoding xanthine dehydrogenase [XDH] located on 2p23-p22), with isolated deficiency of xanthine dehydrogenase; type II, with deficiency of xanthine dehydrogenase and aldehyde oxidase. Only type I patients can metabolize allopurinol. Additionally, xanthinuria occurs in molybdenum cofactor deficiency, where sulfite oxidase (SO) is also inactive.

Diagnosis: Twenty percent of patients are asymptomatic. Symptoms are not specific. Irritability, vomiting, and failure to thrive may be the presenting symptoms. The patient may present at any age with hematuria, pyuria, renal colic, dysuria, urinary frequency, urine incontinence, polyuria, abdominal pain, or symptoms of a urinary tract infection. Laboratory findings include low or absent uric acid replaced by xanthine in concentrations from 10 to 40 μmol/L. Hypoxanthine concentrations are lower than 5 μmol/L. Xanthine and hypoxanthine can be find in the urine, xanthine calculi in the urinary tract, and crystalline deposits in skeletal muscles.

Clinical aspects: Xanthine stones may lead to renal colic, hematuria, voiding dysfunction, irritability, orange-red urinary sediment, hydronephrosis, and pyelonephritis. A unique type of myopathy is associated with crystalline deposits in skeletal muscles. Joint pain and muscle cramps or muscle pain are symptoms of the arthropathy and myopathy.

Precautions before anesthesia: Adequate hydration must be ensured to minimize the urinary concentration of xanthine and hypoxanthine. Evaluate renal function (clinical, echography, laboratory including urea, creatinine, and electrolytes).

Anesthetic considerations: It is essential to maintain adequate hydration and intravascular volume. Succinylcholine should not be used in patients presenting with associated myopathy. Although there are no reports in the literature suggesting that there is an increased risk of hyperkalemia and/or malignant hyperthermia in these patients, the presence of severe muscle cramps may be enough to raise significant concern.

Pharmacological implications: Succinylcholine is best avoided because of myopathy.

Other conditions to be considered:

☞**MOLYBDENUM COFACTOR DEFICIENCY:** Autosomal recessive; present in the neonatal period with microcephaly and central nervous system manifestations. It is caused by a congenital defect of a molybdenum-containing cofactor essential for the function of three distinct enzymes (xanthine dehydrogenase, aldehyde oxidase, sulfite oxidase). Generally lethal in the first year of life because of sulfite oxidase deficiency. Anesthetic implications of this form concern enflurane, which is best avoided because of an increased risk of seizures.

IATROGENIC XANTHINURIA: A medical condition resulting from iatrogenic allopurinol treatment.

REFERENCES:

Chalmers RA, Johnson M, Pallis C, et al: Xanthinuria with myopathy. *Q J Med* 38:493, 1969.

Rytkönen EMK, Halila R, Laan M, et al: The human gene for xanthine dehydrogenase (XDH) is localized on chromosome band 2p22. *Cytogenet Cell Genet* 68:61, 1995.

Sakamoto N, Yamamoto T, Moriwaki Y, et al: Identification of a new point mutation in the human xanthine dehydrogenase gene responsible for a case of classical type I xanthinuria. *Hum Genet* 108(4):279, 2001.

Xeroderma Pigmentosum (XP)

At a glance: A syndrome characterized by a defect in ultraviolet radiation-induced DNA repair mechanisms and by a severe sensitivity to all sources of ultraviolet radiation (especially sunlight). XP is categorized into seven complementation groups according to the capacity of the body to repair DNA. Life-threatening. The DNA damage is cumulative and irreversible. Sometimes lethal in infancy or childhood.

Synonym: Xerodermic Idiocy; Kaposi Disease.

History: A group of rare autosomal recessive inherited disorders that were first described by Ferdinand Ritter von Hebra, Austrian dermatologist, and Moritz Kohn Kaposi, Hungarian dermatologist, in 1874.

Incidence: 1:250,000 in general population; higher in Japan (1:40,000). Sex ratio is about 1.

Genetic inheritance: A rare autosomal recessive genetic defect.

Pathophysiology: Caused by a defect in nucleotide excision repair (NER), leading to an inability to repair DNA damaged by ultraviolet radiation. There are two types of NER: global genome (GG-NER) and transcription coupled (TC-NER). There are seven XP repair genes (XPA to XPG), with seven principal complementation groups of XP corresponding to defects (four other subcategories have been described). Frequency and severity varies among forms; XPA and XPC are the most common.

Diagnosis: Clinically evocated by the skin lesions with a three-stage evolution. Skin is normal at birth. After the age of 6 months, a diffuse erythema, scaling, and freckle-like areas of increased pigmentation, initially on the face can be seen. The second stage is characterized by poikiloderma and the third stage by the appearance of numerous malignancies. Diagnosis may be suspected and can be made during the first stage. It is confirmed in vitro and by a skin biopsy.

Clinical aspects: Normally, it involves the *skin* (photosensitivity, skin hypoplasia, increased patchy skin pigmentation, decreased or increased irregular skin pigmentation, hyperkeratosis, hemangioma capillary, telangiectasia skin, neoplasia), *eyes* (photophobia, optic disc atrophy, conjunctival telangiectasia, paresis of ocular muscles), and *CNS* (more common in XPA and XPD: e.g., abnormality, seizures, areflexia, cerebral cortex atrophy, microcephaly, deafness, and mental retardation). Other possible features include ectopic testes and teeth anomalies.

Precautions before anesthesia: Evaluate the neurological function (clinical, electroencephalogram, CT) and ocular lesions. Avoid radiographs because of photosensitivity.

Anesthetic considerations: Patient behavior in the operating room may be affected by photophobia. It is recommended to dim the light. As with other dermatological illness, intraoperative padding (pressure points) and positioning is very important. Difficult airway management is possible because of skin atrophy, scarring and macroglossia.

Pharmacological implications: The use of inhalational agents is questioned because of their potential interaction with the NER in cells of patients affected with XP, worsening the symptoms of the disease. The interaction between anesthetic drugs and antiepileptic treatment must be considered. Special attention must be given to the administration of new medications and their photosensitivity properties (e.g., antibiotics) medications that might affect DNA must be avoided.

Other conditions to be considered:

☞**DE SANTIS-CACCIONE SYNDROME:** This particular syndrome is usually present in xeroderma pigmentosum group A, and shows, in addition to XP, severe mental deficiency, choreoathetoid neurologic signs (usually), dwarfism, and gonadal hypoplasia.

☞**NETHERTON SYNDROME:** Congenital disorder characterized by abnormal brittle hair (diagnostic sign). Other features include onychodystrophy, cataracts, and teeth problems. Associated with mental retardation, skin sensitivity to light, and skin ichthyosis.

☞**BLOOM SYNDROME:** Cancer-prone genetic disorder inherited as autosomal recessive disease. Patients present with small and short stature, erythematous skin, butterfly facial rash sensitive to sunlight, excessive hypo- and hyperpigmented lesions, and a high rate of bacterial infection as a result of immunodeficiency (requiring antibiotics during surgery). Other features include chronic lung disease and diabetes. Common among Ashkenazi Jews.

☞**COCKAYNE SYNDROME:** The characteristics of this autosomal recessive inherited disease are dwarfism, precociously senile appearance, pigmentary retinal degeneration, optic atrophy, progressive sensorineural deafness, sensitivity to sunlight, and mental retardation. Disproportionately long limbs with large hands and feet and flexion contractures of joints are usual skeletal features.

☞**FANCONI ANEMIA:** Spontaneous chromosomal aberrations associated with hypocellular marrow, pancytopenia, and constitutional aplastic anemia, presenting in the first years of life, and associated with growth retardation.

REFERENCES:

Benhamou S, Sarasin A: ERCC2/XPD gene polymorphisms and cancer risk. *Mutagenesis* 17(6):463, 2002.

Brunner T, Jöhr M: Anesthetic management of a child with xeroderma pigmentosum. *Pediatr Anaesth* 14(8):697, 2004.

Kraemer KH, Lee MM, Scooto J: Xeroderma pigmentosum: Cutaneous, and neurologic abnormalities in 830 published cases. *Arch Dermatol* 123:241, 1987.

Masuda Y, Imaizumi H, Okanuma M, et al: Anesthesia for a patient with xeroderma pigmentosum. *Masui* 51(2):169, 2002.

Xeroderma, Talipes, and Enamel Defect Syndrome

At a glance: Ectodermal dysplasia combined with congenital heart disease.

Synonyms: XTE-Syndrome; Moynahan Syndrome type III.

Incidence and genetic inheritance: This is an extremely rare, autosomal dominant inherited form of ectodermal dysplasia.

Clinical aspects: Characterized by xeroderma, talipes, and tooth enamel defects. Further signs include growth and mild mental retardation, congenital mitral stenosis, cleft palate, absent eyelashes of the lower lid, short-lasting skin vesicles, reduced number of sweat glands associated with hypohidrosis and increased photosensitivity. Hair, finger, and toe nails can be abnormal.

Anesthetic considerations: From an anesthetic point of view, a preoperative echocardiography to assess cardiac function and the degree of mitral stenosis is recommended. Depending on the procedure, patients may need bacterial endocarditis prophylaxis. Xeroderma may also involve the lacrimal system and care must be taken to avoid corneal ulcerations during anesthesia. Vascular access may be challenging in the presence of the skin changes. Environmental temperature must be well controlled to avoid hyperthermia.

Pharmacological implications: In the face of decreased sweating, atropine should not be used and hyperthermia must be avoided.

REFERENCE:

Moynahan EJ: XTE syndrome (xeroderma, talipes and enamel defect): A new heredo-familial syndrome. Two cases. Homozygous inheritance of a dominant gene. *Proc R Soc Med* 63:447, 1970.

X-Linked Adrenoleukodystrophy (XLA)

At a glance: A disorder characterized by progressive demyelinization of the central nervous system and peripheral adrenal insufficiency resulting from adrenal gland atrophy.

Synonyms: Adrenomyeloneuropathy; Addison Disease and Cerebral Sclerosis; Siemerling-Creutzfeldt Disease; Bronze Schilder Disease; Melanodermic Leukodystrophy.

Nature: Genetic disorder, mainly affecting males but 50% of female heterozygotes have symptoms.

Incidence: 1:15,000 to 1:100,000 in general population.

Genetic inheritance: X-linked with six phenotypes, classified according to age of onset, organ involvement, and neurological progression rate. Most common form: *X-adrenoleukodystrophy childhood form:* (most severe); second most common form: *adrenomyeloneuropathy*. Gene locus is the long arm of X chromosome at position 28 (Xq28), which codes for an 80-kDa transmembrane transporter protein. Mutation can be missense, frameshift, nonsense, or deletion. This is distinct from neonatal adrenoleukodystrophy (autosomal recessive).

Pathophysiology: Very-long-chain fatty acids (VLCFA) are metabolized by VLC acyl-CoA synthetases in peroxisomes or mitochondrion. Adrenoleukodystrophy gene mutation may impair the peroxisomal import of this synthetase, leading to VLCFAs (>C22) accumulation. It is uncertain whether these long, rigid, acyl fatty acids reduce membrane fluidity, causing an inflammatory response in the nervous system (demyelination), and reduce steroid synthesis in the adrenal glands.

Diagnosis: Clinical course with demyelinization signs and association of peripheral adrenal insufficiency in 80% of children forms and 65% of adult forms. Diagnosis is confirmed by abnormally high saturated VLCFAs and C26:C22 ratio in blood or accessible tissues. Radiologic imaging reveals symmetrical hypodense corpus callosum and periventricular white matter. Prenatal (chorion villus biopsy) and female heterozygotes (VLCFA profiles) diagnosis available.

Clinical aspects: *X-adrenoleukodystrophy childhood form:* normal childhood development until a mean age of 7 years, followed by parietal-occipital demyelination with rapidly progressive dementia, behavioral changes, visual/auditory defect, and seizures; 90% of patients have an adrenal insufficiency. Average life span is 9.4 years. *Adrenomyeloneuropathy:* milder form with adult onset. Spinal cord involvement (paraparesis/sphincter problems) is more common than cerebral (50% of cases) or adrenal (30% of cases) dysfunction. *Female heterozygotes:* similar clinical picture as adrenomyeloneuropathy; however, presenting normal adrenal glands (99% of cases). Often misdiagnosed as multiple sclerosis.

Precautions before anesthesia: Evaluate the neurological status for evidence of cerebral and spinal demyelination (clinical, EEG, CT/MRI, nerves velocity). Determine if adrenal dysfunction is present and adequately treated. Blood examination: electrolytes, cell blood count, glucose, cortisol levels.

> N.B: Thrombocytopenia is often observed in patients treated with Lorenzo's oil (40% of cases). As well, the use of this oil may cause significant cardiac dysfunction.

Anesthetic considerations: Rapid sequence induction is indicated if airway reflexes are impaired. The presence of dementia as a result of neuronal demyelination may make the patient sensitive to opioids. Regional anesthesia can be difficult (scoliosis) or contraindicated (thrombocytopenia). Osteoporosis (hypogonadism) calls for careful intraoperative positioning.

Pharmacological implications: Succinylcholine should be avoided in the presence of spinal cord compression or acute demyelination. Hypnomidate should also be omitted (depresses adrenal function). Meperidine, ketamine, sevoflurane and enflurane are relative contraindications if seizures are present. Doses and/or concentrations must be carefully selected. Additional steroid stress doses are essential. Consider interaction between anesthetic drugs and antiepileptic treatment.

Other conditions to be considered:

NEONATAL ADRENOLEUKODYSTROPHY: Inherited as an autosomal recessive pattern and rapidly progressive. Both males and females are affected. The abnormalities of the brain and adrenal glands seem different from those caused by other types of adrenoleukodystrophies. Characteristically, the first symptoms begin at birth or shortly after. Mental retardation; facial abnormalities; seizures; polymicrogyria; retinal degeneration; hypotonia; hepatomegaly; and/or adrenal insufficiency. In this form of adrenoleukodystrophy, the demyelinization can affect the gray matter within the spinal cord. Hepatic peroxisomes may be absent or decreased in number in the liver. The concentration of pipecolic acid may be increased in the plasma. Patients with only one of the pair of genes for this disorder typically have no neurological or adrenal symptoms.

☞ALEXANDER SYNDROME: A degenerative and progressive disorder of the nervous system caused by leukodystrophy. Affects mainly males and usually begins at about 6 months of age. Symptoms include mental and physical retardation, enlargement of the brain and head, spasticity (arms and legs), and seizures.

☞ADDISONIAN SYNDROME: Rare disorder associated with chronic and progressive hypofunction of the cortex of the adrenal gland resulting in hypocortisolemia and hypoaldosteronemia. Electrolyte imbalance is the most important consequence of this disease. Hypotension and severe intravascular dehydration can be present if not detected early. The main characteristics are fatigue, weakness, anorexia, frequent diuresis, gastrointestinal discomfort, and changes in skin pigmentation.

☞CANAVAN SYNDROME: Another type of leukodystrophy that affects the central nervous system. Progressive degeneration of nerves within the brain and spinal cord is characteristic of this disorder. The symptoms begin in infancy and are characterized initially by apathy, hypotonia and the loss of previously acquired mental and motor skills and subsequently by hypertonia, spasticity of the arms and legs, poor head control because of lack of muscle atrophy in the neck, megalocephaly, and blindness. Megalocephaly might be present resulting in the development of craniosynostosis and hydrocephaly. The infant may be more susceptible to respiratory tract infections because of the progressive loss of muscle strength in the chest.

☞METACHROMATIC LEUKODYSTROPHY: Rare, inherited form of leukodystrophy described as the accumulation of fat-like substances (sulfatides) in the nervous system and other organs. It is characterized by severe nerve demyelinization. Blindness, seizures, hypertonia, spasticity, paralysis, and dementia are reported. There is an infantile, juvenile, and adult form. The *infantile* form is generally detected in the 2nd year of life, typically before 30 months of age. The *juvenile* form has an onset between the ages of 4 and 10 years. The *adult* usually begins after 16 years of age.

☞PELIZAEUS-MERZBACHER SYNDROME: A very rare slowly progressive demyelinating disease affecting in a diffuse pattern the cerebrum, cerebellum, brainstem, and spinal cord. Two types are described: *X-linked (Infantile form)* and the autosomal dominant *(preadulthood form)*. Clinical features also include: stridor, muscle spasticity, nystagmus. Often fatal in the first year of life from respiratory complications.

☞ZELLWEGER SYNDROME: Rare, hereditary disorder characterized by decreased or missing peroxisomes in the liver, kidney, and brain. It is characterized by facial abnormalities, central nervous system dysfunctions, ocular problems, and hepatomegaly. Most symptoms present in development before birth. Newborns have a typical flat face with a high forehead, hypertelorism, and epicanthal folds. Other symptoms may include hypotonia, dysphagia, seizures, congenital heart defects, hepatomegaly, and/or vision abnormalities such as cataracts.

REFERENCES:

Gartner J, Braun A, Holzinger A, et al: Clinical and genetic aspects of X-linked adrenoleukodystrophy. *Neuropediatrics* 29:3, 1998.

Kindopp AS, Ashbury T: Anaesthetic management of an adult patient with X-linked adrenoleukodystrophy. *Can J Anaesth* 45(10):990, 1998.

X-Linked Hypophosphatemia (XLH)

At a glance: X-Linked Hypophosphatemia (XLH) is characterized by impaired renal phosphate reabsorption and diminished Vitamin-D metabolism. In addition, intestinal calcium and phosphate absorption is also impaired.

Synonyms: Familial Hypophosphatemia; Hypophosphatemic Vitamin D-Resistant Rickets type I; X-Linked Vitamin D-Resistant Rickets; Hereditary Hypophosphatemia type I; Phosphate Diabetes.

Incidence: XLH is the most common form of rickets in industrialized countries. It affects males and females in equal numbers; however, males are usually more severely affected than females. Worldwide approximately 1 in 20,000 live births suffers from the disease.

Genetic inheritance: In most cases, XLH is inherited as a dominant X-linked trait. However, autosomal dominant and recessive traits have also been reported. The X-linked defect seems to be the result of a mutation in the PHEX (X-linked phosphate regulating endopeptidase homolog) gene and has been mapped to Xp22.2-22.1. The autosomal dominant form of familial hypophosphatemia (sometimes associated with decreased glucose tolerance) seems to be caused by a mutation of gene 12p13.3.

Pathophysiology: The two pathogenetic mechanisms involved in this disorder are the failure of the proximal renal tubule to reabsorb phosphate and to convert calcidiol (25-hydroxy-cholecalciferol) to calcitriol (1,25-dihydroxy-choleclaciferol). The defect is characterized by low calcium serum levels in combination with hypophosphatemia not resulting in increased levels of calcitriol. Decreased concentration of inorganic phosphate leads to osteomalacia secondary to impaired function of osteoblasts, since mature bone formation requires the precipitation of hydroxyapatite, which has a high phosphate content (chemical formula $\{Ca[Ca_3(PO_4)_2]_3\}^{2+} \cdot 2\ OH^-$).

Diagnosis: In the absence of a family history of XLH, the diagnosis is made clinically. Nevertheless, the diagnosis is sometimes difficult. This is especially true in the first year of life, since the phosphate levels may be normal even in an infant with an affected parent. In addition, the range of normal serum phosphorus levels in children is significantly higher than in adults. Abnormal bowing of the long bones is usually the first sign, but does not appear before 12 to 18 months of age. Elevated serum alkaline phosphatase levels (often the first laboratory sign), mild hypocalcemia, and moderate hypophosphatemia with significant hyperphosphaturia in the absence of severe secondary hyperparathyroidism are typical. Serum calcitriol levels are inappropriately normal. In contrast to ☞Vitamin D-Resistant Rickets, aminoaciduria and bicarbonaturia are not present.

Clinical aspects: The clinical signs of XLH are quite variable. Major symptoms of XLH include skeletal malformations, bone pain, abnormally bowed legs (see below), and generalized, but usually mild muscle weakness. Affected infants may experience failure to thrive resulting in low weight and a short, stocky stature (with an adult height of usually less than 165 cm). However, most often the symptoms appear at the age of 12 to 18 months and affected infants show a waddling gait, bowing of the legs with coxa vara, genua vara or genus valga (all secondary to the weight-bearing function). Dolichocephaly, ☞Arnold Chiari I malformation, and sensorineural hearing loss because of malformation of the inner ear have been reported. Although serum phosphate levels are equally decreased in affected males and females, the degree of bone involvement in males is significantly more severe. Tetany, rachitic rosary, pectus

deformity, and severe myopathy are usually not features found in these patients. Beside bowing of the long bones (especially of the lower extremities), radiographic features include rachitic changes such as widening, fraying, and cupping of the growth plates (particularly of the tibia, distal femur, radius, and ulna) and overall mild osteopenia. Later on in life, signs of osteoarthritis in the knees and ankles are common and coarsening of the trabecular pattern (consistent with osteomalacia) in combination with Looser transformation zones can be detected and may be associated with fractures and pseudofractures (more common in adults). Dental problems such as cavities because of hypomineralization of the enamel, primary teeth abscesses, but also enlarged pulp chambers and a defect in the calcification of the dentin matrix (called intraglobular dentin) are common findings in these patients. Enthesopathy (the calcification of ligaments, tendons, joint capsules) is common after the age of 40 years and is not only often responsible for the pain, but may also limit joint mobility. Most often this affects elbows, shoulders, hips, (fusion of the sacroiliac joints) or the spine (spinal hyperostosis), where it may result in spinal canal stenosis, scoliosis, and significant disability. Successful treatment consists of oral phosphate supplements along with calcitriol (the active form of vitamin D) to avoid secondary hyperparathyroidism as a consequence of the oral phosphate load. This therapy requires a high compliance from the patient and his/her caregiver, since this means not only taking the medications every 6 hours for many years, but also frequent monitoring. However, phosphate and calcitriol treatment increases the risk of nephrocalcinosis (the risk seems to be correlated with the dose of phosphate administrated) and vitamin D toxicity. Once treatment has been established, growth acceleration and correction of the deformities (to a certain degree) have been described in many patients (with a higher response rate in female patients).

Precautions before anesthesia: Check electrolytes including calcium and phosphate preoperatively and obtain a complete cell blood count. Kidney function should at least be assessed with creatinine, and renal sonography may reveal nephrocalcinosis. Oral phosphate therapy can result in diarrhea (particularly at the beginning of the therapy), if severe, it is important to control the intravascular hydration and acid-base status. Assess spine and neck mobility (possible ankylosis because of spondylophyte and ligamentous calcifications), which may complicate not only central neuraxial anesthesia, but also tracheal intubation.

Anesthetic considerations: Dental anomalies require careful direct laryngoscopy to avoid any damage. Keep the patient well hydrated to maintain good urinary output. Careful positioning and padding is recommended.

Pharmacological implications: Administration of glucose, insulin, glucagon, epinephrine, intravenous sodium chloride, sodium bicarbonate, sodium lactate solutions, diuretics, and corticosteroids may all result in reduced serum phosphate concentrations.

Other conditions to be considered: Rickets may also be found in the following disorders:

☞**ALBRIGHT HEREDITARY OSTEODYSTROPHY:** Round face, short stature and neck, obesity. Intracranial and subcutaneous calcification, neuromuscular problems such as fatigue and muscle cramps. Seizures. Pseudohypoparathyroidism and hypocalcemia. Hypertension. Correction of chronic hypocalcemia is treated by oral calcium and vitamin D. Evaluate for difficult intubation and venous access because of the deformities. Elective surgery should be postponed until serum calcium concentration reaches normal levels. Avoid respiratory or metabolic alkalosis. If surgery cannot be delayed, intravenous calcium therapy must be given with continuous ECG monitoring.

☞**DE TONI DEBRÉ FANCONI SYNDROME:** A rare acquired or inherited condition involving a generalized transport defect in the proximal tubules with renal losses of glucose, phosphate, calcium, uric acid, amino acids, and bicarbonates leading to short stature, osteomalacia, and renal failure.

☞**HEREDITARY VITAMIN D-RESISTANT RICKETS:** A defect in the vitamin D receptor results in hypocalcemia, tetanic seizures, and rickets.

☞**HYPOPHOSPHATASIA:** Variant of the disease in children and adults limited only to dental, without skeletal, problems (premature loss of teeth). Inherited inborn error of metabolism characterized by severe bone disease (similar to vitamin D-resistant rickets), failure to thrive, movement disorders, and low plasma levels of alkaline phosphatase.

☞**LOWE SYNDROME:** Genetically transmitted polymalformative syndrome characterized by the association of ocular problems with renal dysfunction and mental retardation.

☞**METAPHYSEAL CHONDRODYSPLASIA SCHMID TYPE:** A very rare inherited disorder characterized by short stature with abnormally short arms and legs (short-limbed dwarfism). Other physical characteristics may include outward "flaring" of the lower rib cage, genua vara, leg pain, and/or hip deformities (coxa vara). Such abnormalities of the legs and hips typically result in an unusual "waddling" gait.

REFERENCES:

Burnstein MI, Lawson JP, Kottamasu SR, et al: The enthesopathic changes of hypophosphatemic osteomalacia in adults: Radiologic findings. *Am J Roentgenol* 153:785, 1989.

Caldemeyer KS, Boaz JC, Wappner RS, et al: Chiari I malformation: Association with hypophosphatemic rickets and MR imaging appearance. *Radiology* 195:733, 1995.

Tenenhouse HS, Econs MJ: Mendelian hypophosphatemias, in Scriver CR, Beaudet AL, Sly WS, et al. (eds.): *The Metabolic and Molecular Bases of Inherited Disease.* 8th ed. New York, McGraw Hill, 2001; p 5039.

X-Linked Lymphoproliferative (XLP) Syndrome

At a glance: Genetic disorder linked to the long arm of the X-chromosome affecting males and characterized by an extreme sensitivity to Epstein-Barr virus (EBV) infection.

Synonyms: Duncan Disease (named after the last name of a common ancestor of the first described boys by Purtilo); Purtilo Syndrome; Epstein Barr Virus Susceptibility Syndrome.

Incidence: About 350 cases have been described.

Genetic inheritance: X-linked recessive, with gene locus mapping to Xq25. The responsible gene is called SAP/SH2D1A and seems to have a key function in T/B-cell homeostasis. (SAP is the abbreviation for SLAM [signaling lymphocytic activation molecule]-associated protein, and SH2D1A refers to Src homology 2 domain protein 1A).

Pathophysiology: In more than half of these patients, the infection with EBV triggers an infectious mononucleosis that (usually) within a month after onset results in lethal liver failure as a result of fulminant hepatitis with extensive hepatic necrosis. EBV-induced lymphoblasts trigger an abnormal T- and B-cell proliferation, resulting in diffuse infiltration of multiple organs, leading not only to fulminant hepatitis, but also to bone marrow failure with hemophagocytic components. Survivors of this infection initially develop a state of immunodeficiency that can affect all immune cell lines and immunoglobulins and put the patients at high risk for bacterial infections, or develop a malignant lymphoma (see *Clinical Aspects* below) later in life. However, newer studies indicate that dysgammaglobulinemia and lymphoma may occur in these patients even in the absence of a prior EBV infection (sero- and PCR-negative), pointing to a fundamental role of the SAP/SH2D1A gene in the pathogenesis of this syndrome. It has been hypothesized that XLP may be a progressive immunodeficiency disease with manifestation particularly after viral infections.

Diagnosis: Based on clinical criteria, family history, fatal EBV infection, immunodeficiency, aplastic anemia, genotype analysis (SAP/SH2D1A gene), and serology (although not necessarily positive for EBV). DNA probes can reveal the carrier state in females. The definitive diagnosis is made when two or more maternally related males manifest an XLP phenotype following EBV infection. Hyperimmunoglobulinemia A or M (before EBV infection), hyperimmunoglobulinemia G_1 or G_3 (before EBV infection), and inadequate response to EBV infection are considered minor criteria for the diagnosis.

Clinical aspects: The average age at the time of diagnosis is 3 to 5 years. Common presenting symptoms are initially nonspecific, such as fever, nausea, vomiting, and abdominal pain. The three main phenotypes can be distinguished. As mentioned earlier, about half of patients experience a fulminant mononucleosis resulting in liver failure and death. About a quarter of all patients develop a malignant non-Hodgkin lymphoma (often B-cell lymphoma of the Burkitt type) later in life, which may well respond to the initial treatment but seems to have a high relapse rate and ultimately often results in death. The ileocecal area and the central nervous system are the most common primary sites of these lymphomas. About 30% present with dysgammaglobulinemia (variants ranging from agammaglobulinemia over hypogammaglobulinemia [hypo-IgG_1 and IgG_3] to polyclonal hypergammaglobulinemia [hyper-IgA, hyper-IgM] have been described). Other manifestations may include aplastic anemia, vasculitis, and pulmonary lymphomatoid granulomatosis leading to arterial wall destruction and aneurysm formation. Seventy percent of the boys where a follow-up exists (87% of patients) died before the age of 10 years, and only two lived to 40 years. The clinical management includes regular treatment with immunoglobulins containing antibodies against EBV. In patients with hypogammaglobulinemia, immunoglobulins are indicated to prevent recurrent infections. Allogenic bone marrow transplant is a newer and successful treatment option; however, it remains to be seen whether the long-term outcome changes for these patients.

Precautions before anesthesia: Evaluate for cardiac dysfunction, review baseline chest radiographs and ECG. Blood work should include a complete blood cell count, electrolytes, and liver function (e.g., transaminases, coagulation tests, serum proteins). Transfuse as necessary. If major surgery is planned, make sure that irradiated blood products are available. If the patient has had a bone marrow transplant and is on immunosuppressant and cortisone, it is important to evaluate renal function and plan for stress doses of steroids.

Anesthetic considerations: Depending on the manifestations of the disease, these patients may be at a very high risk or at only a slightly increased risk for anesthesia. In the period of acute infectious mononucleosis with liver failure, anesthesia should be restricted to real emergency procedures only. Because the primary site of non-Hodgkin lymphoma is most often extranodal, compression of the airway or major vessels is most likely not present. However, it can result in increased intracranial pressure or ileus, requiring an appropriate anesthesia technique according to the standards. Use a strictly aseptic technique for insertion of any catheters. Avoid regional anesthesia in uncorrected thrombocytopenia.

Pharmacological implications: Parenchymal liver disease alters the metabolism of drugs with high hepatic extraction ratio. Keep in mind that serum protein concentrations may be skewed and the free fraction of highly protein-bound drugs, and their efficacy, can be changed significantly.

Other conditions to be considered: For a summary, see Primary Immunodeficiencies

☞**CHRONIC GRANULOMATOUS DISEASE:** An inherited immune deficiency with abnormality of phagocytic cells that is caused by dysfunctional oxidative metabolism leading to recurrent life-threatening bacterial and fungal infections. Few patients survive into the fourth decade.

☞**OMENN SYNDROME:** An autosomal recessive inherited severe combined immunodeficiency (SCID) secondary to defective T-lymphocytes and a lack of B-lymphocytes.

REFERENCES:

Morra M, Howie D, Grande MS, et al: X-linked lymphoproliferative disease: A progressive immunodeficiency. *Ann Rev Immunol* 19:657, 2001.

Nelson DL, Terhorst C: X-linked lymphoproliferative syndrome. *Clin Exp Immunol* 122:291, 2000.

Seemayer TA, Gross TG, Egeler RM, et al: X-linked lymphoproliferative disease: Twenty-five years after the discovery. *Pediatr Res* 38:471, 1995.

Y

Yellow Nail Syndrome

At a glance: A rare medical condition characterized by the clinical presentation of discolored, hypoplastic nails, recurring pleural effusions, lymphedema, recurrent pneumonia and lymphedema.

Synonym: Lymphedema and Yellow Nails.

Incidence: Unknown (between 1927 and 1960, 10 cases reported in the literature), more frequent in the presence of severe rhinosinusitis symptoms and immunological disorders.

Genetic inheritance: Autosomal dominant.

Pathophysiology: Can be caused by mutation in the forkhead family transcription factor gene MFH1 located on 16q24.3.

Diagnosis: Two of the following criteria must be present: slow-growing nails (89% of cases), lymphedema (80% of cases), pleuropulmonary symptoms (63% of cases) (pleural effusion, recurrent pneumonitis, bronchiectasis, rhinosinusitis).

Clinical aspects: The characteristics of the nails include thickening, diminished growth, and onycholysis. The color may vary from a pale yellow to green. The edema is the initial symptom in one-third of cases. Although it mainly occurs in the lower limb, in time edema also affects the genitalia, hands, face, and vocal cords. Respiratory tract is involved with pleural effusion, restrictive or obstructive defects that are poorly responsive to bronchodilatators. Bronchiectasis, severe rhinosinusitis, and laryngeal edema can also be present. These patients may present chylous ascites and pericardial effusion. Some authors report a lack of IgG2. This illness is well known in adults, often occurring with a late onset. One case report described a nonimmune fetal hydrops and recurrent left chylothorax at 4 weeks of age in an infant with maternal Yellow Nail Syndrome.

Precautions before anesthesia: In the presence of yellow nails, ask about recurrent respiratory infections and watch for the consequences of lymphedema (previous pleural, pericardial or ascitic effusion). Obtain an echocardiography for the exclusion of pericardial effusion. Pulmonary tests are indicated to assess the severity of the respiratory tract involvement. A chest radiograph should be obtained to eliminate the presence of bronchiectasia. Ask about any changes in the voice. If a voice change is present, an orolaryngotracheal examination is useful to assess the extent of the laryngeal edema.

Anesthetic considerations: If an alternative to tracheal intubation is available, it must be considered in the evaluation of the case because of the lymphedematous involvement of each part of the respiratory system. The venous access should prefer large veins and should be maintained for a duration as short as possible because of generalized, congenitally hypoplastic lymphatics. Postoperative chest physiotherapy should be considered. Consider patients as suffering from recurrent airway infection with high respiratory reactivity.

Pharmacological implications: No interactions are known with anesthetic medications. If tracheal intubation is needed, the prophylactic administration of antibiotic is recommended. The use of muscle relaxants should be considered once the airway is secured and lung ventilation confirmed. Anticholinergic agents may make pulmonary secretions more tenacious and difficult to clear.

REFERENCES:

Govaert P, Leroy JG, Pauwels R, et al: Perinatal manifestations of maternal yellow nail syndrome. *Pediatrics* 89:1016, 1992.

Riedel M: Multiple effusions and lymphedema in the yellow nail syndrome. *Circulation* 105(3):E25, 2002.

Young Syndrome

At a glance: Obstructive azoospermia, chronic sinopulmonary infections, and bronchiectasis without ciliary dysfunction. Significant respiratory implications.

Synonyms: Sinusitis Infertility Syndrome; Barry Perkins Young Syndrome; Obstructive Azoospermia and Chronic Sinopulmonary Infections.

Incidence: Probably > to 2:1000 in general population.

Genetic inheritance: Autosomal recessive. High rate of spontaneous mutation.

Pathophysiology: Prolonged mucociliary clearance time (in the presence of normal structure) resulting in chronic sinopulmonary infections. The incidence and severity of infections usually improve after adolescence (unlike with cystic fibrosis). Congenital or acquired obstruction to sperm outflow (between the caput and body of the epididymis) in the presence of normal spermatogenesis results in azoospermia and infertility.

Diagnosis: Combination of azoospermia and chronic sinopulmonary infection in the presence of normal spermatogenesis and hormone function with surgical findings of obstruction to sperm flow are suggestive of the diagnosis.

Clinical aspects: History of recurrent cough and sputum production in childhood. The respiratory symptoms improve after adolescence and only mild residual impairment in pulmonary function, as evidenced by mild decreases in residual volume and peak expiratory flow rate, remain. Chest and sinus radiographic abnormalities consistent with chronic sinopulmonary infections are common. The respiratory tract is not colonized with organisms unlike in cystic fibrosis. These patients most frequently present to infertility clinics later in life.

Precautions before anesthesia: Evaluation of respiratory system is highly indicated. However, clinical evaluation alone may be adequate. If indicated by clinical examination, chest radiography and pulmonary function tests may be required. Important to exclude cystic fibrosis or immotile-cilia syndrome.

Anesthetic considerations: In view of chronic sinopulmonary infections and mild decreases in pulmonary function tests, patients may be at greater risk for postoperative atelectasis. Regional anesthesia may be appropriate for intra- and postoperative pain management. If pulmonary disease is significant, inhalational induction may be prolonged secondary to slow uptake resulting from an abnormal V/Q ratio. Laryngospasm and cough must be expected in Young Syndrome patients. Similar to other patients with chronic airway inflammation, bronchial reactivity is potentially increased. Nasal intubation and nasogastric tubes should probably be avoided because of the presence of sinus infection.

Pharmacological implications: Anticholinergic agents may make pulmonary secretions more tenacious and difficult to clear. Muscle relaxants should be used only with peripheral nerve stimulators because in association with high-dose antibiotics, especially aminoglycosides, the action of nondepolarizing muscle relaxants can be significantly prolonged.

Other conditions to be considered:

☞**IMMOTILE CILIA SYNDROME:** Male infertility and chronic sinopulmonary infections are characteristics of this syndrome. Bronchiectasis is a frequent and intractable problem among Polynesians, specifically New Zealand Maoris and Samoan Islanders. A defect in spermatogenesis is also reported. Several defects in the motor mechanism of cilia can lead to dysfunction or total immotility.

☞**MUCOVISCIDOSIS:** Congenital multiorgan disease affecting mainly the lungs, liver, and pancreas. Frequent lung infections, hemoptysis, intolerance to exercise, presence of clubbing fingers suggesting pulmonary hypertension, rectal prolapse, and nasal polyps.

REFERENCES:
de Iongh R, Ing A, Rutland J: Mucociliary function, ciliary ultrastructure, and ciliary orientation in Young's syndrome. *Thorax* 47:184, 1992.

Handelsman D, Conway A, Boylan L, et al: Young's syndrome: Obstructive azoospermia and chronic sinopulmonary infections. *N Engl J Med* 310:3, 1984.

Yunis-Varon Syndrome

At a Glance: A severe polymalformative syndrome characterized by facial dysmorphism, absent clavicle, and extremity abnormalities. Often lethal within few months because of the failure to thrive and severe cardiorespiratory dysfunction.

Synonym: Cleidocranial Dysplasia with Micrognathia, Absent Thumbs, and Distal Aphalangia.

History: First described by E. Yunis and H. Varon in 1980.

Incidence: Unknown (fewer than 20 case reports worldwide).

Genetic inheritance: Autosomal recessive.

Pathophysiology: Unknown. A lysosomal storage disorder has been evocated.

Diagnosis: Suggested by prenatal ultrasonography, as well as by specific clinical features, including growth retardation prior to and after birth. Defective growth of the bones of the skull along with complete or partial absence of the shoulder blades (cleidocranial dysplasia) associated with characteristic facial features (severe micrognathia) and abnormalities of the fingers and toes complete the diagnosis.

Clinical aspects: Patients have marked psychomotor delay, postnatal failure to thrive, severe feeding problems, and respiratory difficulties. Clinical signs can involve *head and neck* (macrocrania with diastasis of cranial sutures; calvarial dysostosis; sparse scalp hair; hypoplastic facial bones; bitemporal indentations; small eyes; proptosis; low-set, dysplastic ears; anteverted nostrils; narrow and high-arched palate; severe micrognathia; occasional glossoptosis

[moderate]; retracted and poorly delineated lips with diminished nasolabial distance), *skeleton* (absent clavicles; absent sternal ossification; pelvic dysplasia with hip dislocation; hypoplasia of thumbs; middle and distal aphalangia of the other fingers; agenesis of the first metatarsals; hypoplastic proximal phalanges of the big toes; delayed bone maturation; occasional pathological fractures; and nail hypoplasia), *CNS* (arhinencephaly; absent corpus callosum; hypoplasia of the vermis; neuronal loss and vacuolation involving cerebral cortex; basal ganglia; cerebellar dentate nuclei and spinal anterior horns; hypertonia and hypotonia have also been reported), and *heart* (cardiomyopathy, tetralogy of Fallot). The majority of patients die in infancy as a result of severe failure to thrive and recurrent pneumonia.

Precautions before anesthesia: A complete evaluation of the airway is indicated (clinical, radiographs). The cardiac function must be assessed for the potential association of congenital heart defects. An echocardiogram is most useful in this situation. Evaluate neurological function (clinical, CT, EEG). Blood examination must include a complete blood cell count because of frequent infections. Also, the hemoglobin, electrolytes, and glucose must be obtained. If the patient is on parenteral nutrition for failure to thrive, obtain albumin levels, liver enzymes, and bilirubin. Consider sedative premedication in older children with developmental delay.

Anesthetic considerations: There is no literature available about this condition. Because of the presence of facial anomalies suggesting the possibility of difficult airway management, it is recommended to maintain spontaneous ventilation until the airway has been secured and lung ventilation confirmed. The availability of a laryngeal mask airway and/or fiberoptic equipment is required. Particular attention should be given to the positioning of the patient intraoperatively (pathological fractures). Proper padding must be ensured to reduce pressure point complications. Venous access can be difficult because of extremity malformations. Central venous access using the subclavian route should be avoided because of the absence of the clavicle.

Pharmacological implications: In patients affected with muscle hypotonia, it is recommended to avoid succinylcholine because of the risk of sudden severe hyperkalemia. Also, titration of nondepolarizing muscle relaxants is indicated because of the increased sensitivity to their effect and should always be administered while using a nerve stimulator. Hypotonia could be caused by the loss of lower spinal motor neurons with secondary moderate neurogenic muscluar atrophy, as demonstrated in one patient. It is important to consider a potential interaction between anesthetic medications and antiepilepsy treatment. In patients affected with cardiopathy, it is recommended to administer prophylactic antibiotics.

REFERENCES:
Adès LC, Morris LL, Richardson M, et al: Congenital heart malformation in Yunis-Varón syndrome. *J Med Genet* 30:788, 1993.

Walch E, Schmidt M, Brenner RE, et al: Yunis-Varon syndrome: Evidence for a lysosomal storage disease. *Am J Med Genet* 95(2):157, 2000.

Yunis E, Varón H: Cleidocranial dysostosis, severe micrognathism, bilateral absence of thumbs and first metatarsal bone, and distal aphalangia. A new genetic syndrome. *Am J Dis Child* 134:649, 1980.

Z

Zellweger Syndrome

At a glance: A disorder characterized by the congenital absence of functioning peroxisomes (the cellular structures that are responsible for the elimination of toxic substances) resulting in a cerebrohepatorenal syndrome. The disease affects brain development, particularly nerve myelination. Most important features include hepatomegaly, polycystic kidney disease, visual disturbances, and high plasma levels of iron and copper. Other clinical features include muscular hypotonia already noticeable at birth, mental retardation, seizures, coagulopathy, and dysphagia with recurrent aspiration. Congenital heart defects have been described. Life expectancy is approximately 6 months.

Synonym: Cerebro-Hepato-Renal Syndrome.

Genetic inheritance: Autosomal recessive. Gender distribution is equal. Gene map locus is at 7q11.23. There are several phenotypes that are caused by mutations in any of the several different genes involved in peroxisome biogenesis.

Pathophysiology: Thought to be a group of disorders of peroxisomal biogenesis in which the primary defect involves the import mechanisms of matrix enzymes. This results in production of "ghost" organelles that consist of an empty membrane.

Diagnosis: Clinically evocated by aberrant development of the skull, face, ears, eyes, hands, and feet, polycystic kidneys, and intrahepatic biliary dysgenesis. Confirmed by biochemical studies involving blood cells and fibroblasts. The presence of high levels of iron and copper in the blood is characteristic of this disease. There are specific and sensitive biochemical assays of peroxisomal function available, including a decreased dihydroxyacetone phosphate-adenosine triphosphate (DHAP-AT) activity and an increase in very-long-chain fatty acids. Serum iron and iron-binding capacity are high and peroxisomes are abnormal.

Clinical aspects: These infants are subject to early death within a few months (mean = 12.5 weeks). The clinical features involve *head* (high forehead, flat facies, cleft palate, micrognathia, characteristic eye changes, including mongoloid slant, hypertelorism, Brushfield spots, cataracts, pigmentary retinopathy, and optic nerve dysplasia) and central nervous system (CNS) (seizures, absent Moro reflex). Prenatal growth failure, failure to thrive, poor suck, muscular hypotonia, mental retardation, areflexia, deafness and congenital heart defects (patent ductus arteriosus, septal defects, aortic abnormalities) can be observed. Others features include apneas, polycystic kidneys, cryptorchidism, hepatomegaly, jaundice, mitochondrial abnormalities, liver cirrhosis, camptodactyly, talipes equinovarus, and stippled chondral calcification.

Precautions before anesthesia: Full assessment of the disorder and the extent of involvement of neurological, cardiac, respiratory, and hepatic systems. It is recommended to obtain consultation with appropriate specialties, and investigations. Because preoperative fasting is not tolerated by the infant, an endocrine consultation may be required to discuss appropriate intravenous fluids and supplementation. Complete assessment of coagulation. Correct hypoprothrombinemia.

Anesthetic considerations: The usually severe neurological problems may require the insertion of a gastrostomy tube for palliative feeding, which can often be achieved with an eutectic mixture of local anesthetics and infiltration of local anesthesia. The presence of muscular hypotonia must be considered. Ketamine is a useful supplement when general anesthesia not recommended. If anesthesia must be given, considerations include the possibility of a difficult intubation, poor protection of the airway and recurrent pulmonary aspiration, tendency to apnea postoperatively, and complicating factors such as cardiac and hepatic disease.

Pharmacological implications: If anesthesia must be performed, consideration must be given to interactions of the drugs with pre-existing hepatic and renal dysfunction. The use of opiates must be done carefully because of severe neurological defects and tendency to apnea. Prophylactic antibiotics in case of cardiopathy as indicated.

Other conditions to be considered: (An overview table can be found under ☞Leukodystrophies)

☞**ALEXANDER SYNDROME:** A degenerative and progressive disorder of the CNS caused by leukodystrophy. Affects mainly males and usually begins at about 6 months of age. Symptoms include mental and physical retardation, enlargement of the brain and head, spasticity (arms and legs), and seizures.

☞**CANAVAN SYNDROME:** A progressive leukodystrophy caused by spongy degeneration of the central nervous system. It is uniformly fatal within 18 months after onset of symptoms.

☞**METACHROMATIC LEUKODYSTROPHY:** Inherited disorder of myelin metabolism with progressive loss of white matter in the central and peripheral nervous system.

☞**PELIZAEUS-MERZBACHER SYNDROME:** A very rare slowly progressive dysmyelinating disease affecting in a diffuse pattern the cerebrum, cerebellum, brainstem, and spinal cord. Two types are described: X-linked (infantile form) and the autosomal dominant (preadulthood form). Clinical features also include: stridor, muscle spasticity, nystagmus. Often fatal in the first year of life from respiratory complications.

☞**X-LINKED ADRENOLEUKODYSTROPHY:** A disorder characterized by progressive demyelinization of the CNS and peripheral adrenal insufficiency.

☞**SCHILDER SYNDROME:** A rare, progressive and lethal disease of the CNS that affects mostly children and is characterized by adrenal atrophy and diffuse central demyelination. Presents with progressive dementia, spasticity, cortical blindness, deafness, hemiplegia, quadriplegia, ataxia, pyramidal signs, retrobulbar neuritis, and pseudobulbar palsy. Seizures. Onset in late childhood. Most patients die within few months after onset.

☞**CHONDRODYSPLASIA PUNCTATA:** Chondrodysplasia punctata refers to a heterogeneous group of disorders, which have ichthyosis and bony abnormalities probably because of abnormalities of steroidal biosynthesis in common. The international nomenclature and classification of osteochondrodysplasias classified the subtypes of chondrodysplasia punctata as (1) Rhizomelic type, (2) Zellweger Syndrome, (3) Conradi-Hünermann type, (4) X-linked recessive type, (5) Brachytelencephalangic type, (6) Tibial-metacarpal type, (7) Vitamin K-dependent coagulation defect, (8) Other and acquired genetic disorders including warfarin embryopathy. Specific features of the most common individual types of chondrodysplasia punctata are given below.

BENIGN CONGENITAL HYPOTONIA: A nonprogressive neuromuscular disorder that occurs at birth. It is characterized by muscle weakness or "floppiness." It is a disorder of unknown cause and most often considered as a symptom of other neuromuscular diseases.

☞**NEMALINE ROD MYOPATHY:** A hereditary muscular disease characterized by hypotonia. The presence of "nemaline rods" within the muscle fibers (very fine threads) is characteristic of this disease.

INFANTILE MUSCULAR ATROPHY: A severe and usually progressive neuromuscular disorder in infants. This condition is characterized by a generalized hypotonia in the trunk and extremities. It is the result of degenerative changes in the central horn cells of the spinal cord. It is often referred to as "amyotonia congenital syndrome."

REFERENCES:

Brosius U, Gartner J: Cellular and molecular aspects of Zellweger syndrome and other peroxisome biogenesis disorders. *Cell Mol Life Sci* 59:1058, 2002.

Fitzpatrick DR: Zellweger syndrome and associated phenotypes. *J Med Genet* 33:863, 1996.

Suzuki Y, Shimozawa N, Orii T, et al: Genetic and molecular bases of peroxisome biogenesis disorders. *Genet Med* 3:372, 2001.

Zunich Neuroectodermal Syndrome

At a glance: A severe polymalformative syndrome involving early-onset migratory ichthyosiform dermatosis, bilateral ocular coloboma, seizures, and mental retardation. Other features include congenital heart defect (e.g., tetralogy of Fallot, ventricular septal defect, transposition of great vessels), conductive hearing loss, ear defect, and neurological function.

Synonyms: CHIME (*C*olobomas of the Eye, *H*eart Defects, *I*chthyosiform Dermatosis, *M*ental retardation, and *E*ar Defects) Syndrome; CHIME Neuroectodermal Dysplasia; Neuroectodermal Syndrome Zunich type; Zunich-Kaye Syndrome.

Nature: Congenital genetic disorder.

Incidence: Unknown; seven case reports worldwide between 1983 and 1997. There are no new cases reported since.

Genetic inheritance: Autosomal recessive.

Pathophysiology: Unknown.

Diagnosis: Clinically evocated by the association of eye, heart, and ear defect combined with mental retardation and ichthyosis.

Clinical aspects: Patients often have feeding difficulties in their first years of life because of poor coordination of swallowing. Clinical signs can involve *skin* (early onset of migratory ichthyosiform dermatosis, sparse fine hair, thick palms and soles), *head* (brachycephaly, flat and broad nasal root, short philtrum, wide mouth, full lips, widely spaced teeth, occasional cleft palate and bifid uvula), *eyes* (hypertelorism, epicanthic folds, retinal colobomas), *central nervous system (CNS)* (mild cerebral cortical atrophy, mental retardation, seizures and wide-based gait, conductive hearing loss with

abnormal auditory evoked potentials), *heart* (5 of 7 cases between 1983 and 1997 presented with tetralogy of Fallot, transposition of the great arteries, peripheral pulmonary stenosis, or ventricular septal defect), *kidney* (duplicated collecting system, ectopic renal pelvis, ureteropelvic junction obstruction), and *skeleton* (brachydactyly, clinodactyly, broad second toe, occasional club foot). Possible dysregulation of cell division and immunologic dysfunction. After correction of their cardiac defect, their general health is usually satisfactory, except for frequent sinus infections. Exacerbation of seizures and skin rash occur with puberty, and the pruritus associated with the dermatosis has resulted in sudden expression of violent behavior. Mental retardation in the majority of cases, along with the behavioral outbursts, often resulted in the need for constant supervision.

Precautions before anesthesia: A complete medical history and physical examination should be obtained. It is essential to assess the airway and any indications of repetitive pulmonary aspiration and recurrent infections. The presence of associated cardiac defects as well as history of surgical correction must be reviewed. When available, a consultation with a cardiologist must be obtained to assess and determine the cardiac function (e.g., echocardiography and if necessary, cardiac catheterization). The degree of deafness and mental retardation must be evaluated. It is very important to review the treatment and its efficacy in patients affected with epilepsy. Blood examination must include a complete blood cell count because of frequent infections and the possible association with acute lymphocytic leukemia. Hemoglobin, electrolytes, and creatinine (renal function is rarely compromised, but cases of ureteropelvic reflux have been described) must be measured. Depending on the degree of mental retardation, the use of sedative premedication may be indicated. The presence of the patient's care provider in the preoperative area may be helpful when judged appropriate by the anesthesiologist.

Anesthetic considerations: During the first years of life, patients may be at risk for pulmonary aspiration and a rapid-sequence induction is indicated. Anesthetic management should be adapted to each particular heart disease.

Pharmacological implications: In the presence of seizure disorder, avoid potentially epileptogenic drugs such as methohexital, ketamine, enflurane, sevoflurane, atracurium, *cis*-atracurium, and meperidine (these last three, if given in large quantity, because of their respective metabolites, laudanosine and normeperidine). Maintain anticonvulsant therapy perioperatively. In case of cardiopathy antibiotic prophylaxis is required as indicated.

REFERENCES:

Schnur RE, Greenbaum BH, Heymann WR, et al: Acute lymphoblastic leukemia with the CHIME neuroectodermal dysplasia syndrome. *Am J Med Genet* 72:24, 1997.

Zunich J, Kaye CI: New syndrome of congenital ichthyosis with neurologic abnormalities. *Am J Med Genet* 15:331, 1983.

HOW TO USE THE INDEX

Nearly 2000 syndromes are presented in this book. For each, the main heading of an entry represents the most common name for the syndrome. A list of synonyms for each syndrome is also provided, facilitating the identification of each syndrome in different parts of the world.

The category "Other Conditions to Be Considered" indicates potentially related medical conditions that could, from their clinical description (signs and symptoms), be alternative diagnoses in the identification of the patient's condition. For each of these other conditions a list of synonyms is also given.

Some syndromes belong to a larger group of illnesses based on a common physiopathology and require special attention because of their medical implications. These major conditions are presented as an *overview*, and a proper *classification* is detailed for each syndrome member of this larger group.

This comprehensive index takes all these features into account, with helpful icons identifying the type of information found in the main text. It allows the reader to identify the name or potential synonym for the syndrome of interest quickly. Furthermore, the same condition can be cross-referenced easily if listed as an "Other Condition." A series of intuitive typographic features (explained below) will help the user to locate the syndrome, any associated synonyms, or related conditions (Other Conditions to Be Considered) and to distinguish which type of description will be found in the main text.

This index was developed by the authors to meet the needs of our fellow clinicians.

Typographic considerations:

Developed syndrome (main entry)
Other condition to be considered
Synonym of a syndrome
Synonym of another condition not presented as a major syndrome

▭	Icon used to locate an **"Overview"**
▭	Icon used to locate the **"Classification"**
◆	Icon used to locate a **"Synonym"**
⊗	Icon used to locate **"Also mentioned in ..."**

Main Syndrome	🗁 Overview	▥ Classification	♦ *Synonym*	⊗ Also mentioned in . . .

| **Main Syndrome** | ▭ Overview | ▭ Classification | ♦ *Synonym* | ⊗ Also mentioned in . . . |

| **Main Syndrome** | ▱ Overview | ▭ Classification | ♦ *Synonym* | ⊗ Also mentioned in . . . |

Main Syndrome	▭ Overview	▭ Classification	♦ Synonym	⊗ Also mentioned in . . .

Main Syndrome   ▱ Overview   ▱ Classification   ♦ *Synonym*   ⊗ Also mentioned in . . .

| Main Syndrome | 🗁 Overview | ▭ Classification | ♦ *Synonym* | ⊗ Also mentioned in . . . |

Main Syndrome	🗀 Overview	▢ Classification	♦ *Synonym*	⊗ Also mentioned in . . .

Main Syndrome　　　▭ Overview　　　▢ Classification　　　♦ *Synonym*　　　⊗ Also mentioned in . . .

Main Syndrome   ▭ Overview   ▭ Classification   ♦ *Synonym*   ⊗ Also mentioned in . . .

| **Main Syndrome** | 🗁 Overview | 📖 Classification | ♦ *Synonym* | ⊗ Also mentioned in . . . |

Main Syndrome	▭ Overview	▭ Classification	♦ *Synonym*	⊗ Also mentioned in . . .

Main Syndrome	🗀 Overview	📖 Classification	♦ *Synonym*	⊗ Also mentioned in . . .

| Main Syndrome | ⌷ Overview | ⌷ Classification | ♦ Synonym | ⊗ Also mentioned in . . . |

| **Main Syndrome** | 📖 Overview | 📖 Classification | ♦ *Synonym* | ⊗ Also mentioned in . . . |

| **Main Syndrome** | ⌂ Overview | ⊞ Classification | ♦ *Synonym* | ⊗ Also mentioned in . . . |

Main Syndrome	🗁 Overview	📖 Classification	♦ *Synonym*	⊗ Also mentioned in . . .

Main Syndrome		🗁 Overview	📖 Classification	♦ *Synonym*	⊗ Also mentioned in . . .

Main Syndrome	▱ Overview	▱ Classification	♦ *Synonym*	⊗ Also mentioned in . . .

Main Syndrome	▭ Overview	▢ Classification	♦ *Synonym*	⊗ Also mentioned in . . .

| **Main Syndrome** | ▭ Overview | ▢ Classification | ♦ *Synonym* | ⊗ Also mentioned in . . . |

| **Main Syndrome** | ▱ Overview | ▢ Classification | ♦ *Synonym* | ⊗ Also mentioned in . . . |

Main Syndrome	☞ Overview	▭ Classification	♦ *Synonym*	⊗ Also mentioned in . . .

Main Syndrome   🗁 Overview   ▫ Classification   ♦ *Synonym*   ⊗ Also mentioned in . . .

Main Syndrome	▱ Overview	▢ Classification	♦ *Synonym*	⊗ Also mentioned in . . .

| **Main Syndrome** | ▭ Overview | ▭ Classification | ♦ *Synonym* | ⊗ Also mentioned in . . . |

Main Syndrome	▱ Overview	▢ Classification	♦ *Synonym*	⊗ Also mentioned in . . .

Main Syndrome	🗀 Overview	📖 Classification	♦ *Synonym*	⊗ Also mentioned in . . .

Main Syndrome   ▭ Overview   ▦ Classification   ♦ *Synonym*   ⊗ Also mentioned in . . .

| **Main Syndrome** | 🗁 Overview | 📖 Classification | ♦ *Synonym* | ⊗ Also mentioned in . . . |

Main Syndrome	▭ Overview	▢ Classification	♦ *Synonym*	⊗ Also mentioned in . . .

| Main Syndrome | ▭ Overview | ▭ Classification | ♦ *Synonym* | ⊗ Also mentioned in . . . |

Main Syndrome	📂 Overview	📖 Classification	♦ *Synonym*	⊗ Also mentioned in . . .

Main Syndrome	🗁 Overview	▭ Classification	♦ *Synonym*	⊗ Also mentioned in . . .

| **Main Syndrome** | ▭ Overview | ▢ Classification | ♦ *Synonym* | ⊗ Also mentioned in . . . |

Main Syndrome	🗁 Overview	▢ Classification	♦ *Synonym*	⊗ Also mentioned in . . .

Main Syndrome	🗁 Overview	📖 Classification	♦ *Synonym*	⊗ Also mentioned in . . .

Main Syndrome	▱ Overview	▱ Classification	♦ *Synonym*	⊗ Also mentioned in . . .

Main Syndrome	☐ Overview	☐ Classification	♦ *Synonym*	⊗ Also mentioned in . . .

Main Syndrome	◻ Overview	◻ Classification	♦ *Synonym*	⊗ Also mentioned in . . .

Main Syndrome	▭ Overview	▭ Classification	♦ *Synonym*	⊗ Also mentioned in . . .

Main Syndrome	☞ Overview	▥ Classification	♦ *Synonym*	⊗ Also mentioned in . . .

Main Syndrome	▭ Overview	▭ Classification	♦ *Synonym*	⊗ Also mentioned in . . .

Main Syndrome	☞ Overview	▥ Classification	♦ *Synonym*	⊗ Also mentioned in . . .

Main Syndrome	⌂ Overview	▦ Classification	♦ *Synonym*	⊗ Also mentioned in . . .

| **Main Syndrome** | ▱ Overview | ◻ Classification | ◆ *Synonym* | ⊗ Also mentioned in . . . |

Main Syndrome   ⊡ Overview   ▣ Classification   ♦ *Synonym*   ⊗ Also mentioned in . . .

Main Syndrome	⌂ Overview	⊞ Classification	♦ *Synonym*	⊗ Also mentioned in . . .

Main Syndrome	▱ Overview	▭ Classification	♦ *Synonym*	⊗ Also mentioned in . . .

Main Syndrome   ▱ Overview   ▱ Classification   ♦ *Synonym*   ⊗ Also mentioned in . . .

Main Syndrome	📂 Overview	📖 Classification	♦ *Synonym*	⊗ Also mentioned in . . .

Main Syndrome	🗁 Overview	📖 Classification	♦ *Synonym*	⊗ Also mentioned in . . .

Main Syndrome	▷ Overview	▦ Classification	♦ *Synonym*	⊗ Also mentioned in . . .

Main Syndrome	🗁 Overview	🕮 Classification	♦ *Synonym*	⊗ Also mentioned in . . .

Main Syndrome	🗁 Overview	📖 Classification	♦ *Synonym*	⊗ Also mentioned in . . .

Main Syndrome	☞ Overview	▢ Classification	♦ *Synonym*	⊗ Also mentioned in . . .

Main Syndrome	🗁 Overview	⊞ Classification	♦ *Synonym*	⊗ Also mentioned in . . .

Main Syndrome	🗁 Overview	▢ Classification	♦ *Synonym*	⊗ Also mentioned in . . .

Main Syndrome	📂 Overview	📖 Classification	♦ *Synonym*	⊗ Also mentioned in . . .

Main Syndrome	▭ Overview	▣ Classification	♦ *Synonym*	⊗ Also mentioned in . . .

Main Syndrome	⌂ Overview	▥ Classification	♦ *Synonym*	⊗ Also mentioned in . . .

Main Syndrome	▭ Overview	▭ Classification	♦ *Synonym*	⊗ Also mentioned in . . .

| **Main Syndrome** | ▭ Overview | ▭ Classification | ♦ *Synonym* | ⊗ Also mentioned in . . . |

Main Syndrome   ▭ Overview   ▥ Classification   ♦ *Synonym*   ⊗ Also mentioned in . . .

| **Main Syndrome** | 🗁 Overview | 📖 Classification | ♦ *Synonym* | ⊗ Also mentioned in . . . |

| Main Syndrome | ▭ Overview | ▭ Classification | ♦ *Synonym* | ⊗ Also mentioned in . . . |

Main Syndrome	🗁 Overview	⧠ Classification	♦ *Synonym*	⊗ Also mentioned in . . .

Main Syndrome	⌂ Overview	▢ Classification	♦ *Synonym*	⊗ Also mentioned in . . .

Main Syndrome	▭ Overview	▭ Classification	♦ *Synonym*	⊗ Also mentioned in . . .

| **Main Syndrome** | ▭ Overview | ▭ Classification | ♦ *Synonym* | ⊗ Also mentioned in . . . |

Main Syndrome	🖿 Overview	🕮 Classification	♦ *Synonym*	⊗ Also mentioned in . . .

Main Syndrome	📁 Overview	📖 Classification	◊ *Synonym*	⊗ Also mentioned in . . .

| **Main Syndrome** | 🗁 Overview | 📖 Classification | ♦ *Synonym* | ⊗ Also mentioned in . . . |

Main Syndrome	⌂ Overview	⌑ Classification	♦ *Synonym*	⊗ Also mentioned in . . .

| **Main Syndrome** | 🗁 Overview | 📖 Classification | ♦ *Synonym* | ⊗ Also mentioned in . . . |

Main Syndrome	☐ Overview	▭ Classification	♦ *Synonym*	⊗ Also mentioned in . . .

Main Syndrome	▭ Overview	▭ Classification	♦ Synonym	⊗ Also mentioned in . . .